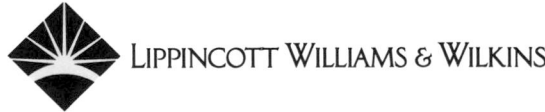

Build your understanding and your confidence with these learning aids!

Study Guide to Accompany Brunner & Suddarth's
Textbook of Medical-Surgical Nursing
Tenth Edition

Mary Jo Boyer, RN, DNSc

The perfect companion to *Brunner & Suddarth's Medical-Surgical Nursing*, this exemplary study tool was developed specifically to help you better understand the concepts, techniques, and disease processes detailed in the textbook.

Look inside and discover...

- Hundreds of exam-style questions prepare you for classroom tests and the NCLEX exam.
- Comprehension, interpretation, and labeling exercises use examples drawn from real clinical applications.
- Learner's self evaluation tools let you check your progress.
- Answers, with rationale, help you understand the reasoning behind correct responses.
- Critical analysis questions help you build vital problem-solving skills.

Handbook for Brunner and Suddarth's
Textbook of Medical-Surgical Nursing
Tenth Edition

Mary Jo Boyer, RN, DNSc

This concise clinical companion to *Brunner and Suddarth's Textbook of Medical-Surgical Nursing*, presents need-to-know information on 200 of the most common medical-surgical disorders encountered in the hospital and community setting. Organized alphabetically, and cross-referenced with the parent text, each entry enables quick access to vital disease information such as: pathophysiology, clinical manifestations, diagnostic evaluation methods, medical and nursing management, diagnoses and interventions.

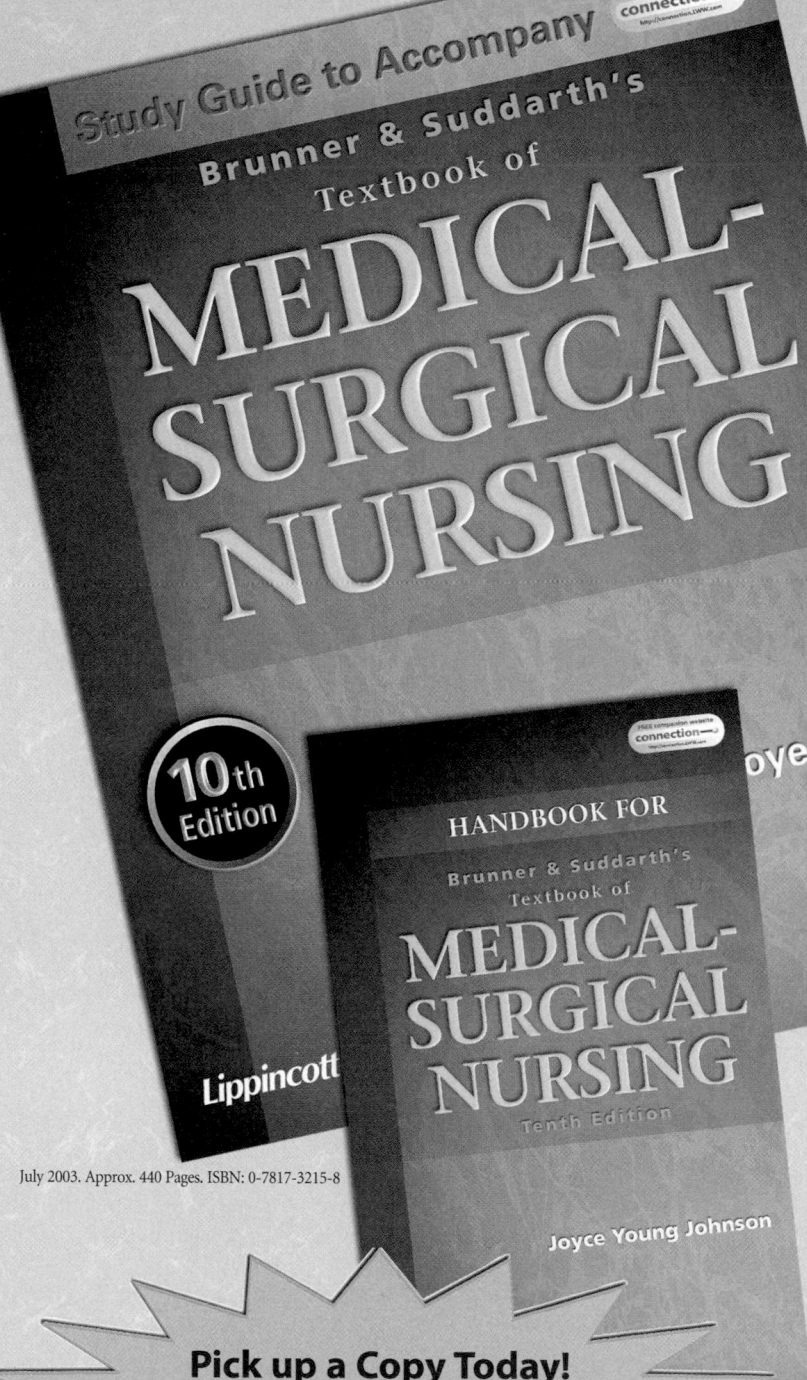

July 2003. Approx. 440 Pages. ISBN: 0-7817-3215-8

Pick up a Copy Today!
Visit Your Health Sciences Bookstore or
Call Toll Free 800-638-3030
Visit us on the Web at LWW.com/nursing

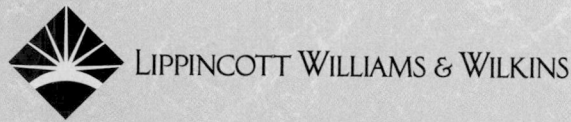
LIPPINCOTT WILLIAMS & WILKINS

July 2003. Approx. 880 Pages. ISBN: 0-7817-4703-1

10th EDITION
Volume 1

Brunner & Suddarth's

Textbook of

MEDICAL-SURGICAL NURSING

Suzanne C. Smeltzer, RN, EdD, FAAN

Professor and Director, Nursing Research
Villanova University College of Nursing
Villanova, Pennsylvania

Brenda G. Bare, RN, MSN

Associate Administrator Patient Care Services/Chief Nurse Executive
Inova Mount Vernon Hospital
Alexandria, Virginia

AND MORE THAN 50 CONTRIBUTORS

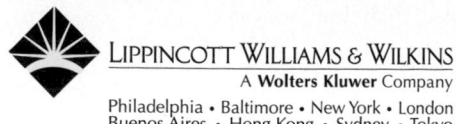

LIPPINCOTT WILLIAMS & WILKINS
A **Wolters Kluwer** Company

Philadelphia • Baltimore • New York • London
Buenos Aires • Hong Kong • Sydney • Tokyo

Senior Acquisitions Editor: Quincy McDonald
Development Editor: Deedie McMahon
Editorial Assistant: Marie Rim
Senior Production Editors: Rosanne Hallowell/Tom Gibbons
Senior Production Manager: Helen Ewan
Managing Editor / Production: Erika Kors
Art Director: Carolyn O'Brien
Illustration Coordinator: Brett MacNaughton
Manufacturing Manager: William Alberti
Indexer: Coughlin Indexing Services, Inc.
Compositor: Circle Graphics
Printer: R. R. Donnelley

Tenth Edition

9   8   7   6   5   4   3

Library of Congress Cataloging-in-Publication Data

Brunner & Suddarth's textbook of medical-surgical nursing.—10th ed. / [edited by]
  Suzanne C. Smeltzer, Brenda G. Bare ; and more than 50 contributors.
     p. ; cm.
  Includes bibliographical references and index.
  ISBN 0-7817-3193-3 (one volume) — ISBN 0-7817-4500-4 (two volumes)
  1. Nursing. 2. Surgical nursing. I. Title: Brunner and Suddarth's textbook of
medical-surgical nursing. II. Title: Textbook of medical-surgical nursing. III. Title:
Medical-surgical nursing. IV. Brunner, Lillian Sholtis. V. Suddarth, Doris Smith. VI.
Smeltzer, Suzanne C. O'Connell. VII. Bare, Brenda G.
  [DNLM: 1. Nursing Care. 2. Perioperative Nursing. WY 150 B8972 2004]
RT41.T46 2004
610.73—dc21
                                                                2003044738

LWW.com

Contributors

Sandra M. Annesi, RN, MSN
Assistant Professor
Nursing Program
Daytona Beach Community College
DeLand, Florida
Chapter 25: Respiratory Care Modalities

Judith C. Bautch, PhD, RN, CS
Professor
Department of Nursing
Winona State University
Winona, Minnesota
*Chapter 54: Assessment and Management of Patients With
Rheumatic Disorders*

Jo Ann Brooks-Brunn, DNS, RN, FAAN, FCCP
Assistant Professor
Thoracic Surgery
Pulmonary and Critical Care Medicine
Indiana University School of Medicine
Indianapolis, Indiana
*Chapter 23: Management of Patients With Chest
and Lower Respiratory Tract Disorders*
*Chapter 24: Management of Patients With Chronic Obstructive
Pulmonary Disease*

Jacqueline Fowler Byers, PhD, RN, CNAA
Associate Professor
School of Nursing
University of Central Florida
Orlando, Florida
Chapter 21: Assessment of Respiratory Function

Kim Cantwell-Gab, BSN, RN, CVN, RVT, RDMS
Vascular Surgery Nurse Specialist
Department of Surgery, Division of Vascular Surgery
University of Washington School of Medicine
Seattle, Washington
*Chapter 31: Assessment and Management of Patients With Vascular
Disorders and Problems of Peripheral Circulation*

Patricia E. Casey, RN, MSN
Director, Regional Cardiovascular Program
Kaiser Permanente Mid-Atlantic Region
Rockville, Maryland
*Chapter 27: Management of Patients With Dysrhythmias
and Conduction Problems*
*Chapter 28: Management of Patients With Coronary
Vascular Disorders*
*Chapter 29: Management of Patients With Structural, Infectious,
and Inflammatory Cardiac Disorders*
*Chapter 30: Management of Patients With Complications
From Heart Disease*

Jill Cash, MSN, APRN, BC
Family Nurse Practitioner
Southern Illinois OB-GYN Associates, SC
Carbondale, Illinois
*Chapter 59: Assessment and Management of Patients With Hearing
and Balance Disorders*

Linda Carman Copel, PhD, RN, CS, CGP, DAPA
Associate Professor
Villanova University College of Nursing
Villanova, Pennsylvania
Chapter 4: Health Education and Health Promotion
Chapter 6: Homeostasis, Stress, and Adaptation
Chapter 7: Individual and Family Considerations Related to Illness

Jullet Corbin, RNC, DNS, FNP
Lecturer
School of Nursing
San Jose State University
San Jose, California
Chapter 10: Chronic Illness

Susanna G. Cunningham, RN, PhD, FAAN, FAHA
Professor
Department of Biobehavioral Nursing and Health Systems
University of Washington School of Nursing
Seattle, Washington
*Chapter 32: Assessment and Management of Patients
With Hypertension*

Lana Currance, RN, BSN, CCRN
Chief Nursing Officer
National Medical Response System
Colorado 2 DMAT/Central U.S. NMRT-Weapons of
Mass Destruction
Parker, Colorado
Chapter 72: Terrorism, Mass Casualty, and Disaster Nursing

Margaret A. Degler, RN, MSN, CRNP, CUNP
Director, Continence Program
West Office of the Center for Urologic Care of Berks County, P.C.
West Reading, Pennsylvania
Chapter 12: Health Care of the Older Adult
Chapter 43: Assessment of Renal and Urinary Tract Function
*Chapter 44: Management of Patients With Upper or Lower Urinary
Tract Dysfunction*
Chapter 45: Management of Patients With Urinary Disorders

Nancy E. Donegan, RN, BS, MPH
Director, Infection Control
Washington Hospital Center
Washington, D.C.
Chapter 70: Management of Patients With Infectious Diseases

Phyllis Dubendorf, RN, MSN, CS-ACNP
Lecturer, Acute Care Nurse Practitioner Program
School of Nursing
University of Pennsylvania
Philadelphia, Pennsylvania
  Chapter 61: Management of Patients With Neurologic Dysfunction

Eleanor Fitzpatrick, RN, MSN, CRNP, CCRN
Clinical Nurse Specialist
Surgical ICU/Intermediate Surgical ICU
Thomas Jefferson University Hospital
Philadelphia, Pennsylvania
  Chapter 39: Assessment and Management of Patients With
    Hepatic Disorders
  Chapter 40: Assessment and Management of Patients With Biliary
    Disorders

Mary Beth Flynn, RN, MS
CNS/Clinical Educator
University of Colorado Hospital
Clinical Faculty
University of Colorado Health Science Center
Denver, Colorado
  Chapter 15: Shock and Multisystem Failure

Kathleen K. Furniss, MSN, APN-C
Nurse Practitioner, Women's Health
Women's Health Initiative
University of Medicine and Dentistry of New Jersey and Associates in
    Women's Health Care
Newark, New Jersey
  Chapter 46: Assessment and Management of Female
    Physiologic Processes
  Chapter 47: Management of Patients With Female
    Reproductive Disorders

Paula Graling, RN, MSN, CNS
Clinical Nurse Specialist
Perioperative Services
Inova Fairfax Hospital
Falls Church, Virginia
  Chapter 18: Preoperative Nursing Management
  Chapter 19: Intraoperative Nursing Management
  Chapter 20: Postoperative Nursing Management

Randolph E. Gross, RN, MS, CS, AOCN
Clinical Nurse Specialist
Evelyn H. Louder Breast Center
Memorial Sloan-Kettering Cancer Center
New York, New York
  Chapter 48: Assessment and Management of Patients
    With Breast Disorders

Doreen Grzelak, RN, MSN, AOCN
Operations Manager
Medical Imaging Center
Department of Radiology
Reston Hospital Center
Reston, Virginia
  Chapter 35: Management of Patients With Oral and Esophageal
    Disorders
  Chapter 37: Management of Patients With Gastric and Duodenal
    Disorders

Janice L. Hinkle, PhD, RN, CNRN
Assistant Professor
Villanova University College of Nursing
Villanova, Pennsylvania
  Chapter 5: Health Assessment
  Chapter 62: Management of Patients With Cerebrovascular Disorders
  Chapter 65: Management of Patient With Oncologic
    and Degenerative Neurologic Disorders

Ryan R. Iwamoto, ARNP, MN, AOCN
Oncology Clinical Coordinator
Genentech BioOncology, Inc.
South San Francisco, California
Nurse Practitioner
Department of Radiation Oncology
Virginia Mason Medical Center
Clinical Instructor
University of Washington and Seattle University
Seattle, Washington
  Chapter 49: Assessment and Management of Problems Related to Male
    Reproductive Processes

Joyce Young Johnson, RN, PhD, CCRN
Assistant Chair
Department of Nursing
Georgia Perimeter College
Clarkston, Georgia
  Chapter 1: Health Care Delivery and Nursing Practice
  Chapter 2: Community-Based Nursing Practice
  Chapter 3: Critical Thinking, Ethical Decision Making,
    and the Nursing Process
  Chapter 8: Perspectives in Transcultural Nursing

Rhonda Kyanko, RN, MS
Nursing Education Coordinator
National Rehabilitation Hospital
Washington, DC
  Chapter 11: Principles and Practices of Rehabilitation

Pamela J. LaBorde, MSN, RN
Clinical Nurse Specialist, Patient Care Services
University of Arkansas Medical Sciences Center
Little Rock, Arkansas
Formerly, Clinical Nurse Specialist, Burn Unit
Orlando Regional Medical Center
Orlando, Florida
  Chapter 57: Management of Patients With Burn Injury

Dale Halsey Lea, RN, MPH, CGC, APGN, FAAN
Assistant Director
Southern Maine Regional Genetics Services
Foundations for Blood Research
Scarborough, Maine
  Chapter 9: Genetics Perspectives in Nursing Practice

Dorothy B. Liddel, RN, MSN, ONC
Associate Professor (Retired)
Department of Nursing
Columbia Union College
Takoma Park, Maryland
  Chapter 66: Assessment of Musculoskeletal Function
  Chapter 67: Musculoskeletal Care Modalities
  Chapter 68: Management of Patients With Musculoskeletal Disorders
  Chapter 69: Management of Patients With Musculoskeletal Trauma

Martha V. Manning, RN, MSN
Nurse Clinician
Inova Emergency Care Center at Fairfax
Fairfax, Virginia
　　Chapter 34: Assessment of Digestive and Gastrointestinal Function
　　Chapter 38: Management of Patients With Intestinal
　　　　and Rectal Disorders

Barbara J. Maschak-Carey, RN, MSN, CDE
Clinical Nurse Specialist
Department of Endocrinology, Diabetes and Metabolism
University of Pennsylvania Health System
Philadelphia, Pennsylvania
　　Chapter 41: Assessment and Management of Patients
　　　　With Diabetes Mellitus

Agnes Masny, RN, MPH, MSN, CRNP
Research Associate/Nurse Practitioner
Population Science Division, Family Risk Assessment Program
Fox Chase Cancer Center
Philadelphia, Pennsylvania
　　Chapter 9: Genetics Perspectives in Nursing

Lou Ann McGinty, MSN, RN
Nurse Science Clinical Specialist
Capitol Health System
Trenton, New Jersey
　　Chapter 64: Management of Patients With Neurologic Infections,
　　　　Autoimmune Disorders, and Neuropathies

Nancy A. Morrissey, RN,C, PhD
Patient Care Director
Mental Health and Behavioral Center
Inova Alexandria Hospital
Alexandria, Virginia
　　Chapter 36: Gastrointestinal Intubation and Special
　　　　Nutritional Modalities

Martha A. Mulvey, CNS,C
Advanced Practice Nurse
Neurosciences
University of Medicine and Dentistry of New Jersey,
　　University Hospital
Newark, New Jersey
　　Chapter 14: Fluids and Electrolytes: Balance and Distribution

Victoria Navarro, RN, MAS, MSN
Director of Clinical Services
Wilmer Eye Institute
The Johns Hopkins Medical Institutions
Baltimore, Maryland
　　Chapter 58: Assessment and Management of Patients With Eye
　　　　and Vision Disorders

Donna Nayduch, RN-CS, MSN, CCRN
Trauma Regional Director
Banner Health
Greeley, Colorado
　　Chapter 71: Emergency Nursing
　　Chapter 72: Terrorism, Mass Casualty, and Disaster Nursing

Kathleen Nokes, PhD, RN, FAAN
Professor
Hunter-Bellevue School of Nursing
New York, New York
　　Chapter 52: Management of Patients With HIV Infection and AIDS

Janet A. Parkosewich, RN, MSN, CCRN
Cardiac Clinical Nurse Specialist
Department of Patient Services
Yale-New Haven Hospital
New Haven, Connecticut
　　Chapter 26: Assessment of Cardiovascular Function

Anne Gallagher Peach, RN, MSN
Chief Operating Officer
M.D. Anderson Cancer Center Orlando
Orlando, Florida
　　Chapter 22: Management of Patients With Upper Respiratory
　　　　Tract Disorders

JoAnne Reifsnyder, PhD, RN, AOCN
Postdoctoral fellow, Psychosocial Oncology
School of Nursing
University of Pennsylvania
Philadelphia, Pennsylvania
　　Chapter 17: End-of-Life Care

Susan A. Rokita, RN, MS, CRNP
Nurse Coordinator, Cancer Center
Oncology Clinical Nurse Specialist
Milton S. Hershey Medical Center of Pennsylvania State University
Hershey, Pennsylvania
　　Chapter 16: Oncology: Nursing Management in Cancer Care

Al Rundio, PhD, RN, ANP
Associate Professor
Medical College of Pennsylvania/Hahnemann University
College of Nursing and Health Professions
Philadelphia, Pennsylvania
　　Chapter 50: Assessment of Immune Function
　　Chapter 51: Management of Patients With Immunodeficiency
　　Chapter 53: Assessment and Management of Patients
　　　　With Allergic Disorders

Catherine Sackett, RN, BS, CANP
Ophthalmic Research Nurse Practitioner
Wilmer Eye Institute
Retinal Vascular Center
The Johns Hopkins Medical Institutions
Baltimore, Maryland
　　Chapter 58: Assessment and Management of Patients With Eye
　　　　and Vision Disorders

Linda Schakenbach, RN, CNS, MSN, CCRN, COCN, CWCN, CS
Clinical Nurse Specialist, Critical Care
Inova Alexandria Hospital
Alexandria, Virginia
　　Chapter 27: Management of Patients With Dysrhythmias
　　　　and Conduction Problems
　　Chapter 28: Management of Patients With Coronary
　　　　Vascular Disorders
　　Chapter 29: Management of Patients With Structural, Infectious,
　　　　and Inflammatory Cardiac Disorders

Margaret A. Spera, NP, APRN
Nurse Practitioner
Family Medical Associates
Ridgefield, Connecticut
Assistant Clinical Professor
Yale University School of Nursing
New Haven, Connecticut
  Chapter 60: Assessment of Neurologic Function

Cindy Stern, RN, MSN
Cancer Network Coordinator
University of Pennsylvania Cancer Center
University of Pennsylvania Health System
Philadelphia, Pennsylvania
  Chapter 16: Oncology: Nursing Management in
    Cancer Care

Christine Tea, RN, MSN, CNA
Patient Care Director
Main OR Perioperative Services
Inova Fairfax Hospital
Falls Church, Virginia
  Chapter 18: Preoperative Nursing Management
  Chapter 19: Intraoperative Nursing Management
  Chapter 20: Postoperative Nursing Management

Mary Laudon Thomas, RN, MS, AOCN
Hematology Clinical Nurse Specialist
Veterans' Administration, Palo Alto Health Care System
Palo Alto, California
  Chapter 33: Assessment and Management of Patients
    With Hematologic Disorders

Dorraine Day Watts, PhD, RN
Interim Director of Research and Education
Inova Health System
Falls Church, Virginia
  Chapter 63: Management of Patients With Neurologic Trauma

Joan Webb, RN, MSN
Instructor
College of Nursing
Widener University
Chester, Pennsylvania
  Chapter 40: Assessment and Management of Patients
    With Biliary Disorders
  Chapter 42: Assessment and Management of Patients
    With Endocrine Disorders

Joyce S. Willens, RN, PhD
Assistant Professor
College of Nursing
Villanova University
Villanova, Pennsylvania
  Chapter 13: Pain Management

Iris Woodard, RN-CS, BSN, ANP
Nurse Practitioner
Department of Dermatology
Kaiser Permanente
Springfield, Virginia
  Chapter 55: Assessment of Integumentary Function
  Chapter 56: Management of Patients With Dermatologic Problems

Consultants and Reviewers

Debbie Amason, BSN, MS, RN
Assistant Professor
Floyd College
Rome, Georgia

William Ames, MSN, RN, FNP
Associate Professor
Elizabethtown Community College
Elizabethtown, Kentucky

Susan Arbogast, MS, RN
Faculty
Maricopa Community College District
    Nursing Program, Phoenix College
    Campus
Phoenix, Arizona

Gail Armstrong, ND, RN
Assistant Professor
University of Colorado School of Nursing
Denver, Colorado

Denise M. Ayers, MSN, RN
Assistant Professor, Nursing
Kent State University at Tuscarawas
New Philadelphia, Ohio

Valerie Benedix, BSN, RN
Nursing Instructor
Clovis Community College
Clovis, New Mexico

Ilene Borze, MS, CEN, RN
Director, Nursing Continuing Education
Faculty
Gateway Community College
Phoenix, Arizona

Donna Bowren, RN, MSN, CNOR, CRNFA
Interim Chairperson, Division of Nursing
    and Allied Health
University of Arkansas Community College
    at Batesville
Batesville, Arkansas

Pat Bradley, RN, MEd MS
Nursing Faculty
Grossmont College
El Cajon, California

Lynn Browning, RN, MSN BC
Assistant Professor of Nursing
Derry Patterson Wingo School of Nursing
Charleston Southern University
Charleston, South Carolina

Elizabeth Bruce, RN, MSN
St. Clair Community College
Chatham, Ontario

Shirley Cantrell, PhD, RN
Associate Professor
Piedmont College
Demorest, Georgia

Donna Cartwright, MS, APRN
Dean, Professional and Applied Technology
    Education
College of Eastern Utah
Price, Utah

Pattie Garrett Clark, MSN, RN
Associate Professor of Nursing
Abraham Baldwin College
Tifton, Georgia

Terry Cicero, MN, CCRN, RN
Instructor, School of Nursing
Seattle University
Seattle, Washington

Tracey D. Cooper, RN, MSN
Director, Nursing Learning Resources Lab
Instructor, South Plains College
Levelland, Texas

Dolly I. Daniel, BSN, CDE, RNC
Diabetes Nurse Specialist
Inova Alexandria Hospital
Alexandria, Virginia

Toni Doherty, MSN, RN
Associate Professor
Department Head, Nursing
Dutchess Community College
Poughkeepsie, New York

Sandra Edwards, BScN, RN
Instructor
Grant MacEwan College
Edmonton, Alberta, Canada

Mary Elliot, BScN, MEd, RN
Professor
Humber College of Applied Arts & Technology
Etobicoke, Ontario, Canada

Cheryl Fenton, BHSc, RN
Professor
Mohawk College
Burlington, Ontario, Canada

Kathie Folsom, RN, BSN, MS
Department Chair
Skagit Valley College
Oak Harbor, Washington

Donna Funk, MN/E ONC, RN
Professor of Nursing
Brigham Young University
Rexburg, Idaho

Vicki Garlock, BSN, MSN, RN
Professor, Nursing Department
Pensacola Junior College
Pensacola, Florida

Mary Catherine Gebhart, MSN, CRRN, RN
Instructor
Georgia State University
Atlanta, Georgia

Donna Gullette, DNS, RN
Associate Professor, Critical Care Chair
Mississippi University for Women
Columbus, Mississippi

Carol Heinrich, PhD, RN
Associate Professor
Department of Nursing
East Stroudsburg University
East Stroudsburg, Pennsylvania

Sandra Hendelman, MS, RN
Adjunct Professor of Nursing
Palm Beach Community College
Lake Worth, Florida
South College

Judith Ann Hughes, EdD, RN
Associate Degree Nursing Coordinator
Southwestern Community College
Sylva, North Carolina

Sadie Pauline Hutson, MSN, RN, CRNP
Cancer Research Training Award
    PreDoctoral Fellow
National Cancer Institute,
    Clinical Genetics Branch
Rockville, MD

Jennifer Johnson, MSN, RN C
Assistant Professor of Nursing
Kent State University, Tuscarawas Campus
New Philadelphia, Ohio

Susan J. Lamanna, MA, MSN, RN, ANP
Associate Professor
Onondaga Community College
Syracuse, New York

Joan Ann Leach, MS, ME, RNC
Professor of Nursing
Capital Community College
Hartford, Connecticut

Gayle Lee, PhD, RN, CCRN
Faculty
Brigham Young University
Rexburg, Idaho

Brenda Lohri-Posey, EdD, RN
Assistant Dean of Learning, Nursing
    & Program Coordination
Belmont Technical College
St. Clairesville, Ohio

Rhonda McLain, MN, RN
Assistant Professor of Nursing
Clayton College & State University
Morrow, Georgia

Pat Nashef, MHSc BA (CPMHN)c, RN
Professional Practice Clinician,
    Mental Health Services

Halton Healthcare Services
Oakville, Ontario
Clinical Faculty
McMaster University School of Nursing
Hamilton, Ontario

Lauren O'Hare, MSN, EdD, RN
Assistant Professor of Nursing
Wagner College
Staten Island, New York

Caroline Ostand, BC, MSN, RN
Clinical Instructor
University of Charleston
Charleston, West Virginia

Thena E. Parrott, PhD, RNCS
Director, Associate Degree Nursing Program
Blinn College
Bryan, Texas

Billie Phillips, PhD, RN, CDFS
Assistant Professor
Tennessee Wesleyan College
Fort Sanders Nursing Department
Athens, Tennessee

Pam Primus, BSN, RN
Nurse Educator
Casper College
Casper, Wyoming

Betty E. Richards, RN, MSN
Professor of Nursing
Middle Georgia College
Cochran, Georgia

Patsy Ruppert Rider, MSN, CS, RN
Clinical Instructor in Nursing
University of Texas at Austin School of Nursing
Austin, Texas

Kathleen L. Russ, MSN, RN
Dean of Student Support/Health Careers
Gateway Technical College
Kenosha, Wisconsin

Esther Salinas, MSN, MSEd, RN
Associate Professor of Nursing
Del Mar College
Corpus Christi, Texas

Marsha Sharp, MSN, RN
Associate Professor
Elizabethtown Community College
Elizabethtown, Kentucky

Kelli Simmons, MS, CS, M-SCNS, RN
Cardiothoracic Clinical Nurse Specialist
University of Missouri Hospitals and Clinics
Columbia, Missouri

Terri Small, MSN, RN C
Assistant Professor of Nursing
Waynesburg College
Waynesburg, Pennsylvania

Darla R. Ura, MA, ANP-CS, RN
Clinical Associate Professor
Emory University
Atlanta, Georgia

Weibin Yang, MD
Assistant Professor of Physical Medicine and
    Rehabilitation Medicine (PM&R)
University of Illinois
Chicago, Illinois

Preface

As the 21st century begins, nurses face a future characterized by changes comparable to those of no preceding century:

- Science and technology have made the world smaller by making it more accessible.
- Mass communication is more widespread, and information is now just an instant away and very easy to obtain.
- Economies are more global than regional.
- Industrial and social changes have made world travel and cultural exchange common.

Today's nurses enter a realm of opportunities and challenges for providing high-quality, evidence-based care in traditional as well as new and innovative health care settings. The rapid changes in health care mandate that nurses be prepared to provide or plan care across the continuum of settings—from hospital or clinic, to home, to community agencies or hospice settings—and during all phases of illness. Recent research has indicated that nurses make significant contributions to the health care outcomes of patients who are hospitalized. Therefore, today's nurses must be prepared to identify patients' short- and long-term needs quickly and to collaborate effectively with patients and families, other members of the health care team, and community agencies to create a seamless system of care. The continued emphasis on health promotion efforts to keep well people healthy and to promote a higher level of well-being among those with acute and chronic illnesses requires today's nurses to assist patients in adopting healthy lifestyles and strategies. Mapping of the human genome and other advances in genetics have moved the issue of genetics to the bedside and increased the need for nurses to become knowledgeable about genetics-related issues.

In preparing for these vast opportunities and responsibilities, today's nurses must be well informed and up-to-date, not only in nursing knowledge and skills but also in research findings, scientific advances, and the ethical dilemmas inherent in many areas of clinical practice. More than ever, today's nurses need to think critically, creatively, and compassionately.

This tenth edition of *Brunner & Suddarth's Textbook of Medical-Surgical Nursing* is designed for the 21st century and nurses' need to be knowledgeable, highly skilled, perceptive, caring, and compassionate. A goal of the textbook is to provide balanced attention to the art and science of adult medical-surgical nursing. It addresses nursing care issues from a physiological, pathophysiological, and psychosocial context and assists the reader to identify priorities of care from that context.

ABOUT THE TENTH EDITION

The tenth edition of *Brunner and Suddarth's Textbook of Medical Surgical Nursing* was constructed to provide today's nursing students with an understanding of the nurse's role in health and illness within evolving practice environments and across the spectrum of health and illness. The textbook's content has been revised and updated by experts in the field to reflect current practice and advances in health care and technology.

NEW CHAPTERS: GENETICS, END-OF-LIFE CARE, AND BIOTERRORISM

Nursing knowledge is constantly expanding. *Chapter 9, Genetics Perspectives in Nursing,* was written in response to genetics information identified during the last few years. Every nurse needs to be aware of the influence of genetics on health and illness, and every nurse needs to have the knowledge and skill to answer patients' questions concerning their heredity and health. In addition to Chapter 9, genetics content has been incorporated into each clinical unit of the textbook.

Chapter 17, End-of-Life Care, also new to the tenth edition, addresses some of the questions posed by technologies that can prolong life, often in the face of insurmountable obstacles. The chapter discusses the nurse's role as it pertains to quality of life, prolongation of dying, pain relief, allocation of resources, ethical issues, communication, healing, spirituality, and patient and family care. It emphasizes the pivotal role of the nurse in providing end-of-life care.

A third new chapter—*Chapter 72, Terrorism, Mass Casualty, and Disaster Nursing*—completes the text by reviewing the nurse's role in relation to patients affected by terrorism and other disasters. Among the issues addressed are emergency preparedness and planning, triage in cases of mass casualty, radiation, chemical and biologic weapons, ethical conflict, stress management, and survival.

NANDA, NIC, NOC: LINKS, LANGUAGES, AND CONCEPT MAPS

Although *Brunner & Suddarth's Textbook of Medical-Surgical Nursing* has long used nursing diagnoses developed by the North American Nursing Diagnosis Association (NANDA), this edition presents the links between the NANDA diagnoses and the Nursing Interventions Classification (NIC) and Nursing-sensitive Outcomes Classification (NOC). The opening page of each unit presents a concept map illustrating these three classification systems and their relationships. Each unit's concept map is accompanied by a case study and a chart presenting examples of actual NANDA, NIC, and NOC terminologies related to the case study. This material is included to introduce the reader to the NIC and NOC language and classifications and bring them to life in the clinical realm. Faculty and students alike may use some of the issues presented in the case studies as a springboard for developing their own concept maps.

RECENT NURSING RESEARCH AND OTHER FEATURES

As before, Nursing Research Profiles included in the chapters identify the implications and applications of recent nursing research findings for nursing practice. The chapters also include charts and text detailing special considerations in caring for the elderly patient and for those with disabilities.

TEACHING TOOLBOX

Each chapter opens with Learning Objectives and a Glossary. Throughout the text the reader will find Nursing Alerts as well as specialized charts focusing on

- Physiology/Pathophysiology
- Risk Factors
- Assessment
- Plans of Nursing Care
- Pharmacology
- Home Care
- Patient Education
- Health Promotion
- Ethics and Related Issues
- Guidelines
- Gerontological Considerations
- Genetics in Nursing Practice

Illustrations, photographs, charts, and tables supplement the text and round out the applied-learning experience. Each chapter concludes with Critical Thinking Exercises, References and Selected Readings, and a list of specialized Resources and Websites.

MANY MORE OF THE LATEST RESOURCES

Additional learning tools accompany the tenth edition and offer visual, tactile, and auditory reinforcement of the text. These resources include:

- **CD-ROM** to help students test their knowledge and enhance their understanding of medical-surgical nursing. This CD includes 500 self-study questions organized by unit; 3000 bonus NCLEX-style cross-disciplinary questions; 3-D animated illustrations that explain common disease processes; and interactive clinical simulations.
- **Student Study Guide** to further enhance the learning experience (available at student bookstores)
- **Instructor's Resource CD-ROM** to help facilitate classroom preparation, with an instructor's manual, test generator, and searchable image collection, among other features
- Supplemental cartridges for **Blackboard** and **WebCT**
- **Connection Website**—Get connected at connection.LWW.com/go/smeltzer.

The tenth edition of *Brunner and Suddarth's Textbook of Medical-Surgical Nursing* continues the tradition of presenting up-to-date content that addresses the art and science of nursing practice. The updating of the material and use of a variety of teaching methods to convey that content are intended to provide the nursing student and other users of the textbook with information needed to provide quality care to patients and families across health care settings and in the home.

Suzanne C. O'Connell Smeltzer, RN, EdD, FAAN
Brenda G. Bare, RN, MSN

Acknowledgments

With great appreciation and respect, the authors acknowledge Lillian S. Brunner, RN, MSN, ScD, LittD, FAAN, and Doris S. Suddarth, RN, BSNE, MSN. The foundation and expertise that they provided for this textbook for many years and the mentoring that they provided to us during earlier editions continue to support us as we strive toward the development of a textbook that encourages students and practitioners of nursing to strive toward excellence in providing skillful and compassionate nursing care.

The authors also gratefully acknowledge the contributions of Janice L. Hinkle, RN, PhD, and Linda Schakenbach, RN, MSN, to this tenth edition of *Brunner and Suddarth's Textbook of Medical-Surgical Nursing*. They have authored chapters of the textbook and guided many contributors in writing and developing chapters throughout the textbook. We greatly appreciate the nursing expertise and experience and the spirit of inquiry that they bring to this tenth edition.

Brunner & Suddarth's
Textbook of Medical-Surgical Nursing
10th edition

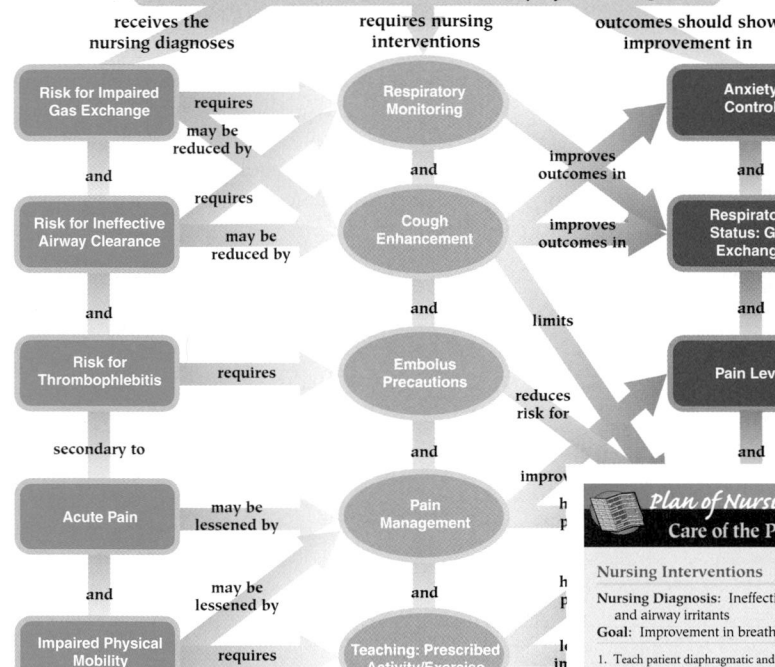

The patient recovering from abdominal surgery with reluctance to move and a history of smoking

◀ **Concept Maps**—with NANDA, NIC, and NOC illustrate reality-based clinical scenarios for the visual learner.

▼ **Plans of Nursing Care**— illustrate applications of the nursing process to diseases and disorders.

Plan of Nursing Care
Care of the Patient With COPD *(Continued)*

Nursing Interventions	Rationale	Expected Outcomes
Nursing Diagnosis: Ineffective breathing pattern related to shortness of breath, mucus, bronchoconstriction, and airway irritants **Goal:** Improvement in breathing pattern		
1. Teach patient diaphragmatic and pursed-lip breathing.	1. Helps patient prolong expiration time and decreases air trapping. With these techniques, patient will breathe more efficiently and effectively.	• Practices pursed-lip and diaphragmatic breathing and uses them when short of breath and with activity • Shows signs of decreased respiratory effort and paces activities
2. Encourage alternating activity with rest periods. Allow patient to make some decisions (bath, shaving) about care based on tolerance level.	2. Pacing activities permits patient to perform activities without excessive distress.	• Uses inspiratory muscle trainer as prescribed
3. Encourage use of an inspiratory muscle trainer if prescribed.	3. Strengthens and conditions the respiratory muscles.	
Nursing Diagnosis: Self-care deficits related to fatigue secondary to increased work of breathing and insufficient ventilation and oxygenation **Goal:** Independence in self-care activities		
1. Teach patient to coordinate diaphragmatic breathing with activity (eg, walking, bending).	1. This will allow the patient to be more active and to avoid excessive fatigue or dyspnea during activity.	• Uses controlled breathing while bathing, bending, and walking • Paces activities of daily living to alternate with rest periods to reduce fatigue and dyspnea
2. Encourage patient to begin to bathe self, dress self, walk, and drink fluids. Discuss energy conservation measures.	2. As condition resolves, patient will be able to do more but needs to be encouraged to avoid increasing dependence.	• Describes energy conservation strategies • Performs same self-care activities as before • Performs postural drainage correctly
3. Teach postural drainage if appropriate.	3. Encourages patient to become involved in own care. Prepares patient to manage at home.	
Nursing Diagnosis: Activity intolerance due to fatigue, hypoxemia, and ineffective breathing patterns		
...tioned consume ...n additional bur-...gh regular, graded ...ups become ...e patient can do ...hort of breath. ...e cycle of		• Performs activities with less shortness of breath • Verbalizes need to exercise daily and demonstrates an exercise plan to be carried out at home • Walks and gradually increases walking time and distance to improve physical condition • Exercises both upper and lower body muscle groups
...ialization, anxiety, depression, lower activity level,		
...s will promote a ...plishment rather ...than defeat and hopelessness.		• Expresses interest in the future • Participates in the discharge plan • Discusses activities or methods that can be performed to ease shortness of breath
2. Encourage activity to level of symptom tolerance.	2. Activity reduces tension and decreases degree of dyspnea as patient becomes conditioned.	• Uses relaxation techniques appropriately • Expresses interest in a pulmonary rehabilitation program

(continued)

Chart 16-5
Home Care Checklist • Chemotherapy Administration

At the completion of the home care instruction, the patient or caregiver will be able to:	Patient	Caregiver
• Demonstrate how to administer the chemotherapy agent in the home.	✓	✓
• Demonstrate safe disposal of needles, syringes, IV supplies, or unused chemotherapy medications.	✓	✓
• List possible side effects of chemotherapeutic agents.	✓	✓
• List complications of medications necessitating a call to the nurse or physician.	✓	✓
• List complications of medications necessitating a visit to the emergency department.	✓	✓
• List names and telephone numbers of resource personnel involved in care (ie, home care nurse, infusion services, IV vendor, equipment company).	✓	✓
• Explain treatment plan (protocol) and importance of upcoming visits to physician.	✓	✓

▲ **Home Care Checklists**—include guidelines on goals and management of home-based patients.

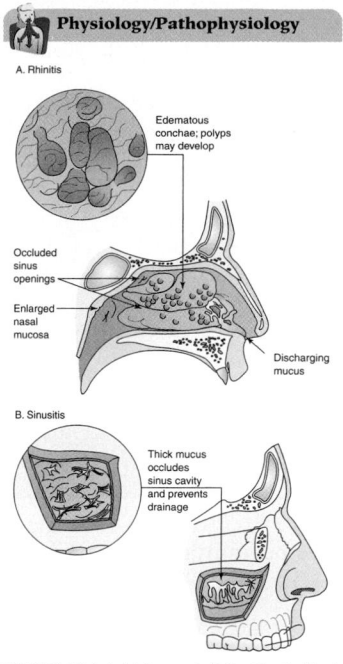

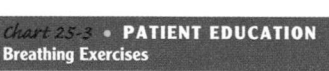

Physiology/Pathophysiology

A. Rhinitis

- Edematous conchae; polyps may develop
- Occluded sinus openings
- Enlarged nasal mucosa
- Discharging mucus

B. Sinusitis

- Thick mucus occludes sinus cavity and prevents drainage

FIGURE 22-1 Pathophysiologic processes in rhinitis and sinusitis. Although pathophysiologic processes are similar in rhinitis and sinusitis, they affect different structures. In rhinitis (A), the mucous membranes lining the nasal passages become inflamed, congested, and edematous. The swollen nasal conchae block the sinus openings, and mucus is discharged from the nostrils. Sinusitis (B) is also marked by inflammation and congestion, with thickened mucous secretions filling the sinus cavities and occluding the openings.

▲ **Pathophysiology Displays**—utilize illustrations and algorithms to demonstrate processes.

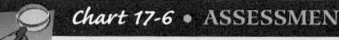

Chart 17-6 • ASSESSMENT

Nursing Assessment of Symptoms Associated With Terminal Illness

- How is this symptom affecting the patient's life?
- What is the meaning of the symptom to the patient? To the family?
- How does the symptom affect physical functioning, mobility, comfort, sleep, nutritional status, elimination, activity level, and relationships with others?
- What makes the symptom better?
- What makes it worse?
- Is it worse at any particular time of the day?
- What are the patient's expectations and goals for m[...] symptom? The family's?
- How is the patient coping with the symptom?
- What is the economic effect of the symptom and it[...] management?

Adapted from Jacox, A., Carr, D. B., & Payne, R. (1994). M[...] *cancer pain.* Rockville, MD: AHCPR.

▲ **Assessment Displays**—provide clinical features of diseases and disorders and include guidelines for assessing health history and exam findings.

Pharmacology Charts—review ▶ recent or common drug therapies with discussion of clinical trials where appropriate.

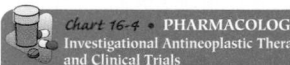

Chart 16-4 • PHARMACOLOGY
Investigational Antineoplastic Therapies and Clinical Trials

Evaluation of the effectiveness and toxic potential of promising new modalities for preventing, diagnosing, and treating cancer is accomplished through clinical trials. Before new chemotherapy agents are approved for clinical use, they are subjected to rigorous and lengthy evaluations to identify beneficial effects, adverse effects, and safety.

- *Phase I* clinical trials determine optimal dosing, scheduling, and toxicity.
- *Phase II* trials determine effectiveness with specific tumor types and further define toxicities. Participants in these early trials are most often those who have not responded to standard forms of treatment. Because phase I and II trials may be viewed as last-chance efforts, patients and families are fully informed about the experimental nature of the trial therapies. Although it is hoped that investigational therapy will effectively treat the disease, the purpose of early phase trials is to gather information concerning maximal tolerated doses, adverse effects, and effects of the antineoplastic agents on tumor growth.
- *Phase III* clinical trials establish the effectiveness of new medications or procedures as compared with conventional approaches. Nurses may assist in the recruitment, consent, and education processes for patients who participate. In many cases, nurses are instrumental in monitoring adherence, assisting patients to adhere to the parameters of the trial, and documenting data describing patients' responses. The physical and emotional needs of patients in clinical trials are addressed in much the same way as those of patients who receive standard forms of cancer treatment.
- *Phase IV* testing further investigates medications in terms of new uses, dosing schedule, and toxicities.

Chart 25-3 • PATIENT EDUCATION
Breathing Exercises

General Instructions
- Breathe slowly and rhythmically to exhale completely and empty the lungs completely.
- Inhale through the nose to filter, humidify, and warm the air before it enters the lungs.
- If you feel out of breath, breathe more slowly by prolonging the exhalation time.
- Keep the air moist with a humidifier.

Diaphragmatic Breathing
Goal: To use and strengthen the diaphragm during breathing
- Place one hand on the abdomen (just below the ribs) and the other hand on the middle of the chest to increase the awareness of the position of the diaphragm and its function in breathing.
- Breathe in slowly and deeply through the nose, letting the abdomen protrude as far as possible.
- Breathe out through pursed lips while tightening (contracting) the abdominal muscles.
- Press firmly inward and upward on the abdomen while breathing out.
- Repeat for 1 minute; follow with a rest period of 2 minutes.
- Gradually increase duration up to 5 minutes, several times a day (before meals and at bedtime).

Pursed-Lip Breathing
Goal: To prolong exhalation and increase airway pressure during expiration, thus reducing the amount of trapped air and the amount of airway resistance.
- Inhale through the nose while counting to 3—the amount of time needed to say "Smell a rose."
- Exhale slowly and evenly against pursed lips while tightening the abdominal muscles. (Pursing the lips increases intratracheal pressure; exhaling through the mouth offers less resistance to expired air.)
- Count to 7 while prolonging expiration through pursed lips—the length of time to say "Blow out the candle."
- While sitting in a chair:
  Fold arms over the abdomen.
  Inhale through the nose while counting to 3.
  Bend forward and exhale slowly through pursed lips while counting to 7.
- While walking:
  Inhale while walking two steps.
  Exhale through pursed lips while walking four or five steps.

Chart 21-8
Risk Factors for Hypoventilation

- Limited neurologic impulses transmitted from the brain to the respiratory muscles, as in spinal cord trauma, cerebrovascular accidents, tumors, myasthenia gravis, Guillain-Barré syndrome, polio, and drug overdose
- Depressed respiratory centers in the medulla, as with anesthesia and drug overdose
- Limited thoracic movement (kyphoscoliosis), limited lung movement (pleural effusion, pneumothorax), or reduced functional lung tissue (chronic pulmonary diseases, severe pulmonary edema)

◀ **Risk Factor Charts**—outline factors that may impair health (eg, carcinogens, environmental factors), and offer preventive measures to sidestep them.

Gerontologic ▶ **Considerations**—provide specific information relevant to the older population.

Gerontologic Considerations
Factors Contributing to Urinary Tract Infection in Older Adults

- High incidence of chronic illness
- Frequent use of antimicrobial agents
- Presence of infected pressure ulcers
- Immobility and incomplete emptying of bladder
- Use of a bedpan rather than a commode or toilet

◀ **Patient Education Boxes**—provide suggestions on such topics as self-care, or how to cope with health challenges.

NURSING ALERT It is the responsibility of all nurses, and particularly perianesthesia and perioperative nurses, to be aware of latex allergies, necessary precautions, and products that are latex-free (Meeker & Rothrock, 1999). Hospital staff are also at risk for developing a latex allergy secondary to repeated exposure to latex products.

▲ **Nursing Alerts**—offer brief tips for clinical practice and red-flag warnings to help students avoid common mistakes.

NURSING RESEARCH PROFILE 12-2
Identification of Agitation in Patients with Alzheimer's Disease

Whall, A. L., Black, M. E. A., Yankou, D. J., et al. (1999). Nurse aides' identification of onset and level of agitation in late stage dementia patients. *American Journal of Alzheimer's Disease, 14*, 202–206.

Purpose
Nursing assistants provide the majority of care to patients in nursing homes. They are vital links in the early identification, and therefore in the treatment, of agitation in patients with Alzheimer's disease. Nurses' aides (NAs) are sometimes characterized as unwilling or unable to manage patients' agitation. This study examines the process by which nurses' aides can successfully identify this agitation.

Design
NAs from five different nursing homes owned by the same corporate entity were asked to participate in the study. Criteria to participate included being employed for at least 1 year. (Rese___ demonstrates that NAs who remain at a facility longer than 1 usually have a commitment to those they serve.) The NAs did receive any additional wages and were only promised a letter t dicate that they had participated in the study. Each NA receive proximately 1 hour of training via audio tapes and conversation nurse experts. Each NA was then paired with a nurse expert t sess his or her skill at appropriately identifying levels of agitatic patients with late-stage Alzheimer's disease.

Conclusions
This study demonstrated that NAs with a minimum of 1 ye employment did an excellent job in acquiring new observa skills with only 1 hour of training and positive reinforcement letter noting their participation in this study. The NAs' assess of signs of agitation agreed with that of the nurse expert more 90% of the time. All the NAs involved reported gaining helpfu sights in managing agitated behavior as a result of participatic the study.

Implications fc
The results of th
observe and rep
session using adu
of their input in
servation and rep
agitation from in

▲ **Glossary**—at the beginning of every chapter, helps students learn vocabulary.

◀ **Nursing Research Profiles**—contain research samples with purpose of research, study sample, and design and findings, and implications for use in evidence-based nursing.

Glossary

adaptation: a change or alteration designed to assist in adapting to a new situation or environment
adrenocorticotropic hormone (ACTH): a hormone produced by the anterior lobe of the pituitary gland that stimulates the secretion of cortisone and other hormones by the adrenal cortex
antidiuretic hormone (ADH): a hormone secreted by the posterior lobe of the pituitary gland that constricts blood vessels, elevates blood pressure, and reduces the excretion of urine
catecholamines: any of the group of amines (such as epinephrine, norepinephrine, or ____ ___ at serve as neurotransmitters ___nitive and behavioral strate__ __anage the stressors that tax a ___urces
___nge in the appearance of a __osure to chronic irritation ___: the group of steroid hor__ __as cortisol, that are produced

by the adrenal cortex; they are involved in carbohydrate, protein, and fat metabolism and have anti-inflammatory properties
gluconeogenesis: the formation of glucose, especially by the liver from noncarbohydrate sources such as amino acids and the glycerol portion of fats
guided imagery: use of the imagination to achieve relaxation or direct attention away from uncomfortable sensations or situations
homeostasis: a steady state within the body; the stability of the internal environment
hyperplasia: an increase in the number of new cells
hypoxia: inadequate supply of oxygen to the cell
infectious agents: biologic agents, such as viruses, bacteria, rickettsiae, mycoplasmas, fungi, protozoa, and nematodes, that cause disease in people
inflammation: a localized, protective reaction of tissue to injury, irritation, or infec-

tion, manifested by pain, redness, heat, swelling, and sometimes loss of function
metabolic rate: the speed at which some substances are broken down to yield energy for bodily processes and other substances are synthesized
metaplasia: a cell transformation in which a highly specialized cell changes to a less specialized cell
negative feedback: feedback that decreases the output of a system
positive feedback: feedback that increases the output of a system
steady state: a stable condition that does not change over time, or when change in one direction is balanced by change in an opposite direction
stress: a disruptive condition that occurs in response to adverse influences from the internal or external environments
vasoconstriction: the narrowing of a blood vessel

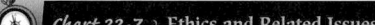

Chart 25-15
GUIDELINES FOR Care of the Patient Being Weaned From Mechanical Ventilation

NURSING INTERVENTIONS	RATIONALE
1. Assess patient for weaning criteria: Vital capacity—10 to 15 mL/kg Maximum inspiratory pressure (MIP) at least –20 cm H_2O Tidal volume—7 to 9 mL/kg Minute ventilation—6 L/min Rapid/shallow breathing index—below 100 breaths/minute/L PaO_2 greater than 60 mm Hg with FiO_2 less than 40%	1. Careful assessment of multiple weaning indices helps to determine readiness for weaning. When the criteria have been met, the patient's likelihood of successful weaning increases.
2. Monitor activity level, assess dietary intake, and monitor results of laboratory tests of nutritional status.	2. Reestablishing independent spontaneous ventilation can be physically exhausting. It is crucial that the patient have enough energy reserves to succeed. Providing periods of rest and recommended nutritional intake can increase the likelihood of successful weaning.
3. Assess the patient's and family's understanding of the weaning process and address any concerns about the process. Explain that the patient may feel short of breath initially and provide encouragement as needed. Reassure the patient that he or she will be attended closely and that if the weaning attempt is not successful, it can be tried again later.	3. The weaning process can be psychologically tiring; emotional support can help promote a sense of security. Explaining that weaning will be attempted again later helps reduce the sense of failure if the first attempts are unsuccessful.
4. Implement the weaning method prescribed: A/C, IMV, SIMV, PSV, PAV, CPAP, or T-piece.	4. The prescribed weaning method should reflect the patient's individualized criteria for weaning and weaning history. By having different methods to choose from, the physician can select the one that best fits the patient.
5. M_____al signs, pulse oximetry, ECG, and respiratory pattern ____or the first 20 to 30 minutes and every 5 minutes after __eaning is complete.	5. Monitoring the patient closely provides ongoing indications of success or failure.
___patent airway; monitor arterial blood gas levels and ___ function tests. Suction the airway as needed.	6. These values can be compared to baseline measurements to evaluate weaning. Suctioning helps to reduce the risk of aspiration and maintain the airway.
___tion with the physician, terminate the weaning process ___actions occur. These include a heart rate increase of __n, systolic blood pressure increase of 20 mm Hg, a ___xygen saturation to less than 90%, respiratory rate __r greater than 20 breaths/minute, ventricular dys___atigue, panic, cyanosis, erratic or labored breathing, __chest movement.	7. These signs and symptoms indicate an unstable patient at risk for hypoxia and ventricular dysrhythmias. Continuing the weaning process can lead to cardiopulmonary arrest.
__ng process continues, measure tidal volume and minute ___very 20 to 30 minutes; compare with the patient's ___es, which have been determined in collaboration ___sician.	8. These values help to determine if weaning is successful and should be continued.
___sychological dependence if the physiologic parameters ___ning is feasible and the patient still resists.	9. Psychological dependence is a common problem after mechanical ventilation. Possible causes include fear of dying and depression from chronic illness. It is important to address this issue before the next weaning attempt.

Chart 22-7   Ethics and Related Issues

Situation
A 68-year-old attorney was diagnosed with cancer of the larynx 8 years ago. He was treated successfully with radiation therapy, resulting in an altered voice quality. Recently, he has complained of shortness of breath and difficulty swallowing. In the past few months, he also has noticed a marked change in his voice and physical condition, which he attributed to "winter colds."

After a complete physical exam and an extensive diagnostic workup and biopsy, it is determined that the cancer has recurred at a new primary site. His health care provider recommends surgery (a total laryngectomy) and chemotherapy as the best options. The patient states that he is not willing to "lose my voice and my livelihood" but instead will "take my chances." He has also expressed concern about his quality of life after surgery. His family has approached you about trying to convince him to have surgery.

Dilemma
The patient's right to refuse treatment conflicts with the family's wishes and recommendation from his health care provider.

Discussion
1. Is the patient making a decision based upon all pertinent information concerning his health status, treatment, options, risk/benefits, and long-term prognosis?
2. What arguments can be made to support the patient's decision to forego treatment?
3. What arguments can be made to question the patient's decision to forego treatment?

▲ **Procedure Guidelines Charts**—offer nursing activities and rationales for important skills.

◀ **Ethics and Related Issues**—showcase brief scenarios and present possible ethical dilemmas for discussion.

Contents

Unit 3

Concepts and Challenges
in Patient Management   214

unit 6

Cardiovascular, Circulatory, and Hematologic Function   644

Unit 8

Metabolic and Endocrine Function   1072

Brunner & Suddarth's
Textbook of
MEDICAL-SURGICAL NURSING

Basic Concepts in Nursing

Applying Concepts from NANDA, NIC, and NOC

A nurse working in an urgent care clinic that serves an economically depressed urban area notes a high incidence of elderly patients with dehydration and heatstroke in the summer months. The nurse verifies the observations by accessing data about hospital admissions for dehydration and heat stroke. The nurse determines that many of the admitted patients live in the area served by the clinic, and that many of the patients live alone and have other chronic illnesses. The nurse sees the need for a plan that includes a community response to this problem. The plan includes arranging an education program about the prevention of dehydration; a community support buddy system in which neighbors or volunteers call or visit homebound elders during critical periods in the summer; and economic support to air condition the senior citizens' center. The concept map illustrates some of the diagnoses, interventions, and outcomes the nurse uses to guide the plan of care.

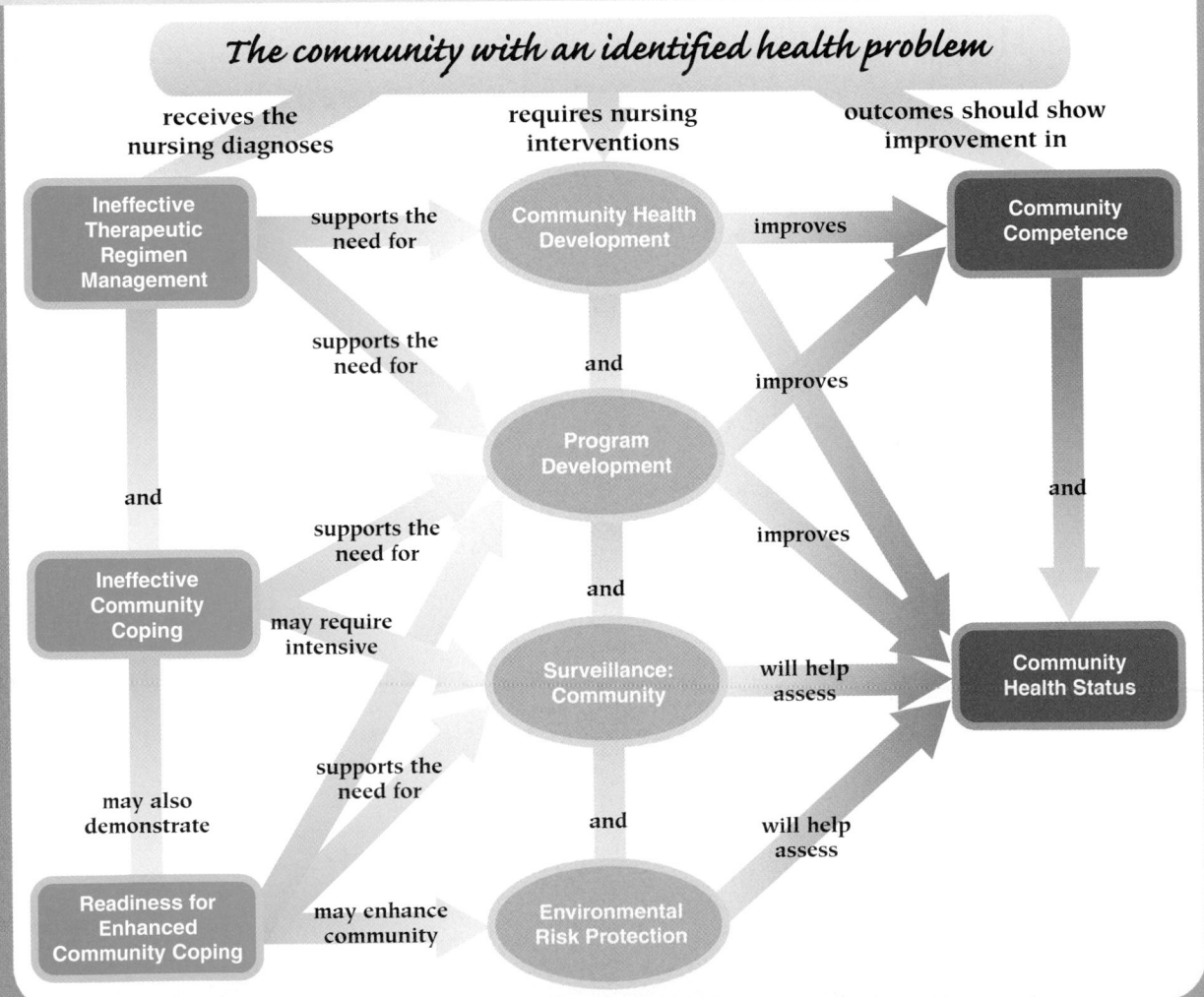

The community with an identified health problem

receives the nursing diagnoses — requires nursing interventions — outcomes should show improvement in

- **Ineffective Therapeutic Regimen Management** — supports the need for → **Community Health Development** — improves → **Community Competence**
- supports the need for
- and
- **Ineffective Community Coping** — supports the need for → **Program Development** — improves
- may require intensive
- and
- **Surveillance: Community** — will help assess → **Community Health Status**
- may also demonstrate — supports the need for
- and
- will help assess
- **Readiness for Enhanced Community Coping** — may enhance community → **Environmental Risk Protection**
- improves
- and

Nursing Classifications and Languages

NANDA
Nursing Diagnoses

Ineffective Community Therapeutic Regimen Management—Pattern of regulating and integrating into community processes programs for treatment of illness and the sequelae of illness that are unsatisfactory for meeting health-related goals

Ineffective Community Coping—A pattern of community activities for adaptation and problem solving that is unsatisfactory for meeting the demands or needs of the community

Readiness for Enhanced Community Coping—Pattern of community activities for adaptation and problem solving that is satisfactory for meeting the demands or needs of the community but can be improved for management of current and future problems/stressors

NIC
Nursing Interventions*

Community Health Development—Facilitating members of a community to identify a community's health concerns, mobilize resources, and implement solutions

Program Development—Planning, implementing, and evaluating a coordinated set of activities designed to enhance wellness, or to prevent, reduce or eliminate one or more health problems of a group or community

Surveillance: Community—Purposeful and ongoing acquisition, interpretation, and synthesis of data for decision making in the community

Environmental Risk Protection—Preventing and detecting disease and injury in populations at risk from environmental hazards

NOC
Nursing Outcomes†

Return to functional baseline status, stabilization of, or improvement in

Community Competence—The ability of a community to collectively problem solve to achieve goals

Community Health Status—The general state of well-being of a community or population

NANDA, North American Nursing Diagnosis Association; NIC, Nursing Interventions Classification; NOC, Nursing Outcomes Classification

*Iowa Intervention Project © 2000. In McCloskey, J. C., & Bulechek, G. M. (2000). *Nursing interventions classification (NIC)* (3rd ed.). St. Louis: Mosby.

†Iowa Outcomes Project © 2000. In Johnson, M., Maas, M., & Moorhead, S. (2000). *Nursing outcomes classification (NOC)* (3rd ed.). St. Louis: Mosby.

Health Care Delivery and Nursing Practice

LEARNING OBJECTIVES

On completion of this chapter, the learner will be able to:

1. Define health and wellness.
2. Describe factors causing significant changes in the health care delivery system and their impact on the health care field and the nursing profession.
3. Describe the practitioner, leadership, and research roles of the nurse.
4. Describe nursing care delivery models.
5. Discuss expanded nursing roles.

*T*he health care industry, like other industries in U.S. society, has experienced profound changes during the past several decades. Nursing, as a health care profession and a major component of the health care delivery system, is significantly affected by shifts in the health care industry. In addition, nursing has been and will continue to be an important force in shaping the future of the health care system.

The Health Care Industry and the Nursing Profession

Although the delivery of nursing care has been affected by changes occurring in the health care system, the definition of nursing has continued to distinguish nursing care and identify the major aspects of nursing care.

NURSING DEFINED

Since the time of Florence Nightingale, who wrote in 1858 that the goal of nursing was "to put the patient in the best condition for nature to act upon him," nursing leaders have described nursing as both an art and a science. However, the definition of nursing has evolved over time. The American Nurses Association (ANA), in its Social Policy Statement (ANA, 1995), defined nursing as "the diagnosis and treatment of human responses to health and illness" and provided the following illustrative list of phenomena that are the focus for nursing care and research:

* Self-care processes
* Physiologic and pathophysiologic processes in areas such as rest, sleep, respiration, circulation, reproduction, activity, nutrition, elimination, skin, sexuality, and communication
* Comfort, pain, and discomfort
* Emotions related to experiences of health and illness
* Meanings ascribed to health and illnesses
* Decision making and ability to make choices
* Perceptual orientations such as self-image and control over one's body and environments
* Transitions across the life span, such as birth, growth, development, and death
* Affiliative relationships, including freedom from oppression and abuse
* Environmental systems

Nurses have a responsibility to carry out their role as defined in the Social Policy Statement, to comply with the nurse practice act of the state where they practice, and to comply with the code for nurses as spelled out by the International Council of Nurses and the ANA. Understanding the needs of health care consumers and the health care delivery system, including the forces that affect nursing and health care delivery, will provide a foundation for examining the delivery of nursing care.

THE PATIENT/CLIENT: CONSUMER OF NURSING AND HEALTH CARE

The central figure in health care services is, of course, the patient. The term *patient,* which is derived from a Latin verb meaning "to suffer," has traditionally been used to describe those who are recipients of care. The connotation commonly attached to the word is one of dependence. For this reason, many nurses prefer to use the term *client,* which is derived from a Latin verb meaning "to lean," connoting alliance and interdependence. For the purposes of this book, the term *patient* will be used throughout, but with the understanding that either term is acceptable.

The patient who seeks care for a health problem or problems (increasing numbers of people have multiple health problems) is also an individual, a member of a family, and a citizen of the community. Patients' needs vary depending on their problem, associated circumstances, and past experiences. One of the nurse's important functions in health care delivery is to identify the patient's immediate needs and take measures to address them.

The Patient's Basic Needs

Certain needs are basic to all people and require satisfaction accordingly. Such needs are addressed on the basis of priority, meaning that some needs are more pressing than others. Once an essential need is met, the person experiences a need on a higher level. Approaching needs according to priority reflects Maslow's hierarchy of needs (Fig. 1-1).

Maslow's Hierarchy

Maslow ranked human needs as follows: physiologic needs; safety and security; belongingness and affection; esteem and self-respect; and self-actualization, which includes self-fulfillment, desire to know and understand, and aesthetic needs. Lower-level needs always remain, but a person's ability to pursue higher-level needs indicates that he or she is moving toward psychological health and well-being. Such a hierarchy of needs is a useful organizational framework that can be applied to the various nursing models for assessment of a patient's strengths, limitations, and need for nursing interventions.

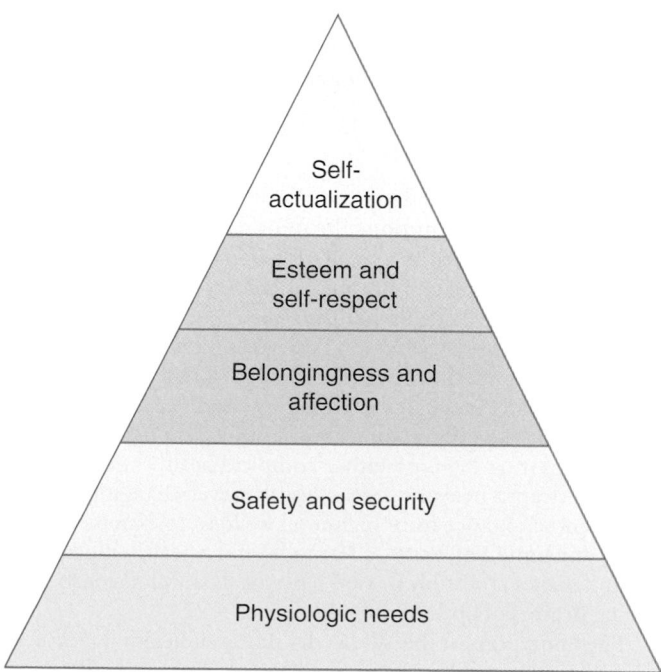

FIGURE 1-1 This scheme of Maslow's hierarchy of human needs shows how a person moves from fulfillment of basic needs to higher levels of needs, with the ultimate goal being integrated human functioning and health.

HEALTH CARE IN TRANSITION

Changes occurring in health care delivery and nursing are the result of societal, economic, technological, scientific, and political forces that have evolved throughout the 20th and into the 21st century. Among the most significant changes are shifts in population demographics, particularly the increase in the aging population and the cultural diversity of the population; changing patterns of diseases; increased technology; increased consumer expectations; the high costs of health care and changes in health care financing; and other health care reform efforts. These changes have led to institutional restructuring, staff downsizing, increased outpatient care services, decreased lengths of hospital stay, and more care being provided in the community and in the home. Such changes are having a dramatic influence on where nurses practice, with an increasing trend for nurses to provide health care in community and home settings. Indeed, these changes have a dynamic influence on our view of health and illness and therefore affect the focus of nursing and health care.

As an increasing proportion of the population reaches age 65 years and older, and with the shift in disease patterns from acute illnesses to chronic illnesses, the traditional disease management and care focus of the health care professions has expanded. There is growing concern about emerging infectious diseases, trauma, and bioterrorism. The health care focus must center more on prevention, health promotion, and management of chronic conditions than in previous times. This shift in focus coincides with a nationwide emphasis on cost control and resource management directed toward providing cost-efficient and cost-effective health care services to the population as a whole.

Health, Wellness, and Health Promotion

The health care system of the United States, which traditionally has been disease oriented, is currently placing greater emphasis on health and its promotion. Similarly, a significant portion of nursing's workforce formerly was focused on the care of patients with acute conditions, but now a growing portion is directing its efforts toward health promotion and disease prevention.

HEALTH

How health is perceived depends on how health is defined. In the preamble to its constitution, the World Health Organization (WHO) defines health as a "state of complete physical, mental, and social well-being and not merely the absence of disease and infirmity" (Hood & Leddy, 2002). Such a definition of health does not allow for any variation in degrees of wellness or illness. On the other hand, the concept of a health–illness continuum allows for a greater range in describing a person's health status. By viewing health and illness on a continuum, it is possible to consider a person as having neither complete health nor complete illness. Instead, a person's state of health is ever-changing and has the potential to range from high-level wellness to extremely poor health and imminent death. The model of the health–illness continuum makes it possible to view a person as simultaneously possessing degrees of both health and illness.

The limitations of the WHO definition of health are clear in relation to chronic illness and disability. A chronically ill person cannot meet the standards of health as established by the WHO definition. However, when viewed from the perspective of the health–illness continuum, people with chronic illness or disability can be understood as having the potential to attain a high level of wellness, if they are successful in meeting their health potential within the limits of their chronic illness or disability.

WELLNESS

Wellness has been defined as being equivalent to health. Cookfair (1996) indicated that wellness "includes a conscious and deliberate approach to an advanced state of physical, psychological, and spiritual health and is a dynamic, fluctuating state of being" (p. 149). Leddy and Pepper (1998) contended that wellness is indicated by the capacity of the person to perform to the best of his or her ability, the ability to adjust and adapt to varying situations, a reported feeling of well-being, and a feeling that "everything is together" and harmonious. With this in mind, it becomes evident that the goal of health care providers is to promote positive changes that are directed toward health and well-being. The fact that the sense of wellness has a subjective aspect emphasizes the importance of recognizing and responding to patient individuality and diversity in health care and nursing.

HEALTH PROMOTION

Today, increasing emphasis is placed on health, health promotion, wellness, and self-care. Health is seen as resulting from a lifestyle that is oriented toward wellness. The result has been the evolution of a wide range of health promotion strategies, including multiphasic screening, genetic testing, lifetime health monitoring programs, environmental and mental health programs, risk reduction, and nutrition and health education. A growing interest in self-care skills is evidenced by the large number of health-related publications, conferences, and workshops designed for the lay public.

Individuals are increasingly knowledgeable about their health and are encouraged to take more interest in and responsibility for their health and well-being. Organized self-care education programs emphasize health promotion, disease prevention, management of illness, self-medication, and judicious use of the professional health care system. In addition, well over 500,000 self-help groups and numerous web sites and chat groups exist for the purpose of sharing experiences and information about self-care with others who have similar conditions, chronic diseases, or disabilities.

Special efforts are being made by health care professionals to reach and motivate members of various cultural and socioeconomic groups concerning lifestyle and health practices. Stress, improper diet, lack of exercise, smoking, drugs, high-risk behaviors (including risky sexual practices), and poor hygiene are all lifestyle behaviors known to have a negative effect on health. Health care professionals are concerned with encouraging behavior that promotes health. The goal is to motivate people to make improvements in the way they live, to modify risky behaviors, and to adopt healthy behaviors.

Influences on Health Care Delivery

The health care delivery system is rapidly changing as the population and its health care needs and expectations change. The shifting demographics of the population, the increase in chronic illnesses and disability, the greater emphasis on economics, and technological advances have resulted in changing emphases in health care delivery and in nursing.

POPULATION DEMOGRAPHICS

Changes in the population in general are affecting the need for and the delivery of health care. The 2000 U.S. census data indicated that there were 281,421,906 people in the country (Pluviose-Fenton, 2001). This population expansion is attributed in part to improved public health services and improved nutrition.

Not only is the population increasing, but the composition of the population is also changing. The decline in birth rate and the increase in life span attributed to improved health care have resulted in fewer school-age children and more senior citizens, most of whom are women. Much of the population resides in highly congested urban areas, with a steady migration of minority groups to the inner cities and a migration of middle-class people to suburban areas. The number of homeless people, including entire families, has increased significantly. The population has become more culturally diverse as increasing numbers of people from different national backgrounds enter the country. Because of such population changes, the need for health care for specific age groups, for women, and for a diverse group of people within specific geographic locations is altering the effectiveness of traditional means of providing health care and is necessitating far-reaching changes in the overall health care delivery system.

Aging Population

The elderly population in the United States has increased significantly and will continue to grow in future years. In 1999, the nation's 34.5 million adults older than 65 years of age constituted 12.7% of the population, with a ratio of 141 older women to 100 older men. The number of people in the United States older than 65 years of age is expected to reach 20% of the population by the year 2030. In addition, persons age 85 years and older constitute one of the fastest-growing segments of the population. According to the U.S. Bureau of the Census (2000), the number of people age 65 to 74 years was 8 times larger in 1999 than in 1900, and the number of people age 75 to 84 years was 16 times larger—but the number of people age 85 years and older was 34 times larger in 1999 than in 1900.

Many elderly people suffer from multiple chronic conditions that are exacerbated by acute episodes. Elderly women, whose conditions are frequently underdiagnosed and undertreated, are of particular concern. There are approximately three women for every two men in the older population, and elderly women are expected to continue to outnumber elderly men. The health care needs of older adults are complex and demand significant investments, both professional and financial, by the health care industry.

Cultural Diversity

An appreciation for the diverse characteristics and needs of individuals from varied ethnic and cultural backgrounds is important in health care and nursing. Some projections indicate that by 2030 racial and ethnic minority groups will comprise 40% of the population of the United States (Gooden, Porter, Gonzalez, & Mims, 2000). With increased immigration, both legal and illegal, this figure could easily increase to more than 50% by the year 2030 or even earlier. As the cultural composition of the population changes, it becomes increasingly important to address cultural considerations in the delivery of health care. Patients from diverse sociocultural groups bring to the health care setting different health care beliefs, values, and practices, as well as different risk factors for some disease conditions and unique reactions to treat-

ment. These factors significantly affect the way an individual responds to health care problems or illness, to those who provide the care, and to the care itself. Unless these factors are understood and respected by health care providers, the care delivered may be ineffective and health care outcomes may be negatively affected.

Culture is defined as learned patterns of behavior, beliefs, and values that can be attributed to a particular group of people. Included among the many characteristics that distinguish cultural groups are the manner of dress, language spoken, values, rules or norms of behavior, gender-specific practices, economics, politics, law and social control, artifacts, technology, dietary practices, and health beliefs and practices.

Health promotion, illness prevention, causes of sickness, treatment, coping, caring, dying, and death are part of the health-related component of every culture. Every person has a unique belief and value system that has been shaped at least in part by his or her cultural environment. This belief and value system is very important and guides the individual's thinking, decisions, and actions. It provides direction for interpreting and responding to illness and to health care.

To promote an effective nurse–patient relationship and positive outcomes of care, nursing care must be culturally competent, appropriate, and sensitive to cultural differences. All attempts should be made to help the individual retain his or her unique cultural characteristics. Providing special foods that have significance and arranging for special religious observances may enable the patient to maintain a feeling of wholeness at a time when he or she may feel isolated from family and community.

Knowing the cultural and social significance that particular situations have for each patient helps the nurse avoid imposing a personal value system when the patient has a different point of view. In most cases, cooperation with the plan of care is greatest when communication among the nurse, the patient, and the patient's family is directed toward understanding the situation or the problem and respecting each other's goals.

CHANGING PATTERNS OF DISEASE

During the past 50 years, the health problems of the American people have changed significantly. Many infectious diseases have been controlled or eradicated; others, such as tuberculosis, acquired immunodeficiency syndrome (AIDS), and sexually transmitted diseases, are on the rise. An increasing number of infectious agents are becoming resistant to antibiotic therapy as a result of widespread inappropriate use of antibiotics. Therefore, conditions that were once easily treated have become complex and more life-threatening than ever before.

The chronicity of illnesses and disability is increasing because of the lengthening life span of Americans and the expansion of successful treatment options for conditions such as cancer, human immunodeficiency virus (HIV) infection, and spina bifida; many people with these conditions live decades longer than in earlier years. Chronically ill people are the largest group of health care consumers in the United States (Davis & Magilvy, 2000). Because the majority of health problems seen today are chronic in nature, many people are learning to protect and maximize their health within the constraints of chronic illness and disability.

As chronic conditions increase, health care broadens from a focus on cure and eradication of disease to include the prevention or rapid treatment of exacerbations of chronic conditions. Nursing, which has always encouraged patients to take control of their conditions, plays a prominent role in the current focus on management of chronic illness and disability.

ADVANCES IN TECHNOLOGY AND GENETICS

Advances in technology and genetics have occurred with greater frequency during the past several decades than in all other periods of civilization. Sophisticated techniques and devices have revolutionized surgery and diagnostic testing, making it possible to perform many procedures and tests on an outpatient basis. Increased knowledge and understanding of genetics has resulted in expanded screening, diagnostic testing, and treatments for a variety of conditions. This is also an era of sophisticated communication systems that connect most parts of the world, with the capability of rapid storage, retrieval, and dissemination of information. Such scientific and technological advances are themselves stimulating brisk change as well as swift obsolescence in health care delivery strategies. The advances in technology and genetics have raised many ethical issues for the health care system, health care providers, and society.

ECONOMIC CHANGES

The philosophy that comprehensive, quality health care should be provided for all citizens prompted governmental concern about spiraling health care costs and wide variations in charges among providers. These concerns led to the Medicare prospective payment system (PPS) and the use of diagnosis-related groups (DRGs).

In 1983, the U.S. Congress passed the most significant health legislation since the Medicare program was enacted in 1965. The government was no longer able to afford to reimburse hospitals for patient care that was delivered without any defined limits or costs. Therefore, it approved a PPS for hospital inpatient services. This system of reimbursement, based on DRGs, set the rates for Medicare payments for hospital services. Hospitals receive payment at a fixed rate for patients with diagnoses that fall into a specific DRG. A fixed payment has been predetermined for more than 470 possible diagnostic categories, covering the majority of medical diagnoses of all patients admitted to the hospital. Hospitals receive the same payment for every patient with a given diagnosis or DRG. If the cost of the patient's care is lower than the payment, the hospital gains a profit; if the cost is higher, the hospital incurs a loss. As a result, hospitals now place greater emphasis on reducing costs, utilization of services, and length of patient stay.

In addition, the Balanced Budget Act of 1997 added new rate requirements for ambulatory payment classifications (APCs) to hospitals and other providers of ambulatory care services. These providers must evaluate all services provided with greater efforts toward cost-effectiveness and reduction of costs.

To qualify for Medicare reimbursement, care providers and hospitals must contract with peer review organizations (PROs) to perform quality and utilization review. The PROs monitor admission patterns, lengths of stay, transfers, and the quality of services and validate the DRG coding. The DRG system has provided hospitals with an incentive to cut costs and discharge patients as quickly as possible.

Nurses in hospitals now care for patients who are older and sicker and require more nursing services; nurses in the community are caring for patients who have been discharged earlier and need acute care services with high-technology and long-term care. The importance of an effective discharge planning program, along with utilization review and a quality improvement program, is unquestionable. Nurses in acute care settings must assume responsibility with other health care team members for maintaining quality care while facing pressures to discharge patients and decrease staffing costs. These nurses must also work with nurses in community settings to ensure continuity of care.

DEMAND FOR QUALITY CARE

The general public has become increasingly interested in and knowledgeable about health care and health promotion. This awareness has been stimulated by television, newspapers, magazines, and other communications media and by political debate. The public has become more health conscious and has in general begun to subscribe strongly to the belief that health and quality health care constitute a basic right, rather than a privilege for a chosen few.

In 1977, the National League for Nursing (NLN) issued a statement on nurses' responsibility to uphold patients' rights. The statement addressed patients' rights to privacy, confidentiality, informed participation, self-determination, and access to health records. This statement also indicated ways in which respect for patients' rights and a commitment to safeguarding them could be incorporated into nursing education programs and upheld and reinforced by those in nursing service. Nurses can directly involve themselves in ensuring specific rights, or they can make their influence felt indirectly (NLN, 1977).

The ANA has worked diligently to promote the delivery of quality health and nursing care. Efforts by the ANA range from assessing the quality of health care provided to the public in these changing times to lobbying legislators to pass bills related to issues such as health insurance or length of hospital stay for new mothers.

Legislative changes have promoted both delivery of quality health care and increased access by the public to this care. The National Health Planning and Resources Act of 1974 emphasized the need for planning and providing quality health care for all Americans through coordinated health services, staffing, and facilities at the national, state, and local levels. Medically underserved populations were the target for the primary care services provided for by this act. By the passage of bills supporting health insurance reform, barring discrimination against individuals with preexisting conditions, and expanding the portability of health care coverage, Congress has acknowledged the needs of consumers for adequate health insurance in this time of longer life spans and chronic illnesses. Efforts in some states to provide full health care coverage for citizens, particularly children, represent measures by state governments to promote access to health care. Legislative support of advanced practice nurses in individual practice is a recognition of the contribution of nursing to the health of consumers, particularly underserved populations.

Quality Improvement and Evidence-Based Practice

In the 1980s, hospitals and other health care agencies implemented ongoing quality assurance (QA) programs. These programs were required for reimbursement for services and for accreditation by the Joint Commission on Accreditation of Healthcare Organizations (JCAHO). QA programs sought to establish accountability on the part of the health professions to society for the quality, appropriateness, and cost of health services provided.

The JCAHO developed a generic model that required monitoring and evaluation of quality and appropriateness of care. The model was implemented in health care institutions and agencies through organization-wide QA programs and reporting systems.

Many aspects of the programs were centralized in a QA department. In addition, each patient care and patient services department was responsible for developing its own plan for monitoring and evaluation. Objective and measurable indicators were used to monitor, evaluate, and communicate the quality and appropriateness of care delivered.

In the early 1990s, it was recognized that quality of care as defined by regulatory agencies continued to be difficult to measure. QA criteria were identified as measures to ensure minimal expectations only; they did not provide mechanisms for identifying causes of problems or for determining systems or processes that need improvement. Continuous quality improvement (CQI) was identified as a more effective mechanism for improving the quality of health care. In 1992, the revised standards of the JCAHO mandated that health care organizations implement a CQI program. Recent amendments to JCAHO standards have specified that patients have the right to care that is considerate and preserves dignity; that respects cultural, psychosocial, and spiritual values; and that is age specific (Krozok & Scoggins, 2001). Quality improvement efforts have focused on ensuring that the care provided meets or exceeds JCAHO standards.

Unlike QA, which focuses on individual incidents or errors and minimal expectations, CQI focuses on the processes used to provide care, with the aim of improving quality by assessing and improving those interrelated processes that most affect patient care outcomes and patient satisfaction. CQI involves analyzing, understanding, and improving clinical, financial, or operational processes. Problems identified as more than isolated events are analyzed, and all issues that may affect the outcome are studied. The main focus is on the processes that affect quality.

As health care agencies continue to implement CQI, nurses have many opportunities to be involved in quality improvement. One such opportunity is through facilitation of evidence-based practice. Evidence-based practice—identifying and evaluating current literature and research and incorporating the findings into care guidelines—has been designated as a means of ensuring quality care. Evidence-based practice includes the use of outcome assessment and standardized plans of care such as clinical guidelines, clinical pathways, or algorithms. Many of these measures are being implemented by nurses, particularly by nurse managers and advanced practice nurses. Nurses directly involved in the delivery of care are engaged in analyzing current data and refining the processes used in CQI. Their knowledge of the processes and conditions that affect patient care is critical in designing changes to improve the quality of the care provided.

Clinical Pathways and Care Mapping

Many hospitals, managed care facilities, and home health services nationwide use clinical pathways or care mapping to coordinate care for a caseload of patients (Klenner, 2000). Clinical pathways serve as an interdisciplinary care plan and as the tool for tracking a patient's progress toward achieving positive outcomes within specified time frames. Clinical pathways have been developed for certain DRGs (eg, open heart surgery, pneumonia with comorbidity, fractured hip), for high-risk patients (eg, those receiving chemotherapy), and for patients with certain common health problems (eg, diabetes, chronic pain). Using current literature and expertise, pathways identify best care. The pathway indicates key events, such as diagnostic tests, treatments, activities, medications, consultation, and education, that must occur within specified times for the patient to achieve the desired and timely outcomes.

A case manager often facilitates and coordinates interventions to ensure that the patient progresses through the key events and achieves the desired outcomes. Nurses providing direct care have an important role in the development and use of clinical pathways through their participation in researching the literature and then developing, piloting, implementing, and revising clinical pathways. In addition, nurses monitor outcome achievement and document and analyze variances. Figure 1-2 presents an example of a clinical pathway. Other examples of clinical pathways can be found in Appendix A.

Care mapping, multidisciplinary action plans (MAPs), clinical guidelines, and algorithms are other evidence-based practice tools that are used for interdisciplinary care planning. These tools are used to move patients toward predetermined outcome markers using phases and stages of the disease or condition. Algorithms are used more often in an acute situation to determine a particular treatment based on patient information or response. Care maps, clinical guidelines, and MAPs (the most detailed of all tools) provide coordination of care and education through hospitalization and after discharge (Cesta & Falter, 1999).

Because care mapping and guidelines are used for conditions in which the patient's progression often defies prediction, specific time frames for achieving outcomes are excluded. Patients with highly complex conditions or multiple underlying illnesses may benefit more from care mapping or guidelines than from clinical pathways, because the use of outcome markers (rather than specific time frames) is more realistic in such cases.

Through case management and the use of clinical pathways or care mapping, patients and the care they receive are continually assessed from preadmission to discharge—and in many cases after discharge in the home care and community settings. These tools are used in hospitals and alternative health care delivery systems to facilitate the effective and efficient care of large groups of patients. The resultant continuity of care, effective utilization of services, and cost containment are expected to be major benefits for society and for the health care system.

ALTERNATIVE HEALTH CARE DELIVERY SYSTEMS

The rising cost of health care over the last few decades has led to the use of managed health care and alternative health care delivery systems, including health maintenance organizations (HMOs) and preferred provider organizations (PPOs).

Managed Care

The PPS has given rise to a much broader pattern of reimbursement and cost control: managed health care. Managed care is an important trend in health care. The failure of the regulatory efforts of past decades to cut costs and the escalation of health care costs to 15% to 22% of the gross domestic product have prompted business, labor, and government to assume greater control over the financing and delivery of health care. The common features that characterize managed care include prenegotiated payment rates, mandatory precertification, utilization review, limited choice of provider, and fixed-price reimbursement. The scope of managed care has expanded from inhospital services; to HMOs or variations such as PPOs; to various ambulatory, long-term, and home care services, as well as related diagnostic and therapeutic services. Over time there has been a significant expansion of managed health care to the point that distinctions among different providers—including HMOs,

(text continues on page 14)

TKR Day of Surgery (date) _____	TKR Post-op Day 1 (date) _____	TKR Post-op Day 2 (date) _____

PHYSICAL ASSESSMENT & TREATMENT

TKR Day of Surgery	TKR Post-op Day 1	TKR Post-op Day 2
___ Possessions labeled and secured	___ AM care completed	___ AM care completed
___ VS Q15 min ×3 until stable, then Q1h×4, then Q4h	___ VS Q4h	___ VS Q4h
___ **VS normal, Temp <101°F**	___ **VS normal, temp <101°F**	___ **VS normal, temp <101°F**
___ Lungs clear, non-productive cough, no dyspnea	___ IS, cough & deep breathing Q1h W/A	___ IS, cough & deep breathing Q4h W/A
___ Oxygen as ordered	___ Lungs clear, non-productive cough, no dyspnea	___ Lungs clear, non-productive cough, no dyspnea
___ IS, cough & deep breathing Q1h W/A	___ Oxygen saturation >92%, oxygen discontinued	___ I/O Q Shift
___ I/O Q Shift	___ I/O Q Shift	___ Saline lock site w/o redness
___ Nausea and vomiting tolerable w or w/o meds	___ IV line converted to saline lock, site w/o redness	___ Wearing TEDs
___ Emesis without blood	___ Nausea and vomiting tolerable w or w/o meds	___ TEDs removed × 1/2 hr, heels w/o redness
___ Wearing TEDs	___ Emesis without blood	___ Skin without breakdown
___ Skin without breakdown	___ Wearing TEDs	___ Pneumatic boots or stockings when in bed
___ Pneumatic boots or stockings on when in bed	___ TEDs removed × 1/2 hr, heels w/o redness	___ CPM settings
___ Begin CPM setting	___ Skin without breakdown	___ Brace applied (if ordered)
___ IV patent, site without redness	___ Pneumatic boots or stockings on when in bed	___ **Alert and Oriented × 3, speech clear**
___ **Alert and Oriented × 3, speech clear**	___ CPM Settings	___ **Normal Neurovascular checks (Q shift)**
___ Normal Neurovascular checks (Q2h)	___ Measured for brace/applied (if ordered)	___ Wound dsg change time:
___ **Hemovac patent and vacuum intact**	___ **Alert and Oriented × 3, speech clear**	___ Staples/sutures intact
___ **Hemovac drainage <500 cc in 8 hrs**	___ **Normal Neurovascular checks (Q shift)**	___ Wound drainage min amt, serous/serosanguinous
___ **Wound bandage clean, dry and intact**	___ Hemovac discontinued	
	___ Wound dsg change time:	
	___ Staples/suture intact	
	___ Wound drainage min amt, serous/serosanguinous	

PSYCHOSOCIAL ASSESSMENT

TKR Day of Surgery	TKR Post-op Day 1	TKR Post-op Day 2
___ Oriented to room		
___ Coping effectively	___ Coping effectively	___ Coping effectively
___ Sleeping well: ❑ with medication ❑ without medication	___ Sleeping well: ❑ with medication ❑ without medication	___ Sleeping well: ❑ with medication ❑ without medication

TESTS/LABS

TKR Day of Surgery	TKR Post-op Day 1	TKR Post-op Day 2
___ Other tests WNL	___ H&H ≥ 9/26	___ H&H ≥ 9/26
	___ Chem 7 WNL	___ Other:
	___ T/K Revision cultures no growth	___ Final T/K Revision cultures without growth
	___ Other:	

PAIN CONTROL/MEDICATION

TKR Day of Surgery	TKR Post-op Day 1	TKR Post-op Day 2
___ IV antibiotics given	___ Transfusion given if ordered ❑ AB ❑ BB ❑ DD	___ **Offer oral meds for pain 30 minutes before therapy prn**
___ Ice pack to surgical site	___ # of transfusions	___ Patient reported pain level ≤ 3 (0–10)
___ Pain control: ❑ Spinal ❑ Epidural ❑ PCA	___ IV Antibiotics completed	
___ Patient reported pain level ≤ 3 (0–10)	___ ❑ Spinal ❑ Epidural ❑ PCA discontinued	
	___ Patient reported pain level ≤ 3 (0–10)	

NUTRITION

TKR Day of Surgery	TKR Post-op Day 1	TKR Post-op Day 2
___ Offered liquids	___ Diet advanced and tolerated	___ No nausea or vomiting, usual diet

(continued)

FIGURE 1-2 A portion of a clinical pathway for Total Knee Replacement (TKR). This section of the pathway indicates the type of clinical treatment or patient care activities to be carried out during the day of surgery and on the first 2 days after surgery for a patient undergoing total knee replacement. The accompanying pathway documentation form is used to document any variances from the pathway that occur. Reproduced with permission from Inova Mount Vernon Hospital, Alexandria, VA.

ELIMINATION

___ Foley catheter in place
___ Urine clear, output ≥30 cc/hr
___ Bowel sounds present, abdomen soft

___ Foley catheter discontinued
___ Voiding QS
___ Bowel sounds present, abdomen soft

___ Voiding QS
___ Normal bowel sounds, abdomen soft

ACTIVITY & THERAPY

___ General plan & comorbidities documented
___ Trapeze in place
___ Heels elevated while in bed
___ Dangled/stood at bedside 6–12 hrs after surgery
___ Ambulate Uni-knee ___

___ Trapeze in place
___ Heels elevated while in bed/knee extended
___ Ambulates to bathroom (BR) with walker or crutches uses 3:1 commode ___
___ PT/OT eval completed, Plan of Care established
___ Goals established (Outcomes/Rehab Rounds Form)
___ Evaluation same as pre-op
___ Chart reviewed

___ Trapeze removed
___ Heels elevated while in bed/knee extended
___ Dressed in gym clothes
___ OOB for 2 of 3 meals
___ Ambulates to BR with walker or crutches/assist:
___ uses 3:1 commode

Instruction and practice:
___ Supine to sit ___
___ Transfers to EOB ___
___ Sit to stand ___

___ Curbs and steps

Tech treatment
___ Gait on level surface ___

___ Device ___
___ Distance ___
___ Toilet transfer
___ Toilet hygiene
___ Grooming
___ Wash UE/trunk/LE
___ Dressing (LE)
___ Dressing (UE)
___ Shoes/socks
___ Brace on/off

Exercises in gym:
___ Ankle pumps, quad/glut sets ___
___ Heelslide ___
___ Straight Leg Raise ___
___ SAQ (right) ___
___ SAQ (left) ___
___ Abduction/adduction

	Extension	HS	Sitting flexion	Quad leg
RK	___	___	___	___
LK	___	___	___	___
Endurance				

___ Instruction in set up of elevated toilet seat

Instruction and practice:
___ Supine to sit ___
___ Transfers to EOB ___
___ Dangle/Stand ___
___ Sit to stand ___
___ OOB in chair
___ Gait on level surface ___

___ Device ___
___ Distance ___

Exercises in gym:
___ Ankle pump, quad/glut sets ___
___ Heelslide ___
___ Straight Leg Raise ___
___ SAQ (right) ___
___ SAQ (left) ___
___ Eval for UE group

	Extension	HS	Sitting flexion	Quad leg
RK	___	___	___	___
LK	___	___	___	___
Endurance				

___ Instruction in set up of elevated toilet seat

Instruction and practice:
___ Ankle pump.
___ Quad/glut sets

FIGURE 1-2 (Continued) *Key:* T/K = total knee; EOB = edge of bed; SAQ = short arc quad; UE = upper extremity; LE = lower extremity; TJR = total joint replacement; RK = right knee; LK = left knee; 3:1 Commode = commode used at bedside, over toilet, and as a shower chair.

(continued)

11

TKR Day of Surgery (date) ___	TKR Post-op Day 1 (date) ___	TKR Post-op Day 2 (date) ___

EDUCATION

TKR Day of Surgery
___ TJR packet given to patient
___ Post do's and don'ts, exercises at bedside
Patient instructed in/demonstrates understanding of
___ IS, cough & deep breathe
___ Weight bearing
___ Bed mobility, use of bedpan
___ Pain management, PCA/CADD

TKR Post-op Day 1
Patient instructed in/demonstrates understanding of
___ IS, cough & deep breathe
___ Ankle pump and quad/glut exercises
___ Pain management
___ Weight bearing
Family teaching scheduled for:

TKR Post-op Day 2
Patient instructed in/demonstrates understanding of
___ IS, cough & deep breathe
___ Pain management
___ Do's and Don'ts
___ Weight bearing
___ Family present for teaching

DISCHARGE PLANNING

TKR Day of Surgery
___ Family Participation reinforced
___ RN completes discharge outcomes form

TKR Post-op Day 1
___ Plan reviewed with patient/family
___ D/C transportation identified ___
___ Discharge orders confirmed

TKR Post-op Day 2
___ Home equipment discussed and ordered
___ Patient adhering to pathway
___ Referrals completed:__ICF __HHC__ OP __Sub acute Rehab

OTHER

SURGEON NOTES

Operative Note in Progress Notes

TKR Post-op Day 1
___ Examination as above, variances noted
___ Reviewed previous day's charting
___ Plan: continue pathway

TKR Post-op Day 2
___ Examination as above, variances noted
___ Reviewed previous day's charting
___ Plan: continue pathway

PATIENT IDENTIFICATION	Initials	Time		Initials	Time		Initials	Time
RN D or A								
RN E								
RN N or P								
PT								
OT								
CM								
Physician								
Tech								
Other								
	TKR POST-OP DAY 1			TKR POST-OP DAY 2				

FIGURE 1-2 (Continued)

(continued)

General Plan

Diagnosis: _____

Knee	☐ Right ☐ Left ☐ Bilateral
	☐ Primary ☐ Revision ☐ Uni-compartmental

Major Releases: _____

Weight bearing status: (with walker or 2 crutches)
☐ Non-weight bearing ☐ 25% ☐ 50% ☐ Full Weight Bearing as tolerated

Brace: _____

CPM _____

Anticoagulation medication: ☐ YES ☐ NO

Variance From General Plan:

☐ **Yes**

See Variance Documentation Pathway

Day _____

Comorbidities: (Date ID/Initials)

_____ Diabetes	_____ Hypertension	_____/_____ HF	_____/_____ CAD
_____ Hypothyroidism	_____ Asthma	_____/_____ BPH	_____/_____ COPD
_____ Obesity	_____ CABG	_____/_____	_____/_____

Date/Time	Pathway Day	Variance/Problem	Action Taken/Outcome	Initials

PATIENT IDENTIFICATION

INOVA JOINT REPLACEMENT CENTER
INOVA MOUNT VERNON HOSPITAL
TOTAL KNEE REPLACEMENT
PATHWAY DOCUMENTATION
DOS, Day 1, Day 2

No. 001150

FIGURE 1-2 (Continued)

13

PPOs, exclusive provider arrangements, managed indemnity plans, and self-insured managed care—are blurring.

Managed care has contributed to a dramatic reduction in inpatient hospital days, continuing expansion of ambulatory care, fierce competition, and marketing strategies that appeal to consumers as well as to insurers and regulators. Hospitals are faced with declining revenues, a declining number of patients, more severely ill patients with shorter lengths of stay, and a need to incorporate cost-effective outpatient or ambulatory care services. As patients return to the community, they have more health care needs, many of which are complex. The demand for home care and community-based services is escalating. Despite their successes, managed care organizations are faced with the challenge of providing quality services under even greater resource constraints. Case management is the methodology used by many organizations to meet this challenge.

Case Management

Case management has become a prominent method for coordinating health care services to ensure cost-effectiveness, accountability, and quality care. The case management process dates back to the public health programs of the early 1900s, in which public health nursing played a dominant role. Over the years, the process has varied in form and function, but the basic theme has remained. The premise of case management is that the responsibility for meeting patient needs rests with one individual or team whose goals are to provide the patient and family with access to required services, to ensure coordination of these services, and to evaluate how effectively these services are delivered.

The reasons case management has gained such prominence can be traced to the decreased cost of care associated with decreased length of hospital stay, coupled with rapid and frequent interunit transfers from specialty to standard care units. The case manager role, instead of focusing on direct patient care, focuses on managing the care of an entire caseload of patients and collaborating with the nurses and other health care personnel who care for the patients. In most instances, the caseload is limited in scope to patients with similar diagnoses, needs, and therapies, and the case managers function across units. They are experts in their specialty areas and coordinate the inpatient and outpatient services needed by patients. The goals of this coordination include quality, appropriateness, and timeliness of services as well as cost reduction. The case manager follows the patient throughout hospitalization and at home after discharge in an effort to promote coordination of health care services that will avert or delay rehospitalization. Evidence-based pathways or similar plans are often used in care management of similar patient populations.

Health Maintenance Organizations

HMOs are prepaid, group health practice systems designed to deliver comprehensive health care services to a defined group of voluntarily enrolled individuals. Members pay premiums as well as designated copayments for services and medications. Individuals receive care from a preselected group of physicians, nurse practitioners (NPs), or other care provider members of the HMO, although some programs allow selection of outside providers for a higher fee. HMOs are based on the holistic concept of care. They provide outpatient (ambulatory) and preventive teaching and health care, as well as inpatient care that meets the health care needs of the whole person. The goal of HMOs is to give comprehensive health care that is of the best quality and quantity for the money available, while eliminating fragmentation and duplication of services. As HMOs have grown, they have expanded to include specialist services and programs for Medicare and Medicaid populations. Some studies show that HMOs are cost-effective and that the quality of care provided by these health care delivery systems is comparable to that provided elsewhere in the same communities. However, concerns have surfaced regarding the limitations on choice of health care provider, diagnostic testing, and length of hospitalization; high case loads; and problematic paperwork that might be imposed by some HMOs (Cesta & Falter, 1999). To address these concerns, some employer and federal health insurance providers offer alternative plans to HMOs.

Preferred Provider Organizations

HMOs have paved the way and served as the model for private fee-for-service (FFS) organizations that offer some choice to consumers. PPOs, point of service (POS) plans, provider service organizations (PSOs), Medicare+Choice plans, and coordinated care plans are some examples of variations on the HMO. These plans allow consumers, including Medicare beneficiaries, to choose their hospitals and physicians and allow providers to be reimbursed on an FFS basis.

In contrast to the HMO, the PPO, POS, or similar organization is not a distinct entity; rather, it is a business arrangement between a group of providers, usually hospitals and physicians, who contract to provide health care to subscribers, usually businesses, for a negotiated fee that often is discounted. Organizations like PPOs allow businesses to decrease their expenses for employee health care benefits, and hospitals and physicians to market their services to employers.

Some advanced practice nurses serve as preferred providers through nursing centers or in individual or joint practice. Advanced practice nurses provide health care delivery that is unique, client-based, and holistic. These nurses often provide care to vulnerable populations, allowing direct access to nursing services. In nursing centers, nurses provide the majority of services, control the budget, and function as chief executive officers. The role of many advanced practice nurses emphasizes primary care with collaborative, interdisciplinary models of practice.

Roles of the Nurse

As stated earlier, nursing is the diagnosis and treatment of human responses to health and illness and therefore focuses on a broad array of phenomena. There are three major roles assumed by the nurse when caring for patients. These roles are often used in concert with one another to provide comprehensive care.

The professional nurse in institutional, community-based or public health, and home care settings has three major roles: the practitioner role, which includes teaching and collaborating; the leadership role; and the research role. Although each role carries specific responsibilities, these roles relate to one another and are found in all nursing positions. These roles are designed to meet the immediate and future health care and nursing needs of consumers who are the recipients of nursing care.

PRACTITIONER ROLE

The practitioner role of the nurse involves those actions that the nurse takes when assuming responsibility for meeting the health care and nursing needs of individual patients, their families, and significant others. This role is the dominant role of nurses in primary, secondary, and tertiary health care settings and in home care and community nursing. It is a role that can be achieved only through use of the nursing process, the basis for all nursing practice. The nurse helps patients meet their needs through direct intervention, by teaching patients and family members to perform care, and by coordinating and collaborating with other disciplines to provide needed services.

LEADERSHIP ROLE

The leadership role of the nurse has traditionally been perceived as a specialized role assumed only by those nurses who have titles that suggest leadership and who are the leaders of large groups of nurses or related health care professionals. However, the constant fluctuation of health care delivery demands and consumers requires a broader definition of nursing leadership, one that identifies the leadership role as inherent within all nursing positions. The leadership role of the nurse involves those actions the nurse executes when assuming responsibility for the actions of others that are directed toward determining and achieving patient care goals.

Nursing leadership is a process involving four components: decision making, relating, influencing, and facilitating. Each of these components promotes change and the ultimate outcome of goal achievement. Basic to the entire process is effective communication, which determines the accomplishment of the process. Leadership in nursing is a process in which the nurse uses interpersonal skills to effect change in the behavior of others. The components of the leadership process are appropriate during all phases of the nursing process and in all settings.

RESEARCH ROLE

The research role of the nurse was traditionally viewed as one carried out only by academicians, nurse scientists, and graduate nursing students. Today, participation in the research process is also considered to be a responsibility of nurses in clinical practice.

The primary task of nursing research is to contribute to the scientific base of nursing practice. Studies are needed to determine the effectiveness of nursing interventions and nursing care. Through such research efforts, the science of nursing will grow and a scientifically based rationale for making changes in nursing practice and patient care will be generated. Evidence-based practice will be facilitated, with a resultant increase in the quality of patient care.

Nurses who have preparation in research methods can use their research knowledge and skills to initiate and implement timely, relevant studies. This is not to say that nurses who do not initiate and implement nursing research studies do not play a significant role in nursing research. Every nurse has valuable contributions to make to nursing research and a responsibility to make these contributions. All nurses must constantly be alert for nursing problems and important issues related to patient care that can serve as a basis for the identification of researchable questions.

Those nurses directly involved in patient care are often in the best position to identify potential research problems and questions. Their clinical insights are invaluable. Nurses also have a responsibility to become actively involved in ongoing research studies. This participation may involve facilitating the data collection process, or it may include actual collection of data. Explaining the study to other health care professionals or to patients and their families is often of invaluable assistance to the nurse who is conducting the study.

Above all, nurses must use research findings in their nursing practice. Research for the sake of research alone is meaningless. As stated previously, evidence-based practice requires the inclusion of valid research. Only with the use and evaluation of research findings in nursing practice will the science of nursing be furthered. Research findings can be substantiated only through use, validation, replication, and dissemination. Nurses must continually be aware of studies that are directly related to their own area of clinical practice and critically analyze those studies to determine the applicability of their conclusions and the implications for specific patient populations. Relevant conclusions and implications can be used to improve patient care.

Models of Nursing Care Delivery

Nursing care can be carried out through a variety of organizational methods. The model of nursing care used varies greatly from one facility to another and from one set of patient circumstances to another. A review of past and current models provides a background for understanding the nursing models and methods needed for today's changing health care delivery system.

TEAM NURSING

Team nursing, which had its origins in the 1950s and 1960s, involved use of a team leader and team members to provide various aspects of nursing care to a group of patients. In team nursing, medications might be given by one nurse while baths and physical care are given by a nursing assistant under the supervision of a nurse team leader. Skill mixes include registered nurses (RNs), often as team leaders; licensed practical nurses; and nursing assistants or unlicensed assistive personnel (UAP). With the current emphasis on cost containment in health care agencies, variations of team nursing are being used, and UAPs are increasingly being included as team members. There has been little substantiation, however, that team nursing is cost-effective. The quality of patient care with this system is questionable, and fragmentation of care is of concern.

PRIMARY NURSING

Primary nursing (not to be confused with primary health care, which pertains to first-contact general health care) refers to comprehensive, individualized care provided by the same nurse throughout the period of care. This type of nursing care allows the nurse to give direct patient care rather than manage and supervise the functions of others who provide direct care for the patient. This care method is rejected by many institutions as too costly; the patient–nurse ratio is small, and a larger professional staff is needed, because the primary nurse is usually an RN. However, primary nursing may provide a foundation for transition to case management in some institutions.

The primary nurse accepts total 24-hour responsibility for a patient's nursing care. Nursing care is directed toward meeting all of the individualized patient needs. The primary nurse is responsible and accountable for involving the patient and family directly in all facets of care and has autonomy in making decisions in this regard. The primary nurse communicates with other members of the health care team regarding the patient's health care. This process promotes continuity of care and collaborative efforts directed toward quality patient care.

During times when the primary nurse is not scheduled to work, an associate nurse or co-nurse assists in overseeing the delivery of care. The associate nurse implements the nursing plan of care and provides feedback to the primary nurse for evaluating the plan of care. The primary nurse assumes responsibility for making appropriate referrals and for ensuring that all relevant information is provided to those who will be involved in the patient's continuing care, including the family.

The long-term survival of primary nursing as it is currently designed is uncertain. As cost-containment measures continue and patient acuity increases, staffing ratios of patients to nurses are increasing. Many nursing service departments and agencies are meeting the increased workload demands by making modifications in their approach to primary nursing or by reverting to team or functional systems for delivering care. Others are changing their staffing mix and redesigning their models of practice to accommodate nurse-extender roles. Still others are changing to more innovative systems such as case management.

COMMUNITY-BASED NURSING AND COMMUNITY HEALTH– PUBLIC HEALTH NURSING

Community-based care and community health–public health (CH-PH) nursing are not new concepts for nursing. Nursing has played a vital role in the community since the middle to late 1800s, as visiting nurses provided care to the sick and poor in their homes and communities and educated patients and family members. Although community health (CH) nursing, public health (PH) nursing, community-based nursing, and home health nursing may be discussed together and aspects of care in each type do overlap, there are distinctions among these terms. Confusion exists regarding the differences, and the similar settings may blur these distinctions (Hunt, 2000; Kovner, 2001). The central idea of CH-PH nursing is that nursing intervention can promote wellness, reduce the spread of illness, and improve the health status of groups of citizens. CH-PH nursing practice is concerned with the general and comprehensive care of the community at large, with emphasis on primary, secondary, and tertiary prevention. Nurses in these settings have traditionally focused on health promotion, maternal and child health, and chronic care.

Community-based nursing occurs in a variety of settings within the community and is directed toward individuals and families (Hunt, 2000). It includes home health care nursing. Most community-based and home health care is directed toward specific patient groups with identified needs; these needs usually relate to illness, injury, or disability resulting most often from advanced age or chronic illness. However, both community-based and CH-PH nurses are now expanding to meet the needs of many groups of patients with a variety of problems and needs. Home health care will be a major aspect of community-based care discussed throughout this text. Home health care services are provided by community-based programs and agencies for specific populations (eg, the elderly, ventilator-dependent patients), as well as by hospital-based home health care agencies, hospices, independent professional nursing practices, and freestanding health care agencies.

As trends continue toward shortened hospital stays and increased use of outpatient health care services, the need for nursing care in the home and community setting has increased dramatically. Because nursing services are being provided outside as well as within the hospital, nurses have a choice of practicing in a variety of health care delivery settings. These settings include acute care medical centers, ambulatory care settings, clinics, urgent care centers, outpatient departments, neighborhood health centers, home health care agencies, independent or group nursing centers, and managed care agencies.

Community nursing centers, which have emerged over the past two decades with the advent of NPs, are nurse managed and provide primary care services that include ambulatory and outpatient care, immunizations, health assessment and screening services, and patient and family education and counseling. The populations that these centers serve are varied, but most typically they include a high proportion of patients who are rural, very young, very old, poor, or members of racial minorities—groups that are generally underserved.

The numbers and kinds of agencies that provide care in the home and community have expanded because of the expanding needs of patients requiring care. Home health care nurses are challenged because patients are discharged from acute care institutions to their homes and communities early in the recovery process and with more complex needs. Many are elderly, and many have multiple medical and nursing diagnoses and multisystem health problems that require acute and intensive nursing care. Medical technologies such as ventilatory support and intravenous or parenteral nutrition therapy, once limited to acute care settings, have been adapted to the home care setting.

As a result, the community-based care setting is becoming one of the largest practice areas for nursing. Home care nursing is now a specialty area that requires advanced knowledge and skills in general nursing practice, with emphasis on community health and acute medical-surgical nursing. Also required are high-level assessment skills, critical thinking, and decision-making skills in a setting where other health care professionals are not available to validate observations, conclusions, and decisions.

Home care nurses often function as acute care nurses in the home, providing "high-tech, high-touch" services to patients with acute health care needs. In addition, they are responsible for patient and family teaching and for contacting community resources and coordinating the continuing care of the patient. For these reasons, the scope of medical-surgical nursing encompasses not only the acute care setting within the hospital but also the acute care setting as it expands into the community and the home. Throughout this textbook, emphasis is placed on the home health care needs of patients, with particular attention given to the teaching, self-care management, and health maintenance needs of patients and their families.

Expanded Nursing Roles

Professional nursing is adapting to meet changing health needs and expectations. One such adaptation is through the expanded role of the nurse, which has developed in response to the need to improve the distribution of health care services and to decrease the cost of health care. NPs, clinical nurse specialists (CNSs), certified nurse-midwives, and certified registered nurse anesthetists are identified as advanced practice nurses. The nurse who functions in an advanced practice role provides direct care to patients through independent practice, practice within a health care agency, or collaboration with a physician. Specialization has evolved within the expanded roles of nursing as a result of the recent explosion of technology and knowledge.

Nurses may receive advanced education in such specialties as family, critical care, coronary care, respiratory care, oncologic care, maternal and child health care, neonatal intensive care, rehabilitation, trauma, rural health, and gerontologic nursing, to name just a few. With the expanded role of the nurse, various titles have emerged that attempt to specify the functions as well as the educational preparation of nurses, although functions are less distinct than in previous years. In medical-surgical nursing, the most significant of these titles are *nurse practitioner* and *clinical nurse specialist,* and the more recent title of *advanced practice nurse,* which encompasses both NPs and CNSs.

Initially the educational preparation for NPs was in certificate programs. Most states now require both NPs and CNSs to have a graduate-level education. The two programs, which originally differed significantly in scope and in their definition of role components, now have many similarities and areas of overlap.

NPs are, for the most part, prepared as generalists (eg, pediatric NP, geriatric NP). They define their role in terms of direct provision of a broad range of primary health care services to patients and families. The focus is on providing primary health care to patients and collaborating with other health professionals. NPs practice in both acute and nonacute care settings. The 1997 Balanced Budget Act provided for NPs to receive direct Medicare reimbursement. In addition, in some states—and with new legislation possibly nationwide—NPs have prescriptive authority (Boyd, 2000).

CNSs, on the other hand, are prepared as specialists who practice within a circumscribed area of care (eg, cardiovascular CNS, oncology CNS). They define their role as having five major components: clinical practice, education, management, consultation, and research. Studies have shown that in reality the CNS focus is often on the education and consultation roles: education and counseling of patients and families and education, counseling, and consultation with nursing staff. Some states have granted CNSs prescriptive authority if they have the required educational preparation. CNSs practice in a variety of settings, including the community and the home, although most practice in acute care settings. Recently, CNSs have been identified by many nursing leaders as ideal case managers. They have the educational background and the clinical expertise to organize and coordinate services and resources to meet the patient's health care needs in a cost-effective and efficient manner.

With advanced practice roles has come a continuing effort by professional nursing organizations to define more clearly the practice of nursing. Nurse practice acts have been amended to give nurses the authority to perform functions that were previously restricted to the practice of medicine. These functions include diagnosis (nursing), treatment, performance of selected invasive procedures, and prescription of medications and treatments. The board of nursing in each state stipulates regulations regarding these functions. The board defines the education and experience required and determines the clinical situations in which a nurse may perform these functions.

In general, initial care, ambulatory health care, and anticipatory guidance are all becoming increasingly important in nursing practice. Advanced practice roles enable nurses to function interdependently with other health care professionals and to establish a more collegial relationship with physicians. As changes in health care continue, the role of advanced practice nurses, especially in primary care settings, is expected to increase in terms of scope, responsibility, and recognition.

COLLABORATIVE PRACTICE

Throughout this chapter we have explored the changing role of nursing. Many references have been made to the significance of the nurse as a member of the health care team. As the unique competencies of nurses are becoming more clearly articulated, there is increasing evidence that nurses provide certain health care services distinct to the profession. However, nursing continues to recognize the importance of collaboration with other health care disciplines in meeting the needs of patients.

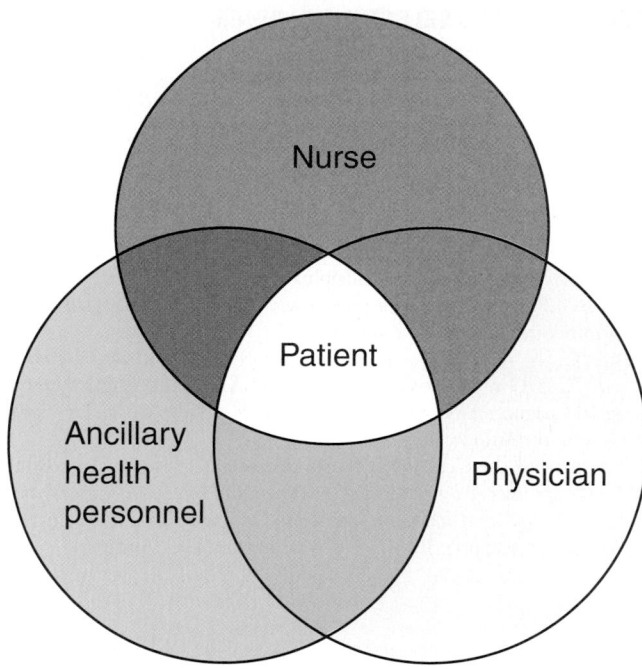

FIGURE 1-3 Collaborative practice model.

Some institutions use the collaborative practice model (Fig. 1-3). Nurses, physicians, and ancillary health personnel function within a decentralized organizational structure, collaboratively making clinical decisions. A joint practice committee, with representation from all care providers, may function at the unit level to monitor, support, and foster collaboration. Collaborative practice is further enhanced with integration of the clinical record and with joint patient care record reviews.

The collaborative model, or a variation of it, should be a primary goal for nursing—a venture that promotes shared participation, responsibility, and accountability in a health care environment that is striving to meet the complex health care needs of the public.

 Critical Thinking Exercises

1. Your clinical assignment is on a cardiac care step-down nursing unit in an acute care hospital. Identify a patient care issue (eg, family support) that could be improved. Describe the mechanism that is available within the hospital to address such quality improvement issues.

2. You are planning the discharge of an elderly patient who has several chronic medical conditions. A case manager has been assigned to this patient. How would you explain the role of the case manager to the patient and her husband?

3. You are assigned to care for a patient who is newly diagnosed with diabetes. The patient's health care is covered by a managed health care plan. How have managed health care plans affected nursing care delivery in acute care hospitals and outpatient settings? How might this specific patient's care be affected?

REFERENCES AND SELECTED READINGS

Books

American Nurses Association. (1995). *Nursing's social policy statement.* Washington, DC: Author.

American Nurses Association. (1991). *Nursing's agenda for health care reform.* Kansas City, MO: Author.

Cookfair, J. M. (1996). *Nursing care in the community.* St. Louis: Mosby–Year Book.

Hood, L., & Leddy, S. K. (2002). *Leddy & Pepper's conceptual bases of professional nursing* (5th ed.). Philadelphia: Lippincott Williams & Wilkins.

Hunt, R. (2000). *Readings in community-based nursing.* Philadelphia: Lippincott Williams & Wilkins.

Krozok, C., & Scoggins, A. (2001). *Patient rights . . . amended to comply with JCAHO standards.* Glendale, CA: CINAHL Information Systems.

National League for Nursing. (1977). *Nursing's role in patients' rights.* New York: Author.

U.S. Bureau of the Census. (Internet release date: January 13, 2000). *Profile of Older Americans: 2000. Population Projections of the United States by Age, Sex, Race, and Hispanic Origin: 1995–2050.* Current Population Reports, P25-1130. Washington, DC: Author.

Journals

Boyd, L. (2000). Advanced practice nursing today. *RN, 63*(9), 57–62.

Cesta, T. G., & Falter, E. J. (1999). Case management. *American Journal of Nursing, 99*(5), 48–51.

Davis, R., & Magilvy, J. K. (2000). Quiet pride: The experience of chronic illness by rural older adults. *Journal of Nursing Scholarship, 32*(4), 386–390.

Gooden, M. B., Porter, C. P., Gonzalez, R. I., & Mims, B. L. (2000). Rethinking the relationship between nursing and diversity. *American Journal of Nursing, 101*(1), 63–65.

Klenner, S. (2000). Mapping out a clinical pathway. *RN, 63*(6), 33–36.

Kovner, C. (2001). Counting nurses: What is community health-public health nursing? *American Journal of Nursing, 101*(1), 59–60.

Pluviose-Fenton, V. (2001). Census 2000 numbers delivered to the president. *Nation's Cities Weekly, 24*(1), 1, 8.

Silver, G. (1997). Editorial: The road from managed care. *American Journal of Public Health, 87*(1), 8–9.

Smith-Campbell, B. (2000). Across to health care: Effects of public funding of the uninsured. *Journal of Nursing Scholarship, 32*(3), 295–300.

Community-Based Nursing Practice

LEARNING OBJECTIVES

On completion of this chapter, the learner will be able to:

1. Discuss the changes in the health care system that have increased the need for medical-surgical nurses to practice in community-based settings.

2. Compare the differences and similarities between community-based and hospital nursing.

3. Describe the discharge planning process in relation to home care preparation.

4. Explain methods for identifying community resources and making referrals.

5. Discuss how to prepare for a home health care visit and how to conduct the visit.

6. Identify personal safety precautions a home care nurse should take when making home visits.

7. Describe the various types of nursing functions provided in ambulatory care facilities, in occupational health and school nursing programs, and to the homeless.

*T*he changes that have occurred in the health care system in the past two decades have increased the need for care in ambulatory settings and in the home. These changes have created a demand for highly skilled and well-prepared nurses to provide community-based care.

The Growing Need for Community-Based Health Care

As described in Chapter 1, the shift in the settings for health care delivery is a result of changes in federal legislation, tighter insurance regulations, decreasing hospital revenues, and the development of alternative health care delivery systems. As a result of federal legislation passed in 1983 and 1997, hospitals and other health care providers are now reimbursed at a fixed rate for patients with the same diagnosis as defined by diagnosis-related groups. Under this system, hospitals and other health care providers can cut costs and earn income by carefully monitoring the types of services they provide and discharging patients as soon as possible. Consequently, patients are being discharged from acute care facilities to their homes or to residential or long-term facilities at much earlier stages of recovery than in the past. Complex technical equipment, such as dialysis machinery, intravenous lines, and ventilators, is often part of home health care (Brown, 2000).

Alternative health care delivery systems, such as health maintenance organizations, preferred provider organizations, and managed health care systems, have also contributed to the drive to control costs and the availability of health care services. These regulations have dramatically reduced the length of hospital stay and have led to patients being treated more frequently in ambulatory care settings and at home. Chapter 1 provides a more thorough discussion of alternative health care delivery systems.

As more health care delivery shifts into the community, more nurses are working in a variety of public health and community-based settings. These settings include public health departments, ambulatory health clinics, long-term care facilities, prenatal and well-baby clinics, hospice agencies, industrial settings (as occupational nurses), homeless shelters and clinics, nursing centers, home health agencies, urgent care centers, same day surgical centers, short-stay facilities, and patients' homes.

Nurses in these settings often deliver care without direct on-site supervision or the support of other health care personnel. They must be self-directed, flexible, adaptable, and tolerant of various lifestyles and living conditions. Expertise in independent decision making, critical thinking, assessment, and health education, and competence in basic nursing care are essential to function effectively in the community-based setting (Brown, 2000; Pierson, 1999).

Community-based nursing is a philosophy of care of individuals and families. The care is provided in a community as the individual or family move among various kinds of service providers outside of hospitals (Hunt, 2000). Although the phrase "community-based nursing" is often interchanged with "community health nursing," a distinction should be made. The phrase "community health nursing" has generally been equated to "public health nursing." Public health nursing is a specialty focused on total populations, although care may be given to individuals. Community-based nursing is broader and may incorporate community health–public health nursing; it is focused on individuals and families rather than total populations. Community-based nursing also includes home health nursing, school health nurs-

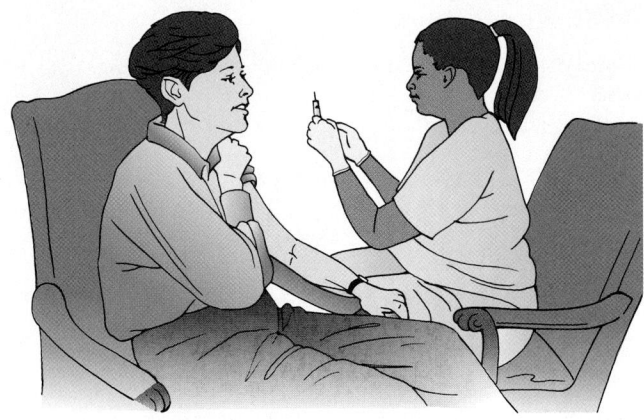

FIGURE 2-1 Community-based nursing takes many forms and focuses. Here the nursing focus is on wellness and the nursing setting is industry. When enlightened employers offer flu vaccines or other health services, the whole community benefits.

ing, and a host of other nursing services provided to individuals and groups in the community (Fig. 2-1).

COMMUNITY-BASED CARE

Community-based nursing practice focuses on promoting and maintaining the health of individuals and groups, preventing and minimizing the progression of disease, and improving quality of life (Hunt, 2000). Although nursing interventions used by public health nurses may involve individuals, families, or small groups, the central focus remains promotion of health and prevention of disease in the entire community. The actions of community health nurses may include provision of direct care to patients and families as well as political advocacy to secure resources for aggregate populations (eg, the aged population). The community health nurse may function as an epidemiologist, a case manager for a group of patients, a coordinator of services provided to an aggregate of patients, an occupational health nurse, a school nurse, a visiting nurse, or a parish nurse. (In parish nursing, the members of the religious community—the parish—are the recipients of care.) The commonality of these various roles is that the nurse maintains a focus on community needs as well as on the needs of the individual patient. Community-based care is generally focused on the individual or family; although efforts may be undertaken to improve the health of the whole community, the individual or family unit is the main focus. The primary concepts of community-based nursing care are self-care and preventive care within the context of culture and community. Two other important concepts are continuity of care and collaboration (Hunt, 2000). Some community-based nursing fields have become specialties in their own right, such as school health nursing and home health nursing.

Primary, secondary, and tertiary levels of preventive care are used by nurses in community-based practice. The focus of primary prevention is on health promotion and prevention of illness or disease, including interventions such as teaching regarding healthy lifestyles (Hunt, 2000). Secondary prevention centers on health maintenance and is aimed at early detection and prompt intervention to prevent or minimize loss of function and independence; it includes interventions such as health screening and health risk appraisal. Tertiary prevention focuses on minimizing deterioration and improving quality of life. Tertiary care may include rehabilitation to assist patients in achieving their maximum potential by working through their physical or psychological challenges (Hunt, 2000).

HOME HEALTH CARE

Home health care is becoming one of the largest practice areas for nurses. Because of the high acuity level of patients, nurses with acute care and high-technology experience are in demand in this field. Tertiary preventive nursing care, which focuses on rehabilitation and restoring maximum health function, is a major goal for home care nurses, although primary and secondary prevention are also included in care. Health care visits may be intermittent or periodic, and telephonic case management may be used to promote communication with home care consumers.

Home care nursing is a unique aspect of community-based nursing. Home care visits are made by nurses who work for home care agencies, public health agencies, and visiting nurse associations; by nurses who are employed by hospitals; and by parish nurses who voluntarily work with the members of their religious communities to promote health. Such visits may also be part of the responsibilities of school nurses, clinic nurses, or occupational health nurses. The type of nursing services provided to patients in their homes varies from agency to agency. Nurses working for home care or hospice agencies make home visits to provide skilled nursing care, follow-up care, and teaching to promote health and prevent complications. Clinic nurses may conduct home visits as part of patient follow-up. Public health, parish, and school nurses may make visits to provide anticipatory guidance to high-risk families and follow-up care to patients with communicable diseases. Many home care patients are acutely ill, and many have chronic health problems and disabilities, requiring nurses to provide more education and monitoring to the patient and family to facilitate compliance.

Holistic care is provided in the home through the collaboration of a multidisciplinary team that includes professional nurses; home health aides; social workers; physical, speech, and occupational therapists; and the physician (Touchard & Berthelot, 1999). The team provides health and social services with oversight of the total health care plan by a case manager, clinical nurse specialist, or nurse practitioner. Parish nurses may work to provide home care training to members of their congregations.

Health care services are provided by official, publicly funded agencies; nonprofit agencies; private businesses; proprietary chains; and hospital-based agencies. Some agencies specialize in high-technology services. Most agencies are reimbursed from a variety of sources, including Medicare and Medicaid programs, private insurance, and direct payments by patients. Each funding source has its own requirements for services rendered, number of visits allowed, and amount of reimbursement the agency will receive. Many home health care expenditures are financed by Medicare and are affected by provisions of the Balanced Budget Act of 1997.

The elderly are the most frequent users of home care services. To be eligible for service, the patient must be acutely ill, homebound, and in need of skilled nursing services. Nursing care includes skilled assessment of the patient's physical, psychological, social, and environmental status. Nursing interventions may include intravenous therapy and injections (Fig. 2-2), parenteral nutrition, venipuncture, catheter insertion, pressure ulcer treatment, wound care, ostomy care, and patient and family teaching. The nurse instructs the patient and family in skills and self-care strategies and in health maintenance and promotion activities (eg, nutritional counseling, exercise programs, stress management).

Medicare allows nurses to manage and evaluate patient care for seriously ill patients who have complex, labile conditions and are at high risk for rehospitalization. The nurse serves as a case

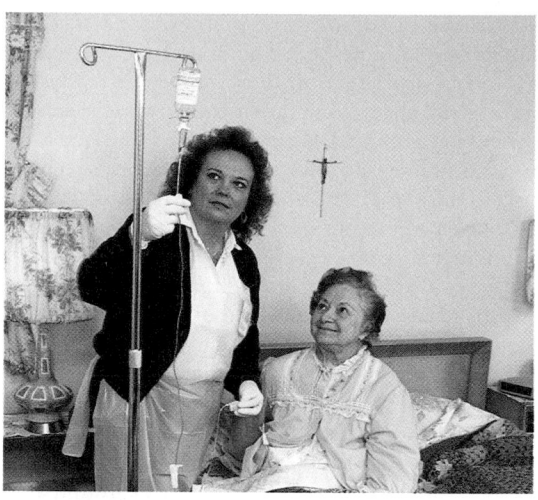

FIGURE 2-2 Intravenous therapy is one of the types of skilled nursing care that may be provided in the home. Courtesy Good Samaritan Certified Home Health Agency, Babylon, New York.

manager and monitors the delivery of care provided to patients in their homes.

Hospital and Community-Based Nursing

Providing nursing care in a patient's home is different from providing care in a hospital. Patients must sign a release form to stay and receive treatment in a hospital. They have little control over what happens to them, and they are expected to comply with the hospital's rules, regulations, and schedule of activities. They sleep in the hospital's beds and often wear hospital gowns or clothes. They are given care, treatments, baths, and medications at times that are usually determined by institutional schedules rather than convenience for the patient. Although hospitalized patients may select meals from a daily menu, there is a limited choice in the type of food they are offered. Family members and friends visit during the hospital's visiting hours.

By contrast, the home care nurse is considered a guest in the patient's home and needs permission to visit and give care. The nurse has minimal control over the lifestyle, living situation, and health practices of the patients he or she visits. This lack of full decision-making authority can create a conflict for the nurse and lead to problems in the nurse–patient relationship. To work successfully with patients, no matter what the setting, it is important for the nurse to be nonjudgmental and to convey respect for the patient's beliefs, even if they differ sharply from the nurse's. This can be difficult when a patient's lifestyle involves activities that the nurse considers harmful or unacceptable, such as smoking, use of alcohol, drug abuse, or overeating.

The cleanliness of a patient's home may not meet the standards of a hospital. Although the nurse can provide teaching points about maintaining clean surroundings, the patient and family determine whether they will implement the nurse's suggestions. The nurse must accept the reality of the situation and deliver the care required regardless of the sanitary conditions of the surroundings.

The kind of equipment and the supplies or resources that usually are available in acute care settings are often unavailable in the patient's home. The nurse has to learn to improvise when providing care, such as when changing a dressing or catheterizing a patient in a regular bed that is not adjustable and lacks a bedside table (Johnson, Smith-Temple, & Carr, 1998).

Infection control is as important in the home as it is in the hospital, but it can be more challenging and requires creative approaches. As in any situation, it is important to cleanse one's hands before and after giving direct patient care, even in a home that does not have running water. If aseptic technique is required, the nurse must have a plan for implementing this technique before going to the home. This applies also to standard precautions, transmission-based precautions, and disposal of bodily secretions and excretions.

If injections are given, the nurse should use a closed container to dispose of syringes. Injectable and other medications must be kept out of the reach of children during visits and must be stored in a safe place if they are to remain in the house. Nurses who perform invasive procedures need to be up-to-date with their immunizations, including hepatitis B and tetanus.

The home environment often has more distractions than a hospital. The home can be filled with background noise and crowded with people and objects. A nurse may have to request that the television be turned down during the visit or that the patient move to a more private place to be interviewed.

Friends, neighbors, or family members may ask the nurse about the patient's condition. A patient has a right to confidentiality, and information should be shared only with the patient's permission. If the nurse carries the patient's medical record into the house, it must be put in a secure place to prevent it from being picked up by others or misplaced.

Discharge Planning for Home Care

To prepare for early hospital discharge and the possible need for follow-up care in the home, discharge planning begins with the patient's admission. Several different personnel or agencies may be involved in the planning process. In hospitals, social workers or nurses may serve as the discharge planners. Some home care agencies have liaison nurses who work with discharge planners to ensure that the patient's needs are met when he or she is released from the hospital. Professionals in ambulatory health care settings may refer patients for home care services to prevent hospitalization. Public health nurses care for patients referred for anticipatory guidance with high-risk families, for case finding, and for follow-up treatment (eg, patients with communicable diseases). Parish nurses may have patients referred, or they may be contacted directly by members of the parish community who need guidance or referrals related to physical or psychosocial health care concerns (Palmer, 2001).

The development of a comprehensive discharge plan requires collaboration with professionals at both the referring agency and the home care agency, public health agency, or other community resource. The process involves identifying the patient's needs and developing a thorough plan to meet them. Communication with and cooperation of the patient and family are essential.

Community Resources and Referrals

Home health nurses and public health nurses act as case managers. After assessing the patient's needs, they may make referrals to other team members, such as home health aides and social workers. They work collaboratively with the health team and the agency or person who referred the patient for service. Continuous coordinated care among all health care providers involved in the patient's care is essential to avoid duplication of effort by the various personnel caring for the patient.

Home care and public health nurses are responsible for providing the patient and family with information about other community resources that are available to meet their needs. During the initial and subsequent visits, they help patients identify these community services and encourage the patient and family to contact the appropriate agencies. When appropriate, the nurse makes the initial contact (Pierson, 1999).

A community-based nurse needs to be knowledgeable about community resources available to patients as well as services provided by local agencies, eligibility requirements, and any possible charges for the services. Most communities have directories of health and social service agencies that the nurse can consult. These directories need to be continually updated as resources change. If a community does not have a resource booklet, the agency may develop one for its staff. It should include the commonly used community resources that patients need, the costs of the services, and eligibility requirements. The patient's place of worship or parish may serve as an important resource for services. The telephone book is often a useful resource for helping patients identify the locations of grocery and drug stores, banks, health care facilities, ambulances, physicians, dentists, pharmacists, social service agencies, and senior citizens programs.

Preparing for a Home Visit

Most agencies have a policy manual that states their philosophy and procedures and defines the services they provide. Becoming familiar with these policies is an essential step before initiating a home visit. It is also important to know the agency's policies and the state law regarding what actions to take if the nurse finds a patient dead, encounters an abusive situation in the family, or determines that a patient cannot safely remain at home.

Before making a home visit, the nurse should review the patient's referral form and other pertinent data concerning the patient. It may be necessary to contact the referring agency if the purpose for the referral is unclear or if important information is missing.

The first step is to call the patient to obtain permission to visit, schedule a time for the visit, and verify the address. This initial phone conversation provides an opportunity to introduce oneself, identify the agency, and explain the reason for the visit.

If a patient does not have a telephone, the nurse should see whether those who made the referral have a number where a phone message can be left for the patient. If an unannounced visit must be made to a patient's home, the nurse should ask permission to come in before entering the house. Explaining the purpose of the referral at the outset and setting up the times for future visits before leaving are also recommended approaches.

Most agencies provide nurses with bags that contain standard supplies and equipment needed during home visits. It is important to keep the bag properly supplied and to bring any additional items that might be needed for the visit. Patients usually do not have the medical supplies they need for treatment.

Conducting a Home Visit

PERSONAL SAFETY PRECAUTIONS

Whenever a nurse makes a home visit, the agency should know the nurse's schedule and the locations of the visits. The nurse should learn about the neighborhood and obtain directions for reaching the expected destination. A plan of action should always be established in case of emergencies.

Nurses are not expected to disregard their personal safety in an effort to make or complete home visits. If nurses encounter dangerous situations during visits, they should return to their agencies and contact their supervisors or law enforcement officials, or both. Suggested precautions to take when making a home visit are presented in Chart 2-1.

INITIAL HOME VISIT

The first visit sets the tone for subsequent visits and is a crucial step in establishing the nurse–patient relationship. The situations encountered can vary depending on numerous factors. Patients may be in pain and unable to care for themselves. Families may be overwhelmed and doubt their ability to care for their loved one. They may not understand why the patient was sent home from the hospital before being totally rehabilitated. They may not comprehend what home care is or why they cannot have 24-hour nursing services. It is critical that the nurse try to convey an understanding of what the patient and family are experiencing and how the illness is affecting their lives.

During the initial home visit, which usually lasts less than an hour, the patient is evaluated and a plan of care is established to be followed or modified on subsequent visits. The nurse informs the patient of the agency's practices, policies, and hours of operation. If the agency is to be reimbursed for the visit, the nurse asks for insurance information, such as a Medicare or Medicaid card.

The initial assessment includes evaluating the patient, the home environment, the patient's self-care abilities or the family's ability to provide care, and the patient's need for additional resources. Identifying possible hazards, such as cluttered walk areas, potential fire risks, air or water pollution, or inadequate sanitation facilities, is also part of the initial assessment.

Documentation considerations for home visits follow fairly specific regulations. The patient's needs and the nursing care given are documented accurately to ensure that the agency will qualify for payment for the visit. Medicare, Medicaid, and third-party payers require documentation of the patient's homebound status and the need for skilled professional nursing care. The medical diagnosis and specific detailed information on the functional limitations of the patient are usually part of the documentation. The goals and the actions appropriate for attaining them need to be identified. Expected outcomes of the nursing interventions must be stated in terms of patient behaviors and must be realistic and measurable. They must reflect the nursing diagnosis or the patient's problems and must specify those actions that are expected to solve the patient's problems. If the documentation is not done correctly, the agency may not be paid for the visit.

DETERMINING THE NEED FOR FUTURE VISITS

While conducting an assessment of the patient's situation, the nurse evaluates the need for future visits and the frequency with which those visits may need to be made. To make these judgments, the nurse may find it helpful to consider the following factors:

- *Current health status:* How well is the patient progressing? How serious are the present signs and symptoms? Has the patient shown signs of progressing as expected, or does it seem that recovery will be delayed?
- *Home environment:* Are worrisome safety factors apparent? Are family or friends available to provide care, or is the patient alone?
- *Level of self-care abilities:* Is the patient capable of self-care? What is the patient's level of independence? Is the patient ambulatory or bedridden? Does the patient have sufficient energy or is he or she frail and easily fatigued?
- *Level of nursing care needed:* What level of nursing care does the patient require? Does the care require basic skills or more complex interventions?
- *Prognosis:* What is the expectation for recovery in this particular instance? What are the chances that complications may develop if nursing care is not provided?
- *Patient education needs:* How well has the patient or family grasped the teaching points made? Is there a need for further follow-up and retraining? What level of proficiency does the patient or family show in carrying out the necessary care?
- *Mental status:* How alert is the patient? Are there signs of confusion or thinking difficulties? Does the patient tend to be forgetful or have a limited attention span?
- *Level of adherence:* Is the patient following the instructions provided? Does the patient seem capable of doing so? Are the family members helpful in this regard, or are they unwilling or unable to assist in caring for the patient as expected?

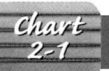

Chart 2-1 Safety Precautions in Home Health Care

- Learn, or preprogram a cellular phone with the telephone numbers of the agency, police, and emergency services.
- Let the agency know your daily schedule and the telephone numbers of your patients so that you can be located if you do not return when expected.
- Know where the patient lives before leaving to make the visit and carry a map for quick referral.
- Keep your car in good working order and have sufficient gas in the tank.
- Park the car near the patient's home and lock it during the visit.
- Do not drive an expensive car or wear expensive jewelry when making visits.
- Know the regular bus schedule and know the routes when using public transportation or walking to the patient's house.
- Carry agency identification and have enough change to make telephone calls in case you get lost or have problems. Most agencies provide cellular phones for their nurses so that the agency can contact the nurse, and so that the nurse can contact the agency in case of an emergency or unexpected situation.
- When making visits in high-crime areas, visit with another person rather than alone.
- Schedule visits only during daylight hours.
- Never walk into a patient's home uninvited.
- If you do not feel safe entering a patient's home, leave the area.
- Become familiar with the layout of the house, including exits from the house.
- If a patient or family member is intoxicated, hostile, or obnoxious, reschedule the visit and leave.
- If a family is having a serious argument or abusing the patient or anyone else in the household, reschedule the visit, contact your supervisor, and report the abuse to the appropriate authorities.

With each subsequent visit, these same factors are evaluated to determine the continuing health needs of the patient. As progress is made and the patient, with or without the help of significant others, becomes more capable of self-care and more independent, the need for home visits may decline.

CLOSING THE VISIT

As the visit comes to a close, it is important to summarize the main points of the visit for the patient and family and to identify expectations for future visits or patient achievements. The following points should be considered at the end of each visit:

- What are the main points the patient or family should remember from the visit?
- What positive attributes have been noted about the patient and the family that will give them a sense of accomplishment?
- What were the main points of the teaching plan or the treatments needed to ensure that the patient and family understand what they must do? A written set of instructions should be left with the patient or family, provided they can read and see (alternative formats include video or audio recordings). Printed material should be in the patient's primary language and in large print when indicated.
- Whom should the patient or family call in case they need to contact someone immediately? Are current emergency telephone numbers readily available? Is telephone service available or can an emergency cell phone service be provided?
- What signs of complications should be reported immediately?
- What is the day and time of the next visit? Will a different nurse make the visit? How frequently will visits be made, and for how long (if determinable at this time)?

Other Community-Based Health Care Settings

AMBULATORY SETTINGS

Ambulatory health care is provided for patients in community or hospital-based settings. The types of agencies that provide ambulatory health care are medical clinics, ambulatory care units, urgent care centers, cardiac rehabilitation programs, mental health centers, student health centers, community outreach programs, and nursing centers. Some ambulatory centers provide care to a specific population, such as migrant workers or Native Americans. Neighborhood health centers provide services to patients who live in a geographically defined area. The centers may operate in freestanding buildings, storefronts, or mobile units. Agencies may provide ambulatory health care in addition to other services, such as offering an adult day care or health program. The kinds of services offered and the patients served depend on the agency's mission.

Nursing responsibilities in ambulatory health care settings include providing direct patient care, conducting patient intake screenings, treating patients with acute or chronic illnesses or emergency conditions, referring patients to other agencies for additional services, teaching patients self-care activities, and offering health education programs that promote health maintenance. A useful tool for the community-based nurse might be the classification scheme developed by the Visiting Nurses Association of Omaha, which contains patient-focused problems that are in one of four domains: environmental, psychosocial, physiologic, and health-related behaviors (Cookfair, 1996).

Nurses also work as clinic managers, direct the operation of clinics, and supervise other health team members. Nurse practitioners, educated in primary care, often practice in ambulatory care settings with a focus on gerontology, pediatrics, family or adult health, or women's health. Constraints imposed by federal legislation and ambulatory payment classifications (APCs) require efficient and effective management of patients in ambulatory settings. Nurses can play an important part in facilitating the function of the ambulatory care facility.

OCCUPATIONAL HEALTH PROGRAMS

Federal legislation, especially the Occupational Safety and Health Act (OSHA), has had a major impact on health conditions in the workplace. The law is directed at creating safer and healthier work conditions. It is in an employer's interest to try to provide a safe working environment, because the result is reduced costs associated with employee absenteeism, hospitalization, and disability.

Occupational nurses may work in solo units in an industrial setting, or they may serve as consultants on a limited or part-time basis. They may also be members of an interdisciplinary team composed of a variety of health care workers such as nurses, physicians, exercise physiologists, health educators, counselors, nutritionists, safety engineers, and industrial hygienists. The occupational health nurse functions in several ways and may provide direct care to employees who become ill or injured, conduct health education programs for company staff members, or set up health programs aimed at establishing specific health behaviors, such as eating properly and getting enough exercise. The nurse must also be knowledgeable about federal regulations pertaining to occupational health and familiar with other pertinent legislation, such as the Americans with Disabilities Act. The occupational health nurse may monitor employees' hearing, vision, blood pressure, or blood glucose levels (Capriotti, Kirby, & Smeltzer, 2000). Exposures to radiation, infectious diseases, and toxic substances are also tracked and reported to government agencies as required.

SCHOOL HEALTH PROGRAMS

School health programs provide valuable services for students and may also serve the school's community. School-age children and adolescents with health problems are at major risk for underachieving or failing in school. The leading health problems of elementary-school children are injuries, infections (including influenza and pneumonia), malnutrition, dental disease, and cancer. The leading problems for high-school students are alcohol and drug abuse, injuries, homicide, pregnancy, sexually transmitted disease, sports injuries, dental disease, and mental and emotional problems. Ideally, school health programs have an interdisciplinary health team consisting of physicians, nurses, dentists, social workers, counselors, school administrators, parents, and students. The school may serve as the site for a family health clinic that offers primary health and mental health services to children and adolescents as well as to all family members in the community. Many school nurses have baccalaureate degrees, and advanced practice nurses are ideally suited to provide the primary care in these settings. Some school nurse programs provide community care. Physical examinations are performed by advanced practice nurses who then diagnose and treat students and families for acute and chronic illnesses. These clinics are cost-effective and are especially beneficial for students from low-income families who lack access to traditional health care or have no health insurance.

The roles of the school nurse are care provider, health educator, consultant, and counselor. The school nurse collaborates with students, parents, administrators, and other health and social service professionals regarding a student's health problems. Nurses perform health screenings, give basic care for minor injuries and complaints, administer medications, monitor the immunization status of students and families, and identify children with health problems. They need to be knowledgeable about state and local regulations affecting school-age children, such as ordinances for excluding students from school because of communicable diseases or parasites such as lice or scabies.

The school nurse is also a health education consultant for teachers. In addition to providing information on health practices, teaching health classes, or participating in the development of the health education curriculum, the school nurse educates the teacher and class when one of the students has a special problem, a disability, or a disease such as hemophilia or acquired immunodeficiency syndrome (AIDS).

CARE FOR THE HOMELESS

No exact figures exist on the number of homeless people in the United States. Homelessness is a growing problem, and the homeless population includes increasing numbers of women with children (often victims of abuse) and elderly people. The homeless are a heterogeneous group, including members of dysfunctional families, the unemployed, and those who cannot find affordable housing. A large number of homeless persons, about 85%, are chronically mentally ill or abuse alcohol or other drugs (Walker, 1998). Some are temporarily homeless as a result of catastrophic natural disasters.

The homeless often have difficulty affording or gaining access to health care. Because of numerous obstacles, they seek health care late in the course of a disease and deteriorate more quickly than other patients. Many of the health problems they experience are related in large part to their living situations. Street life exposes homeless persons to the extremes of hot and cold environments and compounds their health risks.

Homeless persons have high rates of trauma, tuberculosis, upper respiratory tract infections, poor nutrition and anemia, lice, scabies, peripheral vascular problems, sexually transmitted diseases, dental problems, arthritis, hypothermia, skin disorders, and foot problems. Common chronic health problems of the homeless include diabetes, hypertension, heart disease, AIDS, and mental illness. These problems are made more difficult by living on the street and by being discharged to a transitory, homeless situation in which follow-up is unlikely (Hunter, Crosby, Ventura, & Warkentin, 1997; Walker, 1998). Homeless persons who live in shelters frequently encounter overcrowded, unventilated quarters that provide an ideal environment for the spread of communicable diseases such as tuberculosis.

Community-based nurses who work with the homeless must be nonjudgmental, patient, and understanding. They must be proficient in dealing with many different kinds of people who have a wide variety of health problems and needs. Nursing interventions are aimed at attempting to obtain health care services for the homeless and evaluating the health care needs of those who reside in the shelters.

Critical Thinking Exercises

1. Recall a difficult discharge planning situation in which you have been involved. Evaluate the effectiveness of the processes used to accomplish the goals. What changes could have been made that would have improved the processes and the outcomes?

2. A homeless young mother was referred for follow-up home care after discharge from the hospital. During the nurse's initial visit, to the homeless shelter, the patient's daughter asks how often visits will be made and for how long. What assessment criteria would you use to develop answers to these questions? What factors affect the patient's eligibility for home care services versus ambulatory health services?

REFERENCES AND SELECTED READINGS

Books

Cookfair, J. M. (1996). *Nursing care in the community* (2nd ed.). St. Louis: Mosby–Year Book.

Hunt, R. (2000). *Readings in community-based nursing.* Philadelphia: Lippincott, Williams & Wilkins.

Johnson, J. Y., Smith-Temple, A. J., & Carr, P. (1998). *Nurses' guide to home health procedures.* Philadelphia: Lippincott-Raven.

Journals

Allison, D. M. (1997). The nurse practitioner and culturally diverse populations. *Nurse Practitioner Forum, 8*(1), 4.

Brown, S. (2000). The legal pitfalls of home care. *RN, 63*(11), 75–80.

Capriotti, T., Kirby, L. G., & Smeltzer, S. C. (2000). Unrecognized high blood pressure: A major public health issue for the workplace. *AAOHN J, 48*(7), 338–343.

Hunter, J. K., Crosby, F., Ventura, M. R., & Warkentin, L. (1997). Factors limiting evaluation of health care programs for the homeless. *Nursing Outlook, 45*(2), 224–228.

Palmer, J. (2001). Parish nursing: Connecting faith and health. *Reflections on Nursing Leadership, 27*(1), 17–19.

Pierson, C. L. (1999). APNs in home care. *American Journal of Nursing, 99*(10), 22–23.

Touchard, B., & Berthelot, K. (1999). Collaborative home practice: Nursing and occupational therapy ensure appropriate medication administration. *Home Healthcare Nurse, 17*(1), 45–51.

Walker, C. (1998). Homeless people and mental health: A nursing concern. *American Journal of Nursing, 98*(11), 26–32.

RESOURCES AND WEBSITES

Case Management Society of America (CMSA), 8201 Cantrell Road, Suite 230, Little Rock, AR 72227; (501) 225-2229; http://www.cmsa.org.

Centers for Disease Control and Prevention (CDC), 1600 Clifton Road, Atlanta, GA 30333; (800) 311-3435; http://www.cdc.gov.

National Guideline Clearing House (NGC): info@guideline.gov; http://www.guideline.gov.

Joint Commission on Accreditation of Healthcare Organizations (JCAHO), One Renaissance Blvd., Oakbrook Terrace, IL 60181; (630) 792-5000; http://www.jcaho.org.

National Association of School Nurses, Inc., Eastern Office, P.O. Box 1300, Scarborough, ME 04070-1300; (877)-627-6476; http://www.nasn.org.

NurseLinx.com (MDLinx Inc.), 1025 Vermont Avenue, N.W., Suite 810, Washington, DC 20005; (202)543-6544; http://www.nurselinx.com.

Critical Thinking, Ethical Decision Making, and the Nursing Process

On completion of this chapter, the learner will be able to:

1. Define the characteristics of critical thinking and critical thinkers.
2. Describe the critical thinking process.
3. Define ethics and nursing ethics.
4. Identify several ethical dilemmas common to the medical-surgical area of nursing practice.
5. Specify strategies that can be helpful to nurses in ethical decision making.
6. Describe the components of the nursing process.
7. Describe the nursing process.
8. Develop a plan of nursing care for a patient using strategies of critical thinking.

*I*n today's health care arena, the nurse is faced with increasingly complex issues and situations resulting from advanced technology, greater acuity of patients in hospital and community settings, an aging population, and complex disease processes, as well as ethical and cultural factors. Traditionally, nurses have used a problem-solving approach in planning and providing nursing care. Today the decision-making part of problem solving has become increasingly complex and requires critical thinking.

Definition of Critical Thinking

Critical thinking is a multidimensional skill, a cognitive or mental process or set of procedures. It involves reasoning and purposeful, systematic, reflective, rational, outcome-directed thinking based on a body of knowledge, as well as examination and analysis of all available information and ideas. Critical thinking leads to the formulation of conclusions and the most appropriate, often creative, decisions, options, or alternatives (Ignatavicius, 2001; Prideaux, 2000).

Critical thinking includes metacognition, the examination of one's own reasoning or thought processes while thinking, to help strengthen and refine thinking skills (Wilkinson, 2001). Independent judgments and decisions evolve from a sound knowledge base and the ability to synthesize information within the context in which it is presented. Nursing practice in today's society mandates the use of high-level critical thinking skills within the nursing process. Critical thinking enhances clinical decision making, helping to identify patient needs and to determine the best nursing actions that will assist the patient in meeting those needs.

Critical thinking and critical thinkers have distinctive characteristics. As indicated in the above definition, critical thinking is a conscious, outcome-oriented activity; it is purposeful and intentional. The critical thinker is an inquisitive, fair-minded truthseeker with an open-mindedness to the alternative solutions that might surface.

Critical Thinking Process
RATIONALITY AND INSIGHT

Critical thinking is systematic and organized. The skills involved in critical thinking are developed over time through effort, practice, and experience. Skills needed in critical thinking include interpretation, analysis, evaluation, inference, explanation, and self-regulation (Ignatavicius, 2001). Critical thinking requires background knowledge and knowledge of key concepts as well as standards of good thinking (Prideaux, 2000). The critical thinker uses reality-based deliberation to validate the accuracy of data and the reliability of sources, being mindful of and questioning inconsistencies. Interpretation is used to determine the significance of data that are gathered, and analysis is used to identify patient problems indicated by the data. The nurse uses inference to draw conclusions. Explanation is the justification of actions or interventions used to address patient problems and to help a patient move toward desired outcomes. Evaluation is the process of determining whether outcomes have been or are being met, and self-regulation is the process of examining the care provided and adjusting the interventions as needed (Ignatavicius, 2001).

Critical thinking is also reflective, involving metacognition, active evaluation, and refinement of the thinking process. The critical thinker considers the possibility of personal bias when interpreting data and determining appropriate actions. The critical thinker must be insightful and have a sense of fairness and integrity, the courage to question personal ethics, and the perseverance to strive continuously to minimize the effects of egocentricity, ethnocentricity, and other biases on the decision-making process (Alfaro-LeFevre, 1999).

COMPONENTS OF CRITICAL THINKING

Certain cognitive or mental activities can be identified as key components of critical thinking. When thinking critically, a person will do the following:

- Ask questions to determine the reason why certain developments have occurred and to see whether more information is needed to understand the situation accurately.
- Gather as much relevant information as possible to consider as many factors as possible.
- Validate the information presented to make sure that it is accurate (not just supposition or opinion), that it makes sense, and that it is based on fact and evidence.
- Analyze the information to determine what it means and to see whether it forms clusters or patterns that point to certain conclusions.
- Draw on past clinical experience and knowledge to explain what is happening and to anticipate what might happen next, acknowledging personal bias and cultural influences.
- Maintain a flexible attitude that allows the facts to guide thinking and takes into account all possibilities.
- Consider available options and examine each in terms of its advantages and disadvantages.
- Formulate decisions that reflect creativity and independent decision making.

Critical thinking requires going beyond basic problem solving into a realm of inquisitive exploration, looking for all relevant factors that affect the issue, and being an "out-of-the-box" thinker. It includes questioning all findings until a comprehensive picture emerges that explains the phenomenon, possible solutions, and creative methods for proceeding (Wilkinson, 2001). Critical thinking in nursing practice results in a comprehensive patient plan of care with maximized potential for success.

CRITICAL THINKING IN NURSING PRACTICE

Using critical thinking to develop a plan of nursing care requires considering the human factors that might influence the plan. The nurse interacts with the patient, family, and other health care providers in the process of providing appropriate, individualized nursing care. The culture, attitude, and thought processes of the nurse, the patient, and others will affect the critical thinking process from the data-gathering stage through the decision-making stage; therefore, aspects of the nurse-patient interaction must be considered (Wilkinson, 2001). Nurses must use critical thinking skills in all practice settings—acute care, ambulatory care, extended care, and in the home and community. Regardless of the setting, each patient situation is viewed as unique and dynamic. The unique factors that the patient and nurse bring to the health care situation are considered, studied, analyzed, and interpreted. Interpretation of the information presented then allows the nurse to focus on those factors that are most relevant and most significant to the clinical situation. Decisions about what to do and how to do it are then developed into a plan of action.

Fonteyn (1998) identified 12 predominant thinking strategies used by nurses, regardless of their area of clinical practice:

- Recognizing a pattern
- Setting priorities
- Searching for information
- Generating hypotheses
- Making predictions
- Forming relationships
- Stating a proposition ("if–then")
- Asserting a practice rule
- Making choices (alternative actions)
- Judging the value
- Drawing conclusions
- Providing explanations

Fonteyn further identified other, less prominent thinking strategies the nurse might use:

- Pondering
- Posing a question
- Making assumptions (supposing)
- Qualifying
- Making generalizations

These thought processes are consistent with the characteristics of critical thinking and cognitive activities discussed earlier. Fonteyn asserted that exploring how these thinking strategies are used in various clinical situations, and practicing using the strategies, might assist the nurse–learner in examining and refining his or her own thinking skills.

Because developing the skill of critical thinking takes time and practice, critical thinking exercises are offered throughout this book as a means of practicing one's ability to think critically. Additional exercises can be found in the study guide that accompanies the text. The questions listed in Chart 3-1 can serve as a guide in working through the exercises, although it is important to remember that each situation is unique and calls for an approach that fits the particular circumstances being described.

Ethical Nursing Care

In the complex modern world, we are surrounded by ethical issues in all facets of our lives. Consequently, there has been a heightened interest in the field of ethics, in an attempt to gain a better understanding of how these issues influence us. Specifically, in health care the focus on ethics has intensified in response to controversial developments, including advances in technology and genetics, as well as diminished health care and financial resources.

Today, sophisticated technology can prolong life well beyond the time when death would have occurred in the past. Expensive experimental procedures and medications are available for attempting to preserve life, even when such attempts are likely to fail. The development of technological support has had an influence on all stages of life. For example, the prenatal period has been influenced by genetic screening, in vitro fertilization, the harvesting and freezing of embryos, and prenatal surgery. In the early stages of life, premature infants are given a chance for survival by the use of technical support. Children and adults who would have died as a result of organ failure are living longer because of organ transplantation. Technological advances have also contributed to an increase in the average life expectancy. These advances in technology, however, have been a mixed blessing. Questions have been raised about whether, and under what circumstances, it is appropriate to use such technology. Although many individuals are afforded a better quality of life, others face

---

Chart 3-1 The Inquiring Mind: Critical Thinking in Action

Throughout the critical thinking process, a continuous flow of questions evolves in the thinker's mind. Although the questions will vary according to the particular clinical situation, certain general inquiries can serve as a basis for reaching conclusions and determining a course of action.

When faced with a patient situation, it is often helpful to seek answers to some or all of the following questions in an attempt to determine those actions that are most appropriate:

- What relevant assessment information do I need, and how do I interpret this information? What does this information tell me?
- To what problems does this information point? Have I identified the most important ones? Does the information point to any other problems that I should consider?
- Have I gathered all the information I need (signs/symptoms, laboratory values, medication history, emotional factors, mental status)? Is anything missing?
- Is there anything that needs to be reported immediately? Do I need to seek additional assistance?
- Does this patient have any special risk factors? Which ones are most significant? What must I do to minimize these risks?
- What possible complications must I anticipate?
- What are the most important problems in this situation? Do the patient and the patient's family recognize the same problems?
- What are the desired outcomes for this patient? Which have the highest priority? Does the patient see eye to eye with me on these points?
- What is going to be my first action in this situation?
- How can I construct a plan of care to achieve the goals?
- Are there any age-related factors involved, and will they require some special approach? Will I need to make some change in the plan of care to take these factors into account?
- How do the family dynamics affect this situation, and will this have an affect on my actions or the plan of care?
- Are there cultural factors that I must address and consider?
- Am I dealing with an ethical problem here? If so, how am I going to resolve it?
- Has any nursing research been conducted on this subject?

---

extended suffering as a result of efforts to prolong life, usually at great expense. Ethical issues also surround those practices or policies that seem to allocate health care resources unjustly on the basis of age, race, gender, disability, or social mores.

Domain of Nursing Ethics

The ethical dilemmas a nurse may encounter in the medical-surgical arena are numerous and diverse. An awareness of underlying philosophical concepts will help the nurse to reason through these dilemmas. Basic concepts related to moral philosophy, such as ethics terminology, theories, and approaches, are included in this chapter. Understanding the role of the professional nurse in ethical decision making will assist nurses in articulating their ethical positions and in developing the skills needed to make ethical decisions.

ETHICS VERSUS MORALITY

The terms *ethics* and *morality* are used to describe beliefs about right and wrong and to suggest appropriate guidelines for action. In essence, ethics is the formal, systematic study of moral beliefs, whereas morality is the adherence to informal personal values. Because the distinction between the two is slight, they are often used interchangeably.

ETHICS THEORIES

One classic theory in ethics is teleologic theory or consequentialism, which focuses on the ends or consequences of actions. The most well-known form of this theory, utilitarianism, is based on the concept of "the greatest good for the greatest number." The choice of action is clear under this theory, because the action that maximizes good over bad is the correct one. The theory poses difficulty when one must judge intrinsic values and determine whose good is the greatest. Additionally, the question must be asked whether good consequences can justify any amoral actions that might be used to achieve them.

Another theory in ethics is the deontologic or formalist theory, which argues that moral standards or principles exist independently of the ends or consequences. In a given situation, one or more moral principles may apply. The nurse has a duty to act based on the one relevant principle, or the most relevant of several moral principles. Problems arise with this theory when personal and cultural biases influence the choice of the most primary moral principle.

APPROACHES TO ETHICS

Two approaches to ethics are metaethics and applied ethics. An example of metaethics (understanding the concepts and linguistic terminology used in ethics) in the health care environment would be analysis of the concept of informed consent. Nurses are aware that patients must give consent before surgery, but sometimes a question arises as to whether the patient is truly informed. Delving more deeply into the concept of informed consent would be a metaethical inquiry.

Applied ethics is the term used when questions are asked of a specific discipline to identify ethical problems within that discipline's practice. Various disciplines use the frameworks of general ethical theories and moral principles and apply them to specific problems within their domain. Common ethical principles that apply in nursing include autonomy, beneficence, confidentiality, double effect, fidelity, justice, nonmaleficence, paternalism, respect for people, sanctity of life, and veracity. Brief definitions of these important principles can be found in Chart 3-2.

Nursing ethics may be considered a form of applied ethics because it addresses moral situations that are specific to the nursing profession and patient care. Some ethical problems that affect nursing may also apply to the broader area of bioethics and health care ethics. However, the nursing profession is a "caring" rather than

---

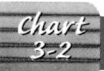 **Chart 3-2** **Common Ethical Principles**

The following common ethical principles may be used to validate moral claims.

Autonomy
This word is derived from the Greek words *autos* ("self") and *nomos* ("rule" or "law"), and therefore refers to self-rule. In contemporary discourse it has broad meanings, including individual rights, privacy, and choice. Autonomy entails the ability to make a choice free from external constraints.

Beneficence
Beneficence is the duty to do good and the active promotion of benevolent acts (eg, goodness, kindness, charity). It may also include the injunction not to inflict harm (see nonmaleficence).

Confidentiality
Confidentiality relates to the concept of privacy. Information obtained from an individual will not be disclosed to another unless it will benefit the person or there is a direct threat to the social good.

Double Effect
This is a principle that may morally justify some actions that produce both good and evil effects.

All four of the following criteria must be fulfilled:

1. The action itself is good or morally neutral.
2. The agent sincerely intends the good and not the evil effect (the evil effect may be foreseen but is not intended).
3. The good effect is not achieved by means of the evil effect.
4. There is proportionate or favorable balance of good over evil.

Fidelity
Fidelity is promise keeping; the duty to be faithful to one's commitments. It includes both explicit and implicit promises to another person.

Justice
From a broad perspective, justice states that like cases should be treated alike. A more restricted version of justice is *distributive justice*,

which refers to the distribution of social benefits and burdens based on various criteria that may include the following:

Equality
Individual need
Individual effort
Societal contribution
Individual merit
Legal entitlement

Retributive justice is concerned with the distribution of punishment.

Nonmaleficence
This is the duty not to inflict harm as well as to prevent and remove harm. Nonmaleficence may be included within the principle of beneficence, in which case nonmaleficence would be more binding.

Paternalism
Paternalism is the intentional limitation of another's autonomy, justified by an appeal to beneficence or the welfare or needs of another. Under this principle, the prevention of evils or harm takes precedence over any potential evils caused by interference with the individual's autonomy or liberty.

Respect for Persons
Respect for persons is frequently used synonymously with *autonomy*. However, it goes beyond accepting the notion or attitude that people have autonomous choice, to treating others in such a way that enables them to make the choice.

Sanctity of Life
This is the perspective that life is the highest good. Therefore, all forms of life, including mere biologic existence, should take precedence over external criteria for judging quality of life.

Veracity
Veracity is the obligation to tell the truth and not to lie or deceive others.

a predominantly "curing" profession; therefore, it is imperative that one not equate nursing ethics solely with medical ethics, because the medical profession has a "cure" focus. Nursing has its own professional code of ethics.

MORAL SITUATIONS

Many situations exist in which ethical analysis is needed. Some are *moral dilemmas,* situations in which a clear conflict exists between two or more moral principles or competing moral claims, and the nurse must choose the lesser of two evils. Other situations represent *moral problems,* in which there may be competing moral claims or principles but one claim or principle is clearly dominant. Some situations result in *moral uncertainty,* when one cannot accurately define what the moral situation is, or what moral principles apply, but has a strong feeling that something is not right. Still other situations may result in *moral distress,* in which the nurse is aware of the correct course of action but institutional constraints stand in the way of pursuing the correct action (Jameton, 1984).

For example, a patient tells a nurse that if he is dying he wants everything possible done. The surgeon and family have made the decision not to tell the patient he is terminally ill and not to resuscitate him if he stops breathing. From an ethical perspective, patients should be told the truth about their diagnoses and should have the opportunity to make decisions about treatments. Ideally, this information should come from the physician, with the nurse present to assist the patient in understanding the terminology and to provide further support, if necessary. A moral problem exists because of the competing moral claims of the family and physician, who wish to spare the patient distress, and the nurse, who wishes to be truthful with the patient as the patient has requested. If the patient's competency were questionable, a moral dilemma would exist because no dominant principle would be evident. The nurse could experience moral distress if the hospital threatens disciplinary action or job termination if the information is disclosed without the agreement of the physician or the family, or both.

It is essential that nurses freely engage in dialogue concerning moral situations, even though such dialogue is difficult for everyone involved. Improved interdisciplinary communication is supported when all members of the health care team can voice their concerns and come to an understanding of the moral situation. The use of an ethics consultant or consultation team could be helpful to assist the health care team, patient, and family to identify the moral dilemma and possible approaches to the dilemma. The nurse should be familiar with agency policy supporting patient self-determination and resolution of ethical issues. The nurse should be an advocate for patient rights in each situation (Trammelleo, 2000).

TYPES OF ETHICAL PROBLEMS IN NURSING

As a profession, nursing is accountable to society. This accountability is spelled out in the American Hospital Association's Patient Care Partnership (Chart 3-3), which reflects social beliefs about health and health care. In addition to accepting this document as one measure of accountability, nursing has further defined its standards of accountability through a formal code of ethics that explicitly states the profession's values and goals. The code (Chart 3-4), established by the American Nurses Association (ANA), consists of ethical standards, each with its own interpretive statements (ANA, 2001). The interpretive statements provide guidance to address and resolve ethical dilemmas by incorporat-

ing universal moral principles (ANA's Code of Ethics Project Task Force, 2000). The code is an ideal framework for nurses to use in ethical decision making.

Ethical issues have always affected the role of the professional nurse. The accepted definition of professional nursing has inspired a new advocacy role for nurses. The ANA, in *Nursing's Social Policy Statement* (1995), defines nursing as "the diagnosis and treatment of human responses to health and illness." This definition supports the claim that nurses must be actively involved in the decision-making process regarding ethical concerns surrounding health care and human responses. Efforts to enact this standard may cause conflict in health care settings in which the traditional roles of the nurse are delineated within a bureaucratic structure. If, however, nurses learn to present ethical conflicts within a logical, systematic framework, struggles over jurisdictional boundaries may decrease. Health care settings in which nurses are valued members of the team promote interdisciplinary communication and may enhance patient care. To practice effectively in these settings, nurses must be aware of ethical issues and assist patients in voicing their moral concerns.

The basic ethical framework of the nursing profession is the phenomenon of human caring. Nursing theories that incorporate the biopsychosocial–spiritual dimensions emphasize a holistic viewpoint, with humanism or caring as the core. As the nursing profession strives to delineate its own theory of ethics, caring is often cited as the moral foundation. For nurses to embrace this professional ethos, it is necessary to be aware not only of major ethical dilemmas but also of those daily interactions with health care consumers that frequently give rise to ethical challenges that are not as easily identified. Although technological advances and diminished resources have been instrumental in raising numerous ethical questions and controversies, including life-and-death issues, nurses should not ignore the many routine situations that involve ethical considerations. Some of the most common issues faced by nurses today include confidentiality, use of restraints, trust, refusing care, genetics, and end-of-life concerns.

Confidentiality

We all need to be aware of the confidential nature of information obtained in daily practice. If information is not pertinent to a case, the nurse should question whether it is prudent to record it in the patient's chart. In the practice setting, discussion of the patient with other members of the health care team is often necessary. These discussions should, however, occur in a private area where it is unlikely that the conversation will be overheard.

Another threat to keeping information confidential is the widespread use of computers and the easy access people have to them. This may increase the potential for misuse of information, which may have negative social consequences (Zolot, 1999). For example, laboratory results regarding testing for human immunodeficiency virus (HIV) infection or genetic screening may lead to loss of employment or insurance if the information is disclosed. Because of these possibilities of maleficence (see Chart 3-2) to the patient, sensitivity to the principle of confidentiality is essential.

Restraints

The use of restraints (including physical and pharmacologic measures) is another issue with ethical overtones. It is important to weigh carefully the risks of limiting a person's autonomy and increasing the risk of injury by using restraints against the risks of not using restraints. Before restraints are used, other strategies, such as

Chart 3-3 The Patient Care Partnership: Understanding Expectations, Rights, and Responsibilities

When you need hospital care, your doctor and the nurses and other professionals at our hospital are committed to working with you and your family to meet your health care needs. Our dedicated doctors and staff serve the community in all its ethnic, religious, and economic diversity. Our goal is for you and your family to have the same care and attention we would want for our families and ourselves.

The sections below explain some of the basics about how you can expect to be treated during your hospital stay. They also cover what we will need from you to care for you better. If you have questions at any time, please ask them. Unasked or unanswered questions can add to the stress of being in the hospital. Your comfort and confidence in your care are very important to us.

What to Expect During Your Hospital Stay

High quality hospital care. Our first priority is to provide you the care you need, when you need it, with skill, compassion, and respect. Tell your caregivers if you have concerns about your care or if you have pain. You have the right to know the identity of doctors, nurses, and others involved in your care, as well as when they are students, residents, or other trainees.

A clean and safe environment. Our hospital works hard to keep you safe. We use special policies and procedures to avoid mistakes in your care and keep you free from abuse or neglect. If anything unexpected and significant happens during your hospital stay, you will be told what happened and any resulting changes in your care will be discussed with you.

Involvement in your care. You and your doctor often make decisions about your care before you go to the hospital. Other times, especially in emergencies, those decisions are made during your hospital stay. When they take place, making decisions should include:

- *Discussing your medical condition and information about medically appropriate treatment choices.* To make informed decisions with your doctor, you need to understand several things:
  - The benefits and risks of each treatment.
  - Whether it is experimental or part of a research study.
  - What you can reasonably expect from your treatment and any long-term effects it might have on your quality of life.
  - What you and your family will need to do after you leave the hospital.
  - The financial consequences of using uncovered services or out-of-network providers.

  Please tell your caregivers if you need more information about treatment choices.
- *Discussing your treatment plan.* When you enter the hospital, you sign a general consent to treatment. In some cases, such as surgery or experimental treatment, you may be asked to confirm in writing that you understand what is planned and agree to it. This process protects your right to consent to or refuse a treatment. Your doctor will explain the medical consequences of refusing recommended treatment. It also protects your right to decide if you want to participate in a research study.
- *Getting information from you.* Your caregivers need complete and correct information about your health and coverage so that they can make good decisions about your care. That includes:

- Past illnesses, surgeries, or hospital stays.
- Past allergic reactions.
- Any medicines or diet supplements (such as vitamins and herbs) that you are taking.
- Any network or admission requirements under your health plan.
- *Understanding your health care goals and values.* You may have health care goals and values or spiritual beliefs that are important to your well-being. They will be taken into account as much as possible throughout your hospital stay. Make sure your doctor, your family, and your care team know your wishes.
- *Understanding who should make decisions when you cannot.* If you have signed a health care power of attorney stating who should speak for you if you become unable to make health care decisions for yourself, or a "living will" or "advance directive" that states your wishes about end-of-life care, give copies to your doctor, your family and your care team. If you or your family need help making difficult decisions, counselors, chaplains and others are available to help.

Protection of your privacy. We respect the confidentiality of your relationship with your doctor and other caregivers, and the sensitive information about your health and health care that are part of that relationship. State and federal laws and hospital operating policies protect the privacy of your medical information. You will receive a Notice of Privacy Practices that describes the ways that we use, disclose and safeguard patient information and that explains how you can obtain a copy of information from our records about your care.

Help preparing you and your family for when you leave the hospital. Your doctor works with hospital staff and professionals in your community. You and your family also play an important role. The success of your treatment often depends on your efforts to follow medication, diet and therapy plans. Your family may need to help care for you at home.

You can expect us to help you identify sources of follow-up care and to let you know if our hospital has a financial interest in any referrals. As long as you agree we can share information about your care with them, we will coordinate our activities with your caregivers outside the hospital. You can also expect to receive information and, where possible, training about the self-care you will need when you go home.

Help with your bill and filing insurance claims. Our staff will file claims for you with health care insurers or other programs such as Medicare and Medicaid. They will also help your doctor with needed documentation. Hospital bills and insurance coverage are often confusing. If you have questions about your bill, contact our business office. If you need help understanding your insurance coverage or health plan, start with your insurance company or health benefits manager. If you do not have health coverage, we will try to help you and your family find financial help or make other arrangements. We need your help with collecting needed information and other requirements to obtain coverage or assistance.

While you are here, you will receive more detailed notices about some of the rights you have as a hospital patient and how to exercise them. We are always interested in improving. If you have questions, comments, or concerns, please contact _____.

Reprinted with permission of the American Hospital Association, copyright 2003.

asking family members to sit with the patient, should be tried (Rogers & Bocchino, 1999). The Joint Commission on Accreditation of Healthcare Organizations (JCAHO) and the Health Care Financing Administration (HCFA) have designated standards for use in care of patients with restraints; these standards are available on the website listed at the end of this chapter (Schiff, 2001).

Trust Issues

Telling the truth (veracity) is one of the basic principles of our culture. Two ethical dilemmas in clinical practice that can directly conflict with this principle are the use of placebos (non-active substances used to treat symptoms) and not revealing a diagnosis to the patient. Both involve the issue of trust, which is an essential element in the nurse–patient relationship. Placebos may be used in experimental research, where the patient is involved in the decision-making process and is aware that placebos are being used in the treatment regimen. However, the use of a placebo as a substitute for an active drug to show that the patient does not have real symptoms is deceptive. This practice may severely undermine the nurse–patient relationship.

Informing patients of their diagnoses when the family and physician have chosen to withhold information is a common ethical situation in nursing practice. The nursing staff often use

American Nurses Association Code of Ethics for Nurses

Chart 3-4

1. The nurse, in all professional relationships, practices with compassion and respect for the inherent dignity, worth, and uniqueness of every individual, unrestricted by considerations of social or economic status, personal attributes, or the nature of health problems.
2. The nurse's primary commitment is to the patient, whether an individual, family, group, or community.
3. The nurse promotes, advocates for, and strives to protect the health, safety, and rights of the patient.
4. The nurse is responsible and accountable for individual nursing practice and determines the appropriate delegation of tasks consistent with the nurse's obligation to provide optimum patient care.
5. The nurse owes the same duties to self as to others, including the responsibility to preserve integrity and safety, to maintain competence, and to continue personal and professional growth.
6. The nurse participates in establishing, maintaining, and improving health care environments and conditions of employment conducive to the provision of quality health care and consistent with the values of the profession through individual and collective action.
7. The nurse participates in the advancement of the profession through contributions to practice, education, administration, and knowledge development.
8. The nurse collaborates with other health professionals and the public in promoting community, national, and international efforts to meet health needs.
9. The profession of nursing, as represented by associations and their members, is responsible for articulating nursing values, for maintaining the integrity of the profession and its practice, and for shaping social policy.

Reprinted with permission from the American Nurses Association, *Code of Ethics for Nurses with Interpretive Statements,* © 2001, American Nurses Publishing, American Nurses Foundation/American Nurses Association, Washington, DC.

---

evasive comments with the patient as a means to maintain professional relationships with other health practitioners. This area is indeed complex because it challenges the nurse's integrity. Trust and connection with the patient play an important part in optimizing care (Day & Stannard, 1999). Strategies the nurse could consider in this situation include the following:

- Not lying to the patient
- Providing all information related to nursing procedures and diagnoses
- Communicating to the family and physician the patient's requests for information

Families often are unaware of the patient's repeated questions to the nurse. With a better understanding of the situation, families may change their perspective. Finally, although providing the information may be the morally appropriate behavior, the manner in which the patient is told is important. Nurses must be compassionate and caring while informing patients; disclosure of information merely for the sake of patient autonomy does not convey respect for others.

Refusing to Provide Care

Any nurse who feels compelled to refuse to provide care for a particular type of patient faces an ethical dilemma. The reasons given for refusal range from a conflict of personal values to fear of personal risk of injury. Such instances have increased since the advent of acquired immunodeficiency syndrome (AIDS) as a major health problem. In one survey, the number of nurses who stated they might refuse to care for a patient with AIDS declined over a 10-year period, from 75% to 20%. The number who might refuse to care for a patient with AIDS who was violent or uncooperative, however, rose from 72% to 82% (Ventura, 1999).

The ethical obligation to care for all patients is clearly identified in the first statement of the Code of Ethics for Nurses. To avoid facing these moral situations, a nurse can follow certain strategies. For example, when applying for a job, one should ask questions regarding the patient population. If one is uncomfortable with a particular situation, then not accepting the position would be an option. Denial of care, or providing substandard nursing care to some members of our society, is not acceptable nursing practice.

End-of-Life Issues

Dilemmas that center on death and dying are prevalent in medical-surgical nursing practice and frequently initiate moral discussion. The dilemmas are compounded by the fact that the idea of curing is paramount in health care. With advanced technology, it may be difficult to accept the fact that nothing more can be done, or that technology may prolong life but at the expense of comfort and quality of life. Focusing on the caring as well as the curing role may assist nurses in dealing with these difficult moral situations. End-of-life issues are discussed in detail in Chapter 17.

PAIN CONTROL

The use of opioids to alleviate a patient's pain may present a dilemma for nurses. Patients with excruciating pain may require large doses of analgesics. Fear of respiratory depression or unwarranted fear of addiction should not prevent nurses from attempting to alleviate pain for the dying patient or for a patient experiencing an acute pain episode. In the case of the terminally ill patient, for example, the actions may be justified by the principle of double effect (see Chart 3-2). The intent or goal of nursing interventions is to alleviate pain and suffering while promoting comfort. The risk of respiratory depression is not the intent of the actions and should not be used as an excuse for withholding analgesia. However, the patient's respiratory status should be carefully monitored and any signs of respiratory depression reported to the physician. The administration of analgesia should be governed by the patient's needs.

DO-NOT-RESUSCITATE ORDERS

The "do not resuscitate" (DNR) order is a controversial issue. When a patient is competent to make decisions, his or her choice for a DNR order should be honored, according to the principles of autonomy or respect for the individual (Trammelleo, 2000). However, a DNR order is at times interpreted to mean that the patient requires less nursing care, when actually these patients may have significant medical and nursing needs, all of which demand attention. Ethically, all patients deserve and should receive appropriate nursing interventions, regardless of their resuscitation status.

LIFE SUPPORT

In contrast to the previous situations are those in which a DNR decision has not been made by or for a dying patient. The nurse may be put in the uncomfortable position of initiating life-support measures when, because of the patient's physical condition, they appear futile. This frequently occurs when the patient is not competent to make the decision and the family (or surrogate decision maker) refuses to consider a DNR order as an option. The nurse may be told to perform a "slow code" (ie, not to rush to resuscitate the patient) or may be given a verbal order not to resuscitate the patient; both are unacceptable medical orders. The best recourse for nurses in these situations is to be aware of hospital policy related to the Patient Self-Determination Act (discussed later) and execution of advance directives. The nurse should communicate with the physician. Discussing the matter with the physician may lead to further communication with the family and to a reconsideration of their decision, especially if they are afraid to let a loved one die with no further efforts to resuscitate (Trammelleo, 2000). Finally, when working with colleagues who are confronting such difficult situations, it helps to talk and listen to their concerns as a way of providing support.

FOOD AND FLUID

In addition to requesting that no heroic measures be taken to prolong life, a dying patient may request that no more food or fluid be administered. Many individuals think that food and hydration are basic human needs, not "invasive measures," and therefore should always be maintained. However, some consider food and hydration as means of prolonging suffering. In evaluating this issue, nurses must take into consideration the potential harm as well as the benefit to the patient of either administering or withdrawing sustenance. Research has not supported the belief that withholding fluids results in a painful death due to thirst (Smith, 1997; Zerwekh, 1997).

Evaluation of harm requires a careful review of the reasons the person has requested the withdrawal of food and hydration. Although the principle of autonomy has considerable merit and is supported by the Code of Ethics for Nurses, there may be situations when the request for withdrawal of food and hydration cannot be upheld. For patients with decreased decision-making capacity, the issues are more complex. Some of these cases have reached courts of law, and different states have different case law precedents forbidding withdrawal of sustenance. Although an advance directive may provide some answers, at present there are no firm guidelines to assist nurses in this area.

Preventive Ethics

As previously mentioned, a dilemma refers to a conflict between two alternatives. In such instances, one's moral decision is to choose the lesser evil of the two. However, various preventive strategies are available to help nurses anticipate or avoid certain kinds of ethical dilemmas.

Frequently, dilemmas occur when the health care practitioners are unsure of the patient's wishes because the person is unconscious or too cognitively impaired to communicate directly. One famous court case in this area of clinical ethics is that of Nancy Cruzan. Cruzan was a young woman involved in a single-car crash, after which she remained in a persistent vegetative state. Her family endured a 3-year legal battle to have her feeding tube removed so that she could be allowed to die. The U.S. Supreme Court decided that a state could require "clear and convincing evidence" of the patient's wishes before withdrawing life support. This ruling and the public response to it served as an impetus for legislation on advance directives, entitled the Patient Self-Determination Act, which became effective in December 1991. The intent of this legislation is to encourage people to prepare advance directives in which they indicate their wishes concerning the degree of supportive care to be provided if they become incapacitated. The regulatory language is quite broad and allows for different institutions to have latitude in implementing the person's directives. This legislation does not require a patient to have an advance directive, but it does require that the patient be informed about them by the staff of the health care facility. Consequently, this is an area where nursing can play a significant role in patient education.

ADVANCE DIRECTIVES

Advance directives are legal documents that specify a patient's wishes before hospitalization and provide valuable information that may assist health care providers in decision making. A living will is one type of advance directive. In most situations, living wills are limited to situations in which the patient's medical condition is deemed terminal. Because it is difficult to define "terminal" accurately, the living will is not always honored. Another potential drawback to the living will is that these documents are frequently written while the person is in good health. It is not unusual for people to change their minds as their illness progresses. Therefore, the patient retains the option to nullify the document.

Another type of advance directive is the durable power of attorney for health care, in which the patient identifies another individual to make health care decisions on his or her behalf. In this type of directive, the patient may have clarified his or her wishes concerning a variety of medical situations. As such, the power of attorney for health care is a less restrictive type of advance directive. Laws concerning advance directives vary among state jurisdictions. Even in states where these documents are not legally binding, however, they provide helpful information and assist health care providers to determine the patient's prior expressed wishes in situations where this information can no longer be obtained directly.

Institutional ethics committees, which exist in many hospitals to assist practitioners with ethical dilemmas, also aid in preventive ethics. The purpose of these multidisciplinary committees varies among institutions. In some hospitals, the committee exists solely for the purpose of developing policies; in others it may have a strong educational or consultation focus. Because these committees usually comprise individuals with some advanced training in ethics, they are important resources to the health care team, patient, and family. Nurses with a particular interest or expertise in the area of ethics are valuable members of ethics committees and can serve as valuable resources for staff nurses.

The heightened interest in ethical decision making has resulted in many continuing education programs, ranging from small seminars or workshops to full-semester courses offered by local colleges or professional organizations. In addition, nursing and medical journals contain articles on ethical issues, and numerous textbooks on clinical ethics or nursing ethics are available. These are valuable resources because they cover the ethical theory and dilemmas of practice in greater depth. The ANA also has publications available to assist nurses with ethical decision making.

Ethical Decision Making

As noted in the preceding discussions, ethical dilemmas are common and diverse in nursing practice. Although the situations vary and experience indicates that there are no clear solutions to these dilemmas, the fundamental philosophical principles are the same, and the process of moral reflection will help nurses to justify their actions. The approach to ethical decision making can follow the steps of the nursing process. Chart 3-5 outlines the steps of an ethical analysis.

Steps of the Nursing Process

The nursing process is a deliberate problem-solving approach for meeting a person's health care and nursing needs. Although the steps of the nursing process have been stated in various ways by different writers, the common components cited are assessment, diagnosis, planning, implementation, and evaluation. The ANA's *Standards of Clinical Nursing Practice* (1998) include an additional component entitled "outcome identification" and establish the sequence of steps in the following order: assessment, diagnosis, outcome identification, planning, implementation, and evaluation. For the purposes of this text, the nursing process will be based on the traditional five steps and will delineate two components in the diagnosis step: nursing diagnoses and collaborative problems. After the diagnoses or problems have been determined, the desired outcomes are often evident. The traditional steps are defined as follows:

1. *Assessment:* The systematic collection of data to determine the patient's health status and identify any actual or potential health problems. (Analysis of data is included as part of the assessment. For those who wish to emphasize its importance, analysis may be identified as a separate step of the nursing process.)

2. *Diagnosis:* Identification of the following two types of patient problems:
   a. *Nursing diagnoses:* Actual or potential health problems that can be managed by independent nursing interventions
   b. *Collaborative problems:* "Certain physiologic complications that nurses monitor to detect onset or changes in status. Nurses manage collaborative problems using physician-prescribed and nursing-prescribed interventions to minimize the complications of the events" (Carpenito, 1999, p. 7).
3. *Planning:* Development of goals and outcomes, as well as a plan of care designed to assist the patient in resolving the diagnosed problems and achieving the identified goals and desired outcomes.
4. *Implementation:* Actualization of the plan of care through nursing interventions.
5. *Evaluation:* Determination of the patient's responses to the nursing interventions and the extent to which the outcomes have been achieved.

Dividing the nursing process into distinct steps serves to emphasize the essential nursing actions that must be taken to resolve the patient's nursing diagnoses and manage any collaborative problems or complications. Dividing the process into separate steps is, however, artificial: the process functions as an integrated whole, with the steps being interrelated, interdependent, and recurrent (Fig. 3-1). Chart 3-6 presents an overview of the nursing activities involved in applying the nursing process.

Using the Nursing Process

ASSESSMENT

Assessment data are gathered through the health history and the physical assessment. In addition, ongoing monitoring is crucial to remain aware of patient needs and the effectiveness of the nursing care that the patient receives.

Chart 3-5 — Steps of an Ethical Analysis

The following are guidelines to assist nurses in ethical decision making. These guidelines reflect an active process in decision making, similar to the nursing process detailed in this chapter.

Assessment
1. Assess the ethical/moral situations of the problem. This step entails recognition of the ethical, legal, and professional dimensions involved.
   a. Does the situation entail substantive moral problems (conflicts among ethical principles or professional obligations)?
   b. Are there procedural conflicts? (For example, who should make the decisions? Any conflicts among the patient, health care providers, family and guardians?)
   c. Identify the significant people involved and those affected by the decision.

Planning
2. Collect information.
   a. Include the following information: the medical facts, treatment options, nursing diagnoses, legal data, and the values, beliefs, and religious components.
   b. Make a distinction between the factual information and the values/beliefs.

   c. Validate the patient's capacity, or lack of capacity, to make decisions.
   d. Identify any other relevant information that should be elicited.
   e. Identify the ethical/moral issues and the competing claims.

Implementation
3. List the alternatives. Compare alternatives with applicable ethical principles and professional code of ethics. Choose either of the frameworks below, or other frameworks, and compare outcomes.
   a. *Utilitarian approach:* Predict the consequences of the alternatives; assign a positive or negative value to each consequence; choose the consequence that predicts the highest positive value or "the greatest good for the greatest number."
   b. *Deontological approach:* Identify the relevant moral principles; compare alternatives with moral principles; appeal to the "higher-level" moral principle if there is a conflict.

Evaluation
4. Decide and evaluate the decision.
   a. What is the best or morally correct action?
   b. Give the ethical reasons for your decision.
   c. What are the ethical reasons against your decision?
   d. How do you respond to the reasons against your decision?

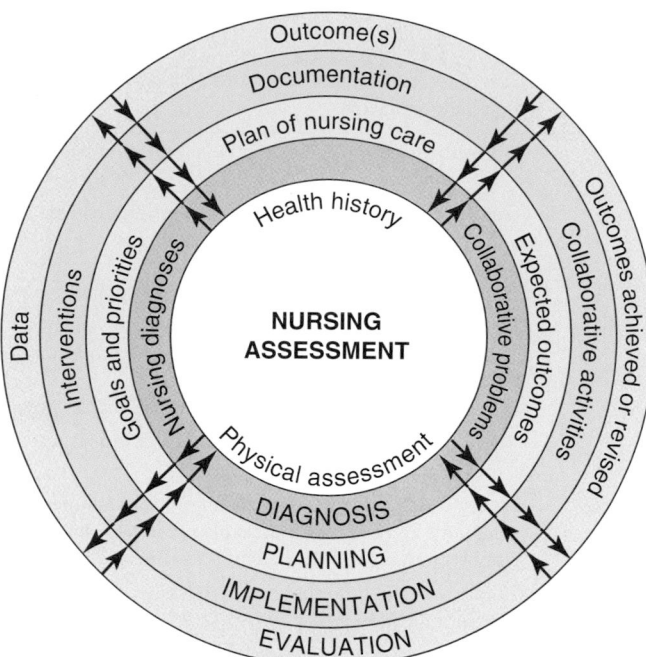

FIGURE 3-1 The nursing process is depicted schematically in this circle. Starting from the innermost circle, nursing assessment, the process moves outward through the formulation of nursing diagnoses and collaborative problems; planning, with setting of goals and priorities in the nursing plan of care; implementation and documentation; and, finally, the ongoing process of evaluation and outcomes.

Health History

The health history is conducted to determine the individual's state of wellness or illness and is best accomplished as part of a planned interview. The interview is a personal dialogue between the patient and the nurse that is conducted in order to obtain information. The nurse's approach to the patient will largely determine the amount and quality of the information that is received. Achieving a relationship of mutual trust and respect requires the ability to communicate a sincere interest in the patient. Examples of effective therapeutic communication techniques that can be used to achieve this goal are found in Table 3-1.

The use of a health history guide may help in obtaining pertinent information and in directing the course of the interview. A variety of health history formats designed to guide the interview are available, but they must be adapted to the responses, problems and needs of the individual. If a previous history is available, it should be used to reduce the need for the patient to repeat information. An experienced interviewer will develop a comfortable style and format for conducting an interview and will be flexible in adapting the format to suit the individual situation, while still obtaining the essential information. Various frameworks are available for acquiring the assessment data, such as functional health patterns, Maslow's hierarchy of needs, and Erikson's "eight stages of man." The information gathered will relate to the patient's physical, psychological, social, emotional, intellectual, developmental, cultural, and spiritual needs.

In some instances, it may be appropriate for the patient to fill out a health history form. When a form is used, the nurse verifies and clarifies the information provided by the patient and seeks any additional information necessary to identify the individual's nursing needs.

Chart 3-6 Steps of the Nursing Process

Assessment
1. Conduct the health history.
2. Perform the physical assessment.
3. Interview the patient's family or significant others.
4. Study the health record.
5. Organize, analyze, synthesize, and summarize the collected data.

Diagnosis
Nursing Diagnosis
1. Identify the patient's nursing problems.
2. Identify the defining characteristics of the nursing problems.
3. Identify the etiology of the nursing problems.
4. State nursing diagnoses concisely and precisely.

Collaborative Problems
1. Identify potential problems or complications that require collaborative interventions.
2. Identify health team members with whom collaboration is essential.

Planning
1. Assign priority to the nursing diagnoses.
2. Specify the goals.
   a. Develop immediate, intermediate, and long-term goals.
   b. State the goals in realistic and measurable terms.
3. Identify nursing interventions appropriate for goal attainment.
4. Establish expected outcomes.
   a. Make sure that the outcomes are realistic and measurable.
   b. Identify critical times for the attainment of outcomes.
5. Develop the written plan of nursing care.
   a. Include nursing diagnoses, goals, nursing interventions, expected outcomes, and critical times.
   b. Write all entries precisely, concisely, and systematically.
   c. Keep the plan current and flexible to meet the patient's changing problems and needs.
6. Involve the patient, family or significant others, nursing team members, and other health team members in all aspects of planning.

Implementation
1. Put the plan of nursing care into action.
2. Coordinate the activities of the patient, family or significant others, nursing team members, and other health team members.
3. Record the patient's responses to the nursing actions.

Evaluation
1. Collect data.
2. Compare the patient's actual outcomes with the expected outcomes. Determine the extent to which the expected outcomes were achieved.
3. Include the patient, family or significant others, nursing team members, and other health care team members in the evaluation.
4. Identify alterations that need to be made in the nursing diagnoses, collaborative problems, goals, nursing interventions, and expected outcomes.
5. Continue all steps of the nursing process: assessment, diagnosis, planning, implementation, and evaluation.

Physical Assessment

A physical assessment may be carried out before, during, or after the health history, depending on the patient's physical and emotional state and the immediate priorities of the situation.

The purpose of the health assessment is to identify those aspects of the patient's physical, psychological, and emotional state that indicate a need for nursing care. It requires the use of sight, hearing, touch, and smell as well as the appropriate interview

Table 3-1 • **Therapeutic Communication Techniques**

TECHNIQUE	DEFINITION	THERAPEUTIC VALUE
Listening	Active process of receiving information and examining one's reactions to the messages received	Nonverbally communicates nurse's interest in patient
Silence	Periods of no verbal communication among participants for therapeutic reasons	Gives patient time to think and gain insights, slows the pace of the interaction, and encourages the patient to initiate conversation, while conveying the nurse's support, understanding, and acceptance
Restating	Repeating to the patient what the nurse believes is the main thought or idea expressed	Demonstrates that the nurse is listening and validates, reinforces, or calls attention to something important that has been said
Reflection	Directing back to the patient his or her feelings, ideas, questions, or content	Validates the nurse's understanding of what the patient is saying and signifies empathy, interest, and respect for the patient
Clarification	Asking the patient to explain what he or she means or attempting to verbalize vague ideas or unclear thoughts of the patient to enhance the nurse's understanding	Helps to clarify the patient's feelings, ideas, and perceptions and to provide an explicit correlation between them and the patient's actions
Focusing	Questions or statements to help the patient develop or expand an idea	Allows the patient to discuss central issues and keeps communication goal-directed
Broad openings	Encouraging the patient to select topics for discussion	Indicates acceptance by the nurse and the value of the patient's initiative
Humor	Discharge of energy through the comic enjoyment of the imperfect	Promotes insight by bringing repressed material to consciousness, resolving paradoxes, tempering aggression, and revealing new options; a socially acceptable form of sublimation
Informing	Providing information	Helpful in health teaching or patient education about relevant aspects of patient's well-being and self-care
Sharing perceptions	Asking the patient to verify the nurse's understanding of what the patient is thinking or feeling	Conveys the nurse's understanding to the patient and has the potential to clarify confusing communication
Theme identification	Underlying issues or problems experienced by the patient that emerge repeatedly during the course of the nurse–patient relationship	Allows the nurse to best promote the patient's exploration and understanding of important problems
Suggesting	Presentation of alternative ideas for the patient's consideration relative to problem solving	Increases the patient's perceived options or choices

Adapted from Stuart, G. W., & Laraia, M. T. (2001). *Stuart and Sundeen's principles and practice of psychiatric nursing* (7th ed., pp. 34–35). St Louis: CV Mosby.

skills and techniques. Physical examination techniques as well as techniques and strategies for assessing behaviors and role changes are discussed in Chapters 5 and 7.

Other Components of the Database

Additional relevant information should be obtained from the patient's family or significant others, from other members of the health team, and from the patient's health record or chart. Depending on the patient's immediate needs, this information may have been obtained before the health history and the physical assessment were done. Whatever the sequence of events, it is important to use all available sources of pertinent data to complete the nursing assessment.

Recording the Database

After the health history and physical assessment are completed, the information obtained is recorded in the patient's permanent record. This record provides a means of communication among members of the health care team and facilitates coordinated planning and continuity of care. The record fulfills other functions as well:

- It serves as the business and legal record for the health care agency and for the professional staff members who are responsible for the patient's care.
- It serves as a basis for evaluating the quality and appropriateness of care and for reviewing the effective use of patient care services.
- It provides data that are useful in research, education, and short- and long-range planning.

A variety of systems are used for documenting patient care, and each health care agency selects the system that best meets its needs. The types of systems available include the problem-oriented health record system, focus charting, patient outcome charting, problem intervention evaluation (PIE) charting, and charting by exception (CBE). In addition, many health care agencies have moved toward computerized documentation systems; these appear to save time, improve the monitoring of quality improvement issues, and make it easier to gain access to patient information.

DIAGNOSIS

The assessment component of the nursing process serves as the basis for identifying nursing diagnoses and collaborative problems. Soon after the completion of the health history and the physical assessment, the nurse organizes, analyzes, synthesizes, and summarizes the data collected and determines the patient's need for nursing care.

Nursing Diagnosis

Nursing, unlike medicine, does not yet have a complete taxonomy, or classification system, of diagnostic labels. Classification of discrete items into meaningful categories organizes components of knowledge into coherent units of related information. Some reasons for establishing taxonomies are to help identify what is known about a field of study, to discover what gaps in knowledge exist, to provide a common language that enhances communication among colleagues, and to facilitate the coding of standardized information for use in databases. Nursing diagnoses, the first taxonomy created in nursing, have fostered the development of autonomy and accountability in nursing and have helped to delineate the scope of practice. Many state nurse practice acts include nursing diagnosis as a nursing function, and nursing diagnosis is included in the ANA's *Standards of Clinical Nursing Practice* and the standards of many nursing specialty organizations.

The official organization that has assumed responsibility for developing the taxonomy of nursing diagnoses and formulating nursing diagnoses acceptable for study is the North American Nursing Diagnosis Association (NANDA). NANDA has grouped diagnoses according to patterns of human responses (Chart 3-7). The diagnostic labels identified by NANDA have been generally accepted but require further validation, refinement, and expansion based on clinical use and research; they are not yet complete or mutually exclusive, and more investigation is needed to determine their validity and clinical applicability.

Choosing a Nursing Diagnosis

When choosing the nursing diagnoses for a particular patient, the nurse must first identify the commonalities among the assessment data collected. These common features lead to the categorization of related data that reveal the existence of a problem and the need for nursing intervention. The patient's identified problems are then defined in the nursing diagnoses. The most commonly selected nursing diagnoses are compiled and categorized by NANDA in a taxonomy that is updated at least every 2 years. It is important to remember that nursing diagnoses are not medical diagnoses; they are not medical treatments prescribed by the physician; and they are not diagnostic studies. Nursing diagnoses are not the equipment used to implement medical therapy, and they are not the problems that the nurse experiences while caring for the patient. They are the patient's actual or potential health problems that independent nursing actions can resolve. Nursing diagnoses that are succinctly stated in terms of the specific problems of the patient will guide the nurse in the development of the nursing plan of care.

To give additional meaning to the diagnosis, the characteristics and the etiology of the problem must be identified and included as part of the diagnosis. For example, the nursing diagnoses and their defining characteristics and etiology for a patient who has rheumatoid arthritis may include

- Impaired physical mobility related to pain and stiffness with joint movement
- Self-care deficits (bathing/hygiene, dressing/grooming, feeding, toileting) related to fatigue and joint stiffness
- Low self-esteem (chronic, situational, risk for situational) related to loss of independence
- Imbalanced nutrition: Less than body requirements related to fatigue and inadequate food intake

Collaborative Problems

In addition to nursing diagnoses and their related nursing interventions, nursing practice involves certain situations and interventions that do not fall within the definition of nursing diagnoses. These activities pertain to potential problems or complications that are medical in origin and require collaborative interventions with the physician and other members of the health care team. The term *collaborative problem* is used to identify these situations.

Collaborative problems are certain physiologic complications that nurses monitor to detect changes in status or onset of complications. Nurses manage collaborative problems using physician-prescribed and nursing-prescribed interventions to minimize complications (Carpenito, 1999, p. 7). A primary focus of the nurse when treating collaborative problems is monitoring the patient for the onset of complications or changes in the status of existing complications. The complications are usually related to the patient's disease process, treatments, medications, or diagnostic studies. The nurse prescribes nursing interventions that are appropriate for managing the complications and implements the treatments prescribed by the physician. Figure 3-2 depicts the differences between nursing diagnoses and collaborative problems. After the nursing diagnoses and collaborative problems have been identified, they are recorded on the plan of nursing care.

PLANNING

Once the nursing diagnoses have been identified, the planning component of the nursing process begins. This phase entails the following:

1. Assigning priorities to the nursing diagnoses and collaborative problems
2. Specifying expected outcomes
3. Specifying the immediate, intermediate, and long-term goals of nursing action
4. Identifying specific nursing interventions appropriate for attaining the outcomes
5. Identifying interdependent interventions
6. Documenting the nursing diagnoses, collaborative problems, expected outcomes, nursing goals, and nursing interventions on the plan of nursing care
7. Communicating to appropriate personnel any assessment data that point to health needs that can best be met by other members of the health care team

Setting Priorities

Assigning priorities to the nursing diagnoses and collaborative problems is a joint effort by the nurse and the patient or family members. Any disagreement about priorities is resolved in a way that is mutually acceptable. Consideration must be given to the

NANDA-Approved Nursing Diagnoses 2001–2002

This list represents the NANDA-approved nursing diagnoses for clinical use and testing.

Pattern 1. Exchanging
- Imbalanced nutrition: More than body requirements
- Imbalanced nutrition: Less than body requirements
- Risk for imbalanced nutrition: More than body requirements
- Risk for infection
- Risk for imbalanced body temperature
- Hypothermia
- Hyperthermia
- Ineffective thermoregulation
- Autonomic dysreflexia
- Risk for autonomic dysreflexia
- Constipation
- Perceived constipation
- Diarrhea
- Bowel incontinence
- Risk for constipation
- Impaired urinary elimination
- Stress urinary incontinence
- Reflex urinary incontinence
- Urge urinary incontinence
- Functional urinary incontinence
- Total urinary incontinence
- Risk for urge urinary incontinence
- Urinary retention
- Ineffective tissue perfusion (specify type: renal, cerebral, cardio-pulmonary, gastrointestinal, peripheral)
- Risk for imbalanced fluid volume
- Excess fluid volume
- Deficient fluid volume
- Risk for deficient fluid volume
- Decreased cardiac output
- Impaired gas exchange
- Ineffective airway clearance
- Ineffective breathing pattern
- Impaired spontaneous ventilation
- Dysfunctional ventilatory weaning response
- Risk for injury
- Risk for falls*
- Risk for suffocation
- Risk for poisoning
- Risk for trauma
- Risk for aspiration
- Risk for disuse syndrome
- Latex allergy response
- Risk for latex allergy response
- Ineffective protection
- Impaired tissue integrity
- Impaired oral mucous membrane
- Impaired skin integrity
- Risk for impaired skin integrity
- Impaired dentition
- Decreased intracranial adaptive capacity
- Disturbed energy field

Pattern 2. Communicating
- Impaired verbal communication

Pattern 3. Relating
- Impaired social interaction
- Social isolation
- Risk for loneliness
- Ineffective role performance
- Impaired parenting
- Risk for impaired parenting

- Risk for impaired parent/infant/child attachment
- Sexual dysfunction
- Interrupted family processes
- Caregiver role strain
- Risk for caregiver role strain
- Dysfunctional family processes: Alcoholism
- Parental role conflict
- Ineffective sexuality patterns

Pattern 4. Valuing
- Spiritual distress
- Risk for spiritual distress
- Readiness for enhanced spiritual well-being

Pattern 5. Choosing
- Ineffective coping
- Impaired adjustment
- Defensive coping
- Ineffective denial
- Disabled family coping
- Compromised family coping
- Readiness for enhanced family coping
- Readiness for enhanced community coping
- Ineffective community coping
- Ineffective therapeutic regimen management
- Noncompliance (specify)
- Ineffective family therapeutic regimen management
- Ineffective community therapeutic regimen management
- Effective therapeutic regimen management
- Decisional conflict (specify)
- Health-seeking behaviors (specify)

Pattern 6. Moving
- Impaired physical mobility
- Risk for peripheral neurovascular dysfunction
- Risk for perioperative-positioning injury
- Impaired walking
- Impaired wheelchair mobility
- Impaired transfer ability
- Impaired bed mobility
- Activity intolerance
- Fatigue
- Risk for activity intolerance
- Disturbed sleep pattern
- Sleep deprivation
- Deficient diversional activity
- Impaired home maintenance
- Ineffective health maintenance
- Delayed surgical recovery
- Adult failure to thrive
- Feeding self-care deficit
- Impaired swallowing
- Ineffective breastfeeding
- Interrupted breastfeeding
- Effective breastfeeding
- Ineffective infant feeding pattern
- Bathing/hygiene self-care deficit
- Dressing/grooming self-care deficit
- Toileting self-care deficit
- Delayed growth and development
- Risk for delayed development
- Risk for disproportionate growth
- Relocation stress syndrome
- Risk for relocation stress syndrome*
- Risk for disorganized infant behavior
- Disorganized infant behavior

(continued)

NANDA-Approved Nursing Diagnoses 2001–2002 (Continued)

- Readiness for enhanced organized infant behavior
- Wandering*

Pattern 7. Perceiving
- Disturbed body image
- Chronic low self-esteem
- Situational low self-esteem
- Risk for situational low self-esteem*
- Disturbed personal identity
- Disturbed sensory perception (specify: visual, auditory, kinesthetic, gustatory, tactile, olfactory)
- Unilateral neglect
- Hopelessness
- Powerlessness
- Risk for powerlessness*

Pattern 8. Knowing
- Deficient knowledge (specify)
- Impaired environmental interpretation syndrome
- Acute confusion
- Chronic confusion
- Disturbed thought processes
- Impaired memory

Pattern 9. Feeling
- Acute pain
- Chronic pain
- Nausea
- Dysfunctional grieving
- Anticipatory grieving
- Chronic sorrow
- Risk for other-directed violence
- Self-mutilation*
- Risk for self-mutilation
- Risk for self-directed violence
- Risk for suicide*
- Post-trauma syndrome
- Rape-trauma syndrome
- Rape-trauma syndrome: Compound reaction
- Rape-trauma syndrome: Silent reaction
- Risk for post-trauma syndrome
- Anxiety
- Death anxiety
- Fear

*New additions to taxonomy.
North American Nursing Diagnosis Association. (2001). *Nursing diagnosis: Definitions and Classification 2001–2002.* Philadelphia: Author.

---

urgency of the problems, with the most critical problems receiving the highest priority. Maslow's hierarchy of needs provides a useful framework for prioritizing problems, with importance being given first to physical needs; once those lower-level needs are met, higher-level needs can be addressed.

Establishing Expected Outcomes

Expected outcomes of the nursing interventions are stated in terms of the patient's behaviors and the time period in which they are to be achieved, as well as any special circumstances related to achieving the outcome (Smith-Temple & Johnson, 2002). These outcomes must be realistic and measurable. The Nursing-Sensitive Outcomes Classification (NOC) (Chart 3-8) and standard outcome criteria for people with specific health problems established by health care agencies are resources for identifying appropriate expected outcomes. These outcomes can be associated with nursing diagnoses and interventions and can be used when appropriate (Aquilino & Keenan, 2000). However, NOC may need to be adapted to establish realistic criteria for the specific patient involved.

The expected outcomes that define the desired behavior of the patient will be used to measure to what extent progress toward resolving the problem has been made. The expected outcomes also serve as the basis for evaluating the effectiveness of the nursing interventions and for deciding whether additional nursing care is needed or whether the plan of care needs to be revised.

Establishing Goals

After the priorities of the nursing diagnoses and expected outcomes have been established, the immediate, intermediate, and long-term goals and the nursing actions appropriate for attaining the goals are identified. The patient and his or her family are included in establishing goals for the nursing actions. Immediate goals are those that can be reached within a short period. Intermediate and long-term goals require a longer time to be achieved and usually involve preventing complications and other health problems and promoting self-care and rehabilitation. For example, goals for a patient with diabetes and a nursing diagnosis of *deficient knowledge related to the prescribed diet* may be stated as follows:

> Immediate goal: Demonstrates oral intake and tolerance of 1500-calorie diabetic diet spaced in three meals and one snack per day
> Intermediate goal: Plans meals for 1 week based on diabetic exchange list
> Long-term goal: Adheres to prescribed diabetic diet

Determining Nursing Actions

In planning appropriate nursing actions to achieve the desired goals and outcomes, the nurse, with input from the patient and significant others, identifies individualized interventions based on the patient's circumstances and preferences that will address each outcome. Interventions should identify the activities needed and who will carry them out. Determination of interdisciplinary activities is made in collaboration with other health care providers as needed.

The nurse identifies and plans patient teaching and return demonstrations as needed to assist the patient in learning self-care activities to be performed. Planned interventions should be ethical and appropriate to the patient's culture, age, and gender. Standardized interventions, such as those found on institutional care plans or in the Nursing Interventions Classification (NIC)

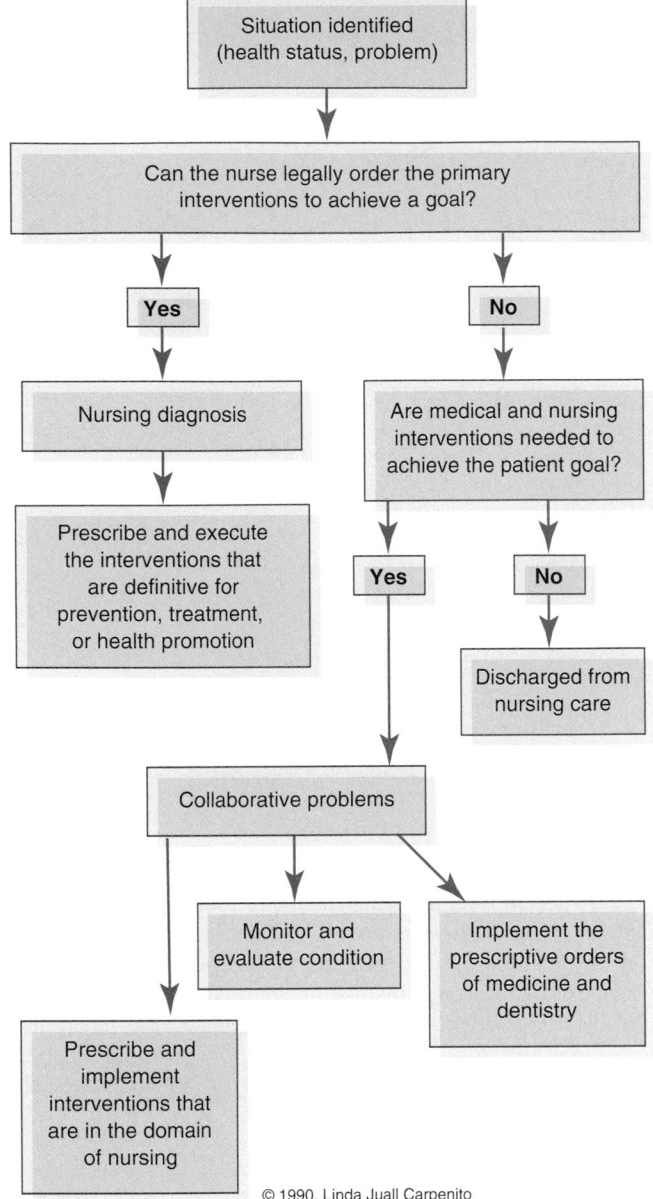

```
┌─────────────────────────────┐
│   Situation identified       │
│  (health status, problem)    │
└─────────────────────────────┘
              │
              ▼
┌─────────────────────────────┐
│ Can the nurse legally order  │
│  the primary interventions   │
│    to achieve a goal?        │
└─────────────────────────────┘
      │                 │
      ▼                 ▼
   [ Yes ]            [ No ]
      │                 │
      ▼                 ▼
┌──────────────┐  ┌──────────────────┐
│   Nursing    │  │ Are medical and  │
│   diagnosis  │  │ nursing          │
└──────────────┘  │ interventions    │
      │           │ needed to achieve│
      ▼           │ the patient goal?│
┌──────────────┐  └──────────────────┘
│ Prescribe and│      │         │
│ execute the  │      ▼         ▼
│ interventions│   [ Yes ]    [ No ]
│ that are     │      │         │
│ definitive   │      │         ▼
│ for          │      │  ┌──────────────┐
│ prevention,  │      │  │ Discharged   │
│ treatment,   │      │  │ from nursing │
│ or health    │      │  │ care         │
│ promotion    │      │  └──────────────┘
└──────────────┘      │
                      ▼
              ┌──────────────────┐
              │  Collaborative   │
              │    problems      │
              └──────────────────┘
                   │        │
                   ▼        ▼
         ┌──────────────┐ ┌──────────────┐
         │ Monitor and  │ │ Implement the│
         │ evaluate     │ │ prescriptive │
         │ condition    │ │ orders of    │
         └──────────────┘ │ medicine and │
              │           │ dentistry    │
              ▼           └──────────────┘
      ┌──────────────┐
      │ Prescribe and│
      │ implement    │
      │ interventions│
      │ that are in  │
      │ the domain   │
      │ of nursing   │
      └──────────────┘

       © 1990, Linda Juall Carpenito
```

FIGURE 3-2 Differentiating nursing diagnoses and collaborative problems. Source: Carpenito, L. J. (2001). *Nursing diagnosis: Application to clinical practice* (8th ed). Philadelphia: Lippincott Williams & Wilkins. Copyright © 1990, Linda Juall Carpenito.

(Aquilino & Keenan, 2000; McCloskey & Bulechek, 2000) can be used. Chart 3-9 describes the NIC system and provides an example of an NIC system intervention. It is important to individualize prewritten interventions to promote optimal effectiveness for each patient.

IMPLEMENTATION

The implementation phase of the nursing process involves carrying out the proposed plan of nursing care. The nurse assumes responsibility for the implementation. Performance of interventions, however, may be carried out by the patient and the family, other members of the nursing team, or other members of the health care team as appropriate. The nurse coordinates the activities of all those involved in implementation so that the schedule of activities facilitates the patient's recovery. The plan of nursing care serves as the basis for implementation:

- The immediate, intermediate, and long-term goals are used as a focus for the implementation of the designated nursing interventions.
- While implementing nursing care, the nurse continually assesses the patient and his or her response to the nursing care.
- Revisions are made in the plan of care as the patient's condition, problems, and responses change and when reassignment of priorities is required

Implementation includes direct or indirect execution of the planned interventions. It is focused on resolving the patient's nursing diagnoses and collaborative problems and achieving expected outcomes, thus meeting the patient's health needs.

Included among nursing interventions are assisting with hygienic care; promoting physical and psychological comfort; supporting respiratory and elimination functions; facilitating the ingestion of food, fluids, and nutrients; managing the patient's immediate surroundings; providing health teaching; promoting a therapeutic relationship; and carrying out a variety of therapeutic nursing activities. Judgment, critical thinking, and good decision-making skills are essential in the selection of appropriate scientifically and ethically based nursing interventions. All nursing interventions are patient-focused and outcome-directed and are implemented with compassion, confidence and a willingness to accept and understand the patient's responses.

Although many nursing actions are independent, others are interdependent, such as carrying out prescribed treatments, administering medications and therapies, and collaborating with other health care team members to accomplish specific expected outcomes and to monitor and manage potential complications. Such interdependent functioning is just that—interdependent. Requests or orders from other health care team members should not be followed blindly but should be assessed critically and questioned when necessary. The implementation phase of the nursing process ends when the nursing interventions have been completed.

EVALUATION

Evaluation, the final step of the nursing process, allows the nurse to determine the patient's response to the nursing interventions and the extent to which the objectives have been achieved. The plan of nursing care is the basis for evaluation. The nursing diagnoses, collaborative problems, priorities, nursing interventions, and expected outcomes provide the specific guidelines that dictate the focus of the evaluation. Through evaluation, the nurse can answer the following questions:

- Were the nursing diagnoses and collaborative problems accurate?
- Did the patient achieve the expected outcomes within the critical time periods?
- Have the patient's nursing diagnoses been resolved?
- Have the collaborative problems been resolved?
- Have the patient's nursing needs been met?
- Should the nursing interventions be continued, revised, or discontinued?

Nursing-Sensitive Outcomes Classification (NOC)

The NOC is a classification of patient outcomes sensitive to nursing interventions. Each outcome is a neutral statement about a variable patient condition, behavior, or perception coupled with a rating scale. The outcome statement and scale can be used to identify baseline functioning, expected outcomes, and actual outcomes for individual patients. The following table is an example of a nursing-sensitive outcome.

Nutritional Status (1004)

Domain—Physiologic Health (II)
Class—Nutrition (K)
Scale—Extremely compromised to Not compromised (a)
Definition   Extent to which nutrients are available to meet metabolic needs

Nutritional Status	Extremely Compromised 1	Substantially Compromised 2	Moderately Compromised 3	Mildly Compromised 4	Not Compromised 5
Indicators					
100401 Nutrient intake	1	2	3	4	5
100402 Food and fluid intake	1	2	3	4	5
100403 Energy	1	2	3	4	5
100404 Body mass	1	2	3	4	5
100405 Weight	1	2	3	4	5
100406 Biochemical measures	1	2	3	4	5
100407 Other _____	1	2	3	4	5
(Specify)					

With permission from Johnson, M., Maas, M., & Moorhead, S. (Eds.). (2000). Nursing outcomes classification [NOC]: Iowa Outcomes Project (2nd ed). St. Louis: Mosby–Year Book.

- Have new problems evolved for which nursing interventions have not been planned or implemented?
- What factors influenced the achievement or lack of achievement of the objectives?
- Do priorities need to be reassigned?
- Should changes be made in the expected outcomes and outcome criteria?

Objective data that provide answers to these questions are collected from all available sources (eg, patient, family, significant others, and health care team members). These data are included in the patient's record and must be substantiated by direct observation of the patient before the outcomes are recorded.

DOCUMENTATION OF OUTCOMES AND REVISION OF PLAN

Outcomes are documented concisely and objectively. Documentation should relate outcomes to the nursing diagnoses and collaborative problems, describe the patient's responses to the interventions, indicate whether the outcomes were met, and include any additional pertinent data (see Plan of Nursing Care).

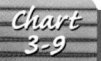

Nursing Interventions Classification (NIC)

The NIC is a standardized classification of nursing treatments (interventions) that includes independent and collaborative interventions. Intervention labels are terms such as hemorrhage control, medication administration, or pain management. Listed under each intervention are multiple discrete nursing actions that together constitute a comprehensive approach to treatment of a particular condition. Not all actions are applicable to every patient; nursing judgment will determine which actions to implement. The following is an example of a nursing intervention:

Weight Management*
Definition: Facilitating maintenance of optimal body weight and percent body fat
Activities:
   Discuss with the patient the relationship between food intake, exercise, weight gain, and weight loss

Discuss with patient the medical conditions that may affect weight
Discuss with patient the habits, customs, and cultural and hereditary factors that influence weight
Discuss risks associated with being overweight or underweight
Determine patient's motivation for changing eating habits
Determine patient's ideal body weight
Determine patient's ideal percent body fat
Develop with patient a method to keep a daily record of intake
Encourage patient to write down realistic weekly goals for food intake and exercise and to display them in a location where they can be reviewed daily
Encourage patient to chart weekly weights, as appropriate
Inform patient about support groups that are available for assistance
Assist in developing well-balanced meal plans consistent with level of energy expenditure

*With permission from McCloskey, J. C., & Bulechek, G. M. (Eds.). (2000). *Nursing interventions classification (NIC): Iowa Interventions Project* (3rd ed). St. Louis: Mosby–Year Book.

Plan of Nursing Care
Example of an Individualized Plan of Nursing Care

Mr. John Lee, a 50-year-old management consultant, was admitted to the nursing unit from his physician's office. A routine physical examination 3 months previously had revealed essential hypertension with BP 170/110 and decreased urine creatinine clearance. During the subsequent 3 months the blood pressure elevation did not respond to diet therapy. Mr. Lee admitted that he had not been successful in adhering to the low-sodium, low-cholesterol weight-reduction diet that had been prescribed for him. He stated, "My life is just too busy—I work all hours of the day and night." He indicated that in addition to his work he and his wife share the responsibility for raising their two teenage daughters. He drinks five to seven cups of coffee daily and drinks alcohol only at social occasions. Admission physical examination revealed BP 194/112, P 96, R 20, T 37°C (98.6°F), height 5'10", weight 210 lbs, and slight edema of the ankles and feet. Mr. Lee stated that his feet are "always puffy at night." There were several darkened areas (2 cm in diameter) on the anterior lower legs bilaterally. A brief hospitalization was planned for thorough evaluation and initiation of therapy. The physician's orders on admission included activity as desired; Lasix, 40 mg bid; monitor vital signs every 4 hours while awake; and 1500 calorie, 1 g sodium, low-cholesterol diet.

Nursing Diagnosis
- Ineffective health maintenance related to hypertension, stress, obesity, and caffeine
- Ineffective coping related to role responsibilities at work and home
- Noncompliance with dietary regimen related to knowledge deficit and lifestyle

Collaborative Problems
1. Ischemic ulcers of lower legs

Goals
Immediate: Gradual decrease in blood pressure
Intermediate: Initiation of lifestyle alterations to decrease stress
Long-term: Alteration of lifestyle to reduce emotional and environmental stressors
      Compliance with dietary regimen
      Absence of ischemic leg ulcers

Nursing Interventions	Expected Outcomes	Outcomes
1. Monitor BP lying, sitting, and standing every 4 h	Experiences no further increase in BP	BP range of 162/112–138/98 since admission No variation greater than 5 mm Hg in systolic or diastolic pressures with position changes No variation between right and left arms Maximum BP from 24 h after admission to time of discharge: 138/98
2. Monitor fluid status: a. I&O	Urinary output adequate in relation to oral intake	Intake: 1850 mL Output: 1685 mL
b. Peripheral edema	No evidence of peripheral edema	Minimal edema of feet late in evening
3. Promote atmosphere conducive to physical and mental rest: a. Encourage alternation of rest and activity	Alternates periods of rest and activity	Rests in bed 1 h in morning and 2 h in afternoon; disconnects phone during rest periods Awake at intervals during night: 8 h of uninterrupted sleep at night after initiation of 30 mg Dalmane at bedtime
b. Encourage limitation of visitors and interactions that are stress-producing	Limits visitors to family in the evenings	Wife and daughters visit 2 h in evening: patient calm and relaxed after visits
	Avoids stress-producing interactions	Wife and daughters aware of need to decrease stress: they consult with patient about regular family activities
4. Assist patient to alter lifestyle to decrease stress a. Discuss relationship between emotional stress and physiologic functioning:	Describes stress as a precursor to alteration in physiologic functioning	Accurately described relationship between stress and hypertension

b. Encourage patient to identify stress-producing stimuli	Identifies lifestyle factors that produce stress	Identified the following stressors:
		  Self-imposed demands of job; unwillingness to refer clients
		  Excessive involvement in daughters' school and recreational activities

(continued)

Plan of Nursing Care
Example of an Individualized Plan of Nursing Care (Continued)

Nursing Interventions	Expected Outcomes	Outcomes
c. Encourage patient to identify adjustments necessary to reduce stress	Identifies lifestyle adjustments necessary to reduce stress Discusses lifestyle adjustments with family	Verbalized plans to make more referrals Identified need to decrease work hours to maximum of 8 h per day Consulted with wife and daughters; will alternate with wife in attending daughters' activities; all family members supportive
5. Encourage patient to identify obesity and caffeine as stressors and aggravators of hypertension; request consultation with dietitian and reinforce instructions given	Identifies harmful effects of obesity and caffeine Makes plans for losing weight Makes plans for decreasing caffeine intake	Accurately described effects of obesity and caffeine on blood pressure Plans to go to Weight Watchers; has had success with this program in the past Drinks 1 cup of coffee for breakfast; uses decaffeinated coffee at mid-morning, lunch, and dinner; expressed satisfaction with this plan
6. Assess for ischemic leg ulcers; report changes in darkened spots on legs to physician	Absence of changes in skin integrity on lower extremities	No changes noted in characteristics of skin of lower legs on days 2 and 3
7. Teach foot care: daily inspection and washing, nail care, avoidance of caustic solutions, lubrication of dry skin, avoidance of heat to feet, well-fitting shoes and socks, avoidance of crossing legs	Describes principles and techniques of proper foot care	Discussed importance of proper foot care; demonstrated proper technique of foot care; shoes and socks fit well; does not cross legs when sitting

The plan of care is subject to change as the patient's needs change, as the priorities of the needs shift, as needs are resolved, and as additional information about the patient's state of health is collected. As the nursing interventions are implemented, the patient's responses are evaluated and documented and the plan of care is revised accordingly. A well-developed, continuously updated plan of care is the greatest assurance that the patient's nursing diagnoses and collaborative problems will be addressed and his or her basic needs will be met.

Critical Thinking Exercises

1. You are an acute care nurse and you have been assigned to the outpatient unit for the shift. How does the approach to critical thinking differ among nursing practice settings (acute care versus ambulatory care settings)?

2. You have just completed the health history for your assigned patient. How would you identify the patient's nursing diagnoses? Describe the kind of resources that are available to help you with identifying these diagnoses.

3. A terminally ill patient's daughter tells you she is not ready to let her father go. The next day you note a "Do Not Resuscitate" order on the chart. Describe which critical thinking skills you could use to address the issue and to develop a plan of care for the patient and family. How did you integrate your critical thinking into the nursing process? What changes might you make in your plan of care consid-

ering the DNR order? What ethical problems or dilemmas might you anticipate?

4. The spouse of your patient tells you information about the patient that the patient has not revealed. How would you determine whether you should communicate this information to the patient's primary nurse?

REFERENCES AND SELECTED READINGS
Books

Alfaro-LeFevre, R. (1999). *Critical thinking in nursing* (2nd ed.). Philadelphia: W. B. Saunders.

American Nurses Association. (2001). *Code of ethics for nurses with interpretive statements.* Washington, DC: American Nurses Publishing.

American Nurses Association. (1995). *Nursing's social policy statement.* Washington, DC: Author.

American Nurses Association. (1998). *Standards of clinical nursing practice* (2nd ed.). Washington, DC: Author.

Bickley, L. S., & Hoekelman, R. A. (1999). *Bates' guide to physical examination and history taking* (7th ed.). Philadelphia: Lippincott Williams & Wilkins.

Carpenito, L. J. (2001). *Nursing diagnosis: Application to clinical practice* (9th ed.). Philadelphia: Lippincott Williams & Wilkins.

Carpenito, L. J. (1999). *Nursing care plan and documentation.* Philadelphia: Lippincott Williams & Wilkins.

Fonteyn, M. E. (1998). *Thinking strategies for nursing practice.* Philadelphia: Lippincott-Raven.

Jameton, A. (1984). *Nursing practice: The ethical issues.* Englewood Cliffs, NJ: Prentice-Hall.

Joint Commission for Accreditation of Hospital Organizations (JCAHO). (1999). *Standards, rights, responsibilities, and ethics.* Oakbrook Terrace, IL: Author.

Johnson, M., & Maas, M. (Eds.). (2000). *Nursing outcomes classification (NOC): Iowa Outcomes Project* (2nd ed.). St. Louis: Mosby–Year Book.

McCloskey, J. C., & Bulechek, G. M. (Eds.). (2000). *Nursing interventions classification (NIC): Iowa Interventions Project* (2nd ed.). St. Louis: Mosby–Year Book.

Smith-Temple, J., & Johnson, J. Y. (2002). *Nurses' guide to clinical procedures* (4th ed.). Philadelphia: Lippincott-Raven.

Stuart, G. W., & Laraia, M. T. (2001). *Stuart and Sundeen's principles and practice of psychiatric nursing.* (7th ed.). St. Louis: Mosby.

Wilkinson, J. M. (2001). *Nursing process and critical thinking.* New Jersey: Prentice-Hall.

Journals

American Nurses Association's Code of Ethics Project Task Force. (2000). A code of ethics for nurses. *American Journal of Nursing, 100*(7), 69, 71–72.

Aquilino, M. L., & Keenan, G. (2000). Having our say: Nursing's standardized nomenclatures. *American Journal of Nursing, 100*(7), 33–38.

Daly, J. M. (1996). A care planning tool that proves what we do. *RN, 59*(6), 26–30.

Day, L. J., & Stannard, D. (1999). Developing trust and connection with patients and their families. *Critical Care Nurse, 19*(3), 66–70.

Haddad, A. (2000). Ethics in action. *RN, 63*(7), 21–22, 24.

Haddad, A. (2001). Ethics in action. *RN, 64*(1), 29–30, 32.

Ignatavicius, D. D. (2001). Six critical thinking skills for at-the-bedside success. *Nursing Management, 32*(1), 37–39.

Prideaux, D. (2000). Do you know? *Medical Teacher, 22*(6), 607.

Rogers, P. D., & Bocchino, N. L. (1999). Restraint-free care: Is it possible? *American Journal of Nursing, 99*(10), 26–33.

Schiff, L. (2001). RN news watch: JCAHO and HCFA now agree on restraint standards. *RN, 64*(1), 14.

Smith, S. A. (1997). Controversies in hydrating the terminally ill patient. *Journal of Intravenous Nursing, 20*(4), 193–200.

Trammelleo, A. D. (2000). Protecting patients' end-of-life choices. *RN, 63*(8), 75, 77, 79.

Ventura, M. J. (1999). Ethics on the job—A survey: The realities of HIV/AIDS. *RN, 62*(4), 26–30.

Zerwekh, J. V. (1997). Do dying patients really need IV fluids? *American Journal of Nursing, 97*(3), 26–31.

Zolot, J. S. (1999). Computer-based patient records. *American Journal of Nursing, 99*(12), 64–69.

RESOURCES AND WEBSITES

Centers for Medicare & Medicaid Services (CMS), 7500 Security Boulevard, Baltimore, MD 21244-1850; (877) 267-2323; http://www.cms.hhs.gov.

Joint Commission on Accreditation of Healthcare Organizations (JCAHO), One Renaissance Blvd., Oakbrook Terrace, IL 60181; (630) 792-5000; http://www.jcaho.org.

Health Education and Health Promotion

LEARNING OBJECTIVES

On completion of this chapter, the learner will be able to:

1. Describe the purposes and significance of health education.
2. Describe the concept of adherence to a therapeutic regimen.
3. Identify variables influencing the elderly person's adherence to a therapeutic regimen.
4. Distinguish the variables that affect learning readiness.
5. Describe strategies that facilitate elderly adults' learning abilities.
6. Describe the relationship of the teaching–learning process to the nursing process.
7. Develop a teaching plan for a patient.
8. Define the concepts of health, wellness, and health promotion.
9. Discuss major health promotion theories.
10. Describe the health promotion principles of self-responsibility, nutrition, stress management, and exercise.
11. Specify the variables that affect health promotion activities for children, young and middle-aged adults, and elderly adults.
12. Describe the role of the nurse in health promotion.

*E*ffective health education lays a solid foundation for individual and community wellness. Teaching is an integral tool that all nurses use to assist patients and families in developing effective health behaviors and in altering lifestyle patterns that predispose people to health risks. Health education is an influential factor directly related to positive patient care outcomes.

Health Education Today

The changes in today's health care environment mandate the use of an organized approach to health education so that patients can meet their specific health care needs. Significant factors for the nurse to consider when planning patient education include the availability of health care outside the conventional hospital setting, the employment of diverse health care providers to accomplish care management goals, and the increased use of alternative strategies rather than traditional approaches to care. The careful consideration of these factors can provide patients with the comprehensive information that is essential for making informed decisions about health care. Demands from consumers for comprehensive information about their health issues throughout the life cycle accentuate the need for holistic health education to occur in every patient–nurse encounter.

The nurse as a teacher is challenged, not only to provide specific patient and family education, but also to focus on the educational needs of communities. Health education is important to nursing care, because it can determine how well individuals and families are able to perform behaviors conducive to optimal self-care.

Teaching, as a function of nursing, is included in all state nurse practice acts and in the *Standards of Clinical Nursing Practice* of the American Nurses Association (ANA, 1998). Health education is an independent function of nursing practice and is a primary responsibility of the nursing profession. All nursing care is directed toward promoting, maintaining, and restoring health; preventing illness; and assisting people to adapt to the residual effects of illness. Many of these nursing activities are accomplished through health education or patient teaching.

Every contact a nurse has with a health care consumer, whether that person is ill or not, should be considered an opportunity for health teaching. Although the person has a right to decide whether or not to learn, the nurse has the responsibility to present information that will motivate the person to recognize the need to learn. Therefore, the nurse must seize opportunities both inside and outside health care settings to facilitate wellness. Educational environments can include homes, hospitals, community health centers, places of business, service organizations, shelters, and consumer action or support groups.

THE PURPOSE OF HEALTH EDUCATION

This emphasis on health education stems in part from the public's right to comprehensive health care, which includes up-to-date health information. It also reflects the emergence of an informed public that is asking more significant questions about health and the health care services it receives. Because of the importance American society places on health and the responsibility each of us has to maintain and promote our own health, members of the health care team, specifically nurses, are obligated to make health education consistently available. Without adequate knowledge and training in self-care skills, consumers cannot make effective decisions about their health.

People with chronic illnesses are among those most in need of health education. As the life span of our population continues to increase, the number of people with such illnesses will also increase. People with chronic illness need health care information to participate actively in and assume responsibility for much of their own care. Health education can help these individuals to adapt to illness, prevent complications, carry out prescribed therapy, and solve problems when confronted with new situations. It can also prevent crisis situations and reduce the potential for rehospitalization resulting from inadequate information about self-care. The goal of health education is to teach people to live life to its healthiest—that is, to strive toward achieving their maximum health potential.

In addition to the public's right to and desire for health education, patient education is also a strategy for reducing health care costs by preventing illness, avoiding expensive medical treatments, decreasing lengthy hospital stays, and facilitating earlier discharge. For health care agencies, offering community wellness programs is a public relations tool for increasing patient satisfaction and for developing a positive image of the institution. Patient education is also a cost-avoidance strategy for those who believe that positive staff–patient relationships avert malpractice suits.

Adherence to the Therapeutic Regimen

One of the goals of patient education is to encourage people to adhere to their therapeutic regimen. Adherence to a therapeutic regimen usually requires that the person make one or more lifestyle changes to carry out specific activities that promote and maintain health. Common examples of behaviors facilitating health include taking prescribed medications, maintaining a healthy diet, increasing daily activities and exercise, self-monitoring for signs and symptoms of illness, practicing specific hygienic measures, seeking periodic health evaluations, and performing other therapeutic and

Glossary

adherence: the process of faithfully following guidelines or directions

community: a group of people living in the same geographical area under the same guidelines

feedback: the return of information about the results of input given to a person or a system

health education: a variety of learning experiences designed to promote behaviors that facilitate health

health promotion: the art and science of assisting people to change their lifestyle toward a higher state of wellness

learning: the act of gaining knowledge and skill

learning readiness: the optimum time for learning to occur; usually corresponds to the learner's perceived need and desire to obtain specific knowledge

nutrition: the science that deals with food and nourishment in humans

physical fitness: the condition of being physically healthy as a result of proper exercise and nutrition

reinforcement: the process of strengthening a given response or behavior to increase

the likelihood that the behavior will continue

self-responsibility: personal accountability for one's actions or behavior

stress management: behaviors and techniques used to strengthen a person's resources against stress

teaching: the imparting of knowledge

therapeutic regimen: a routine that promotes health and healing

wellness: a condition of good physical and emotional health sustained by a healthy lifestyle

preventive measures. The fact that many people do not adhere to their prescribed regimens cannot be ignored or minimized; rates of adherence are generally low, especially when the regimens are complex or of long duration.

Nonadherence to prescribed therapy has been the subject of many studies. For the most part, the findings have been inconclusive, and no one predominant causative factor has been found. Instead, a wide range of variables appears to influence the degree of adherence:

- Demographic variables, such as age, gender, race, socioeconomic status, and level of education
- Illness variables, such as the severity of the illness and the relief of symptoms afforded by the therapy
- Therapeutic regimen variables, such as the complexity of the regimen and uncomfortable side effects
- Psychosocial variables, such as intelligence, availability of significant and supportive people (especially family members), attitudes toward health professionals, acceptance or denial of illness, and religious or cultural beliefs
- Financial variables, especially the direct and indirect costs associated with a prescribed regimen

The nurse's success with health education is determined by ongoing assessment of the variables affecting the patient's capacity to adopt specific behaviors, to obtain resources, and to maintain a helpful social environment (Murray & Zentner, 2001). Teaching programs are more likely to succeed if the variables affecting the patient's adherence are identified and considered in the teaching plan.

The problem of nonadherence to therapeutic regimens is a substantial one that must be remedied before patients can achieve their maximum self-care capabilities and health potential. Surprisingly, a patient's need for knowledge has not been found to be a sufficient stimulus for acquiring knowledge and thereby enabling complete adherence to a health regimen. Teaching programs directed toward stimulating patient motivation produce varying degrees of adherence. The variables of choice, establishment of mutual goals, and the quality of the patient–provider relationship directly influence the behavioral changes that can result from patient education (Rankin & Stallings, 2000). These factors are directly linked to motivation for learning.

Using a learning contract can also be a motivator for learning. Such a contract is based on the assessment of patient needs, health care data, and specific, measurable goals (Redman, 2000). A well-designed learning contract is realistic and positive; it also includes measurable goals, with a specific time frame and reward system for goal achievement. The learning contract is recorded in writing and contains methods for ongoing evaluation.

The value of the contract lies in its clarity, specific delineation of what is to be accomplished, and usefulness for evaluating behavioral change. In a typical learning contract, a series of goals is established, beginning with small, easily attainable objectives and progressing to more advanced goals. Frequent, positive **reinforcement** is provided as the person moves from one goal to the next. An example of incremental goals would be a weight reduction program based on losing 1 to 2 pounds per week rather than one that merely identifies a general goal of losing 30 pounds.

🍃 Gerontologic Considerations

Nonadherence to therapeutic regimens is a significant problem for elderly people, leading to increased morbidity and mortality and increased cost of treatment (U.S. Public Health Service, 2000).

Many nursing home admissions and hospital admissions are linked to nonadherence.

Elderly people frequently have one or more chronic illnesses that are managed with numerous medications and complicated by periodic acute episodes. Elderly people may also have other problems that affect adherence to therapeutic regimens, such as increased sensitivity to medications and their side effects, difficulty in adjusting to change and stress, financial constraints, forgetfulness, inadequate support systems, lifetime habits of self-treatment with over-the-counter medications, visual and hearing impairments, and mobility limitations. To promote adherence among the elderly, time and effort must be taken to assess all variables that may affect health behavior (Fig. 4-1). The nurse must also consider that cognitive deficiencies may be manifested by the elderly person's inability to draw inferences, apply information, or understand the major teaching points (Eliopoulos, 2000). The patient's strengths and limitations must be assessed in order to use existing strengths to compensate for limitations. Above all, health care professionals must work together to provide continuous, coordinated care; otherwise, the efforts of one health care professional may be negated by those of another.

The Nature of Teaching and Learning

Learning can be defined as acquiring knowledge, attitudes, or skills. Teaching is defined as helping another person to learn. These definitions indicate that the teaching–learning process is an active one, requiring the involvement of both teacher and learner in the effort to reach the desired outcome, a change in behavior. The teacher does not simply give knowledge to the learner, but instead serves as a facilitator of learning.

In general, there is no definitive theory about how learning occurs and how it is affected by teaching. However, learning can be affected by factors such as readiness to learn, the learning environment, and the teaching techniques employed (Bastable, 1997; Green & Kreuter, 1999).

LEARNING READINESS

One of the most significant factors influencing learning is the person's learning readiness. For adults, readiness is based on culture, personal values, physical and emotional status, and past experiences

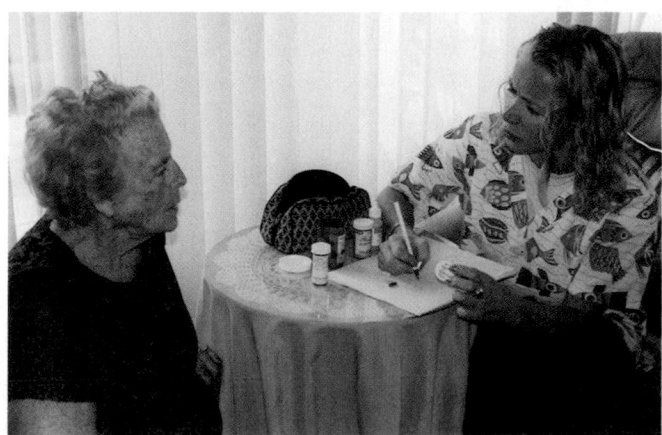

FIGURE 4-1 Taking time to teach patients about their medication and treatment program promotes interest and cooperation. Older adults who are actively involved in learning about their medication and treatment program and the expected effects may be more likely to adhere to the therapeutic regimen.

in learning. The teachable moment for an adult occurs when the content and skills being taught are congruent with the task to be accomplished (Redman, 2000).

Culture encompasses values, ideals, and behaviors, and the traditions within each culture provide the framework for solving the issues and concerns of daily living. Because people with different cultural backgrounds hold different values, lifestyles and choices about health care vary. Culture is a major variable influencing readiness to learn because it affects how a person learns and what information can be learned. Sometimes people will not accept health teaching because it conflicts with culturally mediated values. Before beginning health teaching, the nurse must perform an individual cultural assessment instead of relying only on generalized assumptions about a particular culture. A patient's social and cultural patterns must be appropriately incorporated into the teaching–learning interaction. Chart 4-1 describes cultural assessment components to consider when formulating a teaching plan.

An individual's values include beliefs about what are desirable and undesirable behaviors. The nurse must know what value the patient places on health and health care. In clinical situations, patients express their values through the actions performed and the level of knowledge pursued (Andrews & Boyle, 1998). When the nurse lacks knowledge about the cultural values of the patient being instructed, misunderstanding, lack of cooperation, and negative health outcomes may occur (Leininger, 1991). Each person's values and behaviors can be either an asset or a deficit to the readiness to learn. Therefore, no amount of health education will be accepted by patients unless their values and beliefs about health and illness are respected (Giger & Davidhizar, 1999).

Physical readiness is of vital importance, because until a person is physically capable of learning, attempts at teaching and learning may be both futile and frustrating. For example, someone in acute pain will be unable to focus attention away from the pain long enough to concentrate on learning. Likewise, a person who is short of breath will concentrate on breathing rather than on learning.

Emotional readiness also affects the motivation to learn. A person who has not accepted an existing illness or the threat of illness will not be motivated to learn. People who do not accept a therapeutic regimen, or who view it as conflicting with their present lifestyle, may consciously avoid learning about it. Until a person recognizes the need to learn and demonstrates an ability to learn, teaching efforts may be thwarted. However, it is not always wise to wait for a patient to become emotionally ready to learn, because that time might never come unless efforts are made by the nurse to stimulate the individual's motivation.

Illness and the threat of illness are usually accompanied by anxiety and stress. The nurse who recognizes such reactions can use simple explanations and instructions to alleviate these anxieties and provide further motivation to learn. Because learning involves changes in behavior, it normally produces mild anxiety, which can often be a useful motivating factor.

Emotional readiness can be promoted by creating a warm, accepting, positive atmosphere and by establishing realistic learning goals. When learners achieve success and a feeling of accomplishment, they experience further motivation for participating in additional learning opportunities.

Feedback about progress also motivates learning. Such feedback should be presented in the form of positive reinforcement when learners are successful and in the form of constructive suggestions for improvement when they are unsuccessful.

Experiential readiness refers to past experiences that influence a person's ability to learn. Previous educational experiences and life experiences in general are significant determinants of an individual's approach to learning. A person who has had little or no formal education may not be able to understand the instructional materials presented. A person who has had difficulty learning in the past may be hesitant to try again. Many behaviors required for reaching maximum health potential demand a rather extensive background of knowledge, physical skills, and attitudes. Without this background on which to build, learning may be very difficult and very slow. For example, someone who does not understand the basics of normal nutrition may not be able to understand the restrictions of a specific diet. A person who does not view the desired learning as personally meaningful may reject teaching efforts. A person who is not future-oriented may be unable to appreciate many aspects of preventive health teaching. Experiential readiness is closely related to emotional readiness because motivation tends to be stimulated by an appreciation for the need to learn and by those learning tasks that are familiar, interesting, and meaningful.

Before initiating a teaching–learning program, it is important to assess the learner's physical and emotional readiness to learn, as well as his or her ability to learn what is being taught. This information then becomes the basis for establishing goals that can motivate the person to learn. Involving the learner in the establishment of mutually acceptable goals serves the purpose of encouraging active involvement in the learning process and a willingness to share the responsibility for learning.

THE LEARNING ENVIRONMENT

Although learning can take place without a teacher, most people who are attempting to learn new or altered health behaviors will need the services of a nurse for at least part of the time. The interpersonal interaction between the learner and the nurse who is attempting to meet the individual's learning needs may be formal or informal, depending on the method and techniques of teaching that are found to be most appropriate.

Learning can be optimized by minimizing external variables that interfere with the learning process. For example, the room temperature, lighting, noise levels, and other environmental conditions should be appropriate to the learning situation. Also, the time selected for teaching should be suited to the individual's

---

Chart 4-1

Cultural Assessment Components to Consider When Formulating a Teaching Plan

When formulating a teaching plan, consider the patient's beliefs about

- Body size, shape, boundaries, and functions
- Beauty and strength
- Value of the mind or brain
- Nature and function of blood
- Diet and nutrition
- Communication
- Gender
- Family and social support
- Physical health and illness
- Mental health and illness
- Pain
- Medicine, herbs, and talismans
- Spirituality or religion
- Where a person's essence or soul lies

needs. Scheduling a teaching session at a time of day when the patient is fatigued, uncomfortable, or anxious about a pending diagnostic or therapeutic procedure, or when visitors are present, does not provide an environment conducive to learning. However, if family members are to participate in providing care, the sessions should be timed to take place when the family is present so that they can learn any necessary skills or techniques.

TEACHING TECHNIQUES

Teaching techniques and methods enhance learning if they are appropriate to the individual's needs. Numerous techniques are available, including lectures, group teaching, and demonstrations, all of which can be enhanced with specially prepared teaching materials. The lecture or explanation method of teaching is commonly used but should always be accompanied by discussion. Discussion is important because it affords the learner an opportunity to express feelings and concerns, to ask questions, and to receive clarification.

Group teaching is appropriate for some people because it allows them not only to receive needed information, but also to feel secure as members of a group. Those with similar problems or learning needs have the opportunity to identify with each other and gain moral support and encouragement. However, not everyone relates or learns well in groups, and some people may not benefit from such experiences. Also, if group teaching is used, assessment and follow-up of each individual are imperative to ensure that each has gained sufficient knowledge and skills.

Demonstration and practice are essential ingredients of a teaching program, especially when teaching skills. It is best to demonstrate the skill and then allow the learner ample opportunity for practice. When special equipment is involved, such as syringes for injections, colostomy bags, dialysis equipment, dressings, or suction apparatus, it is important to teach with the same equipment that will be used in the home setting. Learning to perform a skill with one kind of equipment and then having to change to a different kind may lead to confusion, frustration, and mistakes.

Teaching aids that are available to enhance learning include books, pamphlets, pictures, films, slides, audio and video tapes, models, programmed instruction, and computer-assisted learning modules. Such teaching aids are invaluable when used appropriately and can save a significant amount of personnel time and related cost. However, all such aids should be reviewed before use to ensure that they meet the individual's learning needs. Human interaction and discussion cannot be replaced by teaching technologies but may be enhanced by them (Nursing Research Profile 4-1).

Reinforcement and follow-up are important because learning takes time. Allowing ample time to learn and reinforcing what is learned are important teaching strategies; a single teaching session is rarely adequate. Follow-up sessions are imperative to promote learners' confidence in their abilities and to plan for additional teaching sessions. For hospitalized patients who may not be able to transfer what they have learned in the hospital to the home setting, follow-up after discharge is essential to ensure that they have realized the full benefits of a teaching program.

TEACHING PEOPLE WITH DISABILITIES

When providing health information to people who are affected by disabilities, the individual needs of the person must be assessed and incorporated into the teaching plan; teaching techniques and

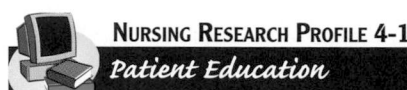

NURSING RESEARCH PROFILE 4-1
Patient Education

Mahon, S. M., & Williams, M. (2000). Information needs regarding menopause. *Cancer Nursing, 23*(3), 176–185.

Purpose
There were two main purposes for conducting this study. The first purpose was to evaluate the relevance and usefulness of a brochure designed to facilitate understanding about menopause and other related female health concerns. The second purpose was to describe the information needs of healthy women at menopause.

Study and Sample Design
The study design was descriptive-correlational and utilized a questionnaire designed by the researchers. Two hundred questionnaires were distributed, and 161 women (ages 26 to 69 years) completed the survey. This convenience sample consisted of women who came to a nurse-managed cancer screening center. These women saw the brochure on display at the center; if they asked for a copy, they were also given a questionnaire to complete and return.

Findings
The participants indicated that they were premenopausal (45%), postmenopausal (40%), or uncertain of menopausal status (15%). Ninety-nine percent of the women said that the brochure was very easy to read and understand. Eighty percent found the information very relevant and important, while 31% found it somewhat relevant and important. Eighty-eight percent thought that the material in the brochure would motivate them to talk with their health care provider, and 10% did not know if it would. The topics most likely to be discussed with a health care provider were hormone replacement therapy, bone mineral density testing, risk and prevention of osteoporosis, and management of menopause.

Nursing Implications
Written educational materials are useful strategies for providing health information. Women want and will seek out information regarding menopause, particularly information that helps them to make menopause management decisions. Nurses need to obtain detailed and accurate health histories from women in order to assist them to determine their menopausal status and other individual health needs.

the imparting of information may need to be altered to accommodate them. Specific groups of people with physical disabilities, emotional disabilities, hearing and visual impairments, learning disabilities, and developmental disabilities require that the nurse be aware of their **health promotion** needs and institute new or modified approaches to teach them about their health. Table 4-1 outlines some of the teaching strategies to use when teaching a person with a disability.

GERONTOLOGIC CONSIDERATIONS

Nurses caring for elderly people must be aware of how the normal changes that occur with aging affect learning abilities and how an elderly person can be assisted to adjust to these changes. Above all, it is important to recognize that just because a person is elderly does not mean that he or she cannot learn. Studies have shown that older adults can learn and remember if information is paced appropriately, is relevant, and is followed by appropriate feedback strategies that apply to all learners (Rankin & Stallings, 2000). Because changes associated with aging vary

TYPE OF DISABILITY	TEACHING STRATEGY
Physical or Emotional Disability	Adapt information to accommodate the person's cognitive, perceptual, and behavior disabilities. Give clear written and oral information. Highlight significant information for easy reference. Avoid medical terminology.
Hearing Impairment	Use slow, directed, deliberate speech. Use sign language if appropriate. Position yourself so that the person can see your mouth if lip reading. Use telecommunication devices for the hearing impaired (TDD). Use written materials and visual aids, such as models and diagrams. Use captioned videos and films. Teach on the side of the "good ear" if unilateral deafness is present.
Visual Impairment	Use optical devices such as a magnifying lens. Use proper lighting and proper contrast of colors on materials and equipment. Use large-print materials. Use Braille materials if appropriate. Convert information to auditory and tactile formats. Obtain audiotapes and talking books. Explain noises associated with procedures, equipment, and treatments. Arrange materials in clockwise pattern.
Learning Disabilities Input disability	If visual perceptual disorder: • Explain information verbally, repeat, and reinforce frequently. • Use audiotapes. • Encourage learner to verbalize information received. If auditory perceptual disorder: • Speak slowly with as few words as possible, repeat, and reinforce frequently. • Use direct eye contact to focus person on task. • Use demonstration and return demonstration such as modeling, role playing, and hands-on experiences. • Use visual tools, written materials, and computers.
Output disability	Use all senses as appropriate. Use written, audiotape, and computer information. Review information and give time to interact and ask questions. Use hand gestures and motions.
Developmental disability	Base information and teaching on developmental stage, not person's age. Use nonverbal cues, gestures, signing, and symbols as needed. Use simple explanations and concrete examples with repetition. Encourage active participation. Demonstrate information and have the person perform return demonstrations.

Table 4-1 • **Teaching People with Disabilities**

significantly among elderly people, the nurse should conduct a thorough assessment of each person's level of physiologic and psychological functioning before teaching begins.

Changes in cognition with age may include slowed mental functioning; decreased short-term memory, abstract thinking, and concentration; and slowed reaction time. These changes are often accentuated by the health problems that cause the elderly to seek health care in the first place. Effective teaching strategies include a slow-paced presentation of small amounts of material at a time, frequent repetition of information, and the use of reinforcement techniques, such as audiovisual and written materials and repeated practice sessions. Distracting stimuli should be minimized as much as possible in the teaching environment.

Sensory changes associated with aging also affect teaching and learning. Teaching strategies to accommodate decreased visual acuity include large-print and easy-to-read materials printed on non-glare paper. Because color discrimination is often impaired, the use of color-coded or highlighted teaching materials may not be effective. To maximize hearing, the teacher must speak distinctly with a normal or lowered pitch, facing the person so that lip reading can occur as needed. Visual cues often help to reinforce verbal teaching.

Family members should be involved in teaching sessions when possible. They provide another source for reinforcement of material and can help the learner to recall instructions later. They can also provide valuable assessment information about the person's living situation and related learning needs.

When the nurse, the family, and other involved health care professionals work collaboratively to facilitate an elderly person's learning, the chances of success will be maximized. Successful learning for the elderly should result in improved self-care management skills, enhanced self-esteem, and a willingness to learn in future sessions.

The Nursing Process in Patient Teaching

The steps of the nursing process—assessment, diagnosis, planning, implementation, and evaluation—are used when constructing a teaching plan to meet an individual's teaching and learning needs (Chart 4-2).

ASSESSMENT

Assessment in the teaching–learning process is directed toward the systematic collection of data about the person's learning needs, the person's readiness to learn, and the family's learning needs. All internal and external variables that affect the patient's readiness to learn are identified. A learning assessment guide may be used for this purpose. Some of the available guides are very general and are directed toward the collection of general health information, whereas others are specific to common medication regimens or disease processes. Such guides facilitate the assessment but must be adapted to the individual's responses, problems, and needs.

As soon as possible after completing the assessment, the nurse organizes, analyzes, synthesizes, and summarizes the data collected and determines the patient's need for teaching.

NURSING DIAGNOSIS

Formulating nursing diagnoses makes educational goals and evaluations of progress more specific and meaningful. Teaching is an integral intervention implied by all nursing diagnoses, and for some diagnoses education is the primary intervention. Ineffective therapeutic regimen management, Impaired home maintenance, Health-seeking behaviors, and Decisional conflict are examples of nursing diagnoses that direct planning for educational needs. The diagnosis "Deficient knowledge" should be used cautiously, because knowledge deficit is not a human response but a factor relating to or causing the diagnosis (eg, Ineffective therapeutic regimen management related to a deficiency of information about wound care is a more appropriate nursing diagnosis than "Deficient knowledge") (Carpenito, 1999). A nursing diagnosis that relates specifically to the patient's and family's learning needs will serve as a guide in the development of the teaching plan.

PLANNING

Once the nursing diagnoses have been identified, the planning component of the teaching–learning process is established in accordance with the steps of the nursing process:

1. Assigning priorities to the diagnoses
2. Specifying the immediate, intermediate, and long-term goals of learning
3. Identifying specific teaching strategies appropriate for attaining goals

---

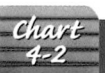

Chart 4-2 **A Guide to Patient Education**

Assessment
1. Assess the person's readiness for health education.
   a. What are the person's health beliefs and behaviors?
   b. What physical and psychosocial adaptations does the person need to make?
   c. Is the learner ready to learn?
   d. Is the person able to learn these behaviors?
   e. What additional information about the person is needed?
   f. Are there any variables (eg, hearing or visual impairment, cognitive issues, literacy issues) that will affect the choice of teaching strategy or approach?
   g. What are the person's expectations?
   h. What does the person want to learn?
2. Organize, analyze, synthesize, and summarize the collected data.

Nursing Diagnosis
1. Formulate the nursing diagnoses that relate to the person's learning needs.
2. Identify the learning needs, their characteristics, and their etiology.
3. State nursing diagnoses concisely and precisely.

Planning and Goals
1. Assign priority to the nursing diagnoses that relate to the individual's learning needs.
2. Specify the immediate, intermediate, and long-term learning goals established by teacher and learner together.
3. Identify teaching strategies appropriate for goal attainment.
4. Establish expected outcomes.
5. Develop the written teaching plan.
   a. Include diagnoses, goals, teaching strategies, and expected outcomes.
   b. Put the information to be taught in logical sequence.
   c. Write down the key points.

d. Select appropriate teaching aids.
e. Keep the plan current and flexible to meet the person's changing learning needs.
6. Involve the learner, family or significant others, nursing team members, and other health care team members in all aspects of planning.

Implementation
1. Put the teaching plan into action.
2. Use language the person can understand.
3. Use appropriate teaching aids and provide Internet resources if appropriate.
4. Use the same equipment that the person will use after discharge.
5. Encourage the person to participate actively in learning.
6. Record the learner's responses to the teaching actions.
7. Provide feedback.

Evaluation
1. Collect objective data.
   a. Observe the person.
   b. Ask questions to determine whether the person understands.
   c. Use rating scales, checklists, anecdotal notes, and written tests when appropriate.
2. Compare the person's behavioral responses with the expected outcomes. Determine the extent to which the goals were achieved.
3. Include the person, family or significant others, nursing team members, and other health care team members in the evaluation.
4. Identify alterations that need to be made in the teaching plan.
5. Make referrals to appropriate sources or agencies for reinforcement of learning after discharge.
6. Continue all steps of the teaching process: assessment, diagnosis, planning, implementation, and evaluation.

4. Specifying the expected outcomes
5. Documenting the diagnoses, goals, teaching strategies, and expected outcomes on the teaching plan

As in the nursing process, the assignment of priorities to the diagnoses should be a joint effort by the nurse and the learner or family members. Consideration must be given to the urgency of the individual's learning needs, with the most critical needs receiving the highest priority.

After the priorities of the diagnoses have been established, the immediate and long-term goals and the teaching strategies appropriate for attaining the goals are identified. Teaching is most effective when the objectives of both the learner and the nurse are in agreement (Lorig, et al., 1996). Learning begins with the establishment of goals that are appropriate to the situation and realistic in terms of the individual's ability and desire to achieve them. Involving the patient and family in establishing goals and subsequently in the planning of teaching strategies promotes their cooperation in the implementation of the teaching plan.

Expected outcomes of teaching strategies can be stated in terms of behaviors of the person, the family, or both. Outcomes should be realistic and measurable, and the critical time periods for attaining them should also be identified. The desired outcomes and the critical time periods will serve as a basis for evaluating the effectiveness of the teaching strategies.

During the planning phase, the nurse must consider the sequence in which the subject matter will be presented in each of the teaching strategies. Critical information (eg, survival skills for the person with diabetes) and material that the person or family identifies to be of particular importance receive high priority. An outline is often helpful for arranging the subject matter and for ensuring that all necessary information is included. Also during this time, appropriate teaching aids to be used in implementing the teaching strategies are prepared or selected.

The entire planning phase of the teaching–learning process is concluded with the formulation of the teaching plan. This teaching plan communicates the following information to all members of the nursing team:

1. The nursing diagnoses that specifically relate to the individual's learning needs and the priorities of these diagnoses
2. The goals of the teaching strategies
3. The teaching strategies, expressed in the form of teaching orders
4. The expected outcomes, which identify the desired behavioral responses of the learner
5. The critical time period within which each outcome is expected to be met
6. The individual's behavioral responses (which must be documented on the teaching plan)

The same rules that apply to writing and revising the plan of nursing care apply to the teaching plan.

IMPLEMENTATION

In the implementation phase of the teaching–learning process, the patient, the family, and other members of the nursing and health care teams carry out the activities outlined in the teaching plan. The nurse coordinates all the activities.

Flexibility during the implementation phase of the teaching–learning process and ongoing assessment of the individual's responses to the teaching strategies support modification of the teaching plan as necessary. Creativity in promoting and sustaining the learner's motivation to learn is essential. New learning needs that may arise after discharge from the hospital or after home care visits have ended should also be taken into account.

The implementation phase is concluded when the teaching strategies have been completed and when the individual's responses to the actions have been recorded. This record serves as the basis for evaluating how well the defined goals and expected outcomes have been achieved.

EVALUATION

Evaluation of the teaching–learning process determines how effectively the person has responded to the teaching strategies and to what extent the goals have been achieved. An important part of the evaluation phase addresses the question, "What can be done to improve the teaching and enhance the learning?" Answers to this question will direct the changes to be made in the teaching plan.

An evaluation must be made of what was done well, and what needs to be changed or reinforced. It cannot be assumed that individuals have learned just because teaching has occurred: learning does not automatically follow teaching. A variety of measurement techniques can be used to identify changes in behavior as evidence that learning has taken place. These techniques include directly observing the behavior; using rating scales, checklists, or anecdotal notes to document the behavior; and indirectly measuring results through oral questioning and written tests. Measurement of actual behavior (direct measurement) is the most accurate and appropriate technique in many patient teaching situations. Nurses often do comparative analysis using patient admission data as the baseline: selected data points observed during the period when nursing care is given and self-care was initiated are compared with the patient's baseline data.

Some examples of indirect measurements are patient satisfaction surveys, attitude surveys, and instruments that evaluate specific health status variables. All direct measurements should be supplemented with indirect measurements whenever possible. Using more than one measuring technique enhances the reliability of the resulting data and decreases the potential for error from a specific measurement strategy.

Measuring is only the beginning of evaluation. It must be followed by interpreting the data and making value judgments about the learning and teaching. Such evaluation should be conducted periodically throughout the teaching–learning program, at its conclusion, and at varying periods after the teaching has ended.

Evaluation of learning after hospitalization is highly desirable, because the analysis of teaching outcomes must extend into home care. With shortened lengths of hospital stay and with short-stay and same-day surgical procedures, follow-up evaluation in the home is especially important. Coordination of efforts and sharing of information between hospital-based and community-based nursing personnel facilitates post-discharge teaching and home care evaluation.

Evaluation is not the end step in the teaching–learning process, but the beginning of a new patient assessment. The information gathered during evaluation should be used to redirect teaching actions, with the goal of improving the learner's responses and outcomes.

Health Promotion

Health teaching and health promotion are linked by a common goal—to encourage people to achieve as high a level of wellness as possible so that they can live maximally healthy lives and avoid preventable illnesses. The call for health promotion has become a cornerstone in health policy because of the need to control costs and reduce unnecessary sickness and death.

The nation's first public health agenda was established in 1979 and set goals for improving the health of all Americans. Additional goals defined as the "1990 Health Objectives" identified improvements to be made in health status, risk reduction, public awareness, health services, and protective measures (U.S. Public Health Service, 1990).

Health goals for the nation were also established in the publication, *Healthy People 2000.* The priorities from this initiative were identified as health promotion, health protection, and the use of preventive services. The most recent publication, *Healthy People 2010,* defines the current national health promotion and disease prevention initiative for the nation. The two essential goals from this report are (1) to increase the quality and years of healthy life for people, and (2) to eliminate health disparities among various segments of the population (U.S. Public Health Service, 2000) (Chart 4-3).

HEALTH AND WELLNESS

The concept of health promotion has evolved because of a changing definition of health and an awareness that wellness exists at many levels of functioning. The definition of health as the mere absence of disease is no longer accepted. Today, health is viewed as a dynamic, ever-changing condition that enables a person to function at an optimum potential at any given time. The ideal health status is one in which people are successful in achieving their full potential regardless of any limitations they might have.

Wellness, as a reflection of health, involves a conscious and deliberate attempt to maximize one's health. Wellness does not just happen; it requires planning and conscious commitment and is the result of adopting lifestyle behaviors for the purpose of attaining one's highest potential for well-being. Wellness is not the same for every person. The person with a chronic illness or disability may still be able to achieve a desirable level of wellness. The key to wellness is to function at the highest potential within the limitations over which there is no control.

A significant amount of information has shown that people, by virtue of what they do or fail to do, influence their own health. Today, many of the major causes of illness are chronic diseases that have been closely related to lifestyle behaviors (eg, heart disease, lung and colon cancer, chronic obstructive pulmonary diseases,

hypertension, cirrhosis, traumatic injury, HIV [human immunodeficiency virus] infection, and acquired immunodeficiency syndrome [AIDS]). Consequently, a person's health status to a large extent is reflective of lifestyle.

HEALTH PROMOTION MODELS

Since the 1950s, many health-promotion models have been constructed to identify health-protecting behaviors and to help explain what makes people engage in these preventive behaviors. A health-protecting behavior is defined as any behavior performed by people, regardless of their actual or perceived health condition, for the purpose of promoting or maintaining their health, whether or not the behavior produces the desired outcome (Downie, Fyfe, & Tannahill, 1990). One framework, the health belief model, was devised to foster understanding of what made some healthy people choose actions to prevent illness while others refused to engage in these protective recommendations (Becker, 1974).

Another model, the resource model of preventive health behavior (Downie, Fyfe, & Tannahill, 1990), addresses the ways that people use resources to promote health. Nurse educators can use this model to assess how demographic variables, health behaviors, and social and health resources influence health promotion. LaLonde's (1977) health determinants model views human biology, environment, lifestyle, and the health care delivery system as the four determinants of a person's health.

A model for promotion of health, designed by Becker and colleagues (1993), is based on the premise that four variables influence the selection and use of health promotion behaviors. The first variable, demographic and disease factors, includes client characteristics such as age, gender, education, employment, severity of illness or disability, and length of illness. Barriers, the next component, are defined as factors that lead to unavailability or difficulty in gaining access to a specific health promotion alternative. The third variable, resources, encompasses such items as financial and social support. The last variable, perceptual factors, consists of how people view their health status, self-efficacy, and the perceived demands of their illness. The developers of this model conducted research to substantiate that these four variables have a positive correlation with a person's quality of life.

The health promotion model developed by Pender (1996), is based on social learning theory and emphasizes the importance of motivational factors that influence the acquiring and sustaining of health-promotion behaviors. This model explores how cognitive-perceptual factors affect one's view of the importance of health. It also examines perceived control of health, self-efficacy, health status, and the benefits and barriers to health promoting behaviors.

These models, along with other examples that can be found in the health promotion literature, can serve as an organizing framework for clinical work and research that supports the enhancement of health. Further efforts, however, are needed to advance understanding of the health promotion behaviors of families and communities.

DEFINITION OF HEALTH PROMOTION

Health promotion can be defined as those activities that assist individuals in developing resources that will maintain or enhance well-being and improve their quality of life. These activities involve a person's efforts to remain healthy in the absence of symptoms and do not require the assistance of a health care team member.

Chart 4-3

Leading Health Indicators to be Used to Measure the Health of the Nation

1. Physical activity
2. Overweight and obesity
3. Tobacco use
4. Substance abuse
5. Responsible sexual behavior
6. Mental health
7. Injury and violence
8. Environmental quality
9. Immunization
10. Access to health care

From U.S. Department of Health & Human Services (2000). *Healthy people 2010.* Washington, DC: U.S. Government Printing Office.

The purpose of health promotion is to focus on a person's potential for wellness and to encourage appropriate alterations in personal habits, lifestyle, and environment in ways that will reduce risks and enhance health and well-being. Health promotion is an active process; that is, it is not something that can be prescribed or dictated. It is up to the individual to decide whether to make the changes that will promote a higher level of wellness. Choices must be made, and only the individual can make these choices.

The concepts of health, wellness, health promotion, and disease prevention have been extensively addressed in the lay literature and news media as well as in professional journals. The result has been a public demand for health information and a response by health care professionals and agencies to provide this information. Health-promotion programs that were once limited to hospital settings have now moved into community settings such as clinics, schools, churches, businesses, and industry. The workplace is quickly becoming an important site for health promotion programs, as employers strive to reduce costs associated with absenteeism, health insurance, hospitalization, disability, excessive turnover of personnel, and premature death.

HEALTH PROMOTION PRINCIPLES

Certain principles underlie the concept of health promotion as an active process: self-responsibility, nutritional awareness, stress reduction and management, and physical fitness.

Self-Responsibility

Taking responsibility for oneself is the key to successful health promotion. The concept of **self-responsibility** is based on the understanding that individuals control their lives. Each of us alone must make those choices that determine how healthy our lifestyle is. As more people recognize the significant effects that lifestyle and behavior have on health, they may assume responsibility for avoiding high-risk behaviors such as smoking, alcohol and drug abuse, overeating, driving while intoxicated, risky sexual practices, and other unhealthy habits. They may also assume responsibility for adopting routines that have been found to have a positive influence on health, such as engaging in regular exercise, wearing a seat belt, and eating a balanced diet.

A variety of different techniques have been used to encourage people to accept responsibility for their health, ranging from extensive educational programs to reward systems. No one technique has been found to be superior to any other. Instead, self-responsibility for health promotion is very individualized and depends on a person's desires and inner motivations. Health promotion programs are important tools for encouraging people to assume responsibility for their health and to develop behaviors that improve health.

Nutrition

Nutrition as a component of health promotion has become the focus of considerable attention and publicity. A vast array of books and magazine articles address the topics of special diets, natural foods, and the hazards of certain substances, such as sugar, salt, cholesterol, artificial colors, and food additives. Good nutrition has been suggested as the single most significant factor in determining health status and longevity.

Nutritional awareness involves an understanding of the importance of a properly balanced diet that supplies all of the essential nutrients. Understanding the relationship between diet and disease is an important facet of a person's self-care. Some clinicians believe that a healthy diet is one that substitutes "natural" foods for processed and refined ones and reduces the intake of sugar, salt, fat, cholesterol, caffeine, alcohol, food additives, and preservatives.

Chapter 5 contains detailed information about the assessment of an individual's nutritional status. The chapter covers physical signs indicating nutritional status, assessment of food intake (food record, 24-hour recall), comparison of food intake with the dietary guidelines outlined in the Food Guide Pyramid, and calculation of ideal body weight.

Stress Management

Stress management and stress reduction are important aspects of health promotion. Studies have shown the negative effects of stress on health and a cause-and-effect relationship between stress and infectious diseases, traumatic injuries (eg, motor vehicle crashes), and some chronic illnesses. Stress has become inevitable in contemporary societies in which demands for productivity have become excessive. More and more emphasis is placed on encouraging people to manage stress appropriately and to reduce stress that is counterproductive. Techniques such as relaxation training, exercise, and modification of stressful situations are often included in health promotion programs that deal with stress. Further information on stress management, including health risk appraisal and stress reduction methods such as biofeedback and the relaxation response, can be found in Chapter 6.

Exercise

Physical fitness is another important component of health promotion. Clinicians and researchers (Anspaugh, Hamrick & Rosata, 1994; Edelman & Mandle, 1998; U.S. Department of Health & Human Services, 1996) examining the relationship between health and physical fitness have found that a regular exercise program can promote health by improving the function of the circulatory system and the lungs, decreasing cholesterol and low-density lipoprotein concentrations, lowering body weight by increasing calorie expenditure, delaying degenerative changes such as osteoporosis, and improving flexibility and overall muscle strength and endurance. On the other hand, exercise can be harmful if it is not started gradually and increased slowly in accordance with the individual's response. An exercise program should be designed specifically for the individual, with consideration given to age, physical condition, and any known cardiovascular or other risk factors. An appropriate exercise program can have a significantly positive effect on the individual's performance capacity, appearance, and general state of physical and emotional health (Nursing Research Profile 4-2).

Health Promotion Throughout the Life Span

Health promotion is a concept and a process that extends throughout the life span. Studies have shown that the health of a child can be affected either positively or negatively by the health practices of the mother during the prenatal period. Therefore, health promotion starts before birth and extends through childhood, adulthood, and old age.

Health promotion includes health screening. The American Academy of Family Physicians has developed recommendations for periodic health examinations that identify the age

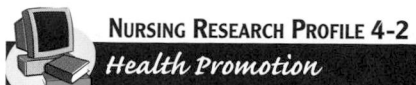

NURSING RESEARCH PROFILE 4-2

Health Promotion

Wall, L. (2000). Changes in hope and power in lung cancer patients who exercise. *Nursing Science Quarterly, 13*(3), 234–242.

Purpose

Cancer is often viewed as a life-threatening disease for which there is little hope for the future and relatively little ability to create change. The purposes of this study were to explore changes in hope and power among lung cancer patients who participated in a preoperative exercise program and to examine hope and power over time.

Sample and Study Design

A sample of 104 preoperative lung cancer patients with a clinical diagnosis of stage IA, IB, IIA, IIB, or IIIA non–small cell carcinoma was recruited for the study. The participants were randomly assigned to the exercise or nonexercise group. To assess for changes in hope and power, the subjects were asked to complete questionnaires on hope (Health Hope Index) and power (Power as Knowing Participation in Change Test) at the time of diagnosis, on the day before surgery, and 4 to 6 days after surgery. The exercise group was instructed about the exercise by the investigator after completion of the first set of questionnaires. The exercise group performed the exercises daily before surgery and recorded their compliance in a journal. The nonexercise group received usual preoperative care that did not include a prescribed exercise program.

Findings

There were no statistically significant relationships between hope or power and the number of days of exercise completed. Both groups had high levels of hope and positive expectations for the future. There were differences in power (defined as the capacity to knowingly participate in change) between the two groups, with power increased in the exercise group compared with the nonexercise group.

Nursing Implications

It is useful for the nurse to understand how patients can effectively participate in change and promote strategies that enhance well-being. By encouraging preoperative exercise, nurses can help patients purposefully participate in change, make decisions about their care, and determine factors that enhance and impede them from taking steps to actively participate in their care.

groups for which specific screening interventions are appropriate. Table 4-2 presents the general population guidelines; specific population standards and guidelines have also been recommended.

CHILDREN AND ADOLESCENTS

Health screening has traditionally been an important aspect of childhood health care. The goal has been to detect health problems at an early age so that they can be treated early in a child's life. Today, health promotion goes beyond the mere screening of children for disabilities and includes extensive efforts to promote positive health practices at a very young age. Because health habits and practices are formed early in life, children should be encouraged to develop positive health attitudes. For this reason, more and more programs are being offered to school-age children and to adolescents to help them develop good health habits. Although the negative results of practices such as smoking, risky sexual activities, alcohol and drug abuse, and poor nutrition are explained in these educational programs, emphasis is also placed on values training, self-esteem, and healthy lifestyle practices. The projects are designed to appeal to

a particular age group, with emphasis on learning experiences that are fun, interesting, and relevant.

YOUNG AND MIDDLE-AGED ADULTS

Young and middle-aged adults represent an age group that not only expresses an interest in health and health promotion but also responds enthusiastically to suggestions that show how lifestyle practices can improve health. Adults are frequently motivated to change their lifestyles in ways that are believed to enhance their health and wellness. Many adults who wish to improve their health turn to health-promotion programs to help them make the desired changes in their lifestyles. They respond in overwhelming numbers to programs that focus on topics such as general wellness, smoking cessation, exercise, physical conditioning, weight control, conflict resolution, and stress management. Because of the nationwide emphasis on health during the reproductive years, young adults actively seek programs that address prenatal health, parenting, family planning, and women's health issues.

Programs that provide health screening, such as those that screen for cancer, high cholesterol, hypertension, diabetes, and hearing impairments, are quite popular with this age group. Programs that cover health promotion for people with specific chronic illnesses such as cancer, diabetes, heart disease, and pulmonary disease are also popular. It is becoming more evident that chronic disease and disability do not preclude health and wellness; rather, positive health attitudes and practices can promote optimal health for people who must live with the limitations imposed by their chronic illnesses and disabilities.

Health-promotion programs can be offered almost anywhere in the community. Common sites include local clinics, elementary schools, high schools, community colleges, recreation centers, churches, and even private homes. Health fairs are frequently held in civic centers and shopping malls. The outreach idea for health-promotion programs has served to meet the needs of many adults who otherwise would not avail themselves of opportunities to strive toward a healthier lifestyle.

The workplace has become a center for health-promotion activity as employers become increasingly concerned about the rising costs of health care insurance to treat illnesses that are related to lifestyle behaviors. They are also concerned about increased absenteeism and lost productivity. For these reasons, many businesses have instituted health-promotion programs in the workplace. Some employ health-promotion specialists to develop and implement the program, and others purchase packaged programs that have already been developed by health care agencies or private health-promotion corporations.

Programs offered at the workplace usually include employee health screening and counseling, physical fitness, nutritional awareness, work safety, and stress management and stress reduction. In addition, efforts are made to promote a safe and healthy work environment. Many large businesses provide exercise facilities for their employees and offer their health-promotion programs to retirees. If employers can show cost-containment benefits from such programs, their dollars will be considered well spent, and more businesses will provide health-promotion programs as a benefit of employment.

ELDERLY ADULTS

Health promotion is as important for the elderly as it is for other age groups. Despite the fact that 80% of people older than 65 years of age have one or more chronic illnesses and about

Table 4-2 • Routine Health Promotion Screening for Adults*	
TYPE OF SCREENING	SUGGESTED TIME FRAME
Routine health examination	Yearly
Blood chemistry profile	Baseline at age 20, then as mutually determined by patient and clinician
Complete blood count	Baseline at age 20, then as mutually determined by patient and clinician
Lipid profile	Baseline at age 20, then as mutually determined by patient and clinician
Hemoccult screening	Yearly after age 50
Electrocardiogram	Baseline at age 40, then as mutually determined by patient and clinician
Blood pressure	Yearly, then as mutually determined by patient and clinician
Tuberculosis skin test	Every 2 years or as mutually determined by patient and clinician
Chest x-ray film	For positive PPD results
Breast self-examination	Monthly
Mammogram	Yearly for women over 40, or earlier or more often if indicated
Clinical breast examination	Yearly
Gynecologic examination	Yearly
Pap test	Yearly
Bone density screening	Based on identification of primary and secondary risk factors (prior to onset of menopause, if indicated)
Nutritional screening	As mutually determined by patient and clinician
Digital rectal examination	Yearly
Sigmoidoscopy	Every 3–5 years after age 50 or as mutually determined by patient and clinician
Prostate examination	Yearly
Prostate-specific antigen	Every 1–2 years after age 50
Testicular examination	Monthly
Skin examination	Yearly or as mutually determined by patient and clinician
Vision screening	Every 2–3 years
Glaucoma	Baseline at age 40, then every 2–3 years until age 70, then yearly
Dental screening	Every 6 months
Hearing screening	As needed
Health risk appraisal	As needed
Adult Immunizations	
Tetanus	Boosters every 10 years
Diphtheria	Boosters every 10 years
Rubella	Given to women of childbearing age if not previously given or if titer is low
Pneumococcal vaccine	Given one time at age 65 or younger if chronic illness or disability is present
Hepatitis B (if not received as a child)	Series of three doses (now, 1 month later, then 5 months after the second date)
Influenza vaccine	Yearly
Lyme disease vaccine, if at risk	Series of three doses (now, 1 month later, and 11 months after the second dose)

*Note: Any of these screenings may be performed more frequently if deemed necessary by the patient or recommended by the health care provider.

50% are limited in their activity, the elderly as a group experience significant gains from health promotion. Clinical work indicates that the elderly are very health-conscious and that most view their health positively and are willing to adopt practices that will improve their health and well-being (Ebersole & Hess, 1997; Staab & Hodges, 1996). Although their chronic illnesses and disabilities cannot be eliminated, these adults can benefit from activities that help them maintain independence and achieve an optimal level of health.

Various health-promotion programs have been developed to meet the needs of older Americans, many of which began within the Department of Health and Human Services. Both public and private organizations continue to be responsive to health promotion, and more programs that serve the elderly are emerging. Many of these programs are offered by health care agencies, churches, community centers, senior citizen residences, and a variety of other organizations. The activities directed toward health promotion for the elderly are the same as those for other age groups: physical fitness and exercise, nutrition, safety, and stress management.

Implications for Nursing

Nurses, by virtue of their expertise in health and health care and their long-established credibility with consumers, play a vital role in health promotion. In many instances they have initiated health-promotion programs or have participated with other health care personnel in developing and providing wellness services in a variety of settings (Fig. 4-2).

As health care professionals, nurses have a responsibility to promote activities that foster well-being, self-actualization, and personal fulfillment. Every interaction with consumers of health care must be viewed as an opportunity to promote positive health attitudes and behaviors.

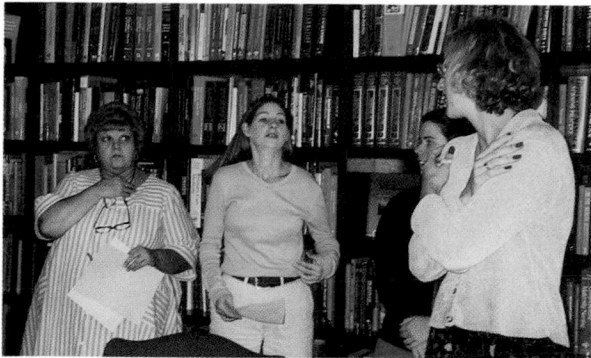

FIGURE 4-2 Teaching aids and demonstrations enhance learning. Here a nurse (*right*) instructs learners during a community health education program. Often generated and developed by nurses, these programs offer the public opportunities to obtain health information about topics ranging from diet, nutrition, and hypercholesterolemia to hypertension, diabetes, cardiopulmonary resuscitation, and others.

 Critical Thinking Exercises

1. You are constructing a patient teaching plan for a mid-life woman who has a diagnosis of multiple sclerosis and is at high risk for development of osteoporosis. Describe the health promotion strategies you would develop for this patient. Indicate the possible variables that could influence the patient's willingness or ability to follow the instructions.

2. You are assigned to teach an elderly patient about the cardiac and diabetic medications that she will be taking at home. How would you assess this patient's condition and psychosocial situation to determine how best to instruct her about her medications? How would you modify your teaching plan if the patient was hard of hearing, visually impaired, or unable to read or write?

3. A neighbor tells you that he has heard about a health fair that is being offered at a nearby civic center. He asks you if you think that he should attend. Describe the reasons you might give for why the neighbor should attend the health fair. He also states that his wife does not need to attend because she is receiving medical care for her arthritis and diabetes. What advice would you offer him about his wife's attending the health fair?

REFERENCES AND SELECTED READINGS

Books

American Nurses Association. (1998). *Standards of clinical nursing practice.* Washington DC: Author.

Andrews, M. M., & Boyle, J. S. (1998). *Transcultural concepts in nursing care* (3rd ed.). Philadelphia: Lippincott Williams & Wilkins.

Anspaugh D. J., Hamrick, M. H., & Rosato, F. D. (1994). *Wellness: Concepts and applications* (2nd ed.). St. Louis: Mosby.

Bastable, S. G. (Ed.). (1997). *Nurse as educator: Principles of teaching and learning.* Boston: Jones & Bartlett.

Becker, M. H. (Ed.). (1974). *The health belief model and personal health behavior.* Thorofare, NJ: Charles B. Slack.

Carpenito, L. J. (1999). *Nursing diagnosis: Application to clinical practice.* Philadelphia: Lippincott Williams & Wilkins.

Downie, R. S., Fyfe, C., & Tannahill, A. (1990). *Health promotion: Models and values.* New York: Oxford University Press.

Doyle, E., & Ward, S. (2001). *The process of community health education and promotion.* Palo Alto, CA: Mayfield Publishing.

Ebersole, P., & Hess, P. (1997). *Toward health aging: Human needs and nursing responses* (5th ed.). Philadelphia: Lippincott-Raven.

Edelman, C., & Mandle, C. L. (1998). *Health promotion throughout the lifespan* (4th ed.). St. Louis: C. V. Mosby.

Eliopoulos, C. (2000). *Gerontological nursing* (5th ed.). Philadelphia: Lippincott Williams & Wilkins.

Giger, J. N., & Davidhizar, R. E. (1999). *Transcultural nursing: Assessment and intervention* (3rd ed.). St. Louis: C. V. Mosby.

Green, L. W., & Kreuter, M. (1999). *Health promotion planning.* Palo Alto, CA: Mayfield Publishing.

Insel, P. M., & Roth, W. T. (2000). *Core concepts in health.* Palo Alto, CA: Mayfield Publishing.

Kreuter, T. L., Farrell, D., Olevitch, L., Brennan, L., & Rimer, B. K. (2000). *Tailoring health messages: Customizing communication with computer technology.* Mahwah, NJ: Lawrence Erlbaum Associates.

LaLonde, M. (1977). *New perspectives on the health of Canadians: A working document.* Ottawa, Canada: Minister of Supply and Services.

Leininger, M. M. (1991). *Culture care diversity and universality: A theory of nursing.* New York: National League of Nursing.

Lorig, K., Stewart, A., Ritter, P., Gonzalez, V., Laurent, D., & Lynch, J. (1996). *Outcome measures for health education and other health care interventions.* Thousand Oaks, CA: Sage.

Marion, L. N. (1996). *Nursing's vision for primary health care in the 21st century.* Washington, DC: ANA Publications.

Murray, R. B., & Zentner, J. P. (2001). *Nursing assessment and health promotion through the life span* (7th ed.). Englewood Cliffs, NJ: Prentice-Hall.

O'Donnell, M. P. (2001). *Health promotion in the workplace.* Albany, NY: Delmar Publishing.

Pender, N. J. (1996). *Health promotion in nursing practice* (3rd ed.). Norwalk, CT: Appleton & Lange.

Rankin, S. H., & Stallings, K. D. (2000). *Patient education: Issues, principles, practices* (4th ed.). Philadelphia: Lippincott Williams & Wilkins.

Redman, B. (2000). *The practice of patient education* (9th ed.). St. Louis: C. V. Mosby.

Staab, A. S., & Hodges, L. C. (1996). *Essentials of gerontological nursing: Adaptation to the aging process.* Philadelphia: Lippincott-Raven.

U.S. Department of Health & Human Services (1996). *Physical activity and health: A report of the Surgeon General.* Atlanta: U.S. Department of Health and Human Services, Centers for Disease Control and Prevention, National Center for Chronic Disease Prevention and Health Promotion.

U.S. Public Health Service. (1990). *Healthy people 2000.* Washington, DC: U.S. Government Printing Office.

U.S. Public Health Service. (1995). *Healthy people 2000: Midcourse review and 1995 revision.* Washington, DC: U.S. Government Printing Office.

U.S. Public Health Service. (2000). *Healthy people 2010: Understanding and improving health.* Washington, DC: U.S. Government Printing Office.

Whitman, T. L. (Ed.). (1999). *Life-span perspectives on health and illness.* Mahwah, NJ: Lawrence Erlbaum Associates.

Woolf, S. H., Jonas, S., & Lawrence, R. S. (1996). *Health promotion and disease prevention in clinical practice.* Baltimore: Williams & Wilkins.

Journals

Asterisks indicate nursing research articles.

Beauchesne, M. A., & Meservey, P. M. (1999). An interdisciplinary community based educational model. *Journal of Professional Nursing, 15*(1), 38–43.

Becker, H. A., Stuifbergen, A. K., Oh, H., & Hall, S. (1993). The self-rated abilities for health practices scale: A health self-efficacy measure. *Health Values, 17,* 42–50.

Campbell, K. N. (1999). Adult education: Helping adults begin the process of learning. *American Association of Occupational Health Nursing, 47*(1), 31–42.

Gray, M., Kanner, S., & Lacey, K. O. (1999). Characteristics of the learner: Children and adolescents. *Diabetes Educator, 25*(6), (Suppl.), 25–33.

Haber, J. (1999). Rx for teaching: Assessing stress. *Home Health Focus, 5*(9), 70–71, 67.

Herje, P. A. (1980). Hows and whys of patient contracting. *Journal of Nursing Education, 5,* 30–34.

Jacubowitz, T. R. (1999). Culturally sensitive care for the elderly. *Nurse Practitioner Forum, 10*(1), 8–11.

Kelleher, C. (1996). Education and training in health promotion: Theory and methods. *Health Promotion International, 11*(1), 47–53.

Lai, S. C., & Cohen, M. N. (1999). Promoting lifestyle changes. *American Journal of Nursing, 99*(4), 63–67.

*Lev, E. L., & Owen, S. V. (1996). A measure of self-care self-efficacy: Strategies used by people to promote health. *Research in Nursing and Health, 19*(5), 421–429.

Lucas, J. A., Orshan, S. A., & Cook, F. (2000). Determinants of health-promoting behaviors among women ages 65 and above living in the community. *Scholarly Inquiry for Nursing Practice, 14*(1), 77–109.

Malone, S. B. (2000). Patient education: Stress management. *Clinical Nurse Specialist, 4*(2), 234–236.

Poss, J. E. (1999). Providing culturally competent care: Is there a role for health promoters? *Nursing Outlook, 47*(1), 30–36.

Robinson, A. W., & Sloan, H. L. (2000). Healthy People 2000: Heart health and old women. *Journal of Gerontological Nursing, 26*(5), 38–45.

Schank, M. J. (1999). Educational innovations—Self-health appraisal: Learning the difficulties of lifestyle change. *Journal of Nursing Education, 38*(1), 10–12.

Schneider, S. L., Richard, M., Huss, K., et al. (1997). Moving health care education into the community. *Nursing Management, 28*(9), 40–43.

Stuifbergen, A. K. (1995). Health-promoting behaviors and quality of life among individuals with multiple sclerosis. *Scholarly Inquiry for Nursing Practice, 9*(1), 31–50.

Wilkinson, J. A. (1999). Understanding patients' health beliefs. *Professional Nurse, 14*(5), 320–322.

Health Assessment

On completion of this chapter, the learner will be able to:

1. Describe the components of the health history.
2. Apply interviewing skills and techniques to conduct a successful interview.
3. Describe the physical examination techniques of inspection, palpation, percussion, and auscultation.
4. Apply the techniques of inspection, palpation, percussion, and auscultation to perform physical assessment of the major body systems.
5. Discuss the techniques of measurement of body mass index, biochemical assessment, clinical examination, and assessment of food intake to assess a person's nutritional status.
6. Identify ethical considerations necessary for protecting the individual's rights related to data collected in the health history or physical examination.
7. Describe factors that may contribute to altered nutritional status in high-risk groups such as adolescents and the elderly.
8. Conduct a health history and physical and nutritional assessment of the patient at home.

*T*he ability to assess the patient is one of the most important skills of the nurse, regardless of the practice setting. In all settings where nurses interact with patients and provide care, eliciting a complete health history and using appropriate assessment skills are critical to identifying physical and psychological problems and concerns experienced by the patient. As the first step in the nursing process, patient assessment is necessary to obtain data that will enable the nurse to make a nursing diagnosis, identify and implement nursing interventions, and assess their effectiveness.

The Role of the Nurse in Assessment

The role of the nurse in health assessment includes obtaining the patient's health history and performing a physical assessment. This role can be carried out in a variety of settings, including the acute care setting, clinic or outpatient office, school, long-term care facility, and the home. A growing list of nursing diagnoses is used by nurses to identify and categorize patient problems that nurses have the knowledge, skills, and responsibility to treat independently. All members of the health care team—physicians, nurses, nutritionists, social workers, and others—use their unique skills and knowledge to contribute to the resolution of patient problems by first obtaining a health history and physical examination. Because the focus of each member of the health care team is unique, a variety of health history and physical examination formats have been developed. Regardless of the format, the database obtained by the nurse is complementary to the databases obtained by other members of the health care team and focuses on nursing's unique concern for the patient.

Basic Guidelines for Conducting a Health Assessment

People who seek health care for a specific problem often feel anxious. Their anxiety may be increased by fear about potential diagnoses, possible disruption of lifestyle, and other concerns. With this in mind, the nurse attempts to establish rapport, put the person at ease, encourage honest communication (Fuller & Schaller-Ayers, 2000), make eye contact, and listen carefully to the person's responses to questions about health issues (Fig. 5-1).

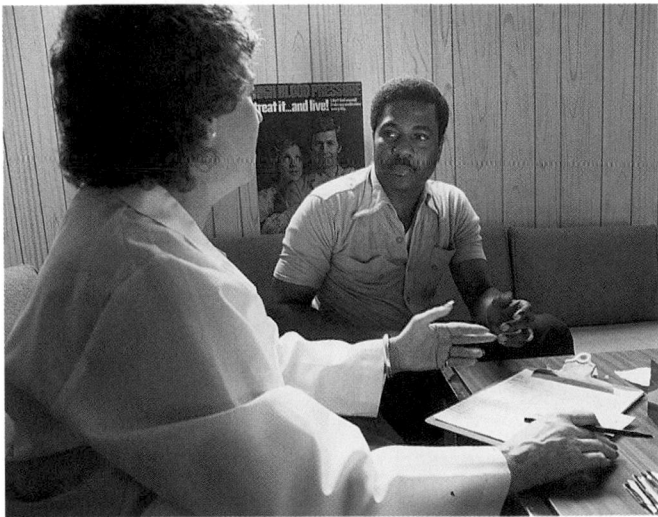

FIGURE 5-1 A comfortable, relaxed atmosphere and an attentive interviewer are essential for a successful clinical interview.

When obtaining the health history or performing the physical examination, the nurse must be aware of his or her own nonverbal communication as well as that of the patient. The nurse takes into consideration the educational and cultural background as well as language proficiency of the patient. Questions and instructions to the patient are phrased in a way that is easily understandable. Technical terms and medical jargon are avoided. In addition, the examiner needs to be aware of the patient's disabilities or impairments (hearing, vision, cognitive, and physical limitations) and takes these into consideration during the history as well as the physical examination. At the end of the assessment, the examiner may summarize and clarify the information obtained and ask if the person has any questions; this provides an opportunity to correct misinformation and add facts that may have been omitted.

Ethical Use of History or Physical Examination Data

A particularly important guideline for use whenever information is elicited from a person through the health history or physical examination is that the person has the right to know why the information is sought and how it will be used. For this reason, it is important to explain what the history and physical examination are, how the information will be obtained, and how it will be used (Fuller & Schaller-Ayers, 2000). It is also important that the individual be aware that the decision to participate is voluntary. A private setting for the history interview and physical examination promotes trust and encourages open, honest communication. After the history collection and examination, the nurse selectively records the data pertinent to the patient's health status. This written record of the patient's history and physical examination findings is then maintained in a secure place and made available only to those health professionals directly involved in the care of the patient. This protects confidentiality and promotes professional conduct.

The Health History

Throughout assessment, and particularly when obtaining the history, attention is focused on the impact of psychosocial, ethnic, and cultural background on the person's health, illness, and health-promotion behaviors. The interpersonal and physical environments, as well as the person's lifestyle and activities of daily living, are explored in depth. Many nurses are responsible for obtaining a detailed history of the person's current health problems, past medical history, family history, and a review of the person's functional status. This results in a total health profile that focuses on health as well as illness and is more appropriately called a health history rather than a medical or a nursing history.

The format of the health history traditionally combines the medical history and the nursing assessment, although formats based on nursing frameworks, such as functional health patterns, have also become a standard. Both the review of systems and patient profile are expanded to include individual and family relationships, lifestyle patterns, health practices, and coping strategies. These components of the health history are the basis of nursing assessment and can be easily adapted to address the needs of any patient population in any setting, institution, or agency.

Combining the information obtained by the physician and the nurse in one health history prevents duplication of information and minimizes efforts on the part of the person to provide this information. This also encourages collaboration among members of the health care team who share in the collection and interpretation of the data (Butler, 1999).

THE INFORMANT

The informant, or the person providing the health history, may not always be the patient, as in the case of a developmentally delayed, mentally impaired, disoriented, confused, unconscious, or comatose patient. The interviewer assesses the reliability of the informant and the usefulness of the information provided. For example, a disoriented patient is often unable to provide a reliable database; people who abuse drugs and alcohol often deny using these substances. The interviewer must make a judgment about the reliability of the information (based on the context of the entire interview), and he or she includes this evaluation in the record.

CULTURAL CONSIDERATIONS

When obtaining the health history, the interviewer takes into account the person's cultural background (Weber & Kelley, 2003). Cultural attitudes and beliefs about health, illness, health care, hospitalization, the use of medications, and the use of complementary therapies are derived from each person's experiences. They vary according to the person's ethnic and cultural background. A person from another culture may have a different view of personal health practices than the health care practitioner.

Similarly, people from some ethnic and cultural backgrounds will not complain of pain, even when it is severe, because outward expressions of pain are considered unacceptable. In some instances they may refuse to take analgesics. Other cultures have their own folklore and beliefs about the treatment of illnesses. All such differences in outlook must be taken into account and accepted when caring for members of other cultures. Attitudes and beliefs about family relationships and the role of women and elderly members of a family must be respected even if those attitudes and beliefs conflict with those of the interviewer.

CONTENT OF THE HEALTH HISTORY

When the patient is seen for the first time by a member of the health care team, the first requirement is a database (except in emergency situations). The sequence and format of obtaining data about the patient vary, but the content, regardless of format, usually addresses the same general topics. A traditional approach includes the following:

- Biographical data
- Chief complaint
- Present health concern (or present illness)
- Past history
- Family history
- Review of systems
- Patient profile

Biographical Data

Biographical information puts the patient's health history in context. This information includes the person's name, address, age, gender, marital status, occupation, and ethnic origins. Some interviewers prefer to ask more personal questions at this part of the interview, while others wait until more trust and confidence have been established or until the patient's immediate or urgent needs

are first addressed. The patient in severe pain or with another urgent problem is unlikely to have a great deal of patience for an interviewer who is more concerned about marital or occupational status than with quickly addressing the problem at hand.

Chief Complaint

The chief complaint is the issue that brings the person to the attention of the health care provider. Questions such as, "Why have you come to the health center today?" or "Why were you admitted to the hospital?" usually elicit the chief complaint. In the home setting, the initial question might be, "What is bothering you most today?" When a problem is identified, the person's exact words are usually recorded in quotation marks (Orient, 2000). However, a statement such as, "My doctor sent me" should be followed up with a question that identifies the probable reason why the person is seeking health care; this reason is then identified as the chief complaint.

Present Health Concern or Illness

The history of the present health concern or illness is the single most important factor in helping the health care team to arrive at a diagnosis or determine the person's needs. The physical examination is helpful but often only validates the information obtained from the history. A careful history assists in correct selection of appropriate diagnostic tests. While diagnostic test results can be helpful, they often support rather than establish the diagnosis.

If the present illness is only one episode in a series of episodes, the entire sequence of events is recorded. For example, a history from a patient whose chief complaint is an episode of insulin shock describes the entire course of the diabetes to put the current episode in context. The details of the health concern or present illness are described from onset until the time of contact with the health care team. These facts are recorded in chronological order, beginning with, for example, "The patient was in good health until . . ." or "The patient first experienced abdominal pain 2 months prior to seeking help."

The history of the present illness or problem includes such information as the date and manner (sudden or gradual) in which the problem occurred, the setting in which the problem occurred (at home, at work, after an argument, after exercise), manifestations of the problem, and the course of the illness or problem. This includes self-treatment (including complementary therapies), medical interventions, progress and effects of treatment, and the patient's perceptions of the cause or meaning of the problem.

Specific symptoms (pain, headache, fever, change in bowel habits) are described in detail, along with the location and radiation (if pain), quality, severity, and duration. The interviewer also asks if the problem is persistent or intermittent, what factors aggravate or alleviate it, and if any associated manifestations exist.

Associated manifestations are symptoms that occur simultaneously with the chief complaint. The presence or absence of such symptoms may shed light on the origin or extent of the problem, as well as on the diagnosis. These symptoms are referred to as significant positive or negative findings and are obtained from a review of systems directly related to the chief complaint. For example, if the person reports a vague symptom such as fatigue or weight loss, all body systems are reviewed and included in this section of the history. If, on the other hand, the person's chief complaint is chest pain, only the cardiopulmonary and gastrointestinal systems may be included in the history of the present illness. In either situation, both positive and negative findings are recorded to define the problem further.

Past Health History

A detailed summary of the person's past health is an important part of the database. After determining the general health status, the interviewer may inquire about immunization status and any known allergies to medications or other substances. The dates of immunization are recorded, along with the type of allergy and adverse reactions. The person is asked to provide information, if known, about his or her last physical examination, chest x-ray, electrocardiogram, eye examination, hearing tests, dental checkup, as well as Papanicolaou (Pap) smear and mammogram (if female), digital rectal examination of the prostate gland (if male), and any other pertinent tests. Previous illnesses are then discussed. Negative as well as positive responses to a list of specific diseases are recorded. Dates, or the age of the patient at the time of illness, as well as the names of the primary health care provider and hospital, the diagnosis, and the treatment are also recorded. A history of the following areas is elicited:

- Childhood illness—rubeola, rubella, polio, whooping cough, mumps, chickenpox, scarlet fever, rheumatic fever, strep throat
- Adult illnesses
- Psychiatric illnesses
- Injuries—burns, fractures, head injuries
- Hospitalizations
- Surgical and diagnostic procedures
- Current medications—prescription, over-the-counter, home remedies, complementary therapies
- Use of alcohol and other drugs

If a particular hospitalization or major medical intervention is related to the present illness, the account of it is not repeated; rather, the report refers to the appropriate part of the report, such as "see history of present illness" or "see HPI" on the data sheet.

Family History

The age and health status, or the age and cause of death, of first-order relatives (parents, siblings, spouse, children) and second-order relatives (grandparents, cousins) are elicited to identify diseases that may be genetic in origin, communicable, or possibly environmental in cause. The following diseases are generally included: cancer, hypertension, heart disease, diabetes, epilepsy, mental illness, tuberculosis, kidney disease, arthritis, allergies, asthma, alcoholism, and obesity. One of the easiest methods of recording such data is by using the family tree or genogram (Fig. 5-2). The results of genetic testing or screening, if known, are recorded. See Chapter 9 for a detailed discussion of genetics.

Review of Systems

The systems review includes an overview of general health as well as symptoms related to each body system. Questions are asked about each of the major body systems in terms of past or present symptoms. Reviewing each body system helps reveal any relevant data. Negative as well as positive answers are recorded. If the patient responds positively to questions about a particular system, the information is analyzed carefully. If any illnesses were previously mentioned or recorded, it is not necessary to repeat them in this part of the history. Instead, reference is made to the appropriate place in the history where the information can be found.

A review of systems can be organized in a formal checklist, which becomes a part of the health history. One advantage of a checklist is that it can be easily audited and is less subject to error than a system that relies heavily on the interviewer's memory.

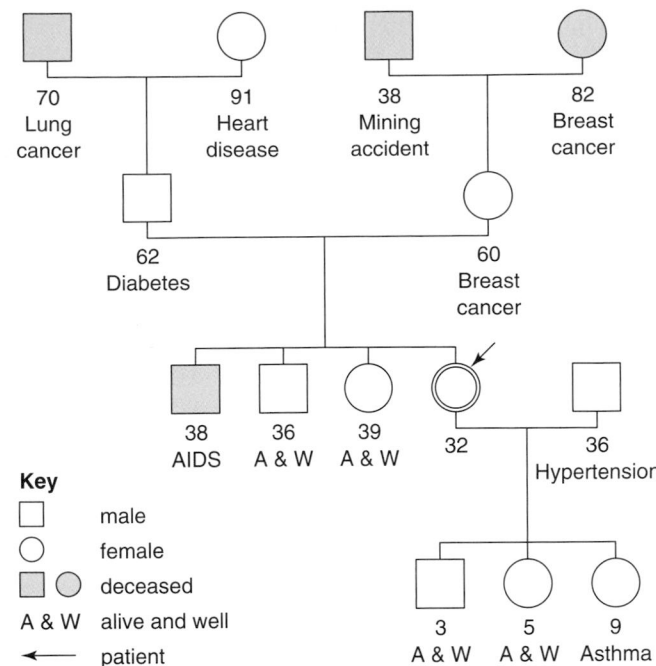

FIGURE 5-2 Diagram (called a genogram) used to record history of family members, including their age and cause of death or, if living, their current health status.

Patient Profile

In the patient profile, more biographical information is gathered. A complete composite, or profile, of the patient is critical to an analysis of the chief complaint and of the person's ability to deal with the problem. A complete patient profile is summarized in Chart 5-1.

The information elicited at this point in the interview is highly personal and subjective. During this stage, the person is encouraged to express feelings honestly and to discuss personal experiences. It is best to begin with general, open-ended questions and to move to direct questioning when specific facts are needed. The patient is often less anxious when the interview progresses from information that is less personal (birthplace, occupation, education) to information that is more personal (sexuality, body image, coping abilities).

A general patient profile consists of the following content areas:

- Past life events related to health
- Education and occupation
- Environment (physical, spiritual, cultural, interpersonal)
- Lifestyle (patterns and habits)
- Presence of a physical or mental disability
- Self-concept
- Sexuality
- Risk for abuse
- Stress and coping response

PAST LIFE EVENTS RELATED TO HEALTH

The patient profile begins with a brief life history. Questions about place of birth and past places of residence help focus attention on the earlier years of life. Personal experiences during childhood or adolescence that have special significance may be elicited by asking, "Was there anything that you experienced as a child or adolescent that would be helpful for me to know about?"

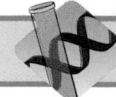

GENETICS IN NURSING PRACTICE

New and exciting discoveries emerging from human genome research are clarifying genetic aspects of health and disease and expanding health opportunities for individuals, families, and communities around the world. These advances call for all nurses to have a heightened awareness of genetics as the core understanding of the mechanisms of disease. Genetics concepts are central to every step of the nursing process.

GENETIC ASPECTS OF HEALTH CARE DELIVERY AND NURSING PRACTICE

Nurses in all areas of practice carry out five main practice activities:

- Help to collect, report, and record genetics information
- Offer genetics information and resources
- Participate in the informed consent process and facilitate informed decision making
- Participate in ongoing management of patients with genetic conditions
- Evaluate and monitor the impact of genetic conditions, testing, and treatment on the individual and family

COMMUNITY-BASED NURSING PRACTICE

Nurses providing community-based care:

- Participate in genetic screening (eg, prenatal screening and newborn screening)
- Provide health care regarding genetic risk factors and management of genetically related disorders in a way that respects the beliefs and concerns of specific ethnic communities
- Educate the public about the contribution of genetics to health and disease
- Engage in dialogue with the public about ethical, legal, and social issues related to genetics discoveries

CRITICAL THINKING AND DECISION MAKING

Nurses use these skills in providing genetic-related health care when they:

- Assess and analyze family history data for genetic risk factors
- Identify those individuals and families in need of referral for genetic testing or counseling
- Ensure the privacy and confidentiality of genetics information

HEALTH EDUCATION AND PROMOTION

Nurses in all settings should be prepared to:

- Inquire about patients' and families' desired health outcomes with regard to genetic-related conditions or risk factors
- Refer patients for genetics services when indicated
- Identify barriers to accessing genetic-related health services
- Offer appropriate genetics information and resources

HEALTH ASSESSMENT

Nurses incorporate a genetics focus into the following health assessments:

- Family history—assess for genetic-related risk factors
- Cultural, social, and spiritual assessment—assess for individual and family perceptions and beliefs around genetics topics
- Physical assessment—assess for clinical features that may suggest a genetic condition is present (eg, unusually tall stature—Marfan syndrome)
- Ethnic background—since many conditions are more common in specific ethnic populations, the nurse gathers information about ethnic background (eg, Tay-Sachs disease in Ashkenazi Jewish populations or thalassemia in Southeast Asian populations)

GENETICS RESOURCES FOR NURSES AND PATIENTS ON THE WEB

Genetic Alliance http://www.geneticalliance.org—a directory of support groups for patients and families with genetic conditions

Gene Clinics http://www.geneclinics.org—a listing of common genetic disorders with up-to-date clinical summaries, genetic counseling and testing information

National Organization of Rare Disorders http://www.rarediseases.org—a directory of support groups and information for patients and families with rare genetic disorders

OMIM: Online Mendelian Inheritance in Man. http://www.ncbi.nlm.nih.gov/omim/stats/html—a complete listing of inherited genetic conditions

---

The interviewer's intent is to encourage the person to make a quick review of his or her earlier life, highlighting information of particular significance. Although many patients may not recall anything significant, others may share information such as a personal achievement, a failure, a developmental crisis, or an instance of physical or emotional abuse.

EDUCATION AND OCCUPATION

Inquiring about current occupation can reveal much about a person's economic status and educational preparation. A statement such as, "Tell me about your job" often elicits information about role, job tasks, and satisfaction with the position. Direct questions about past employment and career goals may be asked if the person does not provide this information.

Asking the person what kind of educational requirements were necessary to attain his or her present job is a more sensitive approach to educational background than asking whether he or she graduated from high school. Information about the patient's general financial status may be obtained by questions such as, "Do you have any financial concerns at this time?" or "Sometimes there just doesn't seem to be enough money to make ends meet. Are you finding this true?" Inquiry about the person's insurance coverage and plans for health care payment is also appropriate.

ENVIRONMENT

The person's physical environment and its potential hazards, spiritual awareness, cultural background, interpersonal relationships, and support system are included in the concept of environment.

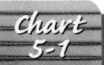

Chart 5-1 Patient Profile

Past Events Related to Health
Place of birth
Places lived
Significant childhood/adolescent experiences

Education and Occupation
Jobs held in past
Current position/job
Length of time at position
Educational preparation
Work satisfaction and career goals

Financial Resources
Income
Insurance coverage

Environment
Physical—living arrangements (type of housing, neighborhood, presence of hazards)
Spiritual—extent to which religion is a part of individual's life; religious beliefs related to perception of health and illness; religious practices
Interpersonal—ethnic background (language spoken, customs and values held, folk practices used to maintain health or to cure illness); family relationships (family structure, roles, communication patterns, support system); friendships (quality of relationship)

Lifestyle Patterns
Sleep (time individual retires, hours per night, comfort measures, awakens rested)
Exercise (type, frequency, time spent)
Nutrition (24-hour diet recall, idiosyncrasies, restrictions)

Recreation (type of activity, time spent)
Caffeine (coffee, tea, cola, chocolate)—kind, amount
Smoking (cigarette, pipe, cigar, marijuana)—kind, amount per day, number of years, desire to quit
Alcohol—kind, amount, pattern over past year
Drugs—kind, amount, route of administration

Physical or Mental Disability
Presence of a disability (physical or mental)
Effect of disability on function and health access
Accommodations needed to support functioning

Self-Concept
View of self in present
View of self in future
Body image (level of satisfaction, concerns)

Sexuality
Perception of self as a man or woman
Quality of sexual relationships
Concerns related to sexuality or sexual functioning

Risk for Abuse
Physical injury in past
Afraid of partner, caregiver, family

Stress and Coping Response
Major concerns or problems at present
Daily "hassles"
Past experiences with similar problems
Past coping patterns and outcomes
Present coping strategies and anticipated outcomes
Individual's expectations of family/friends and health care team in problem resolution

Physical Environment

Information is elicited about the type of housing (apartment, duplex, single-family) in which the person lives, its location, the level of safety and comfort within the home and neighborhood, and the presence of environmental hazards (eg, isolation, potential fire risks, inadequate sanitation). The patient's environment takes on special importance if the patient is homeless or living in a homeless shelter or has a disability.

Spiritual Environment

The term "spiritual environment" refers to the degree to which a person thinks about or contemplates his or her existence, accepts challenges in life, and seeks and finds answers to personal questions. Spirituality may be expressed through identification with a particular religion. Spiritual values and beliefs often direct a person's behavior and approach to health problems and can influence responses to sickness. Illness may create a spiritual crisis and can place considerable stress on a person's internal resources and beliefs. Inquiring about spirituality can identify possible support systems as well as beliefs and customs that need to be considered in planning care. Thus, information is gathered in the following three areas:

- The extent to which religion is a part of the person's life
- Religious beliefs related to the person's perception of health and illness
- Religious practices

The following questions can be used in a spiritual assessment:

- Is religion or God important to you?
- If yes, in what way?
- If no, what is the most important thing in your life?
- Are there any religious practices that are important to you?
- Do you have any spiritual concerns because of your present health problem?

Interpersonal and Cultural Environment

Cultural influences, relationships with family and friends, and the presence or absence of a support system are all a part of one's interpersonal environment. The beliefs and practices that have been shared from generation to generation are known as cultural or ethnic patterns. They are expressed through language, dress, dietary choices, and role behaviors, in perceptions of health and illness, and in health-related behaviors. The influence of these beliefs and customs on how a person reacts to health problems and interacts with health care providers cannot be underestimated (Fuller & Schaller-Ayers, 2000). For this reason, the health history includes information about ethnic identity (cultural and social) and racial identity (biologic). The following questions may assist in obtaining relevant information:

- Where did your parents or ancestors come from? When?
- What language do you speak at home?
- Are there certain customs or values that are important to you?
- Is there anything special you do to keep in good health?
- Do you have any specific practices for treating illness?

Family Relationships and Support System

An assessment of family structure (members, ages, roles), patterns of communication, and the presence or absence of a support system is an integral part of the patient profile. Although the traditional family is recognized as a mother, a father, and children, many different types of living arrangements exist within our society. "Family" may mean two or more people bound by emotional ties or commitments. Live-in companions, roommates, and close friends can all play a significant role in an individual's support system.

LIFESTYLE

The lifestyle section of the patient profile provides information about health-related behaviors. These behaviors include patterns of sleep, exercise, nutrition, and recreation, as well as personal habits such as smoking and the use of drugs, alcohol, and caffeine. Although most people readily describe their exercise patterns or recreational activities, many are unwilling to report their smoking, alcohol use, and drug use; many deny or understate the degree to which they use such substances. Questions such as, "What kind of alcohol do you enjoy drinking at a party?" may elicit more accurate information than, "Do you drink?" The specific type of alcohol (eg, wine, liquor, beer) and the amount ingested per day or per week (eg, 1 pint of whiskey daily for 2 years) are described.

When alcohol abuse is suspected, additional information may be obtained by using common alcohol screening questionnaires such as the CAGE (Cutting down, Annoyance by criticism, Guilty feelings, and Eye-openers), AUDIT (Alcohol Use Disorders Identification Test), TWEAK (Tolerance, Worry, Eye-opener, Amnesia, Kut down), or SMAST (Short Michigan Alcoholism Screening Test). Chart 5-2 shows the CAGE Questions Adapted to Include Drugs (CAGEAID).

Similar questions can be used to elicit information about smoking and caffeine consumption. Questions about drug use follow naturally after questions about smoking, caffeine consumption, and alcohol use. A nonjudgmental approach will make

---

Chart 5-2 — Assessment

Instrument for Assessing Alcohol or Drug Use

CAGE Questions Adapted to Include Drugs (CAGEAID)*
Have you felt you ought to cut down on your drinking *(or drug use)?*
_____Yes _____No
Have people annoyed you by criticizing your drinking *(or drug use)?*
_____Yes _____No
Have you felt bad or guilty about your drinking *(or drug use)?*
_____Yes _____No
Have you ever had a drink *(or used drugs)* **first thing in the morning to steady your nerves or get rid of a hangover** *(or to get the day started)?*
_____Yes _____No

---

*Boldface text shows the original CAGE questions; boldface italic text shows modifications of the CAGE questions used to screen for drug disorders. In a general population, two or more positive answers indicate a need for more in-depth assessment.
From Fleming, M. F., & Barry, K. L. (1992). *Addictive Disorders.* St. Louis: Mosby; and Ewing, J. A. (1984). Detecting alcoholism: The CAGE questionnaire. *Journal of the American Medical Association, 252*(14), 1905–1907.

---

it easier for the person to respond truthfully and factually. If street names or unfamiliar terms are used to describe drugs, the person is asked to define the terms used.

Investigation of lifestyle should also include questions about complementary and alternative therapies. It is estimated that as many as 40% of Americans use some type of complementary or alternative therapies, including special diets, the use of prayer, visualization, or guided imagery, massage, meditation, herbal products, and many others (Evans, 2000; King, Pettigrew & Reed, 1999; Kuhn, 1999). Marijuana is used for symptom management, especially pain, in a number of chronic conditions (Mathre, 2001).

PHYSICAL OR MENTAL DISABILITY

The general patient profile also needs to contain questions about any hearing, vision, cognitive, or physical disability. The presence of an obvious physical deformity—for instance, if the patient walks with crutches or needs a wheelchair to get around—needs further investigation. The etiology of the disability should be elicited; the length of time the patient has had the disability and the impact on function and health access are important to assess.

SELF-CONCEPT

Self-concept refers to one's view of oneself, an image that has developed over many years. To assess self-concept, the interviewer might ask the person how he or she views life: "How do you feel about your life in general?" A person's self-concept can be threatened very easily by changes in physical function or appearance or other threats to health. The impact of certain medical conditions or surgical interventions, such as a colostomy or a mastectomy, can threaten body image. Asking, "Do you have any particular concerns about your body?" may elicit useful information about self-image.

SEXUALITY

No area of assessment is more personal than the sexual history. Interviewers are frequently uncomfortable with such questions and ignore this area of the patient profile or conduct a very cursory interview at this point. Lack of knowledge about sexuality and anxiety about one's own sexuality may hamper the interviewer's effectiveness in dealing with this subject (Ross, Channon-Little & Rosser, 2000).

Sexual assessment can be approached at the end of the interview, at the time interpersonal or lifestyle factors are assessed, or it can be a part of the genitourinary history within the review of systems. For instance, it may be easier to approach a discussion of sexuality after a discussion of menstruation. A similar discussion with the male patient would follow questions related to the urinary system.

Obtaining the sexual history provides an opportunity to discuss sexual matters openly and gives the person permission to express sexual concerns to an informed professional. The interviewer must be nonjudgmental and must use language appropriate to the patient's age and background. It is advisable to begin the assessment with a general question concerning the person's developmental stage and the presence or absence of intimate relationships. Such questions may lead to a discussion of concerns related to sexual expression or the quality of a relationship, or to questions about contraception, risky sexual behaviors, and safer sex practices.

Finding out whether a person is sexually active should precede any attempts to explore issues related to sexuality and sexual function. Care should be taken to initiate conversations about sexuality with elderly patients and not to treat them as asexual beings (Miller, Zylstra & Stranridge, 2000). Questions are worded in such a way that the person feels free to discuss his or her sexuality regardless of marital status or sexual preference. Direct questions are usually less threatening when prefaced with such statements as, "Most people feel that . . ." or "Many people worry about. . . ." This suggests the normalcy of such feelings or behavior and encourages the person to share information that might otherwise be omitted from fear of seeming "different."

If the person answers abruptly or does not wish to carry the discussion any further, then the interviewer should move to the next topic. However, introducing the subject of sexuality indicates to the person that a discussion of sexual concerns is acceptable and can be approached again in the future if so desired. Further discussion of the sexual history is presented in Chapters 46 and 49.

RISK FOR ABUSE

A topic of growing importance in today's society is physical, sexual, and psychological abuse. Such abuse occurs at all ages, to men and women from all socioeconomic, ethnic, and cultural groups (Little, 2000; Marshall, Benton & Brazier, 2000). Few patients, however, will discuss this topic unless they are asked specifically about it. Therefore, it is important to ask direct questions, such as:

- Is anyone physically hurting you?
- Has anyone ever hurt you physically or threatened to do so?
- Are you ever afraid of anyone close to you (your partner, caretaker, or other family members)?

If the person's response indicates that abuse is a risk, further assessment is called for and efforts are made to ensure the person's safety and provide access to appropriate community and professional resources and support systems. Further discussion

Gerontologic Considerations

A health history from the elderly patient should be obtained in a calm, unrushed manner. Because of the increased incidence of impaired hearing and sight in the elderly, lighting should be adequate but not glaring, and distracting noises should be kept to a minimum (Miller, Zylstra & Standridge, 2000). The interviewer should assume a position that enables the person to read lips and facial expressions. People who normally use a hearing aid are asked to use it during the interview. The interviewer should also recognize that there is wide diversity among the elderly population and that differences exist in health, gender, income, and functional status (Bakshi & Miller, 1999; Ludwick, Dieckman & Snelson, 1999).

Elderly people often assume that new physical problems are a result of age rather than a treatable illness. In addition, the signs and symptoms of illness in the elderly are often more subtle than those in younger people and may go unreported. Therefore, the interviewer inquires about subtle physical symptoms and recent changes in function and well-being. Special care is taken in obtaining a complete history of medications used, because many elderly people take many different kinds of prescription and over-the-counter medications (Palmer, 1999). Although elderly people may experience a decline in mental function, it should not be assumed that an elderly person is unable to provide an adequate history. Including a member of the family in the interview process, however (ie, spouse, adult child, sibling, or caretaker), may validate information and provide missing details. Further details about assessment of the elderly are provided in Chapter 12.

of domestic violence and abuse is presented in Chapter 46. When questioned directly, elderly patients rarely admit to abuse (Marshall, Benton & Brazier, 2000). Health care professionals should assess for risk factors, such as high levels of stress or alcoholism in caregivers, evidence of violence, high emotions as well as financial, emotional, or physical dependency. Patients who are elderly or disabled are at increased risk for abuse and should be asked about it as a routine part of assessment.

STRESS AND COPING RESPONSES

Each person handles stress differently. How well we adapt depends on our ability to cope. During a health history, past coping patterns and perceptions of current stresses and anticipated outcomes are explored to identify the person's overall ability to handle stress. It is especially important to identify expectations that the person may have of family, friends, and caregivers in providing financial, emotional, or physical support.

OTHER HEALTH HISTORY FORMATS

The health history format discussed in this chapter is only one possible format that is useful in obtaining and organizing information about a person's health status. Some consider this traditional format to be inappropriate for nurses because it does not focus exclusively on the assessment of human responses to actual or potential health problems. Several attempts have been made to develop an assessment format and database with this focus in mind. One example is the nursing database prototype based on the North American Nursing Diagnosis Association's (NANDA) Unitary Person Framework and its nine human response patterns: exchanging, communicating, relating, valuing, choosing, moving, perceiving, knowing, and feeling. Although there is support in nursing for using this approach, no consensus for its use has been reached.

The National Center for Health Services Research of the U.S. Department of Health and Human Services and other groups from the public and private sectors have focused on assessing not only biologic health but also other dimensions of health. These dimensions include physical, functional, emotional, mental, and social health. Modern efforts to assess health status have focused on the manner in which disease or disability affects the patient's functional status—that is, the ability of the person to function normally and perform his or her usual physical, mental, and social activities. An emphasis on functional assessment is viewed as more holistic than the traditional health or medical history. Instruments to assess health status in these ways may be used by nurses along with their own clinical assessment skills to determine the impact of illness, disease, disability, and health problems on functional status.

Health concerns that are not complex (earache, tonsillectomy) and can be resolved in a short period of time usually do not require the depth or detail that is required when a person is experiencing a major illness or health problem. Additional assessments that go beyond the general patient profile may be used when the patient's health problems are acute and complex or when the illness is chronic. Individuals should be asked about their continuing health promotion and screening practices. Patients who have not been involved in these practices in the past are educated about their importance and are referred to appropriate health care providers.

Regardless of the assessment format used, the nurse's focus during data collection is different from that of the physician and other health team members; however, it complements these approaches and encourages collaboration among the health care providers, as each member brings his or her own expertise and focus to the situation.

Physical Assessment

Physical assessment, or the physical examination, is an integral part of nursing assessment. The basic techniques and tools used in performing a physical examination are described in general in this chapter. The examination of specific systems, including special maneuvers, is described in the appropriate chapters throughout the book. Because the patient's nutritional status is an important factor in health and well-being, a section on nutritional assessment is included in this chapter.

The physical examination is usually performed after the health history is obtained. It is carried out in a well-lighted, warm area. The patient is asked to undress and draped appropriately so that only the area to be examined is exposed. The person's physical and psychological comfort is considered at all times. Procedures and sensations to expect are described to the patient before each part of the examination. The examiner's hands are washed before and immediately after the examination. Fingernails are kept short to avoid injuring the patient. The examiner wears gloves when there is a possibility of coming into contact with blood or other body secretions during the physical examination.

An organized and systematic examination is the key to obtaining appropriate data in the shortest time. Such an approach encourages cooperation and trust on the part of the patient. The individual's health history provides the examiner with a health profile that guides all aspects of the physical examination. Although the sequence of physical examination depends on the circumstances and on the patient's reason for seeking health care, the complete examination usually proceeds as follows:

- Skin
- Head and neck
- Thorax and lungs
- Breasts
- Cardiovascular system
- Abdomen
- Rectum
- Genitalia
- Neurologic system
- Musculoskeletal system

In clinical practice, all relevant body systems are tested throughout the physical examination, not necessarily in the sequence described (Weber & Kelley, 2003). For example, when the face is examined, it is appropriate to check for facial asymmetry and, thus, for the integrity of the seventh cranial nerve; the examiner does not need to repeat this as part of a neurologic examination. When systems are combined in this manner, the patient does not need to change positions repeatedly, which can be exhausting and time-consuming.

A "complete" physical examination is not routine. Many of the body systems are selectively assessed on the basis of the individual's presenting problem. If, for example, a healthy 20-year-old college student requires an examination to play basketball and reports no history of neurologic abnormality, the neurologic assessment is brief. Conversely, a history of transient numbness and diplopia (double vision) usually necessitates a complete neurologic investigation. Similarly, a person with chest pain receives a much more intensive examination of the chest and heart than the person with an earache. In general, the individual's health history guides the examiner in obtaining additional data for a complete picture of the patient's health.

The process of learning physical examination requires repetition and reinforcement in a clinical setting. Only after basic physical assessment techniques are mastered can the examiner tailor the routine screening examination to include thorough assessments of a particular system, including special maneuvers.

The basic tools of the physical examination are vision, hearing, touch, and smell. These human senses may be augmented by special tools (eg, stethoscope, ophthalmoscope, and reflex hammer) that are extensions of the human senses; they are simple tools that anyone can learn to use well. Expertise comes with practice, and sophistication comes with the interpretation of what is seen and heard. The four fundamental techniques used in the physical examination are inspection, palpation, percussion, and auscultation (Weber & Kelley, 2003).

INSPECTION

The first fundamental technique is inspection or observation. General inspection begins with the first contact with the patient. Introducing oneself and shaking hands provide opportunities for making initial observations: Is the person old or young? How old? How young? Does the person appear to be his or her stated age? Is the person thin or obese? Does the person appear anxious or depressed? Is the person's body structure normal or abnormal? In what way, and how different from normal? It is essential to pay attention to the details in observation. Vague, general statements are not a substitute for specific descriptions based on careful observation; for example:

- "The person appears sick." In what way does he or she appear sick? Is the skin clammy, pale, jaundiced, or cyanotic; is the person grimacing in pain; is breathing difficult; does he or she have edema? What specific physical features or behavioral manifestations indicate that the person is "sick"?
- "The person appears chronically ill." In what way does he or she appear chronically ill? Does the person appear to have lost weight? People who lose weight secondary to muscle-wasting diseases (eg, AIDS, malignancy) have a different appearance than those who are merely thin, and weight loss may be accompanied by loss of muscle mass or atrophy. Does the skin have the appearance of chronic illness—that is, is it pale, or does it give the appearance of dehydration or loss of subcutaneous tissue? These important observations are documented in the patient's chart or health record.

Among general observations that should be noted in the initial examination of the patient are posture and stature, body movements, nutrition, speech pattern, and vital signs.

Posture and Stature

The posture that a person assumes often provides valuable information about the illness. Patients who have breathing difficulties (dyspnea) secondary to cardiac disease prefer to sit and may report feeling short of breath lying flat for even a brief time. People with obstructive pulmonary disease not only sit upright but also may thrust their arms forward and laterally onto the edge of the bed (tripod position) to place accessory respiratory muscles at an optimal mechanical advantage. Those with abdominal pain due to peritonitis prefer to lie perfectly still; even slight jarring of the bed will cause agonizing pain. In contrast, patients with abdominal pain due to renal or biliary colic are often restless and may pace the room. Patients with meningeal irritation may experience head or neck pain on bending the head or flexing their knees.

Body Movements

Abnormalities of body movement may be of two general kinds: generalized disruption of voluntary or involuntary movement, and asymmetry of movement. The first category includes tremors of a wide variety; some tremors may occur at rest (Parkinson's disease), whereas others occur only on voluntary movement (cerebellar ataxia). Other tremors may exist during both rest and activity (alcohol withdrawal syndrome, thyrotoxicosis). Some voluntary or involuntary movements are fine, others quite coarse. At the extreme are the convulsive movements of epilepsy or tetanus and the choreiform (involuntary and irregular) movements of patients with rheumatic fever or Huntington's disease. Other aspects of body movement that are noted on inspection include spasticity, muscle spasms, and an abnormal gait.

Asymmetry of movement, in which only one side of the body is affected, may occur with disorders of the central nervous system (CNS), principally in those patients who have had cerebrovascular accidents (strokes). The patient may have drooping of one side of the face, weakness or paralysis of the extremities on one side of the body, and a foot-dragging gait. Spasticity (increased muscle tone) may also be present, particularly in patients with multiple sclerosis.

Nutrition

Nutritional status is important to note. Obesity may be generalized as a result of excessive intake of calories or may be specifically localized to the trunk in those with endocrine disorders (Cushing's disease) or those who have been taking corticosteroids for long periods of time. Loss of weight may be generalized as a result of inadequate caloric intake or may be seen in loss of muscle mass with disorders that affect protein synthesis. Nutritional assessment is discussed in more detail later in this chapter.

Speech Pattern

Speech may be slurred because of CNS disease or because of damage to cranial nerves. Recurrent damage to the laryngeal nerve will produce hoarseness, as will disorders that produce edema or swelling of the vocal cords. Speech may be halting, slurred, or interrupted in flow in some CNS disorders (eg, multiple sclerosis).

Vital Signs

The recording of vital signs is a part of every physical examination. Blood pressure, pulse rate, respiratory rate, and body temperature measurements are obtained and recorded. Acute changes and trends over time are documented; unexpected changes and values that deviate significantly from the patient's normal values are brought to the attention of the patient's primary health care provider. The "fifth vital sign," pain, is also assessed and documented, if indicated.

Fever is an increase in body temperature above normal. A normal oral temperature for most people is an average of 37.0°C (98.6°F); however, some variation is normal. Some people's temperatures are quite normal at 36.6°C (98°F) and others at 37.3°C (99°F). There is a normal diurnal variation of a degree or two in body temperature throughout the day; with temperature usually lowest in the morning and rising during the day to between 37.3° and 37.5°C (99° to 99.5°F), then decreasing again during the night.

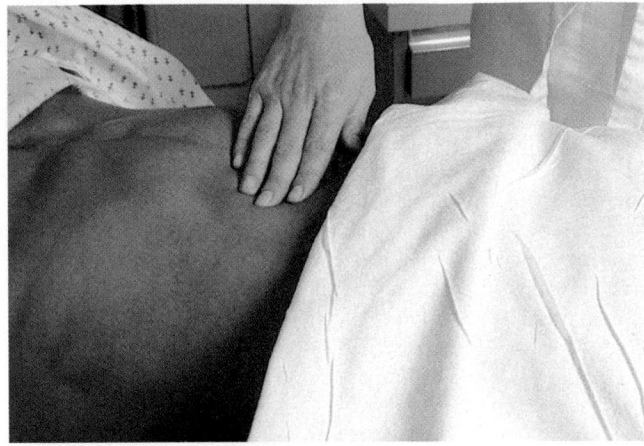

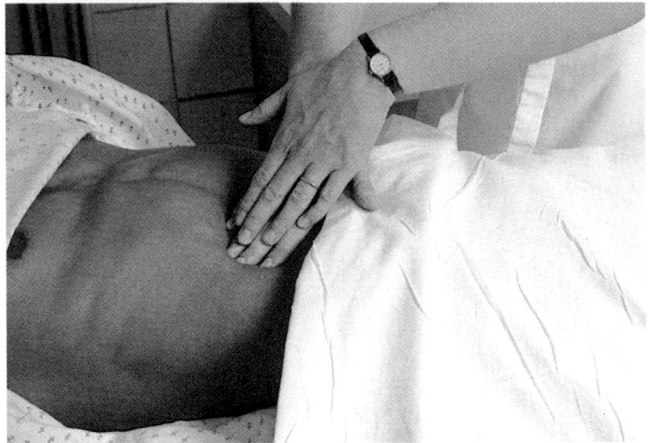

FIGURE 5-3 Light palpation technique (*top*) and deep palpation (*bottom*). Photo © Ken Kasper.

PALPATION

Palpation is a vital part of the physical examination. Many structures of the body, although not visible, may be assessed through the techniques of light and deep palpation (Fig. 5-3). Examples include superficial blood vessels, lymph nodes, the thyroid, the organs of the abdomen and pelvis, and the rectum. When the abdomen is examined, auscultation is performed before palpation and percussion to avoid altering bowel sounds.

Sounds generated within the body, if within specified frequency ranges, also may be detected through touch. Thus, certain murmurs generated in the heart or within blood vessels (thrills) may be detected. Thrills cause a sensation to the hand much like the purring of a cat. Voice sounds are transmitted along the bronchi to the periphery of the lung. These may be perceived by touch and may be altered by disorders affecting the lungs. The phenomenon is called *tactile fremitus* and is useful in assessing diseases of the chest. The significance of these findings is discussed in the relevant chapters of this book.

PERCUSSION

The technique of percussion (Fig. 5-4) translates the application of physical force into sound. It is a skill requiring practice but one that yields much information about disease processes in the chest and abdomen. The principle is to set the chest wall or abdominal wall into vibration by striking it with a firm object. The sound produced reflects the density of the underlying structure. Certain densities produce sounds as percussion notes. These sounds, listed in a se-

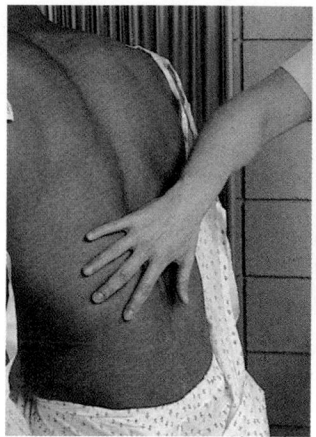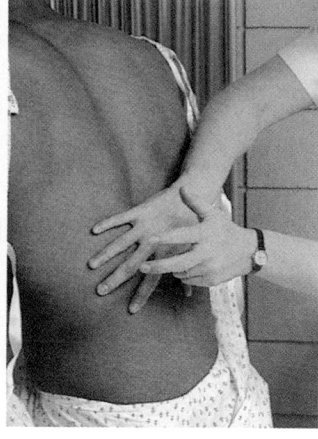

FIGURE 5-4 Percussion technique. The middle finger of one hand strikes the terminal phalanx of the middle finger of the other hand, which is placed firmly against the body. If the action is performed sharply, a brief resonant tone will be produced. The clarity of the tone depends on the brevity of the action. The intensity of the tone varies with the force used. Photo © Ken Kasper.

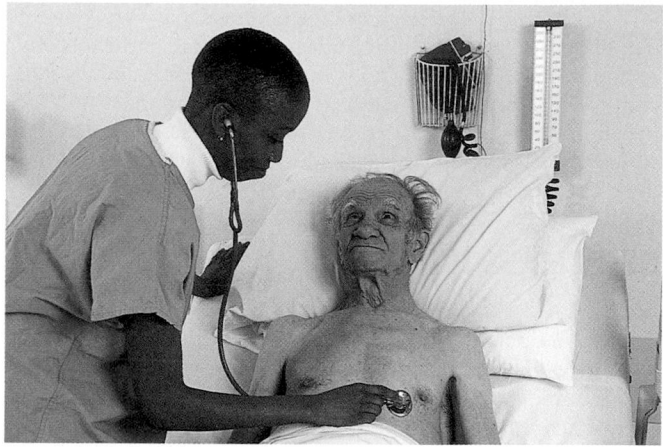

FIGURE 5-5 Technique for auscultating the heart. © B. Proud Photography.

quence that proceeds from the least to the most dense, are called tympany, hyperresonance, resonance, dullness, and flatness. Tympany is the drumlike sound produced by percussing the air-filled stomach. Hyperresonance is audible when one percusses over inflated lung tissue in someone with emphysema. Resonance is the sound elicited over air-filled lungs. Percussion of the liver produces a dull sound, whereas percussion of the thigh results in flatness.

Percussion allows the examiner to assess such normal anatomic details as the borders of the heart and the movement of the diaphragm during inspiration. One may determine the level of pleural effusion (fluid in the pleural cavity) and the location of a consolidated area caused by pneumonia or atelectasis (collapse) of a lobe of the lung. The use of percussion is described further with disorders of the thorax and abdomen.

AUSCULTATION

Auscultation is the skill of listening to sounds produced within the body created by the movement of air or fluid. Examples include breath sounds, the spoken voice, bowel sounds, cardiac murmurs, and heart sounds. Physiologic sounds may be normal (eg, first and second heart sounds) or pathologic (eg, heart murmurs in diastole, or crackles in the lung). Some normal sounds may be distorted by abnormalities of structures through which the sound must travel (eg, changes in the character of breath sounds as they travel through the consolidated lung of the patient with lobar pneumonia).

Sound produced within the body, if of sufficient amplitude, may be detected with the stethoscope, which functions as an extension of the human ear and channels sound. Two end pieces are available for the stethoscope: the bell and the diaphragm. The bell is used to assess very-low-frequency sounds such as diastolic heart murmurs. The entire surface of the bell's disc is placed lightly on the skin surface to avoid flattening the skin and reducing audible vibratory sensations. The diaphragm, the larger disc, is used to assess high-frequency sounds such as heart and lung sounds and is held in firm contact with the skin surface (Fig. 5-5). Touching the tubing or rubbing other surfaces (hair, clothing) during auscultation is avoided to minimize extraneous noises.

Sound produced by the body, like any other sound, is characterized by intensity, frequency, and quality. *Intensity,* or loudness, associated with physiologic sound is low; thus, the use of the stethoscope is needed. *Frequency,* or pitch, of physiologic sound is in reality "noise" in that most sounds consist of a frequency spectrum as opposed to the single-frequency sounds that we associate with music or the tuning fork. The frequency spectrum may be quite low, yielding a rumbling noise, or comparatively high, producing a harsh or blowing sound. *Quality* of sound relates to overtones that allow one to distinguish between different sounds. Sound quality enables the examiner to distinguish between the musical quality of high-pitched wheezing and the low-pitched rumbling of a diastolic murmur.

Nutritional Assessment

An additional area of concern that is often integrated into the health history and physical examination is an in-depth nutritional assessment. Nutrition is important to maintain health and to prevent disease and death (Kant, Schatzkin, Graubard & Schairer, 2000; Landi, Onder, Gambassi et al., 2000; Stampfer, Hu & Manson, 2000). Disorders caused by nutritional deficiency, overeating, or eating poorly balanced meals are among the leading causes of illness and death in the United States today. The three leading causes of death are related, in part, to consequences of unhealthy nutrition: heart disease, cancer, and stroke (Hensrud, 1999). Other examples of health problems associated with poor nutrition include obesity, osteoporosis, cirrhosis, diverticulitis, and eating disorders. When illness or injury occurs, optimal nutrition is an essential factor in promoting healing and resisting infection and other complications (Braunschweig, Gomez & Sheean, 2000). Assessment of a person's nutritional status provides information on obesity, undernutrition, weight loss, malnutrition, deficiencies in specific nutrients, metabolic abnormalities, the effects of medications on nutrition, and special problems of the hospitalized patient and the person who is cared for in the home and in other community settings.

Certain signs and symptoms that suggest possible nutritional deficiency are easy to note because they are specific. Other physical signs may be subtle and must be carefully assessed. A physical sign that suggests a nutritional abnormality should be pursued further. For example, certain signs that may appear to indicate nutritional deficiency may actually reflect other systemic conditions (eg, endocrine disorders, infectious disease). Others may result from impaired digestion, absorption, excretion, or storage of nutrients in the body.

The sequence of assessment of parameters may vary, but evaluation of nutritional status includes one or more of the following methods: measurement of body mass index (BMI) and waist circumference; biochemical measurements (albumin, transferrin, prealbumin, retinol-binding protein, total lymphocyte count, electrolyte levels, creatinine/height index); clinical examination findings; and dietary data.

BODY MASS INDEX

BMI is a ratio based on body weight and height. The obtained value is compared to the established standards; however, trends or changes in values over time are considered more useful than isolated or one-time measurements. BMI (Fig. 5-6) is highly correlated with body fat, but increased lean body mass or a large body frame can also increase the BMI. Individuals who have a BMI below 24 (or who are 80% or less of their desirable body weight for height) are at increased risk for problems associated with poor nutritional status. In addition, a low BMI is associated with higher mortality rates in hospitalized patients and community-dwelling elderly (Landi et al., 2000; Landi, Zuccala, Gambassi et al., 1999).

Those who have a BMI of 25 to 29 are considered overweight; those with a BMI of 30 to 39 are considered obese; above 40 is considered extreme obesity (National Institutes of Health, 2000).

It is important to assess for usual body weight and height. Current weight does not provide information about recent changes in weight; therefore, the patient is asked about his or her usual body weight (Chart 5-3). Decreased height may be due to osteoporosis, an important problem related to nutrition, especially in postmenopausal women. A loss of 2 or 3 inches of height may indicate osteoporosis.

In addition to the calculation of BMI, waist circumference measurement is particularly useful for patients who are catego-

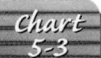

Chart 5-3　Calculating Ideal Body Weight

Women
- Allow 100 lb for 5 feet of height.
- Add 5 lb for each additional inch over 5 feet.
- Subtract 10% for small frame; add 10% for large frame.

Men
- Allow 106 lb for 5 feet of height.
- Add 6 lb for each additional inch over 5 feet.
- Subtract 10% for small frame, add 10% for large frame.

Example: Ideal body weight for a 5′6″ adult is

	Female	Male
5′ of height	100 lb	106 lb
Per additional inch	6″ × 5 lb/inch = 30 lb	6″ × 6 lb/inch = 36 lb
Ideal body weight	130 lb ± 13 lb depending on frame size	142 lb ± 14 lb depending on frame size

Body Mass Index

The body mass index (BMI) is used to determine who is overweight.

$$BMI = \frac{703 \times \text{weight in pounds}}{(\text{height in inches})^2} \quad OR \quad \frac{\text{weight in kilograms}}{(\text{height in meters})^2}$$

BMI score is at the intersection of height and weight. A body mass index score of 25 or more is considered overweight and 30 or more is considered obese.

25 Overweight Limit　　Overweight

Weight	100	105	110	115	120	125	130	135	140	145	150	155	160	165	170	175	180	185	190	195	200	205
Height
5′0″	20	21	21	22	23	24	**25**	26	27	28	29	30	31	32	33	34	35	36	37	38	39	40
5′1″	19	20	21	22	23	24	**25**	26	26	27	28	29	30	31	32	33	34	35	36	37	38	39
5′2″	18	19	20	21	22	23	24	**25**	26	27	27	28	29	30	31	32	33	34	35	36	37	37
5′3″	18	19	19	20	21	22	23	24	**25**	26	27	27	28	29	30	31	32	33	34	35	35	36
5′4″	17	18	19	20	21	21	22	23	24	**25**	26	27	27	28	29	30	31	32	33	33	34	35
5′5″	17	17	18	19	20	21	22	22	23	24	**25**	26	27	27	28	29	30	31	32	32	33	34
5′6″	16	17	18	19	19	20	21	22	23	23	24	**25**	26	27	27	28	29	30	31	31	32	33
5′7″	16	16	17	18	19	20	20	21	22	23	23	24	**25**	26	27	27	28	29	30	31	31	32
5′8″	15	16	17	17	18	19	20	21	21	22	23	24	24	**25**	26	27	27	28	29	30	30	31
5′9″	15	16	16	17	18	18	19	20	21	21	22	23	24	24	**25**	26	27	27	28	29	30	30
5′10″	14	15	16	17	17	18	19	19	20	21	22	22	23	24	24	**25**	26	27	27	28	29	29
5′11″	14	15	15	16	17	17	18	19	20	20	21	22	22	23	24	24	**25**	26	26	27	28	29
6′0″	14	14	15	16	16	17	18	18	19	20	20	21	22	22	23	24	24	**25**	26	26	27	28
6′1″	13	14	15	15	16	16	17	18	18	19	20	20	21	22	22	23	24	24	**25**	26	26	27
6′2″	13	13	14	15	15	16	17	17	18	19	19	20	21	21	22	22	23	24	24	**25**	26	26
6′3″	12	13	14	14	15	16	16	17	17	18	19	19	20	21	21	22	22	23	24	24	**25**	26
6′4″	12	13	13	14	15	15	16	16	17	18	18	19	19	20	21	21	22	23	23	24	24	**25**

Source: Shape Up America. National Institutes of Health

FIGURE 5-6 Body mass index.

rized as of normal weight or overweight. To measure waist circumference, a tape measure is placed in a horizontal plane around the abdomen at the level of the iliac crest. Men who have waist circumferences greater than 40 inches and women who have waist circumferences greater than 35 inches have excess abdominal fat. Those with a high waist circumference are at increased risk of diabetes, dyslipidemias, hypertension, and cardiovascular disease (National Institutes of Health, 2000).

BIOCHEMICAL ASSESSMENT

Biochemical assessment reflects both the tissue level of a given nutrient and any abnormality of metabolism in the utilization of nutrients. These determinations are made from studies of serum (serum protein, serum albumin and globulin, transferrin, retinol-binding protein, hemoglobin, serum vitamin A, carotene, and vitamin C) and studies of urine (creatinine, thiamine, riboflavin, niacin, and iodine). Some of these tests, while reflecting recent intake of the elements detected, can also identify below-normal levels when there are no clinical symptoms of deficiency (see Table 5-1 for a description of serum protein indices).

Low serum albumin and transferrin levels are often used as measures of protein deficits in adults and are expressed as percentages of normal values. Albumin synthesis depends on normal liver function and an adequate supply of amino acids. Because the body stores a large amount of albumin, the serum albumin level may not decrease until malnutrition is severe; thus, its usefulness in detecting recent protein depletion is limited. Decreased albumin levels may be due to overhydration, liver or renal disease, and excessive protein loss because of burns, major surgery, infection, and cancer (Dudek, 2000). Transferrin is a protein that binds and carries iron from the intestine through the serum. Because of its short half-life, decreased transferrin levels respond more quickly to protein depletion than albumin. Serial measurements of these, as well as prealbumin levels, are used to assess the results of nutritional therapy.

Although not available from many laboratories, retinol-binding protein may be a useful means of monitoring acute, short-term changes in protein status.

Reduced total lymphocyte count in people who become acutely malnourished as a result of stress and low-calorie feeding are associated with impaired cellular immunity (Dudek, 2000). Anergy, the absence of an immune response to injection of small concentrations of recall antigen under the skin, may also indicate malnutrition because of delayed antibody synthesis and response.

Serum electrolyte levels provide information about fluid and electrolyte balance and kidney function. The creatinine/height index calculated over a 24-hour period assesses the metabolically active tissue and indicates the degree of protein depletion, comparing expected body mass for height and actual body cell mass. A 24-hour urine sample is obtained, and the amount of creatinine is measured and compared to normal ranges based on the

patient's height and gender. Values less than normal may indicate loss of lean body mass and protein malnutrition.

CLINICAL EXAMINATION

The state of nutrition is often reflected in a person's appearance. Although the most obvious physical sign of good nutrition is a normal body weight with respect to height, body frame, and age, other tissues can serve as indicators of general nutritional status and adequate intake of specific nutrients; these include the hair, skin, teeth, gums, mucous membranes, mouth and tongue, skeletal muscles, abdomen, lower extremities, and thyroid gland (Table 5-2). Specific aspects of clinical examination useful in identifying nutritional deficits include oral examination and assessment of skin for turgor, edema, elasticity, dryness, subcutaneous tone, poorly healing wounds and ulcers, purpura, and bruises. The musculoskeletal examination also provides information about muscle wasting and weakness.

DIETARY DATA

The appraisal of food intake considers the quantity and quality of the diet and also the frequency with which certain food items and nutrients are consumed. Commonly used methods of determining individual eating patterns include the food record and the 24-hour food recall, which can help estimate if the food intake is adequate and appropriate. If these methods are used, instructions about measurement and recording food intake are given when the patient's dietary history is obtained.

Food Record

The food record is used most often in nutritional status studies. The person is instructed to keep a record of food actually consumed over a period of time, varying from 3 to 7 days, and to accurately estimate and describe the specific foods consumed. Food records are fairly accurate if the person is willing to provide factual information and able to estimate food quantities.

24-Hour Recall

The 24-hour recall method is, as the name implies, a recall of food intake over a 24-hour period. The person is asked by the interviewer to recall all food eaten during the previous day and to estimate the quantities of the food consumed. Because information does not always represent usual intake, at the end of the interview the patient is asked if the previous day's food intake was a typical one. To obtain supplementary information about the typical diet, the interviewer also asks how frequently the person eats foods from the major food groups.

CONDUCTING THE DIETARY INTERVIEW

The success of the interviewer in obtaining information for dietary assessment depends on effective communication, which requires that good rapport be established to promote respect and trust. The interviewer explains the purpose of the interview. It is conducted in a nondirective and exploratory way, allowing the respondent to express feelings and thoughts while encouraging him or her to answer specific questions. The manner in which questions are asked will influence the respondent's cooperation. Thus, the interviewer must be nonjudgmental and avoid expressing disapproval, either verbally or by facial expression.

Table 5-1 • **Standard Serum Protein Indices**

SERUM PROTEIN	STANDARD RANGE
Albumin	3.5–5.0 g/dL
Transferrin	>200 mg/dL
Prealbumin	16–30 mg/dL
Retinol-binding protein	2.6–7.7 mg/dL

From Dudek, S. G. (2001). *Nutrition essentials for nursing practice* (4th ed.). Philadelphia: Lippincott Williams & Wilkins.

Table 5-2 • Physical Signs Indicative of Nutritional Status

	SIGNS OF GOOD NUTRITION	SIGNS OF POOR NUTRITION
General appearance	Alert, responsive	Listless, appears acutely or chronically ill
Hair	Shiny, lustrous; firm, healthy scalp	Dull and dry, brittle, depigmented, easily plucked; thin and sparse
Face	Skin color uniform; healthy appearance	Skin dark over cheeks and under eyes, skin flaky, face swollen or hollow/sunken cheeks
Eyes	Bright, clear, moist	Eye membranes pale, dry (xerophthalmia); increased vascularity, cornea soft (keratomalacia)
Lips	Good color (pink), smooth	Swollen and puffy; angular lesion at corners of mouth (cheilosis)
Tongue	Deep red in appearance; surface papillae present	Smooth appearance, swollen, beefy red, sores, atrophic papillae
Teeth	Straight, no crowding, no dental caries, bright	Dental caries, mottled appearance (fluorosis), malpositioned
Gums	Firm, good color (pink)	Spongy, bleed easily, marginal redness, recession
Thyroid	No enlargement of the thyroid	Thyroid enlargement (simple goiter)
Skin	Smooth, good color, moist	Rough, dry, flaky, swollen, pale, pigmented; lack of fat under skin
Nails	Firm, pink	Spoon-shaped, ridged, brittle
Skeleton	Good posture, no malformation	Poor posture, beading of ribs, bowed legs or knock knees
Muscles	Well developed, firm	Flaccid, poor tone, wasted, underdeveloped
Extremities	No tenderness	Weak and tender; edematous
Abdomen	Flat	Swollen
Nervous system	Normal reflexes	Decreased or absent ankle and knee reflexes
Weight	Normal for height, age, and body build	Overweight or underweight

Character of General Intake

Several questions may be necessary to elicit the information needed. When attempting to elicit information about the type and quantity of food eaten at a particular time, the interviewer avoids leading questions, such as, "Do you use sugar or cream in your coffee?" Also, assumptions are not made about the size of servings; instead, questions are phrased so that quantities are more clearly determined. For example, to help determine the size of one hamburger eaten, the patient may be asked, "How many servings were prepared with the pound of meat you bought?" Another approach to determining quantities is to use food models of known sizes in estimating portions of meat, cake, or pie or to record quantities in common measurements, such as cups or spoonfuls (or according to the size of containers, when discussing intake of bottled beverages).

In recording a particular combination dish, such as a casserole, it is useful to ask for the ingredients in the recipe, recording the largest quantities first. When recording quantities of ingredients, one notes whether the food item was raw or cooked and the number of servings provided by the recipe. When the client lists the foods for the recall questionnaire, it may be helpful to read back the list of foods and ask if anything was forgotten, such as fruit, cake, candy, between-meal snacks, or alcoholic beverages.

Additional information obtained during the interview should include methods of preparing food, sources available for food (donated foods, food stamps), food-buying practices, vitamin and mineral supplements, and income range.

Cultural and Religious Considerations

An individual's culture determines to a large extent which foods are eaten and how they are prepared and served. Culture and religious practices together often determine if certain foods are prohibited and if certain foods and spices are eaten on certain holidays or at specific family gatherings. Because of the importance of culture and religious beliefs to many individuals, it is important to be sensitive to these factors when obtaining a dietary history. It

is, however, equally important not to stereotype individuals and assume that because they are from a certain culture or religious group, they adhere to specific dietary customs.

Culturally sensitive materials, such as the food pagoda, are available for making appropriate dietary recommendations (The Chinese Nutrition Society, 1999).

EVALUATING THE DIETARY INFORMATION

After the dietary information has been obtained, the nurse evaluates the patient's dietary intake. If the goal is to determine if the person generally eats a healthful diet, the food intake may be compared to the dietary guidelines outlined in the USDA's Food Guide Pyramid (Fig. 5-7). The pyramid divides foods into five major groups and offers recommendations for variety in the diet, proportion of food from each food group, and moderation in eating fats, oils, and sweets. The person's food intake is compared with recommendations based on various food groups for various age levels.

If the nurse or dietitian is interested in knowing about the intake of specific nutrients, such as vitamin A, iron, or calcium, the patient's food intake is analyzed by consulting a list of foods and their composition and nutrient content. The diet is then analyzed in terms of grams and milligrams of specific nutrients. The total nutritive value is then compared with the recommended dietary allowances that are specific for different age categories, gender, and special circumstances such as pregnancy or lactation (Monsen, 2000). The nurse frequently participates in the nutrition screening of patients and communicates the information to the dietitian and the rest of the team for more detailed assessment and for clinical nutrition intervention.

FACTORS INFLUENCING NUTRITIONAL STATUS IN VARIED SITUATIONS

One sensitive indicator of the body's gain or loss of protein is its nitrogen balance. An adult is said to be in nitrogen equilibrium when the nitrogen intake (from food) equals the nitrogen output

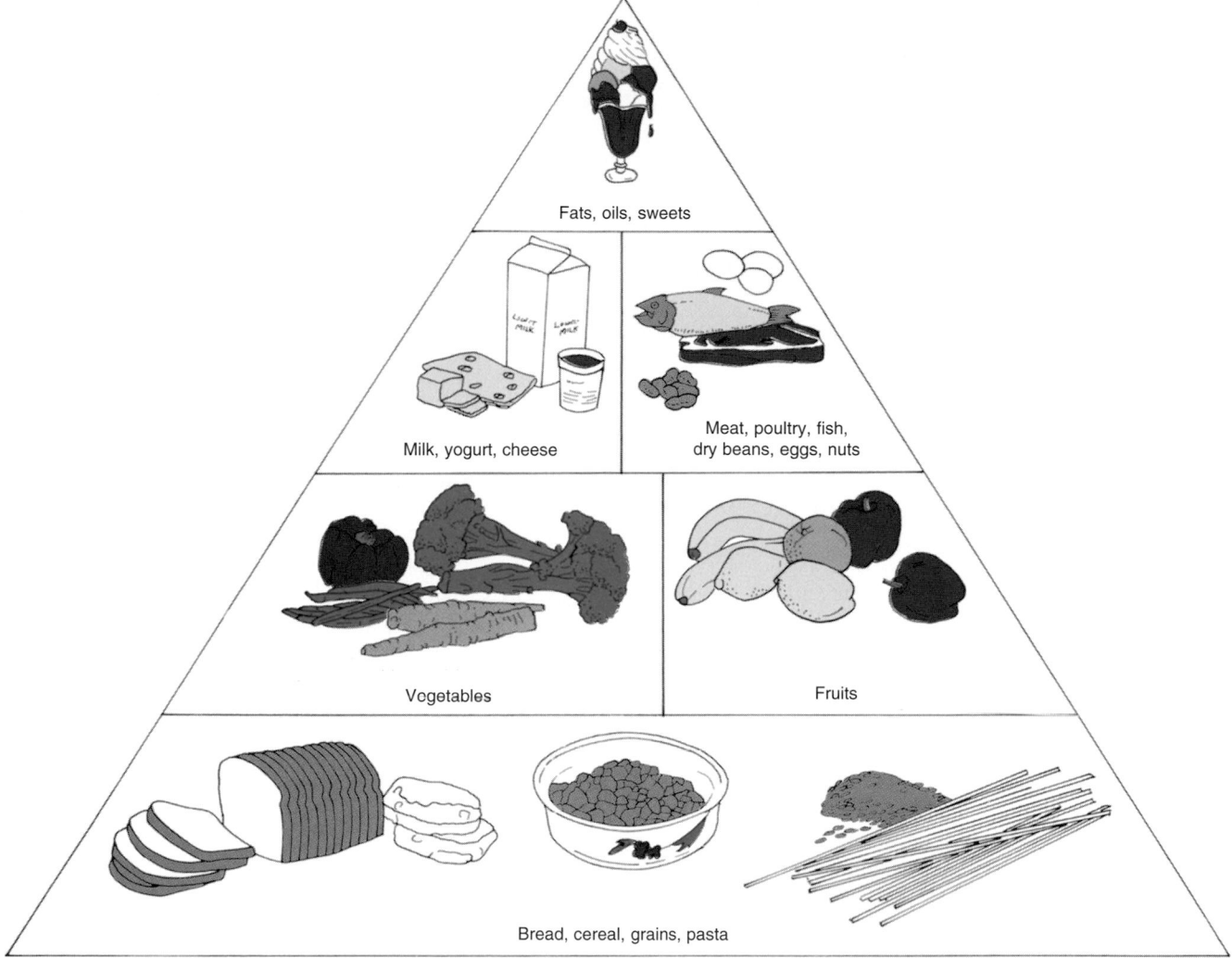

Fats, oils, sweets

Milk, yogurt, cheese

Meat, poultry, fish, dry beans, eggs, nuts

Vegetables

Fruits

Bread, cereal, grains, pasta

FIGURE 5-7 The Food Guide Pyramid emphasizes foods from the five major food groups shown in the three lower sections of the pyramid. Each of these food groups provides some, but not all, of the nutrients an adult needs. Foods in one group cannot replace those in another. No one of these major food groups is more important than another. To receive adequate vitamins, minerals, carbohydrates, and protein, an average adult should eat at least the lowest number of servings from the five major groups. Examples of 1 serving of a food group follow: **Fats and sweets:** use sparingly; **milk, yogurt, cheese** *(dairy)*: 1 C milk or yogurt, 1½ oz natural cheese, 2 oz processed cheese; **meat, poultry, fish, dry beans, eggs, nuts** *(proteins)*: ½ C cooked beans, 1 egg, 2 to 3 oz cooked lean meat, poultry or fish (2 T peanut butter = 1 oz cooked lean meat); **vegetables:** 1 C raw leafy vegetables, ½ C other vegetables (cooked or chopped, raw), ¾ C vegetable juice; **fruits:** 1 medium apple, banana, orange, ½ C chopped or cooked or canned fruit, ¾ C fruit juice; **bread, cereal, rice, pasta:** 1 slice bread, 1 oz ready-to-eat cereal, ½ C cooked cereal, rice or pasta. Source: U.S. Department of Agriculture/U.S. Department of Health and Human Services.

(in urine, feces, and perspiration); it is a sign of health. A positive nitrogen balance exists when nitrogen intake exceeds nitrogen output and indicates tissue growth, such as occurs during pregnancy, childhood, recovery from surgery, and rebuilding of wasted tissue. Negative nitrogen balance indicates that tissue is breaking down faster than it is being replaced. In the absence of an adequate intake of protein, the body converts protein to glucose for energy. This can occur with fever, starvation, surgery, burns, and debilitating diseases. Each gram of nitrogen loss in excess of intake represents the depletion of 6.25 g of protein or 25 g of muscle tissue. Therefore, a negative nitrogen balance of 10 g/day for 10 days could mean the wasting of 2.5 kg (5.5 lb) of muscle tissue as it is converted to glucose for energy.

When conditions that result in negative nitrogen balance are coupled with anorexia (loss of appetite), they can lead to mal-

nutrition. Malnutrition interferes with wound healing, increases susceptibility to infection, and contributes to an increased incidence of complications, longer hospital stay, and prolonged confinement of the patient to bed (Bender, Pusateri, Cook et al., 2000).

The patient who is hospitalized may have an inadequate dietary intake because of the illness or disorder that necessitated the hospital stay or because the hospital's food is unfamiliar or unappealing (Dudek, 2000; Wilkes, 2000). The person who is cared for at home may feel too sick or fatigued to shop and prepare food or may be unable to eat because of other physical problems or limitations. Limited or fixed incomes or the high costs of medications may result in insufficient money to buy nutritious foods. Patients with inadequate housing or inadequate cooking facilities are unlikely to have an adequate nutritional intake.

Because complex treatments (eg, ventilators, intravenous infusions, chemotherapy) once used only in the hospital setting are now being provided in the home and outpatient settings, nutritional assessment of the patient in these settings is an important aspect of home and community-based care as well as hospital-based care (Dabrowski & Rombeau, 2000; Worthington, Gilbert & Wagner, 2000).

Many medications influence nutritional status by suppressing the appetite, irritating the mucosa, or causing nausea and vomiting. Others may influence bacterial flora in the intestine or directly affect nutrient absorption so that secondary malnutrition results. People who must take many medications in a single day often report feeling too full to eat. The person's use of prescription and over-the-counter medications and their effect on appetite and dietary intake are assessed. Many of the factors that contribute to poor nutritional status are identified in Table 5-3.

ANALYSIS OF NUTRITIONAL STATUS

Measurement of BMI and biochemical, clinical, and dietary data are used together to determine the patient's nutritional status. Often the BMI, biochemical measures, and dietary data provide more information about the patient's nutritional status than the clinical examination; the clinical examination may not detect subclinical deficiencies unless such deficiencies become so advanced that overt signs develop. A low intake of nutrients over a period of time may lead to low biochemical levels and without nutritional intervention may result in characteristic and observable signs and symptoms (see Table 5-2). A plan of action for nutritional intervention is based on the results of the dietary assessment and the patient's profile. To be effective, the plan must meet the patient's need for a balanced diet, maintain or control weight, and compensate for increased nutritional needs.

Adolescent Considerations

Adolescence is a time of critical growth and acquisition of lifelong eating habits, and therefore nutritional assessment and analysis are critical. In the past two decades the percentage of adolescents who are overweight has almost tripled (USDHHS, 2001). Despite this, total milk consumption has decreased by 36% compared to prior years (Cavadini, Siega-Riz & Popkin, 2000). Fruit and vegetable consumption is also below the recommended five servings per day.

Adolescent girls are at particular nutritional risk as iron, folate, and calcium intake is below recommended levels (Cavadini, Siega-Riz & Popkin, 2000). Persons with other nutritional disorders, such as anorexia and bulimia, have a better chance for recovery if these disorders are identified in the adolescent years compared to adulthood (Orbanic, 2001).

Assessment in the Home and Community

Assessment of the person in community settings, including the home, consists of collecting information specific to existing health problems, including the patient's physiologic and emotional status, the community and home environment, the adequacy of support systems or care given by family and other care providers, and the availability of needed resources. In addition, the ability of the individual and family to cope with and address their respective needs is evaluated. The physical assessment in the community and home consists of the same techniques used in the

Table 5-3 • Factors Associated With Potential Nutritional Deficits

FACTORS	POSSIBLE CONSEQUENCES
Dental and oral problems (missing teeth, ill-fitting dentures, impaired swallowing or chewing)	Inadequate intake of high-fiber foods
NPO for diagnostic testing	Inadequate caloric and protein intake; dehydration
Prolonged use of glucose and saline IV fluids	Inadequate caloric and protein intake
Nausea and vomiting	Inadequate caloric and protein intake; loss of fluid, electrolytes, and minerals
Stress of illness, surgery, and/or hospitalization	Increased protein and caloric requirement; increased catabolism
Wound drainage	Loss of protein, fluid, electrolytes, and minerals
Pain	Loss of appetite; inability to shop, cook, eat
Fever	Increased caloric and fluid requirement; increased catabolism
Gastrointestinal intubation	Loss of protein, fluid, and minerals
Tube feedings	Inadequate amounts; various nutrients in each formula
Gastrointestinal disease	Inadequate intake and malabsorption of nutrients
Alcoholism	Inadequate intake of nutrients; increased consumption of calories without other nutrients; vitamin deficiencies
Depression	Loss of appetite; inability to shop, cook, eat
Eating disorders (anorexia, bulimia)	Inadequate caloric and protein intake; loss of fluid, electrolytes, and minerals
Medications	Inadequate intake due to medication side effects, such as dry mouth, loss of appetite, decreased taste perception, difficulty swallowing, nausea and vomiting, physical problems that limit shopping, cooking, eating; malabsorption of nutrients
Restricted ambulation or disability	Inability to help self to food, liquids, other nutrients

 *Gerontologic Considerations*

Between 5% and 10% of community-dwelling elderly are estimated to be malnourished, and the prevalence ranges from 30% to 60% in home-bound or elderly living in retirement homes (Griep, Mets, Colly et al., 2000). Elderly people who are malnourished tend to have longer and more expensive hospital stays than those who are adequately nourished; the risk of costly complications is also increased in those who are malnourished (Bender et al., 2000; Braunschweig, Gomez & Sheean, 2000; Cammon & Hackshaw, 2000).

Inadequate dietary intake in the elderly may result from physiologic changes in the gastrointestinal tract, social and economic factors, drug interactions, disease, excessive use of alcohol, and poor dentition or missing teeth. Malnutrition is a common consequence of these factors and in turn leads to illness and frailty of the elderly. Important aspects of care of the elderly in the hospital, home, outpatient setting, or extended care facility include recognizing risk factors and identifying those at risk for inadequate nutrition (Bender et al., 2000; Cammon & Hackshaw, 2000; Morley, 2000).

Many elderly people take excessive and inappropriate medications; this is referred to as polypharmacy. The number of adverse reactions increases proportionately with the number of prescribed and over-the-counter medications taken. Age-related physiologic and pathophysiologic changes may alter the metabolism and elimination of many medications. Medications can influence food intake by producing side effects such as nausea, vomiting, decreased appetite, and changes in sensorium (Morley, 2000). They may also interfere with the distribution, utilization, and storage of nutrients. Disorders affecting any part of the gastrointestinal tract can alter nutritional requirements and health status in people of any age; however, they are likely to occur quickly and more frequently in the elderly.

Nutritional problems in the elderly often occur or are precipitated by such illnesses as pneumonia and urinary tract infections. Acute and chronic diseases may affect the metabolism and utilization of nutrients, which already are altered by the aging process. Flu and pneumonia immunizations, prompt treatment of bacterial infections, and social programs such as Meals on Wheels may reduce the risk of illness-associated malnutrition.

Even the well elderly may be nutritionally at risk because of decreased odor perception, poor dental health, limited ability to shop and cook, financial hardship, and the fact that they often eat alone (Griep, Mets, Colly et al., 2000). Also, reduction in exercise with age without concomitant changes in carbohydrate intake places the elderly at risk for obesity. Nutritional screening in the elderly is a first step in maintaining adequate nutrition and replacing nutrient losses to maintain the individual's health and well being.

hospital, outpatient clinic, or office setting. Privacy is provided and the person is made as comfortable as possible.

A call made to the patient's home before the first home visit lets the patient know when to expect the home care nurse and also provides the opportunity for the patient's primary caregiver to be available. During the home visit, the nurse's assessment is not limited to physical assessment of the patient. Other aspects of assessment include the home environment, safety factors (eg, smoke alarms, obstacles, safety bars in the bathroom), adequacy of facilities required for the patient's care and recovery, food preparation and storage facilities, bathroom facilities, access to a telephone, and the availability of family and community supports. Because patients may have no family members

available to assist them and may live alone in substandard housing or homeless shelters, the nurse needs to be aware of resources available in the community and methods of obtaining those resources for the patient. Figure 5-8 provides an example of a checklist that may be useful in conducting an assessment in the home.

Physical Facilities (check all that apply)
Exterior
- [ ] steps_____
- [ ] unsafe steps_____
- [ ] porch_____
- [ ] litter_____
- [ ] noise_____
- [ ] inadequate lighting_____
- [ ] other_____

Interior
- [ ] accessible bathroom_____
- [ ] level, safe floor surface_____
- [ ] number of rooms_____
- [ ] privacy_____
- [ ] sleeping arrangements_____
- [ ] refrigeration_____
- [ ] trash management_____
- [ ] animals_____
- [ ] adequate lighting_____
- [ ] steps/stairs_____
- [ ] other_____

_____

Safety Hazards found in the patient's current residence (check all that apply)

- [ ] none
- [ ] inadequate floor, roof, or windows
- [ ] inadequate lighting
- [ ] unsafe gas/electric appliances
- [ ] inadequate heating
- [ ] inadequate cooling
- [ ] lack of fire safety devices
- [ ] unsafe floor coverings
- [ ] inadequate stair rails
- [ ] lead-based paint
- [ ] improperly stored hazardous material
- [ ] improper wiring/electrical cords
- [ ] other_____

_____

Safety Factors (check all that apply)
- [ ] smoke/fire detectors_____
- [ ] telephone_____
- [ ] placement of electrical cords_____
- [ ] emergency plan_____

_____
- [ ] emergency phone numbers displayed_____
- [ ] safe portable heaters_____
- [ ] obstacle-free paths_____
- [ ] other_____

_____

FIGURE 5-8 Home assessment checklist.

Critical Thinking Exercises

1. Compare the approach and techniques you would use in assessing a patient who is experiencing severe abdominal pain. How would your approach and technique differ if your patient has dementia? If your patient has dementia and is blind or hard of hearing? If your patient is from a culture with very different values from yours?

2. Your health history and physical examination of an elderly patient alerts you to the possibility of abuse. Explain how you would pursue this further. What assessments are available to assist in assessing this in a more comprehensive manner?

3. You are conducting a health history on a patient who is admitted to the emergency room after he was hit by a car while walking down the center of a major street at 10 PM. He is responsive and able to talk and has no apparent major physical injuries. The ambulance crew that brought him to the emergency room tells you that the patient has probably been drinking. How would this history affect your assessment? How would you assess history of alcohol use in an emergency room setting? How would you do so in a patient in a primary care office? Explain the rationale for your responses.

4. Your nutritional assessment reveals that a female adolescent patient has a high fat intake and minimal calcium intake. What dietary recommendations would you make for this client? What dietary instructions would you develop for her if she is a vegetarian?

5. You have received a referral for home care for a 75-year-old patient who has recently had a stroke and who lives alone in a travel trailer. What physical and environmental factors are important to assess on the initial home visit? Identify the elements in the home that would be safety hazards and those that would be safety factors.

REFERENCES AND SELECTED READINGS

Books and Pamphlets

American Heart Association. (2000). *An eating plan for healthy Americans: Our American Heart Association Diet*. Dallas, TX: Author.

Bickley, L. S., & Szilagyi, P. G. (2003). *Bates' guide to physical examination and history taking* (8th ed.). Philadelphia: Lippincott Williams & Wilkins.

Dudek, S. G. (2001). *Nutrition essentials for nursing practice* (4th ed.). Philadelphia: Lippincott Williams & Wilkins.

Food and Nutrition Board, Institutes of Medicine. (2002). *Dietary reference intakes for energy, carbohydrates, fiber, fat, protein and amino acids (macronutrients): A report of the Panel on Micronutrients, Subcommittees on Upper Reference Levels of Nutrients and Interpretation and Uses of Dietary Reference Intakes, and the Standing Committee on the Scientific Evaluation of Dietary Reference Intakes*. Washington, DC: National Academy Press.

Fuller, J., & Schaller-Ayers, J. (2000). *Health assessment: A nursing approach* (3rd ed.). Philadelphia: Lippincott Williams & Wilkins.

Kuhn, M. (1999). *Complementary therapies for health care providers*. Philadelphia: Lippincott Williams & Wilkins.

National Institutes of Health, National Heart, Lung and Blood Institute, North American Association for the Study of Obesity. (2000). *The practical guide: Identification, evaluation, and treatment of over-*
weight and obesity in adults. NIH Publication Number 00-4084. Bethesda, MD: NIH.

Orient, J. (2000). *Sapira's art and science of bedside diagnosis* (2nd ed.). Philadelphia: Lippincott Williams & Wilkins.

Ross, M., Channon-Little, L., & Rosser, S. (2000). *Sexual health concerns: Interviewing and history taking for health practitioners* (2nd ed.). Philadelphia: F. A. Davis.

United States Department of Agriculture, United States Department of Health and Human Services. *Nutrition and your health: Dietary guidelines for Americans* (5th ed). Bull. No. 232:39.

United States Department of Health and Human Services. (2001). *The Surgeon General's call to action to prevent and decrease overweight and obesity*. Rockville, MD: USDHHS, PHS.

Weber, J., & Kelley, J. (2003). *Health assessment in nursing* (2nd ed.). Philadelphia: Lippincott Williams & Wilkins.

Journals

An asterisk indicates a nursing research article.

General Assessment

Bakshi, S., & Miller, D. (1999). Assessment of the aging man. *Medical Clinics of North America, 83*(5), 1131–1149.

Butler, R. (1999). The 15-minute geriatric assessment. *Geriatrics, 54*(7), 3.

Evans, V. (2000). Herbs and the brain: Friend or foe? *Journal of Neuroscience Nursing, 32*(4), 229–232.

Fiellin, D. A., Reid, M. C., & O'Connor, P. G. Screening for alcohol problems in primary care: A systematic review. *Archives of Internal Medicine, 160*(13), 1977–1989.

Goolsby, M. (2001). Evaluating acute musculoskeletal complaints. *Journal of the American Academy of Nurse Practitioners, 13*(5), 195–199.

Henderson-Martin, B. (2000). No more surprises: Screening patients for alcohol abuse. *American Journal of Nursing, 100*(9), 26–32.

Isaacson, J. H., & Schorling, J. B. (1999). Screening for alcohol problems in primary care. *Medical Clinics of North America, 83*(6), 1547–1563.

King, M., Pettigrew, A., & Reed, F. (1999). Complementary, alternative, integrative: Have nurses kept pace with their clients? *MedSurg Nursing, 8*(4), 239–246.

Kushner, R., & Weinsier, R. (2000). Evaluation of the obese patient. *Medical Clinics of North America, 84*(2), 387–399.

Little, K. (2000). Screening for domestic violence. *Postgraduate Medicine, 108*(2), 135–141.

Ludwick, R., Dieckman, B., & Snelson, C. (1999). Assessment of the geriatric orthopedic trauma patient. *Orthopedic Nursing, 13–18.

Marshall, C., Benton, D., & Brazier, J. (2000). Elder abuse: Using clinical tools to identify clues of mistreatment. *Geriatrics, 55*(2), 42–53.

Mathre, M. L. (2001). Therapeutic cannabis: A patient advocacy issue. *American Journal of Nursing, 101*(4), 61–68.

Miller, K., Zylstra, R., & Standridge, J. (2000). The geriatric patient: A systematic approach to maintaining health. *American Family Physician, 61*(4), 1089–1104

Palmer, R. (1999). Geriatric assessment. *Medical Clinics of North America, 83*(6), 1503–1520.

Walton, J., Miller, J., & Tordecilla, L. (2001). Elder oral assessment and care. *MedSurg Nursing, 10*(1), 37–44.

Nutritional Assessment

Bender, S., Pusateri, M., Cook, A., et al. (2000). Malnutrition: Role of the TwoCal HN med pass program. *MedSurg Nursing, 9*(6), 284–296.

Braunschweig, C., Gomez, S., & Sheean, P. (2000). Impact of declines in nutritional status on outcomes in adult patients hospitalized for more than 7 days. *Journal of the American Dietetic Association, 100*(11), 1316–1322.

Cammon, S., & Hackshaw, H. (2000). Are we starving our patients? *American Journal of Nursing, 100*(5), 43–47.

Cavadini, C., Siega-Riz, A. M., & Popkin, B. (2000). U.S. adolescent food intake trends from 1965 to 1996. *Archives of Diseases of Children, 83*(1), 18–24.

Dabrowski, C., & Rombeau, J. (2000). Practical nutritional management in the trauma intensive care unit. *Surgical Clinics of North America, 80*(3), 921–931.

Dudek, S. (2000). Malnutrition in hospitals: Who's assessing what patients eat? *American Journal of Nursing, 100*(4), 36–43.

*Griep, M., Mets, T., Colly, K., et al. (2000). Risk of malnutrition in retirement homes elderly persons measured by the "Mini-nutritional assessment." *Journal of Gerontology: Medical Sciences, 55A*(2), M57–M63.

Hensrud, D. (1999). Nutrition screening and assessment. *Medical Clinics of North America, 83*(6), 1525–1543.

Kant, A., Schatzkin, A., Graubard, B., & Schairer, C. (2000). A prospective study of diet quality and mortality in women. *JAMA, 283*(16), 2109–2115.

Kennedy, E., & Davis, C. (2000). Dietary guidelines 2000: The opportunity and challenges for reaching the consumer. *Journal of the American Dietetic Association, 100*(12), 1462–1465.

Landi, F., Onder, G., Gambassi, G., et al. (2000). Body mass index and mortality among hospitalized patients. *Archives of Internal Medicine, 160,* 2641–2644.

Landi, F., Zuccala, G., Gambassi, G., et al. (1999). Body mass index and mortality among older people living in the community. *Journal of the American Geriatrics Society, 47,* 1072–1076.

Monsen, E. (2000). Dietary reference intakes for the antioxidant nutrients: Vitamin C, vitamin E, selenium, and carotenoids. *Journal of the American Dietetic Association, 100*(6), 637–640.

Morley, J. (2000). Management of nutritional problems in subacute care. *Clinics in Geriatric Medicine, 16*(4), 817–829.

Orbanic, S. (2001). Understanding bulimia. *American Journal of Nursing, 101*(3), 35–42.

Stampfer, M., Hu, F., Manson, J., et al. (2000). Primary prevention of coronary heart disease in women through diet and lifestyle. *New England Journal of Medicine, 343*(1), 16–22.

The Chinese Nutrition Society. (1999). Dietary guidelines and the food guide pagoda for Chinese residents: Balanced diet, rational nutrition, and health promotion. *Nutrition Today, 34*(3), 106–115.

Wilkes, G. (2000). Nutrition: The forgotten ingredient in cancer care. *American Journal of Nursing, 100*(4), 46–51.

Worthington, P., Gilbert, K., & Wagner, B. (2000). Parenteral nutrition for the acutely ill. *AACN Clinical Issues, 11*(4), 559–579.

RESOURCES AND WEBSITES

The Alliance of Cannabis Therapeutics, http://marijuana-as-medicine.org/alliance.htm.

American Dietetic Association, 216 W. Jackson Blvd., Suite 800, Chicago, IL 60606; Consumer Nutrition Hotline: 800-366-1655; http://www.eatright.org.

American Heart Association, 7320 Greenville Ave., Dallas, TX 75231; National Center: 214-373-6300, Nutrition Information: 214-706-1179; http://www.americanheart.org.

National Cancer Institute, Cancer Information Service, 9000 Rockville Pike, Bldg. 31, Room 10A-24, Bethesda, MD 20892; 1-800-4-CANCER; http://www.nci.nih.gov, http://www.ncu.nih.gov/hpage/cis.htm.

Nutrition Screening Initiative, P.O. Box 753, Waldorf, MD 20604; 202-625-1662, http://www.fiu.edu/~nutreld/NSI.html.

Pennsylvania State Nutrition Center, The Pennsylvania State University, Ruth Building, 417 E. Calder Way, University Park, PA 16802; 814-865-6323.

Biophysical and Psychosocial Concepts in Nursing Practice

Applying Concepts from NANDA, NIC, and NOC

Mr. Hussein is a 38-year-old man who comes to the emergency department (ED) for treatment of high blood pressure. On his previous visit to the ED he reported chest pressure, feelings of numbness and tingling in his arms, and extreme fearfulness that he was having a heart attack. Even though a myocardial infarction was ruled out and subsequent testing revealed that he had no heart disease, Mr. Hussein continues to have feelings of chest pressure and fear that he is having a heart attack. The only abnormal finding has been an elevation of blood pressure (158/88). The nurse interviews Mr. Hussein, who reveals he is under intense financial pressure. The nurse assesses his compliance with his antihypertensive therapy and suggests interventions to help with Mr. Hussein's anxiety. The concept map illustrates the relationships that exist among selected diagnoses, interventions, and outcomes.

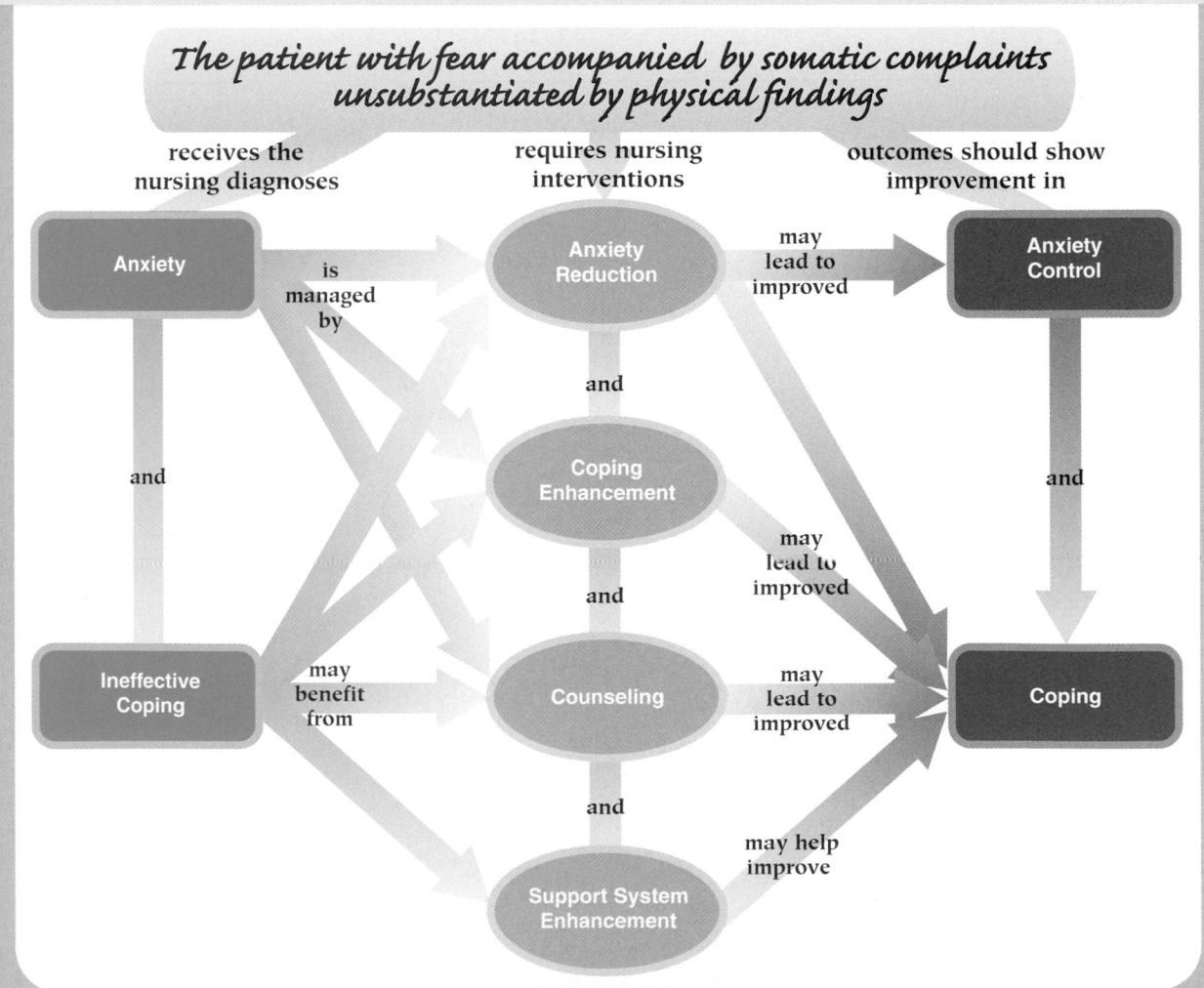

The patient with fear accompanied by somatic complaints unsubstantiated by physical findings

Nursing Classifications and Languages

NANDA
Nursing Diagnoses

Anxiety—Vague uneasy feeling of discomfort or dread accompanied by an autonomic response (the source often nonspecific or unknown to the individual); a feeling of apprehension caused by anticipation of danger. It is an alerting signal that warns of impending danger and enables the individual to take measures to deal with threat.

Ineffective Coping—Inability to perform a valid appraisal of the stressors, inadequate choices of practiced responses, and/or inability to use available resources

NIC
Nursing Interventions*

Anxiety Reduction—Minimizing apprehension, dread, foreboding, or uneasiness related to unidentified source of anticipated danger

Coping Enhancement—Assisting a person to adapt to perceived stressors, changes, or threats that interfere with meeting life demands and roles

Counseling—Use of an interactive helping process focusing on the needs, problems, or feelings of the patient and significant others to enhance or support coping, problem-solving, and interpersonal relationships

Support System Enhancement—Facilitation of support to patient by family, friends, and community

NOC
Nursing Outcomes†

Return to functional baseline status, stabilization of, or improvement in

Anxiety Control—Personal actions to eliminate or reduce feelings of apprehension and tension from an unidentifiable source

Coping—Actions to manage stressors that tax an individual's resources

NANDA, North American Nursing Diagnosis Association; NIC, Nursing Interventions Classification; NOC, Nursing Outcomes Classification

*Iowa Intervention Project © 2000. In McCloskey, J. C., & Bulechek, G. M. (2000). *Nursing interventions classification (NIC)* (3rd ed.). St. Louis: Mosby.

†Iowa Outcomes Project © 2000. In Johnson, M., Maas, M., & Moorhead, S. (2000). *Nursing outcomes classification (NOC)* (3rd ed.). St. Louis: Mosby.

Homeostasis, Stress, and Adaptation

LEARNING OBJECTIVES

On completion of this chapter, the learner will be able to:

1. Relate the principles of internal constancy, homeostasis, stress, and adaptation to the concept of steady state.
2. Identify the significance of the body's compensatory mechanisms in promoting adaptation and maintaining the steady state.
3. Identify physiologic and psychosocial stressors.
4. Compare the sympathetic-adrenal-medullary response to stress to the hypothalamic-pituitary response to stress.
5. Describe the general adaptation syndrome as a theory of adaptation to biologic stress.
6. Describe the relationship of the process of negative feedback to the maintenance of the steady state.
7. Compare the adaptive processes of hypertrophy, atrophy, hyperplasia, dysplasia, and metaplasia.
8. Describe the inflammatory and reparative processes.
9. Assess the health patterns of an individual and determine their effects on maintenance of the steady state.
10. Identify ways in which maladaptive responses to stress can increase the risk of illness and cause disease.
11. Identify measures that are useful in reducing stress.
12. Specify the functions of social networks and support groups in reducing stress.

When the body is threatened or suffers an injury, its response may involve functional and structural changes; these changes may be adaptive (having a positive effect) or maladaptive (having a negative effect). The defense mechanisms that the body exhibits determine the difference between adaptation and maladaptation—health and disease.

Stress and Function

Physiology is the study of the functional activities of the living organism and its parts. Pathophysiology is the study of disordered function of the body. Each different body system performs specific functions to sustain optimal life for the organism. Mechanisms for adjusting internal conditions promote the normal steady state of the organism and ultimately its survival. These mechanisms are compensatory in nature and work to restore balance in the body. An example of this restorative effort is the development of rapid breathing (hyperpnea) after intense exercise in an attempt to compensate for an oxygen deficit and excess lactic acid accumulated in the muscle tissue.

Pathophysiologic processes result when cellular injury occurs at such a rapid rate that the body's compensatory mechanisms can no longer make the adaptive changes necessary to remain healthy. An example of a pathophysiologic change is the development of heart failure: the body reacts by retaining sodium and water and increasing venous pressure, which worsens the condition. These pathophysiologic mechanisms give rise to signs that are observed by the patient, nurse, or other health care provider, or symptoms that are reported by the patient. These observations, plus a sound knowledge of physiologic and pathophysiologic processes, can assist in determining the existence of a problem and can guide the nurse in planning the appropriate course of action.

Dynamic Balance: The Steady State

Physiologic mechanisms must be understood in the context of the body as a whole. The person, as a living system, has both an internal and an external environment, between which information

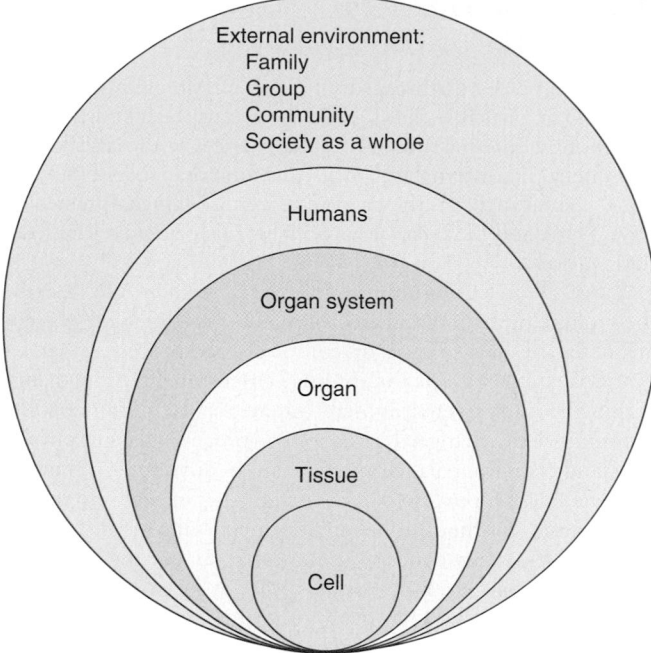

FIGURE 6-1 Constellation of systems. Each system is a subsystem of the larger system (suprasystem) of which it is a part. In this figure the cell is the smallest system, being a subsystem of all other systems.

and matter are continuously exchanged. Within the internal environment each organ, tissue, and cell is also a system or subsystem of the whole, each with its own internal and external environment, each exchanging information and matter (Fig. 6-1). The goal of the interaction of the body's subsystems is to produce a dynamic balance or **steady state** (even in the presence of change), so that all subsystems are in harmony with each other. Four concepts—constancy, homeostasis, stress, and adaptation—enhance the nurse's understanding of steady state.

Glossary

adaptation: a change or alteration designed to assist in adapting to a new situation or environment

adrenocorticotropic hormone (ACTH): a hormone produced by the anterior lobe of the pituitary gland that stimulates the secretion of cortisone and other hormones by the adrenal cortex

antidiuretic hormone (ADH): a hormone secreted by the posterior lobe of the pituitary gland that constricts blood vessels, elevates blood pressure, and reduces the excretion of urine

catecholamines: any of the group of amines (such as epinephrine, norepinephrine, or dopamine) that serve as neurotransmitters

coping: the cognitive and behavioral strategies used to manage the stressors that tax a person's resources

dysplasia: a change in the appearance of a cell after exposure to chronic irritation

glucocorticoids: the group of steroid hormones, such as cortisol, that are produced by the adrenal cortex; they are involved in carbohydrate, protein, and fat metabolism and have anti-inflammatory properties

gluconeogenesis: the formation of glucose, especially by the liver from noncarbohydrate sources such as amino acids and the glycerol portion of fats

guided imagery: use of the imagination to achieve relaxation or direct attention away from uncomfortable sensations or situations

homeostasis: a steady state within the body; the stability of the internal environment

hyperplasia: an increase in the number of new cells

hypoxia: inadequate supply of oxygen to the cell

infectious agents: biologic agents, such as viruses, bacteria, rickettsiae, mycoplasmas, fungi, protozoa, and nematodes, that cause disease in people

inflammation: a localized, protective reaction of tissue to injury, irritation, or infection, manifested by pain, redness, heat, swelling, and sometimes loss of function

metabolic rate: the speed at which some substances are broken down to yield energy for bodily processes and other substances are synthesized

metaplasia: a cell transformation in which a highly specialized cell changes to a less specialized cell

negative feedback: feedback that decreases the output of a system

positive feedback: feedback that increases the output of a system

steady state: a stable condition that does not change over time, or when change in one direction is balanced by change in an opposite direction

stress: a disruptive condition that occurs in response to adverse influences from the internal or external environments

vasoconstriction: the narrowing of a blood vessel

HISTORICAL THEORIES OF THE STEADY STATE

Claude Bernard, a 19th-century French physiologist, developed the biologic principle that for life there must be a constancy or "fixity of the internal milieu" despite changes in the external environment. The internal milieu was the fluid that bathed the cells, and the constancy was the balanced internal state maintained by physiologic and biochemical processes. His principle implied a static process.

Later, Walter Cannon used the term *homeostasis* to describe the stability of the internal environment, which, he said, was coordinated by homeostatic or compensatory processes that responded to changes in the internal environment. Any change within the internal environment initiated a "righting" response to minimize the change. These biologic processes sought physiologic and chemical balance and were under involuntary control.

Rene Jules Dubos (1965) provided further insight into the dynamic nature of the internal environment with his theory that two complementary concepts, homeostasis and adaptation, were necessary for balance. Homeostatic processes occurred quickly in response to stress, rapidly making the adjustments necessary to maintain the internal environment. Adaptive processes resulted in structural or functional changes over time. Dubos also emphasized that acceptable ranges of response to stimuli existed and that these responses varied for different individuals: "Absolute constancy is only a concept of the ideal." Homeostasis and adaptation were both necessary for survival in a changing world.

Homeostasis, then, refers to a steady state within the body. When a change or stress occurs that causes a body function to deviate from its stable range, processes are initiated to restore and maintain the dynamic balance. When these adjustment processes or compensatory mechanisms are not adequate, the steady state is threatened, function becomes disordered, and pathophysiologic mechanisms occur. The pathophysiologic processes can lead to disease and may be active during disease, which is a threat to the steady state. Disease is an abnormal variation in the structure or function of any part of the body. It disrupts function and therefore limits the person's freedom of action.

STRESS AND ADAPTATION

Stress is a state produced by a change in the environment that is perceived as challenging, threatening, or damaging to the person's dynamic balance or equilibrium. The person is, or feels, unable to meet the demands of the new situation. The change or stimulus that evokes this state is the stressor. The nature of the stressor is variable; an event or change that will produce stress in one person may be neutral for another, and an event that produces stress at one time and place for one person may not do so for the same person at another time and place. A person appraises and copes with changing situations. The desired goal is **adaptation**, or adjustment to the change so that the person is again in equilibrium and has the energy and ability to meet new demands. This is the process of **coping** with the stress, a compensatory process with physiologic and psychological components.

Adaptation is a constant, ongoing process that requires a change in structure, function, or behavior so that the person is better suited to the environment; it involves an interaction between the person and the environment. The outcome depends on the degree of "fit" between the skills and capacities of the person, the type of social support available, and the various challenges or stressors being confronted. As such, adaptation is an individual process: each individual has varying abilities to cope or respond. As new challenges are met, this ability to cope and adapt can change, thereby providing the individual with a wide range of adaptive ability. Adaptation occurs throughout the life span as the individual encounters many developmental and situational challenges, especially related to health and illness. The goal of these encounters is to promote adaptation. In situations of health and illness, this goal is realized by optimal wellness.

Because both stress and adaptation may exist at different levels of a system, it is possible to study these reactions at the cellular, tissue, and organ levels. Biologists are concerned mainly with subcellular components or with subsystems of the total body. Behavioral scientists, including many nurse researchers, study stress and adaptation in individuals, families, groups, and societies; they focus on how a group's organizational features are modified to meet the requirements of the social and physical environment in which they exist. Adaptation is a continuous process of seeking harmony in an environment. The desired goals of adaptation for any system are survival, growth, and reproduction.

Stressors: Threats to the Steady State

Each person operates at a certain level of adaptation and regularly encounters a certain amount of change. Such change is expected; it contributes to growth and enhances life. Stressors, however, can upset this equilibrium. A stressor may be defined as an internal or external event or situation that creates the potential for physiologic, emotional, cognitive, or behavioral changes in an individual.

TYPES OF STRESSORS

Stressors exist in many forms and categories. They may be described as physical, physiologic, or psychosocial. Physical stressors include cold, heat, and chemical agents; physiologic stressors include pain and fatigue. Examples of psychosocial stressors are fear of failing an examination and losing a job. Stressors can also occur as normal life transitions that require some adjustment, such as going from childhood into puberty, getting married, or giving birth.

Stressors have also been classified as: (1) day-to-day frustrations or hassles; (2) major complex occurrences involving large groups, even entire nations; and (3) stressors that occur less frequently and involve fewer people. The first group, the day-to-day stressors, includes such common occurrences as getting caught in a traffic jam, experiencing computer downtime, and having an argument with a spouse or roommate. These experiences vary in effect; for example, encountering a rainstorm while one is vacationing at the beach will most likely evoke a more negative response than it might at another time. These less dramatic, frustrating, and irritating events—daily hassles—have been shown to have a greater health impact than major life events because of the cumulative effect they have over time. They can lead to high blood pressure, palpitations, or other physiologic problems (Jalowiec, 1993).

The second group of stressors influences larger groups of people, possibly even entire nations. These include events of history, such as terrorism and war, which are threatening situations when experienced either directly, in the war zone, or indirectly, as through live news coverage. The demographic, economic, and technological changes occurring in society also serve as stressors. The tension produced by any stressor is sometimes a result not only of the change itself, but also of the speed with which the change occurs.

The third group of stressors has been studied most extensively and concerns relatively infrequent situations that directly affect the individual. This category includes the influence of life events such as death, birth, marriage, divorce, and retirement. It also includes the psychosocial crises described by Erikson as occurring in the life cycle stages of the human experience. More enduring chronic stressors have also been placed in this category and may include such things as having a permanent functional disability or coping with the difficulties of providing long-term care to a frail elderly parent.

A stressor can also be categorized according to duration. It may be

- An acute, time-limited stressor, such as studying for final examinations
- A stressor sequence—a series of stressful events that result from an initial event such as job loss or divorce
- A chronic intermittent stressor, such as daily hassles
- A chronic enduring stressor that persists over time, such as chronic illness, a disability, or poverty

STRESS AS A STIMULUS FOR DISEASE

Relating life events to illness (the theoretical approach that defines stress as a stimulus) has been a major focus of psychosocial studies. This can be traced to Adolph Meyer, who in the 1930s observed in "life charts" of his patients a linkage between illnesses and critical life events. Subsequent research revealed that people under constant stress have a high incidence of psychosomatic disease.

Holmes and Rahe (1967) developed life events scales that assign numerical values, called life-change units, to typical life events. Because the items in the scales reflect events that require a change in a person's life pattern, and stress is defined as an accumulation of changes in one's life that require psychological adaptation, one can theoretically predict the likelihood of illness by checking off the number of recent events and deriving a total score. The Recent Life Changes Questionnaire (Tausig, 1982) contains 118 items such as death, birth, marriage, divorce, promotions, serious arguments, and vacations. The events listed include both desirable and undesirable circumstances.

Sources of stress for patients have been well researched (Ballard, 1981; Bryla, 1996; Jalowiec, 1993). People typically experience distress related to alterations in their physical and emotional health status, changes in their level of daily functioning, and decreased social support or the loss of significant others. Fears of immobilization, isolation, loneliness, sensory changes, financial problems, and death or disability increase a person's anxiety level. Loss of one's role or perceived purpose in life can cause intense discomfort. Any of these identified variables plus a myriad of other conditions or overwhelming demands are likely to cause ineffective coping, and a lack of necessary coping skills is often a source of additional distress for an individual. When a person endures prolonged or unrelenting suffering, the outcome is frequently the development of a stress-related illness. Nurses possess the skills to assist people to alter their distressing circumstances and manage their responses to stress.

PSYCHOLOGICAL RESPONSES TO STRESS

After the recognition of a stressor, an individual consciously or unconsciously reacts to manage the situation. This is called the mediating process. A theory developed by Lazarus (1991a) emphasizes cognitive appraisal and coping as important mediators of stress. Appraisal and coping are influenced by antecedent variables that include the internal and external resources of the person.

Appraisal of the Stressful Event

Cognitive appraisal (Lazarus, 1991a; Lazarus & Folkman, 1984) is a process by which an event is evaluated with respect to what is at stake (primary appraisal) and what might and can be done (secondary appraisal). What individuals see as being at stake is influenced by their personal goals, commitments, or motivations. Important factors include how important or relevant the event is to them, whether the event conflicts with what they want or desire, and whether the situation threatens their own sense of strength and ego identity.

As an outcome of primary appraisal, the situation is identified as either nonstressful or stressful. If nonstressful, the situation is irrelevant or benign (positive). A stressful situation may be one of three kinds: (1) one in which harm or loss has occurred; (2) one that is threatening, in that harm or loss is anticipated; and (3) one that is challenging, in that some opportunity or gain is anticipated.

Secondary appraisal is an evaluation of what might and can be done about this situation Actions include assigning blame to those responsible for a frustrating event, thinking about whether one can do something about the situation (coping potential), and determining future expectancy, or whether things are likely to change for better or worse (Lazarus, 1991a, 1991c). A comparison of what is at stake and what can be done about it (a type of risk–benefit analysis) determines the degree of stress.

Reappraisal, a change of opinion based on new information, also occurs. The appraisal process is not necessarily sequential; primary and secondary appraisal and reappraisal may occur simultaneously. Information learned from an adaptational encounter can be stored, so that when a similar situation is encountered again the whole process does not need to be repeated.

The appraisal process contributes to the development of an emotion. Negative emotions such as fear and anger accompany harm/loss appraisals, and positive emotions accompany challenge. In addition to the subjective component or feeling that accompanies a particular emotion, each emotion also includes a tendency to act in a certain way. For example, an unexpected quiz in the classroom might be judged as threatening by unprepared students. They might feel fear, anger, and resentment and might express these emotions outwardly with hostile behavior or comments.

Lazarus (1991a) expanded his former ideas about stress, appraisal, and coping into a more complex model relating emotion to adaptation. He called this model a "cognitive-motivational-relational theory," with the term *relational* "standing for a focus on negotiation with a physical and social world" (p. 13). A theory of emotion was proposed as the bridge to connect psychology, physiology, and sociology: "More than any other arena of psychological thought, emotion is an integrative, organismic concept that subsumes psychological stress and coping within itself and unites motivation, cognition, and adaptation in a complex configuration" (p. 40).

Coping With the Stressful Event

Coping, according to Lazarus, consists of the cognitive and behavioral efforts made to manage the specific external or internal demands that tax a person's resources and may be emotion-focused or problem-focused. Coping that is emotion focused seeks to make the person feel better by lessening the emotional distress felt. Problem-focused coping aims to make direct changes in the environment so that the situation can be managed more effectively. Both types of coping usually occur in a stressful situation. Even if the situation is viewed as challenging or beneficial, coping efforts may be required to develop and sustain the challenge—that is, to maintain the positive benefits of the challenge and to ward off any threats. In harmful or threatening situations, successful coping reduces or eliminates the source of stress and relieves the emotion it generated.

Appraisal and coping are affected by internal characteristics such as health, energy, personal belief systems, commitments or life goals, self-esteem, control, mastery, knowledge, problem-solving skills, and social skills. The characteristics that have been studied most often in nursing research are health-promoting lifestyles and hardiness. A health-promoting lifestyle buffers the effect of stressors. From a nursing practice standpoint, this outcome—buffering the effect of stressors—supports nursing's goal of promoting health. In many circumstances, promoting a healthy lifestyle is more achievable than altering the stressors.

Hardiness is the name given to a general quality that comes from having rich, varied, and rewarding experiences. It is a personality characteristic composed of control, commitment, and challenge. Hardy people perceive stressors as something they can change and therefore control. To them, potentially stressful situations are interesting and meaningful; change and new situations are viewed as challenging opportunities for growth. Some positive support has been found for hardiness as a significant variable that positively influences rehabilitation and overall improvement after an onset of an acute or chronic illness (Felton, 2000; Williams, 2000).

PHYSIOLOGIC RESPONSE TO STRESS

The physiologic response to a stressor, whether it is a physical stressor or a psychological stressor, is a protective and adaptive mechanism to maintain the homeostatic balance of the body. The stress response is a "cascade of neural and hormonal events that have short- and long-lasting consequences for both brain and body . . .; a stressor is an event that challenges homeostasis, with a disease outcome being looked upon as a failure of the normal process of adaptation to the stress" (McEwen & Mendelson, 1993, p. 101).

The General Adaptation Syndrome

Hans Selye developed a theory of adaptation that profoundly influenced the scientific study of stress. In 1936, Selye, experimenting with animals, first described a syndrome consisting of enlargement of the adrenal cortex; shrinkage of the thymus, spleen, lymph nodes, and other lymphatic structures; and the appearance of deep, bleeding ulcers in the stomach and duodenum. He identified this as a nonspecific response to diverse, noxious stimuli. From this beginning, he developed a theory of adaptation to biologic stress that he named the general adaptation syndrome.

PHASES OF THE GENERAL ADAPTATION SYNDROME

The general adaptation syndrome has three phases: alarm, resistance, and exhaustion. During the alarm phase, the sympathetic "fight-or-flight" response is activated with release of **catecholamines** and the onset of the **adrenocorticotropic hormone (ACTH)**–adrenal cortical response. The alarm reaction is defensive and anti-inflammatory but self-limited. Because living in a continuous state of alarm would result in death, the person moves

into the second stage, resistance. During this stage, adaptation to the noxious stressor occurs, and cortisol activity is still increased. If exposure to the stressor is prolonged, exhaustion sets in and endocrine activity increases. This produces deleterious effects on the body systems (especially the circulatory, digestive, and immune systems) that can lead to death. Stages one and two of this syndrome are repeated, in different degrees, throughout life as the person encounters stressors.

Selye compared the general adaptation syndrome with the life process. During childhood, there are too few encounters with stress to promote the development of adaptive functioning, and the child is vulnerable. During adulthood, the person encounters a number of life's stressful events and develops a resistance or adaptation. During the later years, the accumulation of life's stressors and the wear and tear on the organism again deplete the person's ability to adapt, resistance falls, and eventually death occurs.

LOCAL ADAPTATION SYNDROME

According to Selye's theory, a local adaptation syndrome also occurs. This syndrome includes the inflammatory response and repair processes that occur at the local site of tissue injury. The local adaptation syndrome occurs in small, topical injuries, such as contact dermatitis. If the local injury is severe enough, the general adaptation syndrome is activated as well.

Selye emphasized that stress is the nonspecific response common to all stressors, regardless of whether they are physiologic, psychological, or social. The many conditioning factors in each person's environment account for why different demands are interpreted by different people as stressors. Conditioning factors also account for differences in the tolerance of different people for stress: some people may develop diseases of adaptation, such as hypertension and migraine headaches, while others are unaffected.

Interpretation of Stressful Stimuli by the Brain

Physiologic responses to stress are mediated by the brain through a complex network of chemical and electrical messages. The neural and hormonal actions that maintain homeostatic balance are integrated by the hypothalamus, which is located in the center of the brain, surrounded by the limbic system and the cerebral hemispheres. The hypothalamus integrates autonomic nervous system mechanisms that maintain the chemical constancy of the internal environment of the body. Together with the limbic system, it also regulates emotions and many visceral behaviors necessary for survival (eg, eating, drinking, temperature control, reproduction, defense, aggression). The hypothalamus is made up of a number of nuclei; the limbic system contains the amygdala, hippocampus, and septal nuclei, along with other structures.

Literature supports the concept that each of these structures responds differently to stimuli, and each has its own characteristic response (Watkins, 1997). The cerebral hemispheres are concerned with cognitive functions: thought processes, learning, and memory. The limbic system has connections with both the cerebral hemispheres and the brain stem. In addition, the reticular activating system, which is a network of cells that forms a two-way communication system, extends from the brain stem into the midbrain and limbic system. This network controls the alert or waking state of the body.

In the stress response, afferent impulses are carried from sensory organs (eye, ear, nose, skin) and internal sensors (baroreceptors, chemoreceptors) to nerve centers in the brain. The response to the perception of stress is integrated in the hypothalamus, which coordinates the adjustments necessary to return to homeostatic balance. The degree and duration of the response varies; major stress evokes both sympathetic and pituitary adrenal responses.

Neural and neuroendocrine pathways under the control of the hypothalamus are also activated in the stress response. First, there is a sympathetic nervous system discharge, followed by a sympathetic-adrenal-medullary discharge. If the stress persists, the hypothalamic-pituitary system is activated (Fig. 6-2).

SYMPATHETIC NERVOUS SYSTEM RESPONSE

The sympathetic nervous system response is rapid and short-lived. Norepinephrine is released at nerve endings that are in direct contact with their respective end organs to cause an increase in function of the vital organs and a state of general body arousal. The heart rate is increased and peripheral **vasoconstriction** occurs, raising the blood pressure. Blood is also shunted away from abdominal organs. The purpose of these activities is to provide better perfusion of vital organs (brain, heart, skeletal muscles).

Blood glucose is increased, supplying more readily available energy. The pupils are dilated, and mental activity is increased; a greater sense of awareness exists. Constriction of the blood vessels of the skin limits bleeding in the event of trauma. The person is likely to experience cold feet, clammy skin and hands, chills, palpitations, and a knot in the stomach. Typically, the person appears tense, with the muscles of the neck, upper back, and shoulders tightened; respirations may be rapid and shallow, with the diaphragm tense.

SYMPATHETIC-ADRENAL-MEDULLARY RESPONSE

In addition to its direct effect on major end organs, the sympathetic nervous system also stimulates the medulla of the adrenal gland to release the hormones epinephrine and norepinephrine into the bloodstream. The action of these hormones is similar to that of the sympathetic nervous system and have the effect of sustaining and prolonging its actions. Epinephrine and norepinephrine are catecholamines that stimulate the nervous system and produce metabolic effects that increase the blood glucose level

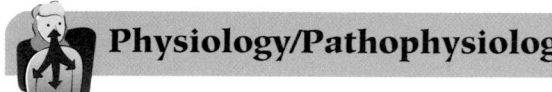

Physiology/Pathophysiology

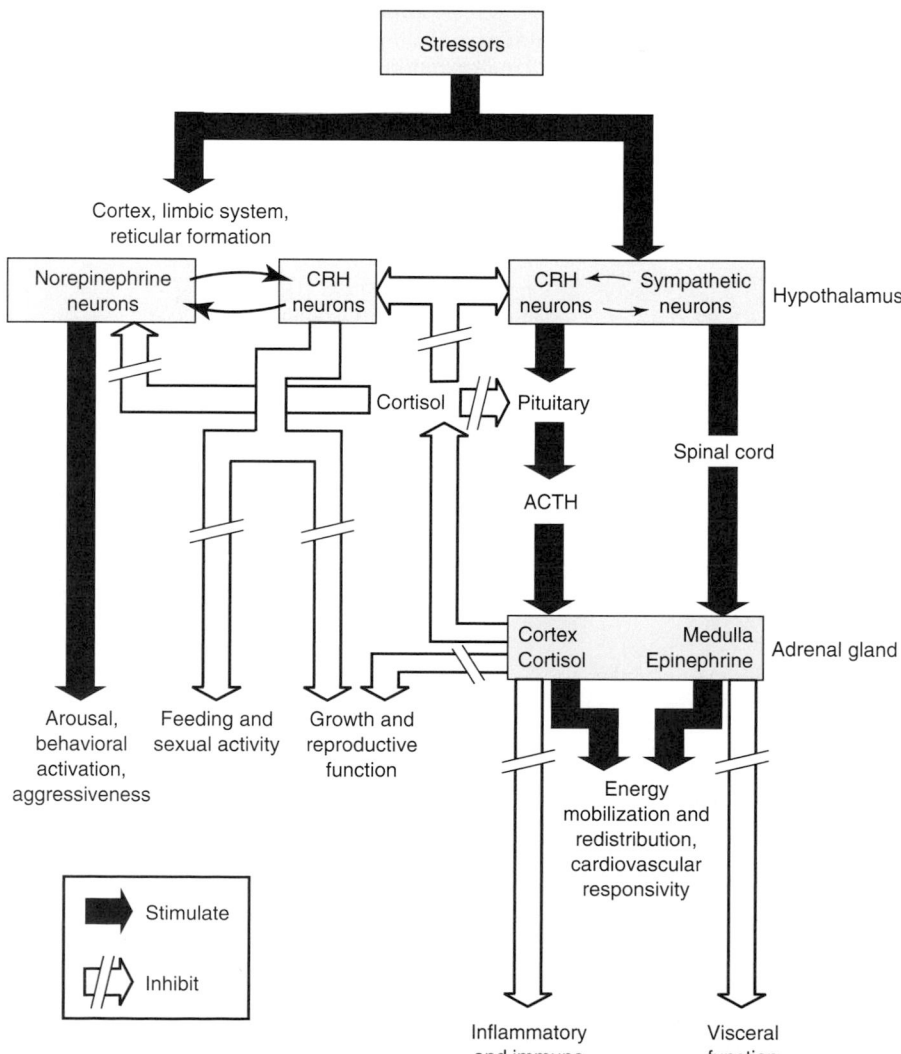

FIGURE 6-2 Integrated responses to stress mediated by the sympathetic nervous system and the hypothalamic–pituitary–adrenocortical axis. The responses are mutually reinforcing, at both the central and peripheral levels. Negative feedback by cortisol also can limit an overresponse that might be harmful to the individual. *Colored arrows,* stimulation; *open arrows,* inhibition; CRH, corticotropin-releasing hormone; ACTH, adrenocorticotropic hormone. Reproduced with permission from Berne, R. M., & Levy, M. N. (1993). *Physiology.* St. Louis: C. V. Mosby.

and increase the **metabolic rate**. The effect of the sympathetic and adrenal-medullary responses is summarized in Table 6-1. This effect is called the "fight-or-flight" reaction.

HYPOTHALAMIC-PITUITARY RESPONSE

The longest-acting phase of the physiologic response, which is more likely to occur in persistent stress, involves the hypothalamic-pituitary pathway. The hypothalamus secretes corticotropin-releasing factor, which stimulates the anterior pituitary to produce ACTH. ACTH in turn stimulates the adrenal cortex to produce **glucocorticoids**, primarily cortisol. Cortisol stimulates protein catabolism, releasing amino acids; stimulates liver uptake of amino acids and their conversion to glucose (**gluconeogenesis**); and inhibits glucose uptake (anti-insulin action) by many body cells but not those of the brain and heart. These cortisol-induced metabolic effects provide the body with a ready source of energy during a stressful situation. This effect has some important implications. For example, a person with diabetes who is under stress, such as that caused by an infection, needs more insulin than usual. Any patient who is under stress (caused, for example, by illness, surgery, trauma or prolonged psychological stress) catabolizes body protein and needs supplements. Children subjected to severe stress have retarded growth.

The actions of the catecholamines (epinephrine and norepinephrine) and cortisol are the most important in the general response to stress. Other hormones released are **antidiuretic hormone (ADH)** from the posterior pituitary and aldosterone from the adrenal cortex. ADH and aldosterone promote sodium and water retention, which is an adaptive mechanism in the event of hemorrhage or loss of fluids through excessive perspiration. ADH has also been shown to influence learning and may thus facilitate coping in new and threatening situations. Secretion of growth hormone and glucagon stimulates the uptake of amino acids by cells, helping to mobilize energy resources. Endorphins, which are endogenous opiates, increase during stress and enhance the threshold for tolerance of painful stimuli. They may also affect mood and have been implicated in the so-called "high" that long-distance runners experience. The secretion of other hormones is also affected, but their adaptive function is less clear.

IMMUNOLOGIC RESPONSE

Research findings show that the immune system is connected to the neuroendocrine and autonomic systems. Lymphoid tissue is richly supplied by autonomic nerves capable of releasing a number of different neuropeptides that can have a direct effect on leukocyte regulation and the inflammatory response. Neuroendocrine hormones released by the central nervous system and endocrine tissues can inhibit or stimulate leukocyte function. The wide variety of stressors people experience may result in different alterations in autonomic activity and subtle variations in neurohormone and neuropeptide synthesis. All of these possible autonomic and neuroendocrine responses can interact to initiate, weaken, enhance, or terminate an immune response (Watkins, 1997).

The study of the relationships among the neuroendocrine system, the central and autonomic nervous systems, and the immune system and the effects of these relationships on overall health outcomes is called *psychoneuroimmunology*. Because one's perception of events and coping styles determine whether, and to what extent, an event activates the stress response system, and because the stress response affects immune activity, one's perceptions, ideas, and thoughts can have profound neurochemical and immunologic consequences. Multiple studies have demonstrated alteration of immune function in people who are under stress, as evidenced by a decrease in the number of leukocytes, impaired immune response to immunizations, and diminished cytotoxic-

Table 6-1 • Sympathetic–Adrenal–Medullary Response to Stress

EFFECT	PURPOSE	MECHANISM
Increased heart rate and blood pressure	Better perfusion of vital organs	Increased cardiac output due to increased myocardial contractility and heart rate; increased venous return (peripheral vasoconstriction)
Increased blood glucose level	Increased available energy	Increased liver and muscle glycogen breakdown; increased breakdown of adipose tissue triglycerides
Mental acuity	Alert state	Increase in amount of blood shunted to the brain from the abdominal viscera and skin
Dilated pupils	Increased awareness	Contraction of radial muscle of iris
Increased tension of skeletal muscles	Preparedness for activity, decreased fatigue	Excitation of muscles; increase in amount of blood shunted to the muscles from the abdominal viscera and skin
Increased ventilation (may be rapid and shallow)	Provision of oxygen for energy	Stimulation of respiratory center in medulla; bronchodilation
Increased coagulability of blood	Prevention of hemorrhage in event of trauma	Vasoconstriction of surface vessels

ity of natural killer cells (Andersen et al., 1998; Constantino, Secula, Rabin, & Stone, 2000; Glaser & Kiecolt-Glaser, 1997; Pike et al., 1997; Robinson, Matthews, & Witek-Janusek, 2000). Other studies have identified certain personality traits, such as optimism and active coping, as having positive effects on health or specific immune measures (Chalfont & Bennett, 1999; Goodkin et al., 1996; Kennedy, 2000; Sergerstrom, Fahey, Kemeny, & Taylor, 1998). As research continues, this new field of study will continue to uncover to what extent and by what mechanisms people can consciously influence their immunity.

MALADAPTIVE RESPONSES TO STRESS

The stress response, which, as indicated earlier facilitates adaptation to threatening situations, has been retained from our evolutionary past. The "fight-or-flight" response, for example, is an anticipatory response that mobilized the bodily resources of our ancestors to deal with predators and other harsh factors in their environment. This same mobilization comes into play in response to emotional stimuli unrelated to danger. For example, a person may get an "adrenaline rush" when competing over a decisive point in a ball game, or when excited about attending a party.

When the responses to stress are ineffective, they are referred to as *maladaptive*. Maladaptive responses are chronic, recurrent responses or patterns of response over time that do not promote the goals of adaptation. The goals of adaptation are somatic or physical health (optimal wellness); psychological health or having a sense of well-being (happiness, satisfaction with life, morale); and enhanced social functioning, which includes work, social life, and family (positive relationships). Maladaptive responses that threaten these goals include faulty appraisals and inappropriate coping (Lazarus, 1991a).

The frequency, intensity, and duration of stressful situations contribute to the development of negative emotions and subsequent patterns of neurochemical discharge. By appraising situations more adequately and coping more appropriately, it is possible to anticipate and defuse some of these situations. For example, frequent potentially stressful encounters (eg, marital discord) might be avoided with better communication and problem solving, or a pattern of procrastination (eg, delaying work on tasks) could be corrected to reduce stress when deadlines approach.

Coping processes that include the use of alcohol or drugs to reduce stress increase the risk of illness. Other inappropriate coping patterns may increase the risk of illness less directly. For example, people who demonstrate "type A" personality behaviors such as impatience, competitiveness, and achievement orientation and have an underlying hostile approach to life are more prone than others to develop stress-related illnesses. Type A behaviors increase the output of catecholamines, the adrenal-medullary hormones, with their attendant effects on the body.

Other forms of inappropriate coping include denial, avoidance, and distancing. Denial may be illustrated by the woman who feels a lump in her breast but downplays its seriousness and delays seeking medical attention. The intent of denial is to control the threat, but it may also endanger life.

Models of illness frequently cite stress and maladaptation as precursors to disease. A general model of illness, based on Selye's theory, suggests that any stressor elicits a state of disturbed physiologic equilibrium. If this state is prolonged or the response is excessive, it will increase the susceptibility of the person to illness. This susceptibility, coupled with a predisposition in the person

(whether from genetic traits, health, or age), leads to illness. If the sympathetic adrenal-medullary response is prolonged or excessive, a state of chronic arousal develops that may lead to high blood pressure, arteriosclerotic changes, and cardiovascular disease. If the production of the ACTH is prolonged or excessive, behavior patterns of withdrawal and depression are seen. In addition, the immune response is decreased, and infections and tumors may develop.

Selye (1976) proposed a list of disorders that he called diseases of maladaptation: high blood pressure, diseases of the heart and blood vessels, diseases of the kidney, hypertension of pregnancy, rheumatic and rheumatoid arthritis, inflammatory diseases of the skin and eyes, infections, allergic and hypersensitivity diseases, nervous and mental diseases, sexual derangements, digestive diseases, metabolic diseases, and cancer.

INDICATORS OF STRESS

Indicators of stress and the stress response include both subjective and objective measures. Chart 6-1 lists signs and symptoms that may be observed directly or reported by the person. They are psychological, physiologic, or behavioral and reflect social behaviors and thought processes. Some of these reactions may be coping behaviors. Over time, each person tends to develop a characteristic pattern of behavior during stress that is a warning that the system is out of balance.

Chart 6-1	**Signs and Symptoms of Stress**

General irritability, hyperexcitation, or depression
Dryness of the throat and mouth
Overpowering urge to cry, scream, or run and hide
Easily fatigued, loss of interest
"Floating anxiety"—do not know exactly why or what
Easily startled
Stuttering or other speech difficulties
Hypermotility: pacing, moving about, cannot sit still
Gastrointestinal signs and symptoms: "butterflies" in the
    stomach, diarrhea, vomiting
Change in menstrual cycle
Loss of or excessive appetite
Increased use of legally prescribed drugs, such as anxiolytics or
    antidepressants
Prone to injuries
Disturbed behavior
Pounding of the heart
Impulsive behavior, emotional instability
Inability to concentrate or think clearly
Feelings of unreality, weakness, or dizziness
Tension, alertness
Trembling, nervous tics
Nervous laughter
Grinding of teeth
Insomnia, nightmares, or other sleep difficulties
Excessive perspiration
Increased frequency of urination
Muscle tension and migraine headaches
Pain in the neck or lower back
Increased smoking
Alcohol and drug addiction

Based on Selye, H. (1976). *Stress in health and disease.* Stoneham, MA: Butterworths. Reprinted with permission of the publisher.

Laboratory measurements of indicators of stress have helped in understanding this complex process. Among the measures, blood and urine analyses can be used to demonstrate changes in hormonal levels and hormonal breakdown products. Reliable measures of stress include blood levels of catecholamines, corticoids, ACTH, and eosinophils. The serum creatine/creatinine ratio and elevations of cholesterol and free fatty acids can also be measured. Immunoglobulin assays may be determined. With greater attention to neuroimmunology, improved laboratory measures are likely to follow. Increases in blood pressure and heart rate can also be measured.

In addition to using laboratory tests, researchers have developed questionnaires to identify and assess stressors, stress, and coping strategies. Many of these are discussed in the research monograph developed by Barnfather and Lyon (1993), which was based on a synthesis conference held by nurse scientists on the state of the science in stress and coping nursing research. Some examples of the research instruments that nurses commonly use to measure levels of client distress and client functioning can be found in a variety of research reports (Cronquist, Wredding, Norlander, Langius, & Bjorvell, 2000; Starzonski & Hilton, 2000). Miller and Smith (1993) provided a stress audit and a stress profile measurement tool that is available in the popular lay literature.

NURSING IMPLICATIONS

It is important for the nurse to realize that the optimal point of intervention to promote health is during the stage when the individual's own compensatory processes are still functioning. Early identification of both physiologic and psychological stressors remains a major role of the nurse, and information on the interrelationships between physical and emotional health can be found in research journals. The nurse should be able to relate the presenting signs and symptoms of distress to the physiology they represent and identify the individual's position on the continuum of function, from health and compensation to pathophysiology and disease. For example, if an anxious middle-aged woman presented for a checkup and was found to be overweight, with a blood pressure of 130/85 mm Hg, the nurse would counsel her with respect to diet, stress management, and activity. The nurse would also encourage weight loss and discuss the woman's intake of salt (which affects fluid balance) and caffeine (which provides a stimulant effect). The patient and the nurse would identify both individual and environmental stressors and discuss strategies to decrease the lifestyle stress, with the ultimate goal being to create a healthy lifestyle and prevent hypertension and its sequelae.

Stress at the Cellular Level

Pathologic processes may occur at all levels of the biologic organism. If the cell is considered the smallest unit or subsystem (tissues being aggregates of cells, organs aggregates of tissues, and so forth), the processes of health and disease or adaptation and maladaptation can all occur at the cellular level. Indeed, pathologic processes are often described by scientists at the subcellular or molecular level.

The cell exists on a continuum of function and structure, ranging from the normal cell, to the adapted cell, to the injured or diseased cell, to the dead cell (Fig. 6-3). Changes from one state to another may occur rapidly and may not be readily de-

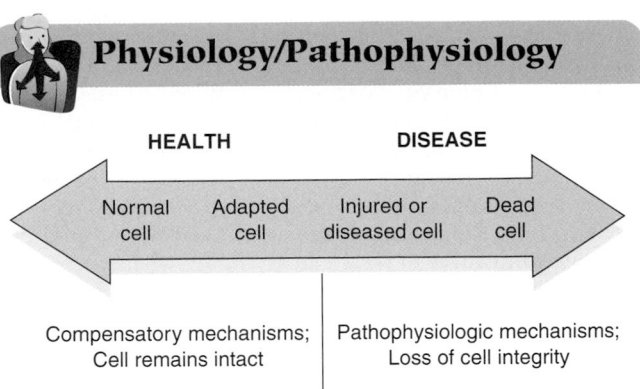

Physiology/Pathophysiology

HEALTH DISEASE

Normal cell | Adapted cell | Injured or diseased cell | Dead cell

Compensatory mechanisms; Cell remains intact | Pathophysiologic mechanisms; Loss of cell integrity

FIGURE 6-3 The cell on a continuum of function and structure. Changes in the cell are not as easily discerned as the diagram depicts. The point at which compensation subsides and pathophysiology begins is not clearly defined.

tectable, because each state does not have discrete boundaries, and disease represents an extension and distortion of normal processes. The earliest changes occur at the molecular or subcellular level and are not perceptible until steady-state functions or structures are altered. With cell injury, some changes may be reversible; in other instances, the injuries are lethal. For example, tanning of the skin is an adaptive, morphologic response to exposure to the rays of the sun. If the exposure is continued, however, sunburn and injury occur, and some cells may die, as evidenced by desquamation ("peeling").

Different cells and tissues respond to stimuli with different patterns and rates of response; some cells are more vulnerable to one type of stimulus or stressor than others. The cell involved, its ability to adapt, and its physiologic state are determinants of the response. For example, cardiac muscle cells respond to **hypoxia** (inadequate oxygenation) more quickly than smooth muscle cells do.

Other determinants of cellular response are the type or nature of the stimulus, its duration, and its severity. For example, neurons that control respiration can develop a tolerance to regular, small amounts of a barbiturate, but one large dose may result in respiratory depression and death.

CONTROL OF THE STEADY STATE

The concept of the cell as existing on a continuum of function and structure includes the relationship of the cell to compensatory mechanisms, which occur continuously in the body to maintain the steady state. Compensatory processes are regulated primarily by the autonomic nervous system and the endocrine system, with control achieved through negative feedback.

Negative Feedback

Negative feedback mechanisms throughout the body monitor the internal environment and restore homeostasis when conditions shift out of the normal range. These mechanisms work by sensing deviations from a predetermined set point or range of adaptability and triggering a response aimed at offsetting the deviation. Blood pressure, acid–base balance, blood glucose level, body temperature, and fluid and electrolyte balance are examples of functions regulated through such compensatory mechanisms.

Most of the human body's control systems are integrated by the brain and influenced by the nervous and endocrine systems. Control activities involve detecting deviations from the predetermined reference point and stimulating compensatory responses in the muscles and glands of the body. The major organs affected are the heart, lungs, kidneys, liver, gastrointestinal tract, and skin. When stimulated, these organs alter their rate of activity or the amount of secretions they produce. Because of this, they have been called the "organs of homeostasis or adjustment."

In addition to the responses controlled by the nervous and endocrine systems, local responses consisting of small feedback loops in a group of cells or tissues are possible. The cells detect a change in their immediate environment and initiate an action to counteract its effect. For example, the accumulation of lactic acid in an exercised muscle stimulates dilation of blood vessels in the area to increase blood flow and improve the delivery of oxygen and removal of waste products.

The net result of the activities of feedback loops is homeostasis. A steady state is achieved by the continuous, variable action of the organs involved in making the adjustments and by the continuous small exchanges of chemical substances among cells, interstitial fluid, and blood. For example, an increase in the carbon dioxide concentration of the extracellular fluid leads to increased pulmonary ventilation, which decreases the carbon dioxide level. On a cellular level, increased carbon dioxide raises the hydrogen ion concentration of the blood. This is detected by chemosensitive receptors in the respiratory control center of the medulla of the brain. The chemoreceptors stimulate an increase in the rate of discharge of the neurons that innervate the diaphragm and intercostal muscles, which increases the rate of respiration. Excess carbon dioxide is exhaled, the hydrogen ion concentration returns to normal, and the chemically sensitive neurons are no longer stimulated.

Positive Feedback

Another type of feedback, **positive feedback**, perpetuates the chain of events set in motion by the original disturbance instead of compensating for it. As the system becomes more unbalanced, disorder and disintegration occur. There are some exceptions to this; blood clotting in humans, for example, is an important positive feedback mechanism.

CELLULAR ADAPTATION

Cells are complex units that dynamically respond to the changing demands and stresses of daily life. They possess a maintenance function and a specialized function. The maintenance function refers to the activities that the cell must perform with respect to itself; specialized functions are those that the cell performs in relation to the tissues and organs of which it is a part. Individual cells may cease to function without posing a threat to the organism. As the number of dead cells increases, however, the specialized functions of the tissues are altered and the individual's health is threatened.

Cells can adapt to environmental stress through structural and functional changes. Some of these adaptations are hypertrophy, atrophy, hyperplasia, dysplasia, and metaplasia (Table 6-2).

Hypertrophy and atrophy lead to changes in the size of cells and hence the size of the organs they form. Compensatory hypertrophy is the result of an enlarged muscle mass and commonly occurs in skeletal and cardiac muscle that experiences a prolonged, increased workload. One example is the bulging muscles of the athlete who engages in body building.

Atrophy can be the consequence of a disease or of decreased use, decreased blood supply, loss of nerve supply, or inadequate nutrition. Disuse of a body part is often associated with the aging

Table 6-2 • Cellular Adaptation to Stressors

ADAPTATION	STIMULUS	EXAMPLE
Hypertrophy—increase in cell size leading to increase in organ size	Increased workload	Leg muscles of runner Arm muscles in tennis player Cardiac muscle in person with hypertension

Atrophy—shrinkage in size of cell, leading to decrease in organ size	Decrease in:
	  Use
	  Blood supply
	  Nutrition
	  Hormonal stimulation
	  Innervation
		Secondary sex organs in aging person
		Extremity immobilized in plaster cast

Hyperplasia—increase in number of new cells (increase in mitosis)	Hormonal influence	Breast changes of a girl in puberty or of a pregnant woman Regeneration of liver cells New red blood cells in blood loss
Dysplasia—change in the appearance of cells after they have been subjected to chronic irritation	Reproduction of cells with resulting alteration of their size and shape	Alterations in epithelial cells of the skin or the cervix, producing irregular tissue changes that could be the precursors of a malignancy
Metaplasia—transformation of one adult cell type to another (reversible)	Stress applied to highly specialized cell	Changes in epithelial cells lining bronchi in response to smoke irritation (cells become less specialized)

process. Cell size and organ size decrease; structures principally affected are the skeletal muscles, the secondary sex organs, the heart, and the brain.

Hyperplasia is an increase in the number of new cells in an organ or tissue. As cells multiply and are subjected to increased stimulation, the tissue mass enlarges. It is a mitotic response (a change occurring with mitosis), but it is reversible when the stimulus is removed. This distinguishes it from neoplasia or malignant growth, which continues after the stimulus is removed. Hyperplasia may be hormonally induced. An example is the increase in the size of the thyroid gland caused by thyroid-stimulating hormone (secreted from the pituitary gland) when a deficit in thyroid hormone is detected.

Dysplasia is the change in the appearance of cells after they have been subjected to chronic irritation. Dysplastic cells have a tendency to become malignant; dysplasia is seen commonly in epithelial cells in the bronchi of smokers.

Metaplasia is a cell transformation in which a highly specialized cell changes to a less specialized cell. This serves a protective function, because the less specialized cell is more resistant to the stress that stimulated the change. For example, the ciliated columnar epithelium lining the bronchi of smokers is replaced by squamous epithelium. The squamous cells can survive; loss of the cilia and protective mucus, however, can have damaging consequences.

These adaptations allow the survival of the organism. They also reflect changes in the normal cell in response to stress. If the stress is unrelenting, the function of the adapted cell may succumb, and cell injury will occur.

CELLULAR INJURY

Injury is defined as a disorder in steady-state regulation. Any stressor that alters the ability of the cell or system to maintain optimal balance of its adjustment processes will lead to injury. Structural and functional damage then occurs, which may be reversible (permitting recovery) or irreversible (leading to disability or death). Homeostatic adjustments are concerned with the small changes within the body's systems. With adaptive changes, compensation occurs and a steady state is achieved, although it may be at new levels. With injury, steady-state regulation is lost, and changes in functioning ensue.

Causes of disorder and injury in the system (cell, tissue, organ, body) may arise from the external or internal environment (Fig. 6-4) and include hypoxia, nutritional imbalance, physical agents, chemical agents, **infectious agents**, immune mechanisms, genetic defects, and psychogenic factors. The most common causes are hypoxia (oxygen deficiency), chemical injury, and infectious agents. In addition, the presence of one injury makes the system more susceptible to another injury. For example, inadequate oxygenation and nutritional deficiencies make the system vulnerable to infection. These agents act at the cellular level by damaging or destroying

- The integrity of the cell membrane, necessary for ionic balance
- The ability of the cell to transform energy (aerobic respiration, production of adenosine triphosphate)
- The ability of the cell to synthesize enzymes and other necessary proteins
- The ability of the cell to grow and reproduce (genetic integrity)

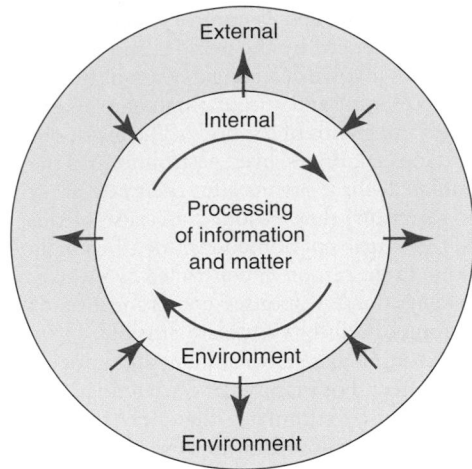

FIGURE 6-4 Influences leading to disorder may arise from the internal environment and the external environment of the system. Excesses or deficits of information and matter may occur, or there may be faulty regulation of processing.

Hypoxia

Inadequate cellular oxygenation (hypoxia) interferes with the cell's ability to transform energy. Hypoxia may be caused by:

- A decrease in blood supply to an area
- A decrease in the oxygen-carrying capacity of the blood (decreased hemoglobin)
- A ventilation/perfusion or respiratory problem that reduces the amount of oxygen available in the blood
- A problem in the cell's enzyme system that makes it unable to use the oxygen delivered to it

The usual cause is ischemia, or deficient blood supply. Ischemia is commonly seen in myocardial cell injury in which arterial blood flow is decreased because of atherosclerotic narrowing of blood vessels. Ischemia also results from intravascular clots (thrombi or emboli) that may form and interfere with blood supply. Thrombi and emboli are common causes of cerebrovascular accidents (strokes). The length of time different tissues can survive without oxygen varies. For example, brain cells may succumb in 3 to 6 minutes, depending on the situation. If the condition leading to hypoxia is slow and progressive, collateral circulation may develop, whereby blood is supplied by other blood vessels in the area. However, this mechanism is not highly reliable.

Nutritional Imbalance

Nutritional imbalance refers to a relative or absolute deficiency or excess of one or more essential nutrients. This may be manifested as undernutrition (inadequate consumption of food or calories) or overnutrition (caloric excess). Caloric excess to the point of obesity overloads cells in the body with lipids. By requiring more energy to maintain the extra tissue, obesity places a strain on the body and has been associated with the development of disease, especially pulmonary and cardiovascular disease.

Specific deficiencies arise when an essential nutrient is deficient or when there is an imbalance of nutrients. Protein deficiencies and avitaminosis (deficiency of vitamins) are typical examples. An energy deficit leading to cell injury can occur if there is insufficient glucose, or insufficient oxygen to transform the glucose into energy. A lack of insulin, or the inability to use insulin, may also prevent glucose from entering the cell from the blood. This occurs in diabetes mellitus, a metabolic disorder that can lead to nutritional deficiency.

Physical Agents

Physical agents, including temperature extremes, radiation, electrical shock, and mechanical trauma, can cause injury to the cells or to the entire body. The duration of exposure and the intensity of the stressor determine the severity of damage.

EXTREMES OF HIGH TEMPERATURE

When a person's temperature is elevated, hypermetabolism occurs and the respiratory rate, heart rate, and basal metabolic rate all increase. With fever induced by infections, the hypothalamic thermostat may be reset at a higher temperature, then return to normal when the fever abates. The increase in body temperature is achieved through physiologic mechanisms. Body temperatures greater than 41°C (106°F) suggest hyperthermia, because the physiologic function of the thermoregulatory center breaks down and the temperature soars. This physiologic condition occurs in people with heat stroke. Eventually, the high temperature causes coagulation of cell proteins, and the cells die. The body must be cooled rapidly to prevent brain damage.

The local response to thermal or burn injury is similar. There is an increase in metabolic activity, and, as heat increases, protein is coagulated, enzyme systems are destroyed, and, in the extreme, charring or carbonization occurs. Burns of the epithelium are classified as partial-thickness burns if epithelializing elements remain to support healing. Full-thickness burns lack such elements and must be grafted for healing. The amount of body surface involved determines the prognosis for the patient. If the injury is severe, the entire body system becomes involved, and hypermetabolism develops as a pathophysiologic response.

EXTREMES OF LOW TEMPERATURE

Extremes of low temperature, or cold, cause vasoconstriction. Blood flow becomes sluggish and clots form, leading to ischemic damage in the involved tissues. With still lower temperatures, ice crystals may form, and the cells may burst.

RADIATION AND ELECTRICAL SHOCK

Radiation is used for diagnosis and treatment of diseases. Ionizing forms of radiation may cause injury by their destructive action. Radiation decreases the protective inflammatory response of the cell, creating a favorable environment for opportunistic infections. Electrical shock produces burns as a result of the heat generated when electrical current travels through the body. It may also abnormally stimulate nerves, leading, for example, to fibrillation of the heart.

MECHANICAL TRAUMA

Mechanical trauma can result in wounds that disrupt the cells and tissues of the body. The severity of the wound, the amount of blood loss, and the extent of nerve damage are significant factors in the outcome.

Chemical Agents

Chemical injuries are caused by poisons, such as lye, which has a corrosive action on epithelial tissue, or by heavy metals, such as mercury, arsenic, and lead, each with its own specific destructive action. Many other chemicals are toxic in specific amounts, in certain people, and in distinctive tissues. Excessive secretion of hydrochloric acid can damage the stomach lining; large amounts of glucose can cause osmotic shifts, affecting the fluid and electrolyte balance; and too much insulin can cause subnormal levels of glucose in the blood (hypoglycemia) and can lead to coma.

Drugs, including prescribed medications, can also cause chemical poisoning. Some individuals are less tolerant of medications than others and manifest toxic reactions at the usual or customary dosages. Aging tends to decrease tolerance to medications. Polypharmacy (taking many medications at one time) also occurs frequently in the aging population and is a problem because of the unpredictable effects of the resulting medication interactions.

Alcohol (ethanol) is also a chemical irritant. In the body, alcohol is broken down into acetaldehyde, which has a direct toxic effect on liver cells that leads to a variety of liver abnormalities, including cirrhosis in susceptible individuals. Disordered liver cell function leads to complications in other organs of the body.

Infectious Agents

Biologic agents known to cause disease in humans are viruses, bacteria, rickettsiae, mycoplasmas, fungi, protozoa, and nematodes. The severity of the infectious disease depends on the number of microorganisms entering the body, their virulence, and the host's defenses (eg, health, age, immune defenses).

Some bacteria, such as those that cause tetanus and diphtheria, produce exotoxins that circulate and create cell damage. Others, such as the gram-negative bacteria, produce endotoxins when they are killed. The tubercle bacillus induces an immune reaction.

Viruses, the smallest living organisms, survive as parasites of the living cells they invade. Viruses infect specific cells. Through a complex mechanism, they replicate within the cells, then invade other cells and continue to replicate. An immune response is mounted by the body to eliminate the viruses, and the cells harboring the viruses can be injured in the process. Typically, an inflammatory response and immune reaction are the physiologic responses of the body to the presence of infection.

Disordered Immune Responses

The immune system is an exceedingly complex system; its purpose is to defend the body from invasion by any foreign object or foreign cell type, such as cancerous cells. This is a steady-state mechanism, but like other adjustment processes it can become disordered, and cell injury will occur. The immune response detects foreign bodies by distinguishing non-self substances from self substances and destroying the non-self entities. The entrance of an antigen (foreign substance) into the body evokes the production of antibodies that attack and destroy the antigen (antigen–antibody reaction).

The immune system can be hypoactive or hyperactive. When it is hypoactive, immunodeficiency diseases occur; when it is hyperactive, hypersensitivity disorders arise. A disorder of the immune system itself can result in damage to the body's own tissues. Such disorders are labeled autoimmune diseases (see Unit 11).

Genetic Disorders

Genetic defects as causes of disease and their effects on genetic structure are of intense research interest. Many of these defects produce mutations that have no recognizable effect, such as lack of a single enzyme; others contribute to more obvious congenital abnormalities, such as Down syndrome. As a result of the Human Genome Project, patients can be genetically assessed for conditions such as sickle cell disease, cystic fibrosis, hemophilia A and B, breast cancer, obesity, cardiovascular disease, phenylketonuria, and Alzheimer's disease. The availability of genetic information and technology enables health care providers to perform screening, testing, and counseling for patients with genetic concerns. Knowledge obtained from the Human Genome Project has also created opportunities for assessing a person's genetic profile and preventing or treating disease. Diagnostic genetics and gene therapy have the potential to identify and modify a gene before it begins to express traits that would lead to disease or disability.

CELLULAR RESPONSE TO INJURY: INFLAMMATION

Cells or tissues of the body may be injured or killed by any of the agents (physical, chemical, infectious) described earlier. When this happens, an inflammatory response (or inflammation) naturally occurs in the healthy tissues adjacent to the site of injury. **Inflammation** is a defensive reaction intended to neutralize, control, or eliminate the offending agent and to prepare the site for repair. It is a nonspecific response (not dependent on a particular cause) that is meant to serve a protective function. For example, inflammation may be observed at the site of a bee sting, in a sore throat, in a surgical incision, and at a burn site. Inflammation also occurs in cell injury events, such as strokes and myocardial infarctions.

Inflammation is not the same as infection. An infectious agent is only one of several agents that may trigger an inflammatory response. An infection exists when the infectious agent is living, growing, and multiplying in the tissues and is able to overcome the body's normal defenses.

Regardless of the cause, a general sequence of events occurs in the local inflammatory response. This sequence involves changes in the microcirculation, including vasodilation, increased vascular permeability, and leukocytic cellular infiltration (Fig. 6-5). As these changes take place, five cardinal signs of inflammation are produced: redness, heat, swelling, pain, and loss of function.

The transient vasoconstriction that occurs immediately after injury is followed by vasodilation and an increased rate of blood flow through the microcirculation. Local heat and redness result. Next, vascular permeability increases, and plasma fluids (including proteins and solutes) leak into the inflamed tissues, producing swelling. The pain produced is attributed to the pressure of fluids or swelling on nerve endings, and to the irritation of nerve endings by chemical mediators released at the site. Bradykinin is one of the chemical mediators suspected of causing pain. Loss of function is most likely related to the pain and swelling, but the exact mechanism is not completely known.

As blood flow increases and fluid leaks into the surrounding tissues, the formed elements (red blood cells, white blood cells, and platelets) remain in the blood, causing it to become more viscous. Leukocytes (white blood cells) collect in the vessels, exit, and migrate to the site of injury to engulf offending organisms and to remove cellular debris in a process called phagocytosis. Fibrinogen in the leaked plasma fluid coagulates, forming fibrin for clot formation, which serves to wall off the injured area and prevent the spread of infection.

Chemical Mediators

Injury initiates the inflammatory response, but chemical substances released at the site induce the vascular changes. Foremost among these chemicals are histamine and the kinins. Histamine

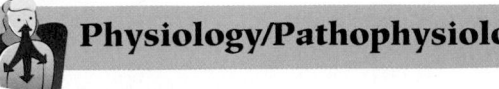

Physiology/Pathophysiology

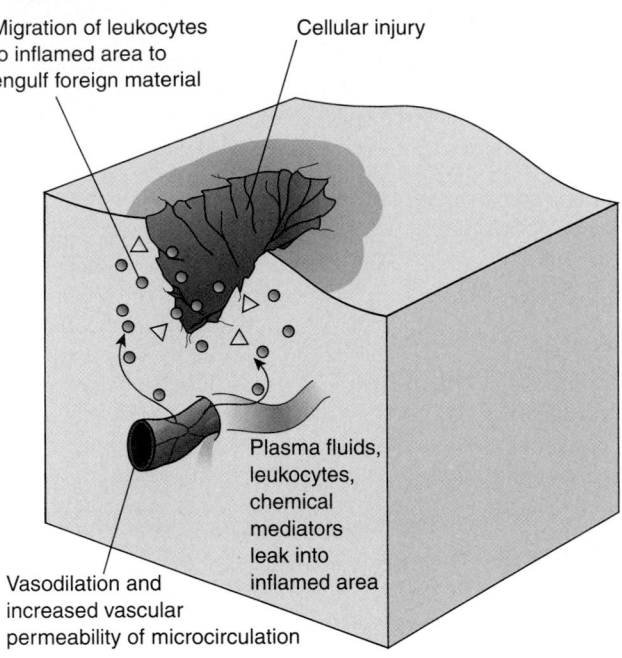

Migration of leukocytes to inflamed area to engulf foreign material

Cellular injury

Plasma fluids, leukocytes, chemical mediators leak into inflamed area

Vasodilation and increased vascular permeability of microcirculation

FIGURE 6-5 Inflammatory response. Chemical, physical, infectious, or other factors cause cellular injury. Vasodilation and release of chemical-mediators, leukocytes, and proteins occur. Leukocytes remove cellular debris. Fibrinogen and plasma coagulate to prevent spread of infection.

is present in many tissues of the body but is concentrated in the mast cells. It is released when injury occurs and is responsible for the early changes in vasodilation and vascular permeability. Kinins increase vasodilation and vascular permeability; they also attract neutrophils to the area. Prostaglandins, another group of chemical substances, are also suspected of causing increased permeability.

Systemic Response to Inflammation

The inflammatory response is often confined to the site, causing only local signs and symptoms. However, systemic responses can also occur. Fever is the most common sign of a systemic response to injury, and it is most likely caused by endogenous pyrogens (internal substances that cause fever) released from neutrophils and macrophages (specialized forms of leukocytes). These substances reset the hypothalamic thermostat, which controls body temperature, and produce fever. Leukocytosis, an increase in the synthesis and release of neutrophils from bone marrow, may occur to provide the body with greater ability to fight infection. During this process, general, nonspecific symptoms develop, including malaise, loss of appetite, aching, and weakness.

Types of Inflammation

Inflammation is categorized primarily by its duration and the type of exudate produced. It may be acute, subacute, or chronic. Acute inflammation is characterized by the local vascular and exudative changes described earlier and usually lasts less than 2 weeks. An acute inflammatory response is immediate and serves a protective function. After the injurious agent is removed, the inflammation subsides and healing takes place with the return of normal or near-normal structure and function.

Chronic inflammation develops if the injurious agent persists and the acute response is perpetuated. Symptoms are present for many months or years. Chronic inflammation may also begin insidiously and never have an acute phase. The chronic response does not serve a beneficial and protective function; on the contrary, it is debilitating and can produce long-lasting effects. As the inflammation becomes chronic, changes occur at the site of injury and the nature of the exudate becomes proliferative. A cycle of cellular infiltration, necrosis, and fibrosis begins, with repair and breakdown occurring simultaneously. Considerable scarring may occur, resulting in permanent tissue damage.

Subacute inflammation falls between acute and chronic inflammation. It includes elements of the active exudative phase of the acute response as well as elements of repair, as in the chronic phase. The term subacute inflammation is not widely used.

CELLULAR HEALING

The reparative process begins at approximately the same time as the injury and is interwoven with inflammation. Healing proceeds after the inflammatory debris has been removed. Healing may occur by regeneration, in which gradual repair of the defect occurs by proliferation of cells of the same type as those destroyed, or by replacement, in which cells of another type, usually connective tissue, fill in the tissue defect and result in scar formation.

Healing by Regeneration

The ability of cells to regenerate depends on whether they are labile, permanent, or stable. Labile cells multiply constantly to replace cells worn out by normal physiologic processes; these include epithelial cells of the skin and those lining the gastrointestinal tract. Permanent cells include neurons—the nerve cell bodies, not their axons. Destruction of a neuron is a permanent loss, but axons may regenerate. If normal activity is to return, tissue regeneration must occur in a functional pattern, especially in the growth of several axons. Stable cells have a latent ability to regenerate. Under normal physiologic processes, they are not shed and do not need replacement, but if they are damaged or destroyed, they are able to regenerate. These include functional cells of the kidney, liver, and pancreas.

Healing by Replacement

Depending on the extent of damage, tissue healing may occur by primary intention or by secondary intention. In primary intention healing, the wound is clean and dry and the edges are approximated, as in a surgical wound. Little scar formation occurs, and the wound is usually healed in a week. In secondary intention healing, the wound or defect is larger and gaping and has necrotic or dead material. The wound fills from the bottom upward with granulation tissue. The process of repair takes longer and results in more scar formation, with loss of specialized function. People who have recovered from myocardial infarction, for example, have abnormal electrocardiographic (ECG) tracings because the electrical signal cannot be conducted through the connective tissue that has replaced the infarcted area.

The condition of the host, the environment, and the nature and severity of the injury affect the processes of inflammation and repair. Any of the injuries previously discussed can lead to death of the cell. Essentially, the cell membrane becomes impaired, resulting in a nonrestricted flow of ions. Sodium and calcium enter the cell, followed by water, which leads to edema, and energy transformation ceases. Nerve impulses are no longer transmitted; muscles no longer contract. As the cells rupture, lysosomal enzymes that destroy tissues escape, and cell death and necrosis occur.

NURSING IMPLICATIONS

In the assessment of the person who seeks health care, both objective signs and subjective symptoms are the primary indicators of the physiologic processes that are occurring. The following questions are addressed during the assessment:

- Are the heart rate, respiratory rate, and temperature normal?
- What emotional distress may be contributing to the patient's health problems?
- Are there other indicators of steady-state deviation?
- What is the person's blood pressure, height, and weight?
- Are there any problems in movement or sensation?
- Does the person demonstrate any problems with affect, behavior, speech, cognitive ability, orientation, or memory?
- Are there obvious impairments, lesions, or deformities?

Further signs of change are indicated in diagnostic studies such as computed tomography (CT), magnetic resonance imaging (MRI), and positron emission tomography (PET). Objective evidence can also be obtained from laboratory data, including electrolytes, blood urea nitrogen (BUN), blood glucose, and urinalysis.

In making a nursing diagnosis, the nurse must relate the symptoms or complaints expressed by the patient to the physical signs that are present. Management of specific biologic disorders is discussed in subsequent chapters; however, the nurse can assist any patient to respond to stress-inducing biologic or psychological disorders with stress-management interventions.

Stress Management: Nursing Interventions

Stress or the potential for stress is ubiquitous; that is, it is everywhere and anywhere at once. Anxiety, frustration, anger, and feelings of inadequacy, helplessness, or powerlessness are emotions often associated with stress. In the presence of these emotions, the customary activities of daily living may be disrupted; for example, a sleep disturbance may be present, eating and activity patterns may be altered, and family processes or role performance may be disrupted.

Many nursing diagnoses are possible for patients suffering from stress. One nursing diagnosis related to stress is Anxiety, which is defined as a vague, uneasy feeling, the source of which may be nonspecific or not known to the person. Stress may also be manifested as ineffective coping patterns, impaired thought processes, or disrupted relationships. These human responses are reflected in the nursing diagnoses of Impaired adjustment, Ineffective coping, Defensive coping, and Ineffective denial, all of which indicate poor adaptive responses. Other possible nursing diagnoses include Social isolation, Risk for impaired parenting, Spiritual distress, Readiness for family coping, Decisional conflict, Situational low self-esteem, and Powerlessness, among others. Because human responses to stress are varied, as are the sources of stress, arriving at an accurate diagnosis allows interventions and goals to be more specific and leads to improved outcomes.

Stress management is directed toward reducing and controlling stress and improving coping. Nurses might use these methods not only with their patients but also in their own lives. The need to prevent illness, improve the quality of life, and decrease the cost of health care makes efforts to promote health essential, and stress control is a significant health-promotion goal. Stress-reduction methods and coping enhancements can derive from either internal or external sources. For example, adopting healthy eating habits and practicing relaxation techniques are internal resources that help to reduce stress; developing a broad social network is an external resource that helps reduce stress. Goods and services that can be purchased are also external resources for stress management, and it is much easier for individuals with adequate financial resources to cope with constraints in the environment, because their sense of vulnerability to threat is decreased.

PROMOTING A HEALTHY LIFESTYLE

An individual's personal resources that aid in coping include health and energy. A health-promoting lifestyle provides these resources and buffers or cushions the impact of stressors. Lifestyles or habits that contribute to the risk of illness can be identified through a health risk appraisal.

A health risk appraisal is an assessment method that is designed to promote health by examining an individual's personal habits and recommending changes when a health risk is identified. Health risk questionnaires estimate the likelihood that a person with a given set of characteristics will become ill. It is hoped that if people are provided with this information, they will alter their activities (eg, stop smoking, have periodic screening examinations) to improve their health. Questionnaires typically address the following information:

1. Demographic data: age, sex, race, ethnic background
2. Personal and family history of diseases and health problems
3. Lifestyle choices
   a. Eating, sleeping, exercise, smoking, drinking, sexual activity, and driving habits
   b. Stressors at home and on the job
   c. Role relationships and associated stressors
4. Physical measurements
   a. Blood pressure
   b. Height, weight
   c. Laboratory analyses of blood and urine
5. Participation in high-risk behaviors

The personal information is compared with average population risk data, and the risk factors are identified and weighted. From this analysis, the person's risks and major health hazards are identified. Further comparisons with population data can estimate how many years will be added to the person's life span if the suggested changes are made. However, research so far has not demonstrated that providing people with such information ensures that they will change their habits. The single most important factor for determining health status is social class, and within a social class the research suggests that the major factor influencing health is level of education (Mickler, 1997).

ENHANCING COPING STRATEGIES

McCloskey and Bulechek (1999) identified "coping enhancement" as a nursing intervention and defined it as "assisting a patient to adapt to perceived stressors, changes, or threats that interfere with meeting life demands and roles" (Chart 6-2). The nurse can build on the patient's existing coping strategies, as identified in the health appraisal, or teach new strategies for coping if necessary.

The five predominant ways of coping with illness identified in a review of 57 nursing research studies were as follows (Jalowiec, 1993):

- Trying to be optimistic about the outcome
- Using social support
- Using spiritual resources
- Trying to maintain control either over the situation or over feelings
- Trying to accept the situation

Other ways of coping included seeking information, reprioritizing needs and roles, lowering expectations, making compromises, comparing oneself to others, planning activities to conserve energy, taking things one step at a time, listening to one's body, and using self-talk for encouragement.

The nurse can implement the coping enhancement interventions and explore methods for improving the patient's coping abilities.

TEACHING RELAXATION TECHNIQUES

Relaxation techniques are a major method used to relieve stress. Commonly used techniques include progressive muscle relaxation, the Benson Relaxation Response, and relaxation with guided imagery. The goal of relaxation training is to produce a response that counters the stress response. When this goal is achieved, the action of the hypothalamus adjusts and decreases the activity of the sympathetic and parasympathetic nervous systems. The sequence of physiologic effects and their signs and symptoms are interrupted, and psychological stress is reduced. This is a learned response and requires practice to achieve.

The different relaxation techniques share four similar elements: (1) a quiet environment, (2) a comfortable position, (3) a passive attitude, and (4) a mental device (something on which to focus the attention, such as a word, phrase, or sound).

Progressive Muscle Relaxation

Progressive muscle relaxation involves tensing and releasing the muscles of the body in sequence and sensing the difference in feeling. It is best if the person lies on a soft cushion on the floor, in a quiet room, breathing easily. Someone usually reads the instructions in a low tone and with a slow and relaxed manner, or a tape of the instructions may be played. The person tenses the muscles in the whole body (one muscle group at a time), holds, senses the tension, and then relaxes. As each muscle group is tensed, the person keeps the rest of the body relaxed. Each time the focus is on feeling the tension and relaxation. When the exercise is completed, the whole body should be relaxed (Benson, 1993; Benson & Stark, 1996).

Benson's Relaxation Response

Benson (1993) describes the following steps of the Benson Relaxation Response:

1. Pick a brief phrase or word that reflects your basic belief system.
2. Choose a comfortable position.
3. Close your eyes.
4. Relax your muscles.

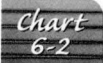

Chart 6-2 Coping Enhancement: Nursing Interventions

Definition

Assisting a patient to adapt to perceived stressors, changes, or threats that interfere with meeting life demands and roles

Activities

Appraise a patient's adjustment to changes in body image as indicated.

Appraise the impact of the patient's life situation on roles and relationships.

Encourage the patient to identify a realistic description of change in role.

Appraise the patient's understanding of the disease process.

Appraise and discuss alternative responses to the situation.

Use a calm, reassuring approach.

Provide an atmosphere of acceptance.

Assist the patient in developing an objective appraisal of the event.

Help the patient to identify the information that he or she is most interested in obtaining.

Provide factual information concerning diagnosis, treatment, and prognosis.

Provide the patient with realistic choices about certain aspects of care.

Encourage an attitude of realistic hope as a way of dealing with feelings of helplessness.

Evaluate the patient's decision-making ability.

Seek to understand the patient's perspective of a stressful situation.

Discourage decision making when the patient is under severe stress.

Encourage gradual mastery of the situation.

Encourage patience in developing relationships.

Encourage relationships with persons who have common interests and goals.

Encourage social and community activities.

Encourage the acceptance of limitations in others.

Acknowledge the patient's spiritual/cultural background.

Encourage the use of spiritual resources if desired.

Explore the patient's previous achievements of success.

Explore the patient's reasons for self-criticism.

Confront the patient's ambivalent (angry or depressed) feelings.

Foster constructive outlets for anger and hostility.

Arrange situations that encourage the patient's autonomy.

Assist the patient in identifying positive responses from others.

Encourage the identification of specific life values.

Explore with the patient previous methods of dealing with life problems.

Introduce the patient to persons (or groups) who have successfully undergone the same experience.

Support the use of appropriate defense mechanisms.

Encourage verbalization of feelings, perceptions, and fears.

Discuss the consequences of not dealing with guilt and shame.

Encourage the patient to identify his or her own strengths and abilities.

Assist the patient in identifying appropriate short- and long-term goals.

Assist the patient in breaking down complex goals into small, manageable steps.

Assist the patient in examining available resources to meet the goals.

Reduce stimuli in the environment that could be misinterpreted as threatening.

Appraise the patient's needs and desires for social support.

Assist the patient to identify available support systems.

Determine the risk of the patient's inflicting self-harm.

Encourage family involvement as appropriate.

Encourage the family to verbalize their feelings about the ill family member.

Provide appropriate social skills training.

Assist the patient to identify positive strategies to deal with limitations and manage needed lifestyle or role changes.

Assist the patient to solve problems in a constructive manner.

Instruct the patient in the use of relaxation techniques as needed.

Assist the patient to grieve and to work through the losses of chronic illness and/or disability if appropriate.

Assist the patient to clarify misconceptions.

Encourage the patient to evaluate his or her own behavior.

Reproduced with permission from McCloskey, J. C., & Bulechek, G. M. (1999). *Nursing intervention classification* (NIC) (3rd ed.) St. Louis: Mosby–Year Book.

---

5. Become aware of your breathing, and start using your selected focus word.
6. Maintain a passive attitude.
7. Continue for a set period of time.
8. Practice the technique twice daily.

This response combines meditation with relaxation. Along with the repeated word or phrase, a passive attitude is essential. If other thoughts or distractions (noises, the pain of an ailment) occur, Benson recommends not fighting the distraction but simply continuing to repeat the focus phrase. The time of day is not important, but the exercise works best on an empty stomach.

Relaxation With Guided Imagery

Simple **guided imagery** is the "purposeful use of imagination to achieve relaxation or direct attention away from undesirable sensations" (McCloskey & Bulechek, 1999, p. 506). The nurse helps the person select a pleasant scene or experience, such as watching the ocean or dabbling the feet in a cool stream. This image serves as the mental device in this technique. As the person sits comfortably and quietly, the nurse guides the individual to review the scene, trying to feel and relive the imagery with all of the senses. A tape recording may be made of the description of the image, or commercial tape recordings for guided imagery and relaxation can be used.

Other relaxation techniques include meditation, breathing techniques, massage, Reiki, music therapy, biofeedback, and the use of humor.

EDUCATING ABOUT STRESS MANAGEMENT

Two commonly prescribed nursing educational interventions—providing sensory information and providing procedural information (eg, preoperative teaching)—have the goal of reducing stress and improving the patient's coping ability. This preparatory education includes giving structured content, such as a lesson in childbirth preparation to expectant parents, a review of cardiovascular anatomy to the cardiac patient, or a description of sensations the patient will experience during cardiac catheterization. These techniques may alter the person–environment relationship such that something that might have been viewed as harmful or a threat will now be perceived more positively. Giving patients information also reduces the emotional response so that they can concentrate and solve problems more effectively (Calvin & Lane, 1999; Millo & Sullivan, 2000).

ENHANCING SOCIAL SUPPORT

The nature of social support and its influence on coping have been studied extensively; social support has been demonstrated to be an effective moderator of life stress. Social support has been found to provide the individual with several different types of emotional information (Heitzman & Kaplan, 1988; Wineman, 1990). The first type of information leads people to believe that they are cared for and loved. This emotional support appears most often in a relationship between two people in which mutual trust and attachment are expressed by helping one another meet their emotional needs. The second type of information leads people to believe that they are esteemed and valued. This is most effective when there is recognition that demonstrates the individual's favorable position in the group. It elevates the person's sense of self-worth and is called esteem support. The third type of information leads people to believe that they belong to a network of communication and mutual obligation. Members of this network share information and make goods and services available to the members on demand.

Social support also facilitates an individual's coping behaviors; this depends, however, on the nature of the social support. People can have extensive relationships and interact frequently, but the necessary support comes only when there is a deep level of involvement and concern, not when people merely touch the surface of each other's lives. The critical qualities within a social network are the exchange of intimate communications and the presence of solidarity and trust.

Emotional support from family and significant others provides a person with love and a sense of sharing the burden. The emotions that accompany stress are unpleasant and often increase in a spiraling fashion if relief is not provided. Being able to talk with someone and express feelings openly may help the person to gain mastery of the situation. Nurses can provide this support; however, it is important to identify the person's social support system and encourage its use. People who are loners, who are isolated, or who withdraw in times of stress have a high risk of coping failure.

Because anxiety can also distort a person's ability to process information, it helps to seek information and advice from others who can assist with analyzing the threat and developing a strategy to manage it. Again, this use of others helps the person to maintain mastery of a situation and to retain self-esteem.

Thus, social networks assist with management of stress by providing the individual with

- A positive social identity
- Emotional support
- Material aid and tangible services
- Access to information
- Access to new social contacts and new social roles

RECOMMENDING SUPPORT AND THERAPY GROUPS

Support groups exist especially for people in similar stressful situations. Groups have been formed by parents of children with leukemia, people with ostomies, mastectomy patients, and those with other kinds of cancer or other serious diseases, chronic illnesses, and disabilities. There are groups for single parents, substance abusers and their family members, and victims of child abuse. Professional, civic, and religious support groups are active in many communities. There are also encounter groups, assertiveness training programs, and consciousness-raising groups to help people modify their usual behaviors in their transactions with their environment. Being a member of a group with similar problems or goals has a releasing effect on a person that promotes freedom of expression and exchange of ideas.

As previously noted, a person's psychological and biologic health, internal and external sources of stress management, and relationships with the environment are predictors of health outcomes. These factors are directly related to the health patterns of the individual. The nurse has a significant role and responsibility in identifying the health patterns of the person receiving care. If those patterns are not achieving physiologic, psychological, and social balance, the nurse is obligated, with the assistance and agreement of the patient, to seek ways to promote balance.

Although this chapter has presented some physiologic mechanisms and perspectives on health and disease, the way that one copes with stress, the way one relates to others, and the values and goals held are also interwoven into those physiologic patterns. To evaluate a patient's health patterns and to intervene if a problem exists requires a total assessment of the person. Specific problems and their nursing management are addressed in greater depth in other chapters.

Critical Thinking Exercises

1. Think about a patient who has survived a major motor vehicle crash and is hospitalized for severe burns, a fractured hip, and multiple lacerations and abrasions. Identify the actual and potential physical, physiological, and psychosocial stressors evident from this person's trauma. Determine nursing strategies to reduce or alleviate these stressors.

2. A 50-year-old woman is diagnosed with osteoporosis after sustaining a rib fracture. The nurse is evaluating the coping style of the woman. What indications would the nurse note in her interactions and follow-up care for this patient that demonstrate that the woman uses problem-focused coping and emotion-focused coping?

3. Select a patient to whom you are assigned who has an acute illness or injury. Describe the manner in which homeostasis has been maintained or disrupted and the compensatory mechanisms that are evident. How does the patient's medical treatment support the compensatory mechanisms? How do you determine the nursing interventions that are appropriate for promoting the healing process?

4. A family composed of two parents, two adolescent male sons, and the maternal grandfather explore with the nurse their health promotion needs. The family's health history reveals that the mother has adult-onset diabetes; the father has coronary artery disease; the sons are somewhat overweight; and the grandfather has mild congestive heart failure. The family has ample resources for making changes in their lifestyle. What interventions would the nurse initiate to promote a healthier lifestyle for this family?

REFERENCES AND SELECTED READINGS

Books

Andreoli, T. E. (Ed.). (1997). *Cecil essentials of medicine* (4th ed.). Philadelphia: W. B. Saunders.

Barnfather, J. S., & Lyon, B. L. (Eds.). (1993). *Stress and coping: State of the science and implications for nursing theory, research and practice.* Indianapolis: Sigma Theta Tau International Inc.

Benson, H. (1993). The relaxation response. In D. Goleman & J. Gurin (Eds.), *Mind-body medicine: How to use your mind for better health* (pp. 125–148). Yonkers, NY: Consumer Reports Books.

Benson, H., & Proctor, W. (1984). *Beyond the relaxation response.* New York: Berkley Books.

Benson, H., & Stark, M. (1996). *Timeless healing.* New York: Scribner.

Copel, L. C. (2000). *Nurse's clinical guide: Psychiatric and mental health care* (2nd ed.). Springhouse, PA: Springhouse.

Dubos, R. (1965). *Man adapting.* New Haven, CT: Yale University Press.

Fauci, A. (Ed.). (1998). *Harrison's principles of internal medicine* (14th ed.). New York: McGraw-Hill.

Guyton, A. C. (1996). *Human physiology: Mechanisms of disease* (6th ed.). Philadelphia: W. B. Saunders.

Guyton, A. C. (1995). *Textbook of medical physiology* (9th ed.). Philadelphia: W. B. Saunders.

Jalowiec, A. (1993). Coping with illness: Synthesis and critique of the nursing literature from 1980–1990. In J. S. Barnfather & B. L. Lyon (Eds.), *Stress and coping: State of the science and implications for nursing theory, research and practice.* Indianapolis: Sigma Theta Tau International Inc.

Lazarus, R. S. (1991a). *Emotion and adaptation.* New York: Oxford University Press.

Lazarus, R. S. (1993). Why we should think of stress as a subset of emotion. In L. Goldberger & S. Breznitz (Eds.), *Handbook of stress* (2nd ed.). New York: The Free Press.

Lazarus, R. S., & Folkman, S. (1984). *Stress, appraisal, and coping.* New York: Springer Publishing Co.

McCloskey, J. C., & Bulechek, G. M. (Eds.). (1999). *Nursing interventions classification (NIC)* (2nd ed.). St. Louis: Mosby–Year Book.

McEwen, B., & Mendelson, S. (1993). Effects of stress on the neurochemistry and morphology of the brain: Counterregulation versus damage. In I. Goldberger & S. Breznitz (Eds.), *Handbook of stress* (2nd ed.). New York: The Free Press.

Mickler, M. (1997). *Community organizing and community building for health.* New Brunswick, NJ: Rutgers University Press.

Miller, L. H., & Smith, A. D. (1993). *The stress solution.* New York: Pocket Books.

North American Nursing Diagnosis Association. (2000). *NANDA nursing diagnoses: Definitions and classifications.* Philadelphia: Author.

Selye, H. (1976). *The stress of life.* (Rev. ed.). New York: McGraw-Hill.

Watkins, A. (Ed.). (1997). *Mind-body medicine: A clinician's guide to psychoneuroimmunology.* New York: Churchill Livingstone.

Journals

Asterisks indicate nursing research articles.

*Almberg, B., Grafstrom, M., & Winblad, B. (1997). Major strain and coping strategies as reported by family members who care for aged demented relatives. *Journal of Advanced Nursing, 26*(4), 683–691.

Anderson, B. L., Farrar, W. B., Golden-Kreutz, D., et al. (1998). Stress and immune responses after surgical treatment for regional breast cancer. *Journal of National Cancer Institute, 90*(1), 30–36.

Baird, C. L. (2000). Living with hurting and difficulty doing: Older women with osteoarthritis. *Clinical Excellence for Nurse Practitioners, 4*(4), 231–237.

Ballard, A. (1981). Identification of environmental stressors for patients in a surgical intensive care unit. *Issues in Mental Health Nursing, 11*(3), 89–100.

Biondi, M., Peronti, M., Pacitti, F., Pancheri, P., Pacifici, R., Altieri, I., Paris, L., & Zuccaro, P. (1994). Personality, endocrine and immune changes after eight months in healthy individuals under normal daily stress. *Psychotherapy and Psychosomatics, 62*(3–4), 176–184.

Black, P. H. (1994). Central nervous system–immune system interactions: Psychoneuroendocrinology of stress and its immune consequences. *Antimicrobial Agents and Chemotherapy, 38*(1), 1–6.

*Brillhart, B., & Johnson, K. (1997). Motivation and the coping process of adults with disabilities: A qualitative study. *Rehabilitation Nursing, 22*(5), 249–256.

Bryla, C. M. (1996). The relationship between stress and the development of breast cancer: A literature review. *Oncology Nursing Forum, 23*(3), 441–448.

Calvin, R. L., & Lane, P. L. (1999). Perioperative uncertainty and state anxiety of orthopedic surgical patients. *Orthopaedic Nursing, 18*(6), 61–66.

Chalfont, L., & Bennett, P. (1999). Personality and coping: Their influence on affect and behavior following myocardial infarction. *Coronary Health Care, 3*(3), 110–116.

Clements, K., & Turpin, G. (2000). Life events exposure, physiological reactivity, and psychological strain. *Journal of Behavioral Medicine, 23*(1), 73–94.

Cohen, J. I. (2000). Stress and mental health: A biobehavioral perspective. *Issues in Mental Health Nursing, 21*(2), 185–202.

*Collins, M. A. (1996). The relation of work stress, hardiness, and burnout among full-time hospital staff nurses. *Journal of Nursing Staff Development, 12*(2), 81–85.

*Constantino, R. E., Sekula, L. K., Rabin, B., & Stone, C. (2000). Negative life experiences, depression, and immune function in abused and non-abused women. *Biological Research in Nursing, 1*(3), 190–198.

Cronquist, A., Wredding, R., Norlander, R., Langius, A., & Bjorvell, H. (2000). Perceived discomfort and related coping phenomenon in patients undergoing percutaneous transluminal coronary angioplasty. *Coronary Health Care, 4*(3), 123–129.

*Fallon, M., Gould, D., & Wainwright, S. P. (1997). Stress and quality of life in the renal transplant patient: A preliminary investigation. *Journal of Advanced Nursing, 25*(3), 562–570.

*Felton, B. S. (2000). Resilience in a multicultural sample of community-dwelling women older than age 85. *Clinical Nursing Research, 9*(2), 102–103.

Glaser, R., & Kiecolt-Glaser, J. K. (1997). Chronic stress modulates the virus-specific immune response to latent herpes simplex virus type 1. *Annals Behavioral Medicine, 19*(2), 78–82.

Goodkin, K., Feaster, D. J., Tuttle, R., Blaney, N. T., Kumar, M., Baum, M. K., Shapshak, P., & Fletcher, M. A. (1996). Bereavement is associated with time-dependent decrements in cellular immune function in asymptomatic human immunodeficiency virus type 1-seropositive homosexual men. *Clinics in Diagnostic Laboratory Immunology, 3*(1), 109–180.

*Hagerty, B. M., Williams, R. A., Coyne, J. C., & Early, M. R. (1996). Sense of belonging and indicators of social and psychological functioning. *Archives of Psychiatric Nursing, 10*(4), 235–244.

Heitzman, C. A., & Kaplan, R. M. (1998). Assessment of methods for measuring social support. *Health Psychology, 7*, 75–109.

Holmes, T. H., & Rahe, R. H. (1967). The social readjustment rating scale. *Journal of Psychosomatic Research, 11*, 213–218.

*Kennedy, J. W. (2000). Women's inner balance: A comparison of stressors, personality traits, and health problems by age groups. *Journal of Advanced Nursing, 31*(3): 639–650.

*Langford, C. P., Bowsher, J., Maloney, J. P., & Lillis, P. P. (1997). Social support: a conceptual analysis. *Journal of Advanced Nursing, 25*(1), 95–100.

Lazarus, R. S. (1991b). Cognition and motivation in emotion. *American Psychologist, 46*(4), 352–367.

Lazarus, R. S. (1991c). Progress on a cognitive-motivational-relational theory of emotion. *American Psychologist, 46*(8), 819–834.

*Mahat, G. (1997). Perceived stressors and coping strategies among individuals with rheumatoid arthritis. *Journal of Advanced Nursing, 25*(6), 1144–1150.

Matthews, K. A., Caggiula, A. R., McAllister, C. G., et al. (1995). Sympathetic reactivity to acute stress and immune response in women. *Psychosomatic Medicine, 57*(6), 564–571.

*Millio, M. E., & Sullivan, K. (2000). Patients with operable esophageal cancer: Their experience of information giving in a regional thoracic unit. *Journal of Clinical Nursing, 9*(2), 236–246.

Morse, D. L. (2000). Continuing care extra: Relocation stress is real. *American Journal of Nursing, 100*(8), 24A–24D.

*Morse, S. R., & Fife, B. (1998). Coping with a partner's cancer, adjustment at four stages of the illness trajectory. *Oncology Nursing Forum, 25*(4), 751–760.

Pike, J. L., Smith, T. L., Hauger, R. L., et al. (1997). Chronic life stress alters sympathetic, neuroendocrine, and immune responsivity to an acute psychological stressor in humans. *Psychosomatic Medicine, 59*(4), 447–457.

Robinson, F. P., Matthews, H. L., Witek-Janusek, L. (2000). Stress reduction and HIV disease: A review of intervention studies using a psychoimmunology framework. *Journal of the Association of Nurses in AIDS Care, 11*(2), 87–96.

*Ryan, M. C. (1996). Loneliness, social support and depression as interactive variables with cognitive status: testing Roy's model. *Nursing Science Quarterly, 9*(3), 107–114.

Schrader, K. A. (1996). Stress and immunity after traumatic injury: The mind–body link. *AACN Clinical Issues in Critical Care Nursing, 7*(3), 351–358.

Seers, K., & Carrol, D. (1998). Relaxation techniques for acute pain management: A systematic review. *Journal of Advanced Nursing, 27*(3), 466–475.

Sergerstrom, S. C., Fahey, J. L., Kemeny, M. E., & Taylor, S. E. (1998). Optimism is associated with mood, coping, and immune change in response to stress. *Journal of Perspectives in Social Psychology, 74*(6), 1646–1655.

Smith, L. L. (2000). Cytokine hypothesis of overtraining: A physiological adaptation to excessive stress? *Medicine and Science in Sports and Exercise, 32*(2), 317–331.

*Starzonski, R., & Hilton, A. (2000). Patient and family adjustment to kidney transplantation with and without an interim period of dialysis. *Nephrology Nursing Journal, 27*(1), 17, 18, 21–33, 52.

Tausig, M. (1982). Measuring life events. *Journal of Health and Social Behavior, 23*(1), 52–64.

Wells-Federman, C. (1996). Awakening the nurse healer within. *Holistic Nursing Practice, 10*(2), 13–29.

*Williams, A. M. (2000). Distress and hardiness: A comparison of African Americans and white caregivers. *Journal of National Black Nurses Association, 11*(1), 21–26.

*Wineman, N. M. (1990). Adaptation to multiple sclerosis: The role of social support, functional disability, and perceived uncertainty. *Nursing Research, 39*, 294–299.

Individual and Family Considerations Related to Illness

On completion of this chapter, the learner will be able to:

1. Describe the holistic approach to sustaining health and well-being.
2. Discuss the concepts of emotional well-being and emotional distress.
3. Identify variables that influence the ability to cope with stress and that are antecedents to emotional disorders.
4. Explain the concepts of anxiety, posttraumatic stress disorder, depression, loss, and grief.
5. Describe a framework for understanding death and dying.
6. Assess the impact of illness on the patient's family and on family functioning.
7. Determine the role of the nurse in identifying substance abuse problems and in assisting the family to cope.
8. Explore the concept of spirituality and address the spiritual needs of patients.
9. Identify nursing actions that promote effective coping for both the patient and the family.

*W*hen people experience threats to their health, they seek out various care providers for the purpose of maintaining or restoring health. In recent years, both the patient and the family have become more involved participants in health care and health promotion activities. At the same time, greater numbers of consumers and practitioners have recognized the interconnectedness of mind, body, and spirit in sustaining well-being and overcoming or coping with illness. This holistic approach to health and wellness and the increased consumer involvement reflect a renewed emphasis on the concepts of choice, healing, and patient–practitioner partnerships. The holistic perspective focuses not only on promoting well-being but also on understanding how one's emotional state contributes to health and illness. By using this knowledge, people are better able to prevent the reoccurrence or exacerbation of problems and to develop strategies to improve their future health status.

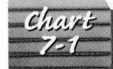

Chart 7-1 Common Complementary and Alternative Therapies

- Alternative medical systems including acupuncture, Ayurveda, homeopathic medicine, and naturopathic medicine
- Mind-body interventions including meditation, certain uses of hypnosis, dance, music, art therapy and prayer
- Biologically based therapies including herbal, special dietary, orthomolecular, and individual biological therapies
- Manipulative and body-based methods including chiropractic and osteopathy
- Energy therapies including Qi gong, Reiki, and therapeutic touch

Reprinted with permission from Dossey, B. M., Guzzetta, C., & Keegan, L. (2002). *Holistic nursing: A handbook for practice.* Gaithersburg, MD: Aspen Publications.

Holistic Approach to Health and Health Care

Since the 1980s, holistic therapies have more frequently accompanied traditional health care. A survey on the use of **holistic health** practices reported that about 34% of the 1539 respondents in a national random sample of adults older than 18 years of age (732 women and 807 men) had consulted with at least one holistic health care practitioner within the past year. The study further noted that although many of the people were also seeing a traditional health care provider, 72% did not inform the physician that they were obtaining holistic treatment (Eisenberg, et al., 1993). Several additional research studies (Sparber, et al., 2000; Wynia, Eisenberg, & Wilson, 1999) support the original work of Eisenberg's group indicating that adult clients, even clients participating in clinical research trials, frequently use **complementary therapies** to assist them in coping with their illnesses and treatments. The need to discuss the use of these adjunct therapies with clients in all settings is imperative. During their clinical assessments, nurses must obtain information about the client's use of complementary therapies. Some of the most commonly used complementary therapies are listed in Chart 7-1.

For some people, the holistic approach is viewed as a way to capitalize on personal strengths and recultivate the values and beliefs about health that were common before the age of technological innovations and the sophistication of biomedical science. A lack of focus on the individual patient, the family, and the environment by some health care providers has created feelings of disillusionment

and depersonalization in many patients. The cost of illness, especially chronic illness care, continues to escalate and accounts for an increasing percentage of health care dollars. At the same time, patient satisfaction with the health care received has decreased.

Active participation of the patient and family in promoting health supports the self-care model historically embraced by the nursing profession. This model is congruent with the philosophy that seeks to balance and integrate the use of crisis medicine and advanced technology with the influence of the mind and spirit on healing. A holistic approach to health reconnects the traditionally separate approaches to mind and body. Factors such as the physical environment, economic conditions, sociocultural issues, emotional state, interpersonal relationships, and support systems can work together or alone to influence health. The connections among physical health, emotional health, and spiritual well-being must be understood and considered when providing health care. It is the nurse's conceptual integration of the physiologic health condition with the emotional and social context, along with the tasks and developments of the patient's life stage, that allows for the development of a holistic plan of nursing care.

The Brain and Physical and Emotional Health

Research on brain structure and function, neurochemical messenger systems (neurotransmitters), and brain–body connections suggests fundamental, delicate, two-way relationships between

---

Glossary

anxiety: an emotional state characterized by feelings of apprehension, discomfort, restlessness, or worry

bereavement: feelings, thoughts, and responses that occur after a loss

complementary therapies: used as an adjunct to traditional health modalities; they typically influence the effects of stress, anxiety, depression, and other physical and emotional states

depression: state in which a person feels sad, distressed, and hopeless, with little to no energy for normal activities

faith: belief and trust in a God or higher power

family: a group whose members are related by reciprocal caring, mutual responsibilities, and loyalties

grief: a universal response to any loss

holistic health: promotion of the total health of mind, body, and spirit

homeopathic medicine: a system of medicine that promotes healing of the whole person by stimulating the natural healing processes within the person

mental disorder: a state in which a person has deficits in functioning, has a distorted sense of self or the world, is unable to sustain relationships, or cannot handle stress or conflict effectively

mental health: a state in which a person can meet basic needs, assume responsibilities, sustain relationships, resolve conflicts, and grow throughout life

posttraumatic stress disorder (PTSD): the development of severe anxiety-type symptoms after the experience of a traumatic life event

substance abuse: a maladaptive pattern of drug use that causes physical and emotional harm with the potential for disruption of daily life

the brain's environment and mood, behavior, and resistance to disease (Cohen & Herbert, 1996). One focus of brain research has been to identify and integrate traditional medical and psychiatric knowledge with new psychobiologic and psychoneuroimmunologic data. Researchers in the field of psychobiology study the biologic basis of mental disturbances and have established some relationships between mental disorders and changes in the structure and function of the brain. Researchers in the field of psychoneuroimmunology study the connections between the emotions, the central nervous system, the neuroendocrine system, and the immune system and have established compelling evidence that psychosocial variables can affect the functioning of the immune system.

As this neuroscientific research continues, data about neurotransmitters and the functioning of the brain will augment existing understanding of emotions, intelligence, memory, and many aspects of general body functioning. In the future, an accepted definition of mental illness may well include biologic information. By enhancing the biologic knowledge base about the brain and nervous system, scientists establish the foundation for breakthroughs in the treatment of both symptoms and illnesses.

These findings suggest that the health care community ought to place as much emphasis on emotional health as it places on physiologic health and ought to recognize how biologic, emotional, and societal problems combine to affect individual patients, families, and communities. Some problems that nurses and other health care providers must address include **substance abuse**, homelessness, family violence, eating disorders, trauma, and chronic **mental health** conditions such as anxiety and depression. To focus attention on these and other mental health problems, the U.S. Department of Health and Human Services initiated a mental health agenda for the nation in the document entitled *Healthy People 2010* (U.S. Public Health Service, 2000). The objectives identified are summarized in Chart 7-2. Nurses in all settings encounter patients with mental health problems and have an integral role in helping to achieve the national goals by recognizing and treating emotional distress and promoting emotional health.

Emotional Health and Emotional Distress

The concept of emotional health encompasses a person's ability to function as comfortably and productively as possible. Typically, people who are mentally healthy are satisfied with themselves and their life situations. In the usual course of living, emotionally healthy people focus on activities geared to meet their needs and attempt to accomplish personal goals while concurrently managing everyday challenges and problems. Often, people must work hard to balance their feelings, thoughts, and behaviors to alleviate emotional distress, and much energy is used to change, adapt, or manage the obstacles inherent in daily living. A mentally healthy person accepts reality and has a positive sense of self. Emotional health is also manifested by having moral and humanistic values and beliefs, having satisfying interpersonal relationships, doing productive work, and maintaining a realistic sense of hope (Chart 7-3).

When people have unmet emotional needs or distress, they experience an overall feeling of unhappiness. As tension escalates, security and survival are threatened. How different people respond to these troublesome situations reflects their level of coping and maturity. Emotionally healthy people endeavor to meet the demands of distressing situations while still facing the typical issues that emerge in their lives. The ways in which people respond to uncomfortable stimuli reflect their exposure to various biologic, emotional, and sociocultural experiences.

When stress interferes with a person's ability to function comfortably and inhibits the effective management of personal needs, that person is at risk for emotional problems. The use of ineffective and unhealthy methods of coping is manifested by dysfunctional behaviors, thoughts, and feelings. These behaviors are aimed at relieving the overwhelming stress, even though they may cause further problems.

Coping ability is strongly influenced by biologic or genetic factors, physical and emotional growth and development, family and childhood experiences, and learning. Typically, a person reverts to the strategies observed early in life that were used by family

---

| Chart 7-2 | **Major Mental Health Objectives for Healthy People in the Year 2010** |

- Reduce the proportion of children and adolescents with disabilities who are reported to be sad, unhappy, or depressed.
- Reduce the proportion of adults with disabilities who report feelings such as sadness, unhappiness, or depression that prevent them from being active
- Increase the proportion of adults with disabilities reporting sufficient emotional support.
- Increase the proportion of adults with disabilities reporting satisfaction with life.
- Reduce the suicide rate.
- Reduce the rate of suicide attempts by adolescents.
- Reduce the proportion of homeless adults who have serious mental illness.
- Increase the proportion of persons with serious mental illness who are employed.
- Reduce the relapse rates for persons with eating disorders including anorexia nervosa and bulimia nervosa.

- Increase the number of persons in primary care who receive mental health screening and assessment.
- Increase the proportion of children with mental health problems who receive treatment.
- Increase the proportion of juvenile justice facilities that screen admissions for mental health problems.
- Increase the proportion of adults with mental disorders who receive treatment.
- Increase the proportion of persons with co-occurring substance abuse and mental disorders who receive treatment for both disorders.
- Increase the number of states and the District of Columbia that track consumer satisfaction with the mental health services they receive.
- Increase the number of states, territories, and the District of Columbia with an operational mental health plan that addresses cultural competence.

U.S. Public Health Service. (2000). *Healthy people 2010: Understanding and improving health.* Washington, DC: U.S. Government Printing Office.

Chart 7-3 Characteristics Associated With Mental Health

- Positive sense of self
- Satisfying interpersonal relationships
- Wide range of appropriate emotions
- Love and care for self and others
- Realistic and responsible behavior
- Effective coping skills
- Ability to negotiate and resolve conflict
- Cooperative and interdependent in working with others
- Engagement in rewarding, productive work
- Adaptable to the daily challenges of life
- Finds meaning and purpose in life
- Has hopes and dreams
- Knowledge of personal strengths and areas needing improvement
- Sense of humor
- Respect for the rights and differences of others

Chart 7-5 Risk Factors for Mental Health Problems

Risk Factors That Cannot Be Changed
Age
Gender
Genetic background
Family history

Risk Factors That Can Be Changed
Marital status
Family environment
Housing problems
Poverty or economic difficulties
Physical health
Nutritional status
Stress level
Social environment and activities
Exposure to trauma
Alcohol and drug use
Environmental toxins or other pollutants
Availability, accessibility, and cost of health services

members, caregivers, and others to solve conflict. If these strategies were not adaptive, the person exhibits a range of painful and nonproductive behaviors. Dysfunctional behavior in one person not only seriously affects that person's emotional health but can also put others at risk for injury or death. As these destructive behaviors are repeated, a cyclic pattern becomes evident: impaired thinking, negative feelings, and more dysfunctional actions that prevent the person from meeting the demands of daily living (Chart 7-4).

No universally accepted definition of what constitutes an emotional disorder exists. But many views and theories share in common the idea that a number of variables can interfere with emotional growth and development and impede successful adaptation to the environment. Most clinicians have adopted the statement from the American Psychiatric Association's *Diagnostic and Statistical Manual of Mental Disorders (DSM-IV TR)*, which defines the term **mental disorder** as a group of behavioral or psychological symptoms or a pattern that manifests itself in significant distress, impaired functioning, or accentuated risk of enduring severe suffering or possible death (American Psychiatric Association, 2000, p. xxi). Risk factors for mental health problems are listed in Chart 7-5.

Patients seen in medical-surgical settings often struggle with psychosocial issues of anxiety, depression, loss, and grief. Abuse, addiction, chemical dependency, body image disturbances, and eating disorders are a few examples of health situations that require extensive physical and emotional care to restore optimal functioning. The dual challenge for the health team is to understand how the patient's emotions influence current physiologic conditions and to identify the best care for the patient experiencing underlying emotional and spiritual distress.

Family Health and Distress

The **family** plays a central role in the life of the patient and is a major part of the context of the patient's life. It is within families that people grow, are nurtured, attain a sense of self, cultivate beliefs and values about life, and progress through life's developmental stages (Chart 7-6). The family is also the first source for socialization and teaching about health and illness. The family prepares the person with strategies for balancing closeness with separateness and togetherness with individuality. A major role of the family is to provide physical and emotional resources to maintain health and a system of support in times of crises, such as in periods of illness. Educating families has been shown to add to their resiliency, adaptation, and adjustment to life stressors (Friedman, 1998).

When a family member becomes ill, all members of the family are affected. Depending on the nature of the health problem, family members may need to make several adaptations to their existing lifestyles or even restructure their lifestyles.

Health problems often have an impact on the family's ability to function. Five family functions described by Wright and Leahey (2000) are viewed as essential to the individual's and family's growth. The first function, management, involves the use of power, decision making about resources, establishment of rules, provision of finances, and future planning—responsibilities assumed by the adults of the family. The second function, boundary setting, makes clear distinctions between the generations and the roles of adults and children within the family structure. Communication is the third function that is important to individual and family growth; healthy families have a full range of clear, di-

Chart 7-4 Characteristics Associated With Mental Disorders

- Severe anxiety
- Severe depression
- Ineffective coping mechanisms
- Extreme feelings of helplessness or powerlessness
- Maladaptive ways of dealing with stress
- Uncomfortable with self and others
- Lack of pleasure from living
- Extreme negative thoughts, feelings, and behaviors
- Disorganized or disturbed thoughts
- Inability to accept reality
- Personality traits that contribute to dysfunctional behaviors
- Desire to hurt self or others
- History of traumatic experience
- Inability to satisfy basic needs
- Lack of a support system
- Physiologic problems resulting from severe, unrelenting stress

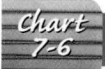

Chart 7-6   Adult Developmental Tasks

Developmental stage and associated tasks can have an impact on how individuals cope with illness.

Young Adult
Establish independence
Establish lifestyle
Develop career
Develop intimate relationships
Marry and start a family

Middle Adult
Establish financial security
Prepare for retirement
Launch children
Refocus on marital relationship
Support growing children and aging parents

Older Adult
Adapt to retirement and alteration in role
Adapt to declining physical stamina
Review life's accomplishments
Prepare for death

---

rect, and meaningful communication among their members. The fourth function is education and support. Education involves modeling skills for living a physically, emotionally, and socially healthy life; support is manifested by actions that tell family members they are cared about and loved. Family support promotes health and is seen as a critical factor in coping with crises and illness situations. The final function is socialization. Families transmit culture and the acceptable behaviors needed to perform adequately in the home and in the world.

NURSING IMPLICATIONS

There are many degrees of family functioning. The nurse assesses family functioning to determine how the family will cope with the impact of the health condition. If the family is chaotic or disorganized, promoting coping skills becomes a priority in the plan of care. The family with preexisting problems may require additional assistance before participating fully in the current health situation. In performing a family assessment, the nurse must evaluate the present family structure and function. Areas of appraisal include demographic data, developmental information (keeping in mind that family members can be in several different developmental stages simultaneously), family structure, family functioning, and coping abilities. The role that the environment plays in family health is also assessed.

Interventions with family members are based on strengthening coping skills through direct care, communication skills, and education. Healthy family communication has a strong influence on the quality of family life and can help the family to make appropriate choices, consider alternative strategies, or persevere through complex circumstances. Within a family system, for example, the identified patient may be undergoing extensive surgery for cancer while the partner has cardiac disease, the adolescent has type 1 diabetes, and the child has a fractured arm. In this situation, there are multiple health concerns along with competing developmental tasks and needs. Despite the obvious concerns of the family members, both individually and collectively, a crisis may or may not be present. This family may be coping effectively; alternatively, the family may be in crisis or may manifest a chronic inability to

handle the situation. The health team conducts a careful and comprehensive family assessment, develops interventions tailored to handle the stressors, implements the specified treatment protocols, and facilitates the construction of social support systems.

The use of existing family strengths, resources, and education is augmented by therapeutic family interventions. The nurse's primary goals are to maintain and improve the patient's present level of health and to prevent physical and emotional deterioration. Next, the nurse intervenes in the cycle that the illness creates: patient illness, stress for other family members, generation of potential for illness in other family members, and additional stress for the patient.

Helping the family members handle the myriad stressors that bombard them daily involves working with family members to develop coping skills. In a 1994 study, Burr and associates identified seven traits that enhance coping of family members under stress. Communication skills and spirituality were the most useful traits. Cognitive abilities, emotional strengths, relationship capabilities, willingness to use community resources, and individual strengths and talents were also associated with effective coping. As nurses work with families, they must not underestimate the impact that their therapeutic interactions, educational information, positive role modeling, provision of direct care, and corrective teaching have on promoting health.

Without the active support of the family members and the health team, the potential for using maladaptive coping mechanisms increases. Often, denial and blaming of individuals occur. Sometimes, physiologic illness, emotional withdrawal, and physical distancing are the results of severe family conflict, violent behaviors, or addiction to drugs and alcohol. Substance abuse is sometimes the outcome for family members who view their ability to cope or solve problems as impossible. Often, people engage in these dysfunctional behaviors when faced with difficult or problematic situations.

Anxiety

All people experience some degree of **anxiety** (a tense emotional state) as they face new, challenging, or threatening life situations. In clinical settings, fear of the unknown, unexpected news about one's health, and any impairment of bodily functions engenders anxiety. Although a mild level of anxiety can mobilize people to take a position, act on the task that needs to be done, or learn to alter lifestyle habits, a more severe level can be almost paralyzing. Anxiety that escalates to a near panic state can be incapacitating. When patients receive unwelcome news about results of diagnostic studies, they are sure to experience anxiety. Different patients manifest the physiologic, emotional, and behavioral signs and symptoms of anxiety in various ways (Nursing Research Profile 7-1).

NURSING IMPLICATIONS

Early clinical observations of guilt or anxiety are an essential component of nursing care (Chart 7-7). A high level of anxiety in a patient will probably exacerbate physiologic distress. For example, a postoperative patient who is in pain may discover that anxiety intensifies the sensation of pain. A patient newly diagnosed with type 1 diabetes mellitus may be worried and fearful and therefore unable to focus on or complete essential self-care activities. The possibility of developing somatic symptoms is high in any patient who is experiencing moderate to severe anxiety.

The *DSM-IV TR* (2000) lists general medical conditions that cause anxiety. They include endocrine diseases, such as hypothyroidism, hyperthyroidism, hypoglycemia, and hyperadrenocor-

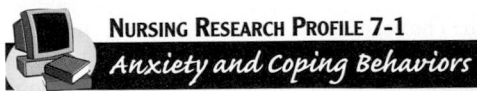

NURSING RESEARCH PROFILE 7-1
Anxiety and Coping Behaviors

Dropkin, M. J. (2001). Anxiety, coping strategies, and coping behaviors in patients undergoing head and neck cancer surgery. *Cancer Nursing, 24*(2), 143–148.

Purpose
This research study described the relationships between preoperative anxiety and the use of coping strategies, and between postoperative self-care and resocialization behaviors, in patients who have facial disfigurement or dysfunction as a result of head and neck cancer surgery.

Study Sample and Design
The sample for this descriptive correlational study consisted of 75 participants (53 men and 22 women) who were about to sustain facial disfigurement and dysfunction as an outcome of head and neck surgery. Subjects were requested to complete the State Trait Anxiety Inventory and the Ways of Coping Questionnaire before their surgery and the Coping Behaviors Score and the Disfigurement/Dysfunction Scale afterward.

Findings
The results of the study revealed no significant correlations between preoperative anxiety and the percentage of problem-focused coping strategies used to handle disfiguring surgery. A high level of anxiety was present, which was equivalent to the anxiety of people admitted to a psychiatric treatment center for an acute anxiety reaction. Although there was low use of problem-focused coping strategies before the surgery, postoperative coping behaviors occurred early in the recovery period. Scores indicated that severe functional impairment was present immediately after surgery. The anxiety scores for these patients decreased over time, but there was no significant correlation between disfigurement/dysfunction and anxiety. The level of anxiety was negatively correlated with self-care after surgery on the fourth and fifth postoperative days. These findings indicate that anxiety is decreased by the performance of self-care behaviors in the early postoperative period.

Nursing Implications
For the nurse caring for a postoperative patient who is undergoing head and neck surgery, it is important to recognize that early participation in self-care behaviors is associated with reduced anxiety in these patients. This relationship between anxiety and self-care increases over time. Therefore, nurses need to facilitate self-care activities in this population, because this intervention can help to promote positive postoperative outcomes.

Chart 7-7 • ASSESSMENT
Assessing Signs and Symptoms of Anxiety

Physiologic Symptoms
Appetite change
Headaches
Muscle tension
Fatigue or lethargy
Weight change
Cold and flu symptoms
Digestive upsets
Grinding teeth
Palpitations
Hypertension
Restlessness
Difficulty sleeping
Skin irritations
Injury prone
Increased use of any alcohol
    or drugs

Emotional Symptoms
Forgetfulness
Low productivity
Feeling dull
Poor concentration
Negative attitude
Confusion
Whirling mind
No new ideas
Boredom
Negative self-talk
Anxiety

Frustration
Depression
Crying periods
Irritability
Worrying
Feeling discouraged
Nervous laughter

Relational Symptoms
Isolation
Intolerance
Resentment
Loneliness
Lashing out
"Clamming up"
Nagging
Distrust
Few friends
No intimacy
Using people

Spiritual Symptoms
Emptiness
Loss of meaning
Doubt
Unforgiving attitude
Martyrdom
Loss of direction
Cynicism
Apathy

Posttraumatic Stress Disorder

In medical-surgical settings, especially in emergency departments, burn units, and rehabilitation centers, nurses care for extremely anxious patients who have experienced devastating events that are typically considered to be outside the realm of normal human experience. Many of these patients suffer from **posttraumatic stress disorder (PTSD)**. PTSD has been described as a

ticism; cardiovascular conditions, such as cardiac dysrhythmia, congestive heart failure, and pulmonary emboli; respiratory problems, such as pneumonia and chronic obstructive pulmonary disease; and neurologic conditions, such as encephalitis and neoplasms.

Every nurse must be vigilant about the patient who worries excessively and demonstrates deterioration in emotional, social, or occupational functioning. If participation in the therapeutic regimen (eg, administration of insulin) becomes a problem because of extreme anxiety, nursing interventions must be immediately initiated. Caring strategies emphasize ways for the patient to verbalize feelings and fears and to identify sources of anxiety. The need to teach and promote effective coping abilities and the use of relaxation techniques are the priorities of care. In some cases, antianxiety medication may be prescribed. Chart 7-8 provides a list of basic nursing principles that are useful for assisting patients to manage severe anxiety. Chapter 6 presents additional information about stress and the relaxation response.

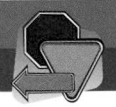

Chart 7-8
GUIDELINES FOR Managing Anxiety

- Listen actively and focus on having the patient discuss personal feelings.
- Use positive remarks and focus on the positive aspects of life in the "here and now."
- Use appropriate touch (with patient permission) to demonstrate support.
- Discuss the importance of safety and the patient's overall sense of well-being.
- Explain all procedures, policies, diagnostic studies, medications, treatments, or protocols for care.
- Explore coping strategies and work with the patient to practice and use them effectively (eg, breathing, progressive relaxation, visualization, imagery).
- Use distraction as indicated to relax and prevent self from being overwhelmed.

condition that generates waves of anxiety, anger, aggression, depression, and suspicion that threaten the person's sense of self and interfere with daily functioning. Specific examples of events that place a person at risk for PTSD are rape, family violence, torture, terrorism, fire, earthquake, and military combat. Patients who have suffered a traumatic event are often frequent users of the health care system by virtue of their extensive injuries, the various treatment modalities that they require, and the overall emotional and physical difficulties experienced.

The physiologic responses noted in people who have been severely traumatized include increased activity of the sympathetic nervous system, increased plasma catecholamine levels, and increased urinary epinephrine and norepinephrine levels. It has been postulated (Gelles, 1997; Gelles & Loseke, 1993) that people with PTSD lose the ability to control their response to stimuli. The resulting excessive arousal can increase overall body metabolism and trigger emotional reactivity. In this situation, the nurse would observe that the patient has difficulty sleeping, has an exaggerated startle response, and is excessively vigilant.

Older people are more susceptible to the physical effects of trauma and the effects of PTSD because of the increased neural inactivation associated with aging. It has also been speculated that when people have a preexisting tendency to become extremely anxious, their vulnerability to PTSD increases (Nursing Research Profile 7-2).

Symptoms of PTSD can occur hours to years after the trauma is experienced. Acute PTSD is defined as the experience of symptoms for less than a 3-month period. Chronic PTSD is defined as the experience of symptoms lasting longer than 3 months. In the case of delayed PTSD, up to 6 months may elapse between the trauma and the manifestation of symptoms (American Psychiatric Association, 2000). For more information see Chart 7-9.

NURSING IMPLICATIONS

It is often thought that the incidence of PTSD is very low in the overall population; when high-risk groups are studied, however, the results indicate that more than 50% of study participants have PTSD (McCann & Pearlman, 1990). Therefore, it is important that nurses consider which of their patients are at risk for PTSD and be knowledgeable about the common symptoms associated with it.

The sensitivity and caring of the nurse creates the interpersonal relationship necessary to work with patients who have PTSD. These patients are physically compromised and are struggling emotionally with situations that are outside the realm of normal human experience–situations that violate the commonly held perceptions of human social justice. Treatment of patients with PTSD includes several essential components: establishing a trusting relationship, addressing and working through the trauma experience, and providing education about the coping skills needed for recovery and self-care. The patient's progress can be influenced by the ability to cope with the various aspects of both the physical and the emotional distress.

Depression

Depression is a common response to health problems and is an often underdiagnosed problem in the patient population. People may become depressed as a result of injury or illness; may be suffering from an earlier loss that is compounded by a new health problem; or they may seek health care for somatic complaints that are bodily manifestations of depression.

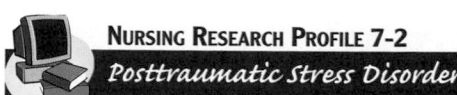

NURSING RESEARCH PROFILE 7-2
Posttraumatic Stress Disorder

Hampton, M. R., & Frombach, I. (2000). Women's experience of traumatic stress in cancer treatment. *Health Care of Women International,* *21*(1), 67–76.

Purpose
A review of literature revealed that few articles in health care journals acknowledge that women's and men's experiences in the health care setting may often be different. The purpose of this study was to examine gender differences in the prevalence and predictors of cancer-related posttraumatic stress disorder (PTSD) in a group of cancer patients.

Study Sample and Design
A total of 225 consecutive patients going to a local cancer clinic were invited to complete a questionnaire packet. The final sample size included 87 patients (59 women and 28 men). Subjects completed the Impact of Events Scale (to measure PTSD), the Appraisal of Life Threat and Treatment Intensity Scale (to differentiate between trauma related to cancer treatment and cancer diagnosis), Ways of Coping—Cancer Version (to measure coping strategies commonly used by cancer patients), and the Meaning of Illness Scale (to assess the meaning the patients constructed out of their experience and three measures of social support).

Findings
The symptoms of PTSD were significantly higher for women than for men ($p > .05$). Major predictors of PTSD for women were perceived intensity of the cancer treatment, problems with health care professionals, and a cognitive avoidance in their coping style. The only predictor of increased PTSD in men was behavioral avoidance. The women reported significantly higher ($p > .05$) levels of treatment intensity, many more types of treatments and number of treatments, and more difficulties with health care professionals. It was further reported by the women that the interpersonal and relational facets of their illnesses were more stressful and were the most difficult aspects of having cancer. Men indicated that their stress was associated with the work role and loss of finances.

Nursing Implications
Some women find the experience of cancer treatment to be very difficult. The intensity of the treatment may place women at risk for development of PTSD. Overall, women need support from health care professionals, additional control over their treatment, opportunity to tell their stories and concerns, support groups, and access to complementary therapies. Having psychosocial resources available could assist in the prevention of, assessment for, and interventions with patients encountering cancer-related PTSD.

Clinical depression is distinguished from everyday feelings of sadness by its duration and severity. Most people occasionally feel down or depressed, but these feelings are short-lived and do not result in impaired functioning. Clinically depressed people usually have had signs of a depressed mood or a decreased interest in pleasurable activities for at least a 2-week period. An obvious impairment in social, occupational, and overall daily functioning occurs in some people. Others function appropriately in their interactions with the outside world by exerting great effort and forcing themselves to mask their distress. Sometimes they are successful at camouflaging their depression for months or years and astonish family members and others when they finally succumb to the problem.

Many people experience depression but seek treatment for somatic complaints. The leading somatic complaints of patients struggling with depression are headache, backache, abdominal

Chart 7-9 • ASSESSMENT

Assessing Physiologic and Psychological Indicators of PTSD

Physiologic Indicators

Dilated pupils
Headaches
Sleep pattern disturbances
Tremors
Elevated blood pressure
Tachycardia or palpitations
Diaphoresis with cold, clammy skin
Hyperventilation
Dyspnea
Smothering or choking sensation
Nausea, vomiting, or diarrhea
Stomach ulcers
Dry mouth
Abdominal pain
Muscle tension or soreness
Exhaustion

Psychological Indicators

Anxiety
Anger
Depression
Fears or phobias
Survivor guilt
Hypervigilance
Nightmares or flashbacks
Intrusive thoughts about the trauma
Impaired memory
Dissociative states
Restlessness or irritability
Strong startle response
Substance abuse
Self-hatred
Feelings of estrangement
Feelings of helplessness, hopelessness, or powerlessness
Lack of interest in life
Inability to concentrate
Difficulty communicating, caring, and expressing love
Problems with relationships
Sexual problems ranging from acting out to impotence
Difficulty with intimacy
Inability to trust
Lack of impulse control
Aggressive, abusive, or violent behavior, including suicide
Thrill-seeking behaviors

Copel, L. C. (2000). *Nurse's clinical guide: Psychiatric and mental health care* (2nd ed.). Springhouse, PA: Springhouse.

about death or suicide or have made suicide attempts (American Psychiatric Association, 2000). A diagnosis of clinical depression is made when a person presents with at least five of nine diagnostic criteria for depression. Chart 7-10 lists these criteria (American Psychiatric Association, 2000). Unfortunately, only one of three depressed people is properly diagnosed and appropriately treated.

In the United States, about 15% of severely depressed people commit suicide, and two-thirds of patients who have committed suicide had been seen by health care practitioners during the month before their death (National Institute of Mental Health, 1999). When patients make statements that are self-deprecating, express feelings of failure, or are convinced that things are hopeless and will not improve, they may be at risk for suicide. Risk factors for suicide include the following:

- Age younger than 20 or older than 45 years, especially older than 65 years
- Gender—women make more attempts, men are more successful
- Dysfunctional family—members have experienced cumulative multiple losses and possess limited coping skills
- Family history of suicide
- Severe depression
- Severe, intractable pain
- Chronic, debilitating medical problems
- Substance abuse
- Severe anxiety
- Overwhelming problems
- Severe alteration in self-esteem or body image
- Lethal suicide plan

NURSING IMPLICATIONS

Because any loss in function, change in role, or alteration in body image is a possible antecedent to depression, nurses in all settings encounter patients who are depressed or who have thought about suicide. Depression is suspected if changes in the patient's thoughts or feelings and a loss of self-esteem are noted. See Chart 7-11 for a list of risk factors for depression. Depression can occur at any age, and it is diagnosed more frequently in women than in men. For elderly patients, the nurse should be aware that decreased mental alertness and withdrawal-type responses may be indicative of de-

Chart 7-10 Diagnostic Criteria for Depression Based on the DSM-IV TR

A person experiences at least five out of nine characteristics, with one of the first two symptoms present most of the time.
1. Depressed mood
2. Loss of pleasure or interest
3. Weight gain or loss
4. Sleeping difficulties
5. Psychomotor agitation or retardation
6. Fatigue
7. Feeling worthless
8. Inability to concentrate
9. Thoughts of suicide or death

American Psychiatric Association. (2000). *Diagnostic and statistical manual of mental disorders (DSM IV-TR)* (4th ed.). Washington, DC: Author.

pain, fatigue, malaise, anxiety, and decreased desire or problems with sexual functioning (Stuart & Laraia, 2000). These sensations are frequently manifestations of depression. The depression is undiagnosed about half of the time and masquerades as physical health problems (Carson, 1999). People with depression also exhibit poor functioning and high rates of absenteeism from work and school.

Specific symptoms of clinical depression include feelings of sadness, worthlessness, fatigue, and guilt and difficulty concentrating or making decisions. Changes in appetite, weight gain or loss, sleep disturbances, and psychomotor retardation or agitation are also common. Often, patients have recurrent thoughts

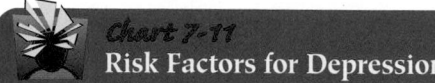

Chart 7-11
Risk Factors for Depression

Family history
Stressful situations
Female gender
Prior episodes of depression
Onset before age 40 years
Medical comorbidity
Past suicide attempts
Lack of support systems
History of physical or sexual abuse
Current substance abuse

NURSING IMPLICATIONS

Substance abuse is encountered in all clinical settings. Intoxication and withdrawal are two common substance abuse problems. Often, the nurse sees patients who have experienced trauma as a result of inebriation. Other patients who are active substance abusers enter the primary care setting with a diagnosis other than that of substance abuse. Many do not disclose the extent of their substance use. The patient's use of denial or lack of knowledge about the devastating effects of psychoactive substances can be detected by the nurse who performs a substance use assessment (Chart 7-12). In addition, the nurse can incorporate tools into the assessment that enable drug use to be detected. Examples of such instruments are the CAGE Questionnaire (Ewing, 1984), the Michigan Alcohol Screening Test (Selzer, 1971), and the Addiction Severity Index (McLellan, Kushner, Metzger, & Peters, 1992). The CAGE Questions Adapted to Include Drugs (CAGEAID) is presented in Chapter 5, Chart 5-2.

Health professionals are in pivotal positions for identifying a substance abuse problem, instituting treatment protocols, and making follow-up referrals. Because substance abuse severely affects the family, the nurse helps the family members confront the situation, decrease their enabling behaviors, and motivate the person to obtain treatment.

Caring for codependent family members is another nursing priority. A codependent person tends to manifest unhealthy patterns in relationships with others. Codependents struggle with a need to be needed, an urge to control others, and a willingness to remain involved and suffer with a person who has a drug problem.

The family may approach the health care team to help set limits on the dysfunctional behavior of a person who abuses substances. At these times, a therapeutic intervention is organized for the purpose of confronting the patient about substance use and the need to obtain drug or alcohol treatment. The nurse or other knowledgeable addiction counselor helps the family present the addicted person with a realistic perspective about the problem, their concerns about and caring for the person, and a specific plan for treatment. This therapeutic intervention works on the premise that honest and caring confrontation can break through the person's denial of the addiction. If the person refuses to participate in the designed plan, the family members define the consequences and state their commitment to follow through with them. This intervention is empowering to the family and usually provides the structure needed to secure treatment.

Even with treatment, however, patients may experience relapse. Nurses work with patients and their families to prevent relapse and to be prepared if relapse occurs. Relapse is considered a

pression. Consultation with the psychiatric liaison nurse to assess and differentiate between dementia-like symptoms and depression is often helpful.

For all patients, talking about their fears, frustration, anger, and despair can help alleviate a sense of helplessness and facilitate the process of obtaining the necessary treatment. Helping patients learn to cope effectively with conflict, interpersonal problems, and grief, and encouraging patients to discuss actual and potential losses may hasten their recovery from depression. Patients can also be helped to identify and decrease negative self-talk and unrealistic expectations and shown how negative thinking contributes to depression. Because physical health and self-care activities are adversely affected by depression, nurses should monitor patients for the onset of new problems. All patients with depression should be evaluated to determine whether they would benefit from antidepressant therapy.

In addition to the measures cited previously for helping patients manage depression, research studies indicate a reduction in distress when anxiety and depression are treated with psychoeducational programs, the establishment of support systems, and counseling (Devine & Westlake, 1995). Referrals to psychoeducational programs can be instrumental in helping patients and their families understand depression, treatment options, and coping strategies. (In crisis situations, it is better to refer the patient to a psychiatrist, psychiatric nurse specialist, or crisis center.) Explaining to patients that depression is a medical illness and not a sign of personal weakness, and that effective treatment will allow them to feel better and stay emotionally healthy, is an important aspect of care (Stuart & Laraia, 2000).

Substance Abuse

Some people use mood-altering substances in an attempt to cope with life's challenges. A person who abuses substances has an inability to make healthy decisions and to solve problems effectively. Typically, people who abuse substances are unable to identify and implement adaptive behaviors and use illegally obtained drugs, prescribed or over-the-counter medications, and alcohol alone or in combination with other drugs in an ineffective attempt to cope with the pressures, strains, and burdens of life. Over time, physiologic, emotional, cognitive, and behavioral problems develop as a result of continuous substance use. These problems cause distress for the individual, the family, and the community. Some people may respond to personal illness or the illness of a loved one by using substances to decrease emotional pain.

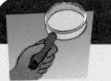

Chart 7-12 • ASSESSMENT
Assessing Substance Abuse

- Past and recurrent use of the substance
- Patient's view of substance use as a problem
- Age when first used and last used substance
- Length and duration of use of substance
- Preferred method of use of substance
- Amount of substance used
- How substance is procured
- Effect of or reaction to substance
- All attempts to cease or decrease substance use

part of the illness process and therefore must be viewed and addressed in the same way that chronic illness is treated.

The nurse who is working with a patient and family struggling with an addiction must dispel the myth that addiction is a defect in character or a moral fault. Views on substance abuse vary within our society. A person's background may help determine whether he or she uses drugs, what drugs are used, and when they are used (Copel, 2000). The combination of variables, such as values and beliefs, family and personal norms, spiritual convictions, and conditions of the current social environment, predisposes a person to the possibility of drug use, motivation for treatment, and continual recovery (Copel, 2000). It has also been said that a person's attitude, especially toward alcohol, reflects the overall beliefs and attitudes of that individual's culture (Giger & Davidhizar, 1999).

Loss and Grief

Loss is a part of the life cycle. All people experience loss in the form of change, growth, and transition. The experience of loss is painful, frightening, and lonely, and it triggers an array of emotional responses (Chart 7-13). People may vacillate between denial, shock, disbelief, anger, inertia, intense yearning, loneliness, sadness, loss of control, depression, and spiritual despair (Brewster, 1999).

In addition to normal losses associated with life cycle stages there are the potential losses of health, a body part, self-image, self-esteem, and even one's life. When loss is not acknowledged or there are multiple losses, anxiety, depression, and health problems may occur. Likewise, people with physical health problems, such as diabetes mellitus, acquired immunodeficiency syndrome (AIDS), cardiac conditions, gastrointestinal disorders, disabilities, and neurologic impairments, tend to respond to these illnesses with feelings of **grief**.

People grieve in different ways, and there is no time line for completing the grief process. The time of grieving often depends on the significance of the loss, the length of time the person was known and loved, the anticipation of or preparation for the loss, the person's emotional stability and maturity, and the person's coping ability (Arnold & Boggs, 1999).

Regardless of the duration of the grieving process, there are two basic goals: (1) healing the self, and (2) recovering from the loss. Other factors that influence grieving are the type of loss, life experiences with various changes and transitions, religious beliefs, cultural background, and personality type (Kemp, 2000). Some patients may resort to abuse of prescription medications, illegal drugs, or alcohol if they find it difficult to cope with the loss; the grief process is then complicated by the use of addictive substances.

NURSING IMPLICATIONS

Nurses identify patients and family members who are grieving and work with them to accomplish the four major tasks of the grief process: (1) acceptance of the loss, (2) acknowledgment of the intensity of the pain, (3) adaptation to life after the loss, and (4) cultivation of new relationships and activities (Worden, 1982). Chart 7-14 outlines nursing care activities useful for those who are bereaved.

Another responsibility of the nurse is to assess and differentiate between grief and depression by knowing the common thoughts, feelings, physical or bodily reactions, and behaviors associated with grief compared with depression (see Chart 7-14). The physical response to grief includes the sensation of somatic distress, a tightness in the throat followed by a choking sensation or shortness of breath, the need to sigh, an empty feeling inside the abdomen, lack of muscle power, and intense disabling distress. Grief can further debilitate an already compromised patient and can have a strong impact on family functioning.

Chart 7-13 • ASSESSMENT

Assessing Signs and Symptoms of Grieving

Physiologic Signs and Symptoms
Heart rate changes
Blood pressure alterations
Gastrointestinal disturbances
Chest discomfort
Shortness of breath
Weakness
Appetite changes
Sleep problems
Vague, but distressing, physical symptoms

Emotional Symptoms
Sadness
Depression
Anger
Social withdrawal
Loneliness
Apathy
Longing for who or what was lost
Blaming of self or others
Questioning of beliefs

Behavioral Symptoms
Slow movements
Forgetfulness
Purposeless activity
Crying
Sighing
Lack of interest
Easily distracted from tasks

Chart 7-14   Caring for the Bereaved

- Have contact physically (with the patient's permission) and emotionally with the person.
- Assess where the person is in the grieving process.
- Demonstrate genuine compassion and caring.
- Give permission to grieve and normalize the grieving process.
- Mention the loss or the deceased person's name.
- Encourage the person to talk about the relationship he or she had with the deceased person.
- Understand that people need to talk about the events and feelings around the death and will repeat themselves.
- Tell the person to expect mood swings, pain, and various life changes.
- Focus on clarifying and using coping skills.
- Allow the person to take a break from grieving and focus on self-care.
- Encourage sources of comfort such as religion or nature.
- Identify secondary losses and unfinished business.
- Acknowledge that there will be eventual recovery.
- Discuss the anniversary phenomenon.
- Encourage medical or psychiatric care as needed.

Death and Dying

Coping with death, one's own or a loved one's, is considered the ultimate challenge. The idea of death is threatening and anxiety-provoking to many people. Kubler-Ross (1975, p. 1) stated, "The key to the question of death unlocks the door of life. . . . For those who seek to understand it, death is a highly creative force." Common fears of dying people are fear of the unknown, pain, suffering, loneliness, loss of the body, and loss of personal control.

In recent years, the process of dying has changed as advances have been made in the care of chronically and terminally ill patients. Technological innovations and modern therapeutic treatments have prolonged the life span, and many deaths are now the result of chronic illnesses that result in physiologic deterioration and subsequent multisystem failure.

Preparation for an impending death can precipitate the experience of anticipatory grieving. Although anticipatory grief can have positive effects on later grief, this does not hold true for all people. For some family members, anticipatory grief is seen as a risk factor for poor early **bereavement** adjustment (Levy, 1991). The nurse must be aware of the uniqueness and individuality inherent in the grieving process and work to meet the needs of those involved in the best way possible.

DEATH AND DYING FRAMEWORKS

Various frameworks for understanding the concept of grief and the stages of death and dying may be useful to the nurse. The stages of bereavement described by Bowlby (1961) are protest, disorganization, and reorganization. Kubler-Ross (1975) conceptualized five stages of grieving: denial, anger, bargaining, depression, and acceptance. Often, the dying person and the survivors do not experience these responses in an orderly or linear fashion; rather, there is random movement between all the stages for differing periods of time. Another model for successful grieving, proposed by Engel (1964), is shock and disbelief, development of awareness, and restitution. The themes common to almost all models of grieving are periods of avoidance, confrontation, and acceptance (Cooley, 1992).

Another framework for understanding the individuality of the dying process is provided by the "patterns of living while dying" described by Martocchio (1982). There are four identified patterns of living based on the clinical trajectories of dying people. The first is referred to as peaks and valleys or periods of hope and periods of depression. Despite the hopeful times, there is still an overall movement toward decline and death. The second pattern is one described as distinct but descending plateaus. This course also reflects a downward trend with progressive debilitation and eventual death. The third pattern is a clear downward slope with many physiologic parameters indicating that death is imminent. This pattern is often observed in the critical care unit when people and families have no time to prepare for the death. The last pattern is a downward slant that reveals a crisis event, such as a severe cerebral hemorrhage with almost no hope of recovery. Often, a patient in this pattern is being maintained on life support systems. The nurse should recognize that a person may experience one or more of these living–dying patterns.

NURSING IMPLICATIONS

Nursing care involves providing comfort, maintaining safety, addressing physical and emotional needs, and teaching coping strategies to terminally ill patients and their families. More than ever, the nurse must explain what is happening to the patient and the family and be a confidante who listens to them talk about dying. Hospice care, attention to family and individual psychosocial issues, and symptom and pain management are all part of the nurse's responsibilities. The nurse must also be concerned with ethical considerations and quality-of-life issues that affect dying people. Of utmost importance to the patient is assistance with the transition from living to dying, maintaining and sustaining relationships, finishing well with the family, and accomplishing what needs to be said and done.

The nurse is the consistent link in promoting understanding of the patient's disease and the dying process and in making the event more manageable for the patient and family, who will require assistance to resolve problems and proceed through the grief work. Retaining as much control as possible during the process of dying allows the patient and family to make as much sense as possible out of an overwhelming situation. In the hospital, in long-term care facilities, and in home settings, the nurse explores choices and end-of-life decisions with the patient and family. Referrals to home care and hospice services, as well as specific referrals appropriate for the management of the situation, are initiated. The nurse is also an advocate for the dying person and works to uphold that person's rights. The use of living wills and advance directives allows the patient to exercise the right to have a "good" death or to die with dignity. Additional information about end-of-life care is presented in Chapter 17.

Spirituality and Spiritual Distress

Spirituality is defined as connectedness with self, others, a life force, or God that allows people to experience self-transcendence and find meaning in life. Spirituality helps people discover a purpose in life, understand the vicissitudes of life, and develop their relationship with God or a Higher Power. Within the framework of spirituality, a person discovers truths about the self, about the world, and about concepts such as love, compassion, wisdom, honesty, commitment, imagination, reverence, and morality. Often, spiritual behavior is expressed through sacrifice, self-discipline, and spending time in activities that focus on the inner self or the soul. Religion and nature are two vehicles that people use to connect themselves with God or a Higher Power; however, bonds to religious institutions, beliefs, or dogma are not required to experience the spiritual sense of self. **Faith,** considered the foundation of spirituality, is a belief in something that a person cannot see (Carson, 1999). The spiritual part of a person views life as a mystery that unfolds over the lifetime, encompassing questions about meaning, hope, relatedness to God, acceptance or forgiveness, and transcendence (Byrd, 1999; Sheldon, 2000; Sussman, Nezami, & Mishra, 1997).

A strong sense of spirituality or religious faith can have a positive impact on health (Dunn & Horgas, 2000; Kendrick & Robinson, 2000; Matthews & Larson, 1995). Spirituality is also a component of hope, and, especially during chronic, serious, or terminal illness, patients and their families often find comfort and emotional strength in their religious traditions or spiritual beliefs. At other times, illness and loss can cause a loss of faith or meaning in life and a spiritual crisis. The nursing diagnosis of spiritual distress is applicable to those who have a disturbance in the belief or value system that provides strength, hope, and meaning in life.

NURSING IMPLICATIONS

Spiritually distressed patients (or family members) may show despair, discouragement, ambivalence, detachment, anger, resentment, or fear. They may question the meaning of suffering, life, and death, and express a sense of emptiness. The nurse assesses spiritual strength by inquiring about the person's sense of spiritual well-being, hope, and peacefulness. Have spiritual beliefs and values changed in response to illness or loss? The nurse assesses current and past participation in religious or spiritual practices and notes the patient's response to questions about spiritual needs— grief, anger, guilt, depression, doubt, anxiety, or calmness—to help determine the patient's need for spiritual care. Another simple assessment technique is to inquire about the patient's and family's desire for spiritual support.

For nurses to provide spiritual care, they must be open to being present and supportive when patients experience doubt, fearfulness, suffering, despair, or other difficult psychological states of being. Interventions that foster spiritual growth or reconciliation include being fully present; listening actively; conveying a sense of caring, respect, and acceptance; using therapeutic communication techniques to encourage expression; suggesting the use of prayer, meditation, or imagery; and facilitating contact with spiritual leaders or performance of spiritual rituals (Sumner, 1998; Sussman, 2000).

Patients with serious, chronic, or terminal illnesses face physical and emotional losses that threaten their spiritual integrity. During acute and chronic illness, rehabilitation, or the dying process, spiritual support can stimulate patients to regain or strengthen their connections with their inner selves, their loved ones, and their God or Higher Power to transcend suffering and find meaning. Nurses can alleviate distress and suffering and enhance wellness by meeting their patients' spiritual needs.

Critical Thinking Exercises

1. A 55-year old man tells the nurse that he is not going to be a part of a clinical drug investigation. He states, "I may not get the drug. I may end up with a placebo. I'm going to try some alternative methods. I feel like traditional medicine is letting me down." How does the nurse handle this situation? What assessment data need to be collected and discussed with other members of the health care team?

2. The nurse is working with a family to develop therapeutic interventions for a family member who has a cocaine and alcohol addiction problem. One family member tells the nurse she will never be able to support the plan decided on by the rest of the family. How would you approach this person? What strategies would be useful for this person and for the entire family?

3. The family of a man who is dying from lung cancer tells the hospice nurse that they are overwhelmed by the hopelessness of their father's situation. What can the nurse do to provide guidance and find hope within terminal illness? How does the nurse assist this family to meet their emotional, social, and spiritual needs?

REFERENCES AND SELECTED READINGS

Books

Aiken, L. (2000). *Dying, death, and bereavement* (4th ed.). Mahwah, NJ: Lawrence Erlbaum.

American Psychiatric Association. (2000). *Diagnostic and statistical manual of mental disorders (DSM IV)* (4th ed.). Washington, DC: Author.

Arnold, E., & Boggs, K. (1999). *Interpersonal relationships: Professional communication skills for nurses* (3rd ed.). Philadelphia: W. B. Saunders.

Barry, P. D. (1998). *Mental health and mental illness* (6th ed.). Philadelphia: Lippincott-Raven.

Bowlby, J. (1961). *Attachment and loss* (Vol. 1). New York: Basic Books.

Boyd-Franklin, N., & Bry, B. H. (2001). *Reaching out in family therapy.* New York: Guilford Press.

Brewster, S. (1999). *To be an anchor in the storm: A guide for families and friends.* New York: Sealpress.

Burr, W., Klein, S., Burr, R., Doxey, C., Haeker, B., Holman, T., Martin, P., McClure, R., Parrish, S., Stuart, D., Taylor, A., & White, M. (1994). *Reexamining family stress: New theory and research.* Thousand Oaks, CA: Sage.

Burr, W., et al. (1993). *Family science.* Pacific Grove, CA: Brooks/Cole.

Carson, V. B. (1999). *Mental health nursing: The nurse-patient journey* (2nd ed.). St. Louis, MO: Mosby.

Copel, L. C. (2000). *Nurse's clinical guide: Psychiatric and mental health care* (2nd ed.). Springhouse, PA: Springhouse.

Feldman, R. (2000). *Development across the life span* (2nd ed.). Upper Saddle River, NJ: Prentice Hall.

Friedman, M. M. (1998). *Family nursing: Research, theory, and practice* (4th ed.). Stamford, CT: Appleton & Lange.

Gelles, J. (1997). *Intimate violence in families.* Thousands Oaks, CA: Sage.

Gelles, J., & Loseke, D. (Eds.) (1993). Current controversies on family violence. Newbury Park, CA: Sage.

Giger, J. N., & Davidhizar, R. E. (1999). *Transcultural nursing: Assessment and intervention* (3rd ed.). St. Louis: C. V. Mosby.

Keegan, L. (2001). *Healing with complementary and alternative therapies.* Albany, NY: Delmar.

Kemp, C. (2000). *Terminal illness.* Philadelphia: Lippincott Williams & Wilkins.

Kubler-Ross, E. (1975). *Death: The final stage of growth.* Englewood Cliffs, NJ: Prentice-Hall.

Kuhn, M. A. (1999). *Complementary therapies for health care providers.* Philadelphia, Lippincott Williams & Wilkins.

Luckmann, J. (1999). *Transcultural communication in nursing.* Albany, NY: Delmar.

Martocchio, B. C. (1982). *Living while dying.* Bowie, MD: Robert J. Brady.

Matthews, D. A., & Larson, D. B. (1995). *The faith factor: An annotated bibliography of clinical research on spiritual subjects* (Vol. 3). Rockville, MD: National Institute for Health Care Research.

McCann, I. J., & Pearlman, L. A. (1990). *Psychological trauma and the adult survivor.* New York: Brunner/Mazel.

McDowell, D. M., & Spitz, H. I. (1999). *Substance abuse: From principles to practice.* Philadelphia: Brunner/Mazel.

Murray, R. B., & Zentner, J. P. (2001). *Health assessment and promotion strategies through the life span* (7th ed.). Stamford, CT: Appleton & Lange.

Nowinski, J. K. (1998). *Family recovery and substance abuse.* Thousand Oaks, CA: Sage.

Rice, F. P. (2001). *Human development: A lifespan approach* (4th ed.). Upper Saddle River, NJ: Prentice Hall.

Rice, V. H. (Ed.) (2000). *Handbook of stress, coping, and health: Implications for nursing research, theory, and practice.* Thousand Oaks, CA: Sage.

Roach, S. S., & Nieto, B. C. (1998). *Healing and the grief process.* Albany, NY: Delmar.

Stanhope, M., & Lancaster, J. (1999). *Community and public health nursing* (7th ed.). St. Louis: C. V. Mosby.

Stuart, G. W., & Laraia, M. T. (2000). *Principles and practice of psychiatric nursing* (7th ed.). St. Louis: C. V. Mosby.

Tucker, J. A., Donovan, D. M., & Marlatt, G. A. (2001). *Changing additive behavior.* NY: Guilford.

U.S. Department of Health & Human Services (1993). *Clinical practice guidelines Agency for Health Care Policy and Research: Number 5. Depression in clinical care: Vol. 1. Detection and diagnosis.* Rockville, MD: U.S. Government Printing Office.

U.S. Department of Health & Human Services (1993). *Clinical practice guidelines Agency for Health Care Policy and Research: Number 5. Depression in primary care: Vol. 2. Treatment of major depression.* Rockville, MD: U.S. Government Printing Office.

U.S. Department of Health & Human Services, Public Health Service, Agency for Health Care Policy and Research. (1993). *Depression in primary care: Vol. 1. Detection and diagnosis.* Clinical Practice Guideline. (AHCPR Publication No. 93-0550). Rockville, MD: U.S. Government Printing Office.

U.S. Department of Health & Human Services, Public Health Service, Agency for Health Care Policy and Research. (1993) *Depression in primary care: Vol. 2, Treatment of major depression.* Clinical Practice Guideline. (AHCPR Publication No. 93-0551). Rockville, MD: U.S. Government Printing Office.

U.S. Public Health Service (2000). *Healthy people 2010: Understanding and improving health.* Washington, DC: U.S. Government Printing Office.

Worden, W. (1982). *Grief counseling and grief therapy: A handbook for the mental health practitioner.* New York: Springer Publishing.

Wright, L. M., & Leahey, M. (2000). *Nurses and families: A guide to family assessment and intervention.* Philadelphia, PA: Davis.

Journals

Asterisks indicate nursing research articles.

General

Cohen, S., & Herbert, T. (1996). Health psychology: Psychological factors and physical disease from the perspective of human psychoneuroimmunology. *Annual Review of Psychology, 47,* 113–142.

Devine, E. C., & Westlake, S. K. (1995). The effects of psychoeducational care provided to adults with cancer: Metaanalysis of 116 studies. *Oncology Nursing Forum, 22*(9), 1369–1376.

Eisenberg, D., Kessler, R., Foster, C., Norlock, F., Calkins, D., & Delbanco, T. (1993). Unconventional medicine in the United States: Prevalence, costs, and patterns of use. *New England Journal of Medicine, 328,* 246–252.

Alternative Therapies

Boutin, P. D., Buchwald, D., Robinson, L., & Collier, A. C. (2000). Use of alternative and complementary therapies among outpatients and physicians at a municipal hospital. *Journal of Alternative and Complementary Medicine, 6*(4), 353–343.

Sparber, A., Wootton, J. C., Bauer, L., Curt, G., Eisenberg, D. M., Levin, T., & Steinberg, S. M. (2000). Use of complementary medicine by adult patients participating in HIV/AIDS clinical trials. *Journal of Alternative and Complementary Medicine, 6*(5), 415–422.

Wolsho, P., Ware, L., Kutner, J., Lin, C., Albertson, G., Cyran, L., Schilling, L., & Anderson, R. J. (2000). Alternative/complementary medicine: Wider usage than generally appreciated. *Journal of Alternative and Complementary Medicine, 6*(4), 321–326.

Wynia, M. K., Eisenberg, D. M., & Wilson, I. B. (1999). Physician-patient communication about complementary and alternative medical therapies: A survey of physicians caring for patients with human immunodeficiency virus infection. *Journal of Alternative and Complementary Medicine, 5*(5), 447–456.

Coping

Backer, J. H. (2000). Stressors, social support, and coping and health dysfunction in individuals with Parkinson's disease. *Journal of Gerontological Nursing, 26*(11), 6–16.

Dzurec, L. C. (2000). Fatigue and relatedness in inordinately tired women. *Journal of Gerontological Nursing, 32*(4), 339–345.

King, K. B., Zewic, J. J., Kimble, L. P., & Rowe, M. A. (1998). Optimism, coping, and long-term recovery from coronary artery surgery in women. *Research in Nursing & Health, 21*(1), 15–26.

Morse, S. R., & Fife, B. (1998). Coping with a partner's cancer: Adjustment at four stages of the illness trajectory. *Oncology Nursing Forum, 25*(4), 751–760.

Schnoll, R. A., Harlow, L. L., & Brower, L. (2000). Spirituality, demographic and disease factors, and adjustment to cancer. *Cancer Practice: A Multidisciplinary Journal of Cancer Care, 8*(6), 298–304.

Twibell, R. S. (1998). Family coping during critical illness. *Dimensions in Critical Care Nursing, 17*(2), 100–112.

Depression

Martin, A. C. (2000). Major depressive illness in women: Assessment and treatment in the primary care setting. *Nurse Practitioner Forum, 11*(3), 179–186.

National Institute of Mental Health. (1992). *Depression awareness, recognition, treatment fact sheet.* DHHS Publication No. [ADM] 92-1680. Rockville, MD: Government Printing Office.

Rasmussen, J. (2000). Treating depression: The continuing challenge of achieving long term recovery. *Mental Health Care and Learning Disabilities, 3*(9), 295–308.

Rogers, J. C., & Holm, M. B. (2000). Daily living skills and habits of older women with depression. *Occupational Therapy Journal of Research, 20*(Suppl. 1), 68S–85S.

Grief, Death, and Dying

Conrad, N. L. (1985). Spiritual support for the dying. *Nursing Clinics of North America, 20*(2), 415–425.

Cooley, M. E. (1992). Bereavement care: A role for nurses. *Cancer Nursing, 15*(2), 125–129.

Fauri, D. P., Ettner, B., & Kovacs, P. T. (2000). Bereavement services in acute care settings. *Death Studies, 24*(1), 51–64.

Engel, G. (1964). Grief and grieving. *American Journal of Nursing, 64*(7), 93–96.

Hallgrinsdottir, E. M. (2000). Accident and emergency nurses' perceptions of caring for families. *Journal of Clinical Nursing, 9*(4), 611–619.

Katz, J., Sedell, M., & Komaromy, C. (2000). Death in homes: Bereavement needs of residents, relatives, and staff. *International Journal of Palliative Nursing, 6*(6), 274–279.

Levy, L. H. (1991). Anticipatory grief: Its measurement and proposed reconceptualization. *Hospice Journal, 7*(4), 1–28.

Nishimoto, P. (1996). Venturing into the unknown: Cultural beliefs about death and dying. *Oncology Nursing Forum, 23*(6), 889–894.

Posttraumatic Stress Disorder

Ellensweig-Tepper, D. (2000). Trauma group therapy for the adolescent female client. *Journal of Child and Adolescent Psychiatric Nursing, 13*(1), 17–28.

McGrath, P. (1999). Posttraumatic stress and the experience of cancer: A literature review. *Journal of Rehabilitation, 65*(3), 17–23.

Miller, J. L. (2000). Post-traumatic stress disorder in primary care. *Journal of the American Academy of Nurse Practitioners, 12*(11), 475–485.

Spirituality

Byrd, E. K. (1999). Spiritual care matters: Application of helping theories and faith in the lives of persons with disabilities. *Journal of Religion, Disability, and Health, 3*(1), 3–13.

Chandler, E. (1999). Spirituality. *Hospice Journal, 14*(3/40), 63–74.

Dunn, K. S., & Horgas, A. L. (2000). The prevalence of prayer as a spiritual self-care modality in elders. *Journal of Holistic Nursing, 18*(4), 337–351.

Dyson, J., Cobb, M. & Forman, D. (1997). The meaning of spirituality: A literature review. *Journal of Advanced Nursing, 26*(6), 1183–1188.

Haln, M. A., Myers, R. N., & Bennetts, P. (2000). Providing spiritual care to cardiac patients: Assessment and implications for practice. *Critical Care Nurse, 20*(4), 54–56, 58, 64, 66–72.

Havranek, J. E. (1999). The role of spirituality in the rehabilitation process. *Journal of Religion, Disability, and Health, 3*(2), 15–35.

*Humphreys, J. (2000). Spirituality and distress in sheltered battered women. *Scholarly Inquiry for Nursing Practice, 14*(2), 115–141.

Kendrick, K. D., & Robinson, S. (2000). Spirituality: Its relevance and purpose for clinical nursing in a new millennium. *Journal of Clinical Nursing, 9*(5), 701–705.

Langer, N. (2000). The importance of spirituality in later life. *Gerontology and Geriatric Education, 20*(3), 41–50.

Sheldon, T. E. (2000). Spirituality as a part of nursing. *Journal of Hospice and Palliative Care, 2*(3), 101–108.

Sherwood, G. D. (2000). The power of nurse-client encounters interpreting spiritual themes. *Journal of Holistic Nursing, 18*(2), 159–175.

Sumner, C. H. (1998). Recognizing and responding to spiritual distress. *American Journal of Nursing, 98*(1), 26–30.

Sussman, D. (2000). A spiritual approach: Nurses and chaplains team up to provide pastoral care. *Healthweek, 5*(17), 12.

Sussman, S., Nezami, E., & Mishra, S. (1997). On operationalizing spiritual experience for health promotion research and practice. *Alternative Therapies in Clinical Practice, 4*(4), 120–125.

Treloar, L. L. (2000). Integration of spirituality into health care practice by nurse practitioners. *Journal of American Academy of Nurse Practitioners, 12*(7), 280–285.

Substance Abuse

Ewing, J. A. (1984). Detecting alcoholism: The CAGE questionnaire. *Journal of American Medical Association, 252*(14), 1906.

McLellan, A. T., Kushner, H., Metzger, D., & Peters, R. (1992). The fifth edition of the addiction severity index. *Journal of Substance Abuse Treatment, 9*(3), 199–213.

Sedlak, C. A., Dokery, M. O., Estok, P. J., & Zeller, R. A. (2000). Alcohol use in women 65 years of age and older. *Health Care of Women International, 21*(7), 567–581.

Selzer, M. L. (1971). The Michigan alcoholism screening test: The quest for a new diagnostic instrument. *American Journal of Psychiatry, 127,* 1653–1658.

Sturn, R., & Sherbourne, C. D. (2000). Data points: Managed care and unmet need for mental health and substance abuse care in 1998. *Psychiatric Services, 51*(2), 177.

RESOURCES AND WEBSITES

Agencies

American Holistic Nurses Association (AHNA), P.O. Box 2130, Flagstaff, AZ 86003-2130; 1-800-278-AHNA; http://www.ahna.org.

Grief Recovery Institute Education Foundation, Inc. (GRIEF), P.O. Box 6061-382, Sherman Oaks, CA 91413; 1-818-907-9600; 1-800-445-4808 (Hotline); http://www.grief.net.

National Hospice Organization (NHO), 1901 North Moore Street, Suite 901, Arlington, VA 22209; 1-703-243-5900.

Aging

American Association of Retired Persons (AARP), 601 "E" Street NW, Washington, DC 20049-0001; 1-202-434-2277; 1-800-424-3410; http://www.aarp.org.

Children of Aging Parents, 1609 Woodbourne Road #302A, Levittown, PA 19057-1511; 1-215-945-6900; 1-800-227-7294.

National Association for Families Caring for their Elders—Eldercare America, 1141 Loxford Terrace, Silver Spring, MD 20901-1130; 1-301-593-1621.

National Council on the Aging, 409 3rd Street SW, Washington, DC 20024; 1-202-424-1200; 1-800-424-9046; info@ncoa.org.

National Office of the Gray Panthers, P.O. Box 214777, Washington, DC 20009; 1-202-466-3132; 1-800-280-5362; dixieh1064@aol.com.

Anxiety

Anxiety Disorders Association of America, 11900 Parklawn Drive #100, Rockville, MD 20852-2624; 1-301-231-9350; anxdis@aol.com.

Bereavement

Compassionate Friends, P.O. Box 3696, Oak Brook, IL 60522-3696; 1-630-990-0010; nationaloffice@compassionatefriends.org; http://www.compassionatefriends.org.

They Help Each Other Spiritually (THEOS), 322 Boulevard of the Allies #105, Pittsburgh, PA 15222-1919; 1-412-471-7779.

Widowed Persons Service, 601 "E" Street NW, Washington, DC 20049-0001; 1-202-434-2260.

Depression

Depression Awareness, Recognition, and Treatment (D/ART), NIMH, 5600 Fishers Lane Room 10-85, Rockville, MD 20857; 1-800-421-4211; 1-301-443-4140.

National Alliance for the Mentally Ill, 200 N. Grebe Road #1015, Arlington, VA 22201-3062; 1-703-524-7600; 1-800-950-NAMI; namioffC@aol.com.

National Mental Health Association, 1021 Prince Street, Alexandria, VA 22314-2971; 1-703-684-7722; 1-800-969-6642; 1-800-433-5959; nmhainfo@aol.com.

Eating Disorders

American Anorexia Bulimia Association Inc., 165 W. 46th Street, #1108, New York, NY 10036-2501; 1-212-575-6200.

National Eating Disorders Association (NEDO), 6655 S. Yale Avenue, Tulsa, OK 74136; 1-918-481-4044.

Posttraumatic Stress Disorder

National Center for PTSD, VA Medical Center (116D), White River Junction, VT 05009; 1-802-296-5132; ncptsd@ncptsd.org.

Substance Abuse

Adult Children of Alcoholics, P.O. Box 3216, Torrence, CA 90510; 1-310-534-1815; http://www.info@adultchildren.org.

Alanon and Alateen Family Group Headquarters Inc., 1600 Corporate Landing Parkway, Virginia Beach, VA 23454-5617; 1-888-4AL-ANON (888-425-2666); http://www.al-anon.org.

Alcoholics Anonymous, Grand Central Station, P.O. Box 459, New York, NY 10163; 1-212-870-3400; http://www.alcoholics-anonymous.org. Children of Alcoholics Foundation, 164 West 74th Street, New York, NY 10115; 1-800-359-2623.

Co-Anon Family Groups, P.O. Box 64742-66, Los Angeles, CA 90064; 1-818-377-4317.

Cocaine Anonymous, 3740 Overland Avenue Suite G, Los Angeles, CA 90034; 1-800-347-8998; http://www.ca.org.

Dual Recovery Anonymous World Services, P.O. Box 8107, Prairie Village, KS 66208; 877-883-2332; http://www.DRAonline.org.

Narcotics Anonymous, P.O. Box 9999, Van Nuys, CA 91409; 1-818-773-9999; http://www.na.org.

Rational Recovery Systems, Box 800, Lotus, CA 95651; 1-530-621-4374.

Secular Organizations for Sobriety (SOS), The Center for Inquiry, 5521 Grosvenor Boulevard, Los Angeles, CA 90066; 1-310-821-8430.

Hotline Numbers

Center for Substance Abuse Prevention Workplace, Hotline 800-WORKPLACE (1-800-967-5752).

Center for Substance Abuse Treatment, National Treatment Hotline 800-662-HELP (1-800-662-4357).

National Alcohol Hotline, Helpline: 1-800-NCA-CALL (1-800-622-2255). National Cocaine Hotline, 1-800-COCAINE (1-800-262-2463).

Perspectives in Transcultural Nursing

LEARNING OBJECTIVES

On completion of this chapter, the learner will be able to:

1. Apply transcultural nursing principles, concepts, and theories when providing nursing care to patients (individuals, families, groups, and communities).

2. Develop strategies for planning, providing, and evaluating culturally competent nursing care for patients from diverse backgrounds.

3. Critically analyze the influence of culture on nursing care decisions and actions for patients.

4. Identify key components of cultural assessment for self and patients.

*I*n the health care delivery system, as in society, the nurse interacts with people of similar and diverse cultural backgrounds. People may have similar or different frames of reference and varied preferences regarding their health and health care needs. Acknowledging and adapting to the cultural needs of the patient and significant others is an important component of nursing care. To plan and deliver culturally competent care, the nurse must understand the definitions of culture and cultural competence and the various aspects of culture that should be explored for each patient.

Definitions of Culture

The concept of culture and its relationship to the health care beliefs and practices of patients and their families and friends provide the foundation for transcultural nursing. This awareness of culture in the delivery of nursing care has been described in different ways, including respect for cultural diversity, culturally sensitive or comprehensive care, and culturally competent or appropriate nursing care (American Association of Colleges of Nursing, 1996; Giger & Davidhizar, 1999; Spector, 2000), or culturally congruent nursing care (Leininger, 2001). Two commonly discussed concepts are cultural diversity and culturally competent care.

The term *culture* was initially defined by the British anthropologist Sir Edward Tylor in 1871 as the knowledge, belief, art, morals, laws, customs, and any other capabilities and habits acquired by humans as members of society. During the past century, and especially during recent decades, hundreds of definitions of culture have been offered that integrate the themes stated by Tylor and the themes of ethnic variations of a population based on race, nationality, religion, language, physical characteristics, and geography (Spector, 2000). To fully appreciate the impact of culture, aspects such as disabilities, gender, social class, physical appearance (eg, weight, height), ideologies (political views), or sexual orientation must be integrated into the definition of culture as well (Gooden, Porter, Gonzalez, & Mims, 2001).

Madeleine Leininger, founder of the specialty called transcultural nursing, indicates that culture involves learned and transmitted knowledge about values, beliefs, rules of behavior, and lifestyle practices that guide designated groups in their thinking and actions in patterned ways (2001). Giger and Davidhizar (1999) state that transcultural nursing is a practice based on the differences and similarities between cultures in relation to health, health care, and illness, with consideration of patient values, beliefs, and practices. Further, culture develops over time as a result of "imprinting the mind through social and religious structures and intellectual and artistic manifestations" (p. 3).

The concept of ethnic culture has four basic characteristics:

- It is learned from birth through language and socialization.
- It is shared by members of the same cultural group, and it includes an internal sense and external perception of distinctiveness.
- It is influenced by specific conditions related to environmental and technical factors and to the availability of resources.
- It is dynamic and ever-changing.

With the exception of the first characteristic, culture related to age, physical appearance, lifestyle, and other less frequently acknowledged aspects also adhere to the above characteristics.

Cultural diversity has also been defined in a number of ways. Often, skin color, religion, and geographic area are the only elements used to identify diversity, with ethnic minorities being considered the primary sources of cultural diversity. As stated earlier, however, there are several other possible sources of cultural diversity. In addition, to truly acknowledge the cultural differences that may influence health care delivery, the nurse must recognize the influence of his or her own culture and cultural heritage (Krumberger, 2000).

Culturally competent nursing care has been defined as effective, individualized care that considers cultural values, is culturally aware and sensitive, and incorporates cultural skills (Hunt, 2000; Krumberger, 2000; Wilkinson, 2001). Culturally competent care is a dynamic process that requires comprehensive knowledge of culture-specific information and an awareness of, and sensitivity to, the effect that culture has on the care situation. It requires the nurse to integrate cultural knowledge, awareness of his or her own cultural perspective, and the patient's cultural perspectives into the plan of care (Giger & Davidhizar, 1999). Exploring one's own cultural beliefs and how they might conflict with the beliefs of the patients being cared for is a first step toward becoming culturally competent (Krumberger, 2000). Understanding the diversity within cultures, such as subcultures, is also important.

SUBCULTURES AND MINORITIES

Although culture is a universal phenomenon, it takes on specific and distinctive features for a particular group, since it encompasses all of the knowledge, beliefs, customs, and skills acquired by the members of that group. When such groups function within a larger cultural group, they are referred to as subcultures.

The term *subculture* is used for relatively large groups of people who share characteristics that enable them to be identified as a distinct entity. Examples of American subcultures based on ethnicity (ie, subcultures with common traits such as physical characteristics, language, or ancestry) include African Americans, Hispanic/Latino Americans, and Native Americans. Each of these subcultures may be further divided; for example, Native Americans consist of American Indians and Alaska Natives, who represent more than 500 federally and state-recognized tribes in addition to an unknown number of tribes that receive no official recognition.

Subcultures may also be based on religion (more than 1200 exist in the United States), occupation (eg, nurses, physicians, other members of the health care team), or shared disability or illness (eg, the Deaf community). In addition, subcultures may be based on age (eg, infants, children, adolescents, adults, older adults), gender (eg, male, female); sexual orientation (eg, homosexual or bisexual men and women), or geographic location (eg, Texans, Southerners, Appalachians).

The nurse should also be sensitive to the intraracial applications of cultural competence. Tensions between subcultures within a designated group could add to the complexity of planning culturally competent care. Some members of one ethnic subculture may be offended or angered if mistaken for members of a different subculture. Similarly, if the attributes of one subculture are mistakenly generalized to a patient belonging to a different subculture, extreme offense could result, as well as inappropriate care planning and implementation (Fields, 2000). It is crucial that nurses refrain from culturally stereotyping a patient in an attempt to be culturally competent. Instead, the patient or significant others should be consulted regarding personal values, beliefs, preferences and cultural identification. This strategy is also applicable for members of nonethnic subcultures.

The term *minority* refers to a group of people whose physical or cultural characteristics differ from the majority of people in a society. At times, minorities may be singled out or isolated from others in society or treated in different or unequal ways. Although there are four federally identified minority groups—Blacks/African Americans, Hispanics, Asian/Pacific Islanders, and Native Americans (Andrews & Boyle, 1999)—the concept of "minority" varies widely and must be understood in a cultural context. For example, men may be considered a minority within the nursing profession, but they constitute a majority within the field of medicine. In addition, Caucasians may be in the minority in some communities in the United States, but they are currently the majority group in the country (although it has been projected that by the middle to late 21st century, Caucasians will be in the minority in the United States). Because at times the term minority connotes inferiority, members of many racial and ethnic groups object to being identified as minorities.

Transcultural Nursing

Transcultural nursing, a term sometimes used interchangeably with cross-cultural, intercultural, or multicultural nursing, refers to a formal area of study and practice that focuses on the cultural care (caring) values, beliefs, and practices of individuals and groups from a particular culture (Giger & Davidhizar, 1999). The underlying focus of transcultural nursing is to provide culture-specific and culture-universal care that promotes the well-being or health of individuals, families, groups, communities, and institutions (Giger & Davidhizar, 1999; Leininger, 2001). When culturally appropriate care is provided, all individuals, and the community or institution at large, benefit. When the care is delivered beyond the nurse's national boundaries, the term international or transnational nursing is often used.

Although many nurses, anthropologists, and others have written about the cultural aspects of nursing and health care, Leininger (2001) developed a comprehensive research-based theory called Culture Care Diversity and Universality. The goal of the theory is to provide culturally congruent nursing care to improve care for people of different or similar cultures. This means promoting recovery from illness, preventing conditions that would limit the patient's health or well-being, or facilitating a peaceful death in ways that are culturally meaningful and appropriate. Nursing care needs to be tailored to fit the patient's cultural values, beliefs, and lifestyle.

Leininger's theory includes providing culturally congruent nursing care (meaningful, beneficial, and satisfying health care tailored to fit the patient's cultural values) through culture care accommodation and culture care restructuring (Fig. 8-1). *Culture care accommodation* refers to those professional actions and decisions that a nurse makes in his or her care to help people of a designated culture achieve a beneficial or satisfying health outcome. *Culture care restructuring* or repatterning refers to those professional actions and decisions that help patients reorder, change, or modify their lifestyles toward new, different, or more beneficial health care patterns. At the same time, the patient's cultural values and beliefs are respected, and a better or healthier lifestyle is provided. Other terms and definitions that provide further insight into culture and health care include the following:

- *Acculturation* is the process by which members of a cultural group adapt to or learn how to take on the behaviors of another group.
- *Cultural blindness* is the inability of a person to recognize his or her own values, beliefs, and practices and those of others because of strong ethnocentric tendencies (the tendency to view one's own culture as superior to others).

- *Cultural imposition* is the tendency to impose one's cultural beliefs, values, and patterns of behavior on a person or persons from a different culture.
- *Cultural taboos* are those activities governed by rules of behavior that are avoided, forbidden, or prohibited by a particular cultural group.

Culturally Competent Nursing Care

Culturally competent or congruent nursing care refers to the complex integration of attitudes, knowledge, and skills (including assessment, decision making, judgments, critical thinking, and evaluation) that enables the nurse to provide care in a culturally sensitive and appropriate manner. Agency and institutional policies are important to achieve culturally competent care.

Policies that promote culturally competent care establish flexible regulations pertaining to visitors (number, frequency, and length of visits), provide translation services for non–English-speaking patients, and train staff to provide care for patients with different cultural values (Suro, 2000). Culturally competent policies also recognize the special dietary needs of patients from selected cultural groups and create an environment in which the traditional healing, spiritual, and religious practices of patients are respected and encouraged.

Giger and Davidhizar (1999) created an assessment model to guide the nurse in exploring cultural phenomena that might affect nursing care. They identified communication, space, time orientation, social organization, environmental control, and biologic variations as relevant phenomena (Giger & Davidhizar, 1999). This model has been used in various patient care settings to provide data essential to the provision of culturally competent care.

CROSS-CULTURAL COMMUNICATION

Establishing an environment of culturally congruent care and respect begins with effective communication, which occurs not only through words, but also through body language and other cues, such as voice, tone, and loudness. Nurse–patient interactions, as well as communications among members of a multicultural health care team, are dependent on the ability to understand and be understood.

Approximately 150 different languages are spoken in the United States, with Spanish accounting for the largest percentage after English. Obviously, nurses cannot become fluent in all languages, but certain strategies for fostering effective cross-cultural communication are necessary when providing care for patients who are not fluent in English. Cultural needs should be considered when choosing an interpreter; fluency in varied dialects, for instance, is beneficial (Suro, 2000). The interpreter's voice quality, pronunciation, use of silence, use of touch, and use of nonverbal communication should also be assessed (Giger & Davidhizar, 1999).

During illness, patients of all ages tend to regress, and the regression often involves language skills. Chart 8-1 summarizes suggested strategies for overcoming language barriers. The nurse should also assess how well the patient and family have understood what has been said. The following cues may signal lack of effective communication:

- Efforts to change the subject. This could indicate that the patient does not understand what you are saying and is attempting to talk about something more familiar.

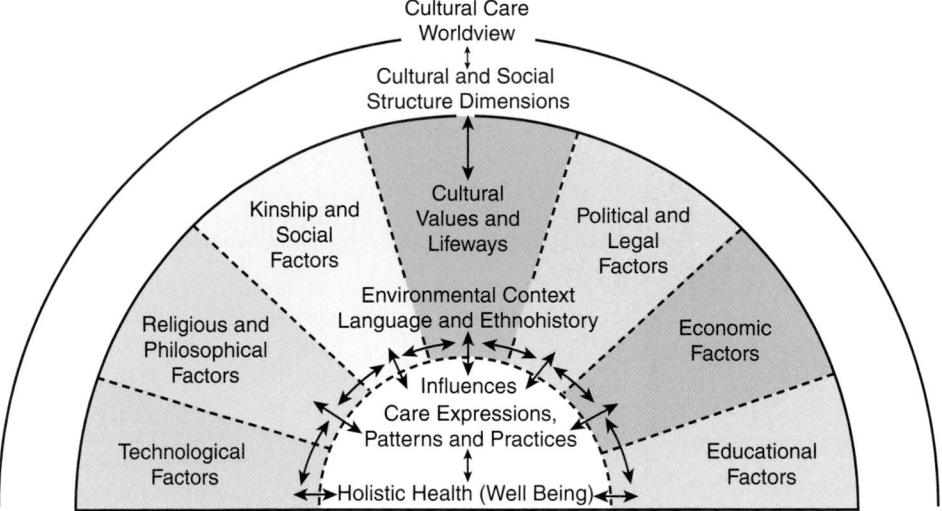

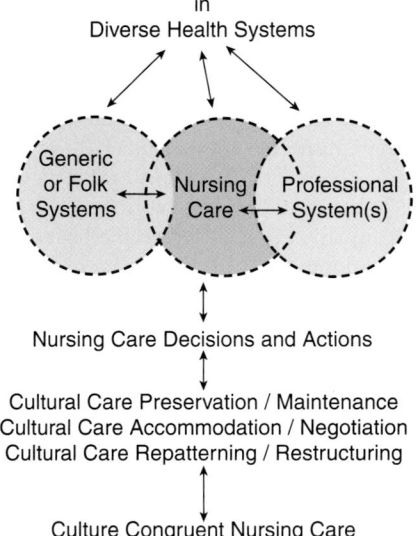

FIGURE 8-1 Leininger's Sunrise Model depicts theory of cultural care diversity and universality. From Leininger, M. M. (Ed.). (2001). *Culture care diversity and university: A theory of nursing.* New York: New York: National League for Nursing Press.

- Absence of questions. Paradoxically, this often means that the listener is not grasping the message and therefore has difficulty formulating questions to ask.
- Inappropriate laughter. A self-conscious giggle may signal poor comprehension and may be an attempt to disguise embarrassment.
- Nonverbal cues. Although a blank expression may signal poor understanding, among some Asian Americans it may reflect a desire to avoid overt expression of emotion. Similarly, avoidance of eye contact may be a cultural expression of respect for the speaker; some Native Americans and Asian Americans use this gesture.

Culturally Mediated Characteristics

Nurses should be aware that patients act and behave in a variety of ways, in part because of the influence of culture on behaviors and attitudes. However, although certain attributes and attitudes are frequently associated with particular cultural groups, as described in the following pages, it is important to remember that not all people from the same cultural background share the same behaviors and views. Although the nurse who fails to consider a patient's cultural preferences and beliefs is considered insensitive and possibly indifferent, the nurse who assumes that all members of any one culture act and behave in the same way runs the risk of stereotyping people. The best way to avoid stereotyping is to view each patient as an individual and to find out the patient's cultural preferences. A thorough culture assessment using a culture assessment tool or questionnaire (see later discussion) is very beneficial.

SPACE AND DISTANCE

People tend to regard the space in their immediate vicinity as an extension of themselves. The amount of space they need between themselves and others to feel comfortable is a culturally determined phenomenon.

Because nurses and patients usually are not consciously aware of their personal space requirements, they frequently have difficulty understanding different behaviors in this regard. For exam-

Chart 8-1 Overcoming Language Barriers

- Greet the patient using the last or complete name. Avoid being too casual or familiar. Point to yourself and say your name. Smile.
- Proceed in an unhurried manner. Pay attention to any effort by the patient or family to communicate.
- Speak in a low, moderate voice. Avoid talking loudly. Remember that there is a tendency to raise the volume and pitch of your voice when the listener appears not to understand. The listener may perceive that you are shouting and/or angry.
- Organize your thoughts. Repeat and summarize frequently. Use audiovisual aids when feasible.
- Use short, simple sentence structure and speak in the active voice.
- Use simple words, such as "pain" rather than "discomfort." Avoid medical jargon, idioms, and slang. Avoid using contractions, such as don't, can't, won't.
- Use nouns repeatedly instead of pronouns. *Example:* Do not say: "He has been taking his medicine, hasn't he?" Do say: "Does Juan take medicine?"
- Pantomime words (use gestures) and simple actions while verbalizing them.
- Give instructions in the proper sequence. *Example:* Do not say: "Before you rinse the bottle, sterilize it." Do say: "First, wash the bottle. Second, rinse the bottle."
- Discuss one topic at a time, and avoid giving too much information in a single conversation. Avoid using conjunctions. *Example:* Do not say: "Are you cold and in pain?" Do say (while pantomiming/gesturing): "Are you cold?" "Are you in pain?"
- Validate whether the person understands by having him or her repeat instructions, demonstrate the procedure, or act out the meaning.
- Use any words you know in the person's language. This indicates that you are aware of and respect the patient's primary means of communicating.
- Try a third language. Many Indo-Chinese speak French. Europeans often know three or four languages. Try Latin words or phrases, if you are familiar with the language.
- Ask who among the patient's family and friends could serve as an interpreter. Be aware of culturally based gender and age differences and diverse socioeconomic, educational, and tribal/regional differences when choosing an interpreter.
- Obtain phrase books from a library or bookstore, make or purchase flash cards, contact hospitals for a list of interpreters, and use both formal and informal networking to locate a suitable interpreter. Although they are costly, some telecommunication companies provide translation services.

ple, one patient may perceive the nurse sitting close to him or her as an expression of warmth and care; another patient may perceive the nurse's act as a threatening invasion of personal space. Research reveals that people from the United States, Canada, and Great Britain require the most personal space between themselves and others, whereas those from Latin America, Japan, and the Middle East need the least amount of space and feel comfortable standing close to others.

If patients appear to position themselves too close or too far away, the nurse should consider cultural preferences for space and distance. Ideally, patients should be permitted to assume a position that is comfortable to them in terms of personal space and distance. Because a significant amount of communication during nursing care requires close physical contact, the nurse should be aware of these important cultural differences and consider them when delivering care (Davidhizar, Dowd, & Newman-Giger, 1999).

EYE CONTACT

Eye contact is also a culturally determined behavior. Although most nurses have been taught to maintain eye contact when speaking with patients, some people from certain cultural backgrounds may interpret this behavior differently. Some Asians, Native Americans, Indo-Chinese, Arabs, and Appalachians, for example, may consider direct eye contact impolite or aggressive, and they may avert their own eyes when talking with nurses and others whom they perceive to be in positions of authority. Some Native Americans stare at the floor during conversations, a cultural behavior conveying respect and indicating that the listener is paying close attention to the speaker. Some Hispanic patients maintain downcast eyes as a sign of appropriate deferential behavior toward others on the basis of age, gender, social position, economic status, and position of authority. Being aware that whether a person makes eye contact may be a result of the culture from which they come will help the nurse understand a patient's behavior and provide an atmosphere in which the patient can feel comfortable.

TIME

Attitudes about time vary widely among cultures and can be a barrier to effective communication between nurses and patients. Views about punctuality and the use of time are culturally determined, as is the concept of waiting. Symbols of time, such as watches, sunrises, and sunsets, represent methods for measuring the duration and passage of time (Giger & Davidhizar, 1999; Spector, 2000).

For most health care providers, time and promptness are extremely important. For example, nurses frequently expect patients to arrive at an exact time for an appointment, despite the fact that the patient is often kept waiting by health care providers who are running late. Health care providers are likely to function according to an appointment system in which there are short intervals of perhaps only a few minutes. For patients from some cultures, however, time is a relative phenomenon, with little attention paid to the exact hour or minute. Some Hispanic people, for example, consider time in a wider frame of reference and make the primary distinction between day and night. Time may also be determined according to traditional times for meals, sleep, and other activities or events. For people from some cultures, the present is of the greatest importance, and time is viewed in broad ranges rather than in terms of a fixed hour. Being flexible in regard to schedules is the best way to accommodate these differences.

Value differences also may influence a person's sense of priority when it comes to time. For example, responding to a family matter may be more important to a patient than meeting a scheduled health care appointment. Allowing for these different views is essential in maintaining an effective nurse-patient relationship. Scolding or acting annoyed at a patient for being late undermines the patient's confidence in the health care system and might result in further missed appointments or indifference to health care suggestions.

TOUCH

The meaning people associate with touching is culturally determined to a great degree. In some cultures (eg, Hispanic, Arab), male health care providers may be prohibited from touching or examining certain parts of the female body. Similarly, it may be inappropriate for females to care for males. Among many Asian Americans, it is impolite to touch a person's head because the spirit is believed to reside there. Therefore, assessment of the head or evaluation of a head injury requires alternative approaches. The patient's culturally defined sense of modesty must also be considered when providing nursing care. For example, some Jewish and Islamic women believe that modesty requires covering their head, arms, and legs with clothing.

COMMUNICATION

Many aspects of care may be influenced by the diverse cultural perspectives held by the health care providers, patient, family, or significant others. One example is the issue of informed consent and full disclosure. In general, a nurse may argue that patients have the right to full disclosure about their disease and prognosis and may feel that advocacy means working to provide that disclosure. Family members of some cultural backgrounds may believe it is their responsibility to protect and spare the patient, their loved one, the knowledge of a terminal illness. Similarly, patients may, in fact, not want to know about their condition and may expect their family members to "take the burden" of that knowledge and related decision-making (Kudzma, 1999). The nurse should not decide that the family or patient is simply wrong or that the patient must know all details of his or her illness. Similar concerns may be noted when patients refuse pain medication or treatment because of cultural beliefs regarding pain or belief in divine intervention or faith healing. Determining the most appropriate and ethical approach to patient care requires an exploration of the cultural aspects of these situations. Self-examination by the nurse and recognition of one's own cultural bias and world view, as discussed earlier, will play a major part in helping the nurse to resolve cultural and ethical conflicts. The nurse must promote open dialogue and work with the patient, family, physician, and other health care providers to reach the culturally appropriate solution for the patient.

OBSERVANCE OF HOLIDAYS

People from all cultures celebrate civil and religious holidays. Nurses should familiarize themselves with major holidays for members of the cultural groups they serve. Information about these important celebrations is available from various sources, including religious organizations, hospital chaplains, and patients themselves. Routine health appointments, diagnostic tests, surgery, and other major procedures should be scheduled to avoid those holidays a patient identifies as significant. Efforts should also be made to accommodate patients and family or significant others, when not contraindicated, as they perform holiday rituals in the health care setting.

DIET

The cultural meanings associated with food vary widely but usually include one or more of the following: relief of hunger; promotion of health and healing; prevention of disease or illness; expression of caring for another; promotion of interpersonal closeness among individuals, families, groups, communities, or nations; and promotion of kinship and family alliances. Food may also be associated with solidification of social ties; celebration of life events (eg, birthdays, marriages, funerals); expression of gratitude or appreciation; recognition of achievement or accomplishment; validation of social, cultural, or religious ceremonial functions; facilitation of business negotiations; and expression of affluence, wealth, or social status.

Culture determines which foods are served and when they are served, the number and frequency of meals, who eats with whom, and who is given the choicest portions. Culture also determines how foods are prepared and served; how they are eaten (with chopsticks, hands, or fork, knife, and spoon); and where people shop for their favorite food items (eg, ethnic grocery stores, specialty food markets).

Religious practices may include fasting (eg, Mormons, Catholics, Buddhists, Jews, Muslims), abstaining from selected foods at particular times (eg, Catholics abstain from meat on Ash Wednesday and on Fridays during Lent), and considerations for medications (eg, Muslims may prefer to use non-pork-derived insulin). Practices may also include the ritualistic use of food and beverages (eg, Passover dinner, consumption of bread and wine during religious ceremonies). Chart 8-2 summarizes some dietary practices of selected religious groups.

Many groups tend to feast, often in the company of family and friends, on selected holidays. For example, many Christians eat large dinners on Christmas and Easter and consume other traditional high-calorie, high-fat foods, such as seasonal cookies, pastries, and candies. These culturally-based dietary practices are especially significant in the care of patients with diabetes, hypertension, gastrointestinal disorders, and other conditions in which diet plays a key role in the treatment and health maintenance regimen.

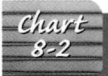

Chart 8-2 **Prohibited Foods and Beverages of Selected Religious Groups**

Hinduism
All meats
Animal shortenings

Islam
Pork
Alcoholic products and beverages (including extracts, such as vanilla and lemon)
Animal shortenings
Gelatin made with pork, marshmallow, and other confections made with gelatin

Judaism
Pork
Predatory fowl
Shellfish and scavenger fish (eg, shrimp, crab, lobster, escargot, catfish). Fish with fins and scales are permissible.
Mixing milk and meat dishes at same meal
Blood by ingestion (eg, blood sausage, raw meat). Blood by transfusion is acceptable.
Note: Packaged foods will contain labels identifying kosher ("properly preserved" or "fitting") and pareve (made without meat or milk) items.

Mormonism (Church of Jesus Christ of Latter-Day Saints)
Alcohol
Tobacco
Beverages containing caffeine stimulants (coffee, tea, colas, and selected carbonated soft drinks)

Seventh-Day Adventism
Pork
Certain seafood, including shellfish
Fermented beverages
Note: Optional vegetarianism is encouraged.

BIOLOGIC VARIATIONS

Along with psychosocial adaptations, nurses must also consider the physiologic impact of culture on patient response to treatment, particularly medications. Data have been collected for many years regarding differences in the effect some medications have on persons of diverse ethnic or cultural origins. Genetic predispositions to different rates of metabolism cause some patients to be prone to overdose reactions to the "normal dose" of a medication, while other patients are likely to experience a greatly reduced benefit from the standard dose of the medication. An antihypertensive agent, for example, may work well for a white male client within a 4-week time span but may take much longer to work or not work at all for an African-American male patient with hypertension. General polymorphism—variation in response to medications resulting from patient age, gender, size, and body composition—has long been acknowledged by the health care community (Kudzma, 1999). Culturally competent medication administration requires that consideration of ethnicity and related factors such as values and beliefs regarding the use of herbal supplements, dietary intake, and genetic factors can affect the effectiveness of treatment and compliance with the treatment regimen (Giger & Davidhizar, 1999; Kudzma, 1999).

COMPLEMENTARY AND ALTERNATIVE THERAPIES

Interventions for alterations in health and wellness vary among cultures. Interventions most commonly used in the United States have been labeled as *conventional medicine* by the National Institutes of Health (n.d.). Other names for conventional medicine were allopathy, Western medicine, regular medicine, mainstream medicine, and biomedicine. Interest in interventions that are not an integral part of conventional medicine prompted the National Institutes of Health to create the Office of Alternative Medicine (OAM) in 1992, and then to establish the National Center for Complementary and Alternative Medicine (NCCAM) in 1999.

The NCCAM grouped complementary and alternative medicine interventions into five main categories: alternative medical systems, mind–body interventions, biologically based therapies, manipulative and body-based methods, and energy therapies (National Institutes for Health, National Center for Complementary and Alternative Medicine, accessed 9/8/01).

- *Alternative medical systems* are defined as complete systems of theory and practice that are different from conventional medicine. Some examples are traditional Eastern medicine (including acupuncture, herbal medicine, oriental massage, and Qi gong); India's traditional medicine, Ayurveda (including diet, exercise, meditation, herbal medicine, massage, exposure to sunlight, and controlled breathing to restore harmony of an individual's body, mind, and spirit); homeopathic medicine (including herbal medicine and minerals); and naturopathic medicine (including diet, acupuncture, herbal medicine, hydrotherapy, spinal and soft-tissue manipulation, electrical currents, ultrasound and light therapy, therapeutic counseling, and pharmacology).
- *Mind–body interventions* are defined as techniques to facilitate the mind's ability to affect symptoms and bodily functions. Some examples are meditation, dance, music, art therapy, prayer, and mental healing.
- *Biologically based therapies* are defined as natural and biologically based practices, interventions, and products. Some examples are herbal therapies (an herb is a plant or plant part that produces and contains chemical substances that act upon the body), special diet therapies (such as those of Drs. Atkins, Ornish, and Pritikin), orthomolecular therapies (magnesium, melatonin, megadoses of vitamins), and biologic therapies (shark cartilage, bee pollen).
- *Manipulative and body-based methods* are defined as interventions based on body movement. Some examples are chiropracty (primarily manipulation of the spine), osteopathic manipulation, massage therapy (soft tissue manipulation), and reflexology.
- *Energy therapies* are defined as interventions that focus on energy fields within the body (biofields) or externally (electromagnetic fields). Some examples are Qi gong, Reiki, therapeutic touch, pulsed electromagnetic fields, magnetic fields, alternating electrical current, and direct electrical current.

A patient may choose to seek an alternative to conventional medical or surgical therapies. Many of these alternative therapies are becoming widely accepted as feasible treatment options. Therapies such as acupuncture and herbal treatments may be recommended by a patient's physician to address aspects of a condition that are unresponsive to conventional medical treatment or to minimize side effects associated with conventional medical therapy. Alternative therapy used to supplement conventional medicine may be referred to as *complementary therapy*.

Physicians and advanced practice nurses may work in collaboration with an herbalist or with a spiritualist or shaman to provide a comprehensive treatment plan for the patient. Out of respect for the way of life and beliefs of patients from different cultures, it is often necessary that the healers and health care providers respect the strengths of each approach (Palmer, 2001). Complementary therapy is becoming more common as health care consumers become more aware of what is available through information in printed media and on the Internet.

As patients become more informed, they are more likely to participate in a variety of therapies in conjunction with their conventional medical treatments. The nurse needs to assess each patient for use of complementary therapies, remain alert to the danger of conflicting treatments, and be prepared to provide information to the patient regarding treatment that may be harmful. The nurse must, however, be accepting of the patient's beliefs and right to control his or her own care. As a patient advocate, the nurse facilitates the integration of conventional medical, complementary, and alternative medical therapies.

Causes of Illness

Three major views, or paradigms, attempt to explain the causes of disease and illness: the biomedical or scientific view, the naturalistic or holistic perspective, and the magico-religious view.

BIOMEDICAL OR SCIENTIFIC

The biomedical or scientific world view prevails in most health care settings and is embraced by most nurses and other health care providers. The basic assumptions underlying the biomedical perspective are that all events in life have a cause and effect, that the human body functions much like a machine, and that all of reality can be observed and measured (eg, blood pressures, PaO_2 levels, intelligence tests). One example of the biomedical or scientific view is the bacterial or viral explanation of communicable diseases.

NATURALISTIC OR HOLISTIC

The second way that some cultures explain the cause of illness is through the naturalistic or holistic perspective, a viewpoint that is found among many Native Americans, Asians, and others. According to this view, the forces of nature must be kept in natural balance or harmony.

One example of a naturalistic belief, held by many Asian groups, is the yin/yang theory, in which health is believed to exist when all aspects of a person are in perfect balance or harmony. Rooted in the ancient Chinese philosophy of Taoism (which translates as "The Way"), the yin/yang theory proposes that all organisms and objects in the universe consist of yin and yang energy. The seat of the energy forces is within the autonomic nervous system, where balance between the opposing forces is maintained during health. Yin energy represents the female and negative forces, such as emptiness, darkness, and cold, whereas the yang forces are male and positive, emitting warmth and fullness. Foods are classified as cold (yin) or hot (yang) in this theory and are transformed into yin and yang energy when metabolized by the body. Cold foods are eaten when the person has a hot illness (eg, fever, rash, sore throat, ulcer, infection), and hot foods are eaten with a cold illness (eg, cancer, headache, stomach cramps, colds). The yin/yang theory is the basis for Eastern or Chinese medicine and is embraced by some Asian Americans.

Many Hispanic, African American, and Arab groups also embrace the hot/cold theory of health and illness. The four humors of the body—blood, phlegm, black bile, and yellow bile—regulate basic bodily functions and are described in terms of temperature and moisture. The treatment of disease consists of adding or subtracting cold, heat, dryness, or wetness to restore the balance of these humors. Beverages, foods, herbs, medicines, and diseases are classified as hot or cold according to their perceived effects on the body, not their physical characteristics. According to the hot/cold theory, the individual as a whole, not just a particular ailment, is significant. Those who embrace the hot/cold theory maintain that health consists of a positive state of total well-being, including physical, psychological, spiritual, and social aspects of the person.

According to the naturalistic world view, breaking the laws of nature creates imbalances, chaos, and disease. People who embrace the naturalistic paradigm use metaphors such as "the healing power of Nature." From the perspective of the Chinese, for example, illness is seen, not as an intruding agent, but as a part of life's rhythmic course and an outward sign of disharmony within.

MAGICO-RELIGIOUS

The third major way in which people view the world and explain the causes of illness is the magico-religious world view. This view's basic premise is that the world is an arena in which supernatural forces dominate and that the fate of the world and those in it depends on the action of supernatural forces for good or evil. Examples of magical causes of illness include belief in voodoo or witchcraft among some African Americans and others from Caribbean countries. Faith healing is based on religious beliefs and is most prevalent among selected Christian religions, including Christian Science, while various healing rituals may be found in many other religions, such as Roman Catholicism and Mormonism (Church of Jesus Christ of Latter Day Saints).

Of course, it is possible to hold a combination of world views, and many patients offer more than one explanation for the cause of their illness. As a profession, nursing largely embraces the scientific or biomedical world view, but some aspects of holism have begun to gain popularity, including a wide variety of techniques for managing chronic pain, such as hypnosis, therapeutic touch, and biofeedback. Belief in spiritual power is also held by many nurses who credit supernatural forces with various unexplained phenomena related to patients' health and illness states.

Regardless of the view held and whether the nurse agrees with the patient's beliefs in this regard, it is important to be aware of how people view their illness and their health and to work within this framework to promote patients' care and well-being.

Folk Healers

Several cultures believe in folk or indigenous healers. The nurse may find some Hispanic patients, for instance, turning to a curandero or curandera, espiritualista (spiritualist), yerbo (herbalist), or sabador (healer who manipulates bones and muscles). Some African American patients may seek assistance from a hougan (voodoo priest or priestess), spiritualist, root doctor (usually a woman who uses magic rituals to treat diseases), or "old lady" (an older woman who has successfully raised a family and who specializes in child care and folk remedies). Native American patients may seek assistance from a shaman or medicine man or woman. Patients of Asian descent may mention that they have visited herbalists, acupuncturists, or bone setters. Several cultures have their own healers, most of whom speak the native tongue of the patient, make house calls, and cost significantly less than healers practicing in the conventional medical health care system.

People seeking complementary and alternative therapies have expanded the practices of folk healers beyond their traditional populations, so the nurse needs to ask patients about participation with folk healers regardless of their cultural background. It is best not to disregard a patient's belief in a folk healer or try to undermine trust in the healer. To do so may alienate and drive the patient away from receiving the care prescribed. A nurse should make an effort to accommodate the patient's beliefs while also advocating the treatment proposed by health science.

Cultural Assessment

Cultural nursing assessment refers to a systematic appraisal or examination of individuals, families, groups, and communities in terms of their cultural beliefs, values, and practices. The purpose of such an assessment is to provide culturally competent care (Giger & Davidhizar, 1999). In an effort to establish a database for determining a patient's cultural background, nurses have developed cultural assessment tools or modified existing assessment tools (Spector, 2000; Leininger, 2001) to ensure that transcultural considerations are included in the plan of care. Giger and Davidhizar's (1999) model has been used to design nursing care from health promotion to nursing skills activities (Giger & Davidhizar, 1999; Smith-Temple & Johnson, 2002). The information presented in this chapter and the following general guidelines can be used to direct the nurse's assessment of culture and its influence on a patient's health beliefs and practices.

- What is the patient's country of origin? How long has the patient lived in this country? What is the primary language and literacy level?
- What is the patient's ethnic background? Does he or she identify strongly with others from the same cultural background?

- What is the patient's religion, and how important is it to his or her daily life?
- Does the patient participate in cultural activities such as dressing in traditional clothing and observing traditional holidays and festivals?
- Are there any food preferences or restrictions?
- What are the patient's communication styles? Is eye contact avoided? How much physical distance is maintained? Is the patient open and verbal about symptoms?
- Who is the head of the family, and is he or she involved in decision making about the patient?
- What does the patient do to maintain his or her health?
- What does the patient think caused the current problem?
- Has the advice of traditional healers been sought?
- Have complementary therapies been utilized?
- What kind of treatment does the patient think will help? What are the most important results he or she hopes to get from this treatment?
- Are there religious rituals related to health, sickness, or death that the patient observes?

Additional Cultural Considerations: Know Thyself

Because the nurse–patient interaction is the focal point of nursing, nurses should consider their own cultural orientation when conducting assessment of the patient and the patient's family and friends.

- Know your own cultural attitudes, values, beliefs, and practices.
- Regardless of "good intention," everyone has cultural "baggage" that ultimately results in ethnocentrism.
- In general, it is easier to understand those whose cultural heritage is similar to our own, while viewing those who are unlike us as strange and different.
- Maintain a broad, open attitude. Expect the unexpected. Enjoy surprises.
- Avoid seeing all people as alike; that is, avoid cultural stereotypes, such as "all Chinese like rice" or "all Italians eat spaghetti."
- Try to understand the reasons for any behavior by discussing commonalities and differences.
- If a patient has said or done something that you do not understand, ask for clarification. Be a good listener. Most patients will respond positively to questions that arise from a genuine concern for and interest in them.
- If at all possible, speak the patient's language (even simple greetings and social courtesies will be appreciated). Avoid feigning an accent or using words that are ordinarily not part of your vocabulary.
- Be yourself. There are no right or wrong ways to learn about cultural diversity.

The Future of Transcultural Nursing Care

By the middle of the 21st century, the average American patient will trace his or her ancestry to Africa, Asia, the Pacific Islands, or the Hispanic or Arab worlds, rather than to Europe (Giger & Davidhizar, 1999). As indicated previously, the concept of culturally competent care applies to health care institutions, which must develop culturally sensitive policies and provide an atmosphere that fosters the provision of culturally competent care by nurses. Those nurses, who reflect the multicultural complexion of our society, must learn to acknowledge and adapt to diversity among their colleagues in the workplace (Davidhizar, Dowd, & Newman-Giger, 1999). In addition, educational institutions must prepare nurses to deliver culturally competent care. Nursing programs, therefore, are exploring creative ways to promote cultural competence in nursing students, including offering multicultural health studies in their curricula (Spector, 2000).

An additional issue related to the provision of culturally competent care is the diversity of the health care delivery workforce. Today more than 80% of all nurses are white women. As the population becomes more culturally diverse, efforts to increase the number of ethnic minority nurses must continue and accelerate. Progress in increasing the percentage of culturally diverse nurses has been significantly slower than the increasing percentage of ethnic minority persons in the United States (Buerhaus & Auerbach, 1999). Efforts must be made to facilitate the recruitment and successful program completion of ethnic minority nursing students.

With increasing frequency, nurses will be expected to provide culturally competent care for patients. Nurses must work effectively with patients, one another, and other health care team members whose ancestry reflects the multicultural complexion of contemporary society in increasing numbers. Cultural diversity remains one of the foremost issues in health care today.

Critical Thinking Exercises

1. You are assigned to care for a hospitalized young male adult whose cultural background is very different from yours. Describe how you would assess his cultural beliefs and practices in developing a plan of nursing care. Explain why it is important to examine your own feelings about his cultural beliefs and practices.

2. An elderly Hispanic female patient who does not speak English is hospitalized after elective surgery. Even though she is progressing well and her discharge has been planned, her family insists on staying with her for as many hours as possible, refusing to leave when visiting hours are over. How can you help the nursing staff to explore the meaning of the family's behavior and to understand their own feelings about this behavior? Devise a strategy that you think will help resolve this situation.

3. You are preparing to discharge an elderly patient who is of foreign origin. The record indicates that she does not speak English and lives alone in a neighborhood where most of the residents are from the same ethnic background as herself. Describe how you would plan discharge teaching to ensure that you can communicate with the patient and family to promote the necessary follow-up care. Explore other aspects of the patient's and family's background that you would want to assess to determine the need for referral to a home health care agency.

REFERENCES AND SELECTED READINGS

Books

American Academy of Nursing, Subpanel on Cultural Competence in Nursing. (1995). *Promoting cultural competence in and through nursing education.* New York: Author.

American Association of Colleges of Nursing. (1996). *Diversity Task Force Report, October 1996.* Washington, D.C.: Author.

Andrews, M. M., & Boyle, J. S. (1999). *Transcultural concepts in nursing care* (3rd ed.). Philadelphia: J. B. Lippincott.

Giger, J. N., & Davidhizar, R. E. (1999). *Transcultural nursing: Assessment and intervention* (3rd ed.). St. Louis: C. V. Mosby.

Hunt, R. (2000). *Readings in community-based nursing.* Philadelphia: Lippincott Williams & Wilkins.

Kuhn, M. A. (1999). *Complementary therapies for health care providers.* Philadelphia: Lippincott Williams & Wilkins.

Leininger, M. M. (Ed.). (2001). *Culture care diversity and universality: A theory of nursing.* New York: National League for Nursing Press.

Smith-Temple, J., & Johnson, J. Y. (2002). *Nurse's guide to clinical procedures.* (4th ed.). Philadelphia: Lippincott Williams & Wilkins.

Spector, R. E. (2000). *Cultural diversity in health and illness.* New Jersey: Prentice-Hall.

Wilkinson, J. M. (2001). *Nursing process and critical thinking.* New Jersey: Prentice-Hall.

Journals

Buerhaus, P. I., & Auerbach, D. (1999). Slow growth in the United States of the number of minorities in the RN workforce. *Image: Journal of Nursing Scholarship, 31*(2), 179–183.

Davidhizar, R., Dowd, S., & Newman-Giger, J. (1999). Managing diversity in the health care workplace. *Health Care Supervisor, 17*(3), 51–62.

Fields, C. D. (2000). Choosing cultural competence over diaspora division. *Black Issues in Higher Education, 17*(16), 6.

Gonzalez, R. I., Gooden, M. B., & Porter, C. P. (2000). Eliminating racial and ethnic disparities in health care. *American Journal of Nursing, 100*(3), 56–58.

Gonzalez, R. (1999). Washington Watch: ANA advocates more diversity in nursing. *American Journal of Nursing, 99*(11), 24.

Gooden, M. B., Porter, C. P., Gonzalez, R. I., & Mims, B. L. (2001). Rethinking the relationship between nursing and diversity. *American Journal of Nursing, 101*(1), 63, 65.

Krumberger, J. M. (2000). Critical care close-up. *RN, 63*(4), 24AC2–24AC3.

Kudzma, E. C. (1999). Culturally competent drug administration. *American Journal of Nursing, 99*(8), 46–51.

Leininger, M. M. (1988). Leininger's theory of nursing: Cultural care diversity and universality. *Nursing Science Quarterly, 1*(4), 152–159.

National Institutes of Health, National Center for Complementary and Alternative Medicine (n.d.). *Major domains of complementary & alternative medicine.* Available at: http://nccam.nih.gov/fcp/classify/. Accessed September 8, 2001.

Palmer, J. (2001). Respecting tradition in healing. *Reflections on Nursing Leadership, 27*(2), 30–31.

Suro, R. (2000). Beyond economics. *American Demographics, 22*(2), 48–55.

RESOURCES AND WEBSITES

Organizations

Asian-Pacific Islander Nurses Association, c/o College of Mount Saint Vincent, 6301 Riverdale Avenue, Riverdale, NY 10471; 1-718-405-3354.

Council on Nursing and Anthropology, c/o Dr. Mildred Roberson, Nursing and Health Sciences, Salisbury State University, Salisbury, MD 21801.

National Alaska–Native American Indian Nurses Association, 3702 South Fife Street #55, K-2, Tacoma, Washington 98408-7318; 1-907-279-3303.

National Association of Hispanic Nurses, 1501 16th Street NW, Washington, DC 20036; 1-202-387-2477; fax 202-483-7183; http://www.thehispanicnurses.org/.

National Black Nurses Association, P.O. Box 1823, Washington, DC 20012-1823; 1-202-393-6870; fax 1-202-347-3808; http://www.nbna.org.

National Gerontological Nursing Association, 7250 Parkway Dr., Suite 510 Hanover, MD 21076; 1-800-723-0560; fax 410-712-4424; e-mail: susan.sibiski@mosby.com.

National Institutes of Health, National Center for Complementary and Alternative Medicine, 6707 Democracy Blvd., Suite 2000, Bethesda, MD 20892-5475; 1-888-644-6226; fax 1-866-464-3616; http://nccam.nih.gov. Accessed 9/8/01.

Office of Minority Health, U.S. Department of Health and Human Services, P.O. Box 37337, Washington, DC 20013-7337; 1-800-444-6472; http://www.omhrc.gov. No cost for accessing database, information specialists, resource network, and publications on major health problems affecting African Americans, Hispanics, Native Americans, and Asian/Pacific Islanders.

Transcultural Nursing Society, c/o Madonna University College of Nursing and Health, 36600 Schoolcraft Road, Livonia MI 48150-1173; 888-432-5470.

Translation Services

AT&T Language Line Services; 1-800-752-6096. Provides written and oral translation in 140 languages.

Genetics Perspectives in Nursing

On completion of this chapter, the learner will be able to:

1. Describe the role of the nurse in integrating genetics in nursing care.
2. Conduct a genetics-based assessment.
3. Identify the common patterns of inheritance of genetic disorders.
4. Identify ethical issues in nursing related to genetics.

*H*uman **genome** discoveries have ushered in a new era of medicine, *genomic medicine,* which recognizes that multiple genes work in concert with environmental influences to cause disease. Genomic medicine aims to improve predictions about individuals' susceptibility to diseases, the time of onset for those diseases, their extent and eventual severity, and which treatments or medications are likely to be most effective or harmful (Billings, 2000). Already, new gene-based strategies for disease detection, management, and treatment have been created, allowing health professionals to tailor care to an individual's particular genetic make-up.

To meet the challenges of genomic medicine, nurses need to understand the new technologies and treatments of gene-based health care. Nurses also must recognize that they are a vital link between patients and health care services; patients often turn to nurses first with questions about family history of risk factors, genetics information, and genetic tests and interpretations. Incorporating genetics into nursing means bringing a genetics framework to health assessments, planning, and interventions that supports identification of and response to individuals' changing genetics-related health needs (Lea, Williams, Jenkins, et al., 2000).

Nurses must learn to recognize patterns of inheritance when obtaining family and medical histories and understand when it is appropriate to consider new gene-based testing and treatment options. This chapter offers a foundation for the clinical applications of genetics principles in medical and surgical nursing, outlines the nurse's role in genetic counseling and evaluation, addresses important ethical issues, and provides genetics resources for nurses and patients.

A Framework for Integrating Genetics Into Nursing Practice

Nursing's unique contribution to genomic medicine is its philosophy of holism. Nurses are ideally positioned to incorporate genetics into their assessments, planning, and interventions for patients at different ages and stages across the lifespan and in all settings. The holistic view that characterizes nursing takes into account each person's intellectual, physical, spiritual, social, cultural, biopsychologic, ethical, and esthetic experiences while ad-

Glossary

allele: any one of two or more alternate forms of a gene at the same location. An allele for each gene is inherited from each parent.

autosome: a single chromosome from any of the 22 pairs of chromosomes not involved in sex determination (XX or XY)

carrier: person who is heterozygous; possessing two different alleles of a gene pair

chromosome: microscopic structures in the cell nucleus that contain genetic information and are constant in number in a species (eg, humans have 46 chromosomes)

deoxyribonucleic acid (DNA): the primary genetic material in humans consisting of nitrogenous bases, a sugar group, and phosphate combined into a double helix

diploid: the number of chromosomes normally present in somatic cells. For humans, that number is 46.

dominant: a genetic trait that is normally expressed when a person has a gene mutation on one of a pair of chromosomes and the "normal" form of the gene is on the other chromosome

genetics: the scientific study of heredity; how specific traits or predispositions are transmitted from parents to offspring

genome: the total genetic complement of an individual genotype

genomics: the study of the human genome, including gene sequencing, mapping, and function

genotype: the genes and the variations therein that a person inherits from his or her parents

haploid: the number of chromosomes present in egg or sperm (gametes); in humans, this is 23

Human Genome Project: an international research effort aimed at identifying and

characterizing the order of every base in the human genome

meiosis: the reduction division of diploid egg or sperm (germ cells) resulting in haploid gametes (having 23 chromosomes each)

mitosis: cell division occurring in somatic cells that normally results in daughter cells with the same number of chromosomes—46 (diploid)

monosomy: missing one of a chromosome pair in normally diploid cells (for example, 45,X females have only one X chromosome)

mutation: a heritable alteration in the genetic material

nondisjunction: the failure of a chromosome pair to separate appropriately during meiosis, resulting in abnormal chromosome numbers in reproductive cells (gametes) or cells

nucleotide: a nucleic acid "building block" composed of a nitrogenous base, a five-carbon sugar, and a phosphate group

pedigree: a diagrammatic representation of a family history

penetrance: the percentage of individuals known to carry the gene for a trait who actually manifest the condition. For example, a trait with 90% penetrance will not be manifested by 10% of persons possessing the gene.

phenotype: a person's entire physical, biochemical, and physiological makeup, as determined by the individual's genotype and environmental factors

polymorphism: a genetic variation with two or more alleles that is maintained in a population

population screening: the application of a test or inquiry to a group to determine if

individuals in the group have an increased likelihood of a genetic condition or a mutation in a specific gene (eg, cholesterol screening for hypercholesterolemia)

predisposition testing: testing that is used to determine the likelihood that a healthy person with or without a family history of a condition will develop the disorder. Having the gene mutation would indicate that the person has an increased susceptibility to the disorder, but this is not a diagnosis. One example is DNA mutation testing for hereditary breast/ovarian cancer.

prenatal screening: testing that is used to identify if a fetus is at risk for a birth defect such as Down syndrome or spina bifida (eg, multiple marker maternal serum screening in pregnancy)

presymptomatic testing: genetic testing that is used to determine whether persons with a family history of a disorder, but no current symptoms, have the gene mutation. An example of this would be Huntington disease.

recessive: a genetic trait that is expressed only when a person has two copies of a mutant autosomal gene or a single copy of a mutant X-linked gene in the absence of another X chromosome

transcription: the process of transforming information from DNA into new strands of messenger RNA

trisomy: the presence of one extra chromosome in an otherwise diploid chromosome complement—for example, trisomy 21 (Down syndrome)

variable expression: variation in the degree to which a trait is manifested; clinical severity

X-linked: located on the X chromosome

dressing genetics information, gene-based testing, diagnosis, and treatments. Thus, knowledge about genetics is basic to nursing practice (Lea, Anderson & Monsen, 1998).

A framework for integrating genetics into nursing practice includes a philosophy of care that recognizes when genetics factors are playing a role or could play a role in an individual's health. This means using family history and the results of genetics tests effectively, informing patients about genetics concepts, understanding the personal and societal impact of genetics information, and valuing the privacy and confidentiality of genetics information.

A person's response to genetics information, genetic testing, or conditions may be either disabling or empowering. Genetics information may stigmatize individuals if it affects how they view themselves or how others view them. Nurses can help individuals and families understand the genetic aspect of themselves and learn how genetic traits and conditions are passed on within families and how genetic and environmental factors influence health and disease (Lea, Anderson & Monsen, 1998; Peters et al., 1999).

Nurses facilitate communication among family members, the health care system, and community resources; they offer valuable support by virtue of their continuity of care with patients and families. All nurses should be able to recognize when a client is asking a question related to genetics information and should know how to obtain genetics information by gathering family and health histories and conducting physical and developmental assessments. Being able to recognize a genetics concern allows the nurse to provide appropriate genetics resources and support to individuals and families (Lea, Jenkins & Francomano, 1998).

Key to nurses' genetics framework is the awareness of one's attitudes, experience, and assumptions about genetics concepts and how these are manifested in one's own practice. Chart 9-1 offers insights on how nurses can conduct periodic self-assessments.

Genetics Concepts

Scientists and philosophers have long speculated about heredity and developed theories to explain how traits are transmitted to offspring. Developments in technology and research have accelerated progress in our understanding of genetics, allowing scientists to better understand relatively rare diseases such as phenylketonuria (PKU) or hemophilia that are related to mutations of a single gene inherited in families. New technologies and tools allow scientists to characterize inherited metabolic variations that interact over time and lead to common diseases such as cancer, heart disease, and dementia. This transition from **genetics** to **genomics** highlights how our understanding of single genes and their individual functions has evolved to understanding how multiple genes act and control biologic processes. Most health conditions are now believed to be the result of a combination of genetic and environmental influences and interactions (Billings, 2000).

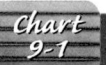 **Chart 9-1**

Examining Our Own Attitudes, Experiences, and Assumptions

Self-knowledge is one of the cornerstones to providing quality nursing care, and as practitioners, our attitudes and experiences have an impact on clinical practice. These attitudes emerge from social, cultural, and religious experiences in one's personal life. Awareness of our own values, beliefs, and cultural perceptions not only is important to the nurse–patient relationship, but it is also the first step in developing a genetics framework.

Periodic self-assessment can help maintain an effective framework as nurses update genetics knowledge and practice. Nurses can develop an awareness of their own attitudes, experiences, and assumptions about genetics concepts by considering the following:

- *One's family's beliefs or values about health.* What are your family, religious, or cultural beliefs about the cause of illness? How have your values or biases influenced your understanding of genetic conditions?
- *One's philosophical, theologic, cultural, and ethical perspectives related to health.* How would these attitudes influence your own use of genetics information or services? What experiences have you had with people from different social, cultural, religious, or ethnic groups? How would you deliver genetics information to individuals from different social, cultural, or ethnic groups? Can you recognize when personal values or biases may affect or interfere with the delivery of genetics information?
- *One's level of genetics expertise.* Can you recognize the limitations of your own genetics experience and know when to refer patients for further genetics work-up?
- *One's experience with birth defects, chronic illnesses, and genetic conditions.* Do you have a family member or friend who has a genetic condition or disorder? Has your experience been that

genetic disorders are disabling or empowering? Do you view a parent "at fault" for having a baby born with a birth defect or genetic condition? Do you advocate for fair access and other rights for individuals who have birth defects, genetic conditions, or other disabilities?
- *One's view of DNA (the most basic concept of who we are, since our genetic makeup is unlike that of any other person except an identical twin).* What are your assumptions about DNA? For example, do you assume that the genetic component of "the self" is a defective self? As another example, healthy carriers of genetic alterations that predispose them to develop certain diseases in the future now belong to a new class of "at risk" individuals. A person who is "at risk" is not ill at present, but may not remain well as long as the "average" person. Is it good to know that you are "at risk" or is this information that should not be identified or revealed because of the risk of potential discrimination?
- *One's beliefs about reproductive options.* What are your beliefs regarding reproductive options such as prenatal diagnosis and pregnancy termination? How might these influence your care of a patient who holds different beliefs?
- *One's view of genetic testing and engineering.* Do you see genetic testing and engineering—the ability to eliminate or enhance certain traits—as a way to create an "ideal genetic self"?
- *One's approach to patients with disabilities.* How are your attitudes made apparent in your practice and practice settings? For example, do you have access to TTY machines and/or interpreters for those who have hearing impairment? Are your intake procedures adapted to meet the needs of an individual with disabilities?

Sources: National Coalition of Health Professional Education in Genetics (2001). *Core competencies;* http://www.nchpeg.org; Kenan, R. (1996). The at-risk health status and technology: A diagnostic invitation and the gift of knowing. *Social Science and Medicine, 42*(11), 1545–1553; Peters, J. A., Djurdjinovic, L. & Baker, D. (1999). The genetic self: The Human Genome Project, genetic counseling and family therapy. *Families, Systems & Health, 17*(1), 5–25.

GENES AND THEIR ROLE IN HUMAN VARIATION

Genes are central components of human health and disease. Work on the **Human Genome Project** (an international research effort to map and sequence the human genome in its entirety) has shown how basic human genetics is to human development, health, and disease. Knowledge that specific genes are associated with specific genetic conditions makes diagnosis possible, even in the unborn. Research continues to demonstrate how many common conditions have genetic causes. Many more associations between genetics, health, and disease will likely be identified as scientists complete and refine human genome mapping and sequencing.

Genes and Chromosomes

A person's unique genetic constitution, called a **genotype**, is made up of some 30,000 to 40,000 genes. A person's **phenotype**, the observable characteristics of his or her genotype, includes physical appearance and other biologic, physiologic, and molecular traits. Environmental influences modify every individual's phenotype, even those with a major genetic component.

Human growth, development, and disease occur as a result of both genetic and environmental influences and interactions. The contribution of genetic factors may be large or small. For example, in a person with cystic fibrosis or PKU, the genetic contribution is significant. In contrast, the genetic contribution underlying a person's response to infection may be less so.

An individual gene is conceptualized as a unit of heredity. A gene is composed of a segment of **deoxyribonucleic acid (DNA)** that contains a specific set of instructions for making the protein or proteins needed by body cells for proper functioning. Genes regulate both the types of proteins made and the rate at which proteins are produced. The structure of the DNA molecule is referred to as the double helix. The essential components of the DNA molecule are sugar-phosphate molecules and pairs of nitrogenous bases. Each **nucleotide** contains a sugar (deoxyribose), a phosphate group, and one of four nitrogenous bases: adenine (A), cytosine (C), guanine (G), and thymine (T). DNA is composed of two-paired strands, each made up of a number of nucleotides. The strands are held together by hydrogen bonds between pairs of bases (Fig. 9-1).

Genes are packaged and arranged in a linear order within **chromosomes**, which are located in the cell nucleus. In humans, 46 chromosomes occur in pairs in all body cells except oocytes (eggs) and sperm, which each contain only 23 chromosomes. Twenty-two pairs of chromosomes, called **autosomes**, are the same in females and males. The 23rd pair is referred to as the sex chromosomes. A female has two X chromosomes, while a male has one X and one Y chromosome. At conception, each parent normally gives one chromosome of each pair to his or her children. As a result, children receive half of their chromosomes from their fathers and half from their mothers (Fig. 9-2).

Careful examination of DNA sequences from many individuals shows that these sequences have multiple versions in a population. These different versions, or sequence variations, are called **alleles**. Sequences found in many forms are said to be polymorphic, meaning that there are at least two common forms of a particular gene.

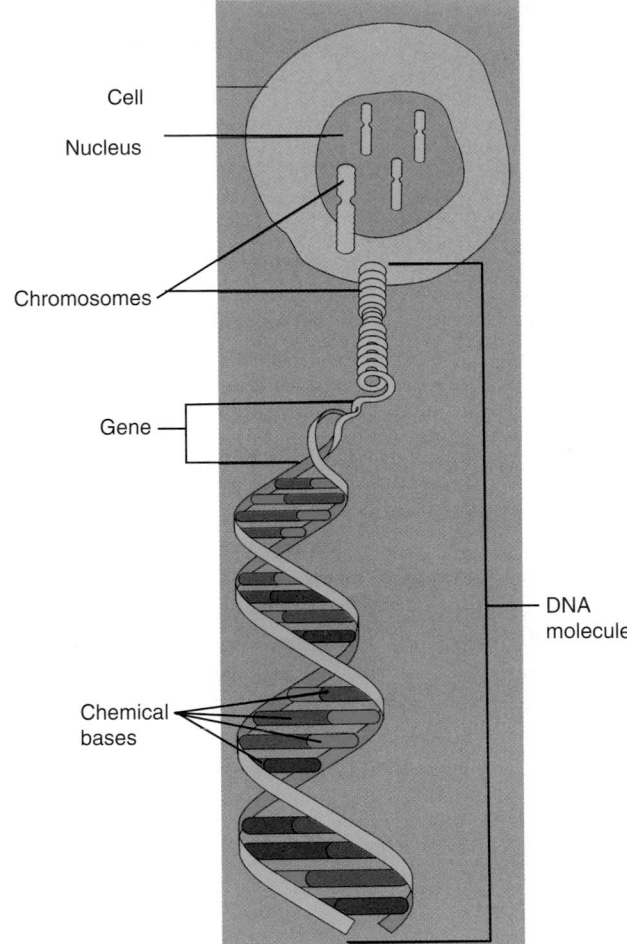

FIGURE 9-1 DNA that carries the instructions that allow cells to make proteins is made up of four chemical bases. Tightly coiled strands of DNA are packaged in units called chromosomes, housed in the cell's nucleus. Working subunits of DNA are known as genes. From the National Institutes of Health and National Cancer Institute. (1995). *Understanding gene testing* (NIH Pub. No. 96-3905). Washington, DC: U.S. Department of Human Services.

Cell Division

The human body grows and develops through a process of cell division. Mitosis and meiosis, two distinctly different types of cell division, contribute to these processes.

Mitosis is the process of cell division involved in cell growth, differentiation, and repair. During mitosis, the chromosomes of each cell duplicate. The result is two cells, called daughter cells, each containing the same number of chromosomes as the parent cell. The daughter cells are said to be **diploid** because they contain 46 chromosomes in 23 pairs. Mitosis occurs in all cells of the body except oocytes (eggs) and sperm.

Meiosis, in contrast, occurs only in reproductive cells and is the process by which oocytes and sperm are formed. During meiosis a reduction in the number of chromosomes takes place, resulting in oocytes or sperm that contain half the usual number or 23 chromosomes. Oocytes and sperm are referred to as **haploid** because they contain a single copy of each chromosome, compared to the usual two chromosomes in all other body cells.

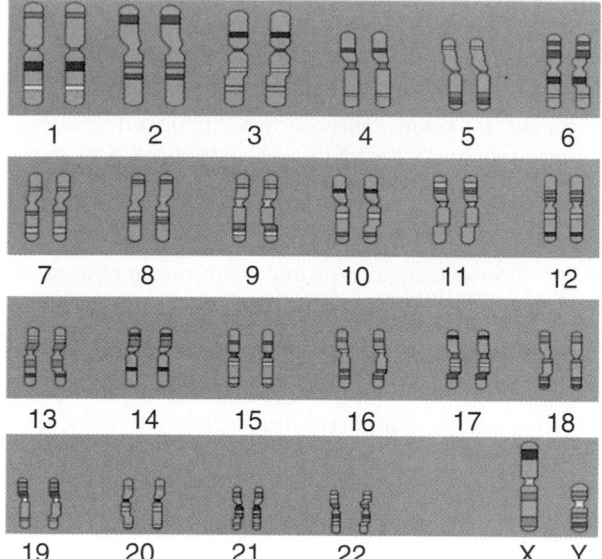

FIGURE 9-2 Each human cell contains 23 pairs of chromosomes, which can be distinguished by size and by unique banding patterns. This set is from a male, since it contains a Y chromosome. Females have two X chromosomes. From the National Institutes of Health and National Cancer Institute. (1995). *Understanding gene testing* (NIH Pub. No. 96-3905). Washington, DC: U.S. Department of Human Services.

During the initial phase of meiosis, paired chromosomes come together in preparation for cell division, portions cross over, and an exchange of genetic material occurs. This event, called recombination, creates greater diversity in the makeup of oocytes and sperm.

During meiosis, a pair of chromosomes may fail to separate completely, creating a sperm or oocyte that contains either two copies or no copy of a particular chromosome. This sporadic event, called **nondisjunction**, can lead to either a trisomy or a monosomy. Down syndrome is an example of **trisomy**. An individual with Down syndrome has three number 21 chromosomes. Turner syndrome is an example of **monosomy**. Girls who have Turner syndrome usually have a single X chromosome, causing them to have short stature and infertility (Lashley, 1998).

Gene Mutations

Within each cell, many intricate and complex interactions regulate and express human genes. Gene structure and function, **transcription** and translation, and protein synthesis are all involved. Alterations in gene structure and function and the process of protein synthesis may influence a person's health. Changes in gene structure, called **mutations**, permanently change the sequence of DNA, which in turn can alter the nature and type of proteins made (Fig. 9-3).

Some gene mutations have no significant effect on the protein product made, while others cause partial or complete changes. How a protein is altered and its importance to proper body functioning determine the mutation's impact. Gene mutations may occur in hormones or enzymes or important protein products, thereby having significant implications for health and disease.

Sickle cell anemia is an example of a genetic condition caused by a small gene mutation that affects protein structure, producing hemoglobin S. A person who inherits two copies of the hemoglobin S gene mutation has the condition sickle cell anemia and experiences the symptoms of severe anemia and thrombotic organ damage resulting from hypoxia (Lashley, 1998; Lea, 2000).

Other gene mutations may be larger, such as a deletion (loss), insertion (addition), duplication (multiplication), or rearrangement (translocation) of a longer DNA segment. Duchenne muscular dystrophy, an inherited form of muscular dystrophy, is an example of a genetic disorder caused by structural gene mutations such as deletions or duplications in the dystrophin gene. Another type of gene mutation, called a triplet or trinucleotide repeat, involves the expansion of more than the usual number of a triplet

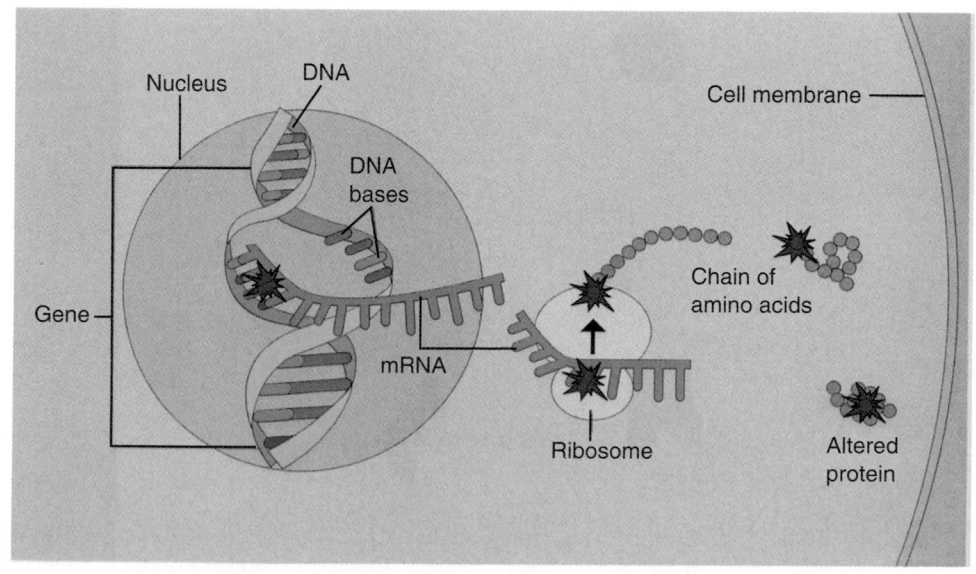

FIGURE 9-3 When a gene contains a mutation, the protein encoded by that gene will be abnormal. Some protein changes are insignificant, others are disabling. From the National Institutes of Health and National Cancer Institute. (1995). *Understanding gene testing* (NIH Pub. No. 96-3905). Washington, DC: U.S. Department of Human Services.

repeat sequence within a gene. Myotonic dystrophy, Huntington disease, and fragile X syndrome are examples of conditions caused by this type of gene mutation.

Gene mutations may be inherited or acquired. Inherited or germ-line gene mutations are present in the DNA of all body cells and are passed on in reproductive cells from parent to child. Germ-line mutations are passed on to all daughter cells when body cells replicate (Fig. 9-4). The gene that causes Huntington disease is one example of a germ-line mutation.

Spontaneous gene mutations take place in individual oocytes or sperm at the time of conception. These mutations are not inherited in other family members. A person who carries the new "spontaneous" mutation, however, may pass on the gene mutation to his or her children. Achondroplasia, Marfan syndrome, and neurofibromatosis type 1 are examples of genetic conditions that may occur in a single family member as a result of spontaneous mutation.

Acquired mutations take place in somatic cells and involve changes in DNA that occur after conception, during a person's lifetime. Acquired mutations develop as a result of cumulative changes in body cells other than reproductive cells (Fig. 9-5). Somatic gene mutations are passed on to the daughter cells derived from that particular cell line.

Gene mutations occur in the human body all the time. Cells have built-in mechanisms by which they can recognize mutations in DNA, and in most situations they correct the change before it is passed on by cell division. However, over time, body cells may lose their ability to repair damage from gene mutations, causing an accumulation of genetic changes that may ultimately result in diseases such as cancer and possibly other conditions of aging, such as Alzheimer's disease (Lashley, 1998).

Genetic Variation

Sorting out the genetic components of complex conditions (eg, heart disease, diabetes, common cancers, psychiatric disorders) that result from the interaction of environment, lifestyle, and the small effects of many genes is ongoing. New studies of genetic variation in humans are underway to develop a map of common DNA variants. Genetic variations occur among individuals of all populations. **Polymorphisms** and single nucleotide polymorphisms (SNPs, pronounced "snips") are the terms used for common genetic variations that occur most frequently throughout the human genome. Some SNPs may contribute directly to a trait or disease expression by altering function. SNPs are becoming increasingly important for the discovery of DNA sequence variations that affect biologic function. Such knowledge will allow clinicians to subclassify diseases and adapt therapies to the individual patient (Collins, 1999; Collins & McKusick, 2001). For example, a polymorphism or SNP can alter a protein or enzyme activity and can thus affect drug efficacy and safety when it occurs in proteins that are targets of medication regimens or that are involved in drug transport or drug metabolism (McCarthy & Hilfiker, 2000; Schafer & Hawkins, 1998).

INHERITANCE PATTERNS IN FAMILIES

Nursing assessment of patients' health includes obtaining and recording family history information. Family history evaluation in the form of a **pedigree** is a first step in establishing the pattern of inheritance. Nurses must become familiar with mendelian patterns of inheritance and pedigree construction and analysis to be able to help identify individuals and families who may benefit from further genetic counseling, testing and therapeutics (Lea, Jenkins & Francomano, 1998; Lea, 2000).

Mendelian conditions are genetic conditions that are inherited in families in fixed proportions among generations. Named after Gregor Mendel, mendelian conditions result from gene mutations present on one or both chromosomes of a pair. An individual gene inherited from one or both parents can cause a mendelian inherited condition. Mendelian conditions are classified according to their pattern of inheritance in families: autosomal dominant, autosomal recessive, and **X-linked**. The terms **dominant** and **recessive** refer to the trait, genetic condition, or phenotype, but not to the genes or alleles that cause the observable characteristics (Thompson et al., 2001).

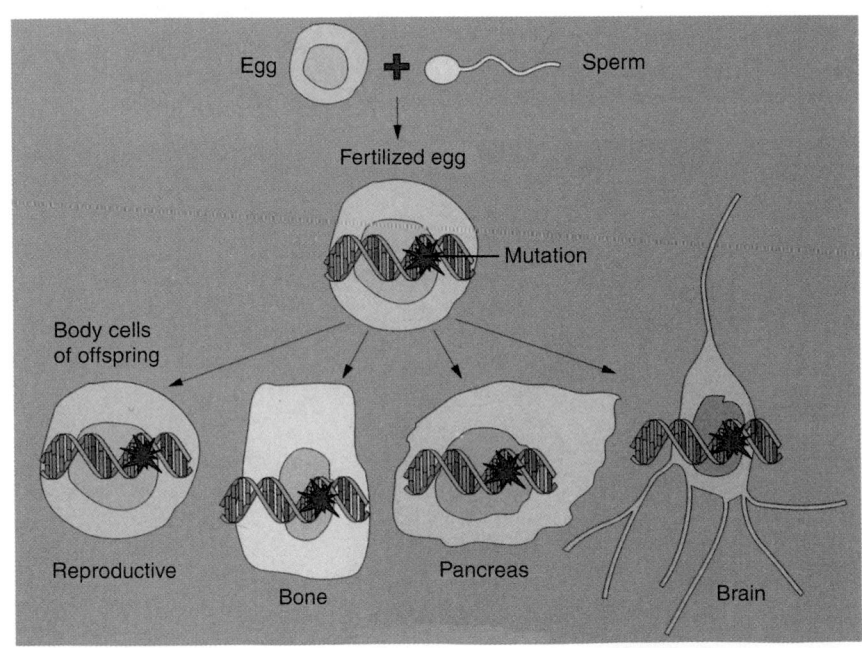

FIGURE 9-4 Hereditary mutations are carried in the DNA of the reproductive cells. When reproductive cells containing mutations combine to produce offspring, the mutation will be present in all of the offspring's body cells. From the National Institutes of Health and National Cancer Institute. (1995). *Understanding gene testing* (NIH Pub. No. 96-3905). Washington, DC: U.S. Department of Human Services.

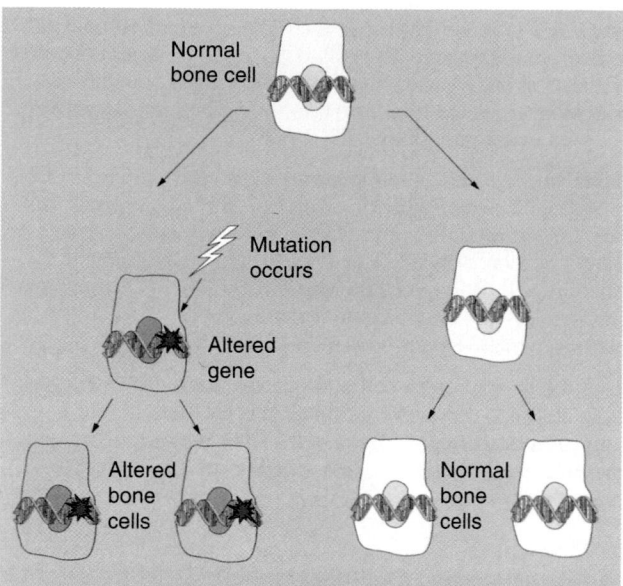

FIGURE 9-5 Acquired mutations develop in DNA during a person's lifetime. If the mutation arises in a body cell, copies of the mutation will exist only in the descendants of that particular cell. From the National Institutes of Health and National Cancer Institute. (1995). *Understanding gene testing* (NIH Pub. No. 96-3905). Washington, DC: U.S. Department of Human Services.

Autosomal Dominant Inheritance

Autosomal dominant inherited conditions affect female and male family members equally and follow a vertical pattern of inheritance in families (Fig. 9-6). An individual who has an autosomal dominant inherited condition carries a gene mutation for that condition on one chromosome of a pair. Each of that individual's offspring has a 50% chance of inheriting the gene mutation for the condition and a 50% chance of inheriting the normal version of the gene. Offspring who do not inherit the gene mutation for the dominant condition will not develop the condition and do not have an increased chance for having chil-

dren with the same condition (Fig. 9-7). Table 9-1 presents characteristics and examples of different patterns of inherited conditions.

Autosomal dominant inherited conditions often present with varying degrees of severity among affected family members and persons. Some individuals with the condition may have significant symptoms, while others may have only mild ones. This characteristic is referred to as **variable expression**; it results from the influences of genetic and environmental factors on clinical presentation.

Another phenomenon observed in autosomal dominant inheritance is **penetrance**, the percentage of persons known to have a particular gene mutation who actually show the trait. Penetrance is observed in conditions such as achondroplasia, in which nearly 100% of persons with the gene mutation typically display traits of the disease. In some conditions, the presence of a gene mutation does not invariably mean that a person will have or develop an autosomal inherited condition. For example, a woman who has the BRCA1 hereditary breast cancer gene mutation has a lifetime risk for breast cancer up to 80%, not 100%. This quality, known as incomplete penetrance, indicates the probability that a given gene will produce disease. In other words, a person may inherit the gene mutation that causes an autosomal dominant condition but may not have any of the observable physical or developmental features of that condition. However, these individuals carry the gene mutation and still have a 50% chance of passing the gene for the condition to each of their children. One of the effects of incomplete penetrance is that the gene appears to "skip" a generation, thus leading to errors in interpreting family history and in genetic counseling. Examples of other genetic conditions with incomplete pene-

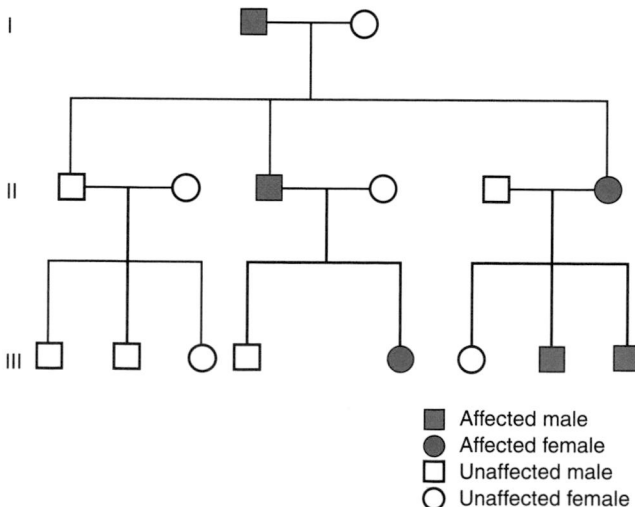

■	Affected male
●	Affected female
□	Unaffected male
○	Unaffected female

FIGURE 9-6 Three-generation pedigree illustrating autosomal dominant inheritance.

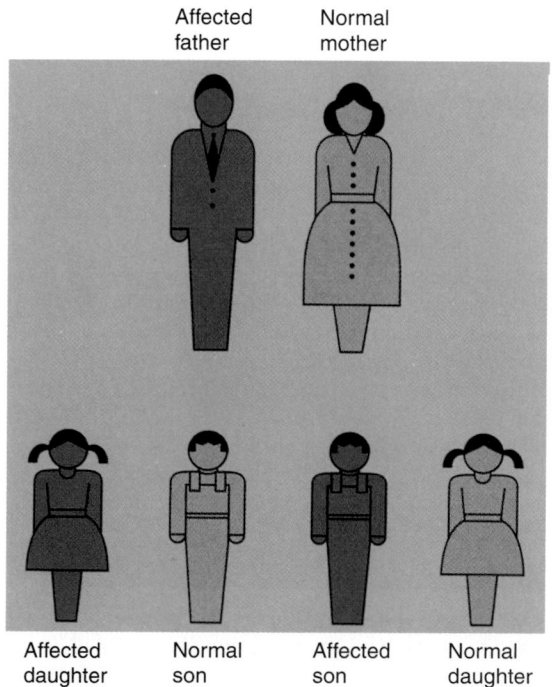

FIGURE 9-7 In dominant genetic disorders, if one affected parent has a disease-causing allele that dominates its normal counterpart, each child in the family has a 50% chance of inheriting the disease allele and the disorder. From the National Institutes of Health and National Cancer Institute. (1995). *Understanding gene testing* (NIH Pub. No. 96-3905). Washington, DC: U.S. Department of Human Services.

Table 9-1 • **Patterns of Mendelian Inheritance**

CHARACTERISTICS	EXAMPLES
Autosomal Dominant Inherited Conditions	
Vertical transmission in families	Hereditary breast/ovarian cancer syndrome
Males and females equally affected	Familial hypercholesterolemia
Variable expression among family members and others with condition	Hereditary non-polyposis colorectal cancer
Reduced penetrance (in some conditions)	Huntington disease
Advanced paternal age associated with sporadic cases	Marfan syndrome
	Neurofibromatosis
Autosomal Recessive Inherited Conditions	
Horizontal pattern of transmission seen in families	Cystic fibrosis
Males and females equally affected	Galactosemia
Associated with consanguinity (genetic relatedness)	Phenylketonuria
Associated with particular ethnic groups	Sickle cell anemia
	Tay-Sachs disease
	Canavan disease
X-Linked Recessive Inherited Conditions	
Vertical transmission in families	Duchenne muscular dystrophy
Males predominantly affected	Hemophilia A and B
	Wiscott-Aldrich syndrome
	Protan and Deutran forms of color blindness
Multifactorial Inherited Conditions	
Occur as a result of genetic and environmental factors combining	Congenital heart defects
May recur in families	Cleft lip and/or palate
Inheritance pattern does not demonstrate the characteristic pattern of inheritance seen with other mendelian inherited conditions	Neural tube defects (anencephaly and spina bifida)
	Diabetes mellitus
	Osteoarthritis
	High blood pressure

Adapted from Lea, D. H., Jenkins, J. F., & Francomano, C. A. (1998). *Genetics in clinical practice: New directions for nursing and health care.* Sudbury, MA: Jones & Bartlett; Lea, D. H. (2002). Genetics. In Maher, A. B., Salmond, S. W., & Pellino, T. A. (Eds.) *Orthopaedic nursing.* Philadelphia: W. B. Saunders.

trance include otosclerosis (40%) and retinoblastoma (80%) (Lashley, 1998).

Autosomal Recessive Inheritance

The pattern of inheritance in autosomal recessive inherited conditions differs from that of autosomal dominant inherited conditions in that it is more horizontal than vertical, with relatives of a single generation tending to have the condition (Fig. 9-8). Genetic conditions inherited in an autosomal recessive pattern are frequently seen among particular ethnic groups and tend to occur more often in children of parents who are related by blood, such as first cousins (see Table 9-1).

In autosomal recessive inheritance, each parent carries a gene mutation on one chromosome of the pair and the normal working copy of the gene on the other chromosome. The parents are said to be **carriers** of the particular gene mutation. Unlike an individual with an autosomal dominant inherited condition, a carrier of a gene mutation for a recessive inherited condition does not have symptoms of the genetic condition. When two carrier parents have children together, they have (with each of their pregnancies) a 25% chance of having a child who inherits the gene mutation from each parent and who will have the condition (Fig. 9-9).

X-Linked Inheritance

X-linked conditions may be inherited in families in recessive or dominant patterns (see Table 9-1). In both, the gene mutation is located on the X chromosome. All males inherit an X chromosome from their mother and a Y chromosome from their father

for a normal sex constitution of 46,XY. Since males have only one X chromosome, they do not have a counterpart for its genes as do females. This means that a gene mutation on their X chromosome is expressed when present in one copy. A female, on the other hand, inherits one X chromosome from each parent for a normal sex constitution of 46,XX. A female may be a carrier of

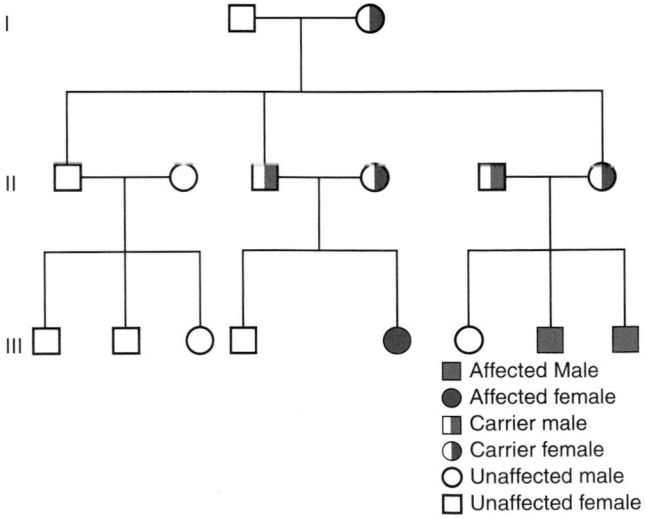

■	Affected Male
●	Affected female
◨	Carrier male
◑	Carrier female
○	Unaffected male
□	Unaffected female

FIGURE 9-8 Three-generation pedigree illustrating autosomal recessive inheritance.

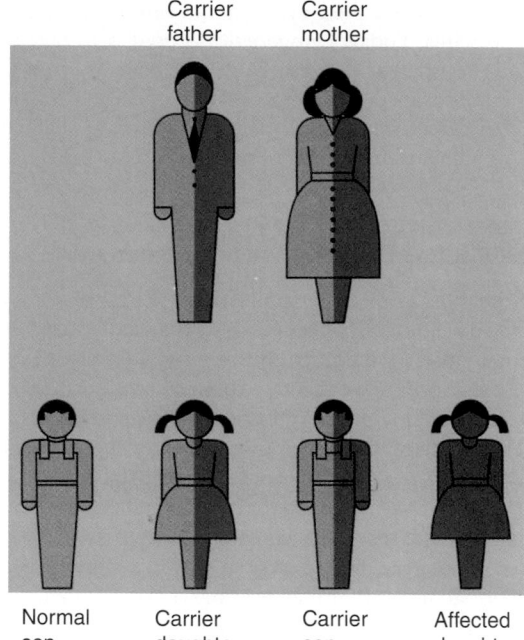

Carrier
father

Carrier
mother

Normal
son

Carrier
daughter

Carrier
son

Affected
daughter

FIGURE 9-9 In diseases associated with altered recessive genes, both parents—though disease-free themselves—carry one normal allele and one altered allele. Each child has one chance in four of inheriting two altered alleles and developing the disorder; one chance in four of inheriting two normal alleles; and two chances in four of inheriting one normal and one altered allele, and being a carrier like both parents. From the National Institutes of Health and National Cancer Institute. (1995). *Understanding gene testing* (NIH Pub. No. 96-3905). Washington, DC: U.S. Department of Human Services.

a gene mutation or affected if the condition results from a gene mutation causing a dominant X-linked condition. Either the X chromosome that a female receives from her mother or the X chromosome she receives from her father may be passed on to her sons, and this is a random occurrence.

The most common pattern of X-linked inheritance is that in which a female is a carrier for a gene mutation on one of her X chromosomes. This is referred to as X-linked recessive inheritance. In X-linked recessive inherited conditions, a female carrier has a 50% chance to pass on the gene mutation to a son, who would be affected, or to a daughter, who would be a carrier like her mother (Fig. 9-10).

Nontraditional Inheritance Patterns

Although mendelian inherited conditions present with a specific pattern of inheritance in some families, many diseases and traits do not follow these simple patterns. A variety of factors influence how a gene performs and is expressed. Different mutations in the same gene can produce variable symptoms in different individuals, as is the case with cystic fibrosis. Different mutations in several genes can lead to the identical outcome, as observed with Alzheimer's disease. Some traits involve the simultaneous mutation in two or more genes. A recently observed phenomenon, imprinting, can determine which pair of genes (the mother's or the father's) will be silenced or activated. This form of inheritance has been observed in Angelman syn-

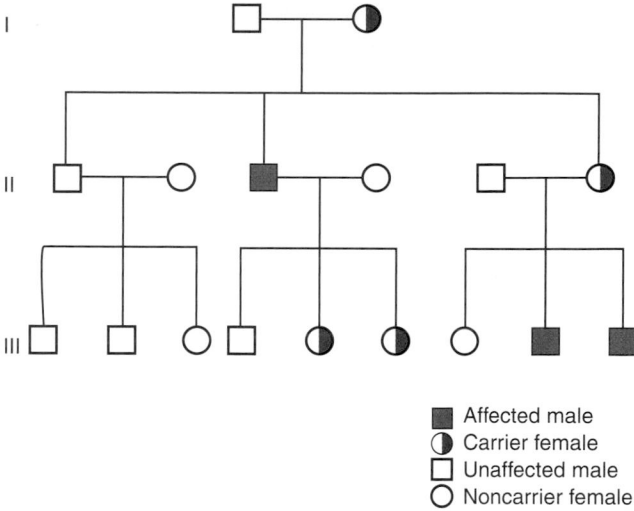

■ Affected male
◖ Carrier female
□ Unaffected male
○ Noncarrier female

FIGURE 9-10 Three-generation pedigree illustrating X-linked recessive inheritance.

drome, a severe form of mental retardation and ataxia (Thompson et al., 2001).

Multifactorial and Complex Genetic Conditions

Many birth defects and common health conditions such as heart disease, high blood pressure, cancer, osteoarthritis, and diabetes occur as a result of interactions of multiple gene mutations and environmental influences, and thus are called multifactorial or complex conditions (see Table 9-1). Multifactorial conditions may cluster in families but do not present with the characteristic pattern of inheritance seen in families having mendelian inherited conditions (Fig. 9-11). Neural tube defects, such as spina bifida and anencephaly, are examples of multifactorial genetic conditions (Chart 9-2).

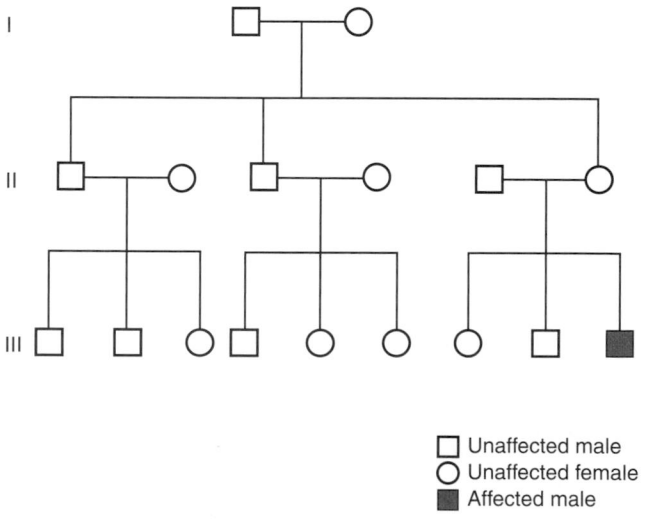

□ Unaffected male
○ Unaffected female
■ Affected male

FIGURE 9-11 Three-generation pedigree illustrating multifactorial conditions.

Chart 9-2 **Neural Tube Defects and Folic Acid**

Most neural tube defects are caused by both genetic and environmental influences that combine during early embryonic development, leading to incomplete closure of the neural tube. More rarely, chromosomal abnormalities such as trisomy 18 or prenatal exposure to certain medications such as valproic acid are the underlying cause of neural tube defects.

Research has shown that folic acid taken in the prescribed amount of 4.0 mg daily prior to conception and during the first 3 months of pregnancy reduces the recurrence of neural tube defects by 70% in women who have had a previously affected pregnancy. It is now recommended that *all* women in childbearing years take folic acid (0.4 mg) daily as part of a multivitamin to decrease the risk for neural tube defects (Centers for Disease Control and Prevention, 1992; Hall & Solehdin, 1998). Folic acid is recognized as an important environmental element that plays a critical role in fetal development and influences the outcome of genetic susceptibility to neural tube defects.

CHROMOSOMAL DIFFERENCES AND GENETIC CONDITIONS

Differences in the number or structure of chromosomes are a major cause of birth defects, mental retardation, and malignancies. Chromosomal differences are present in approximately 1 in every 160 live-born infants and are the cause of greater than 50% of all spontaneous first-trimester pregnancy losses (Lashley, 1998; Thompson et al., 2001). Chromosomal differences most commonly involve an extra or missing chromosome. This is called aneuploidy. Whenever there is an extra or missing chromosome, there is always associated mental or physical disability to some degree.

Down syndrome, or trisomy 21, is a common chromosomal condition that occurs with greater frequency in pregnancies of women who are 35 years or older. A person who has trisomy 21 Down syndrome has a complete extra number 21 chromosome, which causes a particular facial appearance and increased risk for congenital heart defects, thyroid and vision problems, and mental retardation. Other examples of chromosomal differences include trisomy 13 and 18, both more severe than Down syndrome, and conditions involving extra or missing sex chromosomes (eg, Turner syndrome, in which females have only one X chromosome instead of the usual two) (Lashley, 1998).

Chromosomal differences may also involve a structural rearrangement within or between chromosomes. These are less common than chromosomal conditions in which there is an extra or missing chromosome, but occur in 1 in every 500 newborns (Thompson et al., 2001). People who carry "balanced" chromosome rearrangements have all of their chromosomal material, but it is rearranged. A person who carries a balanced chromosomal rearrangement has an increased risk for spontaneous pregnancy loss and for having children with an unbalanced chromosomal arrangement that may result in physical or mental disabilities. Known carriers are therefore offered prenatal counseling and testing.

Chromosome studies may be needed at any age, depending upon the indication. Two common indications are for confirmation of a suspected diagnosis such as Down syndrome, and for a history of two or more unexplained pregnancy losses. Chromosome studies are accomplished by obtaining a tissue sample (eg, blood, skin, amniotic fluid), preparing and staining the chromosomes, and analyzing them under a microscope. The microscopic study of chromosomes is called cytogenetics and is an area that is rapidly evolving. Today, cytogenetics is used with new molecular techniques such as fluorescent in situ hybridization (FISH), which permits more detailed examination of chromosomes. FISH is useful to detect small abnormalities, including characterizing chromosomal rearrangements (Thompson et al., 2001).

Clinical Applications of Genetics

One of the most immediate applications of new genetics discoveries is the development of genetic tests that can be used to detect a trait, diagnose a genetic condition, and identify people who have a genetic predisposition to a disease such as cancer or heart disease. Another emerging application is pharmacogenetics. Pharmacogenetics involves the use of genetic testing to identify genetic variations that relate to the safety and efficacy of medications and gene-based treatments, so that individualized treatment and management plans can be developed. Future applications may include the use of gene chips to map a person's individual genome for genetic variations that may lead to disease. Nurses will be involved in caring for patients who are undergoing genetic testing and gene-based treatments. Knowledge of the clinical applications of modern genetics technologies will prepare nurses to inform and support patients, and to provide high-quality genetics-related health care.

GENETIC TESTING

Genetic tests provide information leading to the diagnosis of inherited conditions or other conditions with a known genetic contribution. Genetic testing involves the use of specific laboratory analyses of chromosomes, genes, or gene products (eg, enzymes, proteins) to learn whether a genetic alteration related to a specific disease or condition is present in an individual. Genetic testing can be DNA-based, chromosomal or biochemical.

There are several important uses for genetic testing, as identified by the Secretary's Advisory Committee on Genetic Testing (SACGT, 2000). Prenatal testing includes all three types of genetic testing (DNA-based, chromosomal and biochemical) and is widely used for prenatal screening and diagnosis of such conditions as Down syndrome. Carrier testing is used to determine carrier status, helping couples or individuals learn whether they carry a recessive allele for an inherited condition (eg, cystic fibrosis, sickle cell anemia, or Tay-Sachs disease) and thus risk passing it on to their children. Genetic testing is also used widely in newborn screening, and in the United States is made available for an increasing number of genetic conditions. Two examples are PKU and galactosemia. Diagnostic testing is used to detect the presence or absence of a particular genetic alteration or allele to identify or confirm a diagnosis of a disease or condition in an affected individual—for example, myotonic dystrophy and fragile X syndrome. In the near future, genetic tests will be increasingly used to identify a person's predisposition to disease and to design specific and individualized treatment and management plans. Examples of current uses of genetic tests are shown in Table 9-2.

Nurses will increasingly participate in genetic testing, especially in the areas of patient education, ensuring informed health choices and consent, advocating for privacy and confidentiality with regard to genetic test results, and assisting patients to understand the complex issues involved in genetic testing (Lea & Williams, 2002).

Table 9-2 • **Genetic Tests: Examples of Current Uses**	
PURPOSE OF GENETIC TEST	TYPE OF GENETIC TEST
Carrier Testing	
Cystic fibrosis	DNA analysis
Tay-Sachs disease	Hexosaminidase A activity testing and DNA analysis
Canavan disease	DNA analysis
Sickle cell anemia	Hemoglobin electrophoresis
Thalassemia	Complete blood count and hemoglobin electrophoresis
Prenatal Diagnosis—amniocentesis is often performed when there is a risk for a chromosomal or genetic disorder:	
Risk for Down syndrome	Chromosomal analysis
Risk for cystic fibrosis	DNA analysis
Risk for Tay-Sachs disease	Hexosaminidase A activity testing and/or DNA analysis
Risk for open neural tube defect	Protein analysis
Diagnosis	
Down syndrome	Chromosomal analysis
Fragile X syndrome	DNA analysis
Myotonic dystrophy	DNA analysis
Presymptomatic Testing	
Huntington disease	DNA analysis
Myotonic dystrophy	DNA analysis
Susceptibility Testing	
Hereditary breast/ovarian cancer	DNA analysis
Hereditary non-polyposis colorectal cancer	DNA analysis

GENETIC SCREENING

Genetic screening, in contrast to genetic testing, is a broader concept and applies to testing of populations or groups independent of a positive family history or symptom manifestation. Genetic screening, as defined in 1975 by the Committee for the Study of Inborn Errors of Metabolism of the National Academy of Sciences (SACGT, 2000), has several major aims. One is management; that is, identifying people with treatable genetic conditions that could prove dangerous to their health if left untreated. An example of this is screening of newborns. A second aim is to provide reproductive options to people with a high probability of having children with severe, untreatable diseases and for whom genetic counseling, prenatal diagnosis, and other reproductive options could be helpful and of interest. This is illustrated by the screening of individuals of Ashkenazi Jewish descent for conditions such Tay-Sachs disease and Canavan disease. A third aim is screening pregnant women to detect birth defects such as neural tube defects and Down syndrome using multiple marker screening. Genetic screening may also be used for public health purposes to determine the incidence and prevalence of a birth defect, or to investigate the feasibility and value of new genetic testing methods.

Most commonly genetic screening occurs in prenatal and newborn programs that involve nurses in various roles and settings. However, it is anticipated that genetic screening will expand in the future to include adult-onset conditions such as cancer, heart disease, diabetes, and hemochromatosis. Table 9-3 gives examples of genetic screening applications.

In the future, population-based (widespread) genetic screening will be applied to help identify people who are predisposed to develop conditions such as breast and colon cancer and heart disease. Nurses will be expected to participate in explaining genetics concepts such as risk and genetic predisposition, supporting informed health decisions and opportunities for prevention and early intervention, and protecting patients' privacy (Lea & Williams, 2002).

TESTING AND SCREENING FOR ADULT-ONSET CONDITIONS

Adult-onset conditions are disorders with a genetic component that are manifested in later life. Often symptoms or clinical manifestations occur only in late adolescence or adulthood, and disease is clearly observed to run in families. Some of these conditions are attributed to specific genetic mutations following either autosomal dominant inheritance or autosomal recessive inheritance. However, the majority of adult-onset conditions are considered to be multifactorial (polygenetic) in nature (eg, heart disease, diabetes, arthritis). Nursing assessment for adult-onset conditions is based on the family history and the identification of diseases or clinical manifestations associated with adult-onset conditions. Knowledge of adult-onset conditions and their genetic basis (ie, mendelian versus multifactorial conditions) influences the nursing considerations for genetic testing. Table 9-4 describes adult-onset conditions, their age of onset, pattern of inheritance, genes involved, and testing availability.

If a single gene accounts for an adult-onset condition in a symptomatic individual, diagnostic testing is used to confirm a diagnosis to assist in the plan of care and management. Diagnostic testing for adult-onset conditions is most frequently used with autosomal dominant conditions, such as Huntington disease or

Table 9-3 • **Applications for Genetic Screening**

TIMING OF SCREENING	PURPOSE	EXAMPLES
Preconception screening	For autosomal recessive inherited genetic conditions that occur with greater frequency among individuals of certain ethnic groups	Cystic fibrosis—all couples, but especially Northern European Caucasian, and Ashkenazi Jewish Tay-Sachs disease—Ashkenazi Jewish Sickle cell anemia—African American, Puerto Rican, Mediterranean, Middle Eastern Alpha-thalassemia—Southeast Asian, African American
Prenatal screening	For genetic conditions that are common and for which prenatal diagnosis is available when a pregnancy is identified at increased risk	Neural tube defects—spina bifida, anencephaly Down syndrome Other chromosomal abnormalities—trisomy 18
Newborn screening	For genetic conditions for which there is specific treatment	Phenylketonuria (PKU) Galactosemia Homocystinuria Biotinidase deficiency

Factor V Leiden thrombophilia, and autosomal recessive conditions, such as hemochromatosis. In families with known adult-onset conditions or with a confirmed genetic mutation in an affected family member, **presymptomatic testing** provides asymptomatic individuals with information about having a genetic mutation and about the likelihood of developing the disease. Huntington disease has served as the model for presymptomatic testing because the presence of the genetic mutation predicts disease onset and progression. Although preventive measures are not yet available for Huntington disease, the genetics information enables health care providers to develop a clinical, supportive, and psychological plan of care. Presymptomatic testing is considered for families with a known adult-onset condition in which either a positive or negative result will affect medical management or in which earlier treatment of a condition is more beneficial than treatment at a later stage. Presymptomatic testing is therefore offered for several adult-onset conditions, such as cancer, thrombophilia, and antitrypsin deficiency.

In the absence of a single disease-causing gene, it is thought that multiple genes are related to the onset of most adult diseases. These susceptibility genes modify or influence the development and severity of disease. Most susceptibility testing is conducted in the research setting to identify candidate genes for disease, such as Alzheimer's, psychiatric conditions, heart disease, hypertension, and hypercholesterolemia. For some diseases, the interaction of several genes and other environmental or metabolic events affect disease onset and progression. Susceptibility testing can help to distinguish variations within the same disease or response to treatment. For example, no single gene is associated with osteoporosis. Several polymorphisms on candidate genes related to the vitamin D receptor, estrogen and androgen receptors, cytokine production and its associated stimulation of osteoclasts, and collagen type 1-alpha 1 are under study to predict bone mineral density and fracture risk. Some susceptibility genes may predict treatment response. For example, individuals can present with similar clinical signs and symptoms of asthma but have different responses to treatment. Susceptibility testing can help classify the asthma as sensitive or resistant to treatment with corticosteroids.

Population screening, the use of genetic testing for large groups or whole populations, to identify late-onset conditions is under development. Currently population screening is offered in some ethnic groups to identify cancer-predisposing genes. For example, Ashkenazi Jewish individuals (Jews of Eastern European origin) have a greater chance of having inherited a specific genetic mutation in the BRCA1 or BRCA2 genes. Individuals with one of these BRCA mutations have approximately a 56% risk for breast cancer, 16% risk for ovarian cancer, and 16% risk for prostate cancer by age 70 (Struewing et al., 1997). Therefore, identifying one of these mutations allows the patient the options of cancer screening as well as other medical management such as chemoprevention or prophylactic mastectomy or oophorectomy in carriers. Population screening is being explored for other adult-onset conditions such as type 2 diabetes and hereditary hemochromatosis (iron overload disorder). For a test to be considered for population screening, there must be: (1) sufficient information about gene distribution within populations, (2) accurate prediction about the development and progression of disease, and (3) appropriate medical management for asymptomatic individuals with a mutation (U.S. Preventive Services Task Force, 1996).

Nursing Considerations for Adult-Onset Conditions

Nurses must be alert for family histories that indicate multiple generations (autosomal dominant inheritance) or multiple siblings (autosomal recessive inheritance) affected with the same condition, or onset of disease earlier than expected in the general population (eg, multiple generations with early-onset hyperlipidemia). Possible adult-onset conditions are discussed with other members of the health care team for appropriate resources and referral.

Information about diagnostic testing is often introduced as part of a diagnostic work-up. The nurse supports the patient in making decisions related to genetic testing and provides referrals for appropriate education and counseling about the adult-onset condition prior to genetic testing. The nurse addresses the patient's questions or concerns about the benefits and limitations of

Table 9-4 • Adult-Onset Disorders

CLINICAL DESCRIPTION	AGE OF ONSET	GENETIC INHERITANCE	TEST AVAILABILITY
Early-onset familial Alzheimer's disease			
Progressive dementia, memory failure, personality disturbance, loss of intellectual functioning associated with cerebral cortical atrophy, beta-amyloid plaque formation and intraneuronal neurofibrillary tangles	<60–65 years and often before 55	A.D.	Presymptomatic
Late-onset familial Alzheimer's disease			
Progressive dementia, cognitive decline	>60–65 years		Presymptomatic
Frontotemporal dementia with parkinsonism—linked to chromosome 17			
Dementia and/or parkinsonism. Slowly progressive behavioral changes, language disturbances and/or extrapyramidal signs and symptoms, rigidity, bradykinesia, and saccadic eye movements	40–60 years	A.D.	Research
Huntington disease			
Widespread degenerative brain change with progressive motor loss both voluntary and involuntary disability, cognitive decline, chorea (involuntary movements) at later stage, psychiatric disturbances	Mean age 35–44 years	A.D.	Diagnostic and presymptomatic
Neuromuscular disorders			
Spinocerebellar ataxia type 6			
Slowly progressive cerebellar ataxia, dysarthria, and nystagmus	Mean age 43–52 years	A.D.	Diagnostic and presymptomatic
Spinocerebellar ataxia type 1			
Ataxia, dysarthria, and bulbar dysfunction	Mean age 30–40 years	A.D.	Diagnostic and presymptomatic
Spinocerebellar ataxia type 2			
Slow saccadic eye movement, peripheral neuropathy, decreased deep tendon reflexes, dementia	Mean age 30–40 years	A.D.	Diagnostic and presymptomatic
Spinocerebellar ataxia type 3			
Progressive cerebellar ataxia and variety of other neurologic symptoms including dystonic-rigid syndrome, parkinsonian syndrome or combined dystonia and peripheral neuropathy	Mean age 30s	A.D.	Diagnostic and presymptomatic
Mild myotonic muscular dystrophy			
Cataracts and myotonia or muscle wasting and weakness, frontal balding, and ECG changes (heart block or arrhythmia), diabetes mellitus in 5% of all cases	20–70 years	A.D. with variable penetrance	Research
Amyotrophic lateral sclerosis (ALS)			
Progressive loss of motor function with predominantly lower motor neuron manifestations	50–70 years	Both A.D. and A.R.	Research
Hematologic conditions			
Hereditary hemochromatosis			
High absorption of iron by GI mucosa resulting in excessive iron storage in liver, skin, pancreas, heart, joints and testes. Abdominal pain, weakness, lethargy, weight loss are early symptoms. Untreated individuals can present with skin pigmentation, diabetes mellitus, hepatic fibrosis or cirrhosis, heart failure, dysrhythmias or arthritis.	40–60 in males; after menopause in females	A.R.	Diagnostic and presymptomatic
Factor V Leiden thrombophilia			
Poor anticoagulant response to activated protein C with increased risk for venous thromboembolism and risk for increased fetal loss during pregnancy	30s; during pregnancy in females	A.D.	Diagnostic and presymptomatic
Polycystic kidney disease dominant			
Most common genetic disease in humans. Manifests with renal cysts, liver cysts, and occasionally intracranial and aortic aneurysm and hypertension. Loss of glomerular filtration can lead to kidney failure.	Variable onset—all carriers have detectable disease by ultrasound at age 30	A.D.	Diagnostic and presymptomatic
Diabetes mellitus type II			
Insulin resistance and impaired glucose tolerance	Variable onset— most often >30	M.F.	Research

(continued)

Table 9-4 • **Adult-Onset Disorders** (Continued)

CLINICAL DESCRIPTION	AGE OF ONSET	GENETIC INHERITANCE	TEST AVAILABILITY
Cardiovascular disease			
Familial hypercholesterolemia. Elevated LDL levels leading to coronary artery disease, xanthomas and corneal arcus.	40–50 years	A.D.	Research
Hyperlipidemia			
Elevated low-density lipoproteins and triglycerides associated with premature coronary disease and peripheral vascular disease	30–40 years		Diagnostic and research
Alpha-1 antitrypsin deficiency			
60–70% small airway and alveolar wall destruction, emphysema especially at bases, COPD	35 yr/smoker 45 yr/nonsmk	M.F. in A.R. fashion	Diagnostic and presymptomatic
Oncology conditions			
Multiple endocrine neoplasia (MEN 2a) (Familial medullary thyroid cancer) Medullary thyroid cancer, pheochromocytoma and parathyroid abnormalities	Early adulthood	A.D.	Diagnostic and presymptomatic
Breast cancer BRCA1, BRCA2 hereditary breast/ovarian cancer Breast, ovarian, prostate and colon (BRCA1) Breast, ovarian and other cancer (BRCA2)	30–70 years often <50 years	A.D.	Predisposition Predisposition
Hereditary non-polyposis colorectal cancer Colorectal, endometrial, bladder, gastric, biliary and renal cell cancers as well as atypical endometrial hyperplasia and uterine leiomyosarcoma	<50 years	A.D.	Predisposition
Li-Fraumeni syndrome Soft tissue sarcoma, breast cancer, leukemia, osteosarcoma, melanoma, and other cancers, often including colon, pancreas, adrenal cortex and brain	Often <40 years	A.D.	Predisposition and research
Cowden syndrome Breast, non-medullary (papillary or follicular) thyroid cancer. Breast fibroadenomas and noncancerous thyroid nodules or goiter. Multiple buccal mucosa papillomas (cobblestone-line papules), facial trichilemmomas, gastrointestinal polyps. High arched palate, thickened furrowed tongue, megaloencephaly and pectus excavatum.	40–50 years for cancer Teens–20s for mucocutaneous lesions	A.D.	Predisposition and research

A.R. = autosomal recessive; A.D. = autosomal dominant; M.F. = multifactorial.
From Cummings, J. L., Vinters, H. V., Cole, G. M., & Khachaturiar, Z. S. (1998). Alzheimer's disease: Etiologies, pathophysiology, cognitive reserve and treatment opportunities. *Neurology, 51(Suppl)*, 2–17; Dik, M. G., Jonker, C., Comijs, H. C., Bouter, L. M., Twisk, J. W., van Kamp, G. J., & Deeg, D. J. (2001). Memory complaints and APOE-epsilon4 accelerate cognitive decline in cognitively normal elderly. *Neurology, 57*(12), 2217–2222; Durr, A., & Brice, A. (2000). Clinical and genetic aspects of spinocerebellar degeneration. *Current Opinions in Neurology, 13*(4), 407–413; GeneTests GeneClinics. (2001). Web site: http://www.genetest.org; Larkin, K., & Fardaei, M. (2001). Myotonic dystrophy—a multigene disorder. *Brain Research Bulletin 2001, 56*(3–4), 389–395; Lindor, N. M., Greene, M. H. and the Mayo Familial Cancer Program. (1998). The concise handbook of familial cancer syndromes. *Journal of the National Cancer Institute, 90*(14), 1039–1071; McIntyre, E. A., & Walker, M. (2002). Genetics of type 2 diabetes and insulin resistance: Knowledge from human studies. *Clinical Endocrinology, 57*(3), 303–311; Pizzuti, A., Friedman, D. L., & Coskey, C. T. (1993). The myotonic dystrophy gene. *Archives of Neurology, 50*(11), 1173–1179; Ridker, P. M., Miletich, J. P., Buring, J. E., Ariyo, A. A., Price, D. T., Manson, J. E., & Hill, J. A. (1998). Factor V Leiden mutation as a risk factor for recurrent pregnancy loss. *Annals of Internal Medicine, 128*(12), 1000–1003; Rogaeva, E. (2002). The solved and unsolved mysteries of the genetics of early-onset Alzheimer's disease. *Neuromolecular Medicine, 2*(1), 1–10; Rosso, S. M., & van Swieten, J. C. (2002). New developments in frontotemporal dementia and parkinsonism linked to chromosome 17. *Current Opinions in Neurology, 15*(4), 423–428.

genetic testing for the individual and the impact on the family. When testing is completed, the nurse provides support for individuals newly diagnosed with an adult-onset condition and provides teaching about the meaning and implications of the test results.

Once a mutation for an adult-onset condition is identified in a family, at-risk family members can be referred for **predisposition testing**. If the patient is found to be the mutation carrier, the nurse provides the patient with information about the risk to other family members. As part of that discussion, the nurse assures the patient that his or her test results are private and confidential and will be shared with others, including family members, only with the patient's permission. If the patient is an unaffected family member, the nurse discusses inheritance and the risk of developing the disease, provides support for the decision-making process, and offers referral for genetics services.

Nursing Care and Interventions in Genetic Counseling and Evaluation

The genetic counseling and evaluation process often involves additional genetic testing and procedures and subsequent decisions for patients and families with regard to reproduction, fertility, testing of children, and management options such as prophylactic surgery. Genetic counseling and evaluation services are traditionally offered at various stages: prenatal or perinatal, newborn or neonatal, childhood, adolescence, and adulthood. Nurses have responsibilities in each of these areas for assessment and providing psychosocial interventions and accurate information as the family members consider their genetic testing and treatment options. In all of these areas, the nurse considers the patient in the context of the family.

When individuals or family members are considering genetic testing, whether it is for prenatal, newborn, childhood or adult-onset conditions, the nurse provides accurate information as they consider their options. For prenatal testing, this would include information and support for subsequent decisions regarding the pregnancy in the event of a prenatal diagnosis of a genetic condition in the fetus. When a genetic diagnosis such as Down syndrome or hereditary breast or ovarian cancer is made, families need information about the range and severity of potential problems, the proportion of individuals with milder aspects of the condition, management options, support organizations, and current understanding of the long-term prognosis (Williams & Lea, 2003).

Decision-making support is an important nursing intervention in many genetic counseling situations. Examples include when a woman or couple considers the options regarding termination of a pregnancy or when individuals are considering presymptomatic testing for conditions such as Huntington disease or predisposition testing for hereditary cancers. The nurse helps the individual and family to acquire information about options, identifies the pros and cons of each option, helps the individual and family to explore their values and beliefs, respects each person's right to receive or not to receive information, and helps the individual to explain the decision to others (McCloskey & Bulechek, 2000).

Other essential components of nursing care and genetic counseling include teaching and an intervention called "coping enhancement." Teaching is needed, for example, when a new genetic diagnosis is made. The family will need information about the range of possible health outcomes in this condition, treatment options, and (in the case of prenatal diagnosis of a genetic condition) management options regarding continuing or ending the pregnancy. "Coping enhancement" involves "assisting a person to adapt to perceived stressors, changes or threats that interfere with meeting life demands and roles" (McCloskey & Bulechek, 2000, p. 234). Coping enhancement is essential throughout the entire genetic counseling, evaluation, and testing process. Indicators of patient knowledge, decision-making, and coping outcomes have been developed (Johnson, Maas, & Moorhead, 2000), and the nurse can use these indicators when documenting nursing care provided to families.

INDIVIDUALIZING GENETIC PROFILES

Information about genes and their variations is helping researchers to identify genetic differences that predispose some individuals or groups to disease and that affect their responses to treatment. The use of individualized genetics information to predict predisposition to common diseases will take considerable time to develop. However, genetic tests for non-disease genes (ie, polymorphisms in detoxifying enzymes, cell or drug receptor variations, or other inherited polymorphisms related to metabolism) are underway. These genetic tests for individual variations or inherited polymorphisms are called genetic profiles. One major effort of genetic profiling is focused on enzyme metabolism. Several polymorphisms related to enzyme metabolism have been identified in the cytochrome P450 family, long known to affect drug metabolism. There are three subcategories of genetic profiles that describe population differences in enzyme metabolism genotypes. These

are based on an individual's genetic make-up for the metabolism of medications or other exogenous compounds into inactive or active metabolites (Norton, 2001b).

The field of pharmacogenetics (the study of gene variations in drug response) is rapidly advancing the way nurses will administer and manage drug treatments. Drug metabolism involves enzyme activity, controlled by genes, for absorption, distribution, and excretion. A single base change, SNPs (single nucleotide polymorphisms), in genes activated for enzyme activity can cause either decreased or increased drug metabolism. Genetic testing for these SNPs will provide a genetic profile, classifying patients according to their drug metabolism type. The SNP classifications of drug metabolism are effective metabolizers (having the expected metabolism), poor metabolizers (lacking the ability to metabolize effectively), and ultra-rapid or rapid metabolizers (having extremely rapid metabolism of drug compounds). Poor metabolizers are most likely to have adverse events due to the prolonged bioavailability of the drug, while ultra-rapid metabolizers have insufficient drug response. Efficient metabolizers can receive the standard expected drug dosage, whereas poor metabolizers need lower doses and ultra-rapid metabolizers need higher doses to obtain a therapeutic effect (Roses, 2000). For example, poor metabolizers of antipsychotic agents are more likely to have oversedation and require dose modification to achieve an expected therapeutic response (Scordo & Spina, 2002).

DNA tests to identify patient-specific genetic profiles will be a treatment priority to assist in planning and evaluating treatment outcomes, to prevent adverse effects, and to improve therapies. Nurses therefore will need to know how polymorphisms affect a patient's susceptibility to disease and treatment response. Understanding the effect of polymorphisms on protein and enzyme function and their distribution in specific populations will be needed for health promotion. Since nurses will provide information about genetic profiles, they will need to know about the impact of genetics on treatment.

Applications of Genetics in Nursing Practice

Nursing practice in genetics-related health care blends the principles of human genetics with nursing care in collaboration with other professionals, including genetics specialists, to foster health improvement, maintenance, and restoration. In any practice setting, nurses will carry out five main activities in genetics-related nursing practice: help collect and interpret relevant family and medical histories; identify patients and families who need further genetic evaluation and counseling and refer them to appropriate genetics services; offer genetics information and resources to patients and families; collaborate with genetics specialists; and participate in the management and coordination of care of patients with genetic conditions. Genetics-related nursing practice includes the care of patients who have genetics conditions, persons who may be predisposed to develop or pass on genetic conditions, and persons who are seeking genetics information and referral for additional genetics services (Lea, Williams, Jenkins, et al., 2000).

Nurses support patients and families with genetics-related health concerns by ensuring that their health choices are informed ones and by advocating for the privacy and confidentiality of genetics information and for equal access to genetic testing and treatments. *The Scope and Standards of Genetics Clinical Nursing Practice,* developed by the International Society of Nurses in Genetics (ISONG, 1998) and published by the American Nurses Association, delineates roles and responsibilities for nurses in providing genetics health care.

GENETICS AND HEALTH ASSESSMENT

Assessment of a person's genetics-related health status is an ongoing process. The nurse collects information that can help identify individuals and families who have actual or potential genetics-related health concerns or who may benefit from further genetics information, counseling, testing, and treatment. This process can begin before conception and continue throughout the lifespan. Nurses evaluate family and past medical histories, including prenatal history, childhood illnesses, developmental history, adult-onset conditions (if adult), past surgeries, treatments, and medications; this information may relate to the genetic condition at hand or being considered. (See Chap. 5 for more information on assessing past medical history.) The nurse also identifies the patient's ethnic background and conducts a physical assessment to gather pertinent genetics information. The assessment also includes the patient's culture, spiritual beliefs, and ancestry. Genetics-related health assessment always includes determining a patient's or family's understanding of actual or potential health concerns related to genetics and understanding how these issues are communicated within a family (ISONG, 1998; Lea, Jenkins & Francomano, 1998).

Family History Assessment

Nurses in any practice setting continuously assess genetic family history to identify the presence of a genetic trait, inherited condition, or predisposition. A questionnaire (Chart 9-3) is often used to identify genetic conditions for which further information, education, testing, or treatment can be offered. In consultation and collaboration with other health care providers and specialists, the nurse can then determine whether further genetic testing and evaluation should be offered for the trait or condition in question. A detailed and accurate family history provides the most complete genetics health information. The family history should include at least three generations, as well as information about the current and past health status of all family members, including the age of onset of any illnesses and cause of death and age at death. The nurse also inquires about medical conditions known to have a heritable component and for which genetic testing may be offered. The nurse obtains information about the presence of birth defects, mental retardation, familial traits, or similarly affected family members (Lashley, 1998; Lea, Jenkins & Francomano, 1998).

The nurse also considers the presence of genetic relatedness (consanguinity) among family members when assessing the risk for genetic conditions in couples or families. For example, when obtaining a preconception or prenatal family history, the nurse asks whether the prospective parents have common ancestors (ie, they are first cousins). This is important to know because individuals who share ancestors have more genes in common than those who are unrelated, thus increasing their chance for having children with an autosomal recessive inherited condition such as cystic fibrosis. The number of shared genes depends upon the degree of relationship. A parent and child, for example, share half of their genes, while first cousins share one in eight of their genes. Ascertaining genetic relatedness gives the nurse the opportunity to offer additional genetic counseling and evaluation. It may also serve as an explanation for families who have a child or individual with a rare autosomal recessive inherited condition (Lea, Jenkins & Francomano, 1998).

When the assessment of family history reveals that the patient has been adopted, genetics-based health assessment becomes more challenging. The nurse and health care team should make all efforts to help the patient obtain as much information as possible about his or her biological parents, including their ethnic backgrounds.

Questions regarding reproductive history (eg, history of miscarriage or stillbirth) are included in genetic family history health assessments to identify possible chromosomal conditions. The nurse also inquires about any history of family members with inherited conditions or birth defects; maternal health conditions such as type 1 diabetes, seizure disorder, or maternal PKU, which may increase the risk for birth defects in children; and exposure to alcohol or other drugs during pregnancy. Maternal age is also noted: women who are 35 years or older who are considering pregnancy and childbearing or who are already pregnant should be offered prenatal diagnosis (eg, testing through amniocentesis) because of the association between advancing maternal age and chromosomal abnormalities such as Down syndrome (Lea, Jenkins & Francomano, 1998).

Ancestry and Ethnicity Assessment

Assessing ancestry and ethnicity helps identify individuals and groups who could benefit from genetic testing for carrier identification, prenatal diagnosis, and susceptibility testing. For example, carrier testing for sickle cell anemia is routinely offered to individuals of African-American heritage, while carrier testing for Tay-Sachs disease and Canavan disease is offered to individuals of Ashkenazi Jewish descent. Professional organizations such as the American College of Obstetrics and Gynecology (ACOG, 2001) recommend that relevant racial and ethnic populations be offered carrier testing. Recently, ACOG and the American College of Medical Genetics (ACMG) recommended that all couples, particularly those of Northern European and Ashkenazi Jewish ancestry, be offered carrier screening for cystic fibrosis (ACOG, 2001). Ideally, carrier testing is offered before conception to allow persons who are carriers to make reproductive decisions. Prenatal diagnosis is offered and discussed when both partners of a couple are found to be carriers.

Inquiring about a patient's ethnic background is also important when assessing for susceptibilities to adult-onset conditions such as hereditary breast or ovarian cancer. For example, a specific BRCA1 cancer-predisposing gene mutation seems to occur more frequently in women of Ashkenazi Jewish descent. Therefore, asking about ethnicity can help identify persons with an increased risk for certain cancer gene mutations (American Medical Association, 2001).

The nurse assesses ancestry and ethnic background to identify individuals who may have an underlying genetic condition that may affect the safety and efficacy of certain medications or treatments. For example, glucose-6-phosphate dehydrogenase deficiency (G6PD) is a common enzyme abnormality that affects millions of people throughout the world, especially those of Mediterranean, Southeast Asian, African, Middle Eastern, and Near Eastern origin. G6PD is transmitted as a gene mutation on the X chromosome. Individuals with a severe deficiency have chronic hemolytic anemia, while others with a milder deficiency develop hemolytic anemia upon exposure to peroxide-producing drugs, infection, exposure to naphthalene in mothballs, or ingestion of the fava (broad) bean (Lashley, 1998).

Assessment of ancestry and ethnic background is also important when considering drug metabolism. The ability to metabolize and eliminate certain medications depends upon acetylation in the liver by the enzyme N-acetyltransferase. Many different versions (polymorphisms) of the gene that codes for N-acetyltransferase

Chart 9-3 Primary Genetic Family History Screening Questionnaire

Question 1

If you, yourself, have, or if a family member in either your family or the family of your partner has, or ever has had, one of the following please circle the check mark under SELF or PARTNER and write in the exact relationship of that person to SELF or PARTNER, i.e., child (born or unborn), partner, sibling, grandparent, cousin, aunt or uncle, niece or nephew.

Condition	Self	Partner	Relationship
Birth defect name?_____	✓	✓	_____
Cancer name?_____	✓	✓	_____
High cholesterol	✓	✓	_____
Cleft lip/cleft palate	✓	✓	_____
Cystic fibrosis (CF)	✓	✓	_____
Down syndrome (DS)	✓	✓	_____
Fragile X syndrome	✓	✓	_____
Gastroschisis (opening in belly at birth)	✓	✓	_____
Hearing loss/deafness (not from aging)	✓	✓	_____
Heart problem (from birth)	✓	✓	_____
Heart disease (early onset)	✓	✓	_____
Hemophilia (slow clotting/heavy bleeding)	✓	✓	_____
Infant death (before one year of age)	✓	✓	_____
Inherited health problems	✓	✓	_____
Kidney problems (other than infection)	✓	✓	_____
Miscarriages	✓	✓	_____
Mental retardation	✓	✓	_____
Muscular weakness (muscular dystrophy)	✓	✓	_____
Pregnancy termination (due to birth defect) _____	✓	✓	_____
Sickle cell anemia	✓	✓	_____
Skin or nerve tumor	✓	✓	_____
Spina bifida (opening in spine, at birth)	✓	✓	_____
Stillbirths	✓	✓	_____
Stroke at an early age (called thrombosis)	✓	✓	_____
Thalassemia	✓	✓	_____
Visual loss/blindness (not from aging)	✓	✓	_____

Note: If you have checked any of these conditions, please talk with your nurse about a genetics referral for counseling and evaluation.

Do you have any other medical problems or issues that are of concern to you?

(Please circle one)   Yes   No

If you circled Yes, please tell your nurse, who may be able to help you or be able to find appropriate support/help for you.

Patient name _____

Date of birth _____

Name of person filling out the form (if different from patient) _____

Relationship to patient _____

Date form filled out _____

Nurse name _____

Date patient seen _____

Courtesy of the Foundation for Blood Research.

---

exist, and these polymorphisms vary among ethnic groups. This is an important consideration, for example, when isoniazid (INH) is prescribed for the treatment of tuberculosis. Patients who are rapid or ultra-rapid metabolizers have a significantly higher risk for developing isoniazid-induced hepatitis; this is especially true for persons of Chinese and Japanese descent (Lashley, 1998).

Physical Assessment

Physical assessment may provide clues that a particular genetic condition is present in an individual and family. Family history assessment may offer initial guidance regarding the particular area for physical assessment. For example, a family history of familial hypercholesterolemia would alert the nurse to assess family members for symptoms of hyperlipidemias (xanthomas, corneal arcus, abdominal pain of unexplained origin). As another example, a family history of neurofibromatosis type I, an inherited condition involving tumors of the central nervous system, would prompt the nurse to carry out a detailed assessment of closely related family members. Skin findings such as café-au-lait spots, axillary freckling, or tumors of the skin (neurofibromas) would warrant referral for further evaluation, including genetic evaluation and counseling (Lea, Jenkins & Francomano, 1998).

When a genetic condition is suspected as a result of a family history or physical assessment, the nurse, in collaboration with the health care team, may initiate further discussion and evaluation. Providing genetics information, offering and discussing genetic tests, and suggesting a referral to a geneticist may be performed (Chart 9-4).

Cultural, Social, and Spiritual Assessment

When collecting and discussing genetics information, the nurse needs to assess the patient's and family's cultural, social, and spiritual orientations. The nurse also needs to consider the patient's views about the significance of a genetic condition and its effect on self-concept, as well as the patient's perception of the role of genetics in health and illness, reproduction, and disability. Patients' social and cultural backgrounds determine their interpretations and values about information obtained from genetic testing and evaluation and thus influence their perceptions of health, illness, and risk. Family structure and decision-making and educational background contribute in the same way (Lea, Jenkins & Francomano, 1998).

Assessing a patient's beliefs, values, and expectations regarding genetic testing and information helps the nurse to provide ap-

propriate information about the specific genetics topic. In some cultures, for example, individuals believe that health means the absence of symptoms and that the cause of illness is supernatural. Patients with these beliefs may initially reject suggestions for presymptomatic or carrier testing. However, by including resources such as family, cultural, and religious community leaders when providing genetics-related health care, the nurse can help ensure that patients receive information in a way that transcends social, cultural, and economic barriers (Lea, Jenkins & Francomano, 1998).

Psychosocial Assessment

Psychosocial assessment is an essential nursing component of the genetics health assessment (Chart 9-5). After conducting an initial psychosocial assessment, the nurse will be aware of the potential impact of new genetic information on the patient and family and how they may cope with this information.

GENETIC COUNSELING AND EVALUATION SERVICES

As the contribution of genetics to the health–illness continuum is recognized, the process of genetic counseling is expected to become a responsibility of all health care professionals in clinical practice. Nurses are obvious and natural providers of genetics services because they are aware of a patient's personal and family history. They assess patients' health and make referrals for specialized diagnosis and treatment. They offer anticipatory guidance by explaining the purpose and goals of a referral. They collaborate with primary care providers and specialists in giving supportive and follow-up counseling. They coordinate follow-up and case management.

Genetics Services

Genetics services provide genetics information, education, and support to patients and families with genetics-related health concerns. Genetics professionals, including medical geneticists,

---

Chart 9-4   Indications for Making a Genetic Referral

Prepregnancy and Prenatal
- Maternal age of 35 years or greater at expected time of delivery
- Previous child with a chromosome problem
- Positive AFP profile screening test
- Previous child with a birth defect or family history of birth defects
- Pregnancy history of two or more unexplained miscarriages
- Maternal conditions such as diabetes, epilepsy, or alcoholism
- Exposures to certain medications or drugs during pregnancy
- Family history of mental retardation

Pediatric
- Positive newborn screening test
- One or more major birth defects
- Unusual (dysmorphic) facial features
- Developmental delay/mental retardation
- Suspicion of a metabolic disorder
- Unusually tall or short stature, or growth delays
- Known chromosomal abnormality

Adult
- Mental retardation without a known cause
- Unexplained infertility or multiple pregnancy losses
- A personal or family history of thrombotic events
- Adult-onset conditions such as hemochromatosis, hearing loss, visual impairment
- Family history of an adult-onset neurodegenerative disorder (eg, Huntington disease)
- Features of a genetic condition such as neurofibromatosis (café-au-lait spots, neurofibromas on the skin), Marfan syndrome (unusually tall stature, dilation of the aortic root), others

Cancer History
- A personal or family history of cancer with a known or suspected inherited predisposition (eg, early-onset breast cancer, colon cancer, ovarian cancer, retinoblastoma)
- Several family members affected by cancer
- A family member with cancer at an unusually young age
- A family member with an unusual type of cancer

Chart 9-5 • ASSESSMENT

Psychosocial Genetic Health Assessment

The nurse assesses:
- Educational level and understanding of the genetic condition or concern in the family.
- Desired goals and health outcomes in relation to genetic condition or concern.
- Family rules regarding disclosure of medical information (eg, some families may not reveal a history of diseases such as cancer or mental illness during the family history assessment).
- Family rules, boundaries, and cultural practices as well as personal preferences about knowing medical information.
- Past coping mechanisms and social support.
- Ability to make an informed decision (eg, is the patient under stress from family situations, acute or chronic illness, or medications that may impair the ability to make an informed decision).

genetics counselors, and advanced practice nurses in genetics, provide specific genetics services to patients and families who are referred by their primary health care providers. A team approach is often used by genetics specialists to obtain and interpret complex family history information, evaluate and diagnose genetic conditions, interpret and discuss complicated genetic test results, support patients throughout the evaluation process, and offer resources for additional professional and family support. Patients participate as team members and decision-makers throughout the process. Genetics services encompass an evaluation and communication process by which individuals and their families come to learn and understand relevant aspects of genetics, to make informed health decisions, and to receive support as they integrate personal and family genetics information into daily living (Lea, Jenkins & Francomano, 1998).

Genetic counseling may take place over an extended period and may entail more than one counseling session, which may include other family members. This allows patients and families to learn and understand genetics information, to receive support and guidance in decision-making, and to obtain comprehensive and coordinated care if they have specific genetic conditions or concerns. The components of genetic counseling are outlined in Chart 9-6. Genetic counseling may be offered at any point during the lifespan, although genetic counseling issues are often relevant to the life stage in which counseling is sought. Some examples are presented in Chart 9-7 (Lea, Jenkins & Francomano, 1998).

Nursing Role in Genetic Counseling

Patients seek genetic counseling for a variety of reasons and at different stages of life. Some are seeking preconception or prenatal information; others are referred following the birth of a child with a birth defect or suspected genetic condition; still others are seeking information for themselves or their families because of the presence or family history of a genetic condition. Regardless of the timing or setting, genetic counseling is offered to all patients who have questions about genetics and their health. In collaboration with the health care team, the nurse considers referring for genetic counseling any patient in whose family a heritable condi-

tion exists and who asks questions such as, "What are my chances for having this condition? Is there a genetic test that will tell me? Is there a genetic treatment or cure? What are my options?" (Lea, Jenkins & Francomano, 1998).

Nurses refer clients, collaborate with genetics specialists, and participate in genetic counseling when they carry out the following activities:

- Provide appropriate genetic information before, during, and in follow-up to genetic counseling
- Help gather relevant family and medical history information
- Offer support to patients and families throughout the genetic counseling process
- Coordinate genetics-related health care with relevant community and national support resources

These activities, carried out in collaboration with patients and families, help ensure that they receive the most benefit from genetic counseling (Lea, Jenkins & Francomano, 1998; Lea, Williams, Jenkins, et al., 2000).

RESPECTING PATIENTS' RIGHTS

Respecting the patient's right to self-determination—that is, supporting decisions that reflect the patient's personal beliefs, values, and interests—is a central principle of how nurses provide genetics information and counseling. Genetics specialists and nurses participating in genetic counseling make every attempt to respect the patient's ability to make autonomous decisions. A first step in providing such nondirective counseling is recognizing one's own values (see Chart 9-1) and how communication of genetics information may be influenced by those values.

Confidentiality of genetics information and respect for privacy are other essential principles underlying genetic counseling. The patient has the right to have testing without having the results divulged to anyone, including insurers or physicians. Some patients pay for testing themselves so that insurers will not learn of the test; others use a different name for testing to protect their privacy. The Health Insurance Portability and Accountability Act (HIPAA) of 1996 prohibits the use of genetics information to establish insurance eligibility. However, it does not prohibit group plans from increasing premiums, excluding coverage for a specific

---

 Chart 9-6 | **Components of Genetic Counseling**

Information and Assessment Sources
- Reason for referral
- Family history
- Medical history/records
- Relevant test results and other medical evaluations
- Social and emotional concerns
- Relevant cultural, educational, and financial factors

Analysis of Data
- Family history
- Physical examination as needed
- Additional laboratory testing and/or procedures (eg, echocardiogram, ophthalmology or neurologic examination)

Communication of Genetic Finding
- Natural history of disorder
- Pattern of inheritance

- Reproductive and family health issues and options
- Testing options
- Management and treatment issues

Counseling and Support
- Identify individual and family questions and concerns.
- Identify existing support systems.
- Provide emotional and social support.
- Refer for additional support and counseling as indicated.

Follow-Up
- Written summary to referring primary care providers and family
- Coordination of care with primary care providers and specialists
- Additional discussions of test results and/or diagnosis

Lea, D. H., Jenkins, J. F., & Francomano, C. A. (1998). *Genetics in clinical practice: New directions for nursing and health care.* Sudbury, MA: Jones & Barlett.

Chart 9-7   Genetic Counseling Across the Lifespan

Prenatal Issues
- Understanding prenatal screening and diagnosis testing
- Implications of reproductive choices
- Potential for anxiety and emotional distress
- Effects on partnership, family and parental–fetal bonding

Newborn Issues
- Understanding newborn screening results
- Potential for disrupted parent–newborn relationship upon diagnosis of a genetic condition
- Parental guilt
- Implications for siblings and other family members
- Coordination and continuity of care

Pediatric Issues
- Caring for children with complex medical needs
- Coordination of care
- Potential for impaired parent–child relationship
- Potential for social stigmatization

Adolescent Issues
- Potential for impaired self-image and decreased self-esteem
- Potential for altered perception of family
- Implications for lifestyle and family planning

Adult Issues
- Potential for ambiguous test results
- Identification of a genetic susceptibility or diagnosis without an existing cure ("therapeutic gap")
- Effect on marriage, reproduction, parenting, and lifestyle
- Potential impact on insurability and employability

Lea, D. H., Jenkins, J. F., & Francomano, C. A. (1998). *Genetics in clinical practice: New directions for nursing and health care.* Sudbury, MA: Jones & Barlett.

condition, or imposing a lifetime cap on benefits. The National Human Genome Research Institute, Policy and Public Affairs and Legislative Activities Branch has a summary of each state's legislation on employment and insurance discrimination (see the resources list at the end of this chapter).

All genetics specialists, including nurses who participate in the genetic counseling process and those with access to individuals' genetic information, must honor the patient's desire for confidentiality. Genetics information should be kept from family members, insurance companies, employers, and schools if the patient desires, even if keeping the information confidential is difficult. The nurse may want to disclose genetics information to family members who could experience significant harm if they do not know such information. However, the patient may have other views and may wish to keep this information from the family, resulting in an ethical dilemma for both patient and nurse. The nurse must honor the patient's wishes while explaining to the patient the potential benefit this information may have to other family members (ISONG, 2002).

PROVIDING PRECOUNSELING INFORMATION
Preparing the patient and family, promoting informed decision-making, and obtaining informed consent are essential in genetic counseling. The nurse assesses the patient's capacity and ability to give voluntary consent. This includes assessment of factors that may interfere with informed consent such as hearing and language deficits, impaired intelligence, and the effects of medica-

tion. The nurse makes sure that the individual's decision to undergo testing is not affected by coercion, persuasion, or manipulation. Because information may need to be repeated over time, the nurse offers follow-up discussion as needed (Bove et al., 1997).

The genetics service to which the nurse refers a patient or family for genetic counseling will ask the nurse to provide background information for evaluation. Genetics specialists need to know the reason for referral, the patient's or family's reason for seeking genetic counseling, and potential genetics-related health concerns. The nurse may refer a family with a new diagnosis of hereditary breast or ovarian cancer, for example, to obtain more information or counseling or to discuss the likelihood of developing the disease and the implications for other family members. The family may have concerns about confidentiality and privacy. Using the nursing assessment, the genetics specialists tailor the genetic counseling to respond to these concerns.

With the patient's permission, the nurse may also provide to the genetics specialists the relevant test results and medical evaluations. The nurse needs to obtain permission from the patient and, if applicable, from other family members to retrieve, review, and transfer medical records that document the genetic condition of concern. In some situations, evaluation of more than one family member may be necessary to establish a diagnosis of a genetic disorder. The nurse can prepare the family for this assessment by explaining that the medical information and evaluation are necessary to ensure that appropriate information and counseling (including risk interpretation) are provided.

The nurse will be asked to provide information about the emotional and social status of the patient and family. Genetics specialists will want to know the coping skills of a family that has recently learned of the diagnosis of a genetic disorder. They will want to be aware of the types of genetics information being sought. The nurse helps to identify cultural and other issues that may influence how information is provided and by whom. For patients with hearing loss, for example, an interpreter's services may have to be arranged. The genetics professional, after determining these issues with the nurse, prepares for the genetic counseling and evaluation with these relevant issues in mind (Lea, Jenkins & Francomano, 1998).

PREPARING THE PATIENT FOR GENETIC EVALUATION
Before the genetic counseling appointment, the nurse discusses with the patient and family the type and nature of family history information that will be collected during the consultation. Family history collection and analysis are comprehensive and focus on information that may be relevant to the specific genetic concern in question. Although targeted to each genetic counseling situation, such analysis always includes assessment for any other potentially inherited conditions for which testing and preventive and treatment measures may be offered.

A physical examination performed by the medical geneticist may be needed to identify specific clinical features that are diagnostic of a genetic condition. The examination also helps to identify whether additional laboratory tests are needed to clarify the diagnosis of a genetic disorder. The detailed physical examination generally involves assessment of all body systems, with a focus on specific physical characteristics considered for diagnosis. The nurse describes the diagnostic evaluations that are part of a genetics consultation and explains their purposes (Lashley, 1998; Lea, Jenkins & Francomano, 1998).

COMMUNICATING GENETICS INFORMATION TO THE PATIENT

After the family history and physical examination are completed, the genetics team reviews the information gathered before beginning genetic counseling with the patient and family. The genetics specialists meet with the patient and family to discuss their findings. When information from family and medical histories and examination confirms the presence of a genetic condition in a family, the genetics specialist discusses with the patient the natural history of the condition, the pattern of inheritance, and the implications of the genetic condition for reproductive and general health. When appropriate, the genetic specialists discuss and describe relevant testing and management options. The nurse assesses the patient's understanding of the genetic consultation and clarifies information given by the specialists.

PROVIDING SUPPORT

The genetics team provides support throughout the counseling session and makes every effort to elicit individual and family concerns. The genetics specialist uses principles of active listening to interpret patient concerns and emotions, seek and provide feedback, and demonstrate understanding of those concerns. When needed, the genetics specialist suggests referral for additional social and emotional support. The genetics specialist discusses pertinent patient and family concerns and needs with the nurse and primary health care team so that they can provide additional support and guidance (Lea, Jenkins & Francomano, 1998). The nurse assesses the patient's understanding of the information given during the counseling session, clarifies information, answers questions, assesses the patient's reactions, and identifies supports.

Providing Follow-Up After Genetic Evaluation

In follow-up to genetic evaluation and counseling, the genetics specialists prepare a written summary of the evaluation and counseling session and, with the patient's permission, send this summary to the primary health care provider as well as all other providers and participants in the patient's care, as identified by the family. The consultation summary outlines the results of family history and physical and laboratory assessments, provides a discussion of the specific diagnosis (when made), reviews the inheritance and associated risk of recurrence for the patient and family, presents reproductive and general health options, and makes recommendations for further testing and management. The summary is also sent to the patient and a copy is retained in the patient's medical records. The nurse has an important role in reviewing the summary with the patient and family and identifying information, education, and counseling for which follow-up genetic counseling may be useful (Lea, Jenkins & Francomano, 1998; Lea & Williams, 2002; Lea & Smith, 2002).

Follow-up genetic counseling is always offered to patients and families, as some may need more time to understand and discuss the specifics of a genetic test or diagnosis or wish to review reproductive options again later when pregnancy is being considered. Follow-up genetic counseling is also offered to clients when further evaluation and counseling of extended family members is recommended (Lea, Jenkins & Francomano, 1998).

As part of follow-up, nurses can educate patients about where to find information about genetics issues. Some resources that provide the most up-to-date and reliable genetics information are available on the Internet. Several of these are listed at the end of the chapter.

Ethical Issues

With recent advances in genetics, nurses must consider their responsibilities in handling genetics information and potential ethical implications such as informed decision-making, privacy and confidentiality of genetics information, and access to and justice in health care. The ethical principles of autonomy, fidelity, and veracity are also important (American Nurses Association, 2001).

Ethical questions relating to genetics occur in various settings and at all levels of nursing practice. At the level of direct patient care, nurses participate in providing genetics information, testing, and gene-based therapeutics. They provide patient care based on the values of self-determination and personal autonomy. The American Nurses Association (2001) states that patients should be as fully involved as possible in the planning and implementation of their own health care; to do so, patients need appropriate, accurate, and complete information given at such a level and in such a form that they and their families can make well-informed personal, medical, and reproductive health decisions. Nurses, as the most accessible health care professionals, are invaluable in the informed consent process. Nurses can help patients clarify values and goals, assess understanding of information, protect the patient's rights, and support their decisions. Nurses can advocate for patient autonomy in health decisions. ISONG's Position Statement "Informed Decision-Making and Consent" (2000) provides support and guidance for nurses who are helping patients who are considering genetic testing.

Nurses need to ensure the privacy and confidentiality of genetics information derived from such sources as the family history, genetic tests, and other genetics-based interventions. Many Americans are increasingly concerned about threats to their personal privacy. Nurses must be aware of the potential ethical issues related to the privacy and confidentiality of genetics information, including conflicts between an individual's privacy versus the family's need for genetics information. ISONG's Position Statement "Privacy and Confidentiality of Genetic Information" (2002) is a useful resource.

An ethical foundation provides nurses with a holistic framework for handling ethical issues with integrity. It also supplies the basis for communicating genetics information to a patient, to a family, to other care providers, to community agencies and organizations, and to society as a whole. In addition, it provides support for nurses facing clinical situations that involve ethical dilemmas. Principle-based ethics offers moral guidelines that nurses can use to justify their nursing practice. The emphasis is on ethical principles of beneficence (to do good) and non-maleficence (to do no harm), as well as autonomy, justice, fidelity, veracity, to help solve ethical dilemmas that may arise in clinical care. Respect for persons is the ethical principle underlying all nursing care. With an ethical foundation that is based on these principles and that incorporates the values of caring, nurses can promote the kind of thoughtful discussions that are useful when patients and families are facing genetics-related health and reproductive decisions and consequences (Scanlon & Fibison, 1995; ISONG, 2000).

Critical Thinking Exercises

1. Your patient, age 53, is recovering from a right mastectomy. She underwent a left mastectomy for breast cancer at age 45. Her daughter, age 31, expresses concern about her own breast cancer risk, telling you that her sister and maternal grandmother have also had breast cancer. What pattern of inheritance is suggested in this family? What genetics information would you provide to this woman?

2. A 48-year-old man is admitted to your medical unit with a new diagnosis of liver cancer. He says he is worried about his children, an 18-year-old boy and a 15-year-old girl: "I don't want them to get this, too." Your nursing assessment reveals a past history of arthritis and diabetes and a family history of "iron overload" in the patient's 40-year-old brother. What adult-onset condition does this history suggest? What nursing action would you take?

3. Your patient has three daughters, ages 25, 30, and 32, and one son, age 22. He also has four sisters, two of whom were diagnosed with breast cancer in their early 40s and chose to have BRCA gene mutation testing. Both were found to carry a BRCA1 gene mutation. The patient's daughters learn of these results and want to be tested to learn of their status. The patient does not want to be tested and tells the nurse at a routine check-up, "I don't want to have testing. I have a right not to be tested, and I don't want to know if I carry that cancer gene. I care about my daughters, but I am afraid to find out for them." How might you respond to the patient? What would you say if one of the patient's daughters calls you and asks for your help? What are the counseling issues for this daughter that are unique to this situation?

REFERENCES AND SELECTED READINGS

Books

American College of Obstetricians and Gynecologists (ACOG). (2001). *Preconception and prenatal carrier screening for cystic fibrosis: Clinical and laboratory guidelines.* Washington, DC: Author.

American Medical Association. (2001). *Identifying and managing hereditary risk for breast and ovarian cancer.* Chicago: Author.

American Nurses Association. (2001). *Code for nurses with interpretive statements.* Washington, DC: Author.

Gardiner, R. R. M., & Sutherland, G. R. (1996). *Chromosome abnormalities and genetic counseling* (2d ed.). New York: Oxford University Press.

Hartl, D., & Jones, E. W. (1998). *Genetics principles and analysis* (4th ed.). Sudbury, MA: Jones & Bartlett Publishing.

ISONG. (1998). *Statement on the scope and standards of genetics clinical nursing practice.* Washington, DC: American Nurses Association.

Iowa Intervention Project. (2000). *Nursing interventions classification* (3rd ed.). St Louis: Mosby.

Iowa Outcomes Project. (2000). *Nursing outcomes classification* (2d ed.) St. Louis: Mosby.

Johnson, M., Maas, M. L., & Moorhead, S. (Eds.) (2000). *Nursing interventions classification.* St. Louis: C.V. Mosby.

Lashley, F. R. (1998). *Clinical genetics in nursing practice* (2d ed.). New York: Springer.

Lea, D. H. (2002). Genetics. In Maher, A. B., Salmond, S. W., & Pellino, T. A. (Eds.) *Orthopaedic nursing.* Philadelphia: W. B. Saunders.

Lea, D. H., Jenkins, J. F., & Francomano, C. A. (1998). *Genetics in clinical practice: New directions for nursing and health care.* Sudbury, MA: Jones & Bartlett.

Lea, D. H., & Smith, R. S. (2002). *Genetics resource guide: A handy reference for public health nurses.* Scarborough, ME: Foundation for Blood Research.

McCloskey, J. C. & Bulechek, G. M. (Eds.). (2000). *Nursing interventions classification (NIC): Iowa Intervention Project* (3rd ed.). St. Louis: C. V. Mosby.

National Academy of Science, Committee for the Study of Inborn Errors of Metabolism. (1975). *Genetic Screening.* Washington, DC: National Academy of Sciences.

National Institutes of Health, National Cancer Institute. (1995). *Understanding gene testing.* Washington, DC: U.S. Department of Health and Human Services, NIH Pub. No. 9603905.

Rimoin, D., Connor, J. M., & Pyeritz, R. (2002). *Emery-Rimoin principles and practice of medical genetics* (4th ed.). New York: Churchill-Livingstone.

Scanlon, C., & Fibison, W. (1995). *Managing genetic information: Implications for nursing practice.* Washington, DC: American Nurses Association.

Secretary's Advisory Committee on Genetic Testing (SACGT). (2000). National Institutes of Health. A public consultation of oversight of genetic tests. Bethesda, MD. Available from http://www4.od.nih.gov/oba/sacgt.htm.

Thompson, M. W., McInnes, R. R., & Willard, H. F. (2001). *Thompson and Thompson's genetics in medicine* (6th ed.). Philadelphia: W. B. Saunders.

U.S. Preventive Services Task Force. (1996). *Guide to clinical preventive services* (2d ed.). Baltimore: Williams & Wilkins.

Williams, J. K., & Lea, D. H. (2003). *Genetic issues for perinatal nurses* (2d ed.). White Plains, NY: March of Dimes.

Journals

ACOG Committee on Genetics. (1996). Screening for Tay-Sachs disease. *International Journal of Gynaecology & Obstetrics, 52*(3), 311–312.

ACOG Committee on Genetics. (1999). Screening for Canavan disease. *International Journal of Gynaecology & Obstetrics, 65*(1), 91–92.

ACOG Committee on Genetics. (2001). Genetic screening for hemoglobinopathies. *International Journal of Gynaecology & Obstetrics, 74*(3), 309–310.

American College of Medical Genetics/American Society of Human Genetics Huntington Disease Genetic Testing Working Group. (1998). ACMG/ASHG statement. Laboratory guidelines for Huntington disease genetic testing. *American Journal of Human Genetics, 62*(5), 1243–1247.

American Society of Clinical Oncology. (1996). Statement of the American Society of Clinical Oncology: Genetic testing for cancer susceptibility. *Journal of Clinical Oncology, 14*(5), 1730–1736.

Anderson, G., Monsen, R. B., Prows, C. A., Tinley, S., & Jenkins, J. (2000). Preparing the nursing profession for participation in a genetic paradigm in health care. *Nursing Outlook, 48*(1), 23–27.

Bartsch, H., Nair, U., Risch, A., et al. (2000). Genetic polymorphism of CYP genes, alone or in combination, as a risk modifier of tobacco-related cancers. *Cancer Epidemiology, Biomarkers and Prevention, 9*(1), 3–28.

Billings, P. R. (2000). Applying advances in genetic medicine: Where do we go from here? *Healthplan, 41*(6), 32–35.

Bove, C. M., Fry, S. T., & MacDonald, D. J. (1997). Presymptomatic and predisposition genetic testing: Ethical and social considerations. *Seminars in Oncology Nursing, 13*(2), 135–140.

Brookes, A. J. (1999). The essence of SNPs. *Gene, 234*(2), 177–186.

Burke, W. (2002). Genetic testing. *New England Journal of Medicine, 347*(23), 1867–1875.

Burke, W., Thomson, E., Khoury, M. J., et al. (1998). Hereditary hemochromatosis: gene discovery and its implications for population-based screening. *Journal of American Medical Association, 280*(2), 172–178.

Centers for Disease Control and Prevention. (1992). Recommendations for the use of folic acid to reduce the number of cases of spina bifida and other neural tube defects. *Morbidity and Mortality Weekly Report, 41*(RR-14), 1–7.

Collins, F. S. (1999). Medical and societal consequences of the Human Genome Project. *New England Journal of Medicine, 341*(1), 28–37.

Collins, F. S., & McKusick, V. A. (2001). Implications of the Human Genome Project for medical science. *Journal of American Medical Association, 285*(5), 540–544.

Cox, N. J., Frigge, M., Nicolae, D. L., et al. (1999). Loci on chromosomes 2 (NIDDM1) and 15 interact to increase susceptibility to diabetes in Mexican Americans. *Nature Genetics, 21*(2), 213–215.

Evans, W. E. & McLeod. (2003). Drug therapy: Pharmacogenomics—Drug disposition, drug targets, and side effects. *New England Journal of Medicine, 348*(6), 538–549.

Evans, W. E., & Relling, M. V. (1999). Pharmacogenomics: Translating functional genomics into rational therapeutics. *Science, 286*(5439), 487–491

Feetham, S. (1999). Families and the genetic revolution. Implications for primary healthcare, education, and research. *Families, Systems & Health, 17*(1), 27–43.

FitzGerald, M. G., MacDonald, D. J., Krainer, M., et al. (1996). Germline BRCA1 mutations in Jewish and non-Jewish women with early-onset breast cancer. *New England Journal of Medicine, 334*(3), 143–149.

Fleisher, L. K., & Cole, J. (2001). Health insurance portability and accountability act is here: What price privacy? *Genetics in Medicine, 3*(4), 286–289.

Ghosh, S., Watanabe, R. M., Valle, T. T., et al. (2000). The Finland-United States Investigation of Non-insulin-dependent Diabetes Mellitus Genetics (FUSION) Study. I. An autosomal genome scan for genes that predispose to type 2 diabetes. *American Journal of Human Genetics, 67*(5), 1174–1185.

Guttmacher, A. E. & Collins, F. S. (2002). Genomic medicine—a primer. *New England Journal of Medicine, 347*(19), 1512–1520.

Hall, J., & Solehdin, M. (1998). Folic acid for the prevention of congenital anomalies. *European Journal of Pediatrics, 157*, 445–450.

Hanis, C. L., Boerwinkle, E., Chakraborty, R., et al. (1996). A genome-wide search for human non-insulin-dependent (type 2) diabetes genes reveals a major susceptibility locus on chromosome 2. *Nature Genetics, 13*(2), 161–166.

ISONG. (2002). Position statement. Privacy and confidentiality of genetic information: The role of the nurse. *MedSurg Nursing, 11*(2), 103. Position statement available on-line: http://www.globalreferrals.com/privacy.htm.

ISONG. (2000). Position statement. Informed decision-making and consent: The role of nursing. *International Society of Nurses in Genetics Newsletter, 11*(3), 7–8. Position statement available on-line: http://www.globalreferrals.com/consent.htm.

ISONG. (2002). Position statement. Genetic counseling for vulnerable populations: The role of nursing. *MedSurg Nursing, 11*(6), 305.

Khoury, M. J., McCabe, L. L., & McCabe, E. R. B. (2003). Population screening in the age of genomic medicine. *New England Journal of Medicine, 348*(1), 50–58.

Lea, D. H., Anderson, G., & Monsen, R. B. (1998). A multiplicity of roles for genetic nursing: Building toward holistic practice. *Holistic Nursing Practice, 12*(3), 77–87.

Lea, D. H. & Williams, J. K. (2002). Genetic testing and screening. *American Journal of Nursing, 102*(7), 36–50.

Lea, D. H., Williams, J. K., Jenkins, J., Jones, S., & Calzone, K. (2000). Genetic health care: Creating interdisciplinary partnerships with nursing in clinical practice. *National Academies of Practice Forum, 2*(3), 177–186.

Lea, D. H. (2000). A clinician's primer in human genetics: What nurses need to know. *Nursing Clinics of North America, 35*(3), 583–614.

McCarthy, J. J., & Hilfiker, R. (2000). The use of single-nucleotide polymorphism maps in pharmacogenomics. *Nature Biotechnology, 18*(5), 505–508.

McKinnon, W. C., Baty, B. J., Bennett, R. L., et al. (1997). Predisposition genetic testing for late-onset disorders in adults. A position paper of the National Society of Genetic Counselors. *Journal of the American Medical Association, 278*(15), 1217–1220.

Nebert, D. W., & Dieter, M. Z. (2000). The evolution of drug metabolism. *Pharmacology, 61*(3), 124–135.

Norton, R. M. (2001*a*). Clinical pharmacogenomics: applications in pharmaceutical R&D. *Drug Discovery Today, 6*(4), 180–185.

Norton, R. M. (2001*b*). Pharmacogenomics: Pharmacogenomics and individualized drug therapy. *Medscape Pharmacotherapy* (http://www.medscape.com).

Peters, J. L., Djurdjinovic, L., & Baker, D. (1999). The genetic self: The Human Genome Project, genetic counseling and family therapy. *Families, Systems & Health, 17*(1), 5–25.

Regaldo, A. (1999). Inventing the pharmacogenomics business. *American Journal of Health Systems Pharmacology, 56*(1), 40–50.

Roses, A. (2000). Pharmacogenetics and future drug development and delivery. *Lancet, 355*(9212), 1358–1361.

Sachidanandam, R., Weissman, D., Schmidt, S. C., et al. (2001). A map of human genome sequence variation containing 1.42 million single nucleotide polymorphisms. *Nature, 409*(6822), 928–933.

Schafer, A. J., & Hawkins, J. R. (1998). DNA variation and the future of human genetics. *Nature Biotechnology, 16*, 33–39.

Scordo, M. G., & Spina, E. (2002). Cytochrome P450 polymorphisms and response to antipsychotic therapy. *Pharmacogenomics, 3*(2), 201–218.

Struewing, J. P., Abeliovich, D., Peretz, T., et al. (1996). The carrier frequency of the BRCA1 185delAG mutation is approximately 1 percent in Ashkenazi Jewish individuals. *Nature Genetics, 12*(1), 198–200.

Struewing, J. P., Hartge, P., Wacholder, S., et al. (1997). The risk of cancer associated with specific mutations of BRCA1 and BRCA2 among Ashkenazi Jews. *New England Journal of Medicine, 336*(20), 1401–1408.

Weinshilboum, R. (2003). Genomic medicine: Inheritance and drug response. *New England Journal of Medicine, 348*(6), 529–537.

RESOURCES AND WEBSITES

Association of Women's Health, Obstetric and Neonatal Nurses, 2000 L. Street, NW, Suite 740, Washington, DC 20036; (202) 261-2400 or (800) 673-8499; fax (202) 728-0575; http://www.awhonn.org/resour/POSITION.

Genetic Alliance, Inc., 4301 Connecticut Ave. NW, Suite 404, Washington, DC 20008-2304; (202) 966-5557; e-mail: info@geneticalliance.org; http://www.geneticalliance.org.

Gene Clinics, University of Washington School of Medicine, 9725 Third Avenue NE, Suite 610, Seattle, WA 98115; (206) 221-4674; fax (206) 221-4679; e-mail: geneclinics@geneclinics.org; http://www.geneclinics.org.

Gene Tests, Children's Hospital and Regional Medical Center, P.O. Box 5371, Seattle, WA 98105-0371; (206) 527-5742; fax (206) 527-5743; e-mail: genetests@genetests.org.

International Society of Nurses in Genetics, Inc. (ISONG), Executive Director Eileen Rawnsley, 7 Haskins Road, Hanover, NH 03755; (603) 643-5706; fax (603) 643-3169; e-mail: Eileen.Rawnsley@valleynet; http://www.nursing.creighton.edu/isong/.

National Coalition for Health Professional Education in Genetics (NCHPEG); 2630 W. Joppa Rd., Suite 320, Lutherville, MD 21093; (410) 583-0600; http://www.nchpeg.org.

National Organization for Rare Disorders, Inc. (NORD), P.O. Box 8923, New Fairfield, CT 06812-8923; (203) 746-6518; fax (203) 746-6481; e-mail: orphan@rarediseases.org.

National Cancer Institute (NCI), Public Inquiries Office, Building, 31, Room 10A03, 31 Center Drive, MSC 2580, Bethesda, MD 20892-2580; (301) 435-3848; http://www.nci.nih.gov.

Online Mendelian Inheritance in Man (OMIM), National Center for Biotechnology Information, National Library of Medicine, Building 38A, Room 8N805, Bethesda, MD 20894; (301) 496-2475; fax (301) 480-9241; http://www.ncbi.nlm.nih.gov/Omim.

Chronic Illness

On completion of this chapter, the learner will be able to:

1. Define "chronic conditions."
2. Identify factors related to the increasing incidence of chronic conditions.
3. Describe characteristics of chronic conditions and implications for people with chronic conditions and for their families.
4. Describe the phases of chronic conditions.
5. Apply the nursing process to the care of the patient with chronic conditions.

Chronic health problems affect people of all ages—they occur in the very young, the middle-aged, and the very old. Chronic conditions do, however, increase in frequency with age, and elderly people often have multiple chronic disorders (Van den Akker, Buntinx, Metsemakers, Roos & Knottnerus, 1998). Chronic illnesses are found in all socioeconomic, ethnic, cultural, and racial groups; certain diseases, however, occur more frequently in some groups than in others (Kington & Smith, 1997). Native Americans between the ages of 45 to 64, for example, have a higher mortality rate from diabetes and cirrhosis than Caucasians in the same age range (Reeves, Remington, Nashold & Pete, 1997). Being poor and lacking adequate health care coverage decreases the likelihood of receiving preventive screening measures such as mammography, cholesterol testing, and routine check-ups (Hagdrup, Simoes & Brownson, 1997). Although some chronic conditions have little effect on quality of life, others have a considerable effect because of related disability (Kempen, Ormel, Brilman & Relyveld, 1997). Certain conditions require advanced technology for survival, as in the late stages of amyotrophic lateral sclerosis or end-stage renal disease. Some people with chronic health conditions and disability function independently with only minor inconvenience to their everyday lives; others require frequent and close monitoring or placement in long-term care facilities.

The Phenomenon of Chronicity

Although each chronic condition has its own specific physiologic characteristics, chronic conditions do share common qualities. Many chronic conditions, for example, have pain and fatigue as associated symptoms. Some degree of disability is usually present in severe or advanced chronic illness, limiting the patient's participation in activities (Collins, 1997). Many chronic conditions require therapeutic regimens to keep them under control. Unlike the term "acute," which implies a curable and relatively short disease course, *chronic* describes a long disease course and conditions that may be incurable. It is this characteristic of duration that often makes managing chronic conditions so difficult for those who must live with them.

Psychological and emotional reactions of patients to acute and chronic conditions and changes in their health status are described in detail in Chapter 7. People who develop chronic conditions may react with shock, disbelief, depression, anger, resentment, or a number of other emotions. How people react and cope with chronic conditions is usually similar to how they react to other events in their lives, depending, in part, on their understanding of the condition and their perceptions of its potential impact on their own and their family's lives. Adjustment to chronic illness is affected by various factors:

- Personality before the illness
- Unresolved anger or grief from the past
- Suddenness, extent, and duration of lifestyle changes necessitated by the illness
- Family and individual resources for dealing with stress
- Stages of individual/family life cycle
- Previous experience with illness and crises
- Codependency in family systems (Lewis, 1998)

Psychological, emotional, and cognitive reactions to chronic conditions are likely to occur at the initial onset, but they may also recur if symptoms worsen or recur after a period of remission. Symptoms associated with chronic illnesses are often unpredictable, and some are perceived as crisis events by patients and their families, who must contend with both the uncertainty of chronic illness and the changes it brings to their lives. This chapter describes some of the problems of living with chronic conditions and offers a guide to nursing assessment and intervention when providing care to people with chronic illness.

DEFINITION OF CHRONIC CONDITIONS

"Chronic conditions" are defined as medical conditions or health problems with associated symptoms or disabilities that require long-term (3 months or longer) management (Robert Wood Johnson Foundation, 1996). The condition may be due to illness, genetic factors, or injury. Management of such conditions includes learning to live with symptoms and/or disabilities and coming to terms with identity changes brought about by having a chronic condition. It also consists of carrying out the lifestyle changes and regimens that are designed to keep symptoms under control and to prevent complications. Although some people take on what might be called a "sick role" identity, most people with chronic conditions do not consider themselves to be sick or ill and try to live as normal a life as is possible. Only when complications develop or when symptoms become severe enough to interfere with performance of daily life activities do most people who are chronically ill think of themselves as being sick or disabled (Nijhof, 1998).

PREVALENCE AND CAUSES OF CHRONIC CONDITIONS

Chronic conditions occur in people of every age group, socioeconomic level, and culture. In 1995, an estimated 99 million people in the United States had chronic conditions, and it has been projected that by the year 2030 about 150 million people will be affected (Robert Wood Johnson Foundation, 1996). Table 10-1 shows the projected increase in rates of people with chronic conditions by year, along with an estimate of the costs to be incurred in managing those conditions.

Not every chronic condition is disabling; some cause only minor inconveniences. Many, however, are severe enough to cause major activity limitations. Figures 10-1 and 10-2 present overviews of the projected number of people in millions with ac-

---

Table 10-1 • **Estimated Number of People and Direct Medical Costs for People With Chronic Conditions, Selected Years, 1995–2050**

	1995	2000	2005	2010	2020	2030	2040	2050
People	99 million	105 million	112 million	120 million	134 million	148 million	158 million	167 million
Dollar costs	$470 billion	$503 billion	$539 billion	$582 billion	$685 billion	$798 billion	$864 billion	$906 billion

With permission from Robert Wood Johnson Foundation. (1996). *Chronic care in America: A 21st century challenge.* Princeton, NJ: Author.

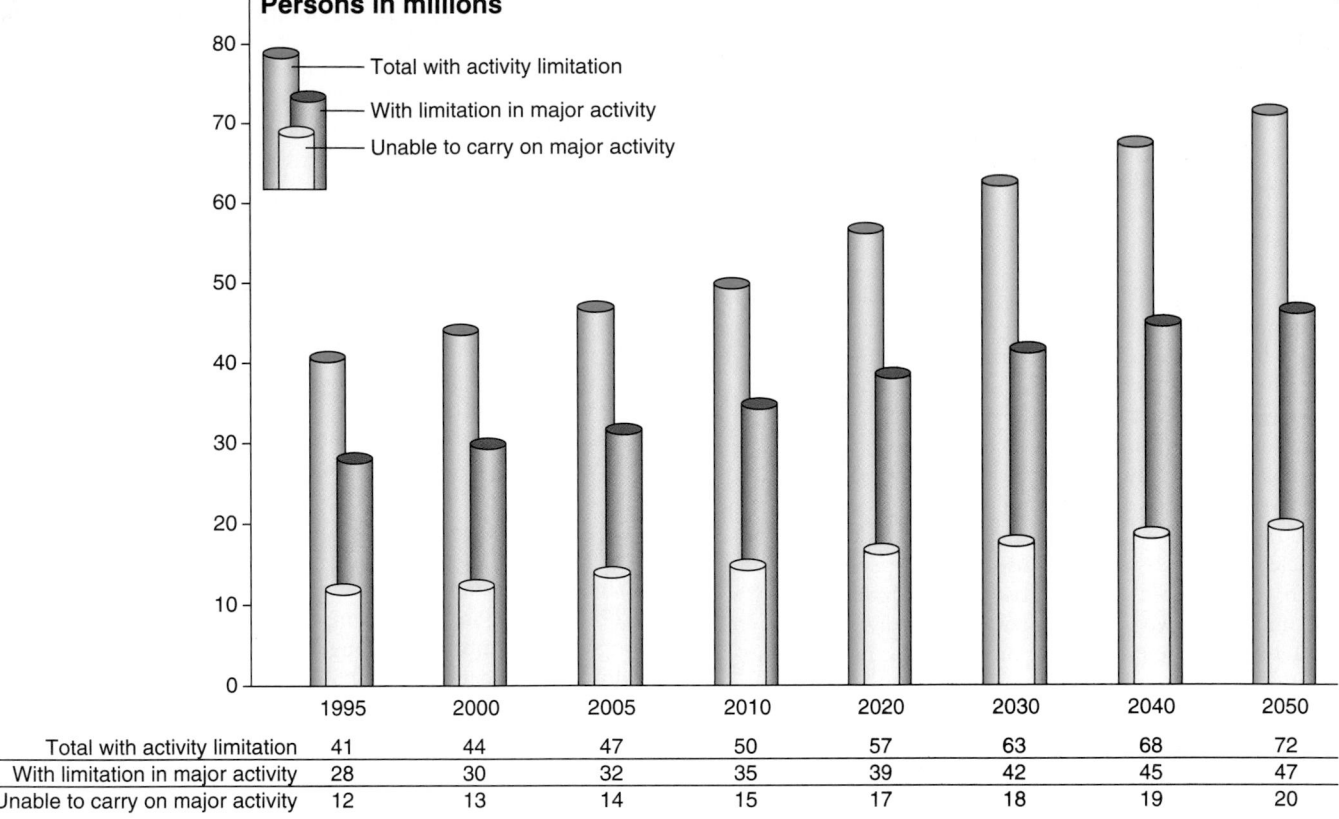

	1995	2000	2005	2010	2020	2030	2040	2050
Total with activity limitation	41	44	47	50	57	63	68	72
With limitation in major activity	28	30	32	35	39	42	45	47
Unable to carry on major activity	12	13	14	15	17	18	19	20

FIGURE 10-1 Projected number of persons by degree of activity limitation due to chronic condition, selected years, 1995–2050. The number of people who will be unable to go to school, to work, or to live independently because of a chronic condition is projected to reach 20 million by 2050. With permission from Robert Wood Johnson Foundation. (1996). *Chronic care in America: A 21st century challenge.* Princeton, NJ: Author.

tivity limitations and the five most disabling chronic conditions. Activity limitations are not limited to adults: an estimated 6.5% of all U.S. children experience some degree of disability. The most common disabling conditions in children are respiratory diseases and mental impairment (Newacheck & Halfon, 1998). People with activity limitations need assistance with their activities of daily living. Figure 10-3 indicates what happens to people with activity limitations whose needs for health care and personal services are not met for various reasons. They may be unable to carry out their therapeutic regimens as prescribed or have their prescriptions filled on time; they may miss physicians' appointments and office visits; and they may be unable to carry out the activities of daily living (Robert Wood Johnson Foundation,

1996). These figures provide an overview of the scope of the problem and are useful in planning health promotion and education programs as well as in allocating resources and services.

Chronic conditions have become the major cause of health-related problems in developed countries, and even developing countries are experiencing an increase in chronic conditions, giving these countries the dual burden of trying to eradicate infectious diseases while learning to manage chronic conditions (Kickbusch, 1997). Some of the reasons that so many people are afflicted with chronic conditions include the following:

- A decrease in mortality from infectious diseases, such as smallpox, diphtheria, and other serious conditions

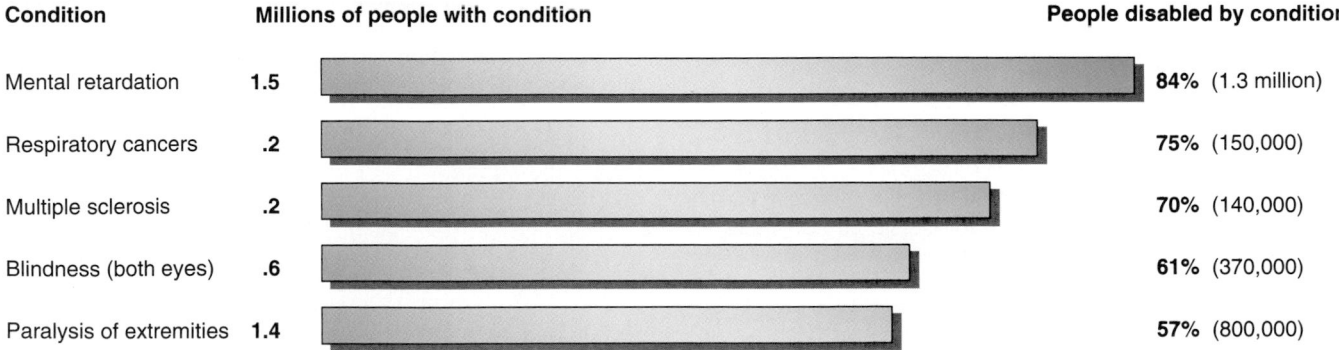

FIGURE 10-2 Five most disabling chronic conditions. With permission from Robert Wood Johnson Foundation. (1996). *Chronic care in America: A 21st century challenge.* Princeton, NJ: Author.

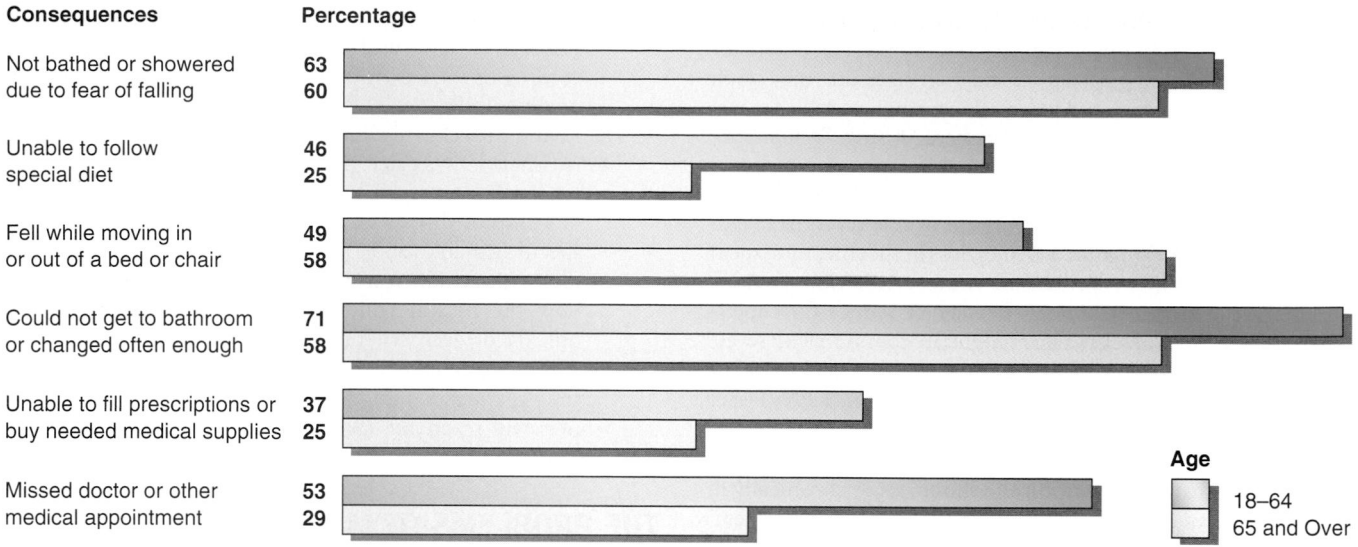

FIGURE 10-3 The consequences of unmet needs for help, by age group. With permission from Robert Wood Johnson Foundation. (1996). *Chronic care in America: A 21st century challenge.* Princeton, NJ: Author.

- Longer life spans because of advances in technology and pharmacology, improved nutrition, safer working conditions, and greater access (for some people) to health care
- Improved screening and diagnostic procedures, enabling early detection and treatment of diseases
- Prompt and aggressive management of acute conditions, such as myocardial infarction and AIDS-related infections
- The tendency to develop single or multiple chronic illnesses with advancing age
- Modern lifestyle factors, such as smoking, chronic stress, and obesity, that increase the risk for chronic illnesses, such as pulmonary disease, hypertension, and cardiovascular disease

A major problem of chronic conditions is that physiologic changes in the body commonly occur before symptomatic manifestations of disease, as in the case of hypertension (Sadowski & Redeker, 1996). Greater emphasis has recently been placed on the adoption of healthy lifestyles, beginning in childhood. Despite the media attention on the benefits of maintaining healthy lifestyles, many Americans are overweight, smoke, and lead sedentary lives. Consequences of unhealthy lifestyles include an alarming increase in the incidence of diabetes, hypertension, obesity, and cardiac and chronic respiratory disorders (Juarbe, 1998; Wing, Goldstein, Acton et al., 2001).

The Characteristics of Chronic Conditions

Sometimes it is difficult for those who are disease-free to understand how lives are changed, often forever, because of chronic conditions. It is also easy for health professionals to focus on treating the illness while overlooking the person who has the disease (Hellstrom, Lindqvist & Mattsson, 1998). In all illnesses, but even more so with chronic conditions, the illness cannot be separated from the person (Soderberg, Lundman & Norberg, 1999). Chronic illness is something that people must contend with on a daily basis. Nurses are unable to relate to what people are facing or plan effective interventions unless they fully understand what it means to have a chronic illness (Carroll, 1998;

Koch, Kralik & Taylor, 2000; Lubkin, 1997). Characteristic effects of chronic illness follow:

1. Managing chronic illness involves more than managing medical problems. Associated psychological and social problems must also be addressed since living for long periods of time with illness symptoms and disability can threaten identity, bring about role changes, alter body image, and disrupt lifestyles (Dean, 1999). This means that continuous adaptation and accommodation are called for, depending upon age and situation in life (Price, 1996; Sidell, 1997). Each major change or decrease in functional ability requires further physical, emotional, and social adaptation for patients and their families (Carroll, 1998; Lewis, 1998; Miller, 1999; Tappan, Williams, Fishman & Theris, 1999).

2. Chronic conditions usually involve many different phases over the course of a person's lifetime. There can be acute periods, stable and unstable periods, flare-ups, and remissions. Each phase brings its own set of physical, psychological, and social problems, and each requires different regimens and types of management (Corbin & Strauss, 1991).

3. Keeping chronic conditions under control requires persistent adherence to therapeutic regimens. Failing to adhere to a treatment plan or to follow a regimen in a consistent manner increases the risks of developing complications and accelerating the disease process. However, the realities of daily life, including the impact of culture, values, and socioeconomic factors, affect the degree to which people adhere to a treatment regimen. Managing a chronic illness takes time, requires knowledge and planning (Baker, 1998), and can be uncomfortable and inconvenient. It is not unusual for patients to discontinue taking medications or to alter dosages because of side effects that are more disturbing or disruptive than illness symptoms. People also frequently cut back on regimens they consider overly time-consuming, fatiguing, or costly (Davis & Magilvy, 2000; Wichowski & Kubsch, 1997).

4. One chronic disease can lead to the development of other chronic conditions. Diabetes, for example, can eventually lead to neurological and vascular changes that may result in vision, cardiac, and kidney disease and erectile dysfunction (Warren-Boulton, Greenberg, Lising & Gallivan, 1999).

5. Chronic illness affects the whole family. Family life can be dramatically altered as a result of role reversals (Saiki-Craighill, 1997), unfilled roles, loss of income, time spent managing illness, decreases in family socialization activities, and the costs of treatment (Dokken & Sydnor-Greenberg, 1998). Stress and caretaker fatigue are common with severe chronic conditions, and the whole family rather than just the individual needs care (Canam & Acorn, 1999; Fisher & Weiks, 2000).

6. The major responsibility for the day-to-day management of illness falls upon the shoulders of chronically ill people and their families. In today's health care system, especially with chronic conditions, day-to-day management, or self-care, has increasingly become a major part of the role of the patient or family. The home, rather than the hospital, is the center of care in chronic conditions since this is where day-to-day management occurs. Hospitals, clinics, doctors' offices, nursing homes, nursing centers, and community agencies (visiting nurse services, social services, and disease-specific associations and societies) are adjuncts or back-up services to that daily home management.

7. The management of chronic conditions is a process of discovery. People can be taught how to manage their conditions. Teaching about symptoms, however, is not the same as experiencing them. Each person must discover how his or her own body reacts under varying conditions—for example, what it is like to be hypoglycemic, what activities are likely to bring on angina, and how these or other conditions can best be prevented and managed.

8. Managing chronic conditions is a collaborative process. The medical, social, and psychological problems associated with chronic problems tend to be complex, especially in severe conditions. The management of chronic conditions should therefore be thought of as a collaborative process that involves many different health care professionals working together with patients and their families to provide the full range of services that are often needed to manage at home (Corbin & Cherry, 1997).

9. The management of chronic conditions is expensive. As indicated in Table 10-1, billions of dollars are spent every year on health care for people with chronic conditions. The money pays for hospitalizations and the purchase of equipment, medications, and supportive services. For example, hospital lengths of stay and charges are higher for acute pediatric conditions if a child also has a chronic condition (Hodgson & Cohen, 1999; Silber, Gleeson & Zhao, 1999). Overall health care costs are not likely to decrease until there is a substantial downward trend in the incidence of chronic conditions and the costs of chronic health care.

10. Chronic conditions raise difficult ethical issues for the patient, health care professionals, and society. No easy solutions exist to problems such as how to establish cost controls, how to allocate scarce resources (eg, kidneys and hearts for transplantation), how to determine what constitutes quality of life, and when to terminate life support. Patients, families, and society respond to ethical issues according to their own moral standards and definitions of quality of life.

11. Living with chronic illness means living with uncertainty (Mishel, 1999; Price, 1996). Although health care professionals have some notion about the usual progression of a chronic disease such as Parkinson's disease, so many specific variables enter into each case that no one can predict with certainty an individual's illness course (that is, how the person will respond to treatment and how quickly or even whether a disease will progress). Even when a patient is "in remission" or "disease-free," he or she experiences a lingering doubt and dread that the illness will reactivate (Smeltzer, 1992; Wiener & Dodd, 1993).

THE PROBLEMS OF MANAGING CHRONIC CONDITIONS

Chronic conditions have implications for everyday living and management problems for individuals and their families as well as for society at large. Most importantly, individual efforts should be directed at preventing chronic conditions since many chronic conditions can be traced, at least in part, to unhealthy lifestyles or behaviors such as smoking and overeating. Thus, changes in lifestyle can result in the prevention of some chronic conditions, or at least a delay in their onset until a later age. Because of the tendency of some people to resist change, however, bringing about alterations in people's lifestyles is one the major challenges facing nurses today.

Once a chronic condition has occurred, the focus shifts from disease prevention to managing symptoms and staying well by avoiding complications (eg, eye problems in the diabetic) and the development of other acute illnesses (eg, pneumonia in a person with chronic obstructive lung disease). Quality of life, often overlooked by health professionals in their approach to care of people with chronic conditions, is also important. Health-promoting behaviors, such as exercise, are essential to quality of life even in people who have chronic illnesses and disabilities because they help to maintain functional status (Stuifbergen & Rogers, 1997). See Nursing Research Profile 10-1 for more information.

Although coworkers, extended family, and health care professionals are affected by the problems of people with chronic illnesses, the problems of living with chronic conditions are most acutely experienced by patients and their immediate families. It is they who feel the greatest impact with lifestyle changes that directly affect quality of life. Nurses provide direct care, especially during acute episodes, but they also provide the teaching and secure the resources and other supports that enable people to integrate their illness into their lives and have some quality of life despite their illness (Michael, 1996). To understand what nursing care is needed, it is important to comprehend the issues that people with chronic illness and their families contend with and manage, often on a daily basis. The challenges of living with chronic conditions can be summarized as follows:

- Alleviating and managing symptoms
- Psychologically adjusting to and physically accommodating disabilities
- Preventing and managing crises and complications
- Carrying out regimens as prescribed
- Validating individual self-worth and family functioning

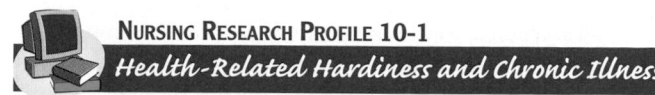

NURSING RESEARCH PROFILE 10-1
Health-Related Hardiness and Chronic Illness

Martin, J. C., Engle, V. F., & Graney, M. J. (1999). Determinants of health-related hardiness among urban older African-American women with chronic illness. *Holistic Nursing Practice, 13*(3), 62–70.

Purpose
Although statistics demonstrated that older African American women experience earlier, more frequent, and more severe limitations from chronic illnesses than any other older adult group, African American women who live beyond the age of 85 usually live longer than their Anglo-American counterparts. Health-related hardiness (HRH), defined as a set of personality characteristics that buffer negative stressful effects associated with living with chronic illness, has been suggested as one factor that contributes to these statistics. The purpose of this study was to identify and quantify the relationship between HRH and function, self-assessed health, morbidity, and health behaviors in urban, older African American women with chronic illness.

Study Sample and Design
A correlational design was used to obtain data about demographic characteristics and the variables of interest among chronically ill older African American women. Questionnaires and structured interviews were used to obtain the data from women during routine appointments at the outpatient clinic of a large urban hospital. Instruments included the Health-Related Hardiness Scale (HRHS), Self-Assess Health (SAH) instrument, Sickness Impact Profile (SIP), and Health Habits Scale. Demographic data obtained included age, education, and marital status of the women.

Findings
The mean age of the sample of 100 women was 68.8 ± 8.6 years. They had a mean of four medical diagnoses and five prescribed daily medications. Hypertension and osteoarthritis were the most common chronic illnesses reported; they occurred in 90% and 74% of the women, respectively. Analysis of data revealed that the women had high levels of HRH, little functional impairment, moderate ratings of the state of their own health, multiple chronic illnesses and use of multiple daily medications, and frequent participation in health behaviors. Significant correlations were found between HRH and years of education and HRH and SIP, which measures the impact of illness on function and performance of activities of daily living. Upon analysis by stepwise multiple linear regression, HRH was best predicted by years of education and function as measured by the SIP.

Nursing Implications
The findings of this study (ie, high levels of HRH, little impairment in function, average levels of self-assessed health, and frequent practice of health behaviors) support the existence of hardiness in older African American women. These findings increase understanding of hardiness as an important variable related to health. Further research is needed to identify factors that will facilitate health promotion and health protection among this group of women.

- Managing threats to identity
- Normalizing individual and family life as much as possible
- Living with altered time, social isolation, and loneliness
- Establishing the networks of support and resources that can enhance quality of life
- Returning to a satisfactory way of life after an acute debilitating episode (another myocardial infarction or stroke) or reactivation of a chronic condition
- Dying with dignity and comfort

IMPLICATIONS FOR NURSING

Working with people with chronic illness or disability requires not just dealing with the medical aspects of their disorder, but also working with the whole person, physically, emotionally, and socially (Dean, 1999). This holistic approach to care requires nurses to draw upon their entire repertoire of knowledge and skills, including knowledge from the social sciences, psychology in particular. People often respond to illness, health teaching, and regimens in ways that are different from the expectations of health care providers. Although quality of life is usually affected by chronic illness, especially if the illness is severe (Schlenk, Erlen, Dunbar-Jacob et al., 1998), patients' perceptions of what constitutes quality of life often drive their management behaviors. Nurses and other health care professionals need to recognize this, even though it may be difficult to see patients make unwise choices and decisions about lifestyles and disease management. Individuals have the right to receive care without fearing ridicule or refusal of treatment, even if they caused their medical conditions through their own indiscretions, such as smoking or failure to follow therapeutic regimens.

As stated previously, chronic conditions have a course, although that course might be too uncertain to predict with any degree of accuracy. An illness course can be thought of as a trajectory— a course—that can be managed or shaped over time to some extent through proper illness management strategies (Robinson, Bevil, Arcangelo et al., 2001; Strauss & Corbin, 1988; Woog, 1992). The trajectory of an illness can also be divided into phases that enable more precise thinking about a person's condition. This enables the nurse to put the present situation into the context of what might have happened to the patient in the past—that is, the life factors and understandings that might have contributed to the present state of the illness. In this way, nurses can more readily address the underlying issues and problems.

Each phase of chronic illness brings with it different problems, both medical and psychosocial. The needs of a stroke patient who is a good candidate for rehabilitation, for example, are very different from those of a patient with terminal cancer. By thinking in terms of phases, and individual patients within a phase, nurses can target their care more specifically to each person. Not every chronic condition is necessarily life-threatening, and not every patient passes through each possible phase of a chronic condition.

PHASES OF CHRONIC ILLNESS

Over the years, chronic conditions can pass through several different phases (Corbin & Cherry, 1997; Strauss & Corbin, 1988). Nine phases have been identified (Chart 10-1):

1. The **pretrajectory phase** describes the stage at which the person is at risk for developing a chronic condition because of genetic factors or lifestyle behaviors that increase susceptibility to chronic illness.
2. The **trajectory phase** is characterized by the onset of symptoms or disability associated with a chronic condition. Since symptoms are being evaluated and diagnostic tests are performed, this phase is often accompanied by uncertainty as the person awaits a diagnosis. Nursing care often involves preparing patients for diagnostic tests and offering emotional support.
3. The **stable phase** of the trajectory indicates that symptoms and disability are being managed adequately. Although the patient is doing well, nursing care is still important at this time to reinforce positive behaviors and to offer ongoing monitoring.

Chart 10-1 · Phases in the Trajectory Model of Chronic Illness

- **Pretrajectory:** Genetic factors or lifestyle behaviors that place an individual or community at risk for the development of a chronic condition
- **Trajectory onset:** Appearance of noticeable symptoms; includes period of diagnostic workup and announcement of diagnosis; may be accompanied by biographic limbo as patient begins to discover and cope with implications of diagnosis
- **Stable:** Illness course and symptoms are under control; biography and everyday life activities are being managed within limitations of illness; illness management centered in the home
- **Unstable:** Period of inability to keep symptoms under control or reactivation of illness; biographic disruption and difficulty in carrying out everyday life activities; adjustments being made in regimen, with care usually taking place at home
- **Acute:** Severe and unrelieved symptoms or the development of illness complications necessitating hospitalization or bed rest to bring illness course under control; biography and everyday life activities temporarily placed on hold or drastically cut back
- **Crisis:** Critical or life-threatening situation requiring emergency treatment or care; biography and everyday life activities suspended until the crisis passes
- **Comeback:** Gradual return to an acceptable way of life within limits imposed by disability or illness; involves physical healing, stretching limitations through rehabilitative procedures, psychosocial coming to terms, and biographic reengagement with adjustments in everyday life activities
- **Downward:** Illness course characterized by rapid or gradual physical decline accompanied by increasing disability or difficulty in controlling symptoms; requires biographic adjustment and alterations in everyday life activities with each major downward step
- **Dying:** Final days or weeks before death; characterized by gradual or rapid shutting down of body processes, biographic disengagement and closure, and relinquishment of everyday life interests and activities

4. The **unstable phase** is characterized by an exacerbation of illness symptoms, development of complications, or reactivation of an illness in remission. During this phase, a person's everyday activities may be temporarily disrupted because symptoms are not well controlled. There may also be more diagnostic tests and a trial of new regimens until some degree of control over symptoms is achieved. During this time of uncertainty, patients look to nurses for guidance and support.

5. The **acute phase** is characterized by sudden onset of severe or unrelieved symptoms or complications that require hospitalization for their management. This phase may require major modification of the person's usual activities for a period of time. Nurses are intensely involved in the care of the chronically ill patient during this period, providing direct care and emotional support to the patient and family members.

6. The **crisis phase** is characterized by a critical or life-threatening situation that requires emergency treatment or care. During this phase patients and their families depend upon the skill, knowledge, and support of nurses and other professionals to stabilize their conditions.

7. The **comeback phase** is the period in the trajectory marked by recovery after an acute period. It includes learning to live with or to overcome disabilities and a return to an acceptable way of life within the limitations imposed by the chronic condition. Although aspects of care may shift to other health care providers during the rehabilitative phase, the role of nurses as organizers of care and collaborators in the recovery of patients is essential.

8. The **downward phase** marks the worsening of a condition. Symptoms and disability continue to progress despite attempts to gain some control through treatment and management regimens. A downward turn does not necessarily mean imminent death; the downward trend can be arrested and an illness restabilized. Since patients are not yet acute or dying but usually are living at home during this time, their contact with nurses is often limited. The supportive presence of nurses is needed, however, because of adjustment issues. Nurses working in clinics and physicians' offices can play an important role in helping patients understand and come to terms with what is happening to them.

9. The **dying phase** is characterized by the gradual or rapid decline in the trajectory despite efforts to halt the disorder or slow the decline through illness management; it is characterized by failure of life-maintaining body functions. During this phase nurses provide direct and supportive care to patients and their families through hospice programs.

Nursing Management

Nursing care of patients with chronic conditions is varied and occurs in an assortment of settings. It can include provision of direct care or supportive care. Such care is often provided in the clinic or physician's office, the hospital, or the patient's home, depending on the status of the illness.

Examples of direct care may include assessing the patient's physical status, providing wound care, managing and overseeing medication regimens, and performing other technical tasks. The availability of this type of nursing care is one of the main reasons patients can remain at home and return to a somewhat normal life after an acute episode of illness.

Because much of the day-to-day responsibility for managing chronic conditions rests with the patient and family, nurses often provide supportive care unless the patient is hospitalized. Supportive care may include ongoing monitoring, teaching, counseling, serving as an advocate for the patient, making referrals, and case-managing. Providing supportive care is just as important as the performance of technical care. For example, through ongoing monitoring that might take place either in the home or a nursing clinic, such as a heart failure clinic, a nurse might detect impending complications, such as signs of heart failure. The nurse might detect these signs before they are noticeable to the patient and could make a referral (call the physician or consult the medical protocol in a clinic) for medical evaluation, thereby preventing a lengthy and costly hospitalization.

CARE BY PHASE: APPLYING THE NURSING PROCESS

The focus of care for patients with chronic conditions is determined largely by illness phase and directed by the nursing process, which includes assessment, diagnosis, planning, implementation, and evaluation.

Step 1: Identifying the Trajectory Phase

The first step is assessment of the patient to determine the specific phase (see Chart 10-1). Assessment enables the nurse to identify the specific medical, social, and psychological problems likely to be encountered in a phase. For instance, the problems of a patient having an acute myocardial infarction are very different from those likely to be encountered with the same patient, 10 years later, dying at home of heart failure. The kinds of direct care, referrals, teaching, and emotional support needed in each situation are different as well.

Step 2: Establishing Goals

Once the phase of illness has been identified for a specific patient, along with the specific medical problems and related social and psychological issues, the next step involves establishing the goals of care. The establishment of goals should be a collaborative effort with the patient, family, and nurse working together, for the attainment of a goal is unlikely if it is primarily the nurse's and not the patient's. The following are two examples of goals to be determined collaboratively, then written in the language of the nursing process.

An elderly man with severe progressive COPD reports increasing difficulty breathing, even with the oxygen level set at 2 liters/min. This interferes with his ability to carry out activities of daily living and has decreased his quality of life. He asks the nurse for help. The nursing diagnosis for this problem might be "Activity intolerance related to less than adequate intake of oxygen secondary to lung disease," and the mutually agreed upon goal of care might be to increase the patient's ability to care for himself. Nursing interventions related to this goal might include teaching the client how to pace his activities and helping him to obtain a home health aide to assist with the most demanding activities of daily living.

In another example, a 45-year-old woman with moderately advanced multiple sclerosis (MS) is hospitalized with a severe bladder infection. She reports that she has problems with self-catheterization because of her disability and that she has difficulty obtaining and consuming adequate fluids during the day. The nursing diagnosis for this problem might be "Toileting self-care deficit (in bladder care) related to decreased functional ability secondary to MS," and the mutual outcomes of care might be to develop strategies to facilitate the self-catheterization process and increase daily fluid intake.

Step 3: Establishing a Plan to Achieve Desired Outcomes

Once goals have been established, the next step consists of establishing a realistic and mutually agreed upon plan for achieving them and identifying specific criteria that can be used to assess the patient's progress. A plan of care for the man with COPD who complains of a decreased ability to care for himself, for example, might include assisting him to prioritize his activities of daily living so he can carry out those that are most important to him before he becomes too short of breath and tired. It might also include exploring how he feels about having someone assist him at home on a regular basis and, if he agrees to having help, checking on the availability and costs of such services. In many cases, people with chronic illness perceive someone helping them as a threat to their independence and self-esteem, the first step to a nursing home or rehabilitation center. Therefore, they are resistant to someone coming into their home to help them. Criteria to measure progress toward goal attainment and strategies to accomplish the goals might include the following:

- At the end of the first nurse–patient session, the patient with COPD will be able to prioritize activities of daily living and agree to look over an information sheet and list of home care agencies provided by the nurse.
- By the second nurse–patient session, the patient will report that he is pacing his activities and is therefore better able to carry out important self-care activities. He will also report that he has read the information provided by the nurse about home care agencies.
- By the third nurse–patient session, the patient will have compiled a list of the self-care activities that are difficult for him to carry out and for which assistance would be beneficial. The patient will also have reviewed his finances and determined how much he can afford to pay for services.
- By the fourth nurse–patient session, the patient will have called a home care agency and made arrangements to have home health services for 2 hours each morning. If the patient cannot make the arrangements, then the nurse would suggest that the family or someone else make them. The goal is to enable the patient to meet basic self-care needs and improve quality of life, thereby having enough time and energy available for other activities. Home health services can help with this. Having the patient make the arrangements for home care promotes a sense of control. People with chronic illness-related disabilities often feel that they have lost a great deal of control over what happens to them; any activities that they can do for themselves, therefore, enhance psychological well being.
- By the fifth home visit the patient will report that all self-care needs are met either by self-pacing of activities or through the assistance of a home health aide.

A plan of care for the woman with MS might be to develop techniques for carrying out self-catheterization within the limitations imposed by her disability and to increase her daily fluid intake to six to eight 8-oz glasses of fluid per day. Indicators that the desired goal has been achieved may include the following:

- By the end of the first nurse–patient session, the patient and nurse will identify with which steps in the self-catheterization procedure the patient is having the most difficulty. The patient will also be able to list three strategies for improving her intake of fluids.
- By the end of the second nurse–patient session, the patient will report that she is performing self-catheterization using the strategies suggested by the nurse for improving her technique. She will also report that she has increased her fluid intake by three glasses.
- By the end of the third nurse–patient session, the patient will report that she can perform self-catheterization three out of four times without difficulty and that her fluid intake is now up to six to eight 8-oz glasses a day.
- By the end of the fourth nurse–patient session, the patient will be ready for discharge with the confidence that she is competent in performing self-catheterization and obtaining adequate fluid intake despite the physical limitations imposed by her illness.

Step 4: Identifying Factors That Facilitate or Hinder Attainment of Goals

The next step involves identifying environmental, social, and psychological factors that might interfere with or facilitate achieving the goal. In the case of the patient with COPD, for example, not having sufficient resources could prevent him from hiring a home health aide. For this reason, the nurse might want to explore carefully the issue of resources with the patient and, if there are financial constraints, enlist the services of a social worker, with the patient's consent, to explore possible community resources. Since the patient is having trouble breathing, the nurse should determine whether the patient is also having difficulty cooking and eating, and whether he is losing weight because of insufficient caloric intake to meet his nutritional needs. If cooking is a problem, then the nurse might look into community resources such as Meals on Wheels. If the patient is losing weight, then the nurse should advise him to eat frequent small meals to lessen the fatigue associated with eating and to supplement meals with high-protein drinks.

In the case of the patient with MS, the nurse might want to explore the extent of the patient's physical limitations, how rapidly the MS seems to be progressing, when during the day she has the most difficulty doing the catheterization, and whether that difficulty might be related to fatigue. If fatigue is a factor, the nurse might explore whether the patient would consider having a home health aide to help her with some of her self-care activities. This would enable the patient to conserve her energy for social activities and personal care, such as self-catheterization. The nurse would also discuss with the patient why she is not taking in an adequate amount of fluids. If the patient is too busy or tired to make frequent trips to the sink or refrigerator to get fluids, the nurse might help the patient develop strategies for saving time and energy. For example, the patient could attach a bottle of water to her wheelchair or walker and carry it around with her, or strategically place bottles of water or other liquids around the house to increase their accessibility. The nurse might also explore with the patient the types of caffeine-free fluids that she enjoys drinking.

Step 5: Implementing Interventions

The fifth step is the intervention phase. Possible interventions include providing direct care, serving as an advocate for the patient, teaching, counseling, making referrals, and case-managing (arranging for resources). For example, if the patient with COPD reports after prioritizing his activities of daily living that showering each morning is the most important self-care activity for him, then having a home health aide come early in the morning to help with the shower would be the best arrangement. The home health aide could also help with breakfast, make the bed, and straighten up the house. In this way, the man would use less energy doing these mundane tasks. After showering and dressing the patient might also want to plan a daily rest period, such as sitting down with a crossword puzzle or reading, that might help him overcome some of his sense of breathlessness and feel more rested.

If spasms or tremors are interfering with the ability of the woman with MS to catheterize herself, then the nurse would want to review the medications she is taking; if, for instance, she is taking antispasmodics, the self-catheterizations could be timed to coincide with the peak medication levels. In an effort to encourage an increased fluid intake, the nurse might want to help the woman build into her daily routine a set time in the morning and afternoon, allowing for flexibility, to take an herbal tea or juice break that would increase the amount of fluids ingested and also provide a rest period. While it is important for a patient with MS to maintain a sense of independence and accomplishment, it is equally important for the patient to learn to recognize his or her limits, through such signs as fatigue, and to manage them through proper planning.

Physicians prescribe therapies, such as medications and diet, and give directions for how much, when, and how they are to be used. Nurses, however, by virtue of their broad knowledge base, can best help patients develop the strategies needed to live with both the symptoms and therapies associated with chronic conditions. Because each patient is an individual, it is important to work individually with each patient and family to identify the best ways to integrate their treatment regimens into their daily living activities. Two tasks are important in managing chronic illness: following regimens to control symptoms and keep the illness stable, and dealing with the psychosocial issues that can hinder illness management and affect quality of life.

Diagnosing and prescribing by physicians are important aspects of chronic illness care, but they represent only half of the battle against disease. The other half includes the teaching, counseling, arranging, and case-managing that enable people to live with their disease and gain independence (Hughes, Hodgson, Muller et al., 2000). Saving the life of a patient with an acute myocardial infarction in the ICU, for example, is a positive outcome, but the patient will have a relapse if he or she is not supported in making the lifestyle changes necessary to reduce the probability of another heart attack. Helping patients and their families to understand and implement regimens and to carry out activities of daily living within the limits of their disabilities is one of the most important aspects of health care delivery—and nursing care—for patients with chronic illnesses and their families.

Step 6: Evaluating the Effectiveness of Interventions

The final step is evaluating the effectiveness of the interventions. In chronic illness, maintaining the stability of the condition while at the same time preserving the patient's control over his or her life and a sense of identity and accomplishment is the primary goal. Success may be defined, however, as merely making progress toward a goal when a patient finds it difficult to implement rapid and drastic changes in the way that he or she does things. Nurses cannot expect that the sedentary person with high blood pressure, for example, is going to develop a sudden passion for exercise. Nor can they expect that working people can easily rearrange their day to accommodate time-consuming regimens such as special diets or complex medication schedules. Bringing about change takes time, patience, creativity, and encouragement from the nurse. Validation by the nurse for each small increment toward goal accomplishment is important for enhancing self-esteem and reinforcing behaviors. If no progress is made or if progress toward goals seems too slow, it may be necessary to redefine the goals or the time frame. The patient may not be ready to progress toward the goals or may be ambivalent about the illness, its treatments, or both (Chin, Polonsky, Thomas & Nerney, 2000). Other conditions such as depression may also interfere with the patient's ability to carry out regimens and make lifestyle changes.

Nurses must also realize that some people will not change. Some people, for example, are unwilling to give up smoking despite advanced COPD. Nor is it unusual to find people with the diagnosis of diabetes failing to adhere completely to their diabetic diets. When patients are having difficulty carrying out regimens or are reluctant to change their lifestyles, nurses should not feel that this is a failure on their part. Patients share responsibility for management of their conditions, and outcomes are as much related to their ability to accommodate the illness and carry out regimens as they are to nursing intervention.

Promoting Home and Community-Based Care

TEACHING PATIENTS SELF-CARE

Since chronic conditions are so costly to individuals, families, and society, one of the major goals of nursing in the 21st century should be the prevention of chronic conditions and the care of people with them. This requires promoting healthy lifestyles and encouraging the use of safety and disease-prevention measures, such as wearing seat belts and obtaining immunizations. Prevention should also begin early in life and continue throughout the life span.

Patient and family teaching is one of the most significant aspects of nursing care and may make the difference in the ability of patients and their families to adapt to chronic health conditions. Well-informed, educated patients are more likely than uninformed patients to be concerned about their health and do what is necessary to maintain it (De Ridder, Depla, Severens & Malsch, 1997). They are also more likely to manage symptoms, recognize the onset of complications, and seek health care early: knowledge is the key to making informed choices and decisions during all phases of the chronic illness trajectory.

Despite the importance of teaching the patient and family, the nurse must recognize that patients recently diagnosed with serious chronic conditions and their families may need time to grasp the significance of their condition and its effect on their life. Teaching should be planned carefully so that it provides information that is important to the patient's well-being at the time without being overwhelming.

The nurse who cares for patients with chronic conditions in the hospital, clinic, or home should assess each patient's knowledge about the illness and its management; the nurse cannot assume that a patient with a long-standing chronic condition has the knowledge necessary to manage the condition. A patient's learning needs change as the trajectory phase and his or her personal situation changes. The nurse must also recognize that patients may know how their body responds under certain conditions and how best to manage their symptoms (Gallo & Knafl, 1998). Contact with patients in the hospital, clinic, or home offers nurses the ideal opportunity to reassess patients' learning needs and to provide additional information about an illness and its management.

CONTINUING CARE

Chronic illness management is a collaborative process between patient, family, nurse, and other health care professionals. Collaboration is not limited to hospital settings; rather, it is important in all settings and throughout the illness trajectory (Corbin & Cherry, 2001). Keeping an illness stable over time requires careful and continued monitoring of symptoms and attention to management regimens. Detecting problems early and assisting patients to develop appropriate management strategies can make a significant difference in outcomes.

Most chronic conditions are managed in the home. Therefore, care and teaching during hospitalization should focus on what the patient needs to know about the condition in order to manage once discharged to home. Nurses in all settings should be aware of the resources and services available in a community and should make the arrangements (before hospital discharge if the patient is hospitalized) necessary to secure those resources and services. When appropriate, home care services are contacted directly. The home care nurse will reassess how the patient and family are adapting to the chronic condition and its treatment and will continue or revise the plan of care accordingly.

Because chronic conditions occur worldwide and the world is increasingly interconnected, nurses should think beyond the individual level to the community and global levels. In terms of illness prevention and health promotion, this entails wide-ranging efforts to assess people for risk factors for chronic illness (eg, blood pressure and diabetes screening, stroke risk assessments) and group teaching related to illness prevention and management.

The nurse should also remind the patient with a chronic illness, and the patient's family, about the need for ongoing health promotion and the screening recommended for all people, as the chronic illness and disability often become the priority to the exclusion of other health-related issues.

NURSING CARE FOR SPECIAL POPULATIONS WITH CHRONIC ILLNESS

When providing care and teaching, the nurse must consider a variety of factors (eg, age, gender, culture, and ethnicity) that influence susceptibility to chronic illness and the ways patients respond to chronic disorders. Certain populations, for example, tend to be more susceptible to certain chronic conditions. Populations at high risk for specific conditions can be targeted for special teaching and monitoring programs. People of different cultures and genders tend to respond to illness differently; being aware of these differences is extremely important (Bates, Rankin-Hill & Sanchez-Ayendez, 1997; Becker, Beyene, Newsom & Rodgers, 1998; Thorne, McCormick & Carty, 1997). For cultures in which patients rely heavily on the support of their families, families must be involved and made part of the nursing care plan. As the United States becomes more multicultural and ethnically diverse, and as the general population ages, nurses need to be aware of how an individual's culture and age facilitate or hinder chronic illness management, and nurses should be prepared to adapt the care they give accordingly (Becker, Beyene, Newsom & Rodgers, 1998; Jennings, 1999; Rehm, 1999).

 Critical Thinking Exercises

1. A 25-year-old graduate student is diagnosed with fibromyalgia after several years of visiting physicians and being told that her symptoms were "all in your mind." Due to chronic fatigue and pain, she often missed days from school and eventually withdrew from school. Her husband is not very supportive because he too thinks the disease is "in her head." How would you help this woman learn to cope with her condition and the damages to her self-esteem? How would you involve her husband in the process?

2. A 19-year-old has been recently diagnosed with diabetes. He is very active in sports and involved with his peers. He says that he is not interested in learning about his condition, refuses to learn to give insulin injections to himself, and eats whatever he wants. How would you approach goal setting and establishing a plan of care with this young adult? What developmental issues will you consider in your teaching?

3. An 85-year-old woman is about to be discharged from the hospital after an acute episode of heart failure. How would the teaching and planning for discharge be different from that of a 45-year-old going home after an acute myocardial infarction?

4. A 43-year-old Native American woman tells you that she is always thirsty and has frequent yeast infections. She also tells you that she has not had a Pap smear or any kind of physical examination since her last child was born 8 years ago because she does not have health insurance and lacks the money to pay for office visits. What would you tell this woman? How would you advise her to find the resources to obtain health care?

5. A 45-year-old African American woman with multiple sclerosis in remission has been advised by her doctor to start a regular exercise program. She asks why she should do exercise since eventually her disease is only going to get worse anyway. She works and has three teenage children at home. How would you explain to her the relationship between health-promotion activities and quality of life? How might you go about establishing with her an exercise plan? How might her family become involved in helping her?

REFERENCES AND SELECTED READINGS

Books

Corbin, J., & Cherry, J. (1997). Caring for the chronically ill elderly in the community. In L. Swanson & T. Tripp-Reiner (Eds.). *Advances in gerontological nursing* (Vol. 2). New York: Springer.

Corbin, J., & Cherry J. (2001). Epilogue: A proactive model of health care. In R. Hyman & J. Corbin (Eds.). *Chronic illness: Research and theory for nursing practice* (pp. 294–299). New York: Springer.

Lubkin, I. M. (1997). *Chronic illness: Impact and interventions.* Boston: Jones & Bartlett.

Robert Wood Johnson Foundation. (1996). *Chronic care in America: A 21st century challenge.* Princeton, NJ: Author.

Robinson, L., Bevil, C., Arcangelo, V., Reifsnyder, J. A., Rothman, N., & Smeltzer, S. (2001). Operationalizing the Corbin and Strauss Trajectory Model for elderly clients with chronic illness. In R. Hyman & J. Corbin (Eds.). *Chronic illness: Research and theory for nursing practice.* New York: Springer.

Smeltzer, S. C. (1992). Use of the trajectory model of nursing in multiple sclerosis. In P. Woog (Ed.). *The chronic illness trajectory framework* (pp. 73–88). New York: Springer.

Strauss, A., & Corbin, J. (1988). *Shaping a new health care system.* San Francisco: Jossey-Bass.

Strauss, A., et al. (1984). *Chronic illness and the quality of life* (2nd ed.). St. Louis: C. V. Mosby.

Woog, P. (Ed.). (1992). *The chronic illness trajectory framework.* New York: Springer.

Journals

Asterisks indicate nursing research articles.

Baker, L. M. (1998). Sense making in multiple sclerosis: The information needs of people during an acute exacerbation. *Qualitative Health Journal, 8*(1), 106–120.

Bates, M. S., Rankin-Hill, L., & Sanchez-Ayendez, M. (1997). The effects of the cultural context of health care on treatment of and response to chronic pain and illness. *Social Science in Medicine, 45*(9), 1333–1347.

Becker, G., Beyene, Y., Newsom, E. M., & Rodgers, D. V. (1998). Knowledge and care of chronic illness in three ethnic minority groups. *Family Medicine, 30*(3), 173–178.

*Canam, C., & Acorn, S. (1999). Quality of life for family caregivers of people with chronic health problems. *Rehabilitation Nursing, 24*(5), 192–196.

Carroll, L. W. (1998). Understanding chronic illness from the patient's perspective. *Radiologic Technology, 70*(1), 37–41.

Chin, M. H., Polonsky, R. S., Thomas, V. D., & Nerney, M. P. (2000). Developing a conceptual framework for understanding illness and attitudes in older, urban African Americans with diabetes. *Diabetes Education, 26*(3), 439–449.

Collins, J. G. (1997). Prevalence of selected chronic conditions: United States, 1990–1992. *Vital Health Statistics, 10*(194), 1–89.

Corbin, J., & Strauss, A. (1991). A nursing model for chronic illness management based upon the trajectory framework. *Scholarly Inquiry for Nursing Practice, 5*(3), 155–174.

*Davis, R. N., & Magilvy, J. K. (2000). Quick Pride: The experience of chronic illness by rural older adults. *Journal of Nursing Scholarship, 32*(4), 385–390.

Dean, P. R. (1999). Personal perception of chronic illness. *Home Care Provider, 4*(2), 54–57.

De Ridder, D., Depla, M., Severens, P., & Malsch, M. (1997). Beliefs on coping with illness: A consumer's perspective. *Social Science in Medicine, 44*(5), 553–559.

Dokken, D. L., & Sydnor-Greenberg, N. (1998). Helping families mobilize their personal resources. *Pediatric Nursing, 24*(1), 66–69.

Fisher, L., & Weiks, K. L. (2000). Can addressing family relationships improve outcomes in chronic disease? Report of the National Working Group on Family-Based Interventions in Chronic Disease. *Journal of Family Practice, 49*(6), 561–566.

*Gallo, A. M., & Knafl, K. A. (1998). Parents' reports of "tricks of the trade" for managing childhood chronic illness. *Journal of the Society of Pediatric Nurses, 3*(3), 93–100.

Hagdrup, N. A., Simoes, E. J., & Brownson, R. C. (1997). Health care coverage: traditional and preventive measures and associations with chronic disease factors. *Journal of Community Health, 22*(5), 387–399.

Hellstrom, O., Lindqvist, P., & Mattsson, B. (1998). A phenomenological analysis of doctor-patient interaction: a case study. *Patient Education & Counseling, 33*(1), 83–89.

Hodgson, R. A., & Cohen, A. J. (1999). Medical care expenditures for diabetes, its chronic complications, and its comorbidities. *Previews in Medicine, 29*(3), 173–186.

*Hough, E. S., Brumitt, G. A., & Templin, T. N. (1999). Social support, demands of illness, and depression in chronically ill urban women. *Health Care for Women International, 20*(4), 349–362.

*Hughes, L. C., Hodgson, N. A., Muller, P., Robinson, L. A., & McCorkle, R. (2000). Information needs of elderly postsurgical cancer patients during the transition from hospital to home. *Journal of Nursing Scholarship, 32*(1), 25–30.

Jennings, A. (1999). The use of available social support networks by older blacks. *Journal of National Black Nurses Association, 10*(2), 4–13.

Juarbe, T. C. (1998). Risk factors for cardiovascular disease in Latina women. *Progress in Cardiovascular Nursing, 13*(2), 17–27.

Kempen, G. I., Ormel, J., Brilman, E. I., & Relyveld, J. (1997). Adaptive responses among Dutch elderly: the impact of eight chronic medical conditions on health-related quality of life. *American Journal of Public Health, 87*(1), 38–44.

Kickbusch, I. (1997). *Think health: what makes the difference?* Paper Presented at the Fourth International Conference on Health Promotion, World Health Organization, Jakarta, July.

Kingston, R. S., & Smith, J. P. (1997). Socioeconomic status and racial and ethnic differences in functional status associated with chronic disease. *American Journal of Public Health, 87*(5), 805–810.

*Koch, T., Kralik, D., & Taylor, J. (2000). Men living with diabetes: minimizing the intrusiveness of the disease. *Journal of Clinical Nursing, 9*(2), 247–254.

Lewis, K. S. (1998). Emotional adjustment to a chronic illness. *Lippincott's Primary Care Practice, 2*(1), 38–51.

*Martin, J. C., Engle, V. F., & Graney, M. J. (1999). Determinants of health-related hardiness among urban older African-American women with chronic illness. *Holistic Nursing Practice, 13*(3), 62–70.

*Michael, S. R. (1996). Integrating chronic illness into one's life: a phenomenological inquiry. *Journal of Holistic Nursing, 14*(3), 251–267.

Miller, M. (1999). Clinical sidebar. *Image: Journal of Nursing Scholarship, 31*(2), 125.

Mishel, M. H. (1999). Uncertainty in chronic illness. *Annual Review of Nursing Research, 17,* 269–294.

Newacheck, P. W., & Halfon, N. (1998). Prevalence and impact of disabling chronic conditions in childhood. *American Journal of Public Health, 88*(4), 610–617.

Nijhof, G. (1998). Heterogeneity in the interpretation of epilepsy. *Qualitative Health Research, 8*(1), 95–105.

Nodhturft, V., Schneider, J. M., Hebert, P. et al. (2000). Chronic disease self-management: improving health outcomes. *Nursing Clinics of North America, 35*(2), 507–518.

*Price, B. (1996). Illness careers: the chronic illness experience. *Journal of Advanced Nursing, 24*(2), 275–279.

Reeves, M. J., Remington, P. L., Nashold, R., & Pete, J. (1997). Chronic disease mortality among Wisconsin Native American Indians, 1984–1993. *Wisconsin Medical Journal, 96*(2), 27–32.

*Rehm, R. S. (1999). Religious faith in Mexican-American families dealing with chronic childhood illness. *Image: Journal of Nursing Scholarship, 31*(1), 33–38.

Sadowski, A. V., & Redeker, N. S. (1996). The hypertensive elder: a review for the primary care provider. *Nurse Practitioner, 21*(5), 105–112.

*Saiki-Craighill, S. (1997). The children's sentinels: mothers and their relationships with health professionals in the context of Japanese health care. *Social Science and Medicine, 44*(3), 291–300.

*Schlenk, E. A., Erlen, J. A., Dunbar-Jacob, J., McDowell, J., Engberg, S., Sereika, S. M., Rohay, J. M., & Bernier, M. J. (1998). Health-related quality of life in chronic disorders: a comparison across studies using the MOS SF-36. *Quality of Life Research, 7*(1), 57–65.

Sidell, N. L. (1997). Adult adjustment to chronic illness: a review of the literature. *Health and Social Work, 22*(1), 5–11.

Silber, J. H., Gleeson, S. P., & Zhao, H. (1999). The influence of chronic disease on resource utilization in common acute pediatric conditions. Financial concerns for children's hospitals. *Archives of Pediatrics and Adolescent Medicine, 153*(2), 169–179.

Soderberg, S., Lundman, B., & Norberg, A. (1999). Struggling for dignity: the meaning of women's experience of living with fibromyalgia. *Qualitative Health Research 9*(5), 575–587.

*Stuifbergen, A. K., & Rogers, S. (1997). Health promotion: an essential component of rehabilitation for people with chronic disabling conditions. *Advances in Nursing Science, 19*(4), 1–20.

*Tappan, R. M., Williams, C., Fishman, S., & Theris, T. (1999). Persistence of self in advanced Alzheimer's disease. *Image: Journal of Nursing Scholarship, 31*(2), 121–125.

*Thorne, S., McCormick, J., & Carty, E. (1997). Deconstructing the gender neutrality of chronic illness and disability. *Health Care Women International, 18*(1), 1–16.

Van den Akker, M., Buntinx, F., Metsemakers, J. F., Roos, S. L, & Knottnerus, J. A. (1988). Multimorbidity in general practice: prevalence, incidence, and determinants of disease. *Journal of Clinical Epidemiology, 51*(5), 367–375.

Warren-Boulton, E., Greenberg, R., Lising, M., & Gallivan, J. (1999). An update on primary care management of type 2 diabetes. *Nurse Practitioner, 24*(12), 14–24.

*Wichowski, H. C., & Kubsch, S. M. (1997). The relationship of self-perception of illness and compliance with health care regimens. *Journal of Advanced Nursing, 25*(3), 548–553.

*Wiener, C., & Dodd, M. J. (1993). Coping amid uncertainty: an illness trajectory perspective. *Scholarly Inquiry for Nursing Practice, 7*(1), 17–35.

Wing, R., Goldstein, M., Acton, K., Birch, L. Jakicic, J., Sallis Jr., J., Smith-West, D., Jeffery, R., & Surwit, R. (2001). Lifestyle changes related to obesity, eating behavior, and physical activity. *Diabetes Care, 24,* 117–123.

RESOURCES AND WEBSITES

ChronicNet: www.chronicnet.org/chronnet/project.htm. This website provides local and national data on chronic care issues and populations.

Robert Wood Johnson Foundation: http://www.rwjf.org. This website has information about health care in the United States, including proceedings of "Patient Education and Consumer Activation in Chronic Disease," July 7, 2000.

Principles and Practices of Rehabilitation

LEARNING OBJECTIVES ●

On completion of this chapter, the learner will be able to:

1. Describe the goals of rehabilitation.
2. Discuss the interdisciplinary approach to rehabilitation.
3. Identify emotional reactions exhibited by patients with disabilities.
4. Use the nursing process as a framework for care of patients with self-care deficits, impaired physical mobility, impaired skin integrity, and altered patterns of elimination.
5. Describe nursing strategies appropriate for promoting self-care through activities of daily living.
6. Describe nursing strategies appropriate for promoting mobility and ambulation and the use of assistive devices.
7. Describe risk factors and related nursing measures to prevent development of pressure ulcers.
8. Incorporate bladder training and bowel training into the plan of care for patients with bladder and bowel problems.
9. Describe the significance of continuity of care from the health care facility to the home or extended care facility for patients who need rehabilitative assistance and services.

*R*ehabilitation is a dynamic, health-oriented process that assists an ill person or a person with **disability** (restriction in performance or function in everyday activities) to achieve the greatest possible level of physical, mental, spiritual, social, and economic functioning. The rehabilitation process helps the patient achieve an acceptable quality of life with dignity, self-respect, and independence and is designed for people with physical, mental, or emotional disabilities. During rehabilitation—sometimes called habilitation—the patient adjusts to the disability by learning how to use resources and to focus on existing abilities. In **habilitation**, abilities, not disabilities, are emphasized.

Rehabilitation is an integral part of nursing because every major illness or injury carries the threat of disability or **impairment**, which involves a loss of function or an abnormality. The principles of rehabilitation are basic to the care of all patients, and rehabilitation efforts should begin during the initial contact with a patient. The goal of rehabilitation is to restore the patient's ability to function independently or at a preillness or preinjury level of functioning as quickly as possible. If this is not possible, the aims of rehabilitation are maximal independence and a quality of life acceptable to the patient. Realistic goals based on individual patient assessment are established with the patient to guide the rehabilitation program.

Rehabilitation services are required by more people than ever before because of advances in technology that save or prolong the lives of seriously ill, injured, and disabled patients. Increasing numbers of patients who are recovering from serious illnesses or injuries are returning to their homes and communities with ongoing needs. Every patient, regardless of age, gender, ethnic group, socioeconomic status, or diagnosis, has a right to rehabilitation services (Chart 11-1).

Approximately 1 in 5 Americans has some form of disability, and 1 in 10 has a severe disability (U.S. Census Bureau, 1997). A person is considered to have a disability, such as a restriction in performance or function in everyday activities, if he or she has difficulty talking, hearing, seeing, walking, climbing stairs, lifting or carrying objects, performing activities of daily living, doing school work, or working at a job. A severe disability is present if a person is unable to perform one or more activities, uses an assistive device for mobility, or needs help from another person to accomplish basic activities. Individuals are also considered severely disabled if they receive federal benefits based on an inability to work.

Approximately 54 million Americans are affected by some form of disability, and this number is expected to increase in the coming decades due to the aging of the population. More than half of

Chart 11-1 • Ethics and Related Issues

Are All Persons Entitled to Rehabilitation?

Situation
You work in an area where many illegal aliens and uninsured residents live. Community violence often creates life-threatening and disabling conditions in members of the population. After a victim of violence has been saved and stabilized, the health care team identifies rehabilitation needs. You are concerned about your patient's inability to perform self-care and to demonstrate safe mobility skills.

Dilemma
As a health care provider, you are concerned about the community as a whole; costs to the community, and the values of the community. You are also aware of client fiduciary responsibility; you recognize costs to your patient when treatment is provided or not provided.

Discussion
Who determines the length of stay and level of care? Who will take care of patients who need rehabilitation but who are unable to pay? Is rehabilitation a basic health care need?

persons with disability are women, and females with disability outnumber males in all age groups except for those 15 to 24 years old (Jans & Stoddard, 1999). One-third of women 75 years of age and older need personal assistance. Currently, more than 10 million people need personal assistance with one or more **activities of daily living (ADLs)**, which include bathing, dressing, feeding, and toileting, or **instrumental activities of daily living (IADLs)**, which include grocery shopping, meal preparation, housekeeping, transportation, and managing finances. About 5 million persons use a cane, more than 2 million use a wheelchair, and at least 1 million use crutches or a walker. Use of these devices and other types of **assistive technology** has increased dramatically due to the aging of the population, technological advances, public policy initiatives, and changes in the delivery and financing of health care (U.S. Census Bureau, 1997).

Americans With Disabilities Act

Among all people age 21 to 64 (the prime employable years), approximately 33% of individuals with a severe disability and 77% of those with a nonsevere disability are employed, compared with

Glossary

activities of daily living (ADLs): Self-care activities including bathing, grooming, dressing, eating, toileting, and bowel and bladder care.

assistive technology: Any item, piece of equipment, or product system—whether acquired commercially, off the shelf, modified, or customized—that is used to improve the functional capabilities of individuals with disabilities.

disability: Restriction or lack of ability to perform an activity in a normal manner; the consequences of impairment in terms of an

individual's functional performance and activity. Disabilities represent disturbances at the level of the person (eg, bathing, dressing, communication, walking, grooming).

habilitation: Making able; learning new skills and abilities to meet maximum potential.

impairment: Loss or abnormality of psychological, physiologic, or anatomic structure or function at the organ level (eg, dysphagia, hemiparesis); an abnormality of body structure, appearance, and organ or system function resulting from any cause.

instrumental activities of daily living (IADLs): Complex aspects of independence including meal preparation, grocery shopping, household management, finances, and transportation.

pressure ulcers: Breakdown of the skin due to prolonged pressure and insufficient blood supply, usually at boney prominences.

rehabilitation: Making able again; relearning skills or abilities or adjusting existing functions.

82% of nondisabled people. The employed person with disability, however, earns less money than the nondisabled person (U.S. Census, 1997). In 1990, the U.S. Congress passed the Americans With Disabilities Act (ADA) (PL 101-336), which constitutes civil rights legislation designed to permit those with disabilities access to job opportunities and to the community. As a result of this act, employers must evaluate an applicant's ability to perform the job and not discriminate on the basis of a disability. Employers must also make "reasonable accommodations," such as equipment or access ramps, to facilitate employment of a person with a disability. The ADA stipulates that communities must provide public transportation that is accessible to people with disabilities. Public facilities (eg, stores, restaurants, hotels) must be accessible and accommodate those with disabilities. Telecommunication providers must offer communication devices for the deaf. A higher quality of life for those with disabilities is an objective of the ADA.

Although the regulations took effect in July 1992, compliance has been slow because the reasonable accommodation "without undue hardship" provisions in the law permit businesses to continue with inaccessible conditions. All new construction and modifications of public facilities, however, must address access by people with disabilities.

Right to Access to Health Care and Health Promotion

For years, people with disabilities have been discriminated against in employment, public accommodations, and public and private services including health care. The needs of the disabled in health care settings produce many challenges to health care providers: how to communicate effectively if there are communication deficits, the additional physical demands for mobility, and time required to provide assistance with self-care routines during hospitalization. Physicians and nurses may not know the specific needs of individuals with disability and may fail to provide services for them. For example, an obstetrician may advise a woman with a spinal cord injury not to become pregnant because the physician lacks experience and knowledge in this area of care. The physician and nurses caring for an expectant woman with disability may not know specific transfer techniques to help her onto an examining table or how to advise her on bowel, bladder, and skin care issues during pregnancy. Before labor and delivery, the medical team needs to be educated about the special needs of a woman with a cervical spinal cord injury in regard to management of autonomic hyperreflexia. Often, the person with disability must educate the health care professionals.

Because of unfavorable interactions with health care providers, including negative attitudes, insensitivity, and lack of knowledge, people with disability may avoid seeking medical intervention or health promotion programs and activities. For this reason, and because the number of individuals with disability is increasing, nurses must acquire knowledge and skills and be accessible to assist these individuals in maintaining a high level of wellness.

Nurses are in key positions to influence the architectural design of health care settings and the selection of equipment that promotes ease of access and health. Padded examination tables that can be raised or lowered make transfers easier for the disabled. Birthing chairs benefit women with disability during yearly pelvic examinations and Pap smears and for urologic evaluations. Ramps, grab bars, and raised and padded toilet seats benefit many persons who have orthopedic disabilities and need routine phys-

ical examination and monitoring (eg, bone density measurements). Just as people without disability should have regular screening tests, such as mammography or testicular and prostate examinations, so should people with disability. The health care professionals who provide these screening and monitoring procedures are in a position to influence decisions about how equipment and procedures can be adapted to meet the special needs of their patients, whether these needs are cognitive, motor, or communicative.

Nurses can provide expert health promotion education classes that are targeted to the disabled. Classes on nutrition and weight management are extremely important to individuals who are wheelchair dependent and need assistance with transfers. Safe sex classes are needed by adolescents and young adults who have spinal cord or traumatic brain injury, because the threats of acquired immunodeficiency syndrome (AIDS) and unplanned pregnancy exist for these populations just as they do for the population in general. Other healthy behaviors about which neurologically disabled persons need education include avoiding alcohol and nonprescription medications while taking antispasmodic and antiseizure medications. Nurses should teach all stroke survivors and patients with diabetes how to monitor their own blood pressure or glucose levels. The warning signs and symptoms of stroke, heart attack, and cancer, as well as how to access help, should also be taught to all disabled persons.

As active members of society, people with disabilities are no longer an invisible minority. An increased awareness of the needs of people with disabilities will bring about changes to improve their access and accommodate their needs. Modification of the physical environment permits access to public and private facilities and services, including health care, and nurses can serve as advocates for the disabled to eliminate discriminatory practices.

Focus of Rehabilitation

Disability can occur at any age and may result from an acute incident, such as stroke or trauma, or from the progression of a chronic condition, such as arthritis or multiple sclerosis. A person with disability experiences many losses, including loss of function, independence, social role, status, and income. A patient and his or her family members experience a range of emotional reactions to these losses. The reactions may progress from disorganization and confusion to denial of the disability, grief over the lost function or body part, depression, anger, and, finally, acceptance of the disability. The reactions may subside over time and may recur at a later time, especially if chronic illness is progressive and results in increasing losses. Not all patients experience all of the stages, although most do exhibit grief. Patients who exhibit grief should not be blithely encouraged to "cheer up." The nurse should show a willingness to listen to the patient talk about the disability and should understand that grief, anger, regret, and resentment are all part of the healing process. See the accompanying Gerontologic Considerations box for concerns unique to older adults.

The patient's preexisting coping abilities play an important role in the adaptation process: one patient may be particularly independent and determined, while another may be dependent and seem to lack personal power. One goal of rehabilitation is to help the patient gain a positive self-image through effective coping. The nurse must recognize different coping abilities and identify when the patient is not coping well or not adjusting to the disability (Nursing Research Profile 11-1). The patient and family may benefit from participating in a support group or talking

Gerontologic Considerations
Concerns of Older Adults Facing Disability

- Loss of independence, which is a source of self-respect and dignity
- Increased potential for discrimination or abuse
- Increased social isolation
- Added burden on spouse who may also have impaired health
- Less access to community services and health care
- Less access to religious institutions
- Increased vulnerability to declining health secondary to other disorders, reduced physiologic reserve, or preexisting impairments of mobility and balance
- Fears and doubts about ability to learn or relearn self-care activities, exercises, and transfer and independent mobility techniques
- Inadequate support system for successful rehabilitation

with a mental health professional to achieve this goal. Refer to Chapter 6 for a detailed discussion of adaptive and maladaptive responses to illness.

The Rehabilitation Team

Rehabilitation is a creative, dynamic process that requires a team of professionals working together with the patient and the family. The team members represent a variety of disciplines, with each health professional making a unique contribution. Each health professional assesses the patient and identifies patient needs within the discipline's domain. Rehabilitative goals are set. Each health professional assesses the patient, identifies patient needs within the discipline's domain, and sets rehabilitative goals. Team members hold group sessions at frequent intervals to collaborate, evaluate progress, and modify goals as needed to facilitate rehabilitation and to promote independence, self-respect, and an acceptable quality of life for the patient.

The patient is the key member of the rehabilitation team. He or she is the focus of the team effort and the one who determines the final outcomes of the process. The patient participates in goal setting, in learning to function using remaining abilities, and in adjusting to living with disabilities.

The patient's family is also incorporated into the team. The family is a dynamic system, so disability of one member affects the other family members. Only by incorporating the family into the rehabilitation process can the family system adapt to the change in one of its members. The family provides ongoing support, participates in problem solving, and learns to provide necessary ongoing care (Nursing Research Profile 11-2).

The rehabilitation nurse develops a therapeutic and supportive relationship with the patient and the family. The nurse always emphasizes the patient's assets and strengths, positively reinforcing his or her efforts to improve self-concept and self-care abilities. During nurse–patient interactions, the nurse actively listens, encourages, and shares the patient's successes.

Using the nursing process, the nurse develops a plan of care designed to facilitate rehabilitation, restore and maintain optimum health, and prevent complications. The nurse helps the patient identify strengths and past successes and develop new goals. Coping with the disability, self-care, mobility, skin care, and bowel and bladder management are frequently areas for nursing intervention. The nurse assumes the roles of caregiver, teacher, counselor, patient advocate, and consultant. The nurse is often the case manager responsible for coordinating the total rehabili-

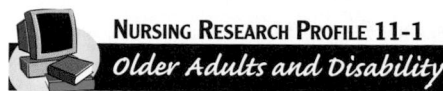
NURSING RESEARCH PROFILE 11-1
Older Adults and Disability

Cataldo, J. (2001). The relationship of hardiness and depression to disability in institutionalized older adults. *Rehabilitation Nursing 26*(1), 28–33.

Purpose
Depression has been linked with disability in several studies of older adults. Hardiness is a personality characteristic that is a buffer in the stress and depression dynamic and increases a person's capability of having a positive psychological reaction to a stressor. Hardiness only partially explains the variance of depression since the hardiest of individuals may become depressed. This study tested two hypotheses: (1) After accounting for the effects of physiologic factors (physical status and length of stay [LOS]), hardiness will significantly contribute to the explanation of disability in a sample of institutionalized elderly people; (2) after accounting for the effects of physical health status, LOS, and hardiness, depression will significantly contribute to the explanation of disability in a sample of institutionalized older people.

Study Sample and Design
A culturally diverse group of 33 women and 25 men ranging in age from 60 to 93 years participated in a 45-minute interview. Hardiness was measured with the Health-Related Hardiness Scale (HRHS) which had 34 items on a 6-point Likert-type scale. The instrument had two dimensions: commitment/challenge and control. High scores indicated higher hardiness. Depression was measured with the Zung Self-Rating Depression Scale (ZSDS), a 22-item screening inventory. High scores indicated a high level of depressive symptomatology. Physical health status was measured with the Clinical Response Scale (CRS), a 56-item generic health index. The items were scored using data from the participants' medical records in a 1-month period. Higher scores indicated worsened health status. LOS data were collected from the facility's computerized system with day of admission being day 1. Disability was measured by the Barthel Activities of Daily Living Index, which had 10 variables related to self-care and mobility. A high score indicated independence, and a low score indicated disability.

Findings
Both hypotheses were supported. The psychological variables of hardiness and depression contributed more than did health status and LOS to explain disability in a sample of elderly nursing home residents. LOS and physical health status accounted for 14.7% of the variance in disability. Hardiness explained 10.5% of the variance, and depression accounted for an additional 7.4% of the variance in disability.

Nursing Implications
Nurses need to guide older persons with disability to develop hardiness. Nurses can encourage them to view the disability as a challenge and to make a commitment to life. The nurse can assist older individuals with disability to take control of their life circumstances (ie, become actively involved in pain management and all daily decision making). Because the level of disability is not exclusively the result of physiologic factors, the nurse should suggest treatment of depression in the older adult with disability.

tative plan, collaborating with and coordinating the services provided by all members of the health care team, including the home care nurse, who is responsible for directing the patient's care after return to the home.

Other members of the rehabilitation team may include a physician, nurse practitioner, physiatrist, physical therapist, occupational therapist, speech-language therapist, psychologist, psychiatric liaison nurse, social worker, vocational counselor,

NURSING RESEARCH PROFILE 11-2
Caregivers

Secrest, J. (2000). Transformation of the relationship: The experience of primary support persons of stroke survivors. *Rehabilitation Nursing* 25(3), 93–99.

Purpose
Most stroke survivors live at home. Effective rehabilitation must include the primary support person (PSP). Nurses teach and counsel the PSP during acute hospitalization, during the rehabilitation phase, and in the home. Understanding the experience of stroke from the PSP's perspective can help nurses design effective interventions for the PSP. The purpose of this study was to investigate the quality, or nature, of life experienced by PSPs of stroke survivors.

Study Sample and Design
The study sample consisted of 8 women and 2 men between the ages of 40 to 72 years. Criteria for inclusion in the study were that (1) the participant was the PSP of a stroke survivor whose stroke occurred at least 6 months previously, and who had completed inpatient rehabilitation and was living at home and (2) the participant was willing and able to articulate the experience. The study design sought to attain a first-person description of the PSP experience. The single interview item was, "Please describe specific experiences you've had since your [significant other's] stroke that stands out for you." The researchers "bracketed" or identified potential biases about the phenomenon being studied so that they would not unduly influence the course of the study. The interview was transcribed verbatim and analyzed by members of the research group.

Findings
Participants rarely spoke of themselves as individuals. Experiences described were in relation to others. They expressed concern about being able to sustain their role over time. Time permeated the interviews: the length of time the couples had been married; changes in the stroke survivor's perception of time; and memory as it is of past time. Memory loss in the stroke survivor was perceived as a loss of an important aspect of the relationship. Other themes emerged. Life was perceived by the PSPs as being fragile. They experienced vigilance as they watched over the stroke victim. The PSP's vigilance did not diminish over time because they were aware of life's fragility and had an increased responsibility in the relationship. A weighty responsibility and a sense of loss were recurrent throughout the transcripts. All participants described the experience of a transformed relationship. The quality was different, but all of the relationships remained intact.

Nursing Implications
Nurses need to assess the pre-stroke relationship of the patient and PSP in order to prepare the PSP for the future. This will enable the nurse to negotiate goals, teach, and counsel the PSP more effectively. Attendance at support groups specifically for the PSP should be encouraged. Nurses are key individuals to organize and maintain support groups. PSPs need permission to focus on themselves, grieve their losses, and find support for their added responsibilities.

orthotist or prosthetist, rehabilitation engineer, and sex counselor or therapist.

Areas of Specialty Practice

Although rehabilitation is a component of every patient's care, there are specialty rehabilitation programs established in general hospitals, free-standing rehabilitation hospitals, and outpatient facilities. The Commission for the Accreditation of Rehabilitation Facilities (CARF) sets standards for these programs and monitors compliance with them.

Specialty rehabilitation programs often meet the needs of patients with neurologic disabilities. Stroke recovery programs and traumatic brain injury rehabilitation emphasize cognitive remediation: assisting patients to compensate for memory, perceptual, judgment, and safety deficits as well as teaching self-care and mobility skills. Other goals include assisting patients to swallow food safely and to communicate effectively. In addition to stroke and brain injury, other neurologic disorders treated include multiple sclerosis, Parkinson's disease, amyotrophic lateral sclerosis, and nervous system tumors.

The number of spinal cord injury rehabilitation programs has increased since World War II. Integral components of the programs include understanding the effects and complications of spinal cord injury; neurogenic bowel and bladder management; sexuality and male fertility enhancement; self-care, including prevention of skin breakdown; bed mobility and transfers; and driving with adaptive equipment. The programs also focus on vocational assessment, training, and reentry into employment and the community.

Orthopedic rehabilitation programs provide comprehensive services to traumatic or nontraumatic amputee patients, patients undergoing joint replacements, and patients with arthritis. Learning to be independent with a prosthesis or a new joint is a major goal of the program. Pain management, energy conservation, and joint protection are other goals.

For patients who have had myocardial infarction, cardiac rehabilitation begins during the acute hospitalization and continues on an outpatient basis. Emphasis is placed on monitored, progressive exercise; nutritional counseling; stress management; and sexuality.

Patients with restrictive or chronic obstructive pulmonary disease or ventilator dependency may be admitted to pulmonary rehabilitation programs. Respiratory therapists help the patient achieve more effective breathing patterns. The programs also teach energy conservation techniques, self-medication, and home ventilatory management.

Comprehensive pain management programs are available for sufferers of chronic pain, especially low back pain. These programs focus on alternative pain treatment modalities, exercise, supportive counseling, and vocational evaluation.

A comprehensive burn rehabilitation program may serve as a step-down unit from an intensive care burn unit. Although rehabilitation strategies are implemented immediately in acute care, a program focused on progressive joint mobility, self-care, and ongoing counseling is imperative for the burn patient.

Children are not exempt from the need for specialized rehabilitation. Pediatric rehabilitation programs meet the needs of children with developmental and acquired disabilities, including cerebral palsy, spina bifida, traumatic brain injuries, and spinal cord injuries.

As in all areas of nursing practice, nurses practicing in the area of rehabilitation must be skilled and knowledgeable about care of patients with substance abuse. For all individuals with disability, including adolescents, the nurse must assess actual or potential substance abuse. Almost 15 million Americans use illicit drugs; approximately 58 million engage in binge or heavy drinking of alcohol; and about 30% of the population uses nicotine products. Parental alcoholism is one of the strongest predictors of substance abuse. Alcohol abuse rates for people with disability may be twice as high as the general population. Forty to eighty percent of spinal cord injuries are related to substance abuse, and 40% to 80% of all traumatic brain injured patients are intoxicated at the time of injury (U.S. Department of Health and Human Services, 2000).

Substance abuse is a critical issue in rehabilitation, especially for disabled individuals who are attempting to gain employment via vocational rehabilitation. Treatment for alcoholism and drug dependencies includes a thorough physical and psychosocial evaluation; detoxification; counseling; medical treatment; psychological assistance for the patient and family; treatment of any coexisting psychiatric illness; and referral to community resources for social, legal, spiritual, or vocational assistance. Length of treatment and the rehabilitation process depends on the individual's needs. Self-help groups are also encouraged, although attendance in such groups (eg, Alcoholics Anonymous, Narcotics Anonymous) poses various challenges for the person who has neurologic deficits, is confined to a wheelchair, or must adapt to encounters with able-bodied attendees who may not understand disability. All specialty areas of rehabilitation require implementation of the nursing process as described in this chapter.

Assessment of Functional Abilities

Comprehensive assessment of functional capacity is the basis for developing a rehabilitation program. Functional capacity measures a person's ability to perform activities of ADLs and IADLs. ADLs include activities performed to meet basic needs, such as personal hygiene, dressing, toileting, eating, and moving. IADLs include activities that are necessary for independent living, such as the ability to shop for and prepare meals, use the telephone, clean, manage finances, and travel.

The nurse observes the patient performing specific activities (eg, eating, dressing) and notes the degree of independence; the time taken; the patient's mobility, coordination, and endurance; and the amount of assistance required. Good joint motion, muscle strength, cardiovascular reserve, and an intact neurologic system are also carefully assessed, because functional ability depends on these factors as well. Observations are recorded on a functional assessment tool. These tools provide a way to standardize assessment parameters and supply a scale or score against which improvements may be measured. They also clearly communicate the patient's level of functioning to all members of the rehabilitation team. Rehabilitation staff use these tools to provide an initial assessment of the patient's abilities and to monitor the patient's progress in independence.

One of the most frequently used tools to assess the patient's level of independence is the Functional Independence Measure (FIM). The FIM is a minimum data set, measuring 18 items. The self-care items measured are eating, bathing, grooming, dressing upper body, dressing lower body, toileting, bladder management, and bowel management. The FIM addresses transfers and the ability to ambulate and climb stairs and also includes communication and social cognition items. A WeeFIM instrument is used for children. For both children and adults, scoring is based on a seven-point scale with items used to assess the patient's level of independence.

The PULSES profile is used to assess physical condition (eg, health/illness status), upper extremity functions (eg, eating, bathing), lower extremity functions (eg, transfer, ambulation), sensory function (eg, vision, hearing, speech), excretory function (ie, control of bowel or bladder), and situational factors (eg, social and financial support). Each of these areas is rated on a scale from one (independent) to four (greatest dependency).

The Barthel Index is used to measure the patient's level of independence in ADLs (feeding, bathing, dressing, grooming), continence, toileting, transfers, and ambulation (or wheelchair mobility). This scale does not address communicative or cognitive abilities.

The Patient Evaluation Conference System (PECS) contains 15 categories. This comprehensive assessment scale includes such areas as medications, pain, nutrition, use of assistive devices, psychological status, vocation, and recreation. There are many other assessment tools designed to evaluate function in persons with specific disabling conditions.

In addition to the detailed functional assessment, the nurse assesses the patient's physical, mental, emotional, spiritual, social, and economic status. Secondary problems related to the disability, such as muscle atrophy and deconditioning, are assessed, as are residual strengths unaffected by disease or disability. Other areas that require nursing assessment include potential for altered skin integrity, altered bowel and bladder control, and sexual dysfunction.

NURSING PROCESS: THE PATIENT WITH SELF-CARE DEFICITS IN ACTIVITIES OF DAILY LIVING

ADLs are those self-care activities that the patient must accomplish each day to meet personal needs. ADLs include personal hygiene/bathing, dressing/grooming, feeding, and toileting. Many patients are unable to perform such activities easily. An ADL program is started as soon as the rehabilitation process begins, because the ability to perform ADLs is frequently the key to independence, return to the home, and reentry into the community.

Assessment

The nurse must observe and assess the patient's ability to perform ADLs to determine the level of independence in self-care and the need for nursing intervention. The activity of bathing requires obtaining bath water and utensils, washing, and drying the body after bathing. Dressing requires getting clothes from the closet, putting on and taking off clothing, and fastening the clothing. Self-feeding requires using utensils to bring food to the mouth, and chewing and swallowing the food. The activity of toileting includes removing clothing to use the toilet, cleansing oneself, and readjusting clothing. Grooming activities include combing hair, brushing teeth, shaving or applying makeup, and washing the hands. Patients who can sit up and raise their hands to their head can begin self-care activities.

In addition, the nurse needs to be aware of the patient's medical conditions, the effect that they have on the ability to perform ADLs, and the family's involvement in the patient's ADLs. This information is valuable in setting goals and developing the plan of care to maximize self-care.

Nursing Diagnosis

Based on the assessment data, major nursing diagnoses for the patient may include the following:

- Self-care deficit: bathing/hygiene, dressing/grooming, feeding, toileting

Planning and Goals

The major goals of the patient include bathing/hygiene independently or with assistance, using adaptive devices as appropriate; dressing/grooming independently or with assistance, using adaptive devices as appropriate; feeding independently or with assistance, using adaptive devices as appropriate; and toileting independently or with assistance, using adaptive devices as appropriate. Another goal is that the patient with a self-care deficit expresses satisfaction with the extent of independence in self-care activities.

Nursing Interventions

FOSTERING SELF-CARE ABILITIES

To learn methods of self-care effectively, the patient must be motivated. An "I'd rather do it myself" attitude is encouraged. The nurse must also help the patient identify the safe limits of independent activity; knowing when to ask for assistance is particularly important.

The nurse teaches, guides, and supports the patient who is learning or relearning how to perform self-care activities. Consistency in instructions and assistance given by health care providers facilitates the learning process. Recording the patient's performance provides data for evaluating progress and may be used as a source for motivation and morale building (Chart 11-2).

Often, a simple maneuver requires concentration and the exertion of considerable effort on the part of the patient with a disability; therefore, self-care techniques need to be adapted to accommodate the individual patient's lifestyle. There is usually more than one way to accomplish a self-care activity, so common sense and a little ingenuity may promote increased independence. For example, a person who cannot quite reach his or her head may be able to do so by leaning forward. Encouraging the patient to participate in a support group may also help the patient to discover inventive or creative solutions to self-care problems.

RECOMMENDING ASSISTIVE DEVICES

If the patient has difficulty in performing an ADL, an adaptive or assistive device (self-help device) may be useful. A large vari-

ety of assistive devices are available commercially or can be fabricated by the nurse, the occupational therapist, the patient, or the family. The nurse should be alert to "gadgets" coming on the market and evaluate their potential for usefulness. Of course, the nurse must exercise professional judgment and caution in recommending devices, because unscrupulous vendors have marketed unnecessary, overly expensive, or useless items to patients in the past.

A wide selection of computerized assistive devices is available, or devices can be designed to help individual patients with severe disabilities to function more independently. The ABLE-DATA project (see Resources list) offers a computerized listing of commercially available aids and equipment for patients with disabilities.

HELPING THE PATIENT ACCEPT LIMITATIONS

If the patient has a severe disability, independent self-care may be an unrealistic goal; in this situation, the rehabilitation nurse teaches the patient how to direct his or her own care. The patient may require a personal attendant to perform ADLs. Family members may not be appropriate for providing bathing/hygiene, dressing/grooming, feeding, and toileting assistance, and a spouse may have difficulty providing bowel and bladder care for the patient and maintaining the role of sexual partner. If a personal caregiver is needed, the disabled person or family members must learn how to manage an employee effectively. The nurse assists the patient in accepting self-care dependency. Independence in other areas, such as social interaction, should be emphasized to promote positive self-concept.

Evaluation

EXPECTED PATIENT OUTCOMES

Expected patient outcomes may include:

1. Demonstrates independent self-care in bathing/hygiene or with assistance, using adaptive devices as appropriate
   a. Bathes self at maximal level of independence
   b. Uses adaptive devices effectively
   c. Reports satisfaction with level of independence in bathing/hygiene
2. Demonstrates independent self-care in dressing/grooming or with assistance, using adaptive devices as appropriate
   a. Dresses/grooms self at maximal level of independence
   b. Uses adaptive devices effectively
   c. Reports satisfaction with level of independence in dressing/grooming
   d. Demonstrates increased interest in appearance
3. Demonstrates independent self-care in feeding or with assistance, using adaptive and assistive devices as appropriate
   a. Feeds self at maximal level of independence
   b. Uses adaptive and assistive devices effectively
   c. Demonstrates increased interest in eating
   d. Maintains adequate nutritional intake
4. Demonstrates independent self-care in toileting or with assistance, using adaptive and assistive devices as appropriate
   a. Toilets self at maximal level of independence
   b. Uses adaptive and assistive devices effectively
   c. Indicates positive feelings regarding level of toileting independence
   d. Experiences adequate frequency of bowel and bladder elimination
   e. Does not experience incontinence, constipation, urinary tract infection, or other complications

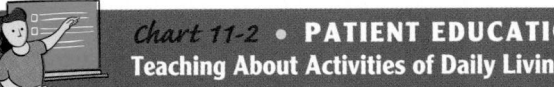

Chart 11-2 • PATIENT EDUCATION
Teaching About Activities of Daily Living

1. Define the goal of the activity with the patient. Be realistic. Set short-term goals that can be accomplished in the near future.
2. Identify several approaches to accomplish the task (eg, there are several ways to put on a given garment).
3. Select the approach most likely to succeed.
4. Specify the approach on the patient's care plan and the patient's level of accomplishment on the progress notes.
5. Identify the motions necessary to accomplish the activity (eg, to pick up a glass, extend arm with hand open; place open hand next to glass; flex fingers around glass; move arm and hand holding glass vertically; flex arm toward body).
6. Focus on gross functional movements initially, and gradually include activities that use finer motions (eg, buttoning clothes, eating with a fork).
7. Encourage the patient to perform the activity up to maximal capacity within the limitations of the disability.
8. Monitor the patient's tolerance.
9. Minimize frustration and fatigue.
10. Support the patient by giving appropriate praise for effort put forth and for acts accomplished.
11. Assist the patient to perform and practice the activity in real-life situations.

NURSING PROCESS: THE PATIENT WITH IMPAIRED PHYSICAL MOBILITY

Patients who are ill or injured are frequently placed on bed rest or have their activities limited. Problems commonly associated with immobility include weakened muscles, joint contracture, and deformity. Each joint of the body has a normal range of motion; if the range is limited, the functions of the joint and of the muscles that move the joint are impaired, and painful deformities may develop. Nurses must identify patients at risk for such complications.

Another problem frequently seen in rehabilitation nursing is an altered ambulatory/mobility pattern. The patient with a disability may be either temporarily or permanently unable to walk independently and unaided. The nurse assesses the mobility of the patient and designs care that promotes independent mobility within the prescribed therapeutic limits.

If a person is not able to exercise and move the joints through their full range of motion, contractures may develop. A contracture is a shortening of the muscle and tendon that leads to deformity and limits joint mobility. When the contracted joint is moved, the patient experiences pain; in addition, more energy is required to move when joints are contracted and deformed.

Assessment

At times, a patient's mobility is restricted because of pain, paralysis, loss of muscle strength, systemic disease, an immobilizing device (eg, cast, brace), or prescribed limits to promote healing. Assessment of the patient's mobility includes positioning, ability to move, muscle strength and tone, joint function, and the prescribed mobility limits. The nurse may need to collaborate with the physical therapist or other team members to assess mobility.

During position change, transfer, and ambulation activities, the nurse assesses the patient's abilities, the extent of disability, and residual capacity for physiologic adaptation. The nurse observes for orthostatic hypotension, pallor, diaphoresis, nausea, tachycardia, and fatigue.

If a patient is not able to ambulate without assistance, the nurse assesses ability to balance, transfer, and use assistive devices (eg, crutches, walker). Crutch walking requires a high energy expenditure and produces considerable cardiovascular stress, so older people with reduced exercise capacity, decreased arm strength, and problems with balance because of old age and multiple diseases may be unable to use them. A walker is more stable and may be a better choice for such patients. The nurse assesses the patient's ability to use various devices that promote mobility. If a patient uses an orthosis, an external appliance that provides support, prevents or corrects deformities, and improves function, the nurse monitors the patient for effective use and potential problems associated with its use.

Nursing Diagnosis

Based on the assessment data, major nursing diagnoses for the patient may include the following:

- Impaired physical mobility
- Activity intolerance
- Risk for injury
- Risk for disuse syndrome
- Impaired walking
- Impaired wheelchair mobility
- Impaired bed mobility

Planning and Goals

The major goals of the patient may include absence of contracture and deformity, maintenance of muscle strength and joint mobility, independent mobility, and increased activity tolerance.

Nursing Interventions

POSITIONING TO PREVENT MUSCULOSKELETAL COMPLICATIONS

Deformities and contractures can often be prevented by proper positioning. Maintaining correct body alignment when the patient is in bed is essential regardless of the position selected. During each contact with the patient, the nurse evaluates the patient's position and assists the patient to achieve proper positioning and alignment. The most common positions that a patient assumes in bed are supine (dorsal), side-lying (lateral), and prone. The nurse helps the patient assume these positions and supports the body in correct alignment with pillows (Chart 11-3). At times, a splint (eg, wrist or hand splint) may be fabricated by the occupational therapist to support a joint and prevent deformity. The nurse must ensure proper use of the splint and provide skin care.

Preventing External Rotation of the Hip

Patients who are in bed for any period of time may develop external rotation deformity of the hip because the ball-and-socket joint of the hip has a tendency to rotate outward when the patient lies on his or her back. A trochanter roll extending from the crest of the ilium to the midthigh prevents this deformity; with correct placement, it serves as a mechanical wedge under the projection of the greater trochanter.

Preventing Footdrop

Footdrop is a deformity in which the foot is plantar flexed (the ankle bends in the direction of the sole of the foot). If the condition continues without correction, the patient will not be able to hold the foot in a normal position and will be able to walk only on his or her toes, without touching the ground with the heel of the foot. The deformity is caused by contracture of both the gastrocnemius and soleus muscles. Damage to the peroneal nerve or loss of flexibility of the Achilles tendon may result in footdrop.

 NURSING ALERT Prolonged bed rest, lack of exercise, incorrect positioning in bed, and the weight of bedding that forces the toes into plantar flexion are factors that contribute to footdrop.

To prevent this disabling deformity, the patient is positioned to sit at 90 degrees in a wheelchair with feet on the footrests or flat on the floor. When the patient is supine in bed, padded splints or protective boots are used to keep the feet at right angles to the legs. Frequent skin inspection of the feet must also be performed to determine whether positioning devices have created any unwanted pressure areas.

The patient is encouraged to perform the following ankle exercises several times each hour: dorsiflexion and plantar flexion of the feet, flexion and extension (curl and stretch) of the toes, and eversion and inversion of the feet at the ankles. The nurse provides frequent passive range-of-motion exercises if the patient is unable to perform active exercises.

MAINTAINING MUSCLE STRENGTH AND JOINT MOBILITY

Optimal function depends on the strength of the muscles and joint motion, and active participation in ADLs promotes main-

Chart 11-3 **Positioning a Patient in Bed**

Supine (Dorsal) Position

1. Align the head with the spine, both laterally and anteroposteriorly.
2. Position the trunk to minimize hip flexion.
3. Flex the arms at the elbow and rest the hands against the lateral abdomen.
4. Extend the legs with a small, firm support under the popliteal area.
5. Support the heels off the mattress with a small pillow or towel roll at the ankles.
6. Point the toes straight up using protective boots to prevent footdrop.
7. Place trochanter rolls under the greater trochanters to prevent external rotation of the hip.

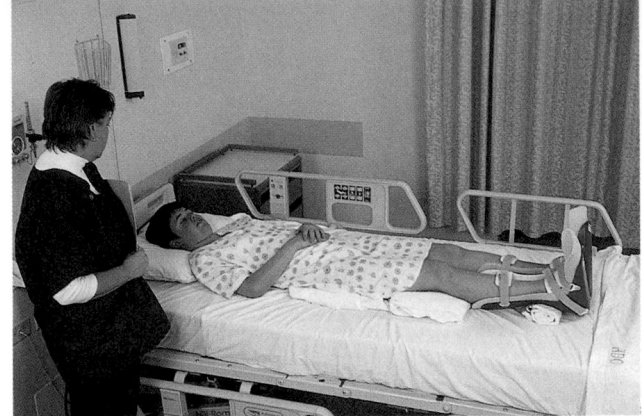

Side-Lying (Lateral Position)

1. Align the head with the spine, and support it with a pillow.
2. Properly align the body; avoid twisting at the shoulders, waist, or hips.
3. Flex shoulders and elbows and support the upper arm with a pillow.
4. Position the uppermost hip joint slightly forward and support the leg in a position of slight abduction by a pillow.
5. Place and support the feet in neutral dorsiflexion.
6. Support the back with a pillow.

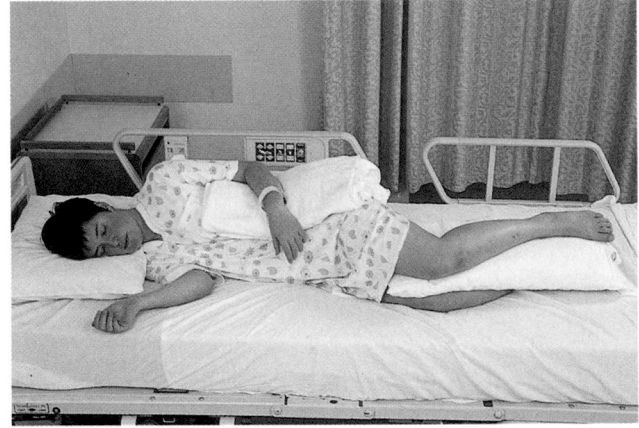

Prone (on Abdomen) Position

1. Turn the head laterally and align it with the rest of the body.
2. Abduct and externally rotate the arms at the shoulder joint; flex the elbows.
3. Place a small, flat support under the pelvis, extending from the level of the umbilicus to the upper third of the thigh.
4. Maintain the lower extremities in a neutral position.
5. Suspend the toes over the edge of the mattress.

Note: Side rails of bed are down for photographic purposes; they should remain raised if the patient is at risk for falling.

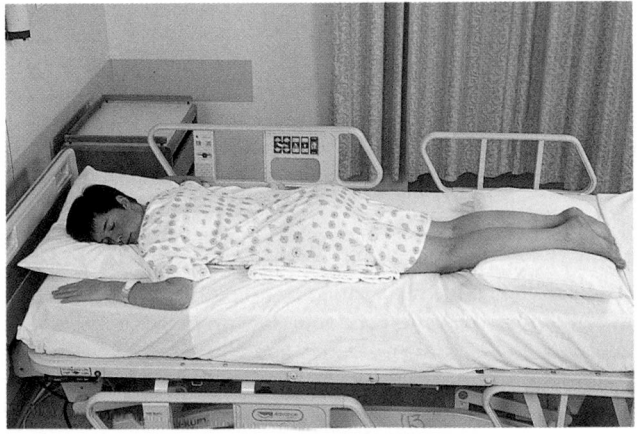

tenance of muscle strength and joint mobility. Range-of-motion exercises and specific therapeutic exercises may be included in the nursing plan of care.

Performing Range-of-Motion Exercises

Range of motion is movement of a joint through its full range in all appropriate planes (Chart 11-4). To maintain or increase the motion of a joint, range-of-motion exercises are initiated as soon as the patient's condition permits. The exercises are planned for the individual to accommodate the wide variation in the degrees of motion that people of varying body builds and age groups can attain (Chart 11-5).

Range-of-motion exercises may be active (performed by the patient under supervision of the nurse), assisted (with the nurse helping if the patient is unable to do the exercise independently), or passive (performed by the nurse). Unless prescribed otherwise, a joint should be moved through its range of motion three times, at least twice a day. The joint to be exercised is supported, the

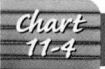

Chart 11-4 **Range-of-Motion Terminology**

Abduction: movement away from the midline of the body

Adduction: movement toward the midline of the body

Flexion: bending of a joint so that the angle of the joint diminishes

Extension: the return movement from flexion; the joint angle is increased

Rotation: turning or movement of a part around its axis

Internal: turning inward, toward the center

External: turning outward, away from the center

Dorsiflexion: movement that flexes or bends the hand back toward the body or the foot toward the leg

Palmar flexion: movement that flexes or bends the hand in the direction of the palm

Plantar flexion: movement that flexes or bends the foot in the direction of the sole

Pronation: rotation of the forearm so that the palm of the hand is down

Supination: rotation of the forearm so that the palm of the hand is up

Opposition: touching the thumb to each fingertip on same hand

Inversion: movement that turns the sole of the foot inward

Eversion: movement that turns the sole of the foot outward

bones above the joint are stabilized, and the body part distal to the joint is moved through the range of motion of the joint. For example, the humerus must be stabilized while the radius and ulna are moved through their range of motion at the elbow joint.

The joint should not be moved beyond its free range of motion; the joint is moved to the point of resistance and stopped at the point of pain. If muscle spasms are present, the joint is moved slowly to the point of resistance. Gentle, steady pressure is then applied until the muscle relaxes, and the motion is continued to the joint's final point of resistance.

To perform assisted or passive range-of-motion exercises, the patient must be in a comfortable supine position with arms at the sides and knees extended. Good body posture is maintained during the exercises. The nurse also uses good body mechanics during the exercise session.

Performing Therapeutic Exercises

Therapeutic exercises are prescribed by the physician and performed with the assistance and guidance of a physical therapist or nurse. Research is also underway to develop computerized robots with gentle, compliant behavior that could be used in the home setting for upper-extremity exercises (Krebs, 2000).

The patient should have a clear understanding of the goal of the prescribed exercise. Written instructions about the frequency, duration, and number of repetitions, as well as simple line drawings of the exercise, help to ensure adherence to the exercise program.

Exercise, when performed correctly, assists in maintaining and building muscle strength, maintaining joint function, preventing deformity, stimulating circulation, developing endurance, and promoting relaxation. Exercise is also valuable in helping to restore motivation and the well-being of the patient. Weight-bearing exercises may slow the bone loss that occurs with disability. There are five types of exercise: passive, active-assistive, active, resistive, and isometric. The description, purpose, and action of each of these exercises are summarized in Table 11-1.

PROMOTING INDEPENDENT MOBILITY

When the patient's condition stabilizes and the physical condition permits, the patient is assisted to sit up on the side of the bed and then to stand. The patient's tolerance of this activity is assessed. Orthostatic (postural) hypotension may develop when the patient assumes a vertical position. Because of inadequate vasomotor reflexes, blood pools in the splanchnic (visceral) area and in the legs, resulting in inadequate cerebral circulation. If indicators of orthostatic hypotension (eg, drop in blood pressure, pallor, diaphoresis, nausea, tachycardia, dizziness) are present, the activity is stopped, and the patient is assisted to a supine position in bed.

Some disabilities, such as spinal cord injury, acute brain injury, and other conditions that require extended periods in the recumbent position, prevent patients from assuming an upright position at the bedside. Several strategies can be used to assist a patient to assume a 90-degree sitting position. First, a reclining wheelchair with elevating leg rests allows a slow and controlled progression from a supine position to a 90-degree sitting position. A tilt table, a board that can be tilted in 5- to 10-degree increments from a horizontal to a vertical position, may also be used. The tilt table promotes vasomotor adjustment to positional changes and helps the patient with limited standing balance and limited weight-bearing activities to avoid the decalcification of bones and low bone mass associated with disuse syndrome and lack of weight-bearing exercise.

Elastic compression stockings are used to prevent venous stasis. For some patients, a compression garment (leotard) or snug-fitting abdominal binder and elastic compression bandaging of the legs are needed to prevent venous stasis and ensuing orthostatic hypotension. When the patient is standing, the feet are protected with a pair of properly fitted shoes. Extended periods of standing are avoided because of venous pooling and pressure on the soles of the feet. The nurse monitors the patient's blood pressure and pulse and observes for signs of orthostatic hypotension and cerebral insufficiency (eg, the patient reports feeling faint and weak), which suggest intolerance of the upright position. If the patient does not tolerate the upright position, the nurse should recline the patient and elevate the patient's legs.

Assisting the Patient With Transfer

A transfer is movement of the patient from one place to another (eg, bed to chair, chair to commode, wheelchair to tub). As soon as the patient is permitted out of bed, transfer activities are started. The nurse assesses the patient's ability to participate actively in the transfer and determines in conjunction with an occupational therapist or physical therapist the required adaptive equipment to promote independence and safety. A lightweight wheelchair with brake extensions, removable and detachable arm rests, and leg rests minimizes structural obstacles during the transfer. Tub seats or benches make transfers in and out of tubs easier and safer. Raised, padded commode seats may also be warranted for patients who must avoid flexing the hips greater than 90 degrees when transferring to a toilet.

It is important that the patient maintain muscle strength and, if possible, perform push-up exercises to strengthen the arm and shoulder extensor muscles. The push-up exercise requires the patient to sit upright in bed; a book is placed under each of the patient's hands to provide a hard surface, and the patient is instructed to push down on the book raising, the body. The nurse should encourage the patient to raise and move the body in different directions by means of these push-up exercises.

The nurse or physical therapist teaches the patient how to transfer. There are several methods of transferring from the bed to the

Chart 11-5   **Performing Range-of-Motion Exercises**

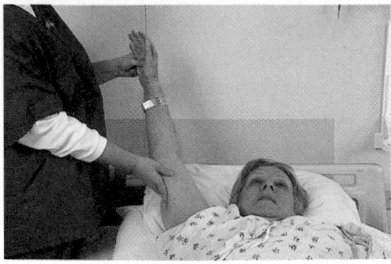

Abduction of shoulder. Move arm from side of body to above the head, then return arm to side of body or neutral position (adduction).

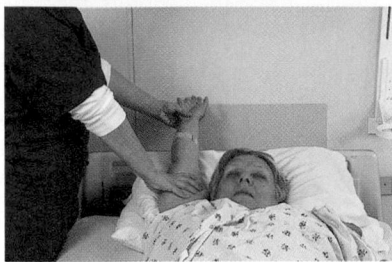

Forward flexion of shoulder. Move arm forward and upward until it is alongside of head.

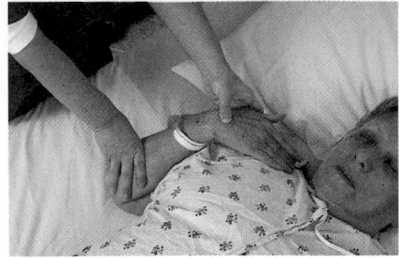

Flexion of elbow. Bend elbow, bringing forearm and hand toward shoulder, then return forearm and hand to neutral position (arm straight).

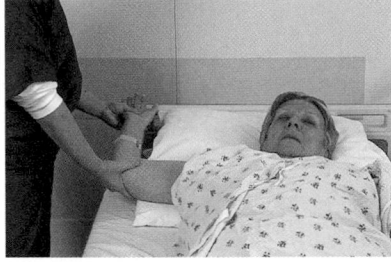

Internal rotation of shoulder. With arm at shoulder height, elbow bent at a 90-degree angle, and palm toward feet, turn upper arm until palm and forearm point backward.

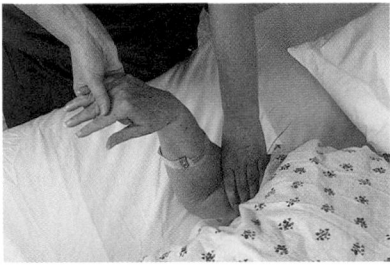

Pronation of forearm. With elbow at waist and bent at a 90-degree angle, turn hand so that palm is facing down.

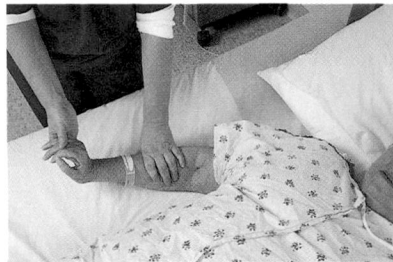

Wrist extension.

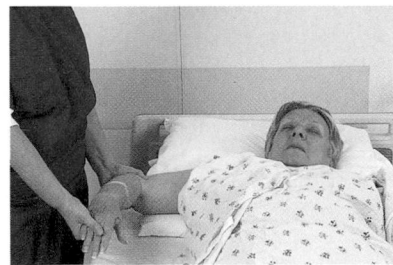

External rotation of shoulder. With arm at shoulder height, elbow bent at a 90-degree angle, and palm toward feet, turn upper arm until the palm and forearm point forward.

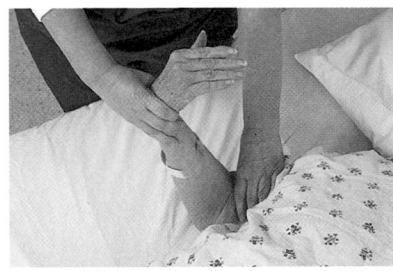

Supination of forearm. With elbow at waist and arm bent at a 90-degree angle, turn hand so that palm is facing up.

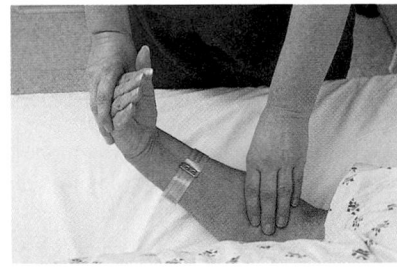

Flexion of wrist. Bend wrist so that palm is toward forearm. Straighten to a neutral position.

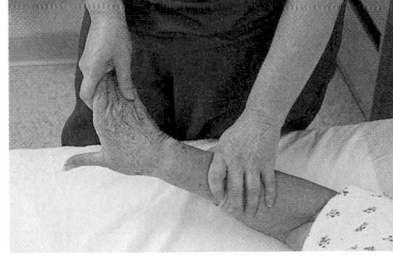

Ulnar deviation. Move hand sideways so that the side of hand on which the little finger is located moves toward forearm.

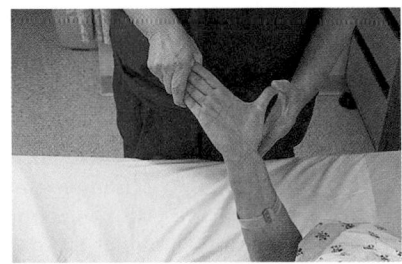

Extension of fingers.

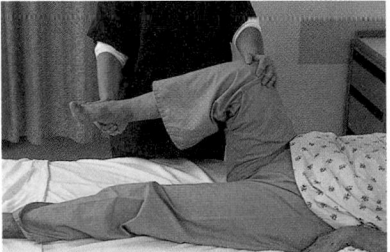

Internal-external rotation of hip. Turn leg in an inward motion so that toes point in. Turn leg in an outward motion so that toes point out.

(continued)

Chart 11-5   Performing Range-of-Motion Exercises (Continued)

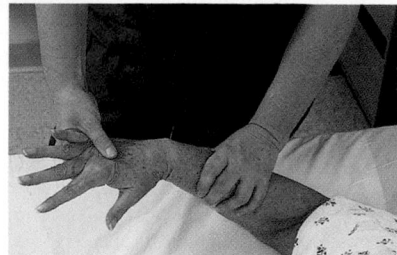

Radial deviation. Move hand sideways so that side of hand on which thumb is located moves toward forearm.

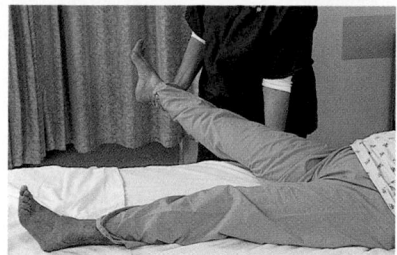

To perform abduction-adduction of hip, move leg outward from the body as far as possible, as shown. Return leg from abducted position to neutral position and across the other leg as far as possible.

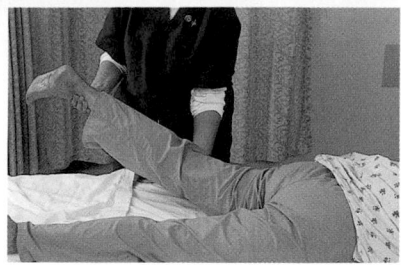

Hyperextension of hip. Place the patient in a prone position, and move leg backward from the body as far as possible.

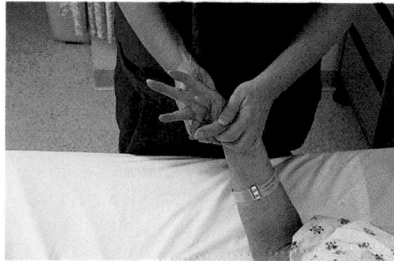

Thumb opposition. Move thumb out and around to touch little finger.

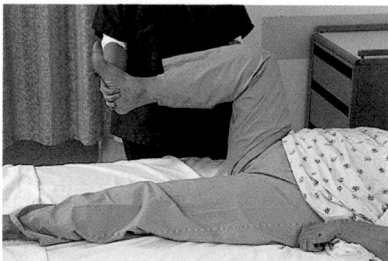

Flexion of the hip and the knee. Bend hip by moving the leg forward as far as possible. Return leg from the flexed position to the neutral position.

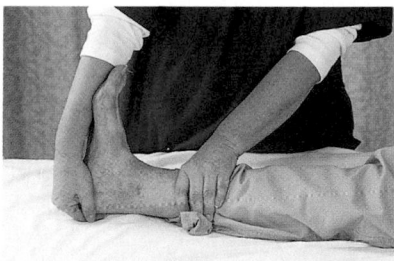

Dorsiflexion of foot. Move foot up and toward the leg. Then move the foot down and away from the leg (plantar flexion).

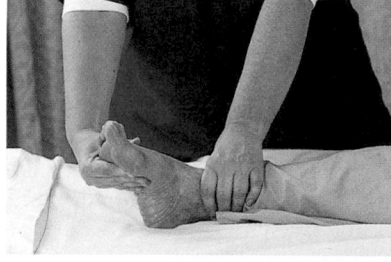

Inversion and eversion of foot. Move foot so that sole is facing outward (eversion). Then move foot so that sole is facing inward (inversion).

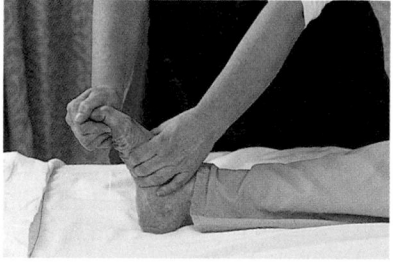

Flexion of toes. Bend the toes toward the ball of foot.

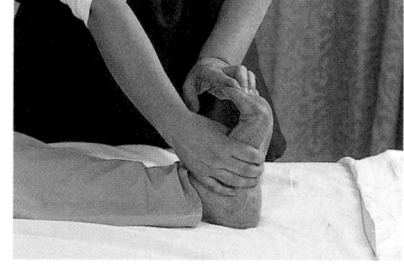

Extension of toes. Straighten toes and pull them toward the leg as far as possible.

wheelchair when the patient is unable to stand, and the technique chosen should be appropriate for the patient, considering his or her abilities and disabilities. It is helpful for the nurse to demonstrate the technique. If the physical therapist is involved in teaching the patient to transfer, the nurse and the physical therapist must collaborate so that consistent instructions are given to the patient. During transfer, the nurse assists and coaches the patient. Figure 11-1 shows weight-bearing and non–weight-bearing transfer.

If the patient's muscles are not strong enough to overcome the resistance of body weight, a polished lightweight board (transfer board, sliding board) may be used to bridge the gap between the bed and the chair. The patient slides across on the board with or without assistance from a caregiver. This board may also be used to transfer the patient from the chair to the toilet or bathtub bench. The nurse should make sure that the patient's fingers do not curl around the edge of the board during the transfer, because the weight of the patient's body can crush them as the patient moves across the board. Safety is a primary concern during a transfer:

- Wheelchairs and beds must be locked before the patient transfers.
- Detachable arm and foot rests are removed to make getting in and out of the chair easier.
- One end of the transfer board is placed under the patient's buttocks and the other end on the surface to which the transfer is being made (eg, the chair).

Table 11-1 • **Therapeutic Exercises**

	DESCRIPTION	PURPOSES	ACTION
Passive	An exercise carried out by the therapist or the nurse without assistance from the patient	To retain as much joint range of motion as possible; to maintain circulation	Stabilize the proximal joint and support the distal part; move the joint smoothly, slowly, and gently through its full range of motion; avoid producing pain.
Active-assistive	An exercise carried out by the patient with the assistance of the therapist or the nurse	To encourage normal muscle function	Support the distal part, and encourage the patient to take the joint actively through its range of motion; give no more assistance than is necessary to accomplish the action; short periods of activity should be followed by adequate rest periods.
Active	An exercise accomplished by the patient without assistance; activities include turning from side to side and from back to abdomen and moving up and down in bed	To increase muscle strength	When possible, active exercise should be performed against gravity; the joint is moved through full range of motion without assistance; make sure that the patient does not substitute another joint movement for the one intended.
Resistive	An active exercise carried out by the patient working against resistance produced by either manual or mechanical means	To provide resistance to increase muscle power	The patient moves the joint through its range of motion while the therapist resists slightly at first and then with progressively increasing resistance; sandbags and weights can be used and are applied at the distal point of the involved joint; the movements should be performed smoothly.
Isometric or muscle setting	Alternately contracting and relaxing a muscle while keeping the part in a fixed position; this exercise is performed by the patient	To maintain strength when a joint is immobilized	Contract or tighten the muscle as much as possible without moving the joint, hold for several seconds, then let go and relax; breathe deeply.

- The patient is instructed to lean forward, push up with his or her hands, and then slide across the board to the other surface.

The nurse frequently assists weak and incapacitated patients out of bed. The nurse supports and gently assists the patient during position changes, protecting the patient from injury. The nurse avoids pulling on the weak or paralyzed upper extremity, to prevent dislocation of the shoulder. The patient is assisted to move toward the stronger side (Chart 11-6).

In the home setting, getting in and out of bed and performing chair, toilet, and tub transfers are difficult for patients with weak musculature and loss of hip, knee, and ankle motion. A rope attached to the headboard of the bed enables the patient to pull toward the center of the bed, and the use of a rope attached to the footboard facilitates getting in and out of bed. The height of a chair can be raised with cushions on the seat or with hollowed-out blocks placed under the chair legs. Grab bars can be attached to the wall near the toilet and tub to provide leverage and stability.

Preparing for Ambulation

Regaining the ability to walk is a prime morale builder. However, to be prepared for ambulation—whether with brace, walker, cane, or crutches—the patient must strengthen the muscles required. Exercise, therefore, is the foundation of preparation. The nurse and physical therapist instruct and supervise the patient in these exercises.

For ambulation, the quadriceps muscles, which stabilize the knee joint, and the gluteal muscles are strengthened. To perform quadriceps-setting exercises, the patient contracts the quadriceps muscle by attempting to push the popliteal area against the mattress and at the same time raising the heel. The patient maintains the muscle contraction until a count of five and relaxes for a count of five. The exercise is repeated 10 to 15 times hourly. Exercising the quadriceps muscles prevents flexion contractures of the knee.

In gluteal setting, the patient contracts or "pinches" the buttocks together to the count of five, relaxes for the count of five, and repeats 10 to 15 times hourly. If ambulatory aids (ie, walker, cane, crutches) are to be used, the muscles of the upper extremities are exercised and strengthened. Push-up exercises are useful. While in a sitting position, the patient raises the body by pushing the hands against the chair seat or mattress. The patient should be encouraged to do push-up exercises while in a prone position also. Pull-up exercises done on a trapeze while lifting the body are also effective for conditioning. The patient is taught to raise the arms above the head and then lower them in a slow, rhythmic manner while holding weights. Gradually, the weight is increased. The hands are strengthened by squeezing a rubber ball.

Typically, the physical therapist designs exercises to help the patient develop the sitting and standing balance, stability, and coordination needed for ambulation. After sitting and standing balance are achieved, the patient uses parallel bars. Under the supervision of the physical therapist, the patient practices shifting weight from side to side, lifting one leg while supporting weight on the other, and then walking between the parallel bars.

A patient who is ready to begin ambulation must be fitted with the appropriate ambulatory aid, instructed about the prescribed weight-bearing limits (eg, non–weight-bearing, partial weight-bearing ambulation), and taught how to use the aid safely. The nurse continually assesses the patient for stability and adherence to weight-bearing precautions and protects the patient from falling. The nurse provides contact guarding by holding on to a gait belt that the patient wears around the waist. The patient should wear sturdy, well-fitting shoes and be advised of the dangers of wet or highly polished floors and throw rugs. The patient should also learn how to ambulate on inclines, uneven surfaces, and stairs.

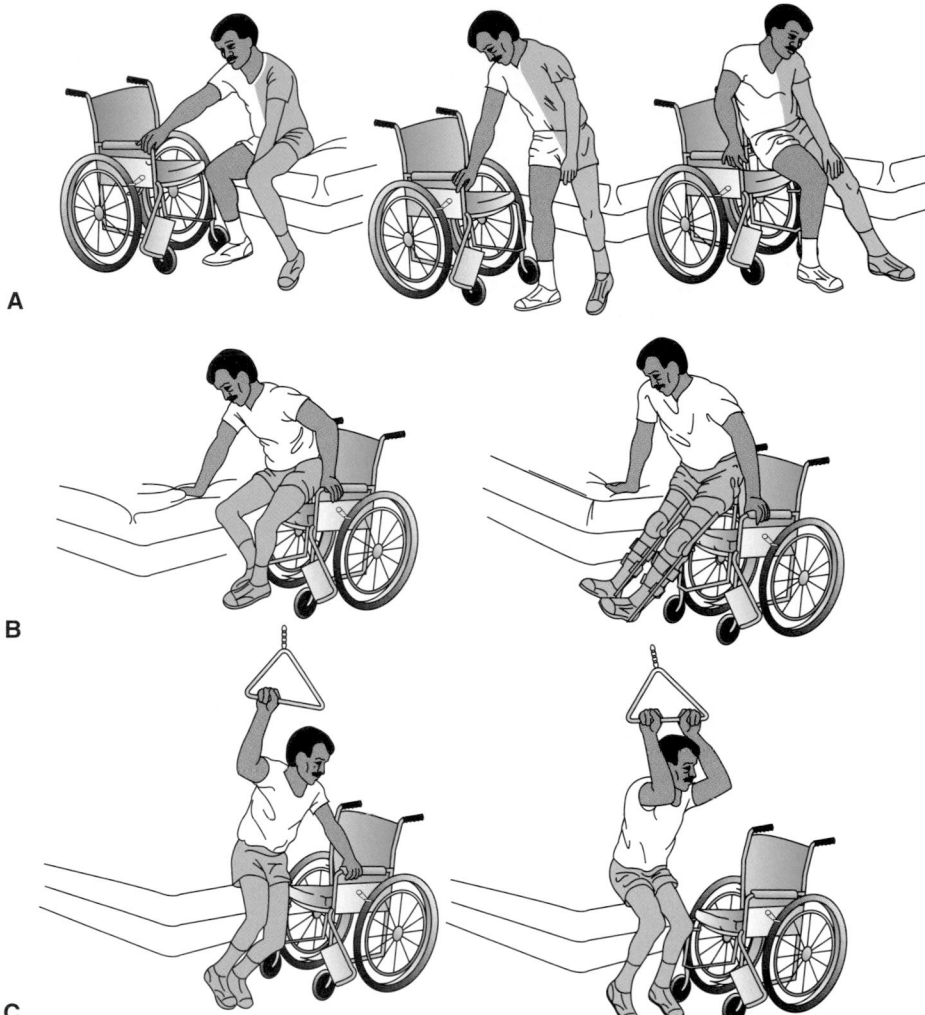

FIGURE 11-1 Methods of patient transfer from the bed to a wheelchair. The wheelchair is in a locked position. Colored areas indicate non wcight-bearing body parts. (**A**) Weight-bearing transfer from bed to chair. The patient stands up, pivots until his back is opposite the new seat, and sits down. (**B**) (*Left*) Non–weight-bearing transfer from chair to bed. (*Right*) With legs braced. (**C**) (*Left*) Non–weight-bearing transfer, combined method. (*Right*) Non–weight-bearing transfer, pull-up method.

Ambulating With Crutches

Patients who are prescribed partial weight-bearing or non–weight-bearing ambulation may use crutches. The nurse or physical therapist should determine whether crutches are appropriate for the patient, because good balance, adequate cardiovascular reserve, strong upper extremities, and erect posture are essential for crutch walking. Ambulating a functional distance (at least the length of a room or house) or maneuvering stairs on crutches requires significant arm strength, because the arms must bear the patient's weight. Muscle groups important for crutch walking include the following:

- Shoulder depressors—to stabilize the upper extremity and prevent shoulder hiking
- Shoulder adductors—to hold the crutch top against the chest wall

---

Chart 11-6 | **Assisting the Patient Out of Bed**

Technique for Moving the Patient to the Edge of the Bed
1. Move head and shoulders of patient toward the edge of the bed.
2. Move feet and legs to the edge of the bed. (The patient is now in a crescent position, which gives good range of motion to the lateral trunk muscles.)
3. Place both arms well under the patient's hips. Next, tighten (set) the muscles of your back and abdomen.
4. Straighten your back while moving the patient toward you.

Technique for Sitting Patient on the Edge of the Bed
1. Place arm and hand under the patient's shoulders.
2. Instruct the patient to push into the bed with the elbow while you lift the patient's shoulders with one arm and swing the legs over the edge of the bed with the other. (Gravity pulls the legs downward, which aids in raising the patient's trunk.)

Technique for Assisting Patient to Stand
1. Position the patient's feet so that they will be well grounded.
2. Face the patient while firmly grasping each side of the patient's rib cage with your hands.
3. Push your knee against one knee of the patient.
4. Rock the patient forward to a standing position. (Your knee is pushed against the patient's knee as he or she comes to the standing position.)
5. Ensure that the patient's knees are "locked" (in full extension) while standing. (Locking the patient's knees is a safety measure for those who are weak or have been in bed for some time.)
6. Give the patient enough time to establish balance.
7. Pivot the patient into a sitting position in the chair.

- Arm flexors, extensors, and abductors (at the shoulder)—to move crutches forward, backward, and sideways
- Forearm extensors—to prevent flexion or buckling; important in raising the body for swinging gait
- Wrist extensors—to enable weight bearing on hand pieces
- Finger and thumb flexors—to grasp the hand piece

Preparing the Patient to Walk With Crutches

Preparatory exercises are prescribed to strengthen the shoulder girdle and upper extremity muscles. Meanwhile, crutches need to be adjusted to the patient before the patient begins ambulating. To determine the approximate crutch length, the patient may be measured standing or lying down. A standing patient is positioned against the wall with the feet slightly apart and away from the wall. Then a distance of 5 cm (2 inches) is marked on the floor, out to the side from the tip of the toe; 15 cm (6 inches) is measured straight ahead from the first mark, and this point is marked on the floor. Next, 5 cm (2 inches) is measured below the axilla to the second mark for the approximate crutch length.

If the patient has to be measured while lying down, he or she is measured from the anterior fold of the axilla to the sole of the foot, and then 5 cm (2 inches) is added. If the patient's height is used, 40 cm (16 inches) is subtracted to obtain the approximate crutch length. The hand piece should be adjusted to allow 20 to 30 degrees of flexion at the elbow. The wrist should be extended and the hand dorsiflexed. A foam rubber pad on the underarm piece is used to relieve pressure of the crutch on the upper arm and thoracic cage. For safety, crutches should have large rubber tips, and the patient should wear firm-soled shoes that fit well.

Teaching Crutch Walking

The nurse or physical therapist explains and demonstrates to the patient how to use the crutches. The patient learns standing balance by standing on the unaffected leg by a chair. To help the patient maintain balance, the nurse holds the patient near the waist or uses a transfer belt.

The patient is taught to support his or her weight on the hand pieces. (For patients who are unable to support their weight through the wrist and hand because of arthritis or fracture, platform crutches that support the forearm and allow the weight to be borne through the elbow are available.) If weight is borne on the axilla, the pressure of the crutch can damage the brachial plexus nerves, producing "crutch paralysis."

For maximum stability, the patient first assumes the tripod position by placing the crutches about 20 to 25 cm (8 to 10 inches) in front and to the side of his or her toes (Fig. 11-2). (This base of support is adjusted according to the height of the patient; a tall person requires a broader base of support than does a short person). In this position, the patient learns how to shift weight and maintain balance.

Before teaching crutch walking, the nurse or therapist determines which gait will be best for the patient. The selection of the crutch gait depends on the type and severity of the disability and on the patient's physical condition, arm and trunk strength, and body balance. The patient should be taught two gaits so that he or she can change from one to another. Shifting crutch gaits relieves fatigue, because each gait requires the use of a different combination of muscles (if a muscle is forced to contract steadily without relaxing, the circulation of the blood to that part is decreased). A faster gait can be used when walking an uninterrupted distance, and a slower gait can be used for short distances or in crowded places. The more common gaits are the four-point, the three-point, the two-point, and the swinging-to and swinging-

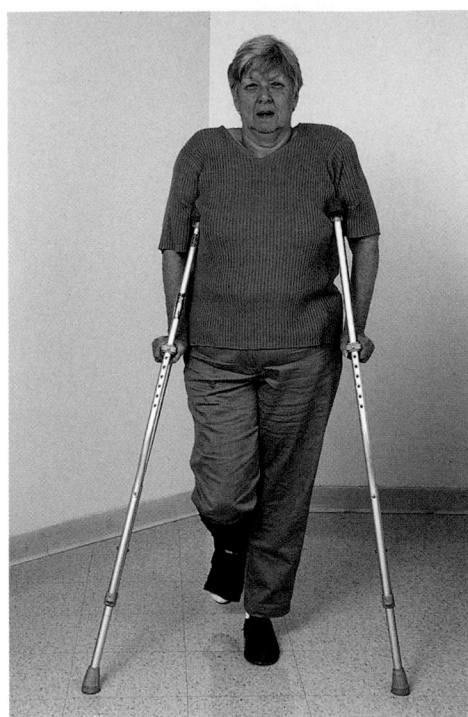

FIGURE 11-2   Crutch walking. The tripod position for basic crutch stance.

through gaits. The sequence of movements for each of these gaits is depicted in Chart 11-7.

The nurse walks with the patient who is just learning how to ambulate with crutches, holding him or her at the waist as needed for balance. During this time, the nurse protects the patient from falls and continually assesses the patient's stability and stamina, since prolonged periods of bed rest and inactivity affect a patient's strength and endurance. Sweating and shortness of breath are indications that crutch-walking practice should be stopped and the patient permitted to rest.

Teaching Maneuvering Techniques

Before a patient is considered to be independent in crutch walking, he or she needs to learn to sit in a chair, stand from sitting, and go up and down stairs.

To sit down:
1. Grasp the crutches at the hand pieces for control.
2. Bend forward slightly while assuming a sitting position.
3. Place the affected leg forward to prevent weight-bearing and flexion.

To stand up:
1. Move forward to the edge of the chair with the strong leg slightly under the seat.
2. Place both crutches in the hand on the side of the affected extremity.
3. Push down on the hand piece while raising the body to a standing position.

To go down stairs:
1. Walk forward as far as possible on the step.
2. Advance crutches to the lower step. The weaker leg is advanced first and then the stronger one. In this way, the stronger extremity shares with the arms the work of raising and lowering the body weight.

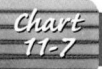

Chart 11-7 Crutch Gaits

Shaded areas are weight-bearing. Arrow indicates advance of foot or crutch. (Read chart from bottom, starting with beginning stance.)

4 POINT GAIT	2 POINT GAIT	3 POINT GAIT	SWING TO	SWING THROUGH
• Partial weight bearing both feet • Maximal support provided • Requires constant shift of weight	• Partial weight bearing both feet • Provides less support • Faster than a 4 point gait	• Non-weight bearing • Requires good balance • Requires arm strength • Faster gait • Can use with walker	• Weight bearing both feet • Provides stability • Requires arm strength • Can use with walker	• Weight bearing • Requires arm strength • Requires coordination/balance • Most advanced gait
4. Advance right foot	4. Advance right foot and left crutch	4. Advance right foot	4. Lift both feet/swing forward/land feet next to crutches	4. Lift both feet/swing forward/land feet in front of crutches
3. Advance left crutch	3. Advance left foot and right crutch	3. Advance left foot and both crutches	3. Advance both crutches	3. Advance both crutches
2. Advance left foot	2. Advance right foot and left crutch	2. Advance right foot	2. Lift both feet/swing forward/land feet next to crutches	2. Lift both feet/swing forward/land feet in front of crutches
1. Advance right crutch	1. Advance left foot and right crutch	1. Advance left foot and both crutches	1. Advance both crutches	1. Advance both crutches
Beginning stance	Beginning stance	Beginning stance	Beginning stance	Beginning stance

To go up stairs:
1. Advance the stronger leg first up to the next step.
2. Advance the crutches and the weaker extremity. Note that the strong leg goes up first and comes down last. A memory device for the patients is, "Up with the good, down with the bad."

AMBULATING WITH A WALKER

A walker provides more support and stability than a cane or crutches. There are two types of walkers: pick-up walkers and rolling walkers. A pick-up walker (one that has to be picked up and moved with each step forward) does not permit a natural walking pattern and is useful for patients who have poor balance or limited cardiovascular reserve or who cannot use crutches. A rolling walker allows automatic walking and is used by patients who cannot lift or who inappropriately carry a pick-up walker. The height of the walker is adjusted to the patient. The patient's arms resting on the walker hand grips should exhibit 20 to 30 degrees of flexion at the elbows. The patient should wear sturdy, well-fitting shoes. The nurse walks with the patient, holds him or her at the waist as needed for balance, continually assesses the patient's stability, and protects the patient from falls.

The patient is instructed to ambulate with a pick-up walker as follows:

1. Push off a chair or bed to come to a standing position. Never pull yourself up using the walker.
2. Hold the walker on the hand grips for stability.
3. Lift the walker, placing it in front of you while leaning your body slightly forward.
4. Walk into the walker, supporting your body weight on your hands when advancing your weaker leg, permitting partial weight bearing or non–weight bearing as prescribed.
5. Balance yourself on your feet.
6. Lift the walker, and place it in front of you again. Continue this pattern of walking.
7. Remember to look up as you walk.

USING A CANE

A cane helps the patient walk with greater balance and support and relieves the pressure on weight-bearing joints by redistributing weight. Quad canes (four-footed canes) provide more stability than straight canes. To fit the patient for a cane, the patient is instructed to flex the elbow at a 30-degree angle, hold the handle of the cane about level with the greater trochanter, and place the tip of the cane 15 cm (6 inches) lateral to the base of the fifth toe. Adjustable canes make individualization easy. The cane should be fitted with a gently flaring tip that has flexible, concentric rings; the tip with its concentric rings provides optimal stability, functions as a shock absorber, and enables the patient to walk with greater speed and less fatigue.

The cane is held in the hand opposite the affected extremity. In normal walking, the opposite leg and arm move together (reciprocal motion); this motion is to be carried through in walking with a cane. The patient is taught to ambulate with a cane as follows:

Cane–foot sequence:
1. Hold the cane in the hand opposite the affected extremity to widen the base of support and to reduce the stress on the involved extremity. If the patient for some reason is unable to use the cane in the opposite hand, the cane may be used on the same side.
2. Advance the cane at the same time the affected leg is moved forward.
3. Keep the cane fairly close to the body to prevent leaning.
4. Bear down on the cane when the unaffected extremity begins the swing phase.

To go up and down stairs using the cane:
1. Step up on the unaffected extremity.
2. Place the cane and affected extremity up on the step.
3. Reverse this procedure for descending steps ("up with the good, down with the bad").

As for all patients beginning ambulation with an ambulatory aid, the nurse continually assesses the patient's stability and protects the patient from falls. The nurse accompanies the patient, holding him or her at the waist as needed for balance. The patient is assessed for tolerance of walking, and rest periods are provided as needed.

ASSISTING THE PATIENT WHO USES AN ORTHOSIS OR PROSTHESIS

Orthoses and prostheses are designed to facilitate mobilization and to maximize the patient's quality of life. An orthosis is an external appliance that provides support, prevents or corrects deformities, and improves function. Orthoses include braces, splints, collars, corsets, or supports that are designed and fitted by an orthotist or prosthetist. Static orthoses (no moving parts) are used to stabilize joints and prevent contractures. Dynamic orthoses are flexible and are used to improve function by assisting weak muscles. A prosthesis is an artificial body part; it may be internal, such as an artificial knee or hip joint, or external, such as an artificial leg or arm.

In addition to learning how to apply and remove the orthosis and maneuver the affected body part correctly, rehabilitation patients must learn how to properly care for the skin that comes in contact with the appliance. Skin problems or **pressure ulcers** may develop if the device is applied too tightly or too loosely, or if it is adjusted improperly. The nurse instructs the patient to clean and inspect the skin daily, to make sure the brace fits snugly without being too tight, to check that the padding distributes pressure evenly, and to wear a cotton garment without seams between the orthosis and the skin.

If the patient has had an amputation, the nurse promotes tissue healing, uses compression dressings to promote residual limb shaping, and minimizes contracture formation. A permanent prosthetic limb cannot be fitted until the tissue has healed completely and the residual limb shape is stable and free of edema. The nurse also helps the patient cope with the emotional issues surrounding loss of a limb and encourages acceptance of the prosthesis. The prosthetist, the nurse, and the physician collaborate to provide instructions related to skin care and care of the prosthesis.

Evaluation

EXPECTED PATIENT OUTCOMES

Expected patient outcomes may include:

1. Demonstrates improved physical mobility
   a. Maintains muscle strength and joint mobility
   b. Does not develop contractures
   c. Participates in exercise program
2. Transfers safely
   a. Demonstrates assisted transfers
   b. Performs independent transfers

3. Ambulates with maximum independence
   a. Uses ambulatory aid safely
   b. Adheres to weight-bearing prescription
   c. Requests assistance as needed
4. Demonstrates increased activity tolerance
   a. Does not experience episodes of orthostatic hypotension
   b. Reports absence of fatigue with ambulatory efforts
   c. Gradually increases distance and speed of ambulation

NURSING PROCESS: THE PATIENT WITH IMPAIRED SKIN INTEGRITY

An estimated 1.5 to 3 million patients develop pressure ulcers annually (Mayo Clinic Rochester, 2001). Both prevention and treatment of pressure ulcers are costly in terms of health care dollars and quality of life for patients at risk. Because the cost in terms of pain and suffering for a person with a pressure ulcer cannot be quantified, all possible efforts should be made to prevent skin breakdown.

Patients confined to bed for long periods, patients with motor or sensory dysfunction, and patients who experience muscular atrophy and reduction of padding between the overlying skin and the underlying bone are prone to pressure ulcers. Pressure ulcers are localized areas of infarcted soft tissue that occur when pressure applied to the skin over time is greater than normal capillary closure pressure, which is about 32 mm Hg. Critically ill patients have a lower capillary closure pressure and are at greater risk for pressure ulcers. The initial sign of pressure is erythema (redness of the skin) caused by reactive hyperemia, which normally resolves in less than 1 hour. Unrelieved pressure results in tissue ischemia or anoxia. The cutaneous tissues become broken or destroyed, leading to progressive destruction and necrosis of underlying soft tissue, and the resulting pressure ulcer is painful and slow to heal.

Assessment

Immobility, impaired sensory perception or cognition, decreased tissue perfusion, decreased nutritional status, friction and shear forces, increased moisture, and age-related skin changes all contribute to the development of pressure ulcers.

IMMOBILITY

When a person is immobile and inactive, pressure is exerted on the skin and subcutaneous tissue by objects on which the person rests, such as a mattress, chair seat, or cast. The development of pressure ulcers is directly related to the duration of immobility: if pressure continues long enough, small vessel thrombosis and tissue necrosis occur, and a pressure ulcer results. Weight-bearing bony prominences are most susceptible to pressure ulcer development because they are covered only by skin and small amounts of subcutaneous tissue. Susceptible areas include the sacrum and coccygeal areas, ischial tuberosities (especially in people who sit for prolonged periods), greater trochanter, heel, knee, malleolus, medial condyle of the tibia, fibular head, scapula, and elbow (Fig. 11-3).

IMPAIRED SENSORY PERCEPTION OR COGNITION

Patients with sensory loss, impaired level of consciousness, or paralysis may not be aware of the discomfort associated with prolonged pressure on the skin and, therefore, may not change their position themselves to relieve the pressure. This prolonged pressure impedes blood flow, reducing nourishment of the skin and underlying tissues. A pressure ulcer may develop in a short period.

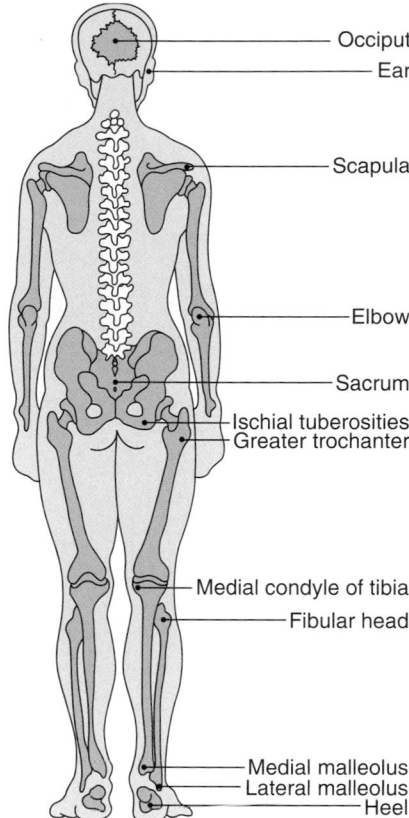

FIGURE 11-3 Areas susceptible to pressure ulcers.

Labels: Occiput, Ear, Scapula, Elbow, Sacrum, Ischial tuberosities, Greater trochanter, Medial condyle of tibia, Fibular head, Medial malleolus, Lateral malleolus, Heel

DECREASED TISSUE PERFUSION

Any condition that reduces the circulation and nourishment of the skin and subcutaneous tissue (altered peripheral tissue perfusion) increases the risk of pressure ulcer development. Patients with diabetes mellitus experience an alteration in microcirculation. Similarly, patients with edema have impaired circulation and poor nourishment of the skin tissue. Obese patients have large amounts of poorly vascularized adipose tissue, which is susceptible to breakdown.

DECREASED NUTRITIONAL STATUS

Nutritional deficiencies, anemias, and metabolic disorders also contribute to pressure ulcer development. Anemia, regardless of its cause, decreases the blood's oxygen-carrying ability and predisposes a patient to pressure ulcer formation. Patients who have low protein levels or who are in a negative nitrogen balance experience tissue wasting and inhibited tissue repair. Serum albumin is a sensitive indicator of protein deficiency; serum albumin levels of less than 3 g/mL are associated with hypoalbuminemic tissue edema and increased risk of pressure ulcers. Specific nutrients, such as vitamin C and trace minerals, are needed for tissue maintenance and repair.

FRICTION AND SHEAR

Mechanical forces also contribute to the development of pressure ulcers. Friction is the resistance to movement that occurs when two surfaces are moved across each other. Shear is created by the interplay of gravitational forces (forces that push the body down) and friction. When shear occurs, tissue layers slide over one another, blood vessels stretch and twist, and the microcirculation of the skin and subcutaneous tissue is disrupted. Evidence of deep tissue damage may be slow to develop and may present through the development of a draining tract. The sacrum and heels are most susceptible to the effects of shear. Pressure ulcers from friction and shear occur when the patient slides down in bed (Fig. 11-4) or when the patient is moved or positioned improperly (eg, dragged up in bed). Spastic muscles and paralysis increase the patient's vulnerability to pressure ulcers related to friction and shear.

INCREASED MOISTURE

Prolonged contact with moisture from perspiration, urine, feces, or drainage produces maceration (softening) of the skin. The skin reacts to the caustic substances in the excreta or drainage and becomes irritated. Moist, irritated skin is more vulnerable to pressure breakdown. Once the skin breaks, the area is invaded by microorganisms (eg, streptococci, staphylococci, *Pseudomonas aeruginosa, Escherichia coli*), and infection occurs. Foul-smelling infectious drainage is present. The lesion may enlarge and allow a continuous loss of serum, which may further deplete the body of essential protein needed for tissue repair and maintenance. The lesion may continue to enlarge and extend deep into the fascia, muscle, and bone, with multiple sinus tracts radiating from the pressure ulcer. With extensive pressure ulcers, systemic infections may develop, frequently from gram-negative organisms.

Gerontologic Considerations

In older adults, the skin has diminished epidermal thickness, dermal collagen, and tissue elasticity. The skin is drier as a result of diminished sebaceous and sweat gland activity. Cardiovascular changes result in decreased tissue perfusion. Muscles atrophy, and bone structures become prominent. Diminished sensory perception and reduced ability to reposition oneself contribute to prolonged pressure on the skin. Therefore, the older adult is more susceptible to pressure ulcers, which cause pain and suffering and reduce quality of life (Agency for Health Care Policy and Research [AHCPR], 1994).

ADDITIONAL RISK FACTORS

In assessing the patient for potential risk for pressure ulcer development, the nurse assesses the patient's mobility, sensory perception, cognitive abilities, tissue perfusion, nutritional status, friction and shear forces, sources of moisture on the skin, and age. The nurse

- Assesses total skin condition at least twice a day
- Inspects each pressure site for erythema
- Assesses areas of erythema for blanching response
- Palpates the skin for increased warmth
- Inspects for dry skin, moist skin, breaks in skin
- Notes drainage and odor
- Evaluates level of mobility
- Notes restrictive devices (eg, restraints, splints)
- Evaluates circulatory status (eg, peripheral pulses, edema)
- Assesses neurovascular status
- Determines presence of incontinence
- Evaluates nutritional and hydration status
- Reviews the patient's record for laboratory studies, including hematocrit, hemoglobin, electrolytes, albumin, transferrin, and creatinine
- Notes present health problems
- Reviews current medications

Scales such as the Braden or Norton scale may be used to facilitate systematic assessment and quantification of a patient's risk for pressure ulcer, although the nurse needs to recognize that the reliability of these scales is not well established. They tend to overestimate those at risk and may promote unwarranted use of costly preventive equipment. See Chart 11-8 for a list of risk factors for development of pressure ulcers.

If a pressure area is noted, the nurse notes its size and location and may use a grading system to describe its severity (see Chart 11-9). Generally, a stage I pressure ulcer is an area of nonblanchable erythema, tissue swelling, and congestion, and the patient complains of discomfort. The skin temperature is elevated because of the increased vasodilation. The redness progresses to a dusky, cyanotic blue-gray appearance, which is the result of skin capillary occlusion and subcutaneous weakening.

A stage II pressure ulcer exhibits a break in the skin through the epidermis or the dermis. An abrasion, blister, or shallow crater may be seen. Necrosis occurs along with venous sludging and thrombosis and edema with cellular extravasation and infiltration.

A stage III pressure ulcer extends into the subcutaneous tissues. Clinically, a deep crater with or without undermining of adjacent tissues is noted.

A stage IV pressure ulcer extends into the underlying structures, including the muscle and, possibly, the bone. The skin lesion may appear insignificant when in reality, beneath the small surface ulcer is a large undermined area of necrotic tissue.

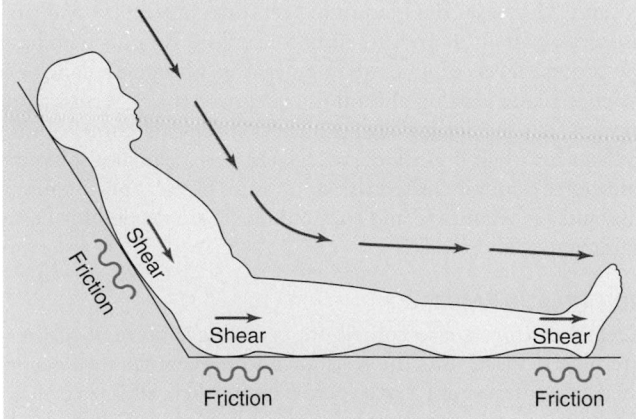

FIGURE 11-4 Mechanical forces contribute to pressure ulcer development. As the person slides down or is improperly pulled up in bed, *friction* resists this movement. *Shear* occurs when one layer of tissue slides over another, disrupting microcirculation of skin and subcutaneous tissue.

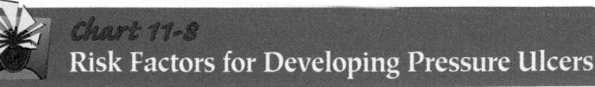

Chart 11-8
Risk Factors for Developing Pressure Ulcers

Prolonged pressure on tissue
Immobility, compromised mobility
Loss of protective reflexes, sensory deficit/loss
Poor skin perfusion, edema
Malnutrition, hypoproteinemia, anemia, vitamin deficiency
Friction, shearing forces, trauma
Incontinence of urine or feces
Altered skin moisture: excessively dry, excessively moist
Advanced age, debilitation
Equipment: casts, traction, restraints

Chart 11-9 • ASSESSMENT

Assessing Pressure Ulcer Stages

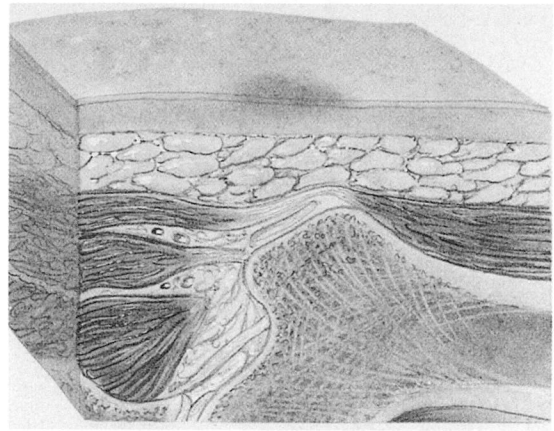

Stage I
- Area of erythema
- Erythema does not blanch with pressure
- Skin temperature elevated
- Tissue swollen and congested
- Patient complains of discomfort
- Erythema progresses to dusky blue-gray

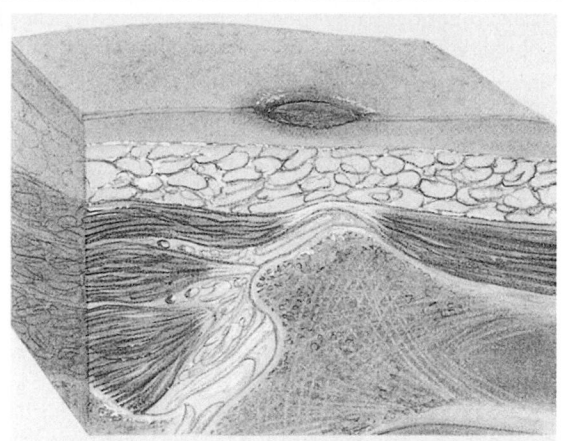

Stage II
- Skin breaks
- Abrasion, blister, or shallow crater
- Edema persists
- Ulcer drains
- Infection may develop

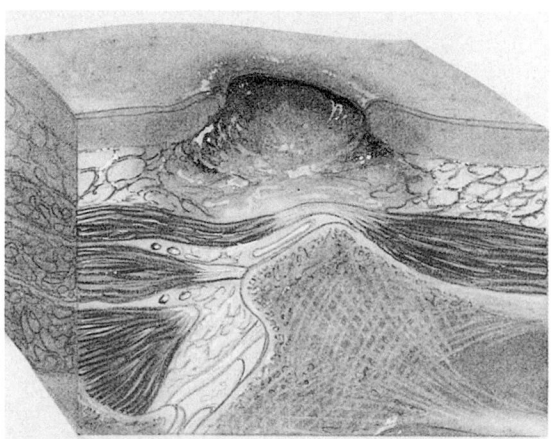

Stage III
- Ulcer extends into subcutaneous tissue
- Necrosis and drainage continue
- Infection develops

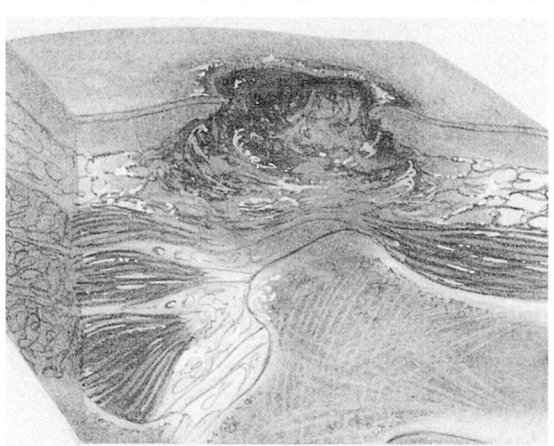

Stage IV
- Ulcer extends to underlying muscle and bone
- Deep pockets of infection develop
- Necrosis and drainage continue

From Weber, J. W., & Kelley, J. (2002). *Health assessment in nursing* (2nd ed.). Philadelphia: Lippincott Williams & Wilkins.

The appearance of purulent drainage or foul odor suggests an infection. With an extensive pressure ulcer, deep pockets of infection are often present. Drying and crusting of exudate may be present. Infection of a pressure ulcer may advance to osteomyelitis, pyarthrosis (pus formation within a joint cavity), sepsis, and septic shock.

Nursing Diagnosis

Based on the assessment data, the nursing diagnoses may include the following:

- Risk for impaired skin integrity

- Impaired skin integrity (related to immobility, decreased sensory perception, decreased tissue perfusion, decreased nutritional status, friction and shear forces, increased moisture, or advanced age)

Planning and Goals

The major goals for the patient may include relief of pressure, improved mobility, improved sensory perception, improved tissue perfusion, improved nutritional status, minimized friction and shear forces, dry surfaces in contact with skin, and healing of pressure ulcer, if present.

Nursing Interventions

RELIEVING PRESSURE

Frequent changes of position are needed to relieve and redistribute the pressure on the patient's skin and to prevent prolonged reduced blood flow to the skin and subcutaneous tissues. This can be accomplished by teaching the patient to change position or by turning and repositioning the patient. The patient's family members should be taught how to position and turn the patient at home to prevent pressure ulcers. Shifting weight allows the blood to flow into the ischemic areas and helps the tissues recover from the effects of pressure. Thus, the patient should be cared for as follows:

- Turned and repositioned at 1-hour to 2-hour intervals
- Encouraged to shift weight actively every 15 minutes

POSITIONING THE PATIENT

The patient should be positioned laterally, prone, and dorsally in sequence unless a position is not tolerated or is contraindicated. The recumbent position is preferred to the semi-Fowler's position because of increased supporting body surface area in this position. In addition to regular turning, there should be small shifts of body weight, such as repositioning of an ankle, elbow, or shoulder. The skin is inspected at each position change and assessed for temperature elevation. If redness or heat is noted or if the patient complains of discomfort, pressure on the area must be relieved.

Another way to relieve pressure over bony prominences is the bridging technique, accomplished through the correct positioning of pillows. Just as a bridge is supported on pillars to allow traffic to move underneath, so can the body be supported by pillows to allow for space between bony prominences and the mattress. A pillow or commercial heel protector may be used to support the heels off the bed when the patient is supine. Placing pillows superior and inferior to the sacrum relieves sacral pressure. Supporting the patient in a 30-degree side-lying position avoids pressure on the trochanter. In the aging patient, frequent small shifts of body weight may be effective. Placing a small rolled towel or sheepskin under a shoulder or hip will allow a return of blood flow to the skin in the area on which the patient is sitting or lying. The towel or sheepskin is moved around the patient's pressure points in a clockwise fashion.

USING PRESSURE-RELIEVING DEVICES

At times, special equipment and beds may be needed to help relieve the pressure on the skin. These are designed to provide support for specific body areas or to distribute pressure evenly.

Patients sitting in wheelchairs for prolonged periods should have wheelchair cushions fitted and adjusted on an individualized basis, using pressure measurement techniques as a guide to selection and fitting. The aim is to redistribute pressure away from areas at risk for ulcers, but no cushion is able to eliminate excessive pressure completely. The patient should be reminded to shift weight frequently and to rise for a few seconds every 15 minutes while sitting in a chair (Fig. 11-5).

Static support devices (such as high-density foam, air, or liquid mattress overlays) distribute pressure evenly by bringing more of the patient's body surface into contact with the supporting surface. Gel-type flotation pads and air-fluidized beds reduce pressure. The weight of a body floating on a fluid system is evenly distributed over the entire supporting surface (according to Pascal's law). Therefore, as the patient's body sinks into the fluid, additional surface becomes available for weight bearing, body

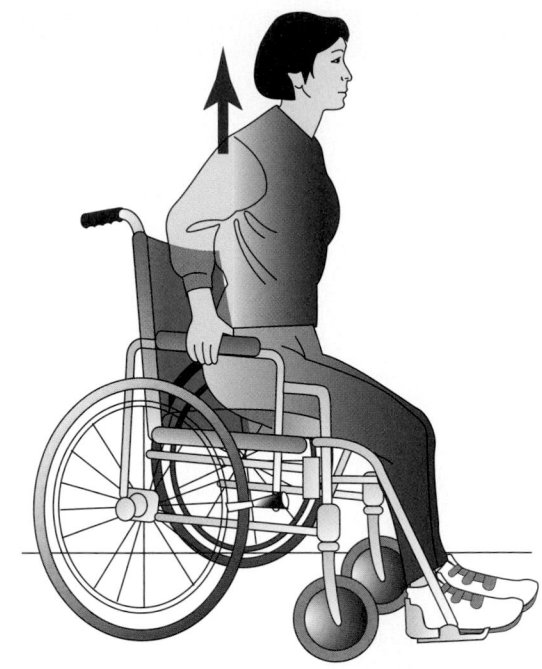

FIGURE 11-5 Wheelchair push-up to prevent ischial pressure ulcers. These push-ups should become an automatic routine (every 15 minutes) for the person with paraplegia. The person should stay up, out of contact with the seat for several seconds. The wheels are kept in the locked position during the exercise.

weight per unit area is decreased, and there is less pressure on the body parts.

Soft, moisture-absorbing padding is also useful because the softness and resilience of padding provides for more even distribution of pressure and the dissipation and absorption of moisture, along with freedom from wrinkles and friction. Bony prominences may be protected by gel pads, sheepskin padding, or soft foam rubber beneath the sacrum, the trochanters, heels, elbows, scapulae, and back of the head when there is pressure on the sites.

Specialized beds have been designed to prevent pressure on the skin. Air-fluidized beds float the patient. Dynamic support surfaces, such as low air-loss pockets, alternately inflate and deflate sections to change support pressure for very high-risk patients who are critically ill and debilitated and cannot be repositioned to relieve pressure. Oscillating or kinetic beds change pressure by means of rocking movements of the bed that redistribute the patient's weight and stimulate circulation. These beds are frequently used with patients who have injuries due to multiple trauma.

IMPROVING MOBILITY

The patient is encouraged to remain active and is ambulated whenever possible. When sitting, the patient is reminded to change positions frequently to redistribute weight. Active and passive exercises increase muscular, skin, and vascular tone. Activity stimulates circulation, which relieves tissue ischemia, the forerunner of pressure ulcers. For the patient at risk for pressure ulcers, turning and exercise schedules are essential: repositioning must occur around the clock.

IMPROVING SENSORY PERCEPTION

The nurse helps the patient recognize and compensate for altered sensory perception. Depending on the origin of the alteration (eg, decreased level of consciousness, spinal cord lesion), specific interventions are selected. Strategies to improve cognition and sensory perception may include stimulating the patient to increase awareness of self in the environment, encouraging the patient to participate in self-care, or supporting the patient's efforts toward active compensation for loss of sensation (eg, a paraplegic patient lifting up from the sitting position every 15 minutes). When decreased sensory perception exists, the patient and caregiver are taught to inspect potential pressure areas visually every morning and evening, using a mirror if necessary, for evidence of pressure ulcer development.

IMPROVING TISSUE PERFUSION

Exercise and repositioning improve tissue perfusion. Massage of erythematous areas is avoided because damage to the capillaries and deep tissue may occur.

 NURSING ALERT Avoid massaging reddened areas, because this may increase the damage to already traumatized skin and tissue.

In patients who have evidence of compromised peripheral circulation (eg, edema), positioning and elevation of the edematous body part to promote venous return and diminish congestion improve tissue perfusion. In addition, the nurse or family must be alert to environmental factors (eg, wrinkles in sheets, pressure of tubes) that may contribute to pressure on the skin and diminished circulation and remove the source of pressure.

IMPROVING NUTRITIONAL STATUS

The patient's nutritional status must be adequate, and a positive nitrogen balance must be maintained, because pressure ulcers develop more quickly and are more resistant to treatment in patients with nutritional disorders. A high-protein diet with protein supplements may be helpful. Iron preparations may be necessary to raise the hemoglobin concentration so that tissue oxygen levels can be maintained within acceptable limits. Ascorbic acid (vitamin C) is necessary for tissue healing. Other nutrients associated with healthy skin include vitamin A, B vitamins, zinc, and sulfur. With balanced nutrition and hydration, the skin is able to remain healthy, and damaged tissues can be repaired (Table 11-2).

To assess nutritional status response to therapeutic strategies, the nurse monitors the patient's hemoglobin, albumin, and body weight weekly. Nutritional assessment is described in further detail in Chapter 5.

REDUCING FRICTION AND SHEAR

Shear occurs when the patient is pulled, is allowed to slump, or moves by digging heels or elbows into the mattress. Raising the head of the bed by even a few centimeters increases the shearing force over the sacral area; therefore, the semireclining position is avoided in patients at risk. Proper positioning with adequate support is also important when a patient is sitting in a chair. Polyester sheepskin pads are thought to reduce shear and friction and may be used with at-risk patients.

 NURSING ALERT To avoid shearing forces when repositioning the patient, the nurse lifts and avoids dragging the patient across a surface.

MINIMIZING IRRITATING MOISTURE

Continuous moisture on the skin must be prevented by meticulous hygienic measures. Perspiration, urine, stool, and drainage must be removed from the skin promptly. The soiled skin should be washed immediately with mild soap and water and blotted dry with a soft towel. The skin may be lubricated with a bland lotion to keep it soft and pliable. Drying agents and powders are avoided. Topical barrier ointments (eg, petroleum jelly) may be helpful in protecting the skin of patients who are incontinent.

Absorbent pads that wick moisture away from the body should be used to absorb drainage. Patients who are incontinent need to be checked *regularly* and have their wet incontinence pads and linens changed promptly. Their skin needs to be cleansed and dried promptly.

PROMOTING PRESSURE ULCER HEALING

Regardless of the stage of the pressure ulcer, the pressure on the area must be eliminated, because the ulcer will not heal until all pressure is removed. The patient must not lie or sit on the pres-

Table 11-2 • Nutritional Requirements to Promote Healing of Pressure Ulcers

NUTRIENT	RATIONALE	RECOMMENDED AMOUNT
Protein	Tissue repair	1.25–1.50 g/kg/day
Calories	Spare protein Restore normal weight	30–35 calories/kg/day
Water	Maintain homeostasis	1 mL/calorie fed or 30 mL/kg/day
Multivitamin	Promote collagen formation	1 daily
Vitamin C	Promote collagen synthesis Support integrity of capillary wall	500–1000 mg daily
Zinc sulfate	Cofactor for collagen formation and protein synthesis Normal lymphocyte and phagocyte response	220 mg daily
Vitamin A	*Caution:* An excess can cause an excessive inflammatory response that could impair healing	—

sure ulcer, even for a few minutes. Individualized positioning and turning schedules must be written in the plan of nursing care and followed meticulously.

In addition, inadequate nutritional status and fluid and electrolyte abnormalities must be corrected to promote healing. Wounds that drain body fluids and protein place the patient in a catabolic state and predispose to hypoproteinemia and serious secondary infections. Protein deficiency must be corrected to heal the pressure ulcer. Carbohydrates are necessary to "spare" the protein and to provide an energy source. Vitamin C and trace elements, especially zinc, are necessary for collagen formation and wound healing.

Stage I Pressure Ulcers

To permit healing of stage I pressure ulcers, the pressure is removed to allow increased tissue perfusion, nutritional and fluid and electrolyte balance are maintained, friction and shear are reduced, and moisture to the skin is avoided.

Stage II Pressure Ulcers

Stage II pressure ulcers have broken skin. In addition to measures listed for stage I pressure ulcers, a moist environment, in which migration of epidermal cells over the ulcer surface occurs more rapidly, should be provided to aid wound healing. The ulcer is gently cleansed with sterile saline solution. Use of a heat lamp to dry the open wound is avoided, as is use of antiseptic solutions that damage healthy tissues and delay wound healing. Semipermeable occlusive dressing, hydrocolloid wafers, or wet saline dressings are helpful in providing a moist environment for healing and in minimizing the loss of fluids and proteins from the body.

Stage III and IV Pressure Ulcers

Stage III and IV pressure ulcers are characterized by extensive tissue damage. In addition to measures listed for stage I, these advanced draining, necrotic pressure ulcers must be cleaned (débrided) to create an area that will heal. Necrotic, devitalized tissue favors bacterial growth, delays granulation, and inhibits healing. Wound cleaning and dressing are uncomfortable; therefore, the nurse must prepare the patient for the procedure by explaining what will occur and administering prescribed analgesia.

Débridement may be accomplished by wet-to-damp dressing changes, mechanical flushing of necrotic and infective exudate, application of prescribed enzyme preparations that dissolve necrotic tissue, or surgical dissection. If an eschar covers the ulcer, it is removed surgically to ensure a clean, vitalized wound. Exudate may be absorbed by dressings or special hydrophilic powders, beads, or gels. Cultures of infected pressure ulcers are obtained to guide selection of antibiotic therapy.

After the pressure ulcer is clean, a topical treatment is prescribed to promote granulation. New granulation tissue must be protected from reinfection, drying, and damage, and care should be taken to prevent pressure and further trauma to the area. Dressings, solutions, and ointments applied to the ulcer should not disrupt the healing process. Multiple agents and protocols are used to treat pressure ulcers, but consistency is an important key to success. Objective evaluation of the pressure ulcer (eg, measurement of the pressure ulcer, inspection for granulation tissue) for response to the treatment protocol must be made every 4 to 6 days. Taking photographs at weekly intervals is a reliable strategy for monitoring the healing process, which may take weeks to months to complete.

Surgical intervention is necessary when the ulcer is extensive, when potential complications (eg, fistula) exist, and when the

ulcer does not respond to treatment. Surgical procedures include débridement, incision and drainage, bone resection, and skin grafting.

PREVENTING RECURRENCE

Recurrence of pressure ulcers should be anticipated; therefore, active, preventive intervention and frequent continuing assessments are essential. The patient's tolerance for sitting or lying on the healed pressure area is increased gradually by increasing the time that pressure is allowed on the area in 5- to 15-minute increments. The patient is taught to increase mobility and to follow a regimen of turning, weight shifting, and repositioning. The patient teaching plan includes instruction on strategies to reduce the risk for development of pressure ulcers and methods to detect, inspect, and minimize pressure areas. Early recognition and intervention are keys to long-term management of potential impaired skin integrity.

Evaluation

EXPECTED PATIENT OUTCOMES

Expected patient outcomes may include:

1. Maintains intact skin
   a. Exhibits no areas of nonblanchable erythema at bony prominences
   b. Avoids massage of bony prominences
   c. Exhibits no breaks in skin
2. Limits pressure on bony prominences
   a. Changes position every 1 to 2 hours
   b. Uses bridging techniques to reduce pressure
   c. Uses special equipment as appropriate
   d. Raises self from seat of wheelchair every 15 minutes
3. Increases mobility
   a. Performs range-of-motion exercises
   b. Adheres to turning schedule
   c. Advances sitting time as tolerated
4. Sensory and cognitive ability improved
   a. Demonstrates improved level of consciousness
   b. Remembers to inspect potential pressure ulcer areas every morning and evening
5. Demonstrates improved tissue perfusion
   a. Exercises to increase circulation
   b. Elevates body parts susceptible to edema
6. Attains and maintains adequate nutritional status
   a. Verbalizes the importance of protein and vitamin C in diet
   b. Eats diet high in protein and vitamin C
   c. Maintains hemoglobin, electrolyte, albumin, transferrin, and creatinine levels at acceptable levels
7. Avoids friction and shear
   a. Avoids semireclining position
   b. Uses sheepskin pad and heel protectors when appropriate
   c. Lifts body instead of sliding across surfaces
8. Maintains clean, dry skin
   a. Avoids prolonged contact with wet or soiled surfaces
   b. Keeps skin clean and dry
   c. Uses lotion to keep skin lubricated
9. Experiences healing of pressure ulcer
   a. Avoids pressure on area
   b. Improves nutritional status
   c. Participates in therapeutic regimen
   d. Demonstrates behaviors to prevent new pressure ulcers
   e. States early indicators of pressure ulcer development

NURSING PROCESS: THE PATIENT WITH ALTERED ELIMINATION PATTERNS

Urinary and bowel incontinence or constipation and impaction are problems that often occur in disabled patients. Incontinence curtails a person's independence, causing embarrassment and isolation. It occurs in up to 15% of the community-based elderly population, and almost half of nursing home residents are bowel or bladder incontinent or both. In addition, constipation may be a problem for patients with disabilities. Complete and predictable evacuation of the bowel is the goal. If a bowel routine is not established, the person may experience abdominal distention; small, frequent oozing of stool; or impaction.

Assessment

Urinary incontinence can be classified as urge, reflex, stress, functional, or total incontinence (AHCPR, 1996). Urge incontinence is involuntary elimination of urine associated with a strong perceived need to void. Reflex (neurogenic) incontinence is associated with a spinal cord lesion that interrupts cerebral control, resulting in no sensory awareness of the need to void. Stress incontinence is associated with weakened perineal muscles that permit leakage of urine when intra-abdominal pressure is increased (eg, with coughing or sneezing). Functional incontinence refers to incontinence in patients with intact urinary physiology who experience mobility impairment, environmental barriers, or cognitive problems and are unable to reach and use the toilet before soiling themselves. Total incontinence occurs in patients who are unable to control excreta because of physiologic or psychological impairment; management of the excreta is the focus of nursing care. Urinary incontinence may result from multiple causes, including urinary tract infection, detrusor instability, bladder outlet obstruction or incompetence, neurologic impairment, bladder spasm or contracture, and inability to reach the toilet in time.

The health history is used to explore bladder and bowel function, symptoms associated with dysfunction, physiologic risk factors for elimination problems, perception of micturition and defecation cues, and functional toileting abilities. Previous and current fluid intake and voiding patterns may be helpful in designing the plan of nursing care. A record of times of voiding and amounts voided is kept for at least 48 hours. In addition, episodes of incontinence and associated activity (eg, coughing, sneezing, lifting), fluid intake time and amount, and medications are recorded. This record is analyzed and used to determine patterns and relationships of incontinence to other activities and factors.

The ability to get to the bathroom, manipulate clothing, and use the toilet are important functional factors that may be related to incontinence. Related cognitive functioning (perception of need to void, verbalization of need to void, and ability to learn to control urination) must also be assessed. In addition, the nurse reviews the results of the diagnostic studies (eg, urinalysis, urodynamic tests, postvoiding residual volumes). See the accompanying Gerontologic Considerations box for factors that affect the older adult.

Bowel incontinence and constipation may result from multiple causes, such as diminished or absent sphincter control, cognitive or perceptual impairment, neurogenic factors, diet, and immobility. The origin of the bowel problem must be determined.

The nurse assesses the patient's normal bowel patterns, nutritional patterns, use of laxatives, gastrointestinal problems (eg, colitis), bowel sounds, anal reflex and tone, and functional abilities.

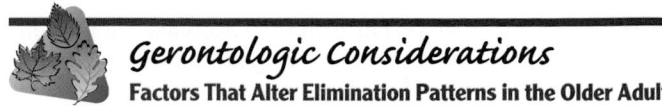

Gerontologic Considerations
Factors That Alter Elimination Patterns in the Older Adult

Decreased bladder capacity
Decreased muscle tone
Increased residual volumes
Delayed perception of elimination cues
Use of medications that alter elimination patterns, such as diuretics (increase volume of urine produced), sedatives (alter bladder sensitivity to cues), and adrenergics or anticholinergics (cause urinary retention)
Functional immobility
Sedentary lifestyle

The character and frequency of bowel movements are recorded and analyzed.

Nursing Diagnosis

Based on the assessment data, major nursing diagnoses for the patient may include the following:

- Impaired bowel elimination
- Impaired urinary elimination

Planning and Goals

The major goals of the patient may include control of urinary incontinence or urinary retention, control of bowel incontinence, and regular elimination patterns.

Nursing Interventions

PROMOTING URINARY CONTINENCE

After the nature of the urinary incontinence has been identified, a nursing plan of care is developed based on analysis of the assessment data. Various approaches to promotion of urinary continence have been designed. Most approaches attempt to condition the body to control urination or to minimize the occurrence of unscheduled urination. Selection of the approach depends on the cause and type of the patient's incontinence. For the program to be successful, the patient's participation and desire to avoid incontinence episodes are crucial, and an optimistic attitude with positive feedback for even slight gains is essential for success. Accurate recording of intake and output and of the response to selected strategies is essential for evaluation.

At no time should the fluid intake be restricted to decrease the frequency of urination. Sufficient fluid intake (2000 to 3000 mL/day according to patient needs) must be ensured. To optimize the likelihood of voiding as scheduled, measured amounts of fluids may be administered about 30 minutes before voiding attempts. In addition, most of the fluids should be consumed before evening to minimize the need to void frequently during the night.

The goal of bladder training is to restore the bladder to normal function. Bladder training can be used with cognitively intact patients experiencing urge incontinence. A voiding and toileting schedule is formulated based on analysis of the assessment data. The schedule specifies times for the patient to try to empty the bladder using a bedpan, toilet, or commode. Privacy should be provided during voiding efforts. The interval between voiding times in the early phase of the bladder training period is short (90 to 120 minutes). The patient is encouraged not to void until the specified voiding time. Voiding success and episodes of incontinence are recorded. As the patient's bladder capacity and control increase, the interval is lengthened. Usually, there is a temporal relationship between drinking, eating, exercising, and voiding. The alert patient can participate in recording intake, activity, and voiding and can plan the schedule to achieve maximum continence. Barrier-free access to the toilet and modification of clothing can help the patient with functional incontinence to achieve self-care in toileting and continence.

Habit training is used to try to keep the patient dry by strict adherence to a toileting schedule and may be successful with stress, urge, or functional incontinence. In the case of a confused person, the caregiver takes the person to the toilet according to the schedule before involuntary voiding occurs. Simple cuing and consistency promote success. Periods of continence and successful voidings are positively reinforced.

Biofeedback is a system through which the patient learns consciously to contract excretory sphincters and control voiding cues. Cognitively intact patients who have stress or urge incontinence may gain bladder control through biofeedback.

Pelvic floor exercises (Kegel exercises) strengthen the pubococcygeus muscle. The patient is instructed to tighten pelvic floor muscles for 4 seconds ten times, and this is repeated four to six times a day. Stopping and starting the stream during urination is recommended to increase control. Daily practice is essential. These exercises are helpful for cognitively intact women who experience stress incontinence.

Suprapubic tapping or stroking of the inner thigh may produce voiding by stimulating the voiding reflex arc in patients with reflex incontinence. This method is not always effective, however, because of detrusor–sphincter dyssynergy. As the bladder reflexively contracts to expel urine, the bladder sphincter reflexively closes, producing a high residual urine volume and an increased incidence of urinary tract infection.

Intermittent self-catheterization is an appropriate alternative for managing reflex incontinence, urinary retention, and overflow incontinence due to an overdistended bladder. The emphasis of patient teaching is on regular emptying of the bladder rather than sterility. Disabled patients reuse and clean catheters with bleach or hydrogen peroxide solutions or soap and water and may use a microwave oven to sterilize catheters. Aseptic intermittent catheterization technique is required in health care institutions because of the potential for bladder infection from resistant organisms. Intermittent self-catheterization may be difficult for patients with limited mobility, dexterity, or vision; however, family members can be taught the procedure.

Indwelling catheters are avoided if at all possible because of the high incidence of urinary tract infections with their use. Short-term use may be needed during treatment of severe skin breakdown due to continued incontinence. Patients with disability who are unable to perform intermittent self-catheterization may elect to use a suprapubic catheter for long-term bladder management. Suprapubic catheters are easier to maintain than indwelling catheters. A fluid intake of 3000 mL/day must be encouraged.

External catheters (condom catheters) and leg bags to collect spontaneous voidings are useful for male patients with reflex or total incontinence. The appropriate design and size must be chosen for maximal success, and the patient or caregiver must be taught how to apply the condom catheter and how to provide daily hygiene, including skin inspection. Instruction on emptying the leg bag must also be provided, and modifications can be made for patients with limited hand dexterity. External collection devices for women do exist, but difficulties with fit have precluded widespread use.

Incontinence pads (briefs) are used only as a last resort, because they only manage rather than solve the incontinence problem. Also, they have a negative psychological effect on the patient because many people think of them as diapers. Every effort should be made to reduce the incidence of incontinence episodes through the other methods that have been described. Incontinence pads may be useful at times for patients with stress or total incontinence to protect clothing, but they should be avoided whenever possible. When incontinence pads are used, they should wick moisture away from the body to minimize contact of moisture and excreta with the skin. Wet incontinence pads must be changed promptly, the skin cleansed, and a moisture barrier applied to protect the skin.

PROMOTING BOWEL CONTINENCE

The goals of a bowel training program are to develop regular bowel habits and to prevent uninhibited bowel elimination. Regular, complete emptying of the lower bowel results in bowel continence. A bowel-training program takes advantage of the patient's natural reflexes. Regularity, timing, nutrition and fluids, exercise, and correct positioning promote predictable defecation.

The nurse records defecation time, character of stool, nutritional intake, cognitive abilities, and functional self-care toileting abilities for 5 to 7 days. Analysis of this record is helpful when designing a bowel program for the patient with fecal incontinence.

Consistency in implementing the plan is essential. A regular time for defecation is established, and attempts at evacuation should be made within 15 minutes of the designated time daily. Natural gastrocolic and duodenocolic reflexes occur about 30 minutes after a meal; therefore, after breakfast is one of the best times to plan for bowel evacuation. If the patient had a previously established habit pattern at a different time of day, however, it should be followed.

The anorectal reflex may be stimulated by rectal suppository (eg, glycerin) or by mechanical stimulation (eg, digital stimulation with a lubricated gloved finger or anal dilator). Mechanical stimulation should be used only in patients with disability who have no voluntary motor function and no sensation as a result of injuries above the sacral segments of the spinal cord, such as quadriplegic, high paraplegic, or severely brain-injured patients. The technique is not effective in patients who do not have an intact sacral reflex arc (eg, those with flaccid paralysis). Mechanical stimulation, suppository insertion, or both should be initiated about 30 minutes before the scheduled bowel elimination time, and the interval between stimulation and defecation is noted for subsequent modification of the bowel program. Once the bowel routine is well established, stimulation with a suppository may not be necessary.

The patient should assume the normal squatting position (knees higher than the hips) and be in a private bathroom for defecation if at all possible, although a padded commode chair or bedside toilet is an acceptable alternative. Seating time is limited in patients who are at risk for skin breakdown. Bedpans should be avoided. A patient with disability who is unable to sit on a toilet should be positioned on the left side with legs flexed and the head of the bed elevated 30 to 45 degrees to increase intra-abdominal pressure. Protective padding is placed behind the buttocks. When possible, the patient is instructed to bear down and to contract the abdominal muscles. Massaging the abdomen from right to left facilitates movement of feces in the lower tract.

PREVENTING CONSTIPATION

The record of bowel elimination, character of stool, food and fluid intake, level of activity, bowel sounds, medications, and other assessment data are reviewed to develop the plan of care. Multiple approaches may be used to prevent constipation. The diet should be well balanced and should include adequate intake of high-fiber foods (vegetables, fruits, bran) to prevent hard stools and to stimulate peristalsis. Fluid intake should be between 2 and 3 L/day unless contraindicated. Prune juice or fig juice (120 mL) taken 30 minutes before a meal once daily is helpful to some cases when constipation is a problem. Physical activity and exercise are encouraged, as is self-care in toileting. The patient is encouraged to respond to the natural urge to defecate. Privacy during toileting is provided. Stool softeners, bulk-forming agents, mild stimulants, and suppositories may be prescribed to stimulate defecation and to prevent constipation.

Evaluation

EXPECTED PATIENT OUTCOMES

Expected patient outcomes may include:

1. Demonstrates control of bowel and bladder function
   a. Experiences no episodes of incontinence
   b. Avoids constipation
   c. Achieves independence in toileting
   d. Expresses satisfaction in level of bowel and bladder control
2. Achieves urinary continence
   a. Uses therapeutic approach appropriate to type of incontinence
   b. Maintains adequate fluid intake
   c. Washes and dries skin after episodes of incontinence
3. Achieves bowel continence
   a. Participates in bowel program
   b. Verbalizes need for regular time for bowel evacuation
   c. Modifies diet to promote continence
   d. Uses bowel stimulants as prescribed and needed
4. Experiences relief of constipation
   a. Uses high-fiber diet, fluids, and exercise to promote defecation
   b. Responds to urge to defecate

Disability and Sexuality Issues

An important issue confronting the patient with a disability, and a vital component of self-concept, is sexuality. Sexuality involves not only biologic sexual activity but also one's concept of masculinity or femininity. It affects the way a person reacts to others and is perceived by them, and it is expressed not only by physical intimacy but also by caring and emotional intimacy.

Sexuality problems faced by patients with disabilities include limited access to information about sexuality, lack of opportunity to form friendships and loving relationships, impaired self-image, and low self-esteem. The person with a disability may have physical and emotional difficulties that interfere with sexual activities. For example, diabetes and spinal cord injury may affect the ability to have an erection. The patient who has suffered a heart attack or stroke may fear having a life-threatening event (eg, another heart attack or stroke) during sexual activity. He or she may fear loss of bowel or bladder control during intimate moments. Changes in desire for sex and in the quality of sexual activities can occur for the patient and the partner, who may be too involved as the caregiver to have desire and energy for sexual activities.

Unfortunately, society and some health care providers contribute to these problems by ignoring patients' sexuality and by viewing disabled persons as asexual. Health care providers' own discomfort and lack of knowledge related to sexuality issues prevent them from providing the patient with disability and his or her partner interventions that promote healthy intimacy. Nurses caring for persons with disability must recognize and address sexual issues in order to promote feelings of self-worth, which are essential to total rehabilitation. The nurse should give the patient "permission" to discuss sexuality concerns and show a willingness to listen and help the patient overcome these concerns. The nurse also has a key role to provide appropriate patient education about how specific disabilities affect sexual function. For example, arthritis produces fatigue and morning stiffness, making planned afternoon sex a better alternative; spinal cord injury impairs erections and ejaculations; and traumatic brain injury may produce an increased or decreased interest in sexual behavior. Classes, books, movies, and support groups are useful tools to help patients learn about sexuality and disability. When open discussion and education about disability and sexuality do not result in a patient's achieving his or her sexuality goals, the nurse should refer the patient for ongoing counseling with a sex counselor or therapist. The patient may need training in communication and in social and assertiveness skills to develop desired relationships.

Fatigue

People with disabilities frequently experience fatigue. Physical and emotional weariness may be caused by discomfort and pain associated with a chronic health problem, deconditioning associated with prolonged periods of bed rest and immobility, impaired motor function requiring excessive expenditure of energy to ambulate, and the frustrations of performing ADLs. Ineffective coping with the disability, unresolved grief, and depression can also contribute to fatigue. The patient can use coping strategies to manage the psychological impact of the disability and pain management techniques to control the associated discomforts (see Chapter 13 for a discussion of pain management). In addition, the nurse can teach the patient to manage fatigue through priority setting and energy-conserving techniques. Special teaching strategies for patients with disabilities are included in Chart 11-10.

Home and Community-Based Care

An important goal of rehabilitation is to assist the person to return to the home environment after learning to manage the disability. A referral system maintains continuity of care when the patient is transferred to the home or to an extended care facility. The plan for discharge is formulated when the patient is first admitted to the hospital, and discharge plans are made with the patient's functional potential in mind.

The patient's support system (family, friends) is assessed. The attitudes of family and friends toward the patient, the disability, and the return home are important in making a successful transition to home. Not all families are able to carry on the arduous programs of exercise, physical training, and personal care that a patient may need. They may not have the resources or stability to care for a severely disabled family member. Even a stable family may be overwhelmed by the physical, emotional, economic, and energy strains of a disabling condition in their family member.

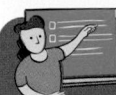

Chart 11-10 • PATIENT EDUCATION
Learning to Cope With Disabilities

The following points may be useful in teaching patients how to reduce their energy output and conserve their strength to achieve a meaningful lifestyle.

Take Control of Your Life
- Face the reality of your disability.
- Emphasize areas of strength.
- Remain outward looking.
- Seek inventive ways to tackle problems.
- Share concerns and frustrations.
- Maintain and improve general health.
- Plan for recreation.

Have Well-Defined Goals and Priorities
- Keep priorities in order; eliminate nonessential activities.
- Plan and pace your activities.

Organize Your Life
- Plan each day.
- Organize work.
- Perform tasks in steps.
- Distribute heavy work throughout the day or week.

Conserve Energy
- Rest before undertaking difficult tasks.
- Stop the activity before fatigue occurs.
- Continue with an exercise conditioning program to strengthen muscles.

Control Your Environment
- Try to be well organized.
- Keep possessions in the same place, so that they can be found with a minimum of effort.
- Store equipment (personal care, crafts, work) in a box or basket.
- Use energy-conservation and work-simplification techniques.
- Keep work within easy reach and in front of you.
- Use adaptive equipment, self-help aids, and labor-saving devices.
- Recruit assistance from others; delegate when necessary.
- Take safety precautions.

Members of the rehabilitation team must not judge the family but rather should provide supportive interventions that help them attain their highest level of function.

The family needs to know as much as possible about the patient's condition and care so that they do not fear the patient's return home. The nurse develops methods for coping with problems that may arise with the patient and family. A skill checklist individualized for the patient and family can be developed to make certain that the family is proficient in assisting the patient with certain tasks. See Chart 11-11 for an example of a home care checklist.

Complementary Therapies

Individuals with disabilities may seek a variety of different therapies. For some, therapeutic horseback riding influences the whole body and has a profound effect on all body systems. Instructors are certified through the North American Riding for the Handicapped Association. Pet therapy and canine companion programs have reduced stress and promoted coping for many disabled persons. Some animals including simian monkeys can pick up the phone, retrieve small assistive devices, assist with drinking beverages, or assist with activating emergency calls. The "working" animals provide companionship as well as physical assistance for elderly persons and persons with disability who may live alone.

Nurses can also encourage persons with disability to take advantage of community programs. T'ai chi classes improve muscle strength, balance, and coordination and can help to prevent falls in the elderly. Disabled persons, including wheelchair users, can participate in T'ai chi classes for improved balance, coordination, muscle strength and control, and a sense of well-being.

Daily journal writing has helped depressed individuals and their families overcome many emotionally draining reactions to adverse circumstances. Nurses are instrumental in teaching patients and family members this cost-effective technique. Relaxation exercises can also be taught by the nurse and encouraged in all settings, including the hospital, rehabilitation setting, outpatient areas, and the home.

Continuing Care

The home care nurse may visit the patient in the hospital, interview the patient and family, and review the ADL sheet to learn which activities the patient can perform. This helps ensure continuity of care and that the patient does not regress but instead maintains the independence gained while in the hospital or rehabilitation setting. The family may need to purchase, borrow, or improvise needed equipment, such as safety rails, a raised toilet seat or commode, or a tub bench. Ramps may need to be built or doorways widened to achieve full access.

Family members are taught how to use equipment and are given a copy of the equipment manufacturer's instruction booklet, the names of resource people, lists of equipment-related supplies, and locations where they may be obtained. A written summary of the care plan is included in family teaching.

A network of support services and communication systems may be required to enhance opportunities for independent living. The nurse uses collaborative, administrative skills to coordinate these activities and to pull together the network of care. The nurse also provides skilled care, initiates additional referrals when indicated, and serves as the patient's advocate and counselor when obstacles are encountered. The nurse continues to reinforce prior teaching and helps the patient to set and achieve attainable goals. The degree to which the patient adapts to the home and community environment depends on the confidence and self-esteem developed during the rehabilitation process and on the acceptance, support, and reactions of the family, employer, and community members.

There is a growing trend toward independent living by people with severe disabilities, either alone or in groups that share resources. Preparation for independent living should include training in managing a household and working with personal care attendants as well as training in mobility. The goal is integration into the community—living and working in the community with accessible housing, employment, public buildings, transportation, and recreation.

State rehabilitation administration agencies provide services to assist people with disability in obtaining the help they need to engage in gainful employment. These services include diagnostic, medical, and mental health services. Counseling, training, placement, and follow-up services are available to help people with disabilities select and attain jobs.

If the patient is transferred to an extended care facility, the transition is planned to promote continued progress. Independence gained continues to be supported, and progress is fostered. Adjustment to the extended care facility is facilitated through communication. The family is encouraged to visit, to be involved, and to take the patient home on weekends and holidays if possible.

Chart 11-11

Home Care Checklist ● **Managing the Therapeutic Regimen at Home**

At the completion of the home care instruction, the patient or caregiver will be able to:	Patient	Caregiver
• State the impact of disability on physiologic functioning.	✓	✓
• State changes in lifestyle necessary to maintain health.	✓	✓
• State the name, dose, side effects, frequency, and schedule for all medications.	✓	✓
• State how to obtain medical supplies after discharge.	✓	✓
• Identify durable medical equipment needs, proper usage, and maintenance necessary for safe utilization:	✓	✓

[ ] Wheelchair—manual/power   [ ] Bedside toilet
[ ] Cushion   [ ] Crutches
[ ] Grab bars   [ ] Walker
[ ] Sliding board   [ ] Prosthesis
[ ] Mechanical lift   [ ] Orthosis
[ ] Raised padded commode seat   [ ] Specialty bed
[ ] Padded commode wheelchair

• Demonstrate usage of adaptive equipment for activities of daily living:	✓	✓

[ ] Long-handled sponge   [ ] Rocker-knife, spork, weighted utensils
[ ] Reacher   [ ] Special closures for clothing
[ ] Universal cuff   [ ] Other
[ ] Plate mat and guard

• Demonstrate mobility skills:	✓	✓

[ ] Transfers: bed to chair; in and out of toilet and tub; in and out of car
[ ] Negotiate ramps, curbs, stairs
[ ] Assume sitting from supine position
[ ] Turn side to side in bed
[ ] Maneuver wheelchair; manage arm and leg rests; lock brakes
[ ] Ambulate safely using assistive devices
[ ] Range-of-motion exercises
[ ] Muscle-strengthening exercises

• Demonstrate skin care:	✓	✓

[ ] Inspect bony prominences every morning and evening
[ ] Identify stage I pressure ulcer and actions to take if present
[ ] Change dressings for stage II to IV pressure ulcers
[ ] State dietary requirements to promote healing of pressure ulcers
[ ] Demonstrate pressure relief at prescribed intervals
[ ] State sitting schedule
[ ] Demonstrate adherence to bed turning schedule, bed positioning, and use of bridging techniques
[ ] Apply and wear protective boots at prescribed times
[ ] Demonstrate correct wheelchair sitting posture
[ ] Demonstrate techniques to avoid friction and shear in bed
[ ] Demonstrate proper hygiene to maintain skin integrity

• Demonstrate bladder care:	✓	✓

[ ] State schedule for voiding, toileting, and catheterization
[ ] Identify relationship of fluid intake to voiding and catheterization schedule
[ ] State how to perform pelvic floor exercises
[ ] Demonstrate clean self-intermittent catheterization and care of catheterization equipment
[ ] Demonstrate indwelling catheter care
[ ] Demonstrate application of external condom catheter
[ ] Demonstrate application, emptying, and cleaning of urinary drainage bag
[ ] Demonstrate application of incontinence pads and performing perineal hygiene
[ ] State signs and symptoms of urinary tract infection

• Demonstrate bowel care	✓	✓

[ ] State optimum dietary intake to promote evacuation
[ ] Identify schedule for optimum bowel evacuation
[ ] Demonstrate techniques to increase intra-abdominal pressure; Valsalva maneuver; abdominal massage; leaning forward
[ ] Demonstrate techniques to stimulate bowel movements: ingesting warm liquids; digital stimulation; insertion of suppositories
[ ] Demonstrate optimum position for bowel evacuation: on toilet with knees higher than hips; left side in bed with knees flexed and head slightly elevated
[ ] Identify complications and corrective strategies for bowel retraining: constipation, impaction, diarrhea, hemorrhoids, rectal bleeding, anal tears

(continued)

Chart 11-11

Home Care Checklist ○ **Managing the Therapeutic Regimen at Home (Continued)**

	Patient	Caregiver
• Identify community resources for peer and family support	✓	✓
[ ] Identify phone numbers for disabled support groups		
[ ] State meeting locations and times		
• Demonstrate how to access transportation	✓	✓
[ ] Identify locations of wheelchair accessibility for public buses or trains		
[ ] Identify phone numbers for private wheelchair van		
[ ] Contact Division of Motor Vehicles for handicapped parking permit		
[ ] Contact Division of Motor Vehicles for driving test when appropriate		
[ ] Identify resources for adapting private vehicle with hand controls or wheelchair lift		
• Identify vocational rehabilitation resources	✓	✓
[ ] State name and phone number of vocational rehabilitation counselor		
[ ] Identify educational opportunities that may lead to future employment		
• Identify community resources for recreation	✓	✓
[ ] State local recreation centers that offer programs for the disabled		
[ ] Identify leisure activities that can be pursued in the community		
• Identify the need for health promotion and screening activities		

Critical Thinking Exercises

1. The patient who has just been admitted to your unit in the rehabilitation hospital is a 58-year-old woman who is recovering from a stroke. She has paralysis on one side, but speech is intact. In discussing the patient's level of functioning with the physical rehabilitation team, describe the kinds of self-care activities that you would assess in developing a rehabilitation plan for the patient.

2. An elderly man who has lost his leg as a result of diabetes is to be discharged to his home, where he will be cared for by his family. The family members are particularly concerned about how to prevent pressure ulcers, because the patient is a diabetic and will be confined primarily to a wheelchair. Describe the instructions you would give them. How might your teaching strategies differ if family members converse primarily in their native tongue, which is not English?

3. You are caring for a young man who has sustained a traumatic brain injury and multiple fractures in a motor vehicle crash. He is ready to return home to continue rehabilitation as an outpatient. You accompany the physical and occupational therapist to assess the patient's home environment in anticipation of his discharge. Compare the types of safety factors that might be considered if the patient lives in a single-story house, in a two-story house, in a two-room apartment in a high-rise building, or on a farm.

REFERENCES AND SELECTED READINGS

Books

Agency for Health Care Policy and Research, Public Health Service, U.S. Department of Health and Human Services. Panel for the Prediction and Prevention of Pressure Ulcers in Adults. (1992). *Pressure ulcers in adults: Prediction and prevention.* Clinical Practice Guideline, Number 3. AHCPR Publication No. 92-0047. Rockville, MD: Author.

Agency for Health Care Policy and Research, Public Health Service, U.S. Department of Health and Human Services. (1994). *Treatment of pressure ulcers.* Clinical Practice Guideline, Number 15. AHCPR Publication No. 95-0652. Rockville, MD: Author.

Agency for Health Care Policy and Research. Public Health Service, U.S. Department of Health and Human Services. Urinary Incontinence Guideline Panel. (1996). *Urinary incontinence in adults: Clinical practice guideline.* AHCPR Pub. No. 96-0682. Rockville, MD: Author.

Alexander, T., Hiduke, R., & Stevens, K. (1999). *Rehabilitation nursing policy and procedure manual* (2nd ed.). Rehabilitation Institute of Chicago. Chicago, IL: McGraw-Hill.

Association of Rehabilitation Nurses. (2000). *Standards and scope of rehabilitation nursing practice.* Glenview, IL: Author.

Association of Rehabilitation Nurses. (2000). *The specialty practice of rehabilitation nursing: A core curriculum* (4th ed.). Skokie, IL: Author.

Association of Rehabilitation Nurses. (1995). *Twenty-one rehabilitation nursing diagnoses: A guide to interventions and outcomes.* Glenview, IL: Author.

Association of Rehabilitation Nurses. (1996). *Scope and standards of advanced clinical practice in rehabilitation nursing.* Glenview, IL: Author.

Association of Rehabilitation Nurses. (1997). *Advanced practice in rehabilitation nursing: A core curriculum.* Glenview, IL: Author.

Derstine, J., & Hargrove, S. (2000). *Comprehensive rehabilitation nursing.* St. Louis, MO: W.B. Saunders.

Dittmar, S., & Gresham, G. (1997). *Functional assessment and outcome measures for the rehabilitation health professional.* Gaithersburg, MD: Aspen.

Easton, K. (1999). *Gerontological rehabilitation nursing.* St. Louis, MO: W. B. Saunders.

Edwards, P., Hertzberg, D., Hays, S., & Youngblood, N. (1999). *Pediatric rehabilitation nursing.* St. Louis, MO: W. B. Saunders.

Hess, C. (1999). *Wound care* (3rd ed.). Springhouse, PA: Springhouse.

Hoeman, S. (1996). *Rehabilitation nursing: Process and application* (2nd ed.). St. Louis, MO: Mosby.

Jans, L., & Stoddard, S. (1999). *Chartbook on women and disability in the United States.* Washington, DC: U.S. National Institute on Disability and Rehabilitation Research.

Krasner, D., & Kane, D. (1997). *Chronic wound care: A clinical source book for healthcare professionals* (2nd ed.). Wayne, PA: Health Management Publications, Inc.

Morrison, M. (2001). *The prevention and treatment of pressure ulcers.* St. Louis, MO: Mosby.

Newman, D. (1999). *The urinary incontinence sourcebook.* Chicago: Lowell House.

Sipski, M., & Alexander, C. (1997). *Sexual function in people with disability and chronic illness: A health professional's guide.* Gaithersburg, MD: Aspen.

Sussman, C., & Bates-Jenson, B. (1998). *Wound care: A collaborative practice manual for physical therapists and nurses.* Gaithersburg, MD: Aspen.

U.S. Census Bureau (1997). *Americans with disabilities, 1997: Household Economic Studies Current Population Reports.* Washington, DC: U.S. Government Printing Office.

U.S. Department of Health and Human Services. (2000, December 14). *HHS Fact Sheet. Substance Abuse—A National Challenge: Prevention, Treatment and Research at HHS.* Washington, DC: U.S. Government Printing Office.

U.S. Department of Justice. (1996). *A guide to disability rights laws.* Washington, DC: U.S. Government Printing Office.

Journals

Asterisks indicate nursing research articles.

Akdolun, N., & Terakye, G. (2001). Sexual problems before and after myocardial infarction: Patients' needs for information. *Rehabilitation Nursing, 26*(4), 152–159.

Beitz, J. (2001). Overcoming barriers to wound care: a systems perspective. *Ostomy/Wound Management, 47*(3), 56–64.

*Cataldo, J. (2001). The relationship of hardiness and depression to disability in institutionalized older adults. *Rehabilitation Nursing, 26*(1), 28–33.

Daly, M. (2000). Rehabilitation in the therapeutic riding arena. *Rehabilitation Nursing, 25*(5), 167–168.

Gray, M. (2000). Urinary retention: management in the acute care setting: Part 1. *American Journal of Nursing, 100*(7), 40–48.

Gray, M. (2000). Urinary retention: management in the acute care setting: Part 2. *American Journal of Nursing, 100*(8), 36–44.

Henderson-Martin, B. (2000). No more surprises: Screening patients for alcohol abuse. *American Journal of Nursing, 100*(9), 26–33.

Hood, P. (2000). Handicapped parking. *American Journal of Nursing, 100*(9), 11.

Krebs, H. (2000). Increasing productivity and quality of care: Robot-aided neuro-rehabilitation. *Journal of Rehabilitation Research and Development, 37*(6), 639–652.

*Masayuki, I. (2000). Prediction of functional outcome after stroke rehabilitation. *American Journal of Physical Medicine and Rehabilitation, 79*(6), 513–518.

Mayo Clinic Rochester (2001). *Geriatric Medicine.* Pressure ulcers: Prevention and management. Available at: http://www.mayo.edu/geriatrics-rst/PU-ToC.html. Accessed August 15, 2001.

*Missik, E. (2001). Women and cardiac rehabilitation: Accessibility issues and policy recommendations. *Rehabilitation Nursing, 26*(4), 141–147.

Modlin, S. (2001). From puppy to service dog: Raising service dogs for the rehabilitation team. *Rehabilitation Nursing, 26*(1), 12–17.

Patel, C. (2000). Vacuum-assisted wound closure. *American Journal of Nursing, 100*(12), 45–48.

Pryor, J. (2000). Creating a rehabilitative milieu. *Rehabilitation Nursing, 25*(4), 141–144.

*Secrest, J. (2000). Transformation of the relationship: The experience of primary support persons of stroke survivors. *Rehabilitation Nursing, 25*(3), 93–99.

Smeltzer, S. C. (2000). Viewpoint: Double jeopardy. The health care system slights women with disabilities. *American Journal of Nursing, 100*(8), 11.

Smith, C., & Holcroft, C. (2000). Journal writing as a complementary therapy for reactive depression: A rehabilitation teaching program. *Rehabilitation Nursing, 25*(5), 170–176.

Sperazza, L. (2001). Rehabilitation options for patients with low vision. *Rehabilitation Nursing, 26*(4), 148–151.

Sullivan, M., & Sharts-Hopko, N. (2000). Preventing the downward spiral: Osteoporosis and MS. *American Journal of Nursing, 100*(8), 26–33.

Thompson, J. (2000). A practical guide to wound care. *RN, 63*(1), 48–58.

Wolf, S., & Barnhardt, H. (1996). Reducing frailty and falls in older persons: An investigation of T'ai chi and computerized balance training. *Journal of American Geriatrics Society, 44,* 489–497.

RESOURCES AND WEBSITES

ABLEDATA, 8401 Colesville Road, Suite 200, Silver Spring, MD 20910; 1-800-227-0216; http://www.abledata.com.

Agency for Healthcare Research and Quality (formerly the Agency for Health Care Policy and Research), 2101 East Jefferson Street, Suite 501; Rockville, MD 20852; 1-800-358-9295; http://www.ahrq.gov.

American Society of Addiction Medicine, 4601 North Park Avenue, Arcade Suite 101, Chevy Chase, MD 20815; 1-301-656-3920; http://www.asam.org.

Assistive Technology Industry Association, 526 Davis Street, Suite 217; Evanston, IL 60201; 1-877-687-2842/847-969-1282; http://www.atia.org.

Association of Rehabilitation Nurses, 4700 W. Lake Avenue, Glenview, IL 60025-1485; 1-800-229-7530; fax 1-847-375-4710; http://www.rehabnurse.org.

Canine Companions for Independence, PO Box 446, Santa Rosa CA 95402-0446; 1-800-572-2275; http://www.caninecompanions.org.

Council for Disability Rights, 205 West Randolph, Suite 1650, Chicago, IL 60606; 1-312-444-9484; http://www.disabilityrights.org.

National Center for Health Statistics, Division of Data Services, Hyattsville, MD 20782-2003; 1-301-458-4636; http://www.cdc.gov/nchs.

National Council on Alcoholism and Drug Dependence, Inc., 20 Exchange Place, Suite 2902, New York, NY 10005; 1-212-269-7797; http://www.ncadd.org.

National Council on Disability, 1331 F Street, NW, Suite 1050, Washington, DC 20004; 1-202-272-2004; http://www.ncd.gov.

National Institute on Disability and Rehabilitation Research (NIDRR), Office of Special Education and Rehabilitation Research, U.S. Department of Education, Washington, DC 20202; 1-202-205-9151; http://www.ed.gov/offices/OSERS/NIDRR.

National Rehabilitation Information Center (NARIC), 1010 Wayne Avenue, Suite 800, Silver Spring, MD 20910; 1-800-346-2742; http://www.naric.com.

Rehabilitation Accreditation Commission, 4891 E. Grant Road, Tucson, AZ 85712.

Sexuality and Information and Education Council of the U.S. (SIECUS), 130 West 42nd Street, Suite 350, New York, NY 10036-7802; 1-212-819-9770; http://www.siecus.org.

Substance Abuse Resources and Disability Issues, Wright State University School of Medicine, Dayton, Ohio 45435; 1-937-259-1384; http://www.med.wright.edu.

U.S. Census Bureau, 4700 Silver Hill Road, Suitland, MD 20746; 1-301-457-4608; http://www.census.gov.

U.S. Department of Health and Human Services, 200 Independence Avenue SW, Washington, DC 20201; 1-202-690-6343; http://www.hhs.gov.

Health Care of the Older Adult

On completion of this chapter, the learner will be able to:

1. Describe the aging American population based on demographic trends and statistical data.
2. Discuss the potential economic effect of the large aging population in America on health care.
3. Identify major legal issues relevant to the care of older people.
4. Compare and contrast the physiologic aspects of aging with those of middle-age adults.
5. Describe the significance of preventive health care and health promotion for the elderly.
6. Identify the important physical and mental health problems of aging and their effects on the functioning of older people and their families.
7. Identify the major geriatric syndromes and their effects on the individual patient.
8. Specify nursing implications related to medication therapy in older people.
9. Examine the concerns of older people and their families in the home and community, in the acute care setting, and in long-term care facilities.
10. Identify the resources available to allow older adults to receive medical and nursing services in their own homes.

$\mathcal{A}$ging, the normal process of time-related change, begins with birth and continues throughout life. The older segment of the American population is growing more rapidly than the rest of the population: the U.S. Census Bureau projects that by the year 2030, there will be more people older than 65 years of age (22%) than people younger than 18 years of age (21%). As the older population increases, the number of people who live to be very old will also increase. Health professionals will be challenged to design strategies that address the higher prevalence of illness within this aging population. Many chronic conditions commonly found among older people can be managed, limited, and even prevented. Older people are more likely to maintain good health and functional independence if appropriate community-based support services are available.

Overview of Aging

DEMOGRAPHICS OF AGING

According to the National Center for Health Statistics, **life expectancy**, the average number of years that a person can be expected to live, has risen dramatically over the past century. In 1900, the average life expectancy was 47.3 years, but by 1998 that figure had increased to 76.7 years. According to data from the National Vital Statistics System, in 1998 a 75-year old man could be expected to live until the age of 85, and a 75-year old woman could be expected to live until the age of 87 (National Center for Health Statistics, 2000).

By 2030, people older than 65 years of age will account for 22% of the population, compared with 13% in 2001 (Fig. 12-1).

More than 70% of elders receive most of their care from informal caregivers. Because many of the baby boomers (those born between 1940 and 1960) tended to have children later in life, these children will face the competing demands of caring for their aging parents while caring for their own dependent children (Spillman, 2001).

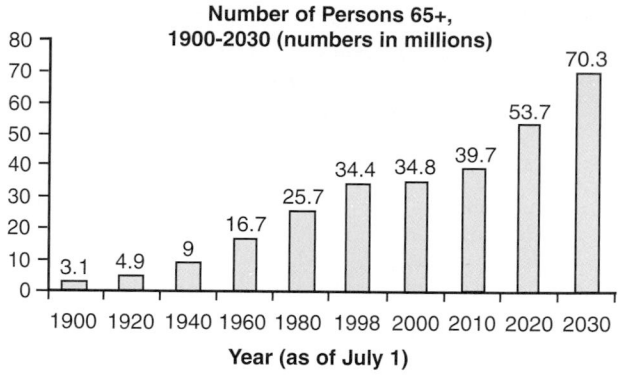

Number of Persons 65+, 1900-2030 (numbers in millions)

FIGURE 12-1 Profile of Americans age 65 years and older based on data from the U.S. Bureau of the Census. Data from year 1900 to present is used to predict millions of Americans aged 65 and older in the year 2030. (http://www.aoa.gov/aoa/stats/profile/default.htm)

Although most older adults enjoy good health, in national surveys as many as 40% of adults age 65 and older report disability. Chronic disease is the major cause of disability, and heart disease, cancer, and stroke continued to be the three most significant causes of death in persons 65 years of age and older in the United States between 1980 and 1998 (Table 12-1). Alzheimer's disease accounted for almost 44,000 deaths in 1999 (National Center for Health Statistics, 2000).

HEALTH CARE COSTS OF AGING

There are serious concerns about whether there will be sufficient health services available as more and more persons in the United States become eligible for publicly funded health programs. The two major health programs in the United States are Medicare and Medicaid, both of which are overseen by the Centers for Medicaid and Medicare Services (CMS), formerly the Health Care Financing Administration (HCFA). Medicare is funded by the Federal gov-

Glossary

ageism: a bias against older people based solely on their chronologic age, without consideration of their functional status

dehydration: condition resulting from excessively low levels of fluid in the body; occurs when fluid output exceeds fluid intake

delirium: an acute, confused state that begins with disorientation but, if not immediately evaluated, can progress to changes in level of consciousness, irreversible brain damage, and sometimes death

dementia: broad term for a syndrome characterized by a general decline in higher brain functioning, such as reasoning, with a pattern of eventual decline in ability to perform even basic activities of daily living, such as toileting and eating

depression: the most common affective (mood) disorder of old age; results from changes in reuptake of the neurochemical serotonin in response to chronic illness

and emotional stresses related to the inevitable physical and social changes associated with the aging process

elder abuse: the physical or emotional harm of an elderly person by one or more of the individual's children, caregivers, or others

geriatrics: the study of old age that includes the physiology, pathology, diagnosis, and management of the disorders and diseases of older adults

gerontology: the combined biologic, psychologic, and sociologic study of older adults within their environment

gerontologic/geriatric nursing: the field of nursing that specializes in the nursing process as it relates to the assessment, nursing diagnosis, planning, implementation, and evaluation of older adults in all environments including acute, intermediate, and skilled care as well as within the community

life expectancy: the average number of years that a person is expected to live

life span: the maximum number of years an individual can be expected to live in the absence of disease or life-threatening trauma

orientation: a term that refers to a person's ability to recognize who and where he or she is in a time continuum; used to evaluate an individual's basic cognitive status

polypharmacy: the administration of multiple medications at the same time; common in older persons with several chronic illnesses

presbycusis: the decreased ability to hear high-pitched tones that naturally begins in midlife as a result of irreversible inner ear changes

presbyopia: the decrease in visual accommodation that occurs with advancing age

urinary incontinence: the unplanned loss of urine, which affects up to 50% of community-residing older adults and approximately 75% to 85% of nursing home residents

Table 12-1 • Annual Deaths and Death Rates for the 10 Leading Causes of Death in People 65 Years and Older*

RANK	CAUSE OF DEATH	NUMBER	RATE[†]
	All causes	1,694,326	5,052.8
1	Heart diseases	615,426	1,835.3
2	Malignant neoplasms, including neoplasms of lymphatic and hematopoietic tissues	381,142	1,136.6
3	Cerebrovascular diseases	138,762	413.8
4	Chronic obstructive pulmonary diseases and allied conditions	88,478	263.9
5	Pneumonia and influenza	74,297	221.6
6	Diabetes mellitus	44,452	132.6
7	Accidents and adverse effects	29,099	86.8
	Motor vehicle crashes	7,626	22.7
	All other accidents and adverse effects	21,473	64.0
8	Alzheimer's disease	20,230	60.3
9	Nephritis, nephrotic syndrome, and nephrosis	20,182	60.2
10	Septicemia	16,899	50.4
	All other causes (residual)	265,359	791.4

*All races, both sexes, United States, 1995.

[†]Rates per 100,000 population.

Anderson, R. N., Kochanek, K. D., & Murphy, S. L. (1997). Report of final mortality statistics, 1995. *Monthly vital statistics report* (Vol. 45, No. 11, Supp. 2, Table 7). Hyattsville, MD: National Center for Health Statistics.

Chart 12-1   **Ethics and Related Issues**

Should a family member who is a durable power of attorney for health care allow her aunt to be given a blood transfusion after hip surgery, when the aunt's hemoglobin suddenly drops? The aunt has clearly stated to the orthopedic surgeon before surgery that she does not want blood products for any reason, even if the situation is life-threatening.

Situation

Mrs. A is an 83-year-old retired teacher who is widowed and a resident of a nursing home. She has a history of Alzheimer's disease, depression, Parkinson's disease, osteoporosis, hypertension, diabetes, and Vitamin B_{12} deficiency. She experienced an unwitnessed fall while walking in the hall with her walker, sustained a hip fracture, and was taken to the hospital. Before this fall she required moderate assistance with activities of daily living, was occasionally incontinent of urine, and ambulated with a walker. After the fracture was confirmed, the risks and benefits of surgical and nonsurgical management were carefully discussed with Mrs. A and her family, including a niece who is her durable power of attorney for health care. During this conversation, Mrs. A consented to surgery but stated that she was a Jehovah's Witness and did not want any blood products, not even for life-threatening situations.

Dilemma

Several ethical issues were relevant to considering a resolution to Mrs. A's situation. The obligation to respect the patient's autonomy in the decision to refuse blood products clearly put Mrs. A's life at risk. Before the surgery, Mrs. A had named her niece responsible for health care decisions; however, she and her niece had conflicting moral viewpoints. Her niece believed it was imperative that Mrs. A receive the transfusion to save her life. The case was taken to the Ethics Committee of the hospital, and a decision was made in favor of the transfusion. After the transfusion, Mrs. A made a quick recovery and was returned to the nursing home. Before leaving the hospital, however, she thanked the staff and her family for honoring her wishes and not giving her any blood products.

Discussion

- What arguments would you offer *against* the transfusion?
- What arguments would you offer *in favor of* the transfusion?
- What arguments would you offer *against* and *in favor of* telling Mrs. A. that she had received a transfusion?

Hofmann, M. T., & Nahass, D. (2001). Case report: The use of an ethics committee regarding the case of an elderly female with blood loss after hip surgery. *Annals of Long-Term Care, 9,* 55–59.

ernment, whereas Medicaid is funded jointly by the Federal and state governments to provide health care for the poor. Medicaid is the dominant public payer of nursing home costs. Eligibility and costs for these services vary from state to state.

Medicare funding covered 32% of the costs of hospital services and 22% of the costs of physician services in the United States in 1998. Nursing home care, in contrast, was financed primarily by Medicaid (46%) and out-of-pocket payments (33%) (National Center for Health Statistics, 2000).

ETHICAL AND LEGAL ISSUES AFFECTING THE OLDER ADULT

Loss of rights, victimization, and other grave problems face the person who has made no plans for personal and property management in the event of disability or death. The advice and services of a competent attorney regarding financial and personal issues can preserve future autonomy and self-determination. The nurse as an advocate can encourage the older person to prepare advance directives for future decision making in the event of incapacitation (Plotkin & Roche, 2000).

A power of attorney is a legal agreement that authorizes a designated person to act in specific, outlined circumstances on behalf of the signer. This is a form of voluntary guardianship, permission for which is freely granted when the older person is competent. Unless stated otherwise, a power of attorney is invalidated on the incapacity of the signer. A durable power of attorney is a similar agreement that continues even if the older person is disabled or incapacitated. This power can include the authorization to make financial or personal decisions, depending on the desires of the signer (Chart 12-1).

A trust is another option that the competent older person can consider. In a trust, the person designates someone to manage his

or her property, stipulates how and under what circumstances the property will be managed, and designates a beneficiary. If incompetency or disability occurs, management of the property is undertaken according to the person's wishes.

If no advance arrangement has been made, and the older person appears unable to make decisions, *anyone* can petition the court for a competency hearing. If the court rules that the person is incompetent, the judge will appoint a guardian—a third party who is given powers by the court to assume responsibility for making financial or personal decisions for that person. There are two kinds of guardians: guardian of the person and guardian of the estate. Because such a court action strips the civil liberties and constitutional rights from the older person, a potential for great harm exists. Safeguards include the following: (1) the older person must be given notice, (2) he or she must be given an opportunity to be legally represented, and (3) medical testimony can be cross-examined. A less restrictive form of guardianship, called limited guardianship, transfers to the appointed guardian only those powers or duties that the older person cannot exercise. Although this alternative is not widely used, it remains an option.

An advance directive is a formal, legally endorsed document that provides instructions for care (living will) or names a proxy decision maker (durable power of attorney) and is to be implemented in the event of the signer's future decision-making incapacity. This written document must be signed by the person and by two witnesses; a copy should be given to the physician and incorporated into the medical record. The person must understand that this document is not meant to be used only when certain (or all) types of medical treatment are withheld; rather, it allows for a detailed description of all health care preferences, including full use of all available medical interventions. The health care proxy has the authority to interpret the patient's wishes on the basis of the medical circumstances of the situation and is not restricted to deciding only whether life-sustaining treatment can be withdrawn or withheld.

In 1990, the Patient Self-Determination Act (PSDA), a federally mandated law, was enacted to require patient education about advance directives at the time of hospital admission, along with documentation of this education. The PSDA is also mandated in nursing homes to enhance resident autonomy by increasing involvement in health care decision making. A growing body of research indicates that nursing homes implement the PSDA more vigorously than hospitals do. In both settings, however, the documentation and placement of advance directives in the medical record varies considerably from facility to facility, as does the education of patients about advance directives. Processes for fulfilling the requirements of the law are continuously being revised in many facilities to promote compliance. The PSDA provides no guidelines regarding how often the advance directives of nursing home residents should be reviewed. Continuing quality improvement programs that establish guidelines for review are more likely to exist in nursing homes in which ethics committees are present. The nurse can play a vital role in advocating for the patient when the patient or a family member is unable to do so.

NURSING CARE OF OLDER ADULTS

Geriatrics, the study of old age, includes the physiology, pathology, diagnosis, and management of the diseases of older adults. The broader field of **gerontology,** or the study of the aging process, draws from the biologic, psychological, and sociologic sciences. Because hospitalized patients are being discharged to home "quicker and sicker" than ever before, nurses in all settings, including hospital, home care, rehabilitation, and outpatient settings, need to be knowledgeable about geriatric nursing principles and skilled in meeting the needs of elderly patients.

Gerontologic or **geriatric nursing** is the field of nursing that specializes in the care of the elderly. The *Standards and Scope of Gerontological Nursing Practice* were originally developed in 1969 by the American Nurses Association; they were revised in 1976 and again in 1987. The nurse gerontologist can be either a specialist or a generalist offering comprehensive nursing care to older persons by combining the basic nursing process of assessment, diagnosis, planning, implementation, and evaluation with a specialized knowledge of aging. Currently, nurses from all nursing programs, including vocational programs (LPN/LVN), traditional hospital programs, and college degree programs (ADN/BSN), as well as master's prepared advanced practice nurses (clinical nurse specialists, nurse practitioners, and nurse anesthetists), care for older adults.

Gerontologic nursing is provided in acute care, skilled and assisted living, community, and home settings. Its goals include promoting and maintaining functional status and helping older adults to identify and use their strengths to achieve optimal independence. The nurse helps the older person to maintain dignity and maximum autonomy despite physical, social, and psychological losses. The nurse who becomes certified in gerontologic nursing has specialized knowledge in the acute and chronic changes specific to older people. The use of advanced practice nurses (APNs) in long-term care has proved to be very effective: when APNs using current scientific knowledge about clinical problems interface with nursing home staff, significantly less deterioration in affect and overall health issues has been demonstrated (Ryden et al., 2000).

Because old age is a normal occurrence that encompasses all experiences of life, care and concern for the elderly cannot be limited to one discipline, but is best provided through a cooperative effort. An interdisciplinary team, through comprehensive geriatric assessment, can combine expertise and resources to provide insight into all aspects of the aging process. Nurses collaborate with the interdisciplinary team to obtain non-nursing services and provide a holistic approach to care.

Normal Age-Related Changes and Health Promotion Activities

Intrinsic aging (from within the person) refers to those changes caused by the normal aging process that are genetically programmed and essentially universal within a species. Universality is the major criterion used to distinguish normal from abnormal aging. Extrinsic aging results from influences outside the person. Illness and disease, air pollution, and sunlight are examples of extrinsic factors that may hasten the aging process and that can be eliminated or reduced through effective health care interventions.

Cellular and extracellular changes of old age cause a change in physical appearance and a decline in function. Measurable changes in shape and body makeup occur. The body's ability to maintain homeostasis becomes increasingly diminished with cellular aging, and organ systems cannot function at full efficiency because of cellular and tissue deficits. Cells become less able to replace themselves, and they accumulate a pigment known as lipofuscin. A degradation of elastin and collagen causes connective tissue to become stiffer and less elastic.

The well-being of an aged person depends on physical, mental, social, and environmental factors. A total assessment includes an evaluation of all major body systems, social and mental status, and the ability of the person to function independently despite a chronic illness. Table 12-2 summarizes the signs and symptoms of age-related changes in the functioning of body systems and suggested nursing interventions.

PHYSICAL ASPECTS OF AGING
Cardiovascular System

Heart disease is the leading cause of death in the aged. The heart valves become thicker and stiffer, and the heart muscle and arteries lose their elasticity. Calcium and fat deposits accumulate within arterial walls, and veins become increasingly tortuous. Although function is maintained under normal circumstances, the cardiovascular system has less reserve and responds less efficiently to stress. The maximum cardiac output decreases by

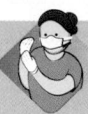

Table 12-2 • Health Promotion:
Age-Related Changes in Body Systems and Health Promotion Strategies

CHANGES	SUBJECTIVE AND OBJECTIVE FINDINGS	HEALTH PROMOTION STRATEGIES
Cardiovascular System Decreased cardiac output; diminished ability to respond to stress; heart rate and stroke volume do not increase with maximum demand; slower heart recovery rate; increased blood pressure	Complaints of fatigue with increased activity Increased heart rate recovery time Normal BP ≤140/90 mm Hg	Exercise regularly; pace activities; avoid smoking; eat a low-fat, low-salt diet; participate in stress-reduction activities; check blood pressure regularly; medication compliance; weight control
Respiratory System Increase in residual lung volume; decrease in vital capacity; decreased gas exchange and diffusing capacity; decreased cough efficiency	Fatigue and breathlessness with sustained activity; impaired healing of tissues as a result of decreased oxygenation; difficulty coughing up secretions	Exercise regularly; avoid smoking; take adequate fluids to liquefy secretions; receive yearly influenza immunization; avoid exposure to upper respiratory tract infections
Integumentary System Decreased protection against trauma and sun exposure; decreased protection against temperature extremes; diminished secretion of natural oils and perspiration	Skin appears thin and wrinkled; complaints of injuries, bruises, and sunburn; complaints of intolerance to heat; bone structure is prominent; dry skin	Avoid solar exposure (clothing, sunscreen, stay indoors); dress appropriately for temperature; maintain a safe indoor temperature; shower preferable to tub bath; lubricate skin
Reproductive System *Female:* Vaginal narrowing and decreased elasticity; decreased vaginal secretions *Male:* Decreased size of penis and testes *Male and female:* Slower sexual response	*Female:* Painful intercourse; vaginal bleeding following intercourse; vaginal itching and irritation; delayed orgasm *Male:* Delayed erection and achievement of orgasm	May require vaginal estrogen replacement; gynecology/urology follow-up; use a lubricant with intercourse
Musculoskeletal System Loss of bone density; loss of muscle strength and size; degenerated joint cartilage	Height loss; prone to fractures; kyphosis; back pain; loss of strength, flexibility, and endurance; joint pain	Exercise regularly; eat a high-calcium diet; limit phosphorus intake; take calcium and vitamin D supplements as prescribed
Genitourinary System *Male:* Benign prostatic hyperplasia	Urinary retention; irritative voiding symptoms including frequency, feeling of incomplete bladder emptying, multiple nighttime voidings	Seek referral to urology specialist; have ready access to toilet; wear easily manipulated clothing; drink adequate fluids; avoid bladder irritants (eg, caffeinated beverages, alcohol, artificial sweeteners); pelvic floor muscle exercises, preferably learned via biofeedback; consider urologic workup
Female: Relaxed perineal muscles, detrusor instability (urge incontinence), urethral dysfunction (stress urinary incontinence)	Urgency/frequency syndrome, decreased "warning time," bathroom mapping; drops of urine lost with cough, laugh, position change	Wear easily manipulated clothing; drink adequate fluids; avoid bladder irritants (eg, caffeinated beverages, alcohol, artificial sweeteners); pelvic floor muscle exercises, preferably learned via biofeedback; consider urologic workup
Gastrointestinal System Decreased salivation; difficulty swallowing food; delayed esophageal and gastric emptying; reduced gastrointestinal motility	Complaints of dry mouth; complaints of fullness, heartburn, and indigestion; constipation, flatulence, and abdominal discomfort	Use ice chips, mouthwash; brush, floss, and massage gums daily; receive regular dental care; eat small, frequent meals; sit up and avoid heavy activity after eating; limit antacids; eat a high-fiber, low-fat diet; limit laxatives; toilet regularly; drink adequate fluids
Nervous System Reduced speed in nerve conduction; increased confusion with physical illness and loss of environmental cues; reduced cerebral circulation (becomes faint, loses balance)	Slower to respond and react; learning takes longer; becomes confused with hospital admission; faintness; frequent falls	Pace teaching; with hospitalization, encourage visitors; enhance sensory stimulation; with sudden confusion, look for cause; encourage slow rising from a resting position

(continued)

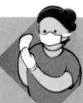

Table 12-2 • Health Promotion:
Age-Related Changes in Body Systems and Health Promotion Strategies (Continued)

CHANGES	SUBJECTIVE AND OBJECTIVE FINDINGS	HEALTH PROMOTION STRATEGIES
Special Senses		
Vision: Diminished ability to focus on close objects; inability to tolerate glare; difficulty adjusting to changes of light intensity; decreased ability to distinguish colors	Holds objects far away from face; complains of glare; poor night vision; confuses colors	Wear eyeglasses, use sunglasses outdoors; avoid abrupt changes from dark to light; use adequate indoor lighting with area lights and nightlights; use large-print books; use magnifier for reading; avoid night driving; use contrasting colors for color coding; avoid glare of shiny surfaces and direct sunlight
Hearing: Decreased ability to hear high-frequency sounds	Gives inappropriate responses; asks people to repeat words; strains forward to hear	Recommend a hearing examination; reduce background noise; face person; enunciate clearly; speak with a low-pitched voice; use nonverbal cues
Taste and smell: Decreased ability to taste and smell	Uses excessive sugar and salt	Encourage use of lemon, spices, herbs

about 25% from age 20 to age 80. Under conditions of stress, both the maximum cardiac output and the maximum HR diminish gradually. The relationship between maximum HR and age is as follows:

$$\text{Normal maximum HR for age} = 220 - \text{age in years}$$

Hypertension has been shown to be a serious risk factor at all ages for cardiovascular disease and stroke. A diagnosis of hypertension is made only after it has been confirmed by at least two subsequent readings. In older people, hypertension is classified as follows:

Isolated systolic hypertension: the systolic reading exceeds 140 mm Hg, and the diastolic measurement is normal or near normal (less than 90 mm Hg)
Primary hypertension: the diastolic pressure is greater than or equal to 90 mm Hg regardless of the systolic pressure
Secondary hypertension: hypertension that can be attributed to an underlying cause

Cardiovascular dysfunction may manifest as congestive heart failure, coronary artery disease, arteriosclerosis, hypertension, intermittent claudication (leg pain caused by walking), peripheral vascular disease, orthostatic hypotension, dysrhythmias, cerebrovascular accidents (strokes), or myocardial infarction (heart attack).

Heart failure (HF) is the number one cause of hospitalization among Medicare recipients and is a major cause of morbidity and mortality among the elderly population in the United States. Older patients often present with different symptoms than those seen in younger patients. Typically, younger persons present for care with the symptoms of exertional dyspnea, orthopnea, and peripheral edema, whereas older patients typically report fatigue, nausea, and abdominal discomfort. In the younger population, men are more prone to HF, but in the elderly population far greater numbers of women develop it. Depending on its cause, HF can require various forms of therapy. The current standard of therapy for HF includes diuretics, angiotensin-converting enzyme inhibitors (ACE inhibitors) and, digoxin. Several large studies have also indicated that carefully monitored, low-dose beta-blockers and spironolactone can decrease mortality (Rittenhouse, 2001).

Cardiovascular health can be promoted by regular exercise, proper diet, weight control, regular blood pressure measurements, stress management, and smoking cessation. To avoid light-headedness, fainting, and possible falls caused by orthostatic hypotension, the older person should be counseled to rise slowly (from a lying, to a sitting, to a standing position); to avoid straining when having a bowel movement; and to consider having five or six small meals each day, rather than three, to minimize the hypotension that can occur after a large meal. Extremes in temperature should be avoided, including hot showers and whirlpool baths. Yard work should be limited to no more than 20 minutes on hot summer days. Exposure to wind or cold weather also should be avoided because of the risk of dizziness or falling associated with slower adjustments of blood pressure. If an individual experiences dependent edema as the day progresses, the use of elastic compression stockings helps to minimize venous pooling.

Respiratory System

Age-related changes in the respiratory system affect lung capacity and function and include increased anteroposterior chest diameter, osteoporotic collapse of vertebrae resulting in kyphosis (increased convex curvature of the spine), calcification of the costal cartilages and reduced mobility of the ribs, diminished efficiency of the respiratory muscles, increased lung rigidity, and decreased alveolar surface area. Increased rigidity or loss of elastic recoil in the lung results in increased residual lung volume and decreased vital capacity. Gas exchange and diffusing capacity are also diminished. Decreased cough efficiency, reduced ciliary activity, and increased respiratory dead space make the older person more vulnerable to respiratory infections.

Health promotion activities that help elderly persons maintain adequate respiratory function include regular exercise, appropriate fluid intake, pneumococcal vaccination, yearly influenza immunizations, and avoidance of people who are ill. As with people of all ages, smoking cessation and frequent hand hygiene are prudent health practices. Hospitalized older adults should be frequently reminded to cough and take deep breaths, particularly postoperatively, because their decreased lung capacity and decreased cough efficiency predispose them to respiratory infections and atelectasis.

Integumentary System

The functions of the skin include protection, temperature regulation, sensation, and excretion. With aging, changes occur that affect the function and appearance of the skin. The epidermis and dermis become thinner. Elastic fibers are reduced in number, and collagen becomes stiffer. Subcutaneous fat diminishes, particularly in the extremities. Decreased numbers of capillaries in the skin result in diminished blood supply. These changes cause a loss of resiliency and wrinkling and sagging of the skin. Hair pigmentation decreases, resulting in gradual graying. The skin becomes drier and susceptible to irritations because of decreased activity of the sebaceous and sweat glands. These changes in the integument reduce tolerance to extremes of temperature and to exposure to the sun.

Strategies to promote healthy skin function include avoiding exposure to the sun, using a lubricating skin cream, avoiding long soaks in the tub, and maintaining adequate intake of water (8 to 10 eight-ounce glasses per day).

Reproductive System

Ovarian production of estrogen and progesterone ceases with menopause. Changes occurring in the female reproductive system include thinning of the vaginal wall, along with a narrowing in size and a loss of elasticity; decreased vaginal secretions, resulting in vaginal dryness, itching, and decreased acidity; involution (atrophy) of the uterus and ovaries; and decreased pubococcygeal muscle tone, resulting in a relaxed vagina and perineum. These changes contribute to vaginal bleeding and painful intercourse.

In older men, the penis and testes decrease in size, and levels of androgens diminish. Erectile dysfunction may develop with concomitant cardiovascular disease, neurologic disorders, diabetes, or even respiratory disease, which limits exercise tolerance.

Sexual desire and activity decline but do not disappear. The use of water-based lubricants can help prevent painful intercourse. Local estrogen replacement intravaginally enhances vaginal tissue without the risks and side effects of oral estrogen. Several modalities are available for treatment of erectile dysfunction, which is linked to cardiovascular, neurologic, endocrine, or occasionally psychological dysfunction. The use of vacuum penile pumps, local injection or placement of vasostimulating medication into the urethral opening, and use of an oral medication, sildenafil citrate (Viagra), have all proved effective for some patients. Sildenafil citrate is contraindicated in patients who are taking oral nitrates.

If significant sexual dysfunction is present, referral to a gynecologist or urologist is warranted. For both men and women, maintenance of a daily physical exercise routine promotes enhanced sexual performance.

Genitourinary System

The genitourinary system continues to function adequately in older people, although there is a decrease in kidney mass, primarily because of a loss of nephrons. Changes in kidney function include a decreased filtration rate, diminished tubular function with less efficiency in resorbing and concentrating the urine, and a slower restoration of acid–base balance in response to stress. Older women often suffer from stress or urge incontinence, or both. Benign prostatic hyperplasia (enlarged prostate gland), which is a common finding in older men, causes a gradual increase in urine retention and overflow incontinence. Prostate cancer, a slow-growing cancer, is most often seen in men older than

70 years of age. Kidney and bladder cancers are most frequently seen after the age of 50 years. Smoking is known to be a primary causative agent of these carcinomas.

Adequate consumption of fluids is important to reduce the risk of bladder infections and urinary incontinence. Other healthy habits include having ready access to toilet facilities and voiding every 2 to 3 hours while awake. Avoidance of bladder-irritating substances—such as caffeinated, carbonated, and acidic beverages, Nutra-sweet, and alcohol—will greatly reduce urinary urgency and frequency. Water intake should be increased to avoid concentrated urine, which causes urinary urgency.

Pelvic floor exercises, first described by Kegel (1948), can also be extremely useful in reducing the symptoms of stress and urge incontinence. Teaching the patient how to do the exercises begins with identifying the pubococcygeus muscle, which is the same muscle used to hold back flatus or to voluntarily stop the flow of urine without contracting the abdomen, buttocks, or inner thigh muscles. The pelvic muscles are first tightened and then relaxed, maintaining a 5-second contraction with 10-second rest intervals. This exercise should be routinely practiced for 30 to 80 repetitions each day; additional repetitions are discouraged because of the risk of fatigue of the muscle. Because achieving better muscle control takes at least several months to accomplish, the elderly person is encouraged to consistently perform the exercises. To maintain pubococcygeus muscle control, these daily exercises must continue indefinitely. The use of biofeedback to confirm the correct execution of these exercises increases their effectiveness significantly.

As menopause approaches, a woman's circulating estrogen decreases, and, as a result, the pelvic floor is deprived of its needed blood supply and nutrients. This causes increasing stress and urge incontinence. Through the use of biofeedback-assisted pelvic muscle exercise, an individual can successfully regain bladder function. These exercises are also recommended for men with dribbling incontinence related to prostatectomy. The nurse instructs the patient to tighten the rectal sphincter until the penis and testes slightly lift. Frequent repetition produces the desired muscle tone.

Constipation can be a major factor contributing to urinary incontinence. The patient is encouraged to eat a high-fiber diet, drink adequate fluids, and increase mobility to promote regular bowel function.

Urinary tract infections are prevalent in older women. The reasons include the effects of decreased estrogen, which shortens the urethral length, allowing easier passage of bacteria into the bladder; less overall fluid consumption, which causes a concentrated urine in which bacteria can proliferate; and the introduction of bacteria from the rectum as a result of poor bathroom hygiene secondary to impaired mobility and joint changes. Limited range of motion of the arm and limited hand dexterity often result in a woman's cleansing the perineal area in a back-to-front motion, causing bacteria such as *Escherichia coli* to be introduced to the urethral meatus and thus into the bladder (Degler, 2000b).

Gastrointestinal System

The older adult is at increased risk for impaired nutrition. Periodontal disease leading to tooth decay and loss of teeth is common. Salivary flow diminishes, and the older person may experience a dry mouth. A preference for sweet and salty foods results from a decrease of taste receptors. Major complaints often center on feelings of fullness, heartburn, and indigestion. Gastric motility may decrease, resulting in delayed emptying of stomach contents.

Diminished secretion of acid and pepsin reduces the absorption of iron, calcium, and vitamin B_{12}. Absorption of nutrients in the small intestine also appears to diminish with age. The function of the liver, gallbladder, and pancreas is generally maintained, although absorption and tolerance to fat may decrease. The incidence of gallstones and common bile duct stones increases progressively with advancing years.

Difficulty in swallowing, or dysphagia, affects 1 in 17 people, including 6.2 million Americans over the age of 60 years, with 300,000 to 600,000 new cases diagnosed each year. It is a serious condition that can be life-threatening. It results from interruption or dysfunction of neural pathways, such as can occur with stroke. It may also develop from dysfunction of the striated and smooth muscles of the gastrointestinal tract in up to 50% of patients with Parkinson's disease and in those with conditions such as multiple sclerosis, poliomyelitis, and amyotrophic lateral sclerosis (Lou Gehrig's disease). Aspiration of food or fluid is the most serious complication and can occur in the absence of coughing or choking (Galvan, 2001).

Constipation is common in aged people. When mild, the symptoms involve abdominal discomfort and flatulence, but more serious consequences include fecal impaction that contributes to diarrhea around the impaction, fecal incontinence, and obstruction. Predisposing factors for constipation include lack of dietary bulk, prolonged use of laxatives, the use of some medications, inactivity, insufficient fluid intake, and excessive dietary fat. Another factor may be ignoring the urge to defecate.

Gastrointestinal health promotion practices include receiving regular dental care; eating small, frequent meals; avoiding heavy activity after eating; eating a high-fiber, low-fat diet; ingesting an adequate amount of fluids; establishing regular bowel habits; and avoiding the use of laxatives and antacids. Understanding that there is a direct correlation between loss of smell and taste perception and food intake helps caregivers to intervene to maintain elderly patients' health.

Nutritional Health

The social, psychological, and physiologic functions of eating influence the dietary habits of the aged person. Decreased physical activity and a slower metabolic rate reduce the number of calories needed by the older adult to maintain an ideal weight. Apathy, immobility, depression, loneliness, poverty, inadequate knowledge, lack of oral health, and lack of taste discrimination also contribute to suboptimal nutrient intake. Budgetary constraints and physical limitations may impair food shopping and meal preparation. Education regarding healthy versus "empty-calorie" foods is helpful.

Health promotion teaching includes encouraging a diet that is low in sodium and saturated fats and high in vegetables, fruits, and fish. The older adult requires a variety of foods to maintain balanced nutrition. No more than 20% to 25% of dietary calories should be consumed as fat. Reducing salt intake is also advocated, because sodium reduction has been shown to correct hypertension in some people. Protein intake should remain the same in later adulthood as in earlier years. Carbohydrates, a major source of energy, should supply the diet with 55% to 60% of the daily calories. Simple sugars should be avoided and complex carbohydrates encouraged. Potatoes, whole grains, brown rice, and fruit provide the person with minerals, vitamins, and fiber and should be encouraged. Drinking 8 to 10 eight-ounce glasses of water per day is recommended unless contraindicated by a medical condition. A multivitamin each day helps to maintain daily nutritional needs.

Sleep

Sleep disturbances frequently occur in older people, affecting more than 50% of adults 65 years of age or older. The elderly often experience variations in their normal sleep–wake cycles, and the lack of quality sleep at night often creates the need for napping during the day. Laboratory screening can help to rule out disease processes that might be affecting an older person's ability to sleep at night. If a spouse notes excessive snoring, a sleep study is indicated to rule out sleep apnea. The nurse can recommend prudent sleep hygiene behaviors such as avoiding daytime napping, eating a light snack before bedtime, and decreasing the overall time in bed to adjust for the fewer hours of sleep needed than when the patient was younger (Grandjean & Gibbons, 2000).

Musculoskeletal System

A gradual, progressive decrease in bone mass begins before the age of 40 years. Excessive loss of bone density results in osteoporosis, which affects both older men and women but is most prevalent in postmenopausal women. It is also seen in older men who are receiving hormone treatments for prostate cancer. A higher incidence is found among northern Europeans and Asians. Its typical form is associated with inactivity, inadequate calcium intake, loss of estrogens, and a history of cigarette smoking. The danger of fracture as a result of bone reabsorption is especially high for the dorsal portion of the vertebra, humerus, radius, femur, and tibia. A loss of height occurs in later life as a result of osteoporotic changes of the spine, kyphosis (excessive convex curvature of the spine), and flexion of the hips and knees. These changes negatively affect mobility, balance, and internal organ function (Fig. 12-2).

The muscles diminish in size and lose strength, flexibility, and endurance with decreased activity and advanced age. Back pain is common. Beginning in middle age, the cartilage of joints progressively deteriorates. Degenerative joint disease is found in everyone past the age of 70 years.

Calcium supplements, vitamin D, fluoride, estrogens, and weight-bearing exercises are often prescribed for the person who is at high risk for or already has osteoporosis. Although osteoporosis cannot be reversed, the disease process can be slowed. A bone density test is the gold standard to assess for osteoporosis. Once it is diagnosed and treatment begun, yearly follow-up determinations of the bone density level are indicated. For skeletal health, the nurse can recommend the following (Scheiber & Torregrosa, 2000):

- A high calcium intake, 1500 mg/day. Dairy products and dark green vegetables are excellent sources, as are soups and broths made with a soup bone and cooked with added vinegar to leach calcium from the bone. Calcium supplements can be recommended to ensure that the daily calcium intake is adequate.
- A low-phosphorus diet. A calcium-to-phosphorus ratio of 1:1 is ideal; red meats, cola drinks, and processed foods that are low in calcium and high in phosphorus are avoided.
- Weight-bearing exercise. The pull of muscle insertions on the long bones strengthens the muscles and retards calcium resorption.
- Reduction of caffeine and alcohol. This assists in stopping further demineralization and renal excretion of calcium.

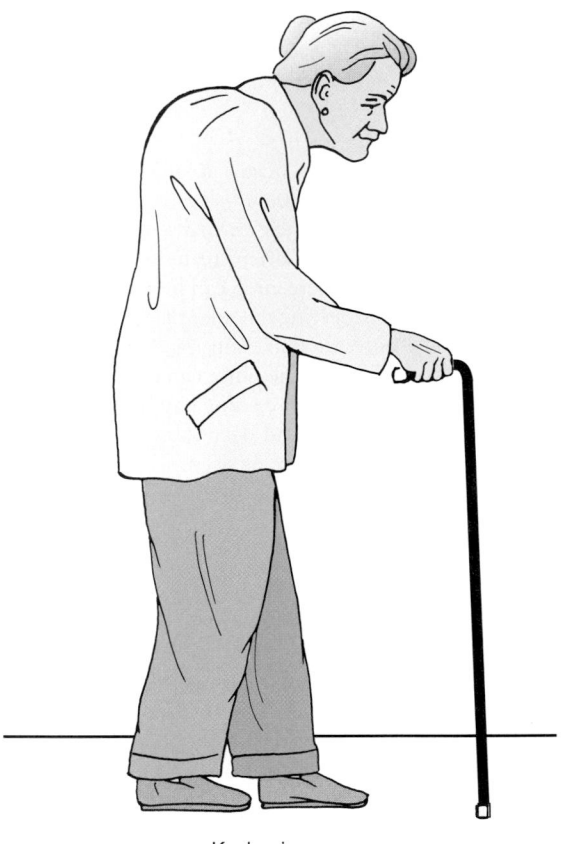

Kyphosis

FIGURE 12-2 Age-related musculoskeletal changes affect posture, stance, and gait.

- Smoking cessation.
- Selective estrogen receptor modulators, such as raloxifene (Evista), preserve bone mineral density without estrogenic effects on the uterus. This medication is indicated for both prevention and treatment of osteoporosis. Although hormone replacement therapy (HRT) has been the mainstay of therapy for perimenopausal women, recent studies have demonstrated greater risks than previously recognized (Chen, Weiss, Newcomb, Barlow & White, 2002).
- The bisphosphate drugs (e.g., Fosamax, Actonel). These drugs bind to mineralized bone surfaces to inhibit osteoclastic activity and promote bone formation.

Muscle strength and flexibility can be enhanced with a program of regular exercise. The axiom "use it or lose it" is very relevant when considering the physical capacity of aged people. The nurse plays an important role by encouraging older adults to participate in a regular exercise program. Regular exercise increases the strength and efficiency of heart contractions, improves oxygen uptake by cardiac and skeletal muscles, reduces fatigue, increases energy, and reduces cardiovascular risk factors. Muscle endurance, strength, and flexibility—all outcomes of regular exercise—also help to promote independence and psychological well-being. Aerobic exercises are the foundation of programs of cardiovascular endurance conditioning. A physical examination by a physician or nurse practitioner is necessary before initiating an exercise program, and older persons should perform exercises in moderation and use short rests to avoid undue fatigue. Swimming and brisk walking are often recommended because they are managed easily and usually are enjoyed by the older person.

Information about the nature and time course of menopause-associated bone loss through early markers may be used to help to preserve bone and thus stop the natural sequelae of osteoporosis. A nurse-led research team used frequent sequential serum markers to confirm these changes and found a correlation with elevated alkaline phosphatase (ALP) and concentrations of follicle-stimulating hormone as a marker for vitamin K status. Therefore, perimenopausal women with elevated ALP can be targeted for health promotion to preserve bone density (Lukacs, 2000). Further information about osteoporosis is presented in Chapter 68.

Nervous System

The structure and function of the nervous system change with advanced age, and a reduction in cerebral blood flow accompanies nervous system changes. The loss of nerve cells contributes to a progressive loss of brain mass, and the synthesis and metabolism of the major neurotransmitters are also reduced. Because nerve impulses are conducted more slowly, older people take longer to respond and react. The autonomic nervous system performs less efficiently, and postural hypotension, which causes the person to lose consciousness or feel lightheaded on standing up quickly, may occur. Cerebral ischemia with related lightheadedness may interfere with mobility and safety. The nurse advises the person to allow a longer time to respond to a stimulus and to move more deliberately. Homeostasis is more difficult to maintain, but in the absence of pathologic changes, the older person functions adequately and retains cognitive and intellectual abilities.

Mental function is threatened by physical or emotional stresses. A sudden onset of confusion may be the first symptom of an infection or change in physical condition (pneumonia, urinary tract infection, medication interactions, **dehydration,** and others).

A slowed reaction time places the older person at risk for falls and injuries, including driving errors. Compared with the per-mile fatality rate for drivers aged 25 to 69 years, that for drivers 70 years of age and older is nine times as high. When an elderly person has been witnessed driving unsafely, he or she should receive a driving fitness evaluation; this is often administered by an occupational therapist in conjunction with a neuropsychologist, who can help with the more detailed cognitive testing (Dolinar, McQuillen, & Ranseen, 2001).

Sensory System

Sensory losses with old age affect all sensory organs and can be devastating to the person who cannot see to read or watch television, hear conversation well enough to communicate, or discriminate taste well enough to enjoy food.

SENSORY LOSSES VERSUS SENSORY DEPRIVATION

Sensory losses can often be helped by assistive devices such as glasses and hearing aids. In contrast, sensory deprivation is the absence of stimuli in the environment or the inability to interpret existing stimuli (perhaps as a result of a sensory loss). This deprivation can lead to boredom, confusion, irritability, disorientation, and anxiety. Meaningful sensory stimulation offered to the older person is often helpful in correcting this problem. One sense can substitute for another in observing and interpreting stimuli. The nurse can enhance sensory stimulation in the environment with colors, pictures, textures, tastes, smells, and sounds. The stimuli are most meaningful if they are interpreted to the older person and if they are changed often. Cognitively impaired persons respond well to touch and to familiar music.

VISION

As new cells form on the outside surface of the lens of the eye, the older central cells accumulate and become yellow, rigid, dense, and cloudy, leaving only the outer portion of the lens elastic enough to change shape (accommodate) and focus at near and far distances. As the lens becomes less flexible, the near point of focus gets farther away. This condition, **presbyopia**, usually begins in the fifth decade of life, and requires the wearing of reading glasses to magnify objects. In addition, the yellowing, cloudy lens causes light to scatter and makes the older person sensitive to glare. The ability to discern blue from green decreases. The pupil dilates slowly and less completely because of increased stiffness of the muscles of the iris, so the older person takes longer to adjust when going to and from light and dark environments or settings and needs brighter light for close vision. Although pathologic visual conditions are not part of normal aging, the incidence of eye disease (most commonly cataracts, glaucoma, diabetic retinopathy, and age-related macular degeneration) increases in older people.

Age-related macular degeneration, in its most severe forms, is the most common cause of blindness in adults older than 55 years of age in the United States, and it is estimated to affect more than 10 million Americans. Risk factors include sunlight exposure, cigarette smoking, and heredity, and people with fair skin and blue eyes are much more prone to the disease. Sunglasses and hats with visors provide some protection. Yearly eye checkups ensure early detection, which makes surgical correction much more successful. Optical aids to magnify print and printed objects may help those already suffering from the effects of macular degeneration to continue to read (Friberg, 2000).

HEARING

Presbycusis, a loss of the ability to hear high-frequency tones attributed to irreversible inner ear changes, occurs in midlife. Older people are often unable to follow conversation because tones of high-frequency consonants (letters f, s, th, ch, sh, b, t, p) all sound alike. Hearing loss may cause the older person to respond inappropriately, misunderstand conversation, and avoid social interaction. This behavior may be erroneously interpreted as confusion. Wax buildup or other correctable problems may also be responsible for major hearing difficulties. A properly prescribed and fitted hearing aid may be useful in reducing hearing deficits.

TASTE AND SMELL

Of the four basic tastes (sweet, sour, salty, and bitter), sweet tastes are particularly dulled in older people. Blunted taste may contribute to the preference for salty, highly seasoned foods, but herbs, onions, garlic, and lemon should be encouraged as substitutes for salt to flavor food.

PSYCHOSOCIAL ASPECTS OF AGING

Successful psychological aging is reflected in the older person's ability to adapt to physical, social, and emotional losses and to achieve contentment, serenity, and life satisfactions. Because changes in life patterns are inevitable over a lifetime, the older person needs resiliency and coping skills when confronting stresses and change. A positive self-image enhances risk taking and participation in new, untested roles.

Although attitudes toward old people differ in ethnic subcultures, a subtle theme of **ageism**—prejudice or discrimination against older people—predominates in our society. It is often based on stereotypes, simplified and often untrue beliefs that reinforce society's negative image of the aged person. Elderly people make up an extremely heterogeneous group, yet negative stereotypes are attributed to all of them.

Fear of aging and the inability of many to confront their own aging process may trigger ageist beliefs. Retirement and perceived nonproductivity are also responsible for negative feelings, since the younger working person may see the older person as not contributing to society and draining economic resources. This negative image is so common in American society that the elderly themselves often believe it. Only through an understanding of the aging process and respect for each person as an individual can the myths of aging be dispelled. If the elderly are treated with dignity and encouraged to maintain autonomy, the quality of their lives will improve.

Stress and Coping in the Older Adult

Coping patterns and the ability to adapt to stress are developed over the course of a lifetime and remain consistent later in life. Experiencing success in younger adulthood helps a person develop a positive self-image that remains solid through even the adversities of old age. A person's abilities to adapt to changes, make decisions, and respond predictably are also determined by past experiences. A flexible, well-functioning person will probably continue as such. Losses may accumulate within a short period of time, however, and become overwhelming. The older person will often have fewer choices and diminished resources to deal with stressful events. Common stressors of old age include normal aging changes that impair physical function, activities, and appearance; disabilities from chronic illness; social and environmental losses related to loss of income and decreased ability to perform previous roles and activities; and the deaths of significant others. Many older adults rely strongly on their spiritual beliefs for comfort during stressful times.

Lack of social engagement (interaction with people within their environment) may be a modifiable risk factor for death in older persons residing in nursing homes. A 5-year study of more than 900 residents of nursing homes, whose average age was 87 years, revealed that those who did not receive social interaction were 2.3 times more likely to die during the follow-up period (Kiely et al., 2000).

Developmental Theories of Aging

Erikson (1963) theorized that a person's life consists of eight stages, each stage representing a crucial turning point in the **life span** stretching from birth to death with its own developmental conflict to be resolved. According to Erikson, the major developmental task of old age is to either achieve ego integrity or suffer despair. Achieving ego integrity requires accepting one's lifestyle, believing that one's choices were the best that could be made at a particular time, and being in control of one's life. Despair results when an older person feels dissatisfied and disappointed with his or her life, and would live differently if given another chance.

Havighurst (1972) also suggested a list of developmental tasks that occur during a lifetime. The tasks of the older person include adjusting to retirement after a lifetime of employment with a possible reduction of income, decreases in physical strength and health, the death of a spouse, establishing affiliation with one's age group, adapting to new social roles in a flexible way, and establishing satisfactory physical living arrangements.

Combining the concepts of both Erikson and Havighurst suggests the following developmental tasks for the older adult: (1) maintenance of self-worth, (2) conflict resolution, (3) adjustment to the loss of dominant roles, (4) adjustment to the deaths of significant others, (5) environmental adaptation, and (6) maintenance of optimal levels of wellness.

Sociologic Theories of Aging

Sociologic theories of aging attempt to predict and explain the social interactions and roles that contribute to the older adult's successful adjustment to old age. The activity theory proposes that life satisfaction in normal aging requires maintaining the active lifestyle of middle age (Havighurst, 1972). The continuity theory proposes that successful adjustment to old age requires continuing life patterns across a lifetime (Atchley, 1989; Neugarten, 1961). Continuity and a connection to the past are maintained through a continuation of well-established habits, values, and interests that are integral to the person's present lifestyle.

COGNITIVE ASPECTS OF AGING

Cognition can be affected by many variables, including sensory impairment, physiologic health, environment, and psychosocial influences. Older adults may experience temporary changes in cognitive function when hospitalized or admitted to skilled nursing facilities, rehabilitation centers, or long-term care facilities. These changes are related to differences in environment or in medical therapy, or to alteration in role performance.

Intelligence

When intelligence test scores from people of all ages are compared (cross-sectional testing), test scores for older adults show a progressive decline beginning in midlife. Research has shown, however, that environment and health have a considerable influence on scores and that certain types of intelligence (eg, spatial perceptions and retention of nonintellectual information) decline, whereas other types do not (problem-solving ability based on past experiences, verbal comprehension, mathematical ability). Cardiovascular health, a stimulating environment, high levels of education, occupational status, and income all appear to have a positive effect on intelligence scores in later life.

Learning and Memory

The ability to learn and acquire new skills and information decreases in the older adult, particularly after the seventh decade of life. Despite this, many older people continue to learn and participate in varied educational experiences. Motivation, speed of performance, and physical status all are important influences on learning.

The components of memory, an integral part of learning, include short-term memory (5 to 30 seconds), recent memory (1 hour to several days), and long-term memory (lifetime). Acquisition of information, registration (recording), retention (storing), and recall (retrieval) are essential components of the memory process. Sensory losses, distractions, and disinterest interfere with acquiring and recording information. Age-related loss occurs more frequently with short-term and recent memory; in the absence of a pathologic process, this is called benign senescent forgetfulness. A nurse considers the process by which older adults learn when he or she uses the following strategies:

- Supplies mnemonics to enhance recall of related data
- Encourages ongoing learning
- Links new information with familiar information
- Uses visual, auditory, and other sensory cues
- Encourages learners to wear prescribed glasses and hearing aids
- Provides glare-free lighting
- Provides a quiet, nondistracting environment
- Sets short-term goals with input from the learner
- Keeps teaching periods short
- Paces learning tasks according to the endurance of the learner
- Encourages verbal participation by learners
- Reinforces successful learning in a positive manner

ENVIRONMENTAL ASPECTS OF AGING

About 95% of the elderly live in the community, and 75% own their homes. In 1991, about 31% of elderly persons were living alone (79% of these were women). In the 65 years and older age group, half as many women as men were married and living with their spouses: 40% of women compared with 74% of men. About 48% of the women older than 65 years of age were widowed, compared with only 15% of the men. This difference in marital status is a result of several factors: women have a longer life expectancy than men do, women tend to marry older men, and women tend to remain widowed, whereas men often remarry (U.S. Bureau of the Census, 2000).

Living Arrangement Options

Ideally, older persons do best in their own, familiar environment. But adjustments to the environment may be required to allow the older adult to remain in his or her own home or apartment. Sometimes, in order to enable them to remain in their own home, an older adult or couple seek out family members who might be willing to live in the home, or agree to board someone in exchange for completion of household chores.

Sometimes older adults or couples agree to move in with adult children. This can be a rewarding experience as the children, their parents, and the grandchildren interact and share household responsibilities. It can also be stressful, depending on the family dynamics. Adult children and their older parents may also choose to pool their financial resources by moving into a house that has an attached "in-law suite." This arrangement provides security for the older adult along with privacy for both families.

Continuing Care Retirement Communities (CCRCs), are becoming more popular as the first of the baby boomers enter their retirement years. CCRCs are retirement communities consisting of single-dwelling houses or apartments for those individuals who are still able to manage all of their day-to-day needs, assisted living apartments for those who need limited assistance with their daily living needs, and skilled nursing services when continuous nursing assistance is required. These communities usually contract for a large down payment before the resident moves into the community. This payment allows the individual or couple the option to reside in the community from the time of total independence through the need for assisted or skilled nursing care. This concept allows for decisions about living arrangements and health care to be made before any decline in health status occurs. A CCRC also provides continuity at a time in an older adult's life when many other factors, such as health status, income, and availability of friends and family members, may be changing.

Assisted living facilities are an option when physical or cognitive changes require at least minimal supervision. Assisted living allows for a degree of independence while providing minimal nursing assistance (eg, administration of medication and coordination of scheduled and acute care medical assistance). Other services, such as laundry, cleaning, and meals, may also be included.

Skilled nursing facilities offer continuous nursing care. Usually, if an older adult suffers a major health event such as a stroke, myocardial infarction, or cancer and is hospitalized, Medicare will cover the cost of the first 30 to 90 days in a skilled nursing facility if ongoing therapy is needed. The stipulation for continued Medicare coverage during this time is documentation of persistent improvement in the required therapies, which most often include physical therapy, occupational therapy, respiratory therapy, and cognitive therapy. Some individuals choose to have nursing home insurance as a means of paying, at least in part, for the cost of these services, should they become necessary. When an individual's financial resources become exhausted as a result of prolonged nursing home care, the family, the institution, or both may apply for Medicaid reimbursement. An increasing number of skilled nursing facilities offer subacute care. This area of the facility offers a high level of nursing care and may either prevent the need for an individual to be transferred to a hospital setting or allow a hospitalized individual to be transferred back to the facility sooner.

Life Care Plans

A life care plan is an individualized document that assesses and evaluates a client's present and future health care and living needs. The typical components of a life care plan are listed in Chart 12-2. Life care plans were originally developed in 1981 as standardized, efficient guidelines for medical and ancillary quality-of-life services. A life care plan provides valuable information regarding factors that can radically affect the individual's health care and quality of life. A life care plan is often requested for individuals with catastrophic injuries or illness (eg, traumatic brain injury, amputation, multiple sclerosis) who will require ongoing rehabilitative and medical services. A life care plan may also serve as the blueprint for what will be expected in long-term care. These plans provide a guideline of anticipated patient care needs for families, insurance companies, attorneys, discharge planners, case managers, and all medical and nursing professionals. The cost of the life care plan varies, depending on the planner, the severity of the injury or illness, and who is paying for the service, but the average cost is currently between $5,000 and $20,000 (Schuman, 2001).

The Role of the Family

Planning for care and understanding the psychosocial issues confronting the older person must be accomplished within the context of the family. If dependency needs occur, the spouse often assumes the role of primary caregiver. In the absence of the surviving spouse, an adult child usually assumes caregiver responsibilities and may eventually need help in providing care and support. Two common myths in American society are that adult children and their aged parents are socially alienated and that adult children abandon their parents when health and other dependency problems arise. Extensive research refutes both of these beliefs. The family is an important source of support for older people (Fig. 12-3). Approximately 81% of elderly persons have living children. Of those elders living alone, two thirds have at least one child living within 30 minutes of their home, and 62% see at least one adult child weekly (U.S. Bureau of the Census, 2000).

Social attitudes and cultural values often dictate that adult children should provide services and financial support and assume the burden of care if their aged parents are unable to care for themselves. Illness creates special problems for people who live alone. If community agencies or adult children are unable to provide care, elders are at high risk for institutionalization.

Regardless of the amount of responsibility and love an adult child exhibits toward dependent elderly parents, strains do develop if care continues for a long period. Research exploring the

Chart 12-2	Life Care Plan Components

Medical history
Social history
Family issues
Vocational/educational history
Projected medical evaluations
Projected physical and occupational therapy needs
Future medical care and medications
Therapeutic supplies
Personal items
Diagnostic testing
Medical equipment and supply needs
Recreational equipment
Aids for independent function
Home/facility care
Transportation needs
Architectural renovations
Potential medical complications
Compromised financial status

Adapted with permission from Schuman, J. (2001). Old concept, new trends: A primer on life care planning. *Long-Term Care Interface, 2*, 28.

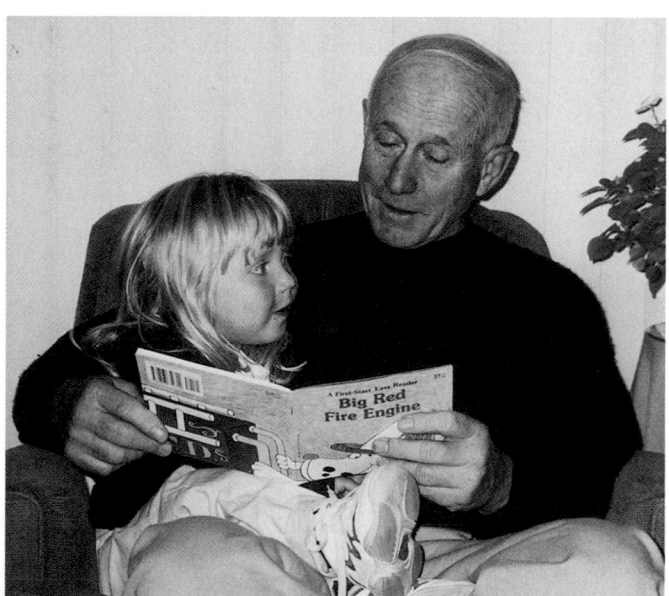

FIGURE 12-3 Families are an important source of psychosocial and physical support for elders and youngsters alike. Caring interaction among grandchildren, grandparents, and other family members typically contributes to the health of all.

relationship between aged parents and their adult children shows that the quality of the parent–child relationship declines with the poor health of the parent. Under certain circumstances of high risk, strains in intergenerational relationships can result in elder abuse (Hoban & Kearney, 2000; Phillips, 2000; Tumolo, 2000).

Elder abuse is an active or passive act or behavior that is harmful to the elderly person. Such behavior includes physical violence, personal neglect, financial exploitation, violation of rights, denial of health care, and self-inflicted abuse. Preventive action should be taken when strains are evident, before elder abuse occurs. Interdisciplinary team members can be enlisted to help the caregiver develop self-awareness, increased insight, and an understanding of the aging process. At the same time, community resources may be useful for both the aged person and the caregiver (Geldmacher, Heck, & O'Toole, 2001).

Community Support Services

Many community supports exist that help the older person maintain independence. Informal sources of help, such as family, friends, the mail carrier, church members, and neighbors, can all keep an informal watch. Area Agencies on Aging perform many community services, including telephone reassurance, friendly visitors, home repair services, and home-delivered meals. Homemaker and chore services can be obtained at an hourly rate through these agencies or through local community nursing services. If a person is unable to pay, these services may be subsidized through local and state funds.

Other community support services are available to help the older person outside the home. Senior centers have social and health promotion activities, and some provide a nutritious noontime meal. Adult day care facilities offer daily nursing care and social opportunities; these services also enable family members to carry on daily activities while the older person is at the day care center.

Home Health Care

Home care is often used as a means to prevent hospitalization for frail, elderly outpatients or to shorten a hospital stay. It can also be used as a high-tech substitute for hospitalization and can include the use of intravenous therapy and other therapies previously delivered in the acute care setting. Home health care was the area of U.S. health care that saw the most rapid rate of growth in the 1990s, and by the end of the 1990s it had come to represent almost one tenth of the total Medicare budget. Rather than viewing home health care as a means of controlling health care costs, the Federal government's Centers for Medicaid and Medicare Services (CMS), formerly the Health Care Financing Administration (HCFA), devised plans to limit the growth of home health care services. The first system put into place to accomplish decreased allocations for home health was called the Prospective Payment System (PPS) for home care, implemented in 2000. Later came a means of quantifying needed home care, called the Outcome and Assessment Information Set (OASIS). The OASIS rates individual consumers of home health care in terms of their ability to perform activities of daily living (ADLs) and instrumental activities of daily living (IADLs). Nursing care and rehabilitation services requiring the expertise of a registered nurse and other health professionals were traditionally paid for by Medicare. With the advent of the PPS, limits on reimbursement may mean consideration of alternative means of reimbursement for such services, including private pay and health insurance products (HCFA, 2000; Plotkin & Roche, 2000; Nus-

baum, 2000). Figure 12-4 shows the estimated growth in Medicare and out-of-pocket annual spending between 2000 and 2025.

Safety and Comfort in the Home Environment

Injuries rank seventh as a cause of death for older people. The nurse can encourage lifestyle and environmental changes that older adults and their families can adopt. Adequate lighting with minimal glare and shadow can be achieved through the use of small area lamps, indirect lighting, sheer curtains to diffuse direct sunlight, dull rather than shiny surfaces, and nightlights. Sharply contrasting colors can be used to mark the edges of stairs. Grab bars by the tub and toilet are useful. Loose clothing, improperly fitting shoes, scatter rugs, small objects, and pets create hazards and increase the risk of falls. A person functions best in familiar settings if furniture and objects remain as unchanged as is safely possible.

Hospice Services

Hospice services are a dignified alternative to the chaos of the acute care setting when a patient with an end-stage disease is not expected to live long. Hospice is a program of supportive and palliative services for dying patients and their families that includes physical, psychological, social, and spiritual dimensions of care. Under Medicare and Medicaid, all needed medical and nursing services are provided to keep the patient as pain free and comfortable as possible. The family must agree to assist in the care of the patient, and services are brought into the home as needed. Hospice services may also be incorporated into the care of residents in long-term care facilities and include care for end-stage dementia.

Hospice services that are provided in a person's home also are rated via the OASIS system. Although this system can be very

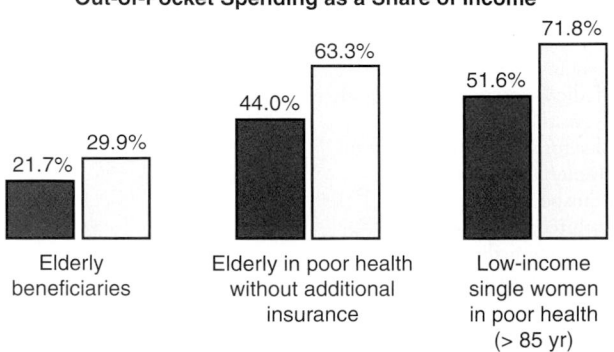

Annual Spending

Out-of-Pocket Spending as a Share of Income

FIGURE 12-4 Medicare beneficiary's out-of-pocket spending.

cumbersome and time-consuming in hospice care because of the many care providers involved, it can serve as an excellent tool with which nurses can assess the effects of particular services on specific patient outcomes (Plotkin & Roche, 2000). For further discussion of hospice care and services see Chapter 17.

Home care and hospice nurses are in a unique position to facilitate early discussions about a patient's wishes and goals at the end of life. Too often, discussion regarding end-of-life care is postponed until a crisis situation occurs, making it difficult or impossible for the patient to be an active participant in the discussion. Home health nurses can assist the patient and family with identifying available options and initiating conversation about preparing an end-of-life plan (Norlander & McSteen, 2000).

PHARMACOLOGIC ASPECTS OF AGING

Older people use more medications than does any other age group: although they comprise only 12.6% of the total population, they use 30% of all prescribed medications and 40% of all over-the-counter medications. Medications have improved the health and well-being of older people by alleviating symptoms of discomfort, treating chronic illnesses, and curing infectious processes. Problems commonly occur, however, because of medication interactions, multiple medication effects, multiple medication use (**polypharmacy**), and noncompliance. Combinations of prescription medications and some over-the-counter medications further complicate the problem.

Any medication is capable of altering nutritional status, which, in the elderly, may already be compromised by a marginal diet or by chronic disease and its treatment. Medications can depress the appetite, cause nausea and vomiting, irritate the stomach, cause constipation or diarrhea, and decrease absorption of nutrients. In addition, they can alter electrolyte balance and carbohydrate and fat metabolism. A few examples of medications capable of altering the nutritional status are antacids, which produce thiamine deficiency; cathartics, which diminish absorption; antibiotics and phenytoin, which reduce utilization of folic acid; and phenothiazines, estrogens, and corticosteroids, which increase food intake and cause weight gain.

Altered Pharmacokinetics

Pharmacokinetics is the study of the actions of medications in the body, including the processes of absorption, distribution, metabolism, and excretion. Variability in these processes in older people (Table 12-3) is caused, in part, by a reduced capacity of the liver and kidneys to metabolize and excrete the medications and by lowered efficiency of the circulatory and nervous systems in coping with the effect of certain medications. Many medications and their metabolites are excreted by the kidney. With advanced age, body weight, total body water, lean body mass, and plasma albumin (protein) all decrease, while body fat increases. Consequently, agents that are highly protein-bound have fewer binding sites and higher pharmacologic activity, whereas fat-soluble agents have more binding sites, and therefore enhanced storage and delayed elimination.

Nursing Implications

The nurse administering medications to older people must be aware of the following:

- Medications removed from the body primarily by renal excretion remain in the body for a longer time in people with decreased renal function. Often dosages must be reduced, because overdosage and medication toxicity at usual therapeutic dosages are common.
- Medications with a narrow safety margin (eg, digitalis glycosides) must be administered cautiously.
- A decline in cardiac output may decrease the delivery rate to the target organ or storage tissue.
- The circulatory and central nervous systems of older people are less able to cope with the effects of certain medications, even when blood levels are normal.
- Idiosyncratic or unusual responses to medications may manifest as toxic reactions and complications.
- As a result of a slowing metabolism, medication levels may increase in the tissues and plasma, leading to prolonged medication action.
- Many elderly people have multiple medical problems that require treatment with one or more medications. The possibility of interactions between medications is further magnified if the older person is also taking one or more over-the-counter medications.
- A high-fiber diet and the use of psyllium (Metamucil) or other laxatives may accelerate gastrointestinal transport and reduce absorption of medications taken concurrently.
- If, for any reason, a patient is not dependable about taking medication, the nurse must be sure that the pill or capsule is actually swallowed and not retained between the cheeks and the gums or teeth.

Teaching self-administration of medication requires asking the patient questions and requesting return demonstrations to ensure that learning has occurred. Sensory and memory losses, as well as decreased manual dexterity, can affect the patient's ability to carry out instructions properly, and the teaching plan will need to be adjusted to meet each patient's needs. The following steps taken by the nurse can help the patient to manage his or her medications and improve compliance:

- Explain the action, side effects, and dosage of each medication.
- Write out the medication schedule.
- Encourage the use of standard containers without safety lids (if there are no children in the household).
- Suggest the use of a multiple-day, multiple-dose medication dispenser to help patients adhere to the medication schedule (Fig. 12-5).
- Destroy old, unused medications.
- Review the medication schedule periodically.
- Discourage the use of over-the-counter medications and herbal agents without consulting a health professional.
- Encourage the patient to take all medications, including over-the-counter medications, with him or her regularly when visiting the primary health care provider.

Physical Health Problems in Older Populations

GERIATRIC SYNDROMES: MULTIPLE PROBLEMS WITH MULTIPLE ETIOLOGIC FACTORS

The frail elderly frequently experience multiple problems, or syndromes. Illness, whether acute or chronic, generally results from several factors rather than from a single cause. When combined with a decrease in host resistance, these factors lead to illness or injury. Although the problems may have developed slowly, the onset of symptoms is often acute. Furthermore, the

Table 12-3 • Altered Drug Responses in Older People

AGE-RELATED CHANGES	EFFECT OF AGE-RELATED CHANGE	APPLICABLE MEDICATIONS
Absorption		
Reduced gastric acid; increased pH (less acid)	Rate of drug absorption—possibly delayed	
Reduced gastrointestinal motility; prolonged gastric emptying	Extent of drug absorption—not affected	
Distribution		

Decreased albumin sites	Serious alterations in drug binding to plasma proteins (the unbound drug gives the pharmacologic response); highly protein-bound medications have fewer binding sites, leading to increased effects and accelerated metabolism and excretion	Selected highly protein-binding medications:
		    Oral anticoagulants (warfarin)
		    Oral hypoglycemic agents (sulfonylureas)
		    Barbiturates
		    Calcium channel blockers
		    Furosemide (Lasix)
		    Nonsteroidal anti-inflammatory drugs (NSAIDs)
		    Sulfonamides
		    Quinidine
		    Phenytoin (Dilantin)

Reduced cardiac output	Decreased perfusion of many bodily organs	
Impaired peripheral blood flow	Decreased perfusion	

Increased percentage of body fat	Proportion of body fat increases with age, resulting in increased ability to store fat-soluble medications; this causes drug accumulation, prolonged storage, and delayed excretion	Selected fat-soluble medications:
		    Barbiturates
		    Diazepam (Valium)
		    Lidocaine
		    Phenothiazines (antipsychotics)
		    Ethanol
		    Morphine

Decreased lean body mass	Decreased body volume allows higher peak levels of medications	
Metabolism		
Decreased cardiac output and decreased perfusion of the liver	Decreased metabolism and delay of breakdown of medications, resulting in prolonged duration of action, accumulation, and drug toxicity	All medications metabolized by the liver
Excretion		

Decreased renal blood flow; loss of functioning nephrons; decreased renal efficiency	Decreased rates of elimination and increased duration of action; danger of accumulation and drug toxicity	Selected medications with prolonged action:
		    Aminoglycoside antibiotics
		    Cimetidine (Tagamet)
		    Chlorpropamide (Diabinase)
		    Digoxin
		    Lithium
		    Procainamide

presenting symptoms may appear in other body systems before becoming apparent in the affected system. The term "frail" is used to describe those elders who are at highest risk for adverse health outcomes or geriatric syndromes. There are no standard clinical criteria for frailty. According to the most widely agreed on definition, frail people are those who are most vulnerable to

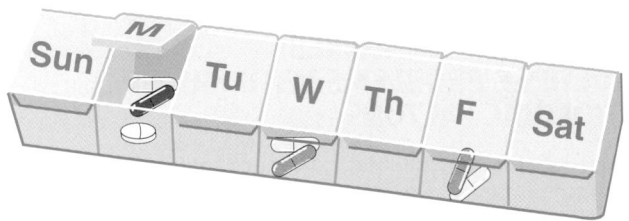

FIGURE 12-5 Commercially available, multiple-dose, multiple-day medication dispensers, such as this one, help older people to follow complex medication regimens safely at home.

significant problems because they meet one or more of the following conditions:

- Being 85 years of age or older
- Being unable to perform IADLs or ADLs independently
- Suffering from multiple chronic diseases

As with specific illnesses, geriatric syndromes are never a normal consequence of aging. Early intervention can prevent further complications and help to maximize the quality of life for many older people (Hazzard et al., 1999).

Impaired Mobility

The causes of decreased mobility are many and varied. Common causes are Parkinson's disease, diabetic neuropathy, cardiovascular compromise, osteoarthritis, osteoporosis, and sensory deficits. Environmental barriers and iatrogenic factors are also significant. Elderly patients should be encouraged to stay as active as possible to avoid the downward spiral of immobility. During illness, bed rest should be kept to a minimum, because even brief periods of bed rest quickly lead to deconditioning and, consequently, to a wide range of complications. When bed rest cannot be avoided, the patient should perform active range-of-motion and strengthening exercises with the unaffected extremities, and the nurse should perform passive range-of-motion exercises on the affected extremities. Frequent position changes help offset the hazards of immobility. Both the staff and the patient's family can assist in maintaining the current level of mobility (Tappen, Roach, Applegate, & Stowell, 2000).

Dizziness

Older people frequently seek help for dizziness, which presents a particular challenge because there are so many possible internal and external causes. For many, the problem is further complicated because of an inability to differentiate between the true dizziness (a sensation of disorientation in relation to position) and vertigo (a spinning sensation). Other similar sensations include near-syncope and disequilibrium. The causes for these sensations range in severity from minor, as in a buildup of ear wax, to severe, as in dysfunction of the cerebral cortex, cerebellum, brain stem, proprioceptive receptors, or the vestibular system. Even a minor reversible cause, such as an ear wax impaction, can result in a loss of balance and a subsequent fall and injury. Because of the many predisposing factors, nurses should seek to identify potentially treatable factors related to the dizziness. This impairment reduction strategy may reduce the vulnerability of older persons to injury (Tinetti, Williams, & Gill, 2000).

Falls and Falling

Falling is a common and preventable source of mortality and morbidity in older adults. As the major cause of trauma in the elderly, falls are not often fatal but do threaten health and the quality of life. Normal and pathologic consequences of aging that contribute to increased falls include visual changes such as loss of depth perception, susceptibility to glare, loss of visual acuity, and difficulty in light accommodation. Neurologic changes include loss of balance, dizziness, loss of position sense, and delayed reaction time (Ruckenstein, 2001). Cardiovascular changes may result in cerebral hypoxia and postural hypotension. Cognitive changes include confusion, loss of judgment, and impulsive behavior. Musculoskeletal changes include altered posture and decreased muscle strength. Use of many medications, medication interactions, and alcohol precipitate falls by causing drowsiness, incoordination, and postural hypotension. Osteoporosis-related fractures can have a negative effect on the individual's ability to maintain an independent living arrangement (Peterson, 2001).

Overall, elderly women who fall sustain a greater degree of injury than do elderly men. The most common fracture occurring from a fall is hip fracture resulting from the combined comorbidities of osteoporosis and the condition or situation that provoked the fall. Studies have shown that elderly people who fall experience a greater decline in their ability to perform ADLs and social activities, have a greater chance of being institutionalized, and use more health care services than elderly people who do not fall (Capezuti, 2000; Tinetti, Williams, & Gill, 2000).

In institutionalized elderly people, restraints in the form of physical modalities (lap belts; geriatric chairs; vest, waist, and jacket restraints) and chemical modalities (medications) are known to precipitate many of the injuries they were meant to prevent. Documented injuries and deaths resulting from these restraints include strangulation, vascular and neurologic damage, pressure ulcers, skin tears, fractures, increased confusion, and significant emotional trauma. The time required to supervise restrained patients adequately is better used addressing the unmet need that provoked the behavior that resulted in the use of restraint. Because of the overwhelming negative consequences of restraint use, the accrediting agencies of nursing homes and acute care facilities now maintain stringent guidelines concerning their use.

Urinary Incontinence

Urinary incontinence can be acute, developing during an illness, or it can develop chronically over a period of years. The older patient often does not report this very common problem unless specifically asked. Transient causes may be attributed to *d*elirium and dehydration; *r*estricted mobility and restraints; *i*nflammation, infection, and impaction; and *p*harmaceuticals and polyuria (use the acronym DRIP to remember them). Once identified, the causative factor can be eliminated. Established incontinence may be a result of neurologic or structural abnormalities (Degler, 2000b).

The pelvic floor serves as the supporting mechanism or "hammock" for the bladder, uterus, and rectum. It may have become weakened as a result of pregnancy, labor and delivery, prior pelvic surgeries, or work that required prolonged standing or lifting. Dysfunction of the pelvic floor can be greatly improved with Kegel exercises. Other measures that help prevent episodes of incontinence include having quick access to toilet facilities and wearing clothing that can be unfastened easily.

The patient with this problem should be urged to seek help from appropriate health personnel, because incontinence can be as emotionally devastating as it is physically debilitating. Nurses who specialize in behavioral approaches to urinary incontinence management are particularly successful in assisting an individual either to regain continence or to significantly improve the level of continence. Although medications such as anticholinergics may decrease some of the symptoms of urge incontinence (detrusor instability), their side effects (dry mouth, slowed gastrointestinal motility, and confusion) may make them inappropriate choices for the elderly. Various surgical procedures are also used to manage urinary incontinence, particularly stress urinary incontinence.

Detrusor hyperactivity with impaired contractility is a type of urge incontinence that is seen predominantly in the elderly population. In this variation of urge incontinence, the patient has absolutely no warning that he or she is about to lose urine. When toileted, the patient often voids only a small volume of urine or none at all, then experiences a large volume of incontinence after leaving the bathroom. The nursing staff should be familiar with this form of incontinence and should not show disapproval to the patient. Many patients with dementia suffer from this type of incontinence because both incontinence and dementia are a result of dysfunction in similar areas of the brain. Prompted, timed voiding can be of assistance to these individuals, although clean intermittent catheterization is the preferred management.

ACQUIRED IMMUNODEFICIENCY SYNDROME IN OLDER ADULTS

Acquired immunodeficiency syndrome (AIDS) is no longer only a disease of young people. It is increasingly recognized that AIDS does not spare the older segment of society. According to a report of the Centers for Disease Control and Prevention, between 1981 to 1989, more than 10% of all AIDS patients nationwide were

50 years of age or older at the time of diagnosis, and about 3% were age 60 years or older. In that report, male homosexual contact and blood transfusions were the predominant modes of transmission among older patients. Transmission by contaminated blood products has declined in recent years, so the predominant mode of transmission in older people now is through sexual contact. The most common AIDS-indicator disease in the older person is *Pneumocystis carinii* pneumonia. Wasting syndrome and HIV encephalopathy are also common in older HIV-infected people. Survival time is significantly shorter in older patients than in younger patients with AIDS (Ory & Mack, 1998).

Common Mental Health Problems in Older Populations

Older adults are less likely than younger people to seek treatment for mental health symptoms, so health professionals are challenged to recognize, assess, refer, collaborate, treat, and support those older adults who exhibit noticeable changes in intellect or affect. In a community setting, the nurse may be the only health care provider who has contact with the person. Symptoms should not be dismissed as age-related changes; a thorough assessment may reveal a treatable, reversible physical or mental condition.

DEPRESSION

Depression is the most common affective or mood disorder of old age and is often responsive to treatment. Its classification and diagnosis vary according to the number, severity, and duration of symptoms. Depression disrupts quality of life, increases the risk of suicide, and becomes self-perpetuating. It may also be an early sign of a chronic illness or the result of physical illness. Signs of depression include feelings of sadness, fatigue, diminished memory and concentration, feelings of guilt or worthlessness, sleep disturbances, appetite disturbances with excessive weight loss or gain, restlessness, impaired attention span, and suicidal ideation.

Although depression among the elderly is widespread, it is often undiagnosed and untreated. Attentive clinical evaluation is essential. Geriatric depression and symptoms of dementia often overlap, so cognitive impairment may be a result of depression rather than dementia. When depression and medical illnesses coexist, as they often do, neglect of the depression can retard physical recovery. Symptoms might be secondary to a medication interaction or an undiagnosed physical condition. Assessing the patient's mental status, including assessing for depression, is vital and must not be overlooked (Charts 12-3 and 12-4).

Depressive illness in late life should be vigorously treated with antidepressants. Psychosocial approaches have also been found to be effective. Selective serotonin reuptake inhibitors, such as paroxetine (Paxil), are clinically useful and exhibit rapid action with a low occurrence of adverse effects. Tricyclic antidepressants, specifically nortriptyline (Aventyl), desipramine (Norpramin), and doxepin (Sinequan), are also clinically effective for depression. Anticholinergic, cardiac, and orthostatic side effects, as well as interactions with other medications, require that these agents be used with care: the dosage must be managed carefully to relieve symptoms and at the same time avoid medication toxicity. It may take 4 to 6 weeks for symptoms to recede, so the

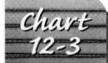

Chart 12-3 Mini-Mental State Examination

Maximum Score

Orientation
5   What is the (year) (season) (date) (day) (month)?
5   Where are we (state) (county) (city) (hospital) (floor)?

Registration
3   Name three objects: One second to say each. Then ask the patient all three after you have said them. Give one point for each correct answer. Repeat them until he learns all three. Count trials and record number. Number of trials: _____.

Attention and calculation
5   Begin with 100 and count backwards by 7 (stop after five answers). Alternatively, spell "world" backwards.

Recall
3   Ask for the three objects repeated above. Give one point for each correct answer.

Language
2   Show a pencil and a watch, and ask subject to name them.
1   Repeat the following: "No 'if's,' 'and's,' or 'but's.' "
3   A three-stage command: "Take a paper in your right hand; fold it in half, and put it on the floor."
1   Read and obey the following: (Show subject the written item.) CLOSE YOUR EYES.
1   Write a sentence.
1   Copy a design (complex polygon as in Bender-Gestalt).
30   **Total score possible**

Reprinted from Folstein, M. F., Folstein, S., & McHugh, P. R. (1975). Mini-mental state: A practical method for grading the cognitive state of patients for the clinician. *Journal of Psychiatric Research, 12,* 189–198. With permission from Pergamon Press Ltd, Headington Hill Hall, Oxford OX3 OBW, UK.

nurse should offer explanations and encouragement during this period.

Alcohol abuse related to depression is significant in the elderly population. Alcohol-related problems in older people often remain hidden, however, since many older adults deny their habit when questioned. Alcohol abuse is especially dangerous in the older person because of changes in renal and liver function as well as the probability of side effects in interactions with prescriptive medications (Adams, Atkinson, Ganz, & O'Conner, 2000).

DELIRIUM

Delirium, often called acute confusional state, begins with confusion and progresses to disorientation. The patient may experience an altered level of consciousness ranging from stupor to excessive activity. Thinking is disorganized, and the attention span is characteristically short. Hallucinations, delusions, fear, anxiety, and paranoia may also be evident. Because of the acute and unexpected onset of symptoms and the unknown underlying cause, delirium is a medical emergency. Delirium occurs secondary to a number of causes, including physical illness, medication or alcohol toxicity, dehydration, fecal impaction, malnutrition, infection, head trauma, lack of environmental cues, and sensory deprivation or overload. Older adults are particularly

Choose the best answer for how you felt this past week.

*1. Are you basically satisfied with your life? YES NO
2. Have you dropped many of your activities and interests? YES NO
3. Do you feel that your life is empty? YES NO
4. Do you often get bored? YES NO
*5. Are you hopeful about the future? YES NO
6. Are you bothered by thoughts you can't get out of your head? YES NO
*7. Are you in good spirits most of the time? YES NO
8. Are you afraid that something bad is going to happen to you? YES NO
*9. Do you feel happy most of the time? YES NO
10. Do you often feel helpless? YES NO
11. Do you often get restless and fidgety? YES NO
12. Do you prefer to stay at home, rather than going out and doing new things? YES NO
13. Do you frequently worry about the future? YES NO
14. Do you feel you have more problems with memory than most? YES NO
*15. Do you think it is wonderful to be alive now? YES NO
16. Do you often feel downhearted and blue? YES NO
17. Do you feel pretty worthless the way you are now? YES NO
18. Do you worry a lot about the past? YES NO
*19. Do you find life very exciting? YES NO
20. Is it hard for you to get started on new projects? YES NO
*21. Do you feel full of energy? YES NO
22. Do you feel that your situation is hopeless? YES NO
23. Do you think that most people are better off than you are? YES NO
24. Do you frequently get upset over little things? YES NO
25. Do you frequently feel like crying? YES NO
26. Do you have trouble concentrating? YES NO
*27. Do you enjoy getting up in the morning? YES NO
28. Do you prefer to avoid social gatherings? YES NO
*29. Is it easy for you to make decisions? YES NO
*30. Is your mind as clear as it used to be? YES NO
Score: _____ (Number of "depressed" answers)*

Norms

Normal: 5 ± 4
Mildly depressed: 15 ± 6
Very depressed: 23 ± 5

*Appropriate (nondepressed) answers = yes; all others = no.

Yesavage, J., et al. (1983). Development and validation of a geriatric screening scale: A preliminary report. *Journal of Psychiatric Research, 17* (1), 37–49. Reprinted with permission from Pergamon Press Ltd., Headington Hill Hall, Oxford OX3 OBW, UK.

vulnerable to acute confusion because of their decreased biologic reserve and the large number of medications that many take. The nurse must recognize the grave implications of the acute symptoms and report them immediately. If the delirium goes unrecognized and the underlying cause is not treated, permanent, irreversible brain damage or death can follow. Delirium is sometimes mistaken for dementia (see Table 12-4 for a comparison of dementia and delirium).

Therapeutic interventions vary, depending on the reason for the symptoms. Because medication interactions and toxicity are often implicated, nonessential medications should be stopped. Nutritional and fluid intake should be supervised and monitored. The environment should be quiet and calm. To increase **orientation** and provide familiar environmental cues, the nurse encourages family members or friends to touch and talk to the patient. It is important to question the family carefully about the patient's prior cognitive state. Ongoing mental status assessments using this baseline are helpful in evaluating responses to treatment and to the hospital or extended care facility admission.

THE DEMENTIAS: MULTI-INFARCT DEMENTIA AND ALZHEIMER'S DISEASE

Dementia reportedly affects 3% to 11% of community-residing adults older than 65 years of age and 20% to 50% of community-residing adults older than age 85. Most of those suffering from dementia who are in the over-85 age group reside in institutional settings. Of those individuals 100 years and older, almost 60% are noted to demonstrate dementia. Despite this high incidence, clinicians fail to detect dementia in 21% to 72% of patients. In order for a diagnosis of dementia to be made, at least two domains of altered function must exist—memory and at least one of the following: language, perception, visuospatial function, calculation, judgment, abstraction, and problem-solving (Mayo Foundation for Medical Education and Research [Mayo], 2001).

Symptoms are usually subtle in onset and often progress slowly until they are obvious and devastating. The changes characteristic of dementia fall into three general categories: cognitive, functional, and behavioral. Reversible causes of dementia include alcohol abuse, medication use (polypharmacy), psychiatric disorders, and normal-pressure hydrocephalus. The three most common nonreversible dementias are Alzheimer's disease, multi-infarct dementia, and mixed Alzheimer's and multi-infarct dementia. Alzheimer's disease accounts for more than 60% of all dementias, and multi-infarct dementia (vascular dementia) accounts for another 5% to 20%. Other non-Alzheimer's dementias include Parkinson's disease, AIDS-related dementia, and Pick's disease. These remaining dementias account for fewer than 15% of cases and are relatively uncommon (National Institute of Neurological Disorders and Stroke, 2000).

Dementia is characterized by an uneven, downward decline in mental function. Multi-infarct dementia is sometimes confused with Alzheimer's disease, paranoia, or delirium because of its unpredictable clinical course. The diagnosis can be even more difficult if the patient is suffering from both Alzheimer's disease and multi-infarct dementia.

Multi-infarct, or vascular dementia, has the following defining characteristics:

- There must be evidence of dementia.
- There must be evidence of cerebrovascular disease (by history, clinical examination, or brain imaging).
- The two disorders must be reasonably related.

Alzheimer's disease is a progressive, irreversible, degenerative neurologic disease that begins insidiously and is characterized by gradual losses of cognitive function and disturbances in behavior and affect. Alzheimer's disease is not found exclusively in the elderly; in 1% to 10% of cases, its onset occurs in middle age. A family history of Alzheimer's disease and the presence of Down syndrome are two established risk factors for Alzheimer's disease. If family members have at least one other relative with Alzheimer's disease, then a familial component, which non-

Table 12-4 • **Summary of Differences Between Dementia and Delirium**

	DEMENTIA		DELIRIUM
	Alzheimer's Disease (AD)	Multi-Infarct Dementia	
Etiology	Familial (genetic [chromosomes 14, 19, 21]) Sporadic	Cardiovascular (CV) disease Cerebrovascular disease Hypertension	Drug toxicity and interactions; acute disease; trauma; chronic disease exacerbation Fluid and electrolyte disorder
Risk factors	Advanced age; genetic factor	Preexisting CV disease	Preexisting cognitive impairment
Occurrence	50%–60% of dementias	20% of dementias	20% of hospitalized older people
Onset	Slow	Often abrupt Follows a stroke or transient ischemic attack	Rapid, acute onset A harbinger of acute medical illness
Age of onset (yr)	Early onset AD: 30s–65 Late onset AD: 65+ Most commonly: 85+	Most commonly 50–70 yr	Any age, but predominantly in older persons
Gender	Males and females equally	Predominantly males	Males and females equally
Course	Chronic, irreversible; progressive, regular, downhill	Chronic, irreversible Fluctuating, stepwise progression	Acute
Duration	2–20 yr	Variable; years	Lasts 1 day to 1 month
Symptom progress	Onset insidious. *Early*—mild and subtle *Middle and late*—intensified Progression to death (infection or malnutrition)	Depends on location of infarct and success of treatment; death due to underlying CV disease	Symptoms are fully reversible with adequate treatment; can progress to chronicity or death if underlying condition is ignored
Mood	Early depression (30%)	Labile: mood swings	Variable
Speech/language	Speech remains intact until late in disease *Early*—mild anomia (cannot name objects); deficits progress until speech lacks meaning; echoes and repeats words and sounds; mutism.	May have speech deficit/aphasia depending on location of lesion	Fluctuating; often cannot concentrate long enough to speak
Physical signs	*Early*—no motor deficits *Middle*—apraxia [70%] (cannot perform purposeful movement) *Late*—Dysarthria (impaired articulation) *End stage*—loss of all voluntary activity; positive neurologic signs	According to location of lesion: focal neurologic signs, seizures Commonly exhibits motor deficits	Signs and symptoms of underlying disease
Orientation	Becomes lost in familiar places (topographic disorientation) Has difficulty drawing three-dimensional objects (visual and spatial disorientation) Disorientation to time, place, and person—with disease progression		May fluctuate between lucidity and complete disorientation to time, place, and person
Memory	Loss is an early sign of dementia; loss of recent memory is soon followed by progressive decline in recent and remote memory		Impaired recent and remote memory; may fluctuate between lucidity and confusion
Personality	Apathy, indifference, irritability *Early disease*—social behavior intact; hides cognitive deficits *Advanced disease*—disengages from activity and relationships; suspicious; paranoid delusions caused by memory loss; aggressive; catastrophic reactions		Fluctuating; cannot focus attention to converse; alarmed by symptoms (when lucid); hallucinations; paranoid
Functional status, activities of daily living	Poor judgment in everyday activities; has progressive decline in ability to handle money, use telephone, function in home and workplace		Impaired
Attention span	Distractable; short attention span		Highly impaired; cannot maintain or shift attention
Psychomotor activity	Wandering, hyperactivity, pacing, restlessness, agitation		Variable; alternates between high agitation, hyperactivity, restlessness, and lethargy
Sleep–wake cycle	Often impaired; wandering and agitation at nighttime		Takes brief naps throughout day and night

specifically includes both environmental triggers and genetic determinants, is said to exist. Genetic studies show that autosomal-dominant forms of Alzheimer's disease are associated with early onset and early death.

In 1987, chromosome 21 was first implicated in early-onset familial Alzheimer's disease. Soon after, the gene coding for amyloid precursor protein (*APP*) was also found to be on chromosome 21. Not until 1991 was an actual mutation in association with familial Alzheimer's disease found in the *APP* gene of chromosome 21. For those with this gene, onset of Alzheimer's disease began in their 50s. Only a few of the cases of familial Alzheimer's disease have been found to involve this genetic mutation. In 1992, chromosome 14 was found to contain an unidentified mutation also linked to familial Alzheimer's disease. Since 1995, molecular biologists have been discovering even more-specific genetic information about the various forms of Alzheimer's disease, including genetic differences between early- and late-onset Alzheimer's disease. These genetic differences are helping to pinpoint risk factors associated with the disease, although the genetic indicators are not specific enough to be used as reliable diagnostic markers (Mayo, 2001).

Pathophysiology

Specific neuropathologic and biochemical changes are found in patients with Alzheimer's disease. These include neurofibrillary tangles (a tangled mass of nonfunctioning neurons) and senile or neuritic plaques (deposits of amyloid protein, part of a larger protein, *APP*) in the brain. This neuronal damage occurs primarily in the cerebral cortex and results in decreased brain size. Similar changes are found to a lesser extent in the normal brain tissue of older adults. Cells that use the neurotransmitter acetylcholine are the ones principally affected by this disease. Biochemically, the enzyme active in producing acetylcholine, which is specifically involved in memory processing, is decreased.

Several theories are currently being tested to explain what predisposes an individual to develop the plaques and neurotangles that can be seen at autopsy on biopsy of the brains of Alzheimer's patients (Mayo, 2001). Scientists continue to increase their understanding of the complex ways in which aging and genetic and nongenetic factors affect and damage brain cells over time and eventually lead to Alzheimer's disease. Researchers have recently discovered how and why amyloid plaques form and cause neuronal death, as well as the possible relationship between various forms of tau protein and impaired function, which leads to neuronal death. The major role of tau protein is to regulate the assembly and stability of neurons. Researchers are also beginning to discover the roles of inflammation and oxidative stress and the contribution of brain infarctions to the disease (Alzheimer's Disease Education and Referral Center, 1999).

Clinical Manifestations

In the early stages of Alzheimer's disease, forgetfulness and subtle memory loss occur. The patient may experience small difficulties in work or social activities but has adequate cognitive function to hide the loss and can function independently. Depression may occur at this time. With further progression of the disease, the deficits can no longer be concealed. Forgetfulness is manifested in many daily actions. These patients may lose their ability to recognize familiar faces, places, and objects and may get lost in a familiar environment. They may repeat the same stories because they forget that they have already told them. Trying to reason with the person and using reality orientation only increase the patient's anxiety without increasing function. Conversation becomes difficult, and there are word-finding difficulties. The ability to formulate concepts and think abstractly disappears; for instance, the patient can interpret a proverb only in concrete terms. The patient is often unable to recognize the consequences of his or her actions and will therefore exhibit impulsive behavior. For example, on a hot day, the patient may decide to wade in the city fountain fully clothed. The patient has difficulty with everyday activities, such as operating simple appliances and handling money.

Personality changes are also usually evident. The patient may become depressed, suspicious, paranoid, hostile, and even combative. Progression of the disease intensifies the symptoms: speaking skills deteriorate to nonsense syllables, agitation and physical activity increase, and the patient may wander at night. Eventually, assistance is needed for most ADLs, including eating and toileting, since dysphagia occurs and incontinence develops. The terminal stage, in which the patient is usually immobile and requires total care, may last for months or years. Occasionally, the patient may recognize family or caretakers. Death occurs as a result of complications such as pneumonia, malnutrition, or dehydration.

Assessment and Diagnostic Findings

The health history, including medical history; family history; social and cultural history; medication history, and the physical examination, including functional and mental health status, are key in the diagnosis of probable Alzheimer's disease. Diagnostic tests, including complete blood count, the Venereal Disease Research Laboratory (VDRL) test for syphilis, HIV testing, chemistry profile, and vitamin B_{12} and thyroid hormone levels, as well as screening with electroencephalography (EEG), computed tomography (CT), magnetic resonance imaging (MRI), and examination of the cerebrospinal fluid may all refute or support a diagnosis of probable Alzheimer's disease.

Depression can closely mimic early-stage Alzheimer's disease and coexists in many patients. A depression scale is helpful in screening for underlying depression. Tests for cognitive function, such as the Mini-Mental State Examination (see Chart 12-3) and the clock-drawing test, are useful for screening. CT and MRI scans of the brain are useful for excluding hematoma, brain tumor, stroke, normal-pressure hydrocephalus, and atrophy but are not reliable in making a definitive diagnosis of Alzheimer's disease. Infections, physiologic disturbances such as hypothyroidism, Parkinson's disease, and vitamin B_{12} deficiency can produce cognitive impairment that may be misdiagnosed as Alzheimer's disease. Biochemical abnormalities can be excluded through examination of the blood and cerebrospinal fluid, but the findings are not specific enough to make the diagnosis. A diagnosis of "probable Alzheimer's disease" is made when the medical history, physical examination, and laboratory tests have excluded all known causes of other dementias. The diagnosis can be confirmed only by cerebral biopsy (Mayo, 2001).

Medical Management

In the fall of 1993, the U.S. Food and Drug Administration approved the first medication for treatment of the symptoms of Alzheimer's disease, tacrine hydrochloride (Cognex). This agent enhances acetylcholine uptake in the brain, thus maintaining memory skills for a period of time. Because this medication can cause liver toxicity, patients must be closely monitored. It was not until early 1997 that donepezil (Aricept), a second medication in this category of acetylcholinesterase inhibitors, was introduced. In 2000, a third medication in this class, rivastigmine (Exelon) was introduced in the United States after completion of research trials conducted in more than 70 countries. These two newer preparations have far fewer side effects, although they continue to require ongoing monitoring. They vary in their level of effectiveness from patient to patient, due in part to their window of effectiveness, which in general is limited to the early stages of dementia (Fillit, 2000).

Nursing Management

Although Alzheimer's disease is the focus of this nursing management discussion, the interventions described apply to all patients with dementia, regardless of the cause. Nursing interventions are aimed at maintaining the patient's physical safety; reducing anxiety and agitation; improving communication; promoting independence in self-care activities; providing for the patient's needs for socialization, self-esteem, and intimacy; maintaining adequate nutrition; managing sleep pattern disturbances; and supporting and educating family caregivers. Research has demonstrated that when

the nurse can provide such support, older adults are able to maintain higher levels of perceived and actual health (Forbes, 2001).

SUPPORTING COGNITIVE FUNCTION

As the patient's cognitive ability declines, the nurse provides a calm, predictable environment that helps the person interpret his or her surroundings and activities. Environmental stimuli are limited, and a regular routine is followed. A quiet, pleasant manner of speaking, clear and simple explanations, and use of memory aids and cues help to minimize confusion and disorientation and give the patient a sense of security. Prominently displayed clocks and calendars may enhance orientation to time. Color-coding the doorway may help the patient who has difficulty locating his or her room. Active participation may help the patient to maintain cognitive, functional, and social interaction abilities for a longer period. Physical activity and communication have also been demonstrated to slow some of the cognitive decline of Alzheimer's disease (Nursing Research Profile 12-1).

PROMOTING PHYSICAL SAFETY

A safe environment allows the patient to move about as freely as possible and relieves the family of constant worry about safety.

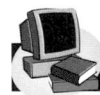

NURSING RESEARCH PROFILE 12-1

The Effect of Conversation on Functional Mobility

Tappen, R., Roach, K., Applegate, E. B., & Stowell, P. (2000). Effect of a combined walking and conversation intervention on functional mobility of nursing home residents with Alzheimer's disease. *Alzheimer Disease and Associated Disorders, 14,* 196–201.

Purpose

Motor loss becomes evident in the later stages of Alzheimer's disease, leading to gait disturbances that predispose the individual to falls and subsequent injuries. The purpose of this study was to assess the effect of a combination of exercise and conversation, compared with walking-only exercise and conversation-only treatments, on the functional mobility of frail nursing home residents with Alzheimer's disease.

Design

A repeated-measures three-group design was used. Sixty-five nursing home residents with Alzheimer's disease were randomly assigned to one of three treatment groups: walking only, having conversation only, or walking and conversing with the study nurses. Treatments were given for 30 minutes three times a week for 16 weeks. The residents' functional mobility was measured before initiation of the treatments and after 16 weeks of intervention. At the end of the intervention period, descriptive statistics, the Student *t* test, analysis of variance (ANOVA) and the chi square test were used to compare the three groups.

Conclusions

As expected, the ambulation function of the participants in the "conversation only" group dropped dramatically. Those participants who were assisted to walk without conversation demonstrated a dramatic drop in ambulation function as well. Of all three groups, the least decline occurred in ambulation function over time in the group of participants with whom the nurses carried on a conversation while these participants were being assisted to walk. This information suggests that while attempting to maintain physical function in the patient with Alzheimer's disease, the nurse can best achieve this goal if socialization is incorporated into exercise sessions.

Implications for Practice

This study demonstrated that assisted walking with conversation can contribute to maintenance of functional mobility in institutionalized patients with Alzheimer's disease. Staff caring for these patients can promote patients' acceptance of assisted walking through the use of effective communication strategies.

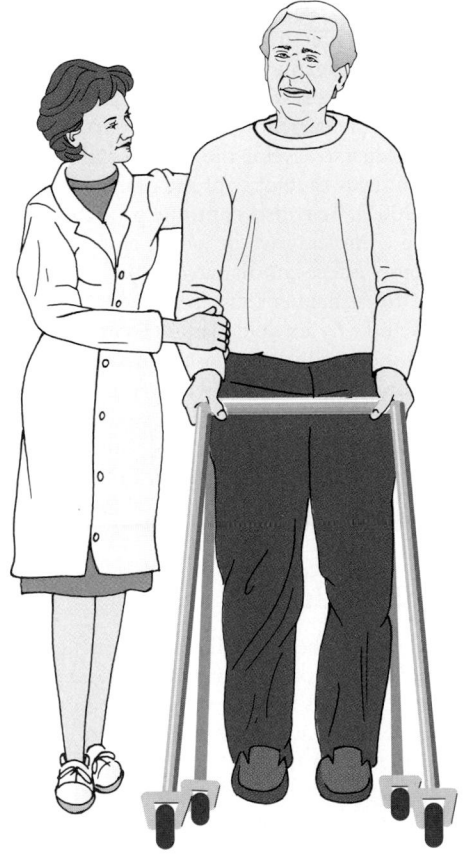

Based on a drawing by Rachel A. Degler.

To prevent falls and other injuries, all obvious hazards are removed. Nightlights are helpful. The patient's intake of medications and food is monitored. Smoking is allowed only with supervision. A hazard-free environment allows the patient maximum independence and a sense of autonomy. Because of a short attention span and forgetfulness, wandering behavior can often be reduced by gently persuading or distracting the patient. Restraints are avoided because they may increase agitation. Doors leading from the house must be secured. Outside the home, all activities must be supervised to protect the patient, and the patient should wear an identification bracelet or neck chain in case he or she becomes separated from the caregiver.

REDUCING ANXIETY AND AGITATION

Despite profound cognitive losses, the patient will, at times, be aware of his or her rapidly diminishing abilities. The patient will need constant emotional support that reinforces a positive self-image. When losses of skills occur, goals are adjusted to fit the patient's declining ability.

The environment should be kept uncluttered, familiar, and noise free. Excitement and confusion can be upsetting and may precipitate a combative, agitated state known as a catastrophic reaction (overreaction to excessive stimulation). During such a reaction, the patient responds by screaming, crying, or becoming abusive (physically or verbally). This may be the patient's only way of expressing an inability to cope with the environment. When this occurs, it is important to remain calm and unhurried. Measures such as listening to music, stroking, rocking, or distraction may quiet the patient. Frequently, the patient forgets what triggered the reaction. Structuring of activities is also helpful. Becoming familiar with the patient's predicted responses to certain stressors helps caregivers to avoid similar situations.

By the time most older persons with dementia have progressed to the late stages of the disease, they typically reside in nursing homes and are predominantly cared for by nurses' aides. Dementia education for caregivers is imperative to minimize patient agitation and is very effectively taught by advanced practice nurse specialists (Nursing Research Profile 12-2).

IMPROVING COMMUNICATION

To promote the patient's interpretation of messages, the nurse remains unhurried and reduces noises and distractions. The nurse uses clear, easy-to-understand sentences to convey messages, because the patient frequently forgets the meaning of words or has difficulty organizing and expressing thoughts. Lists and simple written instructions can serve as reminders to the patient and are often helpful. Sometimes, the patient can point to an object or use nonverbal language to communicate. Tactile stimuli, such as a hug or a hand pat, are usually interpreted as signs of affection, concern, and security.

PROMOTING INDEPENDENCE IN SELF-CARE ACTIVITIES

Pathophysiologic changes in the brain make it difficult for a person with Alzheimer's disease to maintain physical independence. The nurse should help the person remain functionally independent for as long as possible. One way to do this is to simplify daily activities by organizing them into short, achievable steps so that the patient experiences a sense of accomplishment. Frequently, an occupational therapist can suggest ways to simplify tasks or recommend adaptive equipment. Direct patient supervision is sometimes necessary, but maintaining personal dignity and autonomy is important for the person with Alzheimer's disease. He or she is encouraged to make choices when appropriate and to participate in self-care activities as much as possible.

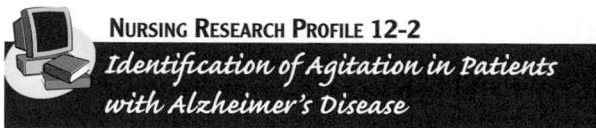

NURSING RESEARCH PROFILE 12-2
Identification of Agitation in Patients with Alzheimer's Disease

Whall, A. L., Black, M. E. A., Yankou, D. J., et al. (1999). Nurse aides' identification of onset and level of agitation in late stage dementia patients. *American Journal of Alzheimer's Disease, 14,* 202–206.

Purpose
Nursing assistants provide the majority of care to patients in nursing homes. They are vital links in the early identification, and therefore in the treatment, of agitation in patients with Alzheimer's disease. Nurses' aides (NAs) are sometimes characterized as unwilling or unable to manage patients' agitation. This study examines the process by which nurses' aides can successfully identify this agitation.

Design
NAs from five different nursing homes owned by the same corporate entity were asked to participate in the study. Criteria to participate included being employed for at least 1 year. (Research demonstrates that NAs who remain at a facility longer than 1 year usually have a commitment to those they serve.) The NAs did not receive any additional wages and were only promised a letter to indicate that they had participated in the study. Each NA received approximately 1 hour of training via audio tapes and conversation with nurse experts. Each NA was then paired with a nurse expert to assess his or her skill at appropriately identifying levels of agitation in patients with late-stage Alzheimer's disease.

Conclusions
This study demonstrated that NAs with a minimum of 1 year of employment did an excellent job in acquiring new observation skills with only 1 hour of training and positive reinforcement via a letter noting their participation in this study. The NAs' assessment of signs of agitation agreed with that of the nurse expert more than 90% of the time. All the NAs involved reported gaining helpful insights in managing agitated behavior as a result of participation in the study.

Implications for Practice
The results of this study support the ability of NAs to accurately observe and report agitated behavior as a result of a brief training session using adult learning principles that stressed the importance of their input into the training and learning objectives. Early observation and reporting of agitated behavior is important to prevent agitation from increasing to the level of physical aggression.

PROVIDING FOR SOCIALIZATION AND INTIMACY NEEDS

Because socialization with old friends can be comforting, visits, letters, and phone calls are encouraged. Visits should be brief and nonstressful; limiting visitors to one or two at a time helps to reduce overstimulation. Because recreation is important, the person is encouraged to enjoy simple activities. Realistic goals that provide satisfaction are appropriate. Hobbies and activities such as walking, exercising, and socializing can improve the quality of life. The nonjudgmental friendliness of a pet may provide a lonely person with stimulation, comfort, and contentment. Care of the pet by the patient can also provide a satisfying activity and an outlet for energy.

Alzheimer's disease does not eliminate the need for intimacy. The patient and his or her spouse may or may not continue to enjoy sexual activity. The spouse should be encouraged to talk about any sexual concerns, and sexual counseling may be suggested if necessary. Simple expressions of love, such as touching and holding, are often meaningful.

PROMOTING ADEQUATE NUTRITION

Mealtime can be a pleasant, social occasion or a time of upset and distress, so it should be kept simple and calm, without confrontations. The patient will prefer familiar foods that look appetizing and taste good. To avoid the patient's "playing" with the food, one dish is offered at a time. Food is cut into small pieces to prevent choking. Liquids may be easier to swallow if they are converted to gelatin. Hot food and beverages are served warm, but the temperature of the foods should be checked to prevent burns.

When lack of coordination interferes with self-feeding, adaptive equipment is helpful. Some patients may do well eating with their fingers. If this is the case, an apron or a smock, rather than a bib, is used to protect clothing. As deficits progress, it may be necessary to feed the patient. Forgetfulness, disinterest, dental problems, incoordination, overstimulation, and choking can all serve as barriers to good nutrition.

PROMOTING BALANCED ACTIVITY AND REST

Many patients with Alzheimer's disease exhibit sleep disturbances, wandering, and behaviors that may be deemed inappropriate. These behaviors are most likely to occur when there are underlying physical or psychological needs that are unmet. It is imperative that caregivers seek to learn the needs of the patient who is exhibiting this type of behavior, because further health decline can ensue if the source of the problem is not corrected. Adequate sleep and physical exercise are essential. If sleep is interrupted or the patient is unable to fall asleep, music, warm milk, or a back rub may help the person relax. During the day, the patient should be given sufficient opportunity to participate in exercise activities, because a regular pattern of activity and rest will enhance nighttime sleep. Long periods of daytime sleeping are discouraged.

SUPPORTING HOME AND COMMUNITY-BASED CARE

The emotional burden placed on the family of a patient with Alzheimer's disease is enormous. The physical health of the patient is often very stable, and the mental degeneration is gradual. Because the diagnosis is not specific, the family may cling to the hope that the diagnosis is incorrect and that the person will improve if he or she tries harder. Aggression and hostility exhibited by the patient are often misunderstood by the caregiver or family, who feel unappreciated, frustrated, and angry. Feelings of guilt, nervousness, and worry contribute to caregiver fatigue, depression, and family dysfunction. In some cases caregivers themselves can become so fatigued as a result of the stress of caregiving that elder neglect or abuse can occur. This has been documented in home situations as well as institutions. If elder neglect or abuse of any kind—including physical, psychological, sexual, or financial abuse—is suspected, the local adult protective services agency must be notified; the role of the nurse is not to prove the neglect or abuse, but to report it (Tumolo, 2000).

The multiple needs of family caregivers have been addressed by the Alzheimer's Association. This national organization is a coalition of family members and professionals who share the goals of family support and service, education, research, and advocacy. Family support groups, respite care, and adult day care are available through the Alzheimer's Association. Concerned volunteers are trained to provide structure to caregiver support groups. Through the use of respite care, a service commonly provided, the caregiver can get away from the home for short periods while someone else is tending to the patient's needs.

The nurse must be sensitive to the highly emotional issues that the family is confronting. Support and education of the caregivers are essential components of care. The family can contact the Alzheimer's Association or a comparable group that provides the opportunity to meet with others who are experiencing similar problems.

The Older Adult in an Acute Care Setting: Altered Responses to Illness

The elderly person entering the acute care setting is at increased risk for complications, infections, and functional decline. The interdisciplinary team and nursing staff can help avert negative outcomes by being knowledgeable about the physiologic and psychological responses of older adults to acute illnesses and by planning and implementing preventive measures. In addition to the interventions discussed in the following paragraphs, general nursing measures that can be taken to avoid complications in the older adult include careful and frequent assessment of vital signs, mental status, fluid balance, and skin integrity; prompt identification and treatment of complications; promotion of independent self-care and mobility; assistance with frequent position changes and deep-breathing exercises; alertness to possible medication reactions; and assistance with ADLs and toileting.

INCREASED SUSCEPTIBILITY TO INFECTION

Infectious diseases present a significant threat of morbidity and mortality to older people, in part because of the blunted response of host defenses caused by a reduction in both cell-mediated and humoral immunity (see Chapters 50 and 51). Age-related loss of physiologic reserve and chronic illnesses also contribute to increased susceptibility. Pneumonia, urinary tract infections, tuberculosis (TB), gastrointestinal infections, and skin infections are some of the commonly occurring infections in older people.

The effects of influenza and pneumococcal infections on older people are also significant. Estimates place the number of deaths from influenza at 10,000 to 40,000 per year. Hospital-acquired pneumonia is responsible for 300,000 deaths annually in the United States, making it the second most common nosocomial infection (after urinary tract infection) and the leading cause of death from hospital-acquired infection. Many of these deaths involve older adults because of their increased vulnerability to infection (Smith-Sims, 2001).

The influenza vaccine is prepared yearly to adjust for the specific immunologic characteristics that are present in the influenza viruses at that time. It is an inactivated preparation that should be taken annually in the fall, preferably in November. The pneumococcal vaccine has 23 type-specific capsular polysaccharides. Protection lasts 4 years or longer. Revaccination is rarely recommended because of the higher incidence of local reaction on subsequent immunizations. Both of these injections can be received at the same time in separate injection sites. The nurse should urge older people to receive these vaccines. All health care providers working with older people or high-risk chronically ill people should also be immunized.

TB significantly affects older adults. Case rates for TB are highest among those who are 65 years of age or older, with the exception of persons with HIV infection. Nursing home residents account for the majority of the cases in the older population. Much of the infection rate is attributed to reactivation of old infection. Pulmonary and extrapulmonary TB often have subtle, nonspecific symptoms. This is of particular concern in the nursing home, because an active case of TB places patients and staff at risk for infection.

The Centers for Disease Control and Prevention (CDC) guidelines suggest that all new admissions to nursing homes receive a Mantoux test (PPD test) unless there is a history of TB or a previous positive response. All patients whose tests are not positive (a positive test is indicated by induration of more than 10 mm at 48 to 72 hours) should receive a second test in 1 week. The first PPD serves to boost the suppressed immune response that may occur with an older person. Chest x-ray studies and possibly sputum studies should be used to follow up on PPD-positive responders and converters. For positive converters, a course of preventive therapy for 6 to 12 months with isoniazid (INH) reduces the risk of active disease by 70%. All negative testers should be periodically retested. The nurse can facilitate this process within the care facility (CDC, 2000).

ALTERED PAIN AND FEBRILE RESPONSES

Many altered physical, emotional, and systemic reactions to disease are attributed to age-related changes in older people. Useful and reliable physical indicators of illness in young and middle-aged people cannot be relied on for the diagnosis of potential life-threatening problems in older adults. The response to pain in older people may be lessened because of reduced acuity of touch, alterations in neural pathways, and diminished processing of sensory data. Research has demonstrated the absence of chest pain in many older adults experiencing a myocardial infarction. Hiatal hernia or upper gastrointestinal distress is often responsible for chest pain in elderly people. Acute abdominal conditions, such as mesenteric infarction and appendicitis, often go unrecognized in elderly people because of atypical signs and absence of pain (Kufrovich, 2001).

The baseline body temperature for older people is about 1°F lower than it is for younger people. In the event of illness, therefore, the body temperature of an older person may not reach a sufficient elevation to qualify as a traditionally defined "fever." A temperature of 37.8°C (100°F), in combination with systemic symptoms, may signal infection. A temperature of 38.3°C (101°F) is almost certainly a serious infection that needs prompt attention. A blunted fever in the face of an infection often indicates a poor prognosis. Elevations in temperature rarely exceed 39.5°C (103°F). The nurse must be alert to other subtle signs of infection: mental confusion, increased respirations, tachycardia, and changed facial appearance and color.

ALTERED EMOTIONAL IMPACT

The emotional component of illness in older people may differ from that in younger people. Many elderly people equate good health with the absence of old age. "You are as old as you feel" is a belief of many. An illness that requires hospitalization or a change in lifestyle is an imminent threat to well-being. Admission to the hospital is often feared and actively avoided. Economic concerns and fear of becoming a burden to the family often lead to high anxiety in older people. The nurse must recognize the implications of fear, anxiety, and dependency in elderly patients. Autonomy and independent decision making are encouraged. A positive and confident demeanor in the nurse and the family promote a positive mental outlook in the elderly patient. In addition to anxiety and fear, older people are at high risk for disorientation, confusion, change in level of consciousness, and other symptoms of delirium if they are admitted to the hospital.

ALTERED SYSTEMIC RESPONSE

The effect of illness on an aged person has far-reaching repercussions. The decline in organ function that occurs in every system of the aging body eventually forces one or more body systems to function at full capacity. Illness places new demands on body systems that have little or no reserve to meet this crisis. Homeostasis, the ability of the body to maintain an internal balance of function and chemical composition, is jeopardized. The older person may be unable to respond effectively to an acute illness or, if a chronic health condition is present, he or she may be unable to sustain appropriate responses over a long period. Furthermore, the older person's ability to respond to definitive treatment is impaired. These altered responses reinforce the need for the nurse to monitor all of the older adult's body system functions closely, being alert to signs of impending systemic complication.

 Critical Thinking Exercises

1. Mrs. C., a 64-year-old woman, arrives at the presurgical admission unit for her scheduled toe amputation; she has chronic arterial insufficiency, secondary to diabetes, with a history of chronic atrial fibrillation. As you review the list of medications that she has brought with her, you discover that she has listed, "Coumadin 3 mg per day", and "Warfarin 1 mg per day." As you question her, she reports that her physician provided a new prescription for her anticoagulation at her preoperative visit last week. She was unaware that Coumadin and warfarin were the same medication and continued on the Coumadin while starting the "new" prescription. What will your first action be?

2. You are working for a home health agency and making regular visits to an 85-year-old widow who recently moved in with her daughter because of declining health. On your first visit since her move, you noted a bruise on the patient's hip. She stated that she had bumped into a chair on the way to the bathroom. On the next visit, you find her in dirty clothing. She stated that the washing machine was broken and her daughter was waiting for the repairman. Today as you visit with the patient, there is a cut on her arm and more bruises. She confides that her daughter is overworked and sometimes gets a bit "impatient" as she is providing care for her. Describe the most appropriate plan of action.

3. As a charge nurse in a skilled nursing facility, your daily assessment of Mr. Jones, a 75-year-old man with late-stage Alzheimer's disease, normally finds him to be medically stable, with a pleasant but confused affect. When you assess him today, his vital signs continue to be stable; however, he angrily yells at you when you speak to him, he is notably agitated, and he cries with pain as he is attempting to void. Based on your understanding of the altered response to acute infection in the elderly, what assessment parameters would you evaluate? What plan of action would you initiate?

REFERENCES AND SELECTED READINGS

Books

Abraham, I. L., & Fulmer, T. (1999). *Geriatric nursing protocols for best practice.* New York: Springer.

Abrams, W. B., Beers, M. H., & Berkow, R. (2000). *Merck manual of geriatrics* (3rd ed.). Whitehouse Station, NJ: Merck & Co.

Alzheimer's Disease Education and Referral (ADEAR) Center. (1999). *Progress report on Alzheimer's Disease.* Silver Springs, MD: U.S. Department of Health and Human Services, Public Health Service, National Institutes of Health, National Institutes of Aging. NIH Pub. No. 99-4664. http://www.alzheimers.org/pubs/prog99.htm.

Burke, M. M., & Laramie, J. A. (2000). *Primary care of the older adult: A multidisciplinary approach.* St. Louis: Mosby.

Centers for Medicare and Medicaid Services. (2002). The Home Health Prospective Payment System (PPS). Baltimore, MD: Author. http://www.cms.hhs.gov/providers/hhapps/default.asp.

Costa, P. T. Jr., Williams, T. F., Somerfield, M., et al. (1996, November). *Recognition and initial assessment of Alzheimer's disease and related dementias: Clinical practice guideline no. 19.* (AHCPR Publication No. 97-0702). Rockville, MD: U.S. Department of Health and Human Services, Public Health Service, Agency for Health Care Policy and Research.

Ebersole, P., & Hess, P. (2001). *Geriatric nursing and healthy aging.* St. Louis: Mosby.

Eliopoulos, C. (2000). *Gerontological nursing* (5th ed.). Philadelphia: Lippincott Williams & Wilkins.

Erikson, E. H. (1963). *Childhood and society* (2nd ed.). New York: W. W. Norton.

Fantl, J. A., Newman, D. K., Colling, J., et al. (1996, March). *Managing acute and chronic urinary incontinence: Clinical practice guideline.* Quick Reference Guide for Clinicians No. 2, 1996 Update. (AHCPR Pub. No. 96-0686). Rockville, MD: U.S. Department of Health and Human Services, Public Health Service, Agency for Health Care Policy and Research.

Gallo, J. J., Fulmer, T., Paveza, G. J., & Reichel, W. (2000). *Handbook of geriatric assessment* (3rd ed.). Gaithersburg, MD: Aspen.

Ham, R. J., & Warshaw G. (2001). *Primary care geriatrics: A case-based approach* (4th ed.). St. Louis: Mosby–Year Book.

Havighurst, R. J. (1972). *Developmental tasks and education* (3rd ed.). New York: McKay.

Hazzard, W. R., Blass, J. P., Ettinger, W. H. Jr., Halter, J. B., & Ouslander, J. G. (1999). *Principles of geriatric medicine and gerontology* (4th ed.). New York: McGraw-Hill.

Health Care Financing Administration Press Office. (2000, January 10). *Health care spending growth rates stay low in 1998: Private spending outpaces public.* Available at: http://www.hhs.gov/news/press/2000pres/20000/10.html.

Health Services Research on Aging. (2000, January). *Building on biomedical and clinical research. Translating research into practice fact sheet.* (AHRQ Publication No. 00-P012). Rockville, MD: Agency for Healthcare Research and Quality. Available at: http://www.ahrq.gov/research/tripage.htm.

Hogstel, M. O. (2001). *Gerontology: Nursing care of the older adult.* Albany: Delmar Publishing.

Holmes, D., Teresi, J. A., & Ory, M. (2000). *Special care units: Research and practice in Alzheimer's disease,* Vol. 4. New York: Springer.

Kane, R. L., Ouslander, J. G., & Abrass, I. B. (1999). *Essentials of clinical geriatrics* (4th ed.). New York: McGraw-Hill.

Lueckenotte, A. G. (2000). *Gerontologic nursing* (2nd ed.). St. Louis: Mosby–Year Book.

Mezey, M. D., Berkman, B. J., & Callahan, C. (2000). *The encyclopedia of elder care: the comprehensive resource on geriatric and social care.* New York: Springer.

National Academy of Social Insurance. (2001). *Financing Medicare's future.* Washington, DC: Author.

National Center for Health Statistics. (2000). *Health, United States, 2000 with adolescent health chartbook.* Hyattsville, Maryland: Author.

Neugarten, B. L. (1961). *Personality in middle and late life.* New York: Atherton Press.

Noelker, L. S., & Harel, Z. (2000). *Linking quality of long term care and quality of life.* New York: Springer.

Roach, S. S. (2000). *Introductory gerontological nursing.* Philadelphia: Lippincott Williams & Wilkins.

Schmidt Luggen, A., Meiner, S. E., & National Gerontological Nursing Association (2000). *NGNA: Core curriculum for gerontological nursing* (2nd ed.). St. Louis: Mosby.

Silin, P. S. (2001). *Nursing homes: The family's journey.* Baltimore: Johns Hopkins University Press.

Strumpf, N. E., Evans, L. K., Wagner, J., & Patterson, J. (1992). *Reducing restraints: Individualized approaches to behavior. A teaching guide.* Huntingdon Valley, PA: Geriatric Research and Training Center.

Takano-Stone, J., Wyman, J. F., & Salisbury, S. S. (1999). *Clinical gerontological nursing: A guide to advanced practice* (2nd ed.). Philadelphia: W. B. Saunders.

U.S. Bureau of the Census. (2000). *Profile of older Americans.* U.S. Department of Health and Human Services Administration on Aging. Available at: http://www.aoa.dhhs.gov/aoa/stats/profile/profile2000.html.

Watson, R. R. (2000). *Handbook of nutrition in the aged* (3rd ed.). Boca Raton, FL: CRC Press.

Zang, S. M., & Allender, J. A. (1999). *Home care of the elderly.* Philadelphia: Lippincott Williams & Wilkins.

Journals

Asterisks indicate nursing research articles.

Adams, W., Atkinson, R., Ganz, S. B., & O'Connor, P. G. (2000). Alcohol problems in the elderly. *Patient Care for the Nurse Practitioner, 3,* 68–89.

*Anderson, M. A., Helms, L. B., Hanson, K. S., & DeVilder, N. W. (1999). Unplanned hospital readmissions: A home care perspective. *Nursing Research, 48,* 299–307.

Atchley, R. C. (1989). Continuity theory of normal aging. *Gerontologist, 29,* 183–190.

*Capezuti, E. (2000). Preventing falls and injuries while reducing side rail use. *Annals of Long Term Care, 8*(6). Available at: http://www.mmhc.com/nhm/v8n6.shtm.

*Capezuti, E., Strumpf, N., Evans, L. K., et al. (1999). Outcomes of nighttime physical restraint removal for severely impaired nursing home residents. *American Journal of Alzheimer's Disease, 14,* 157–164.

Centers for Disease Control and Prevention (Updated October 28, 2000). A strategic plan for the elimination of tuberculosis in the U.S. Available at: http://www.cdc.gov/nchstp/tb/pubs/corecurr/default.htm.

Chen, C. L., Weiss, N. S., Newcome, P., Barlow, W., & White, E. (2002). Hormone replacement therapy in relation to breast cancer. *JAMA, 287*(6), 734–741.

Degler, M. (2000a). Caring for the caregiver. Protocol Driven Healthcare Incorporated. Available at: http://www.MyBladder.com.

Degler, M. (2000b). Reversible causes of urinary incontinence. Protocol Driven Healthcare Incorporated. Available at: http://www.MyBladder.com.

Dolinar, T. M., McQuillen, A. D., Ranseen, J. D., et al. (2001). Health, safety, and the older driver. *Patient Care for the Nurse Practitioner, 4,* 18–32.

Dolinar, T. M., Eisdorfer, C., & Perersen, R. (2001). Strategies for early diagnosis. *Patient Care for the Nurse Practitioner, 4,* 12–22.

Fillet, H. (2000). Improving the quality of managed care for patients with mild to moderate Alzheimer's disease. *CBS HealthWatch by Medscape.* Cliggott Publishing Co., Division of SCP/Cliggott Communications. Available at: http://www.healthwatch.medscape.com.

*Forbes, D. A. (2001). Enhancing mastery and sense of coherence: Important determinants of health in older adults. *Geriatric Nursing, 22,* 29–32.

Friberg, T. (2000). Age-related macular degeneration. *The Clinical Advisor for Nurse Practitioners, 3,* 58–66.

*Galvan, T. J. (2001). Dysphagia: Going down and staying down. *American Journal of Nursing, 101,* 37–42.

Geldmacher, D. S., Heck, E., & O'Toole, E. (2001). Providing for the caregiver. *Patient Care for the Nurse Practitioner, 4,* 36–48.

*Grandjean, C. K., & Gibbons, S. W. (2000). Assessing ambulatory geriatric sleep complaints. *The Nurse Practitioner, 25,* 25–39.

Havighurst, R. J. (1968). Personality and patterns of aging. *Gerontologist, 8,* 20–23.

Hoban, S., & Kearney, K. (2000). Elder abuse and neglect: It takes many forms—If you're not looking, you may miss it. *American Journal of Nursing, 100,* 49–50.

Hofmann, M. T., & Nahass, D. (2001). Case report: The use of an ethics committee regarding the case of an elderly female with blood loss after hip surgery. *Annals of Long-Term Care, 9,* 55–59.

Kegel, A. H. (1948). Progressive resistance exercise in the functional restoration of the perineal muscles. *American Journal of Obstetrics and Gynecology, 56,* 238–248.

Kiely, D. K., Simon, S. E., Jones, R. N., et al. (2000). The protective effect of social engagement on mortality in long-term care. *Journal of the American Geriatrics Society, 48,* 1367–1372.

*Lukacs, J. L., & Reame, N. E. (2000). Concentrations of follicle-stimulating hormone correlate with alkaline phosphatase and a marker for vitamin K status in the perimenopause. *Journal of Women's Health and Gender-Based Medicine, 9,* 731–739.

Mayo Foundation for Medical Education and Research. (2001). *Dementia: Epidemiology.* Geriatric Medicine. Community Internal Medicine Division. Available at: http://www.mayo.edu/geriatrics-rst/Dementia.I.html.

National Institute of Neurological Disorders and Stroke. (Reviewed June 12, 2000). *NINDS Pick's Disease Information Page.* Available at: http://www.ninds.nih.gov/health_and_medical/disorders/picks_doc.htm.

*Naylor, M., Brooten, D., Campbell, R., et al. (1999). Comprehensive discharge planning and home follow-up of hospitalized elders. *Journal of the American Medical Association, 281,* 613–620.

*Norlander, L., & McSteen, K. (2000). The kitchen table discussion: A creative way to discuss end-of-life issues. *Home Healthcare Nurse, 18,* 532–540.

Nusbaum, N. J. (2000). Issues in Home Rehabilitative Care. *Annals of Long-Term Care, 8,* 43–48.

Ory, M. G., & Mack, K. A. (1998). Middle-aged and older people with AIDS: Trends in national surveillance rates, transmission routes and risk factors. *Research on Aging, Special Supplement.*

Patient Self-Determination Act (PSDA). (1990). *Omnibus Budget Reconciliation Act.* Title IV, Sec. 4206. Congress Record 12368, ct 26.

*Pentz, C., & Wilson, A. (2000). Ensuring the quality of OASIS data: One agency's plan. *Home Healthcare Nurse, 19,* 38–42.

*Peterson, J. A. (2001). Osteoporosis overview. *Geriatric Nursing, 22,* 17–23.

*Phillips, L. R. (2000). Domestic violence and aging women. *Geriatric Nursing, 21,* 188–193.

*Plotkin, K., & Roche, J. (2000). The future of home and hospice care: Linking interventions to outcomes home health care. *Home Healthcare Nurse, 18,* 442–450.

*Resnick, B. (2001). Promoting health in older adults: A four-year analysis. *Journal of the American Academy of Nurse Practitioners, 13,* 23–33.

*Rittenhouse, S. K. (2001). Spironolactone for heart failure: A worthy addition to therapy. *Advance for Nurse Practitioners, 9,* 34–40.

Ruckenstein, M. J. (2001). The dizzy patient: How you can help. *Consultant, 41,* 29–34.

*Ryden, M. B., Snyder, M., Gross, C. R., et al. (2000). Value-added outcomes: The lure of advanced practice nurses in long-term care facilities. *Gerontologist, 40,* 654–662.

*Schafer, S. L. (2001). Prescribing for seniors: It's a balancing act. *Journal of the American Academy of Nurse Practitioners, 13,* 108–112.

Scheiber, L. B., & Torregrosa, L. (2000). Osteoporosis: What to tell postmenopausal women about prevention and therapy. *Consultant, 40,* 1021–1028.

Schuman, J. (2001). Old concept, new trends: A primer on life care planning. *Long-Term Care Interface, 2,* 26–29.

*Smith-Sims, K. (2001). Hospital-acquired pneumonia. *American Journal of Nursing, 101,* 24AA–24EE.

Spillman, B. (2001). A conversation with Brenda Spillman, Ph.D.: Interface interview. *Long-Term Care Interface, 2,* 27–29.

*Tappen, R., Roach, K., Applegate, E. B., & Stowell, P. (2000). Effect of a combined walking and conversation intervention on functional mobility of nursing home residents with Alzheimer disease. *Alzheimer Disease and Associated Disorders, 14,* 196–201.

Tinetti, M. E., Williams, C. S., & Gill, T. M. (2000). Dizziness among older adults: A possible geriatric syndrome. *Annals Internal Medicine, 132,* 337–344.

Tumolo, J. (2000). Caregivers who hurt: The tragedy of elder abuse. *Advance for Nurse Practitioners, 8,* 63–65.

Vastag, B. (2002). Hormone replacement therapy falls out of favor with expert committee. *JAMA, 287*(15), 1923–1926.

*Whall, A. L., Black, M. E. A., Yankou, D. J., et al. (1999). Nurses aides' identification of onset and level of agitation in late stage dementia patients. *American Journal of Alzheimer's Disease, 14,* 202–206.

RESOURCES AND WEBSITES

Administration on Aging, 330 Independence Avenue SW, Suite 4760, Washington, DC 20201; 202-619-0724; http://www.aoa.dhhs.gov.

Alzheimer's Association, 919 N. Michigan Avenue, Suite 110, Chicago, IL 60611-1676; 800-272-3900; http://www.alz.org.

Alzheimer's Disease and Related Disorders Association, Inc., 919 N. Michigan Ave., Suite 1000, Chicago, IL 60611-1676; 312-335-8700; 800-272-3900; http://www.alz.org.

Alzheimer's Disease Education and Referral Center (ADEAR), P.O. Box 8250, Silver Spring, MD 20907-8250; 301-495-3311; 800-438-4380; adear@alzheimers.org; http://www.alzheimers.org.

American Association for Geriatric Psychiatry (AAGP), 7910 Woodmont Ave, Suite 1350, Bethesda, MD 20814-3004; 301-654-7850; http://www.aagpgpa.org.

American Association of Homes and Services for the Aging, 901 E Street NW, Suite 500, Washington, DC 20004-2837; 1-202-783-2242; http://www.aahsa.org.

American Association of Retired Persons, 601 E Street NW, Washington, DC 20049; 202-434-2277; 800-424-3410; http://www.aarp.org.

American College of Health Care Administrators, 325 S. Patrick St., Alexandria, VA 22314; 1-703-549-5822; http://www.achca.org.

American Federation for Aging Research (AFAR), 1414 Avenue of the Americas, 18th Floor, New York, NY 10019; 1-212-572-2327; http://www.afar.org.

American Foundation for the Blind, 15 West 16th Street, New York, NY 10011; 212-620-2000; http://www.afb.org.

American Geriatrics Society, Empire State Building, 350 Fifth Ave, Suite 801, New York, NY 10118; 212-308-1414; http://www.americangeriatrics.org.

Association for Gerontology in Higher Education (AGHE), 1001 Connecticut Avenue NW, Suite 410, Washington, DC 20036; 1-202-429-9277; http://www.aghe.org.

Children of Aging Parents (CAPS), Suite 302-A, 16098 Woodbourne Road, Levittown, PA 19057-1511; 215-945-6900; 800-227-7294; http://www.caps4caregivers.org.

Elderhostel, 75 Federal Street, Boston, MA 02110-1941; 617-426-7788; http://www.elderhostel.org.

Family Caregiver Alliance (FCA), 425 Bush St., Suite 500, San Francisco, CA 94108; 415-434-3388; http://www.caregiver.org.

Gerontological Society of America, 1275 K Street NW, Suite 350, Washington, DC 20005-4006; 1-202-842-1275; http://www.geron.org.

Gray Panthers, 2025 Pennsylvania Avenue NW, Suite 821, Washington, DC 20006; 1-202-466-3132; http://www.graypanthers.org.

Legal Services for the Elderly, 17th Floor, 130 West 42nd Street, New York, NY 10036; 1-212-391-0120; http://www.aoa.dhhs.gov/directory/125.html.

National Association for Continence, P.O. Box 8306, Spartanburg, SC 29305-8306; 1-800-BLADDER (1-800-252-3337); http://www.nafc.org.

National Caucus and Center on Black Aged, Inc., Suite 500, 1424 K Street NW, Washington, DC 20005; 1-202-637-8400; http://www.ncba-blackaged.org.

National Center on Elder Abuse (NCEA), 1225 I St NW, Suite 725, Washington, DC 20005; 1-202-898-2586; http://www.health.gov/NHIC/NHICScripts/Entry.cfm?HRCode=HR2395.

National Council on the Aging, Inc., Suite 200, 409 Third Street SW, Washington, DC 20024; 202-479-1200; http://www.ncoa.org.

National Gerontological Nursing Association, 7250 Parkway Drive, Suite 510, Hanover, MD 21076; 1-800-723-0560; http://www.ngna.org.

National Institute on Aging, 31 Center Dr., Room 5C27, Bethesda, MD 20892-2292, 301-496-1752; 800-438-4380; http://www.nih.gov/nia.

Safe Return (program for locating lost patients), Box A-3956, Chicago, IL 60690; 800-572-1122 (to report a lost patient).

Simon Foundation for Continence, P.O. 835, Wilmette, IL 60091; 1-800-237-4666; http://www.simonfoundation.org.

Concepts and Challenges in Patient Management

Applying Concepts from NANDA, NIC, and NOC

Mr. Brandon is a 43-year-old man who sustained a back injury in a work-related incident. He reports severe shooting pains in his lower back and both buttocks. Mr. Brandon is not a candidate for surgery and has undergone physical therapy with little improvement in his pain. He reports that the pain makes it impossible for him to return to his former job, work around the house, or obtain enjoyment from leisure activities. He has been referred to a pain clinic for management. The concept map illustrates the relationships that exist among selected nursing diagnoses, interventions, and outcomes for the patient with chronic pain.

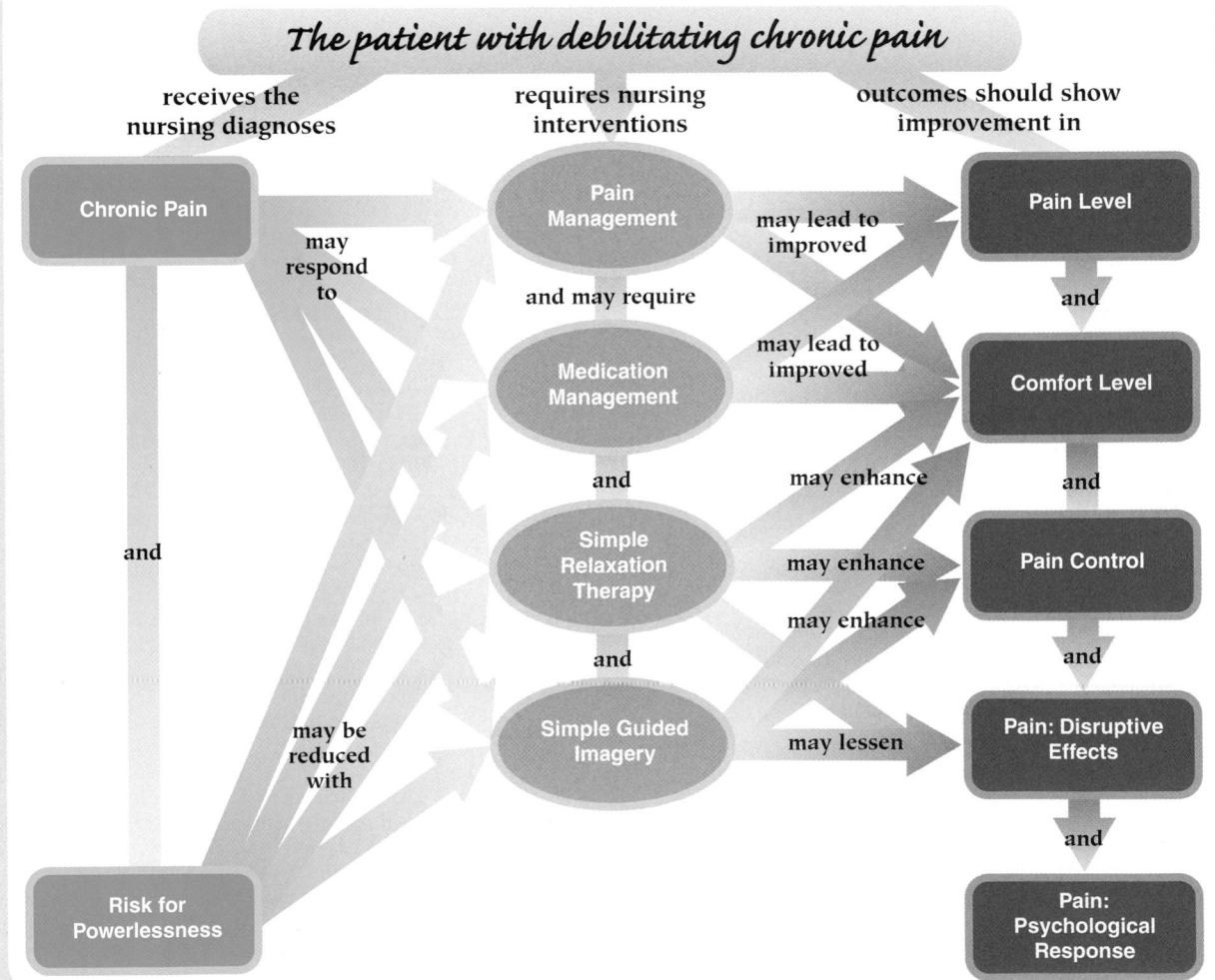

The patient with debilitating chronic pain

receives the nursing diagnoses

requires nursing interventions

outcomes should show improvement in

Chronic Pain

may respond to

Pain Management

may lead to improved

Pain Level

and may require

may lead to improved

Medication Management

and

may enhance

Comfort Level

Simple Relaxation Therapy

may enhance

and

may enhance

Pain Control

and

and

may be reduced with

Simple Guided Imagery

may lessen

Pain: Disruptive Effects

and

Risk for Powerlessness

Pain: Psychological Response

Nursing Classifications and Languages

NANDA
Nursing Diagnoses

Chronic Pain—Unpleasant sensory and emotional experience arising from actual or potential tissue damage or described in terms of such damage; sudden or slow onset of any intensity from mild to severe, constant or recurring, without an anticipated or predictable end and a duration of greater than 6 months

Risk for Powerlessness—At risk for perceived lack of control over a situation and/or one's ability to significantly affect an outcome

NIC
Nursing Interventions*

Pain Management—Alleviation of pain or reduction in pain to a level of comfort that is acceptable to the patient

Medication Management—Facilitation of safe and effective use of prescribed or over-the-counter medicine

Simple Relaxation Therapy—Use of techniques to encourage and elicit relaxation for the purpose of decreasing undesirable signs and symptoms such as pain, muscle tension, or anxiety

Simple Guided Imagery—Purposeful use of imagination to achieve relaxation and/or direct attention away from undesirable sensations

Emotional Support—Provision of reassurance, acceptance, and encouragement during times of stress

Self-Esteem Enhancement—Assisting a patient to increase his or her personal judgment of self-worth

NOC
Nursing Outcomes†

Return to functional baseline status, stabilization of, or improvement in

Pain Level—Severity of reported or demonstrated pain

Comfort Level—Extent of physical and psychological ease

Pain Control—Personal actions to control pain

Pain: Disruptive Effects—Observed or reported disruptive effects of pain on emotions and behavior

Pain: Psychological Response—Cognitive and emotional responses to physical pain

---

NANDA, North American Nursing Diagnosis Association; NIC, Nursing Interventions Classification; NOC, Nursing Outcomes Classification.

*Iowa Intervention Project © 2000. In McCloskey, J. C., & Bulechek, G. M. (2000). *Nursing interventions classification (NIC)* (3rd ed.). St. Louis: Mosby.

†Iowa Outcomes Project © 2000. In Johnson, M., Maas, M., & Moorhead, S. (2000). *Nursing outcomes classification (NOC)* (3rd ed.). St. Louis: Mosby.

Pain Management

LEARNING OBJECTIVES

On completion of this chapter, the learner will be able to:

1. Differentiate between acute pain, chronic pain, and cancer pain.
2. Describe the negative consequences of pain.
3. Describe the pathophysiology of pain.
4. Describe factors that can alter the perception of pain.
5. Demonstrate appropriate use of pain measurement instruments.
6. Explain the physiologic basis of pain relief interventions.
7. Explain the impact of aging on pain.
8. Discuss when opioid tolerance may be a problem.
9. Identify appropriate pain relief interventions for selected groups of patients.
10. Compare the various types of neurosurgical procedures used to treat intractable pain.
11. Develop a plan to prevent and treat the adverse effects of opioid analgesic agents.
12. Use the nursing process as a framework for the care of patients with pain.

*P*ain is an unpleasant sensory and emotional experience associated with actual or potential tissue damage (Merskey & Bogduk, 1994). It is the most common reason for seeking health care. It occurs with many disorders, diagnostic tests, and treatments. It disables and distresses more people than any single disease. Since nurses spend more time with the patient in pain than do other health care providers, nurses need to understand the pathophysiology of pain, the physiologic and psychological consequences of acute and chronic pain, and the methods used to treat pain. Nurses encounter patients in pain in a variety of settings, including acute care, outpatient, and long-term care settings, as well as in the home. Thus, they must have the knowledge and skills to assess pain, to implement pain relief strategies, and to evaluate the effectiveness of these strategies, regardless of setting.

The Fifth Vital Sign

Pain management is considered such an important part of care that the American Pain Society coined the phrase "Pain: The 5th Vital Sign" (Campbell, 1995) to emphasize its significance and to increase the awareness among health care professionals of the importance of effective pain management. Documentation of pain assessment is now as prominent as the documentation of the "traditional" vital signs. Pain assessment and management are also mandated by the Joint Commission on the Accreditation of Healthcare Organizations (JCAHO) (2003).

Calling pain the fifth vital sign suggests that the assessment of pain should be as automatic as taking a patient's blood pressure and pulse. The JCAHO (2003) has incorporated pain and pain management into its standards. JCAHO's standards state that "pain is assessed in all patients" and that "patients have the right to appropriate assessment and management of pain." These standards reflect the importance of pain management.

In health care, the primary care provider's role is to assess and ameliorate pain by administering medications and other treatments. The nurse collaborates with other health care professionals while administering most pain relief interventions, evaluating their effectiveness, and serving as patient advocate when the intervention is ineffective. In addition, the nurse serves as an educator to the patient and family, teaching them to manage the pain relief regimen themselves when appropriate.

The International Association for the Study of Pain definition mentioned earlier encompasses the multidimensional nature of pain (Merskey & Boduck, 1994). A broad definition of pain is "whatever the person says it is, existing whenever the experiencing person says it does" (McCaffery & Beebe, 1989, p.7). This definition emphasizes the highly subjective nature of pain and pain management. The patient is the best authority on the existence of pain. Therefore, validation of the existence of pain is based on the patient's report that it exists.

Although it is important to believe the patient who reports pain, it is equally important to be alert to patients who deny pain in situations where pain would be expected. A nurse who suspects pain in a patient who denies it should explore with the patient the reason for suspecting pain, such as the fact that the disorder or procedure is usually painful or that the patient grimaces when moving or avoids movement. Exploring why the patient may be denying pain is also helpful. Some people deny pain because they fear the treatment that may result if they report or admit pain. Others deny pain for fear of becoming addicted to **opioids** (previously referred to as narcotics) if these medications are prescribed.

Types of Pain

Pain is categorized according to its duration, location, and etiology. Three basic categories of pain are generally recognized: acute pain, chronic (nonmalignant) pain, and cancer-related pain.

Glossary

addiction: a behavioral pattern of substance use characterized by a compulsion to take the drug primarily to experience its psychic effects

agonist: a substance that when combined with the receptor produces the drug effect or desired effect. Endorphins and morphine are agonists on the opioid receptors.

algogenic: causing pain

antagonist: a substance that blocks or reverses the effects of the agonist by occupying the receptor site without producing the drug effect. Naloxone (Narcan) is an opioid antagonist.

balanced analgesia: using more than one form of analgesia concurrently to obtain more pain relief with fewer side effects

breakthrough pain: a sudden and temporary increase in pain occurring in a patient being managed with opioid analgesia

endorphins and **enkephalins:** morphine-like substances produced by the body. Primarily found in the central nervous system, they have the potential to reduce pain.

dependence: occurs when a patient who has been taking opioids experiences a with-

drawal syndrome when the opioids are discontinued; often occurs with opioid tolerance and does not indicate an addiction

nociception: activation of sensory transduction in nerves by thermal, mechanical, or chemical energy impinging on specialized nerve endings. The nerves involved convey information about tissue damage to the central nervous system.

nociceptor: a receptor preferentially sensitive to a noxious stimulus

non-nociceptor: nerve fiber that usually does not transmit pain

opioid: a morphine-like compound that produces bodily effects including pain relief, sedation, constipation, and respiratory depression. This term is preferred over **narcotic.**

pain: an unpleasant sensory and emotional experience resulting from actual or potential tissue damage

pain threshold: the point at which a stimulus is perceived as painful

pain tolerance: the maximum intensity or duration of pain that a person is willing to endure

patient-controlled analgesia (PCA): self-administration of analgesic agents by a patient instructed about the procedure

placebo effect: analgesia that results from the expectation that a substance will work, not from the actual substance itself

prostaglandins: chemical substances that increase the sensitivity of pain receptors by enhancing the pain-provoking effect of bradykinin

referred pain: pain perceived as coming from an area different from that in which the pathology is occurring. An example would be the perception of left arm or jaw pain in a person having a myocardial infarction.

sensitization: a heightened response seen after exposure to a noxious stimulus. Response to the same stimulus is to feel more pain.

tolerance: occurs when a person who has been taking opioids becomes less sensitive to their analgesic properties (and usually side effects). Characterized by the need for increasing doses to maintain the same level of pain relief.

ACUTE PAIN

Usually of recent onset and commonly associated with a specific injury, acute pain indicates that damage or injury has occurred. Pain is significant in that it draws attention to its existence and teaches the person to avoid similar potentially painful situations. If no lasting damage occurs and no systemic disease exists, acute pain usually decreases along with healing. For purposes of definition, acute pain can be described as lasting from seconds to 6 months. However, the 6-month time frame has been criticized (Brookoff, 2000) as inaccurate since many acute injuries heal within a few weeks and most heal by 6 weeks. In a situation where healing is expected in 3 weeks and the patient continues to suffer pain, it should be considered chronic and treated with interventions used for chronic pain. Waiting for the full 6-month time frame in this example could cause needless suffering.

CHRONIC (NONMALIGNANT) PAIN

Chronic pain is constant or intermittent pain that persists beyond the expected healing time and that can seldom be attributed to a specific cause or injury. It may have a poorly defined onset, and it is often difficult to treat because the cause or origin may be unclear. Although acute pain may be a useful signal that something is wrong, chronic pain usually becomes a problem in its own right.

Chronic pain may be defined as pain that lasts for 6 months or longer, although 6 months is an arbitrary period for differentiating between acute and chronic pain. An episode of pain may assume the characteristics of chronic pain before 6 months have elapsed, or some types of pain may remain primarily acute in nature for longer than 6 months. Nevertheless, after 6 months, most pain experiences are accompanied by problems related to the pain itself. Chronic pain serves no useful purpose. If it persists, it may become the patient's primary disorder.

The nurse may come in contact with patients with chronic pain when they are admitted to the hospital for treatment or when they are seen out of the hospital for home care. Frequently the nurse is called on in community-based settings to assist patients in managing pain. For more information on common pain syndromes, see Chart 13-1.

CANCER-RELATED PAIN

Pain associated with cancer may be acute or chronic. Pain resulting from cancer is so ubiquitous that after fear of dying, it is the second most common fear of newly diagnosed cancer patients (Lema, 1997). More than half of the 1,308 cancer patients included in a study conducted by Foley (1999) reported being in moderate to severe pain 50% of the time. Pain in the patient suffering from cancer can be directly associated with the cancer (eg, bony infiltration with tumor cells or nerve compression), a result of cancer treatment (eg, surgery or radiation), or not associated with the cancer (eg, trauma). Most pain associated with cancer, however, is a direct result of tumor involvement. An approach to cancer pain management is illustrated in Figure 13-1. This three-step approach illustrates the types of analgesic medications used for various levels of pain. A cancer pain algorithm developed as a set of analgesic guiding principles appears in Figure 13-2.

PAIN CLASSIFIED BY LOCATION

The previous discussion of acute and chronic pain is an example of the categorization of pain according to duration. Pain is sometimes categorized according to location, such as pelvic pain, head-ache, and chest pain. This type of categorization is helpful in communicating and treating pain. For example, chest pain suggests angina or a myocardial infarction and indicates the need for treatment according to cardiac care standards.

PAIN CLASSIFIED BY ETIOLOGY

Categorizing pain according to etiology is another way to think about pain and its management. Burn pain and postherpetic neuralgia are examples of pain described by their etiology. Clinicians often can predict the course of pain and plan effective treatment using this categorization.

Harmful Effects of Pain

Regardless of its nature, pattern, or cause, pain that is inadequately treated has harmful effects beyond the suffering it causes. For example, unrelieved pain impairs the postoperative patient's ability to sleep (Raymond, Nielsen, Lauigne et al., 2001). Zalon (1997) found that the most common response to severe pain in frail, elderly postoperative women was to lie absolutely still, a response likely to result in postoperative complications.

EFFECTS OF ACUTE PAIN

Unrelieved acute pain can affect the pulmonary, cardiovascular, gastrointestinal, endocrine, and immune systems. The stress response ("neuroendocrine response to stress") that occurs with trauma also occurs with other causes of severe pain. The widespread endocrine, immunologic, and inflammatory changes that occur with stress can have significant negative effects. This is particularly harmful in patients compromised by age, illness, or injury.

The stress response generally consists of increased metabolic rate and cardiac output, impaired insulin response, increased production of cortisol, and increased retention of fluids (see Chap. 6 for details about the stress response). The stress response may increase the patient's risk for physiologic disorders (eg, myocardial infarction, pulmonary infection, thromboembolism, and prolonged paralytic ileus). The patient with severe pain and associated stress may be unable to take a deep breath and may experience increased fatigue and decreased mobility. Although these effects may be tolerated by a young, healthy person, they may hamper recovery in an elderly, debilitated, or critically ill person. Effective pain relief may result in a faster recovery and improved outcomes.

EFFECTS OF CHRONIC PAIN

Like acute pain, chronic pain also has adverse effects. Suppression of the immune function associated with chronic pain may promote tumor growth. Also, chronic pain often results in depression and disability. Although health care providers express concern about the large quantities of opioid medications required to relieve chronic pain in some patients, it is safe to use large doses of these medications to control progressive chronic pain. In fact, failure to administer adequate pain relief may be unsafe because of the consequences of unrelieved pain (McCracken & Iverson, 2001).

Regardless of how the patient copes with chronic pain, pain for an extended period can result in disability. Patients with a number of chronic pain syndromes report depression, anger, and fatigue (Meuser, Pietruck, Radruch et al., 2001; Raymond et al., 2001). The patient may be unable to continue the activities and

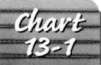

Chart 13-1 Pain Syndromes and Unusual Severe Pain Problems

Complex Regional Pain Syndrome

Complex regional pain syndrome (CRPS) is the name given to a group of conditions previously described as causalgia, reflex sympathetic dystrophy (RSD), and other diagnoses. Complex regional pain syndrome describes a variety of painful conditions that often follow an injury. The magnitude and duration of the pain far exceeds the expected duration and often results in significant impairment of motor function. Reflex sympathetic dystrophy is categorized as CRPS type I and occurs after a relatively minor trauma. Characterized by unexplained diffuse burning pain, usually in the periphery of an extremity, CRPS type I is accompanied by weakness, a skin color and temperature change relative to the other extremity, limited range of motion, hyperesthesia, hypoesthesia, edema, altered hair growth, and sweating (Janig, 2001).

Pain, which worsens with movement, cutaneous stimulation, or stress, often occurs after surgery or trauma to the extremity but is not limited to the area of surgery or trauma. CRPS type I is more common than CRPS type II and is usually managed through a pain clinic. Currently, regional sympathetic blockade and regional IV bretylium offer promise for relief. Tricyclic antidepressants may be tried as well. Complex regional pain syndrome type II refers to causalgia. Type II is more likely to develop after trauma with detectable peripheral nerve lesions (Janig, 2001).

Postmastectomy Pain Syndrome (PMP)

Postmastectomy pain syndrome (PMP) occurs after mastectomy with node dissection but is not necessarily related to the continuation of disease. Characterized by the sensation of constriction accompanied by a burning, prickling, or numbness in the posterior arm, axilla, or chest wall, PMP is often aggravated by movement of the shoulder, resulting in a frozen shoulder from immobilization (Miaskowski & Dibble, 1995).

Post-traumatic headache disorder occurs after trauma to the head and is characterized by daily and persistent headache. It is more likely to follow mild head injury than moderate to severe injury (Uomoto & Esselman, 1993).

Fibromyalgia (Fibrositis)

Fibromyalgia, a chronic pain syndrome characterized by generalized musculoskeletal pain, trigger points, stiffness, fatigability, and sleep disturbances, is aggravated by stress and overexertion. Treatment consists of NSAIDs, trigger point injections with local anesthetics, tricyclic antidepressants, stress reduction, and regular exercise.

Hemiplegia-Associated Shoulder Pain

Hemiplegia-associated shoulder pain is a pain syndrome that affects as many as 80% of stroke patients. It may result from stretching of the shoulder joint due to the uncompensated pull of gravity on the impaired arm. It may be preventable with functional electrical stimulation of involved shoulder muscles.

Pain Associated With Sickle Cell Disease

Pain experienced by patients with sickle cell disease results from venous occlusion caused by the sickle shape of the blood cells, impaired circulation to a muscle or organ, ischemia, and infarction. Acute pain may be managed with IV opioid analgesics administered according to a schedule or by a patient-controlled analgesia (PCA) pump and NSAIDs. Warm soaks and elevating the affected body part may help as well. Meperidine (Demerol) therapy is not recommended in patients with compromised renal function, nor is cold therapy. Patients with sickle cell disease may have a long history of chronic pain. Some issues related to their history include tolerance, possible long-term dependence, racial prejudice, and inadequate pain treatment.

AIDS-Related Pain

As AIDS progresses, so do problems that produce increasing amounts of pain, such as neuropathy, esophagitis, headaches, postherpetic pain, and abdominal, back, bone, and joint pain. Pain relief interventions are individualized and may consist of NSAIDs, long-lasting opioids, such as fentanyl patches, and topical lidocaine. Tricyclic antidepressants may provide comfort in neuropathic and postherpetic pain.

Burn Pain

Possibly the most severe pain, burn pain tends to be underrated by health care professionals the longer they work with burn patients. Besides administration of IV opioid analgesic agents, current therapies to ameliorate pain in burn patients include débridement under general anesthesia; anxiety reduction; intervention with PCA devices, such as hand-held nitrous oxide delivery system; and cognitive techniques, particularly hypnosis.

Guillain-Barré Syndrome and Pain

A progressive, inflammatory disorder of the peripheral nervous system, Guillain-Barré syndrome is characterized by flaccid paralysis accompanied by paresthesia and pain—muscle pain and severe, unrelenting, burning pain. Complaints of severe pain may be difficult to accept in the face of the characteristic flaccid facial response; therefore, the nurse must be sensitive and learn to disregard nonverbal cues that contradict the verbal report of pain. Treatment interventions include NSAIDs for muscle pain and opioids if NSAIDs are ineffective. Causalgia and neurogenic pain may be relieved by systemic or epidural opioids or, possibly, antiseizure agents or tricyclic antidepressants. To relieve the burning, some patients beg to have windows opened and clothing removed, even in cold weather. This suggests that gentle ice massage may help. Research is needed, however, to test this theory.

Opioid Tolerance

Opioid tolerance is common among patients treated for chronic pain, especially patients being treated by multiple health care providers. Opioid tolerance should be suspected when a patient (1) complains of significantly more pain than is usually associated with the condition, (2) requires unusually high doses of opioids to achieve pain relief, or (3) experiences an unusually low incidence and severity of side effects from opioids. Cancer patients also often develop a tolerance to opioids, requiring larger and larger doses of medication to obtain pain relief. In such cases, the nurse must recognize what is happening, seek additional information from the patient or family, and then procure additional prescriptions for analgesics or an alternative intervention. In patients undergoing surgery, epidural local anesthetic agents provide excellent postoperative analgesia, but the problem of opioid tolerance must be elicited from the patient preoperatively.

Occasionally a recovering heroin addict is seen in an acute pain situation (surgery or trauma). This patient may be undergoing treatment with naltrexone (Trexan), a long-acting form of the opioid antagonist naloxone (Narcan). Both the short-acting naloxone and the long-acting naltrexone act by binding to the opioid receptors, so opioids cannot be effective. If surgery is planned, the naltrexone should be discontinued a few days before the procedure. Should a patient receiving naltrexone be in immediate need of pain relief, very high doses of opioids are necessary. Alternative methods of pain relief (local or regional blockade and NSAIDs) should be incorporated in the pain management plan.

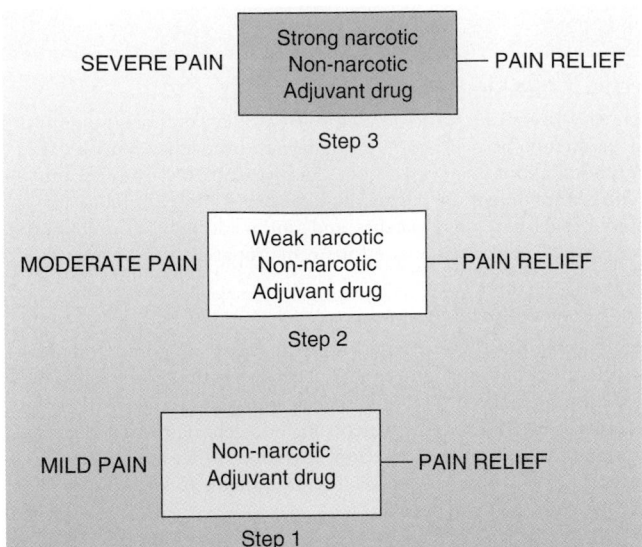

FIGURE 13-1 The World Health Organization three-step ladder approach to relieving cancer pain. Analgesic regimens are based on pain reported as ranging from mild to moderate to severe. Various opioid (narcotic) and nonopioid medications may be combined with other medications to control pain.

interpersonal relationships he or she engaged in before the pain began. Disabilities may range from curtailing participation in physical activities to being unable to take care of personal needs, such as dressing or eating. The nurse needs to understand the effects of chronic pain on the patient and family and needs to be knowledgeable about pain relief strategies and appropriate resources to assist effectively with pain management.

Pathophysiology of Pain

The sensory experience of pain depends on the interaction between the nervous system and the environment. The processing of noxious stimuli and the resulting perception of pain involve the peripheral and central nervous systems.

PAIN TRANSMISSION

Among the nerve mechanisms and structures involved in the transmission of pain perceptions to and from the area of the brain that interprets pain are nociceptors, or pain receptors, and chemical mediators. **Nociceptors** are receptors that are preferentially sensitive to a noxious stimulus. Nociceptors are also called pain receptors, but the former term is preferred.

Nociceptors

Nociceptors are free nerve endings in the skin that respond only to intense, potentially damaging stimuli. Such stimuli may be mechanical, thermal, or chemical in nature. The joints, skeletal muscle, fascia, tendons, and cornea also have nociceptors that have the potential to transmit stimuli that produce pain. However, the large internal organs (viscera) do not contain nerve endings that respond only to painful stimuli. Pain originating in these organs results from intense stimulation of receptors that have other purposes. For example, inflammation, stretching, ischemia, dilation, and spasm of the internal organs all cause an intense response in these multipurpose fibers and can cause severe pain.

Nociceptors are part of complex multidirectional pathways. These nerve fibers branch very near their origin in the skin and send fibers to local blood vessels, mast cells, hair follicles, and sweat glands. When these fibers are stimulated, histamine is released from the mast cells, causing vasodilation. Nociceptors respond to high-intensity mechanical, thermal, and chemical stimuli. Some receptors respond to only one type of stimuli; others, called polymodal nociceptors, respond to all three types of stimuli. These highly specialized neurons transfer the mechanical, thermal, or chemical stimulus into electrical activity or action potentials.

The cutaneous fibers located more centrally further branch and communicate with the paravertebral sympathetic chain of the nervous system and with large internal organs. As a result of the connections between these nerve fibers, pain is often accompanied by vasomotor, autonomic, and visceral effects. In a patient with severe acute pain, for example, gastrointestinal peristalsis may decrease or stop.

Peripheral Nervous System

A number of **algogenic** (pain-causing) substances that affect the sensitivity of nociceptors are released into the extracellular tissue as a result of tissue damage. Histamine, bradykinin, acetylcholine, serotonin, and substance P are chemicals that increase the transmission of pain. The transmission of pain is also referred to as **nociception**. **Prostaglandins** are chemical substances thought to increase the sensitivity of pain receptors by enhancing the pain-provoking effect of bradykinin. These chemical mediators also cause vasodilation and increased vascular permeability, resulting in redness, warmth, and swelling of the injured area.

Once nociception is initiated, the nociceptive action potentials are transmitted by the peripheral nervous system (Porth, 2002). The first-order neurons travel from the periphery (skin, cornea, visceral organs) to the spinal cord via the dorsal horn. There are two main types of fibers involved in the transmission of nociception. Smaller, myelinated Aδ (A delta) fibers transmit nociception rapidly, which produces the initial "fast pain." Type C fibers are larger, unmyelinated fibers that transmit what is called second pain. This type of pain has dull, aching, or burning qualities that last longer than the initial fast pain. The type and concentration of nerve fibers to transmit pain vary by tissue type.

If there is repeated C fiber input, a greater response is noted in dorsal horn neurons, causing the person to perceive more pain. In other words, the same noxious stimulus produces hyperalgesia, and the person reports greater pain than was felt at the first stimulus. For this reason, it is important to treat patients with analgesic agents when they first feel the pain. Patients require less medication and experience more effective pain relief if analgesia is administered before the patient becomes sensitized to the pain.

Chemicals that reduce or inhibit the transmission or perception of pain include **endorphins** and **enkephalins**. These morphine-like neurotransmitters are endogenous (produced by the body). They are examples of substances that reduce nociceptive transmission when applied to certain nerve fibers. The term "endorphin" is a combination of two words: endogenous and morphine. Endorphins and enkephalins are found in heavy concentrations in the central nervous system, particularly the spinal and medullary dorsal horn, the periaqueductal gray matter, hypothalamus, and amygdala. Morphine and other opioid medications act at receptor sites to suppress the excitation initiated by noxious stimuli. The binding of opioids to receptor sites is responsible for the

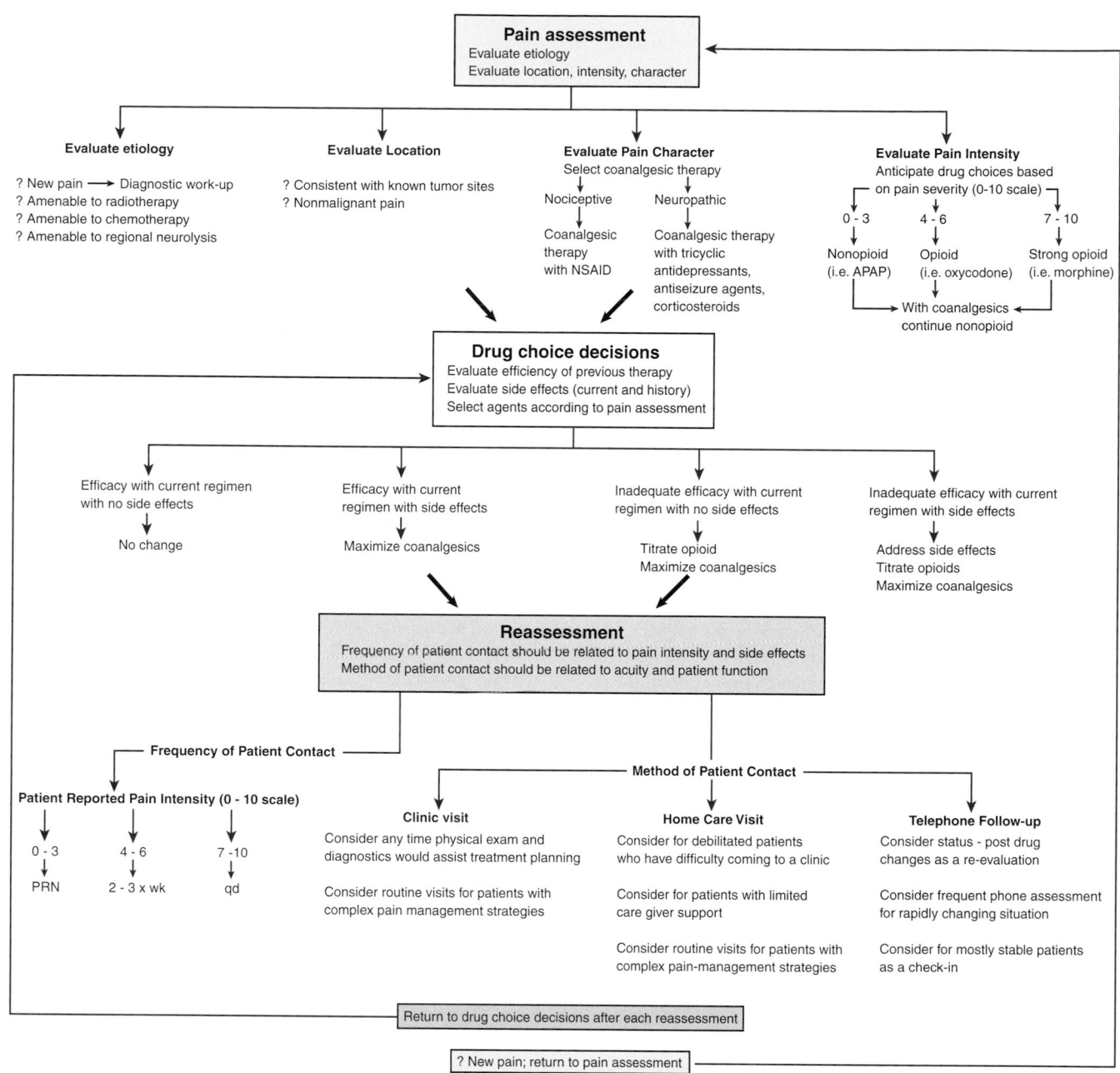

FIGURE 13-2 The cancer pain algorithm (highest level view) is a decision-tree model for pain treatment that was developed as an interpretation of the AHCPR Guideline for Cancer Pain, 1994. Reproduced with permission from DuPen, A. R., DuPen, S., Hansberry, J., et al. (2000). An educational implementation of a cancer pain algorithm for ambulatory care. *Pain Management Nursing, 1* (4), 118.

effects noted after their administration. Each receptor (mu, kappa, delta) responds differently when activated. Table 13-1 summarizes the classification and action of opioid receptors.

Central Nervous System

After tissue injury occurs, nociception (the neurologic transmission of pain impulses) to the spinal cord via the Aδ and C fibers continues. The fibers enter the dorsal horn, which is divided into laminae based on cell type. The laminae II cell type is commonly referred to as the substantia gelatinosa. In the substantia gelatinosa are projections that relay nociception to other parts of the spinal cord (Fig. 13-3).

Nociception continues from the spinal cord to the reticular formation, thalamus, limbic system, and cerebral cortex. Here nociception is localized and its characteristics become apparent to the person, including the intensity. The involvement of the reticular formation, limbic, and reticular activating systems is responsible for the individual variations in the perception of noxious stimuli. Individuals may report the same stimulus differently based on their anxiety, past experiences, and expectations. This is a result of the conscious perception of pain.

For pain to be consciously perceived, neurons in the ascending system must be activated. Activation occurs as a result of input from the nociceptors located in the skin and internal organs. Once activated, the inhibitory interneuronal fibers in the

Table 13-1 • **Opioid Classification and Action**

ORGAN EFFECT	μ	κ	δ
Eye: Pupil	Miosis	Miosis	Mydriasis
Lung: Respiratory rate	Stimulation, then depression	No change	Stimulation
Heart: Rate	Bradycardia	No change	Tachycardia
Body: Temperature	Hypothermia	No change	Unknown
Affect	Indifference	Sedation	Dysphoria
Gastrointestinal system	Constipation	No effects	Nausea

μ = mu; κ = kappa; δ = delta
Willens, J. S. (1994). Pain management in the trauma patient. In V. D. Cardona, P. D. Hurn, P. J. B. Mason, A. M. Scanlon, & S. W. Veise-Berry (Eds.), *Trauma nursing from resuscitation through rehabilitation* (2nd ed., pp 325–362). Philadelphia: W. B. Saunders. With permission of W. B. Saunders. Copyright 1994 by W. B. Saunders.

dorsal horn inhibit or turn off the transmission of noxious stimulating information in the ascending pathway.

Descending Control System

The descending control system is a system of fibers that originate in the lower and midportion of the brain (specifically the periaqueductal gray matter) and terminate on the inhibitory interneuronal fibers in the dorsal horn of the spinal cord. This system is probably always somewhat active; it prevents continuous transmission of stimuli as painful, partly through the action of the endorphins. As nociception occurs, the descending control system is activated to inhibit pain.

Cognitive processes may stimulate endorphin production in the descending control system. The effectiveness of this system is illustrated by the effects of distraction. The distractions of visitors or a favorite TV show may increase activity in the descending control system. Therefore, the person who has visitors may not report pain because activation of the descending control system results in less noxious or painful information being transmitted to consciousness. Once the distraction by the visitors ends, activity in the descending control system decreases, resulting in increased transmission of painful stimuli.

The interconnections between the descending neuronal system and the ascending sensory tract are called inhibitory interneuronal fibers. These fibers contain enkephalin and are primarily activated through the activity of **non-nociceptor** peripheral fibers (fibers that normally do not transmit painful or noxious stimuli) in the same receptor field as the pain receptor, and descending fibers, grouped together in a system called descending control. The enkephalins and endorphins are thought to inhibit pain impulses by stimulating the inhibitory interneuronal fibers, which in turn reduce the transmission of noxious impulses via the ascending system (Puig & Montes, 1998).

The classic gate control theory of pain, described by Melzack and Wall in 1965, was the first to clearly articulate the existence of a pain-modulating system (Melzack, 1996). This theory proposes that stimulation of the skin evokes nervous impulses that are then transmitted by three systems located in the spinal cord. The substantia gelatinosa in the dorsal horn, the dorsal column fibers, and the central transmission cells act to influence nociceptive impulses. The noxious impulses are influenced by a "gating mechanism." Melzack and Wall proposed that stimulation of the large-diameter fibers inhibits the transmission of pain, thus "closing the gate." Conversely, when smaller fibers are stimulated, the gate is opened. The gating mechanism is influenced by nerve impulses that descend from the brain. This theory proposes a specialized system of large-diameter fibers that activate selective cognitive processes via the modulating properties of the spinal gate. Figure 13-4 shows a schematic representation of a gate control system and nociceptive pathways.

The gate control theory was important because it was the first theory to suggest that psychological factors play a role in the perception of pain. The theory guided research toward the cognitive-behavioral approaches to pain management. This theory helps to explain how interventions such as distraction and music therapy provide pain relief.

Melzack (1996) extended the gate control theory after carefully analyzing phantom limb pain. He proposed that a large, widespread network of neurons exists that consists of loops between the thalamus and cortex and between the cortex and the limbic system. Melzack labeled this network the neuromatrix. As

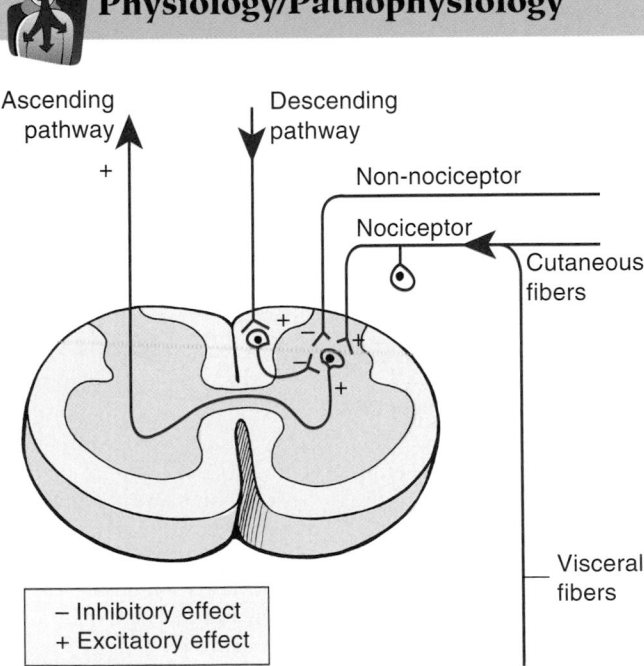

Physiology/Pathophysiology

Ascending pathway
Descending pathway
Non-nociceptor
Nociceptor
Cutaneous fibers
Visceral fibers

− Inhibitory effect
+ Excitatory effect

FIGURE 13-3 Representative nociception system, showing ascending and descending sensory pathways of the dorsal horn.

Physiology/Pathophysiology

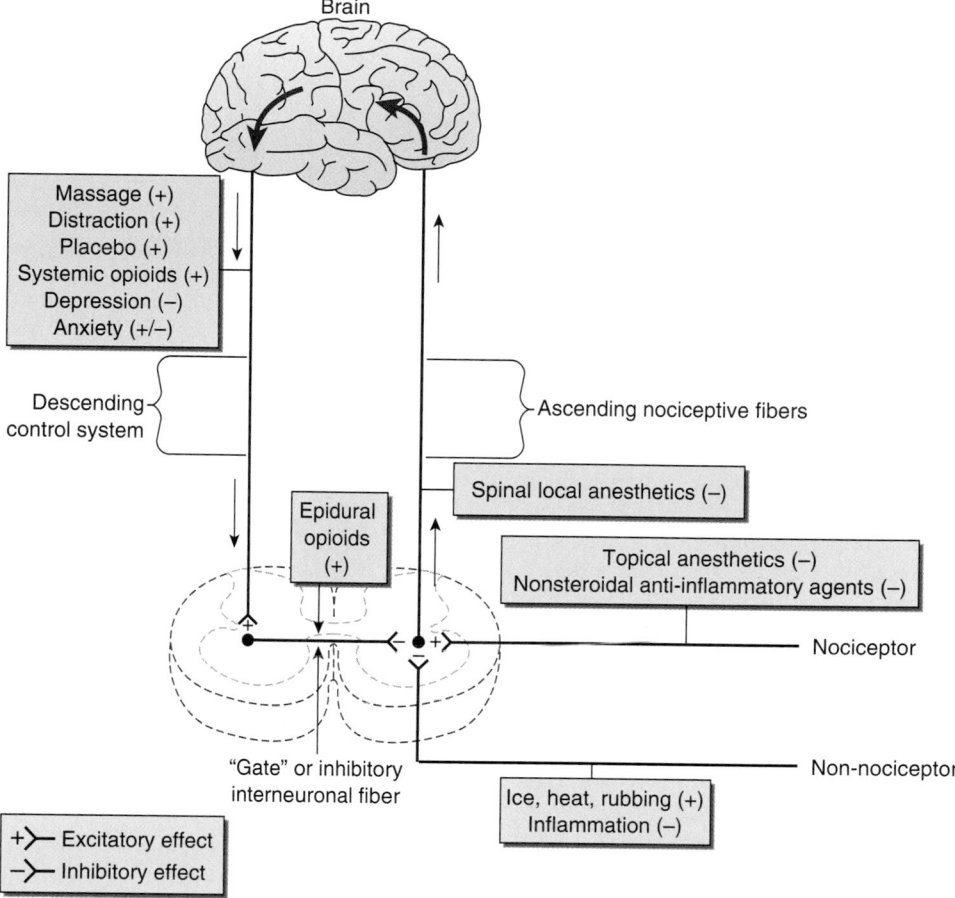

FIGURE 13-4 A schematic representation of the gate control system and aspects of the nociceptive system. The nervous system is made up of stimulatory and inhibitory fibers. For example, stimulation of the nociceptor will result in the transmission of an impulse that will be interpreted as pain. When it is stimulated it will stimulate transmission at the next fiber junction (represented as +>-). The interneuronal fiber is an inhibitory neuron (->-). When it is stimulated it, in turn, inhibits or shuts off transmission at the next junction. So a placebo has a (+) stimulatory effect on the descending control system, which has a stimulatory effect (+) on the interneuronal fiber, which has an inhibitory effect (-) on the ascending control system. A topical anesthetic has an inhibitory effect (-) on nerve transmission at the nociceptor level and a spinal anesthetic has the same impact (-) on the ascending nociceptive fibers.

information is processed in the neuromatrix, a characteristic pattern emerges. This pattern, referred to as the neurosignature, is a continuous outflow from the neuromatrix. Ultimately, the neurosignature output, with a constant stream of input and varying patterns, produces the feelings of the whole body with constantly changing qualities.

Melzack (1996) theorized that in the absence of modulating inputs from the missing limb, the active neuromatrix produces a neurosignature pattern that is perceived as pain. The neuromatrix theory highlights the role of the brain in sustaining the experience of pain. Some researchers have criticized this theory as not adding to the understanding of how psychological factors influence pain (Keefe, Lefebvre & Starr, 1996). While the neuromatrix theory might explain unusual pain phenomena, its contribution to understanding pain management remains to be seen.

FACTORS INFLUENCING THE PAIN RESPONSE

A person's pain experience is influenced by a number of factors, including past experiences with pain, anxiety, culture, age, gender, and expectations about pain relief. These factors may increase or decrease the person's perception of pain, increase or decrease tolerance for pain, and affect the responses to pain.

Past Experience

It is tempting to expect that a person who has had multiple or prolonged experiences with pain would be less anxious and more tolerant of pain than one who has had little pain. For most people, however, this is not true. Often, the more experience a person has had with pain, the more frightened he or she is about subsequent painful events. This person may be less able to tolerate pain; that is, he or she wants relief from pain sooner and before it becomes severe. This reaction is more likely to occur if the person has received inadequate pain relief in the past. A person with repeated pain experiences may have learned to fear the escalation of pain and its inadequate treatment. Once a person experiences severe pain, that person knows just how severe it can be. Conversely, someone who has never had severe pain may have no fear of such pain.

The way a person responds to pain is a result of many separate painful events during a lifetime. For some, past pain may have been constant and unrelenting, as in prolonged or chronic and persistent pain. The individual who has pain for months or years may become irritable, withdrawn, and depressed.

The undesirable effects that may result from previous experience point to the need for the nurse to be aware of the patient's past experiences with pain. If pain is relieved promptly and adequately, the person may be less fearful of future pain and better able to tolerate it.

Anxiety and Depression

Although it is commonly believed that anxiety will increase pain, this is not necessarily true. Research has demonstrated no consistent relationship between anxiety and pain, nor has research shown that preoperative stress reduction training reduces postoperative pain (Keogh, Ellery, Hunt et al., 2001; Rhudy & Meagher, 2000). Postoperative anxiety is most related to preoperative anxiety and postoperative complications. However, anxiety that is relevant or related to the pain may increase the patient's perception of pain. For example, a patient who was treated 2 years ago for breast cancer and now has hip pain may fear that the pain indicates metastasis. In this case, the anxiety may result in increased pain. Anxiety that is unrelated to the pain may distract the patient and may actually decrease the perception of pain. For example, a mother who is hospitalized with complications from abdominal surgery and is anxious about her children may perceive less pain as her anxiety about her children increases.

The routine use of antianxiety medications to treat anxiety in someone with pain may prevent the person from reporting pain because of sedation and may impair the patient's ability to take deep breaths, get out of bed, and cooperate with the treatment plan. The most effective way to relieve pain is by directing the treatment at the pain rather than at the anxiety.

Just as anxiety is associated with pain because of concerns and fears about the underlying disease, depression is associated with chronic pain and unrelieved cancer pain. In chronic pain situations, depression is associated with major life changes due to the limiting effects of the pain, specifically unemployment. Longer durations of pain are associated with an increased incidence of depression (Wall, 1999). Unrelieved cancer pain drastically interferes with the patient's quality of life, and relieving the pain may go a long way toward treating the depression.

Culture

Beliefs about pain and how to respond to it differ from one culture to the next. Early in childhood, individuals learn from those around them what responses to pain are acceptable or unacceptable. For example, a child may learn that a sports injury is not expected to hurt as much as a comparable injury caused by a motor vehicle crash. The child also learns what stimuli are expected to be painful and what behavioral responses are acceptable. These beliefs vary from one culture to another; therefore, people from different cultures who experience the same intensity of pain may not report it or respond to it in the same ways.

Cultural factors must be taken into account to effectively manage pain. Many studies have examined the cultural aspects of pain. Inconsistent results, methodologic weaknesses or flaws (Lasch, 2000), and failure of many researchers to carefully distinguish ethnicity, culture, and race make it difficult to interpret the findings of many of these studies. Factors that help to explain differences in a cultural group include age, gender, education level, and income. In addition, the degree to which a patient identifies with a culture influences the degree to which he or she will adopt new health behaviors or cling to traditional health beliefs and practices. Other factors that affect a patient's response to pain include his or her interaction with the health care system and provider factors (Lasch, Wilkes, Montuori et al., 2000).

The nurse's cultural values may differ from those of other cultures. The nurse's cultural expectations and values may include avoiding exaggerated expressions of pain, such as excessive crying

NURSING RESEARCH PROFILE 13-1

Pain Management Outcomes for Hospitalized Hispanic Patients

McNeill, J. A., Sherwood, G. D., Starck, P. L., & Nieto, B. (2001). Pain management outcomes for hospitalized Hispanic patients. *Pain Management Nursing, 2*(1), 25–36.

Purpose

It has been suggested that members of minority groups are likely to receive inadequate pain management. Hispanics are the fastest-growing ethnic group in the United States, yet few studies have examined pain and its management in this group. The purposes of the study were to describe the experience of acute pain and pain management and outcomes of pain management, and to identify predictors of patient satisfaction in a minority sample.

Study Sample and Design

This cross-sectional, descriptive study explored the outcomes of the pain experience of hospitalized Hispanic patients and identified factors that contribute to patient satisfaction with pain management. The study sample consisted of 104 patients who were postoperative or diagnosed with a painful condition and who were hospitalized for at least 24 hours. The subjects identified themselves as Hispanic and spoke English.

The researchers used the American Pain Society's Patient Outcome Questionnaire–Modified and the Pain Management Index to measure the degree of pain, effectiveness of pain management, and patient satisfaction. Data related to analgesic orders and administration were obtained from the patients' medical records.

Findings

Ninety-eight percent of the patients reported pain in the last 24 hours. The most interference caused by the pain was for participation in activities related to postoperative recovery (mean = 7.1, SD = 2.9) (on a 0–10 numeric scale with higher scores indicating more interference).

The least pain interference was in the area of interpersonal relationships (mean = 3.1, SD = 3.2). The mean score on satisfaction with pain management (on a 1–6 scale with higher scores indicating greater satisfaction) was 4.74 (SD = 1.2). Satisfaction with pain management was inversely and significantly correlated with pain intensity. The lower the patient's pain score, the greater the satisfaction with management of pain. Only 66% of patients who reported pain received an analgesic within the previous 24 hours, although all patients had analgesics prescribed.

The sample was divided into two groups: satisfied (n = 77) and dissatisfied (n = 23) with pain management. The dissatisfied patients reported higher pain now (p = 0.000), higher general pain in the last 24 hours (p = 0.000), and greater interference related to pain for activity (p = 0.000). Seventy-nine (77%) of the patients recalled receiving information about the importance of pain management. This factor did not influence satisfaction.

Nursing Implications

The findings in this study are similar to those noted in a sample of Caucasian patients. The satisfied and dissatisfied groups differed in the areas of pain rating now and general level of pain and interference related to pain regarding sleep, general activity, mood, and relationships. The reason for the reported high degree of satisfaction when those who reported pain and interference with activities is unclear. In spite of the inverse correlation between pain intensity and satisfaction, the satisfaction ratings were high. Further research is needed to identify the factors that determine satisfaction with pain management.

and moaning, seeking immediate relief from pain, and giving complete descriptions of the pain. A patient's cultural expectations may be to moan and complain about pain, to refuse pain relief measures that do not cure the cause of the pain, or to use adjectives such as "unbearable" in describing the pain. A patient from another cultural background may behave in a quiet, stoic manner rather than express the pain loudly. The nurse must react to the person's pain perception and not to the pain behavior because the behavior is different from his or her own culture.

Recognizing the values of one's own culture and learning how these values differ from those of other cultures help to avoid evaluating the patient's behavior on the basis of one's own cultural expectations and values. A nurse who recognizes cultural differences will have a greater understanding of the patient's pain and will be more accurate in assessing pain and behavioral responses to pain, as well as more effective in relieving the pain.

The main issues to consider when caring for patients of a different culture are:

- What does the illness mean to the patient?
- Are there culturally based stigmas related to this illness or pain?
- What is the role of the family in health care decisions?
- Are traditional pain-relief remedies used?
- What is the role of stoicism in that culture?
- Are there culturally determined ways of expressing and communicating pain?
- Does the patient have any fears about the pain?
- Has the patient seen or does the patient want to see a traditional healer?

Regardless of the patient's culture, nurses need to learn about that particular culture and be aware of power and communication issues that will affect care outcomes. Nurses need to avoid stereotyping patients by culture and provide individualized care rather than assuming that a patient of a specific culture will exhibit more or less pain. In addition to avoiding stereotyping, health care providers need to individualize the amount of medications or therapy according to the information provided by the patient. Nurses need to recognize that stereotypes exist and become sensitive to how stereotypes negatively affect care. Patients in turn must be instructed about how and what to communicate about their pain.

Age

Age has long been the focus of research on pain perception and pain tolerance, and again the results have been inconsistent. For example, although some researchers have found that older adults require a higher intensity of noxious stimuli than do younger adults before they report pain (Washington, Gibson & Helme, 2000), others have found no differences in responses of younger and older adults (Edwards & Fillingim, 2000). Other researchers have found that elderly patients (older than 65 years of age) reported significantly less pain than younger patients (Li, Greenwald, Gennis et al., 2001). Experts in the field of pain management have concluded that if pain perception is diminished in the elderly person, it is most likely secondary to a disease process (eg, diabetes) rather than to aging (American Geriatrics Society, 1998). More research is needed in the area of aging and its effects on pain perception to understand what the elderly are experiencing.

Although many elderly people seek health care because of pain, others are reluctant to seek help even when in severe pain because they consider pain to be part of normal aging. Assessment of pain in older adults may be difficult because of the physiologic, psychosocial, and cognitive changes that often accompany aging. In one study, as many as 93% of nursing home residents reported being in pain daily for the past 6 months (Weiner, Peterson, Ladd et al., 1999). Unrelieved pain contributes to the problems of depression, sleep disturbances, delayed rehabilitation, malnutrition, and cognitive dysfunction (Miaskowski, 2000).

The way an older person responds to pain may differ from the way a younger person responds. Because elderly people have a slower metabolism and a greater ratio of body fat to muscle mass than younger people, small doses of analgesic agents may be sufficient to relieve pain, and these doses may be effective longer (Buffum & Buffum, 2000). Elderly patients deal with pain according to their lifestyle, personality, and cultural background, as do younger adults. Many elderly people are fearful of addiction and, as a result, will not report that they are in pain or ask for pain medication. Others fail to seek care because they fear that the pain may indicate serious illness or they fear loss of independence.

Elderly patients must receive adequate pain relief after surgery or trauma. When an elderly person becomes confused after surgery or trauma, the confusion is often attributed to medications, which are then discontinued. However, confusion in the elderly may be a result of untreated and unrelieved pain. In some cases postoperative confusion clears once the pain is relieved. Judgments about pain and the adequacy of treatment should be based on the patient's report of pain and pain relief rather than on age.

Gender

Researchers have studied gender differences in pain levels and in responses to pain. Once again, the results have been inconsistent. In one study, women tended to report higher levels of pain than men and reported their highest intensity of pain during the day, while men reported the highest intensity at night (Morin, Lund, Villarroel et al., 2000). Kelly (1998) reported no gender differences in pain.

Riley, Robinson, Wade et al. (2001) compared pain intensity, pain unpleasantness, and pain-related emotions (depression, anxiety, frustration, fear, and anger) in men and women who were asked to rate their experiences with chronic pain. Women had higher pain intensity, pain unpleasantness, frustration, and fear compared to men. Robinson, Riley, Meyers et al. (2001) reported that men and women are socialized to respond differently and differ in their expectations relative to pain perception. In a study of responses of men and women to chronic pain and anxiety, Edwards, Auguston and Fillingim (2000) noted no difference between genders regarding pain and depression. There was, however, a difference in anxiety and gender, with men being more anxious about their pain.

The pharmacokinetics and pharmacodynamics of opioids differ in men and women and have been attributed to hepatic metabolism, where the microsomal enzyme activity differs (Vallerand & Polomano, 2000). Genetic factors play a role in the varied responses to nonsteroidal anti-inflammatory drugs (NSAIDs) seen in men and women (Buffum & Buffum, 2000).

Placebo Effect

A **placebo effect** occurs when a person responds to the medication or other treatment because of an expectation that the treatment will work rather than because it actually does so. Simply receiving a medication or treatment may produce positive effects. The placebo effect results from the natural (endogenous) production of endorphins in the descending control system. It is a true physiologic response that can be reversed by naloxone, an opioid antagonist (Wall, 1999).

A patient's positive expectations about treatment may increase the effectiveness of a medication or other intervention. Often the more cues the patient receives about the intervention's effectiveness, the more effective it will be. A person who is informed that a medication is expected to relieve pain is more likely to experience pain relief than one who is told that a medication is unlikely to have any effect.

Researchers have shown that different verbal instructions given to patients about therapies affect patient behavior and significantly reduce opioid intake. Pollo, Amanzio, Arslanina et al. (2001) studied the effect of information and expectations in patients who had undergone thoracotomy. Patients in three groups were given an intravenous infusion of normal saline solution and could receive a dose of buprenorphine (Buprenex) on request. One group was given no information about the analgesic effect of the regimen; one group was informed that the infusion received could be an analgesic or a placebo; the third was told that the infusion was a powerful analgesic. Although the three groups did not differ in reported level of pain, the group told that the infusion was a powerful analgesic used less opioid than the other two groups.

A meta-analysis of 114 published research studies comparing placebo with no treatment showed similar results (Hrobjartsson & Gotzsche, 2001). The studies analyzed investigated many clinical conditions; 27 of the 114 trials involved the treatment of pain. Other clinical conditions in the studies included obesity, asthma, hypertension, insomnia, and anxiety. Pain was the only condition in which a placebo effect was demonstrated.

The American Society of Pain Management Nurses (1996) holds the position that placebos (tablets or injections with no active ingredients) should not be used to assess or manage pain in any patient regardless of age or diagnosis. Furthermore, the group recommends that all health care institutions have policies in place prohibiting the use of placebos for this purpose. Educational programs should be conducted to educate providers about effective pain management, and ethics committees should assist in formulating these policies (Chart 13-2).

Chart 13-2 • Ethics and Related Issues

Ethical Administration of Placebos

Because of misperceptions about placebos and the placebo effect, keep in mind some specific principles and guidelines:

- A placebo effect is not an indication that the person does not have pain; rather, it is a true physiologic response.
- Placebos (tablets or injections with no active ingredients) should never be used to test the person's truthfulness about pain or as the first line of treatment.
- A positive response to a placebo (eg, reduction in pain) should never be interpreted as an indication that the person's pain is not real.
- A patient should never be given a placebo as a substitute for an analgesic medication. Although a placebo can produce analgesia, patients receiving a placebo may report that their pain is relieved or that they feel better simply to avoid disappointing the nurse.

Nursing Assessment of Pain

The highly subjective nature of pain makes pain assessment and management challenges for every clinician. The report of pain is a social transaction; thus, assessment and management of pain require a good rapport with the person in pain. In assessing a patient with pain, the nurse reviews the patient's description of the pain and other factors that may influence pain (eg, previous experience, anxiety, and age) as well as the person's response to pain relief strategies. Documentation of the pain level as rated on a pain scale becomes part of the patient's medical record, as does a record of the pain relief obtained from interventions.

Pain assessment includes determining what level of pain relief the acutely ill patient believes is needed to recover quickly or improve function, or what level of relief the chronically or terminally ill patient requires to maintain comfort (Chart 13-3). Part of a thorough pain assessment is to understand the patient's expectations and misconceptions about pain (Chart 13-4). A person who understands that pain relief not only contributes to comfort but also hastens recovery is more likely to request or self-administer treatment appropriately.

CHARACTERISTICS OF PAIN

The factors to consider in a complete pain assessment are the intensity, timing, location, quality, personal meaning, aggravating and alleviating factors, and pain behaviors. The pain assessment begins by observing the patient carefully, noting the patient's overall posture and presence or absence of overt pain behaviors and asking the person to describe, in his or her own words, the specifics of the pain. The words used to describe the pain may point toward the etiology. For example, the classic description of chest pain that results from a myocardial infarction includes pressure or squeezing on the chest. A detailed history should follow the initial description of pain.

Intensity

The intensity of pain ranges from none to mild discomfort to excruciating. There is no correlation between reported intensity and the stimulus that produced it. The reported intensity is influenced by the person's **pain threshold** and **pain tolerance**. Pain threshold is the smallest stimulus for which a person reports pain, and the tolerance is the maximum amount of pain a person can tolerate. To understand variations, the nurse can ask about the present pain intensity as well as the least and the worst pain intensity. Various tools and surveys are helpful to patients trying to describe pain intensity. Examples of pain scales appear in Figure 13-5.

Timing

Sometimes the etiology of pain can be determined when time aspects are known. Therefore, the nurse inquires about the onset, duration, relationship between time and intensity, and whether there are changes in rhythmic patterns. The patient is asked if the pain began suddenly or increased gradually. Sudden pain that rapidly reaches maximum intensity is indicative of tissue rupture, and immediate intervention is necessary. Pain from ischemia gradually increases and becomes intense over a longer time. The chronic pain of arthritis illustrates the usefulness of determining the relationship between time and intensity, because people with arthritis usually report that pain is worse in the morning.

Chart 13-3 Pain at the End of Life

Pain is one of the most feared symptoms at the end of life. Most patients will experience pain as a terminal illness progresses. The inadequate treatment of cancer pain has been well documented (Agency for Health Care Policy and Research, 1994), and in the Study to Understand Prognoses and Preferences for Outcomes and Risks of Treatments (SUPPORT) (1995) investigators noted that nearly 40% of severely chronically ill and older patients who died in hospitals suffered moderate to severe pain in the last 3 days of life. The suffering caused by unrelieved pain touches all aspects of quality of life (activity, appetite, sleep) and can weaken an already fatigued person. Psychologically, unrelieved pain can create anxiety, and depression, negatively affect relationships, and promote thoughts of suicide.

The Joint Commission on Accreditation of Health Care Organizations (JCAHO) implemented pain standards in January 2001. These standards present a unique opportunity to improve care for hospitalized patients. Even though hospices and palliative care agencies are not subject to JCAHO review, many patients with chronic illness who are receiving palliative care may be hospitalized at various times. The standards emphasize pain assessment, patient and family education, continuity of care for symptom management, and evaluation of interventions.

Current barriers to pain management include lack of education, lack of access to opioids, fear of addiction, and legislative issues.

Need for Education
Ferrell et al. (2000) noted that of 45,683 nursing text pages reviewed, 902 were related to pain at the end of life. The end-of-life content constituted 2% of text pages, while the pain content represented only 0.5%. The researchers concluded that more specific content is needed to assist in educating students about pain and pain at the end of life.

Accessibility
The lack of access to opioids is another barrier to adequate pain relief. Patients may have difficulty affording medications. Some pharmacists, fearing crime, paperwork, and regulatory oversight, may not stock opioids or may keep limited quantities on hand. Some insurance companies limit the types of medications and the amount and frequency of renewal of analgesics.

Addiction Fears
The fear of addiction plays a role even at the end of life. Family members may be hesitant to assist the patient in pain management for fear of the social stigma of addiction. This causes needless pain and suffering.

Legal Barriers
Legislative issues play a role in the inadequate management of pain. Many states are enacting Intractable Pain Statutes. These laws aim to reduce physicians' fear of civil or criminal liability or disciplinary action for aggressively managing pain. The tracking system by the Drug Enforcement Agency acts as a deterrent since opioids prescribed by physicians can be tracked. Some physicians fear that prescribing "too many" opioids could be interpreted as treating an addicted patient.

Other Issues
Pain management at the end of life differs little from general pain management. Patients still require comprehensive pain assessment and pain management, even though assessment may be hampered by confusion, delirium, or unconsciousness. Caregivers are taught to observe for signs of restlessness or facial expressions as a "proxy" indicator of pain.

Analgesic agents should be titrated to find the most effective dose and the best tolerated route. The nurse and family members should assess the effectiveness of the current pain therapy. If the pain is not relieved, a larger dose of medication may be necessary. If the pain continues, another medication may be needed or the patient should be given a different analgesic. The titration process requires frequent assessment to effectively manage pain. The analgesic agent or treatment should be appropriate for the type of pain. For example, neuropathic pain, usually described as burning, tingling, numbness, shooting, stabbing or electric, requires a different treatment approach compared to acute pain.

Nonpharmacologic approaches, such as guided imagery and relaxation, can be used to decrease pain and help the patient cope. Careful patient positioning and environmental control are other methods to increase patient comfort.

Respiratory depression should be assessed because over time, patients become tolerant to this side effect. The rate, depth, and level of consciousness should be monitored to determine whether respiratory depression is occurring and requires treatment. A respiratory rate of 6 per minute or greater is usually adequate. If respiratory depression is suspected, a decrease in the opioid dose may be indicated. Frequent stimulation to encourage deep breathing may be required until the opioid is metabolized. In the last few days of life the patient may become restless, which is an indicator of pain. The need to increase the opioid to provide pain relief and the respiratory effects of opioids are considered in decision making. However, comfort should be a priority in the case of a person who clearly is at the end of life, where cure is no longer the goal.

Side effects from analgesics must be managed as in other painful conditions. Tolerance to constipation is rare. Thus, a careful bowel regimen involving diet, bowel stimulants, stool softeners, and/or osmotic agents, must be instituted. Vigilance in the assessment, management, and treatment evaluation of other side effects is similar to that included in previous discussions.

Careful assessment and management of pain at the end of life can make a "good" death possible. Education of health care providers and the family can help patients realize the goal of adequate pain relief throughout the dying process.

Location

The location of pain is best determined by having the patient point to the area of the body involved. Some general assessment forms have drawings of human figures, and the patient is asked to shade in the area involved. This is especially helpful if the pain radiates (**referred pain**). The shaded figures are helpful in determining the effectiveness of treatment or change in the location of pain over time.

Quality

The nurse asks the patient to describe the pain in his or her own words without offering clues. For example, the patient is asked to describe what the pain feels like. Sufficient time must be allowed for the patient to describe the pain and for the nurse to carefully record all words that are used. If the patient cannot describe the quality of the pain, words such as burning, aching, throbbing, or stabbing can be offered. It is important to document the exact words used to describe the pain and which words were suggested by the nurse conducting the assessment.

Personal Meaning

Patients experience pain differently, and the pain experience can mean many different things. It is important to ask how the pain has affected the person's daily life. Some people can continue to

---

Chart 13-4

Common Concerns and Misconceptions About Pain and Analgesia

- Complaining about pain will distract my doctor from his primary responsibility—curing my illness.
- Pain is a natural part of aging.
- I don't want to bother the nurse—he/she is busy with other patients.
- Pain medicine can't really control pain.
- People get addicted to pain medicine easily.
- It is easier to put up with pain than with the side effects that come from pain medicine.
- Good patients avoid talking about pain.
- Pain medicine should be saved in case the pain gets worse.
- Pain builds character. It's good for you.
- Patients should expect to have pain; it's part of almost every hospitalization.

Adapted with permission from Gordon, D. B., & Ward, S. E. (1995). Correcting patient misconceptions about pain. *American Journal of Nursing, 95*(7).

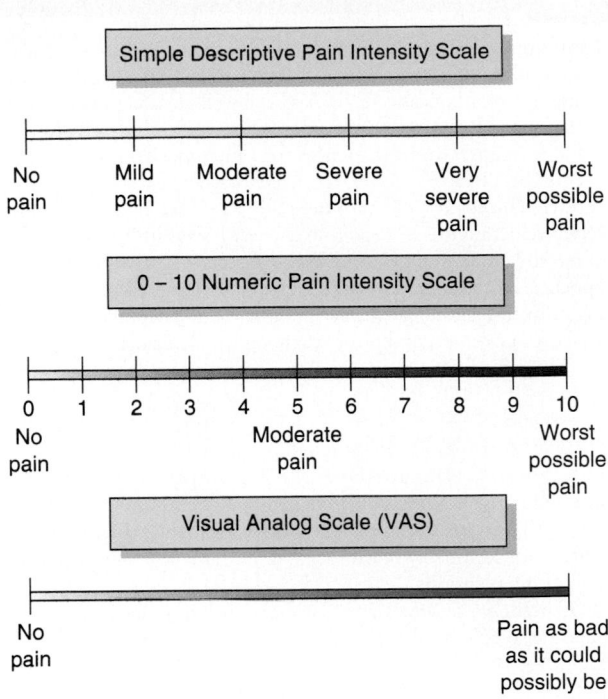

Pain Intensity Scales

A 10-cm baseline is recommended for each of these scales.

FIGURE 13-5 Examples of pain intensity scales.

---

work or study, while others may be disabled. The patient is asked if family finances have been affected. For others, the recurrence of pain may mean worsening of the disease, such as the spread of cancer. The meaning attached to the pain experience helps the nurse understand how the patient is affected and assists in planning treatment.

Aggravating and Alleviating Factors

The nurse asks the patient what if anything makes the pain worse and what makes it better and asks specifically about the relationship between activity and pain. This helps detect factors associated with pain. For example, in a patient with advanced metastatic cancer, pain with coughing may signal spinal cord compression. The nurse ascertains whether environmental factors influence pain since they may easily be changed to help the patient. For example, making the room warmer may help the patient relax and may improve the patient's pain. Finally, the patient is asked if pain is influenced by or affects the quality of sleep or anxiety. Both can significantly affect pain intensity and the quality of life.

Knowledge of alleviating factors assists the nurse in developing a treatment plan. Therefore, it is important to ask about the patient's use of medication (prescribed and over the counter) and the amount and frequency. In addition, the nurse asks if herbal remedies, nonpharmacologic interventions, or alternative therapies have been used with success. This information assists the nurse in determining teaching needs.

Pain Behaviors

When experiencing pain, people express pain with many different behaviors. These nonverbal and behavioral expressions of pain are not consistent or reliable indicators of the quality or intensity of pain, and they should not be used to determine the presence of or the degree of pain experienced. Patients may grimace, cry, rub the affected area, guard the affected area, or immobilize it. Others may moan, groan, grunt, or sigh. Not all patients exhibit the same behaviors, and there may be different meanings associated with the same behavior.

Sometimes in the nonverbal patient, pain behaviors are used as a proxy to assess pain. It is unwise to make judgments and formulate treatment plans based on behaviors that may or may not indicate pain. In the case of an unconscious person, pain should always be assumed to be present and treated. All patients have a right to adequate pain management.

Physiologic responses to pain, such as tachycardia, hypertension, tachypnea, pallor, diaphoresis, mydriasis, hypervigilance, and increased muscle tone, are related to stimulation of the autonomic nervous system. These responses are short-lived as the body adapts to the stress. These physiologic signs could be the result of a change in the patient's condition, such as the onset of hypovolemia. Using physiologic signs to indicate pain is unreliable. Although it is important to observe for any and all pain behaviors, the absence of these behaviors does not indicate an absence of pain.

INSTRUMENTS FOR ASSESSING THE PERCEPTION OF PAIN

Only the patient can accurately describe and assess his or her pain. Clinicians consistently underestimate a patient's level of pain (McCaffery & Ferrell, 1997; McCaffery, Ferrell & Pasaro, 2000; Puntillo, Miaskowski, Kehrle et al., 1997; Thomas et al., 1998). Therefore, a number of pain assessment instruments have been developed to assist in the assessment of a patient's perception of pain (see Fig. 13-5). Such instruments may be used to document the need for intervention, to evaluate the effectiveness of the intervention, and to identify the need for alternative or additional interventions if the initial intervention is ineffective in relieving the pain. For a pain assessment instrument to be useful, it must require little effort on the part of the patient, be easy to understand and use, be easily scored, and be sensitive to small

NURSING RESEARCH PROFILE 13-2

Pain Assessment and Titration of Analgesic Agents

McCaffery, M., Ferrell, B. R., & Pasero, C. (2000). Nurses' personal opinions about patients' pain and their effect on recorded assessments and titration of opioid doses. *Pain Management Nursing, 1*(3), 79–87.

Purpose

Nurses have a key role in pain assessment and management in all areas of clinical practice. Although previous studies have identified lack of knowledge about pain management as a factor contributing to undertreatment of pain, little is known about their personal opinions related to pain management. This study was conducted to explore how nurses' personal opinions about pain intensity influence their decisions about pain assessment and about titration of the prescribed opioid to relieve severe pain.

Study Sample and Design

In this descriptive study, surveys were distributed as a pretest to a convenience sample of nurses attending pain conferences before receiving any information on pain. Data were collected at 20 locations throughout the United States. The surveys presented two vignettes describing patients with postoperative pain. The patients were identical except for their behavior; one patient was smiling and joking while the other remained quiet in bed and grimaced. Nurses were asked to identify their personal opinions about both patients' reported pain intensity, what they would document in the patient record, and what opioid dose they would administer. Patients in both vignettes rated their pain as 8 on a scale of 0 to 10, indicating inadequate pain management and ineffective opioid doses to relieve the severe pain. In both vignettes, it was made clear that increasing the opioid dose would be safe and appropriate. Completed surveys were returned by 1,276 nurses. Of these, a random sample of 100 surveys from each section of the country was

obtained for a total of 400 surveys. Data from the 400 surveys were analyzed.

Findings

Although the nurses who completed the surveys indicated that they would record the patients' pain as 8, fewer nurses believed the smiling patient than the grimacing patient. More nurses (78.3%) believed the grimacing patient's pain intensity and 90% would have documented it correctly. A total of 39% of nurses reported believing the patient who was smiling, and 85.5% stated that they would have documented the reported pain intensity correctly. Nurses were also more likely to correctly increase the opioid dose for the grimacing patient; 62.5% of nurses indicated that they would have increased the dose for the grimacing patient, while only 47.3% reported that they would do so for the smiling patient. Of those nurses who would have increased the opioid dose for the grimacing patient, 16.3% would not do so for the smiling patient.

Nursing Implications

Comparing these results with those of previous studies conducted in 1990 and 1995, the authors noted considerable improvement in assessment and titration of opioids. However, the findings demonstrate that there is a continuing need for education about the different patient responses to pain and the importance of the patient's report of the intensity of pain. More education is needed to address nurses' responsibilities for opioid titration.

---

changes in the characteristic being measured. Figure 13-6 shows a pain assessment algorithm that can be used at the time of assessment to direct clinical decisions for pain management.

Visual Analogue Scales

Visual analogue scales (VAS; see Fig. 13-5) are useful in assessing the intensity of pain. One version of the scale includes a horizontal 10-cm line, with anchors (ends) indicating the extremes of pain. The person is asked to place a mark indicating where the current pain lies on the line. The left anchor usually represents "none" or "no pain," whereas the right anchor usually represents "severe" or "worst possible pain." To score the results, a ruler is placed along the line and the distance the person marked from the left or low end is measured and reported in millimeters or centimeters.

Some patients (eg, children, elderly patients, and visually or cognitively impaired patients) may find it difficult to use an unmarked VAS. In those circumstances, ordinal scales (simple descriptive pain intensity scale, or 0 to 10 numeric pain intensity scale) may be used.

Faces Pain Scale, Revised

This instrument has seven faces depicting expressions that range from contented to obvious distress. The patient is asked to point to the face that most closely resembles the pain intensity felt. Evidence for reliability and validity has been established (Hicks, van Baeyer, Spafford et al., 2001; Hunter, McDowell, Hennessy et al., 2000). Figure 13-7 shows the Faces Pain Scale, Revised.

Guidelines for Using Pain Assessment Scales

Using a written scale to assess pain may not be possible if the person is seriously ill, is in severe pain, or has just returned from surgery. In these cases, the nurse can ask the patient, "On a scale of 0 to 10, 0 being no pain and 10 being pain as bad as it can be, how bad is your pain now?" For patients who have difficulty with a 0 to 10 scale, a 0 to 5 scale may be tried. Whichever scale is used, it should be used consistently. Most patients usually can respond without difficulty. Ideally, the nurse teaches the patient how to use the pain scale before the pain occurs (eg, before surgery). The patient's numerical rating is documented and used to assess the effectiveness of pain relief interventions.

If the person does not speak English or cannot communicate clearly information needed to manage pain, an interpreter, translator, or family member familiar with the person's method of communication should be consulted and a method established for pain assessment. Often a chart can be constructed with English words on one side and the foreign language on the other. The patient can then point to the corresponding word to tell the clinician about the pain.

When a person with pain is cared for at home by family caregivers or the home care nurse, a pain scale may help in assessing the effectiveness of the interventions, if the scale is used before and after the interventions are administered. Scales that address the location and pattern of pain may be useful to the home care nurse in identifying new sources or sites of pain in the chronically or terminally ill patient and in monitoring changes in the patient's level of pain. The patient and family caregivers can be taught to use a pain assessment scale to assess and manage the patient's pain. The home care nurse who sees

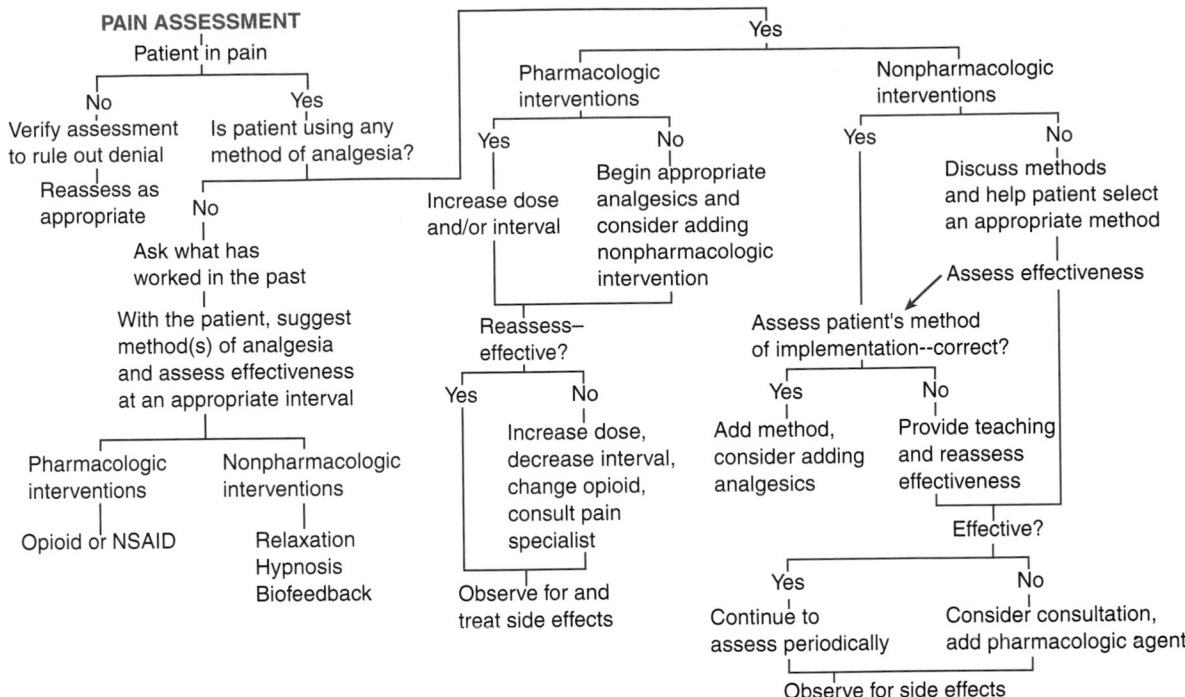

FIGURE 13-6 Pain assessment algorithm. Redrawn with permission from Salerno, E., & Willens, J. S. (1996). *Pain management handbook: An interdisciplinary approach.* St. Louis: C. V. Mosby.

the patient only at intervals may thus benefit from consulting the patient's or family's written record of the pain scores to evaluate how effective the pain management strategies have been over time.

On occasion, a person will deny having pain when most people in similar circumstances would report significant pain. For example, it is not uncommon for a patient recovering from a total joint replacement to deny feeling "pain," but on further questioning will readily admit to having a "terrible ache, but I wouldn't call it pain." From then on, when evaluating this person's pain, the nurse would use the patient's words rather than the word "pain."

NURSE'S ROLE IN PAIN MANAGEMENT

Before discussing what the nurse can do to intervene in the patient's pain, the nurse's role in pain management is reviewed. The nurse helps relieve pain by administering pain-relieving interventions (including both pharmacologic and nonpharmacologic approaches), assessing the effectiveness of those interventions, monitoring for adverse effects, and serving as an advocate for the patient when the prescribed intervention is ineffective in relieving pain. In addition, the nurse serves as an educator to the patient and family to enable them to manage the prescribed intervention themselves when appropriate.

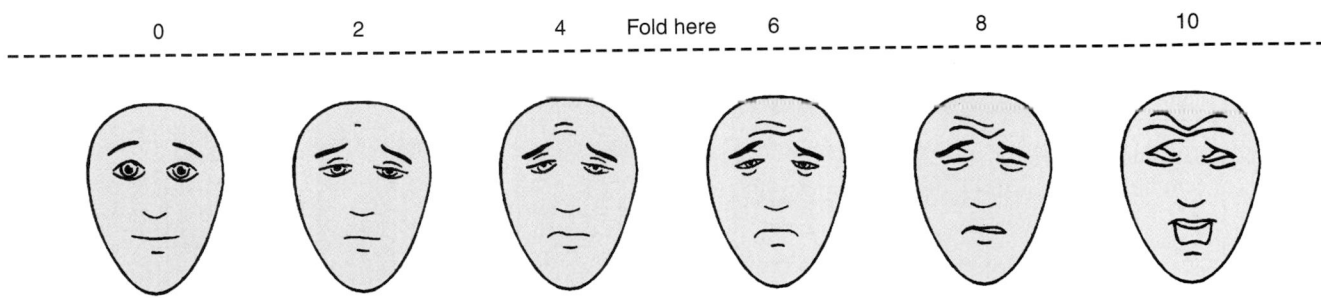

FIGURE 13-7 Faces Pain Scale—Revised. This pain scale is especially suited for helping children describe pain. Instructions for using this scale follow: **"These faces show how much something can hurt. This face** (*point to left-most face*) **shows no pain. The faces show more and more pain** (*point to each from left to right*) **up to this one** (*point to right-most face*). It shows *very much pain.* Point to the face that shows how much you hurt (right now). Score the chosen face *0, 2, 4, 6* or *10*, *counting left to right, so* **0** = *no pain and* **10** = *very much pain. Do not use words like happy or sad. This scale is intended to measure how children feel inside, not how their face looks.* From the *Pediatric Pain Sourcebook.* Original copyright © 2001. Used with permission of the International Association for the Study of Pain and the Pain Research Unit, Sydney Children's Hospital, Randwick NSW 2031, Australia.

Identifying Goals for Pain Management

The information the nurse obtains from the pain assessment is used to identify goals for managing the pain. The goals identified are shared or validated with the patient. For a few patients, the goal may be elimination of the pain. For many, however, this expectation may be unrealistic. Other goals may include a decrease in the intensity, duration, or frequency of pain, and a decrease in the negative effects the pain has on the patient. For example, pain may have a negative effect by interfering with sleep and thereby hampering recovery from an acute illness or decreasing appetite. In such instances, the goals might be to sleep soundly and to take adequate nutrition. Chronic pain may affect the person's quality of life by interfering with work or interpersonal relationships. Thus, a goal may be to decrease time lost from work or to increase the quality of interpersonal relationships.

To determine the goal, a number of factors are considered. The first is the severity of the pain, as judged by the patient. The second factor is the anticipated harmful effects of pain. A high-risk patient is at much greater risk for the harmful effects of pain than a young healthy patient. The third factor is the anticipated duration of the pain. In patients with pain from a disease such as cancer, the pain may be prolonged, possibly for the remainder of the patient's life. Therefore, interventions will be needed for some time and should not detract from the patient's quality of life. A different set of interventions is required if the patient is likely to have pain for only a few days or weeks.

In a study of the dying experience, family members of 2,451 people who had died were interviewed (Lynn, Teno, Phillips et al., 1997). Of these patients, 55% were conscious during their last 3 days of life. Of the conscious patients, 4 in 10 were considered by their family members to be in severe pain most of the time. These findings strongly suggest that pain relief for dying patients should be a primary goal.

The goals for the patient may be accomplished by pharmacologic or nonpharmacologic means, but most success will be achieved with a combination of both. In the acute stages of illness, the patient may be unable to participate actively in relief measures, but when sufficient mental and physical energy is present, the patient may learn self-management techniques to relieve the pain. Thus, as the patient progresses through the stages of recovery, a goal may be to increase the patient's use of self-management pain relief measures.

Establishing the Nurse–Patient Relationship and Teaching

A positive nurse–patient relationship and teaching are key to managing analgesia in the patient with pain, because open communication and patient cooperation are essential to success. A positive nurse–patient relationship characterized by trust is essential. By conveying to the patient the belief that he or she has pain, the nurse often helps reduce the patient's anxiety. Acknowledging to the patient, "I know that you have pain" often eases the patient's mind. Occasionally, patients who fear that no one believes the reported pain feel relieved when they know that the nurse can be trusted to believe the pain exists.

Teaching is equally important, because the patient or family may be responsible for managing the pain at home and preventing or managing side effects. Teaching patients about pain and strategies to relieve it may reduce pain in the absence of other pain relief measures and may enhance the effectiveness of the pain relief measures used.

The nurse also provides information by explaining how pain can be controlled. The patient is informed, for example, that pain should be reported in the early stages. When the patient waits too long to report pain, **sensitization** may occur and the pain may be so intense that it is difficult to relieve. The phenomenon of sensitization is important in effective pain management. Since a heightened response is seen after exposure to a noxious stimulus, the response to that stimulus will be greater, causing the person to feel more pain. When health care providers assess and treat pain before it becomes severe, sensitization is diminished or avoided, and thus less medication is needed.

Providing Physical Care

The patient in pain may be unable to participate in the usual activities of daily living or to perform usual self-care and may need assistance to carry out these activities. The patient is usually more comfortable when physical and self-care needs have been met and efforts have been made to ensure as comfortable a position as possible. A fresh gown and change of bed linens, along with efforts to make the person feel refreshed (eg, brushing teeth, combing hair), often increase the level of comfort and improve the effectiveness of the pain relief measures.

Providing physical care to the patient also gives the nurse (in acute, long-term, and home settings) the opportunity to perform a complete assessment and to identify problems that may contribute to the patient's discomfort and pain. Appropriate and gentle physical touch during care may be reassuring and comforting. If topical treatments such as fentanyl (an opioid analgesic) patches or intravenous or intraspinal catheters are used, the skin around the patch or catheter should be assessed for integrity during physical care.

Managing Anxiety Related to Pain

Anxiety may affect a patient's response to pain. The patient who anticipates pain may become increasingly anxious. Teaching the patient about the nature of the impending painful experience and the ways to reduce pain often decreases anxiety; a person who is experiencing pain will use previously learned strategies to reduce anxiety and pain. Learning about measures to relieve pain may lessen the threat of pain and give the person a sense of control.

What the nurse explains about the available pain relief measures and their effectiveness may also affect the patient's anxiety level. The patient's anxiety may be reduced by explanations that point out the degree of pain relief that can be expected from each measure. For example, the patient who is informed beforehand that an intervention may not eliminate pain completely is less likely to become anxious when a certain amount of pain persists. Anxiety resulting from anticipation of pain or the pain experience itself may often be managed effectively by establishing a relationship with the patient and by patient teaching.

A patient who is anxious about pain may be less tolerant of the pain, which in turn may increase the anxiety level. To prevent the pain and anxiety from escalating, the anxiety-producing cycle must be interrupted. Low levels of pain are easier to reduce or control than are more intense levels. (This concept of sensitization was previously discussed.) Consequently, pain relief measures should be used before pain becomes severe. Many patients believe that they should not request pain relief measures until they cannot tolerate the pain, making it difficult for medications to provide relief. Therefore, it is important to explain to all patients that pain relief or control is more successful if such measures begin before the pain becomes unbearable.

Pain Management Strategies

Reducing pain to a "tolerable" level was once considered the goal of pain management. However, even patients who have described pain relief as adequate often report disturbed sleep and marked distress because of pain. In view of the harmful effects of pain and inadequate pain management, the goal of tolerable pain has been replaced by the goal of relieving the pain. Pain management strategies include both pharmacologic and nonpharmacologic approaches. These approaches are selected on the basis of the patient's requirements and goals. Appropriate analgesic medications are used as prescribed. They are not considered a last resort to be used only when other pain relief measures fail. Any intervention is most successful if initiated before pain sensitization occurs, and the greatest success is usually achieved if several interventions are applied simultaneously.

PHARMACOLOGIC INTERVENTIONS

Managing a patient's pain pharmacologically is accomplished in collaboration with the physician or other primary care provider, the patient, and often the family. The physician or nurse practitioner prescribes specific medications for pain or may insert an intravenous line for administering analgesic medications. Alternatively, an anesthesiologist or nurse anesthetist may insert an epidural catheter for their administration. However, it is the nurse who maintains the analgesia, assesses its effectiveness, and reports if the intervention is ineffective or produces side effects.

The pharmacologic management of pain requires close collaboration and effective communication among health care providers. In the home setting, it is often the family who manages the patient's pain and assesses the effectiveness of pharmacologic interventions, while it is the home care nurse who evaluates the adequacy of pain relief strategies and the family's ability to manage the pain. The home care nurse reinforces teaching and ensures communication among the patient, family care providers, physician, pharmacist, and other health care providers involved in the patient's care.

Premedication Assessment

Before administering any medication, the nurse asks the patient about allergies to medications and the nature of any previous allergic responses. True allergic or anaphylactic responses to opioids are rare, but it is not uncommon for a patient to report an allergy to one of the opioids. On further examination, the nurse often learns that the extent of the allergy was "itching" or "nausea and vomiting." These responses are not allergies; rather, they are side effects that, when necessary, can be managed while the patient's pain is relieved. The patient's description of responses or reactions should be documented and reported before administering the medication.

The nurse obtains the patient's medication history (eg, current, usual, or recent use of prescription or over-the-counter medications or herbal agents), along with a history of health problems. Certain medications or conditions may affect the analgesic medication's effectiveness or the metabolism and excretion of analgesic agents. Before administering analgesic agents, the nurse should assess the patient's pain status, including the intensity of current pain, changes in pain intensity after the previous dose of medication, and side effects of the medication.

Approaches for Using Analgesic Agents

Medications are most effective when the dose and interval between doses are individualized to meet the patient's needs. The only safe and effective way to administer analgesic medications is by asking the patient to rate the pain and by observing the response to medications.

BALANCED ANESTHESIA

Pharmacologic interventions are most effective when a multi-modal or balanced analgesia approach is used. **Balanced analgesia** refers to use of more than one form of analgesia concurrently to obtain more pain relief with fewer side effects. Three general categories of analgesic agents are opioids, NSAIDs, and local anesthetics. These agents work by different mechanisms. Using two or three types of agents simultaneously can maximize pain relief while minimizing the potentially toxic effects of any one agent. When one agent is used alone, it usually must be used in a higher dose to be effective. In other words, although it might require 15 mg morphine to relieve a certain pain, it may take only 8 mg morphine plus 30 mg ketorolac (an NSAID) to relieve the same pain.

PRO RE NATA (PRN)

In the past, the standard method used by most nurses and physicians in administering analgesia was to administer the analgesic *pro re nata* (PRN), or "as needed." The standard practice was for the nurse to wait for the patient to complain of pain and then administer analgesia. As a result, many patients remained in pain because they did not know they needed to ask for medication or waited until the pain became intolerable.

By its very nature, the PRN approach to analgesia leaves the patient sedated or in severe pain much of the time. To receive pain relief from an opioid analgesic, the serum level of that opioid must be maintained at a minimum therapeutic level (Fig. 13-8). By the time the patient complains of pain, the serum opioid level is below the therapeutic level. From the time the patient requests pain medication until the nurse administers the medication, the patient's serum level continues to fall. The lower the serum opioid level, the more difficult it is to achieve the therapeutic level with the next dose. The only way to ensure significant periods of analgesia, using this method, is to give doses large enough to produce periods of sedation.

PREVENTIVE APPROACH

Currently, a preventive approach to relieving pain by administering analgesic agents is considered the most effective strategy because a therapeutic serum level of medication is maintained. With the preventive approach, analgesic agents are administered at set intervals so that the medication acts before the pain becomes severe and before the serum opioid level falls to a subtherapeutic level.

Administering analgesic medication on a time basis, rather than on the basis of the patient's report of pain, prevents the serum drug level from falling to subtherapeutic levels. An example of this would be giving the patient the prescribed morphine or the prescribed NSAID (ibuprofen) every 4 hours rather than waiting until the patient complains of pain. If the patient's pain is likely to occur around the clock or for a great portion of a 24-hour period, a regular around-the-clock schedule of administering analgesia may be indicated. Even if the analgesic is prescribed PRN, it can be administered on a preventive basis before the pa-

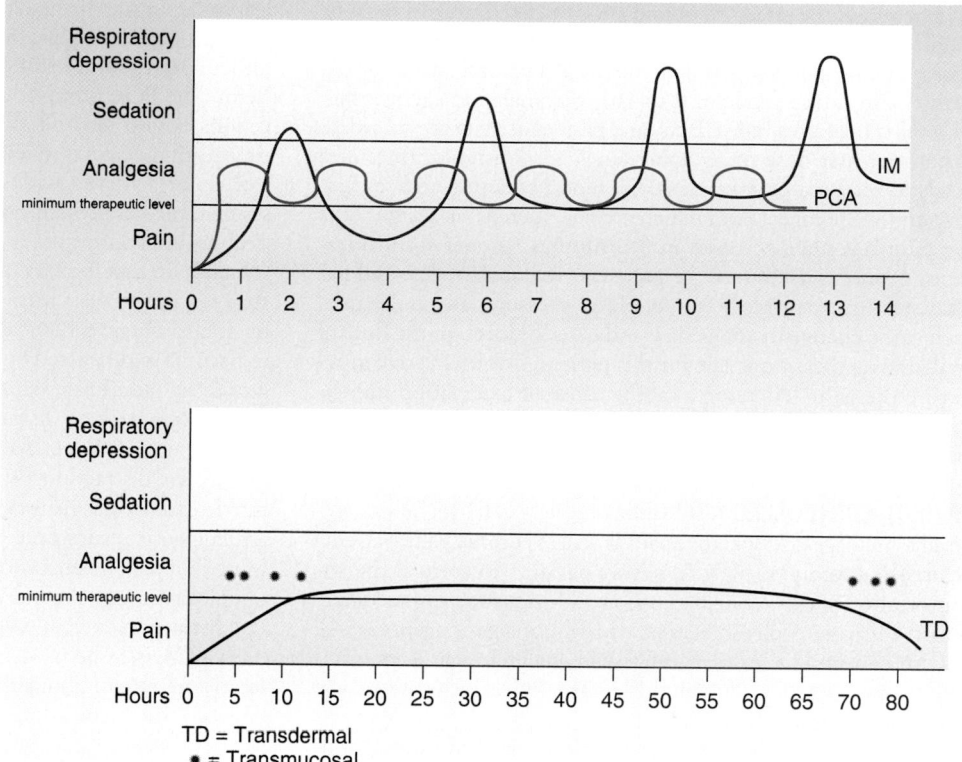

FIGURE 13-8 Relationship of mode of delivery of analgesia to serum analgesic level. *Top:* intramuscular (IM) and intravenous patient-controlled analgesia (PCA); *bottom:* transdermal (TD) and transmucosal (•).

tient is in severe pain, as long as the prescribed interval between doses is observed. The preventive approach reduces the peaks and troughs in the serum level and provides more pain relief for the patient with fewer adverse effects.

Smaller doses of medication are needed with the preventive approach because the pain does not escalate to a level of severe intensity. Thus, a preventive approach may result in the administration of less medication over a 24-hour period, thereby helping prevent tolerance to analgesic agents and decreasing the severity of side effects (eg, sedation and constipation). Better pain control can be achieved with a preventive approach, reducing the amount of time the patient spends in pain.

In using the preventive approach, the nurse assesses the patient for sedation before administering the next dose. The goal is to provide analgesia before the pain becomes severe. It would not be safe to medicate a patient (with an opioid) repeatedly if he or she was sedated or having no pain. It may be necessary to decrease the dosage of the opioid analgesic so that the patient receives pain relief with less sedation.

INDIVIDUALIZED DOSAGE

The dosage and the interval between doses should be based on the patient's requirements rather than on an inflexible standard or routine. People metabolize and absorb medications at different rates and experience different levels of pain. Therefore, one dose of an opioid medication given at specified intervals may be effective for one patient but ineffective for another.

Because of the fear of promoting addiction or causing respiratory depression, health care providers tend to prescribe and administer inadequate dosages of opioid agents to treat acute pain or chronic pain in the terminally ill patient (Chart 13-5). However, even prolonged administration of opioid agents is associated with an extremely low incidence (less than 1%) of addiction. Furthermore, small doses are not necessarily safe doses. For example, some patients receiving a relatively small dose (25 to 50 mg) of meperidine (Demerol) intramuscularly have experienced respiratory depression, whereas other patients have not exhibited any sedation or respiratory depression with very large doses of opioids.

Chart 13-5 • **Ethics and Related Issues**

Inadequate Pain Management

Situation
When taking over the care of ethnic minority patients at the change of shift from a particular colleague, you usually find these patients to be in a great deal of pain. Your nonsystematic observations have led you to conclude these patients receive only a small portion of the analgesia prescribed for them. You have heard a nurse colleague state a belief that people of certain ethnic groups have "no pain tolerance" and are "just looking for drugs."

Dilemma
Racial biases are difficult to change and deal with. To confront this nurse may not alter the behavior but will certainly disrupt the working relationships on the unit. It would be easier to look the other way. On the other hand, you believe that the nurse is giving inadequate and unethical care to selected patients and placing them at greater risk for postoperative complications.

Discussion
• What information would you need to collect before acting?
• From whom could you seek counsel?
• Are the two aspects of the dilemma equally important?

Therefore, the effects of opioid analgesic medications must be monitored, especially when the first dose is given or when the dose is changed or given more frequently. The time, date, the patient's pain rating (scale of 0 to 10), the analgesic agent, other pain relief measures, side effects, and patient activity are recorded. When the first dose of an analgesic is administered, the nurse needs to record a pain rating score, blood pressure, and respiratory and pulse rates (all of which are considered "vital signs"). If the pain has not decreased in 30 minutes (sooner if an intravenous route is used) and the patient is reasonably alert and has a satisfactory respiratory status, blood pressure, and pulse rate, then some change in analgesia is indicated. Although the dose of analgesic medication is safe for this patient, it is ineffective in relieving the pain. Therefore, another dose of medication may be indicated. In such instances, the nurse consults with the physician to determine what further action is warranted.

PATIENT-CONTROLLED ANALGESIA

Used to manage postoperative pain as well as chronic pain, **patient-controlled analgesia** (PCA) allows patients to control the administration of their own medication within predetermined safety limits. This approach can be used with oral analgesic agents as well as with continuous infusions of opioid analgesic agents by intravenous, subcutaneous, or epidural routes. PCA can be used in the hospital or home setting.

The PCA pump permits the patient to self-administer continuous infusions of medication (basal rates) safely and to administer extra medication (bolus doses) with episodes of increased pain or painful activities. A PCA pump is electronically controlled by a timing device. Patients experiencing pain can administer small amounts of medication directly into their intravenous, subcutaneous, or epidural catheter by pressing a button. The pump then delivers a preset amount of medication.

The PCA pump also can be programmed to deliver a constant, background infusion of medication or basal rate and still allow the patient to administer additional bolus doses as needed. The timer can be programmed to prevent additional doses from being administered until a specified time period has elapsed (lock-out time) and until the first dose has had time to exert its maximal effect. Even if the patient pushes the button multiple times in rapid succession, no additional doses are released. If another dose is required at the end of the delay period, the button must be pushed again to receive the dose. Patients who are controlling their own opioid administration usually become sedated and stop pushing the button before any significant respiratory depression occurs. Nevertheless, assessing respiratory status remains a major role for the nurse.

A continuous infusion plus bolus doses may be effective with cancer patients who require large doses of analgesia, or for postsurgical patients. Although this allows more uninterrupted sleep, the risk of sedation increases, especially when the patient has minimal or decreasing pain.

Patients who use PCA achieve better pain relief (Walder, Schafer, Henzi et al., 2001) and often require less pain medication than those who are treated in the standard PRN fashion. Because the patient can maintain a near-constant level of medication, the periods of severe pain and sedation that occur with the traditional PRN regimen are avoided.

To initiate PCA or any analgesia used at home or in the hospital, it is important to avoid playing "catch-up." Pain should be brought under control before PCA starts, often by the use of an initial, larger bolus dose or loading dose. Then, after control is achieved, the pump is programmed to deliver small doses of medication at a time. If the patient with severe pain has a low serum level of opioid analgesic because of an inadequate basal rate, it is difficult to regain control with the small doses available by pump. Before the PCA pump is used, repeated bolus doses of an intravenous opioid may be administered as prescribed over a short time until the pain is relieved. Then PCA is initiated. If pain control is not achieved with the maximal dose of medication prescribed, further prescriptions are obtained. The goal is to achieve a minimum therapeutic level of analgesia and to allow the patient to maintain that level by using the PCA pump. The patient is instructed not to wait until the pain is severe before pushing the button to obtain a bolus dose. The patient is also reminded not to become so distracted by an activity or visitor that he or she forgets to self-administer a prescribed dose of medication. One potential drawback to distraction is that a patient who is using a PCA pump may not self-administer any analgesia during the time of effective distraction. When distraction ends suddenly (eg, the movie ends or the visitors leave), the patient may be left without a therapeutic serum opioid level. When intermittent distraction is used for pain relief, a continuous low-level background infusion of opioid through the PCA pump may be prescribed so that when the distraction ends, it will not be necessary to try to catch up.

If PCA is to be used in the patient's home, the patient and family are taught about the operation of the pump and the side effects of the medication and strategies to manage them.

 NURSING ALERT Family members are cautioned not to push the button for the patient, especially if the patient is asleep, because this overrides some of the safety features of the system.

Local Anesthetic Agents

Local anesthetics work by blocking nerve conduction when applied directly to the nerve fibers. They can be applied directly to the site of injury (eg, a topical anesthetic spray for sunburn) or directly to nerve fibers by injection or at the time of surgery. They can also be administered through an epidural catheter.

TOPICAL APPLICATION

Local anesthetic agents have been successful in reducing the pain associated with thoracic or upper abdominal surgery when injected by the surgeon intercostally. Local anesthetic agents are rapidly absorbed into the bloodstream, resulting in decreased availability at the surgical or injury site and an increased anesthetic level in the blood, increasing the risk of toxicity. Therefore, a vasoconstrictive agent (eg, epinephrine or phenylephrine) is added to the anesthetic agent to decrease its systemic absorption and to maintain its concentration at the surgical or injury site.

A topical anesthetic agent known as eutectic mixture or emulsion of local anesthetics, or EMLA cream, has been effective in preventing the pain associated with invasive procedures such as lumbar puncture or the insertion of intravenous lines. To be effective, EMLA must be applied to the site 60 to 90 minutes before the procedure.

INTRASPINAL ADMINISTRATION

Intermittent or continuous administration of local anesthetic agents through an epidural catheter has been used for years to produce anesthesia during surgery. Although the administration of local anesthetic agents in the spinal canal is still largely confined to acute pain, such as postoperative pain and pain associated with labor and delivery, the epidural administration of local anesthetic agents for pain management is increasing.

A local anesthetic agent administered through an epidural catheter is applied directly to the nerve root. The anesthetic agent can be administered continuously in low doses, intermittently on a schedule, or on demand as the patient requires it, and is often combined with the epidural administration of opioids. Surgical patients treated with this combination experience fewer complications after surgery, ambulate sooner, and have shorter hospital stays than patients receiving standard therapy (Correll, Viscusi, Grunwald et al., 2001).

Opioid Analgesic Agents

Opioids can be administered by various routes, including oral, intravenous, subcutaneous, intraspinal, intranasal, rectal, and transdermal routes. The goal of administering opioids is to relieve pain and improve quality of life; therefore, the route of administration, dose, and frequency of administration are determined on an individual basis. Factors that are considered in determining the route, dose, and frequency of medication include the characteristics of the pain (eg, its expected duration and severity), the overall status of the patient, the patient's response to analgesic medications, and the patient's report of pain. Although the oral route is usually preferred for administering opioids, oral opioids must be given frequently enough and in large enough doses to be effective. Opioid analgesic agents given orally may provide a more consistent serum level than those given intramuscularly.

If the patient is expected to require opioid analgesic agents at home, the patient's and the family's ability to administer opioids as prescribed is considered in planning. Steps are taken to ensure that the medication will be available to the patient. Many pharmacies, especially those in smaller rural areas or inner cities, may be reluctant to stock large amounts of opioids. Therefore, arrangements for obtaining these prescription medications must be made ahead of time.

With the administration of opioids by any route, side effects must be considered and anticipated. Anticipating side effects and taking steps to minimize them increase the likelihood that the patient will receive adequate pain relief without interrupting therapy to treat these effects.

RESPIRATORY DEPRESSION AND SEDATION

Respiratory depression is the most serious adverse effect of opioid analgesic agents administered by intravenous, subcutaneous, or epidural routes. However, it is relatively rare because doses administered through these routes are small, and tolerance to respiratory depressant effects increases if the dose is increased slowly. The risk of respiratory depression increases with age and the concomitant use of other opioids or other central nervous system depressants. The risk of respiratory depression also increases when the catheter is placed in the thoracic area and when the intraabdominal or intrathoracic pressure is increased.

The patient receiving opioids by any route must be assessed frequently for changes in respiratory status. Specific notable changes are decreasing respiratory rate or shallow respirations. Despite the risks associated with their use, intravenous and epidural opioids are considered safe, with the risks related to epidural administration no greater than those related to intravenous or other systemic routes of administration. Sedation, which may occur with any method of administering opioids, is likely to occur when opioid doses are increased. However, the patient often develops tolerance quickly, so that in a short time the patient is no longer sedated by the dose that initially caused sedation. Increasing the time between doses or reducing the dose temporarily, as prescribed, usually prevents deep sedation from occurring. The patient at risk for sedation must be monitored closely for changes in respiratory status. The patient is also at risk for other problems associated with sedation and immobility. Therefore, the nurse must initiate strategies to prevent problems such as skin breakdown.

NAUSEA AND VOMITING

Nausea and vomiting frequently occur with opioid use. Usually these effects occur some hours after the initial injection. Patients, especially postoperative patients, may not think to tell the nurse that they are nauseated, particularly if the nausea is mild. However, the patient receiving an opioid should be assessed for nausea and vomiting, which may be triggered by a position change and may be prevented by having the patient change positions slowly. Adequate hydration and the administration of antiemetic agents may decrease the incidence. Opioid-induced nausea and vomiting often subside within a few days.

CONSTIPATION

Constipation, a common side effect of opioid use, may become so severe that the patient is forced to choose between relief of pain and relief of constipation. This situation can occur in patients after surgery and in patients receiving large doses of opioids to treat cancer-related pain. Preventing constipation must be a high priority in all patients receiving opioids. Whenever a patient receives opioids, a bowel regimen should begin at the same time. Tolerance to this side effect does not occur; rather, it persists even with long-term use of opioids.

Several strategies may help prevent and treat opioid-related constipation. Mild laxatives and a high intake of fluid and fiber may be effective in managing mild constipation. Unless contraindicated, a mild laxative and a stool softener should be administered on a regular schedule. Continued severe constipation, however, often requires the use of a stimulating cathartic agent, such as senna derivatives (Senokot) or bisacodyl (Dulcolax). Oral laxatives and stool softeners may prevent constipation; rectal suppositories may be used if oral agents fail (Plaisance & Ellis, 2002).

INADEQUATE PAIN RELIEF

One factor commonly associated with ineffective pain relief is an inadequate dose of opioid. This is most likely to occur when the caregiver underestimates the patient's pain or the route of administration is changed without the differences in absorption and action being considered. Consequently, the patient receives doses too small to be effective and, possibly, too infrequently to relieve pain. For example, if opioid delivery is changed from the intravenous route to the oral route, the oral dose must be approximately three times greater than that given parenterally to provide relief. Because of differences in absorption of orally administered opioids among individuals, the patient must be assessed carefully to ensure that the pain is relieved.

Table 13-2 lists opioids and dosages that are equivalent to morphine. In general, no recalculation needs to be done when switching from one brand of an agent to another brand of the same medication, with the exception of extended-release oral morphine. Currently, three brands of extended-release morphine (MS Contin, Oramorph, Kadian) are commonly used by cancer patients. Although these agents come in the same dosage form and contain the same drug, they are not considered therapeutically equivalent because they employ different release mechanisms. Patients who need to switch brands should be monitored carefully both for overdose and for inadequate pain relief.

Table 13-2 • **Equianalgesic Conversion Table**

| Drug | ADMINISTRATION ROUTE | | IV:PO Ratio | Half-life (in hours) | Duration (in hours) |
	IV/IM/SQ	PO			
Morphine sulfate	10 mg	30 mg	1:3	2 to 3	2 to 4
Codeine	130 mg	200 mg	NA	2 to 3	2 to 4
Hydromorphone	1.5 mg	7.5 mg	1:5	2 to 3	2 to 4
Levorphanol	2 mg	4 mg	1:2	12 to 15	4 to 6
Meperidine	75 mg	300 mg	1:4	3 to 4	2 to 4
Methadone	10 mg	20 mg	1:2	12 to 190	4 to 8
Oxycodone	NA	20 to 30 mg	NA	2 to 3	2 to 4
Oxymorphone	1 mg or 10-mg suppository	NA	NA	2 to 3	2 to 4
Fentanyl (transdermal)	100-mcg patch = 4 mg/hr v morphine sulphate based on anecdotal experience				

NA = not applicable.
Derby, S. A. (1999). Opioid conversion guidelines for managing adult cancer pain. *American Journal of Nursing, 99*(10), 62–65.

OTHER EFFECTS OF OPIOIDS

During the health history, when asked about drug allergies, patients with previous hospital experience (especially for surgery) may report that they are "allergic" to morphine. This report should be thoroughly investigated. Commonly, this "allergy" will be described as itching only. Pruritus (itching) is a frequent problem associated with opioids administered through any route, but it is not an allergic reaction. Itching can be relieved by administering prescribed antihistamines. Epidurally administered opioids may also cause urinary retention or pruritus. The patient should be monitored and may require urinary catheterization. Small doses of naloxone may be prescribed to relieve these problems in patients who are receiving epidural opioids for the relief of acute postoperative pain.

A number of factors may influence the safety and effectiveness of opioid administration. Opioid analgesic agents are primarily metabolized by the liver and excreted by the kidney. Therefore, metabolism and excretion of analgesic medications will be impaired in patients with liver or kidney disease, increasing the risk of cumulative or toxic effects. In addition, normeperidine, a metabolite of meperidine, may rapidly or unexpectedly accumulate to toxic levels. This is more likely to occur in patients with impaired kidney function and may result in seizures in susceptible patients.

Patients with untreated hypothyroidism are more susceptible to the analgesic effects and side effects of opioids. In contrast, patients with hyperthyroidism may require larger doses for pain relief. Patients with a decreased respiratory reserve from disease or aging may be more susceptible to the depressant effects of opioids and must be carefully monitored for respiratory depression.

Dehydrated patients are at increased risk for the hypotensive effects of opioids. Patients who become hypotensive after the administration of an opioid should be kept recumbent and rehydrated unless fluids are contraindicated. Patients who are dehydrated are also more likely to experience nausea and vomiting with opioid use. Rehydration usually relieves these symptoms.

Patients receiving certain other medications, such as monoamine oxidase (MAO) inhibitors, phenothiazines, or tricyclic antidepressants, may have an exaggerated response to the depressant effects of opioids. Patients taking these medications should receive small doses of opioids and must be monitored closely. Continued pain in these patients indicates that a therapeutic level of the analgesic has not been achieved. The patient must be monitored for sedation even if an analgesic effect has not been obtained.

TOLERANCE AND ADDICTION

There is no maximum safe dosage of opioids, nor is there any easily identifiable therapeutic serum level. Both the maximal safe dosage and therapeutic serum level are relative and individual. **Tolerance** (the need for increasing doses of opioids to achieve the same therapeutic effect) will develop in almost all patients taking opioids over an extended period. Patients requiring opioids over a long term, especially cancer patients, will need increasing doses to relieve pain. After the first few weeks of therapy, the patient's dosing requirements usually level off. Patients who become tolerant to the analgesic effects of large doses of morphine may obtain pain relief by switching to a different opioid. Symptoms of physical *dependence* may occur when the opioids are discontinued; dependence often occurs with opioid tolerance and does not indicate an addiction.

> **NURSING ALERT** Although patients may need increasing levels of opioids, they are not addicted. Physical tolerance usually occurs in the absence of addiction. Tolerance to opioids is common and becomes a problem primarily in terms of delivering or administering the medication (eg, how to administer very large doses of morphine a day to a patient). On the other hand, addiction is rare and should never be the primary concern of the nurse caring for a patient in pain.

Addiction is a behavioral pattern of substance use characterized by a compulsion to take the drug primarily to experience its psychic effects. Fear that patients will become addicted or dependent on opioids has contributed to inadequate treatment of pain. This fear is commonly expressed by health care providers as well as patients and results from lack of knowledge about the low risk of addiction.

In an often-cited classic study (Porter & Jick, 1980) of more than 11,000 patients receiving opioids for a medical indication, only four patients without a history of substance abuse could be identified as becoming addicted. Addiction following therapeutic opioid administration is so negligible that it should not be a consideration when caring for the patient in pain. Thus, patients and health care providers should be dissuaded from withholding pain medication because of concerns about addiction.

Nonsteroidal Anti-inflammatory Drugs

NSAIDs are thought to decrease pain by inhibiting cyclo-oxygenase (COX), the rate-limiting enzyme involved in the production of prostaglandin from traumatized or inflamed tissues. There are two types of COX: COX-1 and COX-2. COX-1 is involved with mediating prostaglandin formation involved in the maintenance of physiologic functions. Some of the physiologic functions include platelet aggregation through the provision of thromboxane precursors and increased gastric mucosal blood flow. This prevents ischemia and promotes mucosal integrity. Inhibition of COX-1 will result in gastric ulceration, bleeding, and renal damage. The second type, COX-2, mediates prostaglandin formation that results in symptoms of pain, inflammation, and fever. Thus, inhibition of COX-2 is desirable. Newer NSAIDs such as celecoxib (Celebrex), rofecoxib (Vioxx), and valdecoxib (Bextra) are COX-2 inhibitors. Ibuprofen (Advil, Motrin), another NSAID, blocks both COX-1 and COX-2 and is effective in relieving mild to moderate pain and has a low incidence of adverse effects. Aspirin, the oldest NSAID, also blocks COX-1 as well as COX-2; however, because it causes frequent and severe side effects, aspirin is infrequently used to treat significant acute or chronic pain.

NSAIDs are very helpful in treating arthritic diseases and may be especially powerful in treating cancer-related bone pain. They have been effectively combined with opioids to treat postoperative and other severe pain. The use of an NSAID with an opioid relieves pain more effectively than the opioid alone. In such cases, the patient may obtain pain relief with less opioid and fewer side effects. It has been shown that intraoperative administration of NSAIDs results in improved postoperative pain control following laparoscopic surgery and in some cases shorter hospital stays (McLaughlin, 1994).

A regimen of a fixed-dose, time-contingent NSAID (eg, every 4 hours) and a separately administered fluctuating dose of opioid may be effective in managing moderate to severe cancer pain. In more severe pain, the opioid dose will also be fixed, with an additional fluctuating dose as needed for **breakthrough pain** (a sudden increase in pain despite the administration of pain-relieving medications). These regimens result in better pain relief with fewer opioid-related side effects.

Most patients tolerate NSAIDs well. However, those with impaired kidney function may require a smaller dose and must be monitored closely for side effects. Patients taking NSAIDs bruise easily because NSAIDs have some anticoagulant effect. Moreover, they may displace other medications, such as warfarin (Coumadin), from serum proteins and increase their effects. High doses or prolonged use can irritate the stomach and in some cases result in gastrointestinal bleeding as well. Thus, monitoring the patient for gastrointestinal bleeding is indicated.

 Gerontologic Considerations Related to Analgesic Agents

Physiologic changes in older adults require that analgesic agents be administered with caution. Drug interactions are more likely to occur in older adults because of the higher incidence of chronic illness and the increased use of prescription and over-the-counter medications. Although the elderly population is an extremely heterogeneous group, differences in response to pain or medications by a patient in this 40-year span (60 to 100 years) are more likely to be due to chronic illness or other individual factors than age. Before administering opioid and nonopioid analgesic agents to elderly patients, the nurse needs to obtain a careful medication history to identify potential drug interactions.

Absorption and metabolism of medications are altered in elderly patients because of decreased liver, renal, and gastrointestinal function. In addition, changes in body weight, protein stores, and distribution of body fluid alter the distribution of medications in the body. As a result, medications are not metabolized as quickly and blood levels of the medication remain higher for a longer period. Elderly patients are more sensitive to medications and at an increased risk for drug toxicity (American Geriatrics Society, 1998).

Opioid and nonopioid analgesic medications can be given effectively to elderly patients but must be used cautiously because of the increased susceptibility to depression of both the nervous and the respiratory systems. Although there is no reason to avoid opioids simply because a person is elderly, meperidine should be avoided because its active and neurotoxic metabolite, normeperidine, is more likely to accumulate in the elderly. In addition, because of decreased binding of meperidine by plasma proteins, blood concentrations of the medication twice those found in younger patients may result.

In many cases, the initial dose of analgesic medication prescribed for an elderly patient may be the same as that for a younger person, or slightly smaller than the normal dose, but because of slowed metabolism and excretion related to aging, the safe interval for subsequent doses may be longer (or prolonged). As always, the best guide to pain management and administration of analgesic agents in all patients regardless of age is what the patient says. The elderly patient may obtain more pain relief for a longer time than a younger patient. As a result, smaller, less frequent doses may be required. The American Geriatrics Society (2002) has published clinical practice guidelines for managing chronic pain in elderly patients.

Tricyclic Antidepressant Agents and Anticonvulsant Medications

Pain of neurologic origin (eg, causalgia, tumor impingement on a nerve, postherpetic neuralgia) is difficult to treat and in general is not responsive to opioid therapy. When these pain syndromes are accompanied by dysesthesia (burning or cutting pain), they may be responsive to a tricyclic antidepressant or an antiseizure agent. When indicated, tricyclic antidepressant agents, such as amitriptyline (Elavil) or imipramine (Tofranil), are prescribed in doses considerably smaller than those generally used for depression. The patient needs to know that a therapeutic effect may not occur before 3 weeks. Antiseizure medications such as phenytoin (Dilantin) or carbamazepine (Tegretol) also are used in doses lower than those prescribed for seizure disorders. Because a variety of medications can be tried, the nurse should be familiar with the possible side effects and should teach the patient and family how to recognize these effects.

ROUTES OF ADMINISTRATION

The route selected for administering an analgesic agent (Table 13-3) depends on the patient's condition and the desired effect of the medication. Analgesic agents can be administered by parenteral, oral, rectal, transdermal, transmucosal, intraspinal, or epidural routes. Each method of administration has advantages and disadvantages. The route chosen should be based on the patient's needs.

Parenteral

Parenteral administration (intramuscular, intravenous, or subcutaneous) of the analgesic medication produces effects more rapidly than oral administration, but these effects are of shorter

Table 13-3 • **Administration Routes for Analgesics**

ROUTE	SITE
Parenteral	Intramuscular (IM)
	Intravenous (IV)
	Subcutaneous (SC)
Gastrointestinal	Oral (PO)
	Rectal (PR)
Transdermal	Skin
Transmucosal	Oral mucosa
	Intranasal mucosa
	Bronchial mucosa
Epidural	Epidural space
Intraspinal	Spinal canal

duration. Parenteral administration may be indicated if the patient is not permitted oral intake or is vomiting. Medication administered by the intramuscular route enters the bloodstream more slowly than medication given intravenously and is metabolized slowly. The rate of absorption may be erratic; it depends on the site selected and the amount of body fat.

The intravenous route is an alternative to intramuscular injection for many but not all analgesic medications. The intravenous route is the preferred parenteral route in most acute care situations because it is much more comfortable for the patient. In addition, peak serum levels and pain relief occur more rapidly and reliably. Because it peaks rapidly (usually within minutes) and is metabolized quickly, an appropriate intravenous dose will be smaller and prescribed at shorter intervals than an intramuscular dose.

Intravenous opioids may be administered by IV push or slow push (eg, over a 5- to 10-minute period) or by continuous infusion with a pump. Continuous infusion provides a steady level of analgesia and is indicated when pain occurs over a 24-hour period (eg, after surgery for the first day or so, or in a patient with prolonged cancer pain who cannot take medication by other routes). The dose of analgesic agent is calculated carefully to relieve pain without producing respiratory depression and other side effects.

The subcutaneous route for infusion of opioid analgesic agents is used for patients with severe pain such as cancer pain; it is particularly useful for patients with limited intravenous access who cannot take oral medications, and patients who are managing their pain at home. The dose of opioid that can be infused through this route is limited because of the small volume that can be administered at one time into the subcutaneous tissue. However, this route is often an effective and convenient way to manage pain.

Oral Route

If the patient can take medication by mouth, oral administration is preferred over parenteral administration because it is easy, noninvasive, and not painful. Severe pain can be relieved with oral opioids if the doses are high enough (see Table 13-2).

In terminally ill patients with prolonged pain, doses may gradually be increased as the disease progresses and causes more pain or as the person builds up a tolerance to the medication. If these higher doses are increased gradually, they usually provide additional pain relief without producing respiratory depression

or sedation. If the route of administration is changed from a parenteral route to the oral route at a dose that is not equivalent in strength (equianalgesic), the smaller oral dose may result in a withdrawal reaction and recurrence of pain.

Rectal Route

The rectal route of administration may be indicated in patients who cannot take medications by any other route. The rectal route may also be indicated for patients with bleeding problems, such as hemophilia. The onset of action of opioids administered rectally is unclear but is delayed compared with other routes of administration. Similarly, the duration of action is prolonged.

Transdermal Route

The transdermal route has been used to achieve a consistent opioid serum level through absorption of the medication via the skin. This route is most often used for cancer patients who are at home or in hospice care and who have been receiving oral sustained-release morphine. Fentanyl (Duragesic) is the only commercially available transdermal medication. The preparation is a patch consisting of a reservoir containing the medication and a membrane.

When the transdermal system is first applied to the skin, the fentanyl, which is fat-soluble, binds to the skin and fat layers. Then it is slowly and systemically absorbed. Therefore, there is a delay in effect while the dermal layer is being saturated. A drug reservoir actually forms in the upper layer of skin. This results in a slowly rising serum level and a slow tapering of the serum level once the patch is removed (see Fig. 13-8). Because it takes 12 to 24 hours for the fentanyl levels to gradually increase from the first patch, the last dose of sustained-release morphine should be given at the same time the first patch is applied (Donner et al., 1996). Transdermal fentanyl is associated with slightly less constipation than oral opioids. Absorption is increased in the febrile patient. A heating pad should never be applied to the area where the patch is applied. Transdermal fentanyl is much more expensive than sustained-release morphine but less costly than methods that deliver parenteral opioids.

Once it is determined that switching from other routes of morphine administration to the patch is appropriate, the correct dosage for the patch must be calculated. If the patient uses an opioid other than morphine, conversion to milligrams of oral morphine is the first step. After determining how many milligrams of morphine (or morphine equivalents) the patient has been using over 24 hours, an initial dose of transdermal fentanyl can be calculated.

Pasaro (1997) suggests one method of calculating the initial dose of fentanyl: the patient's daily dose of morphine is divided by two. Thus, the equivalent of 400 mg morphine used per day would be equivalent to 200 g fentanyl per hour. Patients switched from morphine to fentanyl need to be assessed not only for pain and potential side effects but also for dependence, reflected by withdrawal symptoms, which may consist of shivering, a feeling of coldness, sweating, headache, and paresthesia (Puntillo, Casella et al., 1997). Patients may require short-acting opioids for breakthrough pain before the systemic fentanyl level reaches a therapeutic level.

These conversions and the conversion-type table in the transdermal fentanyl packet insert should be used only to establish the initial dose of fentanyl when the patient switches from oral morphine to fentanyl (and not vice versa). These tables and equations are not meant to be used to determine the dosages of oral morphine for a patient who has been receiving transdermal fentanyl. Many patients will not achieve satisfactory analgesia from the initial dose of transdermal fentanyl and will require an increase in their fentanyl dose to treat breakthrough pain. If the table or equation is used incorrectly to calculate a morphine dose, there is a risk of overdose. If the patient requires a change from transdermal fentanyl back to oral or intravenous morphine (as in the case of surgery), the patch should be removed and intravenous morphine supplied on an assessed need basis.

Before applying a new patch, the patient should be carefully checked for any older, forgotten patches. These should be discarded. Patches should be replaced every 72 hours.

Transmucosal Route

The person with cancer pain who is being cared for at home may be receiving continuous opioids using sustained-release morphine, hydromorphone, oxycodone, transdermal fentanyl, or other medications. These patients often experience short episodes of severe pain (eg, after coughing or moving), or they may experience sudden increases in their baseline pain resulting from a change in their condition. These periods, called breakthrough pain, can be well managed with an oral dose of a short-acting transmucosal opioid that has a rapid onset of action. Currently the only transmucosal opioid available is fentanyl, a lozenge on an applicator stick (often referred to as a lollipop by patients).

Currently the only approved and commercially available transmucosal opioid analgesic agents in a nasal spray form are butorphanol (Stadol) and fentanyl. Butorphanol is a complex medication that simultaneously acts to induce or promote (**agonist**) and inhibit or reverse (**antagonist**) opioid effects. It works like an opioid agonist and an opioid antagonist at the same time. Butorphanol in any form cannot be combined with other opioids (eg, for cancer breakthrough pain) because the antagonist component will block the action of the opioids the patient is already receiving. The principal use of this agent is for brief, moderate to severe pain, such as migraine headaches.

Intranasal fentanyl is useful in cancer-related breakthrough pain. Given in this form, analgesia is achieved within 5 to 10 minutes and was rated as achieving analgesia superior to oral morphine by 50% of patients in one study (Zeppetella, 2000).

Intraspinal and Epidural Routes

Infusion of opioids or local anesthetic agents into the subarachnoid space (intrathecal space or spinal canal) or epidural space has been used for effective control of pain in postoperative patients and those with chronic pain unrelieved by other methods. A catheter is inserted into the subarachnoid or the epidural space at the thoracic or lumbar level for administration of opioid or anesthetic agents (Fig. 13-9). With intrathecal administration, the medication infuses directly into the subarachnoid space and cerebrospinal fluid, which surrounds the spinal cord. With epidural administration, medication is deposited in the dura of the spinal canal and diffuses into the subarachnoid space. It is believed that pain relief from intraspinal administration of opioids is based on the existence of opioid receptors in the spinal cord.

Infusion of opioids and local anesthetic agents through an intrathecal or epidural catheter results in pain relief with fewer side effects, including sedation, than with systemic analgesia. Adverse effects associated with intraspinal administration include spinal headache resulting from loss of spinal fluid when the dura is punctured. This is more likely to occur in younger (less than 40 years of age) patients. The dura must be punctured with the intrathecal route, and dural puncture may occur inadvertently with the epidural route. When dural puncture inadvertently occurs, spinal fluid seeps out of the spinal canal. The resultant headache is likely to be more severe with an epidural needle because it is larger than a spinal needle, and therefore more spinal fluid escapes.

Although respiratory depression generally peaks 6 to 12 hours after epidural opioids are administered, it can occur earlier or up to 24 hours after the first injection. Depending on the lipophilicity (affinity for body fat) of the opioid injected, the time frame for respiratory depression can be short or long. Morphine is hydrophilic, and the time for peak effect is longer compared to fentanyl, which is a lipophilic opioid. All patients should be monitored closely for at least the first 24 hours after the first injection, longer if changes in respiratory status or level of consciousness occur. Opioid antagonist agents such as naloxone must be available for intravenous use if respiratory depression occurs.

The patient is also observed for urinary retention, pruritus, nausea, vomiting, and dizziness. Precautions must be taken to avoid infection at the catheter site and catheter displacement. Only medications without preservatives should be administered

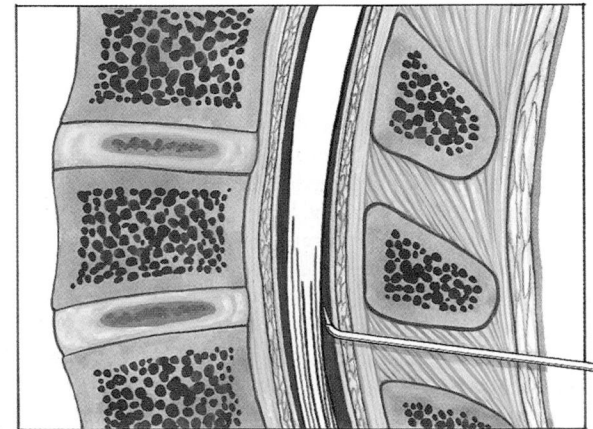
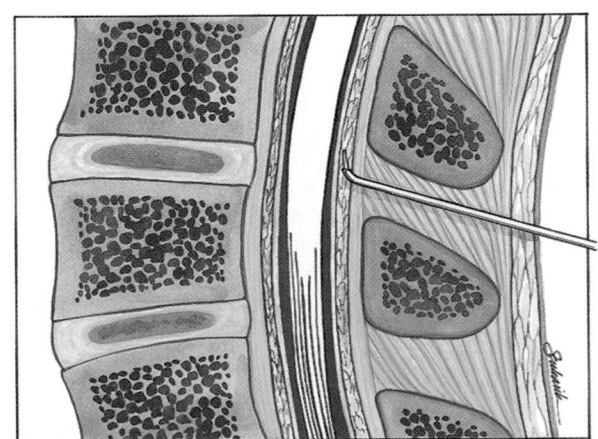

A   **B**

FIGURE 13-9 Placement of intraspinal catheters for administration of analgesic medications: (**A**) intrathecal route, (**B**) epidural route.

into the subarachnoid or epidural space because of the potential neurotoxic effects of preservatives.

During surgery, intrathecal opioids are used almost exclusively after a spinal anesthetic agent is administered. For patients undergoing large abdominal surgical procedures, especially those at risk for postoperative complications, a combination of a general inhaled anesthetic agent for the surgery and a local epidural anesthetic agent and epidural opioids administered after surgery results in excellent pain control with fewer postoperative complications.

Patients who have persistent, severe pain that fails to respond to other treatments, or those who obtain pain relief only with the risk of serious side effects, may benefit from medication administered by a long-term intrathecal or epidural catheter. After the physician tunnels the catheter through the subcutaneous tissue and places the inlet (or port) under the skin, the medication is injected through the skin into the inlet and catheter, which delivers the medication directly into the epidural space. The medication may need to be injected several times a day to maintain an adequate level of pain relief.

In patients who require more frequent doses or continuous infusions of opioid analgesic agents to relieve pain, an implantable infusion device or pump may be used to administer the medication continuously. The medication is administered at a small, constant dose at a preset rate into the epidural or subarachnoid space. The reservoir of the infusion device stores the medication for slow release and needs to be refilled every 1 or 2 months, depending on the patient's needs. This eliminates the need for repeated injections through the skin.

> **NURSING ALERT** An epidural catheter inserted for pain control is usually managed by the nurse. Baseline information necessary to provide safe and effective pain control includes the level or site of catheter insertion, the medications (eg, local anesthetic agents or opioids) that have been administered, and the medications anticipated in the future. The infusion rate is increased with caution when anesthetic agents are combined with opioids. Sensory deficits can occur and patients must be assessed frequently. An infusion with a lower concentration of anesthetic agent allows for administration of a greater concentration of the opioid with a lower risk of sensory deficits.

NURSING MANAGEMENT OF SIDE EFFECTS

Headache resulting from spinal fluid loss may be delayed. Therefore, the nurse needs to assess regularly for headache after either type of catheter is placed. Should headache occur, the patient should remain flat in bed and should be given large amounts of fluids (provided the medical condition allows), and the physician should be notified. An epidural blood patch may be carried out to reduce leakage of spinal fluid.

Cardiovascular effects (hypotension and decreased heart rate) may result from relaxation of the vasculature in the lower extremities. Therefore, the nurse assesses frequently for decreases in blood pressure, pulse rate, and urine output.

For patients experiencing urinary retention and pruritus, the physician may prescribe small doses of naloxone. The nurse administers these doses in a continuous intravenous infusion that is small enough to reverse the side effects of the opioids without reversing the analgesic effects. Diphenhydramine (Benadryl) may also be used to relieve opioid-related pruritus.

PROMOTING HOME AND COMMUNITY-BASED CARE

The patient who receives epidural analgesic agents at home and the family must be taught how to administer the prescribed medication using sterile technique and how to assess for infection. The patient and family also need to learn how to recognize side effects and what to do about them. Although respiratory depression is uncommon, urinary retention may be a problem, and patients and families must be prepared to deal with it if it occurs. Implanted analgesic delivery systems can be safely and confidently used at home only if health care personnel are available for consultation and, possibly, intervention on short notice.

NONPHARMACOLOGIC INTERVENTIONS

Although pain medication is the most powerful pain relief tool available to nurses, it is not the only one. Nonpharmacologic nursing activities can assist in relieving pain with usually low risk to the patient. Although such measures are not a substitute for medication, they may be all that is necessary or appropriate to relieve episodes of pain lasting only seconds or minutes. In instances of severe pain that lasts for hours or days, combining nonpharmacologic interventions with medications may be the most effective way to relieve pain.

Cutaneous Stimulation and Massage

The gate control theory of pain proposes that the stimulation of fibers that transmit nonpainful sensations can block or decrease the transmission of pain impulses. Several nonpharmacologic pain relief strategies, including rubbing the skin and using heat and cold, are based on this theory.

Massage, which is generalized cutaneous stimulation of the body, often concentrates on the back and shoulders. A massage does not specifically stimulate the non-pain receptors in the same receptor field as the pain receptors, but it may have an impact through the descending control system (see earlier discussion). Massage also promotes comfort because it produces muscle relaxation.

Ice and Heat Therapies

Ice and heat therapies may be effective pain relief strategies in some circumstances; however, their effectiveness and mechanism of action need further study. Proponents believe that ice and heat stimulate the non-pain receptors in the same receptor field as the injury.

For greatest effect, ice should be placed on the injury site immediately after injury or surgery. Ice therapy after joint surgery can significantly reduce the amount of analgesic medication required subsequently. Ice therapy may also relieve pain if applied later. Care must be taken to assess the skin prior to treatment and to protect the skin from direct application of the ice. Ice should be applied to an area for no longer than 20 minutes at a time. This prevents the rebound phenomenon that occurs as the body attempts to warm up, rendering the treatment useless. Long applications of ice may result in frostbite or nerve injury. Both ice and heat therapy must be applied carefully and monitored closely to avoid injuring the skin. Neither therapy should be applied to areas with impaired circulation or used with patients with impaired sensation.

Application of heat increases blood flow to an area and contributes to pain reduction by speeding healing. Both dry and moist heat may provide some analgesia, but their mechanisms of action are not well understood. Application of heat to inflamed joints, for example, may provide temporary comfort, but increasing the intra-articular temperature may impair healing (Oosterveld & Rasker, 1994a, 1994b).

Transcutaneous Electrical Nerve Stimulation

Transcutaneous electrical nerve stimulation (TENS) uses a battery-operated unit with electrodes applied to the skin to produce a tingling, vibrating, or buzzing sensation in the area of pain. It has been used in both acute and chronic pain relief and is thought to decrease pain by stimulating the non-pain receptors in the same area as the fibers that transmit the pain. This mechanism is consistent with the gate control theory of pain and explains the effectiveness of cutaneous stimulation when applied in the same area as an injury. For example, when TENS is used in a postoperative patient, the electrodes are placed around the surgical wound.

Another possible explanation for the effectiveness of TENS is the placebo effect (the patient expects it to be effective). In a review of the literature, Carroll, Tramer, McQuay et al. (1996) found that in 15 of 17 studies with randomized control group designs, TENS was ineffective in relieving postoperative pain. In 17 of 19 studies that did not use this design, the authors of these studies concluded that TENS had a positive analgesic effect. The review of these studies suggests that a placebo effect may explain the effectiveness of TENS.

Distraction

Distraction helps relieve both acute and chronic pain (Johnson & Petrie, 1997). Distraction, which involves focusing the patient's attention on something other than the pain, may be the mechanism responsible for other effective cognitive techniques. Distraction is thought to reduce the perception of pain by stimulating the descending control system, resulting in fewer painful stimuli being transmitted to the brain. The effectiveness of distraction depends on the patient's ability to receive and create sensory input other than pain. Distraction techniques may range from simple activities, such as watching TV or listening to music, to highly complex physical and mental exercises. Pain relief generally increases in direct proportion to the person's active participation, the number of sensory modalities used, and the person's interest in the stimuli. Therefore, the stimulation of sight, sound, and touch is likely to be more effective in reducing pain than is the stimulation of a single sense.

Visits from family and friends are effective in relieving pain. Watching an action-packed movie on a large screen with "Surround-Sound" through headphones may be effective (provided the person finds it acceptable). Others may benefit from games and activities (eg, chess) that require concentration. Not all patients obtain pain relief with distraction, especially those in severe pain. With severe pain, the patient may be unable to concentrate well enough to participate in complex physical or mental activities.

Relaxation Techniques

Skeletal muscle relaxation is believed to reduce pain by relaxing tense muscles that contribute to the pain. Considerable evidence supports relaxation as effective in relieving chronic low back pain (NIH Technology Assessment Panel, 1995). Few studies, however, support its effectiveness in reducing postoperative pain. This may be due to the relatively small role skeletal muscles play in postoperative pain, or to the need for the patient to practice the relaxation technique for it to be effective. Practicing the technique may not be possible when it is taught only once, immediately before surgery. A patient who already knows a technique for relaxing may only need to be reminded to use it to reduce or prevent increased pain.

A simple relaxation technique consists of abdominal breathing at a slow, rhythmic rate. The patient may close both eyes and breathe slowly and comfortably. A constant rhythm can be maintained by counting silently and slowly with each inhalation ("in, two, three") and exhalation ("out, two, three"). When teaching this technique, the nurse may count out loud with the patient at first. Slow, rhythmic breathing may also be used as a distraction technique. Relaxation techniques, as well as other noninvasive pain relief measures, may require practice before the patient becomes skilled in using them.

Almost all people with chronic pain can benefit from some method of relaxation. Regular relaxation periods may help to combat the fatigue and muscle tension that occur with and increase chronic pain.

Guided Imagery

Guided imagery is using one's imagination in a special way to achieve a specific positive effect. Guided imagery for relaxation and pain relief may consist of combining slow, rhythmic breathing with a mental image of relaxation and comfort. The nurse instructs the patient to close the eyes and breathe slowly in and out. With each slowly exhaled breath, the patient imagines muscle tension and discomfort being breathed out, carrying away pain and tension and leaving behind a relaxed and comfortable body. With each inhaled breath, the patient imagines healing energy flowing to the area of discomfort.

If guided imagery is to be effective, it requires a considerable amount of time to explain the technique and time for the patient to practice it. Usually, the patient is asked to practice guided imagery for about 5 minutes, three times a day. Several days of practice may be needed before the intensity of pain is reduced. Many patients begin to experience the relaxing effects of guided imagery the first time they try it. Pain relief can continue for hours after the imagery is used. The patient needs to be informed that guided imagery may work only for some people. Guided imagery should be used only in combination with all other forms of treatment that have demonstrated effectiveness.

Hypnosis

Hypnosis, which has been effective in relieving pain or decreasing the amount of analgesic agents required in patients with acute and chronic pain, may promote pain relief in particularly difficult situations (eg, burns). The mechanism by which hypnosis acts is unclear. Its effectiveness depends on the hypnotic susceptibility of the individual (Farthing, Venturino, Brown et al., 1997). In some cases, hypnosis may be effective in the first session, with effectiveness increasing in additional sessions. In other cases, hypnosis does not work at all. Usually, hypnosis must be induced by a specially skilled person (a psychologist or a nurse with specialized training in hypnosis). Sometimes patients learn to perform self-hypnosis.

Neurologic and Neurosurgical Approaches to Pain Management

In some situations, especially with long-term and severe intractable pain, usual pharmacologic and nonpharmacologic methods of pain relief are ineffective. In those situations, neurologic and neurosurgical approaches to pain management may be considered. Intractable pain refers to pain that cannot be relieved satisfactorily by the usual approaches, including medications. Such pain usually is the result of malignancy (especially of the cervix, bladder, prostate, and lower bowel), but it may occur in other conditions, such as postherpetic neuralgia, trigeminal neuralgia, spinal cord arachnoiditis, and uncontrollable ischemia and other forms of tissue destruction.

Neurologic and neurosurgical methods available for pain relief include (1) stimulation procedures (intermittent electrical stimulation of a tract or center to inhibit the transmission of pain impulses), (2) administration of intraspinal opioids (see previous discussion), and (3) interruption of the tracts conducting the pain impulse from the periphery to cerebral integration centers. The latter are destructive or ablative procedures, and their effects are permanent. Ablative procedures are used when other methods of pain relief have failed.

STIMULATION PROCEDURES

Electrical stimulation, or neuromodulation, is a method of suppressing pain by applying controlled low-voltage electrical pulses to the different parts of the nervous system. Electrical stimulation is thought to relieve pain by blocking painful stimuli (the gate control theory). This pain-modulating technique is administered by many modes. TENS and dorsal spinal cord stimulation are the most common types of electrical stimulation used. (See previous discussion of TENS.) In addition, there are also brain-stimulating techniques in which electrodes are implanted in the periventricular area of the posterior third ventricle, allowing the patient to stimulate this area to produce analgesia.

In spinal cord stimulation, a technique used for the relief of chronic, intractable pain, ischemic pain, and pain from angina, a surgically implanted device allows the patient to apply pulsed electrical stimulation to the dorsal aspect of the spinal cord to block pain impulses (Linderoth & Meyerson, 2002). (The largest accumulation of afferent fibers is found in the dorsal column of the spinal cord.) The dorsal column stimulation unit consists of a radiofrequency stimulation transmitter, a transmitter antenna, a radiofrequency receiver, and a stimulation electrode. The battery-powered transmitter and antenna are worn externally; the receiver and electrode are implanted. A laminectomy is performed above the highest level of pain input, and the electrode is placed in the epidural space over the posterior column of the spinal cord. (The placement of the stimulating systems varies.) A subcutaneous pocket is constructed over the clavicular area or some other site for placement of the receiver. The two are connected by a subcutaneous tunnel. Careful patient selection is necessary, and not all patients receive total pain relief.

Deep brain stimulation is performed for special pain problems when the patient does not respond to the usual techniques of pain control. With the patient under local anesthesia, electrodes are introduced through a burr hole in the skull and inserted into a selected site in the brain, depending on the location or type of pain. After the effectiveness of stimulation is confirmed, the implanted electrode is connected to a radiofrequency device or pulse-generator system operated by external telemetry. It is used in neuropathic pain that may occur with damage or injury that occurred following stroke, brain or spinal cord injuries, or phantom limb pain. Use of deep brain stimulation has decreased and may be related to improved pain control and intraspinal therapies (Rezai & Lozano, 2002).

Interruption of Pain Pathways

As described above, stimulation of a peripheral nerve, the spinal cord, or the deep brain using minute amounts of electricity and a stimulating device is used if all other pharmacologic and non-pharmacologic treatments fail to provide adequate relief. These treatments are reversible. If they need to be discontinued, the nervous system continues to function. Treatments that interrupt the pain pathways, however, are permanent.

Pain-conducting fibers can be interrupted at any point from their origin to the cerebral cortex. Some part of the nervous

system is destroyed, resulting in varying amounts of neurologic deficit and incapacity. In time, pain usually returns as a result of either regeneration of axonal fibers or the development of alternative pain pathways.

Destructive procedures used to interrupt the transmission of pain include cordotomy and rhizotomy. These procedures are offered if the patient is thought to be near the end of life and will have an improved quality of life as an outcome (Linderoth & Meyerson, 2002). Often these procedures can provide pain relief for the duration of a patient's life. The use of other methods to interrupt pain transmission is waning since the use of intraspinal therapies and newer pain management treatments are available.

CORDOTOMY

A cordotomy is the division of certain tracts of the spinal cord (Fig. 13-10). It may be performed percutaneously, by the open method after laminectomy, or by other techniques. Cordotomy is performed to interrupt the transmission of pain (Hodge & Christensen, 2002). Care must be taken to destroy only the sensation of pain, leaving motor functions intact.

RHIZOTOMY

Sensory nerve roots are destroyed where they enter the spinal cord. A lesion is made in the dorsal root to destroy neuronal dysfunction and reduce nociceptive input. With the advent of microsurgical techniques, the complications are few, with mild sensory deficits and mild weakness (Fig. 13-11).

Nursing Interventions

With each of these procedures, patients are provided with written and verbal instructions about their expected effect on pain and on possible untoward consequences. The patient is monitored for

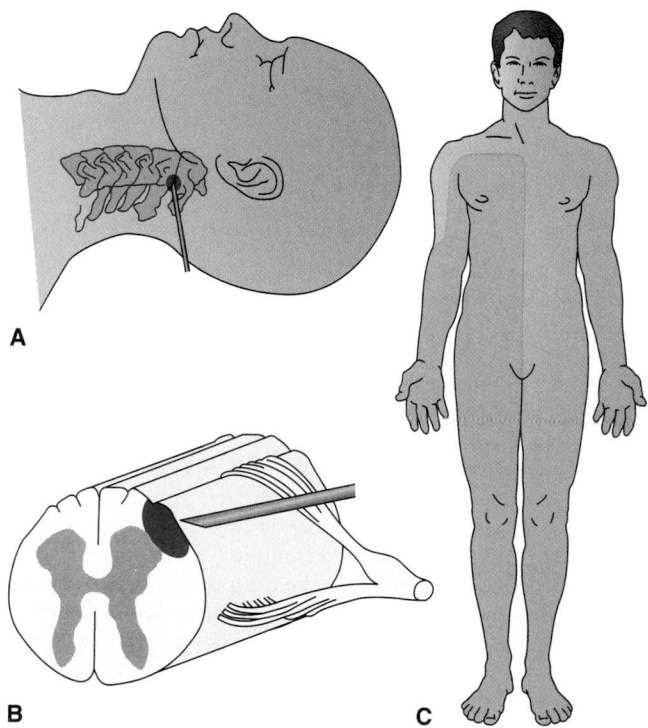

FIGURE 13-10 (**A**) Site of percutaneous C1–C2 cordotomy. (**B**) Lesion produced by percutaneous C1–C2 cordotomy. (**C**) Extent of analgesia produced by left C1–C2 percutaneous cordotomy.

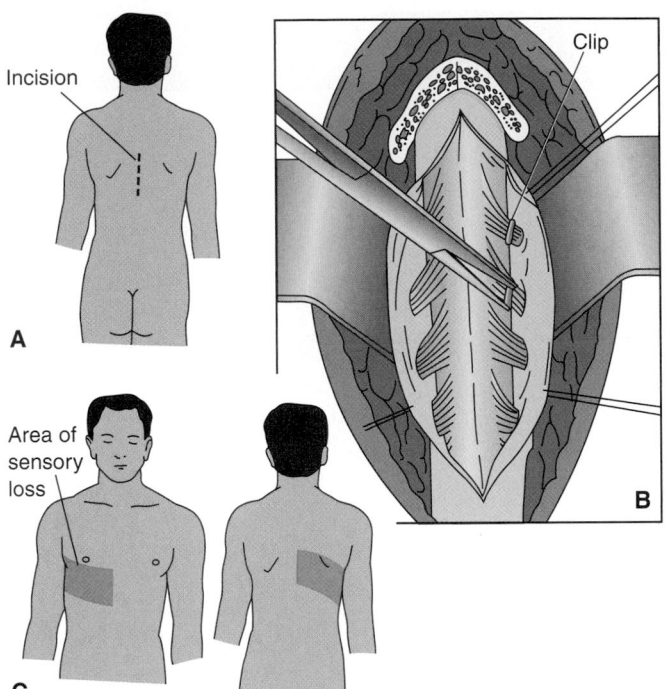

FIGURE 13-11 A rhizotomy may be performed surgically, percutaneously, or chemically, depending on a patient's condition and needs. The procedure is usually done to relieve severe chest pain, for example, from lung cancer. In (**A**) a surgical rhizotomy, (**B**) the spinal roots are divided and banded with a clip to form a lesion and subsequent (**C**) loss of sensation. Adapted with permission from Loeser, J. D. (ed.) (2000). *Bonica's management of pain* (3rd ed.). Philadelphia: Lippincott Williams & Wilkins.

specific effects of each method of pain intervention, both positive and negative. The specific nursing care of patients who undergo neurologic and neurosurgical procedures for the relief of chronic pain depends on the type of procedure performed, its effectiveness in relieving the pain, and the changes in neurologic function that accompany the procedure. After the procedure, the patient's pain level and neurologic function are assessed. Other nursing interventions that may be indicated include positioning, turning and skin care, bowel and bladder management, and interventions to promote patient safety. Pain management remains an important aspect of nursing care with each of these procedures.

ALTERNATIVE THERAPIES

People suffering chronic, debilitating pain are often desperate. Often they will try anything, recommended by anyone, at any price. Information about an array of potential therapies can be found on the Internet and in the self-help section of the bookstore. Therapies specifically recommended for pain from these sources include but are not limited to chelation, therapeutic touch, music therapy, herbal therapy, reflexology, magnetic therapy, electrotherapy, polarity therapy, acupressure, emu oil, pectin therapy, aromatherapy, homeopathy, and macrobiotic dieting. Many of these "therapies" (with the exception of macrobiotic dieting) are probably not harmful. However, they have yet to be proven effective by the standards used to evaluate the effectiveness of medical and nursing interventions. The National Institutes of Health has established an office to examine the effectiveness of alternative therapies.

Despite the lack of scientific evidence that these therapies are effective, a patient may find any one of them helpful via the placebo response. It is important when caring for a patient who is using or considering using untested therapies (often referred to as alternative therapies) not to diminish the patient's hope and potential placebo response. This must be weighed against the professional nurse's responsibility to protect the patient from costly and potentially harmful and dangerous therapies that the patient is not in a position to evaluate scientifically.

Problems arise when patients do not find relief but are deprived of conventional therapy because the alternative therapy "should be helping," or when patients abandon conventional therapy for alternative therapy. In addition, few alternative therapies are free. Desperate patients may risk financial ruin seeking alternative therapies that do not work.

The nurse's role is to help the patient and family understand scientific research and how that differs from anecdotal evidence. Without diminishing the placebo effects the patient may receive, the nurse encourages the patient to assess the effectiveness of the therapy continually using standard pain assessment techniques. In addition, the nurse encourages the patient using alternative therapies to combine them with conventional therapies and to discuss this use with the physician.

Promoting Home and Community-Based Care

In preparing the patient and family to manage pain at home, the patient and family need to be taught and guided about what type of pain or discomfort to expect, how long the pain is expected to last, and when the pain indicates a problem that should be reported. The person who has experienced acute pain as a result of injury, illness, procedure, or surgery will probably receive one or more prescriptions for analgesic medication.

TEACHING PATIENTS SELF-CARE

The patient and family need to understand the purpose of each medication, the appropriate time to use it, the associated side effects, and the strategies that can be used to prevent these problems. The patient and family often need reassurance that pain can be successfully managed at home.

Inadequate control of pain at home is a common reason people seek health care or are readmitted to the hospital. When chronic pain exists, anxiety and fear are often intensified at the time the patient is about to return home. The patient and family are instructed about the techniques for assessing pain, using pain assessment tools, and administering pain medications. These instructions are given verbally and in writing (Chart 13-6).

Opportunities are provided for the patient and family members to practice administering the medication until they are comfortable and confident with the procedure. They are instructed about the risks of respiratory and central nervous system depression associated with opioids and ways to assess for these complications. If the medications cause other predictable effects, such as constipation, the instructions include measures for preventing and treating the problem, as described earlier. Steps are taken to ensure that the needed medications are available from the local pharmacy so that the patient receives the medication when required.

Education for patients and families must stress the need for keeping analgesic agents away from children, who might mistake them for candy. Elderly patients may become lax about this because no children live in the home, but visiting children can be placed at risk. Additionally, analgesic agents must be kept away from other family members who may take them inadvertently.

Chart 13-6 • **PATIENT EDUCATION**
At-Home Pain Management Plan

Pain control plan for
_____

At home, I will take the following medicines for pain control:

Medicine	How to take	How many	How often	Comments
_____	_____	_____	_____	_____
_____	_____	_____	_____	_____
_____	_____	_____	_____	_____

Medicines that you may take to help treat side effects:

Side effect	Medicine	How to take	How many	How often	Comments
_____	_____	_____	_____	_____	_____
_____	_____	_____	_____	_____	_____

Constipation is a very common problem when taking opioid medications. When this occurs, do the following:
- Increase fluid intake (8 to 10 glasses of fluid).
- Exercise regularly.
- Increase fiber in the diet (bran, fresh fruits, vegetables).
- Use a mild laxative, such as milk of magnesia, if no bowel movement in 3 days.
- Take _____ every day at _____ (time) with a full glass of water.
- Use a glycerin suppository every morning (this may help make a bowel movement less painful).

Nondrug pain control methods:
_____
_____

Additional instructions:
_____
_____
_____

Important phone numbers:
Your doctor _____   Your nurse _____
Your pharmacy _____   Emergencies_____
Call your doctor or nurse immediately if your pain increases or if you have a new pain. Also call your doctor early for refill of pain medicines. Do not let your medicines get below 3 or 4 days' supply.
_____

Agency for Health Care Policy and Research. (1994). *Management of cancer pain.* Clinical Practice Guidelines. Rockville, MD: Agency for Health Care Policy and Research, Public Health Service, U.S. Department of Health and Human Services.

Further, analgesic medications should be stored safely and out of sight to prevent others from taking them for their own use or for diverting them to others.

CONTINUING CARE

If the patient is to receive parenteral or intraspinal analgesia at home, a referral to a home care nurse is indicated. The home care nurse makes a home visit to assess the patient and to determine if the pain management program is being implemented and if the technique for injecting or infusing the analgesic agent is being carried out safely and effectively. If the patient has an implanted infusion pump in place, the nurse examines the condition of the pump or injection site and may refill the reservoir with medication as prescribed or may supervise family members in the procedure. Any change in the patient's need for analgesic medications is assessed. In collaboration with the physician, the nurse then assists the patient and family in modifying the medication dose. These efforts enable the patient to obtain adequate pain relief while remaining at home and with family.

As tolerance develops, ever-increasing amounts of opioids are needed. It is important to assure the patient and family that slowly increasing doses will not cause an increased risk of respiratory depression and central nervous system depression, because the patient will become tolerant to these effects also. However, the patient will not become tolerant to the constipating effects of opioids and will require increased efforts to prevent constipation.

Evaluating Pain Management Strategies

An important aspect of caring for the patient in pain is reassessing the pain after the intervention has been implemented. The measure's effectiveness is based on the patient's assessment of pain, as reflected in pain assessment tools. If the intervention was ineffective, the nurse needs to consider other measures. If these are ineffective, the pain relief goals need to be reassessed in collaboration with the physician. The nurse serves as a patient advocate in obtaining additional pain relief.

REASSESSMENTS

After interventions have had a chance to work, the patient is asked to rate the intensity of pain. This assessment is repeated at appropriate intervals after the intervention and compared with the previous rating. These assessments indicate the effectiveness of the pain relief measures and provide a basis for continuing or modifying the plan of care. See the accompanying Plan of Nursing Care for more information.

Evaluation

EXPECTED PATIENT OUTCOMES

Expected patient outcomes may include:

1. Achieves pain relief
   a. Rates pain at a lower intensity (on a scale of 0 to 10) after intervention
   b. Rates pain at a lower intensity for longer periods
2. Patient or family administers prescribed analgesic medications correctly
   a. States correct dose of medication
   b. Administers correct dose using correct procedure
   c. Identifies side effects of medication
   d. Describes actions taken to prevent or correct side effects
3. Uses nonpharmacologic pain strategies as recommended
   a. Reports practice of nonpharmacologic strategies
   b. Describes expected outcomes of nonpharmacologic strategies
4. Reports minimal effects of pain and minimal side effects of interventions
   a. Participates in activities important to recovery (eg, drinking fluids, coughing, ambulating)
   b. Participates in activities important to self and to family (eg, family activities, interpersonal relationships, parenting, social interaction, recreation, work)
   c. Reports adequate sleep and absence of fatigue and constipation

Plan of Nursing Care
Care of the Patient With Pain

Nursing Diagnosis: Pain
Goal: Relief of pain or decrease in intensity of pain

Nursing Interventions	Rationale	Expected Outcomes
1. Reassure patient that you know pain is real and will assist him or her in dealing with it.	1. Fear that pain will not be accepted as real increases tension and anxiety and decreases pain tolerance.	• Reports relief that pain is accepted as real and that he or she will receive assistance in pain relief
2. Use pain assessment scale to identify intensity of pain.	2. Provides baseline for assessing changes in pain level and evaluating interventions	• Reports lower intensity of pain and discomfort after interventions implemented
3. Assess and record pain and its characteristics: location, quality, frequency, and duration.	3. Data assist in evaluating pain and pain relief and identifying multiple sources and types of pain.	• Reports less disruption from pain and discomfort after use of intervention
4. Administer balanced analgesics as prescribed to promote optimal pain relief.	4. Analgesics are more effective if administered early in pain cycle. Simultaneous use of analgesics that work on different portions of the nociceptive system will provide greater pain relief with fewer side effects.	• Uses pain medication as prescribed • Identifies effective pain relief strategies • Demonstrates use of new strategies to relieve pain and reports their effectiveness
5. Readminister pain assessment scale.	5. Permits assessment of effectiveness of analgesia and identifies need for further action if ineffective	• Experiences minimal side effects of analgesia without interruption to treat side effects
6. Document severity of patient's pain on chart.	6. Assists in demonstrating need for additional analgesic or alternative approach to pain management	• Increases interactions with family and friends
7. Obtain additional prescriptions as needed.	7. Inadequate pain relief results in an increased stress response, suffering, and prolonged hospitalizations.	
8. Identify and encourage patient to use strategies that have been successful with previous pain.	8. Encourages use of pain relief strategies familiar to and accepted by patient	
9. Teach patient additional strategies to relieve pain and discomfort: distraction, relaxation, cutaneous stimulation, etc.	9. Use of these strategies along with analgesia may produce more effective pain relief.	
10. Instruct patient and family about potential side effects of analgesics and their prevention and management.	10. Anticipating and preventing side effects enable the patient to continue analgesia without interruption because of side effects.	

Critical Thinking Exercises

1. An 82-year-old woman with cancer has been admitted to a skilled care facility from her home. Her son reports that his mother has become increasingly forgetful and is now unable to manage her medication regimen. He says that she would forget when she took her antidepressant pills and Oxy-Contin. She was so "doped up" that he couldn't bear to see her that way. She is being treated for cancer pain. Two weeks after admission, a pain assessment reveals a pain intensity of 8 on a 0 to 10 scale; she is refusing to get out of bed. Her son is with her and does not want the nurse to give the breakthrough medication or call the physician to titrate the OxyContin for maximal pain relief. Describe the strategies you would use to provide adequate pain management for this patient and the physiologic factors that need to be considered. Identify strategies that you would use to educate her son about her need for pain management. Identify the ethical issues involved in this situation.

2. A 45-year-old patient has just returned from the postanesthesia care unit (PACU) after a laparoscopic cholecystectomy. She has a history of rheumatoid arthritis for which she takes celecoxib (Celebrex) 200 mg bid. She rates her pain intensity from the recent surgery as a 6 (on a 0 to 10 scale) and is complaining of severe pain in multiple joints. Discuss the factors contributing to the pain that this patient is experiencing. What would be the best approach to manage her pain? Analyze the effect of her rheumatoid arthritis and joint pain on her postoperative pain and its management.

3. A 62-year-old man is receiving epidural infusions of an opioid for intractable pain. He will be discharged home, where his daughter will assist in his pain management. Describe the teaching required for the man and his daughter. What side effects should they observe for, and what actions should they take if they occur? How would you modify your discharge teaching plan if the patient lived alone?

4. A 35-year-old patient with a history of heroin use is admitted to the hospital with multiple stab wounds following an altercation. Two days after extensive surgery to repair his wounds, he reports severe, unrelenting pain and reports that the medication he is receiving (ie, an opioid) is ineffective in diminishing his pain. Several staff members believe that he does not have severe pain and only wants more medication because of his history of drug abuse. Describe how you would address pain relief in this patient, and provide rationale for your actions. How would you address the views of the staff members who believe that the patient should not receive additional medication?

REFERENCES AND SELECTED READINGS

Books

Agency for Health Care Policy and Research, Public Health Service, Department of Health and Human Services. (1992). *Acute pain management: Operative or medical procedures and trauma.* Clinical Practice Guidelines. (AHCPR 92-0032). Washington, DC: U.S. Government Printing Office.

Agency for Health Care Policy and Research, Public Health Service, Department of Health and Human Services. (1994). *Management of cancer pain: Adults.* Clinical Practice Guidelines (AHCPR 94-0592). Washington, DC: U.S. Government Printing Office.

American Cancer Society (2001). *American Cancer Society's guide to pain control: Powerful methods to overcome cancer pain.* Atlanta: American Cancer Society.

American Pain Society. (1999). *Principles of analgesic use in the treatment of acute pain and chronic cancer pain* (4th ed.). Skokie, IL: Author.

Benjamin, L. J., Dampier, C. D., Jacox, A., et al. (1999). *Clinical practice guideline for the management of acute and chronic pain in sickle cell disease.* American Pain Society Clinical Practice Guidelines series, No 1. Glenview, IL: American Pain Society.

Bonica, J. J. (2000). *The management of pain* (3d ed.). Philadelphia: Lea & Febiger.

Fillingim, R. B. (2000). *Sex, gender, and pain. Progress in pain research and management*, Vol. 17. Seattle: IASP Press.

Freeman, L. W., & Lawlis, G. F. (2001). *Mosby's complementary and alternative medicine: A research-based approach.* St. Louis: Mosby.

Gatchel, R. J., & Turk, D. C. (Eds.). (1999). *Psychosocial factors in pain.* New York: Guiliford.

Harden, R. N., Baron, R., & Janig, W. (2001). *Complex regional pain syndrome. Progress in pain research and management*, Vol. 22. Seattle: IASP Press.

Hodge, C. J., & Christensen, M. (2002). Anterolateral cordotomy. In K. J. Burchiel (Ed.). *Surgical management of pain.* New York: Thieme.

Janig, W. (2001). CRPS-I and CRPS-II: A strategic view. In R. N. Harden, R. Baron, & W. Janig (Eds.). *Complex regional pain syndrome. Progress in pain research and management*, 22. Seattle: IASP Press.

Joint Commission on Accreditation of Healthcare Organizations. (2003). *Hospital accreditation standards.* Oakbrook Terrace, IL: JCAHO.

Kuhn, M. A. (1999). *Complementary therapies for health care providers.* Philadelphia: Lippincott Williams & Wilkins.

Linderoth, B. & Meyerson, B. A. (2002). Spinal cord stimulation: Mechanisms of action. In K. Burchiel (Ed.). *Surgical management of pain.* New York: Thieme.

McCaffery, M., & Pasaro, C. (1999). *Pain: Clinical manual for nursing practice* (2d ed.). St. Louis: Mosby.

Merskey, H., & Bogduk, N. (Eds.). (1994). *Classification of chronic pain* (2nd ed). International Association for the Study of Pain Taskforce on Taxonomy. Seattle: IASP Press, pp. 209–214.

National Institutes of Health. *Integration of behavioral and relaxation approaches into the treatment of chronic pain and insomnia.* NIH Technology Assessment Statement, Oct. 16–18, 1995.

Porth, C. M. (2002). *Pathophysiology: Concepts of altered health states* (6th ed.). Philadelphia: Lippincott Williams & Wilkins.

Rezai, A. R., & Lozano, A. M. (2002). Deep brain stimulation for chronic pain. In K. J. Burchiel (Ed.). *Surgical management of pain.* New York: Thieme.

Salerno, E., & Willens, J. S. (1996). *Pain management handbook: An interdisciplinary approach.* St. Louis: C. V. Mosby.

Wall, P. D., & Melzack, R. (Eds). (1999). *Textbook of pain* (4th ed.). New York: Churchill Livingstone.

Wall, P. D. (1999). Introduction. In P. D. Wall & R. Melzack (Eds.). *Textbook of pain.* New York: Churchill-Livingstone, pp. 1–8.

Journals

Asterisks indicate nursing research articles.

Altmaier, E. M., Lehmann, T. R., Russell, D. W., et al. (1992). The effectiveness of psychological interventions for the rehabilitation of low back pain: A randomized controlled trial evaluation. *Pain, 49*(3), 329–335.

American Geriatrics Society Panel on Persistent Pain in Older Persons. (2002). The management of persistent pain in older persons. *Journal of the American Geriatrics Society.* 50, 1–20.

American Society of Pain Management Nurses. (1996). ASPMN position statement: Use of placebos for pain management. http://www.aspmn.org/html/Psplacebo.htm (accessed 1/8/02).

Anderson, R., Saiers, J. H., Abram, S., & Schlicht, C. (2001). Accuracy in equianalgesic dosing: Conversion dilemmas. *Journal of Pain and Symptom Management, 21*(5), 397–406.

Brookoff, D. (2000). Chronic pain: 1. A new disease? *Hospital Practice, 35*(7), 42–59.

Buffum, M., & Buffum, J. C. (2000). Nonsteroidal anti-inflammatory drugs in the elderly. *Pain Management Nursing, 1*(2), 40–50.

Campbell, J. (1995). Pain: The fifth vital sign. Presidential Address. American Pain Society, Nov. 11, 1995, Los Angeles.

Carroll, D., Tramer, M., McQuay, H., et al. (1996). Randomization is important in studies with pain outcomes: Systematic review of transcutaneous electrical nerve stimulation in acute postoperative pain. *British Journal of Anaesthesia, 77*(6), 798–803.

Cleeland, C. S., Gonin, R., Baez, L., et al. (1997). Pain and treatment of pain in minority patients with cancer. *Annals of Internal Medicine, 127*(9), 813–816.

*Conner, M., & Deane, D. (1995). Patterns of patient-controlled analgesia and intramuscular analgesia. *Applied Nursing Research, 8*(2), 67–92.

Correll, D. J., Viscusi, E. R., Grunwald, Z., & Moore, J. H. (2001). Epidural analgesia compared with intravenous morphine patient-controlled analgesia: Postoperative outcome measures after mastectomy with immediate TRAM flap breast reconstruction. *Regional Anesthesia Pain Medicine, 26* (5), 444–449.

Derby, S. A. (1999). Opioid conversion guidelines for managing adult cancer pain. *American Journal of Nursing, 99*(10), 62–65.

Donner, B., Zenz, M., Tryba, M., & Strumpf, M. (1996). Direct conversion from oral morphine to transdermal fentanyl: A multicenter study in patients with cancer pain. *Pain, 64*(3), 527–534.

Douglas, D. B. (1999). Hypnosis: Useful, neglected, available. *American Journal of Hospice and Palliative Care, 16* (5), 665–670.

DuPen, A. R., DuPen, S., Hansberry, J., et al. (2000). An educational implementation of a cancer pain algorithm for ambulatory care. *Pain Management Nursing, 1*(4), 116–128.

Edwards, R., Augustson, E. M., & Fillingim, R. (2000). Sex-specific effects of pain related anxiety on adjustment to chronic pain. *Clinical Journal of Pain, 16*(1), 46–53.

Edwards, R. R., & Fillingim, R. B. (2000). Age-associated differences in responses to noxious stimuli. *Journal of Gerontology Series A: Biological Science & Medical Science, 56*(3), M180–185.

Farthing, G. W., Venturino, M., Brown, S. W., & Lazar, J. D. (1997). Internal and external distraction in the control of cold-pressor pain as a function of hypnotizability. *International Journal of Clinical & Experimental Hypnosis, 45*(4), 433–446.

Fenstermaker, R. A. (1999). Neurosurgical invasive techniques for cancer pain: A pain specialist's view. *Current Review of Pain, 3*(3), 190–197.

Ferrell, B. A. (1995). Pain evaluation and management in the nursing home. *Annals of Internal Medicine, 123*(9), 681–687.

*Ferrell, B., Virani, R., Grant, M., & McCaffery, M. (2000). Analysis of pain content in nursing textbooks. *Journal of Pain and Symptom Management, 19*(3), 216–228.

Foley, K. M. (1999). Advances in cancer pain. *Archives of Neurology, 56*(4), 413–417.

Foster, N. E., Baxter, F., Walsh, D. M., et al. (1996). Manipulation of transcutaneous electrical nerve stimulation variables has no effect on two models of experimental pain in humans. *Clinical Journal of Pain, 12*(4), 301–310.

Fries, B. E., Simon, S. E., Morris, J. N., et al. (2001). Pain in U.S. nursing homes: validating a pain scale for the minimum data set. *Gerontologist, 41*(2), 173–179.

Gatchel, R. D., Polatin, P. B., Mayer, T. G., & Carcy, P. D. (1994). Psychopathology and the rehabilitation of patients with chronic low back pain disability. *Archives of Physical Medicine and Rehabilitation, 75*(6), 666–670.

Gordon, D. B., Pellino, T. A., Enloe, M. G., & Foley, D. K. (2000). A nurse-run inpatient pain consultation service. *Pain Management Nursing, 1*(2), 29–33.

Gordon, D. B., & Ward, S. E. (1995). Correcting patient misconceptions about pain. *American Journal of Nursing, 95*(7), 43–45.

Holleran, R. S. (2002). The problem of pain in emergency care. *Nursing Clinics of North America, 37*(1), 67–78.

Hicks, C. L., von Baeyer, C. L., Spafford, P. A., et al. (2001). The Faces Pain Scale-Revised: Toward a common metric in pediatric pain measurement. *Pain, 93*(2), 173–183.

Hrobjartsson, A., & Gotzsche, P. C. (2001). Is placebo powerless? An analysis of clinical trials comparing placebo with no treatment. *New England Journal of Medicine, 344*(21), 1594–1602.

Hunter, M., McDowell, L., Hennessy, R., & Cassey, J. (2000). An evaluation of the Faces Pain Scale with young children. *Journal of Pain and Symptom Management, 20*(2), 122–129.

Janig, W. (2001). CRPS-I and CRPS-II: A strategic view. In Harden, R. N., Baron, R., & Janig, W. (Eds.). *Complex regional pain syndrome. Progress in pain research and management,* Vol. 22. Seattle: IASP Press.

Johnson, M. H., & Petrie, S. M. (1997). The effects of distraction on exercise and cold presser tolerance for chronic low back pain sufferers. *Pain, 69*(1–2), 43–48.

Keefe, F. J., Lefebvre, J. C., & Starr, K. R. (1996). From the gate control theory to the neuromatrix: Revolution or evolution? *Pain Forum, 5*(2), 143–146.

Keefe, F. J., & Williams, D. A. (1990). A comparison of coping strategies in chronic pain in patients in different age groups. *Journal of Gerontology, 45*(4), 161–165.

Kelly, A. M. (1998). Does the clinically significant difference in visual analog scale pain scores vary with gender, age, or cause of pain? *Academy of Emergency Medicine, 5*(11), 1086–1090.

Keogh, E., Ellery, D., Hunt, C., & Hannent, I. (2001). Selective attentional bias for pain-related stimuli amongst fearful individuals. *Pain, 91*(1–2), 91–100.

*Knapp-Spooner, C., Karlik, B. A., Pontieri-Lewis, V., & Yarcheski, A. (1995). Efficacy of patient-controlled analgesia in women cholecystectomy patients. *International Journal of Nursing Studies, 32*(5), 434–442.

Lamberg, L. (1999). Patients in pain need round-the-clock care. *Journal of the American Medical Association, 281*(8), 689–692.

Lasch, K. E. (2000). Culture, pain and culturally sensitive pain care. *Pain Management Nursing, 1*(3), S1, 16–22.

Lasch, K. E., Wilkes, G., Montuori, L. M., et al. (2000). Using focus group methods to develop multicultural cancer patient education materials. *Pain Management Nursing, 1*(4), 129–138.

Li, S. F., Greenwald, P. W., Gennis, P., et al. (2001). Effect of age on acute pain perception of a standardized stimulus in the emergency department. *Annals of Emergency Medicine, 38*(6), 644–647.

Loeb, J. L. (1999). Pain management in long-term care. *American Journal of Nursing, 99*(2), 48–52.

Lynn, J., Teno, J. M., Phillips, R. S., et al. (1997). Perceptions by family members of the dying experience of older and seriously ill patients. *Annals of Internal Medicine, 126*(2), 97–106.

*Malek, C. J. (1996). Pain management: Documenting the decision-making process. *Nursing Case Management, 1*(2), 64–74.

Mayer, D. M., Torma, L., Byock, I., & Norris, K. (2001). Speaking the language of pain. *American Journal of Nursing, 101*(2), 44–49.

McCaffery, M., & Ferrell, B. R. (1997). Nurses' knowledge of pain assessment and management: How much progress have we made? *Journal of Pain Symptom Management, 14*(3), 175–188.

*McCaffery, M., Ferrell, B. R., & Pasaro, C. (2000). Nurses' personal opinions about patients' pain and their effect on recorded assessments and titration of opioid doses. *Pain Management Nursing, 1*(3), 79–87.

McCaffery, M., & Pasero, C. (2001). Stigmatizing patients as addicts. *American Journal of Nursing, 101*(5), 77–79.

McCracken, L. M., & Iverson, G. L. (2001). Predicting complaints of impaired cognitive functioning in patients with chronic pain. *Journal of Pain and Symptom Management, 21*(5), 392–396.

*McNeill, J. A., Sherwood, G. D., Starck, P. L., & Nieto, B. (2001). Pain management outcomes for hospitalized Hispanic patients. *Pain Management Nursing, 2*(4), 25–36.

Melzack, R. (1996). Gate control theory: On the evolution of pain concepts. *Pain Forum, 5*(1), 128–138.

Meuser, T., Pietruck, C., Radruch, L., Stute, P., Lehmann, K. A., & Grond, S. (2001). Symptoms during cancer pain treatment following WHO guidelines: A longitudinal follow-up study of symptom prevalence, severity and etiology. *Pain, 93*(3), 247–257.

Miaskowski, C. (2000). The impact of age on a patient's perception of pain and ways it can be managed. *Pain Management Nursing, 1*(3), S1, 2–7.

*Miaskowski, C., & Dibble, S. L. (1995). The problem of pain in outpatients with breast cancer. *Oncology Nursing Forum, 22*(5), 791–797.

Morin, C., Lund, J. P., Villarroel, T., et al. (2000). Differences between the sexes in post-surgical pain. *Pain, 85*(1–2), 79–85.

National Institutes of Health. (1997). Acupuncture. _NIH Consensus Statement, 15_(5), 1–34.

NIH Technology Assessment Panel on Integration of Behavioral and Relaxation Approaches into the Treatment of Chronic Pain and Insomnia. (1995). Integration of behavioral and relaxation approaches into the treatment of chronic pain and insomnia. _Journal of the American Medical Association, 276_(4), 313–318.

North, R., & Levy R. (1994). Consensus conference on the neurosurgical management of pain. _Neurosurgery, 34_(4), 756–760.

Oosterveld, F. G. & Rasker, J. J. (1994a). Effects of local heat and cold treatment on surface and articular temperature of arthritic knees. _Arthritis & Rheumatism, 37_(11), 1578–582.

Oosterveld, F. G. & Rasker, J. J. (1994b). Treating arthritis with locally applied heat or cold. _Seminars in Arthritis & Rheumatism, 24_(2), 82–90.

Panke, J. T. (2002). Difficulties in managing pain at the end of life. _American Journal of Nursing, 102_(7), 26–33.

Pasaro, C. L. (1997). Using the Faces scale to assess pain. _American Journal of Nursing, 97_(7), 19–20.

Pasaro, C., & McCaffery, M. (2001). The lidocaine patch. _American Journal of Nursing, 101_(3), 22–23.

Pasaro, C., & McCaffery, M. (2001). Selective COX-2 inhibitors. _American Journal of Nursing, 101_(4), 55–56.

Pasaro, C., & McCaffery, M. (2002). Monitoring sedation _American Journal of Nursing, 102_(2), 67–69.

Pasaro, C. (2002). Subcutaneous opioid infusion. _American Journal of Nursing, 102_(7), 61–62.

Pasaro, C., & Montgomery, R. (2002). Intravenous fentanyl. _American Journal of Nursing, 102_(4), 73–76.

Peloso, P. M. (2000). NSAIDs: A Faustian bargain. _American Journal of Nursing, 100_(6), 34–39.

Perez, R. S. G. M., Kwakkel, G., Zuurmond, W. W. A., & de Lange, J. J. (2001). Treatment of reflex sympathetic dystrophy (CRPS type I): A research synthesis of 21 randomized clinical trials. _Journal of Pain and Symptom Management, 21_(6), 511–526.

Perin, M. L. (2000). Corticosteroids for cancer pain. _American Journal of Nursing, 100_(4), 15–16.

Plaisance, L., & Ellis, J. A. (2002). Opioid-induced constipation. _American Journal of Nursing, 102_(3), 72–73.

Pollo, A., Amanzio, M., Arslanina, A., et al. (2001). Response expectancies in placebo analgesia and their clinical relevance. _Pain, 93_(1), 77–84.

Porter, J., & Jick, H. (1980). Addiction rare in patients treated with narcotics. _New England Journal of Medicine, 302_(2), 123.

Puig, M. M., & Montes, A. (1998). Opioids: From receptors to clinical application. _Current Review of Pain, 2_(4), 243–241.

*Puntillo, K., Casella, W., & Reid, M. (1997). Opioid and benzodiazepine tolerance and dependence: Application of theory to critical care practice. _Heart & Lung, 26_(4), 317–324.

*Puntillo, K. A., Miaskowski, C., Kehrle, K., et al. (1997). Relationship between behavioral and physiological indicators of pain, critical care patients' self-reports of pain, and opioid administration. _Critical Care Medicine, 25_(7), 1159–1166.

Raymond, I., Nielsen, T. A., Lauigne, G., et al. (2001). Quality of sleep and its daily relationship to pain intensity in hospitalized adult burn patients. _Pain, 92_(3), 381–388.

Rhiner, M., & Kedziera, P. (1999). Managing breakthrough pain. A new approach. _American Journal of Nursing, 99_(3), Supplement, 1–12.

Rhudy, J. L., & Meagher, M. W. (2000). Fear and anxiety: Divergent effects on human pain thresholds. _Pain, 84_(1), 65–75.

Riley, J. L., Robinson, M. E., Wade, J. B., et al. (2001). Sex differences in negative emotional response to chronic pain. _Journal of Pain, 2_(6), 354–359.

Robinson, M. E., Riley, J. L., Meyers, C. D., et al. (2001). Gender role expectations of pain. Relationship to sex differences in pain. _Journal of Pain, 2_(5), 251–257.

*Simpson, T., Lee, E. R., & Cameron, C. (1996). Relationships among sleep dimensions and factors that impair sleep after cardiac surgery. _Research in Nursing & Health, 19_(3), 213–223.

Slaughter, A., Pasaro, C., & Manworren, R. (2002). Unacceptable pain levels. _American Journal of Nursing, 102_(5), 75–77.

SUPPORT Principal Investigators. (1995). A controlled trial to improve care for seriously ill hospitalized patients: The study to understand prognoses and preferences for outcomes and risks of treatments (SUPPORT). _Journal of the American Medical Association, 274_(20), 1591–1598.

Thomas, T., Robinson, C., Champion, D., et al. (1998). Prediction and assessment of the severity of post-operative pain and of satisfaction with management. _Pain, 75_(2–3), 177–185.

Tucker, K. L. (2001). Deceptive placebo administration. _American Journal of Nursing, 101_(8), 55–56.

Uomoto, J. M., & Esselman, P. C. (1993). Traumatic brain injury and chronic pain: Differential types and rates by head injury severity. _Archives of Physical Medicine and Rehabilitation, 74_(1), 61–64.

Unruh, A. M., Ritchie, J., & Merskey, H. (1999). Does gender affect appraisal of pain and pain coping strategies? _Clinical Journal of Pain, 15_(1), 31–40.

Vallerand, A. H., & Polomano, R. C. (2000). The relationship of gender to pain. _Pain Management Nursing, 1_(3, suppl), 8–15.

Walker, B., Shafer, M., Henzi, I. & Tramer, M. R. (2002). Efficacy and safety of patient-controlled opioid analgesia for postoperative pain. A quantitative systematic review. _Acta Anaesthesiology Scandinavia, 45_(7), 795–804.

*Ward, S. E., Berry, P. E., & Misiewicz, H. (1996). Concerns about analgesia among patients and family caregivers in a hospice setting. _Research in Nursing & Health, 19_(3), 205–211.

Washington, L. L., Gibson, S. J., & Helme, R. D. (2000). Age-related differences in endogenous analgesic response to repeated cold water immersion in human volunteers. _Pain, 89_(1), 89–96.

*Watt-Watson, J., Garfinkel, P., Gallop, R., et al. (2000). The impact of nurses' empathetic responses on patients' pain management in acute care. _Nursing Research, 49_(4), 191–200.

Weiner, D., Peterson, B., Ladd, K., McConnell, E., & Keefe, F. (1999). Pain in nursing home residents: An exploration of prevalence, staff perspectives, and practical aspects of measurement. _Clinical Journal of Pain, 15_(2), 92–101.

*Zalon, M. L. (1997). Pain in frail, elderly women after surgery. _Image: Journal of Nursing Scholarship, 29_(1), 21–26.

Zeppetella, G. (2000). An assessment of the safety, efficacy, and acceptability of intranasal fentanyl citrate in the management of breakthrough pain: A pilot study. _Journal of Pain and Symptom Management, 20_(4), 253–258.

RESOURCES AND WEBSITES

American Academy of Pain Management, 13947 Mono Way #A, Sonora, CA 95370; (209) 533-9744; http://www.aapainmanage.org.

American Chronic Pain Association, P.O. Box 850, Rocklin, CA 95677; (800) 533-3231; http://www.theacpa.org.

American Pain Foundation, 201 N. Charles Street, Suite 710, Baltimore, MD 21201; (888) 615-7246; http://www.painfoundation.org.

American Pain Society, 4700 W. Lake Street, Glenview, IL 60025; (847) 375-4715; http://www.ampainsoc.org.

American Society of Pain Management Nurses, 7794 Grow Drive, Pensacola, FL 32514; (222) 34ASPMN; fax (850) 484-8762; http://www.aspmn.org.

International Pain Foundation, 909 NE 43rd St., Room 306, Seattle, WA 98105-6020; (206) 547-6409; fax (206) 547-1703; http://dasnetO2.dokkyomed.ac.ip/IASPM/IASP.html; e-mail: IASP@locke.hs. washington.ed.

Last Acts: an initiative for care and caring at the end of life. Includes "Innovations in End-of-Life Care," an international journal and on-line forum: http://www.lastacts.org.

National Hospice Organization, Suite 901, 1901 N. Moore St., Arlington, VA 22209; (703) 243-5900; http://www.nho.org.

"Pain Control," a monthly column in American Journal of Nursing.

Fluid and Electrolytes: Balance and Distribution

LEARNING OBJECTIVES

On completion of this chapter, the learner will be able to:

1. Differentiate between osmosis, diffusion, filtration, and active transport.

2. Describe the role of the kidneys, lungs, and endocrine glands in regulating the body's fluid composition and volume.

3. Identify the effects of aging on fluid and electrolyte regulation.

4. Plan effective care of patients with the following imbalances: fluid volume deficit and fluid volume excess; sodium deficit (hyponatremia) and sodium excess (hypernatremia); potassium deficit (hypokalemia) and potassium excess (hyperkalemia).

5. Describe the etiology, clinical manifestations, management, and nursing interventions for the following imbalances: calcium deficit (hypocalcemia) and calcium excess (hypercalcemia); magnesium deficit (hypomagnesemia) and magnesium excess (hypermagnesemia); phosphorus deficit (hypophosphatemia) and phosphorus excess (hyperphosphatemia); chloride deficit (hypochloremia) and chloride excess (hyperchloremia).

6. Explain the role of the lungs, kidneys, and chemical buffers in maintaining acid–base balance.

7. Compare metabolic acidosis and alkalosis with regard to causes, clinical manifestations, diagnosis, and management.

8. Compare respiratory acidosis and alkalosis with regard to causes, clinical manifestations, diagnosis, and management.

9. Interpret arterial blood gas measurements.

10. Demonstrate a safe and effective procedure of venipuncture.

11. Describe measures used for preventing complications of intravenous therapy.

Fluid and electrolyte balance is a dynamic process that is crucial for life. Potential and actual disorders of fluid and electrolyte balance occur in every setting, with every disorder, and with a variety of changes that affect well people (eg, increased fluid and sodium loss with strenuous exercise and high environmental temperature; inadequate intake of fluid and electrolytes) as well as those who are ill.

Fundamental Concepts

The nurse needs to understand the physiology of fluid and electrolyte balance and acid–base balance to anticipate, identify, and respond to possible imbalances in each. The nurse also must use effective teaching and communication skills to help prevent and treat various fluid and electrolyte disturbances.

AMOUNT AND COMPOSITION OF BODY FLUIDS

Approximately 60% of a typical adult's weight consists of fluid (water and electrolytes). Factors that influence the amount of body fluid are age, gender, and body fat. In general, younger people have a higher percentage of body fluid than older people, and men have proportionately more body fluid than women. Obese people have less fluid than thin people because fat cells contain little water.

Body fluid is located in two fluid compartments: the intracellular space (fluid in the cells) and the extracellular space (fluid outside the cells). Approximately two thirds of body fluid is in the intracellular fluid (ICF) compartment and is located primarily in the skeletal muscle mass.

The extracellular fluid (ECF) compartment is further divided into the intravascular, interstitial, and transcellular fluid spaces. The intravascular space (the fluid within the blood vessels) contains plasma. Approximately 3 L of the average 6 L of blood volume is made up of plasma. The remaining 3 L is made up of erythrocytes, leukocytes, and thrombocytes. The interstitial space contains the fluid that surrounds the cell and totals about 11 to 12 L in an adult. Lymph is an example of interstitial fluid. The transcellular space is the smallest division of the ECF compartment and contains approximately 1 L of fluid at any given time. Examples of transcellular fluid are cerebrospinal, pericardial, synovial, intraocular, and pleural fluids; sweat; and digestive secretions.

Body fluid normally shifts between the two major compartments or spaces in an effort to maintain an equilibrium between the spaces. Loss of fluid from the body can disrupt this equilibrium. Sometimes fluid is not lost from the body but is unavailable for use by either the ICF or ECF. Loss of ECF into a space that does not contribute to equilibrium between the ICF and the ECF is referred to as a third-space fluid shift, or "third spacing" for short.

An early clue of a third-space fluid shift is a decrease in urine output despite adequate fluid intake. Urine output decreases because fluid shifts out of the intravascular space; the kidneys then receive less blood and attempt to compensate by decreasing urine output. Other signs and symptoms of third spacing that indicate an intravascular fluid volume deficit include increased heart rate, decreased blood pressure, decreased central venous pressure, edema, increased body weight, and imbalances in fluid intake and output (I&O). Third-space shifts occur in ascites, burns, peritonitis, bowel obstruction, and massive bleeding into a joint or body cavity.

Electrolytes

Electrolytes in body fluids are active chemicals (cations, which carry positive charges, and anions, which carry negative charges). The major cations in body fluid are sodium, potassium, calcium, magnesium, and hydrogen ions. The major anions are chloride, bicarbonate, phosphate, sulfate, and proteinate ions.

These chemicals unite in varying combinations. Therefore, electrolyte concentration in the body is expressed in terms of milliequivalents (mEq) per liter, a measure of chemical activity, rather than in terms of milligrams (mg), a unit of weight. More specifically, a milliequivalent is defined as being equivalent to the electrochemical activity of 1 mg of hydrogen. In a solution, cations and anions are equal in mEq/L.

Electrolyte concentrations in the ICF differ from those in the ECF, as reflected in Table 14-1. Because special techniques are

Glossary

acidosis: an acid–base imbalance characterized by an increase in H^+ concentration (decreased blood pH). A low arterial pH due to reduced bicarbonate concentration is called metabolic acidosis; a low arterial pH due to increased PCO_2 is respiratory acidosis

active transport: physiologic pump that moves fluid from an area of lower concentration to one of higher concentration; active transport requires adenosine triphosphate (ATP) for energy

alkalosis: an acid–base imbalance characterized by a reduction in H^+ concentration (increased blood pH). A high arterial pH with increased bicarbonate concentration is called metabolic alkalosis; a high arterial pH due to reduced PCO_2 is respiratory alkalosis

diffusion: the process by which solutes move from an area of higher concentration to one of lower concentration; does not require expenditure of energy

hydrostatic pressure: the pressure created by the weight of fluid against the wall that contains it. In the body, hydrostatic pressure in blood vessels results from the weight of fluid itself and the force resulting from cardiac contraction.

hypertonic solution: a solution with an osmolality higher than that of serum

hypotonic solution: a solution with an osmolality lower than that of serum

isotonic solution: a solution with the same osmolality as serum and other body fluids. Osmolality falls within normal range for serum (280–300 mOsm/kg).

osmolality: the number of osmoles (the standard unit of osmotic pressure) per kilogram of solution. Expressed as mOsm/kg. Used more often in clinical practice than the term *osmolarity* to evaluate serum and urine. In addition to urea and glucose, sodium contributes the largest number of particles to osmolality.

osmolarity: the number of osmoles, the standard unit of osmotic pressure per liter of solution. It is expressed as milliosmoles per liter (mOsm/L); describes the concentration of solutes or dissolved particles.

osmosis: the process by which fluid moves across a semipermeable membrane from an area of low solute concentration to an area of high solute concentration; the process continues until the solute concentrations are equal on both sides of the membrane.

tonicity: the measurement of the osmotic pressure of a solution; another term for osmolality

ELECTROLYTES	MEQ/L
Extracellular Fluid (Plasma)	
Cations	
Sodium (Na)	142
Potassium (K)	5
Calcium (Ca++)	5
Magnesium (Mg++)	2
Total cations	154
Anions	
Chloride (Cl−)	103
Bicarbonate (HCO3−)	26
Phosphate (HPO4−−)	2
Sulfate (SO4−−)	1
Organic acids	5
Proteinate	17
Total anions	154
Intracellular Fluid	
Cations	
Potassium (K+)	150
Magnesium (Mg++)	40
Sodium (Na+)	10
Total cations	200
Anions	
Phosphates and sulfates	150
Bicarbonate (HCO3−)	10
Proteinate	40
Total anions	200

Table 14-1 • **Approximate Major Electrolyte Content in Body Fluid**

required to measure electrolyte concentrations in the ICF, it is customary to measure the electrolytes in the most accessible portion of the ECF, namely the plasma.

Sodium ions, which are positively charged, far outnumber the other cations in the ECF. Because sodium concentration affects the overall concentration of the ECF, sodium is important in regulating the volume of body fluid. Retention of sodium is associated with fluid retention, and excessive loss of sodium is usually associated with decreased volume of body fluid.

As shown in Table 14-1, the major electrolytes in the ICF are potassium and phosphate. The ECF has a low concentration of potassium and can tolerate only small changes in potassium concentrations. Therefore, release of large stores of intracellular potassium, typically caused by trauma to the cells and tissues, can be extremely dangerous.

The body expends a great deal of energy maintaining the high extracellular concentration of sodium and the high intracellular concentration of potassium. It does so by means of cell membrane pumps that exchange sodium and potassium ions. Normal movement of fluids through the capillary wall into the tissues depends on **hydrostatic pressure** (the pressure exerted by the fluid on the walls of the blood vessel) at both the arterial and the venous ends of the vessel and the osmotic pressure exerted by the protein of plasma. The direction of fluid movement depends on the differences in these two opposing forces (hydrostatic versus osmotic pressure).

In addition to electrolytes, the ECF transports other substances, such as enzymes and hormones. It also carries blood components, such as red and white blood cells, throughout the body.

REGULATION OF BODY FLUID COMPARTMENTS

Osmosis and Osmolality

When two different solutions are separated by a membrane that is impermeable to the dissolved substances, fluid shifts through the membrane from the region of low solute concentration to the region of high solute concentration until the solutions are of equal concentration; this diffusion of water caused by a fluid concentration gradient is known as **osmosis** (Fig. 14-1*A*). The magnitude of this force depends on the number of particles dissolved in the solutions, not on their weights. The number of dissolved particles contained in a unit of fluid determines the osmolality of a solution, which influences the movement of fluid between the fluid compartments. **Tonicity** is the ability of all the solutes to cause an osmotic driving force that promotes water movement from one compartment to another (Porth, 2002). The control of tonicity determines the normal state of cellular hydration and cell size. Sodium, mannitol, glucose, and sorbitol are effective osmoles (capable of affecting water movement). Three other terms are associated with osmosis: osmotic pressure, oncotic pressure, and osmotic diuresis.

- Osmotic pressure is the amount of hydrostatic pressure needed to stop the flow of water by osmosis. It is primarily determined by the concentration of solutes.
- Oncotic pressure is the osmotic pressure exerted by proteins (eg, albumin).
- Osmotic diuresis occurs when the urine output increases due to the excretion of substances such as glucose, mannitol, or contrast agents in the urine.

Diffusion

Diffusion is the natural tendency of a substance to move from an area of higher concentration to one of lower concentration (see Fig. 14-1*B*). It occurs through the random movement of ions and molecules. Examples of diffusion are the exchange of oxygen and carbon dioxide between the pulmonary capillaries and alveoli and the tendency of sodium to move from the ECF compartment, where the sodium concentration is high, to the ICF, where its concentration is low.

Filtration

Hydrostatic pressure in the capillaries tends to filter fluid out of the vascular compartment into the interstitial fluid. Movement of water and solutes occurs from an area of high hydrostatic pressure to an area of low hydrostatic pressure. Filtration allows the kidneys to filter 180 L of plasma per day. Another example of filtration is the passage of water and electrolytes from the arterial capillary bed to the interstitial fluid; in this instance, the hydrostatic pressure is furnished by the pumping action of the heart.

Sodium–Potassium Pump

As stated earlier, the sodium concentration is greater in the ECF than in the ICF, and because of this, sodium tends to enter the cell by diffusion. This tendency is offset by the sodium–potassium pump, which is located in the cell membrane and actively moves sodium from the cell into the ECF. Conversely, the high intracellular potassium concentration is maintained by pumping potassium into the cell. By definition, **active transport** implies that

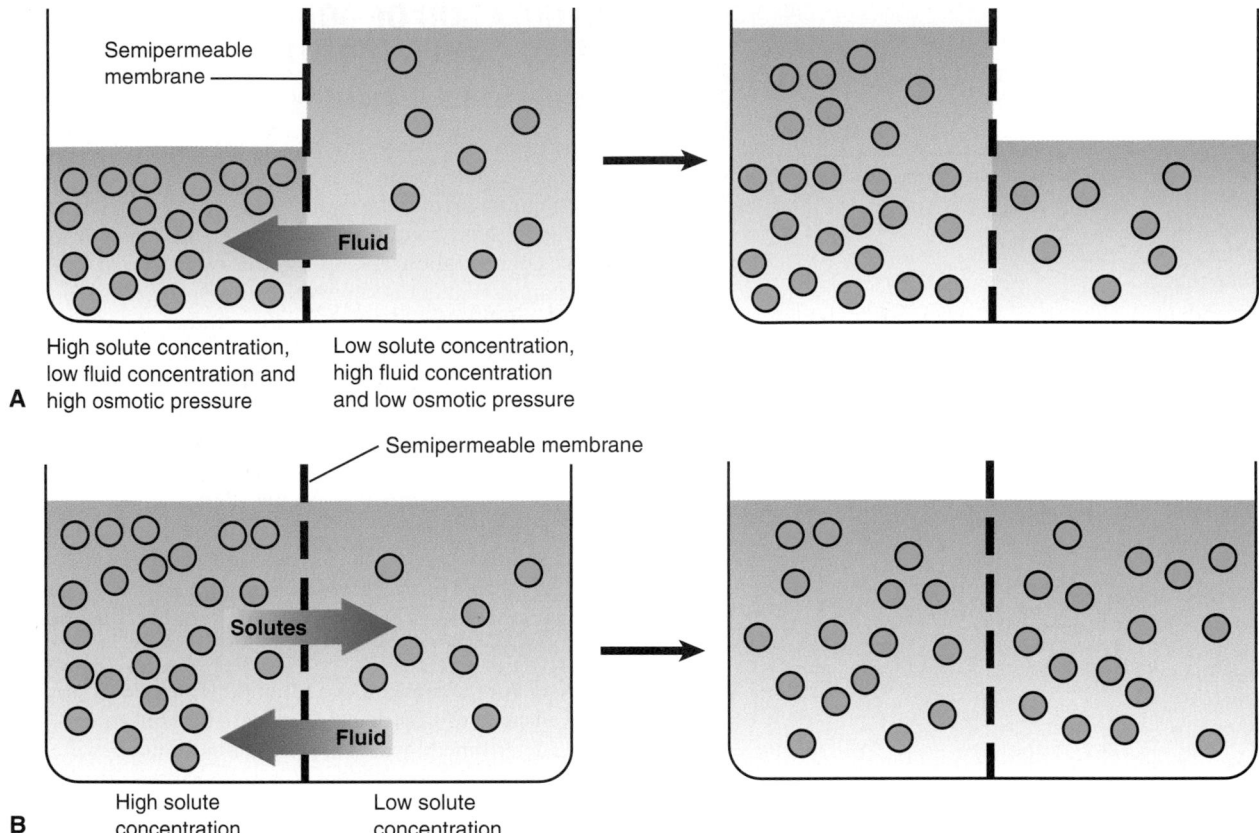

FIGURE 14-1 (**A**) Osmosis: movement of fluid to area of high solute concentration and eventual equalization of solute concentration. (**B**) Diffusion: movement of fluid and solutes and equalization of solute concentration.

energy must be expended for the movement to occur against a concentration gradient.

ROUTES OF GAINS AND LOSSES

Water and electrolytes are gained in various ways. A healthy person gains fluids by drinking and eating. In patients with some disorders, fluids may be provided by the parenteral route (intravenously or subcutaneously) or by means of an enteral feeding tube in the stomach or intestine.

 **NURSING ALERT** When fluid balance is critical, all routes of gain and all routes of loss must be recorded and all volumes compared. Organs of fluid loss include the kidneys, skin, lungs, and gastrointestinal (GI) tract.

Kidneys

The usual daily urine volume in the adult is 1 to 2 L. A general rule is that the output is approximately 1 mL of urine per kilogram of body weight per hour (1 mL/kg/h) in all age groups.

Skin

Sensible perspiration refers to visible water and electrolyte loss through the skin (sweating). The chief solutes in sweat are sodium, chloride, and potassium. Actual sweat losses can vary from 0 to 1,000 mL or more every hour, depending on the environmental

temperature. Continuous water loss by evaporation (approximately 600 mL/day) occurs through the skin as insensible perspiration, a nonvisible form of water loss. Fever greatly increases insensible water loss through the lungs and the skin, as does loss of the natural skin barrier (through major burns, for example).

Lungs

The lungs normally eliminate water vapor (insensible loss) at a rate of approximately 400 mL every day. The loss is much greater with increased respiratory rate or depth, or in a dry climate.

GI Tract

The usual loss through the GI tract is only 100 to 200 mL daily, even though approximately 8 L of fluid circulates through the GI system every 24 hours (called the GI circulation). Because the bulk of fluid is reabsorbed in the small intestine, diarrhea and fistulas cause large losses. In healthy people, the daily average intake and output of water are approximately equal (Table 14-2).

LABORATORY TESTS FOR EVALUATING FLUID STATUS

Osmolality reflects the concentration of fluid that affects the movement of water between fluid compartments by osmosis. Osmolality measures the solute concentration per kilogram in blood and urine. It is also a measure of a solution's ability to cre-

Table 14-2 • Average Daily Intake and Output in an Adult

INTAKE		OUTPUT	
Oral liquids	1,300 mL	Urine	1,500 mL
Water in food	1,000 mL	Stool	200 mL
Water produced	300 mL	Insensible	
by metabolism		Lungs	300 mL
		Skin	600 mL
Total gain*	2,600 mL	Total loss*	2,600 mL

*Approximate volumes

ate osmotic pressure and affect the movement of water. Serum osmolality primarily reflects the concentration of sodium. Urine osmolality is determined by urea, creatinine, and uric acid. When measured with serum osmolality, urine osmolality is the most reliable indicator of urine concentration. Osmolality is reported as milliosmoles per kilogram of water (mOsm/kg).

Osmolarity, another term that describes the concentration of solutions, is measured in milliosmoles per liter (mOsm/L). The term "osmolality," however, is used more often in clinical practice. Normal serum osmolality is 280 to 300 mOsm/kg, and normal urine osmolality is 250 to 900 mOsm/kg. Sodium predominates in ECF osmolality and holds water in this compartment.

Factors that increase and decrease serum and urine osmolality are identified in Table 14-3. Serum osmolality may be measured directly through laboratory tests or estimated at the bedside by doubling the serum sodium level or by using the following formula:

$$Na^+ \times 2 = \frac{Glucose}{18} + \frac{BUN}{3} = \text{Approximate value of serum osmolality}$$

The calculated value usually is within 10 mOsm of the measured osmolality.

Urine specific gravity measures the kidneys' ability to excrete or conserve water. The specific gravity of urine is compared to the weight of distilled water, which has a specific gravity of 1.000. The normal range of specific gravity is 1.010 to 1.025. Urine specific gravity can be measured at the bedside by placing a calibrated

hydrometer or urinometer in a cylinder of approximately 20 mL of urine. Specific gravity can also be assessed with a refractometer or dipstick with a reagent for this purpose. Specific gravity varies inversely with urine volume; normally, the larger the volume of urine, the lower the specific gravity. Specific gravity is a less reliable indicator of concentration than urine osmolality; increased glucose or protein in urine can cause a falsely high specific gravity. Factors that increase or decrease urine osmolality are the same for urine specific gravity.

Blood urea nitrogen (BUN) is made up of urea, an end product of metabolism of protein (from both muscle and dietary intake) by the liver. Amino acid breakdown produces large amounts of ammonia molecules, which are absorbed into the bloodstream. Ammonia molecules are converted to urea and excreted in the urine. The normal BUN is 10 to 20 mg/dL (3.5–7 mmol/L). The BUN level varies with urine output. Factors that increase BUN include decreased renal function, GI bleeding, dehydration, increased protein intake, fever, and sepsis. Those that decrease BUN include end-stage liver disease, a low-protein diet, starvation, and any condition that results in expanded fluid volume (eg, pregnancy).

Creatinine is the end product of muscle metabolism. It is a better indicator of renal function than BUN because it does not vary with protein intake and metabolic state. The normal serum creatinine is approximately 0.7 to 1.5 mg/dL (SI: 60–130 mmol/L); however, its concentration depends on lean body mass and varies from person to person. Serum creatinine levels increase when renal function decreases.

Hematocrit measures the volume percentage of red blood cells (erythrocytes) in whole blood and normally ranges from 44% to 52% for males and 39% to 47% for females. Conditions that increase the hematocrit value are dehydration and polycythemia; those that decrease hematocrit are overhydration and anemia.

Urine sodium values change with sodium intake and the status of fluid volume (as sodium intake increases, excretion increases; as the circulating fluid volume decreases, sodium is conserved). Normal urine sodium levels range from 50 to 220 mEq/24 h (50–220 mmol/24 h). A random specimen usually contains more than 40 mEq/L of sodium. Urine sodium levels are used to assess volume status and are useful in the diagnosis of hyponatremia and acute renal failure.

HOMEOSTATIC MECHANISMS

The body is equipped with remarkable homeostatic mechanisms to keep the composition and volume of body fluid within narrow limits of normal. Organs involved in homeostasis include the kidneys, lungs, heart, adrenal glands, parathyroid glands, and pituitary gland.

Kidney Functions

Vital to the regulation of fluid and electrolyte balance, the kidneys normally filter 170 L of plasma every day in the adult, while excreting only 1.5 L of urine. They act both autonomously and in response to blood-borne messengers, such as aldosterone and antidiuretic hormone (ADH). Major functions of the kidneys in maintaining normal fluid balance include the following:

- Regulation of ECF volume and osmolality by selective retention and excretion of body fluids
- Regulation of electrolyte levels in the ECF by selective retention of needed substances and excretion of unneeded substances

Table 14-3 • Comparison of Serum and Urine Osmolality

FLUID	FACTORS INCREASING OSMOLALITY	FACTORS DECREASING OSMOLALITY
Serum (275–300 mOsm/kg)	Free water loss Diabetes insipidus Sodium overload Hyperglycemia Uremia	SIADH Renal failure Diuretic use Adrenal insufficiency
Urine (250–900 mOsm/kg)	Fluid volume deficit SIADH HF Acidosis	Fluid volume excess Diabetes insipidus

SIADH, syndrome of inappropriate antidiuretic hormone; HF, heart failure.

- Regulation of pH of the ECF by retention of hydrogen ions
- Excretion of metabolic wastes and toxic substances

Given these functions, it is readily apparent that renal failure will result in multiple fluid and electrolyte problems. Renal function declines with advanced age, as do muscle mass and daily exogenous creatinine production. Thus, high-normal and minimally elevated serum creatinine values may indicate substantially reduced renal function in the elderly.

Heart and Blood Vessel Functions

The pumping action of the heart circulates blood through the kidneys under sufficient pressure to allow for urine formation. Failure of this pumping action interferes with renal perfusion and thus with water and electrolyte regulation.

Lung Functions

The lungs are also vital in maintaining homeostasis. Through exhalation, the lungs remove approximately 300 mL of water daily in the normal adult. Abnormal conditions, such as hyperpnea (abnormally deep respiration) or continuous coughing, increase this loss; mechanical ventilation with excessive moisture decreases it. The lungs also have a major role in maintaining acid–base balance. Changes from normal aging result in decreased respiratory function, causing increased difficulty in pH regulation in older adults with major illness or trauma.

Pituitary Functions

The hypothalamus manufactures ADH, which is stored in the posterior pituitary gland and released as needed. ADH is sometimes called the water-conserving hormone because it causes the body to retain water. Functions of ADH include maintaining the osmotic pressure of the cells by controlling the retention or excretion of water by the kidneys and by regulating blood volume (Fig. 14-2).

Adrenal Functions

Aldosterone, a mineralocorticoid secreted by the zona glomerulosa (outer zone) of the adrenal cortex, has a profound effect on fluid balance. Increased secretion of aldosterone causes sodium retention (and thus water retention) and potassium loss. Conversely, decreased secretion of aldosterone causes sodium and water loss and potassium retention.

Cortisol, another adrenocortical hormone, has only a fraction of the mineralocorticoid potency of aldosterone. When secreted in large quantities, however, it can also produce sodium and fluid retention and potassium deficit.

Parathyroid Functions

The parathyroid glands, embedded in the thyroid gland, regulate calcium and phosphate balance by means of parathyroid hormone (PTH). PTH influences bone resorption, calcium absorption from the intestines, and calcium reabsorption from the renal tubules.

Other Mechanisms

Changes in the volume of the interstitial compartment within the ECF can occur without affecting body function. The vascular compartment, however, cannot tolerate change as readily and must be carefully maintained to ensure that tissues receive adequate nutrients.

BARORECEPTORS

The baroreceptors are small nerve receptors that detect changes in pressure within blood vessels and transmit this information to the central nervous system. They are responsible for monitoring the circulating volume, and they regulate sympathetic and parasympathetic neural activity as well as endocrine activities. They are categorized as low-pressure and high-pressure baroreceptor systems. Low-pressure baroreceptors are located in the cardiac atria, particularly the left atrium. The high-pressure baroreceptors are nerve endings in the aortic arch and in the cardiac sinus. Another high-pressure baroreceptor is located in the afferent arteriole of the juxtaglomerular apparatus of the nephron.

As arterial pressure decreases, baroreceptors transmit fewer impulses from the carotid sinuses and the aortic arch to the vasomotor center. A decrease in impulses stimulates the sympathetic nervous system and inhibits the parasympathetic nervous system. The outcome is an increase in cardiac rate, conduction, and contractility and in circulating blood volume. Sympathetic stimulation constricts renal arterioles; this increases the release of aldosterone, decreases glomerular filtration, and increases sodium and water reabsorption.

RENIN–ANGIOTENSIN–ALDOSTERONE SYSTEM

Renin is an enzyme that converts angiotensinogen, an inactive substance formed by the liver, into angiotensin I. Renin is released by the juxtaglomerular cells of the kidneys in response to decreased renal perfusion. Angiotensin-converting enzyme (ACE) converts angiotensin I to angiotensin II. Angiotensin II, with its vasoconstrictor properties, increases arterial perfusion pressure and stimulates thirst. As the sympathetic nervous system is stimulated, aldosterone is released in response to an increased release of renin. Aldosterone is a volume regulator and is also released as serum potassium increases, serum sodium decreases, or adrenocorticotropic hormone increases.

ADH AND THIRST

ADH and the thirst mechanism have important roles in maintaining sodium concentration and oral intake of fluids. Oral intake is controlled by the thirst center located in the hypothalamus. As serum concentration or osmolality increases or blood volume decreases, neurons in the hypothalamus are stimulated by intracellular dehydration; thirst then occurs, and the person increases oral intake of fluids. Water excretion is controlled by ADH, aldosterone, and baroreceptors, as mentioned previously. The presence or absence of ADH is the most significant factor in determining whether the urine that is excreted is concentrated or dilute.

OSMORECEPTORS

Located on the surface of the hypothalamus, osmoreceptors sense changes in sodium concentration. As osmotic pressure increases, the neurons become dehydrated and quickly release impulses to the posterior pituitary, which increases the release of ADH. ADH travels in the blood to the kidneys, where it alters permeability to water, causing increased reabsorption of water and decreased urine output. The retained water dilutes the ECF and returns its concentration to normal. Restoration of normal osmotic pressure provides feedback to the osmoreceptors to inhibit further ADH release (see Fig. 14-2).

RELEASE OF ATRIAL NATRIURETIC PEPTIDE

Atrial natriuretic peptide (ANP) is released by cardiac cells in the atria of the heart in response to increased atrial pressure. Any dis-

Physiology/Pathophysiology

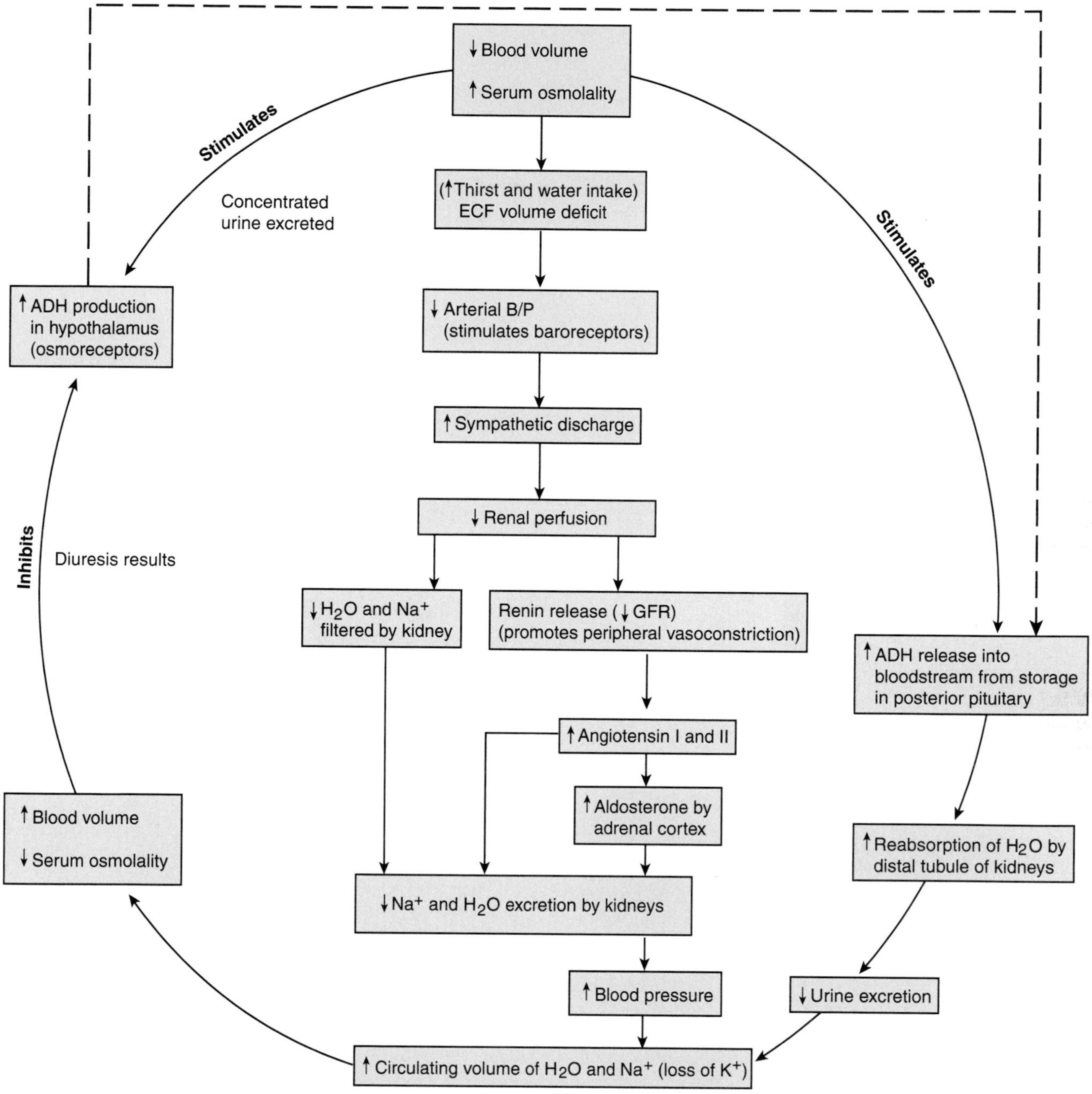

FIGURE 14-2 Fluid regulation cycle.

order that results in volume expansion or increased cardiac filling pressures (eg, high sodium intake, heart failure, chronic renal failure, atrial tachycardia, or use of vasoconstrictor agents) will increase the release of ANP. The action of ANP is the direct opposite of the renin–angiotensin–aldosterone system and decreases blood pressure and volume (Fig. 14-3). The ANP measured in plasma is normally 20 to 77 pg/mL (20—77 ng/L). This level increases in acute heart failure, paroxysmal atrial tachycardia, hyperthyroidism, subarachnoid hemorrhage, and small cell lung cancer.

The level decreases in chronic heart failure and with the use of medications such as urea (Ureaphil) and prazosin (Minipress).

Gerontologic Considerations

Normal physiologic changes of aging, including reduced renal and respiratory function and reserve and alterations in the ratio of body fluids to muscle mass, may alter the responses of an elderly person to fluid and electrolyte changes and acid–base disturbances. In

Physiology/Pathophysiology

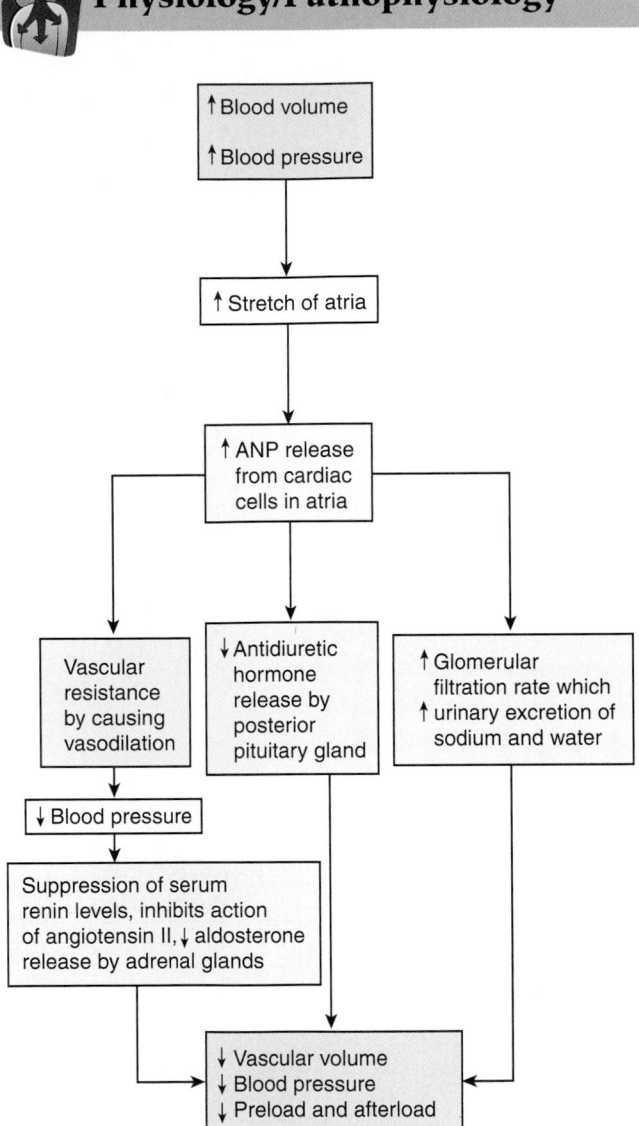

FIGURE 14-3 Role of atrial natriuretic peptide (ANP) in maintenance of fluid balance.

addition, the frequent use of medications in older adults can affect renal and cardiac function and fluid balance, thereby increasing the likelihood of fluid and electrolyte disturbances. Routine procedures, such as the vigorous administration of laxatives before colon x-ray studies, may produce a serious fluid volume deficit, necessitating the use of intravenous (IV) fluids to prevent hypotension and other effects of hypovolemia.

Alterations in fluid and electrolyte balance that may produce minor changes in young and middle-aged adults have the potential to produce profound changes in older adults, accompanied by a rapid onset of signs and symptoms. In other elderly patients, the clinical manifestations of fluid and electrolyte disturbances may be subtle or atypical. For example, fluid deficit or reduced sodium levels (hyponatremia) may cause confusion in the elderly person, whereas in young and middle-aged people the first sign commonly is increased thirst. Rapid infusion of an excessive volume of IV fluids may produce fluid overload and cardiac failure

in the elderly patient. These reactions are likely to occur more quickly and with the administration of smaller volumes of fluid than in healthy young and middle-aged adults because of the decreased cardiac reserve and reduced renal function that accompany aging.

Increased sensitivity to fluid and electrolyte changes in the elderly patient requires careful assessment, with attention to intake and output of fluids from all sources and to changes in daily weight; careful monitoring of side effects and interactions of medications; and prompt reporting and management of disturbances. Additional gerontologic considerations relating to specific fluid and electrolyte disturbances are discussed later in this chapter.

Fluid Volume Disturbances

FLUID VOLUME DEFICIT (HYPOVOLEMIA)

Fluid volume deficit (FVD) occurs when loss of extracellular fluid volume exceeds the intake of fluid. It occurs when water and electrolytes are lost in the same proportion as they exist in normal body fluids, so that the ratio of serum electrolytes to water remains the same. Fluid volume deficit (hypovolemia) should not be confused with the term *dehydration,* which refers to loss of water alone with increased serum sodium levels. FVD may occur alone or in combination with other imbalances. Unless other imbalances are present concurrently, serum electrolyte concentrations remain essentially unchanged.

Pathophysiology

FVD results from loss of body fluids and occurs more rapidly when coupled with decreased fluid intake. FVD can develop from inadequate intake alone if the decreased intake is prolonged. Causes of FVD include abnormal fluid losses, such as those resulting from vomiting, diarrhea, GI suctioning, and sweating, and decreased intake, as in nausea or inability to gain access to fluids (Beck, 2000).

Additional risk factors include diabetes insipidus, adrenal insufficiency, osmotic diuresis, hemorrhage, and coma. Third-space fluid shifts, or the movement of fluid from the vascular system to other body spaces (eg, with edema formation in burns or ascites with liver dysfunction), also produce FVD.

Clinical Manifestations

FVD can develop rapidly and can be mild, moderate, or severe, depending on the degree of fluid loss. Important characteristics of FVD include acute weight loss; decreased skin turgor; oliguria; concentrated urine; postural hypotension; a weak, rapid heart rate; flattened neck veins; increased temperature; decreased central venous pressure; cool, clammy skin related to peripheral vasoconstriction; thirst; anorexia; nausea; lassitude; muscle weakness; and cramps.

Assessment and Diagnostic Findings

Laboratory data useful in evaluating fluid volume status include BUN and its relation to the serum creatinine concentration. A volume-depleted patient has a BUN elevated out of proportion to the serum creatinine level (a ratio greater than 20:1). The cause of hypovolemia may be determined through the health history and physical examination. The BUN can be elevated due to dehydration or decreased renal perfusion and function. Also, the hematocrit level is greater than normal because the red blood cells become suspended in a decreased plasma volume.

Serum electrolyte changes may also exist. Potassium and sodium levels can be reduced (hypokalemia, hyponatremia) or elevated (hyperkalemia, hypernatremia).

- Hypokalemia occurs with GI and renal losses.
- Hyperkalemia occurs with adrenal insufficiency.
- Hyponatremia occurs with increased thirst and ADH release.
- Hypernatremia results from increased insensible losses and diabetes insipidus.

Urine specific gravity is increased in relation to the kidneys' attempt to conserve water and decreased with diabetes insipidus. Urine osmolality is greater than 450 mOsm/Kg, since the kidneys try to compensate by conserving water. Normal values for these tests are listed in Table 14-4.

 ## Gerontologic Considerations

Elderly patients have special nursing care needs because of their propensity for developing fluid and electrolyte imbalances (Beck, 2000; Kugler & Hustead, 2000). Fluid balance in the elderly patient is often marginal at best because of certain physiologic changes associated with the aging process. Some of these changes include reduction in total body water (associated with increased body fat content and decreased muscle mass); reduction in renal function, resulting in decreased ability to concentrate urine; de-creased cardiovascular and respiratory function; and disturbances in hormonal regulatory functions. Although these changes are viewed as normal in the aging process, they must be considered when the elderly person becomes ill because age-related changes predispose the person to fluid and electrolyte imbalances. These physiologic changes must be considered during assessment of the elderly patient as well as before initiating treatment for fluid and electrolyte imbalances.

Assessment of the elderly patient should be modified some-what from that of younger adults. For example, skin turgor is less valid in the assessment of elderly patients because their skin has lost some of its elasticity; therefore, other assessment measures (eg, slowness in filling of veins of the hands and feet) become more important in detecting FVD. In the elderly patient, skin turgor is best tested over the forehead or the sternum, because al-terations in skin elasticity are less marked in these areas. As in any patient, skin turgor should be monitored serially to detect subtle changes.

The nurse should perform a functional assessment of the aged person's ability to determine fluid and food needs and to obtain adequate intake. For example, is the patient mentally clear? Is the patient able to ambulate and use both arms and hands to reach fluids and foods? Is the patient able to swallow? All of these ques-tions have a direct bearing on how patients will be able to meet their own need for fluids and foods. During an elderly patient's hospital stay, the nurse must provide fluids for any patient who is unable to carry out self-care activities.

Table 14-4 • Laboratory Values Used In Evaluating Fluid and Electrolyte Status in Adults

TEST	USUAL REFERENCE RANGE	SI UNITS
Serum sodium	135–145 mEq/L	135–145 mmol/L
Serum potassium	3.5–5.3 mEq/L	3.5–5.3 mmol/L
Total serum calcium	8.6–10. mg/dL (approx. 50% in ionized form)	2.15–2.5 mmol/L
Serum magnesium	1.3–2.5 mEq/L	0.65–1.25 mmol/L
Serum phosphorus	2.5–4.5 mg/dL	0.87–1.45 mmol/L
Serum chloride	97–107 mEq/L	97–107 mmol/L
Carbon dioxide content	22–30 mEq/L	22–30 mmol/L
Serum osmolality	280–300 mOsm/kg H_2O	280–300 mmol/kg H_2O
Blood urea nitrogen (BUN)	5–20 mg/dL	1.8–7.1 mmol/L
Serum creatinine	Females: 0.5–1.1 mg/dL Males: 0.6–1.2 mg/dL	44–97 mmol/L 53–105 mmol/L
BUN to creatinine ratio	10:1–15:1	—
Hematocrit	Males: 42–52% Females: 35–47%	Volume fraction: 0.42–0.52 Volume fraction: 0.35–0.47
Serum glucose	70–105 mg/dL	3.9–5.8 mmol/L
Serum albumin	3.5–5.0 g/dL	3.5–5.0 g/L
Urinary sodium	75–220 mEq/day	75–220 mmol/day
Urinary potassium (intake-dependent)	25–123 mEq/day	25–123 mmol/day
Urinary chloride	110–250 mEq/24 h	110–250 mmol/24 h
Urine specific gravity	1.016–1.022	1.016–1.022
Urine osmolality	250–900 mOsm/kg H_2O	250–900 mmol/kg H_2O
Urinary pH	Random: 4.5–8.0 Typical urine <5–6	4.5–8.0 <5–6

Another concern is that some elderly patients deliberately restrict their fluid intake to avoid embarrassing episodes of incontinence. In this situation, the nurse also identifies interventions to deal with the incontinence, such as encouraging the patient to wear protective clothing or devices, carry a urinal in the car, or pace fluid intake to allow access to toilet facilities during the day. Elderly people without cardiovascular or renal dysfunction should be reminded to drink adequate fluids.

Medical Management

When planning the correction of fluid loss for the patient with FVD, the health care provider considers the usual maintenance requirements of the patient and other factors (such as fever) that can influence fluid needs. When the deficit is not severe, the oral route is preferred, provided the patient can drink. When fluid losses are acute or severe, however, the IV route is required. Isotonic electrolyte solutions (eg, lactated Ringer's or 0.9% sodium chloride) are frequently used to treat the hypotensive patient with FVD because they expand plasma volume. As soon as the patient becomes normotensive, a hypotonic electrolyte solution (eg, 0.45% sodium chloride) is often used to provide both electrolytes and water for renal excretion of metabolic wastes. These and additional fluids are listed in Table 14-5.

Accurate and frequent assessments of intake and output, weight, vital signs, central venous pressure, level of consciousness, breath sounds, and skin color should be performed to determine when therapy should be slowed to avoid volume overload. The rate of fluid administration is based on the severity of loss and the patient's hemodynamic response to volume replacement.

If the patient with severe FVD is not excreting enough urine and is therefore oliguric, the health care provider needs to determine whether the depressed renal function is the result of reduced renal blood flow secondary to FVD (prerenal azotemia) or, more seriously, to acute tubular necrosis from prolonged FVD. The test used in this situation is referred to as a fluid challenge test. During a fluid challenge test, volumes of fluid are administered at specific rates and intervals while the patient's hemodynamic response to this treatment is monitored (ie, vital signs, breath sounds, sensorium, central venous pressure, urine output).

A typical example of a fluid challenge involves administering 100 to 200 mL of normal saline solution over 15 minutes. The goal is to provide fluids rapidly enough to attain adequate tissue perfusion without compromising the cardiovascular system. The response by a patient with FVD but normal renal function will be increased urine output and an increase in blood pressure and central venous pressure.

Shock can occur when the volume of fluid lost exceeds 25% of the intravascular volume, or when fluid loss is rapid. Shock and its causes and treatment are discussed in detail in Chapter 15.

Nursing Management

To assess for FVD, the nurse monitors and measures fluid intake and output at least every 8 hours, and sometimes hourly. As FVD develops, body fluid losses exceed fluid intake. This loss may be in the form of excessive urination (polyuria), diarrhea, vomiting, and so on. Later, after FVD fully develops, the kidneys attempt to conserve needed body fluids, leading to a urine output of less than 30 mL/h in an adult. Urine in this instance is concentrated and represents a healthy renal response. Daily body weights are monitored; an acute loss of 0.5 kg (1 lb) represents a fluid loss of approximately 500 mL. (One liter of fluid weighs approximately 1 kg, or 2.2 lb.)

Vital signs are closely monitored. The nurse observes for a weak, rapid pulse and postural hypotension (ie, a drop in systolic pressure exceeding 15 mm Hg when the patient moves from a lying to a sitting position). A decrease in body temperature often accompanies FVD, unless there is a concurrent infection.

Skin and tongue turgor is monitored on a regular basis. In a healthy person, pinched skin immediately returns to its normal position when released. This elastic property, referred to as turgor, is partially dependent on interstitial fluid volume. In a person with FVD, the skin flattens more slowly after the pinch is released. When FVD is severe, the skin may remain elevated for many seconds. Tissue turgor is best measured by pinching the skin over the sternum, inner aspects of the thighs, or forehead.

NURSING ALERT The skin turgor test is not as valid in elderly people as in younger people because skin elasticity decreases with age; therefore, other assessment parameters must be considered.

Evaluating tongue turgor, which is not affected by age, may be more valid than evaluating skin turgor. In a normal person, the tongue has one longitudinal furrow. In the person with FVD, there are additional longitudinal furrows and the tongue is smaller, because of fluid loss. The degree of oral mucous membrane moisture is also assessed; a dry mouth may indicate either FVD or mouth breathing.

Urinary concentration is monitored by measuring the urine specific gravity. In a volume-depleted patient, the urinary specific gravity should be above 1.020, indicating healthy renal conservation of fluid.

Mental function is eventually affected in severe FVD as a result of decreasing cerebral perfusion. Decreased peripheral perfusion can result in cold extremities. In patients with relatively normal cardiopulmonary function, a low central venous pressure is indicative of hypovolemia. Patients with acute cardiopulmonary decompensation require more extensive hemodynamic monitoring of pressures in both sides of the heart to determine if hypovolemia exists.

PREVENTING FVD

To prevent FVD, the nurse identifies patients at risk and takes measures to minimize fluid losses. For example, if the patient has diarrhea, diarrhea control measures should be implemented and replacement fluids administered. These measures may include administering antidiarrheal medications and small volumes of oral fluids at frequent intervals.

CORRECTING FVD

When possible, oral fluids are administered to help correct FVD, with consideration given to the patient's likes and dislikes. Also, the type of fluid the patient has lost is considered, and attempts are made to select fluids most likely to replace the lost electrolytes. If the patient is reluctant to drink because of oral discomfort, the nurse assists with frequent mouth care and provides nonirritating fluids. The patient may be offered small volumes of fluids at frequent intervals rather than a large volume all at once. If nausea is present, antiemetics may be needed before oral fluid replacement can be tolerated.

If the patient cannot eat and drink, the nurse may need to administer fluid by an alternative route (enteral or parenteral) prescribed to prevent renal damage related to prolonged FVD.

Table 14-5 • Selected Water and Electrolyte Solutions

SOLUTION	COMMENTS
Isotonic Solutions	
0.9% NaCl (isotonic, also called normal saline) Na^+ 154 mEq/L Cl^- 154 mEq/L (308 mOsm/L) Also available with varying concentrations of dextrose (the most frequently used is a 5% dextrose concentration)	• An isotonic solution that expands the extracellular fluid volume, used in hypovolemic states, resuscitative efforts, shock, diabetic ketoacidosis, metabolic alkalosis, hypercalcemia, mild Na^+ deficit • Supplies an excess of Na^+ and Cl^-; can cause fluid volume excess and hyperchloremic acidosis if used in excessive volumes, particularly in patients with compromised renal function, heart failure, or edema • Not desirable as a routine maintenance solution, as it provides only Na^+ and Cl^- (and these are provided in excessive amounts) • When mixed with 5% dextrose, the resulting solution becomes hypertonic in relation to plasma and, in addition to the above described electrolytes, provides 170 calories/L • Only solution that may be administered with blood products
Lactated Ringer's solution (Hartmann's solution) Na^+ 130 mEq/L K^+ 4 mEq/L Ca^{++} 3 mEq/L Cl^- 109 mEq/L Lactate (metabolized to bicarbonate) 28 mEq/L (274 mOsm/L) Also available with varying concentrations of dextrose (the most common is 5% dextrose)	• An isotonic solution that contains multiple electrolytes in roughly the same concentration as found in plasma (note that solution is lacking in Mg^{++}): provides 9 calories/L • Used in the treatment of hypovolemia, burns, fluid lost as bile or diarrhea, and for acute blood loss replacement • Lactate is rapidly metabolized into HCO_3^- in the body. Lactated Ringer's solution should not be used in lactic acidosis because the ability to convert lactate into HCO_3^- is impaired in this disorder. • Not to be given with a pH > 7.5, as bicarbonate is formed as lactate breaks down, causing alkalosis • Should not be used in renal failure because it contains potassium and can cause hyperkalemia • Similar to plasma
5% dextrose in water (D_5W) No electrolytes 50 g of dextrose	• An isotonic solution that supplies 170 calories/L and free water to aid in renal excretion of solutes • Used in treatment of hypernatremia, fluid loss, and dehydration • Should not be used in excessive volumes in the early postoperative period (when ADH secretion is increased due to stress reaction) • Should not be used solely in treatment of fluid volume deficit, because it dilutes plasma electrolyte concentrations • Contraindicated in head injury because it may cause increased intracranial pressure • Should not be used for fluid resuscitation as it can cause hyperglycemia • Should be used with caution in patients with renal or cardiac disease because of risk of fluid overload • Electrolyte-free solutions may cause peripheral circulatory collapse, anuria in patients with sodium deficiency, and increased body fluid loss. • Converts to hypotonic solution as dextrose is metabolized by body. Over time, D_5W without NaCl can cause water intoxication (intracellular FVE) as the solution is hypotonic.
Hypotonic Solutions	
0.45% NaCl (half-strength saline) Na^+ 77 mEq/L Cl^- 77 mEq/L (154 mOsm/L) Also available with varying concentrations of dextrose (the most common is a 5% concentration)	• Provides Na^+, Cl^-, and free water • Free water is desirable to aid the kidneys in elimination of solute. • Lacking in electrolytes other than Na^+ and Cl^- • When mixed with 5% dextrose, the solution becomes slightly hypertonic to plasma and in addition to the above-described electrolytes provides 170 calories. • Used to treat hypertonic dehydration, Na^+ and Cl^- depletion, and gastric fluid loss • Not indicated for third-space fluid shifts or increased intracranial pressure • Administer cautiously, as it can cause fluid shifts from vascular system into cells, resulting in cardiovascular collapse and increased intracranial pressure.
Hypertonic Solutions	
3% NaCl (hypertonic saline) Na^+ 513 mEq/L Cl^- 513 mEq/L (1,026 mOsm/L)	• Highly hypertonic solution used only in critical situations to treat hyponatremia • Must be administered slowly and cautiously, as it can cause intravascular volume overload and pulmonary edema • Supplies no calories • Assists in removing intracellular fluid excess
5% NaCL (hypertonic solution) Na^+ 855 mEq/L Cl^- 855 mEq/L (1,710 mOsm/L)	• Highly hypertonic solution used to treat symptomatic hyponatremia • Administered slowly and cautiously, as it can cause intravascular volume overload and pulmonary edema • Supplies no calories
Colloid Solutions	
Dextran 40 in NS or 5% D_5W	• Colloid solution used as volume/plasma expander for intravascular part of ECF • Affects clotting by coating platelets and decreasing ability to clot • Remains in circulatory system for 6 hours • Used to treat hypovolemia in early shock to increase pulse pressure, cardiac output, and arterial blood pressure • Improves microcirculation by decreasing RBC aggregation • Contraindicated in hemorrhage, thrombocytopenia, renal disease, and severe dehydration

FLUID VOLUME EXCESS (HYPERVOLEMIA)

Fluid volume excess (FVE) refers to an isotonic expansion of the ECF caused by the abnormal retention of water and sodium in approximately the same proportions in which they normally exist in the ECF. It is always secondary to an increase in the total body sodium content, which, in turn, leads to an increase in total body water. Because there is isotonic retention of body substances, the serum sodium concentration remains essentially normal.

Pathophysiology

FVE may be related to simple fluid overload or diminished function of the homeostatic mechanisms responsible for regulating fluid balance. Contributing factors can include heart failure, renal failure, and cirrhosis of the liver. Another contributing factor is consumption of excessive amounts of table or other sodium salts. Excessive administration of sodium-containing fluids in a patient with impaired regulatory mechanisms may predispose him or her to a serious FVE as well (Beck, 2000).

Clinical Manifestations

Clinical manifestations of FVE stem from expansion of the ECF and include edema, distended neck veins, and crackles (abnormal lung sounds). Other manifestations include tachycardia; increased blood pressure, pulse pressure, and central venous pressure; increased weight; increased urine output; and shortness of breath and wheezing.

Assessment and Diagnostic Findings

Laboratory data useful in diagnosing FVE include BUN and hematocrit levels. In FVE, both of these values may be decreased because of plasma dilution. Other causes for abnormalities in these values include low protein intake and anemia. In chronic renal failure, both serum osmolality and the sodium level are decreased due to excessive retention of water. The urine sodium level is increased if the kidneys are attempting to excrete excess volume. Chest x-rays may reveal pulmonary congestion. Hypervolemia occurs when aldosterone is chronically stimulated (ie, cirrhosis, heart failure, and nephrotic syndrome). Urine sodium levels, therefore, will not rise in these conditions.

Medical Management

Management of FVE is directed at the causes. When the fluid excess is related to excessive administration of sodium-containing fluids, discontinuing the infusion may be all that is needed. Symptomatic treatment consists of administering diuretics and restricting fluids and sodium.

PHARMACOLOGIC THERAPY

Diuretics are prescribed when dietary restriction of sodium alone is insufficient to reduce edema by inhibiting the reabsorption of sodium and water by the kidneys. The choice of diuretic is based on the severity of the hypervolemic state, the degree of impairment of renal function, and the potency of the diuretic. Thiazide diuretics block sodium reabsorption in the distal tubule, where only 5% to 10% of filtered sodium is reabsorbed. Loop diuretics, such as furosemide (Lasix), bumetanide (Bumex), or torsemide (Demadex), can cause a greater loss of both sodium and water because they block sodium reabsorption in the ascending limb of the loop of Henle, where 20% to 30% of filtered sodium is normally reabsorbed. Generally, thiazide diuretics, such as hydrochlorothiazide (HydroDIURIL), trichlormethiazide (Diurese), and methyclothiazide (Enduron), are prescribed for mild to moderate hypervolemia and loop diuretics for severe hypervolemia.

Electrolyte imbalances may result from the effect of the diuretic. Hypokalemia can occur with all diuretics except those that work in the last distal tubule of the nephrons (eg, spironolactone). Potassium supplements can be prescribed to avoid this complication. Hyperkalemia can occur with diuretics that work in the last distal tubule, especially in patients with decreased renal function. Hyponatremia occurs with diuresis due to increased release of ADH secondary to reduction in circulating volume. Decreased magnesium levels occur with administration of loop and thiazide diuretics due to decreased reabsorption and increased excretion of magnesium by the kidney.

Azotemia (increased nitrogen levels in the blood) can occur with FVE when urea and creatinine are not excreted due to decreased perfusion by the kidneys and decreased excretion of wastes. High uric acid levels (hyperuricemia) can also occur from increased reabsorption and decreased excretion of uric acid by the kidneys.

HEMODIALYSIS

When renal function is so severely impaired that pharmacologic agents cannot act efficiently, other modalities are considered to remove sodium and fluid from the body. Hemodialysis or peritoneal dialysis may be used to remove nitrogenous wastes and control potassium and acid–base balance, and to remove sodium and fluid. Continuous renal replacement therapy may also be considered. See Chapter 44 for discussion of these treatment modalities.

NUTRITIONAL THERAPY

Treatment of FVE usually involves dietary restriction of sodium. An average daily diet not restricted in sodium contains 6 to 15 g of salt, whereas low-sodium diets can range from a mild restriction to as little as 250 mg of sodium per day, depending on the patient's needs. A mild sodium-restricted diet allows only light salting of food (about half the amount as usual) in cooking and at the table, and no addition of salt to commercially prepared foods that are already seasoned. Of course, foods high in sodium must be avoided. It is the sodium salt, sodium chloride, rather than sodium itself that contributes to edema. Therefore, patients need to read food labels carefully to determine salt content.

Because about half of ingested sodium is in the form of seasoning, seasoning substitutes can play a major role in decreasing sodium intake. Lemon juice, onions, and garlic are excellent substitute flavorings, although some patients prefer salt substitutes. Most salt substitutes contain potassium and must therefore be used cautiously by patients taking potassium-sparing diuretics (eg, spironolactone, triamterene, amiloride). They should not be used at all in conditions associated with potassium retention, such as advanced renal disease. Salt substitutes containing ammonium chloride can be harmful to patients with liver damage.

In some communities, the drinking water may contain too much sodium for a sodium-restricted diet. Depending on its source, water may contain as little as 1 mg or more than 1,500 mg per quart. Patients may need to use distilled water when the local water supply is very high in sodium. Also, patients on sodium-restricted diets should be cautioned to avoid water softeners that add sodium to water in exchange for other ions, such as calcium.

Nursing Management

To assess for FVE, the nurse measures intake and output at regular intervals to identify excessive fluid retention. The patient is weighed daily and acute weight gain is noted. An acute weight gain of 0.9 kg (about 2 lb) represents a gain of approximately 1 L of fluid. The nurse also needs to assess breath sounds at regular intervals in at-risk patients, particularly when parenteral fluids are being administered. The nurse monitors the degree of edema in the most dependent parts of the body, such as the feet and ankles in ambulatory patients and the sacral region in bedridden patients. The degree of pitting edema is assessed, and the extent of peripheral edema is monitored by measuring the circumference of the extremity with a tape marked in millimeters.

PREVENTING FVE

Specific interventions vary somewhat with the underlying condition and the degree of FVE. Most patients, however, require sodium-restricted diets in some form, and adherence to the prescribed diet is encouraged. The patient is instructed to avoid over-the-counter medications without first checking with a health care provider because these substances may contain sodium. When fluid retention persists despite adherence to a prescribed diet, hidden sources of sodium, such as the water supply or use of water softeners, should be considered.

DETECTING AND CONTROLLING FVE

Detecting FVE is of primary importance before the condition becomes critical. Interventions include promoting rest, restricting sodium intake, monitoring parenteral fluid therapy, and administering appropriate medications.

Some patients benefit from regular rest periods, as bed rest favors diuresis of edema fluid. The mechanism is probably related to diminished venous pooling and the subsequent increase in effective circulating blood volume and renal perfusion. Sodium and fluid restriction should be instituted as indicated. Because most patients with FVE require diuretics, the patient's response to these agents is monitored. The rate of parenteral fluids and the patient's response to these fluids are also closely monitored. If dyspnea or orthopnea is present, the patient is placed in a semi-Fowler's position to promote lung expansion. The patient is turned and positioned at regular intervals because edematous tissue is more prone to skin breakdown than normal tissue.

Because conditions predisposing to FVE are likely to be chronic, the patient is taught to monitor his or her response to therapy by documenting fluid intake and output and body weight changes. The importance of adhering to the treatment regimen is emphasized.

TEACHING PATIENTS ABOUT EDEMA

Because edema is a common manifestation of FVE, patients need to recognize its symptoms and importance. The nurse gives special attention to edema when teaching patients with FVE. Edema can occur from increased capillary fluid pressure, decreased capillary oncotic pressure, or increased interstitial oncotic pressure, thus expanding the interstitial fluid compartment. Edema can be localized (eg, in the ankle, as in rheumatoid arthritis) or generalized (as in cardiac and renal failure). Severe generalized edema is called anasarca.

Edema occurs when there is a change in the capillary membrane, increasing the formation of interstitial fluid or decreasing the removal of interstitial fluid. Sodium retention is a frequent cause of the increased extracellular fluid volume. Burns and infec-

tion are examples of conditions associated with increased interstitial fluid volume. Obstruction to lymphatic outflow, a plasma albumin level less than 1.5 to 2 g/dL, or a decrease in plasma oncotic pressure contributes to increased interstitial fluid volume. The kidneys retain sodium and water when there is decreased extracellular volume as a result of decreased cardiac output from heart failure. A thorough medication history is necessary to identify any medications that may cause edema, such as nonsteroidal anti-inflammatory drugs (NSAIDs), estrogens, corticosteroids, or antihypertensives.

Ascites is a form of edema in which fluid accumulates in the peritoneal cavity; it results from nephrotic syndrome or cirrhosis. Patients commonly report shortness of breath and a sense of pressure because of pressure on the diaphragm.

Edema usually affects dependent areas. It can be seen in the ankles, sacrum, scrotum, or the periorbital region of the face. Pitting edema is so named because a pit forms after a finger is pressed into edematous tissue. In pulmonary edema, the amount of fluid in the pulmonary interstitium and the alveoli increases. Manifestations include shortness of breath, increased respiratory rate, diaphoresis, and crackles and wheezing on auscultation of the lungs.

Decreased hematocrit resulting from hemodilution, arterial blood gas results indicative of respiratory **alkalosis** and hypoxemia, and decreased serum sodium and osmolality from retention of fluid may occur with edema. BUN and creatinine levels increase, urine specific gravity decreases as the kidneys attempt to excrete excess water, and the urine sodium level drops due to increased aldosterone production.

The goal of treatment is to preserve or restore the circulating intravascular fluid volume. In addition to treating the cause, other treatments may include diuretic therapy, restriction of fluids and sodium, elevation of the extremities, application of elastic compression stockings, paracentesis, dialysis, or continuous arteriovenous hemofiltration in cases of renal failure or life-threatening fluid volume overload.

Electrolyte Imbalances

Disturbances in electrolyte balances occur in clinical practice and must be corrected for the patient's health and safety. Table 14-6 summarizes the major fluid and electrolyte imbalances that are described in the text. An example of an electrolyte imbalance is an altered sodium balance.

SIGNIFICANCE OF SODIUM

Sodium is the most abundant electrolyte in the ECF; its concentration ranges from 135 to 145 mEq/L (135—145 mmol/L). Consequently, sodium is the primary determinant of ECF osmolality. Decreased sodium is associated with parallel changes in osmolality. The fact that sodium does not easily cross the cell wall membrane, plus its abundance or high concentration, accounts for its primary role in controlling water distribution throughout the body. In addition, sodium is the primary regulator of ECF volume. A loss or gain of sodium is usually accompanied by a loss or gain of water. Sodium also functions in establishing the electrochemical state necessary for muscle contraction and the transmission of nerve impulses.

Sodium imbalance occurs frequently in clinical practice and can develop under simple and complex circumstances. Sodium deficit and excess are the two most common sodium imbalances.

Table 14-6 • **Major Fluid and Electrolyte Imbalances**

IMBALANCE	CONTRIBUTING FACTORS	SIGNS/SYMPTOMS AND LABORATORY FINDINGS
Fluid volume deficit (hypovolemia)	Loss of water and electrolytes, as in vomiting, diarrhea, fistulas, fever, excess sweating, burns, blood loss, gastrointestinal suction, and third-space fluid shifts; and decreased intake, as in anorexia, nausea, and inability to gain access to fluid. Diabetes insipidus and uncontrolled diabetes mellitus also contribute to a depletion of extracellular fluid volume.	Acute weight loss, decreased skin turgor, oliguria, concentrated urine, weak rapid pulse, capillary filling time prolonged, low central venous pressure (CVP), ↓ blood pressure, flattened neck veins, dizziness, weakness, thirst and confusion, ↑ pulse, muscle cramps. *Labs indicate:* ↑ hemoglobin and hematocrit, ↑ serum and urine osmolality and specific gravity, ↓ urine sodium, ↑ BUN and creatinine
Fluid volume excess (hypervolemia)	Compromised regulatory mechanisms, such as renal failure, heart failure, and cirrhosis; and overzealous administration of sodium-containing fluids. Prolonged corticosteroid therapy, severe stress, and hyperaldosteronism augment fluid volume excess.	Acute weight gain, edema, distended jugular veins, crackles, and elevated CVP, shortness of breath, ↑ blood pressure, bounding pulse and cough. *Labs indicate:* ↓ hemoglobin and hematocrit, ↓ serum and urine osmolality, ↓ urine sodium and specific gravity
Sodium deficit (hyponatremia) Serum sodium <135 mEq/L	Loss of sodium, as in use of diuretics, loss of GI fluids, renal disease, and adrenal insufficiency. Gain of water, as in excessive administration of D_5W and water supplements for patients receiving hypotonic tube feedings; disease states associated with SIADH such as head trauma and oat-cell lung tumor; and medications associated with water retention (oxytocin and certain tranquilizers). Hyperglycemia and heart failure cause a loss of sodium.	Anorexia, nausea and vomiting, headache, lethargy, confusion, muscle cramps and weakness, muscular twitching, seizures, papilledema, dry skin, ↑ pulse, ↓ BP *Labs indicate:* ↓ serum and urine sodium, ↓ urine specific gravity and osmolality
Sodium excess (hypernatremia) Serum sodium >145 mEq/L	Water deprivation in patients unable to drink at will, hypertonic tube feedings without adequate water supplements, diabetes insipidus, heatstroke, hyperventilation, and watery diarrhea. Excess corticosteroid, sodium bicarbonate, and sodium chloride administration, and salt water near-drowning victims.	Thirst, elevated body temperature, swollen dry tongue and sticky mucous membranes, hallucinations, lethargy, restlessness, irritability, focal or grand mal seizures, pulmonary edema, hyperreflexia, twitching, nausea, vomiting, anorexia, ↑ pulse, and ↑ BP. *Labs indicate.* ↑ serum sodium, ↓ urine sodium, ↑ urine specific gravity and osmolality
Potassium deficit (hypokalemia) Serum potassium <3.5 mEq/L	Diarrhea, vomiting, gastric suction, corticosteroid administration, hyperaldosteronism, carbenicillin, amphotericin B, bulimia, osmotic diuresis, alkalosis, starvation, diuretics, and digoxin toxicity	Fatigue, anorexia, nausea and vomiting, muscle weakness, polyuria, decreased bowel motility, ventricular asystole or fibrillation, paresthesias, leg camps, ↓ BP, ileus, abdominal distention, hypoactive reflexes, *ECG:* flattened T waves, prominent U waves, ST depression, prolonged PR interval.
Potassium excess (hyperkalemia) Serum potassium >5.0 mEq/L	Pseudohyperkalemia, oliguric renal failure, use of potassium-conserving diuretics in patients with renal insufficiency, metabolic acidosis, Addison's disease, crush injury, burns, stored bank blood transfusions, and rapid IV administration of potassium	Vague muscular weakness, tachycardia → bradycardia, dysrhythmias, flaccid paralysis, paresthesias, intestinal colic, cramps, irritability, anxiety. *ECG:* tall tented T waves, prolonged PR interval and QRS duration, absent P waves, ST depression.
Calcium deficit (hypocalcemia) Serum calcium <8.5 mg/dL	Hypoparathyroidism (may follow thyroid surgery or radical neck dissection), malabsorption, pancreatitis, alkalosis, vitamin D deficiency, massive subcutaneous infection, generalized peritonitis, massive transfusion of citrated blood, chronic diarrhea, decreased parathyroid hormone, and diuretic phase of renal failure	Numbness, tingling of fingers, toes, and circumoral region; positive Trousseau's sign and Chvostek's sign; seizures, carpopedal spasms, hyperactive deep tendon reflexes, irritability, bronchospasm, anxiety, impaired clotting time, ↓ prothrombin, *ECG:* prolonged QT interval and lengthened ST.
Calcium excess (hypercalcemia) Serum calcium >10.5 mg/dL	Hyperparathyroidism, malignant neoplastic disease, prolonged immobilization, overuse of calcium supplements, vitamin D excess, oliguric phase of renal failure, acidosis, corticosteroid therapy, thiazide diuretic use, increased parathyroid hormone, and digoxin toxicity	Muscular weakness, constipation, anorexia, nausea and vomiting, polyuria and polydipsia, hypoactive deep tendon reflexes, lethargy, deep bone pain, pathologic fractures, flank pain, and calcium stones. *ECG:* shortened QT interval, bradycardia, heart blocks.
Magnesium deficit (hypomagnesemia) Serum magnesium <1.8 mg/dL	Chronic alcoholism, hyperparathyroidism, hyperaldosteronism, diuretic phase of renal failure, malabsorptive disorders, diabetic ketoacidosis, refeeding after starvation, parenteral nutrition, chronic laxative use, diarrhea, acute myocardial infarction, heart failure, decreased serum K^+ and Ca^{++} and certain pharmacologic agents (such as gentamicin, cisplatin, and cyclosporine)	Neuromuscular irritability, positive Trousseau's and Chvostek's signs, insomnia, mood changes, anorexia, vomiting, increased tendon reflexes, and ↑ BP. *ECG:* PVCs, flat or inverted T waves, depressed ST segment.

(continued)

Table 14-6 • **Major Fluid and Electrolyte Imbalances** (Continued)

IMBALANCE	CONTRIBUTING FACTORS	SIGNS/SYMPTOMS AND LABORATORY FINDINGS
Magnesium excess (hypermagnesemia) Serum magnesium >2.7 mg/dL	Oliguric phase of renal failure (particularly when magnesium-containing medications are administered), adrenal insufficiency, excessive IV magnesium administration, and DKA	Flushing, hypotension, drowsiness, hypoactive reflexes, depressed respirations, cardiac arrest and coma, diaphoresis. *ECG:* tachycardia → bradycardia, prolonged PR interval and QRS.
Phosphorus deficit (hypophosphatemia) Serum phosphorus <2.5 mg/dL	Refeeding after starvation, alcohol withdrawal, diabetic ketoacidosis, respiratory alkalosis, ↓ magnesium, ↓ potassium, hyperparathyroidism, vomiting, diarrhea, hyperventilation, vitamin D deficiency associated with malabsorptive disorders, burns, acid–base disorders, parenteral nutrition, and diuretic use	Paresthesias, muscle weakness, bone pain and tenderness, chest pain, confusion, cardiomyopathy, respiratory failure, seizures, tissue hypoxia, and increased susceptibility to infection
Phosphorus excess (hyperphosphatemia) Serum phosphorus >4.5 mg/dL	Acute and chronic renal failure, excessive intake of phosphorus, vitamin D excess, respiratory acidosis, hypoparathyroidism, volume depletion, leukemia/lymphoma treated with cytotoxic agents, increased tissue breakdown, rhabdomyolysis	Tetany, tachycardia, anorexia, nausea and vomiting, muscle weakness, signs and symptoms of hypocalcemia
Chloride excess (hyperchloremia) Serum chloride >108 mEq/L	Excessive sodium chloride infusions with water loss, head injury (sodium retention), hypernatremia, renal failure, corticosteroid use, dehydration, severe diarrhea (loss of bicarbonate), respiratory alkalosis, administration of diuretics, overdose of salicylates, Kayexalate, acetazolamide, phenylbutazone and ammonium chloride use, hyperparathyroidism, metabolic acidosis	Tachypnea, lethargy, weakness, deep rapid respirations, decline in cognitive status, decreased cardiac output, dyspnea, tachycardia, pitting edema, dysrhythmias, coma *Labs indicate:* increased serum chloride, increased serum sodium, decreased serum pH, decreased serum bicarbonate, normal anion gap, increased urinary chloride level
Chloride deficit (hypochloremia) Serum chloride <96 mEq/L	Addison's disease, reduced chloride intake or absorption, untreated diabetic ketoacidosis, chronic respiratory acidosis, excessive sweating, vomiting, gastric suction, diarrhea, sodium and potassium deficiency, metabolic alkalosis, loop, osmotic, or thiazide diuretic use, overuse of bicarbonate, rapid removal of ascitic fluid with a high sodium content, intravenous fluids that lack chloride (dextrose and water), draining fistulas and ileostomies, heart failure, cystic fibrosis	Agitation, irritability, tremors, muscle cramps, hyperactive deep tendon reflexes, hypertonicity, tetany, slow, shallow respirations, seizures, dysrhythmias, coma *Labs indicate:* ↓ serum chloride, ↓ serum sodium, ↑ pH, ↑ serum bicarbonate, ↑ total carbon dioxide content, ↓ urine chloride level

SODIUM DEFICIT (HYPONATREMIA)

Hyponatremia refers to a serum sodium level that is below normal (less than 135 mEq/L [135 mmol/L]). Plasma sodium concentration represents the ratio of total body sodium to total body water. A decrease in this ratio can occur from a low quantity of total body sodium with a lesser reduction in total body water, normal total body sodium content with excess total body water, and an excess of total body sodium with an even greater excess of total body water. However, a hyponatremic state can be superimposed on an existing FVD or FVE.

Sodium may be lost by way of vomiting, diarrhea, fistulas, or sweating, or it may be associated with the use of diuretics, particularly in combination with a low-salt diet. A deficiency of aldosterone, as occurs in adrenal insufficiency, also predisposes the patient to sodium deficiency.

Dilutional Hyponatremia

In water intoxication (dilutional hyponatremia), the patient's serum sodium level is diluted by an increase in the ratio of water to sodium. This causes water to move into the cell, so that the patient develops an ECF volume excess. Predisposing conditions for this type of hyponatremia include syndrome of inappropriate antidiuretic hormone (SIADH), hyperglycemia, and increased water intake through the administration of electrolyte-poor parenteral fluids, the use of tap-water enemas, or the irrigation of nasogastric tubes with water instead of normal saline solution.

Water may be gained abnormally by the excessive parenteral administration of dextrose and water solutions, particularly during periods of stress. It may also be gained by compulsive water drinking (psychogenic polydipsia).

SIADH

The basic physiologic disturbances in SIADH are excessive ADH activity, with water retention and dilutional hyponatremia, and inappropriate urinary excretion of sodium in the presence of hyponatremia. SIADH can be the result of either sustained secretion of ADH by the hypothalamus or production of an ADH-like substance from a tumor (aberrant ADH production).

Conditions associated with SIADH include oat-cell lung tumors, head injuries, endocrine and pulmonary disorders, physiologic or psychological stress, and the use of medications such as oxytocin, cyclophosphamide, vincristine, thioridazine, and amitriptyline. SIADH is discussed in more detail in Chapter 42.

Clinical Manifestations

Clinical manifestations of hyponatremia depend on the cause, magnitude, and speed with which the deficit occurs. Poor skin turgor, dry mucosa, decreased saliva production, orthostatic fall in blood pressure, nausea, and abdominal cramping occur. Neurologic changes, including altered mental status, are probably related to the cellular swelling and cerebral edema associated with hyponatremia. As the extracellular sodium level decreases, the cellular fluid becomes relatively more concentrated and pulls water into the cells (Fig. 14-4). In general, patients with an acute decrease in serum sodium levels have more severe symptoms and higher mortality rates than do those with more slowly developing hyponatremia.

Features of hyponatremia associated with sodium loss and water gain include anorexia, muscle cramps, and a feeling of exhaustion. When the serum sodium level drops below 115 mEq/L (115 mmol/L), signs of increasing intracranial pressure, such as lethargy, confusion, muscle twitching, focal weakness, hemiparesis, papilledema, and seizures, may occur.

Assessment and Diagnostic Findings

Regardless of the cause of hyponatremia, the serum sodium level is less than 135 mEq/L; in SIADH it may be quite low, such as 100 mEq/L (100 mmol/L) or less. Serum osmolality is also decreased, except in azotemia or ingestion of toxins. When hyponatremia is due primarily to sodium loss, the urinary sodium content is less than 20 mEq/L (20 mmol/L), suggesting increased proximal reabsorption of sodium secondary to ECF volume depletion; the specific gravity is low, such as 1.002 to 1.004. When hyponatremia is due to SIADH, however, the urinary sodium content is greater than 20 mEq/L and the urine specific gravity is usually over 1.012. Although the patient with SIADH retains water abnormally and thus gains body weight, there is no peripheral edema; instead, fluid accumulates inside the cells. This phenomenon is sometimes manifested as "fingerprinting" when the finger is pressed over a bony prominence, such as the sternum.

Medical Management

The key to treating hyponatremia is assessment; this includes the speed with which hyponatremia occurred rather than relying only on the patient's actual serum sodium value (Fall, 2000).

SODIUM REPLACEMENT

The obvious treatment for hyponatremia is careful administration of sodium by mouth, nasogastric tube, or the parenteral route. For patients who can eat and drink, sodium is easily replaced, because sodium is consumed abundantly in a normal diet. For those who cannot consume sodium, lactated Ringer's solution or isotonic saline (0.9% sodium chloride) solution may be prescribed. Serum sodium must not be increased by greater than 12 mEq/L in 24 hours, to avoid neurologic damage due to osmotic demyelination. This condition may occur when the serum sodium concentration is overcorrected (above 140 mEq/L) too rapidly or in the presence of hypoxia or anoxia (Pirzada & Imran, 2001). It may produce lesions in the pons that cause paraparesis, dysarthria, dysphagia, and coma. Table 14-5 describes the components of selected water and electrolyte solutions. The usual daily sodium requirement in adults is approximately 100 mEq, provided there are no abnormal losses.

In SIADH, the administration of hypertonic saline solution alone cannot change the plasma sodium concentration. Excess sodium would be excreted rapidly in a highly concentrated urine. With the addition of the diuretic furosemide (Lasix), urine is not concentrated and isotonic urine is excreted to effect a change in water balance. In patients with SIADH, in whom water restriction is difficult, lithium or demeclocycline can antagonize the osmotic effect of ADH on the medullary collecting tubule.

WATER RESTRICTION

In a patient with normal or excess fluid volume, hyponatremia is treated by restricting fluid to a total of 800 mL in 24 hours. This is far safer than sodium administration and is usually effective. When neurologic symptoms are present, however, it may be necessary to administer small volumes of a hypertonic sodium solution, such as 3% or 5% sodium chloride. Incorrect use of these fluids is extremely dangerous because 1 L of 3% sodium chloride solution contains 513 mEq of sodium, and 1 L of 5% sodium chloride solution contains 855 mEq of sodium. If edema exists alone, sodium is restricted; if edema and hyponatremia occur together, both sodium and water are restricted.

> **NURSING ALERT** Highly hypertonic sodium solutions (3% and 5% sodium chloride) should be administered only in intensive care settings under close observation, because only small volumes are needed to elevate the serum sodium level from a dangerously low value. These fluids are administered slowly and in small volumes, and the patient is monitored closely for fluid overload. The purpose is to relieve acute manifestations of cerebral edema and to prevent neurologic complications rather than to correct the sodium concentration specifically. Along with the sodium solution, the patient may receive a loop diuretic to prevent ECF volume overload and to increase water excretion.

Nursing Management

The nurse needs to identify patients at risk for hyponatremia so that they can be monitored. Early detection and treatment of this disorder are necessary to prevent serious consequences. For patients at risk, the nurse monitors fluid intake and output as well as daily body weights. Abnormal losses of sodium or gains of water are noted. GI manifestations, such as anorexia, nausea, vomiting, and abdominal cramping, are also noted. The nurse must be particularly alert for central nervous system changes, such as lethargy, confusion, muscle twitching, and seizures. In

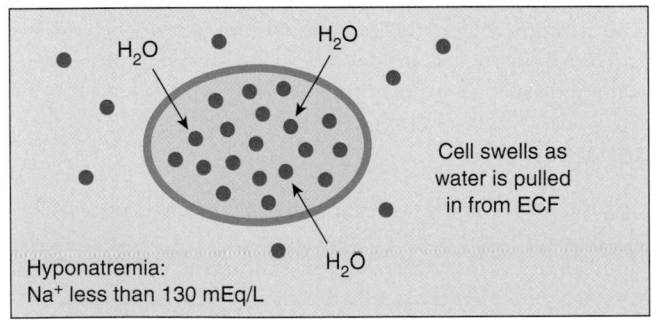

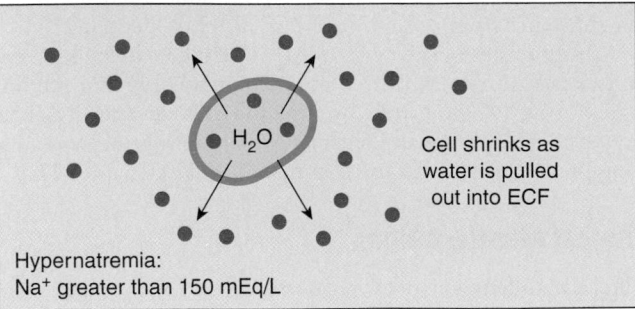

FIGURE 14-4 Effect of extracellular sodium level on cell size.

general, more severe neurologic signs are associated with very low sodium levels that have fallen rapidly because of fluid overloading. Serum sodium levels are monitored very closely in patients at risk for hyponatremia; when indicated, urinary sodium levels and specific gravity are also monitored.

Hyponatremia is a frequently overlooked cause of confusion in elderly patients. The elderly are at increased risk for hyponatremia because of changes in renal function and subsequent decreased ability to excrete excessive water loads. Administration of medications causing sodium loss or water retention is a predisposing factor.

DETECTING AND CONTROLLING HYPONATREMIA

For patients experiencing abnormal losses of sodium who can consume a general diet, the nurse encourages foods and fluids with a high sodium content. For example, broth made with one beef cube contains approximately 900 mg of sodium; 8 oz of tomato juice contains approximately 700 mg of sodium. The nurse also needs to be familiar with the sodium content of parenteral fluids (see Table 14-5).

> **NURSING ALERT** When administering fluids to patients with cardiovascular disease, the nurse assesses for signs of circulatory overload (eg, cough, dyspnea, puffy eyelids, dependent edema, or weight gain in 24 hours). The lungs are auscultated for crackles. Extreme care is taken when administering highly hypertonic sodium (eg, 3% or 5% sodium chloride) fluids, because these fluids can be lethal if infused carelessly.

For patients taking lithium, the nurse observes for lithium toxicity, particularly when sodium is lost by an abnormal route. In such instances, supplemental salt and fluid are administered. Because diuretics promote sodium loss, patients taking lithium are instructed not to use diuretics without close medical supervision. For all patients on lithium therapy, adequate salt intake should be ensured.

Excess water supplements are avoided in patients receiving isotonic or hypotonic enteral feedings, particularly if abnormal sodium loss occurs or water is being abnormally retained (as in SIADH). Actual fluid needs are determined by evaluating fluid intake and output, urine specific gravity, and serum sodium levels.

RETURNING SODIUM LEVEL TO NORMAL

When the primary problem is water retention, it is safer to restrict fluid intake than to administer sodium. Administering sodium to a patient with normovolemia or hypervolemia predisposes the patient to fluid volume overload. As stated previously, the nurse must monitor patients with cardiovascular disease very closely.

In severe hyponatremia, the aim of therapy is to elevate the serum sodium level only enough to alleviate neurologic signs and symptoms. It is generally recommended that the serum sodium concentration be raised no higher than 125 mEq/L (125 mmol/L) with a hypertonic saline solution.

SODIUM EXCESS (HYPERNATREMIA)

Hypernatremia is a higher-than-normal serum sodium level (exceeding 145 mEq/L [145 mmol/L]) (Adrogue & Madias, 2000a). It can be caused by a gain of sodium in excess of water or by a loss of water in excess of sodium. It can occur in patients with normal fluid volume or in those with FVD or FVE. With a water loss, the patient loses more water than sodium; as a result, the serum

sodium concentration increases and the increased concentration pulls fluid out of the cell. This is both an extracellular and intracellular FVD. In sodium excess, the patient ingests or retains more sodium than water.

Pathophysiology

A common cause of hypernatremia is fluid deprivation in unconscious patients who cannot perceive, respond to, or communicate their thirst (Adrogue & Madias, 2000a). Most often affected in this regard are very old, very young, and cognitively impaired patients. Administration of hypertonic enteral feedings without adequate water supplements leads to hypernatremia, as does watery diarrhea and greatly increased insensible water loss (eg, hyperventilation, denuding effects of burns).

Diabetes insipidus, a deficiency of ADH from the posterior pituitary gland, leads to hypernatremia if the patient does not experience, or cannot respond to, thirst or if fluids are excessively restricted. Less common causes are heat stroke, near-drowning in sea water (which contains a sodium concentration of approximately 500 mEq/L), and malfunction of either hemodialysis or peritoneal dialysis proportioning systems. IV administration of hypertonic saline or excessive use of sodium bicarbonate also causes hypernatremia.

Clinical Manifestations

The clinical manifestations of hypernatremia are primarily neurologic and are presumably the consequence of cellular dehydration (Adrogue & Madias, 2000a). Hypernatremia results in a relatively concentrated ECF, causing water to be pulled from the cells (see Fig. 14-4). Clinically, these changes may be manifested by restlessness and weakness in moderate hypernatremia and by disorientation, delusions, and hallucinations in severe hypernatremia. Dehydration (resulting in hypernatremia) is often overlooked as the primary reason for behavioral changes in the elderly patient. If hypernatremia is severe, permanent brain damage can occur (especially in children). Brain damage is apparently due to subarachnoid hemorrhages that result from brain contraction.

A primary characteristic of hypernatremia is thirst. Thirst is so strong a defender of serum sodium levels in healthy people that hypernatremia never occurs unless the person is unconscious or is denied access to water. Unfortunately, ill people may have an impaired thirst mechanism. Other signs include a dry, swollen tongue and sticky mucous membranes. Flushed skin, peripheral and pulmonary edema, postural hypotension, and increased muscle tone and deep tendon reflexes are additional signs and symptoms of hypernatremia. Body temperature may rise mildly but returns to normal when the hypernatremia is corrected.

Assessment and Diagnostic Findings

In hypernatremia, the serum sodium level exceeds 145 mEq/L (145 mmol/L) and the serum osmolality exceeds 295 mOsm/kg (295 mmol/L). The urine specific gravity and urine osmolality are increased as the kidneys attempt to conserve water (provided the water loss is from a route other than the kidneys) (Fall, 2000).

Medical Management

Hypernatremia treatment consists of a gradual lowering of the serum sodium level by the infusion of a hypotonic electrolyte solution (eg, 0.3% sodium chloride) or an isotonic nonsaline solution (eg, dextrose 5% in water [D_5W]). D_5W is indicated when water needs to be replaced without sodium. Many clinicians consider a hypotonic sodium solution to be safer than D_5W because it allows a gradual reduction in the serum sodium level and thereby decreases the risk of cerebral edema. It is the solution of choice in severe hyperglycemia with hypernatremia. A rapid reduction in the serum sodium level temporarily decreases the plasma osmolality below that of the fluid in the brain tissue, causing dangerous cerebral edema. Diuretics also may be prescribed to treat the sodium gain.

There is no consensus about the exact rate at which serum sodium levels should be reduced. As a general rule, the serum sodium level is reduced at a rate no faster than 0.5 to 1 mEq/L to allow sufficient time for readjustment through diffusion across fluid compartments. Desmopressin acetate (DDAVP) may be prescribed to treat diabetes insipidus if it is the cause of hypernatremia.

Nursing Management

As in hyponatremia, fluid losses and gains are carefully monitored in patients at risk for hypernatremia. The nurse should assess for abnormal losses of water or low water intake and for large gains of sodium, as might occur with ingestion of over-the-counter medications with a high sodium content (such as Alka-Seltzer). Also, it is important to obtain a medication history because some prescription medications have a high sodium content. In addition, the nurse notes the patient's thirst or elevated body temperature and evaluates it in relation to other clinical signs. The nurse monitors for changes in behavior, such as restlessness, disorientation, and lethargy.

PREVENTING HYPERNATREMIA

The nurse attempts to prevent hypernatremia by offering fluids at regular intervals, particularly in debilitated patients unable to perceive or respond to thirst. If fluid intake remains inadequate, the nurse consults with the physician to plan an alternate route for intake, either by enteral feedings or by the parenteral route. If enteral feedings are used, sufficient water should be administered to keep the serum sodium and BUN within normal limits. As a rule, the higher the osmolality of the enteral feeding, the greater the need for water supplementation.

For patients with diabetes insipidus, adequate water intake must be ensured. If the patient is alert and has an intact thirst mechanism, merely providing access to water may be sufficient. If the patient has a decreased level of consciousness or other disability interfering with adequate fluid intake, parenteral fluid replacement may be prescribed. This therapy can be anticipated in patients with neurologic disorders, particularly in the early postoperative period.

CORRECTING HYPERNATREMIA

When parenteral fluids are necessary for managing hypernatremia, the nurse monitors the patient's response to the fluids by reviewing serial serum sodium levels and by observing for changes in neurologic signs. With a gradual decrease in the serum sodium level, the neurologic signs should improve. As stated in the discussion on management, too-rapid reduction in the serum sodium level renders the plasma temporarily hypo-osmotic to the fluid in the brain tissue, causing movement of fluid into brain cells and dangerous cerebral edema (Adrogue & Madias, 2000a).

SIGNIFICANCE OF POTASSIUM

Potassium is the major intracellular electrolyte; in fact, 98% of the body's potassium is inside the cells. The remaining 2% is in the ECF, and it is this 2% that is important in neuromuscular function. Potassium influences both skeletal and cardiac muscle activity. For example, alterations in its concentration change myocardial irritability and rhythm. Under the influence of the sodium–potassium pump and based on the body's needs, potassium is constantly moving in and out of cells. The normal serum potassium concentration ranges from 3.5 to 5.5 mEq/L (3.5–5.5 mmol/L), and even minor variations are significant. Potassium imbalances are commonly associated with various diseases, injuries, medications (diuretics, laxatives, antibiotics), and special treatments, such as parenteral nutrition and chemotherapy (Cohn et al., 2000).

To maintain potassium balance, the renal system must function because 80% of the potassium is excreted daily from the body by way of the kidneys; the other 20% is lost through the bowel and in sweat. The kidneys are the primary regulators of potassium balance and accomplish this by adjusting the amount of potassium that is excreted in the urine. As serum potassium levels increase, so does the potassium level in the renal tubular cell. A concentration gradient occurs, favoring the movement of potassium into the renal tubule with the loss of potassium in the urine. Aldosterone also increases the excretion of potassium by the kidney. Because the kidneys do not conserve potassium as well as they conserve sodium, potassium may still be lost in urine in the presence of a potassium deficit.

POTASSIUM DEFICIT (HYPOKALEMIA)

Hypokalemia (below-normal serum potassium concentration) usually indicates an actual deficit in total potassium stores. Hypokalemia may occur in patients with normal potassium stores; however, when alkalosis is present, a temporary shift of serum potassium into the cells occurs (see discussion of alkalosis later in this chapter).

As stated earlier, hypokalemia is a common imbalance (Gennari, 1998). GI loss of potassium is probably the most common cause of potassium depletion. Vomiting and gastric suction frequently lead to hypokalemia, partly because potassium is actually lost when gastric fluid is lost, but more so because potassium is lost through the kidneys in association with metabolic alkalosis. Because relatively large amounts of potassium are contained in intestinal fluids, potassium deficit occurs frequently with diarrhea. Intestinal fluid may contain as much potassium as 30 mEq/L. Potassium deficit also occurs from prolonged intestinal suctioning, recent ileostomy, and villous adenoma (a tumor of the intestinal tract characterized by excretion of potassium-rich mucus).

Alterations in acid–base balance have a significant effect on potassium distribution. The mechanism involves shifts of hydrogen and potassium ions between the cells and the ECF. Hypokalemia can cause alkalosis, and in turn alkalosis can cause hypokalemia. For example, hydrogen ions move out of the cells in alkalotic states to help correct the high pH, and potassium ions move in to maintain an electrically neutral state. (This is discussed further in the section on acid–base balance.)

Hyperaldosteronism increases renal potassium wasting and can lead to severe potassium depletion. Primary hyperaldosteronism is seen in patients with adrenal adenomas. Secondary hyperaldosteronism occurs in patients with cirrhosis, nephrotic syndrome, heart failure, and malignant hypertension (Wilcox, 1999).

Potassium-losing diuretics, such as the thiazides (eg, chlorothiazide [Diuril] and polythiazide [Renese]), can induce hypokalemia, particularly when administered in large doses to patients with inadequate potassium intake. Other medications that can lead to hypokalemia include corticosteroids, sodium penicillin, carbenicillin, and amphotericin B (Cohn et al., 2000; Gennari, 1998).

Because insulin promotes the entry of potassium into skeletal muscle and hepatic cells, patients with persistent insulin hypersecretion may experience hypokalemia, which is often the case in patients receiving high-carbohydrate parenteral fluids (as in parenteral nutrition).

Patients who are unable or unwilling to eat a normal diet for a prolonged period are at risk for hypokalemia. This may occur in debilitated elderly people, alcoholics, and patients with anorexia nervosa. In addition to poor intake, people with bulimia frequently suffer increased potassium loss through self-induced vomiting and laxative and diuretic abuse.

Magnesium depletion causes renal potassium loss and must be corrected first; otherwise, urine loss of potassium will continue. Penicillins may produce renal potassium loss by acting as poorly reabsorbable anions and thus increasing distal sodium delivery and sodium-potassium loss.

Clinical Manifestations

Potassium deficiency can result in widespread derangements in physiologic function. Severe hypokalemia can cause death through cardiac or respiratory arrest. Clinical signs rarely develop before the serum potassium level has fallen below 3 mEq/L (3 mmol/L) unless the rate of fall has been rapid. Manifestations of hypokalemia include fatigue, anorexia, nausea, vomiting, muscle weakness, leg cramps, decreased bowel motility, paresthesias (numbness and tingling), dysrhythmias, and increased sensitivity to digitalis (Gennari, 1998). If prolonged, hypokalemia can lead to an inability of the kidneys to concentrate urine, causing dilute urine (resulting in polyuria, nocturia) and excessive thirst. Potassium depletion depresses the release of insulin and results in glucose intolerance.

Assessment and Diagnostic Findings

In hypokalemia, the serum potassium concentration is less than the lower limit of normal. Electrocardiographic (ECG) changes can include flat T waves and/or inverted T waves, suggesting ischemia, and depressed ST segments (Fig. 14-5). An elevated U wave is specific to hypokalemia. Hypokalemia increases sensitivity to digitalis, predisposing the patient to digitalis toxicity at lower digitalis levels. Metabolic alkalosis is commonly associated with hypokalemia. This is discussed further in the section on acid–base disturbances.

The source of the potassium loss is usually evident from a careful history. When this is not the case, however, and the etiology of the loss is unclear, a 24-hour urinary potassium excretion test can be performed to distinguish between renal and extrarenal loss. Urinary potassium excretion exceeding 20 mEq/24 h with hypokalemia suggests that renal potassium loss is the cause.

Medical Management

If hypokalemia cannot be prevented by conventional measures such as increased intake in the daily diet, it is treated with oral or IV replacement therapy (Gennari, 1998). Potassium loss must be corrected daily; administration of 40 to 80 mEq/day of potas-

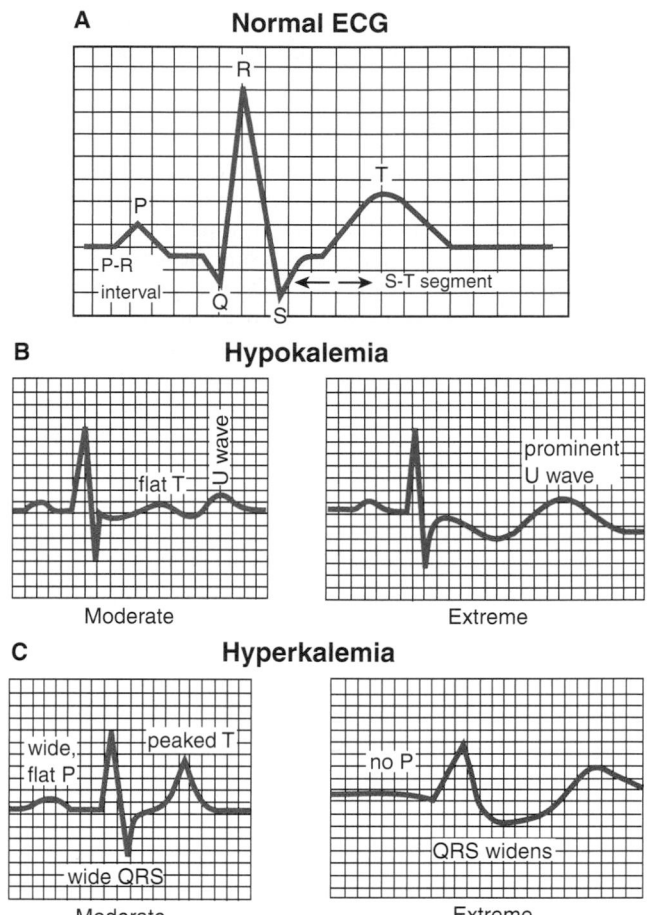

FIGURE 14-5 Effect of potassium on ECG. (**A**) Normal tracing. (**B**) Hypokalemia: serum potassium level below normal. Figure on *left* illustrates flattening of the T wave and the appearance of a U wave. Figure on *right* illustrates further flattening with prominent U wave. (**C**) Hyperkalemia: serum potassium level above normal. Figure on *left* illustrates moderate elevation with wide, flat P wave, wide QRS complex, and peaked T wave. Figure on *right* illustrates ECG changes seen with extreme potassium elevation: widening of QRS complex and absence of P wave.

sium is adequate in the adult if there are no abnormal losses of potassium.

For patients at risk for hypokalemia, a diet containing sufficient potassium should be provided. Dietary intake of potassium in the average adult is 50 to 100 mEq/day. Foods high in potassium include fruits (especially raisins, bananas, apricots, and oranges), vegetables, legumes, whole grains, milk, and meat.

When dietary intake is inadequate for any reason, the physician may prescribe oral or IV potassium supplements (Gennari, 1998). Many salt substitutes contain 50 to 60 mEq of potassium per teaspoon and may be sufficient to prevent hypokalemia.

 NURSING ALERT Oral potassium supplements can produce small bowel lesions; therefore, the patient must be assessed for and cautioned about abdominal distention, pain, or GI bleeding.

When oral administration of potassium is not feasible, the IV route is indicated. The IV route is mandatory for patients with severe hypokalemia (eg, a serum level of 2 mEq/L). Although potassium chloride is usually used to correct potassium deficits, the physician may prescribe potassium acetate or potassium phosphate.

Nursing Management

Because hypokalemia can be life-threatening, the nurse needs to monitor for its early presence in patients at risk. Fatigue, anorexia, muscle weakness, decreased bowel motility, paresthesias, and dysrhythmias are signals that warrant assessing the serum potassium concentration. When available, the ECG may provide useful information. For example, patients receiving digitalis who are at risk for potassium deficiency should be monitored closely for signs of digitalis toxicity, because hypokalemia potentiates the action of digitalis. Physicians usually prefer to keep the serum potassium level above 3.5 mEq/L (3.5 mmol/L) in patients receiving digitalis medications such as digoxin.

PREVENTING HYPOKALEMIA

Measures are taken to prevent hypokalemia when possible (Gennari, 1998). Prevention may involve encouraging the patient at risk to eat foods rich in potassium (when the diet allows). Sources of potassium include fruit and fruit juices (bananas, melon, citrus fruit), fresh and frozen vegetables, fresh meats, and processed foods. When hypokalemia is due to abuse of laxatives or diuretics, patient education may help alleviate the problem. Part of the health history and assessment should be directed at identifying problems amenable to prevention through education. Careful monitoring of fluid intake and output is necessary because 40 mEq of potassium is lost for every liter of urine output. The ECG is monitored for changes, and arterial blood gas values are checked for elevated bicarbonate and pH levels.

CORRECTING HYPOKALEMIA

Great care should be exercised when administering potassium, particularly in older adults, who have lower lean body mass and total body potassium levels and therefore lower potassium requirements. Additionally, with the physiologic loss of renal function with advancing years, potassium may be retained more readily in older than in younger people.

ADMINISTERING IV POTASSIUM

Potassium should be administered only after adequate urine flow has been established. A decrease in urine volume to less than 20 mL/h for 2 consecutive hours is an indication to stop the potassium infusion until the situation is evaluated. Potassium is primarily excreted by the kidneys; therefore, when oliguria occurs, potassium administration can cause the serum potassium concentration to rise dangerously.

 NURSING ALERT Potassium is never administered IV push or intramuscularly. IV potassium must be administered using an infusion pump to avoid replacing potassium too quickly.

Each health care facility has its own standard of care, which should be consulted; however, IV potassium should not be administered faster than 20 mEq/h or in concentrations greater than 30 to 40 mEq/L unless hypokalemia is severe, because this can cause life-threatening dysrhythmias. When prepared for IV infusions, the fluid should be agitated well to prevent bolus doses that can result when the potassium concentrates at the bottom of the IV container.

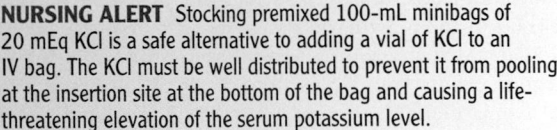 **NURSING ALERT** Stocking premixed 100-mL minibags of 20 mEq KCl is a safe alternative to adding a vial of KCl to an IV bag. The KCl must be well distributed to prevent it from pooling at the insertion site at the bottom of the bag and causing a life-threatening elevation of the serum potassium level.

When potassium is administered through a peripheral vein, the rate of administration must be decreased to avoid irritating the vein and causing a burning sensation during administration. In general, concentrations greater than 60 mEq/L are not administered in peripheral veins because venous pain and sclerosis may occur. For routine maintenance needs, potassium is suitably diluted and administered at a rate no faster than 10 mEq/h. In critical situations, more concentrated solutions (such as 40 mEq/L) may be administered through a central line. Even in extreme hypokalemia, however, potassium should be administered no faster than 20 to 40 mEq/h (suitably diluted). In such a situation, the patient must be monitored by ECG and observed closely for other signs and symptoms, such as changes in muscle strength.

POTASSIUM EXCESS (HYPERKALEMIA)

Hyperkalemia (greater-than-normal serum potassium concentration) seldom occurs in patients with normal renal function. Like hypokalemia, hyperkalemia is often due to iatrogenic (treatment-induced) causes. Although less common than hypokalemia, hyperkalemia is usually more dangerous because cardiac arrest is more frequently associated with high serum potassium levels.

A variation of hyperkalemia, pseudohyperkalemia has a number of causes The most common causes are the use of a tight tourniquet around an exercising extremity while drawing a blood sample and hemolysis of the sample before analysis. Other causes include marked leukocytosis (white blood cell count exceeding 200,000) or thrombocytosis (platelet count exceeding 1 million), drawing blood above a site where potassium is infusing, and familial pseudohyperkalemia, where potassium leaks out of the red blood cells while the blood is awaiting analysis. Failure to be aware of these causes of pseudohyperkalemia can lead to aggressive treatment of a nonexistent hyperkalemia, resulting in serious lowering of serum potassium levels. Thus, measurements of grossly elevated levels should be verified.

The major cause of hyperkalemia is decreased renal excretion of potassium. Thus, significant hyperkalemia is commonly seen in patients with untreated renal failure, particularly those in whom potassium levels rise as a result of infection or excessive intake of potassium in food or medications. In addition, patients with hypoaldosteronism and Addison's disease are at risk for hyperkalemia because these conditions are characterized by deficient adrenal hormones, leading to sodium loss and potassium retention.

Medications have been identified as a probable contributing factor in more than 60% of hyperkalemic episodes. Medications commonly implicated are potassium chloride, heparin, ACE inhibitors, captopril, NSAIDs, and potassium-sparing diuretics. In most such cases, potassium regulation is compromised by renal insufficiency (Perazella, 2000).

Although a high intake of potassium can cause severe hyperkalemia in patients with impaired renal function, hyperkalemia rarely occurs in people with normal renal function. For all patients, however, improper use of potassium supplements predisposes them to hyperkalemia, especially when salt substitutes are used. Not all patients receiving potassium-losing diuretics require potassium supplements, and patients receiving potassium-conserving diuretics should not receive supplements.

> **NURSING ALERT** Potassium supplements are extremely dangerous when patients have impaired renal function and thus decreased ability to excrete potassium. Even more dangerous is the IV administration of potassium to such patients, as serum levels can rise very quickly. Aged (stored) blood should not be administered to patients with impaired renal function because the serum potassium concentration of stored blood increases as the storage time increases, a result of red blood cell deterioration. It is possible to exceed the renal tolerance of any patient with rapid IV potassium administration, as well as when large amounts of oral potassium supplements are ingested.

In **acidosis**, potassium moves out of the cells into the ECF. This occurs as hydrogen ions enter the cells, a process that buffers the pH of the ECF (acidosis is discussed later in this chapter). An elevated extracellular potassium level should be anticipated when extensive tissue trauma has occurred, as in burns, crushing injuries, or severe infections. Similarly, it can occur with lysis of malignant cells after chemotherapy.

Clinical Manifestations

The most important consequence of hyperkalemia is its effect on the myocardium. Cardiac effects of an elevated serum potassium level are usually not significant below a concentration of 7 mEq/L (7 mmol/L), but they are almost always present when the level is 8 mEq/L (8 mmol/L) or greater. As the plasma potassium level rises, disturbances in cardiac conduction occur. The earliest changes, often occurring at a serum potassium level greater than 6 mEq/L (6 mmol/L), are peaked, narrow T waves; ST-segment depression; and a shortened QT interval. If the serum potassium level continues to rise, the PR interval becomes prolonged and is followed by disappearance of the P waves. Finally, there is decomposition and prolongation of the QRS complex (see Fig. 14-5). Ventricular dysrhythmias and cardiac arrest may occur at any point in this progression.

Severe hyperkalemia causes skeletal muscle weakness and even paralysis, related to a depolarization block in muscle. Similarly, ventricular conduction is slowed. Although hyperkalemia has marked effects on the peripheral nervous system, it has little effect on the central nervous system. Rapidly ascending muscular weakness leading to flaccid quadriplegia has been reported in patients with very high serum potassium levels. Paralysis of respiratory and speech muscles can also occur. Additionally, GI manifestations, such as nausea, intermittent intestinal colic, and diarrhea, may occur in hyperkalemic patients.

Assessment and Diagnostic Findings

Serum potassium levels and ECG changes are crucial to the diagnosis of hyperkalemia, as discussed above. Arterial blood gas analysis may reveal metabolic acidosis; in many cases, hyperkalemia occurs with acidosis.

Medical Management

An immediate ECG should be obtained to detect changes. Shortened repolarization and peaked T waves are seen initially. It is prudent as well to obtain a repeat serum potassium level from a vein without an IV infusion containing potassium to verify results.

In nonacute situations, restriction of dietary potassium and potassium-containing medications may suffice. For example, eliminating the use of potassium-containing salt substitutes in the patient taking a potassium-conserving diuretic may be all that is needed to deal with mild hyperkalemia.

Prevention of serious hyperkalemia by the administration, either orally or by retention enema, of cation exchange resins (eg, Kayexalate) may be necessary in patients with renal impairment. Cation exchange resins cannot be used if the patient has a paralytic ileus because intestinal perforation can occur. Kayexalate can bind with other cations in the GI tract and contribute to the development of hypomagnesemia and hypocalcemia; it may also cause sodium retention and fluid overload (Karch, 2002).

EMERGENCY PHARMACOLOGIC THERAPY

When serum potassium levels are dangerously elevated, it may be necessary to administer IV calcium gluconate. Within minutes after administration, calcium antagonizes the action of hyperkalemia on the heart. Infusion of calcium does not reduce the serum potassium concentration but immediately antagonizes the adverse cardiac conduction abnormalities. Calcium chloride and calcium gluconate are not interchangeable: calcium gluconate contains 4.5 mEq of calcium and calcium chloride contains 13.6 mEq of calcium; therefore, caution must be used.

Monitoring the blood pressure is essential to detect hypotension, which may result from the rapid IV administration of calcium gluconate. The ECG should be continuously monitored during administration; the appearance of bradycardia is an indication to stop the infusion. The myocardial protective effects of calcium are transient, lasting about 30 minutes. Extra caution is required if the patient has been "digitalized" (received accelerated dosages of a digitalis-based cardiac glycoside to reach a desired serum digitalis level rapidly) because parenteral administration of calcium sensitizes the heart to digitalis and may precipitate digitalis toxicity.

IV administration of sodium bicarbonate may be necessary to alkalinize the plasma and cause a temporary shift of potassium into the cells. Also, sodium bicarbonate furnishes sodium to antagonize the cardiac effects of potassium. Effects of this therapy begin within 30 to 60 minutes and may persist for hours; however, they are temporary.

IV administration of regular insulin and a hypertonic dextrose solution causes a temporary shift of potassium into the cells. Glucose and insulin therapy has an onset of action within 30 minutes and lasts for several hours.

Beta-2 agonists also move potassium into the cells and may be used in the absence of ischemic cardiac disease. These stopgap measures only temporarily protect the patient from hyperkalemia. If the hyperkalemic condition is not transient, actual removal of potassium from the body is required; this may be accomplished by using cation exchange resins, peritoneal dialysis, hemodialysis or other forms of renal replacement therapy.

Nursing Management

Patients at risk for potassium excess, for example those with renal failure, should be identified so they can be monitored closely for signs of hyperkalemia. The nurse observes for signs of muscle weakness and dysrhythmias. The presence of paresthesias is noted, as are GI symptoms such as nausea and intestinal colic. For patients at risk, serum potassium levels are measured periodically.

Elevated serum potassium levels may be erroneous; thus, highly abnormal levels should always be verified. To avoid false reports of hyperkalemia, prolonged use of a tourniquet while drawing the blood sample is avoided, and the patient is cautioned not to exercise the extremity immediately before the blood sample is obtained. The blood sample is delivered to the laboratory as soon as possible, because hemolysis of the sample results in a falsely elevated serum potassium level.

PREVENTING HYPERKALEMIA

Measures are taken to prevent hyperkalemia in patients at risk, when possible, by encouraging the patient to adhere to the prescribed potassium restriction. Potassium-rich foods to be avoided include coffee, cocoa, tea, dried fruits, dried beans, and whole-grain breads. Milk and eggs also contain substantial amounts of potassium. Conversely, foods with minimal potassium content include butter, margarine, cranberry juice or sauce, ginger ale, gumdrops or jellybeans, hard candy, root beer, sugar, and honey.

CORRECTING HYPERKALEMIA

As stated earlier, it is possible to exceed the tolerance for potassium in any person if it is administered rapidly by the IV route. Therefore, great care should be taken to monitor potassium solutions closely, paying close attention to the solution's concentration and rate of administration. When potassium is added to parenteral solutions, the potassium is mixed with the fluid by inverting the bottle several times. Potassium chloride should never be added to a hanging bottle because the potassium might be administered as a bolus (potassium chloride is heavy and settles to the bottom of the container).

It is important to caution patients to use salt substitutes sparingly if they are taking other supplementary forms of potassium or potassium-conserving diuretics. Also, potassium-conserving diuretics, such as spironolactone (Aldactone), triamterene (Dyrenium), and amiloride (Midamor); potassium supplements; and salt substitutes should not be administered to patients with renal dysfunction. Most salt substitutes contain approximately 50–60 mEq of potassium per teaspoon.

SIGNIFICANCE OF CALCIUM

More than 99% of the body's calcium is located in the skeletal system; it is a major component of bones and teeth. About 1% of skeletal calcium is rapidly exchangeable with blood calcium; the rest is more stable and only slowly exchanged. The small amount of calcium located outside the bone circulates in the serum, partly bound to protein and partly ionized. Calcium plays a major role in transmitting nerve impulses and helps to regulate muscle contraction and relaxation, including cardiac muscle. Calcium is instrumental in activating enzymes that stimulate many essential chemical reactions in the body, and it also plays a role in blood coagulation. Because many factors affect calcium regulation, both hypocalcemia and hypercalcemia are relatively common disturbances.

The normal total serum calcium level is 8.5 to 10.5 mg/dL (2.1–2.6 mmol/L). It exists in plasma in three forms: ionized, bound, and complexed. About 50% of the serum calcium exists in an ionized form that is physiologically active and important for neuromuscular activity and blood coagulation. The normal ionized serum calcium level is 4.5 to 5.1 mg/dL (1.1–1.3 mmol/L) and is the only form that is physiologically and clinically significant. Less than half of the plasma calcium is bound to serum proteins, primarily albumin. The remainder is combined with nonprotein anions: phosphate, citrate, and carbonate.

Calcium is absorbed from foods in the presence of normal gastric acidity and vitamin D. Calcium is excreted primarily in the feces, the remainder in urine. The serum calcium level is controlled by PTH and calcitonin. As ionized serum calcium decreases, the parathyroid glands secrete PTH. This event then increases calcium absorption from the GI tract, increases calcium reabsorption from the renal tubule, and releases calcium from the bone. The increase in calcium ion concentration suppresses PTH secretion. When calcium increases excessively, the thyroid gland secretes calcitonin. It briefly inhibits calcium reabsorption from bone and decreases the serum calcium concentration.

CALCIUM DEFICIT (HYPOCALCEMIA)

Hypocalcemia (lower-than-normal serum concentration of calcium) occurs in a variety of clinical situations. A patient may have a total body calcium deficit (as in osteoporosis) but a normal serum calcium level. Elderly people with osteoporosis, who spend an increased amount of time in bed, are at increased risk for hypocalcemia as bed rest increases bone resorption.

Several factors can cause hypocalcemia. Primary hypoparathyroidism results in this disturbance, as does surgical hypoparathyroidism. The latter is far more common. Not only is hypocalcemia associated with thyroid and parathyroid surgery, but it can also occur after radical neck dissection and is most likely in the first 24 to 48 hours after surgery. Transient hypocalcemia can occur with massive administration of citrated blood (as in exchange transfusions in newborns), because citrate can combine with ionized calcium and temporarily remove it from the circulation.

Inflammation of the pancreas causes the breakdown of proteins and lipids. It is thought that calcium ions combine with the fatty acids released by lipolysis, forming soaps. As a result of this process, hypocalcemia occurs and is common in pancreatitis. It has also been suggested that hypocalcemia might be related to excessive secretion of glucagon from the inflamed pancreas, resulting in increased secretion of calcitonin (a hormone that lowers serum calcium).

Hypocalcemia is common in patients with renal failure because these patients frequently have elevated serum phosphate levels. Hyperphosphatemia usually causes a reciprocal drop in the serum calcium level. Other causes of hypocalcemia include inadequate vitamin D consumption, magnesium deficiency, medullary thyroid carcinoma, low serum albumin levels, alkalosis, and alcohol abuse. Medications predisposing to hypocalcemia include aluminum-containing antacids, aminoglycosides, caffeine, cisplatin, corticosteroids, mithramycin, phosphates, isoniazid, and loop diuretics.

Osteoporosis is associated with prolonged low intake of calcium and represents a total body calcium deficit, even though serum calcium levels are usually normal. This disorder occurs in millions of Americans and is most common in postmenopausal women. It is characterized by loss of bone mass, causing bones to become porous and brittle and therefore susceptible to fracture. See Chapter 68 for further discussion of osteoporosis.

Clinical Manifestations

Tetany is the most characteristic manifestation of hypocalcemia and hypomagnesemia. Tetany refers to the entire symptom complex induced by increased neural excitability. These symptoms are due to spontaneous discharges of both sensory and motor fibers in peripheral nerves. Sensations of tingling may occur in the

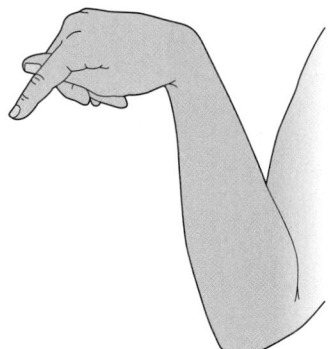

FIGURE 14-6 Trousseau's sign. Ischemia-induced carpal spasm can occur with hypocalcemia or hypomagnesemia.

tips of the fingers, around the mouth, and less commonly in the feet. Spasms of the muscles of the extremities and face may occur. Pain may develop as a result of these spasms.

Trousseau's sign (Fig. 14-6) can be elicited by inflating a blood pressure cuff on the upper arm to about 20 mm Hg above systolic pressure; within 2 to 5 minutes, carpopedal spasm (an adducted thumb, flexed wrist and metacarpophalangeal joints, extended interphalangeal joints with fingers together) will occur as ischemia of the ulnar nerve develops. Chvostek's sign consists of twitching of muscles supplied by the facial nerve when the nerve is tapped about 2 cm anterior to the earlobe, just below the zygomatic arch.

Seizures may occur because hypocalcemia increases irritability of the central nervous system as well as of the peripheral nerves. Other changes associated with hypocalcemia include mental changes such as depression, impaired memory, confusion, delirium, and even hallucinations. A prolonged QT interval is seen on the ECG due to prolongation of the ST segment; a form of ventricular tachycardia called torsades de pointes may occur.

Assessment and Diagnostic Findings

When evaluating serum calcium levels, one must consider several other variables, such as the serum albumin level and arterial pH. Because abnormalities in serum albumin levels may affect interpretation of the serum calcium level, it may be necessary to calculate the corrected serum calcium if the serum albumin level is abnormal. For every decrease in serum albumin of 1 g/dL below 4 g/dL, the total serum calcium level is underestimated by approximately 0.8 mg/dL. The following is a quick method to calculate the corrected serum calcium level:

$$\text{Measured total serum } Ca^{++} \text{ level (mg/dL)} + 0.8$$
$$\times (4.0 - \text{measured albumin level [g/dL]})$$
$$= \text{corrected total calcium concentration (mg/dL)}.$$

An example of the calculations needed to obtain the corrected total serum calcium level is as follows:

A patient's reported serum albumin level is 2.5 g/dL; the reported serum calcium level is 10.5 mg/dL.

- The decrease in serum albumin level from normal level (difference from normal albumin of 4 g/dL) is calculated: 4 g/dL − 2.5 g/dL = 1.5 g/dL
- The following ratio is calculated:
  0.8 mg/dL: 1 g/dL = ? mg/dL: 1.5 mg/dL
  ? = 0.8 mg × 1.5
  ? = 1.2 mg/dL calcium

- Add 1.2 to 10.5 mg (reported serum calcium level) to obtain the corrected total serum calcium level of 11.7 mg/dL.
  1.2 + 10.5 mg = 11.7 mg/dL

Clinicians often ignore a low serum calcium level in the presence of a similarly low serum albumin level. The ionized calcium level is usually normal in patients with reduced total serum calcium levels and concomitant hypoalbuminemia. When the arterial pH increases (alkalosis), more calcium becomes bound to protein. As a result, the ionized portion decreases. Symptoms of hypocalcemia may occur with alkalosis. Acidosis (low pH) has the opposite effect—that is, less calcium is bound to protein and thus more exists in the ionized form. However, relatively small changes in serum calcium levels occur in these acid–base abnormalities.

Ideally, the laboratory should measure the ionized level of calcium. In many laboratories, however, only the total calcium level is reported; thus, concentration of the ionized fraction must be estimated by simultaneous measurement of the serum albumin level. PTH levels are decreased in hypoparathyroidism. Magnesium and phosphorus levels need to be assessed to identify possible causes of decreased calcium.

Medical Management

Acute symptomatic hypocalcemia is life-threatening and requires prompt treatment with IV administration of calcium (Marx, 2000). Parenteral calcium salts include calcium gluconate, calcium chloride, and calcium gluceptate. Although calcium chloride produces a significantly higher ionized calcium level than calcium gluconate, it is not used as often because it is more irritating and can cause sloughing of tissue if it infiltrates. Too-rapid IV administration of calcium can cause cardiac arrest, preceded by bradycardia. IV calcium administration is particularly dangerous in patients receiving digitalis-derived medications because calcium ions exert an effect similar to that of digitalis and can cause digitalis toxicity, with adverse cardiac effects. IV calcium should be diluted in D_5W and given as a slow IV bolus or a slow IV infusion using a volumetric infusion pump. The IV site must be observed often for any evidence of infiltration because of the risk for sloughing of tissues with calcium infusions. A 0.9% sodium chloride solution should not be used with calcium because it will increase renal calcium loss. Solutions containing phosphates or bicarbonate should not be used with calcium because they will cause precipitation when calcium is added. The nurse must clarify with the physician which calcium salt to administer, because calcium gluconate yields 4.5 mEq of calcium and calcium chloride provides 13.6 mEq of calcium. Calcium can cause postural hypotension; therefore, the patient is kept in bed for IV replacement and blood pressure is monitored.

Vitamin D therapy may be instituted to increase calcium absorption from the GI tract. Aluminum hydroxide, calcium acetate, or calcium carbonate antacids may be prescribed to decrease elevated phosphorus levels before treating hypocalcemia for the patient with chronic renal failure. Increasing the dietary intake of calcium to at least 1,000 to 1,500 mg/day in the adult is recommended (eg, milk products; green, leafy vegetables; canned salmon; sardines; fresh oysters). Because hypomagnesemia can also cause tetany, if the tetany responds to IV calcium, then a low magnesium level is explored as a possible cause in chronic renal failure.

Nursing Management

It is important to observe for hypocalcemia in patients at risk. Seizure precautions are initiated when hypocalcemia is severe. The status of the airway is closely monitored because laryngeal stridor can occur. Safety precautions are taken, as indicated, if confusion is present.

People at high risk for osteoporosis are instructed about the need for adequate dietary calcium intake; if not consumed in the diet, calcium supplements should be considered. Also, the value of regular weight-bearing exercise in decreasing bone loss should be emphasized, as should the effect of medications on calcium balance. For example, alcohol and caffeine in high doses inhibit calcium absorption, and moderate cigarette smoking increases urinary calcium excretion. Additional teaching topics may involve discussion of medications such as alendronate (Fosamax), risedronate (Actonel), raloxifene (Evista), and calcitonin to reduce the rate of bone loss. Teaching also addresses strategies to reduce risk for falls.

CALCIUM EXCESS (HYPERCALCEMIA)

Hypercalcemia (excess of calcium in the plasma) is a dangerous imbalance when severe; in fact, hypercalcemic crisis has a mortality rate as high as 50% if not treated promptly.

The most common causes of hypercalcemia are malignancies and hyperparathyroidism. Malignant tumors can produce hypercalcemia by a variety of mechanisms. The excessive PTH secretion associated with hyperparathyroidism causes increased release of calcium from the bones and increased intestinal and renal absorption of calcium. Calcifications of soft tissue occur when the calcium–phosphorus product exceeds 70 (serum calcium [mg/dL] × serum phosphorus [mg/dL]) (Marx, 2000).

Bone mineral is lost during immobilization, sometimes causing elevation of total (and especially ionized) calcium in the bloodstream. Symptomatic hypercalcemia from immobilization, however, is rare; when it does occur, it is virtually limited to people with high calcium turnover rates (eg, adolescents during a growth spurt). Most cases of hypercalcemia secondary to immobility occur after severe or multiple fractures or spinal cord injury.

Thiazide diuretics may cause a slight elevation in serum calcium levels because they potentiate the action of PTH on the kidneys, reducing urinary calcium excretion. The milk-alkali syndrome can occur in patients with peptic ulcer treated for a prolonged period with milk and alkaline antacids, particularly calcium carbonate. Vitamin A and D intoxication, as well as the use of lithium, can cause calcium excess.

Clinical Manifestations

As a rule, the symptoms of hypercalcemia are proportional to the degree of elevation of the serum calcium level. Hypercalcemia reduces neuromuscular excitability because it suppresses activity at the myoneural junction. Symptoms such as muscle weakness, incoordination, anorexia, and constipation may be due to decreased tone in smooth and striated muscle. Cardiac standstill can occur when the serum calcium level is about 18 mg/dL (4.5 mmol/L). The inotropic effect of digitalis is enhanced by calcium; therefore, digitalis toxicity is aggravated by hypercalcemia.

Anorexia, nausea, vomiting, and constipation are common symptoms of hypercalcemia. Dehydration occurs with nausea, vomiting, anorexia, and calcium reabsorption at the proximal renal tubule. Abdominal and bone pain may also be present. Abdominal distention and paralytic ileus may complicate severe hypercalcemic crisis. Excessive urination due to disturbed renal tubular function produced by hypercalcemia may be present. Severe thirst may occur secondary to the polyuria caused by the high solute (calcium) load. Patients with chronic hypercalcemia may develop symptoms similar to those of peptic ulcer because hypercalcemia increases the secretion of acid and pepsin by the stomach.

Confusion, impaired memory, slurred speech, lethargy, acute psychotic behavior, or coma may occur. The more severe symptoms tend to appear when the serum calcium level is approximately 16 mg/dL (4 mmol/L) or above. However, some patients become profoundly disturbed with serum calcium levels of only 12 mg/dL (3 mmol/L). These symptoms resolve as serum calcium levels return to normal after treatment.

Hypercalcemic crisis refers to an acute rise in the serum calcium level to 17 mg/dL (4.3 mmol/L) or higher. Severe thirst and polyuria are characteristically present. Other findings may include muscle weakness, intractable nausea, abdominal cramps, obstipation (very severe constipation) or diarrhea, peptic ulcer symptoms, and bone pain. Lethargy, confusion, and coma may also occur. This condition is very dangerous and may result in cardiac arrest.

Assessment and Diagnostic Findings

The serum calcium level is greater than 10.5 mg/dL (2.6 mmol/L). Cardiovascular changes may include a variety of dysrhythmias and shortening of the QT interval and ST segment. The PR interval is sometimes prolonged. The double-antibody PTH test may be used to differentiate between primary hyperparathyroidism and malignancy as a cause of hypercalcemia: PTH levels are increased in primary or secondary hyperparathyroidism and suppressed in malignancy. X-rays may reveal the presence of osteoporosis, bone cavitation, or urinary calculi. The Sulkowitch urine test analyzes the amount of calcium in the urine; in hypercalcemia, dense precipitation is observed due to hypercalciuria.

Medical Management

Therapeutic aims in hypercalcemia include decreasing the serum calcium level and reversing the process causing hypercalcemia. Treating the underlying cause (eg, chemotherapy for a malignancy or partial parathyroidectomy for hyperparathyroidism) is essential.

PHARMACOLOGIC THERAPY

General measures include administering fluids to dilute serum calcium and promote its excretion by the kidneys, mobilizing the patient, and restricting dietary calcium intake. IV administration of 0.9% sodium chloride solution temporarily dilutes the serum calcium level and increases urinary calcium excretion by inhibiting tubular reabsorption of calcium. Administering IV phosphate can cause a reciprocal drop in serum calcium. Furosemide (Lasix) is often used in conjunction with administration of a saline solution; in addition to causing diuresis, furosemide increases calcium excretion.

Calcitonin can be used to lower the serum calcium level and is particularly useful for patients with heart disease or renal failure who cannot tolerate large sodium loads. Calcitonin reduces bone resorption, increases the deposit of calcium and phosphorus in the bones, and increases urinary excretion of calcium and phosphorus. Although available in several forms, calcitonin derived from salmon is commonly used. Skin testing for allergy to salmon calcitonin is necessary before the hormone is administered. Systemic allergic reactions are possible since this hormone is a protein; resistance to the medication may develop later because of antibody formation. Calcitonin is administered by intramuscular injection rather than subcutaneously because patients with hypercalcemia have poor perfusion of subcutaneous tissue.

For patients with cancer, treatment is directed at controlling the condition by surgery, chemotherapy, or radiation therapy. Corticosteroids may be used to decrease bone turnover and tubular reabsorption for patients with sarcoidosis, myelomas, lymphomas, and leukemias; patients with solid tumors are less responsive. The bisphosphonates inhibit osteoclast activity. Pamidronate (Aredia) is the most potent of these agents and is given IV; it causes a transient, mild pyrexia, decreased white blood cell count, and myalgia. Etidronate (Didronel) is another bisphosphonate that is given IV, but its action is slower. Mithramycin, a cytotoxic antibiotic, inhibits bone resorption and thus lowers the serum calcium level. This agent must be used cautiously because it has significant side effects, including thrombocytopenia, nephrotoxicity, rebound hypercalcemia when discontinued, and hepatotoxicity. Inorganic phosphate salts can be administered orally or by nasogastric tube (in the form of Phospho-Soda or Neutra-Phos), rectally (as retention enemas), or IV. IV phosphate therapy is used with extreme caution in the treatment of hypercalcemia because it can cause severe calcification in various tissues, hypotension, tetany, and acute renal failure.

Nursing Management

It is important to monitor for hypercalcemia in patients at risk. Interventions such as increasing patient mobility and encouraging fluids can help prevent hypercalcemia, or at least minimize its severity. Hospitalized patients at risk for hypercalcemia are encouraged to ambulate as soon as possible; outpatients and those cared for in their homes are informed of the importance of frequent ambulation.

When encouraging oral fluids, the nurse considers the patient's likes and dislikes. Fluids containing sodium should be administered unless contraindicated by other conditions, because sodium favors calcium excretion. Patients are encouraged to drink 3 to 4 quarts of fluid daily. Adequate fiber should be provided in the diet to offset the tendency for constipation. Safety precautions are taken, as necessary, when mental symptoms of hypercalcemia are present. The patient and family are informed that these mental changes are reversible with treatment. Increased calcium potentiates the effects of digitalis; therefore, the patient is assessed for signs and symptoms of digitalis toxicity. ECG changes (premature ventricular contractions, paroxysmal atrial tachycardia, and heart block) can occur; therefore, the cardiac rate and rhythm are monitored for any abnormalities.

SIGNIFICANCE OF MAGNESIUM

Next to potassium, magnesium is the most abundant intracellular cation. It acts as an activator for many intracellular enzyme systems and plays a role in both carbohydrate and protein metabolism. Magnesium balance is important in neuromuscular function. Because magnesium acts directly on the myoneural junction, variations in the serum concentration of magnesium affect neuromuscular irritability and contractility. For example, an excess of magnesium diminishes the excitability of the muscle cells, whereas a deficit increases neuromuscular irritability and contractility.

Magnesium produces its sedative effect at the neuromuscular junction, probably by inhibiting the release of the neurotransmitter acetylcholine. It also increases the stimulus threshold in nerve fibers.

Magnesium exerts effects on the cardiovascular system, acting peripherally to produce vasodilation. Magnesium is thought to have a direct effect on peripheral arteries and arterioles, which results in a decreased total peripheral resistance. Magnesium disorders include hypomagnesemia and hypermagnesemia.

MAGNESIUM DEFICIT (HYPOMAGNESEMIA)

Hypomagnesemia refers to a below-normal serum magnesium concentration. The normal serum magnesium level is 1.5 to 2.5 mEq/L (or 1.8–3.0 mg/dL; 0.8–1.2 mmol/L). Approximately one third of serum magnesium is bound to protein; the remaining two thirds exists as free cations (Mg^{++}). Like calcium, it is the ionized fraction that is primarily involved in neuromuscular activity and other physiologic processes. As with calcium levels, magnesium levels should be evaluated in combination with albumin levels. Low serum albumin levels decrease total magnesium.

Hypomagnesemia is a common yet often overlooked imbalance in acutely and critically ill patients. It may occur with withdrawal from alcohol and administration of tube feedings or parenteral nutrition.

An important route for magnesium loss is the GI tract. Loss of magnesium from the GI tract may occur with nasogastric suction, diarrhea, or fistulas. Because fluid from the lower GI tract has a higher concentration of magnesium (10–14 mEq/L) than fluid from the upper tract (1–2 mEq/L), losses from diarrhea and intestinal fistulas are more likely to induce magnesium deficit than are those from gastric suction. Although magnesium losses are relatively small in nasogastric suction, hypomagnesemia will occur if losses are prolonged and magnesium is not replaced through IV infusion. Because the distal small bowel is the major site of magnesium absorption, any disruption in small bowel function, as in intestinal resection or inflammatory bowel disease, can lead to hypomagnesemia.

Alcoholism is currently the most common cause of symptomatic hypomagnesemia in the United States. Hypomagnesemia is particularly troublesome during treatment of alcohol withdrawal. Therefore, the serum magnesium level should be measured at least every 2 or 3 days in patients going through withdrawal from alcohol. The serum magnesium level may be normal on admission but fall as a result of metabolic changes, such as the intracellular shift of magnesium associated with IV glucose administration.

During nutritional repletion, the major cellular electrolytes move from the serum to newly synthesized cells. Thus, if the enteral or parenteral feeding formula is deficient in magnesium content, serious hypomagnesemia will occur. Because of this, serum magnesium levels should be measured at regular intervals in patients who are receiving parenteral nutrition and enteral feedings, especially those who have undergone a period of starvation. Other causes of hypomagnesemia include the administration of aminoglycosides, cyclosporine, cisplatin, diuretics, digitalis, and amphotericin and the rapid administration of citrated blood, especially to patients with renal or hepatic disease. Magnesium deficiency often occurs in diabetic ketoacidosis, secondary to increased renal excretion during osmotic diuresis and shifting of magnesium into the cells with insulin therapy. Other contributing causes are sepsis, burns, and hypothermia.

Clinical Manifestations

Clinical manifestations of hypomagnesemia are largely confined to the neuromuscular system. Some of the effects are due directly to the low serum magnesium level; others are due to secondary changes in potassium and calcium metabolism. Symptoms do not usually occur until the serum magnesium level is less than 1 mEq/L (0.5 mmol/L).

Among the neuromuscular changes are hyperexcitability with muscle weakness, tremors, and athetoid movements (slow, involuntary twisting and writhing). Others include tetany, generalized tonic-clonic or focal seizures, laryngeal stridor, and positive Chvostek's and Trousseau's signs (see earlier discussion in this chapter), which occur, in part, because of accompanying hypocalcemia.

Magnesium deficiency can disturb the ECG by prolonging the QRS, depressing the ST segment, and predisposing to cardiac dysrhythmias, such as premature ventricular contractions, supraventricular tachycardia, torsades de pointes (a form of ventricular tachycardia), and ventricular fibrillation. Increased susceptibility to digitalis toxicity is associated with low serum magnesium levels. This is important because patients receiving digoxin are also likely to be receiving diuretic therapy, predisposing them to renal loss of magnesium.

Hypomagnesemia may be accompanied by marked alterations in mood. Apathy, depression, apprehension, and extreme agitation have been noted, as well as ataxia, dizziness, insomnia, and confusion. At times, delirium, auditory or visual hallucinations, and frank psychoses may occur.

Assessment and Diagnostic Findings

On laboratory analysis, the serum magnesium level is less than 1.5 mEq/L or 1.8 mg/dL (0.75 mmol/L). Hypomagnesemia is frequently associated with hypokalemia and hypocalcemia. About 25% of magnesium is protein-bound, principally to albumin. A decreased serum albumin level can, therefore, reduce the measured total magnesium concentration; however, it does not reduce the ionized plasma magnesium concentration. ECG evaluations reflect magnesium, calcium, and potassium deficiencies, tachydysrhythmias, prolonged PR and QT intervals, widening QRS, ST segment depression, flattened T waves, and a prominent U wave. Torsades de pointes is associated with a low magnesium level. Premature ventricular contractions, paroxysmal atrial tachycardia, and heart block may also occur. Urinary magnesium levels may be helpful in identifying causes of magnesium depletion and are measured after a loading dose of magnesium sulfate is administered. Two newer diagnostic techniques (nuclear magnetic resonance spectroscopy and the ion selective electrode) are sensitive and direct means to measure ionized serum magnesium levels.

Medical Management

Mild magnesium deficiency can be corrected by diet alone. Principal dietary sources of magnesium are green leafy vegetables, nuts, legumes, whole grains, and seafood. Magnesium is also plentiful in peanut butter and chocolate. When necessary, magnesium salts can be administered orally to replace continuous excessive losses. Diarrhea is a common complication of excessive ingestion of magnesium. Patients receiving parenteral nutrition require magnesium in the IV solution to prevent hypomagnesemia. IV administration

of magnesium sulfate must be given by an infusion pump and at a rate not to exceed 150 mg/min. A bolus dose of magnesium sulfate given too rapidly can produce cardiac arrest. Vital signs must be assessed frequently during magnesium administration to detect changes in cardiac rate or rhythm, hypotension, and respiratory distress. Monitoring urine output is essential before, during, and after magnesium administration; the physician is notified if urine volume decreases to less than 100 mL over 4 hours. Calcium gluconate must be readily available to treat hypocalcemic tetany or hypermagnesemia.

Overt symptoms of hypomagnesemia are treated with parenteral administration of magnesium. Magnesium sulfate is the most commonly used magnesium salt. Serial magnesium concentrations can be used to regulate the dosage.

Nursing Management

The nurse should be aware of patients at risk for hypomagnesemia and observe for its signs and symptoms. Patients receiving digitalis are monitored closely because a deficit of magnesium can predispose them to digitalis toxicity. When hypomagnesemia is severe, seizure precautions are implemented. Other safety precautions are instituted, as indicated, if confusion is observed.

Because difficulty in swallowing (dysphagia) may occur in magnesium-depleted patients, the ability to swallow should be tested with water before oral medications or foods are offered. Dysphagia is probably related to the athetoid or choreiform (rapid, involuntary, and irregular jerking) movements associated with magnesium deficit. To determine neuromuscular irritability, the nurse needs to assess and grade deep tendon reflexes (see Chap. 60 for discussion of assessment and grading reflexes).

Teaching plays a major role in treating magnesium deficit, particularly that resulting from abuse of diuretic or laxative medications. In such cases, the nurse can instruct the patient about the need to consume magnesium-rich foods. For patients experiencing hypomagnesemia from abuse of alcohol, the nurse can provide teaching, counseling, support, and possible referral to alcohol abstinence programs or other professional help.

MAGNESIUM EXCESS (HYPERMAGNESEMIA)

Hypermagnesemia is a greater-than-normal serum concentration of magnesium. A serum magnesium level can appear falsely elevated when blood specimens are allowed to hemolyze or are drawn from an extremity with a tourniquet that was applied too tightly.

By far the most common cause of hypermagnesemia is renal failure. In fact, most patients with advanced renal failure have at least a slight elevation in serum magnesium levels. This condition is aggravated when such patients receive magnesium to control seizures or inadvertently take one of the many commercial antacids that contain magnesium salts.

Hypermagnesemia can occur in a patient with untreated diabetic ketoacidosis when catabolism causes the release of cellular magnesium that cannot be excreted because of profound fluid volume depletion and resulting oliguria. An excess of magnesium can also result from excessive magnesium administered to treat hypertension of pregnancy and to lower serum magnesium levels. Increased serum magnesium levels can also occur in adrenocortical insufficiency, Addison's disease, or hypothermia. Excessive use of antacids (eg, Maalox, Riopan, Mylanta) and laxatives (Milk of Magnesia) also increases serum magnesium levels.

Clinical Manifestations

Acute elevation of the serum magnesium level depresses the central nervous system as well as the peripheral neuromuscular junction. At mildly elevated levels, there is a tendency for lowered blood pressure because of peripheral vasodilation. Nausea, vomiting, soft tissue calcifications, facial flushing, and sensations of warmth may also occur. At higher magnesium concentrations, lethargy, difficulty speaking (dysarthria), and drowsiness can occur. Deep tendon reflexes are lost, and muscle weakness and paralysis may develop. The respiratory center is depressed when serum magnesium levels exceed 10 mEq/L (5 mmol/L). Coma, atrioventricular heart block, and cardiac arrest can occur when the serum magnesium level is greatly elevated and not treated.

Assessment and Diagnostic Findings

On laboratory analysis, the serum magnesium level is greater than 2.5 mEq/L or 3.0 mg/dL (1.25 mmol/L). ECG findings may include a prolonged PR interval, tall T waves, and a widened QRS. ECG findings demonstrate a prolonged QT interval and atrioventricular blocks.

Medical Management

Hypermagnesemia can be prevented by avoiding the administration of magnesium to patients with renal failure and by carefully monitoring seriously ill patients who are receiving magnesium salts. In patients with severe hypermagnesemia, all parenteral and oral magnesium salts are discontinued. In emergencies, such as respiratory depression or defective cardiac conduction, ventilatory support and IV calcium are indicated. In addition, hemodialysis with a magnesium-free dialysate can reduce the serum magnesium to a safe level within hours. Loop diuretics and 0.45% sodium chloride (half-strength saline) solution enhance magnesium excretion in patients with adequate renal function. IV calcium gluconate (10 mL of a 10% solution) antagonizes the neuromuscular effects of magnesium.

Nursing Management

Patients at risk for hypermagnesemia are identified and assessed. When hypermagnesemia is suspected, the nurse monitors the vital signs, noting hypotension and shallow respirations. The nurse also observes for decreased patellar reflexes and changes in the level of consciousness. Medications that contain magnesium are not given to patients with renal failure or compromised renal function, and patients with renal failure are cautioned to check with their health care providers before taking over-the-counter medications. Caution is essential when preparing and administering magnesium-containing fluids parenterally because available parenteral magnesium solutions (eg, 2-mL ampules or 50-mL vials) differ in concentration.

SIGNIFICANCE OF PHOSPHORUS

Phosphorus is a critical constituent of all the body's tissues. It is essential to the function of muscle and red blood cells, the formation of adenosine triphosphate (ATP) and 2,3-diphospho-glycerate, and the maintenance of acid–base balance, as well as to the nervous system and the intermediary metabolism of carbohydrate, protein, and fat. The normal serum phosphorus level is 2.5 to 4.5 mg/dL (0.8–1.5 mmol/L) and may be as high as 6 mg/dL (1.94 mmol/L) in infants and children. Serum phosphorus levels are presumably greater in children because of the high rate of skeletal growth. Phosphorus is the primary anion of the ICF. About 85% of phosphorus is located in bones and teeth, 14% in soft tissue, and less than 1% in the ECF. Phosphorus is critical to nerve and muscle function and provides structural support to bones and teeth. Phosphorus levels decrease with age.

PHOSPHORUS DEFICIT (HYPOPHOSPHATEMIA)

Hypophosphatemia is a below-normal serum concentration of inorganic phosphorus. Although it often indicates phosphorus deficiency, hypophosphatemia may occur under a variety of circumstances in which total body phosphorus stores are normal. Conversely, phosphorus deficiency is an abnormally low content of phosphorus in lean tissues and may exist in the absence of hypophosphatemia.

Hypophosphatemia may occur during the administration of calories to patients with severe protein-calorie malnutrition. It is most likely to occur with overzealous intake or administration of simple carbohydrates. This syndrome can be induced in anyone with severe protein-calorie malnutrition (eg, patients with anorexia nervosa or alcoholism, or elderly debilitated patients unable to eat). As many as 50% of patients hospitalized because of chronic alcoholism have hypophosphatemia.

Marked hypophosphatemia may develop in malnourished patients who receive parenteral nutrition if the phosphorus loss is not adequately corrected. Other causes of hypophosphatemia include prolonged intense hyperventilation, alcohol withdrawal, poor dietary intake, diabetic ketoacidosis, and major thermal burns. Low magnesium levels, low potassium levels, and hyperparathyroidism related to increased urinary losses of phosphorus contribute to hypophosphatemia. Respiratory alkalosis can cause a decrease in phosphorus because of an intracellular shift of phosphorus.

Excess phosphorus binding by antacids containing magnesium, calcium, or albumin may decrease the phosphorus available from the diet to amounts below that required to maintain serum phosphorus balance. The degree of hypophosphatemia depends on the amount of phosphorus in the diet compared to the dose of antacid. Vitamin D regulates intestinal ion absorption; therefore, a deficiency of vitamin D may cause decreased calcium and phosphorus levels, which may lead to osteomalacia (softened, brittle bones).

Clinical Manifestations

Most of the signs and symptoms of phosphorus deficiency appear to result from a deficiency of ATP, 2,3-diphosphoglycerate, or both. ATP deficiency impairs cellular energy resources; diphosphoglycerate deficiency impairs oxygen delivery to tissues.

A wide range of neurologic symptoms may occur, such as irritability, fatigue, apprehension, weakness, numbness, paresthesias, confusion, seizures, and coma. Low levels of diphosphoglycerate may reduce the delivery of oxygen to peripheral tissues, resulting in tissue anoxia. Hypoxia then leads to an increase in respiratory rate and respiratory alkalosis, causing phosphorus to move into the cells and potentiating hypophosphatemia.

It is thought that hypophosphatemia predisposes a person to infection. In laboratory animals, hypophosphatemia is associated with depression of the chemotactic, phagocytic, and bacterial activity of granulocytes.

Muscle damage may develop as the ATP level in the muscle tissue declines. Clinical manifestations are muscle weakness, muscle pain, and at times acute rhabdomyolysis (disintegration of striated muscle). Weakness of respiratory muscles may greatly impair ventilation. Hypophosphatemia also may predispose a person to insulin resistance and thus hyperglycemia. Chronic loss of phosphorus can cause bruising and bleeding from platelet dysfunction.

Assessment and Diagnostic Findings

On laboratory analysis, the serum phosphorus level is less than 2.5 mg/dL (0.80 mmol/L) in adults. When reviewing laboratory results, the nurse should keep in mind that glucose or insulin administration causes a slight decrease in the serum phosphorus level. PTH levels are increased in hyperparathyroidism. Serum magnesium may decrease due to increased urinary excretion of magnesium. Alkaline phosphatase is increased with osteoblastic activity. X-rays may show skeletal changes of osteomalacia or rickets.

Medical Management

Prevention of hypophosphatemia is the goal. In patients at risk for hypophosphatemia, serum phosphate levels should be closely monitored and correction initiated before deficits become severe. Adequate amounts of phosphorus should be added to parenteral solutions, and attention should be paid to the phosphorus levels in enteral feeding solutions.

Severe hypophosphatemia is dangerous and requires prompt attention. Aggressive IV phosphorus correction is usually limited to patients whose serum phosphorus levels fall below 1 mg/dL (0.3 mmol/L) and whose GI tract is not functioning. Possible dangers of IV phosphorus administration include tetany from hypocalcemia and metastatic calcification from hyperphosphatemia. The rate of phosphorus administration should not exceed 10 mEq/h, and the site should be carefully monitored because tissue sloughing and necrosis can occur with infiltration. In less acute situations, oral phosphorus replacement is usually adequate.

Nursing Management

The nurse identifies patients at risk for hypophosphatemia and monitors for it. Because malnourished patients receiving parenteral nutrition are at risk when calories are introduced too aggressively, preventive measures involve gradually introducing the solution to avoid rapid shifts of phosphorus into the cells.

For patients with documented hypophosphatemia, careful attention is given to preventing infection because hypophosphatemia may alter the granulocytes. In patients requiring correction of phosphorus losses, the nurse frequently monitors serum phosphorus levels and documents and reports early signs of hypophosphatemia (apprehension, confusion, change in level of consciousness). If the patient experiences mild hypophosphatemia, foods such as milk and milk products, organ meats, nuts, fish, poultry, and whole grains should be encouraged. With moderate hypophosphatemia, supplements such as Neutra Phos capsules (250 mg phosphorus/capsule) or Fleets Phospho Soda (815 mg phosphorus/5 mL) may be prescribed (Metheny, 2000).

PHOSPHORUS EXCESS (HYPERPHOSPHATEMIA)

Hyperphosphatemia is a serum phosphorus level that exceeds normal. Various conditions can lead to this imbalance, but the most common is renal failure. Other causes include chemotherapy for neoplastic disease, hypoparathyroidism, respiratory acidosis or diabetic ketoacidosis, high phosphate intake, profound muscle necrosis, and increased phosphorus absorption. The primary complication of increased phosphorus is metastatic calcification (soft tissue, joints, and arteries), which results when the calcium–magnesium product (calcium × magnesium) exceeds 70 mg/dL.

Clinical Manifestations

An elevated serum phosphorus level causes few symptoms. Symptoms that do occur usually result from decreased calcium levels and soft tissue calcifications. The most important short-term consequence is tetany. Because of the reciprocal relationship between phosphorus and calcium, a high serum phosphorus level tends to cause a low serum calcium concentration. Tetany can result, causing tingling sensations in the fingertips and around the mouth. Anorexia, nausea, vomiting, muscle weakness, hyperreflexia, and tachycardia may occur.

The major long-term consequence is soft tissue calcification, which occurs mainly in patients with a reduced glomerular filtration rate. High serum levels of inorganic phosphorus promote precipitation of calcium phosphate in nonosseous sites, decreasing urine output, impairing vision, and producing palpitations.

Assessment and Diagnostic Findings

On laboratory analysis, the serum phosphorus level exceeds 4.5 mg/dL (1.5 mmol/L) in adults. Serum phosphorus levels are normally higher in children, presumably because of the high rate of skeletal growth. The serum calcium level is useful also for diagnosing the primary disorder and assessing the effects of treatments. X-ray studies may show skeletal changes with abnormal bone development. PTH levels are decreased in hypoparathyroidism. BUN and creatinine levels are used to assess renal function.

Medical Management

When possible, treatment is directed at the underlying disorder. For example, hyperphosphatemia may be related to volume depletion or respiratory or metabolic acidosis. In renal failure, elevated PTH production contributes to a high phosphorus level and bone disease. Measures to decrease the serum phosphate level in these patients include vitamin D preparations such as calcitol (Rocaltrol, in oral preparation), Calcijex (for IV administration), or paricalcitol (Zemplar). Vitamin D does not increase the serum calcium, thus permitting more aggressive treatment of hyperphosphatemia with calcium-binding antacids, phosphate-binding gels or antacids, restriction of dietary phosphate, and dialysis.

Nursing Management

The nurse monitors patients at risk for hyperphosphatemia. When a low-phosphorus diet is prescribed, the patient is instructed to avoid phosphorus-rich foods such as hard cheese, cream, nuts, whole-grain cereals, dried fruits, dried vegetables, kidneys, sardines, sweetbreads, and foods made with milk. When appropriate, the nurse instructs the patient to avoid phosphate-containing substances such as laxatives and enemas that contain phosphate. The nurse also teaches the patient to recognize the signs of impending hypocalcemia and to monitor for changes in urine output.

SIGNIFICANCE OF CHLORIDE

Chloride, the major anion of the ECF, is found more in interstitial and lymph fluid compartments than in blood. Chloride is also contained in gastric and pancreatic juices and sweat. Sodium and chloride in water make up the composition of the ECF and assist in determining osmotic pressure.

The serum level of chloride reflects a change in dilution or concentration of the ECF and does so in direct proportion to sodium. Aldosterone secretion increases sodium reabsorption, thereby increasing chloride reabsorption. The choroid plexus, where cerebrospinal fluid forms in the brain, depends on sodium and chloride to attract water to form the fluid portion of the cerebrospinal fluid. Bicarbonate has an inverse relationship with chloride. As chloride moves from plasma into the red blood cells (called the chloride shift), bicarbonate moves back into the plasma. Hydrogen ions are formed, which then help to release oxygen from hemoglobin. When the level of one of these three electrolytes (sodium, bicarbonate, or chloride) is disturbed, the other two will be affected as well.

CHLORIDE DEFICIT (HYPOCHLOREMIA)

Chloride control depends on the intake of chloride and the excretion and reabsorption of its ions in the kidneys. Chloride is produced in the stomach as hydrochloric acid; a small amount of chloride is lost in the feces. Chloride-deficient formulas, salt-restricted diets, GI tube drainage, and severe vomiting and diarrhea are risk factors for hypochloremia. As chloride decreases (usually because of volume depletion), sodium and bicarbonate ions are retained by the kidney to balance the loss. Bicarbonate accumulates in the ECF, which raises the pH and leads to hypochloremic metabolic alkalosis.

Clinical Manifestations

The signs and symptoms of hypochloremia are those of acid–base and electrolyte imbalances. The signs and symptoms of hyponatremia, hypokalemia, and metabolic alkalosis may also be noted. Metabolic alkalosis is a disorder that results in a high pH and a high serum bicarbonate level as a result of excess alkali intake or loss of hydrogen ions. With compensation, the $PaCO_2$ increases to 50 mm Hg. Hyperexcitability of muscles, tetany, hyperactive deep tendon reflexes, weakness, twitching, and muscle cramps may result. Hypokalemia can cause hypochloremia, resulting in cardiac dysrhythmias. In addition, because low chloride levels parallel low sodium levels, a water excess may occur. Hyponatremia can cause seizures and coma.

Assessment and Diagnostic Findings

The normal serum chloride level is 96 to 106 mEq/L (96–106 mmol/L). Inside the cell, the chloride level is 4 mEq/L. In addition to the chloride level, sodium and potassium levels are also evaluated because these electrolytes are lost along with chloride. Arterial blood gas analysis identifies the acid–base imbalance, which is usually metabolic alkalosis. The urine chloride level, which is also measured, decreases in hypochloremia.

Medical Management

Treatment involves correcting the cause of hypochloremia and contributing electrolyte and acid–base imbalances. Normal saline (0.9% sodium chloride) or half-strength saline (0.45% sodium chloride) solution is administered IV to replace the chloride. The physician may reevaluate whether patients receiving diuretics (loop, osmotic, or thiazide) should discontinue these medications or change to another diuretic.

Foods high in chloride are provided; these include tomato juice, salty broth, canned vegetables, processed meats, and fruits. A patient who drinks free water (water without electrolytes) or bottled water will excrete large amounts of chloride; therefore, this kind of water should be avoided. Ammonium chloride, an acidifying agent, may be prescribed to treat metabolic alkalosis; the dosage depends on the patient's weight and serum chloride level. This agent is metabolized by the liver, and its effects last for about 3 days.

Nursing Management

The nurse monitors intake and output, arterial blood gas values, and serum electrolyte levels, as well as the patient's level of consciousness and muscle strength and movement. Changes are reported to the physician promptly. Vital signs are monitored and respiratory assessment is carried out frequently. The nurse teaches the patient about foods with high chloride content.

CHLORIDE EXCESS (HYPERCHLOREMIA)

Hyperchloremia exists when the serum level exceeds 106 mEq/L (106 mmol/L). Hypernatremia, bicarbonate loss, and metabolic acidosis can occur with high chloride levels. Hyperchloremic metabolic acidosis is also known as normal anion gap acidosis (see discussion in Acid–Base Disturbances section of this chapter). It is usually caused by the loss of bicarbonate ions via the kidney or the GI tract with a corresponding increase in chloride ions. Chloride ions in the form of acidifying salts accumulate and acidosis occurs with a decrease in bicarbonate ions.

Clinical Manifestations

The signs and symptoms of hyperchloremia are the same as those of metabolic acidosis, hypervolemia, and hypernatremia. Tachypnea; weakness; lethargy; deep, rapid respirations; diminished cognitive ability; and hypertension occur. If untreated, hyperchloremia can lead to a decrease in cardiac output, dysrhythmias, and coma. A high chloride level is accompanied by a high sodium level and fluid retention.

Assessment and Diagnostic Findings

The serum chloride level is 108 mEq/L (108 mmol/L) or greater, the serum sodium level is greater than 145 mEq/L (145 mmol/L), the serum pH is less than 7.35, the serum bicarbonate level is less than 22 mEq/L (22 mmol/L), and there is a normal anion gap of 8 to 12 mEq/L (8–12 mmol/L). Urine chloride excretion increases.

Calculation of the serum anion gap is important in analyzing acid–base disorders. The sum of all negatively charged electrolytes (anions) equals the sum of all positively charged electrolytes (cations) with several anions that are not routinely measured leading to an anion gap. It is based primarily on three electrolytes: sodium, chloride, and bicarbonate or serum CO_2. A low anion gap may be attributed to hypoproteinemia, while an elevated anion gap can be due to metabolic acidosis.

Medical Management

Correcting the underlying cause of hyperchloremia and restoring electrolyte, fluid, and acid–base balance are essential. Lactated Ringer's solution may be prescribed to convert lactate to bicarbonate in the liver, which will increase the base bicarbonate level and correct the acidosis. Sodium bicarbonate may be given IV to increase bicarbonate levels, which leads to the renal excretion of chloride ions as bicarbonate and chloride compete for combination with sodium. Diuretics may be administered to eliminate chloride as well. Sodium, fluids, and chloride are restricted.

Nursing Management

Monitoring vital signs, arterial blood gas values, and intake and output is important to assess the patient's status and the effectiveness of treatment. Assessment findings related to respiratory, neurologic, and cardiac systems are documented and changes discussed with the physician. The nurse teaches the patient about the diet that should be followed to manage hyperchloremia.

Acid–Base Disturbances

Acid–base disturbances are commonly encountered in clinical practice. Identification of the specific acid–base imbalance is important in identifying the underlying cause of the disorder and in determining appropriate treatment (Kraut & Madias, 2001).

Plasma pH is an indicator of hydrogen ion (H^+) concentration. Homeostatic mechanisms keep pH within a normal range (7.35–7.45). These mechanisms consist of buffer systems, the kidneys, and the lungs. The H^+ concentration is extremely important: the greater the concentration, the more acidic the solution and the lower the pH. The lower the H^+ concentration, the more alkaline the solution and the higher the pH. The pH range compatible with life (6.8–7.8) represents a tenfold difference in H^+ concentration in plasma.

BUFFER SYSTEMS

Buffer systems prevent major changes in the pH of body fluids by removing or releasing H^+; they can act quickly to prevent excessive changes in H^+ concentration. Hydrogen ions are buffered by both intracellular and extracellular buffers. The body's major extracellular buffer system is the bicarbonate-carbonic acid buffer system. This is the system that is assessed when arterial blood gases are measured. Normally, there are 20 parts of bicarbonate (HCO_3^-) to one part of carbonic acid (H_2CO_3). If this ratio is altered, the pH will change. It is the ratio of HCO_3^- to H_2CO_3 that is important in maintaining pH, not absolute values. Carbon dioxide (CO_2) is a potential acid; when dissolved in water, it becomes carbonic acid ($CO_2 + H_2O = H_2CO_3$). Thus, when CO_2 is increased, the carbonic acid content is also increased, and vice versa. If either bicarbonate or carbonic acid is increased or decreased so that the 20:1 ratio is no longer maintained, acid–base imbalance results.

Less important buffer systems in the ECF include the inorganic phosphates and the plasma proteins. Intracellular buffers include proteins, organic and inorganic phosphates, and, in red blood cells, hemoglobin.

Kidneys

The kidneys regulate the bicarbonate level in the ECF; they can regenerate bicarbonate ions as well as reabsorb them from the renal tubular cells. In respiratory acidosis and most cases of metabolic acidosis, the kidneys excrete hydrogen ions and conserve bicarbonate ions to help restore balance. In respiratory and metabolic alkalosis, the kidneys retain hydrogen ions and excrete bicarbonate ions to help restore balance. The kidneys obviously cannot compensate for the metabolic acidosis created by renal failure. Renal compensation for imbalances is relatively slow (a matter of hours or days).

Lungs

The lungs, under the control of the medulla, control the CO_2 and thus the carbonic acid content of the ECF. They do so by adjusting ventilation in response to the amount of CO_2 in the blood. A rise in the partial pressure of CO_2 in arterial blood ($PaCO_2$) is a powerful stimulant to respiration. Of course, the partial pressure of oxygen in arterial blood (PaO_2) also influences respiration. Its effect, however, is not as marked as that produced by the $PaCO_2$.

In metabolic acidosis, the respiratory rate increases, causing greater elimination of CO_2 (to reduce the acid load). In metabolic alkalosis, the respiratory rate decreases, causing CO_2 to be retained (to increase the acid load).

ACUTE AND CHRONIC METABOLIC ACIDOSIS (BASE BICARBONATE DEFICIT)

Metabolic acidosis is a clinical disturbance characterized by a low pH (increased H^+ concentration) and a low plasma bicarbonate concentration. It can be produced by a gain of hydrogen ion or a loss of bicarbonate (Swenson, 2001). It can be divided clinically into two forms, according to the values of the serum anion gap: high anion gap acidosis and normal anion gap acidosis. The anion gap reflects normally unmeasured anions (phosphates, sulfates, and proteins) in plasma. Measuring the anion gap is essential in analyzing acid–base disorders correctly. The anion gap can be calculated by either one of the following equations:

$$\text{Anion gap} = Na^+ + K^+ - (Cl^- + HCO_3^-)$$
$$\text{Anion gap} = Na^+ - (Cl^- + HCO_3^-)$$

Potassium is often omitted from the equation because of its low level in the plasma; thus, the second equation is used more often than the first.

The normal value for an anion gap is 8 to 12 mEq/L (8–12 mmol/L) without potassium in the equation. The normal value for the anion gap if including potassium in the equation is 12 to 16 mEq/L (12–16 mmol/L). The unmeasured anions in the serum normally account for less than 16 mEq/L of the anion production. An anion gap greater than 16 mEq (16 mmol/L) suggests excessive accumulation of unmeasured anions. An anion gap occurs because not all electrolytes are measured. More anions are left unmeasured than cations.

Normal anion gap acidosis results from the direct loss of bicarbonate, as in diarrhea, lower intestinal fistulas, ureterostomies, and use of diuretics; early renal insufficiency; excessive administration of chloride; and the administration of parenteral nutrition without bicarbonate or bicarbonate-producing solutes (eg, lactate).

Normal anion gap acidosis is also referred to as hyperchloremic acidosis. A reduced or negative anion gap is primarily caused by hypoproteinemia. Disorders that cause a decreased or negative anion gap are rare compared to those related to an increased or high anion gap (Rose & Post, 2001).

High anion gap acidosis results from excessive accumulation of fixed acid. If it is increased to 30 mEq/L (30 mmol/L) or more, then a high anion gap metabolic acidosis is present regardless of what the pH and the HCO_3^- are. High ion gap occurs in ketoacidosis, lactic acidosis, the late phase of salicylate poisoning, uremia, methanol or ethylene glycol toxicity, and ketoacidosis with starvation. The hydrogen is buffered by HCO_3^-, causing the bicarbonate concentration to fall. In all of these instances, abnormally high levels of anions flood the system, increasing the anion gap above normal limits.

Clinical Manifestations

Signs and symptoms of metabolic acidosis vary with the severity of the acidosis. They may include headache, confusion, drowsiness, increased respiratory rate and depth, nausea, and vomiting. Peripheral vasodilation and decreased cardiac output occur when the pH falls below 7. Additional physical assessment findings include decreased blood pressure, cold and clammy skin, dysrhythmias, and shock (Swenson, 2001).

Chronic metabolic acidosis is usually seen with chronic renal failure. The bicarbonate and pH decrease slowly; thus, the patient is asymptomatic until the bicarbonate is approximately 15 mEq/L or less.

Assessment and Diagnostic Findings

Arterial blood gas measurements are valuable in diagnosing metabolic acidosis (Swenson, 2001). Expected blood gas changes include a low bicarbonate level (less than 22 mEq/L) and a low pH (less than 7.35). The cardinal feature of metabolic acidosis is a decrease in the serum bicarbonate level. Hyperkalemia may accompany metabolic acidosis as a result of the shift of potassium out of the cells. Later, as the acidosis is corrected, potassium moves back into the cells and hypokalemia may occur. Hyperventilation decreases the CO_2 level as a compensatory action. As stated previously, calculation of the anion gap is helpful in determining the cause of metabolic acidosis. An ECG will detect dysrhythmias caused by the increased potassium.

Medical Management

Treatment is directed at correcting the metabolic defect (Swenson, 2001). If the problem results from excessive intake of chloride, treatment is aimed at eliminating the source of the chloride. When necessary, bicarbonate is administered if the pH is less than 7.1 and the bicarbonate level is less than 10. Although hyperkalemia occurs with acidosis, hypokalemia may occur with reversal of the acidosis and subsequent movement of potassium back into the cells. Therefore, the serum potassium level is monitored closely and hypokalemia is corrected as acidosis is reversed.

In chronic metabolic acidosis, low serum calcium levels are treated before treating chronic metabolic acidosis to avoid tetany resulting from an increase in pH and a decrease in ionized calcium. Alkalyzing agents may be given if the serum bicarbonate level is less than 12 mEq/L. Treatment modalities may also include hemodialysis or peritoneal dialysis.

ACUTE AND CHRONIC METABOLIC ALKALOSIS (BASE BICARBONATE EXCESS)

Metabolic alkalosis is a clinical disturbance characterized by a high pH (decreased H^+ concentration) and a high plasma bicarbonate concentration. It can be produced by a gain of bicarbonate or a loss of H^+ (Khanna & Kurtzman, 2001).

Probably the most common cause of metabolic alkalosis is vomiting or gastric suction with loss of hydrogen and chloride ions. The disorder also occurs in pyloric stenosis, in which only gastric fluid is lost. Gastric fluid has an acid pH (usually 1–3); therefore, loss of this highly acidic fluid increases the alkalinity of body fluids. Other situations predisposing to metabolic alkalosis include those associated with loss of potassium, such as diuretic therapy that promotes excretion of potassium (eg, thiazides, furosemide), and excessive adrenocorticoid hormones (as in hyperaldosteronism and Cushing's syndrome).

Hypokalemia produces alkalosis in two ways: (1) the kidneys conserve potassium, and thus H^+ excretion increases; and (2) cellular potassium moves out of the cells into the ECF in an attempt to maintain near-normal serum levels (as potassium ions leave the cells, hydrogen ions must enter to maintain electroneutrality). Excessive alkali ingestion from antacids containing bicarbonate or from using sodium bicarbonate during cardiopulmonary resuscitation can also cause metabolic alkalosis.

Chronic metabolic alkalosis can occur with long-term diuretic therapy (thiazides or furosemide), villous adenoma, external drainage of gastric fluids, significant potassium depletion, cystic fibrosis, and the chronic ingestion of milk and calcium carbonate.

Clinical Manifestations

Alkalosis is primarily manifested by symptoms related to decreased calcium ionization, such as tingling of the fingers and toes, dizziness, and hypertonic muscles. The ionized fraction of serum calcium decreases in alkalosis as more calcium combines with serum proteins. Because it is the ionized fraction of calcium that influences neuromuscular activity, symptoms of hypocalcemia are often the predominant symptoms of alkalosis. Respirations are depressed as a compensatory action by the lungs. Atrial tachycardia may occur. As the pH increases above 7.6 and hypokalemia develops, ventricular disturbances may occur. Decreased motility and paralytic ileus may also occur.

Symptoms of chronic metabolic alkalosis are the same as for acute metabolic alkalosis, and as potassium decreases, frequent premature ventricular contractions or U waves are seen on the ECG.

Assessment and Diagnostic Findings

Evaluation of arterial blood gases reveals a pH greater than 7.45 and a serum bicarbonate concentration greater than 26 mEq/L. The $PaCO_2$ increases as the lungs attempt to compensate for the excess bicarbonate by retaining CO_2. This hypoventilation is more pronounced in semiconscious, unconscious, or debilitated patients than in alert patients. The former may develop marked hypoxemia as a result of hypoventilation. Hypokalemia may accompany metabolic alkalosis.

Urinary chloride levels may help to identify the cause of metabolic alkalosis if the patient's history provides inadequate information. Metabolic alkalosis is the setting in which urine chloride concentration may be a more accurate estimate of volume than is the urine sodium concentration. Urine chloride concentrations help to differentiate between vomiting or diuretic ingestion or one of the causes of mineralocorticoid excess. Hypovolemia and hypochloremia in patients with vomiting or cystic fibrosis, those receiving nutritional repletion, or those taking diuretics produce urine chloride concentrations less than 25 mEq/L. Signs of hypovolemia are not present and the urine chloride concentration exceeds 40 mEq/L in patients with mineralocorticoid excess or alkali loading; these patients usually have expanded fluid volume. The urine chloride concentration should be less than 15 mEq/L when decreased chloride levels and hypovolemia occur.

Medical Management

Treatment of metabolic alkalosis is aimed at reversing the underlying disorder (Khanna & Kurtzman, 2001).

Sufficient chloride must be supplied for the kidney to absorb sodium with chloride (allowing the excretion of excess bicarbonate). Treatment also includes restoring normal fluid volume by administering sodium chloride fluids (because continued volume depletion serves to maintain the alkalosis). In patients with hypokalemia, potassium is administered as KCl to replace both K^+ and Cl^- losses. Histamine-2 receptor antagonists, such as cimetidine (Tagamet), reduce the production of gastric HCl, thereby decreasing the metabolic alkalosis associated with gastric suction. Carbonic anhydrase inhibitors are useful in treating metabolic alkalosis in patients who cannot tolerate rapid volume expansion (eg, patients with heart failure). Because of volume depletion from GI loss, the patient's fluid intake and output must be monitored carefully. Management of chronic metabolic alkalosis is aimed at correcting the underlying acid–base disorder.

ACUTE AND CHRONIC RESPIRATORY ACIDOSIS (CARBONIC ACID EXCESS)

Respiratory acidosis is a clinical disorder in which the pH is less than 7.35 and the $PaCO_2$ is greater than 42 mm Hg. It may be either acute or chronic.

Respiratory acidosis is always due to inadequate excretion of CO_2 with inadequate ventilation, resulting in elevated plasma CO_2 levels and thus elevated carbonic acid (H_2CO_3) levels (Epstein & Singh, 2001). In addition to an elevated $PaCO_2$, hypoventilation usually causes a decrease in PaO_2. Acute respiratory acidosis occurs in emergency situations, such as acute pulmonary edema, aspiration of a foreign object, atelectasis, pneumothorax, overdose of sedatives, sleep apnea syndrome, administration of oxygen to a patient with chronic hypercapnia (excessive CO_2 in the blood), severe pneumonia, and acute respiratory distress syndrome. Respiratory acidosis can also occur in diseases that impair respiratory muscles, such as muscular dystrophy, myasthenia gravis, and Guillain-Barré syndrome.

Mechanical ventilation can be associated with hypercapnia if the rate of effective alveolar ventilation is inadequate. Ventilation is fixed in these patients, and CO_2 may be retained if the rate of CO_2 production is increased.

Clinical Manifestations

Clinical signs in acute and chronic respiratory acidosis vary. Sudden hypercapnia (elevated $PaCO_2$) can cause increased pulse and respiratory rate, increased blood pressure, mental cloudiness, and feeling of fullness in the head. An elevated $PaCO_2$ causes cerebrovascular vasodilation and increased cerebral blood flow, particularly when it is higher than 60 mm Hg. Ventricular fibrillation may be the first sign of respiratory acidosis in anesthetized patients.

If respiratory acidosis is severe, intracranial pressure may increase, resulting in papilledema and dilated conjunctival blood vessels. Hyperkalemia may result as hydrogen concentration overwhelms the compensatory mechanisms and moves into cells, causing a shift of potassium out of the cell.

Chronic respiratory acidosis occurs with pulmonary diseases such as chronic emphysema and bronchitis, obstructive sleep apnea, and obesity. As long as the $PaCO_2$ does not exceed the body's ability to compensate, the patient will be asymptomatic. However, if the $PaCO_2$ rises rapidly, cerebral vasodilation will increase intracranial pressure; cyanosis and tachypnea will develop. Patients with chronic obstructive pulmonary disease who gradually accumulate CO_2 over a prolonged period (days to months) may not develop symptoms of hypercapnia because compensatory renal changes have had time to occur.

> **NURSING ALERT** When the $PaCO_2$ is chronically above 50 mm Hg, the respiratory center becomes relatively insensitive to CO_2 as a respiratory stimulant, leaving hypoxemia as the major drive for respiration. Oxygen administration may remove the stimulus of hypoxemia, and the patient develops "carbon dioxide narcosis" unless the situation is quickly reversed. Therefore, oxygen is administered only with extreme caution.

Assessment and Diagnostic Findings

Arterial blood gas evaluation reveals a pH less than 7.35, a $PaCO_2$ greater than 42 mm Hg, and a variation in the bicarbonate level, depending on the duration of the acidosis in acute respiratory acidosis. When compensation (renal retention of bicarbonate) has fully occurred, the arterial pH may be within the lower limits of normal. Depending on the cause of respiratory acidosis, other diagnostic measures would include monitoring of serum electrolyte levels, chest x-ray for determining any respiratory disease, and a drug screen if an overdose is suspected. An ECG to identify any cardiac involvement as a result of chronic obstructive pulmonary disease may be indicated as well.

Medical Management

Treatment is directed at improving ventilation (Epstein & Singh, 2001); exact measures vary with the cause of inadequate ventilation. Pharmacologic agents are used as indicated. For example, bronchodilators help reduce bronchial spasm, antibiotics are used for respiratory infections, and thrombolytics or anticoagulants are used for pulmonary emboli.

Pulmonary hygiene measures are initiated, when necessary, to clear the respiratory tract of mucus and purulent drainage. Adequate hydration (2–3 L/day) is indicated to keep the mucous membranes moist and thereby facilitate the removal of secretions. Supplemental oxygen is used as necessary.

Mechanical ventilation, used appropriately, may improve pulmonary ventilation. Inappropriate mechanical ventilation (eg, increased dead space, insufficient rate or volume settings, high fraction of inspired oxygen [FiO_2] with excessive CO_2 production) may cause such rapid excretion of CO_2 that the kidneys will be unable to eliminate excess bicarbonate quickly enough to prevent alkalosis and seizures. For this reason, the elevated $PaCO_2$ must be decreased slowly. Placing the patient in a semi-Fowler's position facilitates expansion of the chest wall. Treatment of chronic respiratory acidosis is the same as for acute respiratory acidosis.

ACUTE AND CHRONIC RESPIRATORY ALKALOSIS (CARBONIC ACID DEFICIT)

Respiratory alkalosis is a clinical condition in which the arterial pH is greater than 7.45 and the $PaCO_2$ is less than 38 mm Hg. As with respiratory acidosis, acute and chronic conditions can occur.

Respiratory alkalosis is always due to hyperventilation, which causes excessive "blowing off" of CO_2 and, hence, a decrease in the plasma carbonic acid concentration. Causes can include extreme anxiety, hypoxemia, the early phase of salicylate intoxication, gram-negative bacteremia, and inappropriate ventilator settings that do not match the patient's requirements.

Chronic respiratory alkalosis results from chronic hypocapnia, and decreased serum bicarbonate levels are the consequence. Chronic hepatic insufficiency and cerebral tumors are predisposing factors.

Clinical Manifestations

Clinical signs consist of lightheadedness due to vasoconstriction and decreased cerebral blood flow, inability to concentrate, numbness and tingling from decreased calcium ionization, tinnitus, and at times loss of consciousness. Cardiac effects of respiratory alkalosis include tachycardia and ventricular and atrial dysrhythmias (Foster et al., 2001).

Assessment and Diagnostic Findings

Analysis of arterial blood gases assists in the diagnosis of respiratory alkalosis. In the acute state, the pH is elevated above normal as a result of a low $PaCO_2$ and a normal bicarbonate level. (The kidneys cannot alter the bicarbonate level quickly.) In the compensated state, the kidneys have had sufficient time to lower the bicarbonate level to a near-normal level. Evaluation of serum electrolytes is indicated to identify any decrease in potassium as hydrogen is pulled out of the cells in exchange for potassium; decreased calcium, as severe alkalosis inhibits calcium ionization, resulting in carpopedal spasms and tetany; or decreased phosphate due to alkalosis, causing an increased uptake of phosphate by the cells. A toxicology screen should be performed to rule out salicylate intoxication.

Patients with chronic respiratory alkalosis are usually asymptomatic, and the diagnostic evaluation and plan of care are the same as for acute respiratory alkalosis.

Medical Management

Treatment depends on the underlying cause of respiratory alkalosis (Foster et al., 2001). If the cause is anxiety, the patient is instructed to breathe more slowly to allow CO_2 to accumulate or to breathe into a closed system (such as a paper bag). A sedative may be required to relieve hyperventilation in very anxious patients. Treatment for other causes of respiratory alkalosis is directed at correcting the underlying problem.

MIXED ACID–BASE DISORDERS

At times patients can simultaneously experience two or more independent acid–base disorders. A normal pH in the presence of changes in the $PaCO_2$ and plasma HCO_3^- concentration immediately suggests a mixed disorder. The only mixed disorder that cannot occur is a mixed respiratory acidosis and alkalosis, because it is impossible to have alveolar hypoventilation and hyperventilation at the same time. An example of a mixed disorder is the simultaneous occurrence of metabolic acidosis and respiratory acidosis during respiratory and cardiac arrest.

COMPENSATION

Generally, the pulmonary and renal systems compensate for each other to return the pH to normal. In a single acid–base disorder, the system not causing the problem will try to compensate by returning the ratio of bicarbonate to carbonic acid to the normal 20:1. The lungs compensate for metabolic disturbances by changing CO_2 excretion. The kidneys compensate for respiratory disturbances by altering bicarbonate retention and H^+ secretion.

In respiratory acidosis, excess hydrogen is excreted in the urine in exchange for bicarbonate ions. In respiratory alkalosis, the renal excretion of bicarbonate increases, and hydrogen ions are retained. In metabolic acidosis, the compensatory mechanisms increase the ventilation rate and the renal retention of bicarbonate.

In metabolic alkalosis, the respiratory system compensates by decreasing ventilation to conserve CO_2 and raise the $PaCO_2$. Because the lungs respond to acid–base disorders within minutes, compensation for metabolic imbalances occurs faster than compensation for respiratory imbalances. Table 14-7 summarizes compensation effects.

BLOOD GAS ANALYSIS

Blood gas analysis is often used to identify the specific acid–base disturbance and the degree of compensation that has occurred. The analysis is usually based on an arterial blood sample, but when an arterial sample cannot be obtained, a mixed venous sample may be used. Results of arterial blood gas analysis provide information about alveolar ventilation, oxygenation, and acid–base balance. It is necessary to evaluate the serum electrolytes (sodium, potassium, and chloride) and carbon dioxide along with arterial blood gas data as they are often the first sign of an acid–base disorder. The health history, physical examination, previous blood gas results, and serum electrolytes should always be part of the assessment used to determine the cause of the acid–base disorder (Kraut & Madias, 2001). Treatment of the underlying condition usually corrects most acid–base disorders. Table 14-8 compares normal ranges of venous and arterial blood gas values. See also Chart 14-1.

Table 14-7 • **Acid–Base Disturbances and Compensation**

DISORDER	INITIAL EVENT	COMPENSATION
Respiratory acidosis	↑ $PaCO_2$, ↑ or normal HCO_3^-, ↓ pH	Kidneys eliminate H^+ and retain HCO_3^-
Respiratory alkalosis	↓ $PaCO_2$, ↓ or normal HCO_3^-, ↑ pH	Kidneys conserve H^+ and excrete HCO_3^-
Metabolic acidosis	↓ or normal $PaCO_2$, ↓ HCO_3^-, ↓ pH	Lungs eliminate CO_2, conserve HCO_3^-
Metabolic alkalosis	↑ or normal $PaCO_2$, ↑ HCO_3^-, ↑ pH	Lungs ↓ ventilation to ↑ PCO_2, kidneys conserve H^+ to excrete HCO_3^-

Table 14-8 • **Normal Values: Arterial and Venous Blood**

PARAMETER	ARTERIAL SAMPLE	VENOUS SAMPLE
pH	7.35–7.45	7.33–7.41
PaCO$_2$	35–45 mm Hg	35–40 mmHg
Oxygen saturation	93–98%	65–75%
Base excess or deficit	+/− 2 mmol/L	+/− 4 mmol/L
HCO$_3^-$	22–26 mEq/L	24–28 Eq/L

Parenteral Fluid Therapy

IV fluid administration is performed in the hospital, outpatient diagnostic and surgical settings, clinics, and home to replace fluids, administer medications, and provide nutrients when no other route is available.

PURPOSE

The choice of an IV solution depends on the purpose of its administration. Generally, IV fluids are administered to achieve one or more of the following goals:

- To provide water, electrolytes, and nutrients to meet daily requirements
- To replace water and correct electrolyte deficits
- To administer medications and blood products

IV solutions contain dextrose or electrolytes mixed in various proportions with water. Pure, electrolyte-free water can never be administered IV because it rapidly enters red blood cells and causes them to rupture.

TYPES OF IV SOLUTIONS

Solutions are often categorized as **isotonic, hypotonic,** or **hypertonic,** according to whether their total osmolality is the same as, less than, or greater than that of blood (see the section Laboratory Tests for Evaluating Fluid Status for a discussion of osmolality).

Electrolyte solutions are considered isotonic if the total electrolyte content (anions + cations) is approximately 310 mEq/L. They are considered hypotonic if the total electrolyte content is less than 250 mEq/L and hypertonic if the total electrolyte content exceeds 375 mEq/L. The nurse must also consider a solution's osmolality, keeping in mind that the osmolality of plasma is approximately 300 mOsm/L (300 mmol/L). For example, a 10% dextrose solution has an osmolality of approximately 505 mOsm/L.

Chart 14-1 • **ASSESSMENT**

Arterial Blood Gases

The following steps are recommended to evaluate arterial blood gas values. They are based on the assumption that the average values are:
pH = 7.4
PaCO$_2$ = 40 mm Hg
HCO$_3^-$ = 24 mEq/L
1. *First, note the pH.* It can be high, low, or normal, as follows:
    pH > 7.4 (alkalosis)
    pH < 7.4 (acidosis)
    pH = 7.4 (normal)
A normal pH may indicate perfectly normal blood gases, *or* it may be an indication of a *compensated* imbalance. A compensated imbalance is one in which the body has been able to correct the pH by either respiratory or metabolic changes (depending on the primary problem). For example, a patient with primary metabolic acidosis starts out with a low bicarbonate level but a normal CO$_2$ level. Soon afterward, the lungs try to compensate for the imbalance by exhaling large amounts of CO$_2$ (hyperventilation). As another example, a patient with primary respiratory acidosis starts out with a high CO$_2$ level; soon afterward, the kidneys attempt to compensate by retaining bicarbonate. If the compensatory mechanism is able to restore the bicarbonate to carbonic acid ratio back to 20:1, full compensation (and thus normal pH) will be achieved.
2. The next step is to determine the primary cause of the disturbance. This is done by evaluating the PaCO$_2$ and HCO$_3^-$ in relation to the pH.
Example: pH > 7.4 (alkalosis)
a. If the PaCO$_2$ is < 40 mm Hg, the primary disturbance is respiratory alkalosis. (This situation occurs when a patient hyperventilates and "blows off" too much CO$_2$. Recall that CO$_2$ dissolved in water becomes carbonic acid, the acid side of the "carbonic acid–bicarbonate buffer system.")
b. If the HCO$_3^-$ is >24 mEq/L, the primary disturbance is metabolic alkalosis. (This situation occurs when the body gains too

much bicarbonate, an alkaline substance. Bicarbonate is the basic or alkaline side of the "carbonic acid–bicarbonate buffer system.")
Example: pH < 7.4 (acidosis)
a. If the PaCO$_2$ is >40 mm Hg, the primary disturbance is respiratory acidosis. (This situation occurs when a patient hypoventilates and thus retains too much CO$_2$, an acidic substance.)
b. If the HCO$_3^-$ is <24 mEq/L, the primary disturbance is metabolic acidosis. (This situation occurs when the body's bicarbonate level drops, either because of direct bicarbonate loss or because of gains of acids such as lactic acid or ketones.)
3. The next step involves determining if compensation has begun. This is done by looking at the value other than the primary disorder. If it is moving in the same direction as the primary value, compensation is underway. Consider the following gases:
pH	PaCO$_2$	HCO$_3^-$
(1) 7.20	60 mm Hg	24 mEq/L
(2) 7.40	60 mm Hg	37 mEq/L
The first set (1) indicates acute respiratory acidosis without compensation (the PaCO$_2$ is high, the HCO$_3^-$ is normal). The second set (2) indicates chronic respiratory acidosis. Note that compensation has take place; that is, the HCO$_3^-$ has elevated to an appropriate level to balance the high PaCO$_2$ and produce a normal pH.
4. Two distinct acid–base disturbances may occur simultaneously. These can be identified when the pH does not explain one of the changes.
Example: Metabolic and respiratory acidosis
a. pH	7.21	decreased acid
b. PaCO$_2$	52	increased acid
c. HCO$_3$	13	decreased acid
This is an example of metabolic and respiratory acidosis.

When administering parenteral fluids, the nurse monitors the patient's response to the fluids, considering the fluid volume, the content of the fluid, and the patient's clinical status.

Isotonic Fluids

Fluids that are classified as isotonic have a total osmolality close to that of the ECF and do not cause red blood cells to shrink or swell. The composition of these fluids may or may not approximate that of the ECF. Isotonic fluids expand the ECF volume. One liter of isotonic fluid expands the ECF by 1 L; however, it expands the plasma by only 0.25 L because it is a crystalloid fluid and diffuses quickly into the ECF compartment. For the same reason, 3 L of isotonic fluid is needed to replace 1 L of blood loss. Because these fluids expand the intravascular space, patients with hypertension and heart failure should be carefully monitored for signs of fluid overload.

D₅W

A solution of D_5W has a serum osmolality of 252 mOsm/L. Once administered, the glucose is rapidly metabolized, and this initially isotonic solution then disperses as a hypotonic fluid, one-third extracellular and two-thirds intracellular. It is essential to consider this action of D_5W, especially if the patient is at risk for increased intracranial pressure. During fluid resuscitation, this solution should not be used because it can cause hyperglycemia. Therefore, D_5W is used mainly to supply water and to correct an increased serum osmolality. About 1 L of D_5W provides fewer than 200 kcal and is a minor source of calories for the body's daily requirements.

NORMAL SALINE SOLUTION

Normal saline (0.9% sodium chloride) solution has a total osmolality of 308 mOsm/L. Because the osmolality is entirely contributed by electrolytes, the solution remains within the ECF. For this reason, normal saline solution is often used to correct an extracellular volume deficit. Although referred to as "normal," it contains only sodium and chloride and does not actually simulate the ECF. It is used with administration of blood transfusions and to replace large sodium losses, as in burn injuries. It is not used for heart failure, pulmonary edema, renal impairment, or sodium retention. Normal saline does not supply calories.

OTHER ISOTONIC SOLUTIONS

Several other solutions contain ions in addition to sodium and chloride and are somewhat similar to the ECF in composition. Lactated Ringer's solution contains potassium and calcium in addition to sodium chloride. It is used to correct dehydration and sodium depletion and replace GI losses. Lactated Ringer's solution contains bicarbonate precursors as well. These solutions are marketed, with slight variations, under various trade names.

Hypotonic Fluids

One purpose of hypotonic solutions is to replace cellular fluid, because it is hypotonic as compared with plasma. Another is to provide free water for excretion of body wastes. At times, hypotonic sodium solutions are used to treat hypernatremia and other hyperosmolar conditions. Half-strength saline (0.45% sodium chloride) solution, with an osmolality of 154 mOsm/L, is frequently used. Multiple-electrolyte solutions are also available. Excessive infusions of hypotonic solutions can lead to intravascular fluid depletion, decreased blood pressure, cellular edema, and cell damage. These solutions exert less osmotic pressure than the ECF.

Hypertonic Fluids

When normal saline solution or lactated Ringer's solution contains 5% dextrose, the total osmolality exceeds that of the ECF. The dextrose is quickly metabolized, however, and only the isotonic solution remains. Therefore, any effect on the intracellular compartment is temporary. Similarly, with hypotonic multiple-electrolyte solutions containing 5% dextrose, once the dextrose is metabolized, these solutions disperse as hypotonic fluids.

Higher concentrations of dextrose, such as 50% dextrose in water, are administered to help meet caloric requirements. These solutions are strongly hypertonic and must be administered into central veins so that they can be diluted by rapid blood flow.

Saline solutions are also available in osmolar concentrations greater than that of the ECF. These solutions draw water from the ICF to the ECF and cause cells to shrink. If administered rapidly or in large quantity, they may cause an extracellular volume excess and precipitate circulatory overload and dehydration. As a result, these solutions must be administered cautiously and usually only when the serum osmolality has decreased to dangerously low levels. Hypertonic solutions exert an osmotic pressure greater than that of the ECF.

Other IV Substances

When the patient's GI tract is unable to tolerate food, nutritional requirements are often met using the IV route. Parenteral solutions may include high concentrations of glucose, protein, or fat to meet nutritional requirements. The parenteral route may also be used to administer colloids, plasma expanders, and blood products. Examples of blood products include whole blood, packed red blood cells, albumin, and cryoprecipitate; these are discussed in more detail in Chapter 33.

Many medications are also delivered by the IV route, either by infusion or directly into the vein. Because IV medications enter the circulation rapidly, administration by this route is potentially very hazardous. All medications can produce adverse reactions; however, medications given by the IV route can cause these reactions within 15 minutes after administration because the medications are delivered directly into the bloodstream. Administration rates and recommended dilutions for individual medications are available in specialized texts pertaining to IV medications and in manufacturers' package inserts; these should be consulted to ensure safe IV administration of medications.

> **NURSING ALERT** The nurse must assess the patient for a history of allergic reactions to medications; although this is important when any medication is to be administered, it is even more important with IV administration because the medication is delivered directly into the bloodstream.

Nursing Management of the Patient Receiving IV Therapy

Venipuncture, or the ability to gain access to the venous system for administering fluids and medications, is an expected nursing skill in many settings. This responsibility includes selecting the appropriate venipuncture site and type of cannula and being proficient in the technique of vein entry.

PREPARING TO ADMINISTER IV THERAPY

Before performing venipuncture, the nurse carries out hand hygiene, applies gloves, and informs the patient about the procedure. Next the nurse selects the most appropriate insertion site and type of cannula for a particular patient. Factors influencing these choices include the type of solution to be administered, the expected duration of IV therapy, the patient's general condition, and the availability of veins. The skill of the person initiating the infusion is also an important consideration.

CHOOSING AN IV SITE

Many sites can be used for IV therapy, but ease of access and potential hazards vary. Veins of the extremities are designated as peripheral locations and are ordinarily the only sites used by nurses. Because they are relatively safe and easy to enter, arm veins are most commonly used (Fig. 14-7). The metacarpal, cephalic, basilic, and median veins as well as their branches are recommended sites because of their size and ease of access. More distal sites should be used first, with more proximal sites used subsequently. Leg veins should rarely, if ever, be used because of the high risk of thromboembolism. Additional sites to avoid include veins distal to a previous IV infiltration or phlebitic area, sclerosed or thrombosed veins, an arm with an arteriovenous shunt or fistula, or an arm affected by edema, infection, blood clot, or skin breakdown. The arm on the side of a mastectomy is avoided because of impaired lymphatic flow.

Central veins commonly used by physicians include the subclavian and internal jugular veins. It is possible to gain access to (or cannulate) these larger vessels even when peripheral sites have collapsed, and they allow for the administration of hyperosmolar solutions. Hazards are much greater, however, and may include inadvertent entry into an artery or the pleural space.

Ideally, both arms and hands are carefully inspected before choosing a specific venipuncture site that does not interfere with mobility. For this reason, the antecubital fossa is avoided, except as a last resort. The most distal site of the arm or hand is generally used first so that subsequent IV access sites can be moved progressively upward. The following are factors to consider when selecting a site for venipuncture:

- Condition of the vein
- Type of fluid or medication to be infused
- Duration of therapy
- Patient's age and size
- Whether the patient is right- or left-handed
- Patient's medical history and current health status
- Skill of the person performing the venipuncture

After applying a tourniquet, the nurse palpates and inspects the vein. The vein should feel firm, elastic, engorged, and round, not hard, flat, or bumpy. Because arteries lie close to veins in the antecubital fossa, the vessel should be palpated for arterial pulsation (even with a tourniquet on), and cannulation of pulsating vessels should be avoided. General guidelines for selecting a cannula include:

- Length: ¾ to 1.25 inches long
- Diameter: narrow diameter of the cannula to occupy minimal space within the vein
- Gauge: 20 to 22 gauge for most IV fluids; a larger gauge for caustic or viscous solutions; 14 to 18 gauge for blood administration and for trauma patients and those undergoing surgery

Hand veins are easiest to cannulate. Cannula tips should not rest in a flexion area (eg, the antecubital fossa) as this could inhibit the IV flow.

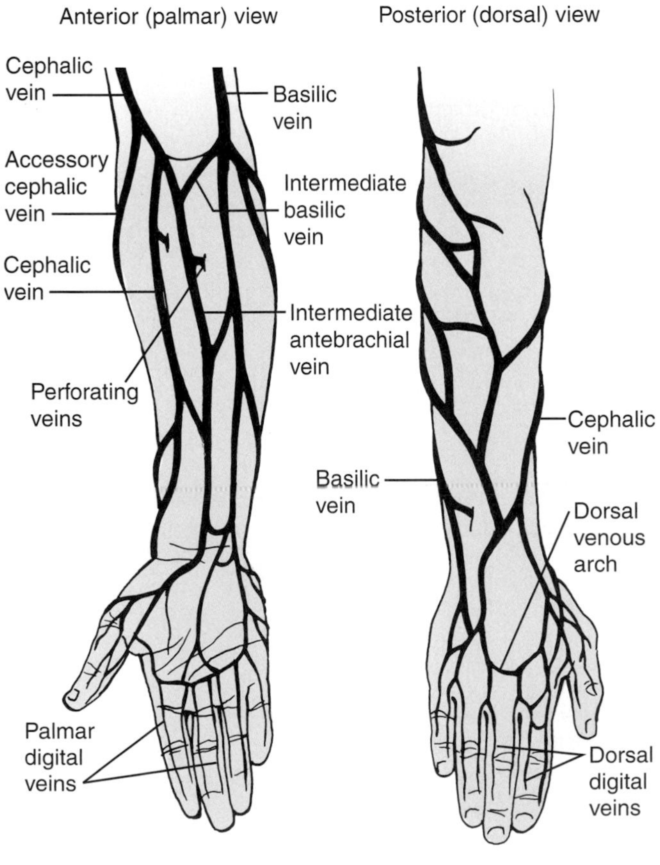

SELECTING VENIPUNCTURE DEVICES

Equipment used to gain access to the vasculature includes cannulas, needleless IV delivery systems, and peripherally inserted central catheter or midline catheter access lines.

Cannulas. Most peripheral access devices are cannulas. They have an obturator inside a tube that is later removed. "Catheter" and "cannula" are terms that are used interchangeably. The main types of cannula devices available are those referred to as winged infusion sets (butterfly) with a steel needle or as an over-the-needle catheter with wings, indwelling plastic cannulas inserted over a steel needle, and indwelling plastic cannulas inserted through a steel needle. Scalp vein or butterfly needles are short steel needles with plastic wing handles. These are easy to insert, but because they are small and nonpliable, infiltration occurs easily. The use of these needles should be limited to obtaining blood specimens or administering bolus injections or infusions lasting only a few hours, as they increase the risk for vein injury and infiltration. Insertion of an over-the-needle catheter requires the additional step of advancing the catheter into the vein after venipuncture. Because these devices are less likely to cause infiltration, they are frequently preferred over winged infusion sets.

Anterior (palmar) view   Posterior (dorsal) view

Cephalic vein
Basilic vein
Accessory cephalic vein
Intermediate basilic vein
Cephalic vein
Intermediate antebrachial vein
Perforating veins
Cephalic vein
Basilic vein
Dorsal venous arch
Palmar digital veins
Dorsal digital veins

FIGURE 14-7 Site selection for peripheral cannulation of veins: anterior (palmar) veins at *left,* posterior (dorsal) veins at *right.*

Plastic cannulas inserted through a hollow needle are usually called intracatheters. They are available in long lengths and are well suited for placement in central locations. Because insertion requires threading the cannula through the vein for a relatively long distance, these can be difficult to insert. The most commonly used infusion device is the over-the-needle catheter. A hollow metal stylet is preinserted into the catheter and extends through the distal tip of the catheter to allow puncture of the vessel, in an effort to guide the catheter as the venipuncture is performed. The vein is punctured and a flashback of blood appears in the closed chamber behind the catheter hub. The catheter is threaded through the stylet into the vein and the stylet is then removed. There are many safety over-the-needle catheter designs available with retracting stylets to protect health care workers from needlestick injuries.

Many types of cannulas are available for IV therapy. Some of the variations in these cannulas include the thickness of the cannula wall (affects rate of flow), the sharpness of the insertion needles (determines needle insertion technique), the softening properties of the cannula (influences the length of time the cannula can remain in place), safety features (minimizes risk of needlestick injuries and blood-borne exposure), and the number of lumens (determines the number of solutions that can be infused simultaneously). Cannula systems that help prevent needlesticks and transmission of blood-borne diseases are discussed below. Most standard peripheral catheters are composed of some form of plastic. Teflon (polytetrafluoroethylene)–coated catheters have less thrombogenic properties and are less inflammatory than polyurethane or PVC. Catheter size for steel needles can range from $\frac{3}{8}$ to 1.5 inches in length and 27 to 13 gauge. Plastic catheters range in length from $\frac{5}{8}$ to 2 inches or as long as 12 inches. The size of the catheter ranges from 27 to 12 gauge.

To select the ideal product for use, consideration should be given to which product provides the greatest patient satisfaction and offers quality, cost-effective infusion care. All devices should be radiopaque to determine catheter location by x-ray, if indicated. All catheters are thrombogenic and differ only in their degree of thrombus occurrence. Biocompatibility, another characteristic of a catheter, ensures that inflammation and irritation do not occur. Silicone catheters are the most bioinert catheter available today.

Needleless IV Delivery Systems. In an effort to decrease needlestick injuries and exposure to HIV, hepatitis, and other blood-borne pathogens, agencies have implemented needleless IV delivery systems. These systems have built-in protection against needlestick injuries and provide a safe means of using and disposing of an IV administration set (which consists of tubing, an area for inserting the tubing into the container of IV fluid, and an adapter for connecting the tubing to the needle). Numerous companies produce needleless components. IV line connectors allow the simultaneous infusion of IV medications and other intermittent medications (known as a piggyback delivery) without the use of needles (Fig. 14-8). Technology is advancing and moving away from use of the traditional stylet. An example is a self-sheathing stylet that is recessed into a rigid chamber at the hub of the catheter when its insertion is complete. Other designs have placed the stylet at the end of a flexible wire to avoid needlesticks.

Many examples of these devices are on the market. Each institution must evaluate products to determine its own needs based on OSHA guidelines and the institution's policies and procedures.

Peripherally Inserted Central Catheter or Midline Catheter Access Lines. Patients who need moderate- to long-term parenteral therapy often receive a peripherally inserted central

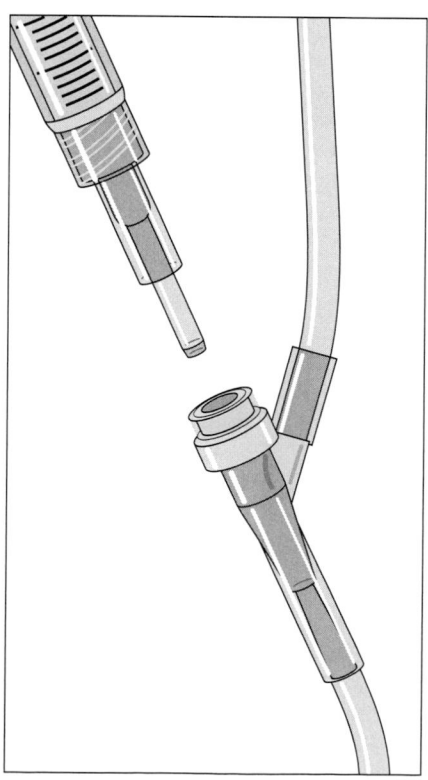

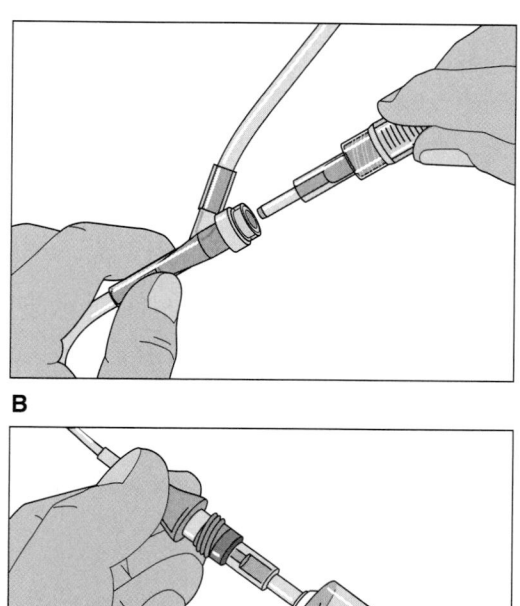

FIGURE 14-8 One example of a needleless IV access device (InterLink Syringe Cannula, Baxter Healthcare Corp., Becton Dickinson Division) (**A**) designed to prevent needlesticks and other accidents. After drawing medication into a syringe according to manufacturer's guidelines and swabbing the Y-site intersection with antiseptic, the nurse can insert the syringe-cannula apparatus into the Y site (**B**) and deliver bolus dose medications. If a blood tube holder (**C**) is attached to the cannula, blood can be withdrawn safely without fear of contact or spills. **A**

B

C

catheter or a midline catheter. These catheters are also used for patients with limited peripheral access (eg, obese or emaciated patients, IV/injection drug users) who require IV antibiotics, blood, and parenteral nutrition. For these devices to be used, the median cephalic, basilic, and cephalic veins must be pliable (not sclerosed or hardened) and not subject to repeated puncture. If these veins are damaged, then central venous access via the subclavian or internal jugular vein, or surgical placement of an implanted port or a vascular access device, must be considered as an alternative. Table 14-9 compares peripherally inserted central and midline catheter lines.

The principles for inserting these lines are much the same as those for inserting peripheral catheters; however, their insertion should be undertaken only by those who are experienced and specially skilled in inserting IV lines.

The physician prescribes the line and the solution to be infused. Insertion of either line requires sterile technique. The size of the catheter lumen chosen is based on the type of solution, the size of the patient, and the vein to be used. The patient's consent is obtained before use of these catheters. Use of the dominant arm is recommended as the site for inserting the cannula into the superior vena cava to ensure adequate arm movement, which encourages blood flow and reduces the risk of dependent edema.

TEACHING THE PATIENT

Except in emergency situations, a patient should be prepared in advance for an IV infusion. The venipuncture, the expected length of infusion, and activity restrictions are explained. Then the patient should have an opportunity to ask questions and voice concerns. For example, some patients believe they will die if small bubbles in the tubing enter their veins. After acknowledging this fear, the nurse can explain that usually only relatively large volumes of air administered rapidly are dangerous.

PREPARING THE IV SITE

Before preparing the skin, the nurse should ask the patient if he or she is allergic to latex or iodine, products commonly used in preparing for IV therapy. Excessive hair at the selected site may be removed by clipping to increase the visibility of the veins and to facilitate insertion of the cannula and adherence of dressings to the IV insertion site. Because infection can be a major complication of IV therapy, the IV device, the fluid, the container, and the tubing must be sterile. The insertion site is scrubbed with a sterile pad soaked in 10% povidone–iodine (Betadine) or chlorhexidine gluconate solution for 2 to 3 minutes, working from the center of the area to the periphery and allowing the area to air dry. The site should not be wiped with 70% alcohol because the alcohol negates the effect of the disinfecting solution. (Alcohol pledgets are used for 30 seconds instead, only if the patient is allergic to iodine.) The nurse must perform hand hygiene and put on gloves. Nonsterile disposable gloves must be worn during the venipuncture procedure because of the likelihood of coming into contact with the patient's blood.

PERFORMING VENIPUNCTURE

Guidelines and a suggested sequence for venipuncture are presented in Chart 14-2. For veins that are very small or particularly fragile, modifications in the technique may be necessary. Alternative methods can be found in journal articles or in specialized textbooks of IV therapy. Institutional policies and procedures determine whether all nurses must be certified to perform veni-

puncture. A nurse certified in IV therapy or an IV team can be consulted to assist with initiating IV therapy.

MAINTAINING THERAPY

Maintaining an existing IV infusion is a nursing responsibility that demands knowledge of the solutions being administered and the principles of flow. In addition, patients must be assessed carefully for both local and systemic complications.

FACTORS AFFECTING FLOW

The flow of an IV infusion is governed by the same principles that govern fluid movement in general.

- Flow is directly proportional to the height of the liquid column. Raising the height of the infusion container may improve a sluggish flow.
- Flow is directly proportional to the diameter of the tubing. The clamp on IV tubing regulates the flow by changing the tubing diameter. In addition, the flow is faster through large-gauge rather than small-gauge cannulas.
- Flow is inversely proportional to the length of the tubing. Adding extension tubing to an IV line will decrease the flow.
- Flow is inversely proportional to the viscosity of a fluid. Viscous IV solutions, such as blood, require a larger cannula than do water or saline solutions.

MONITORING FLOW

Because so many factors influence gravity flow, a solution does not necessarily continue to run at the speed originally set. Therefore, the nurse monitors IV infusions frequently to make sure that the fluid is flowing at the intended rate. The IV container should be marked with tape to indicate at a glance whether the correct amount has infused. The flow rate is calculated when the solution is originally started, then monitored at least hourly. To calculate the flow rate, the nurse determines the number of drops delivered per milliliter; this varies with equipment and is usually printed on the administration set packaging. A formula that can be used to calculate the drop rate is:

$$\text{gtt/mL of infusion set} / 60 \ (\text{min in hr}) \times \text{total hourly vol} = \text{gtt/min}$$

Flushing of a vascular device is performed to ensure patency and prevent the mixing of incompatible medications or solutions. This procedure should be carried out at established intervals, according to hospital policy and procedure, especially for intermittently used catheters. Most manufacturers and researchers (LeDuc, 1997) suggest the use of saline for flushing. The volume of the flush solution should be equal to at least twice the volume capacity of the catheter. The catheter should be clamped before the syringe is completely empty and withdrawn to prevent reflux of blood into the lumen, which could cause catheter clotting.

A variety of electronic infusion devices are available to assist in IV fluid delivery. These devices allow more accurate administration of fluids and medications than is possible with routine gravity-flow setups. A pump is a positive-pressure device that uses pressure to infuse fluid at a pressure of 10 psi. Newer models use a pressure of 5 psi. The pressure exerted by the pump overrides vascular resistance (increased tubing length, low height of the IV container).

Volumetric pumps calculate the volume delivered by measuring the volume in a reservoir that is part of the set and calibrated in mL/h. A controller is an infusion assist device that relies on gravity for infusion; the volume is calibrated in drops/min. A controller

Table 14-9 • **Comparison of Peripherally Inserted Central and Midline Catheters**

	PERIPHERALLY INSERTED CENTRAL CATHETER	MIDLINE CATHETER
Indications	Parenteral nutrition; IV fluid replacement; administration of chemotherapy agents, analgesics, and antibiotics; removal of blood specimens	Parenteral nutrition; IV fluid replacement; administration of analgesics and antibiotics (no solution or medications with a pH <5 or >9 or osmolarity >500 mOsm/L); removal of blood specimens
Features	Single- and double-lumen catheters available 40–60 cm long; gauge variable (16–24 g)	Single- and double-lumen catheters available (16–24 g) 7.5–20 cm in length. Can increase two gauges in size as it softens
Material	Radiopaque, polymer (polyurethane), Silastic materials. Flexible.	Silicone, polyurethane and their derivatives
Insertion sites	Venipuncture performed in the antecubital fossa, above or below it into the basilic, cephalic, or axillary veins of the dominant arm. The median basilic is the ideal insertion site.	Venipuncture performed 2–3 fingerbreadths above the antecubital fossa or 1 fingerbreadth below the antecubital fossa into the cephalic, basilic, or median cubital vein
Catheter placement	The tip of the catheter lies in the superior vena cava or the brachiocephalic vein.	Between the antecubital area and the head of the clavicle (tip in axilla region). The tip terminates in the proximal portion of the extremity below axilla and proximal to central veins and is advanced 3–10 inches.
Insertion method	Through-the-needle technique, with or without a guidewire, breakaway needle with introducer or cannula with introducer (peelaway sheath). (A peripherally inserted central catheter can also be used as a midline catheter.) Insertion can be accomplished at the bedside using sterile technique. Arm to be used should be positioned in abduction to 90-degree angle. Consent is required. Catheter may stay in place for up to 12 months or as long as required without complications.	No separate guidewire or introducer is needed. Stiff catheter is passed using the catheter advancement tab. Insertion can be accomplished at the bedside using sterile technique. Arm to be used should be positioned in abduction to 45-degree angle. Consent is required. Catheter may stay in place for 2–4 weeks.
Potential complications	Malposition, pneumothorax, hemothorax, hydrothorax, dysrhythmias, nerve or tendon damage, respiratory distress, catheter embolism, thrombophlebitis, or catheter occlusion. Compared with centrally placed catheters, venipuncture in the antecubital space reduces risk of insertion complications.	Thrombosis, phlebitis, air embolism, infection, vascular perforation, bleeding, catheter transection, occlusion
Contraindications	Dermatitis, cellulitis, burns, high fluid volume infusions, rapid bolus injections, hemodialysis, and venous thrombosis. No clamping of this catheter or splinting of the arm permitted. No blood pressure or tourniquets to be used on extremity where PICC is inserted.	Dermatitis, cellulitis, burns, high fluid volume infusions, rapid bolus injection, hemodialysis, and venous thrombosis. No blood pressure or tourniquet to be used on extremity where midline catheter is placed.
Catheter maintenance	Sterile dressing changes according to agency policy and procedures. Generally, dressing is changed 2 or 3 ×/week or when wet, soiled, or nonocclusive. Line is flushed every 12 hours with 3 mL normal saline followed by heparin 3 mL (100 U/mL) per lumen.	Sterile dressing changes according to policy and procedures. Generally the dressing should be changed 2 or 3 ×/week or when wet, soiled, or nonocclusive. Line is flushed after each infusion or every 12 hours with 5–10 mL normal saline followed by 1 mL of heparin (100 U/mL). Catheter must be anchored securely to prevent its dislodgment.
Postplacement	Chest x-ray needed to confirm placement	Chest x-ray to assess placement may be obtained if unable to flush catheter, if no free flow blood return, if difficulty with catheter advancement, or if guidewire difficult to remove or bent on removal.
Assessment	Daily measurement of arm circumference (4″ above insertion site) and length of exposed catheter	Daily measurement of arm circumference (4″ above insertion site) and length of exposed catheter
Removal	Catheter should be removed when no longer indicated for use, if contaminated, or if complications occur. Arm is abducted during removal. Pressure is applied on removal with a sterile dressing and antiseptic ointment to site. Dressing is changed every 24 hours until epithelialization occurs.	Catheter should be removed when no longer indicated for use, if contaminated, or if complications occur. Arm is abducted during removal. Pressure is applied on removal with a sterile dressing and antiseptic ointment to site. Dressing is changed every 24 hours until epithelialization occurs.
Advantages	Reduces cost and avoids repeated venipunctures compared with centrally placed catheters. Decreases incidence of catheter-related infections.	Reduces cost and avoids repeated venipunctures compared with centrally placed catheters. Decreases incidence of catheter-related infections.

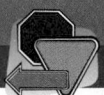

Chart 14-2

GUIDELINES FOR Starting an Intravenous Infusion

NURSING ACTION	RATIONALE
Preparation	
1. Verify prescription for IV therapy, check solution label, and identify patient.	1. Serious errors can be avoided by careful checking.
2. Explain procedure to patient.	2. Knowledge increases patient comfort and cooperation.
3. Carry out hand hygiene and put on disposable nonlatex gloves.	3. Asepsis is essential to prevent infection. Prevents exposure of nurse to patient's blood and of patient and nurse to latex.
4. Apply a tourniquet 4–6 inches above the site and identify a suitable vein.	4. This will distend the veins and allow them to be visualized.
5. Choose site. Use distal veins of hands and arms first.	5. Careful site selection will increase likelihood of successful venipuncture and preservation of vein. Using distal sites first preserves sites proximal to the previously cannulated site for subsequent venipunctures. Veins of feet and lower extremity should be avoided due to risk of thrombophlebitis. (In consultation with the physician, the saphenous vein of the ankle or dorsum of the foot may occasionally be used.)
6. Choose IV cannula or catheter.	6. Length and gauge of cannula should be appropriate for both site and purpose of infusion. The shortest gauge and length needed to deliver prescribed therapy should be used.
7. Connect infusion bag and tubing, and run solution through tubing to displace air; cover end of tubing.	7. Prevents delay; equipment must be ready to connect immediately after successful venipuncture to prevent clotting
8. Raise bed to comfortable working height and position for patient; adjust lighting. Position patient's arm below heart level to encourage capillary filling. Place protective pad on bed under patient's arm.	8. Proper positioning will increase likelihood of success and provide comfort for patient.
Procedure	
1. Depending on agency policy and procedure, lidocaine 1% (without epinephrine) 0.1–0.2 mL may be injected locally to the IV site or a transdermal analgesic cream (EMLA) may be applied to the site 60 minutes before IV placement or blood withdrawal. Intradermal injection of bacteriostatic 0.9% sodium chloride may have a local anesthetic effect.	1. Reduces pain locally from procedure and decreases anxiety about pain
2. Question the patient carefully about sensitivity to latex; use blood-pressure cuff rather than latex tourniquet if there is possibility of sensitivity.	2. Reduces risk of allergic reaction
3. Apply a new tourniquet for each patient or a blood pressure cuff 15 to 20 cm (6–8 in) above injection site. Palpate for a pulse distal to the tourniquet. Ask patient to open and close fist several times or position patient's arm in a dependent position to distend a vein.	3. The tourniquet distends the vein and makes it easier to enter; it should never be tight enough to occlude arterial flow. If a radial pulse cannot be palpated distal to the tourniquet, it is too tight. A new tourniquet should be used for each patient to prevent the transmission of microorganisms. A blood pressure cuff may be used for elderly patients to avoid rupture of the veins. A clenched fist encourages the vein to become round and turgid. Positioning the arm below the level of the patient's heart promotes capillary filling. Warm packs can promote vasodilation as well.
4. Ascertain if the patient is allergic to iodine. Prepare site by scrubbing with chlorhexidine gluconate or povidone–iodine swabs for 2–3 min in circular motion, moving outward from injection site. Allow to dry. a. If the site selected is excessively hairy, clip hair. (Check agency's policy and procedure about this practice.) b. 70% isopropyl alcohol is an alternative solution that may be used.	4. Strict asepsis and careful site preparation are essential to prevent infection.
5. With hand not holding the venous access device, steady patient's arm and use finger or thumb to pull skin taut over vessel.	5. Applying traction to the vein helps to stabilize it.
6. Holding needle bevel up and at 5°–25° angle, depending on the depth of the vein, pierce skin to reach but not penetrate vein.	6. Bevel-up position usually produces less trauma to skin and vein. A superficial vein needs a smaller cannula angle and a vein deeper in subcutaneous tissue requires a greater cannula angle.
7. Decrease angle of needle further until nearly parallel with skin, then enter vein either directly above or from the side in one quick motion.	7. Two-stage procedure decreases chance of thrusting needle through posterior wall of vein as skin is entered. No attempt should be made to reinsert the stylet because of risk of severing or puncturing the catheter.

(continued)

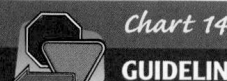

Chart 14-2

GUIDELINES FOR Starting an Intravenous Infusion (Continued)

NURSING ACTION	RATIONALE
8. If backflow of blood is visible, straighten angle and advance needle. Additional steps for catheter inserted over needle: a. Advance needle 0.6 cm (¼–½ in) after successful venipuncture. b. Hold needle hub, and slide catheter over the needle into the vein. Never reinsert needle into a plastic catheter or pull the catheter back into the needle. c. Remove needle while pressing lightly on the skin over the catheter tip; hold catheter hub in place.	8. Backflow may not occur if vein is small; this position decreases chance of puncturing posterior wall of vein. a. Advancing the needle slightly makes certain the plastic catheter has entered the vein. b. Reinsertion of the needle or pulling the catheter back can sever the catheter, causing catheter embolism. c. Slight pressure prevents bleeding before tubing is attached.
9. Release tourniquet and attach infusion tubing; open clamp enough to allow drip.	9. Infusion must be attached promptly to prevent clotting of blood in cannula. After two unsuccessful attempts at venipuncture, assistance by a more experienced health care provider is recommended to avoid unnecessary trauma to the patient and the possibility of limiting future sites for vascular access.
10. Slip a sterile 2-in × 2-in gauze pad under the catheter hub.	10. The gauze acts as a sterile field.
11. Anchor needle firmly in place with tape.	11. A stable needle is less likely to become dislodged or to irritate the vein.
12. Cover the insertion site with a transparent dressing, bandage, or sterile gauze; tape in place with nonallergenic tape but do not encircle extremity.	12. Tape encircling extremity can act as a tourniquet.
13. Tape a small loop of IV tubing onto dressing.	13. The loop decreases the chance of inadvertent cannula removal if the tubing is pulled.
14. Cover the insertion site with a dressing according to hospital policy and procedure. A gauze or transparent dressing may be used.	14. Transparent dressings allow assessment of the insertion site for phlebitis, infiltration, and infection without removing the dressing.
15. Label dressing with type and length of cannula, date, time, and initials.	15. Labeling facilitates assessment and safe discontinuation.
16. A padded, appropriate-length arm board may be applied to an area of flexion (neurovascular checks should be performed frequently).	16. Secures cannula placement and allows correct flow rate (neurovascular checks assess nerve, muscle, and vascular function to be sure function is not affected by immobilization)
17. Calculate infusion rate and regulate flow of infusion. For hourly IV rate use the following formula: gtt/mL of infusion set/60 (min in hr) × total hourly vol = gtt/min	17. Infusion must be regulated carefully to prevent overinfusion or underinfusion. Calculation of the IV rate is essential for the safe delivery of fluids. Safe administration requires knowledge of the volume of fluid to be infused, total infusion time, and the calibration of the administration set (found on the IV tubing package; 10, 12, 15, or 60 drops to deliver 1 mL of fluid).
18. Document site, cannula size and type, the number of attempts at insertion, time, solution, IV rate, and patient response to procedure.	18. Documentation is essential to promote continuity of care.

uses a drop sensor to monitor the flow. Factors essential for the safe use of pumps include alarms to signify the presence of air in the IV line and occlusion. The standard for the accurate delivery of fluid or medication via an electronic IV infusion pump is plus or minus 5%. The manufacturer's directions must be read carefully before using any infusion pump or controller, because there are many variations in available models. Use of these devices does not eliminate the need for the nurse to monitor the infusion and the patient frequently.

DISCONTINUING AN INFUSION

The removal of an IV catheter is associated with two possible dangers: bleeding and catheter embolism. To prevent excessive bleeding, a dry, sterile pressure dressing should be held over the site as the catheter is removed. Firm pressure is applied until hemostasis occurs.

If a plastic IV catheter is severed, the loose fragment can travel to the right ventricle and block blood flow. To detect this com-

plication when the catheter is removed, the nurse compares the expected length of the catheter with its actual length. Plastic catheters should be withdrawn carefully and their length measured to make certain that no fragment has broken off.

Great care must be exercised when using scissors around the dressing site. If the catheter clearly has been severed, the nurse can attempt to occlude the vein above the site by applying a tourniquet to prevent the catheter from entering the central circulation (until surgical removal is possible). As always, however, it is better to prevent a potentially fatal problem than to deal with it after it has occurred. Fortunately, catheter embolism can be prevented easily by following simple rules:

- Avoid using scissors near the catheter.
- Avoid withdrawing the catheter through the insertion needle.
- Follow the manufacturer's guidelines carefully (eg, cover the needle point with the bevel shield to prevent severance of the catheter).

MANAGING SYSTEMIC COMPLICATIONS

IV therapy predisposes the patient to numerous hazards, including both local and systemic complications. Systemic complications occur less frequently but are usually more serious than local complications. They include circulatory overload, air embolism, febrile reaction, and infection.

Fluid Overload.   Overloading the circulatory system with excessive IV fluids causes increased blood pressure and central venous pressure. Signs and symptoms of fluid overload include moist crackles on auscultation of the lungs, edema, weight gain, dyspnea, and respirations that are shallow and have an increased rate. Possible causes include rapid infusion of an IV solution or hepatic, cardiac, or renal disease. The risk for fluid overload and subsequent pulmonary edema is especially increased in elderly patients with cardiac disease; this is referred to as circulatory overload.

The treatment for circulatory overload is decreasing the IV rate, monitoring vital signs frequently, assessing breath sounds, and placing the patient in a high Fowler's position. The physician is contacted immediately. This complication can be avoided by using an infusion pump for infusions and by carefully monitoring all infusions. Complications of circulatory overload include heart failure and pulmonary edema.

Air Embolism.   The risk of air embolism is rare but ever-present. It is most often associated with cannulation of central veins. Manifestations of air embolism include dyspnea and cyanosis; hypotension; weak, rapid pulse; loss of consciousness; and chest, shoulder, and low back pain. Treatment calls for immediately clamping the cannula, placing the patient on the left side in the Trendelenburg position, assessing vital signs and breath sounds, and administering oxygen. Air embolism can be prevented by using a Luer-Lok adapter on all lines, filling all tubing completely with solution, and using an air detection alarm on an IV pump. Complications of air embolism include shock and death. The amount of air necessary to induce death in humans is not known; however, the rate of entry is probably as important as the actual volume of air.

Septicemia and Other Infection.   Pyrogenic substances in either the infusion solution or the IV administration set can induce a febrile reaction and septicemia. Signs and symptoms include an abrupt temperature elevation shortly after the infusion is started, backache, headache, increased pulse and respiratory rate, nausea and vomiting, diarrhea, chills and shaking, and general malaise. In severe septicemia, vascular collapse and septic shock may occur. Causes of septicemia include contamination of the IV product or a break in aseptic technique, especially in immunocompromised patients. Treatment is symptomatic and includes culturing of the IV cannula, tubing, or solution if suspect and establishing a new IV site for medication or fluid administration. See Chapter 15 for a discussion of septic shock.

Infection ranges in severity from local involvement of the insertion site to systemic dissemination of organisms through the bloodstream, as in septicemia. Measures to prevent infection are essential at the time the IV line is inserted and throughout the entire infusion. Prevention includes:

- Careful hand hygiene before every contact with any part of the infusion system or patient
- Examining the IV containers for cracks, leaks, or cloudiness, which may indicate a contaminated solution
- Using strict aseptic technique

- Firmly anchoring the IV cannula to prevent to-and-fro motion
- Inspecting the IV site daily and replacing a soiled or wet dressing with a dry sterile dressing. (Antimicrobial agents that should be used for site care include 2% tincture of iodine, 10% povidone–iodine, alcohol, or chlorhexidine, used alone or in combination.)
- Removing the IV cannula at the first sign of local inflammation, contamination, or complication
- Replacing the peripheral IV cannula every 48 to 72 hours, or as indicated
- Replacing the IV cannula inserted during emergency conditions (with questionable asepsis) as soon as possible
- Using a 0.2-micron air-eliminating and bacteria/particulate retentive filter with non-lipid-containing solutions that require filtration. The filter can be added to the proximal or distal end of the administration set. If added to the proximal end between the fluid container and the tubing spike, the filter ensures sterility and particulate removal from the infusate container and prevents inadvertent infusion of air. If added to the distal end of the administration set, it filters air particles and contaminants introduced from add-on devices, secondary administration sets, or interruptions to the primary system.
- Replacing the solution bag and administration set in accordance with agency policy and procedure
- Infusing or discarding medication or solution within 24 hours of its addition to an administration set
- Changing primary and secondary continuous administration sets every 72 hours, or immediately if contamination is suspected
- Changing primary intermittent administration sets every 24 hours, or immediately if contamination is suspected

MANAGING LOCAL COMPLICATIONS

Local complications of IV therapy include infiltration and extravasation, phlebitis, thrombophlebitis, hematoma, and clotting of the needle.

Infiltration and Extravasation.   Infiltration is the unintentional administration of a nonvesicant solution or medication into surrounding tissue. This can occur when the IV cannula dislodges or perforates the wall of the vein. Infiltration is characterized by edema around the insertion site, leakage of IV fluid from the insertion site, discomfort and coolness in the area of infiltration, and a significant decrease in the flow rate. When the solution is particularly irritating, sloughing of tissue may result. Closely monitoring the insertion site is necessary to detect infiltration before it becomes severe.

Infiltration is usually easily recognized if the insertion area is larger than the same site of the opposite extremity; however, it is not always so obvious. A common misconception is that a backflow of blood into the tubing proves that the catheter is properly placed within the vein. If the catheter tip has pierced the wall of the vessel, however, IV fluid will seep into tissues as well as flow into the vein. Although blood return occurs, infiltration has occurred as well. A more reliable means of confirming infiltration is to apply a tourniquet above (or proximal to) the infusion site and tighten it enough to restrict venous flow. If the infusion continues to drip despite the venous obstruction, infiltration is present.

As soon as the nurse notes infiltration, the infusion should be stopped, the IV discontinued, and a sterile dressing applied to the site after careful inspection to determine the extent of infiltration. The infiltration of any amount of blood product, irritant, or vesicant is considered the most severe.

The IV infusion should be started in a new site or proximal to the infiltration if the same extremity is used. A warm compress may be applied to the site if small volumes of noncaustic solutions have infiltrated over a long time, and the affected extremity should be elevated to promote the absorption of fluid. If the infiltration is recent, a cold compress may be applied to the area. Infiltration can be detected and treated early by inspecting the site every hour for redness, pain, edema, blood return, coolness at the site, and IV fluid draining from the IV site. Using the appropriate size and type of cannula for the vein prevents this complication. According to the Infusion Nursing Standards of Practice, a standardized infiltration scale should be used to document the infiltration (Alexander, 2000):

0 = No symptoms
1 = Skin blanched, edema less than 1 inch in any direction, cool to touch, with or without pain
2 = Skin blanched, edema 1 to 6 inches in any direction, cool to touch, with or without pain
3 = Skin blanched, translucent, gross edema greater than 6 inches in any direction, cool to touch, mild to moderate pain, possible numbness
4 = Skin blanched, translucent, skin tight, leaking, skin discolored, bruised, swollen, gross edema greater than 6 inches in any direction, deep pitting tissue edema, circulatory impairment, moderate to severe pain, infiltration of any amount of blood products, irritant, or vesicant

Extravasation is similar to infiltration, with an inadvertent administration of vesicant or irritant solution or medication into the surrounding tissue. Medications such as dopamine, calcium preparations, and chemotherapeutic agents can cause pain, burning, and redness at the site. Blistering, inflammation, and necrosis of tissues can occur. The extent of tissue damage is determined by the concentration of the medication, the quantity that extravasated, the location of the infusion site, the tissue response, and the duration of the process of extravasation.

The infusion must be stopped and the physician notified promptly. The agency's protocol for extravasation is initiated; the protocol may specify specific treatments, including antidotes specific to the medication that extravasated, and may indicate whether the IV line should remain in place or be removed before treatment. The protocol often specifies that the infusion site be infiltrated with an antidote prescribed after assessment by the physician and application of warm or cold compresses, depending on the medication infusing. This extremity should not be used for further cannula placement. Thorough neurovascular assessments of the affected extremity must be performed frequently.

Reviewing the institution's IV policy and procedures and incompatibility charts and checking with the pharmacist before administering any IV medication, whether given peripherally or centrally, is a prudent way to determine incompatibilities and vesicant potential to prevent extravasation. Careful, frequent monitoring of the IV site, avoiding insertion of IV devices in areas of flexion, securing the IV line, and using the smallest catheter possible that accommodates the vein help minimize the incidence and severity of this complication. In addition, when vesicant medication is administered by IV push, it should be given through a side port of an infusing IV solution to dilute the medication and decrease the severity of tissue damage if extravasation oc-

curs. Extravasation should always be rated as a grade 4 on the infiltration scale.

Phlebitis. Phlebitis is defined as inflammation of a vein related to a chemical or mechanical irritation, or both. It is characterized by a reddened, warm area around the insertion site or along the path of the vein, pain or tenderness at the site or along the vein, and swelling. The incidence of phlebitis increases with the length of time the IV line is in place, the composition of the fluid or medication infused (especially its pH and tonicity), the size and site of the cannula inserted, ineffective filtration, improper anchoring of the line, and the introduction of microorganisms at the time of insertion. The Intravenous Nursing Society has identified specific standards for assessing phlebitis (Alexander, 2000); these appear in Chart 14-3.

Treatment consists of discontinuing the IV and restarting it in another site, and applying a warm, moist compress to the affected site. Phlebitis can be prevented by using aseptic technique during insertion, using the appropriate-size cannula or needle for the vein, considering the composition of fluids and medications when selecting a site, observing the site hourly for any complications, anchoring the cannula or needle well, and changing the IV site according to agency policy and procedures.

Thrombophlebitis. Thrombophlebitis refers to the presence of a clot plus inflammation in the vein. It is evidenced by localized pain, redness, warmth, and swelling around the insertion site or along the path of the vein, immobility of the extremity because of discomfort and swelling, sluggish flow rate, fever, malaise, and leukocytosis.

Treatment includes discontinuing the IV infusion, applying a cold compress first to decrease the flow of blood and increase platelet aggregation followed by a warm compress, elevating the extremity, and restarting the line in the opposite extremity. If the patient has signs and symptoms of thrombophlebitis, the IV line should not be flushed (although flushing may be indicated in

Chart 14-3 • ASSESSMENT

Phlebitis

According to the Infusion Nurses Society, documentation of phlebitis should be standardized. Phlebitis should be graded according to the most severe presenting indication

Grade	Clinical Criteria
0	No clinical symptoms
1	Erythema at access site with or without pain
2	Pain at access site Erythema, edema, or both
3	Pain at access site Erythema, edema, or both Streak formation Palpable venous cord (1 in. or shorter)
4	Pain at access site with erythema Streak formation Palpable venous cord (longer than 1 in.) Purulent drainage

Note: If this scale is not being used in an institution, then the description associated with the number can be used to describe the assessment.
From Infusion Nursing Standards of Practice (2000). *Journal of Intravenous Nursing.* 23(6S), S56–S69.

the absence of phlebitis to ensure cannula patency and to prevent mixing incompatible medications and solutions).

Thrombophlebitis can be prevented by avoiding trauma to the vein at the time the IV is inserted, observing the site every hour, and checking medication additives for compatibility.

Hematoma. Hematoma results when blood leaks into tissues surrounding the IV insertion site. Leakage can result from perforation of the opposite vein wall during venipuncture, the needle slipping out of the vein, and insufficient pressure applied to the site after removing the needle or cannula. The signs of a hematoma include ecchymosis, immediate swelling at the site, and leakage of blood at the site.

Treatment includes removing the needle or cannula and applying pressure with a sterile dressing; applying ice for 24 hours to the site to avoid extension of the hematoma and then a warm compress to increase absorption of blood; assessing the site; and restarting the line in the other extremity if indicated. A hematoma can be prevented by carefully inserting the needle and using diligent care when a patient has a bleeding disorder, takes anticoagulant medication, or has advanced liver disease.

Clotting and Obstruction. Blood clots may form in the IV line as a result of kinked IV tubing, a very slow infusion rate, an empty IV bag, or failure to flush the IV line after intermittent medication or solution administrations. The signs are decreased flow rate and blood backflow into the IV tubing.

If blood clots in the IV line, the infusion must be discontinued and restarted in another site with a new cannula and administration set. The tubing should not be irrigated or milked. Neither the infusion rate nor the solution container should be raised, and the clot should not be aspirated from the tubing. Clotting of the needle or cannula may be prevented by not permitting the IV solution bag to run dry, taping the tubing to prevent kinking and maintain patency, maintaining an adequate flow rate, and flushing the line after intermittent medication or other solution administration. In some cases, a specially trained nurse or physician may inject a thrombolytic agent into the catheter to clear an occlusion resulting from fibrin or clotted blood.

PROMOTING HOME AND COMMUNITY-BASED CARE

Teaching Patients Self-Care. At times, IV therapy must be administered in the home setting, in which case much of the daily management rests with the patient and family. Teaching becomes essential to ensure that the patient and family can manage the IV fluid and infusion properly and avoid complications. Written instructions as well as demonstration and return demonstration help reinforce the key points for all these functions.

Continuing Care. Home infusion therapies cover a wide range of treatments, including antibiotic, analgesic, and antineoplastic medications; blood or blood component therapy; and parenteral nutrition. When direct nursing care is necessary, arrangements can be made to have an infusion nurse visit the home and administer the IV therapy as prescribed. In addition to implementing and monitoring the IV therapy, the nurse carries out a comprehensive assessment of the patient's condition and continues to teach the patient and family about the skills involved in overseeing the IV therapy setup. Any dietary changes that may be necessary because of fluid or electrolyte imbalances are explained or reinforced during such sessions.

Periodic laboratory testing may be necessary to assess the effects of IV therapy and the patient's progress. Blood specimens may be obtained by a laboratory near the patient's home, or a home visit may be arranged to obtain blood specimens for analysis.

The nurse collaborates with the case manager in assessing the patient, family, and home environment; developing a plan of care in accordance with the patient's treatment plan and level of ability; and arranging for appropriate referral and follow-up if necessary. Any necessary equipment may be provided by the agency or purchased by the patient, depending on the terms of the home care arrangements. Appropriate documentation is necessary to assist in obtaining third-party payment for the service provided.

Critical Thinking Exercises

1. A 40-year-old man with peptic ulcer disease reports vomiting, nausea, dry mucous membranes, and abdominal pain for the last 2 days. His BP is 92/64 and pulse is 120. His laboratory results show a serum sodium level of 125 mEq/L, urine sodium level of 5 mEq/L, and measured serum osmolality of 270 mOsm/L. What IV solution do you anticipate will be prescribed for him? Provide a rationale for its use, and discuss the nursing actions relevant to its administration.

2. A 30-year-old woman comes into the emergency department with a temperature of 39.4°C (103°F). For the last 4 days she has had a productive cough and has experienced dyspnea increasing in severity. Her serum laboratory results are as follows: WBC = 20,000, pH = 7.59, $PaCO_2$ = 26, PaO_2 = 40, SaO_2 = 80, HCO_3 = 20, Na^+ = 140, K^+ = 4.2, Cl^- = 106, CO_2 = 20. What is the acid–base disorder? What treatments and relevant nursing actions related to the underlying disorder and its treatment should the nurse anticipate?

3. A 48-year-old woman reports shortness of breath that has been increasing in the last 3 months so much so that she is no longer able to use her treadmill. She is a nonsmoker. Her chest x-ray is negative. She does not take any medications. Her arterial blood gases are as follows: pH = 7.41, $PaCO_2$ = 37 mm Hg, PaO_2 = 94 mm Hg, HCO_3 = 23 mmHg, pulse oximetry = 98%. What is your interpretation of her blood gas values? What action is indicated by these results?

4. An obtunded 84-year-old man is admitted to the hospital from the nursing home with a high fever. The following clinical data are obtained on admission: temperature 39.4°C (102°F); BP 150/90; pulse rate of 110; dry, mucous membranes. Laboratory test results include the following: serum Na^+ = 184 mEq/L, urine osmolality – 640 mOsm/kg; urine culture and sensitivity shows pyuria and many bacteria. His peripheral IV at the site of the right dorsal metacarpal vein is infiltrated. What method of administering IV fluids would the nurse anticipate? What factors are probably contributing to his hypernatremia? What nursing actions should be taken in assisting with treatment of this patient's fluid and electrolyte imbalance?

5. A 65-year-old patient with severe, long-standing COPD is admitted to the hospital for treatment of impending renal failure. Explain the effects of his pulmonary disorder on the acid–base disturbances that commonly occur with renal failure. What are the nursing observations and assessment that are indicated because of the occurrence of these two disorders?

REFERENCES AND SELECTED READINGS

Books

Chernecky, C. C., & Berger, B. J. (2001) *Laboratory tests and diagnostic procedures* (3d ed.). Philadelphia: W. B. Saunders.

Guyton, A. C. (2000). *Textbook of medical physiology* (10th ed.). Philadelphia: W. B. Saunders.

Hankins, J., Lonsway-Waldman, R., Hedrick, C., & Perdue, M. B. (2001). *Infusion therapy in clinical practice* (2d ed.). Philadelphia: W. B. Saunders.

Heitz, U., & Horne, M. (2001). *Pocket guide to fluid, electrolyte, and acid-base balance* (4th ed.). St. Louis: Mosby.

Karch, A. M. (2002). *Lippincott's nursing drug guide.* Philadelphia: Lippincott Williams & Wilkins.

Kee, J., & Paulanka, B. (2000). *Handbook of fluid, electrolyte and acid-base imbalances.* Albany, NY: Delmar Publishers.

Martin, L. (1999). *All you need to know to interpret arterial blood gases* (2d ed.). Philadelphia: Lippincott Williams & Wilkins.

Metheny, N. M. (2000). *Fluid and electrolyte balance: Nursing considerations* (4th ed.). Philadelphia: Lippincott Williams & Wilkins.

Otto, S. E. (2001). *Pocket guide to intravenous therapy* (4th ed.). St. Louis: C. V. Mosby.

Porth, C. M. (2002). *Pathophysiology: Concepts of altered health states* (6th ed.). Philadelphia: Lippincott Williams & Wilkins.

Price, S. A., & Wilson, L. M. (2003). *Pathophysiology. Clinical concepts of disease processes.* St. Louis: Mosby–Year Book.

Rose, B., & Post, T. (2001). *Clinical physiology of acid–base and electrolyte disorders* (5th ed.). New York: McGraw-Hill.

Weinstein, S. (2001). *Plumer's principles and practice of intravenous therapy.* Philadelphia: Lippincott Williams & Wilkins.

Journals

Asterisks indicate nursing research articles.

Fluid and Electrolyte Balances

Adrogue, H. J., & Madias, N. E. (2000*a*). Hyponatremia. *New England Journal of Medicine, 342*(21), 1581–1589.

Adrogue, H. J., & Madias, N. E. (2000*b*). Hypernatremia. *New England Journal of Medicine, 342*(20),1493–1499.

Anonymous. (2000). Part 1: Introduction to the International Guidelines 2000 for CPR and ECC: A consensus on science. *Circulation, 102*(8 Suppl), I1–I11.

Beck, L. H. (2000). The aging kidney. Defending a delicate balance of fluid and electrolytes. *Geriatrics, 55*(4), 26–28, 31–32.

Brater, D. C. (1998). Diuretic therapy. *New England Journal of Medicine, 339*(6), 387–395.

Carlstedt, F., & Lind, L. (2001). Hypocalcemic syndromes. *Critical Care Clinics, 17*(1), 139–153, vii–viii.

Castiglione, V. (2000). Emergency: Hyperkalemia. *American Journal of Nursing, 100*(1), 55–56.

Clayton, K. (1997). Cancer-related hypercalcemia: How to spot it, how to manage it. *American Journal of Nursing, 97*(5), 42–49.

Cohn, J. N., Kowey, P. R., Whelton, P. K., & Prisant, L. M. (2000). New guidelines for potassium replacement in clinical practice: A contemporary review by the National Council on Potassium in Clinical Practice. *Archives of Internal Medicine, 160*(16), 2429–2436.

Fall, P. J. (2000). Hyponatremia and hypernatremia. A systematic approach to causes and their correction. *Postgraduate Medicine, 107*(5), 75–82.

Fulop, M. (1998). Algorithms for diagnosing some electrolyte disorders. *American Journal of Emergency Medicine, 16*(1), 76–84.

Gross, P. (2001). Correction of hyponatremia. *Seminars in Nephrology, 21*(3), 269–272.

Gennari, F. J. (1998). Hypokalemia. *New England Journal of Medicine, 339*(7), 451–458.

Goldhill, D. R. (1997). Calcium and magnesium. *Care of the Critically Ill, 13*(3), 112–115.

Kreimeier, U. (2000). Pathophysiology of fluid imbalance. *Critical Care (London), 4*, Suppl 2:S3–S7.

Kugler, J. P., & Hustead, T. (2000). Hyponatremia and hypernatremia in the elderly. *American Family Physician, 61*(12), 3623–3630.

Lee, C. T., Guo, H. R., & Chen, J. B. (2000). Hyponatremia in the emergency department. *American Journal of Emergency Medicine, 18*(3), 264–268.

Lilly, L. L., & Guanci, R. (1997). Persistent potassium problems. *American Journal of Nursing, 97*(6), 14.

Marx, S. J. (2000). Hyperparathyroid and hypoparathyroid disorders. *New England Journal of Medicine, 343*(25), 1863–1875.

Nayback, A. M. (2000). Hyponatremia as a consequence of acute adrenal insufficiency and hypothyroidism. *Journal of Emergency Nursing, 26*(2), 130–133.

Oster, J. R., & Singer, I. (1999). Hyponatremia, hypoosmolality, and hypotonicity. *Archives of Internal Medicine, 159*(4), 333–336.

Perazella, M. A. (2000). Drug-induced hyperkalemia: Old culprits and new offenders. *American Journal of Medicine, 109*(4), 307–314.

Pirzada, N. A., & Ali, I. I. (2001). Central pontine myelinolysis. *Mayo Clinic Proceedings, 76*(5), 559–562.

*Rateau, M. R. (2000). Confusion and aggression in restrained elderly persons undergoing hip repair surgery. *Applied Nursing Research, 13*(1), 50–54.

Schmidt, T. C. (2000). Assessing a sodium and fluid imbalance. *Nursing, 30*(1), 18.

Suhayda, R. & Walton, J. C. (2002). Preventing and managing dehydration. *MedSurg Nursing, 11*(6), 267–278.

Terpstra, T. L., & Terpstra, T. L. (2000). Syndrome of inappropriate antidiuretic hormone: Recognition and management. *MedSurg Nursing, 9*(2). 61–68.

Toto, K. H. (1998). Fluid balance assessment. *Critical Care Nursing Clinics of North America, 10*(4), 383–400.

Wilcox, C. S. (1999). Metabolic and adverse effects of diuretics. *Seminars in Nephrology, 19*(6), 557–568.

Acid–Base Balance

Adrogue, H. E., & Adrogue, H. J. (2001). Acid-base physiology. *Respiratory Care, 46*(4), 328–341.

Epstein, S. K., & Singh, N. (2001). Respiratory acidosis. *Respiratory Care, 46*(4), 366–383.

Foster, G. T., Vaziri, N. D., & Sassoon, C. S. (2001). Respiratory alkalosis. *Respiratory Care, 46*(4), 384–391.

Horne, C., & Derrico, D. (1999). Mastering the art of arterial blood gas measurement. *American Journal of Nursing, 99*(8), 26–32.

Khanna, A., & Kurtzman, N. A. (2001). Metabolic alkalosis. *Respiratory Care, 46*(4), 354–365.

Kraut, J. A., & Madias, N. E. (2001). Approach to patients with acid-base disorders. *Respiratory Care, 46*(4), 392–403.

Sassoon, C. S., & Arruda, J. A. (2001). Acid-base disturbance. *Respiratory Care, 46*(4), 327.

Shoulders-Odom, B. (2000). Using an algorithm to interpret arterial blood gases. *Dimensions of Critical Care Nursing, 19*(1), 36–41.

Swenson, E. R. (2001). Metabolic acidosis. *Respiratory Care, 46*(4), 342–353.

Wallace, L. S. (2000). Using color to simplify ABG interpretation. *MedSurg Nursing, 9*(4), 205–207.

Williams, A. (1998). ABC of oxygen. Assessing and interpreting arterial blood gases and acid-base balance. *British Medical Journal, 317*(7167), 1213–1216.

Wong, F. W. H. (1999). A new approach to ABG interpretation. *American Journal of Nursing, 99*(8), 26–32.

Intravenous Administration

Alexander, M. (2000). Infusion Nursing Standards of Practice. *Journal of Intravenous Nursing, 23*(6), Suppl. S5–S88.

Andrews, C. M. (2002). Emergency: Preventing air embolism. *American Journal of Nursing, 102*(1), 34–36.

Andris, D. A., & Jrzywda, E. A. (1999). Central venous catheter occlusion: Successful management strategies. *MedSurg Nursing, 8*(4), 229–236.

Aschenbrenner, D. A. (2000). Skin preps and protocols. *American Journal of Nursing, 100*(4), 78.

Carlson, K. (1999). Correct utilization and management of peripherally inserted central catheters and midline catheters in the alternate care setting. *Journal of Intravenous Nursing, 22*(6), Suppl. S46–S50.

Driscoll, M., et al. (1997). Inserting and maintaining peripherally inserted central catheters. *MedSurg Nursing, 6*(6), 350–358.

*Fetzer, S. J. (2002). Reducing venipuncture and intravenous insertion pain with eutectic mixture of local anesthetic. A meta-analysis. *Nursing Research, 51*(2), 119–124.

*Fry, C. & Aholt, D. (2001). Local anesthesia prior to the insertion of peripherally inserted central catheters. *Journal of Infusion Nursing, 24*(6), 404–408.

Hadaway, L. C. (1999). Vascular access devices: Meeting patients' needs. *MedSurg Nursing, 8*(5), 296–303.

Intravenous Nurses Society. (1997). Position paper: Midline and midclavicular catheters. *Journal of Intravenous Nursing, 20*(4), 175–178.

Intravenous Nurses Society. (1997). Position paper: Peripherally inserted central catheters. *Journal of Intravenous Nursing, 20*(4), 172–174.

Krzywda, E. A. (1998). Central venous access—catheters, technology, and physiology. *MedSurg Nursing, 7*(3), 132–139.

Kupensky, D. (1998). Applying current research to influence clinical practice. *Journal of Intravenous Nursing, 21*(5), 271–274.

LeDuc, K. (1997) Efficacy of normal saline solution versus heparin solution for maintaining patency of peripheral intravenous catheters in children. *Journal of Emergency Nursing, 23*(4), 306–309.

Macklin, D. (2000). Removing a PICC. *American Journal of Nursing, 100*(1), 52–54.

Millam, D. (2000). On the road to successful venipuncture. *Nursing, 30*(4), 34–48.

Moureau, N., & Zonderman, A. (2000) Does it always have to hurt? Premedications for adults and children for use with intravenous therapy. *Journal of Intravenous Nursing, 23*(4), 213–219.

RESOURCES AND WEBSITES

Infusion Nurses Society, 220 Norwood Park South, Norwood, MA 02062; (781) 440-9408; http://www.ins1.org.

Shock and Multisystem Failure

LEARNING OBJECTIVES ●

On completion of this chapter, the learner will be able to:

1. Describe shock and its underlying pathophysiology.
2. Compare clinical findings of the compensatory and progressive stages of shock.
3. Describe organ damage that may occur with shock.
4. Compare hypovolemic, cardiogenic, and circulatory shock in terms of causes, pathophysiologic effects, and medical and nursing management.
5. Describe indications for varying types of fluid replacement.
6. Identify vasoactive medications used in treating shock, and describe nursing implications associated with their use.
7. Discuss the importance of nutritional support in all forms of shock.
8. Discuss the role of the nurse in psychosocial support of both the patient experiencing shock and the family.
9. Discuss the syndrome of multiple organ dysfunction.

Shock is a life-threatening condition with a variety of underlying causes. It is characterized by inadequate tissue perfusion that, if untreated, results in cell death. The nurse caring for the patient with shock or at risk for shock must understand the underlying mechanisms of shock and recognize its subtle as well as more obvious signs. Rapid assessment and response are essential to the patient's recovery.

Shock can best be defined as a condition in which systemic blood pressure is inadequate to deliver oxygen and nutrients to support vital organs and cellular function (Mikhail, 1999). Adequate blood flow to the tissues and cells requires the following components: adequate cardiac pump, effective vasculature or circulatory system, and sufficient blood volume. When one component is impaired, blood flow to the tissues is threatened or compromised. Without treatment, inadequate blood flow to the tissues results in poor delivery of oxygen and nutrients to the cells, cellular starvation, cell death, organ dysfunction progressing to organ failure, and eventual death.

Significance of Shock

Shock affects all body systems. It may develop rapidly or slowly, depending on the underlying cause. During shock, the body struggles to survive, calling on all its homeostatic mechanisms to restore blood flow and tissue perfusion. Any insult to the body can create a cascade of events resulting in poor tissue perfusion. Therefore, almost any patient with any disease state may be at risk for developing shock.

Nursing care of the patient with shock requires ongoing systematic assessment. Many of the interventions required in caring for the patient with shock call for close collaboration with other members of the health care team and a physician's orders. The nurse must anticipate such orders because they need to be executed with speed and accuracy.

Conditions Precipitating Shock

CLASSIFICATION OF SHOCK

Shock can be classified by etiology and may be described as (1) **hypovolemic shock**, (2) **cardiogenic shock**, or (3) **circulatory** or **distributive shock**. Some authors identify a fourth category, obstructive shock, that results from disorders that cause mechanical obstruction to blood flow through the central circulatory system despite normal myocardial function and intravascular volume.

Examples include pulmonary embolism, cardiac tamponade, dissecting aortic aneurysm, and tension pneumothorax. In this discussion, obstructive disorders are discussed as examples of noncoronary cardiogenic shock. Hypovolemic shock occurs when there is a decrease in the intravascular volume. Cardiogenic shock occurs when the heart has an impaired pumping ability; it may be of coronary or noncoronary origin. Circulatory shock results from a maldistribution or mismatch of blood flow to the cells.

NORMAL CELLULAR FUNCTION

Energy metabolism occurs within the cell, where nutrients are chemically broken down and stored in the form of adenosine triphosphate (ATP). Cells use this stored energy to perform necessary functions, such as active transport, muscle contraction, and biochemical synthesis, as well as specialized cellular functions, such as the conduction of electrical impulses. ATP can be synthesized aerobically (in the presence of oxygen) or anaerobically (in the absence of oxygen). Aerobic metabolism yields far greater amounts of ATP per mole of glucose than does anaerobic metabolism and, therefore, is a more efficient and effective means of producing energy. Additionally, anaerobic metabolism results in the accumulation of the toxic end product lactic acid, which must be removed from the cell and transported to the liver for conversion into glucose and glycogen.

PATHOPHYSIOLOGY

In shock, the cells lack an adequate blood supply and are deprived of oxygen and nutrients; therefore, they must produce energy through anaerobic metabolism. This results in low energy yields from nutrients and an acidotic intracellular environment. Because of these changes, normal cell function ceases (Fig. 15-1). The cell swells and the cell membrane becomes more permeable, allowing electrolytes and fluids to seep out of and into the cell. The sodium-potassium pump becomes impaired; cell structures, primarily the mitochondria, are damaged; and death of the cell results.

Vascular Responses

Oxygen attaches to the hemoglobin molecule in red blood cells, and the blood carries it to body cells. The amount of oxygen that is delivered to cells depends both on blood flow to a specific area and on blood oxygen concentration. Blood is continuously re-

---

Glossary

anaphylactic shock: circulatory shock state resulting from a severe allergic reaction producing an overwhelming systemic vasodilation and relative hypovolemia

biochemical mediators: messenger substances that may be released by a cell to create an action at that site or be carried by the bloodstream to a distant site before being activated; also called cytokines

cardiogenic shock: shock state resulting from impairment or failure of the myocardium

colloids: intravenous solutions that contain molecules that are too large to pass through capillary membranes

crystalloids: electrolyte solutions that move freely between the intravascular compartment and interstitial spaces

circulatory shock: shock state resulting from displacement of blood volume creating a relative hypovolemia and inadequate delivery of oxygen to the cells; also called distributive shock

hypovolemic shock: shock state resulting from decreased intravascular volume due to fluid loss

neurogenic shock: shock state resulting from loss of sympathetic tone causing relative hypovolemia

septic shock: circulatory shock state resulting from overwhelming infection causing relative hypovolemia

shock: physiologic state in which there is inadequate blood flow to tissues and cells of the body

systemic inflammatory response syndrome (SIRS): overwhelming inflammatory response in the absence of infection causing relative hypovolemia and decreased tissue perfusion

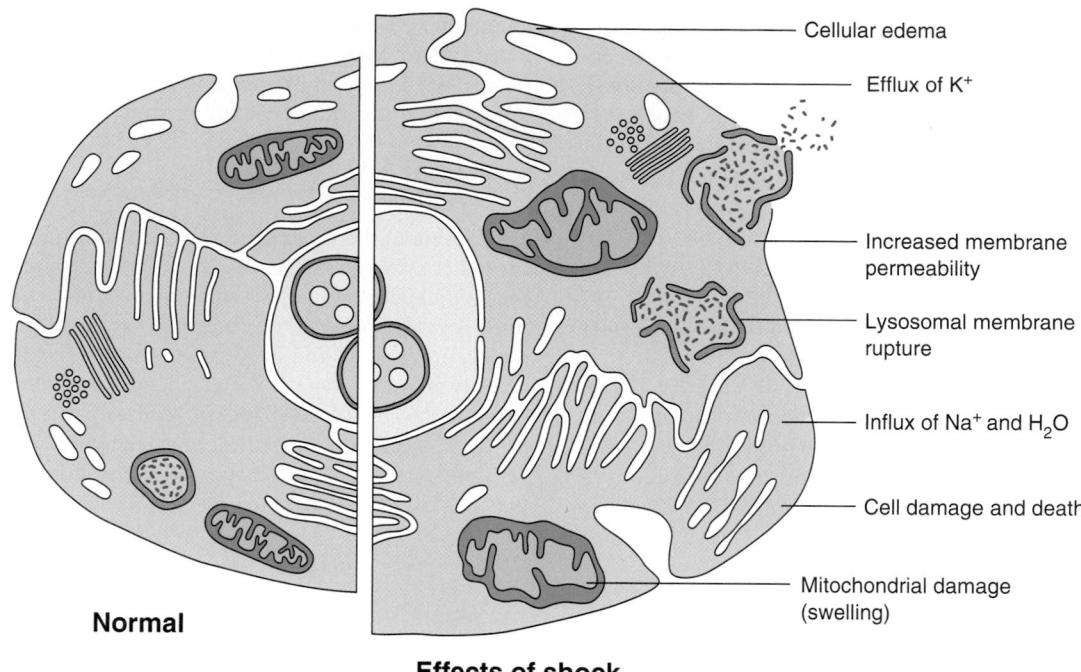

Normal   **Effects of shock**

FIGURE 15-1 Cellular effects of shock. The cell swells and the cell membrane becomes more permeable, and fluids and electrolytes seep from and into the cell. Mitochondria and lysosomes are damaged, and the cell dies.

cycled through the lungs to be reoxygenated and to eliminate end products of cellular metabolism, such as carbon dioxide. The heart muscle is the pump that propels the freshly oxygenated blood out to the body tissues. This process of circulation is facilitated through an elaborate and dynamic vasculature consisting of arteries, arterioles, capillaries, veins, and venules. The vasculature can dilate or constrict based on central and local regulatory mechanisms. Central regulatory mechanisms stimulate dilation or constriction of the vasculature to maintain an adequate blood pressure. Local regulatory mechanisms, referred to as autoregulation, stimulate vasodilation or vasoconstriction in response to biochemical mediators (also called cytokines) released by the cell, communicating its need for oxygen and nutrients (Jindal, Hollenberg & Dellinger, 2000) A biochemical mediator is a substance released by a cell or immune cells such as polymorphonuclear leukocytes (PMNs) or macrophages; the substance triggers an action at a cell site or travels in the bloodstream to a distant site, where it triggers action.

Blood Pressure Regulation

Three major components of the circulatory system—blood volume, the cardiac pump, and the vasculature—must respond effectively to complex neural, chemical, and hormonal feedback systems to maintain an adequate blood pressure and ultimately perfuse body tissues.

Blood pressure is regulated through a complex interaction of neural, chemical, and hormonal feedback systems affecting both cardiac output and peripheral resistance. This relationship is expressed in the following equation:

Mean arterial blood pressure = cardiac output × peripheral resistance

Cardiac output is determined by stroke volume (the amount of blood ejected at systole) and heart rate. Peripheral resistance is determined by the diameter of the arterioles.

Tissue perfusion and organ perfusion depend on mean arterial pressure (MAP). The MAP is the average pressure at which blood moves through the vasculature. Although true MAP can be calculated only by complex methods, Chart 15-1 displays a convenient formula for clinical use in estimating MAP. MAP should exceed 70 to 80 mm Hg for cells to receive the oxygen and nutrients needed to metabolize energy in amounts sufficient to sustain life (Balk, 2000a).

Blood pressure is regulated by the baroreceptors (pressure receptors) located in the carotid sinus and aortic arch. These pressure receptors convey impulses to the sympathetic nervous center in the medulla of the brain. When blood pressure drops, catecholamines (epinephrine and norepinephrine) are released from the adrenal medulla of the adrenal glands. This increases heart rate and vasoconstriction, thus restoring blood pressure. Chemoreceptors, also located in the aortic arch and carotid arteries, regulate blood pressure and respiratory rate using much the same mechanism in response to changes in oxygen and carbon dioxide concentrations in the blood. These primary regulatory mechanisms can respond to changes in blood pressure on a moment-to-moment basis.

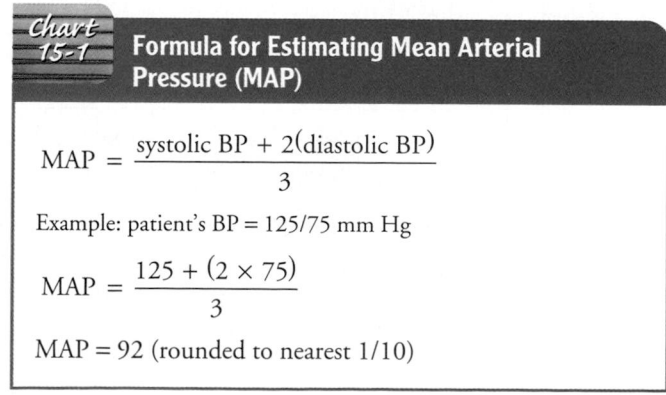

Chart 15-1

Formula for Estimating Mean Arterial Pressure (MAP)

$$MAP = \frac{\text{systolic BP} + 2(\text{diastolic BP})}{3}$$

Example: patient's BP = 125/75 mm Hg

$$MAP = \frac{125 + (2 \times 75)}{3}$$

MAP = 92 (rounded to nearest 1/10)

The kidneys also play an important role in blood pressure regulation. They regulate blood pressure by releasing renin, an enzyme needed for the conversion of angiotensin I to angiotensin II, a potent vasoconstrictor. This stimulation of the renin-angiotensin mechanism and resulting vasoconstriction indirectly lead to the release of aldosterone from the adrenal cortex, which promotes the retention of sodium and water. The increased concentration of sodium in the blood then stimulates the release of antidiuretic hormone (ADH) by the pituitary gland. ADH causes the kidneys to retain water further in an effort to raise blood volume and blood pressure. These secondary regulatory mechanisms may take hours or days to respond to changes in blood pressure.

To summarize, adequate blood volume, an effective cardiac pump, and an effective vasculature are necessary to maintain blood pressure and tissue perfusion. When one of the three components of this system begins to fail, the body is able to compensate through increased work by the other two (Fig. 15-2). When compensatory mechanisms can no longer compensate for the failed system, body tissues are inadequately perfused, and shock occurs. Without prompt intervention, shock progresses, resulting in organ dysfunction, organ failure, and death.

Stages of Shock

Some think of the shock syndrome as a continuum along which the patient struggles to survive. A convenient way to understand the physiologic responses and subsequent clinical signs and symptoms is to divide the continuum into separate stages: compensatory, progressive, and irreversible. (Although some authorities identify an initial stage of shock, changes attributed to this stage occur at the cellular level and are generally not detectable clinically.) The earlier that medical management and nursing interventions can be initiated along this continuum, the greater the patient's chance of survival.

Physiology/Pathophysiology

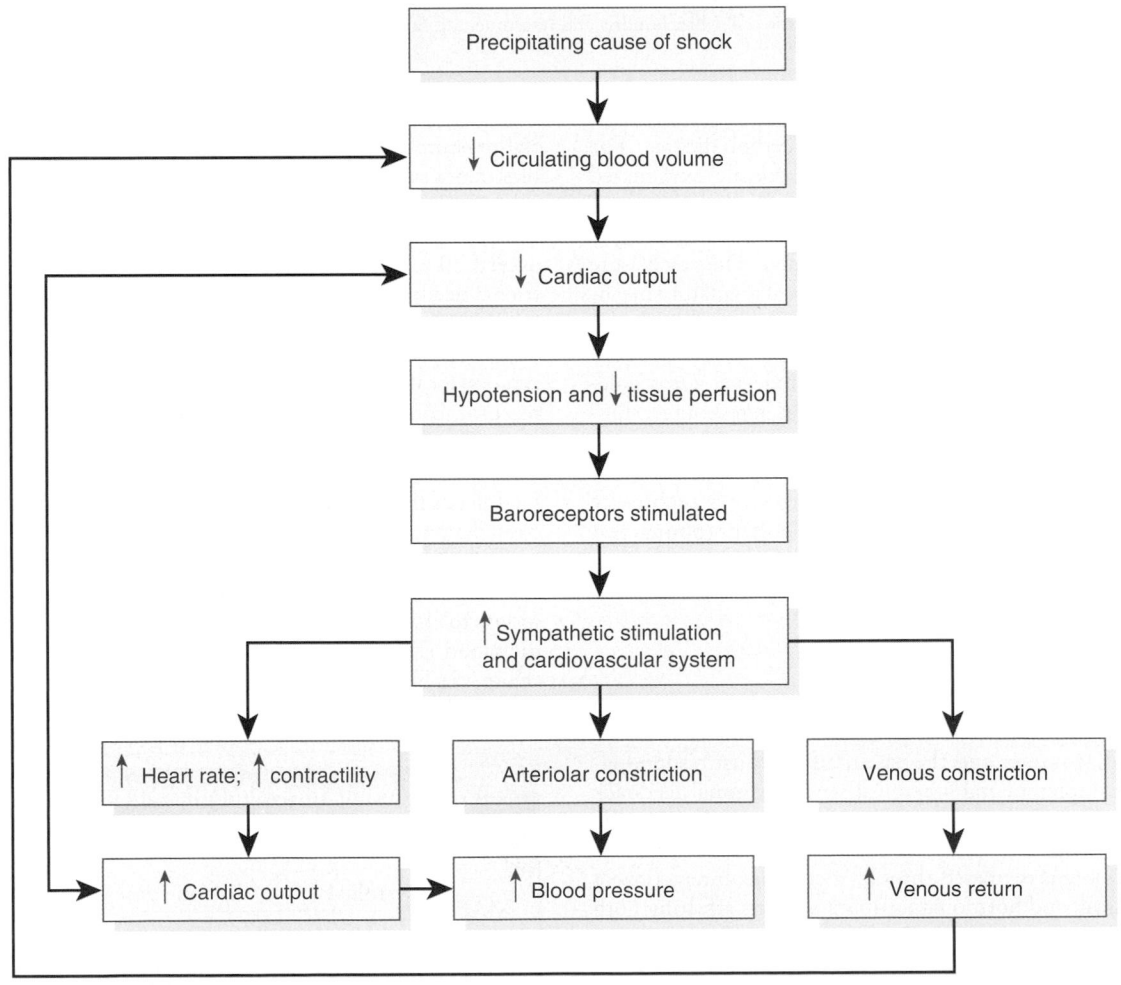

FIGURE 15-2 Compensatory mechanisms for the restoration of circulatory blood volume in shock. Adapted with permission from Jones, K. (1996). Shock. In J. M. Clochesy, C. Breu, et al. (Eds.). *Critical care nursing* (2nd ed.). Philadelphia: W. B. Saunders Company.

COMPENSATORY STAGE

In the compensatory stage of shock, the patient's blood pressure remains within normal limits. Vasoconstriction, increased heart rate, and increased contractility of the heart contribute to maintaining adequate cardiac output. This results from stimulation of the sympathetic nervous system and subsequent release of catecholamines (epinephrine and norepinephrine). The patient displays the often-described "fight or flight" response. The body shunts blood from organs such as the skin, kidneys, and gastrointestinal tract to the brain and heart to ensure adequate blood supply to these vital organs. As a result, the patient's skin is cold and clammy, bowel sounds are hypoactive, and urine output decreases in response to the release of aldosterone and ADH.

Clinical Manifestations

Despite a normal blood pressure, the patient shows numerous clinical signs indicating inadequate organ perfusion (Chart 15-2). The result of inadequate perfusion is anaerobic metabolism and a buildup of lactic acid, producing metabolic acidosis. The respiratory rate increases in response to metabolic acidosis. This rapid respiratory rate facilitates removal of excess carbon dioxide but raises the blood pH and often causes a compensatory respiratory alkalosis. The alkalotic state causes mental status changes, such as confusion or combativeness, as well as arteriolar dilation. If treatment begins in this stage of shock, the prognosis for the patient is good.

Medical Management

Medical treatment is directed toward identifying the cause of the shock, correcting the underlying disorder so that shock does not progress, and supporting those physiologic processes that thus far have responded successfully to the threat. Because compensation cannot be effectively maintained indefinitely, measures such as fluid replacement and medication therapy must be initiated to maintain an adequate blood pressure and reestablish and maintain adequate tissue perfusion.

Nursing Management

Early intervention along the continuum of shock is the key to improving the patient's prognosis. Therefore, the nurse needs to assess systematically those patients at risk for shock to recognize the subtle clinical signs of the compensatory stage before the patient's blood pressure drops.

MONITORING TISSUE PERFUSION

In assessing tissue perfusion, the nurse observes for changes in level of consciousness, vital signs (including pulse pressure), urinary output, skin, and laboratory values. In the compensatory stage of shock, serum sodium and blood glucose levels are elevated in response to the release of aldosterone and catecholamines.

The role of the nurse at the compensatory stage of shock is to monitor the patient's hemodynamic status and promptly report deviations to the physician, assist in identifying and treating the underlying disorder by continuous in-depth assessment of the patient, administer prescribed fluids and medications, and promote patient safety. Vital signs are key indicators of the patient's hemodynamic status; however, blood pressure is an indirect method of monitoring tissue hypoxia. Pulse pressure correlates well to stroke volume, the amount of blood ejected from the heart with systole. Pulse pressure is calculated by subtracting the diastolic measurement from the systolic measurement; the difference is the pulse pressure. Normally, the pulse pressure is 30 to 40 mm Hg (Mikhail, 1999). Narrowing or decreased pulse pressure is an earlier indicator of shock than a drop in systolic blood pressure. Decreased or narrowing pulse pressure, an early indication of decreased stroke volume, is illustrated in the following example:

Systolic blood pressure − diastolic blood pressure = pulse pressure

Normal pulse pressure:
Systolic BP **Diastolic BP** **Pulse Pressure**
120 mg Hg − 80 mm Hg = 40 mm Hg

Narrowing of pulse pressure:
Systolic BP **Diastolic BP** **Pulse Pressure**
90 mm Hg − 70 mm Hg = 20 mm Hg

Elevation in the diastolic blood pressure with release of catecholamines and attempts to increase venous return through vasoconstriction is an early compensatory mechanism in response to decreased stroke volume, blood pressure, and overall cardiac output.

NURSING ALERT By the time blood pressure drops, damage has already been occurring on the cellular and tissue levels. Therefore, the patient at risk for shock must be assessed and monitored closely before the blood pressure falls.

Although treatments are prescribed and initiated by the physician, the nurse usually implements them, operates and troubleshoots equipment used in treatment, monitors the patient's status during treatment, and assesses the immediate effects of treatment. Additionally, the nurse assesses the response of the patient and the family to the crisis and to treatment.

Chart 15-2 • ASSESSMENT
Clinical Findings in Stages of Shock

Finding	Compensatory	Progressive	Irreversible
Blood pressure	Normal	Systolic <80–90 mm Hg	Requires mechanical or pharmacologic support
Heart rate	>100 bpm	>150 bpm	Erratic or asystole
Respiratory status	>20 breaths/min	Rapid, shallow respirations; crackles	Requires intubation
Skin	Cold, clammy	Mottled, petechiae	Jaundice
Urinary output	Decreased	0.5 mL/kg/hr	Anuric, requires dialysis
Mentation	Confusion	Lethargy	Unconscious
Acid–base balance	Respiratory alkalosis	Metabolic acidosis	Profound acidosis

REDUCING ANXIETY

While experiencing a major threat to health and well-being and being the focus of attention of many health care providers, the patient often becomes anxious and apprehensive. Providing brief explanations about the diagnostic and treatment procedures, supporting the patient during those procedures, and providing information about their outcomes are usually effective in reducing stress and anxiety and thus promoting the patient's physical and mental well-being.

PROMOTING SAFETY

Another nursing intervention is monitoring potential threats to the patient's safety, because a high anxiety level and altered mental status typically impair a person's judgment. In this stage, patients who were previously cooperative and followed instructions may now disrupt intravenous lines and catheters and complicate their condition. Therefore, close monitoring is essential.

PROGRESSIVE STAGE

In the progressive stage of shock, the mechanisms that regulate blood pressure can no longer compensate and the MAP falls below normal limits, with an average systolic blood pressure of less than 90 mm Hg (Abraham et al., 2000).

Pathophysiology

Although all organ systems suffer from hypoperfusion at this stage, two events perpetuate the shock syndrome. First, the overworked heart becomes dysfunctional; the body's inability to meet increased oxygen requirements produces ischemia; and biochemical mediators cause myocardial depression (Kumar, Haery & Parrillo, 2000; Price, Anning, Mitchell et al., 1999). This leads to failure of the cardiac pump, even if the underlying cause of the shock is not of cardiac origin. Second, the autoregulatory function of the microcirculation fails in response to numerous biochemical mediators released by the cells, resulting in increased capillary permeability, with areas of arteriolar and venous constriction further compromising cellular perfusion. At this stage, the patient's prognosis worsens. The relaxation of precapillary sphincters causes fluid to leak from the capillaries, creating interstitial edema and return of less fluid to the heart. Even if the underlying cause of the shock is reversed, the breakdown of the circulatory system itself perpetuates the shock state, and a vicious circle ensues.

Assessment and Diagnostic Findings

Chances of survival depend on the patient's general health before the shock state as well as the amount of time it takes to restore tissue perfusion. As shock progresses, organ systems decompensate.

RESPIRATORY EFFECTS

The lungs, which become compromised early in shock, are affected at this stage. Subsequent decompensation of the lungs increases the likelihood that mechanical ventilation will be needed if shock progresses. Respirations are rapid and shallow. Crackles are heard over the lung fields. Decreased pulmonary blood flow causes arterial oxygen levels to decrease and carbon dioxide levels to increase. Hypoxemia and biochemical mediators cause an intense inflammatory response and pulmonary vasoconstriction, perpetuating the pulmonary capillary hypoperfusion and hypoxemia. The hypoperfused alveoli stop producing surfactant and

subsequently collapse. Pulmonary capillaries begin to leak their contents, causing pulmonary edema, diffusion abnormalities (shunting), and additional alveolar collapse. Interstitial inflammation and fibrosis are common as the pulmonary damage progresses (Fein & Calalang-Colucci, 2000). This condition is sometimes referred to as acute respiratory distress syndrome (ARDS), acute lung injury (ALI), shock lung, or noncardiogenic pulmonary edema. Further explanation of ARDS, as well as its nursing management, can be found in Chapter 23.

CARDIOVASCULAR EFFECTS

A lack of adequate blood supply leads to dysrhythmias and ischemia. The patient has a rapid heart rate, sometimes exceeding 150 bpm. The patient may complain of chest pain and even suffer a myocardial infarction. Cardiac enzyme levels (eg, lactate dehydrogenase, CPK-MB, and cTn-I) rise. In addition, myocardial depression and ventricular dilation may further impair the heart's ability to pump enough blood to the tissues to meet oxygen requirements.

NEUROLOGIC EFFECTS

As blood flow to the brain becomes impaired, the patient's mental status deteriorates. Changes in mental status occur as a result of decreased cerebral perfusion and hypoxia; the patient may initially exhibit confusion or a subtle change in behavior. Subsequently, lethargy increases and the patient begins to lose consciousness. The pupils dilate and are only sluggishly reactive to light.

RENAL EFFECTS

When the MAP falls below 80 mm Hg (Guyton & Hall, 2000), the glomerular filtration rate of the kidneys cannot be maintained, and drastic changes in renal function occur. Acute renal failure (ARF) can develop. ARF is characterized by an increase in blood urea nitrogen (BUN) and serum creatinine levels, fluid and electrolyte shifts, acid–base imbalances, and a loss of the renal-hormonal regulation of blood pressure. Urinary output usually decreases to below 0.5/mL/kg per hour (or below 30 mL per hour) but can be variable depending on the phase of ARF. For further information about ARF, see Chapter 45.

HEPATIC EFFECTS

Decreased blood flow to the liver impairs the liver cells' ability to perform metabolic and phagocytic functions. Consequently, the patient is less able to metabolize medications and metabolic waste products, such as ammonia and lactic acid. The patient becomes more susceptible to infection as the liver fails to filter bacteria from the blood. Liver enzymes (aspartate aminotransferase [AST], formerly serum glutamic-oxaloacetic transaminase [SGOT]; alanine aminotransferase [ALT], formerly serum glutamate pyruvate transaminase [SGPT]; lactate dehydrogenase) and bilirubin levels are elevated, and the patient appears jaundiced.

GASTROINTESTINAL EFFECTS

Gastrointestinal ischemia can cause stress ulcers in the stomach, placing the patient at risk for gastrointestinal bleeding. In the small intestine, the mucosa can become necrotic and slough off, causing bloody diarrhea. Beyond the local effects of impaired perfusion, gastrointestinal ischemia leads to bacterial toxin translocation, in which bacterial toxins enter the bloodstream through the lymph system. In addition to causing infection, bacterial toxins can cause cardiac depression, vasodilation, increased capillary permeability, and an intense inflammatory response with activation of additional biochemical mediators. The net result is interference with healthy cells and their ability to metabolize nutrients (Balk, 2000b; Jindal et al., 2000).

HEMATOLOGIC EFFECTS

The combination of hypotension, sluggish blood flow, metabolic acidosis, and generalized hypoxemia can interfere with normal hemostatic mechanisms. Disseminated intravascular coagulation (DIC) can occur either as a cause or as a complication of shock. In this condition, widespread clotting and bleeding occur simultaneously. Bruises (ecchymoses) and bleeding (petechiae) may appear in the skin. Coagulation times (prothrombin time, partial thromboplastin time) are prolonged. Clotting factors and platelets are consumed and require replacement therapy to achieve hemostasis. Further discussion of disseminated intravascular coagulation appears in Chapter 33.

Medical Management

Specific medical management in the progressive stage of shock depends on the type of shock and its underlying cause. It is also based on the degree of decompensation in the organ systems. Medical management specific to each type of shock is discussed in later sections of this chapter. Although there are several differences in medical management by type of shock, some medical interventions are common to all types. These include use of appropriate intravenous fluids and medications to restore tissue perfusion by (1) optimizing intravascular volume, (2) supporting the pumping action of the heart, and (3) improving the competence of the vascular system. Other aspects of management may include early enteral nutritional support and use of antacids, histamine-2 blockers, or antipeptic agents to reduce the risk of gastrointestinal ulceration and bleeding.

Nursing Management

Nursing care of the patient in the progressive stage of shock requires expertise in assessing and understanding shock and the significance of changes in assessment data. The patient in the progressive stage of shock is often cared for in the intensive care setting to facilitate close monitoring (hemodynamic monitoring, electrocardiographic monitoring, arterial blood gases, serum electrolyte levels, physical and mental status changes), rapid and frequent administration of various prescribed medications and fluids, and possibly intervention with supportive technologies, such as mechanical ventilation, dialysis, and intra-aortic balloon pump.

Working closely with other members of the health care team, the nurse carefully documents treatments, medications, and fluids that are administered by members of the team, recording the time, dosage or volume, and the patient's response. Additionally, the nurse coordinates both the scheduling of diagnostic procedures that may be carried out at the bedside and the flow of health care personnel involved in the patient's care.

PREVENTING COMPLICATIONS

If supportive technologies are used, the nurse helps reduce the risk of related complications and monitors the patient for early signs of complications. Monitoring includes evaluating blood levels of medications, observing invasive vascular lines for signs of infection, and checking neurovascular status if arterial lines are inserted, especially in the lower extremities. Simultaneously, the nurse promotes the patient's safety and comfort by ensuring that all procedures, including invasive procedures and arterial and venous punctures, are carried out using correct aseptic techniques and that venous and arterial puncture and infusion sites are maintained with the goal of preventing infection. Positioning and repositioning the patient to promote comfort, prevent pulmonary complications, and maintain skin integrity are integral to caring for the patient in shock.

PROMOTING REST AND COMFORT

Efforts are made to minimize the cardiac workload by reducing the patient's physical activity and fear or anxiety. Promoting rest and comfort is a priority in the patient's care. To ensure that the patient gets as much uninterrupted rest as possible, the nurse performs only essential nursing activities. To conserve the patient's energy, the nurse protects the patient from temperature extremes (excessive warmth or shivering cold), which can increase the metabolic rate and subsequently the cardiac workload. The patient should not be warmed too quickly, and warming blankets should not be applied because they can cause vasodilation and a subsequent drop in blood pressure.

SUPPORTING FAMILY MEMBERS

Because the patient in shock is the object of intense attention by the health care team, the family members may feel neglected; however, they may be reluctant to ask questions or seek information for fear that they will be in the way or will interfere with the attention given to the patient. The nurse should make sure that the family is comfortably situated and kept informed about the patient's status. Often, family members need advice from the health care team to get some rest; they are more likely to take this advice if they feel that the patient is being well cared for and that they will be notified of any significant changes in the patient's status. A visit from the hospital chaplain may be comforting to the family and provides some attention to the family while the nurse concentrates on the patient.

IRREVERSIBLE STAGE

The irreversible (or refractory) stage of shock represents the point along the shock continuum at which organ damage is so severe that the patient does not respond to treatment and cannot survive. Despite treatment, blood pressure remains low. Complete renal and liver failure, compounded by the release of necrotic tissue toxins, creates an overwhelming metabolic acidosis. Anaerobic metabolism contributes to a worsening lactic acidosis. Reserves of ATP are almost totally depleted, and mechanisms for storing new supplies of energy have been destroyed. Multiple organ dysfunction progressing to complete organ failure has occurred, and death is imminent. Multiple organ dysfunction can occur as a progression along the shock continuum or as a syndrome unto itself and is further described later in this chapter.

Medical Management

Medical management during the irreversible stage of shock is usually the same as for the progressive stage. Although the patient's condition may have progressed from the progressive to the irreversible stage, the judgment that the shock is irreversible can be made only retrospectively on the basis of the patient's failure to respond to treatment. Strategies that may be experimental (ie, investigational medications, such as antibiotic agents and immunomodulation therapy) may be tried to reduce or reverse the severity of shock.

Nursing Management

As in the progressive stage of shock, the nurse focuses on carrying out prescribed treatments, monitoring the patient, preventing complications, protecting the patient from injury, and providing comfort. Offering brief explanations to the patient about what is happening is essential even if there is no certainty that the patient hears or understands what is being said.

As it becomes obvious that the patient is unlikely to survive, the family needs to be informed about the prognosis and likely outcomes. Opportunities should be provided, throughout the patient's care, for the family to see, touch, and talk to the patient. A close family friend or spiritual advisor may be of comfort to the family in dealing with the inevitable death of the patient. Whenever possible and appropriate, the family should be approached regarding any living will, advance directive, or other written or verbal wishes the patient may have shared in the event that he or she cannot participate in end-of-life decisions. In some cases, ethics committees may assist the family and health care team in making difficult decisions.

During this stage of shock, families may misinterpret the actions of the health care team. They have been told that nothing has been effective in reversing the shock and that the patient's survival is very unlikely, yet the health care team continues to work feverishly on the patient. A distraught, grieving family may interpret this as a chance for recovery when none exists. As a result, family members may become angry when the patient dies. Conferences with all members of the health care team and the family will promote better understanding by the family of the patient's prognosis and the purpose for the measures being taken. During these conferences, it is essential to explain that the equipment and treatments being provided are for the patient's comfort and do not suggest that the patient will recover. Families should be encouraged to express their wishes concerning the use of life-support measures.

Overall Management Strategies in Shock

As described previously and in the discussion of types of shock to follow, management in all types and all phases of shock includes the following:

- Fluid replacement to restore intravascular volume
- Vasoactive medications to restore vasomotor tone and improve cardiac function
- Nutritional support to address the metabolic requirements that are often dramatically increased in shock

Therapies described in this section require collaboration among all members of the health care team to ensure that the manifestations of shock are quickly identified and that adequate and timely treatment is instituted to achieve the best outcome possible.

FLUID REPLACEMENT

Fluid replacement is administered in all types of shock. The type of fluids administered and the speed of delivery vary, but fluids are given to improve cardiac and tissue oxygenation, which in part depends on flow. The fluids administered may include **crystalloids** (electrolyte solutions that move freely between intravascular and interstitial spaces), **colloids** (large-molecule intravenous solutions), or blood components.

Crystalloid and Colloid Solutions

The best fluid to treat shock remains controversial. In emergencies, the "best" fluid is often the fluid that is readily available. Both crystalloids and colloids, as described later, can be given to restore intravascular volume. Blood component therapy is used most frequently in hypovolemic shock.

Crystalloids are electrolyte solutions that move freely between the intravascular compartment and the interstitial spaces. Isotonic crystalloid solutions are often selected because they contain the same concentration of electrolytes as the extracellular fluid and therefore can be given without altering the concentrations of electrolytes in the plasma.

Common intravenous fluids used for resuscitation in hypovolemic shock include 0.9% sodium chloride solution (normal saline) and lactated Ringer's solution (Choi et al., 1999). Ringer's lactate is an electrolyte solution containing the lactate ion, which should not be confused with lactic acid. The lactate ion is converted to bicarbonate, which helps to buffer the overall acidosis that occurs in shock.

A disadvantage of using isotonic crystalloid solutions is that three parts of the volume are lost to the interstitial compartment for every one part that remains in the intravascular compartment. This occurs in response to mechanisms that store extracellular body fluid. Diffusion of crystalloids into the interstitial space necessitates that more fluid be administered than the amount lost (Choi et al., 1999).

Care must be taken when rapidly administering isotonic crystalloids to avoid causing excessive edema, particularly pulmonary edema. For this reason, and depending on the cause of the hypovolemia, a hypertonic crystalloid solution, such as 3% sodium chloride, is sometimes administered in hypovolemic shock. Hypertonic solutions produce a large osmotic force that pulls fluid from the intracellular space to the extracellular space to achieve a fluid balance (Choi et al., 1999; Fein & Calalang-Colucci, 2000). The osmotic effect of hypertonic solutions results in fewer fluids being administered to restore intravascular volume. Complications associated with use of hypertonic saline solution include excessive serum osmolality, hypernatremia, hypokalemia, and altered thermoregulation.

Generally, intravenous colloidal solutions are considered to be plasma proteins, which are molecules that are too large to pass through capillary membranes. Colloids expand intravascular volume by exerting oncotic pressure, thereby pulling fluid into the intravascular space. Colloidal solutions have the same effect as hypertonic solutions in increasing intravascular volume, but less volume of fluid is required than with crystalloids. Additionally, colloids have a longer duration of action than crystalloids because the molecules remain within the intravascular compartment longer.

An albumin solution is commonly used to treat hypovolemic shock. Albumin is a plasma protein; an albumin solution is prepared from human plasma and is heated to reduce its potential to transmit disease. The disadvantages of albumin are its high cost and limited availability, which depends on blood donors. Synthetic colloid preparations, such as hetastarch and dextran solution, are now widely used. Dextran, however, may interfere with platelet aggregation and therefore is not indicated if hemorrhage is the cause of the hypovolemic shock or if the patient has a coagulation disorder (coagulopathy).

 **NURSING ALERT** With all colloidal solutions, side effects include the rare occurrence of anaphylactic reactions, for which the nurse must monitor the patient closely.

Complications of Fluid Administration

Close monitoring of the patient during fluid replacement is necessary to identify side effects and complications. The most common and serious side effects of fluid replacement are cardiovascular overload and pulmonary edema.

Patients receiving fluid replacement must be monitored frequently for adequate urinary output, changes in mental status, skin perfusion, and changes in vital signs. Lung sounds are auscultated frequently to detect signs of fluid accumulation. Adventitious lung sounds, such as crackles, may indicate pulmonary edema.

Often a right atrial pressure line (also known as a central venous pressure line) is inserted. In addition to physical assessment, the right atrial pressure value helps in monitoring the patient's response to fluid replacement. A normal right atrial pressure value is 4 to 12 mm Hg or cm H_2O. Several readings are obtained to determine a range, and fluid replacement is continued to achieve a pressure within normal limits. Hemodynamic monitoring with arterial and pulmonary artery lines may be implemented to allow close monitoring of the patient's perfusion and cardiac status as well as response to therapy.

VASOACTIVE MEDICATION THERAPY

Vasoactive medications are administered in all forms of shock to improve the patient's hemodynamic stability when fluid therapy alone cannot maintain adequate MAP. Specific medications are selected to correct the particular hemodynamic alteration that is impeding cardiac output. Specific vasoactive medications are prescribed for the patient in shock because they can support the patient's hemodynamic status. These medications help to increase the strength of myocardial contractility, regulate the heart rate, reduce myocardial resistance, and initiate vasoconstriction.

Vasoactive medications are selected for their action on receptors of the sympathetic nervous system. These receptors are known as alpha-adrenergic and beta-adrenergic receptors. Beta-adrenergic receptors are further classified as beta$_1$- and beta$_2$-adrenergic receptors. When alpha-adrenergic receptors are stimulated, blood vessels constrict in the cardiorespiratory and gastrointestinal systems, skin, and kidneys. When beta$_1$-adrenergic receptors are stimulated, heart rate and myocardial contraction increase. When beta$_2$-adrenergic receptors are stimulated, vasodilation occurs in the heart and skeletal muscles, and the bronchioles relax. The medications used in treating shock consist of various combinations of vasoactive medications to maximize tissue perfusion by stimulating or blocking the alpha- and beta-adrenergic receptors.

When vasoactive medications are administered, vital signs must be monitored frequently (at least every 15 minutes until stable, or more often if indicated). Vasoactive medications should be administered through a central venous line because infiltration and extravasation of some vasoactive medications can cause tissue necrosis and sloughing. An intravenous pump or controller should be used to ensure that the medications are delivered safely and accurately.

Individual medication dosages are usually titrated by the nurse, who adjusts the intravenous drip rates based on the physician's prescription and the patient's response. Dosages are changed to maintain the MAP (usually above 80 mm Hg) at a physiologic level that ensures adequate tissue perfusion.

> **NURSING ALERT** Vasoactive medications should never be stopped abruptly because this could cause severe hemodynamic instability, perpetuating the shock state.

Dosages of vasoactive medications should be tapered and the patient should be weaned from the medication with frequent monitoring (every 15 minutes) of blood pressure. Table 15-1 presents some of the commonly prescribed vasoactive medications used in treating shock.

NUTRITIONAL SUPPORT

Nutritional support is an important aspect of care for the patient with shock. Increased metabolic rates during shock increase energy requirements and therefore caloric requirements. The patient in shock requires more than 3,000 calories daily.

The release of catecholamines early in the shock continuum causes glycogen stores to be depleted in about 8 to 10 hours. Nutritional energy requirements are then met by breaking down lean body mass. In this catabolic process, skeletal muscle mass is broken down even when the patient has large stores of fat or adipose tissue. Loss of skeletal muscle can greatly prolong the recovery

Table 15-1 • Vasoactive Agents Used in Treating Shock

MEDICATION	DESIRED ACTION IN SHOCK	DISADVANTAGES
Sympathomimetics Amrinone (Inocor) Dobutamine (Dobutrex) Dopamine (Intropin) Epinephrine (Adrenalin) Milrinone (Primacor)	Improve contractility, increase stroke volume, increase cardiac output	Increase oxygen demand of the heart
Vasodilators Nitroglycerine (Tridil) Nitroprusside (Nipride)	Reduce preload and afterload, reduce oxygen demand of heart	Cause hypotension
Vasoconstrictors Norepinephrine (Levophed) Phenylephrine (Neo-Synephrine) Vasopressin (Pitressin)	Increase blood pressure by vasoconstriction	Increase afterload, thereby increasing cardiac workload; compromise perfusion to skin, kidneys, lungs, GI tract

time for the patient in shock. Parenteral or enteral nutritional support should be initiated as soon as possible, with some form of enteral nutrition always being administered. The integrity of the gastrointestinal system depends on direct exposure to nutrients. Additionally, glutamine (an essential amino acid during stress) is important in the immunologic function of the gastrointestinal tract, providing a fuel source for lymphocytes and macrophages. Glutamine can be administered through enteral nutrition (Rauen & Munro, 1998).

Stress ulcers occur frequently in acutely ill patients because of the compromised blood supply to the gastrointestinal tract. Therefore, antacids, histamine-2 blockers (eg, famotidine [Pepcid], ranitidine [Zantac]), and antipeptic agents (eg, sucralfate [Carafate]) are prescribed to prevent ulcer formation by inhibiting gastric acid secretion or increasing gastric pH.

Hypovolemic Shock

In addition to caring for the patient through different stages of shock, the nurse needs to tailor interventions to the type of shock, whether it is hypovolemic, cardiogenic, or circulatory shock.

Hypovolemic shock, the most common type of shock, is characterized by a decreased intravascular volume. Body fluid is contained in the intracellular and extracellular compartments. Intracellular fluid accounts for about two thirds of the total body water. The extracellular body fluid is found in one of two compartments: intravascular (inside blood vessels) or interstitial (surrounding tissues). The volume of interstitial fluid is about three to four times that of intravascular fluid. Hypovolemic shock occurs when there is a reduction in intravascular volume of 15% to 25%. This would represent a loss of 750 to 1,300 mL of blood in a 70-kg (154-lb) person.

Pathophysiology

Hypovolemic shock can be caused by external fluid losses, such as traumatic blood loss, or by internal fluid shifts, as in severe dehydration, severe edema, or ascites (Chart 15-3). Intravascular volume can be reduced both by fluid loss and fluid shifting between the intravascular and interstitial compartments.

The sequence of events in hypovolemic shock begins with a decrease in the intravascular volume. This results in decreased venous return of blood to the heart and subsequent decreased ventricular filling. Decreased ventricular filling results in decreased stroke volume (amount of blood ejected from the heart) and decreased cardiac output. When cardiac output drops, blood pressure drops and tissues cannot be adequately perfused (Fig. 15-3).

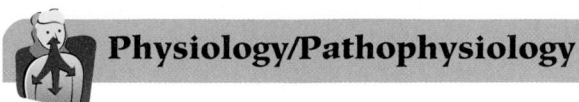

Physiology/Pathophysiology

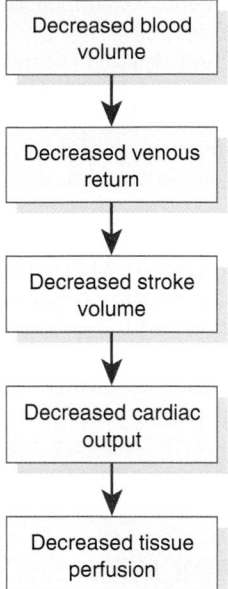

FIGURE 15-3 Pathophysiologic sequence of events in hypovolemic shock.

Medical Management

Major goals in treating hypovolemic shock are to (1) restore intravascular volume to reverse the sequence of events leading to inadequate tissue perfusion, (2) redistribute fluid volume, and (3) correct the underlying cause of the fluid loss as quickly as possible. Depending on the severity of shock and the patient's condition, it is likely that efforts will be made to address all three goals simultaneously.

TREATMENT OF THE UNDERLYING CAUSE

If the patient is hemorrhaging, efforts are made to stop the bleeding. This may involve applying pressure to the bleeding site or surgery to stop internal bleeding. If the cause of the hypovolemia is diarrhea or vomiting, medications to treat diarrhea and vomiting are administered as efforts are made simultaneously to identify and treat the cause. In the elderly patient, dehydration may be the cause of hypovolemic shock.

FLUID AND BLOOD REPLACEMENT

Beyond reversing the primary cause of the decreased intravascular volume, fluid replacement (also referred to as fluid resuscitation) is of primary concern. At least two large-gauge intravenous lines are inserted to establish access for fluid administration. Two intravenous lines allow simultaneous administration of fluid, medications, and blood component therapy if required. Because the goal of the fluid replacement is to restore intravascular volume, it is necessary to administer fluids that will remain in the intravascular compartment and thus avoid creating fluid shifts from the intravascular compartment into the intracellular compartment. Table 15-2 summarizes the fluids commonly used in treating shock.

Chart 15-3
Risk Factors for Hypovolemic Shock

External: Fluid Losses	Internal: Fluid Shifts
Trauma	Hemorrhage
Surgery	Burns
Vomiting	Ascites
Diarrhea	Peritonitis
Diuresis	Dehydration
Diabetes insipidus	

Table 15-2 • **Fluid Replacement in Shock**

FLUIDS	ADVANTAGES	DISADVANTAGES
Crystalloids		
0.9% sodium chloride (normal saline solution)	Widely available, inexpensive	Requires large volume of infusion; can cause pulmonary edema
Lactated Ringer's	Lactate ion helps buffer metabolic acidosis	Requires large volume of infusion; can cause pulmonary edema
Hypertonic saline (3%, 5%, 7.5%)	Small volume needed to restore intra-vascular volume	Danger of hypernatremia
Colloids		
Albumin (5%, 25%)	Rapidly expands plasma volume	Expensive; requires human donors; limited supply; can cause heart failure
Dextran (40, 70)	Synthetic plasma expander	Interferes with platelet aggregation; not recommended for hemorrhagic shock
Hetastarch	Synthetic; less expensive than albumin; effect lasts up to 36 h	Prolongs bleeding and clotting times

Lactated Ringer's and 0.9% sodium chloride solutions are isotonic crystalloid fluids commonly used in treating hypovolemic shock (Jindal et al., 2000). Large amounts of fluid must be administered to restore intravascular volume because isotonic crystalloid solutions move freely between the fluid compartments of the body and do not remain in the vascular system.

Colloids (eg, albumin, hetastarch, and dextran) may also be used. Dextran is not indicated if the cause of the hypovolemic shock is hemorrhage because it interferes with platelet aggregation.

Blood products, also colloids, may need to be administered, particularly when the cause of the hypovolemic shock is hemorrhage. Because of the risk of transmitting bloodborne viruses and the scarcity of blood products, however, these products are used only if other alternatives are unavailable or blood loss is extensive and rapid. Packed red blood cells are administered to replenish the patient's oxygen-carrying capacity in conjunction with other fluids that will expand volume. Current recommendations are to base the need for transfusions on the patient's oxygenation needs, which are determined by vital signs, blood gas values, and clinical appearance rather than using an arbitrary laboratory value. Synthetic forms of blood (ie, compounds capable of carrying oxygen in the same way that blood does) are potential alternatives.

REDISTRIBUTION OF FLUID

In addition to administering fluids to restore intravascular volume, positioning the patient properly assists fluid redistribution. A modified Trendelenburg position (Fig. 15-4) is recommended in hypovolemic shock. Elevating the legs promotes the return of venous blood. Positioning the patient in a full Trendelenburg position, however, makes breathing difficult and therefore is not recommended.

PHARMACOLOGIC THERAPY

If fluid administration fails to reverse hypovolemic shock, then the same medications given in cardiogenic shock are used because unreversed hypovolemic shock progresses to cardiogenic shock (the vicious circle).

If the underlying cause of the hypovolemia is dehydration, medications are also administered to reverse the cause of the dehydration. For example, insulin is administered if dehydration is secondary to hyperglycemia; desmopressin (DDAVP) is administered for diabetes insipidus, antidiarrheal agents for diarrhea, and antiemetic medications for vomiting.

Nursing Management

Primary prevention of shock is an essential focus of nursing intervention. Hypovolemic shock can be prevented in some instances by closely monitoring patients who are at risk for fluid deficits and assisting with fluid replacement before intravascular volume is depleted. In other circumstances, hypovolemic shock cannot be prevented, and nursing care focuses on assisting with treatment targeted at treating its cause and restoring intravascular volume.

General nursing measures include ensuring safe administration of prescribed fluids and medications and documenting their administration and effects. Another important nursing role is monitoring for signs of complications and side effects of treatment and reporting these signs early in treatment.

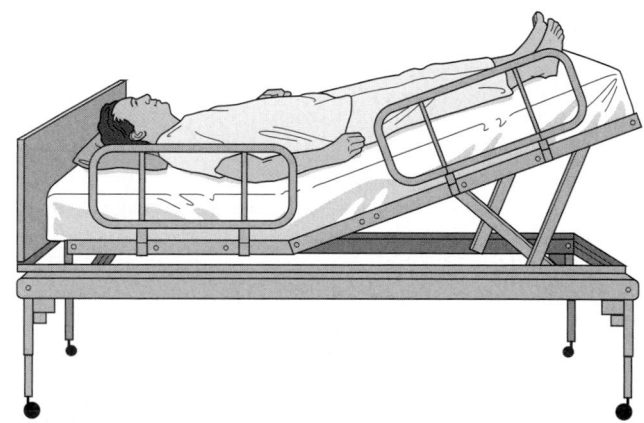

FIGURE 15-4 Proper positioning (modified Trendelenburg) for the patient who shows signs of shock. The lower extremities are elevated to an angle of about 20 degrees; the knees are straight, the trunk is horizontal, and the head is slightly elevated.

ADMINISTERING BLOOD AND FLUIDS SAFELY

Administering blood transfusions safely is a vital nursing role. In emergency situations, it is important to obtain blood specimens quickly to obtain a baseline complete blood count and to type and cross-match the blood in anticipation of blood transfusions. The patient who receives a transfusion of blood products must be monitored closely for adverse effects (see Chap. 33).

Fluid replacement complications can occur, often when large volumes are administered rapidly. Therefore, the nurse monitors the patient closely for cardiovascular overload and pulmonary edema. The risk of these complications is increased in the elderly and in patients with pre-existing cardiac disease. Hemodynamic pressure, vital signs, arterial blood gases, hemoglobin and hematocrit levels, and fluid intake and output are among the parameters monitored. The patient's temperature should also be monitored closely to ensure that rapid fluid resuscitation does not precipitate hypothermia. Intravenous fluids may need to be warmed during the administration of large volumes. Physical assessment focuses on observing the jugular veins for distention and monitoring jugular venous pressure. Jugular venous pressure is low in hypovolemic shock; it increases with effective treatment and is significantly increased with fluid overload and heart failure. The nurse needs to monitor cardiac and respiratory status closely and report changes in blood pressure, pulse pressure, heart rate, rhythm, and lung sounds to the physician.

IMPLEMENTING OTHER MEASURES

Oxygen is administered to increase the amount of oxygen carried by available hemoglobin in the blood. A patient who is confused may feel apprehensive with an oxygen mask or cannula in place, and frequent explanations about the need for the mask may reduce some of the patient's fear and anxiety. Simultaneously, the nurse must direct efforts to the safety and comfort of the patient.

Cardiogenic Shock

Cardiogenic shock occurs when the heart's ability to contract and to pump blood is impaired and the supply of oxygen is inadequate for the heart and tissues. The causes of cardiogenic shock are known as either coronary or noncoronary. Coronary cardiogenic shock is more common than noncoronary cardiogenic shock and is seen most often in patients with myocardial infarction. Coronary cardiogenic shock occurs when a significant amount of the left ventricular myocardium has been destroyed (Price et al., 1999). Patients experiencing an anterior wall myocardial infarction are at the greatest risk for developing cardiogenic shock because of the potentially extensive damage to the left ventricle caused by occlusion of the left anterior descending coronary artery (Chart 15-4). Non-coronary causes can be related to

severe metabolic problems (severe hypoxemia, acidosis, hypoglycemia, and hypocalcemia) and tension pneumothorax.

Pathophysiology

In cardiogenic shock, cardiac output, which is a function of both stroke volume and heart rate, is compromised. When stroke volume and heart rate decrease or become erratic, blood pressure drops and tissue perfusion is compromised. Along with other tissues and organs being deprived of adequate blood supply, the heart muscle itself receives inadequate blood. The result is impaired tissue perfusion. Because impaired tissue perfusion weakens the heart and impairs its ability to pump blood forward, the ventricle does not fully eject its volume of blood at systole. As a result, fluid accumulates in the lungs. This sequence of events can occur rapidly or over a period of days (Fig. 15-5).

Clinical Manifestations

Patients in cardiogenic shock may experience angina pain and develop dysrhythmias and hemodynamic instability.

Medical Management

The goals of medical management are to (1) limit further myocardial damage and preserve the healthy myocardium and (2) improve the cardiac function by increasing cardiac contractility, decreasing ventricular afterload, or both (Price et al., 1999). In general, these goals are achieved by increasing oxygen supply to the heart muscle while reducing oxygen demands.

CORRECTION OF UNDERLYING CAUSES

As with all forms of shock, the underlying cause of cardiogenic shock must be corrected. It is necessary first to treat the oxygenation needs of the heart muscle to ensure its continued ability to pump blood to other organs. In the case of coronary cardiogenic shock, the patient may require thrombolytic therapy, angioplasty, or coronary artery bypass graft surgery. In the case of noncoronary cardiogenic shock, the patient may require a cardiac valve replacement or correction of a dysrhythmia. For further explanation of these procedures, refer to Chapters 27 and 28.

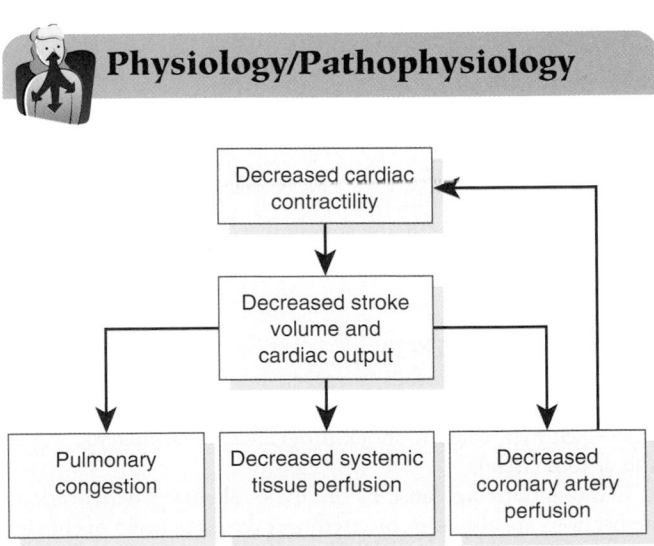

Physiology/Pathophysiology

FIGURE 15-5 Pathophysiologic sequence of events in cardiogenic shock.

Chart 15-4
Risk Factors for Cardiogenic Shock

Coronary Factors	Non-coronary Factors
Myocardial infarction	Cardiomyopathies
	Valvular damage
	Cardiac tamponade
	Dysrhythmias

INITIATION OF FIRST-LINE TREATMENT

First-line treatment of cardiogenic shock involves the following actions:

- Supplying supplemental oxygen
- Controlling chest pain
- Providing selected fluid support
- Administering vasoactive medications
- Controlling heart rate with medication or by implementation of a transthoracic or intravenous pacemaker
- Implementing mechanical cardiac support (intra-aortic balloon counterpulsation therapy, ventricular assist systems, or extracorporeal cardiopulmonary bypass)

Oxygenation. In the early stages of shock, supplemental oxygen is administered by nasal cannula at a rate of 2 to 6 L/min to achieve an oxygen saturation exceeding 90%. Monitoring arterial blood gas values and pulse oximetry values helps to indicate whether the patient requires a more aggressive method of oxygen delivery.

Pain Control. If the patient experiences chest pain, morphine sulfate is administered intravenously for pain relief. In addition to relieving pain, morphine dilates the blood vessels. This reduces the workload of the heart by both decreasing the cardiac filling pressure (preload) and reducing the pressure against which the heart muscle has to eject blood (afterload). Morphine also relieves the patient's anxiety. Cardiac enzyme (CPK-MB and cTn-I) levels are measured, and serial 12-lead electrocardiograms are obtained to assess the degree of myocardial damage.

Hemodynamic Monitoring. Hemodynamic monitoring is initiated to assess the patient's response to treatment. In many institutions, this is performed in the intensive care unit, where an arterial line can be inserted. The arterial line enables accurate and continuous monitoring of blood pressure and provides a port from which to obtain frequent arterial blood samples without having to perform repeated arterial punctures. A multilumen pulmonary artery catheter is inserted to allow measurement of the pulmonary artery pressures, myocardial filling pressures, cardiac output, and pulmonary and systemic resistance. For more information, see Chapter 30.

PHARMACOLOGIC THERAPY

Vasoactive medication therapy consists of multiple pharmacologic strategies to restore and maintain adequate cardiac output. In coronary cardiogenic shock, the aims of vasoactive medication therapy are improved cardiac contractility, decreased preload and afterload, or stable heart rate.

Because improving contractility and decreasing cardiac workload are opposing pharmacologic actions, two classifications of medications may be administered in combination: sympathomimetic agents and vasodilators. Sympathomimetic medications increase cardiac output by mimicking the action of the sympathetic nervous system through vasoconstriction, resulting in increased preload, and by increasing myocardial contractility (inotropic action) or increasing the heart rate (chronotropic action). Vasodilators are used to decrease preload and afterload, thus reducing the workload of the heart and the oxygen demand. Medications commonly combined to treat cardiogenic shock include dobutamine, dopamine, and nitroglycerin (see Table 15-1).

Dobutamine. Dobutamine (Dobutrex) produces inotropic effects by stimulating myocardial beta receptors, increasing the strength of myocardial activity and improving cardiac output. Myocardial alpha-adrenergic receptors are also stimulated, resulting in decreased pulmonary and systemic vascular resistance (decreased afterload). Dobutamine enhances the strength of cardiac contraction, improving stroke volume ejection and overall cardiac output (Jindal et al., 2000; Price et al., 1999).

Nitroglycerin. Intravenous nitroglycerin (Tridil) in low doses acts as a venous vasodilator and therefore reduces preload. At higher doses, nitroglycerin causes arterial vasodilation and therefore reduces afterload as well. These actions, in combination with medium-dose dopamine, increase cardiac output while minimizing cardiac workload. Additionally, vasodilation enhances blood flow to the myocardium, improving oxygen delivery to the weakened heart muscle (Price et al., 1999).

Dopamine. Dopamine (Intropin) is a sympathomimetic agent that has varying vasoactive effects depending on the dosage. It may be used with dobutamine and nitroglycerine to improve tissue perfusion. Low-dose dopamine (0.5 to 3.0 μg/kg/min) increases renal and mesenteric blood flow, thereby preventing ischemia of these organs because shock causes blood to be shunted away from the kidneys and the mesentery. This dosage, however, does not improve cardiac output. Medium-dose dopamine (4 to 8 μg/kg/min) has sympathomimetic properties and improves contractility (inotropic action) and slightly increases the heart rate (chronotropic action). At this dosage, dopamine increases cardiac output and therefore is desirable. High-dose dopamine (8 to 10 μg/kg/min) predominantly causes vasoconstriction, which increases afterload and thus increases cardiac workload. Because this effect is undesirable in patients with cardiogenic shock, dopamine dosages must be carefully titrated. Once the patient's blood pressure stabilizes, low-dose dopamine may be continued for its effect of promoting renal perfusion in particular. In severe metabolic acidosis, which occurs in the later stages of shock, dopamine's effectiveness is diminished. To maximize the effectiveness of any vasoactive agent, metabolic acidosis must first be corrected. The physician may prescribe intravenous sodium bicarbonate to treat the acidosis (Jindal et al., 2000).

Other Vasoactive Medications. Additional vasoactive agents that may be used in managing cardiogenic shock include norepinephrine (Levophed), epinephrine (Adrenalin), milrinone (Primacor), amrinone (Inocor), vasopressin (Pitressin), and phenylephrine (Neo-Synephrine). Each of these medications stimulates different receptors of the sympathetic nervous system. A combination of these medications may be prescribed, depending on the patient's response to treatment. All vasoactive medications have adverse effects, making specific medications more useful than others at different stages of shock. Diuretics such as furosemide (Lasix) may be administered to reduce the workload of the heart by reducing fluid accumulation (see Table 15-1).

Antiarrhythmic Medications. Antiarrhythmic medication is also part of the medication regimen in cardiogenic shock. Multiple factors, such as hypoxemia, electrolyte imbalances, and acid–base imbalances, contribute to serious cardiac dysrhythmias in all patients with shock. Additionally, as a compensatory response to decreased cardiac output and blood pressure, the heart rate increases beyond normal limits. This impedes cardiac output further by shortening diastole and thereby decreasing the time for ventricular filling. Consequently, antiarrhythmic medications are required to stabilize the heart rate. For a full discussion of cardiac dysrhythmias as well as commonly prescribed medications, see Chapter 27. General principles regarding the administration of vasoactive medications are discussed later in this chapter.

Fluid Therapy. In addition to medications, appropriate fluid is necessary in treating cardiogenic shock. Administration of fluids must be monitored closely to detect signs of fluid overload. Incremental intravenous fluid boluses are cautiously administered to determine optimal filling pressures for improving cardiac output. A fluid bolus should never be given quickly because rapid fluid administration in patients with cardiac failure may result in acute pulmonary edema.

MECHANICAL ASSISTIVE DEVICES

If cardiac output does not improve despite supplemental oxygen, vasoactive medications, and fluid boluses, mechanical assistive devices are used temporarily to improve the heart's ability to pump. Intra-aortic balloon counterpulsation is one means of providing temporary circulatory assistance (see Chap. 30). A polyurethane balloon catheter is inserted percutaneously through the common femoral artery and advanced into the descending thoracic aorta. The balloon catheter is connected to a console containing a gas-filled pump. The timing of the balloon inflation is synchronized electrocardiographically with the beginning of diastole, and the balloon deflation occurs just before systole. The goals of intra-aortic balloon counterpulsation include the following:

- Increased stroke volume
- Improved coronary artery perfusion
- Decreased preload
- Decreased cardiac workload
- Decreased myocardial oxygen demand (Kumar et al., 2000)

Other means of mechanical assistance include left and right ventricular assist devices and total artificial hearts. These devices are electrical pumps or pumps driven by air. They assist or replace the ventricular pumping action of the heart. Human heart transplantation may be the only option remaining for a patient who has cardiogenic shock and who cannot be weaned from mechanical assistive devices. (Mechanical assistive devices and heart transplantation are discussed in Chap. 30.)

Another short-term means of providing cardiac or pulmonary support to the patient in cardiogenic shock is through an extracorporeal device similar to the cardiopulmonary bypass (CPB) used in open-heart surgery. The CPB system requires systemic anticoagulation, arterial and venous cannulation of the femoral artery and vein, and connection to a centrifugal, oxygenated pump. The catheter tip is advanced into the right atrium. This system lowers left and right ventricular pressures, reducing the workload and oxygen needs of the heart. Complications of CPB include coagulopathies, myocardial ischemia, infection, and thromboembolism. CPB is used only in emergency situations until definitive treatment, such as heart transplantation, can be initiated.

Nursing Management

PREVENTING CARDIOGENIC SHOCK

In some circumstances, identifying patients at risk early and promoting adequate oxygenation of the heart muscle and decreasing cardiac workload can prevent cardiogenic shock. This can be accomplished by conserving the patient's energy, promptly relieving angina, and administering supplemental oxygen. Often, however, cardiogenic shock cannot be prevented. In such in-

stances, nursing management includes working with other members of the health care team to prevent shock from progressing and to restore adequate cardiac function and tissue perfusion.

MONITORING HEMODYNAMIC STATUS

A major role of the nurse is monitoring the patient's hemodynamic and cardiac status. Arterial lines and electrocardiographic monitoring equipment must be maintained and functioning properly. The nurse anticipates the medications, intravenous fluids, and equipment that might be used and is ready to assist in implementing these measures. Changes in hemodynamic, cardiac, and pulmonary status are documented and reported promptly. Additionally, adventitious breath sounds, changes in cardiac rhythm, and other abnormal physical assessment findings are reported immediately.

ADMINISTERING MEDICATIONS AND INTRAVENOUS FLUIDS

The nurse has a critical role in safe and accurate administration of intravenous fluids and medications. Fluid overload and pulmonary edema are risks because of ineffective cardiac function and accumulation of blood and fluid in the pulmonary tissues. The nurse documents and records medications and treatments that are administered as well as the patient's response to treatment.

The nurse needs to be knowledgeable about the desired effects as well as the side effects of medications. For example, it is important to monitor the patient for decreased blood pressure after administering morphine or nitroglycerin. The patient receiving thrombolytic therapy must be monitored for bleeding. Arterial and venous puncture sites must be observed for bleeding and pressure must be applied at the sites if bleeding occurs. Neurologic assessment is essential after the administration of thrombolytic therapy to assess for the potential complication of cerebral hemorrhage associated with the therapy. Intravenous infusions must be observed closely because tissue necrosis and sloughing may occur if vasopressor medications infiltrate the tissues. Urine output, BUN, and serum creatinine levels are monitored to detect decreased renal function secondary to the effects of cardiogenic shock or its treatment.

MAINTAINING INTRA-AORTIC BALLOON COUNTERPULSATION

The nurse plays a critical role in caring for the patient receiving intra-aortic balloon counterpulsation (see Chap. 30). The nurse makes ongoing timing adjustments of the balloon pump to maximize its effectiveness by synchronizing it with the cardiac cycle. The patient is at great risk for circulatory compromise to the leg on the side where the catheter for the balloon has been placed; therefore, the nurse must frequently check the neurovascular status of the lower extremities.

ENHANCING SAFETY AND COMFORT

Throughout care, the nurse must take an active role in safeguarding the patient, enhancing comfort, and reducing anxiety. This includes administering medication to relieve chest pain, preventing infection at the multiple arterial and venous line insertion sites, protecting the skin, and monitoring respiratory function. Proper positioning of the patient promotes effective breathing without decreasing blood pressure and may also increase the patient's comfort while reducing anxiety.

Brief explanations about procedures that are being performed and the use of comforting touch often provide reassurance to the patient and family. Families are usually anxious and benefit from opportunities to see and talk to the patient. Explanations of treatments and the patient's response to them are often comforting to family members.

Circulatory Shock

Circulatory or distributive shock occurs when blood volume is abnormally displaced in the vasculature—for example, when blood volume pools in peripheral blood vessels. The displacement of blood volume causes a relative hypovolemia because not enough blood returns to the heart, which leads to subsequent inadequate tissue perfusion. The ability of the blood vessels to constrict helps return the blood to the heart. Thus, the vascular tone is determined both by central regulatory mechanisms, as in blood pressure regulation, and by local regulatory mechanisms, as in tissue demands for oxygen and nutrients. Therefore, circulatory shock can be caused either by a loss of sympathetic tone or by release of biochemical mediators from cells.

The varied mechanisms leading to the initial vasodilation in circulatory shock further subdivide this classification of shock into three types: (1) **septic shock**, (2) **neurogenic shock**, and (3) **anaphylactic shock**.

The different types of circulatory shock cause variations in the pathophysiologic chain of events and are explained here separately. In all types of circulatory shock, massive arterial and venous dilation allows blood to pool peripherally. Arterial dilation reduces systemic vascular resistance. Initially, cardiac output can be high in circulatory shock, both from the reduction in afterload (systemic vascular resistance) and from the heart muscle's increased effort to maintain perfusion despite the incompetent vasculature secondary to arterial dilation. Pooling of blood in the periphery results in decreased venous return. Decreased venous return results in decreased stroke volume and decreased cardiac output. Decreased cardiac output, in turn, causes decreased blood pressure and ultimately decreased tissue perfusion. Figure 15-6 presents the pathophysiologic sequence of events in circulatory shock.

SEPTIC SHOCK

Septic shock is the most common type of circulatory shock and is caused by widespread infection (Chart 15-5). Despite the increased sophistication of antibiotic therapy, the incidence of septic shock has continued to rise during the past 60 years. It is the most common cause of death in noncoronary intensive care units in the United States and the 13th leading cause of death in the U.S. population (Balk, 2000a). Elderly patients are at particular risk for sepsis because of decreased physiologic reserves and an aging immune system (Balk, 2000a; Vincent & Ferreira, 2000). Toxic shock syndrome, a specific form of septic shock, is described in Chapter 47.

Nosocomial infections (infections occurring in the hospital) in critically ill patients most frequently originate in the bloodstream, lungs, and urinary tract (in decreasing order of frequency) (Richards, Edwards, Culver et al., 1999). The source of infection is an important determinant of the clinical outcome. The greatest risk of sepsis occurs in patients with bacteremia (bloodstream) and pneumonia (Simon & Trenholme, 2000). Other infections that may progress to septic shock include intra-abdominal infections, wound infections, bacteremia associated with intravascular catheters (Eggimann & Pittet, 2001), and indwelling urinary catheters. Additional risk factors that contribute to the growing incidence of septic shock are the increased awareness and identi-

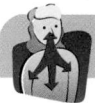 **Physiology/Pathophysiology**

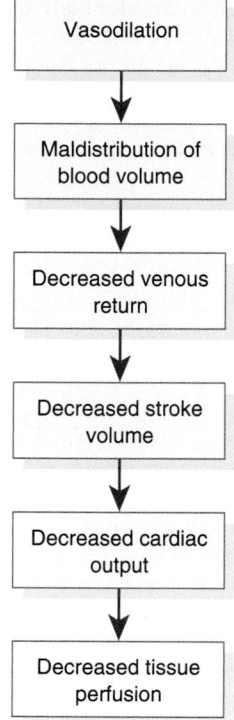

FIGURE 15-6 Pathophysiologic sequence of events in circulatory shock.

fication of septic shock; the increased number of immunocompromised patients (due to malnutrition, alcoholism, malignancy, and diabetes mellitus); the increased incidence of invasive procedures and indwelling medical devices; the increased number of resistant microorganisms; and the increasingly older population (Balk, 2000a). The incidence of septic shock can be reduced by débriding wounds to remove necrotic tissue and carrying out infection control practices, including the use of meticulous aseptic technique, properly cleaning and maintaining equipment, and using thorough hand-hygiene techniques.

The most common causative microorganisms of septic shock are the gram-negative bacteria; however, there is also an increased

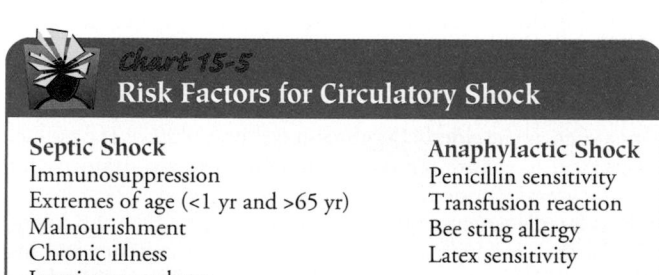

Chart 15-5
Risk Factors for Circulatory Shock

Septic Shock	**Anaphylactic Shock**
Immunosuppression	Penicillin sensitivity
Extremes of age (<1 yr and >65 yr)	Transfusion reaction
Malnourishment	Bee sting allergy
Chronic illness	Latex sensitivity
Invasive procedures	

Neurogenic Shock
Spinal cord injury
Spinal anesthesia
Depressant action of medications
Glucose deficiency

incidence of gram-positive bacterial infections. Currently, gram-positive bacteria are responsible for 50% of bacteremic events (Simon & Trenholme, 2000). Other infectious agents such as viruses and funguses also can cause septic shock.

When a microorganism invades body tissues, the patient exhibits an immune response. This immune response provokes the activation of biochemical mediators associated with an inflammatory response and produces a variety of effects leading to shock. Increased capillary permeability, which leads to fluid seeping from the capillaries, and vasodilation are two such effects that interrupt the ability of the body to provide adequate perfusion, oxygen, and nutrients to the tissues and cells.

Septic shock typically occurs in two phases. The first phase, referred to as the hyperdynamic, progressive phase, is characterized by a high cardiac output with systemic vasodilation. The blood pressure may remain within normal limits. The heart rate increases, progressing to tachycardia. The patient becomes hyperthermic and febrile, with warm, flushed skin and bounding pulses. The respiratory rate is elevated. Urinary output may remain at normal levels or decrease. Gastrointestinal status may be compromised as evidenced by nausea, vomiting, diarrhea, or decreased bowel sounds. The patient may exhibit subtle changes in mental status, such as confusion or agitation.

The later phase, referred to as the hypodynamic, irreversible phase, is characterized by low cardiac output with vasoconstriction, reflecting the body's effort to compensate for the hypovolemia caused by the loss of intravascular volume through the capillaries. In this phase, the blood pressure drops and the skin is cool and pale. Temperature may be normal or below normal. Heart and respiratory rates remain rapid. The patient no longer produces urine, and multiple organ dysfunction progressing to failure develops.

Systemic inflammatory response syndrome (SIRS) presents clinically like sepsis. The only difference between SIRS and sepsis is that there is no identifiable source of infection. SIRS stimulates an overwhelming inflammatory immunologic and hormonal response, similar to that seen in septic patients. Despite an absence of infection, antibiotic agents may still be administered because of the possibility of unrecognized infection. Additional therapies directed to the support of the patient with SIRS are similar to those for sepsis. If the inflammatory process progresses, septic shock may develop.

Medical Management

Current treatment of septic shock involves identifying and eliminating the cause of infection. Specimens of blood, sputum, urine, wound drainage, and invasive catheter tips are collected for culture using aseptic technique.

Any potential routes of infection must be eliminated. Intravenous lines are removed and reinserted at other body sites. Antibiotic-coated intravenous central lines may be placed to decrease the risk of invasive line-related bacteremia in high-risk patients, such as the elderly (Eggimann & Pittet, 2001). If possible, urinary catheters are removed. Any abscesses are drained and necrotic areas débrided.

Fluid replacement must be instituted to correct the hypovolemia that results from the incompetent vasculature and inflammatory response. Crystalloids, colloids, and blood products may be administered to increase the intravascular volume.

PHARMACOLOGIC THERAPY

If the infecting organism is unknown, broad-spectrum antibiotic agents are started until culture and sensitivity reports are received (Simon & Trenholme, 2000). A third-generation cephalosporin plus an aminoglycoside may be prescribed initially. This combination works against most gram-negative and some gram-positive organisms. When culture and sensitivity reports are available, the antibiotic agent may be changed to one that is more specific to the infecting organism and less toxic to the patient.

Research efforts show promise for improving the outcomes of septic shock. Although past treatments focused on destroying the infectious organism, emphasis is now on altering the patient's immune response to the organism. The cell walls of gram-negative bacteria contain a lipopolysaccharide, an endotoxin released during phagocytosis (Abraham et al., 2001). Endotoxin and/or gram-positive cell wall products interact with inflammatory biochemical mediators, initiating an intense inflammatory response and systemic effects that lead to shock. Current research focuses on the development of medications that will inhibit or modulate the effects of biochemical mediators, such as endotoxin and procalcitonin (Bernard, Vincent, Laterre, et al., 2001). The focus on immunotherapy in treating septic shock is expected to shed light on how the cellular response to infection leads to shock.

Recombinant human activated protein C (APC), or drotrecogin alfa (Xigris), has recently been demonstrated to reduce mortality in patients with severe sepsis (Bernard, Artigas, Dellinger et al., 2001). It has been approved by the U.S. Food and Drug Administration for treatment of adults with severe sepsis and resulting acute organ dysfunction who are at high risk of death. It acts as an antithrombotic, anti-inflammatory, and profibrinolytic agent. Its most common serious side effect is bleeding. Therefore, it is contraindicated in patients with active internal bleeding, recent hemorrhagic stroke, intracranial surgery, or head injury.

NUTRITIONAL THERAPY

Aggressive nutritional supplementation is critical in the management of septic shock because malnutrition further impairs the patient's resistance to infection. Nutritional supplementation should be initiated within the first 24 hours of the onset of shock (Mizock, 2000). Enteral feedings are preferred to the parenteral route because of the increased risk of iatrogenic infection associated with intravenous catheters; however, enteral feedings may not be possible if decreased perfusion to the gastrointestinal tract reduces peristalsis and impairs absorption.

Nursing Management

The nurse caring for any patient in any setting must keep in mind the risks of sepsis and the high mortality rate associated with septic shock. All invasive procedures must be carried out with aseptic technique after careful hand hygiene. Additionally, intravenous lines, arterial and venous puncture sites, surgical incisions, traumatic wounds, urinary catheters, and pressure ulcers are monitored for signs of infection in all patients. The nurse identifies patients at particular risk for sepsis and septic shock (ie, elderly and immunosuppressed patients or patients with extensive trauma or burns or diabetes), keeping in mind that these high-risk patients may not develop typical or classic signs of infection and sepsis. Confusion, for example, may be the first sign of infection and sepsis in elderly patients.

When caring for the patient with septic shock, the nurse collaborates with other members of the health care team to identify the site and source of sepsis and the specific organisms involved. Appropriate specimens for culture and sensitivity are often obtained by the nurse.

Elevated body temperature (hyperthermia) is common with sepsis and raises the patient's metabolic rate and oxygen consumption. Fever is one of the body's natural mechanisms for fighting infections. Thus, an elevated temperature may not be treated unless it reaches dangerous levels (more than 40°C [104°F]) or unless the patient is uncomfortable. Efforts may be made to reduce the temperature by administering acetaminophen or applying hypothermia blankets. During these therapies, the nurse monitors the patient closely for shivering, which increases oxygen consumption. Efforts to increase comfort are important if the patient experiences fever, chills, or shivering.

The nurse administers prescribed intravenous fluids and medications, including antibiotic agents and vasoactive medications to restore vascular volume. Because of decreased perfusion to the kidneys and liver, serum concentrations of antibiotic agents that are normally cleared by these organs may increase and produce toxic effects. Therefore, the nurse monitors blood levels (antibiotic agent, BUN, creatinine, white blood count) and reports increased levels to the physician.

As with other types of shock, the nurse monitors the patient's hemodynamic status, fluid intake and output, and nutritional status. Daily weights and close monitoring of serum albumin levels help determine the patient's protein requirements.

NEUROGENIC SHOCK

In neurogenic shock, vasodilation occurs as a result of a loss of sympathetic tone. This can be caused by spinal cord injury, spinal anesthesia, or nervous system damage. It can also result from the depressant action of medications or lack of glucose (eg, insulin reaction or shock).

Neurogenic shock may have a prolonged course (spinal cord injury) or a short one (syncope or fainting). It is characterized by dry, warm skin rather than the cool, moist skin seen in hypovolemic shock. Another characteristic is bradycardia, rather than the tachycardia that characterizes other forms of shock.

Medical Management

Treatment of neurogenic shock involves restoring sympathetic tone either through the stabilization of a spinal cord injury or, in the instance of spinal anesthesia, by positioning the patient properly. Specific treatment of neurogenic shock depends on its cause. Further discussion of managing the patient with a spinal cord injury is presented in Chapter 63. If hypoglycemia (insulin shock) is the cause, glucose is rapidly administered. Hypoglycemia and the insulin reaction are described further in Chapter 41.

Nursing Management

It is important to elevate and maintain the head of the bed at least 30 degrees to prevent neurogenic shock when a patient is receiving spinal or epidural anesthesia. Elevation of the head of the bed helps to prevent the spread of the anesthetic agent up the spinal cord. In suspected spinal cord injury, neurogenic shock may be prevented by carefully immobilizing the patient to prevent further damage to the spinal cord.

Nursing interventions are directed toward supporting cardiovascular and neurologic function until the usually transient episode of neurogenic shock resolves. Applying elastic compression stockings and elevating the foot of the bed may minimize pooling of blood in the legs. Pooled blood increases the risk for thrombus formation. Therefore, the nurse needs to check the patient daily for any redness, tenderness, warmth of the calves, and positive Homans' sign (calf pain on dorsiflexion of the foot). To elicit Homans' sign, the nurse lifts the patient's leg, flexing it at the knee and dorsiflexing the foot. If the patient complains of pain in the calf, the sign is positive and suggestive of deep vein thrombosis.

Administering heparin or low-molecular-weight heparin (Lovenox) as prescribed, applying elastic compression stockings, or initiating pneumatic compression of the legs may prevent thrombus formation. Performing passive range of motion of the immobile extremities helps promote circulation.

Patients who have experienced a spinal cord injury may not report pain caused by internal injuries. Therefore, in the immediate postinjury period, the nurse must monitor the patient closely for signs of internal bleeding that could lead to hypovolemic shock.

ANAPHYLACTIC SHOCK

Anaphylactic shock is caused by a severe allergic reaction when a patient who has already produced antibodies to a foreign substance (antigen) develops a systemic antigen–antibody reaction. This process requires that the patient has previously been exposed to the substance. An antigen–antibody reaction provokes mast cells to release potent vasoactive substances, such as histamine or bradykinin, that cause widespread vasodilation and capillary permeability. Anaphylactic shock occurs rapidly and is life-threatening. Because anaphylactic shock occurs in patients already exposed to an antigen who have developed antibodies to it, it can often be prevented. Therefore, patients with known allergies need to understand the consequences of subsequent exposure to the antigen and should wear medical identification that lists their sensitivities. This could prevent inadvertent administration of a medication that would lead to anaphylactic shock. Additionally, the patient and family need instruction about emergency use of medications to treat anaphylaxis.

Medical Management

Treatment of anaphylactic shock requires removing the causative antigen (eg, discontinuing an antibiotic agent), administering medications that restore vascular tone, and providing emergency support of basic life functions. Epinephrine is given for its vasoconstrictive action. Diphenhydramine (Benadryl) is administered to reverse the effects of histamine, thereby reducing capillary permeability. These medications are given intravenously. Nebulized medications, such as albuterol (Proventil), may be given to reverse histamine-induced bronchospasm.

If cardiac arrest and respiratory arrest are imminent or have occurred, cardiopulmonary resuscitation is performed. Endotracheal intubation or tracheotomy may be necessary to establish an airway. Intravenous lines are inserted to provide access for administering fluids and medications. Anaphylaxis and specific chemical mediators are discussed further in Chapter 53.

Nursing Management

The nurse has an important role in preventing anaphylactic shock: assessing all patients for allergies or previous reactions to antigens (eg, medications, blood products, foods, contrast agents, latex) and communicating the existence of these allergies or reactions to others. Additionally, the nurse assesses the patient's understanding of previous reactions and steps taken by the patient and family to prevent further exposure to antigens. When new allergies are identified, the nurse advises the patient to wear or carry identification that names the specific allergen or antigen.

When administering any new medication, the nurse observes the patient for an allergic reaction. This is especially important with intravenous medications. Allergy to penicillin is one of the most common causes of anaphylactic shock. Patients who have a penicillin allergy may also develop an allergy to similar medications. For example, they may react to cefazolin sodium (Ancef) because it has a similar antimicrobial action of attaching to the penicillin-binding proteins found on the walls of infectious organisms. Previous adverse drug reactions increase the risk that an elderly patient will develop an undesirable reaction to a new medication. If the elderly patient reports an allergy to a medication, the nurse must be aware of the risks involved in the administration of similar medications.

In the hospital and outpatient diagnostic testing sites, the nurse must identify patients at risk for anaphylactic reactions to contrast agents (radiopaque, dye-like substances that may contain iodine) used for diagnostic tests. These include patients with a known allergy to iodine or fish or those who have had previous allergic reactions to contrast agents. This information must be conveyed to the staff at the diagnostic testing site, including x-ray personnel.

The nurse must be knowledgeable about the clinical signs of anaphylaxis, must take immediate action if signs and symptoms occur, and must be prepared to begin cardiopulmonary resuscitation if cardiorespiratory arrest occurs. In addition to monitoring the patient's response to treatment, the nurse assists with intubation if needed, monitors the hemodynamic status, ensures intravenous access for administration of medications, administers prescribed medications and fluids, and documents treatments and their effects.

Community health and home care nurses whose role includes administering medications, including antibiotic agents, in the patient's home or other settings must be prepared to administer epinephrine subcutaneously or intramuscularly in the event of an anaphylactic reaction.

After recovery from anaphylaxis, the patient and family require an explanation of the event. Further, the nurse provides instruction about avoiding future exposure to antigens and administering emergency medications to treat anaphylaxis (see Chap. 53).

Multiple Organ Dysfunction Syndrome

Multiple organ dysfunction syndrome (MODS) is altered organ function in an acutely ill patient that requires medical intervention to support continued organ function. The disorder can be further categorized as primary or secondary MODS.

Pathophysiology

Primary MODS is the result of direct tissue insult, which then leads to impaired perfusion or ischemia. Secondary MODS is most often a complication of septic shock or SIRS. However, MODS may be a complication of any form of shock because of inadequate tissue perfusion. As previously described, in shock all organ systems suffer damage from a lack of adequate perfusion that can result in organ failure. A syndrome of sequential organ failure has been further observed. The exact mechanism that triggers this syndrome is unknown.

Although various causes of MODS have been identified, including dead or injured tissue, infection, and perfusion deficits, it is not yet possible to predict which patients will develop MODS. This is partly because much of the organ damage occurs at the cellular level and therefore cannot be directly observed or measured. The organ failure usually begins in the lungs and is followed by failure of the liver, gastrointestinal system, and kidneys (Balk, 2000b). Advanced age, malnutrition, and coexisting diseases appear to increase the risk of MODS in an acutely ill patient.

Clinical Manifestations

The clinical course of MODS follows one of two patterns. In both patterns, there is an initial event that results in low blood pressure. The cause of the drop in blood pressure is treated, and the patient appears to respond. In the first pattern of MODS (primary MODS), which occurs most often when the initiating event is a pulmonary one such as lung injury, the patient experiences respiratory compromise that necessitates intubation. This usually occurs within 72 hours of the initiating event. Respiratory failure leads rapidly to MODS, resulting in a mortality rate of 30% to 75% (Fein & Calalang-Colucci, 2000).

In secondary MODS, the pattern is more insidious. It occurs most often in the patient with septic shock and progressively unfolds over about 1 month. The patient also experiences respiratory failure and requires intubation. The patient remains hemodynamically stable for about 7 to 14 days. Despite this apparent stability, the patient exhibits a hypermetabolic state characterized by hyperglycemia (elevated blood glucose level), hyperlacticacidemia (excess of lactic acid in the blood), and polyuria (excessive urinary output). The metabolic rate is 1.5 to 2 times basal metabolic rate. Infection is usually present, and skin breakdown begins to occur. During this stage, there is a severe loss of skeletal muscle mass (autocatabolism). If the hypermetabolic phase can be reversed, patients may survive with some damage to affected organ systems (Mizock, 2000). If the hypermetabolic process cannot be halted and cells do not receive adequate oxygen and nutrients, irreversible organ failure and death occur.

If the hypermetabolic phase cannot be reversed, MODS progresses and is characterized by jaundice, hyperbilirubinemia (liver failure), and oliguria progressing to anuria (renal failure), often requiring dialysis. The patient becomes less hemodynamically stable and begins to require vasoactive medications and fluid support. Because of a lack of consistent definitions to describe organ failure, the exact incidence of MODS is hard to define (Balk, 2000b; Vincent & Ferreira, 2000). However, it is reasonable to say that the onset of organ dysfunction is an ominous prognostic sign; the more organs that fail, the worse the outcome.

Medical Management

Prevention remains the top priority in managing MODS. Elderly patients are at increased risk of MODS because of the lack of physiologic reserve associated with aging and the natural degenerative process, especially immune compromise (Balk, 2000b). Early detection and documentation of initial signs of infection are essential in managing elderly patients with MODS. Subtle changes in mentation and a gradual rise in temperature are early warning signs. Other patients at risk of MODS are those with chronic illness, malnutrition, immunosuppression, and surgical or traumatic wounds.

If preventive measures fail, treatment measures to reverse MODS are aimed at (1) controlling the initiating event, (2) promoting adequate organ perfusion, and (3) providing nutritional support.

Nursing Management

The general plan of nursing care for the patient with MODS is the same as that for the patient in septic shock. Primary nursing interventions are aimed at supporting the patient and monitoring organ perfusion until primary organ insults are halted. Providing information and support to family members is a critical role of the nurse in caring for patients with MODS. Addressing end-of-life decisions is an important role of the health care team to ensure that supportive therapies are congruent with the patient's wishes.

Gerontologic Considerations

The population as a whole is aging: the most rapidly growing population group consists of people over 65 years of age. The physiologic changes associated with aging, coupled with pathologic and chronic disease states, place the older individual at increased risk of developing a state of shock and possibly MODS. Medications such as beta-blocking agents (metoprolol [Lopressor]) used to treat hypertension may mask tachycardia, a primary compensatory mechanism to increase cardiac output, during hypovolemic states. The aging immune system may not mount a truly febrile response (temperature more than 40°C), but an increasing trend in body temperature should be addressed. The heart does not function well in hypoxemic states, and the aging heart may respond to decreased myocardial oxygenation with dysrhythmias that may be misinterpreted as a normal part of the aging process. Lastly, changes in mentation may be inappropriately misinterpreted as dementia. The older individual with a sudden change in mentation should be aggressively treated for the presence of infection and organ hypoperfusion. The elderly patient can overcome shock states if signs and symptoms are treated early with aggressive and supportive therapies. Nurses play an essential role in assessing and interpreting subtle changes in the older patient's response to illness.

PROMOTING COMMUNICATION

The nurse encourages frequent and open communication about treatment modalities and options to ensure that the patient's wishes regarding medical management are met. For patients who survive MODS, communicating the goals of rehabilitation and informing the patient of progress toward those goals are essential, as the massive loss of skeletal muscle mass makes rehabilitation a long, slow process. A strong nurse–patient relationship built on effective communication will provide needed encouragement during this phase of recovery.

PROMOTING HOME AND COMMUNITY-BASED CARE

Teaching Patients Self-Care. The patient who experiences and survives shock may have been unable to get out of bed for an extended period of time and is likely to have a slow, prolonged recovery. The patient and family are instructed about strategies to prevent further episodes of shock by identifying the factors implicated in the initial episode. In addition, the patient and family require instruction about assessments needed to identify the complications that may occur after the patient is discharged from the hospital. Depending on the type of shock and its management, the patient or family may require instruction about treatment modalities such as emergency administration of medications, intravenous therapy, parenteral nutrition, skin care, exercise, and ambulation. The patient and family are also instructed about the need for gradual increases in ambulation and other activity. The need for adequate dietary intake is another crucial aspect of teaching.

Continuing Care in the Home and Community. Because of the physical toll associated with recovery from shock, the patient may be cared for in an extended care facility or rehabilitation setting after hospital discharge. Alternatively, a referral may be made for home care. The home care nurse assesses the patient's physical status and monitors recovery. The nurse also assesses the adequacy of treatments that are continued at home and the ability of the patient and family to cope with these treatments. The patient is likely to require close medical supervision until complete recovery occurs. The home care nurse reinforces the importance of continuing medical care and assists the patient and family to identify and mobilize community resources.

 Critical Thinking Exercises

1. A new nurse on your medical unit tells you that she believes a patient with a myocardial infarction is going into shock. She does not know if the patient is experiencing anaphylactic shock related to a medication he received or cardiogenic shock due to his cardiac disorder. How would you differentiate between anaphylactic and cardiogenic shock, and what medical treatments would you anticipate?

2. An elderly man is admitted from a nursing home with a recent onset of confusion and combative behavior. You know that sudden changes in mental status may be an early sign of sepsis in the elderly. How would you assess this patient for the possibility of septic shock, and how would the management of the elderly patient differ from that of a younger patient?

3. While driving through a rural area, you see a crash and stop to help. Two passengers who have been removed from the cars by passersby are seriously injured. One is bleeding profusely; the other is clutching his abdomen and chest because of severe pain. Describe the type of shock that is most likely in each of these individuals. What actions would you take at the scene to prevent shock or prevent it from progressing?

4. A patient who has used a wheelchair for the last 10 years because of a spinal cord injury was burned when her clothing caught fire as she prepared dinner. Her burns are extensive but limited to her upper body. What types of shock are possible in this patient? What therapy directed at prevention or treatment of shock would you anticipate? Describe the rationale for the therapies that you have identified. How would this patient's disability affect management?

REFERENCES AND SELECTED READINGS

Books
Baldwin, K. M., Davey, S. S., Morris, S. E., & Burger, M. (1998). Shock, multiple organ dysfunction syndrome, and burns in adults. In K. L. McCance & S. E. Huether (Eds.), *Pathophysiology: The biologic basis for disease in adults and children* (3d ed.). St. Louis: Mosby.
Guyton, A. C., & Hall, J. E. (Eds.). (2000). *Textbook of medical physiology* (10th ed.). Philadelphia: W. B. Saunders

Harvey, M. A. (1998). Systemic inflammatory response syndrome and multiorgan dysfunction syndrome. In M. R. Kinney, S. B. Dunbar, J. A. Brooks-Brunn, N. Molter, & J. M. Vitello-Cicciu (Eds.), *AACN's clinical reference for critical care nursing* (4th ed.). St. Louis: Mosby.

McKinley, M. G. (2001). Shock. In M. L. Sole, M. L. Lamborn & J. C. Hartshorn (Eds.), *Introduction to critical care nursing* (3d ed.). Philadelphia: W. B. Saunders.

Rauen, C. A., & Munro, N. (1998). Shock. In M. R. Kinney, S. B. Dunbar, J. A. Brooks-Brunn, N. Moleter, & J. M. Vitello-Cicciu (Eds.), *AACN's clinical reference for critical care nursing* (4th ed.). St. Louis: Mosby.

Journals

Abraham, E., Matthay, M. A., Dinarello, C. A., et al. (2000). Consensus conference definitions for sepsis, septic shock, acute lung injury, and acute respiratory distress syndrome: Time for a reevaluation. *Critical Care Medicine, 28* (1), 232–235.

Balk, R. A. (2000*a*). Severe sepsis and septic shock: Definitions, epidemiology, and clinical manifestations. *Critical Care Clinics, 16*(2), 179–192.

Balk, R. A. (2000*b*). Pathogenesis and management of multiple organ dysfunction or failure in severe sepsis and septic shock. *Critical Care Clinics, 16*(2), 337–351.

Bernard, G. R., Vincent, J. L., Laterre, R. F., et al. (2001). Efficacy and safety of recombinant human activated protein C for severe sepsis. *New England Journal of Medicine, 344*(10), 699–707.

Bernard, G., Artigas, A., Dellinger, P., et al. (2001). Clinical expert roundtable discussion (session 3) at the Margaux Conference on Critical Illness: The role of activated protein C in severe sepsis. *Critical Care Medicine, 29*(7): Suppl 1:S75–S77.

Bochud, P. Y., Glauser, M. P., & Calandra, T. (2001) International Sepsis Forum. Antibiotics in sepsis. *Intensive Care Medicine, 27,* Suppl 1:S33–48.

Choi, P. T., Yip, G., Quinonez, L. G., & Cook, D. J. (1999). Crystalloids vs colloids in fluid resuscitation: A systematic review. *Critical Care Medicine, 27*(1), 200–209.

Eggimann, P., & Pittet, D. (2001). Catheter-related infections in intensive care units: An overview with special emphasis on prevention. *Advances in Sepsis, 1*(1), 2–13.

Fein, A. M., & Calalang-Colucci, M. G. (2000). Acute lung injury and acute respiratory distress syndrome in sepsis and septic shock. *Critical Care Clinics, 16*(2), 289–313.

International Sepsis Forum. (2001). Guidelines for the management of severe sepsis and septic shock. *Intensive Care Medicine, 27,* Suppl 1:S1–134.

Jindal, N., Hollenberg, S. M., & Dellinger, R. P. (2000). Pharmacologic issues in the management of septic shock. *Critical Care Clinics, 16*(2), 233–248.

Kirschenbaum, L. A., Astiz, M. E., Rackow, E. C., et al. (2000). Microvascular response in patients with cardiogenic shock. *Critical Care Medicine, 28*(5), 1290–1294.

Kumar, A., Haery, C., & Parrillo, J. E. (2000). Myocardial dysfunction in septic shock. *Critical Care Clinics, 16*(2), 251–281.

Manns, B. J., Lee. H., Doig, C. J., et al. (2002). An economic evaluation of activated protein C treatment for severe sepsis. *New England Journal of Medicine, 347*(13), 993–1000.

Matthay, M. A. (2001). Severe sepsis: A new treatment with both anticoagulant and anti-inflammatory properties. *New England Journal of Medicine, 344*(10), 759–762.

Matot, I., & Sprung, C. L. (2001). Definition of sepsis. *Intensive Care Medicine, 27,* Suppl 1:S3–9.

Mikhail, J. (1999). Resuscitation endpoints in trauma. *AACN Clinical Issues, 10*(1), 10–21.

Mizock, B. A. (2000). Metabolic derangements in sepsis and septic shock. *Critical Care Clinics, 16*(2), 319–333.

Price, S., Anning, P. B., Mitchell, J. A., & Evans, T. W. (1999). Myocardial dysfunction in sepsis: Mechanisms and therapeutic implications. *European Heart Journal, 20*(10), 715–724.

Richards, M. J., Edwards, J. R., Culver, D. H., & Gaynes, R. P. (1999). Nosocomial infections in medical intensive care units in the United States. *Critical Care Medicine, 27*(5), 887–892.

Rivers, E., Nguyen, B., Savstad, S., et al. (2001). Early goal-directed therapy in the treatment of severe sepsis and septic shock. *New England Journal of Medicine, 345*(19), 1368–1377.

Simon, D., & Trenholme, G. (2000). Antibiotic selection for patients with septic shock. *Critical Care Clinics, 16*(2), 215–229.

Vincent, J. L., & Ferreira, F. L. (2000). Evaluation of organ failure: We are making progress. *Intensive Care Medicine, 26*(6), 1023–1024.

Vincent, J. L. (2001). International Sepsis Forum. Hemodynamic support in septic shock. *Intensive Care Medicine, 27,* Suppl 1:S80–92.

Oncology: Nursing Management in Cancer Care

On completion of this chapter, the learner will be able to:

1. Compare the structure and function of the normal cell and the cancer cell.
2. Differentiate between benign and malignant tumors.
3. Identify agents and factors that have been found to be carcinogenic.
4. Describe the significance of health education and preventive care in decreasing the incidence of cancer.
5. Differentiate among the purposes of surgical procedures used in cancer treatment, diagnosis, prophylaxis, palliation, and reconstruction.
6. Describe the roles of surgery, radiation therapy, chemotherapy, bone marrow transplantation, and other therapies in treating cancer.
7. Describe the special nursing needs of patients receiving chemotherapy.
8. Describe common nursing diagnoses and collaborative problems of patients with cancer.
9. Use the nursing process as a framework for care of patients with cancer.
10. Describe the concept of hospice in providing care for patients with advanced cancer.
11. Discuss the role of the nurse in assessment and management of common oncologic emergencies.

*C*ancer nursing practice covers all age groups and nursing specialties and is carried out in a variety of health care settings, including the home, community, acute care institutions, and rehabilitation centers. The scope, responsibilities, and goals of cancer nursing, also called **oncology** nursing, are as diverse and complex as those of any nursing specialty. Because many people associate cancer with pain and death, nurses need to identify their own reactions to cancer and set realistic goals to meet the challenges inherent in caring for patients with cancer.

In addition, the cancer nurse must be prepared to support the patient and family through a wide range of physical, emotional, social, cultural, and spiritual crises. Chart 16-1 identifies major areas of responsibility for nurses caring for patients with cancer.

Epidemiology

Although cancer affects every age group, most cancers occur in people older than 65 years of age. Overall, the incidence of cancer is higher in men than in women and higher in industrialized sectors and nations.

More than 1.2 million Americans are diagnosed each year with a cancer affecting one of various body sites (Fig. 16-1). Cancer is second only to cardiovascular disease as a leading cause of death in the United States. Each year, more than 550,000 Americans die of a malignant process. In order of frequency, the leading causes of cancer deaths in the United States are lung, prostate, and colorectal cancer in men and lung, breast, and colorectal cancer in women (Jemal, Thomas, Murray & Thun, 2002).

Relative 5-year survival rates for African Americans are lower for every cancer site when compared to whites. In the United States, cancer mortality in African Americans is higher than in any other racial group. This finding is related to the higher incidence and later stage of diagnosis among African Americans. The increased cancer morbidity and mortality for this group are largely related to economic factors, education, and barriers to health care rather than to racial characteristics (Greenlee et al., 2000).

Pathophysiology of the Malignant Process

Cancer is a disease process that begins when an abnormal cell is transformed by the genetic mutation of the cellular DNA. This abnormal cell forms a clone and begins to proliferate abnormally, ignoring growth-regulating signals in the environment surrounding the cell. The cells acquire invasive characteristics, and changes occur in surrounding tissues. The cells infiltrate these tissues and gain access to lymph and blood vessels, which carry the cells to other areas of the body. This phenomenon is called **metastasis** (cancer spread to other parts of the body).

Cancer is not a single disease with a single cause; rather, it is a group of distinct diseases with different causes, manifestations, treatments, and prognoses.

PROLIFERATIVE PATTERNS

During the life span, various body tissues normally experience periods of rapid or proliferative growth that must be distinguished from malignant growth activity. Several patterns of cell growth exist: **hyperplasia, metaplasia, dysplasia, anaplasia,** and **neoplasia** (see Glossary).

Cancerous cells are described as **malignant** neoplasms. They demonstrate uncontrolled cell growth that follows no physiologic

Glossary

alopecia: hair loss

anaplasia: cells that lack normal cellular characteristics and differ in shape and organization with respect to their cells of origin; usually, anaplastic cells are malignant.

biologic response modifier (BRM) therapy: use of agents or treatment methods that can alter the immunologic relationship between the tumor and the host to provide a therapeutic benefit

biopsy: a diagnostic procedure to remove a small sample of tissue to be examined microscopically to detect malignant cells

brachytherapy: delivery of radiation therapy through internal implants

cancer: a disease process whereby cells proliferate abnormally, ignoring growth-regulating signals in the environment surrounding the cells

carcinogenesis: process of transforming normal cells into malignant cells

chemotherapy: use of drugs to kill tumor cells by interfering with cellular functions and reproduction

control: containment of the growth of cancer cells

cure: prolonged survival and disappearance of all evidence of disease so that the patient has the same life expectancy as anyone else in his or her age group

cytokines: substances produced by cells of the immune system to enhance production and functioning of components of the immune system

dysplasia: bizarre cell growth resulting in cells that differ in size, shape, or arrangement from other cells of the same type of tissue

extravasation: leakage of medication from the veins into the subcutaneous tissues

grading: identification of the type of tissue from which the tumor originated and the degree to which the tumor cells retain the functional and structural characteristics of the tissue of origin

hyperplasia: increase in the number of cells of a tissue; most often associated with periods of rapid body growth

malignant: having cells or processes that are characteristic of cancer

metaplasia: conversion of one type of mature cell into another type of cell

metastasis: spread of cancer cells from the primary tumor to distant sites

myelosuppression: suppression of the blood cell–producing function of the bone marrow

nadir: lowest point of white blood cell depression after therapy that has toxic effects on the bone marrow

neoplasia: uncontrolled cell growth that follows no physiologic demand

neutropenia: abnormally low absolute neutrophil count

oncology: field or study of cancer

palliation: relief of symptoms associated with cancer

radiation therapy: use of ionizing radiation to interrupt the growth of malignant cells

stomatitis: inflammation of the oral tissues, often associated with some chemotherapeutic agents

staging: process of determining the size and spread, or metastasis, of a tumor

thrombocytopenia: decrease in the number of circulating platelets; associated with the potential for bleeding

tumor-specific antigen (TSA): protein on the membrane of cancer cells that distinguishes the malignant cell from a benign cell of the same tissue type

vesicant: substance that can cause tissue necrosis and damage, particularly when extravasated

xerostomia: dry oral cavity resulting from decreased function of salivary glands

Responsibilities of the Nurse in Cancer Care

- Support the idea that cancer is a chronic illness that has acute exacerbations rather than one that is synonymous with death and suffering.
- Assess own level of knowledge relative to the pathophysiology of the disease process.
- Make use of current research findings and practices in the care of the patient with cancer and his or her family.
- Identify patients at high risk for cancer.
- Participate in primary and secondary prevention efforts.
- Assess the nursing care needs of the patient with cancer.
- Assess the learning needs, desires, and capabilities of the patient with cancer.
- Identify nursing problems of the patient and the family.
- Assess the social support networks available to the patient.
- Plan appropriate interventions with the patient and the family.
- Assist the patient to identify strengths and limitations.
- Assist the patient to design short-term and long-term goals for care.
- Implement a nursing care plan that interfaces with the medical care regimen and that is consistent with the established goals.
- Collaborate with members of a multidisciplinary team to foster continuity of care.
- Evaluate the goals and resultant outcomes of care with the patient, the family, and members of the multidisciplinary team.
- Reassess and redesign the direction of the care as determined by the evaluation.

demand. Benign and malignant growths are classified and named by tissue of origin, as described in Table 16-1.

Benign and malignant cells differ in many cellular growth characteristics, including the method and rate of growth, ability to metastasize or spread, general effects, destruction of tissue, and ability to cause death. These differences are summarized in Table 16-2. The degree of anaplasia (lack of differentiation of cells) ultimately determines the malignant potential.

CHARACTERISTICS OF MALIGNANT CELLS

Despite their individual differences, all cancer cells share some common cellular characteristics in relation to the cell membrane, special proteins, the nuclei, chromosomal abnormalities, and the rate of mitosis and growth. The cell membranes are altered in cancer cells, which affects fluid movement in and out of the cell. The cell membrane of malignant cells also contains proteins called **tumor-specific antigens** (for example, carcinoembryonic antigen and prostate-specific antigen), which develop as they become less differentiated (mature) over time. These proteins distinguish the malignant cell from a benign cell of the same tissue type. They may be useful in measuring the extent of disease in a person and in tracking the course of illness during treatment or relapse. Malignant cellular membranes also contain less fibronectin, a cellular cement. They are therefore less cohesive and do not adhere to adjacent cells readily.

Leading Sites of New Cancer Cases and Deaths—2002 Estimates*

Cancer Cases by Site and Sex

Male

Prostate
189,000 (30%)

Lung & bronchus
90,200 (14%)

Colon & rectum
72,600 (11%)

Urinary bladder
41,500 (7%)

Melanoma of the skin
30,100 (5%)

Non-Hodgkin's lymphoma
28,200 (4%)

Kidney
19,100 (3%)

Oral cavity
18,900 (3%)

Leukemia
17,600 (3%)

Pancreas
14,700 (2%)

All sites
637,500 (100%)

Female

Breast
203,500 (31%)

Lung & bronchus
79,200 (12%)

Colon & rectum
75,700 (12%)

Uterine corpus
39,300 (6%)

Non-Hodgkin's lymphoma
25,700 (4%)

Melanoma of the skin
23,500 (4%)

Ovary
23,300 (4%)

Thyroid
15,800 (2%)

Pancreas
15,600 (2%)

Urinary bladder
15,000 (2%)

All sites
647,400 (100%)

Cancer Deaths by Site and Sex

Male

Lung & bronchus
89,200 (31%)

Prostate
30,200 (11%)

Colon & rectum
27,800 (10%)

Pancreas
14,500 (5%)

Non-Hodgkin's lymphoma
12,700 (5%)

Leukemia
12,100 (4%)

Esophagus
9,600 (3%)

Liver
8,900 (3%)

Urinary bladder
8,600 (3%)

Kidney
7,200 (3%)

All sites
288,200 (100%)

Female

Lung & bronchus
65,700 (25%)

Breast
39,600 (15%)

Colon & rectum
28,800 (11%)

Pancreas
15,200 (6%)

Ovary
13,900 (5%)

Non-Hodgkin's lymphoma
11,700 (4%)

Leukemia
9,600 (4%)

Uterine corpus
6,600 (2%)

Brain
5,900 (2%)

Multiple myeloma
5,300 (2%)

All sites
267,300 (100%)

*Excludes basal and squamous cell skin cancers and in situ carcinoma except urinary bladder.
Percentages may not total 100% due to rounding.

©2002, American Cancer Society, Inc., Surveillance Research

FIGURE 16-1 Estimated leading sites of cancer incidences and deaths, 2002. *Cancer Facts and Figures, 2002.* American Cancer Society, Atlanta, Georgia.

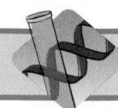

GENETICS IN NURSING PRACTICE—Concepts and Challenges in Patient Management

Cancer is a genetic disease. Every phase of carcinogenesis is affected by multiple genetic mutations. Some of these mutations are inherited (present in germ-line cells), but most (90%) are somatic mutations that are acquired mutations in specific cells.

EXAMPLES OF CANCERS INFLUENCED BY GENETIC FACTORS

- Cowden syndrome
- Familial adenomatous polyposis
- Familial melanoma syndrome
- Hereditary breast and ovarian cancer
- Hereditary non-polyposis colon cancer
- Neurofibromatosis type 1
- Retinoblastoma

NURSING ASSESSMENTS

FAMILY HISTORY

- Obtain information about both maternal and paternal sides of family.
- Obtain cancer history of at least three generations.
- Look for clustering of cancers that occur at earlier ages, multiple primary cancers in one individual, cancer in paired organs, and two or more close relatives with the same type of cancer suggestive of hereditary cancer syndromes.

PHYSICAL ASSESSMENT

- Physical findings that may predispose the patient to cancer, such as multiple colonic polyps, suggestive of a polyposis syndrome
- Skin findings, such as atypical moles, that may be related to familial melanoma syndrome
- Multiple café au lait spots, axillary freckling, and two or more neurofibromas associated with neurofibromatosis type I
- Facial trichilemmomas, mucosal papillomatosis, multinodular thyroid goiter or thyroid adenomas, macrocephaly, fibrocystic breasts and other fibromas or lipomas related to Cowden syndrome

MANAGEMENT ISSUES SPECIFIC TO GENETICS

- Assess patient's understanding of genetic factors related to his or her cancer.
- Refer for cancer risk assessment when a hereditary cancer syndrome is suspected so that patient and family can discuss inheritance, risk with other family members and availability of genetic testing.
- Offer appropriate genetics information and resources.
- Assess patient's understanding of genetics information.
- Provide support to patient and families with known genetic test results for hereditary cancer syndromes.
- Participate in the management and coordination of risk-reduction measures for those with known genetic mutations.

RESOURCES AND WEBSITES

American Cancer Society http://www.cancer.org—offers general information about cancer and support resources for families

Gene Clinics http://www.geneclinics.org—a listing of common genetic disorders with up-to-date clinical summaries, genetic counseling, and testing information

National Organization of Rare Disorders http://www.rarediseases.org—a directory of support groups and information for patients and families with rare genetic disorders

National Cancer Institute http://www.cancernet.nci.nih.gov—a listing of cancers with clinical summaries and treatment reviews, information on genetic risks for cancer, listing of cancer centers providing genetic cancer risk assessment services

Genetic Alliance http://www.geneticalliance.org—a directory of support groups for patients and families with genetic conditions

OMIM: Online Mendelian Inheritance in Man http://www.ncbi.nlm.nih.gov/omim/stats/html—a complete listing of known inherited genetic conditions

---

Typically, nuclei of cancer cells are large and irregularly shaped (pleomorphism). Nucleoli, structures within the nucleus that house ribonucleic acid (RNA), are larger and more numerous in malignant cells, perhaps because of increased RNA synthesis. Chromosomal abnormalities (translocations, deletions, additions) and fragility of chromosomes are commonly found when cancer cells are analyzed.

Mitosis (cell division) occurs more frequently in malignant cells than in normal cells. As the cells grow and divide, more glucose and oxygen are needed. If glucose and oxygen are unavailable, malignant cells use anaerobic metabolic channels to produce energy, which makes the cells less dependent on the availability of a constant oxygen supply.

INVASION AND METASTASIS

Malignant disease processes have the ability to allow the spread or transfer of cancerous cells from one organ or body part to another by invasion and metastasis. Patterns of metastasis can be partially explained by circulatory patterns and by specific affinity for certain malignant cells to bind to molecules in specific body tissue.

Invasion, which refers to the growth of the primary tumor into the surrounding host tissues, occurs in several ways. Mechanical pressure exerted by rapidly proliferating neoplasms may force fingerlike projections of tumor cells into surrounding tissue and interstitial spaces. Malignant cells are less adherent and may break off from the primary tumor and invade adjacent structures. Malignant cells are thought to possess or produce specific destructive enzymes (proteinases), such as collagenases (specific to collagen), plasminogen activators (specific to plasma), and lysosomal hydrolyses. These enzymes are thought to destroy surrounding tissue, including the structural tissues of the vascular basement membrane, facilitating invasion of malignant cells. The mechanical pressure of a rapidly growing tumor may enhance this process.

Metastasis is the dissemination or spread of malignant cells from the primary tumor to distant sites by direct spread of tumor cells to body cavities or through lymphatic and blood circulation. Tumors growing in or penetrating body cavities may shed cells or emboli that travel within the body cavity and seed the surfaces of other organs. This can occur in ovarian cancer when malignant cells enter the peritoneal cavity and seed the peritoneal surfaces of such abdominal organs as the liver or pancreas.

Table 16-1 • Tumors and Tissue Types

TISSUE TYPE	BENIGN TUMORS	MALIGNANT TUMORS
Epithelial		
Surface	Papilloma	Squamous cell carcinoma
Glandular	Adenoma	Adenocarcinoma
Connective		
Fibrous	Fibroma	Fibrosarcoma
Adipose	Lipoma	Liposarcoma
Cartilage	Chondroma	Chondrosarcoma
Bone	Osteoma	Osteosarcoma
Blood vessels	Hemangioma	Hemangiosarcoma
Lymph vessels	Lymphangioma	Lymphangiosarcoma
Lymph tissue		Lymphosarcoma
Muscle		
Smooth	Leiomyoma	Leiomyosarcoma
Striated	Rhabdomyoma	Rhabdomyosarcoma
Neural Tissue		
Nerve cell	Neuroma	Neuroblastoma
Glial tissue	Glioma (benign)	Glioblastoma, astrocytoma, medulloblastoma, oligodendroglioma
Nerve sheaths	Neurilemmoma	Neurilemmal sarcoma
Meninges	Meningioma	Meningeal sarcoma
Hematologic		
Granulocytic		Myelocytic leukemia
Erythrocytic		Erythrocytic leukemia
Plasma cells		Multiple myeloma
Lymphocytic		Lymphocytic leukemia or lymphoma
Monocytic		Monocytic leukemia
Endothelial Tissue		
Blood vessels	Hemangioma	Hemangiosarcoma
Lymph vessels	Lymphangioma	Lymphangiosarcoma
Endothelial lining		Ewing's sarcoma

Reproduced with permission from Porth, C. M. (2002). *Pathophysiology: Concepts of altered health states* (6th ed.). Philadelphia: Lippincott Williams & Wilkins.

Table 16-2 • Characteristics of Benign and Malignant Neoplasms

CHARACTERISTICS	BENIGN	MALIGNANT
Cell characteristics	Well-differentiated cells that resemble normal cells of the tissue from which the tumor originated	Cells are undifferentiated and often bear little resemblance to the normal cells of the tissue from which they arose
Mode of growth	Tumor grows by expansion and does not infiltrate the surrounding tissues; usually encapsulated	Grows at the periphery and sends out processes that infiltrate and destroy the surrounding tissues
Rate of growth	Rate of growth is usually slow	Rate of growth is variable and depends on level of differentiation; the more anaplastic the tumor, the faster its growth
Metastasis	Does not spread by metastasis	Gains access to the blood and lymphatic channels and metastasizes to other areas of the body
General effects	Is usually a localized phenomenon that does not cause generalized effects unless its location interferes with vital functions	Often causes generalized effects, such as anemia, weakness, and weight loss
Tissue destruction	Does not usually cause tissue damage unless its location interferes with blood flow	Often causes extensive tissue damage as the tumor outgrows its blood supply or encroaches on blood flow to the area; may also produce substances that cause cell damage
Ability to cause death	Does not usually cause death unless its location interferes with vital functions	Usually causes death unless growth can be controlled

Reproduced with permission from Porth, C. M. (2002). *Pathophysiology: Concepts of altered health states* (6th ed.). Philadelphia: Lippincott Williams & Wilkins.

Metastatic Mechanisms

Lymph and blood are key mechanisms by which cancer cells spread. Angiogenesis, a mechanism by which the tumor cells are ensured a blood supply, is another important process.

LYMPHATIC SPREAD

The most common mechanism of metastasis is lymphatic spread, which is transport of tumor cells through the lymphatic circulation. Tumor emboli enter the lymph channels by way of the interstitial fluid that communicates with lymphatic fluid. Malignant cells also may penetrate lymphatic vessels by invasion. After entering the lymphatic circulation, malignant cells either lodge in the lymph nodes or pass between lymphatic and venous circulation. Tumors arising in areas of the body with rapid and extensive lymphatic circulation are at high risk for metastasis through lymphatic channels. Breast tumors frequently metastasize in this manner through axillary, clavicular, and thoracic lymph channels.

HEMATOGENOUS SPREAD

Another metastatic mechanism is hematogenous spread, by which malignant cells are disseminated through the bloodstream. Hematogenous spread is directly related to the vascularity of the tumor. Few malignant cells can survive the turbulence of arterial circulation, insufficient oxygenation, or destruction by the body's immune system. In addition, the structure of most arteries and arterioles is far too secure to permit malignant invasion. Those malignant cells that do survive this hostile environment are able to attach to endothelium and attract fibrin, platelets, and clotting factors to seal themselves from immune system surveillance. The endothelium retracts, allowing the malignant cells to enter the basement membrane and secrete lysosomal enzymes. These enzymes then destroy surrounding body tissues and thereby allow implantation.

ANGIOGENESIS

Malignant cells also have the ability to induce the growth of new capillaries from the host tissue to meet their needs for nutrients and oxygen. This process is referred to as angiogenesis. It is through this vascular network that tumor emboli can enter the systemic circulation and travel to distant sites. Large tumor emboli that become trapped in the microcirculation of distant sites may further metastasize to other sites. Research into ways to prevent angiogenesis is ongoing.

Carcinogenesis

Malignant transformation, or **carcinogenesis**, is thought to be at least a three-step cellular process: initiation, promotion, and progression.

In *initiation,* the first step, initiators (carcinogens), such as chemicals, physical factors, and biologic agents, escape normal enzymatic mechanisms and alter the genetic structure of the cellular DNA. Normally, these alterations are reversed by DNA repair mechanisms, or the changes initiate programmed cellular suicide (apoptosis). Occasionally, cells escape these protective mechanisms, and permanent cellular mutations occur. These mutations usually are not significant to cells until the second step of carcinogenesis.

During *promotion,* repeated exposure to promoting agents (co-carcinogens) causes the expression of abnormal or mutant genetic information even after long latency periods. Latency periods for the promotion of cellular mutations vary with the type of agent and the dosage of the promoter as well as the innate characteristics of the target cell.

Cellular oncogenes, present in all mammalian systems, are responsible for the vital cellular functions of growth and differentiation. Cellular proto-oncogenes are present in cells and act as an "on switch" for cellular growth. Similarly, cancer suppressor genes "turn off" or regulate unneeded cellular proliferation. When the suppressor genes become mutated, rearranged, or amplified or lose their regulatory capabilities, malignant cells are allowed to reproduce. The p53 gene is a tumor suppressor gene that is frequently mutated in many human cancers. This gene regulates whether cells will repair or die after DNA damage. Mutant p53 gene is associated with a poor prognosis and may be associated with determining response to treatment. Once this genetic expression occurs in cells, the cells begin to produce mutant cell populations that are different from their original cellular ancestors.

Progression is the third step of cellular carcinogenesis. The cellular changes formed during initiation and promotion now exhibit increased malignant behavior. These cells now show a propensity to invade adjacent tissues and to metastasize. Agents that initiate or promote cellular transformation are referred to as carcinogens.

ETIOLOGY

Certain categories of agents or factors implicated in carcinogenesis include viruses and bacteria, physical agents, chemical agents, genetic or familial factors, dietary factors, and hormonal agents.

Viruses and Bacteria

Viruses as a cause of human cancers are hard to determine because viruses are difficult to isolate. Infectious causes are considered or suspected, however, when specific cancers appear in clusters. Viruses are thought to incorporate themselves in the genetic structure of cells, thus altering future generations of that cell population—perhaps leading to a cancer. For example, the Epstein-Barr virus is highly suspect as a cause in Burkitt's lymphoma, nasopharyngeal cancers, and some types of non-Hodgkin's lymphoma and Hodgkin's disease.

Herpes simplex virus type II, cytomegalovirus, and human papillomavirus types 16, 18, 31, and 33 are associated with dysplasia and cancer of the cervix. The hepatitis B virus is implicated in cancer of the liver; the human T-cell lymphotropic virus may be a cause of some lymphocytic leukemias and lymphomas; and the human immunodeficiency virus (HIV) is associated with Kaposi's sarcoma. The bacterium *Helicobacter pylori* has been associated with an increased incidence of gastric malignancy, perhaps secondary to inflammation and injury of gastric cells.

Physical Agents

Physical factors associated with carcinogenesis include exposure to sunlight or radiation, chronic irritation or inflammation, and tobacco use.

Excessive exposure to the ultraviolet rays of the sun, especially in fair-skinned, blue- or green-eyed people, increases the risk for skin cancers. Factors such as clothing styles (sleeveless shirts or shorts), use of sunscreens, occupation, recreational habits, and environmental variables, including humidity, altitude, and latitude, all play a role in the amount of exposure to ultraviolet light.

Exposure to ionizing radiation can occur with repeated diagnostic x-ray procedures or with radiation therapy used to treat disease. Fortunately, improved x-ray equipment appropriately minimizes the risk for extensive radiation exposure. Radiation therapy used in disease treatment or exposure to radioactive materials at nuclear weapon manufacturing sites or nuclear power plants is associated with a higher incidence of leukemias, multiple myeloma, and cancers of the lung, bone, breast, thyroid, and other tissues. Background radiation from the natural decay processes that produce radon has also been associated with lung cancer. Homes with high levels of trapped radon should be ventilated to allow the gas to disperse into the atmosphere.

Chemical Agents

About 75% of all cancers are thought to be related to the environment. Tobacco smoke, thought to be the single most lethal chemical carcinogen, accounts for at least 30% of cancer deaths (Heath & Fontham, 2001). Smoking is strongly associated with cancers of the lung, head and neck, esophagus, pancreas, cervix, and bladder. Tobacco may also act synergistically with other substances, such as alcohol, asbestos, uranium, and viruses, to promote cancer development.

Chewing tobacco is associated with cancers of the oral cavity and primarily occurs in men younger than 40 years of age. Many chemical substances found in the workplace have proved to be carcinogens or co-carcinogens. The extensive list of suspected chemical substances continues to grow and includes aromatic amines and aniline dyes; pesticides and formaldehydes; arsenic, soot, and tars; asbestos; benzene; betel nut and lime; cadmium; chromium compounds; nickel and zinc ores; wood dust; beryllium compounds; and polyvinyl chloride.

Most hazardous chemicals produce their toxic effects by altering DNA structure in body sites distant from chemical exposure. The liver, lungs, and kidneys are the organ systems most often affected, presumably because of their roles in detoxifying chemicals.

Genetic and Familial Factors

Almost every cancer type has been shown to run in families. This may be due to genetics, shared environments, cultural or lifestyle factors, or chance alone. Genetic factors play a role in cancer cell development. Abnormal chromosomal patterns and cancer have been associated with extra chromosomes, too few chromosomes, or translocated chromosomes. Specific cancers with underlying genetic abnormalities include Burkitt's lymphoma, chronic myelogenous leukemia, meningiomas, acute leukemias, retinoblastomas, Wilms' tumor, and skin cancers, including malignant melanoma.

Approximately 5% to 10% of cancers of adulthood and childhood display a familial predisposition. Inherited cancer syndromes, such as premenopausal breast cancer, tend to occur at an early age and at multiple sites in one organ or pair of organs. In cancers with a familial predisposition, individuals may develop multiple cancers; commonly, two or more first-degree relatives share the same cancer type. Cancers associated with familial inheritance include retinoblastomas, nephroblastomas, pheochromocytomas, malignant neurofibromatosis, and breast, ovarian, endometrial, colorectal, stomach, prostate, and lung cancers. In 1994, the BRCA-1 gene was identified; it is linked to breast and ovarian cancer syndrome. The BRCA-2 gene, which has also been identified, is associated with early-onset breast cancer (Nogueira & Appling, 2000). Work continues to identify other specific genes related to cancer incidence (Greco, 2000).

Dietary Factors

Dietary factors are thought to be related to 35% of all environmental cancers (Heath & Fontham, 2001). Dietary substances can be proactive (protective), carcinogenic, or co-carcinogenic. The risk for cancer increases with long-term ingestion of carcinogens or co-carcinogens or chronic absence of proactive substances in the diet.

Dietary substances associated with an increased cancer risk include fats, alcohol, salt-cured or smoked meats, foods containing nitrates and nitrites, and a high caloric dietary intake. Food substances that appear to reduce cancer risk include high-fiber foods, cruciferous vegetables (cabbage, broccoli, cauliflower, Brussels sprouts, kohlrabi), carotenoids (carrots, tomatoes, spinach, apricots, peaches, dark-green and deep-yellow vegetables), and possibly vitamins E and C, zinc, and selenium.

Obesity is associated with endometrial cancer and possibly postmenopausal breast cancers. Obesity may also increase the risk for cancers of the colon, kidney, and gallbladder.

Hormonal Agents

Tumor growth may be promoted by disturbances in hormonal balance either by the body's own (endogenous) hormone production or by administration of exogenous hormones. Cancers of the breast, prostate, and uterus are thought to depend on endogenous hormonal levels for growth. Diethylstilbestrol (DES) has long been recognized as a cause of vaginal carcinomas. Oral contraceptives and prolonged estrogen replacement therapy are associated with increased incidence of hepatocellular, endometrial, and breast cancers, whereas they appear to decrease the risk for ovarian and endometrial cancers. The combination of estrogen and progesterone appears safest in decreasing the risk for endometrial cancers. Hormonal changes with reproduction are also associated with cancer incidence. Increased numbers of pregnancies are associated with a decreased incidence of breast, endometrial, and ovarian cancers.

ROLE OF THE IMMUNE SYSTEM

In humans, malignant cells are capable of developing on a regular basis. Some evidence indicates, however, that the immune system can detect the development of malignant cells and destroy them before cell growth becomes uncontrolled. When the immune system fails to identify and stop the growth of malignant cells, clinical cancer develops.

Patients who for various reasons are immunoincompetent have been shown to have an increased incidence of cancer. Organ transplant recipients who receive immunosuppressive therapy to prevent rejection of the transplanted organ have an increased incidence of lymphoma, Kaposi's sarcoma, squamous cell cancer of the skin, and cervical and anogenital cancers. Patients with immunodeficiency diseases, such as AIDS, have an increased incidence of Kaposi's sarcoma, lymphoma, and rectal and head and neck cancers. Some patients who have received alkylating chemotherapeutic agents to treat Hodgkin's disease have an increased incidence of secondary malignancies. Autoimmune diseases, such as rheumatoid arthritis and Sjögren's syndrome, are associated with increased cancer development. Finally, age-related changes, such as declining organ function, increased incidence of chronic diseases, and diminished immunocompetence, may contribute to an increased incidence of cancer in older people.

Normal Immune Responses

Normally, an intact immune system has the ability to combat cancer cells in several ways. Usually, the immune system recognizes as foreign certain antigens on the cell membranes of many cancer cells. These antigens are known as tumor-associated antigens (also called tumor cell antigens) and are capable of stimulating both cellular and humoral immune responses.

Along with the macrophages, T lymphocytes, the soldiers of the cellular immune response, are responsible for recognizing tumor-associated antigens. When T lymphocytes recognize tumor antigens, other T lymphocytes that are toxic to the tumor cells are stimulated. These lymphocytes proliferate and are released into the circulation. In addition to possessing cytotoxic (cell-killing) properties, T lymphocytes can stimulate other components of the immune system to rid the body of malignant cells.

Certain lymphokines, which are substances produced by lymphocytes, are capable of killing or damaging various types of malignant cells. Other lymphokines can mobilize other cells, such as macrophages, that disrupt cancer cells. Interferon (IFN), a substance produced by the body in response to viral infection, also possesses some antitumor properties. Antibodies produced by B lymphocytes, associated with the humoral immune response, also defend the body against malignant cells. These antibodies act either alone or in combination with the complement system or the cellular immune system.

Natural killer (NK) cells are a major component of the body's defense against cancer. NK cells are a subpopulation of lymphocytes that act by directly destroying cancer cells or by producing lymphokines and enzymes that assist in cell destruction.

Immune System Failure

How is it, then, that malignant cells can survive and proliferate despite the elaborate immune system defense mechanisms? Several theories suggest how tumor cells can evade an apparently intact immune system. If the body fails to recognize the malignant cell as different from "self" (non-self or foreign), the immune response may not be stimulated. When tumors do not possess tumor-associated antigens that label them as foreign, the immune response is not alerted. The failure of the immune system to respond promptly to the malignant cells allows the tumor to grow too large to be managed by normal immune mechanisms.

Tumor antigens may combine with the antibodies produced by the immune system and hide or disguise themselves from normal immune defense mechanisms. These tumor antigen–antibody complexes can suppress further production of antibodies. Tumors are also capable of changing their appearance or producing substances that impair usual immune responses. These substances not only promote tumor growth but also increase the patient's susceptibility to infection by various pathogenic organisms. As a result of prolonged contact with a tumor antigen, the patient's body may be depleted of the specific lymphocytes and no longer able to mount an appropriate immune response.

Abnormal concentrations of host suppressor T lymphocytes may play a role in developing cancers. Suppressor T lymphocytes normally assist in regulating antibody production and diminishing immune responses when they are no longer required. Low levels of serum antibodies and high levels of suppressor cells have been found in patients with multiple myeloma, a cancer associated with hypogammaglobulinemia (low amounts of serum antibodies). Carcinogens, such as viruses and certain chemicals, including chemotherapeutic agents, may weaken the immune system and ultimately enhance tumor growth.

Detection and Prevention of Cancer

Nurses and physicians have traditionally been involved with tertiary prevention, the care and rehabilitation of the patient after cancer diagnosis and treatment. In recent years, however, the American Cancer Society, the National Cancer Institute, clinicians, and researchers have placed greater emphasis on primary and secondary prevention of cancer. Primary prevention is concerned with reducing the risks of cancer in healthy people. Secondary prevention involves detection and screening to achieve early diagnosis and prompt intervention to halt the cancer process.

PRIMARY PREVENTION

By acquiring the knowledge and skills necessary to educate the community about cancer risk, nurses in all settings play a key role in cancer prevention. Assisting patients to avoid known carcinogens is one way to reduce the risk for cancer. Another way involves adopting dietary and various lifestyle changes that epidemiologic and laboratory studies show influence the risk for cancer. Several clinical trials have been undertaken to identify medications that may help to reduce the incidence of certain types of cancer. Recently, a breast cancer prevention study supported by the National Cancer Institute was conducted at multiple medical centers throughout the country. The results of this study indicated that the medication tamoxifen can reduce the incidence of breast cancer by 49% in postmenopausal women identified as at high risk for breast cancer (Fisher et al., 1998). Nurses can use their teaching and counseling skills to encourage patients to participate in cancer prevention programs and to promote healthful lifestyles.

SECONDARY PREVENTION

The evolving understanding of the role of genetics in cancer cell development has contributed to prevention and screening efforts. Individuals who have inherited specific genetic mutations have an increased susceptibility to cancer. For example, individuals who have familial adenomatosis polyposis have an increased risk for colon cancer. Women in whom the BRCA-1 and BRCA-2 genes have been identified have an increased risk for breast and ovarian cancer. To provide individualized education and recommendations for continued surveillance and care in high-risk populations, nurses need to be familiar with ongoing developments in the field of genetics and cancer (Greco, 2000). Many centers across the country are offering innovative cancer risk evaluation programs that provide in-depth screening and follow-up for individuals who are found to be at high risk for cancer.

Numerous factors, such as race, cultural influences, access to care, physician–patient relationship, level of education, income, and age, influence the knowledge, attitudes, and beliefs people have about cancer. These factors also influence the type of health-promoting behaviors they practice. For example, Phillips, Cohen, and Moses (1999) examined beliefs, attitudes, and practices related to breast cancer and breast cancer screening in African American women (Nursing Research Profile 16-1). They found that cultural, spiritual, and socioeconomic factors seen in the women studied could be identified as barriers to breast health screening behaviors. Nurses can use this type of information in planning education, prevention, and screening programs.

Public awareness about health-promoting behaviors can be increased in a variety of ways. Health education and health maintenance programs are sponsored by community organizations such as churches, senior citizen groups, and parent–teacher associations. Although primary prevention programs may focus on the hazards of tobacco use or the importance of nutrition, secondary prevention programs may promote breast and testicular self-examination and Papanicolaou (Pap) tests. Many organizations conduct cancer screening events that focus on cancers with the highest incidence rates or those that have improved survival rates if diagnosed early, such as breast or prostate cancers. These events offer education and examinations such as mammograms, digital rectal examinations, and prostate-specific antigen blood tests for minimal or no cost. Programs of this nature are often targeted to individuals who lack access to health care or cannot afford to participate on their own.

Similarly, nurses in all settings can develop programs that identify risks for patients and families and that incorporate teaching and counseling into all educational efforts, particularly for patients and families with a high incidence of cancer. The American Cancer Society has developed a public education program, "Taking Control," that integrates diet, exercise, and general health habit tips that people can follow to reduce their risk for cancer (Chart 16-2). Nurses and physicians can encourage individuals to comply with detection efforts as suggested by the American Cancer Society (Table 16-3).

Diagnosis of Cancer and Related Nursing Considerations

A cancer diagnosis is based on assessment for physiologic and functional changes and results of the diagnostic evaluation. Patients with suspected cancer undergo extensive testing to (1) determine the presence of tumor and its extent, (2) identify possible spread (metastasis) of disease or invasion of other body tissues, (3) evaluate the function of involved and uninvolved body systems and organs, and (4) obtain tissue and cells for analysis, including evaluation of tumor stage and grade. The diagnostic evaluation is guided by information obtained through a complete history and physical examination. Knowledge of suspicious symptoms and of the behavior of particular types of cancer assists in determining which diagnostic tests are most appropriate (Table 16-4).

A patient undergoing extensive testing is usually fearful of the procedures and anxious about the possible test results. The nurse can help relieve fear and anxiety by explaining the tests to be performed, the sensations likely to be experienced, and the patient's role in the test procedures. The nurse encourages the patient and family to voice their fears about the test results, supports the patient and family throughout the test period, and reinforces and clarifies information conveyed by the physician. The nurse also

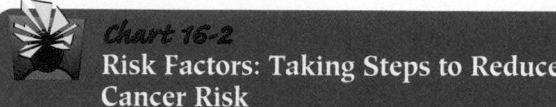

Chart 16-2

Risk Factors: Taking Steps to Reduce Cancer Risk

When teaching individual patients or groups, nurses can recommend the following cancer prevention strategies:

1. Increase consumption of fresh vegetables (especially those of the cabbage family) because studies indicate that roughage and vitamin-rich foods help to prevent certain kinds of cancer.
2. Increase fiber intake because high-fiber diets may reduce the risk for certain cancers (eg, breast, prostate, and colon).
3. Increase intake of vitamin A, which reduces the risk for esophageal, laryngeal, and lung cancers.
4. Increase intake of foods rich in vitamin C, such as citrus fruits and broccoli, which are thought to protect against stomach and esophageal cancers.
5. Practice weight control because obesity is linked to cancers of the uterus, gallbladder, breast, and colon.
6. Reduce intake of dietary fat because a high-fat diet increases the risk for breast, colon, and prostate cancers.
7. Practice moderation in consumption of salt-cured, smoked, and nitrate-cured foods; these have been linked to esophageal and gastric cancers.
8. Stop smoking cigarettes and cigars, which are carcinogens.
9. Reduce alcohol intake because drinking large amounts of alcohol increases the risk of liver cancer. (*Note:* People who drink heavily and smoke are at greater risk for cancers of the mouth, throat, larynx, and esophagus.)
10. Avoid overexposure to the sun, wear protective clothing, and use a sunscreen to prevent skin damage from ultraviolet rays that increase the risk of skin cancer.

Adapted from the "Taking Control" program of the American Cancer Society.

encourages the patient and family members to communicate and share their concerns and to discuss their questions and concerns with each other.

TUMOR STAGING AND GRADING

A complete diagnostic evaluation includes identifying the stage and grade of the tumor. This is accomplished before treatment begins to provide baseline data for evaluating outcomes of therapy and to maintain a systematic and consistent approach to ongoing diagnosis and treatment. Treatment options and prognosis are determined on the basis of staging and grading.

Staging determines the size of the tumor and the existence of metastasis. Several systems exist for classifying the anatomic extent of disease. The TNM system is frequently used. In this system, T refers to the extent of the primary tumor, N refers to lymph node involvement, and M refers to the extent of metastasis (Chart 16-3). A variety of other staging systems are used to describe the extent of cancers, such as central nervous system cancers, hematologic cancers, and malignant melanoma, that the TNM system does not describe appropriately. Staging systems also provide a convenient shorthand notation that condenses lengthy descriptions into manageable terms for comparisons of treatments and prognoses.

Grading refers to the classification of the tumor cells. Grading systems seek to define the type of tissue from which the tumor originated and the degree to which the tumor cells retain the

Table 16-3 • **American Cancer Society Recommendations for Early Detection of Cancer in Asymptomatic, Average-Risk People**

SITE	GENDER	AGE	EVALUATION	FREQUENCY
Breast	F	20–39	Clinical breast examination (CBE)	Every 3 years
			Breast self-examination (BSE)	Every month
		≥ 40	Clinical breast examination (CBE)	Every year
			Breast self-examination (BSE)	Every month
			Mammogram	Every year
Colon/rectum	M/F	≥ 50	Fecal occult blood test	Every year
			and	
			Flexible sigmoidoscopy	Every 5 years
			or	
			Colonoscopy	Every 10 years
			or	
			Double-contrast barium enema	Every 5 years
Prostate	M	≥ 50 (or <50 if at high risk)	Prostate-specific antigen and digital rectal examination (DRE)	Every year
Cervix	F	≥ 18 (or younger if sexually active)	Papanicolaou (Pap) test*	Every year
			Pelvic examination	Every year
Cancer-related checkups	M/F	≥20–39	Checkup that includes examination for cancers of the thyroid, testicles, ovaries, lymph nodes, oral cavity, and skin	Every 3 years
		40+	as well as counseling about health practices and risk factors	Every year

*After 3 or more consecutive satisfactory normal examinations, the Pap test may be performed less frequently at the discretion of the physician.
Adapted from American Cancer Society (2001). *American Cancer Society's guidelines for the early detection of cancer.* Atlanta: American Cancer Society, Inc.

Table 16-4 • **Imaging Tests Used to Detect Cancer**

TEST	DESCRIPTION	DIAGNOSTIC USES
Tumor marker identification	Analysis of substances found in blood or other body fluids that are made by the tumor or by the body in response to the tumor	Breast, colon, lung, ovarian, testicular, prostate cancers
Magnetic resonance imaging (MRI)	Use of magnetic fields and radiofrequency signals to create sectioned images of various body structures	Neurologic, pelvic, abdominal, thoracic cancers
Computed tomography (CT scan)	Use of narrow beam x-ray to scan successive layers of tissue for a cross-sectional view	Neurologic, pelvic, skeletal, abdominal, thoracic cancers
Fluoroscopy	Use of x-rays that identify contrasts in body tissue densities; may involve the use of contrast agents	Skeletal, lung, gastrointestinal cancers
Ultrasonography (ultrasound)	High-frequency sound waves echoing off body tissues are converted electronically into images; used to assess tissues deep within the body	Abdominal and pelvic cancers
Endoscopy	Direct visualization of a body cavity or passageway by insertion of an endoscope into a body cavity or opening; allows tissue biopsy, fluid aspiration and excision of small tumors; both diagnostic and therapeutic	Bronchial, gastrointestinal cancers
Nuclear medicine imaging	Uses intravenous injection or ingestion of radioisotope substances followed by imaging of tissues that have concentrated the radioisotopes	Bone, liver, kidney, spleen, brain, thyroid cancers
Positron emission tomography (PET scan)	Computed cross-sectional images of increased concentration of radioisotopes in malignant cells provide information about biologic activity of malignant cells; help distinguish between benign and malignant processes and responses to treatment	Lung, colon, liver, pancreatic, breast, esophagus cancers; Hodgkin's and non-Hodgkin's lymphoma and melanoma
Radioimmunoconjugates	Monoclonal antibodies are labeled with a radioisotope and injected intravenously into the patient; the antibodies that aggregate at the tumor site are visualized with scanners	Colorectal, breast, ovarian, head and neck cancers; lymphoma and melanoma

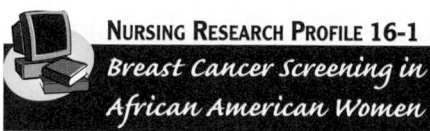

NURSING RESEARCH PROFILE 16-1
Breast Cancer Screening in African American Women

Phillips, J. P., Cohen, M. Z., & Moses, G. (1999). Breast cancer screening and African American women: Fear, fatalism, and silence. *Oncology Nursing Forum, 26*(3), 561–571.

Purpose
African American women are more likely to develop breast cancer and to be diagnosed later in the disease than Caucasian women. This qualitative study explored beliefs, attitudes, and practices related to breast cancer among African American women.

Study Sample and Design
Three focus groups were conducted with 26 African American women recruited from three employment groups to represent different socioeconomic groups. The focus group discussions were guided by a semistructured guide developed from the literature on breast cancer screening and the Health Belief Model. Topics included African American women and health, breast health, breast cancer beliefs, breast cancer screening, and health-seeking behavior. Women in the focus groups were also asked their opinions of how best to inform African American women about breast cancer screening. Focus group discussions, lasting 90 minutes, were audiotaped and the tapes of the focus groups were transcribed verbatim. The transcriptions were analyzed for themes and for similarities and differences among the three different socioeconomic groups: employed middle-income women, employed low-income women, and unemployed low-income women.

Findings
All three groups spoke of panic and fear as the predominant feelings associated with breast cancer, and all groups associated breast cancer with death. Only the middle-income women identified early detection as useful. Fear, pessimism, and belief that breast cancer is inevitable were common feelings and beliefs that can serve as barriers among African American women to participation in cancer screening. Cost of mammography, problems with transportation, and pain were also identified as barriers to screening. Although unemployed women believed that they were likely to develop breast cancer, the employed low-income women and middle-income women felt that they were somewhat likely and not very likely to develop breast cancer, respectively. The belief that breast cancer is inevitable may contribute to failure to seek screening or early treatment. All three groups indicated that there is limited discussion of breast cancer within the African American community.

Nursing Implications
The results of this study demonstrate the need to consider the beliefs and concerns of African American women when developing education and implementing screening programs. Further, health care providers need to understand the cultural and socioeconomic factors that influence screening in African American women. The findings of the study demonstrate that differences in beliefs and knowledge occur and that stereotyping by culture or ethnic group should be avoided.

Chart 16-3 · TNM Classification System

T The extent of the primary tumor
N The absence or presence and extent of regional lymph node metastasis
M The absence or presence of distant metastasis

The use of numerical subsets of the TNM components indicates the progressive extent of the malignant disease.

Primary Tumor (T)
TX Primary tumor cannot be assessed
T0 No evidence of primary tumor
Tis Carcinoma in situ
T1, T2, T3, T4 Increasing size and/or local extent of the primary tumor

Regional Lymph Nodes (N)
NX Regional lymph nodes cannot be assessed
N0 No regional lymph node metastasis
N1, N2, N3 Increasing involvement of regional lymph nodes

Distant Metastasis (M)
MX Distant metastasis cannot be assessed
M0 No distant metastasis
M1 Distant metastasis

Green, F., et al. (Eds) (2002). *AJCC cancer staging manual* (6th ed.). New York: Springer-Verlag.

---

functional and histologic characteristics of the tissue of origin. Samples of cells to be used to establish the grade of a tumor may be obtained through cytology (examination of cells from tissue scrapings, body fluids, secretions, or washings), biopsy, or surgical excision.

This information assists the health care team to predict the behavior and prognosis of various tumors. The tumor is assigned a numeric value ranging from I to IV. Grade I tumors, also known as well-differentiated tumors, closely resemble the tissue

of origin in structure and function. Tumors that do not clearly resemble the tissue of origin in structure or function are described as poorly differentiated or undifferentiated and are assigned grade IV. These tumors tend to be more aggressive and less responsive to treatment than well-differentiated tumors.

Management of Cancer

Treatment options offered to cancer patients should be based on realistic and achievable goals for each specific type of cancer. The range of possible treatment goals may include complete eradication of malignant disease (**cure**), prolonged survival and containment of cancer cell growth (**control**), or relief of symptoms associated with the disease (**palliation**).

The health care team, the patient, and the patient's family must have a clear understanding of the treatment options and goals. Open communication and support are vital as the patient and family periodically reassess treatment plans and goals when complications of therapy develop or disease progresses.

Multiple modalities are commonly used in cancer treatment. A variety of therapies, including surgery, radiation therapy, chemotherapy, and biologic response modifier (BRM) therapy, may be used at various times throughout treatment. Understanding the principles of each and how they interrelate is important in understanding the rationale and goals of treatment.

SURGERY

Surgical removal of the entire cancer remains the ideal and most frequently used treatment method. The specific surgical approach, however, may vary for several reasons. Diagnostic surgery is the definitive method of identifying the cellular characteristics that influence all treatment decisions. Surgery may be the primary method of treatment, or it may be prophylactic, palliative, or reconstructive.

Diagnostic Surgery

Diagnostic surgery, such as a **biopsy**, is usually performed to obtain a tissue sample for analysis of cells suspected to be malignant. In most instances, the biopsy is taken from the actual tumor. The three most common biopsy methods are the excisional, incisional, and needle methods.

Excisional biopsy is most frequently used for easily accessible tumors of the skin, breast, upper and lower gastrointestinal tract, and upper respiratory tract. In many cases, the surgeon can remove the entire tumor and surrounding marginal tissues as well. This removal of normal tissue beyond the tumor area decreases the possibility that residual microscopic disease cells may lead to a recurrence of the tumor. This approach not only provides the pathologist who stages and grades the cells with the entire tissue specimen but also decreases the chance of seeding the tumor (disseminating cancer cells through surrounding tissues).

Incisional biopsy is performed if the tumor mass is too large to be removed. In this case, a wedge of tissue from the tumor is removed for analysis. The cells of the tissue wedge must be representative of the tumor mass so that the pathologist can provide an accurate diagnosis. If the specimen does not contain representative tissue and cells, negative biopsy results do not guarantee the absence of cancer.

Excisional and incisional approaches are often performed through endoscopy. Surgical incision, however, may be required to determine the anatomic extent or stage of the tumor. For example, a diagnostic or staging laparotomy, the surgical opening of the abdomen to assess malignant abdominal disease, may be necessary to assess malignancies such as gastric cancer.

Needle biopsies are performed to sample suspicious masses that are easily accessible, such as some growths in the breasts, thyroid, lung, liver, and kidney. Needle biopsies are fast, relatively inexpensive, and easy to perform and usually require only local anesthesia. In general, the patient experiences slight and temporary physical discomfort. In addition, the surrounding tissues are disturbed only minimally, thus decreasing the likelihood of seeding cancer cells. Needle aspiration biopsy involves aspirating tissue fragments through a needle guided into an area suspected of bearing disease. Occasionally, radiologic imaging or magnetic resonance imaging is used to help locate the suspected area and guide the placement of the needle. In some instances, the aspiration biopsy does not yield enough tissue to permit accurate diagnosis. A needle core biopsy uses a specially designed needle to obtain a small core of tissue. Most often, this specimen is sufficient to permit accurate diagnosis.

In some situations, it is necessary to biopsy lymph nodes that are near the suspicious tumor. It is well known that many cancers can spread (metastasize) from the primary site to other areas of the body through the lymphatic circulation. Knowing whether adjacent lymph nodes contain tumor cells helps physicians plan for systemic therapies instead of, or in addition to, surgery in order to combat tumor cells that have gone beyond the primary tumor site. The use of injectable dyes and nuclear medicine imaging can assist the surgeon in identifying lymph nodes (sentinel nodes) that process lymphatic drainage for the involved area. This procedure is used in patients with melanoma and is being used with increasing frequency in patients with cancers of the breast, colon, and vulva, although it is still considered investigational.

The choice of biopsy method is based on many factors. Of greatest importance is the type of treatment anticipated if the cancer diagnosis is confirmed. Definitive surgical approaches include the original biopsy site so that any cells disseminated during the biopsy are excised at the time of surgery. Nutrition and hematologic, respiratory, renal, and hepatic function are considered in determining the method of treatment as well. If the biopsy requires general anesthesia and if subsequent surgery is likely, the effects of prolonged anesthesia on the patient are considered.

The patient and family are given an opportunity to discuss the options before definitive plans are made. The nurse, as the patient's advocate, serves as a liaison between the patient and the physician to facilitate this process. Time should be set aside to minimize interruptions. Time should be provided for the patient to ask questions and for thinking through all that has been discussed.

Surgery as Primary Treatment

When surgery is the primary approach in treating cancer, the goal is to remove the entire tumor or as much as is feasible (a procedure sometimes called debulking) and any involved surrounding tissue, including regional lymph nodes.

Two common surgical approaches used for treating primary tumors are local and wide excisions. Local excision is warranted when the mass is small. It includes removal of the mass and a small margin of normal tissue that is easily accessible. Wide or radical excisions (en bloc dissections) include removal of the primary tumor, lymph nodes, adjacent involved structures, and surrounding tissues that may be at high risk for tumor spread. This surgical method can result in disfigurement and altered functioning. Wide excisions are considered, however, if the tumor can be removed completely and the chances of cure or control are good.

In some situations, video-assisted endoscopic surgery is replacing surgeries associated with long incisions and extended recovery periods. In these procedures, an endoscope with intense lighting and an attached multichip minicamera is inserted through a small incision into the body. The surgical instruments are inserted into the surgical field through one or two additional small incisions, each about 3 cm long. The camera transmits the image of the involved area to a monitor so the surgeon can manipulate the instruments to perform the necessary procedure. This type of procedure is now being used for many thoracic and abdominal surgeries.

Salvage surgery is an additional treatment option that uses an extensive surgical approach to treat the local recurrence of the cancer after a less extensive primary approach is used. A mastectomy to treat recurrent breast cancer after primary lumpectomy and radiation is an example of salvage surgery.

In addition to the use of surgical blades or scalpels to excise the mass and surrounding tissues, several other types of surgical interventions are available. Electrosurgery makes use of electrical current to destroy the tumor cells. Cryosurgery uses liquid nitrogen to freeze tissue to cause cell destruction. Chemosurgery uses combined topical chemotherapy and layer-by-layer surgical removal of abnormal tissue. Laser surgery (*l*ight *a*mplification by *s*timulated *e*mission of *r*adiation) makes use of light and energy aimed at an exact tissue location and depth to vaporize cancer cells. Stereotactic radiosurgery (SRS) is a single and highly precise administration of high-dose radiation therapy used in some types of brain and head and neck cancers. This type of radiation has such a dramatic effect on the target area that the changes are considered to be comparable to more traditional surgical approaches (International Radiosurgery Support Association, 2000). (Radiation therapy is discussed later in this chapter.)

A multidisciplinary approach to patient care is essential during and after any type of surgery. The effects of surgery on the patient's body image, self-esteem, and functional abilities are addressed. If necessary, a plan for postoperative rehabilitation is made before the surgery is performed.

The growth and dissemination of cancer cells may have produced distant micrometastases by the time the patient seeks treatment. Therefore, attempting to remove wide margins of tissue in the hope of "getting all the cancer cells" may not be feasible. This reality substantiates the need for a coordinated multidisciplinary approach to cancer therapy. Once the surgery has been completed, one or more additional (or adjuvant) modalities may be chosen to increase the likelihood of destroying the cancer cells. However, some cancers that are treated surgically in the very early stages are considered to be curable (eg, skin cancers, testicular cancers).

Prophylactic Surgery

Prophylactic surgery involves removing nonvital tissues or organs that are likely to develop cancer. The following factors are considered when electing prophylactic surgery:

- Family history and genetic predisposition
- Presence or absence of symptoms
- Potential risks and benefits
- Ability to detect cancer at an early stage
- Patient's acceptance of the postoperative outcome

Colectomy, mastectomy, and oophorectomy are examples of prophylactic operations. Recent developments in the ability to identify genetic markers indicative of a predisposition to develop some types of cancer may play a role in decisions concerning prophylactic surgeries. Some controversy, however, exists about adequate justification for prophylactic surgical procedures. For example, a strong family history of breast cancer, positive BRCA-1 or BRCA-2 findings, an abnormal physical finding on breast examination such as progressive nodularity and cystic disease, a proven history of breast cancer in the opposite breast, abnormal mammography findings, and abnormal biopsy results may be factors considered in making the decision to proceed with a prophylactic mastectomy (Houshmand, Campbell, Briggs, McFadden & Al-Tweigeri, 2000; Zimmerman, 2002).

Because the long-term physiologic and psychological effects are unknown, prophylactic surgery is offered selectively to patients and discussed thoroughly with the patient and family. Preoperative teaching and counseling, as well as long-term follow-up, are provided.

Palliative Surgery

When cure is not possible, the goals of treatment are to make the patient as comfortable as possible and to promote a satisfying and productive life for as long as possible. Whether the period is extremely brief or lengthy, the major goal is a high quality of life—with quality defined by the patient and family. Honest and informative communication with the patient and family about the goal of surgery is essential to avoid false hope and disappointment.

Palliative surgery is performed in an attempt to relieve complications of cancer, such as ulcerations, obstructions, hemorrhage, pain, and malignant effusions (Table 16-5).

Reconstructive Surgery

Reconstructive surgery may follow curative or radical surgery and is carried out in an attempt to improve function or obtain a more desirable cosmetic effect. It may be performed in one operation

Table 16-5 • Indications for Palliative Surgical Procedures

PROCEDURE	INDICATIONS
Pleural drainage tube placement	Pleural effusion
Peritoneal drainage tube placement (Tenckoff catheter)	Ascites
Abdominal shunt placement (Levine shunt)	Ascites
Pericardial drainage tube placement	Pericardial effusion
Colostomy or ileostomy	Bowel obstruction
Gastrostomy, jejunostomy tube placement	Upper gastrointestinal tract obstruction
Biliary stent placement	Biliary obstruction
Ureteral stent placement	Ureteral obstruction
Nerve block	Pain
Cordotomy	Pain
Venous access device placement (for administering parenteral analgesics)	Pain
Epidural catheter placement (for administering epidural analgesics)	Pain
Hormone manipulation (removal of ovaries, testes, adrenals, pituitary)	Tumors that depend on hormones for growth

or in stages. Patients are instructed about possible reconstructive surgical options before the primary surgery by the surgeon who will perform the reconstruction. Reconstructive surgery may be indicated for breast, head and neck, and skin cancers.

The nurse must recognize the patient's needs and the impact that altered functioning and altered body image may have on quality of life. Providing the patient and family with opportunities to discuss these issues is imperative. The needs of the individual must be accurately assessed and validated in each situation for any type of reconstructive surgery.

Nursing Management in Cancer Surgery

The patient undergoing surgery for cancer requires general perioperative nursing care, as described in Unit 4, along with specific care related to the patient's age, organ impairment, nutritional deficits, disorders of coagulation, and altered immunity that may increase the risk for postoperative complications. Combining other treatment methods, such as radiation and chemotherapy, with surgery also contributes to postoperative complications, such as infection, impaired wound healing, altered pulmonary or renal function, and the development of deep vein thrombosis. In these situations, the nurse completes a thorough preoperative assessment for all factors that may affect patients undergoing surgical procedures.

The patient undergoing surgery for the diagnosis or treatment of cancer is often anxious about the surgical procedure, possible findings, postoperative limitations, changes in normal body functions, and prognosis. The patient and family require time and assistance to deal with the possible changes and outcomes resulting from the surgery.

The nurse provides education and emotional support by assessing patient and family needs and exploring with the patient and family their fears and coping mechanisms, encouraging them to take an active role in decision making when possible. When the patient or family asks about the results of diagnostic testing and surgical procedures, the nurse's response is guided by the information the physician previously conveyed to them. The patient and family may also ask the nurse to explain and clarify information that the physician initially provided but that they did not grasp because they were anxious at the time. It is important for the nurse to communicate frequently with the physician and other health care team members to be certain that the information provided is consistent.

After surgery, the nurse assesses the patient's responses to the surgery and monitors for possible complications, such as infection, bleeding, thrombophlebitis, wound dehiscence, fluid and electrolyte imbalance, and organ dysfunction. The nurse also provides for patient comfort. Postoperative teaching addresses wound care, activity, nutrition, and medication information.

Plans for discharge, follow-up and home care, and treatment are initiated as early as possible to ensure continuity of care from hospital to home or from a cancer referral center to the patient's local hospital and health care provider. Patients and families are also encouraged to use community resources such as the American Cancer Society or Make Today Count for support and information.

RADIATION THERAPY

In **radiation therapy**, ionizing radiation is used to interrupt cellular growth. More than half of patients with cancer receive a form of radiation therapy at some point during treatment. Radiation may be used to cure the cancer, as in Hodgkin's disease, testicular seminomas, thyroid carcinomas, localized cancers of the head and neck, and cancers of the uterine cervix. Radiation therapy may also be used to control malignant disease when a tumor cannot be removed surgically or when local nodal metastasis is present, or it can be used prophylactically to prevent leukemic infiltration to the brain or spinal cord.

Palliative radiation therapy is used to relieve the symptoms of metastatic disease, especially when the cancer has spread to brain, bone, or soft tissue, or to treat oncologic emergencies, such as superior vena cava syndrome or spinal cord compression.

Two types of ionizing radiation—electromagnetic rays (x-rays and gamma rays) and particles (electrons [beta particles], protons, neutrons, and alpha particles)—can lead to tissue disruption. The most harmful tissue disruption is the alteration of the DNA molecule within the cells of the tissue. Ionizing radiation breaks the strands of the DNA helix, leading to cell death. Ionizing radiation can also ionize constituents of body fluids, especially water, leading to the formation of free radicals and irreversibly damaging DNA. If the DNA is incapable of repair, the cell may die immediately, or it may initiate cellular suicide (apoptosis), a genetically programmed cell death.

Cells are most vulnerable to the disruptive effects of radiation during DNA synthesis and mitosis (early S, G2, and M phases of the cell cycle). Therefore, those body tissues that undergo frequent cell division are most sensitive to radiation therapy. These tissues include bone marrow, lymphatic tissue, epithelium of the gastrointestinal tract, hair cells, and gonads. Slower-growing tissues or tissues at rest are relatively radioresistant (less sensitive to the effects of radiation). Such tissues include muscle, cartilage, and connective tissues.

A radiosensitive tumor is one that can be destroyed by a dose of radiation that still allows for cell regeneration in the normal tissue. Tumors that are well oxygenated also appear to be more sensitive to radiation. In theory, therefore, radiation therapy may be enhanced if more oxygen can be delivered to tumors. In addition, if the radiation is delivered when most tumor cells are cycling through the cell cycle, the number of cancer cells destroyed (cell-killing) is maximal.

Certain chemicals, including chemotherapy agents, act as radiosensitizers and sensitize more hypoxic (oxygen-poor) tumors to the effects of radiation therapy. Radiation is delivered to tumor sites by external or internal means.

External Radiation

If external radiation therapy is used, one of several delivery methods may be chosen, depending on the depth of the tumor. Depending on the amount of energy they contain, x-rays can be used to destroy cancerous cells at the skin surface or deeper in the body. The higher the energy, the deeper the penetration into the body. Kilovoltage therapy devices deliver the maximal radiation dose to superficial lesions, such as lesions of the skin and breast, whereas linear accelerators and betatron machines produce higher-energy x-rays and deliver their dosage to deeper structures with less harm to the skin and less scattering of radiation within the body tissues. Gamma rays are another form of energy used in radiation therapy. This energy is produced from the spontaneous decay of naturally occurring radioactive elements such as cobalt 60. The gamma rays also deliver this radiation dose beneath the skin surface, sparing skin tissue from adverse effects.

Some centers nationwide treat more hypoxic, radiation-resistant tumors with particle-beam radiation therapy. This type of therapy accelerates subatomic particles (neutrons, pions, heavy ions) through body tissue. This therapy, which is also known as high linear energy transfer radiation, damages target cells as well as cells in its pathway.

A few centers are using intraoperative radiation therapy (IORT), which involves delivering a single dose of high-fraction radiation therapy to the exposed tumor bed while the body cavity is open during surgery. Cancers for which IORT is being used include gastric, pancreatic, colorectal, bladder, and cervical cancers and sarcomas. Toxicity with IORT is minimized because the radiation is precisely targeted to the diseased areas, and exposure to overlying skin and structures is avoided.

Internal Radiation

Internal radiation implantation, or **brachytherapy**, delivers a high dose of radiation to a localized area. The specific radioisotope for implantation is selected on the basis of its half-life, which is the time it takes for half of its radioactivity to decay. This internal radiation can be implanted by means of needles, seeds, beads, or catheters into body cavities (vagina, abdomen, pleura) or interstitial compartments (breast). Brachytherapy may also be administered orally as with the isotope I^{131}, used to treat thyroid carcinomas.

Intracavitary radioisotopes are frequently used to treat gynecologic cancers. In these malignancies, the radioisotopes are inserted into specially positioned applicators after the position is verified by x-ray. These radioisotopes remain in place for a prescribed period and then are removed. Patients are maintained on bed rest and log-rolled to prevent displacement of the intracavitary delivery device. An indwelling urinary catheter is inserted to ensure that the bladder remains empty. Low-residue diets and antidiarrheal agents, such as diphenoxylate (Lomotil), are provided to prevent bowel movement during therapy, to prevent the radioisotopes from being displaced.

Interstitial implants, used in treating such malignancies as prostate, pancreatic, or breast cancer, may be temporary or permanent, depending on the radioisotopes used. These implants usually consist of seeds, needles, wires, or small catheters positioned to provide a local radiation source and are less frequently dislodged. With internal radiation therapy, the farther the tissue is from the radiation source, the lower the dosage. This spares the noncancerous tissue from the radiation dose.

Because patients receiving internal radiation emit radiation while the implant is in place, contacts with the health care team are guided by principles of time, distance, and shielding to minimize exposure of personnel to radiation. Safety precautions used in caring for the patient receiving brachytherapy include assigning the person to a private room, posting appropriate notices about radiation safety precautions, having staff members wear dosimeter badges, making sure that pregnant staff members are not assigned to this patient's care, prohibiting visits by children or pregnant visitors, limiting visits from others to 30 minutes daily, and seeing that visitors maintain a 6-foot distance from the radiation source.

Radiation Dosage

The radiation dosage is dependent on the sensitivity of the target tissues to radiation and on the tumor size. The lethal tumor dose is defined as that dose that will eradicate 95% of the tumor yet preserve normal tissue. The total radiation dose is delivered over several weeks to allow healthy tissue to repair and to achieve greater cell kill by exposing more cells to the radiation as they begin active cell division. Repeated radiation treatments over time (fractionated doses) also allow for the periphery of the tumor to be reoxygenated repeatedly because tumors shrink from the outside inward. This increases the radiosensitivity of the tumor, thereby increasing tumor cell death.

Toxicity

Toxicity of radiation therapy is localized to the region being irradiated. Toxicity may be increased when concomitant chemotherapy is administered. Acute local reactions occur when normal cells in the treatment area are also destroyed and cellular death exceeds cellular regeneration. Body tissues most affected are those that normally proliferate rapidly, such as the skin, the epithelial lining of the gastrointestinal tract, including the oral cavity, and the bone marrow. Altered skin integrity is a common effect and can include alopecia (hair loss), erythema, and shedding of skin (desquamation). After treatments have been completed, reepithelialization occurs.

Alterations in oral mucosa secondary to radiation therapy include stomatitis, **xerostomia** (dryness of the mouth), change and loss of taste, and decreased salivation. The entire gastrointestinal mucosa may be involved, and esophageal irritation with chest pain and dysphagia may result. Anorexia, nausea, vomiting, and diarrhea may occur if the stomach or colon is in the irradiated field. Symptoms subside and gastrointestinal reepithelialization occurs after treatments are complete.

Bone marrow cells proliferate rapidly, and if bone marrow–producing sites are included in the radiation field anemia, leukopenia (decreased white blood cells [WBCs]), and **thrombocytopenia** (a decrease in platelets) may result. Patients are then at increased risk for infection and bleeding until blood cell counts return to normal. Chronic anemia may occur. Research continues to develop radioprotective agents that can protect normal tissue from radiation damage.

Certain systemic side effects are also commonly experienced by patients receiving radiation therapy. These manifestations, which are generalized, include fatigue, malaise, and anorexia. This syndrome may be secondary to substances released when tumor cells break down. The effects are temporary and subside with the cessation of treatment.

Late effects of radiation therapy may also occur in various body tissues. These effects are chronic, usually produce fibrotic changes secondary to a decreased vascular supply, and are irreversible. These late effects can be most severe when they involve vital organs such as the lungs, heart, central nervous system, and bladder. Toxicities may intensify when radiation is combined with other treatment modalities.

Nursing Management in Radiation Therapy

The patient receiving radiation therapy and the family often have questions and concerns about its safety. To answer questions and allay fears about the effects of radiation on others, on the tumor, and on the patient's normal tissues and organs, the nurse can explain the procedure for delivering radiation and describe the equipment, the duration of the procedure (often minutes only), the possible need for immobilizing the patient during the procedure, and the absence of new sensations, including pain, during the procedure. If a radioactive implant is used, the nurse informs the patient and family about the restrictions placed on visitors and health care personnel and other radiation precautions. Patients also need to understand their own role before, during, and after the procedure. See Chapter 47 for further discussion of radiation treatment for gynecologic cancers.

PROTECTING THE SKIN AND ORAL MUCOSA

The nurse assesses the patient's skin, nutritional status, and general feeling of well-being. The skin and oral mucosa are assessed frequently for changes (particularly if radiation therapy is directed to these areas). The skin is protected from irritation, and the patient is instructed to avoid using ointments, lotions, or powders on the area.

Gentle oral hygiene is essential to remove debris, prevent irritation, and promote healing. If systemic symptoms, such as weakness and fatigue, occur, the patient may need assistance with activities of daily living and personal hygiene. Additionally, the nurse offers reassurance by explaining that these symptoms are a result of the treatment and do not represent deterioration or progression of the disease.

PROTECTING THE CAREGIVERS

When a patient has a radioactive implant in place, nurses and other health care providers need to protect themselves as well as the patient from the effects of radiation. Specific instructions are usually provided by the radiation safety officer from the x-ray department. The instructions identify the maximum time that can be spent safely in the patient's room, the shielding equipment to be used, and special precautions and actions to be taken if the implant is dislodged. The nurse should explain the rationale for these precautions to keep the patient from feeling unduly isolated.

CHEMOTHERAPY

In **chemotherapy**, antineoplastic agents are used in an attempt to destroy tumor cells by interfering with cellular functions and reproduction. Chemotherapy is used primarily to treat systemic disease rather than lesions that are localized and amenable to surgery or radiation. Chemotherapy may be combined with surgery or radiation therapy, or both, to reduce tumor size preoperatively, to destroy any remaining tumor cells postoperatively, or to treat some forms of leukemia. The goals of chemotherapy (cure, control, palliation) must be realistic because they will define the medications to be used and the aggressiveness of the treatment plan.

Cell Kill and the Cell Cycle

Each time a tumor is exposed to a chemotherapeutic agent, a percentage of tumor cells (20% to 99%, depending on dosage) is destroyed. Repeated doses of chemotherapy are necessary over a prolonged period to achieve regression of the tumor. Eradication of 100% of the tumor is nearly impossible, but a goal of treatment is to eradicate enough of the tumor so that the remaining tumor cells can be destroyed by the body's immune system.

Actively proliferating cells within a tumor (growth fraction) are the most sensitive to chemotherapeutic agents. Nondividing cells capable of future proliferation are the least sensitive to antineoplastic medications and consequently are potentially dangerous. The nondividing cells must be destroyed, however, to eradicate a cancer completely. Repeated cycles of chemotherapy are used to kill more tumor cells by destroying these nondividing cells as they begin active cell division.

Reproduction of both healthy and malignant cells follows the cell cycle pattern (Fig. 16-2). The cell cycle time is the time required for one tissue cell to divide and reproduce two identical daughter cells. The cell cycle of any cell has four distinct phases, each with a vital underlying function:

1. G_1 phase—RNA and protein synthesis occur.
2. S phase—DNA synthesis occurs.

3. G_2 phase—premitotic phase; DNA synthesis is complete, mitotic spindle forms.
4. Mitosis—cell division occurs.

The G_0 phase, the resting or dormant phase of cells, can occur after mitosis and during the G_1 phase. In the G_0 phase are those dangerous cells that are not actively dividing but have the potential for replicating. The administration of certain chemotherapeutic agents (as well as administration of some other forms of therapy) is coordinated with the cell cycle.

Classification of Chemotherapeutic Agents

Certain chemotherapeutic agents (cell cycle–specific drugs) destroy cells actively reproducing by means of the cell cycle. Many of these agents are specific to certain phases of the cell cycle. Most affect cells in the S phase by interfering with DNA and RNA synthesis. Others, such as the vinca or plant alkaloids, are specific to the M phase, where they halt mitotic spindle formation.

Chemotherapeutic agents that act independently of the cell cycle phases are termed cell cycle–nonspecific agents. These agents usually have a prolonged effect on cells, leading to cellular damage or death. Many treatment plans combine cell cycle–specific and cell cycle–nonspecific agents to increase the number of vulnerable tumor cells killed during a treatment period.

Chemotherapeutic agents are also classified according to various chemical groups, each with a different mechanism of action. These include the alkylating agents, nitrosureas, antimetabolites, antitumor antibiotics, plant alkaloids, hormonal agents, and miscellaneous agents. The classification, mechanism of action, common drugs, cell cycle specificity, and common side effects of antineoplastic agents are listed in Table 16-6.

Chemotherapeutic agents from each category may be used to enhance the tumor cell kill during therapy by creating multiple cellular lesions. Combined medication therapy relies on medications of differing toxicities and with synergistic actions. Using combination drug therapy also prevents development of drug-resistant mechanisms.

Combining older medications with other agents, such as levamisole, leucovorin, hormones, or interferons (IFN), has shown some benefit in combating resistance of cells to chemotherapeutic agents. Newer investigational agents are being studied for effectiveness in resistant tumor lines. For more information about investigative drugs, see Chart 16-4.

Administration of Chemotherapeutic Agents

Chemotherapeutic agents may be administered in the hospital, clinic, or home setting by topical, oral, intravenous, intramuscular, subcutaneous, arterial, intracavitary, and intrathecal routes. The administration route usually depends on the type of agent, the required dose, and the type, location, and extent of tumor being treated. Guidelines for the administration of chemotherapy have been developed by the Oncology Nursing Society. Patient education is essential to maximize safety if chemotherapy is administered in the patient's home (Chart 16-5).

DOSAGE

Dosage of antineoplastic agents is based primarily on the patient's total body surface area, previous response to chemotherapy or radiation therapy, and major organ function.

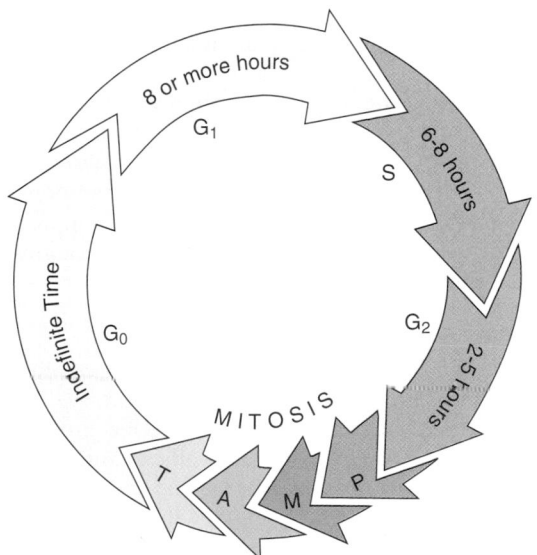

FIGURE 16-2 Phases of the cell cycle extend over the interval between the midpoint of mitosis to the subsequent end point in mitosis in a daughter cell. G_1 is the postmitotic phase during which ribonucleic acid (RNA) and protein synthesis are increased and cell growth occurs. G_0 is the resting, or dormant, phase of the cell cycle. In the S phase, nucleic acids are synthesized and chromosomes replicated in preparation for cell mitosis. During G_2, RNA and protein synthesis occurs as in G_1. (P = prophase, M = metaphase, A = anaphase, T = telophase.) From Porth, C. M. (2002). *Pathophysiology: Concepts of altered health states* (6th ed). Philadelphia: Lippincott Williams & Wilkins.

Table 16-6 • Antineoplastic Agents

DRUG CLASS AND EXAMPLES	MECHANISM OF ACTION	CELL CYCLE SPECIFICITY	COMMON SIDE EFFECTS
Alkylating Agents busulfan, carboplatin, chlorambucil, cisplatin, cyclophosphamide, dacarbazine, hexamethyl melamine, ifosfamide, melphalan, nitrogen mustard, thiotepa	Alter DNA structure by misreading DNA code, initiating breaks in the DNA molecule, cross-linking DNA strands	Cell cycle–nonspecific	Bone marrow suppression, nausea, vomiting, cystitis (cyclophosphamide, ifosfamide), stomatitis, alopecia, gonadal suppression, renal toxicity (cisplatin)
Nitrosureas carmustine (BCNU), lomustine (CCNU), semustine (methyl CCNU), streptozocin	Similar to the alkylating agents; cross the blood–brain barrier	Cell cycle–nonspecific	Delayed and cumulative myelosuppression, especially thrombocytopenia; nausea, vomiting
Topoisomerase I Inhibitors irinotecan, topotecan	Induce breaks in the DNA strand by binding to enzyme topoisomerase I, preventing cells from dividing	Cell cycle–specific	Bone marrow suppression, diarrhea, nausea, vomiting, hepatotoxicity
Antimetabolites 5-azacytadine, cytarabine, edatrexate fludarabine, 5-fluorouracil (5-FU), FUDR, gemcitabine, hydroxyurea, leustatin, 6-mercaptopurine, methotrexate, pentostatin, 6-thioguanine	Interfere with the biosynthesis of metabolites or nucleic acids necessary for RNA and DNA synthesis	Cell cycle–specific (S phase)	Nausea, vomiting, diarrhea, bone marrow suppression, proctitis, stomatitis, renal toxicity (methotrexate), hepatotoxicity
Antitumor Antibiotics bleomycin, dactinomycin, daunorubicin, doxorubicin (Adriamycin), idarubicin, mitomycin, mitoxantrone, plicamycin	Interfere with DNA synthesis by binding DNA; prevent RNA synthesis	Cell cycle–nonspecific	Bone marrow suppression, nausea, vomiting, alopecia, anorexia, cardiac toxicity (daunorubicin, doxorubicin)
Mitotic Spindle Poisons *Plant alkaloids:* etoposide, teniposide, vinblastine, vincristine (VCR), vindesine, vinorelbine *Taxanes:* paclitaxel, docetaxel	Arrest metaphase by inhibiting mitotic tubular formation (spindle); inhibit DNA and protein synthesis	Cell cycle–specific (M phase)	Bone marrow suppression (mild with VCR), neuropathies (VCR), stomatitis
	Arrest metaphase by inhibiting tubulin depolymerization	Cell cycle–specific (M phase)	Bradycardia, hypersensitivity reactions, bone marrow suppression, alopecia, neuropathies
Hormonal Agents androgens and antiandrogens, estrogens and antiestrogens, progestins and antiprogestins, aromatase inhibitors, luteinizing hormone–releasing hormone analogs, steroids	Bind to hormone receptor sites that alter cellular growth; block binding of estrogens to receptor sites (antiestrogens); inhibit RNA synthesis; suppress aromatase of P450 system, which decreases estrogen level	Cell cycle–nonspecific	Hypercalcemia, jaundice, increased appetite, masculinization, feminization, sodium and fluid retention, nausea, vomiting, hot flashes, vaginal dryness
Miscellaneous Agents asparaginase, procarbazine	Unknown or too complex to categorize	Varies	Anorexia, nausea, vomiting, bone marrow suppression, hepatotoxicity, anaphylaxis, hypotension, altered glucose metabolism

SPECIAL PROBLEMS: EXTRAVASATION

Special care must be taken whenever intravenous vesicant agents are administered. **Vesicants** are those agents that, if deposited into the subcutaneous tissue (**extravasation**), cause tissue necrosis and damage to underlying tendons, nerves, and blood vessels. Although the complete mechanism of tissue destruction is unclear, it is known that the pH of many antineoplastic drugs is responsible for the severe inflammatory reaction as well as the ability of these drugs to bind to tissue DNA. Sloughing and ulceration of the tissue may be so severe that skin grafting may be necessary. The full extent of tissue damage may take several weeks to become apparent. Medications classified as vesicants include dactinomycin,

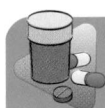

Chart 16-4 • PHARMACOLOGY
Investigational Antineoplastic Therapies and Clinical Trials

Evaluation of the effectiveness and toxic potential of promising new modalities for preventing, diagnosing, and treating cancer is accomplished through clinical trials. Before new chemotherapy agents are approved for clinical use, they are subjected to rigorous and lengthy evaluations to identify beneficial effects, adverse effects, and safety.

- *Phase I* clinical trials determine optimal dosing, scheduling, and toxicity.
- *Phase II* trials determine effectiveness with specific tumor types and further define toxicities. Participants in these early trials are most often those who have not responded to standard forms of treatment. Because phase I and II trials may be viewed as last-chance efforts, patients and families are fully informed about the experimental nature of the trial therapies. Although it is hoped that investigational therapy will effectively treat the disease, the purpose of early phase trials is to gather information concerning maximal tolerated doses, adverse effects, and effects of the antineoplastic agents on tumor growth.
- *Phase III* clinical trials establish the effectiveness of new medications or procedures as compared with conventional approaches. Nurses may assist in the recruitment, consent, and education processes for patients who participate. In many cases, nurses are instrumental in monitoring adherence, assisting patients to adhere to the parameters of the trial, and documenting data describing patients' responses. The physical and emotional needs of patients in clinical trials are addressed in much the same way as those of patients who receive standard forms of cancer treatment.
- *Phase IV* testing further investigates medications in terms of new uses, dosing schedule, and toxicities.

daunorubicin, doxorubicin (Adriamycin), nitrogen mustard, mitomycin, vinblastine, vincristine, and vindesine.

Only specially trained physicians and nurses should administer vesicants. Careful selection of peripheral veins, skilled venipuncture, and careful administration of medications are essential. Indications of extravasation during administration of vesicant agents include the following:

- Absence of blood return from the intravenous catheter
- Resistance to flow of intravenous fluid
- Swelling, pain, or redness at the site

If extravasation is suspected, the medication administration is stopped immediately, and ice is applied to the site (unless the extravasated vesicant is a vinca alkaloid). The physician may aspirate any infiltrated medication from the tissues and inject a neutralizing solution into the area to reduce tissue damage. Selection of the neutralizing solution depends on the extravasated agent. Examples of neutralizing solutions include sodium thiosulfate, hyaluronidase, and sodium bicarbonate. Recommendations and guidelines for managing vesicant extravasation have been issued by individual medication manufacturers, pharmacies, and the Oncology Nursing Society, and they differ from one medication to the next.

When frequent, prolonged administration of antineoplastic vesicants is anticipated, right atrial Silastic catheters or venous access devices may be inserted to promote safety during medication administration and reduce problems with access to the circulatory system (Figs. 16-3 and 16-4). Complications associated with their use include infection and thrombosis.

TOXICITY

Toxicity associated with chemotherapy can be acute or chronic. Cells with rapid growth rates (eg, epithelium, bone marrow, hair follicles, sperm) are very susceptible to damage, and various body systems may be affected as well.

Gastrointestinal System. Nausea and vomiting are the most common side effects of chemotherapy and may persist for up to 24 hours after its administration. The vomiting centers in the brain are stimulated by (1) activation of the receptors found in the chemoreceptor trigger zone (CTZ) of the medulla; (2) stimulation of peripheral autonomic pathways (gastrointestinal tract and pharynx); (3) stimulation of the vestibular pathways (inner ear imbalances, labyrinth input); (4) cognitive stimulation (central nervous system disease, anticipatory nausea and vomiting); and (5) a combination of these factors.

Medications that can decrease nausea and vomiting include serotonin blockers, such as ondansetron, granisetron, and dolasetron, which block serotonin receptors of the gastrointestinal tract and CTZ, and dopaminergic blockers, such as metoclopramide (Reglan), which block dopamine receptors of the CTZ. Phenothiazines, sedatives, corticosteroids, and histamines are used in combination with serotonin blockers with the more emetogenic chemotherapeutic regimens (Bremerkamp, 2000).

Chart 16-5
Home Care Checklist • Chemotherapy Administration

At the completion of the home care instruction, the patient or caregiver will be able to:	Patient	Caregiver
• Demonstrate how to administer the chemotherapy agent in the home.	✓	✓
• Demonstrate safe disposal of needles, syringes, IV supplies, or unused chemotherapy medications.	✓	✓
• List possible side effects of chemotherapeutic agents.	✓	✓
• List complications of medications necessitating a call to the nurse or physician.	✓	✓
• List complications of medications necessitating a visit to the emergency department.	✓	✓
• List names and telephone numbers of resource personnel involved in care (ie, home care nurse, infusion services, IV vendor, equipment company).	✓	✓
• Explain treatment plan (protocol) and importance of upcoming visits to physician.	✓	✓

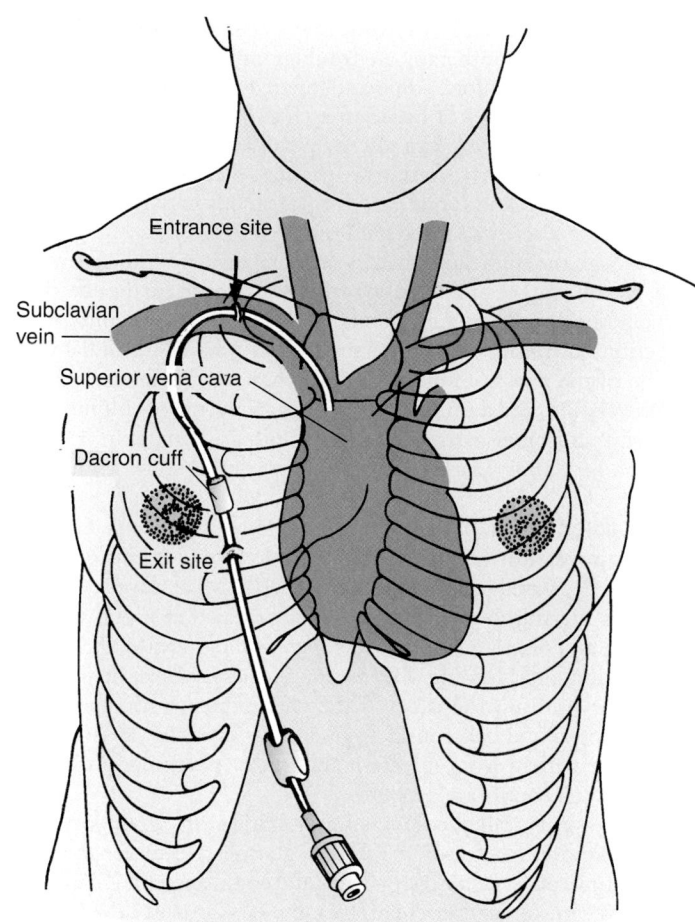

FIGURE 16-3 Right atrial catheter. The right atrial catheter is inserted into the subclavian vein and advanced until its tip lies in the superior vena cava just above the right atrium. The proximal end is then tunneled from the entry site through the subcutaneous tissue of the chest wall and brought out through an exit site on the chest. The Dacron cuff anchors the catheter in place and serves as a barrier to infection.

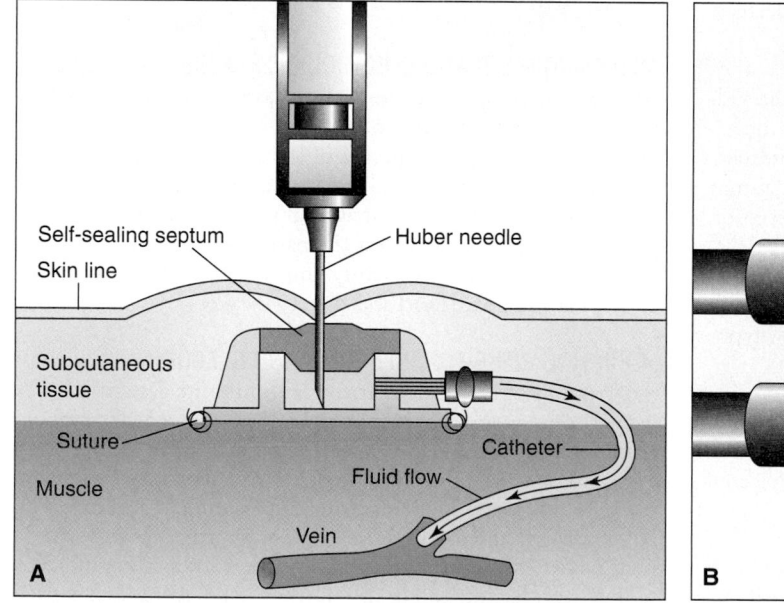

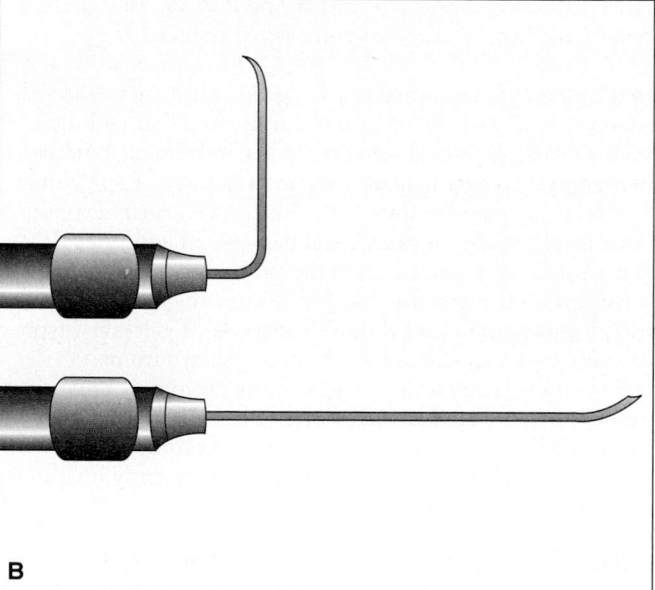

FIGURE 16-4 Implanted vascular access device. (**A**) A schematic diagram of an implanted vascular access device used for administering medication, fluids, blood products, and nutrition. The self-sealing septum permits repeated puncture by Huber needles without damage or leakage. (**B**) Two Huber needles used to enter the implanted vascular port. The 90-degree needle is used for top-entry ports for continuous infusions.

Delayed nausea and vomiting that occur later than 48 to 72 hours after chemotherapy are troublesome for some patients. To minimize discomfort, some antiemetic medications are necessary for the first week at home after chemotherapy. Relaxation techniques and imagery can also help to decrease stimuli contributing to symptoms. Altering the patient's diet to include small frequent meals, bland foods, and comfort foods may reduce the frequency or severity of these symptoms.

Although the epithelium that lines the oral cavity quickly renews itself, its rapid rate of proliferation makes it susceptible to the effects of chemotherapy. As a result, stomatitis and anorexia are common. The entire gastrointestinal tract is susceptible to mucositis (inflammation of the mucosal lining), and diarrhea is a common result. Antimetabolites and antitumor antibiotics are the major culprits in mucositis and other gastrointestinal symptoms. Irinotecan is responsible for causing diarrhea, which can be severe in some patients.

Hematopoietic System. Most chemotherapeutic agents cause **myelosuppression** (depression of bone marrow function), resulting in decreased production of blood cells. Myelosuppression decreases the number of WBCs (leukopenia), red blood cells (anemia), and platelets (thrombocytopenia) and increases the risk for infection and bleeding. Depression of these cells is the usual reason for limiting the dose of the chemotherapeutic agents. Monitoring blood cell counts frequently is essential, as is protecting the patient from infection and injury, particularly while the blood cell counts are depressed.

Other agents, called colony-stimulating factors (granulocyte colony-stimulating factor [G-CSF], granulocyte-macrophage colony-stimulating factor [GM-CSF], and erythropoietin [EPO]), can be administered after chemotherapy. G-CSF and GM-CSF stimulate the bone marrow to produce WBCs, especially neutrophils, at an accelerated rate, thus decreasing the duration of neutropenia. The colony-stimulating factors decrease the episodes of infection and the need for antibiotics and allow for more timely cycling of chemotherapy with less need to reduce the dosage. EPO stimulates red blood cell production, thus decreasing the symptoms of chronic administered anemia.

Renal System. Chemotherapeutic agents can damage the kidneys because of their direct effects during excretion and the accumulation of end products after cell lysis. Cisplatin, methotrexate, and mitomycin are particularly toxic to the kidneys. Rapid tumor cell lysis after chemotherapy results in increased urinary excretion of uric acid, which can cause renal damage. In addition, intracellular contents are released into the circulation, resulting in excessive levels of potassium and phosphates (hyperkalemia and hyperphosphatemia) and diminished levels of calcium (hypocalcemia). (See later discussion of tumor lysis syndrome.)

Monitoring blood urea nitrogen, serum creatinine, creatinine clearance, and serum electrolyte levels is essential. Adequate hydration, alkalinization of the urine to prevent formation of uric acid crystals, and the use of allopurinol are frequently indicated to prevent these side effects.

Cardiopulmonary System. Antitumor antibiotics (daunorubicin and doxorubicin) are known to cause irreversible cumulative cardiac toxicities, especially when total dosage reaches 550 mg/m². Cardiac ejection fraction (volume of blood ejected from the heart with each beat) and signs of congestive heart failure must be monitored closely. Bleomycin, carmustine (BCNU), and busulfan are known for their cumulative toxic effects on lung function. Pulmonary fibrosis can be a long-term effect of prolonged dosage with these agents. Therefore, the patient is monitored closely for changes in pulmonary function, including pulmonary function test results. Total cumulative doses of bleomycin are not to exceed 400 units.

Reproductive System. Testicular and ovarian function can be affected by chemotherapeutic agents, resulting in possible sterility. Normal ovulation, early menopause, or permanent sterility may result. In men, temporary or permanent azoospermia (absence of spermatozoa) may develop. Reproductive cells may be damaged during treatment, resulting in chromosomal abnormalities in offspring. Banking of sperm is recommended for men before treatments are initiated to protect against sterility or any mutagenic damage to sperm.

Patients and their partners need to be informed about potential changes in reproductive function resulting from chemotherapy. They are advised to use reliable methods of birth control while receiving chemotherapy and not to assume that sterility has resulted.

Neurologic System. The taxanes and plant alkaloids, especially vincristine, can cause neurologic damage with repeated doses. Peripheral neuropathies, loss of deep tendon reflexes, and paralytic ileus may occur. These side effects are usually reversible and disappear after completion of chemotherapy. Cisplatin is also responsible for peripheral neuropathies; hearing loss due to damage to the acoustic nerve can also occur.

Miscellaneous. Fatigue is a distressing side effect for most patients that greatly affects quality of life. Fatigue can be debilitating and last for months after treatment.

Nursing Management in Chemotherapy

The nurse has an important role in assessing and managing many of the problems experienced by the patient undergoing chemotherapy. Because of the systemic effects on normal as well as malignant cells, these problems are often widespread, affecting many body systems.

ASSESSING FLUID AND ELECTROLYTE STATUS

Anorexia, nausea, vomiting, altered taste, and diarrhea put the patient at risk for nutritional and fluid and electrolyte disturbances. Changes in the mucosa of the gastrointestinal tract may lead to irritation of the oral cavity and intestinal tract, further threatening the patient's nutritional status. Therefore, it is important for the nurse to assess the patient's nutritional and fluid and electrolyte status frequently and to use creative ways to encourage an adequate fluid and dietary intake.

MODIFYING RISKS FOR INFECTION AND BLEEDING

Suppression of the bone marrow and immune system is an expected consequence of chemotherapy and frequently serves as a guide in determining appropriate chemotherapy dosage. However, this effect also increases the risk for anemia, infection, and bleeding disorders. Therefore, nursing assessment and care focus on identifying and modifying factors that further increase the patient's risk. Aseptic technique and gentle handling are indicated to prevent infection and trauma. Laboratory test results, particularly blood cell counts, are monitored closely. Untoward changes in blood test results and signs of infection and bleeding must be reported promptly. The patient and family members are instructed about measures to prevent these problems at home (see Plan of Nursing Care for more information).

(text continues on page 343)

Plan of Nursing Care
The Patient With Cancer

Nursing Interventions	Rationale	Expected Outcomes

Nursing Diagnosis: Risk for infection related to altered immunologic response
Goal: Prevention of infection

Nursing Interventions	Rationale	Expected Outcomes
1. Assess patient for evidence of infection: a. Check vital signs every 4 hours. b. Monitor WBC count and differential each day. c. Inspect all sites that may serve as entry ports for pathogens (intravenous sites, wounds, skin folds, bony prominences, perineum, and oral cavity). 2. Report fever ≥38.3°C (101°F), chills, diaphoresis, swelling, heat, pain, erythema, exudate on any body surfaces. Also report change in respiratory or mental status, urinary frequency or burning, malaise, myalgias, arthralgias, rash, or diarrhea. 3. Obtain cultures and sensitivities as indicated before initiation of antimicrobial treatment (wound exudate, sputum, urine, stool, blood). 4. Initiate measures to minimize infection. a. Discuss with patient and family (1) Placing patient in private room if absolute WBC count <1,000/mm³ (2) Importance of patient avoiding contact with people who have known or recent infection or recent vaccination b. Instruct all personnel in careful hand hygiene before and after entering room. c. Avoid rectal or vaginal procedures (rectal temperatures, examinations, suppositories; vaginal tampons). d. Use stool softeners to prevent constipation and straining. e. Assist patient in practice of meticulous personal hygiene. f. Instruct patient to use electric razor. g. Encourage patient to ambulate in room unless contraindicated. h. Avoid fresh fruits, raw meat, fish, and vegetables if absolute WBC count <1,000/mm³; also remove fresh flowers and potted plants. i. Each day: change drinking water, denture cleaning fluids, and respiratory equipment containing water. 5. Assess intravenous sites every day for evidence of infection: a. Change intravenous sites every other day.	1. Signs and symptoms of infection may be diminished in the immunocompromised host. Prompt recognition of infection and subsequent initiation of therapy will reduce morbidity and mortality associated with infection. 2. Early detection of infection facilitates early intervention. 3. These tests identify the organism and indicate the most appropriate antimicrobial therapy. Use of inappropriate antibiotics enhances proliferation of additional flora and encourages growth of antibiotic-resistant organisms. 4. Exposure to infection is reduced. a. Preventing contact with pathogens helps prevent infection. b. Hands are significant source of contamination. c. Incidence of rectal and perianal abscesses and subsequent systemic infection is high. Manipulation may cause disruption of membrane integrity and enhance progression of infection. d. This minimizes trauma to tissues. e. This prevents skin irritation. f. Minimizes skin trauma. g. Minimizes chance of skin breakdown and stasis of pulmonary secretions. h. Fresh fruits and vegetables harbor bacteria not removed by ordinary washing. Flowers and potted plants are also sources of organisms. i. Stagnant water is a source of infection. 5. Nosocomial staphylococcal septicemia is closely associated with intravenous catheters. a. Incidence of infection is increased when catheter is in place >72 hr.	• Demonstrates normal temperature and vital signs. • Exhibits absence of signs of inflammation: local edema, erythema, pain, and warmth. • Exhibits normal breath sounds on auscultation. • Takes deep breaths and coughs every 2 hours to prevent respiratory dysfunction and infection. • Exhibits absence of pathologic bacteria on cultures. • Avoids contact with others with infections. • Avoids crowds. • All personnel carry out hand hygiene after each voiding and bowel movement. • Excoriation and trauma of skin are avoided. • Trauma to mucous membranes is avoided (avoidance of rectal thermometers, suppositories, vaginal tampons, perianal trauma). • Uses recommended procedures and techniques if participating in management of invasive lines or catheters. • Uses electric razor. • Is free of skin breakdown and stasis of secretions. • Adheres to dietary and environmental restrictions. • Exhibits no signs of septicemia or septic shock. • Exhibits normal vital signs, cardiac output, and arterial pressures when monitored. • Demonstrates ability to administer colony-stimulating factor.

(continued)

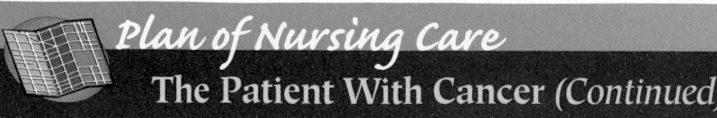

Plan of Nursing Care

The Patient With Cancer *(Continued)*

Nursing Interventions	Rationale	Expected Outcomes
b. Cleanse skin with povidone-iodine before arterial puncture or venipuncture.	b. Povidone-iodine is effective against many gram-positive and gram-negative pathogens.	
c. Change central venous catheter dressings every 48 hours.	c. Allows observation of site and removes source of contamination.	
d. Change all solutions and infusion sets every 48 hours.	d. Once introduced into the system, microorganisms are capable of growing in infusion sets despite replacement of container and high flow rates.	
6. Avoid intramuscular injections.	6. Reduces risk for skin abscesses.	
7. Avoid insertion of urinary catheters; if catheters are necessary, use strict aseptic technique.	7. Rates of infection *greatly* increase after urinary catheterization.	
8. Teach patient or family member to administer granulocyte (or granulocyte-macrophage) colony-stimulating factor when prescribed.	8. Granulocyte colony-stimulating factor decreases the duration of neutropenia and the potential for infection.	

Nursing Diagnosis: Impaired skin integrity: erythematous and wet desquamation reactions to radiation therapy
Goal: Maintenance of skin integrity

1. In erythematous areas: a. Avoid the use of soaps, cosmetics, perfumes, powders, lotions and ointments, deodorants. b. Use only lukewarm water to bathe the area. c. Avoid rubbing or scratching the area. d. Avoid shaving the area with a straight-edged razor. e. Avoid applying hot-water bottles, heating pads, ice, and adhesive tape to the area. f. Avoid exposing the area to sunlight or cold weather. g. Avoid tight clothing in the area. Use cotton clothing. h. Apply vitamin A&D ointment to the area.	1. Care to the affected areas must focus on preventing further skin irritation, drying, and damage g. Allows air circulation to affected area. h. Aids healing.	• Avoids use of soaps, powders, and other cosmetics on site of radiation therapy. • States rationale for special care of skin. • Exhibits minimal change in skin. • Avoids trauma to affected skin region (avoids shaving, constricting and irritating clothing, extremes of temperature, and use of adhesive tape). • Reports change in skin promptly. • Demonstrates proper care of blistered or open areas. • Exhibits absence of infection of blistered and opened areas.
2. If wet desquamation occurs: a. Do not disrupt any blisters that have formed. b. Avoid frequent washing of the area. c. Report any blistering. d. Use *prescribed* creams or ointments. e. If area weeps, apply a thin layer of gauze dressing.	2. Open weeping areas are susceptible to bacterial infection. Care must be taken to prevent introduction of pathogens. d. Decreases irritation and inflammation of the area. e. Enhances drying.	

Nursing Diagnosis: Impaired oral mucous membrane: stomatitis
Goal: Maintenance of intact oral mucous membranes

1. Assess oral cavity daily.	1. Provides baseline for later evaluation.	• States rationale for frequent oral assessment and hygiene.
2. Instruct patient to report oral burning, pain, areas of redness, open lesions on the	2. Identification of initial stages of stomatitis will facilitate prompt interventions,	

(continued)

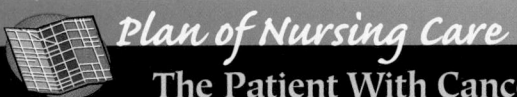

Plan of Nursing Care

The Patient With Cancer *(Continued)*

Nursing Interventions	Rationale	Expected Outcomes
lips, pain associated with swallowing, or decreased tolerance to temperature extremes of food. 3. Encourage and assist in oral hygiene. **Preventive** 　a. Avoid commercial mouthwashes. 　b. Brush with soft toothbrush; use non-abrasive toothpaste after meals and bedtime; floss every 24 h unless painful or platelet count falls below 40,000 cu/mm. **Mild stomatitis** (generalized erythema, limited ulcerations, small white patches: *Candida*) 　c. Use normal saline mouth rinses every 2 h while awake; every 6 h at night. 　d. Use soft toothbrush or toothette. 　e. Remove dentures except for meals; be certain dentures fit well. 　f. Apply lip lubricant. 　g. Avoid foods that are spicy or hard to chew and those with extremes of temperature. **Severe stomatitis** (confluent ulcerations with bleeding and white patches covering more than 25% of oral mucosa) 　h. Obtain tissue samples for culture and sensitivity tests of areas of infection. 　i. Assess ability to chew and swallow; assess gag reflex. 　j. Use oral rinses as prescribed or place patient on side and irrigate mouth; have suction available (may combine in solution saline, anti-*Candida* agent, such as Mycostatin, and topical anesthetic agent as described below). 　k. Remove dentures. 　l. Use toothette or gauze soaked with solution for cleansing. 　m. Use lip lubricant. 　n. Provide liquid or pureed diet. 　o. Monitor for dehydration. 4. Minimize discomfort. 　a. Consult physician for use of topical anesthetic, such as dyclonine and diphenhydramine, or viscous lidocaine. 　b. Administer systemic analgesics as prescribed. 　c. Perform mouth care as described.	including modification of treatment as prescribed by physician. 　a. Alcohol content of mouthwashes will dry oral tissues and potentiate breakdown. 　b. Limits trauma and removes debris. 　c. Assists in removing debris, thick secretions, and bacteria. 　d. Minimizes trauma. 　e. Minimizes friction and discomfort. 　f. Promotes comfort. 　g. Prevents local trauma. 　h. Assists in identifying need for antimicrobial therapy. 　i. Patient may be in danger of aspiration. 　j. Facilitates cleansing, provides for safety and comfort. 　k. Prevents trauma from ill-fitting dentures. 　l. Limits trauma, promotes comfort. 　m. Promotes comfort. 　n. Ensures intake of easily digestible foods. 　o. Decreased oral intake and ulcerations potentiate fluid deficits. 　a. Alleviates pain and increases sense of well-being; promotes participation in oral hygiene and nutritional intake. 　c. Promotes removal of debris, healing, and comfort.	• Identifies signs and symptoms of stomatitis to report to nurse or physician. • Participates in recommended oral hygiene regimen. • Avoids mouthwashes with alcohol. • Brushes teeth and mouth with soft toothbrush. • Uses lubricant to keep lips soft and non-irritated. • Avoids hard-to-chew, spicy, and hot foods. • Exhibits clean, intact oral mucosa. • Exhibits no ulcerations or infections of oral cavity. • Exhibits no evidence of bleeding. • Reports absent or decreased oral pain. • Reports no difficulty swallowing. • Exhibits healing (reepithelialization) of oral mucosa within 5 to 7 days (mild stomatitis). • Exhibits healing of oral tissues within 10 to 14 days (severe stomatitis). • Exhibits no bleeding or oral ulceration. • Consumes adequate fluid and food. • Exhibits absence of dehydration and weight loss.

(continued)

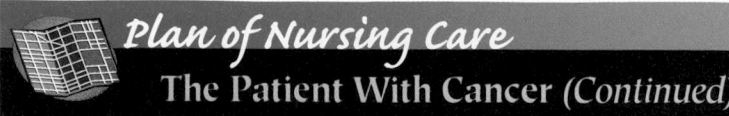

Plan of Nursing Care
The Patient With Cancer *(Continued)*

Nursing Interventions	Rationale	Expected Outcomes

Nursing Diagnosis: Impaired tissue integrity: alopecia
Goal: Maintenance of tissue integrity; coping with hair loss

Nursing Interventions	Rationale	Expected Outcomes
1. Discuss potential hair loss and regrowth with patient and family.	1. Provides information so patient and family can begin to prepare cognitively and emotionally for loss.	• Identifies alopecia as potential side effect of treatment.
2. Explore potential impact of hair loss on self-image, interpersonal relationships, and sexuality.	2. Facilitates coping.	• Identifies positive and negative feelings and threats to self-image.
3. Prevent or minimize hair loss through the following:	3. Retains hair as long as possible.	• Verbalizes meaning that hair and possible hair loss have for him or her.
a. Use scalp hypothermia and scalp tourniquets, if appropriate.	a. Decreases hair follicle uptake of chemotherapy (not used for patients with leukemia or lymphoma because tumor cells may be present in blood vessels or scalp tissue).	• States rationale for modifications in hair care and treatment. • Uses mild shampoo and conditioner and shampoos hair only when necessary.
b. Cut long hair before treatment.	b–e. Minimizes hair loss due to the weight and manipulation of hair.	• Avoids hair dryer, curlers, sprays, and other stresses on hair and scalp.
c. Use mild shampoo and conditioner, gently pat dry, and avoid excessive shampooing.		• Wears hat or scarf over hair when exposed to sun.
d. Avoid electric curlers, curling irons, dryers, clips, barrettes, hair sprays, hair dyes, and permanent waves.		• Takes steps to deal with possible hair loss before it occurs; purchases wig or hairpiece.
e. Avoid excessive combing or brushing; use wide-toothed comb.		• Maintains hygiene and grooming.
4. Prevent trauma to scalp.	4. Preserves tissue integrity.	• Interacts and socializes with others.
a. Lubricate scalp with vitamin A&D ointment to decrease itching.	a. Assists in maintaining skin integrity.	• States that hair loss and necessity of wig are temporary.
b. Have patient use sunscreen or wear hat when in the sun.	b. Prevents ultraviolet light exposure.	
5. Suggest ways to assist in coping with hair loss:	5. Minimizes change in appearance.	
a. Purchase wig or hairpiece before hair loss.	a. Wig that closely resembles hair color and style is more easily selected if hair loss has not begun.	
b. If hair loss has occurred, take photograph to wig shop to assist in selection.	b. Facilitates adjustment.	
c. Begin to wear wig before hair loss.		
d. Contact the American Cancer Society for donated wigs, or a store that specializes in this product.		
e. Wear hat, scarf, or turban.	e. Conceals loss.	
6. Encourage patient to wear own clothes and retain social contacts.	6. Assists in maintaining personal identity.	
7. Explain that hair growth usually begins again once therapy is completed.	7. Reassures patient that hair loss is usually temporary.	

Nursing Diagnosis: Imbalanced nutrition, less than body requirements, related to nausea and vomiting
Goal: Fewer episodes of nausea and vomiting before, during, and after chemotherapy

Nursing Interventions	Rationale	Expected Outcomes
1. Assess the patient's previous experiences and expectations of nausea and vomiting, including causes and interventions used.	1. Identifies patient concerns, misinformation, potential strategies for intervention. Also gives patient sense of empowerment and control.	• Identifies previous triggers of nausea and vomiting. • Exhibits decreased apprehension and anxiety.
2. Adjust diet before and after drug administration according to patient preference and tolerance.	2. Each patient responds differently to food after chemotherapy. A diet containing foods that relieve the patient's nausea or vomiting is most helpful.	• Identifies previously used successful interventions for nausea and vomiting. • Reports decrease in nausea.

(continued)

Plan of Nursing Care

The Patient With Cancer *(Continued)*

Nursing Interventions	Rationale	Expected Outcomes
3. Prevent unpleasant sights, odors, and sounds in the environment.	3. Unpleasant sensations can stimulate the nausea and vomiting center.	• Reports decrease in incidence of vomiting.
4. Use distraction, music therapy, biofeedback, self-hypnosis, relaxation techniques, and guided imagery before, during, and after chemotherapy.	4. Decreases anxiety, which can contribute to nausea and vomiting. Psychological conditioning may also be decreased.	• Consumes adequate fluid and food when nausea subsides. • Demonstrates use of distraction, relaxation, and imagery when indicated.
5. Administer prescribed antiemetics, sedatives, and corticosteroids before chemotherapy and afterward as needed.	5. Administration of antiemetic regimen before onset of nausea and vomiting limits the adverse experience and facilitates control. Combination drug therapy reduces nausea and vomiting through various triggering mechanisms.	• Exhibits normal skin turgor and moist mucous membranes. • Reports no additional weight loss.
6. Ensure adequate fluid hydration before, during, and after drug administration; assess intake and output.	6. Adequate fluid volume dilutes drug levels, decreasing stimulation of vomiting receptors.	
7. Encourage frequent oral hygiene.	7. Reduces unpleasant taste sensations.	
8. Provide pain relief measures, if necessary.	8. Increased comfort increases physical tolerance of symptoms.	
9. Assess other causes of nausea and vomiting, such as constipation, gastrointestinal irritation, electrolyte imbalance, radiation therapy, medications, and central nervous system metastasis.	9. Multiple factors may cause nausea and vomiting.	

Nursing Diagnosis: Imbalanced nutrition: less than body requirements, related to anorexia, cachexia, or malabsorption

Goal: Maintenance of nutritional status and of weight within 10% of pretreatment weight

1. Teach patient to avoid unpleasant sights, odors, sounds in the environment during mealtime.	1. Anorexia can be stimulated or increased with noxious stimuli.	• Exhibits weight loss no greater than 10% of pretreatment weight. • Reports decreasing anorexia and increased interest in eating.
2. Suggest foods that are preferred and well tolerated by the patient, preferably high-calorie and high-protein foods. Respect ethnic and cultural food preferences.	2. Foods preferred, well tolerated, and high in calories and protein maintain nutritional status during periods of increased metabolic demand.	• Demonstrates normal skin turgor. • Identifies rationale for dietary modifications. • Participates in calorie counts and diet histories.
3. Encourage adequate fluid intake, but limit fluids at mealtime.	3. Fluids are necessary to eliminate wastes and prevent dehydration. Increased fluids with meals can lead to early satiety.	• Uses appropriate relaxation and imagery before meals.
4. Suggest smaller, more frequent meals.	4. Smaller, more frequent meals are better tolerated because early satiety does not occur.	• Exhibits laboratory and clinical findings indicative of adequate nutritional intake: normal serum protein and transferrin levels; normal serum iron levels; normal hemoglobin, hematocrit, and lymphocyte levels; normal urinary creatinine levels.
5. Promote relaxed, quiet environment during mealtime with increased social interaction as desired.	5. A quiet environment promotes relaxation. Social interaction at mealtime increases appetite.	
6. If possible, serve wine at mealtime with foods.	6. Wine often stimulates appetite and adds calories.	• Consumes diet high in required nutrients. • Carries out oral hygiene before meals.
7. Consider cold foods, if desired.	7. Cold, high-protein foods are often more tolerable and less odorous than hot foods.	• Reports that pain does not interfere with meals.
8. Advocate nutritional supplements and high-protein foods between meals.	8. Supplements and snacks add protein and calories to meet nutritional requirements.	• Reports decreasing episodes of nausea and vomiting.
9. Encourage frequent oral hygiene.	9. Oral hygiene stimulates appetite and increases saliva production.	• Participates in increasing levels of activity.
10. Provide pain relief measures.	10. Pain impairs appetite.	• States rationale for use of tube feedings or hyperalimentation.
11. Provide control of nausea and vomiting.	11. Nausea and vomiting increase anorexia.	• Participates in management of tube feedings or parenteral nutrition, if prescribed.
12. Increase activity level as tolerated.	12. Increased activity promotes appetite.	

(continued)

Plan of Nursing Care
The Patient With Cancer *(Continued)*

Nursing Interventions	Rationale	Expected Outcomes
13. Decrease anxiety by encouraging verbalization of fears, concerns; use of relaxation techniques; imagery at mealtime.	13. Relief of anxiety may increase appetite.	
14. Position patient properly at mealtime.	14. Proper body position and alignment are necessary to aid chewing and swallowing.	
15. For collaborative management, provide enteral tube feedings of commercial liquid diets, elemental diets, or blenderized foods as prescribed.	15. Tube feedings may be necessary in the severely debilitated patient who has a functioning gastrointestinal system.	
16. Provide parenteral nutrition with lipid supplements as prescribed.	16. Parenteral nutrition with supplemental fats supplies needed calories and proteins to meet nutritional demands, especially in the nonfunctional gastrointestinal system.	
17. Administer appetite stimulants as prescribed by physician.	17. Although the mechanism is unclear, medications such as megestrol acetate (Megace) have been noted to improve appetite in patients with cancer and HIV infection.	

Nursing Diagnosis: Fatigue
Goal: Increased activity tolerance and decreased fatigue level

Nursing Interventions	Rationale	Expected Outcomes
1. Encourage several rest periods during the day, especially before and after physical exertion.	1. During rest, energy is conserved and levels are replenished. Several shorter rest periods may be more beneficial than one longer rest period.	• Reports decreasing levels of fatigue. • Increases participation in activities gradually. • Rests when fatigued. • Reports restful sleep.
2. Increase total hours of nighttime sleep.	2. Sleep helps to restore energy levels.	• Requests assistance with activities appropriately.
3. Rearrange daily schedule and organize activities to conserve energy expenditure.	3. Reorganization of activities can reduce energy losses and stressors.	• Reports adequate energy to participate in activities important to him or her
4. Encourage patient to ask for others' assistance with necessary chores, such as housework, child care, shopping, cooking.	4. Conserves energy.	(eg, visiting with family, hobbies).
5. Encourage reduced job workload, if possible, by reducing number of hours worked per week.	5. Reducing workload decreases physical and psychological stress and increases periods of rest and relaxation.	• Consumes diet with recommended protein and caloric intake. • Uses relaxation exercises and imagery to decrease anxiety and promote rest.
6. Encourage adequate protein and calorie intake.	6. Protein and calorie depletion decreases activity tolerance.	• Participates in planned exercise program gradually.
7. Encourage use of relaxation techniques, mental imagery.	7. Promotion of relaxation and psychological rest decreases physical fatigue.	• Reports no breathlessness during activities.
8. Encourage participation in planned exercise programs.	8. Proper exercise programs increase endurance and stamina.	• Exhibits acceptable hemoglobin and hematocrit levels.
9. For collaborative management, administer blood products as prescribed.	9. Lowered hemoglobin and hematocrit predispose patient to fatigue due to decreased oxygen availability.	• Exhibits normal fluid and electrolyte balance. • Reports decreased discomfort.
10. Assess for fluid and electrolyte disturbances.	10. May contribute to altered nerve transmission and muscle function.	• Exhibits improved mobility.
11. Assess for sources of discomfort.	11. Coping with discomfort requires energy expenditure.	
12. Provide strategies to facilitate mobility.	12. Impaired mobility requires increased energy expenditure.	

Nursing Diagnosis: Chronic Pain
Goal: Relief of pain and discomfort

Nursing Interventions	Rationale	Expected Outcomes
1. Use pain scale to assess pain and discomfort characteristics: location, quality, frequency, duration, etc.	1. Provides baseline for assessing changes in pain level and evaluation of interventions.	• Reports decreased level of pain and discomfort on pain scale.

(continued)

Plan of Nursing Care
The Patient With Cancer (Continued)

Nursing Interventions	Rationale	Expected Outcomes
2. Assure patient that you know that pain is real and will assist him or her in reducing it.	2. Fear that pain will not be considered real increases anxiety and reduces pain tolerance.	• Reports less disruption from pain and discomfort.
3. Assess other factors contributing to patient's pain: fear, fatigue, anger, etc.	3. Provides data about factors that decrease patient's ability to tolerate pain and increase pain level.	• Explains how fatigue, fear, anger, etc., contribute to severity of pain and discomfort.
4. Administer analgesics to promote optimum pain relief within limits of physician's prescription.	4. Analgesics tend to be more effective when administered early in pain cycle.	• Accepts pain medication as prescribed. • Exhibits decreased physical and behavioral signs of pain and discomfort in acute pain (no grimacing, crying, moaning; displays interest in surroundings and activities around him).
5. Assess patient's behavioral responses to pain and pain experience.	5. Provides additional information about patient's pain.	• Takes an active role in administration of analgesia.
6. Collaborate with patient, physician, and other health care team members when changes in pain management are necessary.	6. New methods of administering analgesia must be acceptable to patient, physician, and health care team to be effective; patient's participation decreases the sense of powerlessness.	• Identifies additional effective pain relief strategies. • Uses alternative pain relief strategies appropriately.
7. Encourage strategies of pain relief that patient has used successfully in previous pain experience.	7. Encourages success of pain relief strategies accepted by patient and family.	• Reports effective use of new pain relief strategies and decrease in pain intensity.
8. Teach patient new strategies to relieve pain and discomfort: distraction, imagery, relaxation, cutaneous stimulation, etc.	8. Increases number of options and strategies available to patient.	• Reports that decreased level of pain permits participation in other activities and events.

Nursing Diagnosis: Anticipatory grieving related to loss; altered role functioning
Goal: Appropriate progression through grieving process

1. Encourage verbalization of fears, concerns, and questions regarding disease, treatment, and future implications.	1. An increased and accurate knowledge base decreases anxiety and dispels misconceptions.	• The patient and family progress through the phases of grief as evidenced by increased verbalization and expression of grief.
2. Encourage active participation of patient or family in care and treatment decisions.	2. Active participation maintains patient independence and control.	• The patient and family identify resources available to aid coping strategies during grieving.
3. Visit family frequently to establish and maintain relationships and physical closeness.	3. Frequent contacts promote trust and security and reduce feelings of fear and isolation.	• The patient and family use resources and supports appropriately.
4. Encourage ventilation of negative feelings, including projected anger and hostility, within acceptable limits.	4. This allows for emotional expression without loss of self-esteem.	• The patient and family discuss the future openly with each other.
5. Allow for periods of crying and expression of sadness.	5. These feelings are necessary for separation and detachment to occur.	• The patient and family discuss concerns and feelings openly with each other.
6. Involve clergy as desired by the patient and family.	6. This facilitates the grief process and spiritual care.	• The patient and family use nonverbal expressions of concern for each other.
7. Advise professional counseling as indicated for patient or family to alleviate pathologic grieving.	7. This facilitates the grief process.	
8. Allow for progression through the grieving process at the individual pace of the patient and family.	8. Grief work is variable. Not every person uses every phase of the grief process, and the time spent in dealing with each phase varies with every person. To complete grief work, this variability must be allowed.	

Nursing Diagnosis: Disturbed body image and situational low self-esteem related to changes in appearance, function, and roles
Goal: Improved body image and self-esteem

1. Assess patient's feelings about body image and level of self-esteem.	1. Provides baseline assessment for evaluating changes and assessing effectiveness of interventions.	• Identifies concerns of importance. • Takes active role in activities. • Maintains previous role in decision making.

(continued)

Plan of Nursing Care
The Patient With Cancer (*Continued*)

Nursing Interventions	Rationale	Expected Outcomes
2. Identify potential threats to patient's self-esteem (eg, altered appearance, decreased sexual function, hair loss, decreased energy, role changes). Validate concerns with patient.	2. Anticipates changes and permits patient to identify importance of these areas to him or her.	• Verbalizes feelings and reactions to losses or threatened losses.
3. Encourage continued participation in activities and decision making.	3. Encourages and permits continued control of events and self.	• Participates in self-care activities. • Permits others to assist in care when he or she is unable to be independent.
4. Encourage patient to verbalize concerns.	4. Identifying concerns is an important step in coping with them.	• Exhibits interest in appearance and uses aids (cosmetics, scarves, etc.) appropriately.
5. Individualize care for the patient.	5. Prevents or reduces depersonalization and emphasizes patient's self-worth.	• Participates with others in conversations and social events and activities.
6. Assist patient in self-care when fatigue, lethargy, nausea, vomiting, and other symptoms prevent independence.	6. Physical well-being improves self-esteem.	• Verbalizes concern about sexual partner and/or significant others.
7. Assist patient in selecting and using cosmetics, scarves, hair pieces, and clothing that increase his or her sense of attractiveness.	7. Promotes positive body image.	• Explores alternative ways of expressing concern and affection.
8. Encourage patient and partner to share concerns about altered sexuality and sexual function and to explore alternatives to their usual sexual expression.	8. Provides opportunity for expressing concern, affection, and acceptance.	

Collaborative Problem: Potential complication: risk for bleeding problems
Goal: Prevention of bleeding

Nursing Interventions	Rationale	Expected Outcomes
1. Assess for potential for bleeding: monitor platelet count.	1. Mild risk: 50,000–100,000/mm³ $(0.05–0.1 \times 10^{12}/L)$ Moderate risk: 20,000–50,000/mm³ $(0.02–0.05 \times 10^{12}/L)$ Severe risk: less than 20,000/mm³ $(0.02 \times 10^{12}/L)$	• Signs and symptoms of bleeding are identified. • Exhibits no blood in feces, urine, or emesis. • Exhibits no bleeding of gums or of injection or venipuncture sites. • Exhibits no ecchymosis (bruising).
2. Assess for bleeding:	2. Early detection promotes early intervention.	• Patient and family identify ways to prevent bleeding.
a. Petechiae or ecchymosis	a. Indicates injury to microcirculation and larger vessels.	• Uses recommended measures to reduce risk of bleeding (uses soft toothbrush, shaves with electric razor only).
b. Decrease in hemoglobin or hematocrit	b. Indicates blood loss.	• Exhibits normal vital signs.
c. Prolonged bleeding from invasive procedures, venipunctures, minor cuts or scratches		• Reports that environmental hazards have been reduced or removed.
d. Frank or occult blood in any body excretion, emesis, sputum		• Consumes adequate fluid. • Reports absence of constipation.
e. Bleeding from any body orifice		• Avoids substances interfering with clotting.
f. Altered mental status	f. Indicates neurologic involvement.	• Absence of tissue destruction.
3. Instruct patient and family about ways to minimize bleeding:	3. Patient can participate in self-protection.	• Exhibits normal mental status and absence of signs of intracranial bleeding.
a. Use soft toothbrush or toothette for mouth care.	a. Prevents trauma to oral tissues.	• Avoids medications that interfere with clotting (eg, aspirin).
b. Avoid commercial mouthwashes.	b. Contain high alcohol content that will dry oral tissues.	• Absence of epistaxis and cerebral bleeding.
c. Use electric razor for shaving.	c. Prevents trauma to skin.	
d. Use emery board for nail care.	d. Reduces risk of trauma to nailbeds.	
e. Avoid foods that are difficult to chew.	e. Prevents oral tissue trauma.	
4. Initiate measures to minimize bleeding.	4. Preserves circulating blood volume.	
a. Draw all blood for lab work with one daily venipuncture.	a. Minimizes trauma and blood loss.	
b. Avoid taking temperature rectally or administering suppositories and enemas.	b. Prevents trauma to rectal mucosa.	

(*continued*)

Plan of Nursing Care
The Patient With Cancer *(Continued)*

Nursing Interventions	Rationale	Expected Outcomes
c. Avoid intramuscular injections; use smallest needle possible.	c. Prevents intramuscular bleeding.	
d. Apply direct pressure to injection and venipuncture sites for at least 5 min.	d. Minimizes blood loss.	
e. Lubricate lips with petrolatum.	e. Prevents skin from drying.	
f. Avoid bladder catheterizations; use smallest catheter if catheterization is necessary.	f. Prevents trauma to urethra.	
g. Maintain fluid intake of at least 3 L/24 h unless contraindicated.	g. Hydration helps to prevent skin drying.	
h. Use stool softeners or increase bulk in diet.	h. Prevents constipation and straining that may injure rectal tissue.	
i. Avoid medications that will interfere with clotting (eg, aspirin).	i. Minimizes risk of bleeding.	
j. Recommend use of water-based lubricant before sexual intercourse.	j. Prevents friction and tissue trauma.	
5. When platelet count is less than 20,000/mm³, institute the following:	5. Platelet count of less than 20,000/mm³ $(0.02 \times 10^{12}/L)$ is associated with increased risk of spontaneous bleeding.	
a. Bed rest with padded side rails	a. Reduces risk of injury	
b. Avoidance of strenuous activity	b. Increases intracranial pressure and risk of cerebral hemorrhage.	
c. Platelet transfusions as prescribed; administer prescribed diphenhydramine hydrochloride (Benadryl) or hydrocortisone sodium succinate (Solu-Cortef) to prevent reaction to platelet transfusion.	c. Allergic reactions to blood products are associated with antigen–antibody reaction that causes platelet destruction.	
d. Supervise activity when out of bed.		
e. Caution against forceful nose blowing.	e. Prevents trauma to nasal mucosa and increased intracranial pressure.	

ADMINISTERING CHEMOTHERAPY

The local effects of the chemotherapeutic agent are also of concern. The patient is observed closely during its administration because of the risk and consequences of extravasation (particularly of vesicant agents, which may produce necrosis if deposited in the subcutaneous tissues). Local difficulties or problems with administration of chemotherapeutic agents are brought to the attention of the physician promptly so that corrective measures can be taken immediately to minimize local tissue damage.

IMPLEMENTING SAFEGUARDS

Nurses involved in handling chemotherapeutic agents may be exposed to low doses of the drugs by direct contact, inhalation, and ingestion. Urinalyses of personnel repeatedly exposed to cytotoxic agents demonstrate mutagenic activity. Although not all mutagens are carcinogenic, they can produce permanent inheritable changes in the genetic material of cells.

Although long-term studies of nurses handling chemotherapeutic agents have not been conducted, it is known that chemotherapeutic agents are associated with secondary formation of cancers and chromosome abnormalities. Additionally, nausea, vomiting, dizziness, alopecia, and nasal mucosal ulcerations have been reported in health care personnel who have handled chemotherapeutic agents.

Because of known and potential hazards associated with handling chemotherapeutic agents, the Occupational Safety and Health Administration, Oncology Nursing Society, hospitals, and other health care agencies have developed specific precautions for those involved in the preparation and administration of chemotherapy (Chart 16-6).

BONE MARROW TRANSPLANTATION

Although surgery, radiation therapy, and chemotherapy have resulted in improved survival rates for cancer patients, many cancers that initially respond to therapy recur. This is true of hematologic cancers that affect the bone marrow and solid tumor cancers treated with lower doses of antineoplastics to spare the bone marrow from larger, ablative doses of chemotherapy or radiation therapy.

The role of bone marrow transplantation (BMT) for malignant as well as some nonmalignant diseases continues to grow. Types of BMT based on the source of donor cells include:

1. Allogeneic (from a donor other than the patient): either a related donor (ie, family member) or a matched unrelated donor (national bone marrow registry, cord blood registry)

Chart 16-6 **Safety in Administering Chemotherapy**

Safety recommendations from the Occupational Safety and Health Administration (OSHA), Oncology Nursing Society (ONS), hospitals, and other health care agencies for the preparation and handling of antineoplastic agents follow:

- Use a biologic safety cabinet for the preparation of all chemotherapy agents.
- Wear surgical gloves when handling antineoplastic agents and the excretions of patients who received chemotherapy.
- Wear disposable, long-sleeved gowns when preparing and administering chemotherapy agents.
- Use Luer-Lok fittings on all intravenous tubing used to deliver chemotherapy.
- Dispose of all equipment used in chemotherapy preparation and administration in appropriate, leak-proof, puncture-proof containers.
- Dispose of all chemotherapy wastes as hazardous materials.

When followed, these precautions greatly minimize the risk of exposure to chemotherapy agents.

2. Autologous (from patient)
3. Syngeneic (from an identical twin)

The process of obtaining donor cells has evolved over the years. Donor cells can be obtained by the traditional harvesting of large amounts of bone marrow tissue under general anesthesia in the operating room. A newer method, referred to as peripheral blood stem cell transplant (PBSCT), is gaining widespread use. This method of collection uses apheresis of the donor to collect stem cells for reinfusion. It is considered to be a safer and more cost-effective means of collection than the traditional harvesting of marrow.

Allogeneic BMT, used primarily for disease of the bone marrow, depends on the availability of a human leukocyte antigen–matched donor. This greatly limits the number of transplants possible. An advantage to allogeneic BMT is that the transplanted cells should not be immunologically tolerant of the patient's malignancy and should cause a lethal graft-versus-disease effect to the malignant cells. The recipient must undergo ablative doses of chemotherapy and possibly total body irradiation to destroy all existing bone marrow and malignant disease. The harvested donor marrow is infused intravenously into the recipient and travels to sites in the body where it produces bone marrow and establishes itself. This establishment of the new bone marrow is known as engraftment. Once engraftment is complete (2 to 4 weeks, sometimes longer), the new bone marrow becomes functional and begins producing red blood cells, WBCs, and platelets.

Before engraftment, patients are at a high risk for infection, sepsis, and bleeding. Side effects of the high-dose chemotherapy and total body irradiation can be acute and chronic. Acute side effects include alopecia, hemorrhagic cystitis, nausea, vomiting, diarrhea, and severe stomatitis. Chronic side effects include sterility, pulmonary dysfunction, cardiac dysfunction, and liver disease. Patients receive immunosuppressant drugs, such as cyclosporine, tacrolimus (FK 506), or azathioprine (Imuran), to prevent graft-versus-host disease (GVHD). In allogeneic transplant recipients, GVHD occurs when the T lymphocytes from the transplanted donor marrow become activated and mount an immune response against the recipient's tissues (skin, gastrointestinal tract, liver). T lymphocytes respond in this manner because they view the recipient's tissue as "foreign," immunologically differing from what

they recognize as "self" in the donor. GVHD may occur acutely or chronically. The first 100 days or so after allogeneic transplantation are crucial for BMT patients until the immune system and blood-making capacity (hematopoiesis) have recovered sufficiently to prevent infection and hemorrhage. Most acute side effects, such as nausea, vomiting, and mucositis, also resolve in the initial 100 days after transplantation. Patients are also at risk for development of venous occlusive disease (VOD), a vascular injury to the liver from the high-dose chemotherapy occurring in the first 100 days or so after BMT. VOD can lead to acute liver failure and death.

Autologous BMT is considered for patients with disease of the bone marrow who do not have a suitable donor for allogeneic BMT and for patients who have healthy bone marrow but require bone marrow–ablative doses of chemotherapy to cure an aggressive malignancy. Stem cells are collected from the patient and preserved for reinfusion and, if necessary, treated to kill any malignant cells within the marrow. The patient is treated with ablative chemotherapy and, possibly, total body irradiation to eradicate any remaining tumor. The stem cells are then reinfused and engraft. Until engraftment occurs in the bone marrow sites of the body, the patient is at high risk for infection, sepsis, and bleeding. Acute and chronic toxicities from chemotherapy and radiation therapy may be severe. The risk of VOD is also present after an autologous transplant. No immunosuppressant medications are necessary after autologous BMT because the patient did not receive foreign tissue. A disadvantage of autologous transplantation is the risk that viable tumor cells may remain in the bone marrow despite conditioning regimens (high-dose chemotherapy).

Syngeneic BMT is the least common type of transplantation because it requires an identical sibling for harvest. Syngeneic transplantations result in fewer complications and no marrow rejection because the donor is an identical tissue match to the recipient. The transplantation and collection processes are the same with syngeneic BMT as with allogeneic BMT.

Nursing Management in Bone Marrow Transplantation

Nursing care of patients undergoing BMT is complex and demands a high level of skill. Transplantation nursing can be extremely rewarding yet extremely stressful. The success of BMT is greatly influenced by nursing care throughout the transplantation process.

IMPLEMENTING PRETRANSPLANTATION CARE

All patients must undergo extensive pretransplantation evaluations to assess the current clinical status of the disease. Nutritional assessments, extensive physical examinations and organ function tests, and psychological evaluations are conducted. Blood work includes assessing past antigen exposure (for example, to hepatitis virus, cytomegalovirus, herpes simplex virus, HIV, and syphilis). The patient's social support systems and financial and insurance resources are also evaluated. Informed consent and patient teaching about the procedure and pretransplantation and posttransplantation care are vital.

PROVIDING CARE DURING TREATMENT

Skilled nursing care is required during the treatment phase of BMT when high-dose chemotherapy (conditioning regimen) and total body irradiation are administered. The acute toxicities of nausea, diarrhea, mucositis, and hemorrhagic cystitis require close monitoring and constant attention by the nurse.

Nursing management during the bone marrow or stem cell infusions consists of monitoring the patient's vital signs and blood oxygen saturation; assessing for adverse effects, such as fever, chills, shortness of breath, chest pain, cutaneous reactions, nausea, vomiting, hypotension or hypertension, tachycardia, anxiety, and taste changes; and providing ongoing support and patient teaching.

Throughout the period of bone marrow aplasia until engraftment of the new marrow occurs, patients are at high risk for dying of sepsis and bleeding. Patients require support with blood products and hemopoietic growth factors. Potential infection may be bacterial, viral, fungal, or protozoan in origin. Renal complications arise from the nephrotoxic chemotherapy agents used in the conditioning regimen or those used to treat infection (amphotericin B, aminoglycosides). Tumor lysis syndrome and acute tubular necrosis are also risks after BMT.

GVHD requires skillful nursing assessment to detect early effects on the skin, liver, and gastrointestinal tract. VOD resulting from the conditioning regimens used in BMT can result in fluid retention, jaundice, abdominal pain, ascites, tender and enlarged liver, and encephalopathy. Pulmonary complications, such as pulmonary edema, interstitial pneumonia, and other pneumonias, often complicate the recovery after BMT.

Providing Posttransplantation Care

Ongoing nursing assessment in follow-up visits is essential to detect late effects of therapy in BMT patients. Late complications are those that occur 100 days or more after BMT. Late effects include infections, such as varicella zoster infection, restrictive pulmonary abnormalities, and recurrent pneumonias. Sterility often results. Chronic GVHD involves the skin, liver, intestine, esophagus, eye, lungs, joints, and vaginal mucosa. Cataracts may also develop after total body irradiation.

Psychosocial assessments by nursing staff must be ongoing. In addition to the stressors affecting patients at each phase of the transplantation experience, marrow donors and family members also have psychosocial needs that must be addressed.

CARING FOR THE DONORS

Donors commonly experience mood alterations, decreased self-esteem, and guilt from feelings of failure if the transplantation fails. Family members must be educated and supported to reduce anxiety and promote coping during this difficult time. Family members must also be assisted to maintain realistic expectations of themselves as well as of the patient.

As BMT becomes more prevalent, many moral and ethical issues become apparent, including those related to informed consent, allocation of resources, and quality of life.

HYPERTHERMIA

Hyperthermia (thermal therapy), the generation of temperatures greater than physiologic fever range (above 41.5°C [106.7°F]), has been used for many years to destroy tumors in human cancers. Malignant cells may be more sensitive than normal cells to the harmful effects of high temperatures for several reasons. Malignant cells lack the repair mechanisms necessary to repair cell damage by elevated temperatures. Most tumor cells lack an adequate blood supply to provide needed oxygen during periods of increased cellular demand, such as during hyperthermia. Cancerous tumors lack blood vessels of adequate size for dissipation of heat. In addition, the body's immune system may be indirectly stimulated when hyperthermia is used.

Hyperthermia is most effective when combined with radiation therapy, chemotherapy, or biologic therapy. Hyperthermia and radiation therapy are thought to work well together because hypoxic tumor cells and cells in the S phase of the cell cycle are more sensitive to heat than radiation; the addition of heat damages tumor cells so that they cannot repair themselves after radiation therapy. Hyperthermia is thought to alter cellular membrane permeability when used with chemotherapy, allowing for an increased uptake of the chemotherapeutic agent. Hyperthermia may enhance function of immune system cells, such as macrophages and T cells, which are stimulated by many biologic agents.

Heat can be produced by using radiowaves, ultrasound, microwaves, magnetic waves, hot-water baths, or even hot-wax immersions. Hyperthermia may be local or regional, or it may include the whole body. Local or regional hyperthermia may be delivered to a cancerous extremity (for malignant melanoma) by regional perfusion, in which the affected extremity is isolated by a tourniquet and an extracorporeal circulator heats the blood flowing through the affected part. Hyperthermia probes may also be inserted around a tumor in a local area and attached to a heat source during treatment. Chemotherapeutic agents, such as melphalan (Alkeran), may also be heated and instilled into the region's circulating blood. Local or regional hyperthermia may also include infusion of heated solutions into cancerous body organs. Whole-body hyperthermia to treat disseminated disease may be achieved by extracorporeal circulation, immersion of patients in heated water or paraffin, or enclosure in heated suits.

Side effects of hyperthermic treatments include skin burns and tissue damage, fatigue, hypotension, peripheral neuropathies, thrombophlebitis, nausea, vomiting, diarrhea, and electrolyte imbalances. Resistance to hyperthermia may develop during the treatment because cells adapt to repeated thermal insult. Research into the effectiveness of hyperthermia, methods of delivery, and side effects is ongoing.

Nursing Management in Hyperthermia

Although hyperthermia has been used for many years, many patients and their families are unfamiliar with this cancer treatment. Consequently, they need explanations about the procedure, its goals, and its effects. The patient is assessed for adverse effects, and efforts are made to reduce their occurrence and severity. Local skin care at the site of the implanted hyperthermic probes is also required.

BIOLOGIC RESPONSE MODIFIERS

Biologic response modifier (BRM) therapy involves the use of naturally occurring or recombinant (reproduced through genetic engineering) agents or treatment methods that can alter the immunologic relationship between the tumor and the cancer patient (host) to provide a therapeutic benefit. Although the mechanisms of action vary with each type of BRM, the goal is to destroy or stop the malignant growth. The basis of BRM treatment lies in the restoration, modification, stimulation, or augmentation of the body's natural immune defenses against cancer.

Nonspecific Biologic Response Modifiers

Some of the early investigations of the stimulation of the immune system involved nonspecific agents such as Bacille Calmette-Guérin (BCG) and *Corynebacterium parvum*. When injected into the patient, these agents serve as antigens that stimulate an immune response. The hope is that the stimulated immune system will then eradicate malignant cells. Extensive animal and human investigations with BCG have shown promising results, especially in treating localized malignant melanoma. Additionally, BCG is considered to be a standard form of treatment for localized bladder cancer. Use of nonspecific agents in advanced cancer remains limited, however, and research is continuing in an effort to identify other uses and other agents.

Monoclonal Antibodies

Monoclonal antibodies (MoAbs), another type of BRM, became available through technological advances, enabling investigators to grow and produce specific antibodies for specific malignant cells. Theoretically, this type of specificity allows the MoAb to destroy the cancer cells and spare normal cells. The production of MoAbs involves injecting tumor cells that act as antigens into mice. Antibodies made in response to injected antigens can be found in the spleen of the mouse. Antibody-producing spleen cells are combined with a cancer cell that has the ability to grow indefinitely in culture medium and continue producing more antibodies. The combination of spleen cells and the cancer cells is referred to as a hybridoma. From hybridomas that continue to grow in the culture medium, the desired antibodies are harvested, purified, and prepared for diagnostic or therapeutic use (Fig. 16-5). Alternative methods of producing MoAbs using human or genetically engineered sources are under investigation.

MoAbs are being used as aids in diagnostic evaluation. By attaching a radioactive substance to the MoAb, physicians can detect both primary and metastatic tumors through radiologic techniques. This process is referred to as radioimmunodetection. OncoScint (Cytogen Corp., Princeton, NJ) is a U.S. Food and Drug Administration (FDA)-approved MoAb that is used to assist in diagnosing ovarian and colorectal cancers. The use of MoAbs in detecting breast, gastric, and prostate cancers and lymphoma is under investigation. MoAbs are also used in purging residual tumor cells from the bone marrow or peripheral blood of patients who are undergoing BMT for peripheral stem cell rescue after high-dose cytotoxic therapy.

Several MoAbs have been approved for treatment in cancer. Rituximab (Rituxan) is used for the treatment of relapsed or refractory non-Hodgkin's lymphoma (Kosits & Callaghan, 2000). Trastuzumab (Herceptin) is approved as a single agent or given in addition to chemotherapy for the treatment of some types of metastatic breast cancer (Yarbro, 2000). Alemtuzumab (Campath) is used in the treatment of some forms of leukemia (Seeley & DeMeyer, 2002). Gemtuzumab ozogomicin (Mylotarg) is a combination of a MoAb and the antitumor antibiotic calicheamicin, which is used for the treatment of a specific type of acute myeloid leukemia (Sorokin, 2000). Gemtuzumab ozogomicin is an example of immunoconjugate therapy or a "magic bullet" that transports cancer-killing substances to the cancer cells. Ibritumomab-tiuxetan (Zevalin) is another form of immunoconjugate therapy that combines a monoclonal antibody and a radioactive source for the treatment of specific types of non-Hodgkin's lymphoma. The monoclonal antibody delivers the radioactive source to the malignant cells, causing the cells to be destroyed by both radioactivity and normal immune responses (Estes, 2002). Researchers are continuing to explore the development and use of other MoAbs either alone or in combination with other substances such as radioactive materials, chemotherapeutic agents, toxins, hormones, or other BRMs.

Cytokines

Cytokines, substances produced by cells of the immune system to enhance the production and functioning of components of the immune system, are also the focus of cancer treatment research. Cytokines are grouped into families, such as interferons, interleukins, colony-stimulating factors, and tumor necrosis factors (TNFs).

INTERFERON

Interferons (IFNs) are examples of cytokines with both antiviral and antitumor properties. When stimulated, all nucleated cells are capable of producing these glycoproteins, which are classified according to their biologic and chemical properties: IFN-α is produced by leukocytes, IFN-β is produced by fibroblasts, and IFN-γ is produced by lymphocytes.

Although the exact antitumor effects of IFNs have not been thoroughly established, it is thought that they either stimulate the immune system or assist in preventing tumor growth. The antitumor effects are dependent on the type of IFN and the disease for which IFN is being used. IFNs enhance both lymphocyte and antibody production. They also facilitate the cytolytic or cell destruction role of macrophages and natural killer cells. Additionally, IFNs can inhibit cell multiplication by increasing the duration of various phases of the cell cycle.

The effects of IFN have been demonstrated in a variety of malignancies. IFN-α has been approved by the FDA for treating hairy-cell leukemia, Kaposi's sarcoma, chronic myelogenous leukemia, high-grade non-Hodgkin's lymphoma, and melanoma. Other positive responses have been seen in hematologic malignancies and renal carcinomas. IFN-α, IFN-β, and IFN-γ have been approved by the FDA for the treatment of several nonmalignant diseases. IFN is administered through subcutaneous, intramuscular, intravenous, and intracavitary routes. Efforts are underway to establish the effectiveness of IFN for various malignancies in combination with other treatment regimens.

INTERLEUKINS

Interleukins are a subgroup of cytokines known as lymphokines and monokines because they are primarily produced by lymphocytes and monocytes. About 15 different interleukins have been identified. They act by signaling and coordinating other cells of the immune system. The FDA has approved interleukin-2 (IL-2) as a treatment option for renal cell cancer and metastatic melanoma in adults. Originally referred to as T-cell growth factor, IL-2 is known to stimulate the production and activation of several different types of lymphocytes. In addition, IL-2 enhances the production of other types of cytokines and plays a role in influencing both humoral and cell-mediated immunity.

Clinical trials are being conducted on IL-2 as well as other interleukins, such as IL-1, IL-4, and IL-6, for their roles in treating other cancers. Some early-stage clinical trials are assessing the effects of interleukins in combination with chemotherapy. In addition, interleukins are being investigated for their role as growth factors for treating myelosuppression after the use of some forms of chemotherapy.

HEMATOPOIETIC GROWTH FACTORS (COLONY-STIMULATING FACTORS)

Hematopoietic growth factors, also known as colony-stimulating factors, are hormone-like substances naturally produced by cells within the immune system. Hematopoietic growth factors of different types regulate the production of all cells in the blood, including neutrophils, macrophages, monocytes, red blood cells, and platelets. FDA approval of GM-CSF, G-CSF, IL-11, and EPO (Epogen) has contributed significantly to the supportive care of patients with cancer.

Although these agents do not treat the underlying malignancy, they do target the effects of myelotoxic cancer therapies

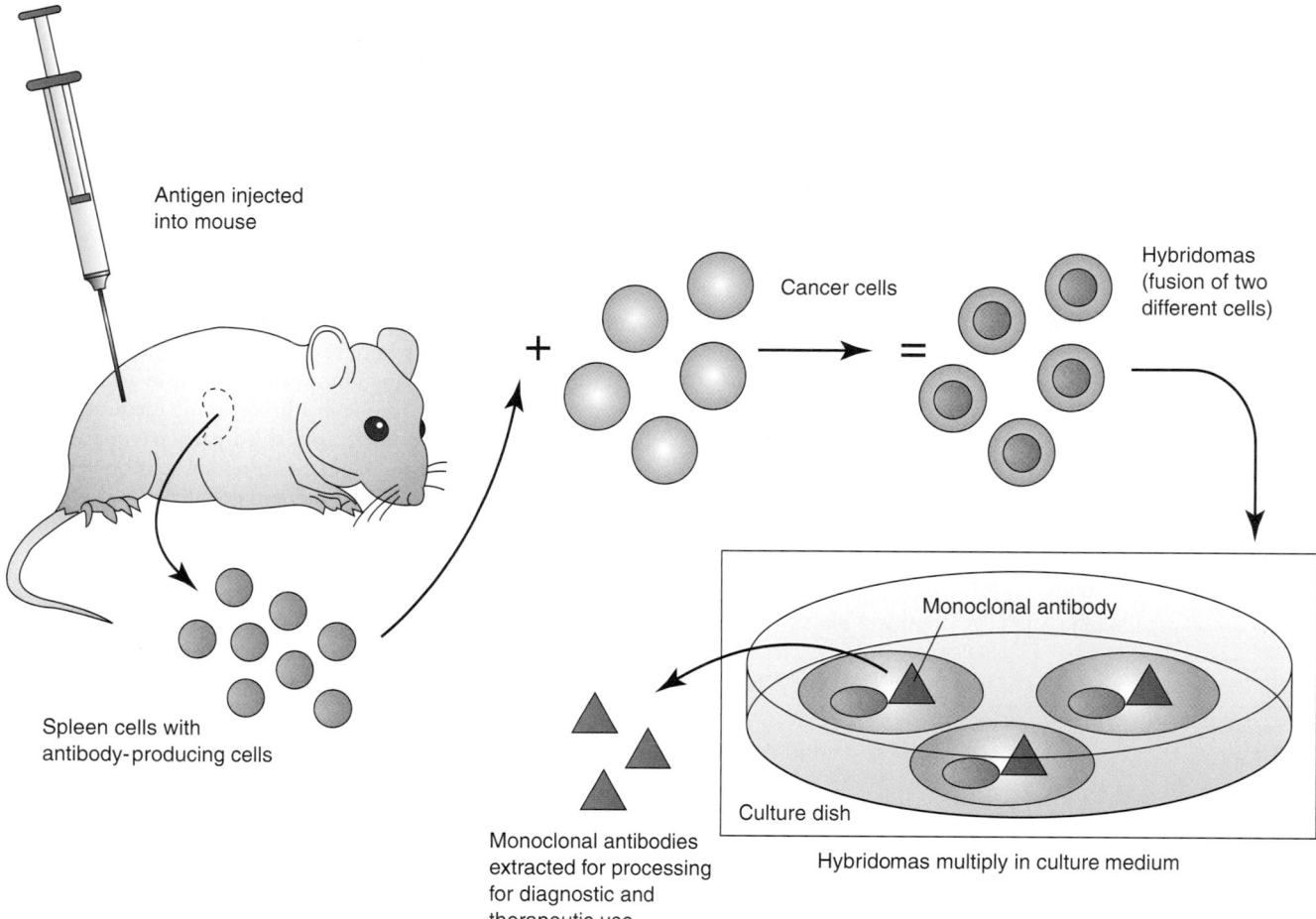

FIGURE 16-5 Antibody-producing spleen cells are fused with cancer cells. This process produces cells called hybridomas. These cells, which can grow indefinitely in a culture medium, produce antibodies that are harvested, purified, and prepared for diagnostic or treatment purposes.

(adversely affecting the bone marrow), such as radiation and chemotherapy. Previously, the myelotoxic or bone marrow suppressive effects of chemotherapy had imposed limits on some chemotherapy agents and contributed to the development of life-threatening infections.

GM-CSF is used to treat the **neutropenia** (decreased numbers of neutrophils in the blood) associated with BMT. G-CSF is used to treat neutropenia associated with chemotherapy for solid tumor malignancies. IL-11 is used to prevent severe thrombocytopenia and reduce the need for platelet transfusions in patients following myelosuppressive therapy for nonmyeloid cancers. EPO is used to treat anemia in cancer patients as well as in patients with chronic renal disease and in patients with HIV infection with zidovudine-induced anemia. Other growth factors, such as macrophage colony-stimulating factor and IL-3, are being investigated.

TUMOR NECROSIS FACTOR

TNF is a cytokine naturally produced by macrophages, lymphocytes, astrocytes, and microglial cells of the brain. The exact role of TNF is still under investigation. In vitro studies have shown TNF to stimulate other cells of the immune response; in animal studies it has been shown to have direct tumor-killing activity. Clinical trials using systemic TNF have been halted because of severe toxicities (Pazadur, Coia, Hoskins & Wagman, 2001). Current clinical trials are examining local administration of TNF for patients with sarcomas and melanomas of the extremities.

Retinoids

Retinoids are vitamin A derivatives (retinol, all-*trans*-retinoic acid, and 13-*cis*-retinoic acid) that play a role in growth, reproduction, epithelial cell differentiation, and immune function. All-*trans*-retinoic acid (tretinoin) has been granted FDA approval for treating acute promyelocytic leukemia, a rare form of leukemia. Retinoids are being tested for treating both hematologic cancers and solid tumors and for preventing a variety of cancers (Evans & Kaye, 1999; Kelloff, 2000; Kurie, 1999).

Nursing Management in Biologic Response Modifier Therapy

Patients receiving BRM therapy have many of the same needs as cancer patients undergoing other treatment approaches. However, some BRM therapies are still investigational and considered a last-chance effort by many patients who have not responded to standard treatments. Consequently, it is essential that the nurse assess the need for education, support, and guidance for both the patient and family and assist in planning and evaluating patient care.

MONITORING THERAPEUTIC AND ADVERSE EFFECTS

Nurses need to be familiar with each agent given and the potential effects (Table 16-7). Adverse effects, such as fever, myalgia, nausea, and vomiting, as seen with IFN therapy, may not be life-threatening. However, nurses must be aware of the impact of these side effects on the patient's quality of life. Other life-threatening adverse effects (eg, capillary leak syndrome, pulmonary edema, and hypotension) may occur with IL-2 therapy. Nurses must work closely with physicians to assess and manage potential toxicities of BRM therapy. Because of the investigational nature of many of these agents, the nurse will be administering them in a research setting. Accurate observations and careful documentation are essential components of patient assessment and data collection.

PROMOTING HOME AND COMMUNITY-BASED CARE

Teaching Patients Self-Care. Some BRMs, such as IFN, EPO, and G-CSF, can be administered by the patient or family in the home. Nurses teach patients and families, as needed, how to administer these agents through subcutaneous injections. Further, they provide instructions about side effects and assist patients and families to identify strategies to manage many of the common side effects of BRM therapy, such as fatigue, anorexia, and flu-like symptoms.

Continuing Care. Referral for home care is usually indicated to monitor the patient's responses to treatment and continue and reinforce teaching. During home visits, the nurse assesses the patient's and family's technique in administering medications. The nurse collaborates with physicians, third-party payors, and pharmaceutical companies to help patients obtain reimbursement for home administration of BRM therapies. The nurse also reminds

Table 16-7 • Side Effects of FDA-Approved Biologic Response Modifiers

AGENT	SELECTED SIDE EFFECTS
Monoclonal Antibodies	
Rituximab	Allergic/anaphylactic reactions; fever; chills; nausea; headache; abdominal pain; decreased lymphocyte, white blood cell, platelet, and red blood cell counts; back pain; night sweats; itching; cough; infection
Trastuzumab	Allergic/anaphylactic reactions, hypotension, fever, chills, heart failure, stroke, diarrhea, infection, rash, nausea, vomiting, anorexia, insomnia, dizziness, headache, chills, back pain, weakness, rhinitis, pharyngitis, cough
Gemtuzumab	Allergic/anaphylactic reactions; fever; chills; weakness; abdominal pain; headache; dyspnea; epistaxis; cough; tachycardia; hemorrhage; local skin reaction; rash; petechiae; peripheral edema; nausea; vomiting; diarrhea; anorexia; stomatitis; constipation; indigestion; dizziness; decreased platelet, white and red blood cell counts; increased bilirubin, potassium, and LDH values
Alemtuzumab	Allergic/anaphylactic reactions, fever, chills, rash, hives, itching, sweating, nausea, vomiting, diarrhea, stomatitis, abdominal pain, indigestion, infection, headache, dizziness, muscle pain, insomnia, dyspnea, cough, bronchitis/pneumonitis, pharyngitis, fatigue, skeletal pain, anorexia, weakness, peripheral edema, decreased white, platelet, and red blood cell counts
Ibritumomab	Decreased platelets, white blood cell and red blood cell counts, weakness, chills, abdominal pain, fever, difficulty breathing, nausea and vomiting
Cytokines	
Interferon alfa	Flu-like symptoms (fever, chills, weakness, muscle and joint pain, headaches); fatigue; anorexia; mental status changes; rash; pruritus; hair loss; abdominal pain; nausea; constipation; diarrhea; irritation at the injection site; depression; irritability; insomnia; cough; decreased white blood cell, red blood cell, and platelet counts; abnormal liver function values
Interleukin-2	Flu-like symptoms (fever, chills, weakness, muscle and joint pain, headaches); fatigue; anorexia; nausea; vomiting; diarrhea; capillary leak syndrome; edema and fluid retention; hypotension; tachycardia; skin rash; erythema; desquamation; irritation at the injection site; weight gain during therapy due to fluid retention; weight loss after therapy related to anorexia with long-term therapy; decreased white blood cell, red blood cell, and platelet counts; abnormal liver function values
Filgrastim (granulocyte growth factor)	Bone pain, malaise, fever, fatigue, headache, skin rash, weakness
Sargranstim (granulocyte-macrophage growth factor)	Allergic/anaphylactic reaction with first dose, bone pain, fever, fatigue, headache, weakness, chills, skin rash, infection
Epoetin alfa (erythrocyte growth factor)	Fever, fatigue, weakness, bone pain, diarrhea, dizziness, nausea, edema, shortness of breath
Oprelvekin (platelet growth factor)	Edema, fever, headache, rash, chills, bone pain, fatigue, nausea, vomiting, abdominal pain, constipation, rhinitis, cough, arrhythmia, skin discoloration, bleeding, dehydration, amblyopia, dermatitis
Retinoids	
Retinoic acid	Headache, fever, skin and mucous membrane dryness, bone pain, nausea and vomiting, dyspnea, pleural and pericardial effusions, malaise, chills, bleeding, heart failure, mental status changes, depression, abnormal liver function tests

patients about the importance of keeping follow-up appointments with the physician and assesses the patient's need for changes in care.

PHOTODYNAMIC THERAPY

Photodynamic therapy, or phototherapy, is an investigational cancer treatment that uses photosensitizing agents, such as porfimer (Photofrin). When administered intravenously, these agents are retained in higher concentrations in malignant tissue than in normal tissue. They are then activated by a light source, usually laser light, which penetrates body tissue. The light-activated agent then creates activated singlet oxygen molecules that are cytotoxic or harmful to body tissue cells. Because most of the photosensitizing agent has been retained in malignant tissue, a selective cytotoxicity can be achieved with minimal destruction to normal tissues.

Cancers treated with phototherapy include esophageal cancers, endobronchial tumors, skin cancers, breast cancers, intraperitoneal tumors, and malignant central nervous system disease. The major side effect of therapy is photosensitivity for 4 to 6 weeks after treatment. Patients must protect themselves from direct and indirect sunlight to prevent skin burns. In addition, local reactions are observed in the area treated. Liver and renal function should also be monitored for transient abnormalities. As with any investigational treatment, emotional support and education are vital to assist the patient and family.

GENE THERAPY

As early as 1914, the somatic mutation theory of cancer suggested that cancer develops as a result of inherited or acquired genetic mutations that lead to a disturbance in the normal chromosomal balance regulating cell growth and reproduction. Technological advances and information gained through intense study of genetics have assisted researchers and clinicians in predicting, diagnosing, and treating cancer. Gene therapy includes approaches that correct genetic defects or manipulate genes to induce tumor cell destruction in the hope of preventing or combating disease. Somatic cell (any cell not contained in an embryo or destined to become an egg or sperm) gene therapy is the only publicly funded form of gene therapy in the United States. This type of therapy involves the insertion of a desired gene into the targeted cells. Human germ cell manipulation is considered by many to be controversial and a potential source of bioethical concerns (Frankel & Chapman, 2000).

Although gene therapy is currently investigational, researchers predict it will have a profound impact on medical and health care in the 21st century. More than 100 clinical trials for gene therapy in treating cancer have been initiated. An example of one such trial involves inserting the p53 tumor suppressor gene into cancer cells. Normally this gene is responsible for repairing damaged cells or causing cell death when the cell cannot be repaired. Many types of cancer cells have mutated p53 genes that then lead to uncontrolled cell growth. Insertion of normal p53 genes can lead to either cancer cell death or slowing of tumor growth. This approach has been tested in lung, head and neck, and colon cancers (Wasil & Buchbinder, 2000). In another clinical trial, a "suicide gene" is inserted into tumor cells to facilitate cell death. When the gene for herpes simplex virus thymidine kinase is inserted into malignant cells, those cells become infected with the virus and susceptible to destruction by antiviral drugs, such as ganciclovir. This approach has been tried in treating brain, ovar-

ian, and breast cancers (Fibison, 2000). For more information about investigational therapies, see Chart 16-4.

UNPROVEN AND UNCONVENTIONAL THERAPIES

A diagnosis of cancer evokes many emotions in patients and families, including feelings of fear, frustration, and loss of control. Despite increasing 5-year survival rates with the use of traditional methods of treatment, a significant number of patients use or seriously consider using some form of unconventional treatment. Hopelessness, desperation, unmet needs, lack of factual information, and family or social pressures are major factors that motivate patients to seek unconventional methods of treatment and allow them to fall prey to deceptive practices and quackery. Although research is scant and accuracy of reporting may be questionable, it is estimated that 30% to 50% of patients with cancer may be using a complementary or alternative method of treatment.

Caring for patients who choose unconventional methods may place members of the health care team in difficult situations professionally, legally, and ethically. Nurses must keep in mind those ethical principles that help guide professional practice, such as autonomy, beneficence, nonmaleficence, and justice.

Unconventional treatments have not demonstrated scientifically, in an objective, reproducible method, the ability to cure or control cancer. In addition to being ineffective, some unconventional treatments may also be harmful to patients and may cost thousands of dollars. Most unproven cancer treatments can be categorized as machines and devices, drugs and biologicals, metabolic and dietary regimens, or mystical and spiritual approaches.

Machines and Devices

Electrical gadgets and devices are commonly reputed to cure cancers. Most are operated by people with questionable training who report unrealistic and unlikely success stories. Such machines are often decorated with elaborate lights and dials and produce vibrations or other sensations.

Drugs and Biologicals

Medicinal agents, herbs, proteins (such as shark cartilage), megavitamins (including vitamin C therapy), immune therapy, vaccines, enzymes, hydrogen peroxide, and sera have been frequent components of fraudulent cancer therapy. These agents have included oral, intravenous, and external medications derived from weeds, flowers, and herbs and the blood and urine of patients and animals. Many of these agents, especially in megadoses, can be toxic and can have untoward interactions with concomitant medications. Herbs commonly used by individuals with cancer include echinacea, essiac, ginseng, green tea, pau d'arco, and hoxsey (Montbriand, 1999). Many of these treatments are costly.

Metabolic and Dietary Regimens

Metabolic and dietary regimens emphasize the ingestion of only natural substances to purify the body and retard cancerous growth. These regimens include the grape diet, the carrot juice diet, garlic, onions, various teas, coffee enemas, and raw liver intake. Laetrile (vitamin B, amygdalin), one of the best-known forms of cancer quackery, was advocated as an agent to kill tumor cells by releasing cyanide, which is especially toxic to malignant cells. The National Cancer Institute, in response to public demand, investigated the effects of laetrile and reported no therapeutic benefits with its use; indeed, many toxic effects (cyanide poisoning, fever, rash, headache, vomiting, diarrhea, and hypotension) were reported. Macrobiotic diets have also been advocated as a cancer treatment to reestablish balance between the major forces in the universe, yin and yang. People who adhere to macrobiotic diets tend to develop vitamin, mineral, and protein deficiencies; experience additional weight loss due to decreased calorie intake; and receive no therapeutic benefits from the diet.

Mystical and Spiritual Approaches

Traditional Chinese medicine attempts to balance chi forces in order to heal the body. Mystical or spiritual approaches to cancer therapy include such techniques as psychic surgery, faith healing, "laying on of hands," prayer groups, and invocation of mystical universal powers to kill cancerous growths. These techniques are difficult to disclaim because they are based on faith.

Nursing Management in Unconventional Therapies

A trusting relationship, supportive care, and promotion of hope in the patient and family are the most effective means of protecting them from fraudulent therapy and questionable cancer cures. Truthful responses given in a nonjudgmental manner to questions and inquiries about unproven methods of cancer treatments may alleviate the fear and guilt on the part of the patient and family that they are not "doing everything we can" to obtain a cure. The nurse may inform the patient and family of the characteristics common to fraudulent therapy so that they will be informed and cautious when evaluating other forms of "therapy." The nurse should encourage any patient who uses unconventional therapies to inform the physician about such use. Knowing this information can help prevent interactions with medications and other therapies that may be prescribed and avoid attributing the side effects of unconventional therapies to prescribed medications.

NURSING PROCESS: THE PATIENT WITH CANCER

The outlook for patients with cancer has greatly improved because of scientific and technological advances. As a result of the underlying disease or various treatment modalities, however, the patient with cancer may experience a variety of secondary problems, such as infection, reduced WBC counts, bleeding, skin problems, nutritional problems, pain, fatigue, and psychological stress.

Assessment

Regardless of the type of cancer treatment or prognosis, many patients with cancer are susceptible to the following problems and complications. An important role of the nurse on the oncology team is to assess the patient for these problems and complications.

INFECTION

In all stages of cancer, the nurse assesses factors that can promote infection. Infection is the leading cause of death in cancer patients. Factors predisposing patients to infection are summarized in

Table 16-8. The nurse monitors laboratory studies to detect early changes in WBC counts. Common sites of infection, such as the pharynx, skin, perianal area, urinary tract, and respiratory tract, are assessed frequently. The typical signs of infection (swelling, redness, drainage, and pain), however, may not occur in the immunosuppressed patient due to a diminished local inflammatory response. Fever may be the only sign of infection that the patient exhibits. The nurse also monitors the patient for sepsis, particularly if invasive catheters or infusion lines are in place.

WBC function is often impaired in cancer patients. A decrease in circulating WBCs is referred to as leukopenia or granulocytopenia. There are three types of WBCs: neutrophils, basophils, and eosinophils. The neutrophils, totaling 60% to 70% of all the body's WBCs, play a major role in combating infection by engulfing and destroying infective agents in a process called phagocytosis. Both the total WBC count and the concentration of neutrophils are important in determining the patient's ability to fight infection.

A differential WBC count identifies the relative numbers of WBCs and permits tabulation of polymorphonuclear neutrophils (mature neutrophils, reported as "polys," PMNs, or "segs") and immature forms of neutrophils (reported as bands, metamyelocytes, and "stabs"). These numbers are compiled and reported as the absolute neutrophil count (ANC). The ANC is calculated by the following formula:

$$ANC = \frac{(\text{Total WBC count} \times [\% \text{ segmented neutrophils} + \% \text{ bands}])}{100}$$

For example, if the patient's total WBC count is 6,000, with segmented neutrophils 25% and bands 25%, the ANC would be 3,000.

Neutropenia, an abnormally low ANC, is associated with an increased risk for infection. The risk for infection rises as the ANC decreases and persists. An ANC of less than 1,000 cells/mm³ reflects a severe risk for infection. **Nadir** is the lowest ANC after myelosuppressive chemotherapy or radiation therapy. Therapies that suppress bone marrow function are called myelosuppressive. Febrile patients who are neutropenic are assessed for infection through cultures of blood, sputum, urine, stool, catheter, or wounds, if appropriate. In addition, a chest x-ray is often included to assess for pulmonary infections.

BLEEDING

The nurse assesses cancer patients for factors that may contribute to bleeding. These include bone marrow suppression from radiation, chemotherapy, and other medications that interfere with coagulation and platelet functioning, such as aspirin, dipyridamole (Persantine), heparin, or warfarin (Coumadin). Common bleeding sites include skin and mucous membranes; the intestinal, urinary, and respiratory tracts; and the brain. Gross hemorrhage, as well as blood in the stools, urine, sputum, or vomitus (melena, hematuria, hemoptysis, hematemesis), oozing at injection sites, bruising (ecchymosis), petechiae, and changes in mental status, are monitored and reported.

SKIN PROBLEMS

The integrity of skin and tissue is at risk in cancer patients because of the effects of chemotherapy, radiation therapy, surgery, and invasive procedures carried out for diagnosis and therapy. As part of the assessment, the nurse identifies which of these predisposing factors are present and assesses the patient for other risk factors, including nutritional deficits, bowel and bladder incontinence, immobility, immunosuppression, multiple skin folds,

FACTORS	UNDERLYING MECHANISMS
Table 16-8 • Factors Predisposing Cancer Patients to Infection	
1. Impaired skin and mucous membrane integrity	• Loss of body's first line of defense against invading organisms.
2. Chemotherapy	• Many agents cause suppression of bone marrow, resulting in decreased production and function of white blood cells. Chemotherapy agents that cause mucositis impair skin and mucous membrane integrity. Organ damage associated with certain agents may also predispose patients to infection. Organ damage such as pulmonary fibrosis or cardiomyopathy that is associated with certain agents may also predispose patients to infection.
3. Radiation therapy	• Radiation involving sites of bone marrow production may result in bone marrow suppression. May also lead to impaired tissue integrity.
4. Biologic response modifiers	• Some biologic response modifiers may cause bone marrow suppression and organ dysfunction.
5. Malignancy	• Malignant cells may infiltrate the bone marrow and interfere with production of white blood cells and lymphocytes. Hematologic malignancies (leukemias and lymphomas) are associated with impaired function and production of blood cells.
6. Malnutrition	• Results in impaired function and production of cells of the immune response. May contribute to impaired skin integrity.
7. Medications	• Antibiotics disturb the balance of normal flora, allowing them to become pathogenic. This process occurs most commonly in the gastrointestinal tract. Corticosteroids and nonsteroidal anti-inflammatory drugs mask inflammatory responses.
8. Urinary catheter	• Creates port and mechanism of entry for organisms.
9. Intravenous catheter	• Results in impaired skin integrity and site of entry for organisms.
10. Other invasive procedures (surgery, paracentesis, thoracentesis, drainage tubes, endoscopies, mechanical ventilation)	• Creates port of entry and possible introduction of exogenous organisms into the system.
11. Contaminated equipment	• Environmental objects such as stagnant water in oxygen equipment are associated with growth of microorganisms.
12. Age	• Increasing age associated with declining organ function. Also associated with decreased production and functioning of the cells of the immune system.
13. Chronic illness	• Associated with impaired organ function and altered immune responses.
14. Prolonged hospitalization	• Allows increased exposure to nosocomial infection and colonization of new organisms.

and changes related to aging. Skin lesions or ulcerations secondary to the tumor are noted. Alterations in tissue integrity throughout the gastrointestinal tract are particularly bothersome to the patient. Any lesions of the oral mucous membranes are noted, as are their effects on the patient's nutritional status and comfort level.

HAIR LOSS

Alopecia (hair loss) is another form of tissue disruption common to cancer patients who receive radiation therapy or chemotherapy. In addition to noting hair loss, the nurse also assesses the psychological impact of this side effect on the patient and the family.

NUTRITIONAL CONCERNS

Assessing the patient's nutritional status is an important nursing role. Impaired nutritional status may contribute to disease progression, immune incompetence, increased incidence of infection, delayed tissue repair, diminished functional ability, and decreased capacity to continue antineoplastic therapy. Altered nutritional status, weight loss, and cachexia (muscle wasting, emaciation) may be secondary to decreased protein and caloric intake, metabolic or mechanical effects of the cancer, systemic disease, side effects of the treatment, or the emotional status of the patient.

The patient's weight and caloric intake are monitored on a consistent basis. Other information obtained through assessment includes diet history, any episodes of anorexia, changes in appetite, situations and foods that aggravate or relieve anorexia, and medication history. Difficulty in chewing or swallowing is determined and the occurrence of nausea, vomiting, or diarrhea is noted.

Clinical and laboratory data useful in assessing the patient's nutritional status include anthropometric measurements (triceps skin fold and middle-upper arm circumference), serum protein levels (albumin and transferrin), serum electrolytes, lymphocyte count, skin response to intradermal injection of antigens, hemoglobin levels, hematocrit, urinary creatinine levels, and serum iron levels.

PAIN

Pain and discomfort in cancer may be related to the underlying disease, pressure exerted by the tumor, diagnostic procedures, or the cancer treatment itself. As in any other situation involving pain, cancer pain is affected by both physical and psychosocial influences.

In addition to assessing the source and site of pain, the nurse also assesses those factors that increase the patient's perception of pain, such as fear and apprehension, fatigue, anger, and social isolation. Pain assessment scales (see Chap. 13) are useful in assessing the patient's pain level before pain-relieving interventions are instituted and in evaluating their effectiveness.

FATIGUE

Acute fatigue, which occurs after an energy-demanding experience, serves a protective function; chronic fatigue, however, does not. It is often overwhelming, excessive, and not responsive to rest, and it seriously affects quality of life. Fatigue is the most commonly reported side effect in patients who receive chemotherapy and radiation therapy. The nurse assesses for feelings of weariness, weakness, lack of energy, inability to carry out necessary and valued daily functions, lack of motivation, and inability to concentrate. Patients may become less verbal and appear pallid, with relaxed facial musculature. The nurse assesses physiologic and psychological stressors that can contribute to fatigue, including pain, nausea, dyspnea, constipation, fear, and anxiety. (See Nursing Research Profile 16-2.)

PSYCHOSOCIAL STATUS

Nursing assessment also focuses on the patient's psychological and mental status as the patient and the family face this life-threatening experience, unpleasant diagnostic tests and treatment modalities, and progression of disease. The patient's mood and emotional reaction to the results of diagnostic testing and prognosis are assessed, along with evidence that the patient is progressing through the stages of grief and can talk about the diagnosis and prognosis with the family.

BODY IMAGE

Cancer patients are forced to cope with many assaults to body image throughout the course of disease and treatment. Entry into the health care system is often accompanied by depersonalization. Threats to self-concept are enormous as patients face the realization of illness, possible disability, and death. To accommodate treatments or because of the disease, many cancer patients are forced to alter their lifestyles. Priorities and values change when body image is threatened. Disfiguring surgery, hair loss, cachexia, skin changes, altered communication patterns, and sexual dysfunction are some of the devastating results of cancer and its treatment that threaten the patient's self-esteem and body image. The nurse identifies these potential threats and assesses the patient's ability to cope with these changes.

Diagnosis

NURSING DIAGNOSES

Based on the assessment data, nursing diagnoses of the patient with cancer may include the following:

- Impaired oral mucous membrane
- Impaired tissue integrity
- Impaired tissue integrity: alopecia
- Impaired tissue integrity: malignant skin lesions
- Imbalanced nutrition, less than body requirements
- Anorexia
- Malabsorption
- Cachexia
- Chronic pain
- Fatigue
- Disturbed body image
- Anticipatory grieving

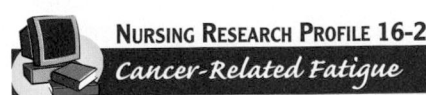

NURSING RESEARCH PROFILE 16-2
Cancer-Related Fatigue

Berger, A. M., & Farr, L. (1999). The influence of daytime inactivity and nighttime restlessness on cancer-related fatigue. *Oncology Nursing Forum,* *26*(10), 1663–1671.

Purpose

Negative, long-term consequences of chemotherapy, including fatigue, have been reported. Many women report fatigue during and following breast cancer treatment; however, perceptions of fatigue have not been objectively quantified. The purpose of this study was to identify relationships between circadian activity/rest indicators and fatigue experienced by women during the first three chemotherapy cycles for stage I/II breast cancer.

Study Sample and Design

A prospective, descriptive, repeated-measures study was conducted over a 12-month period. Seventy-two participants were recruited for the study; 12 withdrew, leaving a sample of 60 women. To be eligible for the study, women had to be 33 to 69 years of age, diagnosed for the first time with stage I/II breast cancer, scheduled to begin one of three intravenous chemotherapy regimens following recent modified radical mastectomy or breast-conservation surgery, English-speaking, and able to complete the research instruments.

A wrist actigraph was used for continuous monitoring of body movement over time, providing data for analysis of circadian activity/rest cycles; relative activity within days and across days; and the timing, duration, and disruption of sleep. Data were collected for 96 hours at the start of each treatment and for 72 hours at the midpoint of each chemotherapy cycle. Data from the actigraph were downloaded to a software program. The Piper Fatigue scale was used to measure participants' subjective perception of fatigue shortly after each chemotherapy treatment and on the midpoint days of each cycle coinciding with the actigraph measurements.

Findings

Analysis of data revealed that participants who were less active during the day and had more nighttime awakenings consistently reported higher levels of cancer-related fatigue (CRF) at the midpoint of each chemotherapy cycle. The number of night awakenings had the strongest association with CRF. Decreased daytime activity and nighttime restlessness were associated with higher CRF. Participants who were more active maintained more distinctive circadian activity/rest rhythms.

Nursing Implications

The findings of this study demonstrate that women whose sleep is disrupted at midpoints of chemotherapy cycles are at risk for CRF. Higher CRF levels are associated with the cumulative effects of less daytime activity, more daytime sleep, and night awakenings. Sedentary lifestyles in response to fatigue result, in turn, in increased fatigue. These findings suggest the need to assist women with developing a balance of activity and rest; advising women to "take it easy" during chemotherapy may result in decreased activity and increased fatigue.

COLLABORATIVE PROBLEMS/ POTENTIAL COMPLICATIONS

Based on the assessment data, potential complications that may develop include the following:

- Infection and sepsis
- Hemorrhage
- Superior vena cava syndrome
- Spinal cord compression
- Hypercalcemia
- Pericardial effusion

- Disseminated intravascular coagulation
- Syndrome of inappropriate secretion of antidiuretic hormone
- Tumor lysis syndrome

See the later section, Oncologic Emergencies, for more information.

Planning and Goals

The major goals for the patient may include management of stomatitis, maintenance of tissue integrity, maintenance of nutrition, relief of pain, relief of fatigue, improved body image, effective progression through the grieving process, and absence of complications.

Nursing Interventions

The patient with cancer is at risk for various adverse effects of therapy and complications. The nurse in all health care settings, including the home, assists the patient and family in managing these problems.

MANAGING STOMATITIS

Stomatitis, an inflammatory response of the oral tissues, commonly develops within 5 to 14 days after the patient receives certain chemotherapeutic agents, such as doxorubicin and 5-fluorouracil, and BRMs, such as IL-2 and IFN. As many as 40% of patients receiving chemotherapy experience some degree of stomatitis during treatment. Patients receiving dose-intensive chemotherapy (considerably higher doses than conventional dosing), such as those undergoing BMT, are at increased risk for stomatitis. Stomatitis may also occur with radiation to the head and neck. Stomatitis is characterized by mild redness (erythema) and edema or, if severe, by painful ulcerations, bleeding, and secondary infection. In severe cases of stomatitis, cancer therapy may be temporarily halted until the inflammation decreases.

As a result of normal everyday wear and tear, the epithelial cells that line the oral cavity undergo rapid turnover and slough off routinely. Chemotherapy and radiation interfere with the body's ability to replace those cells. An inflammatory response develops as denuded areas appear in the oral cavity. Poor oral hygiene, existing dental disease, use of other medications that dry mucous membranes, and impaired nutritional status contribute to morbidity associated with stomatitis. Radiation-induced xerostomia (dry mouth) associated with decreased function of the salivary glands may contribute to stomatitis in patients who have received radiation to the head and neck.

Myelosuppression (bone marrow depression) resulting from underlying disease or its treatment predisposes the patient to oral bleeding and infection. Pain associated with ulcerated oral tissues can significantly interfere with nutritional intake, speech, and a willingness to maintain oral hygiene.

Although multiple studies on stomatitis have been published, the optimal prevention and treatment approaches have not been identified. However, most clinicians agree that good oral hygiene that includes brushing, flossing, and rinsing is necessary to minimize the risk for oral complications associated with cancer therapies. Soft-bristled toothbrushes and nonabrasive toothpaste prevent or reduce trauma to the oral mucosa. Oral swabs with spongelike applicators may be used in place of a toothbrush for painful oral tissues. Flossing may be performed unless it causes pain or unless platelet levels are below 40,000/mm³ (0.04 × 10^{12}/L). Oral rinses with saline solution or tap water may be nec-

essary for patients who cannot tolerate a toothbrush. Products that irritate oral tissues or impair healing, such as alcohol-based mouth rinses, are avoided. Foods that are difficult to chew or are hot or spicy are avoided to minimize further trauma. The patient's lips are lubricated to keep them from becoming dry and cracked. Topical anti-inflammatory and anesthetic agents may be prescribed to promote healing and minimize discomfort. Products that coat or protect oral mucosa are used to promote comfort and prevent further trauma. The patient who experiences severe pain and discomfort with stomatitis requires systemic analgesics.

Adequate fluid and food intake is encouraged. In some instances, parenteral hydration and nutrition are needed. Topical or systemic antifungal and antibiotic medications are prescribed to treat local or systemic infections.

MAINTAINING TISSUE INTEGRITY

Some of the most frequently encountered disturbances of tissue integrity, in addition to stomatitis, include skin and tissue reactions to radiation therapy, alopecia, and metastatic skin lesions.

The patient who is experiencing skin and tissue reactions to radiation therapy requires careful skin care to prevent further skin irritation, drying, and damage. The skin over the affected area is handled gently; rubbing and use of hot or cold water, soaps, powders, lotions, and cosmetics are avoided. The patient may avoid tissue injury by wearing loose-fitting clothes and avoiding clothes that constrict, irritate, or rub the affected area. If blistering occurs, care is taken not to disrupt the blisters, thus reducing the risk of introducing bacteria. Moisture- and vapor-permeable dressings, such as hydrocolloids and hydrogels, are helpful in promoting healing and reducing pain. Aseptic wound care is indicated to minimize the risk for infection and sepsis. Topical antibiotics, such as 1% silver sulfadiazine cream (Silvadene), may be prescribed for use on areas of moist desquamation (painful, red, moist skin).

ASSISTING PATIENTS TO COPE WITH ALOPECIA

The temporary or permanent thinning or complete loss of hair is a potential adverse effect of various radiation therapies and chemotherapeutic agents. The extent of alopecia depends on the dose and duration of therapy. These treatments cause alopecia by damaging stem cells and hair follicles. As a result, the hair is brittle and may fall out or break off at the surface of the scalp. Loss of other body hair is less frequent. Hair loss usually begins within 2 to 3 weeks after the initiation of treatment; regrowth begins within 8 weeks after the last treatment. Some patients who undergo radiation to the head may sustain permanent hair loss. Many health care providers view hair loss as a minor problem when compared with the potentially life-threatening consequences of cancer. For many patients, however, hair loss is a major assault on body image, resulting in depression, anxiety, anger, rejection, and isolation. To patients and families, hair loss can serve as a constant reminder of the challenges cancer places on their coping abilities, interpersonal relationships, and sexuality.

The nurse's role is to provide information about alopecia and to support the patient and family in coping with disturbing effects of therapy, such as hair loss and changes in body image. Patients are encouraged to acquire a wig or hairpiece before hair loss occurs so that the replacement matches their own hair. Use of attractive scarves and hats may make the patient feel less conspicuous. Nurses can refer patients to supportive programs, such as "Look Good, Feel Better," offered by the American Cancer Society. Knowledge that hair usually begins to regrow after completing therapy may comfort some patients, although the color and texture of the new hair may be different.

MANAGING MALIGNANT SKIN LESIONS

Skin lesions may occur with local extension of the tumor or embolization of the tumor into the epithelium and its surrounding lymph and blood vessels. Secondary growth of cancer cells into the skin may result in redness (erythematous areas) or can progress to wounds involving tissue necrosis and infection. The most extensive lesions tend to disintegrate and are purulent and malodorous. In addition, these lesions are a source of considerable pain and discomfort. Although this type of lesion is most often associated with breast cancer and head and neck cancers, it can also occur with lymphoma, leukemia, melanoma, and cancers of the lung, uterus, kidney, colon, and bladder. The development of severe skin lesions is usually associated with a poor prognosis for extended survival.

Ulcerating skin lesions usually indicate widely disseminated disease unlikely to be eradicated. Managing these lesions becomes a nursing priority. Nursing care includes carefully assessing and cleansing the skin, reducing superficial bacteria, controlling bleeding, reducing odor, and protecting the skin from pain and further trauma. The patient and family require assistance and guidance to care for these skin lesions at home. Referral for home care is indicated.

PROMOTING NUTRITION

Most cancer patients experience some weight loss during their illness. Anorexia, malabsorption, and cachexia are examples of nutritional problems that commonly occur in cancer patients; special attention is needed to prevent weight loss and promote nutrition.

Anorexia

Among the many causes of anorexia in the cancer patient are alterations in taste, manifested by increased salty, sour, and metallic taste sensations, and altered responses to sweet and bitter flavors, leading to decreased appetite, decreased nutritional intake, and protein-calorie malnutrition. Taste alterations may result from mineral (eg, zinc) deficiencies, increases in circulating amino acids and cellular metabolites, or the administration of chemotherapeutic agents. Patients undergoing radiation therapy to the head and neck may experience "mouth blindness," which is a severe impairment of taste.

Alterations in the sense of smell also alter taste; this is a common experience of patients with head and neck cancers. Anorexia may occur because the person feels full after eating only a small amount of food. This sense of fullness occurs secondary to a decrease in digestive enzymes, abnormalities in the metabolism of glucose and triglycerides, and prolonged stimulation of gastric volume receptors, which convey the feeling of being full. Psychological distress, such as fear, pain, depression, and isolation, throughout illness may also have a negative impact on appetite. The person may develop an aversion to food because of nausea and vomiting after treatment.

Malabsorption

Many cancer patients are unable to absorb nutrients from the gastrointestinal system as a result of tumor activity and cancer treatment. Tumors can affect the gastrointestinal activity in several ways. They may impair enzyme production or produce fistulas. They secrete hormones and enzymes, such as gastrin; this leads to increased gastrointestinal irritation, peptic ulcer disease, and decreased fat digestion. They also interfere with protein digestion.

Chemotherapy and radiation can irritate and damage mucosal cells of the bowel, inhibiting absorption. Radiation therapy can cause sclerosis of the blood vessels in the bowel and fibrotic changes in the gastrointestinal tissue. Surgical intervention may change peristaltic patterns, alter gastrointestinal secretions, and reduce the absorptive surfaces of the gastrointestinal mucosa, all leading to malabsorption.

Cachexia

Cachexia is common in patients with cancer, especially in advanced disease. Cancer cachexia is related to inadequate nutritional intake along with increasing metabolic demand, increased energy expenditure due to anaerobic metabolism of the tumor, impaired glucose metabolism, competition of the tumor cells for nutrients, altered lipid metabolism, and a suppressed appetite. It is characterized by loss of body weight, adipose tissue, visceral protein, and skeletal muscle. Patients who are cachectic complain of loss of appetite, early satiety, and fatigue. As a result of protein losses they are often anemic and have peripheral edema.

General Nutritional Considerations

Whenever possible, every effort is used to maintain adequate nutrition through the oral route. Food should be prepared in ways that make it appealing. Unpleasant smells and unappetizing-looking foods are avoided. Family members are included in the plan of care to encourage adequate food intake. The patient's preferences, as well as physiologic and metabolic requirements, are considered when selecting foods. Small, frequent meals are provided, with supplements between meals. Patients often tolerate larger amounts of food earlier in the day rather than later, so meals can be planned accordingly. Patients should avoid drinking fluids while eating, to avoid early satiety. Oral hygiene before mealtime often makes meals more pleasant. Pain, nausea, and other symptoms that may interfere with nutrition are assessed and managed. Medications such as corticosteroids or progestational agents such as megestrol acetate have been used successfully as appetite stimulants.

If adequate nutrition cannot be maintained by oral intake, nutritional support via the enteral route may be necessary. Short-term nutritional supplementation may be provided through a nasogastric tube. However, if nutritional support is needed beyond several weeks, a gastrostomy or jejunostomy tube may be inserted. Patients and families are taught to administer enteral nutrition in the home setting.

If malabsorption is a problem, enzyme and vitamin replacement may be instituted. Additional strategies include changing the feeding schedule, using simple diets, and relieving diarrhea. If malabsorption is severe, parenteral nutrition (PN) may be necessary. PN can be administered in several ways: by a long-term venous access device, such as a right atrial catheter, an implanted venous port, or a peripherally inserted central catheter (Fig. 16-6). The nurse teaches the patient and family to care for venous access devices and to administer PN. Home care nurses may assist with or supervise PN in the home.

Interventions to reduce cachexia usually do not prolong survival but may improve the patient's quality of life. Before invasive nutritional strategies are instituted, the nurse should assess the patient carefully and discuss the options with the patient and family. Creative dietary therapies, enteral (tube) feedings, or PN may be necessary to ensure adequate nutrition. Nursing care is

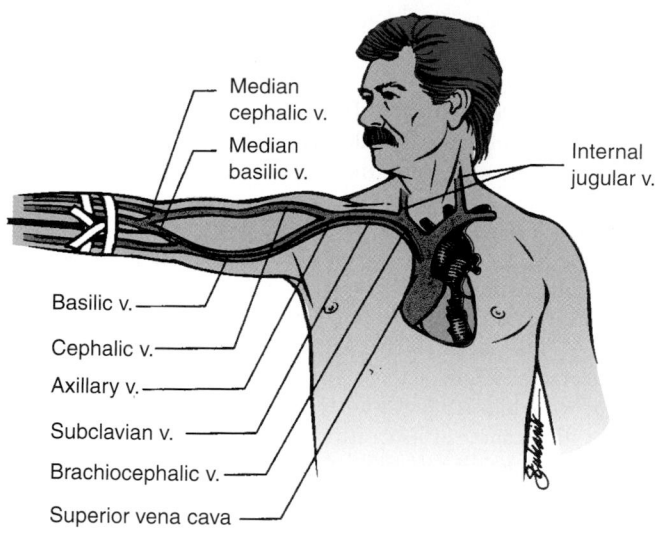

Median cephalic v.
Median basilic v.
Internal jugular v.
Basilic v.
Cephalic v.
Axillary v.
Subclavian v.
Brachiocephalic v.
Superior vena cava

FIGURE 16-6 A peripherally inserted central catheter (PICC) is advanced through the cephalic or basilic vein to the axillary, subclavian, or brachiocephalic vein or the superior vena cava.

also directed toward preventing trauma, infection, and other complications that increase metabolic demands.

RELIEVING PAIN

Of all patients with progressive cancer, more than 75% experience pain (Yarbro, Hansen-Frogge & Goodman, 1999). Although patients with cancer may have acute pain, their pain is more frequently characterized as chronic. (For more information on cancer-related pain, see Chap. 13.) As in other situations involving pain, the experience of cancer pain is influenced by both physical and psychosocial factors.

Cancer can cause pain in various ways (Table 16-9). Pain is also associated with various cancer treatments. Acute pain is linked with trauma from surgery. Occasionally, chronic pain syndromes, such as postsurgical neuropathies (pain related to nerve tissue injury), occur. Some chemotherapeutic agents cause tissue necrosis, peripheral neuropathies, and stomatitis—all potential sources of pain—whereas radiation therapy can cause pain secondary to skin or organ inflammation. Cancer patients may have other sources of pain, such as arthritis or migraine headaches, that are unrelated to the underlying cancer or its treatment.

In today's society, most people expect pain to disappear or resolve quickly, and in fact it usually does. Although controllable, cancer pain is commonly irreversible and not quickly resolved.

For many patients, pain is a signal that the tumor is growing and that death is approaching. As the patient anticipates the pain and anxiety increases, pain perception heightens, producing fear and further pain. Chronic cancer pain, then, can be best described as a cycle progressing from pain to anxiety to fear and back to pain again.

Pain tolerance, the point past which pain can no longer be tolerated, varies among people. Pain tolerance is decreased by fatigue, anxiety, fear of death, anger, powerlessness, social isolation, changes in role identity, loss of independence, and past experiences. Adequate rest and sleep, diversion, mood elevation, empathy, and medications such as antidepressants, antianxiety agents, and analgesics enhance tolerance to pain.

Inadequate pain management is most often the result of misconceptions and insufficient knowledge about pain assessment and pharmacologic interventions on the part of patients, families, and health care providers. Successful management of cancer pain is based on thorough and objective pain assessment that examines physical, psychosocial, environmental, and spiritual factors. A multidisciplinary team approach is essential to determine optimal management of the patient's pain. Unlike instances of chronic nonmalignant pain, systemic analgesics play a central role in managing cancer pain.

The World Health Organization (Dalton & Youngblood, 2000) advocates a three-step approach to treating cancer pain (see Chap. 13). Analgesics are administered based on the patient's level of pain. Nonopioid analgesics (eg, acetaminophen) are used for mild pain; weak opioid analgesics (eg, codeine) are used for moderate pain; and strong opioid analgesics (eg, morphine) are used for severe pain. If the patient's pain escalates, the strength of the analgesic medication is increased until the pain is controlled. Adjuvant medications are also administered to enhance the effectiveness of analgesics and to manage other symptoms that may contribute to the pain experience. Examples of adjuvant medications include antiemetics, antidepressants, anxiolytics, antiseizure agents, stimulants, local anesthetics, radiopharmaceuticals (radioactive agents that may be used to treat painful bone tumors), and corticosteroids.

Preventing and reducing pain help to decrease anxiety and break the pain cycle. This can be accomplished best by administering analgesics on a regularly scheduled basis as prescribed (the preventive approach to pain management), with additional analgesics administered for breakthrough pain as needed and as prescribed.

Various pharmacologic and nonpharmacologic approaches offer the best methods of managing cancer pain. No reasonable approaches, even those that may be invasive, should be over-

Table 16-9 • Sources of Cancer Pain

SOURCE	DESCRIPTIONS	UNDERLYING CANCER
Bone metastasis	Throbbing, aching	Breast, prostate, myeloma
Nerve compression, infiltration	Burning, sharp, tingling	Breast, prostate, lymphoma
Lymphatic or venous obstruction	Dull, aching, tightness	Lymphoma, breast, Kaposi's sarcoma
Ischemia	Sharp, throbbing	Kaposi's sarcoma
Organ obstruction	Dull, crampy, gnawing	Colon, gastric
Organ infiltration	Distention, crampy	Liver, pancreatic
Skin inflammation, ulceration, infection, necrosis	Burning, sharp	Breast, head and neck, Kaposi's sarcoma

looked because of a poor or terminal prognosis. Nurses help patients and families to take an active role in managing pain. Nurses provide education and support to correct fears and misconceptions about opioid use. Inadequate pain control leads to suffering, anxiety, fear, immobility, isolation, and depression. Improving a patient's quality of life is as important as preventing a painful death.

DECREASING FATIGUE

In recent years, fatigue has been recognized as one of the most significant and frequent symptoms experienced by patients receiving cancer therapy. Nurses help the patient and family to understand that fatigue is usually an expected and temporary side effect of the cancer process and of many treatments used. Fatigue also stems from the stress of coping with cancer. It does not always signify that the cancer is advancing or that the treatment is failing. Potential sources of fatigue are summarized in Chart 16-7.

Nursing strategies are implemented to minimize fatigue or assist the patient to cope with existing fatigue. Helping the patient to identify sources of fatigue aids in selecting appropriate and individualized interventions. Ways to conserve energy are developed to help the patient plan daily activities. Alternating periods of rest and activity are beneficial. Regular, light exercise may decrease fatigue and facilitate coping, whereas lack of physical activity and "too much rest" can actually contribute to deconditioning and associated fatigue.

Patients are encouraged to maintain as normal a lifestyle as possible by continuing with those activities they value and enjoy. Prioritizing necessary and valued activities can assist patients in planning for each day. Both patients and families are encouraged to plan to reallocate responsibilities, such as attending to child care, cleaning, and preparing meals. Patients who are employed full-time may need to reduce the number of hours worked each week. The nurse assists the patient and family in coping with these changing roles and responsibilities.

Nurses also address factors that contribute to fatigue and implement pharmacologic and nonpharmacologic strategies to manage pain. Nutrition counseling is provided to patients who are not eating enough calories or protein. Small, frequent meals require less energy for digestion. Serum hemoglobin and hematocrit levels are monitored for deficiencies, and blood products or EPO are administered as prescribed. Patients are monitored for alterations in oxygenation and electrolyte balances. Physical therapy and assistive devices are beneficial for patients with impaired mobility.

IMPROVING BODY IMAGE AND SELF-ESTEEM

A positive approach is essential when caring for the patient with an altered body image. To help the patient retain control and positive self-esteem, it is important to encourage independence and continued participation in self-care and decision making. The patient should be assisted to assume those tasks and participate in those activities that are personally of most value. Any negative feelings that the patient has or threats to body image should be identified and discussed. The nurse serves as a listener and counselor to both the patient and the family. Referral to a support group can provide the patient with additional assistance in coping with the changes resulting from cancer or its treatment. In many cases, a cosmetologist can provide ideas about hair or wig styling, make-up, and the use of scarves and turbans to help with body image concerns.

Patients who experience alterations in sexuality and sexual function are encouraged to discuss concerns openly with their partner. Alternative forms of sexual expression are explored with the patient and partner to promote positive self-worth and acceptance. The nurse who identifies serious physiologic, psychological, or communication difficulties related to sexuality or sexual function is in a key position to assist the patient and partner to seek further counseling if necessary.

ASSISTING IN THE GRIEVING PROCESS

A cancer diagnosis need not indicate a fatal outcome. Many forms of cancer are curable; others may be cured if treated early. Despite these facts, many patients and their families view cancer as a fatal disease that is inevitably accompanied by pain, suffering, debility, and emaciation. Grieving is a normal response to these fears and to the losses anticipated or experienced by the patient with cancer. These may include loss of health, normal sensations, body image, social interaction, sexuality, and intimacy. The patient, family, and friends may grieve for the loss of quality time to spend with others, the loss of future and unfulfilled plans, and the loss of control over one's own body and emotional reactions.

The patient and family just informed of the cancer diagnosis frequently respond with shock, numbness, and disbelief. It is often during this stage that the patient and family are called on to make important initial decisions about treatment. They require the support of the physician, nurse, and other health care team members to make these decisions. An important role of the nurse is to answer any questions the patient and family have and clarify information provided by the physician.

In addition to assessing the response of the patient and family to the diagnosis and planned treatment, the nurse assists them in framing their questions and concerns, identifying resources and support people (eg, spiritual advisor, counselor), and communicating their concerns with each other. Support groups for patients and families are available through hospitals and various community organizations. These groups provide direct assistance, advice, and emotional support.

As the patient and family progress through the grieving process, they may express anger, frustration, and depression. During this time, the nurse encourages the patient and family to verbalize their feelings in an atmosphere of trust and support. The nurse continues to assess their reactions and provides assistance and support as they confront and learn to deal with new problems.

If the patient enters the terminal phase of disease, the nurse may realize that the patient and family members are at different stages of grief. In such cases, the nurse assists the patient and family to ac-

---

Chart 16-7

Sources of Fatigue in Cancer Patients

Pain, pruritus
Imbalanced nutrition related to anorexia, nausea, vomiting, cachexia
Electrolyte imbalance related to vomiting, diarrhea
Ineffective protection related to neutropenia, thrombocytopenia, anemia
Impaired tissue integrity related to stomatitis, mucositis
Impaired physical mobility related to neurologic impairments, surgery, bone metastasis, pain, and analgesic use
Deficient knowledge related to disease process, treatment
Anxiety related to fear, diagnosis, role changes, uncertainty of future
Ineffective breathing patterns related to cough, shortness of breath, and dyspnea
Disturbed sleep pattern related to cancer therapies, anxiety, and pain

knowledge and cope with their reactions and feelings. Nurses also assist patients and families to explore preferences for issues related to end-of-life care such as withdrawal of active disease treatment, desire for the use of life support measures, and symptom management. Support, which can be as simple as holding the patient's hand or just being with the patient at home or at the bedside, often contributes to peace of mind. Maintaining contact with the surviving family members after the death of the cancer patient may help them to work through their feelings of loss and grief. See Chapter 17 for further discussion of end-of-life issues.

MONITORING AND MANAGING POTENTIAL COMPLICATIONS

Despite advances in cancer care, infection remains the leading cause of death. In the cancer patient, defense against infection is compromised in many different ways. The integrity of the skin and mucous membrane, the body's first line of defense, is challenged by multiple invasive diagnostic and therapeutic procedures, by adverse effects of radiation and chemotherapy, and by the detrimental effects of immobility.

Impaired nutrition resulting from anorexia, nausea, vomiting, diarrhea, and the underlying disease alters the body's ability to combat invading organisms. Medications such as antibiotics disturb the balance of normal flora, allowing the overgrowth of pathogenic organisms. Other medications can also alter the immune response (see Chap. 50). Cancer itself may be immunosuppressive. Cancers such as leukemia and lymphoma are often associated with defects in cellular and humoral immunity. Advanced cancer can lead to obstruction by the tumor of the hollow viscera (such as the intestines), blood vessels, and lymphatic vessels, creating a favorable environment for proliferation of pathogenic organisms. In some patients, tumor cells infiltrate bone marrow and prevent normal production of WBCs. Most often, however, a decrease in WBCs is a result of bone marrow suppression after chemotherapy or radiation therapy.

The use of the hematopoietic growth factors, also called colony-stimulating factors (see the previous discussion of BRM therapy), has reduced the severity and duration of neutropenia associated with myelosuppressive chemotherapy and radiation therapy. The administration of these factors assists in reducing the risk for infection and, possibly, in maintaining treatment schedules, drug dosages, treatment effectiveness, and the quality of life.

Infection

Gram-positive organisms, such as *Streptococcus* and *Staphylococcus* species, are the most frequently isolated causes of infection. Gram-negative organisms, such as *Escherichia coli* and *Pseudomonas aeruginosa,* and fungal organisms, such as *Candida albicans,* also contribute to the incidence of serious infection.

Fever is probably the most important sign of infection in the immunocompromised patient. Although fever may be related to a variety of noninfectious conditions, including the underlying cancer, any temperature of 38.3°C (101°F) or higher is reported and dealt with promptly.

Antibiotics may be prescribed to treat infections after cultures of wound drainage, exudate, sputum, urine, stool, or blood are obtained. Patients with neutropenia are treated with broad-spectrum antibiotics before the infecting organism is identified because of the high incidence of mortality associated with untreated infection. Broad-spectrum antibiotic coverage or empiric therapy most often includes a combination of medications to

defend the body against the major pathogenic organisms. An important component of the nurse's role is to administer these medications promptly according to the prescribed schedule to achieve adequate blood levels of the medications.

Strict asepsis is essential when handling intravenous lines, catheters, and other invasive equipment. Exposure of the patient to others with an active infection and to crowds is avoided. Patients with profound immunosuppression, such as BMT recipients, may need to be placed in a protective environment where the room and its contents are sterilized and the air is filtered. These patients may also receive low-bacteria diets, avoiding fresh fruits and vegetables. Hand hygiene and appropriate general hygiene are necessary to reduce exposure to potentially harmful bacteria and to eliminate environmental contaminants. Invasive procedures, such as injections, vaginal or rectal examinations, rectal temperatures, and surgery, are avoided. The patient is encouraged to cough and perform deep-breathing exercises frequently to prevent atelectasis and other respiratory problems. Prophylactic antimicrobial therapy may be used for patients who are expected to be profoundly immunosuppressed and at risk for certain infections. The nurse teaches the patient and family to recognize signs and symptoms of infection to report, perform effective hand hygiene, use antipyretics, maintain skin integrity, and administer hematopoietic growth factors when indicated.

Septic Shock

The nurse assesses the patient frequently for infection and inflammation throughout the course of the disease. Septicemia and septic shock are life-threatening complications that must be prevented or detected and treated promptly. Patients with signs and symptoms of impending sepsis and septic shock require immediate hospitalization and aggressive treatment.

Signs and symptoms of septic shock (see Chap. 15) include altered mental status, either subnormal or elevated temperature, cool and clammy skin, decreased urine output, hypotension, dysrhythmias, electrolyte imbalances, and abnormal arterial blood gas values. The patient and family members are instructed about signs of septicemia, methods for preventing infection, and actions to take if infection or septicemia occurs.

Septic shock is most often associated with overwhelming gram-negative bacterial infections. The nurse monitors the blood pressure, pulse rate, respirations, and temperature of the patient with shock every 15 to 30 minutes. Neurologic assessments are carried out to detect changes in orientation and responsiveness. Fluid and electrolyte status is monitored by measuring fluid intake and output and serum electrolytes. Arterial blood gas values and pulse oximetry are monitored to determine tissue oxygenation. The nurse administers intravenous fluids, blood products, and vasopressors as prescribed to maintain the patient's blood pressure and tissue perfusion. Supplemental oxygen is often necessary. Broad-spectrum antibiotics are administered as prescribed to combat the underlying infection (see Chap. 15).

Bleeding and Hemorrhage

Thrombocytopenia, a decrease in the circulating platelet count, is the most common cause of bleeding in cancer patients and is usually defined as a count of less than 100,000/mm³ (0.1 × 10¹²/L). When the count falls between 20,000 and 50,000/mm³ (0.02 to 0.05 × 10¹²/L), the risk for bleeding increases. Counts under 20,000/mm³ (0.02 × 10¹²/L) are associated with an increased risk for spontaneous bleeding, for which the patient requires a platelet transfusion. Platelets are essential for normal blood clotting and coagulation (hemostasis).

Thrombocytopenia often results from bone marrow depression after certain types of chemotherapy and radiation therapy. Tumor infiltration of the bone marrow can also impair the normal production of platelets. In some cases, platelet destruction is associated with an enlarged spleen (hypersplenism) and abnormal antibody function that occur with leukemia and lymphoma.

In addition to monitoring laboratory values, the nurse continues to assess the patient for bleeding. The nurse also takes steps to prevent trauma and minimize the risk for bleeding by encouraging the patient to use a soft, not stiff, toothbrush and an electric, not straight-edged, razor. Additionally, the nurse avoids unnecessary invasive procedures (eg, rectal temperatures, intramuscular injections, and catheterization) and assists the patient and family to identify and remove environmental hazards that may lead to falls or other trauma. Soft foods, increased fluid intake, and stool softeners, if prescribed, may be indicated to reduce trauma to the gastrointestinal tract. The joints and extremities are handled and moved gently to minimize the risk for spontaneous bleeding. The nurse may administer IL-11, which has been approved by the FDA (Rust, Wood & Battiato, 1999) to prevent severe thrombocytopenia and to reduce the need for platelet transfusions following myelosuppressive chemotherapy in patients with nonmyeloid malignancies. In some instances, the nurse teaches the patient or family member to administer IL-11 in the home.

Hemorrhage may be related to various underlying abnormalities, such as thrombocytopenia and coagulation disorders. These clinical situations are often associated with the cancer itself or the adverse effects of cancer treatments. Sites of hemorrhage may include the gastrointestinal, respiratory, and genitourinary tracts and the brain. Blood pressure and pulse and respiratory rates are monitored every 15 to 30 minutes when hospitalized patients experience bleeding.

Serum hemoglobin and hematocrit are monitored carefully for changes indicating blood loss. The nurse tests all urine, stool, and emesis for occult blood. Neurologic assessments are performed to detect changes in orientation and behavior. The nurse administers fluids and blood products as prescribed to replace any losses. Vasopressor agents are administered as prescribed to maintain blood pressure and ensure tissue oxygenation. Supplemental oxygen is used as necessary.

PROMOTING HOME AND COMMUNITY-BASED CARE

Teaching Patients Self-Care

Patients with cancer usually return home from acute care facilities or receive treatment in the home or outpatient area rather than acute care facilities. The shift from the acute care setting also shifts the responsibility for care to the patient and family. As a result, families and friends must assume increased involvement in patient care, which requires teaching that enables them to provide care. Teaching initially focuses on providing information needed by the patient and family to address the most immediate care needs likely to be encountered at home.

Side effects of treatments and changes in the patient's status that should be reported are reviewed verbally and reinforced with written information. Strategies to deal with side effects of treatment are discussed with the patient and family. Other learning needs are identified based on the priorities conveyed by the patient and family as well as on the complexity of care provided in the home.

Technological advances allow home administration of chemotherapy, PN, blood products, parenteral antibiotics, and parenteral analgesics; management of symptoms; and care of vascular access devices. Although home care nurses provide care and support for patients receiving this advanced technical care, the patient and family need instruction and ongoing support that allow them to feel comfortable and proficient in managing these treatments at home. Follow-up visits and telephone calls from the nurse are often reassuring to the patient and family and increase their comfort in dealing with complex and new aspects of care. Continued contact facilitates evaluation of the patient's progress and ongoing needs.

Continuing Care

Referral for home care is often indicated for the patient with cancer. The responsibilities of the home care nurse include assessing the home environment, suggesting modifications in the home or in care to assist the patient and family in addressing the patient's physical needs, providing physical care, and assessing the psychological and emotional impact of the illness on the patient and family.

Assessing changes in the patient's physical status and reporting relevant changes to the physician help to ensure that appropriate and timely modifications in therapy are made. The home care nurse also assesses the adequacy of pain management and the effectiveness of other strategies to prevent or manage the side effects of treatment modalities.

The patient's and family's understanding of the treatment plan and management strategies is assessed, and previous teaching is reinforced. The nurse often facilitates the coordination of patient care by maintaining close communication with all health care providers involved in the patient's care. The nurse may make referrals and coordinate available community resources (eg, local office of the American Cancer Society, home aides, church groups, parish nurses, and support groups) to assist patients and caregivers.

Evaluation

EXPECTED PATIENT OUTCOMES

For specific patient outcomes, see the Plan of Nursing Care. Expected patient outcomes may include:

1. Maintains integrity of oral mucous membranes
2. Maintains adequate tissue integrity
3. Maintains adequate nutritional status
4. Achieves relief of pain and discomfort
5. Demonstrates increased activity tolerance and decreased fatigue
6. Exhibits improved body image and self-esteem
7. Progresses through the grieving process
8. Experiences no complications, such as infection, or sepsis, and no episodes of bleeding or hemorrhage

Cancer Rehabilitation

Many cancer patients, including those who receive primary surgical treatment and adjuvant chemotherapy or radiation therapy, return to work and their usual activities of daily living. These patients may encounter a variety of problems, including changes in their functional abilities and in the attitudes of employers, coworkers, and family members who still view cancer as a terminal, debilitating disease. Nurses play an important role in the rehabilitation of the cancer patient. Both the patient and family are included as part of any rehabilitation effort because cancer affects not only the patient but also the family members. In addition, with the shift away from inpatient care, many families are caring for patients at home. To maximize beneficial outcomes, evaluation of the patient's needs related to cancer rehabilitation begins early in cancer treatment (Table 16-10).

Assessment for body image changes as a result of disfiguring treatments is necessary to facilitate the patient's adjustment to changes in appearance or functional abilities. The nurse can refer the patient and family to a variety of support groups sponsored by the American Cancer Society, such as those for people who have had laryngectomies or mastectomies. Nurses also collaborate with physical, occupational, and enterostomal therapists in improving the patient's abilities in the use of prosthetic and assistive devices, and in altering the home environment as needed.

Patients often experience distress (eg, pain, nausea) related to the underlying cancer or treatments. These symptoms may interfere with work and quality of life. Nurses assess for these problems and assist the patient in identifying strategies for coping with them. For patients with gastrointestinal disturbances after chemotherapy, altering work hours or receiving treatments in the evenings may prove helpful. Collaboration with physicians and pharmacists is helpful in identifying appropriate interventions.

Nurses collaborate with dietitians to help patients plan meals that will be acceptable and meet nutritional requirements. Nurses are also involved in the ongoing assessment of patients to detect any long-term consequences of cancer treatment.

Although the Americans With Disabilities Act of 1990 was intended to protect patients with disabling disorders against discrimination, recovering cancer patients have reported instances of unfair practices and discrimination in the workplace. Some employers do not understand that different kinds of cancers have different prognoses and different effects on functional ability. As a result, employers may hesitate to hire or continue to employ people with cancer, especially if ongoing treatment regimens require adjustments in work schedules. Employers, coworkers, and families may continue to view the person as "sick" despite ongoing recovery or completion of treatment. Attitudes of coworkers can be a problem when the patient has a communication impairment, as may occur in some head and neck cancers. The patient may benefit from vocational rehabilitation services of the American Cancer Society or other agencies.

Nurses can participate in efforts to educate employers and the public in general to ensure that the rights of patients with cancer are maintained. Whenever possible, nurses assist patients and families to resume preexisting roles. Psychologists and clergy or spiritual advisors are consulted to assist with psychosocial and spiritual concerns. Rehabilitation shifts the focus from what has been lost to what can be done with existing strengths and abilities. In that spirit, nurses encourage patients to regain the highest level of function and independence possible.

 Table 16-10 • Assessing Patient Needs for Cancer Rehabilitation

AREA OF NEED	FACTORS TO ASSESS
Functional	
Activities of daily living	Mobility
	Cognitive impairment
	Sensory impairments
	Communication barriers
Physiologic	
Nutrition	Need for enteral or parenteral nutrition
Elimination	Alterations in bowel and bladder function
Symptoms related to disease or treatment	Pain
	Nausea, vomiting, diarrhea
	Dyspnea, fatigue
	Skin impairment, alopecia
Psychosocial Resources	
Family	Availability of caregiver, home physical environment
	Availability of private transportation; affordability of transportation
Community	Availability of public transportation; affordability of transportation
	Availability and access to community organizations for assistance and support
Personal	Spiritual concerns
	Family relationships
	Body image
	Coping abilities
	Sexuality
Financial	Job security for patient and family members
	Need for vocational training

Gerontologic Considerations

As a result of an increased life expectancy and an increased risk for cancer with age, nurses are providing cancer-related care for growing numbers of elderly patients. More than 58% of all cancers occur in people older than 65 years of age, and about two thirds of all cancer deaths occur in people 65 years of age and older. Nursing care of this population addresses special needs, including physical, psychosocial, and financial concerns.

Oncology nurses working with the elderly population need to understand the normal physiologic changes that occur with aging. These changes include decreased skin elasticity; decreased skeletal mass, structure, and strength; decreased organ function and structure; impaired immune system mechanisms; alterations in neurologic and sensory functions; and altered drug absorption, distribution, metabolism, and elimination. These changes ultimately influence the elderly patient's ability to tolerate cancer treatment. In addition, many elderly patients have other chronic diseases and associated treatments that may limit tolerance to cancer treatments (Table 16-11).

Potential chemotherapy-related toxicities, such as renal impairment, myelosuppression, fatigue, and cardiomyopathy, may increase as a result of declining organ function and diminished physiologic reserves. The recovery of normal tissues after radiation therapy may be delayed, and the patient may experience more severe adverse effects, such as mucositis, nausea and vomiting, and myelosuppression. Because of decreased tissue healing capacity and declining pulmonary and cardiovascular functioning, the older patient is slower to recover from surgery. Elderly patients are also at increased risk for complications such as atelectasis, pneumonia, and wound infections.

Table 16-11 • **Age-Related Changes and Their Effects on Patients with Cancer**

AGE-RELATED CHANGES	IMPLICATIONS
Impaired immune system	Use special precautions to avoid infection; monitor for atypical signs and symptoms of infection.
Altered drug absorption, distribution, metabolism, and elimination	Mandates careful calculation of chemotherapy and frequent assessment for drug response and side effects.
Increased prevalence of other chronic diseases	Monitor for effect of cancer or its treatment on patient's other chronic diseases; monitor patient's tolerance for cancer treatment.
Diminished renal, respiratory, and cardiac reserve	Be proactive in prevention of decreased renal function, atelectasis, pneumonia, and cardiovascular compromise.
Decreased skin and tissue integrity; reduction in body mass; delayed healing	Prevent pressure ulcers secondary to immobility. Monitor skin and mucous membranes for changes related to radiation or chemotherapy. Prevent wound infection.
Decreased musculoskeletal strength	Prevent falls; encourage use of hip protectors if indicated.
Decreased neurosensory functioning: loss of vision, hearing, and distal extremity tactile senses	Provide teaching and instructions modified for patient's hearing and vision loss; provide instruction concerning safety and skin care for distal extremities.
Potential changes in cognitive and emotional capacity	Provide teaching and support modified for patient's level of functioning.

Access to cancer care for elderly patients may be limited by discriminatory or fatalistic attitudes of health care providers, caregivers, and patients themselves. Issues such as the gradual loss of supportive resources, declining health or loss of a spouse, and unavailability of relatives or friends may result in limited access to care and unmet needs for assistance with activities of daily living. In addition, the economic impact of health care may be difficult for those living on fixed incomes.

The nurse must be aware of the special needs of the aging population. Cancer prevention, detection, and screening efforts are directed toward the elderly as well as the younger population. Nurses carefully monitor elderly patients receiving cancer treatments for signs and symptoms of adverse effects. In addition, the elderly patient is instructed to report all symptoms to the physician. It is not uncommon for the elderly patient to delay reporting symptoms, attributing them to "old age." Many elderly people do not want to report illness for fear of losing their independence or financial security. Sensory losses (eg, hearing and visual losses) and memory deficits are considered when planning patient education because they may affect the patient's ability to process and retain information. In such cases, the nurse needs to act as a patient advocate, encouraging independence and identifying resources for support when indicated.

Care of the Patient with Advanced Cancer

The patient with advanced cancer is likely to experience many of the problems previously described, but all to a greater degree. Symptoms of gastrointestinal disturbances, nutritional problems, weight loss, and cachexia make the patient more susceptible to skin breakdown, fluid and electrolyte problems, and infection.

Although not all cancer patients experience pain, those who do commonly fear that it will not be adequately treated. Although treatment at this stage of illness is likely to be palliative rather than curative, prevention and appropriate management of problems can improve the quality of the patient's life considerably. For example, use of analgesia at set intervals rather than on an "as needed" basis usually breaks the cycle of tension and anxiety associated with waiting until pain becomes so severe that pain relief is inadequate once the analgesic is given. Working with the patient and family, as well as with other health care providers, on a pain-management program based on the patient's requirements frequently increases the patient's comfort and sense of control. In addition, the dose of opioid analgesic required is often reduced as pain becomes more manageable and other medications (eg, sedatives, tranquilizers, muscle relaxants) are added to assist in relieving pain.

If the patient is a candidate for radiation therapy or surgical intervention to relieve severe pain, the consequences of these procedures (eg, percutaneous nerve block, cordotomy) are explained to the patient and family, and measures are taken to prevent complications resulting from altered sensation, immobility, and changes in bowel and bladder function.

With the appearance of each new symptom, the patient may experience dread and fear that the disease is progressing. However, one cannot assume that all symptoms are related to the cancer. The new symptoms and problems are evaluated and treated aggressively if possible to increase the patient's comfort and improve quality of life.

Weakness, immobility, fatigue, and inactivity typically occur in the advanced stages of cancer as a result of the tumor, treatment, inadequate nutritional intake, or shortness of breath. The nurse works with the patient to set realistic goals and to provide rest balanced with planned activities and exercise. Other measures include assisting the patient in identifying energy-conserving methods for accomplishing tasks and promoting activities that the patient values the most.

Efforts are made throughout the course of the disease to provide the patient with as much control and independence as desired, but with assurance that support and assistance are available when needed. Additionally, the health care team works with the patient and family to ascertain and comply with the patient's wishes about treatment methods and care as the terminal phase of illness and death approach.

HOSPICE

For many years, society was unable to cope appropriately with patients in the most advanced stages of cancer, and patients died in acute care settings rather than at home or in facilities designed to meet their needs. The needs of patients with terminal illnesses are best met by a comprehensive multidisciplinary program that focuses on quality of life, palliation of symptoms, and provision of psychosocial and spiritual support for the patient and family when cure and control of the disease are no longer possible. The concept of hospice, which originated in Great Britain, best addresses these needs. Most important, the focus of care is on the family, not just the patient. Hospice care can be provided in several settings: free-standing, hospital-based, and community or home-based settings.

Because of the high costs associated with maintaining free-standing hospices, care is often delivered by coordinating services provided by both the hospital and community. Although physi-cians, social workers, clergy, dietitians, pharmacists, physical therapists, and volunteers are involved in patient care, nurses are most often the coordinators of all hospice activities. It is essential that home care and hospice nurses possess advanced skills in assessing and managing pain, nutrition, dyspnea, bowel dysfunction, and skin impairments.

In addition, hospice programs facilitate clear communication among family members and health care providers. Most patients and families are informed of the prognosis and are encouraged to participate in decisions regarding pursuing or terminating cancer treatment. Through collaboration with other support disciplines, nurses assist patients and families to cope with changes in role identity, family structure, grief, and loss. Hospice nurses are actively involved in bereavement counseling. In many instances, family support for survivors continues for about 1 year. See Chapter 17 for detailed discussion of end-of-life care.

Oncologic Emergencies

For information about these emergencies, see Table 16-12.

Table 16-12 • Oncologic Emergencies: Manifestations and Management

EMERGENCY	CLINICAL MANIFESTATIONS AND DIAGNOSTIC FINDINGS	MANAGEMENT
Superior Vena Cava Syndrome (SVCS) Compression or invasion of the superior vena cava by tumor, enlarged lymph nodes, intraluminal thrombus that obstructs venous circulation, or drainage of the head, neck, arms, and thorax. Typically associated with lung cancer, SVCS can also occur with lymphoma and metastases. If untreated, SVCS may lead to cerebral anoxia (because not enough oxygen reaches the brain), laryngeal edema, bronchial obstruction, and death.	*Clinical* Gradually or suddenly impaired venous drainage giving rise to • Progressive shortness of breath (dyspnea), cough, and facial swelling • Edema of the neck, arms, hands, and thorax and reported sensation of skin tightness and difficulty swallowing • Possibly engorged and distended jugular, temporal, and arm veins • Dilated thoracic vessels causing prominent venous patterns on the chest wall • Increased intracranial pressure, associated visual disturbances, headache, and altered mental status *Diagnostic* Diagnosis is confirmed by • Clinical findings • Chest x-ray • Thoracic CT scan • MRI Intraluminal thrombosis is identified by venogram.	*Medical* • Radiation therapy to shrink tumor size and relieve symptoms • Chemotherapy for radiation-resistant tumor (eg, lymphoma or small cell lung cancer) or when the mediastinum has been irradiated to maximum tolerance • Anticoagulant or thrombolytic therapy for intraluminal thrombosis • Surgery (less common), eg, vena cava bypass graft (synthetic or autologous) to redirect blood flow around the obstruction • Supportive measures such as oxygen therapy, corticosteroids, and diuretics *Nursing* • Identify patients at risk for SVCS. • Monitor and report clinical manifestations of SVCS. • Monitor cardiopulmonary and neurologic status. • Facilitate breathing by positioning the patient properly. This helps to promote comfort and reduce anxiety produced by difficulty breathing resulting from progressive edema. • Promote energy conservation to minimize shortness of breath. • Monitor the patient's fluid volume status and administer fluids cautiously to minimize edema. • Assess for thoracic radiation-related problems such as dysphagia (difficulty swallowing) and esophagitis. • Monitor for chemotherapy-related problems, such as myelosuppression. • Provide postoperative care as appropriate.

(continued)

Table 16-12 • Oncologic Emergencies: Manifestations and Management (Continued)

EMERGENCY	CLINICAL MANIFESTATIONS AND DIAGNOSTIC FINDINGS	MANAGEMENT
Spinal Cord Compression Potentially leading to permanent neurologic impairment and associated morbidity and mortality, compression of the cord and its nerve roots may result from tumor, lymphomas, or intervertebral collapse. The prognosis depends on the severity and rapidity of onset. About 70% of compressions occur at the thoracic level, 20% in the lumbosacral level, and 10% in the cervical region. Metastatic cancers (breast, lung, kidney, prostate, myeloma, lymphoma) and related bone erosion are associated with spinal cord compression.	*Clinical* • Local inflammation, edema, venous stasis, and impaired blood supply to nervous tissues • Local or radicular pain along the dermatomal areas innervated by the affected nerve root (eg, thoracic radicular pain extends in a band around the chest or abdomen) • Pain exacerbated by movement, coughing, sneezing, or the Valsalva maneuver • Neurologic dysfunction, and related motor and sensory deficits (numbness, tingling, feelings of coldness in the affected area, inability to detect vibration, loss of positional sense) • Motor loss ranging from subtle weakness to flaccid paralysis • Bladder and/or bowel dysfunction depending on level of compression (above S2, overflow incontinence; from S3 to S5, flaccid sphincter tone and bowel incontinence) *Diagnostic* • Percussion tenderness at the level of compression • Abnormal reflexes • Sensory and motor abnormalities • MRI, myelogram, spinal cord x-rays, bone scans, and CT scan	*Medical* • Radiation therapy to reduce tumor size to halt progression and corticosteroid therapy to decrease inflammation and swelling at the compression site • Surgery only if symptoms progress despite radiation therapy or if vertebral fracture leads to additional nerve damage • Chemotherapy as adjuvant to radiation therapy for patients with lymphoma or small cell lung cancer • *Note:* Despite treatment, patients with poor neurologic function before treatment are less likely to regain complete motor and sensory function; patients who develop complete paralysis usually do not regain all neurologic function. *Nursing* • Perform ongoing assessment of neurologic function to identify existing and progressing dysfunction. • Control pain with pharmacologic and non-pharmacologic measures. • Prevent complications of immobility resulting from pain and decreased function (eg, skin breakdown, urinary stasis, thrombophlebitis, and decreased clearance of pulmonary secretions). • Maintain muscle tone by assisting with range-of-motion exercises in collaboration with physical and occupational therapists. • Institute intermittent urinary catheterization and bowel training programs for patients with bladder or bowel dysfunction. • Provide encouragement and support to patient and family coping with pain and altered functioning, lifestyle, roles, and independence.
Hypercalcemia In patients with cancer, hypercalcemia is a potentially life-threatening metabolic abnormality resulting when the calcium released from the bones is more than the kidneys can excrete or the bones can reabsorb. It may result from: • Bone destruction by tumor cells and subsequent release of calcium • Production of prostaglandins and osteoclast-activating factor, which stimulate bone breakdown and calcium release • Tumors that produce parathyroid-like substances that promote calcium release • Excessive use of vitamins and minerals and conditions unrelated to cancer, such as dehydration, renal impairment, primary hyperparathyroidism, thyrotoxicosis, thiazide diuretics, and hormone therapy	*Clinical* Fatigue, weakness, confusion, decreased level of responsiveness, hyporeflexia, nausea, vomiting, constipation, polyuria (excessive urination), polydipsia (excessive thirst), dehydration, and dysrhythmias *Diagnostic* Serum calcium level exceeding 11 mg/dL (2.74 mmol/L)	*Medical* See Chapter 14. *Nursing* • Identify patients at risk for hypercalcemia and assess for signs and symptoms of hypercalcemia. • Educate patient and family; prevention and early detection can prevent fatality. • Teach at-risk patients to recognize and report signs and symptoms of hypercalcemia. • Encourage patients to consume 2 to 3 L of fluid daily unless contraindicated by existing renal or cardiac disease. • Explain the use of dietary and pharmacologic interventions such as stool softeners and laxatives for constipation. • Advise patients to maintain nutritional intake without restricting normal calcium intake. • Discuss antiemetic therapy if nausea and vomiting occur. • Promote mobility by emphasizing its importance in preventing demineralization and breakdown of bones.

(continued)

Table 16-12 • Oncologic Emergencies: Manifestations and Management (Continued)

EMERGENCY	CLINICAL MANIFESTATIONS AND DIAGNOSTIC FINDINGS	MANAGEMENT
Pericardial Effusion and Cardiac Tamponade Cardiac tamponade is an accumulation of fluid in the pericardial space. The accumulation compresses the heart and thereby impedes expansion of the ventricles and cardiac filling during diastole. As ventricular volume and cardiac output fall, the heart pump fails, and circulatory collapse develops. With gradual onset, fluid accumulates gradually, and the outer layer of the pericardial space stretches to compensate for rising pressure. Large amounts of fluid accumulate before symptoms of heart failure occur. With rapid onset, pressures rise too quickly for the pericardial space to compensate. Cancerous tumors, particularly from adjacent thoracic tumors (lung, esophagus, breast cancers), and cancer treatment are the most common causes of cardiac tamponade. Radiation therapy of 4,000 cGy or more to the mediastinal area has also been implicated in pericardial fibrosis, pericarditis, and resultant cardiac tamponade. Untreated pericardial effusion and cardiac tamponade lead to circulatory collapse and cardiac arrest.	*Clinical* • Neck vein distention during inspiration (Kussmaul's sign) • Pulsus paradoxus (systolic blood pressure decrease exceeding 10 mm Hg during inspiration; pulse gets stronger on expiration) • Distant heart sounds, rubs and gallops, cardiac dullness • Compensatory tachycardia (heart beats faster to compensate for decreased cardiac output) • Increased venous and vascular pressures *Diagnostic* • ECG helps diagnose pericardial effusion. • In small effusion, chest x-rays show small amounts of fluid in the pericardium; in large effusions, x-ray films disclose "water-bottle" heart (obliteration of vessel contour and cardiac chambers). • ECG and CT scans help diagnose pleural effusions and evaluate effect of treatment. • Narrow pulse pressure • Shortness of breath and tachypnea • Weakness, chest pain, orthopnea, anxiety, diaphoresis, lethargy, and altered consciousness from decreased cerebral perfusion	*Medical* • Pericardiocentesis (the aspiration or withdrawal of the pericardial fluid by a large-bore needle inserted into the pericardial space). In malignant effusions, pericardiocentesis provides only temporary relief; fluid usually reaccumulates. Windows or openings in the pericardium can be created surgically as a palliative measure to drain fluid into the pleural space. Catheters may also be placed in the pericardial space and sclerosing agents (such as tetracycline, talc, bleomycin, 5-fluorouracil, or thiotepa) injected to prevent fluid from reaccumulating. • Radiation therapy or antineoplastic agents, depending on how sensitive the primary tumor is to these treatments. In mild effusions, prednisone and diuretic medications may be prescribed and the patient's status carefully monitored. *Nursing* • Monitor vital signs and oxygen saturation frequently. • Assess for pulsus paradoxus. • Monitor ECG tracings. • Assess heart and lung sounds, neck vein filling, level of consciousness, respiratory status, and skin color and temperature. • Monitor and record intake and output. • Review laboratory findings (eg, arterial blood gas and electrolyte levels). • Elevate the head of the patient's bed to ease breathing. • Minimize patient's physical activity to reduce oxygen requirements; administer supplemental oxygen as prescribed. • Provide frequent oral hygiene. • Reposition and encourage the patient to cough and take deep breaths every 2 hours. • As needed, maintain patent IV access, reorient the patient, and provide supportive measures and appropriate patient instruction.
Disseminated Intravascular Coagulation (DIC, also called consumption coagulopathy) Complex disorder of coagulation or fibrinolysis (destruction of clots), which results in thrombosis or bleeding. DIC is most commonly associated with hematologic cancers (leukemia); cancer of prostate, GI tract, and lungs; chemotherapy (methotrexate, prednisone, L-asparaginase, vincristine, and 6-mercaptopurine), and disease processes, such as sepsis, hepatic failure, and anaphylaxis. Blood clots form when normal coagulation mechanisms are triggered. Once activated, the clotting cascade continues to consume clotting factors and platelets faster than the body can re-	*Clinical* *Chronic DIC:* Few or no observable symptoms or easy bruising, prolonged bleeding from venipuncture and injection sites, bleeding of the gums, and slow GI bleeding *Acute DIC:* life-threatening hemorrhage and infarction; clinical symptoms of this syndrome are varied and depend on the organ system involved in thrombus and infarction or bleeding episodes *Diagnostic* • Prolonged prothrombin time (PT or protime) • Prolonged partial thromboplastin time (PTT) • Prolonged thrombin time (TT) • Decreased fibrinogen level • Decreased platelet level • Decrease in clotting factors	*Medical* • Chemotherapy, biologic response modifier therapy, radiation therapy, or surgery is used to treat the underlying cancer. • Antibiotic therapy is used for sepsis. • Anticoagulants, such as heparin or antithrombin III, decrease the stimulation of the coagulation pathways. • Transfusion of fresh-frozen plasma or cryoprecipitates (which contain clotting factors and fibrinogen), packed red blood cells, and platelets may be used as replacement therapy to prevent or control bleeding. • Although controversial, antifibrinolytic agents such as aminocaproic acid (Amicar), which is associated with increased thrombus formation, may be used.

(continued)

Table 16-12 • Oncologic Emergencies: Manifestations and Management (Continued)

EMERGENCY	CLINICAL MANIFESTATIONS AND DIAGNOSTIC FINDINGS	MANAGEMENT
place them. Clots are deposited in the microvasculature, placing the patient at great risk for impaired circulation, tissue hypoxia, and necrosis. In addition, fibrinolysis occurs, breaking down clots and increasing the circulating levels of anticoagulant substances, thereby placing the patient at risk for hemorrhage.	• Decreased hemoglobin • Decreased hematocrit • Elevated fibrin split products • Positive protamine sulfate precipitation test (thrombin activation test)	*Nursing* • Monitor vital signs. • Measure and document intake and output. • Assess skin color and temperature; lung, heart, and bowel sounds; level of consciousness, headache, visual disturbances, chest pain, decreased urine output, and abdominal tenderness. • Inspect all body orifices, tube insertion sites, incisions, and bodily excretions for bleeding. • Review laboratory test results. • Minimize physical activity to decrease injury risks and oxygen requirements. • Prevent bleeding; apply pressure to all venipuncture sites, and avoid nonessential invasive procedures; provide electric rather than straight-edged razors; avoid tape on the skin and advise gentle but adequate oral hygiene. • Assist the patient to turn, cough, and take deep breaths every 2 hours. • Reorient the patient, if needed; maintain a safe environment; and provide appropriate patient education and supportive measures.
Syndrome of Inappropriate Secretion of Antidiuretic Hormone (SIADH) The continuous, uncontrolled release of antidiuretic hormone (ADH), produced by tumor cells or by the abnormal stimulation of the hypothalmic–pituitary network, leads to increased extracellular fluid volume, water intoxication, hyponatremia, and increased excretion of urinary sodium. As fluid volume increases, stretch receptors in the right atrium respond by releasing a second hormone, atrial naturetic factor (ANF). The release of ANF causes increased renal excretion of sodium, which worsens hyponatremia. The most common cause of SIADH is cancer, especially small cell cancers of the lung. Antineoplastics—vincristine, vinblastine, cisplatin, and cyclophosphamide—and morphine also stimulate ADH secretion, which promotes conservation and reabsorption of water by the kidneys. As more fluid is absorbed, the circulatory volume increases, ANF is released, and sodium is actively excreted by the kidneys in compensation.	*Clinical* *Serum sodium levels below 120 mEq/L* (SI: 120 mmol/L): symptoms of hyponatremia including personality changes, irritability, nausea, anorexia, vomiting, weight gain, fatigue, muscular pain (myalgia), headache, lethargy, and confusion. *Serum sodium levels below 110 mEq/L* (SI: 110 mmol/L): seizure, abnormal reflexes, papilledema, coma, and death. Edema is rare. *Diagnostic* • Decreased serum sodium level • Increased urine osmolality • Increased urinary sodium level • Decreased BUN, creatinine, and serum albumin levels secondary to dilution • Abnormal water load test results	*Medical* Fluid intake range limited to 500 to 1,000 mL/day to increase the serum sodium level and decrease fluid overload. If water restriction alone is not effective in correcting or controlling serum sodium levels, demeclocycline is often prescribed to interfere with the antidiuretic action of ADH and ANF. When neurologic symptoms are severe, parenteral sodium replacement and diuretic therapy are indicated. Electrolyte levels are monitored carefully to detect secondary magnesium, potassium, and calcium imbalances. After the symptoms of SIADH are controlled, the underlying cancer is treated. If water excess continues despite treatment, pharmacologic intervention (urea and furosemide) may be indicated. *Nursing* • Maintain intake and output measurements. • Assess level of consciousness, lung and heart sounds, vital signs, daily weight, and urine specific gravity; also assess for nausea, vomiting, anorexia, edema, fatigue, and lethargy. • Monitor laboratory test results, including serum electrolyte levels, osmolality, and blood urea nitrogen, creatinine, and urinary sodium levels. • Minimize the patient's activity; provide appropriate oral hygiene; maintain environmental safety; and restrict fluid intake if necessary. • Reorient the patient and provide instruction and encouragement as needed.
Tumor Lysis Syndrome Potentially fatal complication associated with radiation- or chemotherapy-induced cell destruction of large or rapidly growing cancers such as leukemia, lymphoma, and small cell lung cancer. The release of intracellular contents from the tumor cells, leads to electrolyte imbalances—hyperkalemia,	*Clinical* Clinical manifestations depend on the extent of metabolic abnormalities. • Neurologic: Fatigue, weakness, memory loss, altered mental status, muscle cramps, tetany, paresthesias (numbness and tingling), seizures • Cardiac: Elevated blood pressure, shortened QT complexes, widened QRS waves, dysrhythmias, cardiac arrest	*Medical* • To prevent renal failure and restore electrolyte balance, aggressive fluid hydration is initiated 48 hours before and after the initiation of cytotoxic therapy to increase urine volume and eliminate uric acid and electrolytes. Urine is alkalinized by adding sodium bicarbonate to IV fluid to maintain a urine pH of 7 or more; this prevents renal failure secondary to uric acid precipitation in the kidneys.

(continued)

Table 16-12 • Oncologic Emergencies: Manifestations and Management (Continued)

EMERGENCY	CLINICAL MANIFESTATIONS AND DIAGNOSTIC FINDINGS	MANAGEMENT
hypocalcemia, hyperphosphatemia, and hyperuricemia—because the kidneys can no longer excrete large volumes of the released intracellular metabolites.	• GI: Anorexia, nausea, vomiting, abdominal cramps, diarrhea • Renal: Flank pain, oliguria, anuria, renal failure, acidic urine pH *Diagnostic* Electrolyte imbalances identified by laboratory test results	• Diuretic therapy, with a carbonic anhydrase inhibitor or acetazolamide, to alkalinize the urine • Allopurinol therapy to inhibit the conversion of nucleic acids to uric acid • Administration of a cation-exchange resin, such as sodium polystyrene sulfonate (Kayexalate) to treat hyperkalemia by binding and eliminating potassium through the bowel • Administration of hypertonic dextrose and regular insulin temporarily shifts potassium into cells and lowers serum potassium levels. • Administration of phosphate-binding gels, such as aluminum hydroxide, to treat hyperphosphatemia by promoting phosphate excretion in the feces. • Hemodialysis when patients are unresponsive to the standard approaches for managing uric acid and electrolyte abnormalities *Nursing* • Identify at-risk patients, including those in whom tumor lysis syndrome may develop up to 1 week after therapy has been completed. • Institute essential preventive measures (eg, fluid hydration and allopurinol). • Assess patient for signs and symptoms of electrolyte imbalances. • Assess urine pH to confirm alkalization. • Monitor serum electrolyte and uric acid levels for evidence of fluid volume overload secondary to aggressive hydration. • Instruct patients to report symptoms indicating electrolyte disturbances.

 Critical Thinking Exercises

1. You are seeing a married couple in their 70s in the clinic for blood pressure checks. What questions regarding cancer screening are appropriate for them? How would you respond if your suggestions for cancer screening are met with the answer that they are too old to worry about cancer? What special considerations are there if the woman has a physical disability that requires her to use a wheelchair?

2. A 54-year-old woman with bone metastases secondary to breast cancer has been admitted to the hospital with a diagnosis of hypercalcemia. Describe the underlying cause of hypercalcemia and the medical and nursing management strategies that are anticipated. What patient monitoring would be essential before and after treatment of hypercalcemia?

3. One of your home care patients, a 42-year-old executive of a major corporation, has a nonresectable malignant brain tumor for which she is receiving radiation therapy. She is being discharged from the hospital and will continue therapy as an outpatient. She and her husband are concerned about her future and survival and are also concerned about the impact of the diagnosis on the couple's 10-year-old twins. She is also concerned about her ability to carry out her executive responsibilities. What assessment by the nurse is indicated at this point, and what actions would be warranted by the nurse to help the patient and her husband deal with their concerns?

4. A 70-year-old man with advanced cancer living at home with his wife has been experiencing increasingly severe pain for which an oral opioid analgesic has recently been prescribed. What nursing assessments are essential for the home care nurse? What teaching will be indicated for the patient and family? How would you modify your teaching if the patient and his wife understand little English?

REFERENCES AND SELECTED READINGS

Books

Abeloff, M. D., Armitage, J. D., Lichter, A., & Niederhuber, J. E. (Eds). (2000). *Clinical oncology* (2nd ed.). Philadelphia: Churchill Livingstone.

Abrahm, J. L. (2000). *A physician's guide to pain and symptom management in cancer patients*. Baltimore: The Johns Hopkins University Press.

Agency for Health Care Policy and Research, Public Health Service, Department of Health and Human Services. (1992). *Acute pain management: Operative or medical procedures and trauma.* Clinical Practice Guideline (AHCPR 92-0032). Washington, DC: U.S. Government Printing Office.

Agency for Health Care Policy and Research, Public Health Service, Department of Health and Human Services. (1994). *Management of cancer pain: adults.* Clinical Practice Guideline (AHCPR 94-0592). Washington, DC: U.S. Government Printing Office.

American Cancer Society (2002). *Cancer facts and figures 2002.* Atlanta: American Cancer Society.

American Pain Society. (1999). *Principles of analgesic use in the treatment of acute pain and chronic cancer pain: A concise guide to medical practice* (4th ed.). Skokie, IL: American Pain Society.

Barraclough, J. (1999). *Cancer and emotion: A practical guide to psychooncology* (3rd ed.). West Sussex: John Wiley and Sons.

Boik, J. (1995). *Cancer and natural medicine: A textbook of basic science and clinical research.* Princeton, MN: Oregon Medical Press.

DeVita, V. T., Hellman, S., & Rosenberg, S. A. (Eds.). (1995). *Biologic therapy of cancer* (2nd ed.). Philadelphia: J. B. Lippincott.

Green, F., et al. (2002). *AJCC cancer staging manual* (6th ed.). New York: Springer-Verlag.

Groenwald, S., Hansen-Frogge, M., Goodman, M., & Henke Yarbro, C. (Eds.). (1998). *Comprehensive cancer nursing review* (4th ed.). Boston: Jones and Bartlett.

Heath, C. W., & Fontham, E. (2001). Cancer etiology. In: *Clinical oncology.* Atlanta: American Cancer Society.

Huber, E. B., & Magrath, I. (Eds.) (1998). *Gene therapy in treatment of cancer: Progress and prospects.* New York: Cambridge University Press.

Lenhard, R. E., Osteen, R. T., & Gansler, T. (Eds.). (2001). *Clinical oncology.* Atlanta: American Cancer Society.

Loeser, J. D. (Ed.) (2001). *Bonica's management of pain* (3d ed.). Philadelphia: Lippincott Williams & Wilkins.

Miaskowski, C. (1997). *Oncology nursing: An essential guide for patient care.* Philadelphia: W. B. Saunders.

Pazadur, R., Coia, L. R., Hoskins, W. J., & Wagman, L. D. (Eds.). (2001). *Cancer management: A multidisciplinary approach.* Melville, NY: PRR, Inc.

Perry, M. C. (Ed.). (1997). *The chemotherapy source book* (2nd ed.). Baltimore: Williams & Wilkins.

Ratain, M. J., Tempero, M., & Skosey, C. (2001). *Outline of oncology therapeutics.* Philadelphia: Saunders.

Winningham, M. L., & Barton-Burke, M. (Eds.) (2000). *Fatigue in cancer: A multidisciplinary approach.* Sudbury, MA: Jones & Bartlett.

Yarbro, C., Hansen-Frogge, M., & Goodman, M. (Eds.) (1999). *Cancer symptom management* (2d ed.). Sudbury, MA: Jones & Bartlett.

Yarbro, C. H. (Ed.) (2000). *Cancer: Principles and practice* (5th ed). Sudbury, MA: Jones & Bartlett.

Yokes, E. F., & Golomb, H. M. (Eds.). (1999). *Oncologic therapies.* New York: Springer.

Journals

General

Asterisks indicate nursing research articles.

Balducci, L., & Extermann, M. (2000). Management of cancer in the older person: A practical approach. *The Oncologist, 5*(3), 224–237.

*Berger, A. M., & Farr, L. (1999). The influence of daytime inactivity and nighttime restlessness on cancer-related fatigue. *Oncology Nursing Forum, 26*(10), 1663–1671.

Brown, J. K. (2002). A systematic review of the evidence on symptom management of cancer-related anorexia and cachexia. *Oncology Nursing Forum, 29*(3), 517–532.

Brown, P. A. (1999). Nutrition and cancer. *MedSurg Nursing, 8*(6), 333–345.

Carroll-Johnson, R. M. (Ed.). (2000). Cancer prevention and early detection: Oncology nursing's next frontier. *Oncology Nursing Forum, 27*(9) supplement, 1–63.

Cassileth, B. R. (1999). Evaluating complementary and alternative therapies for cancer patients. *CA: Cancer Journal for Clinicians, 49*(6), 362–375.

Chernecky, C., & Shelton, B. (2001). Pulmonary complications in patients with cancer. *American Journal of Nursing, 101*(5), 24A, 24E, 24G, 24H.

Cunningham, R. S. (Ed.). (2000). Nutrition and cancer. *Seminars in Oncology Nursing, 16*(2), 1–173.

Daniel, B. T. (Ed). (2001). Palliative and supportive care of advanced cancer. *Nursing Clinics of North America, 36*(4), 631–869.

Finley, J. P. (2000). Management of cancer cachexia. *AACN Clinical Issues, 11*(4), 590–603.

Fisher, B., et al. (1998). Tamoxifen for prevention of breast cancer: Report of the National Surgical Adjuvant Breast and Bowel Project P-1 study. *Journal of National Cancer Institute, 90*(18), 1371–1388.

Grant, M., & Kravits, K. (2000). Symptoms and their impact on nutrition. *Seminars in Oncology Nursing, 16*(2), 113–121.

Greenlee, R. T., Murray, T., Bolden, S., et al. (2000). Cancer statistics, 2000. *CA: Cancer Journal for Clinicians, 50*, 7–30.

Haisfield-Wolfe, M. E., & Baxendale-Cox, L. (1999). Staging of malignant and cutaneous wounds: A pilot study. *Oncology Nursing Forum, 22*(6), 1055–1064.

*Howell, D., Butler, L., Vincent, L., Watt-Watson, J., & Stearns, N. (2000). Influencing nurses' knowledge, attitudes and practice in cancer pain management. *Cancer Nursing, 23*(1), 55–63.

Houshmand, S. L., Campbell, C. T., Briggs, S. E., McFadden, A. W. J., & Al-Tweigeri, T. (2000). Prophylactic mastectomy and genetic testing: An update. *Oncology Nursing Forum, 27*(10), 1537–1547.

Hsueh, E. C., Hansen, N., & Giulaino, A. E. (2000). Intraoperative lymphatic mapping and sentinel lymph node dissection in breast cancer. *CA: Cancer Journal for Clinicians, 50*(3), 279–291.

International Radiosurgery Support Association (2000). Stereotactic radiosurgery overview. Retrieved from the World Wide Web: http://www.irsa.org/srs.html Jan. 25, 2002.

Jemal, A., Thomas, A., Murray, T., & Thun, M. (2002). Cancer statistics, 2002. *CA: Cancer Journal for Clinicians, 52*(1), 23–47.

Jennings, M. (Ed.) (2001). Treatment advances in surgical oncology. *Nursing Clinics of North America, 36*(3), 499–623.

Kelly, L. D. (1999). Nursing assessment and patient management. *Seminars in Oncology Nursing, 15*(4), 282–291.

Kurtz, M. E., Kurtz, J. C., Stommel, M., Given, C. W., & Given, B. (2001). Physical functioning and depression among older persons with cancer. *Cancer Practice, 9*(1), 11–18.

Letizia, M. (2001). Addressing alopecia: Helping patients with cancer deal with hair loss. *American Journal of Nursing, 101*(4), 24LL.

Messner, C., & Patterson, D. (2001). The challenge of cancer in the workplace. *Cancer Practice, 9*(1), 50–51.

Montbriand, M. J. (1999). Past and present herbs used to treat cancer: Medicine, magic, or poison? *Oncology Nursing Forum, 26*(1), 49–59.

Moore, S. (2002). Cutaneous metastatic breast cancer. *Clinical Journal of Oncology Nursing, 6*(5), 255–260

Nail, L. M. (2002). Fatigue in patients with cancer. *Oncology Nursing Forum, 29*(3), 537–546.

*Phillips, M. P., Cohen, M. Z., & Moses, G. (1999). Breast cancer screening and African American women: Fear, fatalism and silence. *Oncology Nursing Forum, 26*(3), 561–571.

Rust, D. M., Wood, L. S., & Battiato, L. A. (1999). Oprelvekin: an alternative treatment for thrombocytopenia. *Clinical Journal of Oncology Nursing, 3*(2), 57–62.

Shih, A., Misakowski, C., Dodd, M. L., et al. (2002). A research review of current treatment for radiation-induced oral mucositis in patients with head and neck cancer. *Oncology Nursing Forum, 29*(7), 1063–1080.

Sonis, S. T., et al. (2001). Oral mucositis and the clinical and economic outcomes of hematopoietic stem-cell transplantation. *Journal of Clinical Oncology, 19*(8), 2201–2205.

Smith, R. A., et al. (2001). American Cancer Society guidelines for the early detection of cancer: Update of early detection guidelines for prostate, colorectal and endometrial cancers. *CA: Cancer Journal for Clinicians, 51*(1), 38–76.

*Sparber, A., Bauer, L., Curt, G., Eisenberg, D., Levin, T., Parks, S., Steinberg, S. M., & Wooten, J. (2000). Use of complementary medicine by adult patients participating in cancer clinical trials. *Oncology Nursing Forum, 27*(4), 623–630.

Whitman, M. M. (2000). The starving patient: Supportive care for people with cancer. *Clinical Journal of Oncology Nursing, 4*(3), 121–125.

Wilson, R. L. (2000). Optimizing nutrition for patients with cancer. *Clinical Journal of Oncology Nursing, 4*(1), 23–28.

Wojtaszek, C. (2000). Management of chemotherapy-induced stomatitis. *Clinical Journal of Oncology Nursing, 4*(6), 263–270.

Yeager, K. A., Webster, J., Crain, M., Kasow, J., & McGuire, D. B. (2000). Implementation of an oral care standard for leukemia and transplantation patients. *Cancer Nursing, 23*(1), 40–47.

Zimmerman, V. L. (2002). BRCA gene mutations and cancer. *American Journal of Nursing, 102*(8), 28–36.

Biologic Response Modifiers

Buchsel, P. C., Forgey, A., Grape, F. B., & Hamann, S. S. (2002) Granulocyte macrophage colony-stimulating factor: Current practice and novel approaches. *Clinical Journal of Oncology Nursing, 6*(4), 198–205.

Buchsel, P. C., Murph, B. S., & Newton, S. A. (2002). Epoetin alpha: Current and future indications and nursing implications. *Clinical Journal of Oncology Nursing, 6*(5), 261–267.

Capriotti, T. (2001). Monoclonal antibodies: Drugs that combine pharmacology and biotechnology. *MedSurg Nursing, 10*(2), 89–95.

Estes, J. (Ed.) (2002). New approaches to the management of non-Hodgkin's lymphoma. A continuing education activity. *Seminars in Oncology Nursing, 18*(1), supplement, 1–33.

Evans, T. R., & Kaye, S. B. (1999). Retinoids: Present role and future potential. *British Journal of Cancer, 800*(1–2), 1–8.

Kelloff, G. J. (2000). Perspectives on cancer chemoprevention research and drug development. *Advances in Cancer Research, 78*(2000), 199–334.

Kosits, C., & Callaghan, S. (2000). Rituximab: A new monoclonal antibody therapy for non-Hodgkin's lymphoma. *Oncology Nursing Forum, 27*(1), 51–59.

Kurie, J. M. (1999). The biologic basis for the use of retinoids in cancer prevention and treatment. *Current Opinion in Oncology, 11*(6), 497–502.

Moldawer, N., & Carr, E. (2000). The promise of recombinant interleukin-2. *American Journal of Nursing, 100*(5), 35–39.

Peyrot, J. (1999). Herceptin. *Oncology Nursing Forum, 26*(3), 515–516.

Seeley, K. & DeMeyer, E. (2002). Nursing care of patients receiving Campath. *Clinical Journal of Oncology Nursing, 6*(3), 138–143.

Sorokin, P. (2000). Mylotarg approved for patients with CD33⁺ acute myeloid leukemia. *Clinical Journal of Oncology Nursing, 4*(5), 279–280.

Sorokin, P. (2002). New agents and future directions in biotherapy. *Clinical Journal of Oncology Nursing, 6*(1), 19–24.

Weiner, L. M. (1999). An overview of monoclonal antibody therapy of cancer. *Seminars in Oncology, 26*(4) supplement 12, 41–50.

Yarbro, C. (Ed.). (2000). A new biologic approach for the treatment of metastatic breast cancer. *Seminars in Oncology Nursing, 16*(4) supplement 1, 1–38.

Bone Marrow Transplantation

Alcoser, P. W., & Burchett, S. (1999). Bone marrow transplantation: Immune system suppression and reconstitution. *American Journal of Nursing, 99*(6), 26–31.

Applebaum, F. R. (1996). The use of bone marrow and peripheral blood cell transplantation in the treatment of cancer. *CA: Cancer Journal for Clinicians, 46*(3), 142–164.

Buchsel, P. C., & Kapustay, P. M. (1995). Peripheral stem cell transplantation. *Oncology Nursing Update: Patient Treatment and Support, 2*(2), 1–14.

Buchsel, P. C., et al. (1996). Delayed complications of bone marrow transplantation: An update. *Oncology Nursing Forum, 23*(8), 1267–1291.

Hurley, C. (1997). Ambulatory care after bone marrow or peripheral blood stem cell transplantation. *Clinical Journal of Oncology Nursing, 1*(1), 19–21.

Poliquin, C. M. (1997). Overview of bone marrow and peripheral blood stem cell transplantation. *Clinical Journal of Oncology Nursing, 1*(1), 11–17.

Carcinogenesis and Risk Factors

Foltz, A. T., & Mahon, S. M. (2000). Application of carcinogenesis theory to primary prevention. *Oncology Nursing Forum, 27*(9), supplement, 5–11.

Fraser, M. C., et al. (1997). Familial cancers: Evolving challenges for nursing practice. *Oncology Nursing Update: Patient Treatment and Support, 4*(3), 1–18.

Greco, K. E. (2000). Cancer genetics nursing: Impact of the double helix. *Oncology Nursing Forum, 27*(9), supplement, 29–36.

Kobayashi, A., Miaskowski, C., Wallhagen, M., & Smith-McCune, K. (2000). Recent developments in understanding the immune response to human papilloma virus infection and cervical neoplasia. *Oncology Nursing Forum, 27*(4), 643–651.

Lessick, M., Wickham, R., Chapman, D., et al. (2001). Advances in genetic testing for cancer risk. *MedSurg Nursing, 10*(3), 123–127.

Stillman, J. M., & Stillman, S. D. (1996). Cancer and the workplace. *CA: Cancer Journal for Clinicians, 46*(2), 70–92.

Chemotherapy

Anastasia, P. J. (2000). Effectiveness of oral 5-HT3 receptor antagonists for emetogenic chemotherapy. *Oncology Nursing Forum, 277*(3), 483–493.

Bremerkamp, M. (2000). Mechanisms of action of 5-HT3 receptor antagonists: Clinical overview and nursing implications. *Clinical Journal of Oncology Nursing, 4*(5), 201–207.

Dodd, M. J., Dibble, S. L., Miaskowski, C., et al. (2000). Randomized clinical trial of the effectiveness of 3 commonly used mouthwashes to treat chemotherapy-induced mucositis. *Oral Surgery Oral Medicine Oral Pathology Oral Radiology & Endodontics, 90*(1), 39–47.

Doherty, K. M. (1999). Closing the gap in prophylactic antiemetic therapy: Patient factors in calculating the emetogenic potential of chemotherapy. *Clinical Journal of Oncology Nursing, 3*(3), 113–119.

Line, L. G., Campbell, J. M., & Kinion, E. S. (2001). Infections in patients receiving cytotoxic chemotherapy. *MedSurg Nursing, 10*(2), 61–68.

Rogers, B. B. (2001). Mucositis in the oncology patient. *Nursing Clinics of North America, 36*(4), 745–760.

Schulmeister, L., & Camp-Sorrell, D. (2000). Chemotherapy extravasation from implanted ports. *Oncology Nursing Forum, 27*(3), 531–538.

Gene Therapy

Fibison, W. J. (2000). Gene therapy. *Nursing Clinics of North America, 35*(3), 757–773.

Frankel, M. S., & Chapman, A. R. (2000). Human inheritable genetic modifications: Assessing scientific, ethical, religious and policy issues. *American Association for the Advancement of Science,* 1–82.

Johnson, K. J., & Brensinger, J. D. (2000). Genetic counseling and testing: Implications for clinical practice. *Nursing Clinics of North America, 35*(3), 615–626.

Lea, D. H. (2000). A clinician's primer in human genetics. *Nursing Clinics of North America, 35*(3), 583–614.

Nogueira, S. M., & Appling, S. E. (2000). Breast cancer: Genetics, risks and strategies. *Nursing Clinics of North America, 35*(3), 663–669.

Olsen, S. J., & Zawaacki, K. (2000). Hereditary colorectal cancer. *Nursing Clinics of North America, 35*(3), 671–685.

Wasil, T., & Buchbinder, A. (2000). Gene therapy in human cancer: Report of Human Clinical Trials. *Cancer Investigation, 18*(8), 740–746.

Oncologic Emergencies

Barnett, M. L. (1999). Hypercalcemia. *Seminars in Oncology Nursing, 15*(3), 190–201.

Beauchamp, K. A. (1998). Pericardial tamponade: An oncologic emergency. *Clinical Journal of Oncology Nursing, 2*(3), 85–95.

Bucholtz, J. D. (1999). Metastatic epidural spinal cord compression. *Seminars in Oncology Nursing, 15*(3), 150–159.

Ezzone, S. A. (1999). Tumor lysis syndrome. *Seminars in Oncology Nursing, 15*(3), 190–201.

Gardner, C. M. (1999). Cancer-related spinal cord compression. *American Journal of Nursing, 99*(7), 34–35.

Haapoja, I. S., & Blendowski, C. (1999). Superior vena cava syndrome. *Seminars in Oncology Nursing, 15*(3), 183–189.

Holmes Gobel, B. (Ed.). (1999). Oncologic emergencies. *Seminars in Oncology Nursing, 15*(3), 149–234.

Schindler, N., & Vogelzang, R. L. (1999). Superior vena cava: Experience with endovascular stents and surgical treatment. *Surgical Clinics of North America, 79*(3), 683–694.

Terpstra, T. L., & Terpstra, T. L. (2000). Syndrome of inappropriate antidiuretic hormone secretion: Recognition and management. *MedSurg Nursing, 9*(2), 61–68.

Wheeler, A. P., & Gordon, B. R. (1999). Current concepts: Treating patients with severe sepsis. *New England Journal of Medicine, 340*(3), 207–214.

Pain

Chang, H. M. (1999). Cancer pain management. *Medical Clinics of North America, 83*(3), 711–736.

Ciezki, J. P., Komurcy, S., & Macklis, R. M. (2000). Palliative radiotherapy. *Seminars in Oncology, 27*(1), 90–93.

Dalton, J. A. & Youngblood, R. (2000). Clinical application of the WHO analgesic ladder. *Journal of Intravenous Nursing, 23*(2), 118–124.

Easley, M. K., & Elliott, S. (2001). Managing pain at the end of life. *Nursing Clinics of North America, 36*(4), 779–794.

Grossman, S. A., Benditti, C., Payne, R., & Syrjala, K. (1999). NCCN practice guidelines for cancer pain. *Oncology, 13*(11A), 1–4.

Pargeon, K. L., & Hailey, B. J. (1999). Barriers to effective cancer pain management. *Journal of Pain and Symptom Management, 18*(5), 358–368.

Radiation Therapy

Abel, L. J., Blatt, H. J., Stipetich, R. L., et al. (2000). The role of urinary assessment scores in the nursing management of patients receiving prostate brachytherapy. *Clinical Journal of Oncology Nursing, 4*(3), 126–129.

Blackman, A. (1997). Radiation-induced skin alterations. *MedSurg Nursing, 6*(3), 172–175.

Cash, J. C., & Dattoli, M. J. (1997). Management of patients receiving trans-perineal Palladium-103 prostate implants. *Oncology Nursing Forum, 24*(8), 1361–1367.

*Christman, N. J., Oakley, M. G., & Cronin, S. N. (2001). Developing and using preparatory information for women undergoing radiation therapy for cervical or uterine cancer. *Oncology Nursing Forum, 28*(1), 93–98.

Iwamoto, R. R., & Maher, K. E. (2001). Radiation therapy for prostate cancer. *Seminars in Oncology Nursing, 17*(2), 90–100.

Stajduhar, K. I., Neithercut, J., Chu, E., Pham, P., Rohde, J., Sicotte, A., & Young, K. (2000). Thyroid cancer patients' experiences of receiving iodine-131 therapy. *Oncology Nursing Forum, 27*(8), 1213–1218.

*Velji, K., & Fitch, M. (2001). The experience of women receiving brachytherapy for gynecologic cancer. *Oncology Nursing Forum, 28*(4), 743–751.

RESOURCES AND WEBSITES

Professional Organizations

American Society of Clinical Oncology (ASCO), 1900 Duke Street, Suite 200, Alexandria, VA 22314; (703) 299-0150, Fax: (703) 299-1044; http://www.asco@asco.org.

National Comprehensive Cancer Network, 50 Huntingdon Pike, Suite 200, Rockledge, PA 19046; (215) 728-4788, Fax: (215) 728-3877, (888) 909-NCCN, (888) 909-6226; http://www.nccn.org.

Oncology Nursing Society (ONS), 510 Holiday Drive, Pittsburgh, PA 15220-2749; (412) 921-7373; http://www.ons.org.

Patient/Family Support and Education

American Brain Tumor Association, 2720 River Road, Des Plaines, IL 60018; (847) 827-9910, Fax: (847) 827-9918, Patient Line: (800) 886-2282; http://www.abta.org.

American Cancer Society (ACS), 1599 Clifton Road NE, Atlanta, GA 30329; (800)-ACS-2345 (check your local directory for the unit of division nearest you); http://www.cancer.org.

Cancer Care, Inc., National Office, 275 7th Ave., New York, NY 10001; Services: (212) 302-2400, (800)-813-HOPE (4673); http://www.info@cancercare.org.

Cancer Information Network: http://www.cancernetwork.com.

CancerNet (a service of the National Cancer Institute): cancernet-staff@mail.nih.gov; http://cancernet.nci.nih.gov/index.html.

CancerSource World Headquarters, 40 Tall Pine Drive, Sudbury, MA 01776; http://www.cancersource.com.

Make Today Count, 1235 East Cherokee Street, Springfield, MO 85804; (407) 885-3324 or (800) 432-2273.

National Alliance of Breast Cancer Organizations (NABCO), 9 East 37th Street, 10th Floor, New York, NY 10016; (888) 806-2226; http://www.nabo.org:80/index.html.

The National Cancer Institute Public Inquiries Office, Building, 31, Room 10A31, 31 Center Drive, MSC 2580, Bethesda, MD 20892-2580; (800)-4-CANCER; http://rex.nci.nih.gov.

National Coalition for Cancer Survivorship, 1010 Wayne Avenue, Suite 770, Silver Spring, MD 20910-5600; (301) 650-9127 or (877) NCCS-YES (877-622-7937); Fax: (301) 565-9670; http://www.cansearch.org.

The National Hospice and Palliative Care Organization, 1700 Diagonal Road, Suite 300, Alexandria, VA 22314; (703) 837-1500; http://info@nhpco.org.

Oncolink; the University of Pennsylvania Cancer Center, 3400 Spruce St., Philadelphia, PA 19104; http://www.oncolink.upenn.edu.

The Wellness Community, 35 E. Seventh St., Suite 412, Cincinnati, OH 45202; (513) 421-7111, Fax (513) 421-7119, (888)-793-WELL; http://www.wellness-community.org.

End-of-Life Care

On completion of this chapter, the learner will be able to:

1. Discuss the historical, legal, and sociocultural perspectives of palliative and end-of-life care in the United States.
2. Define palliative care.
3. Compare and contrast the settings where palliative care and end-of-life care are provided.
4. Describe the principles and components of hospice care.
5. Identify barriers to improving care at the end of life.
6. Reflect on personal experience with and attitudes toward death and dying.
7. Apply skills for communicating with terminally ill patients and their families.
8. Provide culturally and spiritually sensitive care to terminally ill patients and their families.
9. Implement nursing measures to manage physiologic responses to terminal illness.
10. Support actively dying patients and their families.
11. Identify components of uncomplicated grief and mourning and implement nursing measures to support the patient and family.

Nursing and End-of-Life Care

One of the most difficult realities that nurses face is that, despite our very best efforts, some patients will die. Although we cannot change this fact, we can have a significant and lasting effect on the way in which patients live until they die, the manner in which the death occurs, and the enduring memories of that death for the families. Nursing has a long history of holistic, person- and family-centered care. Indeed, the definition of nursing offered by the American Nurses Association (ANA) highlights nursing's commitment to the diagnosis and treatment of human responses to illness (ANA, 1995). There is perhaps no setting or circumstance in which care—that is, attention to the human responses—is more important than in caring for the dying patient.

Knowledge about end-of-life decisions and principles of care is essential to supporting patients during decision making and in end-of-life closure in ways that recognize their unique responses to illness and that support their values and goals. Education, clinical practice, and research concerning end-of-life care are evolving, and the need to prepare nurses and other health care professionals to care for the dying has emerged as a priority. The National Institute for Nursing Research has taken the lead in coordinating research related to end-of-life care within the National Institutes of Health (Grady, 1999). At no time in nursing's history has there been a greater opportunity to bring research, education, and practice together to change the culture of dying, bringing much-needed improvement to care that is relevant across practice settings, age groups, cultural backgrounds, and illnesses.

THE CONTEXT FOR DEATH AND DYING IN AMERICA

In the past three decades there has been a surge of interest in the care of the dying, with an emphasis on the settings in which death occurs, the technologies used to sustain life, and the challenges of trying to improve end-of-life care. The focus on care of the dying has been motivated by the aging of the population, the prevalence of and publicity surrounding life-threatening illnesses such as cancer and AIDS, and the efforts of health care providers to build a continuum of service that spans the lifetime from birth until death (Lesparre & Matherlee, 1998). Although there are more

opportunities than ever before to allow a peaceful death, the knowledge and technologies available to health care providers have made the process of dying anything but peaceful. According to Callahan (1993a), Americans view death as what happens when medicine fails, an attitude that often places the study of death and improvement of the dying process outside of the focus of modern medicine and health care. Numerous initiatives aimed at improving end-of-life care have been launched in recent years, spurred by a widespread call for substantive change in the way Americans deal with death.

The Palliative Care Task Force of the Last Acts Campaign (Last Acts, 1997) identified the following as precepts or principles underlying a more comprehensive and humane approach to care of the dying:

- Respecting patients' goals, preferences, and choices
- Attending to the medical, emotional, social, and spiritual needs of the dying person
- Using strengths of interdisciplinary resources
- Acknowledging and addressing caregiver concerns
- Building mechanisms and systems of support

TECHNOLOGY AND END-OF-LIFE CARE

In the last century, chronic, degenerative diseases replaced communicable diseases as the major causes of death. Although technological advances in health care have extended and improved the quality of life for many, the ability of technologies to prolong life beyond the point that some would consider meaningful has raised troubling ethical issues. In particular, the use of technology to sustain life has raised perplexing issues with regard to quality of life, prolongation of dying, adequacy of pain relief and symptom management, and allocation of scarce resources. The major ethical question that has emerged concerning the use of technology to extend life is: Because we can prolong life through a particular intervention, does it necessarily follow that we must do so? In the latter half of the 20th century a "technological imperative" practice pattern among health care professionals emerged, along with an expectation among patients and families that every available means to extend life must be tried.

Decisions to apply every available technology to extend life have contributed to the shift in the place of death from the home to the hospital or extended care facility. In the earlier part of the last

---

Glossary

assisted suicide: use of pharmacological agents to hasten the death of a terminally ill patient; illegal in most states

autonomy: self-determination; in the health care context, the right of the individual to make choices about the use and discontinuation of medical treatment

bereavement: period during which mourning for a loss takes place

euthanasia: Greek for "good death;" has evolved to mean the intentional killing by act or omission of a dependent human being for his or her alleged benefit

grief: the personal feelings that accompany an anticipated or actual loss

hospice: a coordinated program of interdisciplinary care and services provided pri-

marily in the home to terminally ill patients and their families

interdisciplinary collaboration: members of diverse health care disciplines jointly plan, implement, and evaluate care

Medicare Hospice Benefit: a Medicare entitlement that provides for comprehensive, interdisciplinary palliative care and services for eligible beneficiaries who have a terminal illness and a life expectancy of less than 6 months

mourning: individual, family, group, and cultural expressions of grief and associated behaviors

palliative care: comprehensive care for patients whose disease is not responsive to cure; care also extends to patients' families

palliative sedation: use of pharmacological agents, at the request of the terminally ill patient, to induce sedation when symptoms have not responded to other management measures. The purpose is not to hasten the patient's death but to relieve intractable symptoms.

spirituality: personal belief systems that focus on a search for meaning and purpose in life, intangible elements that impart meaning and vitality to life, and a connectedness to a higher or transcendent dimension

terminal illness: progressive, irreversible illness that despite cure-focused medical treatment will result in the patient's death

century, most deaths occurred at home. Because of this, most families had direct experience "being with" death, providing care to family members at the end of life and mourning for the loss of loved ones. As the place of death shifted to the hospital, families became increasingly distanced from the death experience. By the early 1970s, when hospice care was just beginning in this country, technology had become the expected companion of the critically and terminally ill (Wentzel, 1981). The implications of technological intervention at the end of life continue to be profound, affecting a societal view of death that influences how clinicians care for the dying, how family and friends participate in care, how patients and families understand and choose among end-of-life care options, how families prepare for **terminal illness** and death, and how they heal following the death of a loved one.

SOCIOCULTURAL CONTEXT

Although each individual experiences terminal illness uniquely, such illness is also shaped substantially by the social and cultural contexts in which it occurs. In the United States, life-threatening illness, life-sustaining treatment decisions, dying, and death occur in a social environment where illness is largely considered a foe and where battles are either lost or won (Benoliel, 1993). A care/cure dichotomy has emerged in which health care providers may view cure as the ultimate good and care as second best, a good only when cure is no longer possible (Benoliel, 1993; Gadow, 1988). In such a model of health or medical care, alleviating suffering is not as valued as curing disease, and patients who cannot be cured feel distanced from the health care team, concluding that when treatment has failed, they too have failed. Patients and families who have internalized the socially constructed meaning of care as second best may fear that any shift from curative goals in the direction of comfort-focused care will result in no care or poorer-quality care, and that the clinicians on whom they have come to rely will abandon them if they withdraw from the battle for cure.

The reduction of patients to their diseases is exemplified in the frequently relayed message in late-stage illness that "nothing more can be done." This all-too-frequently used statement communicates the belief of many clinicians that there is nothing of value to offer patients who are beyond cure. In a care-focused perspective, mind, body, and spirit are inextricable, and treating the body without attending to the other components is considered inadequate to evoke true healing (Upledger, 1989; Wendler, 1996). This expanded notion of healing as care, along with and beyond cure, implies that healing can take place throughout life and outside the boundaries of contemporary medicine. In this expanded definition, healing is transcendent and its boundaries are unlimited, even as body systems begin to fail at the end of life (Byock, 1997).

Clinicians' Attitudes Toward Death

Clinicians' attitudes toward the terminally ill and dying remain the greatest barrier to improving care at the end of life. Kübler-Ross illuminated the concerns of the seriously ill and dying in her seminal work *On Death and Dying,* published in 1969. At that time, it was common for patients to be kept uninformed about life-threatening diagnoses, particularly cancer, and for physicians and nurses to avoid open discussion of death and dying with their patients (Krisman-Scott, 2000; Seale, 1991). Kübler-Ross taught the health care community that having open discussion about life and death issues did not harm patients, and that the patients in fact welcomed such openness. She was openly critical of what she called "a new but depersonalized science in the service of prolonging life rather than diminishing human suffering" (Kübler-Ross, 1969, p. 20). She taught the health care community that healing could not take place in a conspiracy of silence, and that as clinicians break the silence and enter the patient's world, they too can be healed by their struggles and strengths. Her work revealed that, given adequate time and some help in working through the process, patients could reach a stage of acceptance where they were neither angry nor depressed about their fate (Kübler-Ross, 1969).

Clinicians' reluctance to discuss disease and death openly with patients stems from their own anxieties about death as well as misconceptions about what and how much patients want to know about their illnesses. In an early study of care of the dying in hospital settings, sociologists Glaser and Strauss (1965) discovered that health care professionals in hospital settings avoided direct communication about dying in hope that the patient would discover it on his or her own. They identified four "awareness contexts," described as the patient's, physician's, family's, and other health care professionals' awareness of the patient's status and their recognition of each other's awareness:

1. Closed awareness: The patient is unaware of his or her terminal state while others are aware. Closed awareness may be characterized by families and health care professionals conspiring to guard the "secret," fearing that the patient would not be able to cope with full disclosure about his or her status, and the patient's acceptance of others' accounts of his or her "future biography" as long as they give him or her no reason to be suspicious.
2. Suspected awareness: The patient suspects what others know and attempts to find out. Suspected awareness may be triggered by inconsistencies in families' and clinicians' communication and behavior, discrepancies between clinicians' accounts of the seriousness of the patient's illness, or a decline in the patient's condition or other environmental cues.
3. Mutual pretense awareness: The patient, the family, and the health care professionals are aware that the patient is dying but all pretend otherwise.
4. Open awareness: All are aware that the patient is dying and are able to openly acknowledge that reality.

Glaser and Strauss (1965) also identified a pattern of clinician behavior in which those who feared or were uncomfortable discussing death developed and substituted "personal mythologies" for appraisals of what level of disclosure patients actually wanted. For example, clinicians avoided direct communication with patients about the seriousness of their illness based on their beliefs that (1) patients already knew the truth or would ask if they wanted to know, or (2) patients would subsequently lose all hope, give up, or be psychologically harmed by disclosure.

Glaser and Strauss' findings were published more than 35 years ago, yet their observations remain valid today. Although a growing number of health care providers are becoming comfortable with assessing patients' and families' information needs and disclosing honest information about the seriousness of illness, many still avoid the topic of death in hopes that the patient will ask or find out on his or her own. Despite progress on many health care fronts, those who work with dying patients have identified the persistence of a "conspiracy of silence" about dying (Stanley, 2000, p. 34).

Patient and Family Denial

Denial on the part of the patient and family about the seriousness of terminal illness also has been cited as a barrier to discussion about end-of-life treatment options. Kübler-Ross (1969) was one of the first to examine patient denial and expose it as a useful coping mechanism that enables patients to gain temporary emotional distance from something that is too painful to contemplate fully. Patients who are characterized as being in denial may be using that strategy to preserve important interpersonal relationships, to protect others from the emotional effects of their illness, or to protect themselves because of fears of abandonment.

Connor (1992) studied a small group of terminally ill cancer patients who were characterized by their use of denial as a coping mechanism. Participants in the experimental group were questioned in structured interviews about their perceptions of the most difficult aspects of having cancer and those actions that they or others take that make these difficulties easier or more difficult to bear. They were offered psychosocial intervention that consisted largely of therapeutic communication followed by a postintervention assessment of their use of denial as a defense mechanism. The use of denial by patients in a control group was also assessed, but these patients did not receive the psychosocial intervention. The researcher concluded that terminally ill patients using denial respond favorably to sensitive psychosocial intervention, as indicated by decreased scores on an instrument to measure denial. Connor acknowledged, however, that additional research is needed to gauge the timing of such interventions according to some measure of patient readiness.

In a more recent study, researchers reported that while the majority of a sample of 200 patients with advanced cancer in their final weeks of life were completely aware of their medical prognosis, a combined total of 26.5% were either unaware or only partially aware (Chochinov, Tataryn, Wilson, Ennis & Lander, 2000). Depression was nearly three times greater in those patients who were unaware of their prognosis. The researchers concluded that denial of prognosis is more likely in patients with underlying psychological or emotional distress. Similarly, Chow and colleagues (2001) reported that many patients surveyed about their understanding of palliative radiation therapy for advanced cancer believed that their disease was curable, that the radiation therapy would cure their cancer, or that the therapy would prolong their lives. Importantly, most also reported that they were unfamiliar with the concept of radiation therapy, were not given information, or were not satisfied with the information their physicians had provided. Clearly, further research is needed to examine the complex interplay between patients' misconceptions about advanced illness, their underlying psychological states, and clinicians' persistent lack of candor in discussing treatment expectations and prognosis.

The question of how to communicate with patients in a way that acknowledges where they are on the continuum of acceptance, while providing them with unambiguous information, remains a challenge. Zerwekh (1994) analyzed stories from 32 hospice nurses and concluded that nurses in a hospice setting were adept at interventions deemed important in care of the dying, namely truth telling and encouraging patient **autonomy**. Although she acknowledged that each individual views "truth" differently, she observed that hospice nurses participating in the study used communication skills to assist the patient and family to discuss end-of-life issues. Hospice nurses deliberately spoke about sensitive matters that were usually avoided and gave patients and families truthful representations of their status when patients were in transition from curative to palliative care. Although timing of the questions takes experience, speaking the truth can be a relief to patients and families, enhancing their autonomy by making way for truly informed consent as the basis for decision making.

Assisted Suicide

The assisted suicide debate has aimed a spotlight on the adequacy and quality of end-of-life care in the United States. **Assisted suicide** refers to providing another person the means to end his or her own life. Physician-assisted suicide involves the prescription by a physician of a lethal dose of medication for the purpose of ending someone's life (not to be confused with the ethically and legally supported practices of withholding or withdrawing medical treatment in accordance with the wishes of the terminally ill individual).

Judeo-Christian beliefs support the view that suicide is a violation of natural law and the law of God (Helm, 1984; Sorenson, 1991). However, there have recently been calls for the legalization of assisted suicide. Although the preference to take one's own life over awaiting death has been evident through the ages, these recent efforts to legalize assisted suicide underscore the need for changes in the ways individuals with terminal illnesses are cared for and treated at the end of their lives. This is further emphasized by the efforts of groups such as the Hemlock Society to have physician-assisted suicide legalized and the Hemlock Society's publication of information to the public describing methods for ending one's own life when such assistance from physicians is not available.

Although assisted suicide is expressly prohibited under statutory or common law in the majority of states, the calls for legalized assisted suicide have highlighted inadequacies in the care of the dying. In 1990, Dr. Jack Kevorkian, a retired pathologist, assisted a 54-year-old woman with early Alzheimer's disease to end her life using a device that he had devised to allow a patient to control the infusion of a lethal dose of potassium chloride. In 1999, after 130 deaths and nine trials, Kevorkian was convicted on second-degree murder charges in the death of a 52-year-old man with amyotrophic lateral sclerosis and is currently serving a 10 - to 25-year prison sentence in Michigan. In a telephone poll conducted the week following the conviction, 55% of respondents disagreed with the verdict (Langer, 1999).

Meanwhile, public support for physician-assisted suicide has resulted in a number of state ballot initiatives. In 1994, voters approved the Oregon Death with Dignity Act, the first such legislative initiative to pass. This law provides for terminally ill patients' access to physician-assisted suicide under very controlled circumstances. After numerous challenges, a majority of Oregonians voted against an attempted repeal, and the law was implemented in 1997. The most recent challenges to the law included the 1999 federal Pain Relief Promotion Act, a bill designed to derail the implementation of the Oregon law by prohibiting the use of federally controlled substances for physician-assisted suicide, and a 2001 directive from Attorney General John Ashcroft to the Drug Enforcement Agency to track and prosecute physicians who prescribe under the Oregon law. There is an ongoing battle in the courts over this issue, and while Oregon is currently the only state with a statute legalizing physician-assisted suicide, it is likely that the issue will be pursued in the courts and through ballot measures in other states.

Whereas proponents of physician-assisted suicide argue that terminally ill individuals should have a legally sanctioned right to make independent decisions about the value of their lives and the timing and circumstances of their deaths, its opponents argue for greater access to symptom management and psychosocial support for individuals approaching the end of life. Numerous ethical and legal issues have been raised, including voluntariness and authenticity of requests in relation to the mental competence and decision-making capacity of patients who request physician-assisted suicide, the existence of underlying untreated clinical depression or other suffering, and issues of overt or perceived coercion. Assisted suicide is opposed by nursing and medical organizations as a violation of the ethical traditions of nursing and medicine. The ANA Position Statement on Assisted Suicide acknowledges the complexity of the assisted suicide debate but clearly states that nursing participation in assisted suicide is a violation of the Code for Nurses. The ANA Position Statement further stresses the important role of the nurse in supporting effective symptom management, contributing to the creation of environments for care that honor the patient's and family's wishes, and ascertaining and addressing their concerns and fears (ANA, 1994).

Settings for End-of-Life Care: Palliative Care Programs and Hospice

PALLIATIVE CARE

As concerns have grown about the poor quality of life patients experience during progressive illness, broadening the concept of palliative care beyond the hospice has begun to take hold in health care settings across the country (Jones, 1997). **Palliative care** is an approach to care for the seriously ill that has long been a part of cancer care. Both palliative care and hospice have been recognized as important bridges between the compulsion for cure-oriented care and physician-assisted suicide (Saunders & Kastenbaum, 1997). Advocates for improved care for the dying have stated that acceptance, management, and understanding of death should become fully integrated concepts in mainstream health care (Callahan, 1993a; Morrison, Siu, Leipzig et al., 2000). Increasingly, palliative care is being offered to patients with noncancer chronic illnesses, where comprehensive symptom management and psychosocial and spiritual support can enhance the patient's and family's quality of life.

While hospice care is considered by many to be the "gold standard" for palliative care, the term **hospice** is generally associated with palliative care that is delivered at home or in special facilities to patients who are approaching the end of life. Palliative care is conceptually broader than hospice care, defined as the active, total care of patients whose disease is not responsive to treatment (World Health Organization, 1990).

Palliative care emphasizes management of psychological, social, and spiritual problems in addition to control of pain and other physical symptoms. As the definition suggests, palliative care is not care that begins when cure-focused treatment ends. The goal of palliative care is to improve the patient's and family's quality of life, and many aspects of this type of comprehensive, comfort-focused approach to care are applicable earlier in the process of life-threatening disease in conjunction with cure-focused treatment. However, definitions of palliative care, the services that are part of it, and the clinicians who provide it are evolving steadily.

Some would argue that palliative care is no different from comprehensive nursing, medical, social, and spiritual care and that patients should not have to be labeled as "dying" to receive person-focused care and symptom management. In addition to a focus on the multiple dimensions of the illness experience for both patients and their families, palliative care emphasizes the interdisciplinary collaboration that is necessary to bring about the desired outcomes for patients and their families. **Interdisciplinary collaboration** is distinguished from multidisciplinary practice in that the former is based on communication and cooperation among the various disciplines; each member of the team contributes to a single care plan that addresses the needs of the patient and family.

Palliative Care at the End of Life

As discussed above, palliative care is broadly conceptualized as comprehensive, person- and family-centered care when disease is not responsive to treatment. The broadening of the concept of palliative care actually followed the development of hospice services in the United States. Hospice care is in fact palliative care. The difference is that hospice care is associated with the end of life, and although it focuses on quality of life, hospice care by necessity usually includes realistic emotional, social, spiritual, and financial preparation for death. In the mid-1970s, when hospice care was introduced in the United States, it was more broadly conceived as care that addressed the whole person—physical, social, emotional, and spiritual—and was available to patients earlier in the process of life-threatening illness. After hospice care was recognized as a distinct program of services under Medicare in the early 1980s, organizations providing hospice care were able to receive Medicare reimbursement if they could demonstrate that the hospice program met the Medicare "conditions of participation," or regulations, for hospice providers.

While Medicare reimbursement resulted in new rules for hospices, it also defined when Medicare beneficiaries are able to use their **Medicare Hospice Benefit**. In most programs, the Medicare definitions for patient eligibility are used to guide all enrollment decisions. According to Medicare, the patient who wishes to use his or her Medicare Hospice Benefit must be certified by a physician as terminally ill, with a life expectancy of 6 months or less if the disease follows its natural course. Thus, hospice has come to be defined as care provided to terminally ill persons and their families in the last 6 months of the patient's life. Because of additional Medicare rules concerning completion of all cure-focused medical treatment before the Medicare Hospice Benefit may be accessed, many patients delay enrollment in hospice programs until very close to the end of life.

The reasons for late referral to hospice and the underuse of hospice services are complex. They may include values and attitudes of health care providers, the inadequate dissemination of existing knowledge about pain and symptom management, health care providers' difficulties in effectively communicating with terminally ill individuals, and insufficient attention to palliative care concepts in health care providers' education and training.

Hospices care for approximately 29% of patients who are eligible (National Hospice and Palliative Care Organization, 2001). For the most part, the remainder of terminally ill patients die in hospitals and long-term care facilities. It is clear that better care for the dying is urgently needed in hospitals, long-term care facilities, home care agencies, and outpatient settings. At the same time, many chronic diseases do not have a predictable "end stage" that fits hospice eligibility criteria, meaning that many patients die after a long, slow, and often painful decline, without the benefit of the coordinated palliative care that is unique to hospice programs. The palliative approach to care could benefit many more patients if it were available across settings for care and earlier in the disease process. In an attempt to make this valuable approach to care more widely available, palliative care programs are being developed in other settings for patients who are either not eligible for hospice or are "not ready" to enroll in a formal hospice program. As yet, there is no dedicated reimbursement to providers for palliative care services when they are delivered outside of the hospice setting, making the sustainability of such programs challenging.

Palliative Care in the Hospital Setting

Since the advent of diagnosis-related groups (DRGs) as the basis for prospective payment for hospital services in the 1980s, there has been a financial incentive for hospitals to transfer patients with terminal illnesses who were no longer in need of acute-level care to other settings, such as long-term care facilities and home, to receive care (Field & Cassel, 1997). Despite the economic and human costs associated with death in the hospital setting, as many as 50% of all deaths occur in acute care settings (Hogan et al., 2000). The landmark Study to Understand Prognoses and Preferences for Outcomes and Risks of Treatments (SUPPORT, 1995) documented troubling deficiencies in the care of the dying in hospital settings:

- Many patients received unwanted care at the end of life.
- Clinicians were not aware of patient preferences for life-sustaining treatment, even when preferences were documented in the clinical record.
- Pain was often poorly controlled at the end of life.
- Efforts to enhance communication were ineffective.

It is clear that many patients will continue to opt for hospital care or by default will find themselves in hospital settings at the end of life. Increasingly, hospitals are conducting system-wide assessments of end-of-life care practices and outcomes and are developing innovative models for delivering high-quality, person-centered care to patients approaching the end of life. Hospitals cite considerable financial barriers to providing high-quality palliative care in an acute care setting (Cassel, Ludden & Moon, 2000). Public policy changes have been called for that would provide reimbursement to hospitals for care delivered via designated hospital-wide palliative care beds, clustered palliative care units, or palliative care consultation services in acute care settings.

Palliative Care in Long-Term Care Facilities

The place of death for a growing number of Americans after the age of 65 is the long-term care facility (Alliance for Aging Research, 1997) As many as one third of all Medicare beneficiaries who die in any given year spend all or part of their last year of life in a long-term care facility (Hogan et al., 2000). The trend favoring care of dying patients in long-term care facilities will continue as the population ages and as managed care payors pressure health care providers to minimize costs (Field & Cassel, 1997). Yet residents of long-term care facilities reportedly have poor access to high-quality palliative care. Regulations that govern how care in these facilities is organized and reimbursed tend to emphasize restorative measures and fail to reward palliative care (Zerzan, Stearns & Hanson, 2000). Although home hospice programs have been permitted since 1986 to enroll long-term care facility residents in hospice programs and provide interdisciplinary services to residents who qualify for hospice care, the Office of the Inspector General, an oversight arm of the federal government, has questioned whether such services are an unnecessary duplication of services already provided by facility staff (Office of the Inspector General, 1997). While there has been regulatory scrutiny on the one hand, long-term care facilities of all types are under increasing public pressure to improve care of the dying and are beginning to develop palliative care units or services, contract with home hospice programs to provide hospice care in the facilities, and educate staff, residents, and their families about pain and symptom management and end-of-life care.

HOSPICE CARE

Hospice in the United States is not a place, but a concept of care in which the end of life is viewed as a developmental stage. The root of the word hospice is *hospes,* meaning "host." Historically, hospice has referred to a shelter or way station for weary travelers on a pilgrimage (Bennahum, 1996). In the years that followed Kübler-Ross's groundbreaking work, the concept of hospice care as an alternative to depersonalized death in institutions began as a grassroots movement. Her work, and the development of the concept of hospice in England by Dr. Cicely Saunders, resulted in recognition of gaps in the existing system of care for the terminally ill (Amenta, 1986). Hospice care began in response to "noticeable gaps . . . (1) between treating the disease and treating the person, (2) between technological research and psycho-social support, and (3) between the general denial of the fact of death in our society and the acceptance of death by those who face it" (Wentzel, 1981, p. 11). According to Saunders, who founded the world-renowned St. Christopher's Hospice in London (Bennahum, 1996), the principles underlying hospice are as follows:

- Death must be accepted.
- The patient's total care is best managed by an interdisciplinary team whose members communicate regularly with each other.
- Pain and other symptoms of terminal illness must be managed.
- The patient and family should be viewed as a single unit of care.
- Home care of the dying is necessary.
- Bereavement care must be provided to family members.
- Research and education should be ongoing.

Hospice Care in the United States

Although the concept dates to ancient times, hospice as a way of caring for those at the end of life did not emerge in the United States until the 1960s (Hospice Association of America, 2001). The hospice movement in the United States is based on the belief that meaningful living is achievable during terminal illness, and that it is best supported in the home, free from technological interventions to prolong physiologic dying (Amenta, 1986). After the first U.S. hospice was founded in Connecticut in 1974, the concept quickly spread and the number of hospice programs in the United States has grown dramatically. In the years between 1984 and 1996, which followed the creation of the Medicare Hospice Benefit, there was a 70-fold increase in the number of hospices participating in Medicare (Hospice Association of America, 2001).

Despite more than 25 years of existence in the United States, hospice remains an option for end-of-life care that has not been fully integrated into mainstream health care. Although hospice care is available to persons with any life-limiting condition, it has primarily been used by patients with advanced cancer, where the disease staging and trajectory lend themselves to more reliable prediction about the end of life (Boling & Lynn, 1998; Christakis & Lamont, 2000). Many reasons have been proposed for the reluctance of physicians to refer patients to hospice and the reluctance of patients to accept this form of care. These include the difficulties in making a terminal prognosis, the strong association of hospice with death, advances in "curative" treatment options in late-stage illness, and financial pressures on health care providers that may cause them to retain rather than refer hospice-eligible patients. The result is that patients who could benefit from the comprehensive, interdisciplinary support offered by hospice programs frequently do not enter hospice care until their final days (or hours) of life (Christakis & Lamont, 2000).

Hospice is a coordinated program of interdisciplinary services provided by professional caregivers and trained volunteers to patients with serious, progressive illnesses that are not responsive to cure. In hospice settings, the patient and family together are the unit of care. The goal of hospice care is to enable the patient to remain at home, surrounded by the people and objects that have been important to him or her throughout life. Hospice care does not seek to hasten death, nor does it encourage the prolongation of life through artificial means. Hospice care hinges on the competent patient's full or "open" awareness of dying; it embraces a realism about death, such that the patient and family are assisted to understand the dying process and can live each moment as fully as possible.

Although most hospice care is provided in the patient's own home, some hospice programs have developed inpatient facilities or residences where terminally ill patients without family support or those who desire inpatient care may receive hospice services.

Eligibility criteria for hospice vary depending on the hospice program, but generally patients must have a progressive, irreversible illness and limited life expectancy and have opted for palliative care rather than cure-focused treatment. Although hospices have historically served cancer patients, patients with any life-limiting illness are eligible.

Medicare Hospice Benefit

In 1983, the Medicare Hospice Benefit was implemented to cover hospice care for Medicare beneficiaries. State Medical Assistance (Medicaid) also provides coverage for hospice care, as do most commercial insurers. Federal reimbursement for hospice care ushered in a new era in hospice in which program standards developed and published by the federal government codified what had formerly been a grassroots, loosely organized and defined ideal for care at the end of life. To receive Medicare dollars for hospice services, programs are required to comply with conditions of participation promulgated by the Centers for Medicare and Medicaid Services. Medicare standards have come to largely define hospice philosophy and services. Eligibility criteria for hospice coverage under the Medicare Hospice Benefit are specified in Chart 17-1. Federal rules for hospices require that the patient's continuing eligibility for hospice care is reviewed periodically. There is no limit to the length of time that an eligible patient may continue to receive hospice care. Patients who live longer than 6 months under hospice care are not discharged if their physician and the hospice medical director continue to certify that the patient is terminally ill with a life expectancy of 6 months or less, assuming that the disease continues its expected course. The hospice certification and review process and the open-ended benefit structure are intended to address the difficulty physicians face in predicting how long a patient will live, so that patients are not restricted to a lifetime limit on the number of hospice days they may receive.

Chart 17-1

Eligibility Criteria for Hospice Care

General
- Serious, progressive illness
- Limited life expectancy
- Informed choice of palliative care over cure-focused treatment

Hospice-Specific
- Presence of a family member or other caregiver continuously in the home when the patient is no longer able to safely care for him/herself (some hospices have created special services within their programs for patients who live alone, but this varies widely)

Medicare and Medicaid Hospice Benefits
- Medicare Part A; Medical Assistance eligibility
- Waiver of traditional Medicare/Medicaid benefits for the terminal illness
- Life expectancy of 6 months or less
- Physician certification of terminal illness
- Care must be provided by a Medicare-certified hospice program

---

To use hospice benefits under Medicare or Medicaid, the patient must meet eligibility criteria and "elect" to use the hospice benefit in place of traditional Medicare or Medicaid benefits for the terminal illness. Once the patient elects the benefit, the Medicare-certified hospice program assumes responsibility for providing and paying for the care and treatment related to the underlying illness for which hospice care was elected. The Medicare-certified hospice is paid a predetermined dollar amount for each day of hospice care each patient receives. Four levels of hospice care are covered under Medicare and Medicaid hospice benefits:

- Routine home care: All services provided are included in the daily rate to the hospice.
- Inpatient respite care: A 5-day inpatient stay, provided on an occasional basis to relieve the family caregivers
- Continuous care: Continuous nursing care provided in the home for management of a medical crisis. Care reverts to the routine home care level when the crisis is resolved. (For example, the patient develops seizure activity and a nurse is placed in the home continuously to monitor the patient and administer medications. After 72 hours the seizure activity is under control, the family has been instructed how to care for the patient, and the continuous nursing care is stopped.)
- General inpatient care: Inpatient stay for symptom management that cannot be provided in the home; not subject to the guidelines for a standard hospital inpatient stay.

Most hospice care is provided at the "routine home care" level and includes the services depicted in Chart 17-2. According to federal guidelines, hospices may provide no more than 20% of the aggregate annual patient days at the inpatient level. Patients may "revoke" their hospice benefits at any time, resuming traditional coverage under Medicare or Medicaid for the terminal illness. They may also re-elect their hospice benefits at a later time after reassessment for eligibility according to these criteria

Nursing Care of the Terminally Ill Patient

Many patients suffer unnecessarily when they do not receive adequate attention for the symptoms accompanying serious illness. Careful evaluation of the patient should include not only the physical problems but also the psychosocial and spiritual dimen-

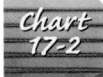

Chart 17-2 Home Hospice Services Covered Under the Medicare / Medicaid Hospice Benefit Routine Home Care Level

- Nursing care: Provided by or under the supervision of a registered nurse, available 24 hours a day
- Medical social services
- Physician's services
- Counseling services, including dietary counseling
- Home health aide/homemaker
- Physical/occupational/speech therapists
- Volunteers
- Bereavement follow-up (for up to 13 months following the death of the patient)
- Medical supplies for the palliation of the terminal illness
- Medical equipment for the palliation of the terminal illness
- Medications for the palliation of the terminal illness

Chart 17-3 Methods of Stating End-of-Life Preferences

Advance directives—Written documents that allow the individual of sound mind to document preferences regarding end-of-life care that should be followed when the signer is terminally ill and unable to verbally communicate his/her wishes. The documents are generally completed in advance of or during serious illness. The most common types are the living will (also known as a medical directive) and a proxy directive (also known as a durable power of attorney for health care).

Proxy directive—The appointment and authorization of another individual to make medical decisions on behalf of the person who created an advance directive when he/she is no longer able to speak for him/herself. This is also known as a health care power of attorney or durable power of attorney for health care.

Living will—Also known as a medical directive. A type of advance directive in which the individual of sound mind documents treatment preferences. Provides instructions for care in the event that the signer is terminally ill and not able to communicate wishes directly. Often accompanied by a proxy directive (also known as a health care power of attorney).

Durable power of attorney for health care—A legal document that enables the signer to designate another individual to make health care decisions on his/her behalf when he/she is unable to do so.

sions of the patient's and family's experience of serious illness. This approach contributes to a more comprehensive understanding of how the patient's and family's life has been affected by the illness and will lead to nursing care that addresses the needs in every dimension.

PSYCHOSOCIAL ISSUES

Nurses are responsible for educating patients about the possibilities and probabilities inherent in their illness and their life with the illness, and for supporting them as they conduct life review, values clarification, treatment decision making, and end-of-life closure. The only way to do this effectively is to try to appreciate and understand the illness from the patient's perspective.

Kübler-Ross's (1969) work revealed that patients in the final stages of life can and will talk openly about their experiences, exposing as a myth the view that patients will be harmed by honest discussion with their caregivers about death. Despite the continued reluctance of health care providers to engage in open discussion about end-of-life issues, studies have confirmed that patients want information about their illness and end-of-life choices are not harmed by open discussion about death (McSkimming, Super, Driever et al., 1997; Virmani, Schneiderman & Kaplan, 1994).

At the same time, nurses need to be both culturally aware and sensitive in their approaches to communication with patients and families about death. Attitudes toward open disclosure about terminal illness vary widely among different cultures, and direct communication to the patient about such matters may be viewed as harmful (Blackhall, Murphy, Frank et al., 1995). To provide effective patient- and family-centered care at the end of life, nurses must be willing to set aside their assumptions so that they can discover what type and amount of disclosure is most meaningful to each patient and family within their unique belief systems.

The social and legal evolution of advance directive documents represents some progress in our willingness to both contemplate and communicate our wishes surrounding the end of life (Chart 17-3). Now legally sanctioned in every state and federally sanctioned through the Patient Self-Determination Act (PSDA) of 1990, advance directives are written documents that allow the individual who is of sound mind to document his or her preferences regarding the use or nonuse of medical treatment at the end of life, specify the preferred setting for care, and communicate other valuable insights into his or her values and beliefs. The addition

of a proxy directive (the appointment and authorization of another individual to make medical decisions on behalf of the person who created the advance directive when he or she can no longer speak for himself or herself) is an important addition to the "living will" or medical directive that specifies the signer's preferences. Although these documents are widely available from health care providers, community organizations, bookstores, and the Internet, their underuse reflects society's continued discomfort with openly confronting the subject of death. Further, the existence of a properly executed advance directive does not reduce the complexity of end-of-life decisions. The advance directive should not be considered an adequate substitute for ongoing communication between health care provider, patient, and family as the end of life approaches (Lynn, 1991).

COMMUNICATION

As has been discussed, remarkable strides have been made in the ability to prolong life, but attention to care for the dying lags behind (Callahan, 1993b). On one level, this comes as no surprise. Each of us will eventually face death, and most would agree that one's own demise is a subject he or she would prefer not to contemplate. Indeed, Glaser and Strauss (1965) noted that unwillingness in our culture to talk about the process of dying is tied to our discomfort with the notion of particular deaths—those of our patients' and our own—rather than talking about death in the abstract, which is more comfortable. Finucane (1999) observed that our struggle to stay alive is a prerequisite to being human. Confronting death in our patients uncovers our own deeply rooted fears.

To develop a level of comfort and expertise in communicating with seriously and terminally ill patients and their families, nurses and other clinicians need to first consider their own experiences with and values concerning illness and death. Reflection, reading, and talking with family members, friends, and colleagues can assist the nurse to examine beliefs about death and dying. Talking with individuals from differing cultural backgrounds can assist the nurse to view personally held beliefs through a different lens, and can help to sensitize the nurse to death-related beliefs and practices in other cultures. Discussion with nursing and non-nursing colleagues can also be useful to reveal the values shared by many health care professions and identify diversity in the values of patients in their care. Values clarification and personal death awareness exercises can provide a starting point for self-discovery and discussion.

Skills for Communicating With the Seriously Ill

Nurses need to develop skill and comfort in assessing patients' and families' responses to serious illness and planning interventions that will support their values and choices throughout the continuum of care. Patients and families need ongoing assistance: telling a patient something once is not teaching, and hearing the patient's words is not the same as active listening. Throughout the course of a serious illness, patients and their families will encounter complicated treatment decisions, bad news about disease progression, and recurring emotional responses. In addition to the time of initial diagnosis, lack of response to the treatment course, decisions to continue or withdraw particular interventions, and decisions about hospice care are examples of critical points on the treatment continuum that demand patience, empathy, and honesty from the nurse. Discussing sensitive issues such as serious illness, hopes for survival, and fears associated with death is never easy. However, the art of therapeutic communication can be learned and, like other skills, must be practiced to gain expertise. Similar to other skills, communication should be practiced in a "safe" setting, such as a classroom or clinical skills laboratory with other students or clinicians.

Although communication with each patient and family should be tailored to their level of understanding and values concerning disclosure, general guidelines for the nurse include the following (Addington, 1991):

- Deliver and interpret the technical information necessary for making decisions without hiding behind medical terminology.
- Realize that the best time for the patient to talk may be when it is least convenient for you.
- Being fully present during any opportunity for communication is often the most helpful form of communication.
- Allow the patient and family to set the agenda regarding the depth of the conversation.

Nursing Interventions When the Patient and Family Receive Bad News

Communicating about a life-threatening diagnosis or about disease progression is best accomplished by the interdisciplinary team in any setting—a physician, nurse, and social worker should be present whenever possible to provide information, facilitate discussion, and address concerns. Most importantly, the presence of the team conveys caring and respect for the patient and family. Creating the right setting is particularly important. If the patient wishes to have family present for the discussion, arrangements should be made to have the discussion at a time that is best for the patient and family. A quiet area with a minimum of disturbances should be used. Each clinician who is present should turn off beepers or other communication devices for the duration of the meeting and should allow sufficient time for the patient and family to

absorb and respond to the news. Finally, the space in which the meeting takes place should be conducive to seating all of the participants at eye level. It is difficult enough for patients and families to be the recipients of bad news without having an array of clinicians standing uncomfortably over them at the foot of the patient's bed.

After an initial discussion of a life-threatening illness or progression of a disease, patients and their families will have many questions and may need to be reminded of factual information. Coping with news about a serious diagnosis or poor prognosis is an ongoing process. The nurse needs to be sensitive to these ongoing needs and may need to repeat previously provided information or simply be present while the patient and family react emotionally. The most important intervention the nurse can provide is listening empathetically. Seriously ill patients and their families need time and support to cope with the changes brought about by serious illness and the prospect of impending death. The nurse who is able to sit comfortably with another's suffering, time and time again, without judgment and without the need to solve the patient's and family's problems provides an intervention that is a gift beyond measure. Keys to effective listening include the following:

- Resist the impulse to fill the "empty space" in communication with talk.
- Allow the patient and family sufficient time to reflect and respond after asking a question.
- Prompt gently: "Do you need more time to think about this?"
- Avoid distractions (noise, interruptions).
- Avoid the impulse to give advice.
- Avoid canned responses: "I know just how you feel."
- Ask questions.
- Assess understanding—your own and the patient's—by restating, summarizing, and reviewing.

Responding With Sensitivity To Difficult Questions

Patients will often direct questions or concerns to nurses before they have been able to fully discuss the details of their diagnosis and prognosis with the physician or the entire health care team. Using open-ended questions allows the nurse to elicit the patient's and family's concerns, explore misconceptions and needs for information, and form the basis for collaboration with the physician and other team members. For example, the seriously ill patient may ask the nurse, "Am I dying?" The nurse should avoid making unhelpful responses that dismiss the patient's real concerns or defer the issue to another care provider. Nursing assessment and intervention are always possible, even when a need for further discussion with the physician is clearly indicated. Whenever possible, discussions in response to the patient's concerns should occur when the patient expresses a need, although it may be the least convenient time for the nurse (Addington, 1991). Creating an uninterrupted space of just 5 minutes can do much to identify the source of the concern, allay anxieties, and plan for follow-up. For example, in response to the question, "Am I dying?" the nurse could establish eye contact and follow with a statement acknowledging the patient's fears ("This must be very difficult for you") and an open-ended statement or question ("Tell me more about what is on your mind."). The nurse then needs to listen intently, ask additional questions for clarification, and provide reassurance only when it is realistic. In this example, the nurse might quickly ascertain that the patient's question emanates from a need for specific information—about diagnosis and prognosis from the physician, about the physiology of the dying process from the nurse, or perhaps about financial implications for the family from the social worker. The chaplain may also be called upon to talk with the patient about existential concerns.

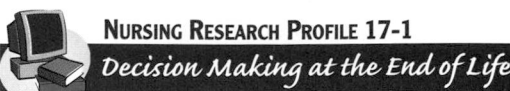

NURSING RESEARCH PROFILE 17-1
Decision Making at the End of Life

Tilden, V. P., Tolle, S. W., Nelson, C. A., & Fields, J. (2001). Family decision-making to withdraw life-sustaining treatments from hospitalized patients. *Nursing Research, 50*(2), 105–115.

Purpose
Although participation of family members in end-of-life decision making is increasing, little is known about the stress associated with their participation. Further, it is not known how families' reasoning processes compare to those of clinicians. The purpose of this study was to assess factors that affect family stress associated with withdrawal of life-sustaining treatment from their dying, hospitalized relatives. Investigators also compared family members and clinicians on their reasoning about the decision.

Study Sample and Design
A descriptive quantitative study was conducted in four large tertiary-care centers. Family members who had participated in the decision to withdraw life-sustaining treatment from patients who had been unable to make their own decisions were invited to participate.

Seventy-four family members of 51 patients participated in the study and were interviewed for data collection 1 to 2 months after the death of the patient; 65 family members were interviewed again 7 to 8 months later. Clinician data about the families' decision making were obtained from physicians (n = 21) and nurses (n = 24) 2 months after patients' deaths.

The Horowitz Impact of Events Scale and the mental/emotional state scale of the Rand 36-item Health Survey 1.0 was used to measure family stress. The researchers measured the importance of each of three factors (quality of life, patient preference, and prolongation of life) to family and clinician reasoning about treatment decisions by single-item indicators scaled on a 0 to 100-mm visual analog scale (VAS). The VAS scores indicated the likelihood that the respective factors would be considered in reaching a decision.

Findings
High levels of family stress were found 1 month and 7 to 8 months after the death, although stress levels at 7 to 8 months were lower. Patient/family characteristics that were associated with increased stress included the absence of advance directives (ADs), being an ethnic minority, and having a longer commuting distance to the hospital during the decedent's hospitalization. Families were more likely than clinicians to prioritize life prolongation over quality of life, particularly in the absence of an AD. Family members described their participation in decision making about withdrawing life support as one of the most difficult things they had ever had to do.

Nursing Implications
It is important for health care providers to recognize the impact of participation in end-of-life decision making on family members and to support them at this time. The study underscores the importance of assisting families to identify patients' preferences for end-of-life care and the importance of ADs in easing the process for family members. Further research is needed to compare the effect of having a written AD to guide family members versus patients' informal conversations about treatment preferences on family stress levels.

As a member of the interdisciplinary team caring for the patient at the end of life, the nurse fills an important role in facilitating the team's understanding of the patient's values and preferences, the family dynamics concerning decision making, and the patient's and family's response to treatment and changing health status. Many dilemmas in patient care at the end of life are related to poor communication between team members and the patient and family and failure of team members to communicate effectively with each other. Regardless of the care setting, the nurse can ensure a proactive approach to the psychosocial care of the patient and family. Periodic, structured assessments provide an opportunity for all parties to consider their priorities and plan for an uncertain future. The nurse can assist the patient and family to clarify their values and preferences concerning end-of-life care by using a structured approach. Sufficient time must be devoted to each step, so that the patient and family have time to process new information, formulate questions, and consider their options. The nurse may need to plan several meetings to accomplish the four steps described in Table 17-1.

PROVIDING CULTURALLY SENSITIVE CARE AT THE END OF LIFE

Although death, grief, and mourning are universally accepted aspects of living, values, expectations, and practices during serious illness, as death approaches, and following death are culturally bound and expressed. Health care providers may share very similar values concerning end-of-life care and may find that they are inadequately prepared to assess for and implement care plans that support culturally diverse perspectives. Historical mistrust of the health care system and unequal access to even basic medical care may underlie the beliefs and attitudes among ethnically diverse populations (Crawley, Payne, Bolden et al., 2000; Phipps, True & Pomerantz, 2000). In addition, lack of education or knowledge concerning end-of-life care treatment options and language barriers influence decisions among many socioeconomically disadvantaged groups.

Much of the formal structure concerning health care decisions in the United States is rooted in the Western notions of autonomy, truth telling, and the acceptability of withdrawing or withholding life-prolonging medical treatment at the end of life. Yet in many cultures, interdependence is valued over autonomy, leading to decision and communication styles that favor relinquishment of decision making to family members or to a perceived authority figure, such as the physician (Blackhall et al., 1995; Ersek, Kagawa-Singer, Barnes et al., 1998). In addition, there is variation in preference regarding the use of life-prolonging medical treatments such as cardiopulmonary resuscitation and artificially provided nutrition and hydration at the end of life; some groups are less likely to agree with withholding or withdrawing such life support in terminal illness (Caralis, Davis, Wright et al., 1993).

The nurse's role is to assess the values, preferences, and practices of every patient, regardless of ethnicity, socioeconomic status, or background. The nurse can share knowledge about the patient's and family's cultural beliefs and practices with the health care team and facilitate the adaptation of the care plan to accommodate these practices. For example, the nurse may find that a patient prefers to have his eldest son make all of his care decisions. Institutional practices and laws governing informed consent are also rooted in the Western notion of autonomous decision making

Table 17-1 • Discussing End-of-Life Care

STEPS	ACTIONS
1. Initiate discussion	• Establish a supportive relationship with patient and family 　• State the purposes of the patient/family–health care team conference: 　　• To ensure that the plan of care is consistent with patient and family values and preferences 　　• To find out how best to support this patient and family 　• Inquire if the patient or family have questions or concerns that they want to express • Elicit values and preferences concerning: 　• Patient and family decision-making roles 　　• How have major decisions been made in the past? 　　• How have treatment/care decisions been made during the course of the illness? 　　• Has the patient appointed a surrogate? 　　　• Formal (Durable Power of Attorney) 　　　• Informal 　　• How does the patient/family want decisions to be structured from this point on? 　• Setting for receiving care at the end of life 　　• Home 　　• Home with hospice care 　　• Assisted living or long-term care with/without hospice 　　• Disposition when unable to care for self independently (plan for how and where the patient prefers to receive care when he/she can no longer live independently) 　• Family involvement in care provision
2. Clarify understanding of the medical treatment plan and prognosis	• Identify what the patient and family understand • Identify gaps in knowledge, need for consultation with other members of the health care team • Use simple, everyday language
3. Identify end-of-life priorities	• Facilitate open discussion about priorities 　• "What is most important to you now?" 　• "How can (I/we) best help you to meet your goals?" • Allow sufficient time for emotional response
4. Contribute to the interdisciplinary care plan	• Provide guidance and/or referral for understanding medical options • Make recommendations for referrals to other disciplines or services (eg, spiritual care, support groups, community resources) • Identify need for patient/family teaching • Develop a plan for follow-up: 　• Schedule (frequency, time, place) 　• Participants 　• Tasks/assignments 　• Communication that needs to occur before the next meeting • Family member responsible for coordination

Adapted with permission from Balaban, R. B. (2000). A physician's guide to talking about end-of-life care. *Journal of General Internal Medicine, 15(3)*, 195–200. Oxford: Blackwell Science Ltd.

and informed consent. If a patient who wishes to defer decisions to his son, the nurse can work with the team to negotiate informed consent, respecting the patient's right not to participate in decision making and honoring his family's cultural practices (Ersek et al., 1998).

The nurse should assess and document the patient's and family's specific beliefs, preferences, and practices regarding end-of-life care, preparation for death, and after-death rituals. Chart 17-4 identifies topics that the nurse should cover and questions that the nurse may use to elicit the information. The nurse must use judgment and discretion about the timing and setting for eliciting this information. Some patients may wish to have a family member speak for them or because of advanced illness may be unable to provide information. The nurse should give the patient and family a context for the discussion, such as "It is very important to us to provide care that addresses your needs and the needs of your family. We want to honor and support your wishes, and want you to feel free to tell us how we are doing, and what we could do to better meet your needs. I'd like to ask you some questions; what you tell me will help me to understand and support what is most important to you at this time. You don't need to answer anything that makes you uncomfortable. Is it all right to ask some questions?" The assessment of end-of-life beliefs, preferences, and practices will probably need to be carried out in short segments over a period of time (for example, across multiple days of an inpatient hospital stay or in conjunction with multiple patient visits to an outpatient setting). The novice nurse's discomfort with asking questions and discussing this type of sensitive content can be reduced by prior practice in a classroom or clinical skills laboratory, observation of interviews conducted by experienced nurses, and partnering with an experienced nurse during the first few assessments.

Chart 17-4 • ASSESSMENT

Nursing Assessment of End-of-Life Care Beliefs, Preferences, and Practices

- *Disclosure/truth telling:* "Tell me how you/your family talk about very sensitive or serious matters."
  - Content: "Are there any topics that you or your family are uncomfortable discussing?"
  - Person responsible for disclosure: "Is there one person in the family who assumes responsibility for obtaining and sharing information?"
  - Disclosure practices regarding children: "What kind of information may be shared with children in your family, and who is responsible for communicating with the children?"
  - Sharing of information within the family or community group: "What kind/how much information should be shared with your immediate family? Your extended family? Others in the community (for example, members of a religious community)?"
- *Decision-making style:* "How are decisions made in your family? Who would you like to be involved in decisions about your treatment or care?"
  - Individual
  - Family-centered
  - Family elder or patriarch/matriarch
  - Deference to authority (such as the physician)
- *Symptom management:* "How would you like us to help you to manage the physical effects of your illness?"
  - Acceptability of medications used for symptom relief
  - Beliefs regarding expression of pain and other symptoms
  - Degree of symptom management desired
- *Life-sustaining treatment expectations:* "Have you thought about what type of medical treatment you/your loved one want(s) as the

end of life is nearing? Do you have an advanced directive (living will and/or durable power of attorney)?"
  - Nutrition/hydration at the end of life
  - Cardiopulmonary resuscitation
  - Ventilator
  - Dialysis
  - Antibiotics
  - Medications to treat infection
- *Desired location of dying:* "Do you have a preference about being at home or in some other location when you die?"
  - Desired role for family members in providing care: "Who do you want to be involved in caring for you at the end of life?"
  - Gender-specific prohibitions: "Are you uncomfortable having either males or females provide your care or your loved one's personal care?"
- *Spiritual/religious practices and rituals:* "Is there anything that we should know about your spiritual or religious beliefs about death? Are there any practices that you would like us to observe as death is nearing?"
- *Care of the body after the death:* "Is there anything that we should know about how a body/your body should be treated after death?"
- *Expression of grief:* "What types of losses have you and your family experienced? How do you and your family express grief?"
- *Funeral and burial practices:* "Are there any rituals or practices associated with funerals or burial that are especially important to you?"
- *Mourning practices:* "How have you and your family carried on after a loss in the past? Are their particular behaviors or practices that are expected or required?"

GOAL SETTING IN PALLIATIVE CARE AT THE END OF LIFE

As the treatment goals begin to shift in the direction of comfort care over aggressive disease-focused treatment, symptom relief and patient/family-defined quality of life assume greater prominence in treatment decision making. Patient, family, and clinicians may all be accustomed to an almost automatic tendency to pursue exhaustive diagnostic testing to locate and treat the source of the patient's illness or symptoms. Each decision to withdraw treatment or discontinue diagnostic testing will be an extremely emotional one for the patient and family. They may fear that the support from health care providers on which they have come to rely will be withdrawn along with the treatment.

Throughout the course of the illness, and especially as the patient's functional status and symptoms indicate approaching death, clinicians need to assist the patient and family to weigh the benefits of continued diagnostic testing and disease-focused medical treatment against the burdens of those activities. Patients and their families may be extremely reluctant to forego monitoring that has become routine throughout the illness (such as blood testing, x-rays) but that may contribute little to a primary focus on comfort. Likewise, health care providers from other disciplines may have difficulty discontinuing such diagnostic testing or medical treatment. The nurse should collaborate with other members of the interdisciplinary team to share assessment findings and develop a coordinated plan of care (Fig. 17-1). In addition, the nurse may assist the patient and family to clarify their goals, expected outcomes, and values as they consider treatment options

(Chart 17-5). The nurse needs to work with interdisciplinary colleagues to ensure that the patient and family are referred for continuing psychosocial support, symptom management, and assistance with other care-related challenges (eg, arranging for home care or hospice support, referrals for financial assistance).

SPIRITUAL CARE

Attention to the spiritual component of the patient's and family's illness experience is not new within the context of nursing care, yet many nurses lack the comfort or skills to assess and intervene in this dimension. **Spirituality** contains features of religiosity, but the two concepts are not interchangeable (Highfield, 2000). Spirituality involves the "search for meaning and purpose in life and relatedness to a transcendent dimension" (Hermann, 2001, p. 67). For most people, contemplating their own deaths raises many issues, such as the meaning of existence, the purpose of suffering, and the existence of an afterlife. In a national survey on spiritual beliefs and the dying process conducted by Gallup for the Nathan Cummings Foundation and Fetzer Institute in 1996 and published in 1997, respondents' greatest worries about death included the following:

- The medical matter of greatest worry was the possibility of being vegetable-like for some period of time (73%).
- The emotional matter of greatest worry was not having the chance to say goodbye to someone (73%) or the possibility of having great physical pain before death (67%).
- The practical matter of greatest worry was how family or loved ones will be cared for (65%) or thinking that death

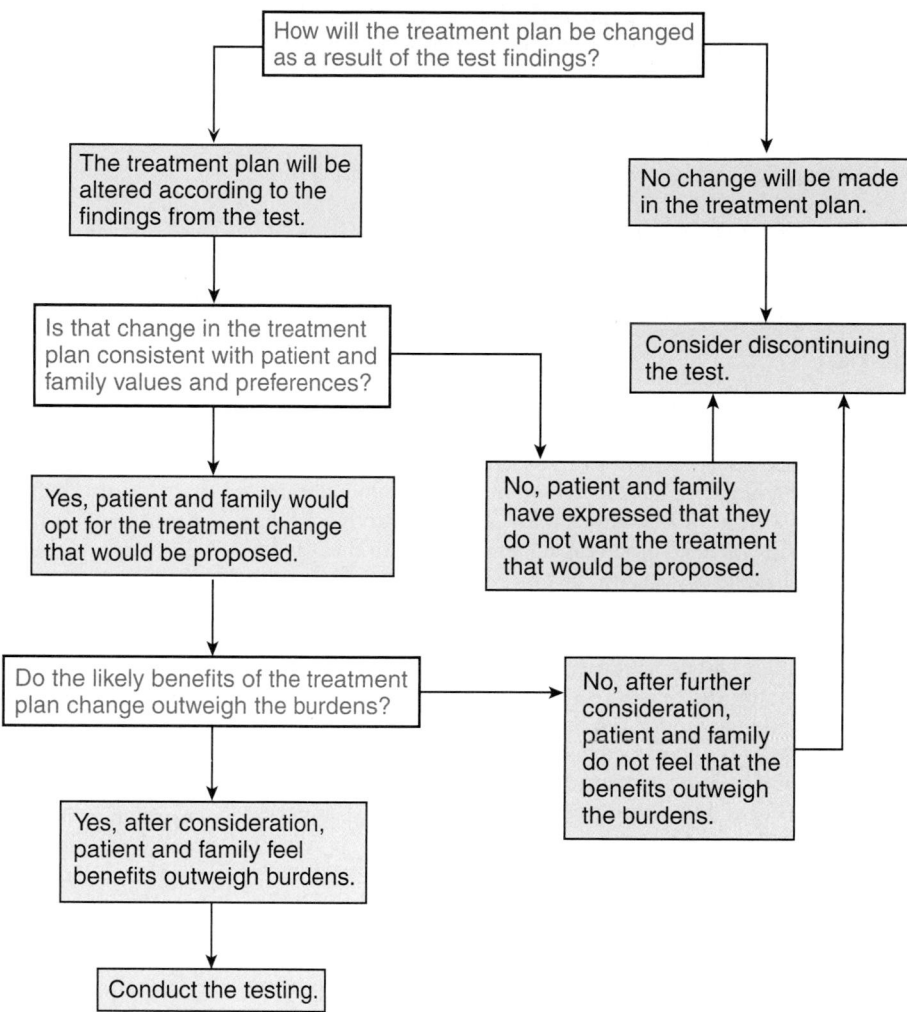

FIGURE 17-1 An algorithm for decision making about diagnostic testing at the end of life.

will be a cause of inconvenience and stress for those who love them (64%).

- The spiritual matter of greatest worry was not being forgiven by God (56%) or dying when removed or cut off from God or a higher power (51%).

The spiritual assessment is a key component of comprehensive nursing assessment for terminally ill patients and their families. Although the nursing assessment should include religious affiliation, spiritual assessment is conceptually much broader than religion and thus is relevant regardless of the patient's expression of religious preference or affiliation. In addition to assessment of the role of religious faith and practices, important religious rituals, and connection to a religious community, the nurse should further explore:

- The harmony or discord between the patient's and family's beliefs
- Other sources of meaning, hope, and comfort
- The presence or absence of a sense of peace of mind and purpose in life
- Spiritually or religiously based beliefs about illness, medical treatment, care of the sick

---

Chart 17-5 • ASSESSMENT

Nursing Assessment of the Patient and Family Perspective: Goal Setting in Palliative Care

- Patient and family
  - Awareness of diagnosis, illness stage, and prognosis
    - "Tell me your understanding of your illness right now."
  - Values
    - "Tell me what is most important to you as you are thinking about the treatment options available to you/your loved one."
  - Preferences
    - "You've said that being comfortable and pain-free is most important to you right now. Where would you like to receive

care (home, hospital, long-term care facility, doctor's office), and how can I help?"
- Expected/desired outcomes
  - "What are your hopes and expectations for this (diagnostic test [eg, CT scan] or treatment)?"
- Benefits and burdens
  - "Is there a point at which you would say that the testing or treatment is outweighed by the burdens it is causing you (eg, getting from home to the hospital, pain, nausea, fatigue, interference with other important activities)?"

Maugans (1996) created the useful mnemonic "SPIRIT" to assist health care professionals to include spiritual assessment in their practice:

- *S*piritual belief system
- *P*ersonal spirituality
- *I*ntegration and involvement with others in a spiritual community
- *R*itualized practices and restrictions
- *I*mplications for medical care
- *T*erminal events planning

HOPE

Kübler-Ross maintained that hope persisted across every stage of terminal illness, noting that "even the most accepting, the most realistic patients left the possibility open for some cure, for the discovery of a new drug, or the 'last-minute success in a research project' " (1969, p. 139). Viktor Frankl (1984), a survivor of the Holocaust, described a human capacity for optimism that can be maintained in spite of the possibility or even certainty of pain and death. In terminal illness, hope represents patients' imagined future, forming the basis of a positive, accepting attitude and providing their lives with meaning, direction and optimism (Hickey, 1986). When hope is viewed this way, it is not limited to cure of the disease, and instead focuses on what is achievable in the time remaining. Many patients find hope in working on important relationships and creating legacies. The terminally ill patient can be extremely resilient, reconceptualizing hope repeatedly as he or she approaches the end of life.

The concept of hope has been delineated and studied by numerous nurse researchers, and its presence has been related to concepts such as spirituality, quality of life, and transcendence. Morse and Doberneck (1995) defined hope as a multidimensional construct that provides comfort to the individual as he or she endures life threats and personal challenges. These authors identified seven universal components of hope from their study of patients who had survived serious illness:

- Realistic initial assessment of the threat
- Envisioning alternatives and setting goals
- Bracing for negative outcomes
- Realistic assessment of resources
- Solicitation of mutually supportive relationships
- Continuous evaluation for signs reinforcing the goals
- Determination to endure

The nurse can support the patient and family by using effective listening and communication skills and encouraging realistic hope that is specific to the patient's and family's needs for information, expectations for the future, and values and preferences concerning the end of life. It is important for the nurse to engage in self-reflection and identify her or his own biases and fears concerning illness, life, and death. As nurses become more skilled in working with seriously ill patients, they can become less determined to "fix" and more willing to listen, more comfortable with silence, grief, anger, and sadness, and more fully present with patients and their families.

Nursing interventions for enabling and supporting hope include:

- Listening attentively
- Encouraging sharing of feelings
- Providing accurate information
- Encouraging and supporting patient control over his or her circumstances, choices, and environment whenever possible
- Assisting the patient to explore ways for finding meaning in his or her life
- Encouraging realistic goals
- Facilitating effective communication within the family
- Making referrals for psychosocial and spiritual counseling
- Assisting with the development of supports in the home or community when none exist

MANAGING PHYSIOLOGIC RESPONSES TO ILLNESS

Patients approaching the end of life experience many of the same symptoms, regardless of their underlying disease processes. Symptoms in terminal illness may be caused by the disease, either directly (eg, dyspnea due to chronic obstructive lung disease) or indirectly (eg, nausea and vomiting related to pressure in the gastric area), by the treatment for the disease, or by a coexisting disorder that is unrelated to the disease. Chapter 13 presents assessment principles for pain that include identifying the effect of the pain on the patient's life, the importance of believing the patient's report of the pain and its effect, and the importance of systematic assessment of pain. Similarly, symptoms such as dyspnea, nausea, weakness, and anxiety should be as carefully and systematically assessed and managed. Questions that guide the assessment of symptoms are listed in Chart 17-6.

The goals of symptom management at the end of life are to completely relieve the symptom when possible, or to decrease the symptom to a level that the patient can tolerate when it cannot be completely relieved. Medical interventions may be aimed at treating the underlying causes of the symptoms. Pharmacologic and nonpharmacologic methods for symptom management may be used in combination with medical interventions to modify the physiologic causes of symptoms. For example, some patients who develop pleural effusion secondary to metastatic cancer may experience temporary relief of the associated dyspnea following thoracentesis, an invasive medical procedure in which fluid is drained from the pleural space. In addition, pharmacologic management with low-dose oral morphine is very effective in relieving dyspnea, and guided relaxation may reduce the anxiety associated with the sensation of breathlessness. As with pain, the principles

Chart 17-6 • ASSESSMENT

Nursing Assessment of Symptoms Associated With Terminal Illness

- How is this symptom affecting the patient's life?
- What is the meaning of the symptom to the patient? To the family?
- How does the symptom affect physical functioning, mobility, comfort, sleep, nutritional status, elimination, activity level, and relationships with others?
- What makes the symptom better?
- What makes it worse?
- Is it worse at any particular time of the day?
- What are the patient's expectations and goals for managing the symptom? The family's?
- How is the patient coping with the symptom?
- What is the economic effect of the symptom and its management?

Adapted from Jacox, A., Carr, D. B., & Payne, R. (1994). *Management of cancer pain*. Rockville, MD: AHCPR.

of pharmacologic symptom management are the smallest dose of the medication to achieve the desired effect, avoidance of polypharmacy, anticipation and management of medication side effects, and creation of a therapeutic regimen that is acceptable to the patient based on his or her goals for maximizing quality of life.

As with pain management, patients may elect to tolerate higher symptom levels in exchange for greater independence, mobility, alertness, or other priorities. Anticipating and planning interventions for symptoms that have not yet occurred is a cornerstone of end-of-life care. Both patients and family members cope more effectively with new symptoms and exacerbations of existing symptoms when they know what to expect and how to manage it. Hospice programs typically provide "emergency kits" containing ready-to-administer doses of a variety of medications that are useful to treat symptoms in advanced illness. Family members can be instructed to administer a prescribed dose from the emergency kit, often avoiding prolonged suffering for the patient as well as rehospitalization for symptom management.

Pain

Pain and suffering are among the most feared consequences of cancer (Roth & Breitbart, 1996). Pain is a significant symptom for many cancer patients throughout their treatment and disease course; it results both from the disease and the modalities used to treat it. Numerous studies have indicated that patients with advanced illness, particularly cancer, experience considerable pain (Field & Cassel, 1997; Jacox, Carr, & Payne, 1994). While the means to relieve pain have existed for many years, the continued, pervasive undertreatment of pain has been well documented (American Pain Society, 1999; Jacox et al., 1994). It is estimated that as many of 70% of patients with advanced cancer experience severe pain (Jacox et al., 1994; World Health Organization, 1990). The impact of poorly managed pain on patients' psychological, emotional, social, and financial well-being has attracted considerable research interest, but practice has been slow to change (Spross, 1992).

Patients who have an established regimen of analgesics should continue to receive those medications as they approach the end of life. Inability to communicate pain should not be equated with the absence of pain. While most pain can be managed effectively using the oral route, as the end of life nears patients may be less able to swallow oral medications due to somnolence or nausea. Patients who have been receiving opioids should continue to receive equianalgesic doses via the rectal or sublingual routes. Concentrated morphine solution can be very effectively delivered by the sublingual route, as the small liquid volume is well tolerated even when the patient cannot swallow. As long as the patient continues to receive opioids, a regimen to combat constipation must be implemented. If the patient cannot swallow laxatives or stool softeners, rectal suppositories or enemas may be necessary.

The nurse should teach the family about continuation of comfort measures as the patient approaches the end of life, how to administer analgesics via alternate routes, and how to assess for pain when the patient cannot verbally report pain intensity. Because the analgesics administered orally or rectally are short-acting, typically scheduled as frequently as every 3 to 4 hours around the clock, there is always a strong possibility that the patient approaching the end of life will die in close proximity to the time of analgesic administration. If the patient is at home, family members administering analgesics need to be prepared for this possibility. They will need reassurance that they did not "cause" the death of the patient by administering a dose of analgesic medication (see Chart 13-3).

Dyspnea

Dyspnea is an uncomfortable awareness of breathing that is common in patients approaching the end of life (Brant, 1998). Dyspnea is a highly subjective symptom that often is not associated with visible signs of distress, such as tachypnea, diaphoresis, or cyanosis. Patients with primary lung tumors, lung metastases, pleural effusion, and restrictive lung disease may experience significant dyspnea. Although the underlying cause of the dyspnea can be identified and treated in some cases, the burdens of additional diagnostic evaluation and treatment aimed at the physiological problem may outweigh the benefits. The treatment of dyspnea varies depending on the patient's general physical condition and imminence of death. For example, a blood transfusion may provide temporary symptom relief for the anemic patient earlier in the disease process; however, as the patient approaches the end of life the benefits are typically short-lived or absent.

NURSING ASSESSMENT AND INTERVENTION

As is true in pain assessment and management, the patient's report of dyspnea must be believed. Also like the experience of physical pain, the meaning of the dyspnea to the patient may increase his or her suffering. For example, the patient may interpret increasing dyspnea as a sign that death is approaching. For some patients, sensations of breathlessness may invoke frightening images of drowning or suffocation, and the resulting cycle of fear and anxiety may create even greater sensations of breathlessness. Therefore, the nurse should conduct a careful assessment of the psychosocial and spiritual components of the symptom (see Chart 17-5). Physical assessment parameters include:

- Symptom intensity, distress, and interference with activities (scale of 0 to 10)
- Auscultation of lung sounds
- Assessment of fluid balance
- Measurement of dependent edema (circumference of lower extremities)
- Measurement of abdominal girth
- Temperature
- Skin color
- Sputum quantity and character
- Cough

To determine the intensity of the symptom and its interference with daily activities, patients can be asked to self-report using a scale of 0 to 10, where 0 is no dyspnea and 10 is the worst imaginable dyspnea. Measurement of the patient's baseline before treatment and subsequent measures during exacerbation of the symptom, periodically during treatment, and whenever the treatment plan changes will provide ongoing objective evidence for the efficacy of the treatment plan. In addition, physical assessment findings may assist in locating the source of the dyspnea and selecting nursing interventions to relieve the symptom. The components of the assessment will change as the patient's condition changes. For example, when the patient who has been on daily weights can no longer get out of bed, the goal of comfort may outweigh the benefit of continued weights. Like other symptoms at the end of life, dyspnea can be managed effectively in the absence of assessment and diagnostic data (ie, arterial blood gases) that are standard when the patient's illness or symptom is reversible.

Nursing management of dyspnea at the end of life is directed toward administering medical treatment for the underlying pathology, monitoring the patient's response to treatment, assisting the patient and family to manage anxiety (which exacerbates dyspnea), altering the perception of the symptom, and conserving energy (Chart 17-7). Pharmacologic intervention is aimed at modifying lung physiology and improving performance as well as altering the perception of the symptom. Bronchodilators and corticosteroids are examples of medications used to treat underlying obstructive pathology, thereby improving overall lung function. Low doses of opioids are very effective in relieving dyspnea, although the mechanism of relief is not entirely clear. Although dyspnea in terminal illness is typically not associated with diminished blood oxygen saturation, low-flow oxygen often provides psychological comfort to the patient and the family, particularly in the home setting.

As discussed above, dyspnea may be exacerbated by anxiety, and anxiety may trigger episodes of dyspnea, setting off a respiratory crisis in which patient and family may panic. For patients receiving care at home, patient and family instruction should include anticipation and management of crisis situations and a clearly communicated emergency plan. Patients and families should be instructed about medication administration, condition changes that should be reported to the physician and nurse, and strategies for coping with diminished reserves and increasing symptomatology as the disease progresses. The patient and family need reassurance that the symptom can be effectively managed at home without the need for activation of the emergency medical services or hospitalization and that a nurse will be available at all times via telephone or to conduct a visit.

Nutrition and Hydration at the End of Life

ANOREXIA

Anorexia and cachexia are common problems in the seriously ill. The profound changes in the patient's appearance and his or her concomitant lack of interest in the socially important rituals of mealtime are particularly disturbing to families. The approach to the problem varies depending on the patient's stage of illness, level of disability associated with the illness, and desires. The anorexia-cachexia syndrome is characterized by disturbances in carbohydrate, protein, and fat metabolism, endocrine dysfunction, and anemia. The syndrome results in severe asthenia (loss of energy). Although causes of anorexia may be controlled for a period of time, progressive anorexia is an expected and natural part of the dying process. Anorexia may be related to or exacerbated by situational variables (eg, the ability to have meals with the family versus eating alone in the "sick room"), progression of the disease, treatment for the disease, or psychological distress. The patient and family should be instructed in strategies to manage the variables associated with anorexia. Table 17-2 summarizes nursing measures and patient and family teaching for managing anorexia.

USE OF PHARMACOLOGIC AGENTS TO STIMULATE APPETITE IN THE TERMINALLY ILL

A number of pharmacologic agents are commonly used to stimulate appetite in anorectic patients. Commonly used medications for appetite stimulation include dexamethasone (Decadron), cyproheptadine (Periactin), megestrol acetate (Megace), and dronabinol (Marinol). Dexamethasone initially increases appetite and may provide short-term weight gain in some patients. However, therapy may need to be discontinued in the patient with a longer life expectancy, as after 3 to 4 weeks corticosteroids interfere with the synthesis of muscle protein. Cyproheptadine may be used when corticosteroids are contraindicated, such as when the patient is diabetic. It promotes mild appetite increase but no appreciable weight gain. Megestrol acetate produces temporary weight gain of primarily fatty tissue, with little effect on protein balance. Because of the time required to see any effect from this agent, therapy should not be initiated if life expectancy is less than 30 days. Finally, dronabinol is a psychoactive compound found in cannabis that may be helpful in reducing nausea and vomiting, appetite loss, pain, and anxiety, thereby improving intake in some patients. However, dronabinol is not as effective as the other agents for appetite stimulation in most patients. Although the use of these agents may cause temporary weight gain, their use is not associated with an increase in lean body mass in the terminally ill. Therapy should be tapered or discontinued after 4 to 8 weeks if there is no response (Wrede-Seaman, 1999).

CACHEXIA

Cachexia refers to severe muscle wasting and weight loss associated with illness. Although anorexia may exacerbate cachexia, it is not the primary cause. Cachexia is associated with changes in metabolism that include hypertriglyceridemia, lipolysis, and accelerated protein turnover, leading to depletion of fat and protein stores (Plata-Salaman, 1997). However, the pathophysiology of cachexia in terminal illness is not well understood. In terminal illness, the severity of tissue wasting is greater than would be expected from reduced food intake alone, and typically increasing appetite or food intake does not reverse cachexia in the terminally ill.

Anorexia and cachexia differ from starvation (simple food deprivation) in several important ways. Appetite is lost early in the process, the body becomes catabolic in a dysfunctional way, and supplementation by gastric feeding (tube feeding) or parenteral nutrition in advanced disease does not replenish lost lean body mass. At one time it was believed that cancer patients with rapidly growing tumors developed cachexia because the

---

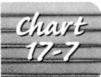

Chart 17-7 **Palliative Nursing Interventions for Dyspnea**

Decrease Anxiety
- Administer prescribed anxiolytic medications as indicated for anxiety or panic associated with dyspnea.
- Assist with relaxation techniques, guided imagery.
- Provide patient with a means to call for assistance (call bell/light within reach in a hospital or long-term care facility; hand-held bell or other device for home).

Treat Underlying Pathology
- Administer prescribed bronchodilators and corticosteroids (obstructive pathology).
- Administer blood products, erythropoietin as prescribed (typically not beneficial in advanced disease).
- Administer prescribed diuretics and monitor fluid balance.

Alter Perception of Breathlessness
- Administer prescribed oxygen therapy via nasal cannula, if tolerated; masks may not be well tolerated.
- Administer prescribed low-dose opioids via oral route (morphine sulfate is used most commonly).
- Provide air movement in the patient's environment with a portable fan.

Reduce Respiratory Demand
- Teach patient and family to implement energy conservation measures.
- Place needed equipment, supplies, and nourishment within reach.
- For home or hospice care, offer bedside commode, electric bed (with head that elevates).

Table 17-2 • Measures for Managing Anorexia

NURSING INTERVENTIONS	PATIENT AND FAMILY TEACHING TIPS
Initiate measures to ensure adequate dietary intake without adding stress to the patient at mealtimes.	Reduce the focus on "balanced" meals; offer the same food as often as the patient desires it.
Assess the impact of medications (eg, chemotherapy, antiretrovirals) or other therapies (radiation therapy, dialysis) that are being used to treat the underlying illness.	Increase the nutritional value of meals. For example, add dry milk powder to milk, and use this fortified milk to prepare cream soups, milkshakes, and gravies.
Administer and monitor effects of prescribed treatment for nausea, vomiting, and delayed gastric emptying.	
Encourage patient to eat when effects of medications have subsided.	Allow and encourage the patient to eat when hungry, regardless of usual meal times.
Assess and modify environment to eliminate unpleasant odors and other factors that cause nausea, vomiting, and anorexia.	Eliminate or reduce noxious cooking odors, pet odors, or other odors that may precipitate nausea, vomiting, or anorexia.
Remove items that may reduce appetite (soiled tissues, bedpans, emesis basins, clutter).	Keep patient's environment clean, uncluttered, and comfortable.
Assess and manage anxiety and depression to the extent possible.	Make mealtime a shared experience away from the "sick" room whenever possible.
	Reduce stress at mealtimes.
	Avoid confrontations about the amount of food consumed.
	Reduce or eliminate routine weighing of the patient.
Position to enhance gastric emptying.	Encourage patient to eat in a sitting position; elevate the head of the patient's bed.
	Plan meals (food selection and portion size) that the patient desires.
	Provide small frequent meals if they are easier for patient to eat.
Assess for constipation and/or intestinal obstruction.	Ensure that patient and family understand that prevention of constipation is essential, even when the patient's intake is minimal.
Prevent and manage constipation on an ongoing basis, even when the patient's intake is minimal.	Encourage adequate fluid intake, dietary fiber, and use of bowel program to prevent constipation.
Provide frequent mouth care, particularly following nourishment.	Assist the patient to rinse after every meal. Avoid mouthwashes that contain alcohol or glycerine, which dry mucous membranes.
Ensure that dentures fit properly.	Weight loss may cause dentures to loosen and cause irritation. Remove them to inspect the gums and to provide oral care.
Administer and monitor effects of topical and systemic treatment for oropharyngeal pain.	Patient's comfort may be enhanced if pain medications given on an as-needed basis for breakthrough pain are administered before mealtimes.

tumor created an excessive nutritional demand and diverted nutrients from the rest of the body. Recent research links cytokines produced by the body in response to a tumor to a complex inflammatory-immune response present in patients whose tumors have metastasized, leading to anorexia, weight loss, and altered metabolism. An increase in cytokines occurs not only in cancer but also in AIDS and many other chronic diseases (Plata-Salaman, 1997).

ARTIFICIAL NUTRITION AND HYDRATION IN TERMINAL ILLNESS

Along with breathing, eating and drinking are essential to survival throughout one's lifetime. As patients near the end of life, their bodies' nutritional needs change, their desire for food and fluid may diminish, and they may no longer be able to use, eliminate, or store nutrients and fluids adequately. Eating, feeding, and sharing meals are important social activities in families and communities, and food preparation and enjoyment are linked to happy memories, strong emotions, and hopes for survival. For the patient with serious illness, food preparation and mealtimes often become battlegrounds where well-meaning family members argue, plead, and cajole to encourage the ill person to eat. It is not unusual for seriously ill patients to lose their appetites entirely, to develop

strong aversions for foods they have enjoyed in the past, or to crave a particular food to the exclusion of all other foods.

Although nutritional supplementation may be an important part of the treatment plan in early or chronic illness, unintended weight loss and dehydration are expected sequelae of progressive illness. As illness progresses, patients, families, and clinicians may believe that without artificial nutrition and hydration, the terminally ill patient will "starve," causing profound suffering and hastened death. However, starvation should not be viewed as the failure to implant tubes for nutritional supplementation or hydration of terminally ill patients with irreversible progression of disease. Studies have demonstrated that terminally ill patients who were hydrated had neither improved biochemical parameters nor improved states of consciousness (Waller, Hershkowitz & Adunsky, 1994). Similarly, survival was not increased when terminally ill patients with advanced dementia received enteral feeding (Meier, Ahronheim, Morris et al., 2001). Further, in patients who are close to death there are beneficial effects to withholding or withdrawing artificial nutrition and hydration, such as decreased urine output and incontinence, decreased gastric fluids and emesis, decreased pulmonary secretions and respiratory distress, and decreased edema and pressure discomfort (Zerwekh, 1987).

As the patient approaches the end of life, families and health care providers should offer the patient what he or she desires and can most easily tolerate. Nurses should instruct the family how to separate feeding from caring by demonstrating love, sharing, and caring by being with the loved one in other ways. Preoccupation with appetite, feeding, and weight loss diverts energy and time that the patient and family could use in other meaningful activities. The following are tips to promote nutrition for the terminally ill patient:

- Offer small portions of favorite foods.
- Do not be overly concerned about a "balanced" diet.
- Cool foods may be better tolerated than hot foods.
- Offer cheese, eggs, peanut butter, mild fish, chicken, or turkey. Meat (especially beef) may taste bitter and unpleasant.
- Add milkshakes, "Instant Breakfast" drinks, or other liquid supplements.
- Add dry milk powder to milkshakes and cream soups to increase protein and calorie content.
- Place nutritious foods at the bedside (fruit juices, milkshakes in insulated drink containers with straws).
- Schedule meals when family members can be present to provide company and stimulation.
- Avoid arguments at mealtime.
- Assist the patient to maintain a schedule of oral care. Rinse the mouth after each meal or snack. Avoid mouthwashes that contain alcohol. Use a soft toothbrush. Treat ulcers or lesions. Make sure dentures fit well.
- Treat pain and other symptoms.
- Offer ice chips made from frozen fruit juices.
- Allow the patient to refuse foods and fluids.

Delirium

Many patients may remain alert, arousable, and able to communicate until very close to death. Others may sleep for long intervals and awaken only intermittently, with eventual somnolence until death. Delirium refers to concurrent disturbances in level of consciousness, psychomotor behavior, memory, thinking, attention, and sleep-wake cycle (Brant, 1998). In some patients, a period of agitated delirium may precede death, sometimes causing families to be hopeful that the suddenly active patient may be getting better. Confusion may be related to underlying, treatable conditions such as medication side effects or interactions, pain or discomfort, hypoxia or dyspnea, a full bladder or impacted stool. In patients with cancer, confusion may be secondary to brain metastases. Delirium may also be related to metabolic changes, infection, and organ failure.

The patient with delirium may become hypoactive or hyperactive, restless, irritable, and fearful. Sleep deprivation and hallucinations may occur. If treatment of the underlying factors contributing to these symptoms bring no relief, a combination of pharmacologic intervention with neuroleptics or benzodiazepines may be effective in decreasing distressing symptoms. Haloperidol (Haldol) may reduce hallucinations and agitation. Benzodiazepines (eg, lorazepam [Ativan]) can reduce anxiety but will not clear the sensorium and may contribute to worsening cognitive impairment if used alone.

Nursing interventions are aimed at identifying the underlying causes of delirium, acknowledging the family's distress over its occurrence, reassuring them about what is normal, teaching the family how to interact with and ensure safety for the patient with delirium, and monitoring the effects of medications used to treat severe agitation, paranoia, or fear. Confusion may mask the patient's unmet spiritual needs and fears about dying. Spiritual intervention, music therapy, gentle massage, and therapeutic touch may provide some relief. Reducing environmental stimuli, avoiding harsh lighting or very dim lighting (which may produce disturbing shadows), the presence of familiar faces, and gentle reorientation and reassurance are also helpful.

Depression

Clinical depression should not be accepted as an inevitable consequence of dying, nor should it be confused with sadness and anticipatory grieving, which are normal reactions to the losses associated with impending death. Emotional and spiritual support and control of disturbing physical symptoms are appropriate interventions for situational depression associated with terminal illness. The psychological sequelae of cancer pain have been linked to suicidal thought and less frequently to carrying out a planned suicide (Ripamonti, Filiberti, Totis et al., 1999). Cancer patients with advanced disease are especially vulnerable to delirium, depression, suicidal ideation, and severe anxiety (Roth & Breitbart, 1996). Higher levels of debilitation predict higher levels of pain and depressive symptoms, and the presence of pain doubles the likelihood of developing major psychiatric complications of illness (Roth & Breitbart, 1996). Patients and their families must be given space and time to experience sadness and to grieve, but patients should not have to endure untreated depression at the end of their lives. An effective combined approach to clinical depression includes relief of physical symptoms, attention to emotional and spiritual distress, and pharmacologic intervention with psychostimulants, selective serotonin reuptake inhibitors (SSRIs), and tricyclic antidepressants (Block, 2000).

PALLIATIVE SEDATION AT THE END OF LIFE

Effective control of symptoms can be achieved under most conditions, but some patients may experience distressing, intractable symptoms. Although its use remains controversial, **palliative sedation** is offered in some settings to patients who are close to death, who have symptoms that do not respond to conventional pharmacologic and nonpharmacologic approaches, and as a result are experiencing unrelieved suffering. Palliative sedation is distinguished from **euthanasia** or physician-assisted suicide in that the intent of palliative sedation is to palliate the symptoms, not to hasten the patient's death. Palliative sedation is most commonly used when the patient exhibits intractable pain, dyspnea, seizures, or delirium. It is generally considered appropriate in only the most difficult cases. Before implementing palliative sedation, the care team should assess for the presence of underlying and treatable causes of suffering, such as depression or spiritual pain. Finally, patients and families should be fully informed about the use of this treatment and alternatives.

Palliative sedation is accomplished through infusion of a benzodiazepine or barbiturate in doses adequate to induce sleep and eliminate signs of discomfort (Quill & Byock, 2000). The nurse acts as a collaborating member of the interdisciplinary team, providing emotional support to the patient and family, facilitating clarification of values and preferences, and providing comfort-focused physical care. Once sedation has been induced, the nurse will need to continue comfort care, monitor the physiologic effects of the sedation, support the family during the final hours or days of the patient's life, and ensure communication within the care team and between the team and family.

Nursing Care of the Patient Who Is Close to Death

Providing care to the patient who is close to death and being present at the time of death can be one of the most rewarding experiences a nurse can have. Patients and their families are understandably fearful of the unknown, and the approach of death may prompt new concerns or cause previous fears or issues to resurface. It has often been said that as we age and as we approach death, we do not become different people, just more like ourselves. Families that have always had difficulty communicating or in which there are old resentments and hurts may experience heightened difficulty as their loved one nears death. In contrast, the time at the end of life can also afford the family the opportunity to resolve old hurts and learn new ways of being a family. Regardless of the setting, dying patients can be made comfortable, space can be made for their loved ones to remain present when they wish, and the opportunity to experience growth and healing can be facilitated by skilled practitioners. Likewise, regardless of setting, patients' and families' apprehension surrounding the time of death may be diminished if they know what to expect as death nears and how to respond.

EXPECTED PHYSIOLOGIC CHANGES WHEN THE PATIENT IS CLOSE TO DEATH

Observable, expected changes in the body take place as the patient approaches death and organ systems begin to fail. Nursing care measures aimed at patient comfort should be continued: pain medications (administered rectally or sublingually), turning, mouth care, eye care, positioning to facilitate draining of secretions, and measures to protect the skin from incontinence should be continued. The nurse should consult with the physician about discontinuing measures that no longer contribute to patient comfort such as drawing blood, administering tube feedings, suctioning (in most cases), and invasive monitoring. The nurse should prepare the family for the normal, expected changes that accompany the period immediately preceding death. Although the exact time of death cannot be predicted, it is often possible to identify when a patient is very close to death. Hospice programs frequently provide written information for families so they know what to expect and what to do as death nears (Chart 17-8).

If they have been prepared for the time of death, families are less likely to panic and will be better able to be with their loved one in a meaningful way. Noisy, gurgling breathing or moaning is generally most distressing to the family. In most cases, the sounds of breathing at the end of life are related to oropharyngeal relaxation and diminished awareness. Family members may have difficulty believing that the patient is not in pain or that his or her breathing could not be improved by suctioning secretions. Patient positioning and family reassurance are the most helpful responses to these symptoms.

Terminal "Bubbling"

When death is imminent, the patient may become increasingly somnolent and unable to clear sputum or oral secretions, which may lead to further impairment of breathing from pooled and/or dried and crusted secretions. The sound and appearance of the secretions are often more distressing to the family than is the presence of the secretions to the patient. Family distress over the changes in patient condition may be eased by supportive nursing care. Continuation of comfort-focused interventions and reassurance that the patient is not in any distress can do much to ease family concerns. Gentle mouth care with a moistened swab or very soft toothbrush will help to maintain the integrity of the patient's mucous membranes. In addition, gentle oral suctioning, positioning to enhance drainage of secretions, and sublingual or transdermal administration of anticholinergic drugs (Table 17-3) to reduce the production of secretions will provide comfort to the patient and support to the family. Deeper suctioning may cause significant discomfort to the dying patient and is rarely of any benefit, as secretions will reaccumulate rapidly.

THE DEATH VIGIL

Although every death is unique, it is often possible for the experienced clinician to assess that the patient is "actively" or imminently dying and to prepare the family in the final days or hours leading to death. As death nears, the patient may withdraw, sleep for longer intervals, or become somnolent. The family should be encouraged to be with the patient, to speak and reassure him or her of their presence, to stroke or touch him or her, or to lie alongside him or her (even in the hospital or long-term care facility) if they are comfortable with this degree of closeness and can do so without causing discomfort to the patient.

Family members may have gone to great lengths to ensure that their loved one will not die alone. However, despite the best intentions and efforts of families and clinicians, the patient's death may occur at a time when no one is present. In any setting, it is unrealistic for family members to be at the patient's bedside 24 hours a day, and it is not unusual for patients to die when the family has stepped away from the bedside just briefly. Experienced hospice clinicians have observed and reported that some patients appear to "wait" until family members are away from the bedside to die, perhaps to spare their loved ones the pain of being present at the time of death. The nurse can reassure family members throughout the death vigil by being present intermittently or continuously, modeling behaviors (such as touching and speaking to the patient), providing encouragement in relation to family caregiving, providing reassurance about normal physiologic changes, and encouraging family rest breaks. When the patient dies while the family is away from the bedside, the family may express feelings of guilt and profound grief and will need emotional support.

AFTER-DEATH CARE

The time of death is generally preceded by a period of gradual diminishment of bodily functions in which increasing intervals between respirations, a weakened and irregular pulse, diminishing blood pressure, and skin color changes or mottling may be observed. For the patient who has received adequate management of symptoms and for the family who has received adequate preparation and support, the actual time of death is commonly peaceful and occurs without struggle. The nurse may or may not be present at the time of the patient's death. In many states, the certifying physician may authorize the nurse to make the pronouncement of death and sign the death certificate. The determination of death is made through a physical examination that includes auscultation for the absence of breathing and heart sounds. Home care or hospice programs in which the nurse makes the time-of-death visit and pronouncement of death will have policies and procedures to guide the nurse's actions during this visit. Immediately upon cessation of vital functions the body will begin

Chart 17-8 Signs of Approaching Death

The person will show less interest in eating and drinking. For many patients, refusal of food is an indication that they are ready to die. Fluid intake may be limited to that which will keep their mouths from feeling too dry.

- What you can do: Offer, but do not force, fluids and medication. Sometimes, pain or other symptoms that have required medication in the past may no longer be present. For most patients, pain medications will still be needed, and can be provided by concentrated oral solutions placed under the tongue or by rectal suppository.

Urinary output may decrease in amount and frequency.

- What you can do: No response is needed unless the patient expresses a desire to urinate and cannot. Call the hospice nurse for advice if you are not sure.

As the body weakens, the patient will sleep more and begin to detach from the environment. He or she may refuse your attempts to provide comfort.

- What you can do: Allow your loved one to sleep. You may wish to sit with him or her, play soft music, or hold hands. Your loved one's withdrawal is normal and is not a rejection of your love.

Mental confusion may become apparent, as less oxygen is available to supply the brain. The patient may report strange dreams or visions.

- What you can do: As he or she awakens from sleep, remind him or her of the day and time, where he or she is, and who is present. This is best done in a casual, conversational way.

Vision and hearing may become somewhat impaired and speech may be difficult to understand.

- What you can do: Speak clearly but no more loudly than necessary. Keep the room as light as the patient wishes, even at night. Carry on all conversations as if they can be heard, since hearing may be the last of the senses to cease functioning. Many patients are able to talk until minutes before death and are reassured by the exchange of a few words with a loved one.

Secretions may collect in the back of the throat and rattle or gurgle as the patient breathes though the mouth. He or she may try to cough, and his or her mouth may become dry and encrusted with secretions.

- What you can do: if the patient is trying to cough up secretions and is experiencing choking or vomiting, call the hospice nurse for assistance.
Secretions may drain from the mouth if you place the patient on his/her side and provide support with pillows.

Cleansing the mouth with moistened mouth swabs will help to relieve the dryness that occurs with mouth breathing.
Offer water in small amounts to keep the mouth moist. A straw with one finger placed over the end can be used to transfer sips of water to the patient's mouth.

Breathing may become irregular with periods of no breathing (apnea). The patient may be working very hard to breathe and may make a moaning sound with each breath. As the time of death nears, the breathing remains irregular and may become more shallow and mechanical.

- What you can do: Raising the head of the bed may help the patient to breathe more easily. The moaning sound does not mean that the patient is in pain or other distress; it is the sound of air passing over very relaxed vocal cords.

As the oxygen supply to the brain decreases, the patient may become restless. It is not unusual to pull at the bed linens, to have visual hallucinations, or even to try to get out of bed at this point.

- What you can do: Reassure the patient in a calm voice that you are there. Prevent him/her from falling by trying to get out of bed. Soft music or a back rub may be soothing.

The patient may feel hot one moment and cold the next as the body loses its ability to control the temperature. As circulation slows, the arms and legs may become cool and bluish. The underside of the body may darken. It may be difficult to feel a pulse at the wrist.

- What you can do: Provide and remove blankets as needed. Avoid using electric blankets, which may cause burns because the patient cannot tell you if he or she is too warm.
Sponge the patient's head with a cool cloth if this provides comfort.

Loss of bladder and bowel control may occur around the time of death.

- What you can do: Protect the mattress with waterproof padding and change the padding as needed to keep the patient comfortable.

As people approach death, many times they report seeing gardens, libraries, or family or friends who have died. They may ask you to pack their bags and find tickets or a passport. Sometimes they may become insistent and attempt to do these chores themselves. They may try getting out of bed (even if they have been confined to bed for a long time) so that they can "leave."

- What you can do: Reassure the patient that it is all right; he or she can "go" without getting out of bed. Stay close, share stories, and be present.

Used with permission from the Family Home Hospice of the Visiting Nurse Association of Greater Philadelphia.

---

to change. The body will become dusky or bluish, waxen-appearing, and cool, blood will darken and pool in dependent areas of the body (such as the back and sacrum if the body is in a supine position), and urine and stool may be evacuated.

Immediately following the death, the family should be allowed and encouraged to spend time with the deceased. Normal responses of family members at the time of death vary widely and range from quiet expressions of grief to overt expressions that include wailing and prostration. Families' desires for privacy during their time with the deceased should be honored. Family members may wish to independently manage or assist with care of the body after death. If the death occurs in a

Table 17-3 • Pharmacologic Management of Excess Oral/Respiratory Secretions When Death is Imminent

MEDICATION	DOSE
Atropine sulfate ophthalmic drops	1 or 2 drops 1% oral/sublingual tid prn or around the clock (ATC)
Glycopyrrolate (Robinul®)	1–2 mg oral/rectal/sublingual tid prn or ATC
Hyoscyamine (Levsin®)	0.125 mg oral/sublingual q 6 h prn or ATC
Scopolamine (Transderm Scop®)	1 patch q 3 days

Reprinted with permission from ExcelleRx, Inc. (2000). *Hospice Pharmacia Pharmaceutical Care ToolKit* (3rd Ed.). Philadelphia: Author.

long-term care facility, the nurse follows the facility's procedure for preparation of the body and transportation to the facility's morgue. However, the family's needs to remain with the deceased, to wait until other family members arrive before the body is moved, and to perform after-death rituals should be honored. When an expected death occurs in the home setting, the body is often transported directly to the funeral home by the funeral director.

GRIEF, MOURNING, AND BEREAVEMENT

A wide range of feelings and behaviors are normal, adaptive, and healthy reactions to the loss of a loved one. **Grief** refers to the personal feelings that accompany an anticipated or actual loss. **Mourning** reflects the individual, family, group, and cultural expressions of grief and associated behaviors. **Bereavement** refers to the period of time during which mourning takes place. Both grief reactions and mourning behaviors change over time as the individual learns to live with the loss. Although the pain of the loss may be tempered by the passage of time, recent conceptualizations of loss as an ongoing developmental process maintain that time does not heal the bereaved individual completely (Silverman, 2001); that is, the bereaved do not get over a loss entirely, nor do they return to who they were before the loss. Rather, they develop a new sense of who they are and where they fit in a world that has changed dramatically and permanently.

Anticipatory Grief and Mourning

Denial, sadness, anger, fear, and anxiety are normal grief reactions in the individual with life-threatening illness and those close to him or her. Kübler-Ross (1969) described five common emotional reactions to dying that are applicable to the experience of any loss (Table 17-4). Although useful in understanding the overall experience of the dying process, the stages that Kübler-Ross described have been misinterpreted as following a linear, expected trajectory. Not every patient or family member experiences every stage, many patients never reach a stage of acceptance, and patients and families fluctuate on a sometimes day-to-day basis in their emotional responses. Further, while impending loss stresses the patient, those who are close to him or her, and the functioning of the family unit, awareness of dying also provides a unique opportunity for family members to reminisce, resolve relationships, plan for the future, and say goodbye.

Individual and family coping with the anticipation of death is complicated by the varied and conflicting trajectories that grief and mourning may assume in the family. For example, while the patient may be experiencing sadness while contemplating role changes that have been brought about by the illness, the patient's spouse or partner may be expressing or holding in feelings of anger about the current changes in role and impending loss of the relationship; others in the family may be engaged in denial (eg, "Dad will get better; he just needs to eat more."), fear ("Who will take care of us?" or "Will I get sick too?"), or profound sadness

Table 17-4 • Kübler-Ross's Five Stages of Dying

STAGE	NURSING IMPLICATIONS
Denial: "This cannot be true." Feelings of isolation. May search for another health care professional who will give a more favorable opinion. May seek unproven therapies.	Denial can be an adaptive response, providing a buffer after bad news. It allows time to mobilize defenses, but can be maladaptive when it prevents the patient or family from seeking help and when denial behaviors cause more pain or distress than the illness or interfere with everyday functions. Nurses should assess the patient's and family's coping style, information needs, and understanding of the illness and treatment to establish a basis for empathetic listening, education, and emotional support. Rather than confronting the patient with information he or she is not ready to hear, the nurse can encourage him or her to share fears and concerns. Open-ended questions or statements such as "Tell me more about how you are coping with this new information about your illness" can provide a springboard for expression of concerns.
Anger: "Why me?" Feelings of rage, resentment or envy directed at God, health care professionals, family, others.	Anger can be very isolating, and loved ones or clinicians may withdraw. Nurses should allow the patient and family to express anger, treating them with understanding, respect, and knowledge that the root of the anger is grief over impending loss.
Bargaining: "I just want to see my grandchild's birth, then I'll be ready. . . ." Patient and/or family plead for more time to reach an important goal. Promises are sometimes made with God.	Terminally ill patients are sometimes able to outlive prognoses and achieve some future goal. Nurses should be patient, allow expression of feelings, and support realistic and positive hope.
Depression: "I just don't know how my kids are going to get along after I'm gone." Sadness, grief, mourning for impending losses.	Normal and adaptive response. Clinical depression should be assessed and treated when present. Nurses should encourage the patient and family to express their sadness fully. Insincere reassurance or encouragement of unrealistic hopes should be avoided.
Acceptance: "I've lived a good life, and I have no regrets." Patient and/or family are neither angry nor depressed.	The patient may withdraw as his or her circle of interest diminishes. The family may feel rejected by the patient. Nurses need to support the family's expression of emotions and encourage them to continue to be present for the patient.

and withdrawal. Although each of these behaviors is normal, tension may arise when one or more family members perceive that others are less caring, too emotional, or too detached.

The nurse needs to assess the characteristics of the family system and intervene in a manner that supports and enhances the cohesion of the family unit. Parameters for assessing the family facing life-threatening illness are identified in Chart 17-9. The nurse can patiently guide family members to talk about their feelings and understand them in the broader context of anticipatory grief and mourning. Acknowledging and expressing feelings, continuing to interact with the patient in meaningful ways, and planning for the time of death and bereavement are adaptive family behaviors. Professional support provided by grief counselors in the community, at a local hospital, in the long-term care facility, or associated with a hospice program can help both the patient and family to sort out and acknowledge feelings and make the end of life as meaningful as possible.

Grief and Mourning After Death

When a loved one dies, the family members enter a new phase of grief and mourning as they begin to accept the loss, feel the pain of permanent separation, and prepare to live a life without the deceased. Even if the loved one died after a long illness, preparatory grief experienced during the terminal illness will not preclude the

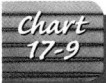

Assessing Anticipatory Mourning in the Family Facing Life-Threatening Illness

- Family constellation
  - Identify the members who constitute the patient's family.
    - Who is important to the patient?
  - Identify roles and relationships among the family members.
    - Who is the primary caregiver?
    - By what authority is this person the primary caregiver?
- Cohesion and boundaries
  - How autonomous/interdependent are family members?
    - Degree of involvement with each other as individuals and as a family
    - Degree of bonding between family members
    - Degree of "teamwork" in the family
    - Degree of reliance on individual family members for specific tasks/roles
  - How do family members differ in:
    - Personality?
    - World view?
    - Priorities?
  - What are the implicit and explicit expectations or "rules" for behavior within the family?
- Flexibility and adaptability
  - What is the family's ability to integrate new information?
  - How does the family manage change?
  - How able are the family members to assume new roles and responsibilities?
- Communication
  - What is the style of communication in the family, in terms of:
    - Openness?
    - Directness?
    - Clarity?
  - What are the constraints on communication?
  - What topics are avoided?

grief and mourning that follow the death. Following the patient's death after a long or difficult illness, family members may experience conflicting feelings of relief that the loved one's suffering has ended, compounded by guilt and grief related to unresolved issues or the circumstances of death. Grief work may be especially difficult if the patient's death was painful, prolonged, accompanied by unwanted interventions, or unattended. Families who had no preparation or support during the period of imminence and death may have a more difficult time finding a place for the painful memories.

Although some family members may experience prolonged or complicated mourning, most grief reactions fall within a "normal" range. The feelings are often profound, but the bereaved individual eventually reconciles the loss and finds a way to re-engage with his or her life. Grief and mourning are affected by individual characteristics, coping skills, and experiences with illness and death; the nature of the relationship to the deceased; factors surrounding the illness and the death; family dynamics; social support; and cultural expectations and norms. After-death rituals, including preparation of the body, funeral practices, and burial rituals, are socially and culturally significant ways that members of a family begin to accept the reality and finality of death. Preplanning of funerals is becoming increasingly common, and hospice professionals in particular assist families to make plans for death, often involving the patient who may wish to take an active planning role. Preplanning the funeral relieves the family of the decision burden in the intensely emotional period following a death. Uncomplicated grief and mourning are characterized by emotional feelings of sadness, anger, guilt, and numbness; physical sensations such as hollowness in the stomach and tightness in the chest, weakness, and lack of energy; cognitions that include preoccupation with the loss and a sense of the deceased as still present; and behaviors such as crying, visiting places that are reminders of the deceased, social withdrawal, and restless overactivity (Worden, 1991).

In general, the period of mourning is an adaptive response to loss during which the mourner comes to accept the loss as real and permanent, acknowledges and experiences the painful emotions that accompany the loss, experiences life without the deceased, overcomes impediments to adjustment, and finds a new way of living in a world without the loved one. Particularly immediately following the death, the mourner begins to recognize the reality and permanence of the loss by talking about the deceased and telling and retelling the story of the illness and death. Societal norms in the United States are frequently at odds with the normal grieving processes of individuals, where time excused from work obligations is typically measured in days and mourners are often expected to get over the loss quickly and get on with life.

In reality, the work of grief and mourning takes time, and avoiding grief work following the death often leads to long-term adjustment difficulties. According to Rando (2000), mourning for a loss involves the "undoing" of psychosocial ties that bind the mourner to the deceased, personal adaptation to the loss, and learning to live in the world without the deceased. Six key processes of mourning allow the individual to accommodate to the loss in a healthy way: recognition of the loss; reaction to the separation, experiencing and expressing the pain of the loss; recollection and re-experiencing the deceased, the relationship, and the associated feelings; relinquishing old attachments to the deceased; readjustment to adapt to the new world without forgetting the old; and reinvestment (Rando, 2000). Similarly, Worden (1991) described four tasks of mourning: acceptance of the reality of the loss, working through the pain of grief, adjusting to the environment in which the deceased is gone, and emotional "relocation" of the deceased in order to move on with life.

Although many individuals complete the work of mourning with the informal support of family and friends, many find that talking with others who have had a similar experience, such as in formal support groups, normalizes the feelings and experiences and provides a framework for learning new skills to cope with the loss and create a new life. Bereavement support groups are often sponsored by hospitals, hospices, and other community organizations. Groups for parents who have lost a child, children who have lost a parent, widows, widowers, and gay men and lesbians who have lost a life partner are some examples of specialized support groups available in many communities. Nursing interventions for those experiencing grief and mourning are identified in Chart 17-10.

Complicated Grief and Mourning

Complicated grief and mourning are characterized by prolonged feelings of sadness and feelings of general worthlessness or hopelessness that persist long after the death, prolonged symptoms that interfere with activities of daily living (anorexia, insomnia, fatigue, panic), or self-destructive behaviors such as alcohol or substance abuse and suicidal ideation or attempts. Complicated grief and mourning require professional assessment and can be treated with pharmacologic and psychological interventions.

Coping With Death and Dying: Professional Caregiver Issues

Whether practicing in the trauma center, intensive care unit or other acute care setting, home care, hospice, long-term care, or the many locations where patients and their families receive ambulatory services, nurses are closely involved with complex and emotionally laden issues surrounding loss of life. To be most effective and satisfied with the care they provide, nurses need to at-

tend to their own emotional responses to the losses they witness every day. Well before the nurse exhibits symptoms of stress or burnout, he or she should acknowledge the difficulty of coping with others' pain on a daily basis and put healthy practices in place that will guard against emotional exhaustion. In hospice settings, where death, grief, and loss are expected outcomes of patient care, interdisciplinary colleagues rely on each other for support, using meeting time to express frustration, sadness, anger, and other emotions; to learn coping skills from each other; and to speak about how they were affected by the lives of those patients who have died since the last meeting. In many settings, staff members organize or attend memorial services to support families and other caregivers, who find comfort in joining each other to remember and celebrate the lives of patients. Finally, healthy personal habits, including diet, exercise, stress reduction activities (such as dance, yoga, t'ai chi, meditation), and sleep, will help guard against the detrimental effects of stress.

Critical Thinking Exercises

1. Your patient, age 70, has metastatic prostate cancer and is receiving home hospice care. In the past, he has received transfusions of packed red blood cells to treat anemia associated with bone marrow involvement. He has received only temporary benefit from the transfusions. The patient's wife has asked that her husband's hemoglobin continue to be checked weekly because she is concerned about his increasing weakness and exertional dyspnea. The interdisciplinary team is meeting to discuss the patient's treatment plan. The team consensus is that he is unlikely to live more than a few days or weeks. What additional assessment data are needed to determine the wishes and expectations of the patient? Of the wife? What are the team's options for intervention? What are the pros and cons associated with each option?

2. You are conducting your first home care visit to an 88-year-old woman who has been hospitalized three times in the last 4 months with heart failure. She is short of breath, although she uses oxygen continuously. She is confined to bed and is incontinent and has a stage III pressure ulcer on her coccyx. She is not interested in eating and has lost 30 lb in the last 4 months. She is becoming progressively weaker. Her husband, also 88, has limited mobility due to arthritis. He has a history of colon cancer and has had a colostomy for the last 10 years. Although he tries to take care of her, it is becoming increasingly difficult for him to do so. They have been married for almost 70 years and are very devoted to each other. What assessments would you carry out and what strategies would you implement to (1) relieve some of the patient's symptoms and discomfort, (2) assist her husband in management of her care, and (3) prepare both of them for her inevitable death?

3. You have been assigned to care for a 34-year-old father of three in the end stages of ALS. He was discharged home from the hospital yesterday and is being admitted to the local visiting nurse association's home palliative care program. During the admission assessment, when you ask him about his religion and beliefs as part of the spiritual assessment that is performed at the time of admission, he says to

---

<table>
<tr><td>Chart 17-10</td><td>Nursing Interventions for Grief and Mourning</td></tr>
</table>

- Support the expression of feelings.
  - Encourage the telling of the story using open-ended statements or questions (eg, "Tell me about your husband").
  - Assist the mourner to find an outlet for his/her feelings: talking, attending a support group, keeping a journal, finding a safe outlet for angry feelings (writing letters that will not be mailed, physical activity)
  - Assess emotional affect and reinforce the normalcy of feelings.
- Assess for guilt and regrets.
  - Are you especially troubled by a certain memory or thought?
  - How do you manage those memories?
- Assess for the presence of social support.
  - Do you have someone to whom you can talk about your husband?
  - Can I help you to find someone you can talk to?
- Assess coping skills.
  - How are you managing day to day?
  - Have you experienced other losses? How did you manage those?
  - Are there things you are having trouble doing?
  - Do you have/need help with specific tasks?
- Assess for signs of complicated grief and mourning and offer professional referral.

you, "I don't go to church anymore and I really don't have time for people who want to talk about religion." Should you respond to his comment? If not, why? If so, what will you say? Should you continue with part or all of a spiritual assessment? Explain your rationale. If you continue with the spiritual assessment, what questions would you use in the assessment? Discuss your plan for follow-up.

REFERENCES AND SELECTED READINGS

Books and Monographs

Addington, T. G. (1991). *Communication and cancer.* Hershey, PA: Central Pennsylvania Oncology Group.

Alliance for Aging Research. (1997). *Seven deadly myths: Uncovering the facts about the high cost of the last year of life.* Washington, DC: Author.

Amenta, M. O. (1986). The hospice movement. In M. O. Amenta & N. L. Bohnet (Eds.)., *Nursing care of the terminally ill* (pp. 49–64). Boston: Little Brown.

American Nurses Association. (1995). *Nursing's social policy statement.* Washington, DC: Author.

American Nurses Association (1994). Position statement on assisted suicide [On-line]. Available: http://nursingworld.org/readroom/position/ethics/etsuic.htm.

American Pain Society. (1999). *Principles of analgesic use in the treatment of acute pain and cancer pain* (4th ed.). Glenview, IL: Author.

Barnard, D., Towers, A., Boston, P., & Lambrinidou, Y. (2000). *Crossing over: narratives of palliative care.* New York: Oxford.

Bennahum, D. A. (1996). The historical development of hospice and palliative care. In D. C. Sheehan & W. B. Forman (Eds.), *Hospice and palliative care: Concepts and practice* (pp. 1–10). Boston: Jones & Bartlett.

Byock, I. (1997). *Dying well: The prospect for growth at the end of life.* New York: Riverhead.

Callahan, D. (1993b). *The troubled dream of life.* New York: Simon & Schuster.

Doyle, D., Hanks, G. W. C., & MacDonald, N. (Eds.). (1998). *Oxford textbook of palliative medicine* (2d Ed.). New York: Oxford.

ExcelleRx, Inc. (2000). *Hospice Pharmacia Pharmaceutical Care ToolKit* (3d Ed.). Philadelphia: Author.

Family Home Hospice of the Visiting Nurse Association of Greater Philadelphia. (1999). *Signs of approaching death.* Philadelphia: Author.

Ferrell, B. R., & Coyle, N. (Eds.). (2001). *Textbook of palliative nursing.* New York: Oxford.

Field, M. J., & Cassel, C. K. (Eds.). (1997). *Approaching death: Improving care at the end of life.* Washington, DC: National Academy Press.

Frankl, V. E. (1984). *Man's search for meaning.* New York: Washington Square.

Gadow, S. (1988). Covenant without cure: Letting go and holding on in chronic illness. In J. Watson & M. A. Ray (Eds.). *The ethics of cure and the ethics of care.* New York: NLN

George H. Gallup International Institute (1997). *Spiritual beliefs and the dying process.* Princeton, NJ: Author.

Glaser, B. G., & Strauss, A. (1965). *Awareness of dying.* Chicago: Aldine.

Hogan, C., Lynn, J., Gabel, J., Lunney, J., O'Mara, A., & Wilkinson, A. (2000, May 1). *Medicare beneficiaries' costs and use of care in the last year of life.* Washington, DC: MedPAC.

Hospice Association of America. (2001). *Hospice facts & statistics.* Washington, DC: Author.

Jacox, A., Carr, D. B., & Payne, R. (1994). *Management of cancer pain.* Clinical practice guideline No. 9 (AHCPR Publication No. 94-0592). Washington, DC: Agency for Health Care Policy and Research, United States Department of Health and Human Services, Public Health Service.

Kübler-Ross, E. (1969). *On death and dying.* New York: MacMillan.

Lesparre, M., & Matherlee, K. (1998). *Delivering and financing care at the end of life.* Issue Brief (No. 711). Washington, DC: The George Washington University.

Lynn, J., Schuster, J. L., & Kabcenell, A. (2000). *Improving care for the end of life: A sourcebook for health care managers and clinicians.* New York: Oxford.

Matzo, M. L., & Sherman, D. W. (Eds.). (2001). *Palliative care nursing: Quality care to the end of life.* New York: Springer.

McSkimming, S. A., Super, A., Driever, M. J., Schoessler, M., Franey, S. G., & Fonner, E. (1997). *Living and healing during life-threatening illness.* Portland, OR: Supportive Care of the Dying.

National Hospice and Palliative Care Organization. (2001). *Facts and figures on hospice care in America.* Alexandria, VA: Author.

Occupational Home Economics Education Series (1977). Attitudes toward death. In *Care and independent living services for the aging* (Section III-A22). Washington, DC: U.S. Government Printing Office.

Office of the Inspector General, Department of Health and Human Services. (1997). *Hospice patients in nursing homes* (DHHS Publication No. OEI-05-95-00250). Washington, DC: U.S. Government Printing Office.

Plata-Salaman, C. (1997). Symptoms in terminal illness: A research workshop. Cachexia or wasting: basic perspective [On-line]. Available: http://www.nih.gov/ninr/end-of-life.htm.

Rando, T. A. (2000). Promoting healthy anticipatory mourning in intimates of the life-threatened or dying person. In T. A. Rando (Ed.), *Clinical dimensions of anticipatory mourning* (pp. 307–378). Champaign, IL: Research Press.

Saunders, C., & Kastenbaum, R. (Eds.). (1997). *Hospice care on the international scene.* New York: Springer.

Smith, S. A. (2000). *Hospice concepts: A guide to palliative care in terminal illness.* Champaign, IL: Research Press.

Tilly, J., & Wiener, J. (2001). *Medicaid and end-of-life care.* Washington, DC: Last Acts.

Wentzel, K. B. (1981). *To those who need it most, hospice means hope.* Boston: Charles River.

World Health Organization. (1990). *Cancer pain relief and palliative care: Report of a WHO expert committee.* World Health Organization Technical Report Series, 804, 1–75.

Worden, J. W. (1991). *Grief counseling and grief therapy.* New York: Springer.

Wrede-Seaman, L. (1999). *Symptom management algorithms: A handbook for palliative care.* Yakima, WA: Intellicard.

Journals

Ameling, A., & Povilonis, M. (2002). Spirituality, meaning, mental health, and nursing. *Journal of Psychosocial Nursing and Mental Health Services, 39*(4), 14–20.

Balaban, R. B. (2000). A physician's guide to talking about end-of-life care. *Journal of General Internal Medicine, 15,* 195–200.

Benoliel, J. Q. (1993). The moral context of oncology nursing. *Oncology Nursing Forum (Supplement), 20*(10), 5–12.

Blackhall, L. J., Murphy, S. T., Frank, G., Michel, V., & Azen, S. (1995). Ethnicity and attitudes toward patient autonomy. *Journal of the American Medical Association, 274*(10), 820–825.

Block, S. D. (2000). Assessing and managing depression in the terminally ill patient. *Annals of Internal Medicine, 132*(3), 209–218.

Boling, A., & Lynn, J. (1998). Hospice: Current practice, future possibilities. *Hospice Journal, 13*(1/2), 29–36.

Brant, J. M. (1998). The art of palliative care: Living with hope, dying with dignity. *Oncology Nursing Forum, 25*(96), 995–1004.

Brinson, S. V., & Brunk, Q. (2000). Hospice family caregivers: An experience in coping. *The Hospice Journal, 15*(3), 1–12.

Buchanan, J., Borland, R., Cosolo, W., Millership, R., Haines, I., Zimet, A., & Zalcberg, J. (1996). Patients' beliefs about cancer management. *Supportive Care in Cancer, 4*(2), 110–117.

Callahan, D. (1993a). Pursuing a peaceful death. *Hastings Center Report, 23*(4), 33–38.

Campbell, M. L., & Field, B. E. (1991). Management of the patient with do not resuscitate status: Compassion and cost containment. *Heart & Lung, 20*(4), 345–348.

Caralis, P. V., Davis, B., Wright, K., & Marcial, E. (1993). The influence of ethnicity and race on attitudes toward advance directives, life-prolonging treatments and euthanasia. *Journal of Clinical Ethics, 4*(2), 155–165.

Cassel, C. K., Ludden, J. M., & Moon, G. M. (2000). Perceptions of barriers to high-quality palliative care in hospitals. *Health Affairs, 19*(5), 166–172.

Chochinov, H. M., Tataryn, D. J., Wilson, K. G., Ennis, M., & Lander S. (2000). Prognostic awareness and the terminally ill. *Psychosomatics, 41* (6), 500–504.

Chow, E., Anderson, L., Wong, R., et al. (2001). Patients with advanced cancer: A survey of the understanding of their illness and expectations from palliative radiotherapy for symptomatic metastases. *Clinical Oncology, 13*(3), 204–208.

Christakis, N. A., & Lamont, E. B. (2000) Extent and determinants of error in doctors' prognoses in terminally ill patients: Prospective cohort study. *British Medical Journal, 320,* 469–473.

Connor, S. R. (1992). Denial in terminal illness: To intervene or not to intervene. *Hospice Journal, 8*(4), 1–15.

Crawley, L., Payne, R., Bolden, J., Payne, T., Washington, P., & Williams, S. (2000). Palliative and end-of-life care in the African American community. *Journal of the American Medical Association, 284*(19), 2518–2521.

Eiser, A. R., & Weiss, M. D. (2001). The underachieving advance directive: Recommendations for increasing advance directive completion. *American Journal of Bioethics Online, 1*(2). Available: http://www.ajobonline.com/online_carticles/oa03.php.

Ersek, M., Kagawa-Singer, M., Barnes, D., Blackhall, L., & Koenig, B. A. (1998). Multicultural considerations in the use of advance directives. *Oncology Nursing Forum, 25*(10), 1683–1690.

Ferrell, B. R. & Coyle, N. (2002). An overview of palliative nursing care. *American Journal of Nursing, 102*(5), 26–31.

Ferrell, B., Virani, R., Grant, M., Coyne, P., & Uman, G. (2000). Beyond the Supreme Court decision: Nursing perspectives on end-of-life care. *Oncology Nursing Forum, 27*(3), 445–455.

Fetters, M. D., Churchill, L., & Danis, M. (2001). Conflict resolution at the end of life. *Critical Care Medicine, 29*(5), 921–925.

Finucane, T. (1999) How gravely ill becomes dying. *Journal of the American Medical Association, 282*(17), 1670–1672.

Gbrich, C. (2001). The emotions and coping strategies of caregivers of family members with a terminal cancer. *Journal of Palliative Care, 17*(1), 30–36.

Grady, P. A. (1999). Improving care at the end of life: Research issues. *Journal of Hospice and Palliative Nursing, 1*(94), 151–155.

Helm, A. (1984). Debating euthanasia: An international perspective. *Journal of Gerontological Nursing, 10*(11), 20–24.

Hermann, C. P. (2001). Spiritual needs of dying patients: A qualitative study. *Oncology Nursing Forum, 28*(91), 67.

Hermann, C., & Looney, S. (2001). The effectiveness of symptom management in hospice patients during the last seven days of life. *Journal of Hospice and Palliative Nursing, 3*(3), 88–96.

Hickey, S. S. (1986). Enabling hope. *Cancer Nursing, 9,* 133–137.

Highfield, M. E. F. (2000). Providing spiritual care to patients with cancer. *Clinical Journal of Oncology Nursing, 4*(3), 115–120.

*Jezuit, D. L. (2000). Suffering of critical care nurses with end-of-life decisions. *MedSurg Nursing, 9*(3). 145–152.

Jones, D. (1997). Issues and trends affecting the nation's hospices. *Caring, 16*(11), 14–24.

Kagawa-Singer, M., & Blackhall, L. J. (2001). Negotiating cross-cultural issues at the end of life. *Journal of the American Medical Association, 286*(23), 2993–3001.

*Kirchhoff, K. T., Spuhler, V., Walker, L. et al. (2000). Intensive care nurses' experiences with end-of-life care. *American Journal of Critical Care 9*(1), 36–42.

Krisman-Scott, M. A. (2000). An historical analysis of disclosure of terminal status. *Journal of Nursing Scholarship, 32*(1), 47–52.

LaDuke, S. (2001). Terminal dyspnea and palliative care. *American Journal of Nursing 101*(11), 26–31.

Langer, G. (1999). Kevorkian verdict unpopular. [Online]. Available: http://abcnews.go.com/sections/us/DailyNews/kevorkian_poll990327.html.

Last Acts Palliative Care Task Force. (1997). Precepts of palliative care [On-line]. Available: http://www.lastacts.org/docs/profprecepts.pdf

Lynn, J. (1991). Why I don't have a living will. *Law, Medicine & Health Care, 19*(1–2), 101–104.

Maugans, T. A. (1996). The SPIRITual history. *Archives of Family Medicine, 5*(1), 11–16.

Meier, D. E., Ahronheim, J. C., Morris, J., Baskin-Lyons, S., & Morrison, S. (2001). High short-term mortality in hospitalized patients with advanced dementia. *Archives of Internal Medicine, 161,* 594–599.

Morrison, R. S., Siu, A. L., Leipzig, R. M., Cassel, C. K., & Meier, D. E. (2000). The hard task of improving care at the end of life. *Archives of Internal Medicine, 160,* 743–747.

Morse, J. M. (2000). On comfort and comforting. *American Journal of Nursing, 100*(9), 34–37.

Morse, J. M., & Doberneck, B. (1995). Delineating the concept of hope. *Image: Journal of Nursing Scholarship, 27,* 283–291.

Patrick, D. L., Engelberg, R. A., & Curtis, J. R. (2001) Evaluating the quality of dying and death. *Journal of Pain and Symptom Management, 22*(3), 717–726.

Phipps, E., True, G., & Pomerantz, S. (2000). Approaches to end-of-life care in culturally diverse communities [On-line]. Available: http://www.lastacts.org/statsite/3770la%5Feln%5Fnewsletter.htm.

Post-White, J., Ceronsky, C., Kreitzer, M. J., Nickelson, K., Drew, D., Mackey, K. W., Koopmeiners, L., & Gutknecht, S. (1996). Hope, spirituality, sense of coherence, and quality of life in patients with cancer. *Oncology Nursing Forum, 23*(10), 1571–1579.

Quill, T. E., & Byock, I. R. (2000). Responding to intractable terminal suffering: The role of terminal sedation and voluntary refusal of foods and fluids. *Annals of Internal Medicine, 132*(5), 408–414.

Raudonis, B. M. (1992). Ethical considerations in qualitative research with hospice patients. *Qualitative Health Research, 2*(2), 238–249.

Ripamonti, C., Filiberti, A., Totis, A., DeConno, F., & Tamburini, M. (1999). Suicide among patients with cancer cared for at home by palliative care teams. *Lancet, 354*(9193), 1877–1878.

Roth, A. J., & Breitbart, W. (1996). Psychiatric emergencies in terminally ill cancer patients. *Hematology/Oncology Clinics of North America, 10*(1), 235–258.

Seale, C. (1991). Communication and awareness about death: A study of a random sample of dying people. *Social Science and Medicine, 32*(8), 943–952.

Silverman, P. R. (2001). Living with grief, rebuilding a world. *Innovations in End-of-Life Care* [On-line serial], 3(3). Available: http://www2.edc.org/lastaacts/editorail.asp.

Sorenson, B. F. (1991). Euthanasia: the "good death"? *Surgical Neurology, 35,* 827–830.

Spross, J. A. (1992). Cancer pain relief: An international perspective. *Oncology Nursing Forum, 19*(7), 5–19.

Stanley, K. J. (2000). Silence is not golden: Conversations with the dying. *Clinical Journal of Oncology Nursing, 4*(1), 34–40.

Steinhauser, K. E., Christakis, N. A., Clipp, E. C., McNeilly, M., Grambow, S., Parker, J., & Tulsky, J. A. (2001). Preparing for the end of life: Preferences of patients, families, physicians and other care providers. *Journal of Pain and Symptom Management, 22*(3), 727–737.

SUPPORT Principal Investigators. (1995). A controlled trial to improve care for seriously ill hospitalized patients. *Journal of the American Medical Association, 274*(20), 1591–1598.

Teno, J. M., Fisher, E. S., Hamel, M. B., Coppola, K., & Dawson, N. V. (2002). Medical care inconsistent with patients' treatment goals: Association with 1-year Medicare resource use and survival. *Journal of American Geriatrics Society, 50*(3), 496–500.

Tilden, V. P. (2000). Policy perspectives: Advance directives. *American Journal of Nursing, 100*(12), 49–51.

Tolle, S. W., Tilden, V. P., Rosenfeld, A. G., & Hickman, S. E. (2000). Family reports of barriers to optimal care of the dying. *Nursing Research, 49*(6), 310–317.

Upledger, J. E. (1989). Self-discovery and self-healing. In R. Carlson & B. Shield (Eds.), *Healers on healing* (pp. 67–72). Los Angeles: Tarcher.

Virmani, J., Schneiderman, L. J., & Kaplan, R. M. (1994). Relationship of advance directives to physician-patient communication. *Archives of Internal Medicine, 154,* 909–913.

Waller, A., Hershkowitz, M., & Adunsky, A. (1994). The effects of intravenous fluid infusion on blood and urine parameters of hydration and on state of consciousness in terminally ill patients. *American Journal of Hospice and Palliative Care, 26*–29.

Wendler, M. C. (1996). Understanding healing: A conceptual analysis. *Journal of Advanced Nursing, 24*(4), 836–842.

Wenrich, M. D., Curtis, J. R., Shannon, S. E., Carline, J. D., Ambrozy, D. M., & Ramsey, P. G. (2001). Communicating with dying patients within the spectrum of medical care from terminal diagnosis to death. *Archives of Internal Medicine, 161*(6), 868–874.

Yedidia, M. J., & MacGregor, B. (2001). Confronting the prospect of dying: Reports of terminally ill patients. *Journal of Pain and Symptom Management, 22*(4), 807–819.

Zerwekh, J. V. (1987). Should fluid and nutrition support be withheld from terminally ill patients? *American Journal of Hospice & Palliative Care, 4*(4), 37–38.

Zerwekh, J. (1994). The truth tellers: How hospice nurses help patients confront death. *American Journal of Nursing, 94*(2), 31–34.

Zerwekh, J. V. (1997). Do dying patients really need IV fluids? *American Journal of Nursing, 97*(3), 26–30.

Zerzan, J., Stearns, S., & Hanson, L. (2000). Access to palliative care and hospice in nursing homes. *Journal of the American Medical Association, 284*(19), 2489–2493.

RESOURCES AND WEBSITES

American Academy of Hospice & Palliative Medicine, 4700 West Lake Avenue, Glenview, IL 60025-1485; 847-375-4712; http://www.aahpm.org.

Americans for Better Care of the Dying (ABCD), 4125 Albemarle Street NW, Suite 210, Washington, DC 20016; (202) 895-9485, http://www.abcd-caring.org.

American Hospice Foundation, 2120 L Street NW, Suite 200, Washington, DC 20037; 202-223-0204; Fax 202-223-0208; E-mail: ahf@msn.com; http://www.americanhospice.org/.

Center to Improve Care of the Dying (at George Washington University). Offices located at the RAND Corporation, 1200 South Hayes Street, Arlington, VA 22202-5050; 703-413-1100; http://www.gwu.edu/~cicd/.

Children's Hospice International, 2202 Mount Vernon Avenue, Suite 3C, Alexandria, VA 22301; 800-24-CHILD; http://www.chionline.org.

Choice in Dying, Inc., 1035 30th Street NW, Washington, DC 20016; 202-338-9790; http://www.choices.org.

Compassion in Dying, 6312 SW Capital Highway, Suite 415, Portland, OR 97201; 503-221-9556; http://www.compassionindying.org/.

Department of Pain Medicine and Palliative Care at Beth Israel Medical Center, 1st Avenue at 16th Street, 12 Baird Hall, New York, NY 10003; 212-844-1472; http://www.stoppain.org.

Growthhouse, Inc. (provides information and referral services for agencies working with death and dying issues), San Francisco, CA; 415-863-3045; http://www.growthhouse.org.

HMS Center for Palliative Care (Harvard Medical School), Massachusetts General Hospital, Founders House 606, 55 Fruit Street, Boston, MA 02114; 617-724-9509; http://www.hms.harvard.edu/cdi/pallcare/.

Hospice Association of America, National Association for Home Care, 228 Seventh Street SE, Washington, DC 20003; (202) 547-7424; http://www.nahc.org/.

Hospice Education Institute, 190 Westbrook Road, Essex, CT 06426; (800) 331-1620; http://www.hospiceworld.org/.

Hospice Foundation of America, 2001 S St. NW #300, Washington, DC 20009; (800) 854-3402; http://www.hospicefoundation.org.

Hospice Net, http://www.hospicenet.org/index.html.

Hospice and Palliative Nurses Association (HPNA), Penn Center West One, Suite 229, Pittsburgh, PA 15276; (412) 787-9301; http://www.hpna.org.

Hospice Web (links to other resources), http://www.hospiceweb.com/links.htm.

Innovations in End-of-Life Care (online journal), http://www2.edc.org/lastacts/.

Last Acts Campaign to Improve End-of-Life Care, Located at Partnership for Caring, Inc., 1620 Eye Street NW, Suite 202, Washington, DC 20006; 202-296-8071; http://www.lastacts.org.

National Hospice and Palliative Care Organization, National Hospice Foundation, 1700 Diagonal Rd, Suite 300, Alexandria, VA 22314; 703-516-4928; http://www.nhpco.org.

Palliative Care Nursing, http://www.palliativecarenursing.net/index.html.

Partnership for Caring: America's Voices for the Dying, National Office, 1620 Eye Street NW, Suite 202, Washington, DC 20006; 202-296-8071; http://www.partnershipforcaring.org.

Project on Death in America, Open Society Institute, 400 West 59th Street, New York, NY 10019; 212-548-0150; http://www.soros.org/death.html.

Supportive Care of the Dying: A Coalition for Compassionate Care, For more information, contact Sylvia McSkimming, PhD, RN, Executive Director c/o Providence Health System, 4805 NE Glisan Street, 2E07, Portland, OR 97213; (503) 215-5053; http://www.careofdying.org.

The Center to Advance Palliative Care at The Mount Sinai School of Medicine, 1255 5th Avenue, Suite C-2, New York, NY, 10029-6574; Main line: (212) 201-2670; http://www.capcmssm.org.

Toolkit of Instruments to Measure End-of-life care (TIME; Dr. Joan Teno at Brown University): http://www.chcr.brown.edu/pcoc/toolkit.htm.

Perioperative Concepts and Nursing Management

Applying Concepts from NANDA, NIC, and NOC

Mr. Ott, a 54-year-old smoker, was admitted to the surgical unit 5 hours ago after colon resection for cancer. He is groggy but easily arousable. He can move all extremities with equal strength, but feels better lying still. In the last 4 hours, 125 mL of greenish material has drained from his nasogastric tube (NGT), which is connected to low intermittent suction. His abdomen is mildly distended; bowel sounds are absent. The large abdominal dressing has a reconstitutable bulb drain with 30mL of serosanguineous drainage; the dressing's minimal visible drainage has not increased in several hours. A peripheral IV of D5W 1/2NS with 20 mEq of KCl is running at 125 mL/h. Mr. Ott has voided 600 mL of clear urine. Vital signs are: Temp 97°F; HR 82, B/P 112/70; Resp 12 and shallow. Lung auscultation reveals scattered crackles throughout and a weak cough. After a 50-mg morphine injection, Mr. Ott ranks his pain at 3 (down from 7). He is reluctant to use his incentive spirometer for fear of more pain. The concept map illustrates the relationships among the nursing diagnoses, interventions, and outcomes.

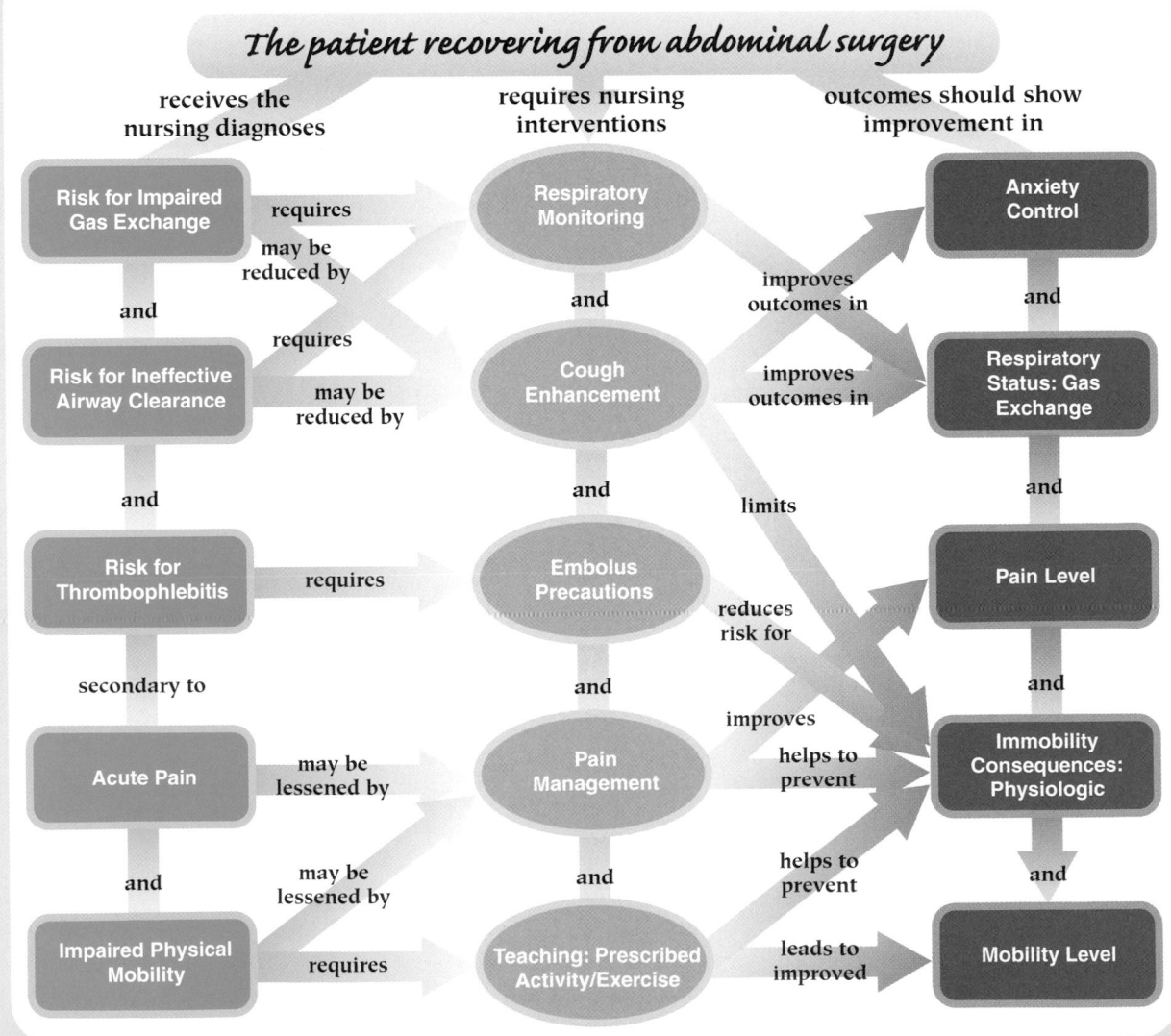

The patient recovering from abdominal surgery

receives the nursing diagnoses → requires nursing interventions → outcomes should show improvement in

Nursing Diagnoses		Nursing Interventions		Outcomes
Risk for Impaired Gas Exchange	requires / may be reduced by	Respiratory Monitoring	improves outcomes in	Anxiety Control
and	requires	and		and
Risk for Ineffective Airway Clearance	may be reduced by	Cough Enhancement	improves outcomes in	Respiratory Status: Gas Exchange
and		and	limits	and
Risk for Thrombophlebitis	requires	Embolus Precautions	reduces risk for	Pain Level
secondary to		and	improves	and
Acute Pain	may be lessened by	Pain Management	helps to prevent	Immobility Consequences: Physiologic
and	may be lessened by	and	helps to prevent	and
Impaired Physical Mobility	requires	Teaching: Prescribed Activity/Exercise	leads to improved	Mobility Level

Nursing Classifications and Languages

NANDA
Nursing Diagnoses

Risk for Impaired Gas Exchange—At risk for excess or deficit in oxygenation and/or carbon dioxide elimination at the alveolar-capillary membrane

Risk for Ineffective Airway Clearance—At risk for inability to clear secretions or obstructions from the respiratory tract to maintain a clear airway

Risk for Thrombophlebitis—At risk for clot formation in the deep veins of the legs

Acute Pain—Unpleasant sensory and emotional experience arising from actual or potential tissue damage or described in terms of such damage

Impaired Physical Mobility—Limitation in independent, purposeful physical movement of the body or of one or more extremities

NIC
Nursing Interventions*

Respiratory Monitoring—Collection and analysis of patient data to ensure airway patency and adequate gas exchange

Cough Enhancement—Promotion of deep inhalation by the patient with subsequent generation of high intrathoracic pressures and compression of underlying lung parenchyma for the forceful expulsion of air

Embolus Precautions—Reduction of the risk of embolus in a patient with thrombi or at risk for developing thrombi

Pain Management—Alleviation of pain or reduction in pain to a level of comfort that is acceptable to the patient

Teaching: Prescribed Activity/ Exercise—Preparing a patient to achieve and/or maintain a prescribed level of activity

NOC
Nursing Outcomes†

Return to functional baseline status, stabilization of, or improvement in

Anxiety Control—Personal actions to eliminate or reduce feelings of apprehension and tension from an unidentifiable source

Respiratory Status: Gas Exchange—The alveolar exchange of O_2 or CO_2 to maintain arterial blood gas concentrations; measured on a scale of extremely compromised to not compromised

Pain Level—Severity of reported or demonstrated pain

Immobility Consequences: Physiologic—Extent of compromise in physiologic functioning due to impaired physical mobility

Mobility Level—Ability to move purposefully

NANDA, North American Nursing Diagnosis Association; NIC, Nursing Interventions Classification; NOC, Nursing Outcomes Classification.

*Iowa Intervention Project © 2000. In McCloskey, J. C., & Bulechek, G. M. (2000). *Nursing interventions classification (NIC)* (3rd ed.). St. Louis: Mosby.

†Iowa Outcomes Project © 2000. In Johnson, M., Maas, M., & Moorhead, S. (2000). *Nursing outcomes classification (NOC)* (3rd ed.). St. Louis: Mosby.

Preoperative Nursing Management

On completion of this chapter, the learner will be able to:

1. Define the three phases of the perioperative period.
2. Describe a comprehensive preoperative assessment to identify surgical risk factors.
3. Identify the causes of preoperative anxiety and describe nursing measures to alleviate it.
4. Identify legal and ethical considerations related to informed consent.
5. Describe preoperative nursing measures that decrease the risk for infection and other postoperative complications.
6. Describe the immediate preoperative preparation of the patient.
7. Develop a preoperative teaching plan designed to promote the patient's recovery from anesthesia and surgery, thus preventing postoperative complications.

Surgery, whether elective or emergent, is a stressful, complex event. Today, as a result of advances in surgical techniques and instrumentation as well as in anesthesia, many surgical procedures that were once performed in an inpatient setting now take place in an ambulatory or outpatient setting. Approximately 60% of elective surgeries are now performed in an ambulatory or outpatient setting (Russell, Williams & Bulstrode, 2000). This trend has increased the acuity and complexity of surgical patients and procedures. The number of surgical patients admitted for overnight hospital stays is expected to continue to decrease.

In the past, the patient scheduled for elective surgery would be admitted to the hospital at least 1 day before surgery for evaluation and preparation; these activities are now completed before the patient is admitted to the hospital. Today, many patients arrive at the hospital the morning of surgery and go home after recovering in the postanesthesia care unit (PACU) from the anesthesia. Often, surgical patients who require hospital stays are trauma patients, acutely ill patients, patients undergoing major surgery, patients who require emergency surgery, and patients with a concurrent medical disorder. Although each setting offers its own unique advantages for the delivery of patient care, all require a comprehensive preoperative nursing assessment and nursing intervention to prepare the patient and family before surgery.

Today's technology has led to more complex procedures, more complicated microsurgical and laser technology, more sophisticated bypass equipment, increased use of laparoscopic surgery, and more sensitive monitoring devices. Surgery might now involve the transplantation of multiple human organs, the implantation of mechanical devices, the reattachment of body parts, and the use of robots and minimally invasive procedures in the operating room (Mack, 2002). Advances in anesthesia have kept pace with these surgical technologies. More sophisticated monitoring and new pharmacologic agents, such as short-acting anesthetics and more effective antiemetics, have improved postoperative pain management, reduced postoperative nausea and vomiting, and shortened procedure and recovery times.

Concurrent with technologic advances have been changes in the delivery of and payment for health care. Pressure to reduce hospital stays and contain costs has resulted in patients undergoing diagnostic **preadmission testing (PAT)** and preoperative preparation before admission to the hospital. Many facilities have a presurgical services department to facilitate testing and to initiate the nursing assessment process, which may focus on patient demographics, health history, and other information pertinent to the surgical procedure. The increasing use of **ambulatory or same-day surgery** means that patients leave the hospital sooner, which increases the need for teaching, discharge planning, preparation for self-care, and referral for home care and rehabilitation

services. Competent care of ambulatory or same-day surgical patients requires a sound knowledge of all aspects of perioperative and perianesthesia nursing practice.

Perioperative and Perianesthesia Nursing

The special field known as perioperative and perianesthesia nursing includes a wide variety of nursing functions associated with the patient's surgical experience during the perioperative period. **Perioperative** and perianesthesia nursing addresses the nursing roles relevant to the three phases of the surgical experience: **preoperative**, **intraoperative**, and **postoperative**. As shown in Chart 18-1, each phase begins and ends at a particular point in the sequence of events that constitutes the surgical experience, and each includes a wide range of activities the nurse performs using the nursing process and based on the standards of practice (American Society of PeriAnesthesia Nurses, 2000; Litwack, 1999; Quinn, 1999).

PREOPERATIVE PHASE

The **preoperative phase** begins when the decision to proceed with surgical intervention is made and ends with the transfer of the patient onto the operating room table. The scope of nursing activities during this time can include establishing a baseline evaluation of the patient before the day of surgery by carrying out a preoperative interview (which includes not only a physical but also an emotional assessment, previous anesthetic history, and identification of known allergies or genetic problems that may affect the surgical outcome), ensuring that necessary tests have been or will be performed (preadmission testing), arranging appropriate consultative services, and providing preparatory education about recovery from anesthesia and postoperative care. On the day of surgery, patient teaching is reviewed, the patient's identity and the surgical site are verified, informed consent is confirmed, and an intravenous infusion is started. If the patient is going home the same day, the availability of safe transport and the presence of an accompanying responsible adult is verified. Depending on when the preadmission evaluation and testing were done, the nursing activities on the day of surgery may be as basic as performing or updating the preoperative patient assessment and addressing questions the patient or family may have.

INTRAOPERATIVE PHASE

The **intraoperative phase** begins when the patient is transferred onto the operating room table and ends when he or she is admitted to the postanesthesia care unit (PACU). In this

---

Glossary

ambulatory surgery: may include *outpatient (or same-day)* surgery that does not require an overnight hospital stay or *short stay,* with admission to an inpatient hospital setting for less than 24 hours

informed consent: the patient's autonomous decision about whether to undergo a surgical procedure; based on the nature of the condition, the treatment options, and the risks and benefits involved

intraoperative phase: period of time from when the patient is transferred to the operating room table to when he or she is admitted to the postanesthesia care unit (PACU)

perioperative phase: period of time that constitutes the surgical experience; includes the preoperative, intraoperative, and postoperative phases of nursing care

postoperative phase: period of time that begins with the admission of the patient

to the PACU and ends after a follow-up evaluation in the clinical setting or home

preadmission testing (PAT): diagnostic testing performed before admission to the hospital

preoperative phase: period of time from when the decision for surgical intervention is made to when the patient is transferred to the operating room table

Chart 18-1 Examples of Perioperative Nursing Activities

Preoperative Phase

Preadmission Testing
1. Initiates initial preoperative assessment
2. Initiates teaching appropriate to patient's needs
3. Involves family in interview
4. Verifies completion of preoperative testing
5. Verifies understanding of surgeon-specific preoperative orders (eg, bowel preparation, preoperative shower)
6. Assesses patient's need for postoperative transportation and care

Admission to Surgical Center or Unit
1. Completes preoperative assessment
2. Assesses for risks for postoperative complications
3. Reports unexpected findings or any deviations from normal
4. Verifies that operative consent has been signed
5. Coordinates patient teaching with other nursing staff
6. Reinforces previous teaching
7. Explains phases in perioperative period and expectations
8. Answers patient's and family's questions
9. Develops a plan of care

In the Holding Area
1. Assesses patient's status; baseline pain and nutritional status
2. Reviews chart
3. Identifies patient
4. Verifies surgical site and marks site per institutional policy
5. Establishes intravenous line
6. Administers medications if prescribed
7. Takes measures to ensure patient's comfort
8. Provides psychological support
9. Communicates patient's emotional status to other appropriate members of the health care team

Intraoperative Phase

Maintenance of Safety
1. Maintains aseptic, controlled environment
2. Effectively manages human resources, equipment, and supplies for individualized patient care
3. Transfers patient to operating room bed or table
4. Positions the patient
   • Functional alignment
   • Exposure of surgical site
5. Applies grounding device to patient
6. Ensures that the sponge, needle, and instrument counts are correct
7. Completes intraoperative documentation

Physiologic Monitoring
1. Calculates effects on patient of excessive fluid loss or gain
2. Distinguishes normal from abnormal cardiopulmonary data
3. Reports changes in patient's vital signs
4. Institutes measures to promote normothermia

Psychological Support (Before Induction and When Patient Is Conscious)
1. Provides emotional support to patient
2. Stands near or touches patient during procedures and induction
3. Continues to assess patient's emotional status

Postoperative Phase

Transfer of Patient to Postanesthesia Care Unit
1. Communicates intraoperative information
   • Identifies patient by name
   • States type of surgery performed
   • Identifies type of anesthetic used
   • Reports patient's response to surgical procedure and anesthesia
   • Describes intraoperative factors (eg, insertion of drains or catheters; administration of blood, analgesic agents, or other medications during surgery; occurrence of unexpected events)
   • Describes physical limitations
   • Reports patient's preoperative level of consciousness
   • Communicates necessary equipment needs
   • Communicates presence of family and/or significant others

Postoperative Assessment Recovery Area
1. Determines patient's immediate response to surgical intervention
2. Monitors patient's physiologic status
3. Assesses patient's pain level and administers appropriate pain relief
4. Maintains patient's safety (airway, circulation, prevention of injury)
5. Administers medications, fluid, and blood component therapy, if prescribed
6. Provides oral fluids if prescribed for ambulatory surgery patient
7. Assesses patient's readiness for transfer to in-hospital unit or for discharge home based on institutional policy (eg, Alderete score, see Chap. 20)

Surgical Unit
1. Continues close monitoring of patient's physical and psychological response to surgical intervention
2. Assesses patient's pain level and administers appropriate pain relief measures
3. Provides teaching to patient during immediate recovery period
4. Assists patient in recovery and preparation for discharge home
5. Determines patient's psychological status
6. Assists with discharge planning

Home or Clinic
1. Provides follow-up care during office or clinic visit or by telephone contact
2. Reinforces previous teaching and answers patient's and family's questions about surgery and follow-up care
3. Assesses patient's response to surgery and anesthesia and their effects on body image and function
4. Determines family's perception of surgery and its outcome

---

phase, the scope of nursing activity can include providing for the patient's safety, maintaining an aseptic environment, ensuring proper function of equipment, providing the surgeon with specific instruments and supplies for the surgical field, and completing appropriate documentation. In some instances, the nursing activities can encompass providing emotional support by holding the patient's hand during general anesthesia induction, assisting in positioning the patient on the operating room table using basic principles of body alignment, or acting as scrub nurse, circulating nurse, or registered nurse first assistant (RNFA).

POSTOPERATIVE PHASE

The **postoperative phase** begins with the admission of the patient to the PACU and ends with a follow-up evaluation in the clinical setting or at home. The scope of nursing care covers a wide range of activities during this period. In the immediate postoperative phase, the focus includes maintaining the patient's airway, monitoring vital signs, assessing the effects of the anesthetic agents, assessing the patient for complications, and providing comfort and pain relief. Nursing activities then focus on promoting the patient's recovery and initiating the teaching, follow-up

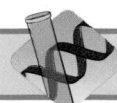

GENETICS IN NURSING PRACTICE—Perioperative Nursing

Nurses who are caring for patients undergoing surgery need to take various genetic considerations into account when assessing patients throughout the perioperative experience. For example, surgical outcomes may be altered by genetic conditions that may cause complications with anesthesia, including the following:

- Malignant hyperthermia
- Central core disease (CCD)
- Duchenne muscular dystrophy
- Hyperkalemic periodic paralysis
- King-Denborough

NURSING ASSESSMENTS

PREOPERATIVE FAMILY HISTORY ASSESSMENT

- Obtain a thorough assessment of personal and family history, inquiring about prior problems with surgery or anesthesia with specific attention to complications such as fever, rigidity, dark urine, unexpected reactions.
- Inquire about any history of musculoskeletal complaints, history of heat intolerance, fevers of unknown origin, or unusual drug reaction.
- Assess for family history of any sudden or unexplained death, especially during participation in athletic events.

PHYSICAL ASSESSMENT

- Assess for subclinical muscle weakness.
- Assess for other physical features suggestive of an underlying genetic condition, such as contractures, kyphoscoliosis, and pterygium with progressive weakness.

MANAGEMENT ISSUES SPECIFIC TO GENETICS

- Inquire whether DNA mutation or other genetic testing has been performed on an affected family member.
- If indicated, refer for further genetic counseling and evaluation so that family members can discuss inheritance, risk to other family members, availability of diagnostic/genetic testing.
- Offer appropriate genetics information and resources.
- Assess patient's understanding of genetics information.
- Provide support to families with newly diagnosed malignant hyperthermia.
- Participate in management and coordination of care of patients with genetic conditions and individuals predisposed to develop or pass on a genetic condition.

GENETICS RESOURCES FOR NURSES AND THEIR PATIENTS ON THE WEB

Genetic Alliance: http://www.geneticalliance.org—a directory of support groups for patients and families with genetic conditions

Gene Clinics: http://www.geneclinics.org—a listing of common genetic disorders with up-to-date clinical summaries, genetic counseling and testing information

International Council of Nurses http://www.icn.ch/matters_genetics.htm—ICN's statement re: genetics and nursing.

National Organization of Rare Disorders: http://www.rarediseases.org—a directory of support groups and information for patients and families with rare genetic disorders

OMIM: Online Mendelian Inheritance in Man: http://www.ncbi.nlm.nih.gov/omim/stats/html—a complete listing of inherited genetic conditions

---

care, and referrals essential for recovery and rehabilitation after discharge. Each phase is reviewed in more detail in the three chapters of this unit.

Historically, the perioperative nurse's practice environment has been isolated, consisting of the area behind the double doors of the surgical suite. Although the nursing process guided nursing care, the fundamentals of assessment, diagnosis, planning, intervention, and evaluation were often misunderstood by practitioners unfamiliar with the delivery of surgical care. In recent years, the acceptance of a conceptual model for patient care, published by the Association of PeriOperative Registered Nurses, formerly known as the Association of Operating Room Nurses (still abbreviated AORN), has helped to delineate the relationship of various components of nursing practice and the effect on patient outcomes (Beyea, 2000). The Perioperative Nursing Data Set (PNDS) is a language that describes the practice of perioperative nursing practice in four domains: safety, physiologic responses, behavioral responses, and health care systems (Fig. 18-1). The first three domains reflect phenomena of concern to perioperative nurses and are composed of nursing diagnoses, interventions, and outcomes that surgical patients and their families experience. The fourth domain, the health care system, comprises structural data elements and focuses on clinical processes and outcomes. The model is used to depict the relationship of nursing process components to the achievement of optimal patient outcomes.

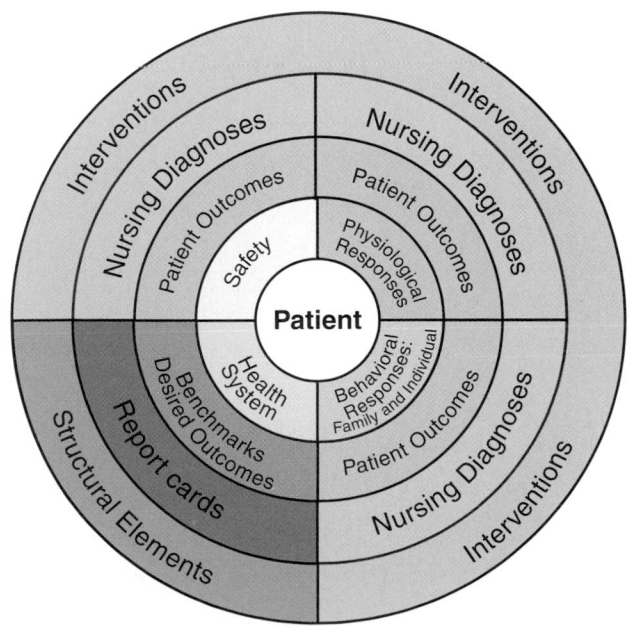

FIGURE 18-1 Perioperative patient-focused model. © With permission from Association of PeriOperative Registered Nurses, Inc., Denver, CO.

Surgical Classifications

Surgery may be performed for various reasons. A surgical procedure may be diagnostic (eg, biopsy or exploratory laparotomy). It may be curative (eg, excision of a tumor or an inflamed appendix) or reparative (eg, multiple wound repair). Surgery may be reconstructive or cosmetic (eg, mammoplasty or a facelift), or it may be palliative (eg, to relieve pain or correct a problem; for instance, a gastrostomy tube may be inserted to compensate for the inability to swallow food). Surgery may also be classified according to the degree of urgency involved: emergent, urgent, required, elective, and optional. These terms are defined in Table 18-1.

Preparation for Surgery

INFORMED CONSENT

Voluntary and written **informed consent** from the patient is necessary before nonemergent surgery can be performed. Such written consent protects the patient from unsanctioned surgery and protects the surgeon from claims of an unauthorized operation. In the best interests of all parties concerned, sound medical, ethical, and legal principles are followed. The nurse may ask the patient to sign the form and may witness the patient's signature. It is the physician's responsibility to provide appropriate information. Chart 18-2 lists the criteria for a valid informed consent.

Many ethical principles are integral to informed consent (see Chap. 3). Before the patient signs the consent form, the surgeon must provide a clear and simple explanation of what the surgery will entail. The surgeon must also inform the patient of the benefits, alternatives, possible risks, complications, disfigurement, disability, and removal of body parts as well as what to expect in the early and late postoperative periods. If the patient needs additional information to make his or her decision, the nurse notifies the physician about this. Also, the nurse ascertains that the consent form has been signed before administering psychoactive premedication, because the consent may not be valid if it was obtained while the patient was under the influence of medications that can affect judgment and decision-making

| Chart 18-2 | **Criteria for Valid Informed Consent** |

Voluntary Consent
Valid consent must be freely given, without coercion.

Incompetent Patient
Legal definition: individual who is *not* autonomous and cannot give or withhold consent (eg, individuals who are mentally retarded, mentally ill, or comatose)

Informed Subject
Informed consent should be in writing. It should contain the following:
- Explanation of procedure and its risks
- Description of benefits and alternatives
- An offer to answer questions about procedure
- Instructions that the patient may withdraw consent
- A statement informing the patient if the protocol differs from customary procedure

Patient Able to Comprehend
Information must be written and delivered in language understandable to the patient. Questions must be answered to facilitate comprehension if material is confusing.

capacity. Informed consent is necessary in the following circumstances:

- Invasive procedures, such as a surgical incision, a biopsy, a cystoscopy, or paracentesis
- Procedures requiring sedation and/or anesthesia (see Chap. 19 for a discussion of levels of sedation and anesthesia)
- A nonsurgical procedure, such as an arteriography, that carries more than slight risk to the patient
- Procedures involving radiation

The patient personally signs the consent if he or she is of legal age and is mentally capable. When the patient is a minor or unconscious or incompetent, permission must be obtained from a responsible family member (preferably next of kin) or legal guardian. An emancipated minor (married or independently earning his or her own living) may sign his or her own consent form. State regulations and agency policy must be followed. In

---

Table 18-1 • **Categories of Surgery Based on Urgency**

CLASSIFICATION	INDICATIONS FOR SURGERY	EXAMPLES
I. Emergent—Patient requires immediate attention; disorder may be life-threatening	Without delay	Severe bleeding Bladder or intestinal obstruction Fractured skull Gunshot or stab wounds Extensive burns
II. Urgent—Patient requires prompt attention	Within 24–30 h	Acute gallbladder infection Kidney or ureteral stones
III. Required—Patient needs to have surgery	Plan within a few weeks or months	Prostatic hyperplasia without bladder obstruction Thyroid disorders Cataracts
IV. Elective—Patient should have surgery	Failure to have surgery not catastrophic	Repair of scars Simple hernia Vaginal repair
V. Optional—Decision rests with patient	Personal preference	Cosmetic surgery

an emergency, it may be necessary for the surgeon to operate as a lifesaving measure without the patient's informed consent. Every effort, however, must be made to contact the patient's family. In such a situation, contact can be made by telephone, telegram, fax, or other electronic means.

When the patient has doubts and has not had the opportunity to investigate alternative treatments, a second opinion may be requested. No patient should be urged or coerced to sign an operative permit. Refusing to undergo a surgical procedure is a person's legal right and privilege. However, such information must be documented and relayed to the surgeon so that other arrangements can be made. For example, additional explanations may be provided to the patient and family, or the surgery may be rescheduled.

The consent process can be improved by providing audiovisual materials to supplement discussion, by ensuring that the wording of the consent form is understandable, and by using other strategies and resources as needed to help the patient understand its content.

NURSING ALERT The signed consent form is placed in a prominent place on the patient's chart and accompanies the patient to the operating room.

ASSESSMENT OF HEALTH FACTORS THAT AFFECT PATIENTS PREOPERATIVELY

The overall goal in the preoperative period is for the patient to have as many positive health factors as possible. Every attempt is made to stabilize those conditions that otherwise hinder a smooth recovery. When negative factors dominate, the risks of surgery and postoperative complications increase.

Before any surgical treatment is initiated, a health history is obtained, a physical examination is performed during which vital signs are noted, and a database is established for future comparisons (Meeker & Rothrock, 1999). During the physical examination, many factors are considered that have the potential to affect the patient undergoing surgery. Health care providers should be alert for signs of abuse that can occur at all ages and to men and women from all socioeconomic, ethnic, and cultural groups (Little, 2000; Marshall, Benton & Brazier, 2000). Findings need to be reported accordingly (see Chap. 5 for further discussion of signs of abuse).

Blood tests, x-rays, and other diagnostic tests are prescribed when specifically indicated by information obtained from a thorough history and physical examination (King, 2000). These preliminary contacts with the health care team provide the patient with opportunities to ask questions and to become acquainted with those who may be providing care during and after surgery.

Nutritional and Fluid Status

Optimal nutrition is an essential factor in promoting healing and resisting infection and other surgical complications (Braunschweig, Gomez & Sheean, 2000). Assessment of a patient's nutritional status provides information on obesity, undernutrition, weight loss, malnutrition, deficiencies in specific nutrients, metabolic abnormalities, the effects of medications on nutrition, and special problems of the hospitalized patient (Quinn, 1999). Nutritional needs may be determined by measurement of body mass index and waist circumference (National Institutes of Health, 2000). See Chapter 5 for further discussion of nutritional assessment.

Any nutritional deficiency, such as malnutrition, should be corrected before surgery so that enough protein is available for tissue repair (King, 2000; Russell, Williams & Bulstrode, 2000). The nutrients needed for wound healing are summarized in Table 18-2.

Dehydration, hypovolemia, and electrolyte imbalances can lead to significant problems in patients with comorbid medical conditions or in elderly patients. The severity of fluid and electrolyte imbalances is often difficult to determine. Mild volume deficits may be treated during surgery; however, additional time may be needed to correct pronounced fluid and electrolyte deficits to promote the best possible preoperative condition.

Drug or Alcohol Use

People who abuse drugs or alcohol frequently deny or attempt to hide it. In such situations, the nurse who is obtaining the patient's health history needs to ask frank questions with patience, care, and a nonjudgmental attitude. See Chapter 5 for an assessment of alcohol and drug use.

Because acutely intoxicated persons are susceptible to injury, surgery is postponed in these patients if possible. If emergency surgery is required, local, spinal, or regional block anesthesia is used for minor surgery. Otherwise, to prevent vomiting and potential aspiration, a nasogastric tube is inserted before administering general anesthesia.

The person with a history of chronic alcoholism often suffers from malnutrition and other systemic problems that increase the surgical risk. Additionally, alcohol withdrawal delirium (delirium tremens) may be anticipated up to 72 hours after alcohol withdrawal. Delirium tremens is associated with a significant mortality rate when it occurs postoperatively.

Chart 18-3 gives more information about risk factors that may lead to complications.

Respiratory Status

The goal for potential surgical patients is optimal respiratory function. Patients are taught breathing exercises and use of an incentive spirometer if indicated. Because adequate ventilation is potentially compromised during all phases of surgical treatment, surgery is usually postponed when the patient has a respiratory infection. Patients with underlying respiratory disease (eg, asthma, chronic obstructive pulmonary disease) are assessed carefully for current threats to their pulmonary status. Patients' use of medications that may affect recovery is also assessed (King, 2000; Smetana, 1999).

Patients who smoke are urged to stop 2 months before surgery (King, 2000), although many do not do so. These patients should be counseled to stop smoking at least 24 hours prior to surgery. Research suggests that counseling has a positive effect on the patient's smoking behavior 24 hours preceding surgery, helping reduce the potential for adverse effects associated with smoking such as increased airway reactivity, decreased mucociliary clearance, as well as physiologic changes in the cardiovascular and immune systems (Shannon-Cain, Webster & Cain, 2002).

Cardiovascular Status

The goal in preparing any patient for surgery is to ensure a well-functioning cardiovascular system to meet the oxygen, fluid, and nutritional needs of the perioperative period. If the patient has

Table 18-2 • **Nutrients Important for Wound Healing**

NUTRIENT	RATIONALE FOR INCREASED NEED	POSSIBLE DEFICIENCY OUTCOME
Protein	To replace the lean body mass lost during the catabolic phase after stress To restore blood volume and plasma proteins lost through exudates, bleeding from the wound, and possible hemorrhage To replace losses resulting from immobility (increased excretion) To meet the increased needs for tissue repair and resistance to infection	Significant weight loss Impaired/delayed wound healing Shock related to decreased blood volume Edema related to decreased serum albumin Diarrhea related to decreased albumin Anemia Increased risk of infection related to decreased antibodies, impaired tissue integrity Decreased lipoprotein synthesis → fatty infiltration of the liver → liver damage Increased mortality
Calories	To replace losses related to lack of oral intake and hypermetabolism during catabolic phase after stress To spare protein To restore normal weight	Signs and symptoms of protein deficiency due to use of protein to meet energy requirements Extensive weight loss
Water	To replace fluid lost through vomiting, hemorrhage, exudates, fever, drainage, diuresis To maintain homeostasis	Signs, symptoms, and complications of dehydration, such as poor skin turgor, dry mucous membranes, oliguria, anuria, weight loss, increased pulse rate, decreased central venous pressure
Vitamin C	Important for capillary formation, tissue synthesis, and wound healing through collagen formation Needed for antibody formation	Impaired/delayed wound healing related to impaired collagen formation and increased capillary fragility and permeability Increased risk of infection related to decreased antibodies
Thiamine, niacin, riboflavin	Requirements increase with increased metabolic rate	Decreased enzymes available for energy metabolism
Folic acid, vitamin B_{12}	Needed for cell proliferation and therefore tissue synthesis Important for maturation of red blood cells Impaired folic acid synthesis associated with the use of some antibiotics; impaired vitamin B_{12} absorption associated with the use of some antibiotics	Decreased or arrested cell division Megaloblastic anemia
Vitamin A	Important for tissue synthesis, wound healing, and immune function Enhances resistance to infection	Impaired/delayed wound healing related to decreased collagen synthesis; impaired immune function Increased risk of infection
Vitamin K	Important for normal blood clotting Impaired intestinal synthesis associated with the use of antibiotics	Prolonged prothrombin time
Iron	To replace iron lost through blood loss	Signs, symptoms, and complications of iron deficiency anemia, such as fatigue, weakness, pallor, anorexia, dizziness, headaches, stomatitis, glossitis, cardiovascular and respiratory changes, possible cardiac failure
Zinc	Needed for protein synthesis and wound healing Needed for normal lymphocyte and phagocyte response	Impaired/delayed wound healing Impaired immune response

Reproduced with permission from Dudek, S. G. (Ed.). (2001). *Nutrition essentials for nursing practice* (4th ed.). Philadelphia: Lippincott Williams & Wilkins.

uncontrolled hypertension, surgery may be postponed until the blood pressure is under control.

Because cardiovascular disease increases the risk for complications, patients with these conditions require greater-than-usual diligence during all phases of nursing management and care (King, 2000). Depending on the severity of the symptoms, surgery may be deferred until medical treatment can be instituted to improve the patient's condition. At times, surgical treatment can be modified to meet the cardiac tolerance of the patient. For example, in a patient with obstruction of the descending colon and coronary artery disease, a temporary simple colostomy may be performed rather than a more extensive colon resection that would require a prolonged period of anesthesia.

Hepatic and Renal Function

The presurgical goal is optimal function of the liver and urinary systems so that medications, anesthetic agents, body wastes, and toxins are adequately processed and removed from the body.

The liver is important in the biotransformation of anesthetic compounds. Therefore, any disorder of the liver has an effect on how anesthetic agents are metabolized. Because acute liver disease is associated with high surgical mortality, preoperative improvement in liver function is a goal. Careful assessment is made with the help of various liver function tests (see Chap. 39).

Because the kidneys are involved in excreting anesthetic drugs and their metabolites and because acid–base status and metabolism

Chart 18-3
Risk Factors for Surgical Complications

Hypovolemia
Dehydration or electrolyte imbalance
Nutritional deficits
Extremes of age (very young, very old)
Extremes of weight (emaciation, obesity)
Infection and sepsis
Toxic conditions
Immunologic abnormalities
Pulmonary disease
    Obstructive disease
    Restrictive disorder
    Respiratory infection
Renal or urinary tract disease
    Decreased renal function
    Urinary tract infection
    Obstruction
Pregnancy
    Diminished maternal physiologic reserve
Cardiovascular disease
    Coronary artery disease or previous myocardial infarction
    Cardiac failure
    Dysrhythmias
    Hypertension
    Prosthetic heart valve
    Thromboembolism
    Hemorrhagic disorders
    Cerebrovascular disease
Endocrine dysfunction
    Diabetes mellitus
    Adrenal disorders
    Thyroid malfunction
Hepatic disease
    Cirrhosis
    Hepatitis
Preexisting mental or physical disability

are also important considerations in anesthesia administration, surgery is contraindicated when a patient has acute nephritis, acute renal insufficiency with oliguria or anuria, or other acute renal problems. The exception is surgery that is performed as a lifesaving measure or that is necessary to improve urinary function, as in the case of an obstructive uropathy.

Endocrine Function

The patient with diabetes who is undergoing surgery is at risk for hypoglycemia and hyperglycemia. Hypoglycemia may develop during anesthesia or postoperatively from inadequate carbohydrates or from excessive administration of insulin. Hyperglycemia, which may increase the risk for surgical wound infection, may result from the stress of surgery, which may trigger increased levels of catecholamine. Other risks are acidosis and glucosuria. Although the surgical risk in the patient with controlled diabetes is no greater than in the nondiabetic patient, the goal is to maintain the blood glucose level at less than 200 mg/dL. Frequent monitoring of blood glucose levels is important before, during, and after surgery (see Chap. 41 for discussion of the patient with diabetes undergoing surgery).

Patients who have received corticosteroids are at risk for adrenal insufficiency. Therefore, the use of corticosteroids for any purpose during the preceding year must be reported to the anesthesiologist or anesthetist and surgeon. Additionally, the patient is monitored for signs of adrenal insufficiency.

Patients with uncontrolled thyroid disorders are at risk for thyrotoxicosis (with hyperthyroid disorders) and respiratory failure (with hypothyroid disorders). Therefore, the patient is assessed for a history of these disorders.

Immune Function

An important function of the preoperative assessment is to determine the existence of allergies, including the nature of previous allergic reactions. It is especially important to identify and document any sensitivity to medications and past adverse reactions to these agents. The patient is asked to identify any substances that precipitated previous allergic reactions, including medications, blood transfusions, contrast agents, latex, and food products, and to describe the signs and symptoms produced by these substances. A sample latex allergy screening questionnaire is shown in Figure 18-2.

Immunosuppression is common with corticosteroid therapy, renal transplantation, radiation therapy, chemotherapy, and disorders affecting the immune system, such as acquired immunodeficiency syndrome (AIDS) and leukemia. The mildest symptoms or slightest temperature elevation must be investigated. Because patients who are immunosuppressed are highly susceptible to infection, great care is taken to ensure strict asepsis.

Previous Medication Use

A medication history is obtained from each patient because of the possible effects of medications on the patient's perioperative and perianesthesia course and the possibility of drug interactions (Quinn, 1999). Any medication the patient is using or has used in the past is documented, including over-the-counter (OTC) preparations and herbal agents and the frequency with which they are used. Potent medications have an effect on physiologic functions; interactions of such medications with anesthetic agents can cause serious problems, such as arterial hypotension and circulatory collapse.

The potential effects of prior medication therapy are evaluated by the anesthesiologist or anesthetist, who considers the length of time the patient has used the medications, the physical condition of the patient, and the nature of the proposed surgery. Medications that cause particular concern are listed in Table 18-3.

Many patients take self-prescribed or OTC medications in addition to those listed in Table 18-3. Aspirin is a common OTC medication prescribed by physicians or taken independently by patients to prevent myocardial infarction, stroke, and other disorders (Karch, 2002). Because of the effects of aspirin or other OTC medications and possible interactions with other medications and anesthetic agents, it is important to ask a patient about their use. The information is noted in the patient's chart and conveyed to the anesthesiologist or anesthetist and surgeon.

The use of herbal medications is widespread among patients. Approximately 15 million Americans report their use (Ang-Lee, Moss & Yuan, 2001; Karch, 2002; Lyons, 2002). Patients with chronic illnesses may be using herbal medications to supplement their prescribed medications or in place of them. Certain herbal medications, such as echinacea, ephedra, garlic (*Allium sativum*), ginkgo, ginseng, kava kava (*Piper methysticum*), St. John's wort

Ask the patient the following questions. Check "Yes" or "No" in the box.	YES	NO
1. Has a doctor ever told you that you are allergic to latex?		
2. Do you have on-the-job exposure to latex?		
3. Were you born with problems involving your spinal cord?		
4. Have you ever had allergies, asthma, hay fever, eczema or problems with rashes?		
5. Have you ever had respiratory distress, rapid heart rate or swelling?		
6. Have you ever had swelling, itching, hives or other symptoms after contact with a balloon?		
7. Have you ever had swelling, itching, hives or other symptoms after a dental examination or procedure?		
8. Have you ever had swelling, itching, hives or other symptoms following a vaginal or rectal examination or after contact with a diaphragm or condom?		
9. Have you ever had swelling, itching, hives or other symptoms during or within one hour after wearing rubber gloves?		
10. Have you ever had a rash on your hands that lasted longer than one week?		
11. Have you ever had swelling, itching, hives, runny nose, eye irritation, wheezing, or asthma after contact with any latex or rubber product?		
12. Have you ever had swelling, itching, hives or other symptoms after being examined by someone wearing rubber or latex gloves?		
13. Are you allergic to bananas, avocados, kiwi or chestnuts?		
14. Have you ever had an unexplained anaphylactic episode?		

Pre-op RN Signature: _____

Patient Name: _____

Procedure: _____

FIGURE 18-2   Example of a latex allergy assessment form. Courtesy of Inova Fairfax Hospital, Falls Church, VA.

(*Hypericum perforatum*), licorice (*Glycyhiza glabra*), and valerian (*Valeriana officinalis*) have been identified as the most commonly used herbal medications that may cause concern during the perioperative period (Ang-Lee, Moss & Yuan, 2001; Kuhn, 1999; Lyons, 2002). Because of the potential effects of herbal medications on coagulation and potential interactions with other medications, the nurse must ask surgical patients explicitly about the use of these agents, document their use, and inform the surgical team and anesthesiologist or anesthetist (Brumly, 2000).

NURSING ALERT Because of possible adverse interactions, the nurse must assess and document the patient's use of prescription medications, OTC medications (especially aspirin), and herbal medications. The nurse must clearly communicate this information to the anesthesiologist or anesthetist.

Psychosocial Factors

All patients have some type of emotional reaction before any surgical procedure, be it obvious or hidden, normal or abnormal. For example, preoperative anxiety may be an anticipatory response to an experience the patient views as a threat to his or her customary role in life, body integrity, or life itself. Psychological distress directly influences body functioning. Therefore, it is imperative to identify any anxiety the patient is experiencing.

By taking a careful health history, the nurse elicits patient concerns that can have a bearing on the course of the surgical experience (Quinn, 1999). Undoubtedly, a patient about to undergo surgery is faced with various fears, including fears of the unknown, of death, of anesthesia, pain, or cancer. Concerns about loss of work time, loss of job, increased responsibilities or burden on family members, and the threat of permanent incapacity further

Table 18-3 • Medications With the Potential to Affect the Surgical Experience

AGENT (GENERIC AND TRADE EXAMPLE)	EFFECT OF INTERACTION WITH ANESTHETICS
Corticosteroids Prednisone (Deltasone)	Cardiovascular collapse can occur if discontinued suddenly. Therefore, a bolus of corticosteroid may be administered intravenously immediately before and after surgery.
Diuretics Hydrochlorothiazide (HydroDIURIL)	During anesthesia, may cause excessive respiratory depression resulting from an associated electrolyte imbalance
Phenothiazines Chlorpromazine (Thorazine)	May increase the hypotensive action of anesthetics
Tranquilizers Diazepam (Valium)	May cause anxiety, tension, and even seizures if withdrawn suddenly
Insulin	Interaction between anesthetics and insulin must be considered when a patient with diabetes is undergoing surgery.
Antibiotics Erythromycin (Ery-Tab)	When combined with a curariform muscle relaxant, nerve transmission is interrupted and apnea from respiratory paralysis may result.
Anticoagulants Warfarin (Coumadin)	Can increase the risk of bleeding during the intraoperative and postoperative periods; should be discontinued in anticipation of elective surgery. The surgeon will determine how long before the elective surgery the patient should stop taking an anticoagulant, depending on the type of planned procedure and the medical condition of the patient.
Antiseizure Medications Phenytoin (Dilantin)	An intravenous route of medication may need to be administered to keep the patient seizure-free in the intraoperative and postoperative periods.
Monoamine Oxidase (MAO) Inhibitors Phenelzine sulfate (Nardil)	May increase the hypotensive action of anesthetics

contribute to the emotional strain created by the prospect of surgery. Less obvious concerns may occur because of previous experiences with the health care system and people the patient has known with the same condition.

People express fear in different ways. For example, one patient may repeatedly ask a lot of questions, even though answers were given previously. Another person may withdraw, deliberately avoiding communication, perhaps by reading or watching television. Still others may talk about trivialities. Consequently, the nurse must be empathetic, listen well, and provide information that helps alleviate concerns.

An important outcome of the psychosocial assessment is the determination of the extent and role of the patient's support network. The value and reliability of all available support systems are assessed. Other information, such as usual level of functioning and typical daily activities, may assist in the patient's care and rehabilitation plans. Assessing the patient's readiness to learn and determining the best approach to maximize comprehension will provide the basis for preoperative patient education.

Spiritual and Cultural Beliefs

Spiritual beliefs play an important role in how people cope with fear and anxiety. Regardless of the patient's religious affiliation, spiritual beliefs can be as therapeutic as medication. Every attempt must be made to help the patient obtain the spiritual help that he or she requests. Faith has great sustaining power. Thus, the beliefs of each patient should be respected and supported. Some

nurses avoid the subject of a clergy visit lest the suggestion alarm the patient. Asking if the patient's spiritual advisor knows about the impending surgery is a caring, nonthreatening approach.

Showing respect for a patient's cultural values and beliefs facilitates rapport and trust. Some areas of assessment include identifying the ethnic group to which the patient relates and the customs and beliefs the patient holds about illness and health care providers. For example, patients from some cultural groups are unaccustomed to expressing feelings openly. Nurses need to consider this pattern of communication when assessing pain. As a sign of respect, people from other cultural groups may not make direct eye contact with others. The nurse needs to know that this lack of eye contact is not avoidance or a lack of interest.

Perhaps the most valuable skill at the nurse's disposal is listening carefully to the patient, especially when obtaining the history. Invaluable information and insights may be gained by engaging in conversation and using communication and interviewing skills. An unhurried, understanding, and caring nurse invites confidence on the part of the patient.

Special Considerations

In the preoperative period, attention needs to be paid to patients with special considerations. These may include the patient who is undergoing ambulatory surgery, the geriatric patient, the patient who is obese, the patient with a disability, and the patient undergoing emergency surgery.

THE AMBULATORY SURGERY PATIENT

The brief time the patient and family spend in the ambulatory setting is an important factor in the preoperative period. The nurse must quickly and comprehensively assess and anticipate the patient's needs and at the same time begin planning for discharge and follow-up home care.

The nurse needs to be sure that the patient and family understand that the patient will go first to the preoperative holding area before going to the operating room for the surgical procedure and then will spend some time in the PACU before being discharged home with the family later that day. Other preoperative teaching content should also be verified (see the section later in this chapter on instructing the ambulatory surgery patient) and reinforced as needed. The nurse should ensure that any plans for follow-up home care are in place if needed (Quinn, 1999).

ELDERLY PATIENTS

The older person undergoing surgery may have a combination of chronic illnesses and health problems in addition to the specific one for which surgery is indicated. Elderly people frequently do not report symptoms, perhaps because they fear a serious illness may be diagnosed or because they accept such symptoms as part of the aging process. Subtle clues alert the nurse to underlying problems.

Health care staff must remember that the hazards of surgery for the aged are proportional to the number and severity of coexisting health problems and the nature and duration of the operative procedure. The underlying principle that guides the preoperative assessment, surgical care, and postoperative care is that the aged patient has less physiologic reserve (the ability of an organ to return to normal after a disturbance in its equilibrium) than the younger patient. Cardiac reserves are lower; renal and hepatic functions are depressed; and gastrointestinal activity is likely to be reduced. Dehydration, constipation, and malnutrition may be evident. Sensory limitations, such as impaired vision or hearing and reduced tactile sensitivity, are often the reasons for falls and burns. Therefore, the nurse must be alert to maintaining a safe environment. Arthritis is common in older people and may affect mobility, making it difficult for the patient to turn from one side to the other or ambulate without discomfort. Protective measures include adequate padding for tender areas, moving the patient slowly, protecting bony prominences from prolonged pressure, and providing gentle massage to promote circulation.

The condition of the mouth is important to assess. Dental caries, dentures, and partial plates are particularly significant to the anesthesiologist or anesthetist because decayed teeth or dental prostheses may become dislodged during intubation and occlude the airway.

An additional area to assess in elderly patients is the preoperative level of activity. Research suggests that elderly patients who had hip replacement surgery and who reported performing greater physical activities (including heavy chores) preoperatively can walk greater distances postoperatively than elderly patients who are less physically active prior to surgery (Whitney & Parkman, 2002).

As the body ages, its ability to perspire decreases. Because decreased perspiration leads to dry, itchy skin, which becomes fragile and is easily abraded, precautions are taken when moving an elderly person. Decreased subcutaneous fat makes older people more susceptible to temperature changes. A lightweight cotton blanket is an appropriate cover when an elderly patient is moved to and from the operating room.

Most elderly people have experienced personal illnesses and possibly life-threatening illnesses of friends and family. Such experiences may result in fears about the surgery and about the future. Providing the patient with an opportunity to express these fears enables the patient to gain some peace of mind and a sense of being understood.

Preoperative pain assessment and teaching are important with elderly patients. It is important for nurses to incorporate pain management information and pain communication skills when teaching elderly persons how to obtain greater postoperative pain relief (McDonald, Freeland, Thomas & Moore, 2001).

Because the elderly patient may have greater risks during the perioperative period, the following are critical: (1) skillful preoperative assessment and treatment, (2) skillful anesthesia and surgery, and (3) meticulous and competent postoperative and postanesthesia management.

OBESE PATIENTS

Like age, obesity increases the risk and severity of complications associated with surgery (National Institutes of Health, 2000). During surgery, fatty tissues are especially susceptible to infection. Additionally, obesity increases technical and mechanical problems related to surgery. Therefore, dehiscence (wound separation) and wound infections are more common. Moreover, the obese patient may be more difficult to care for because of the added weight; the patient tends to breathe poorly when supine, which increases the risk of hypoventilation and postoperative pulmonary complications. In addition, abdominal distention, phlebitis, and cardiovascular, endocrine, hepatic, and biliary diseases occur more readily in obese patients (Dudek, 2001). It has been estimated that for each 30 pounds of excess weight, about 25 additional miles of blood vessels are needed, and this places increased demands on the heart.

PATIENTS WITH DISABILITIES

Special considerations for patients with a mental or physical disability include the need for assistive devices, modifications in preoperative teaching, additional assistance with and attention to positioning or transferring, and the effects of the disability on surgery and anesthesia (Quinn, 1999).

Assistive devices include hearing aids, eyeglasses, braces, prostheses, and other devices. Individuals who are hearing-impaired may need a translator or some alternative communication system perioperatively. If they rely on signing or speech (lip) reading, and if their eyeglasses or contact lenses are removed or if health care staff wear surgical masks, these patients will need an alternative method of communication. These needs must be identified as a factor in the preoperative evaluation and clearly communicated to personnel. Specific strategies for accommodating the patient's needs must be identified ahead of time. Ensuring the safety of assistive devices is important; these devices are expensive and likely to be lost.

Most patients are directed to move from the stretcher to the operating room table and back again. In addition to being unable to see or hear instructions, patients with a disability may be unable to move without special devices or a great deal of assistance. The patient with a disability that affects body position (eg, cerebral palsy, post-polio syndrome, and other neuromuscular disorders) may need special positioning during surgery to prevent pain and injury. Moreover, these patients may be unable to sense whether their extremities are positioned incorrectly.

Patients with respiratory problems related to a disability (eg, multiple sclerosis, muscular dystrophy) may experience difficulties unless the problems are made known to the anesthesiologist or anesthetist and adjustments are made. These factors need to be clearly identified in the preoperative period and communicated to the appropriate personnel.

PATIENTS UNDERGOING EMERGENCY SURGERY

Emergency surgeries are unplanned and occur with little time for preparation (Meeker & Rothrock, 1999). The unpredictable nature of trauma and emergency surgery poses unique challenges to the nurse throughout the perioperative period.

All of the previously discussed factors that affect patients preparing to undergo surgery apply to these patients, usually in a very condensed time frame. The preoperative assessment may actually coincide with resuscitation efforts in the emergency department (Meeker & Rothrock, 1999). For the unconscious patient, informed consent and essential information, such as pertinent past medical history and allergies, need to be obtained from a family member, if one is available. A quick visual survey of the patient is essential to identify all sites of injury when the emergency surgery is due to trauma (see Chap. 71 for more information).

The psychological status of the patient undergoing emergency surgery should be assessed quickly if the patient is awake (Meeker & Rothrock, 1999). The patient may have undergone a very frightening experience and may need extra support and explanation of the surgery.

Preoperative Nursing Interventions

PREOPERATIVE TEACHING

Nurses have long recognized the value of preoperative instruction (Fitzpatrick, 1998). Each patient is taught as an individual, with consideration for any unique concerns or needs; the program of instruction should be based on the individual's learning needs (Quinn, 1999). Multiple teaching strategies should be used (eg, verbal, written, return demonstration), depending on the patient's needs and abilities. Preoperative teaching is initiated as soon as possible. It should start in the physician's office and continue until the patient arrives in the operating room.

When and What to Teach

Ideally, instruction is spaced over a period of time to allow the patient to assimilate information and ask questions as they arise. Frequently, teaching sessions are combined with various preparation procedures to allow for an easy and timely flow of information. The nurse should guide the patient through the experience and allow ample time for questions. Some patients may feel too many descriptive details will increase their anxiety level, and the nurse should respect their wish for less detail.

Teaching should go beyond descriptions of the procedure and should include explanations of the sensations the patient will experience. For example, telling the patient only that preoperative medication will relax him or her before the operation is not as effective as also noting that the medication may result in light-

headedness and drowsiness. Knowing what to expect will help the patient anticipate these reactions and thus attain a higher degree of relaxation than might otherwise be expected.

The ideal timing for preoperative teaching is not on the day of surgery but during the preadmission visit when diagnostic tests are performed. At this time, the nurse or resource person answers questions and provides important patient teaching. During this visit, the patient can meet and ask questions of the perioperative nurse, view audiovisuals, receive written materials, and be given the telephone number to call as questions arise closer to the date of surgery. Most institutions provide written instructions (designed to be copied and given to patients) about many types of surgery (Economou & Economou, 1999).

Deep-Breathing, Coughing, and Incentive Spirometers

One goal of preoperative nursing care is to teach the patient how to promote optimal lung expansion and consequent blood oxygenation after anesthesia. The patient assumes a sitting position to enhance lung expansion. The nurse then demonstrates how to take a deep, slow breath and how to exhale slowly. After practicing deep breathing several times, the patient is instructed to breathe deeply, exhale through the mouth, take a short breath, and cough from deep in the lungs (Chart 18-4). The nurse also demonstrates how to use an incentive spirometer, a device that provides measurement and feedback related to breathing effectiveness. In addition to enhancing respiration, these exercises may help the patient to relax.

If there will be a thoracic or abdominal incision, the nurse demonstrates how the incision line can be splinted to minimize pressure and control pain. The patient should put the palms of both hands together, interlacing the fingers snugly. Placing the hands across the incisional site acts as an effective splint when coughing. Additionally, the patient is informed that medications are available to relieve pain and should be taken regularly for pain relief so that effective deep-breathing and coughing exercises can be performed. The goal in promoting coughing is to mobilize secretions so they can be removed. Deep breathing before coughing stimulates the cough reflex. If the patient does not cough effectively, atelectasis (lung collapse), pneumonia, and other lung complications may occur.

Mobility and Active Body Movement

The goals of promoting mobility postoperatively are to improve circulation, prevent venous stasis, and promote optimal respiratory function.

The nurse explains the rationale for frequent position changes after surgery and then shows the patient how to turn from side to side and how to assume the lateral position without causing pain or disrupting intravenous lines, drainage tubes, or other equipment. Any special position the individual patient will need to maintain after surgery (eg, adduction or elevation of an extremity) is discussed, as is the importance of maintaining as much mobility as possible despite restrictions. Reviewing the process before surgery is helpful because the patient may be too uncomfortable after surgery to absorb new information.

Exercises of the extremities include extension and flexion of the knee and hip joints (similar to bicycle riding while lying on the side). The foot is rotated as though tracing the largest possible circle with the great toe (see illustrations in Chart 18-4). The elbow and shoulder are also put through range of motion. At first,

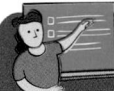

Chart 18-4 • PATIENT EDUCATION
Preoperative Instructions to Prevent Postoperative Complications

Preoperative teaching for patients undergoing surgery includes instruction in breathing and leg exercises used to prevent postoperative complications, such as pneumonia and deep vein thrombosis. These exercises may be performed in the hospital or at home.

Diaphragmatic Breathing
Diaphragmatic breathing refers to a flattening of the dome of the diaphragm during inspiration, with resultant enlargement of the upper abdomen as air rushes in. During expiration, the abdominal muscles contract.
1. Practice in the same position you would assume in bed after surgery: a semi-Fowler's position, propped in bed with the back and shoulders well supported with pillows.
2. With your hands in a loose-fist position, allow the hands to rest lightly on the front of the lower ribs, with your fingertips against lower chest to feel the movement.

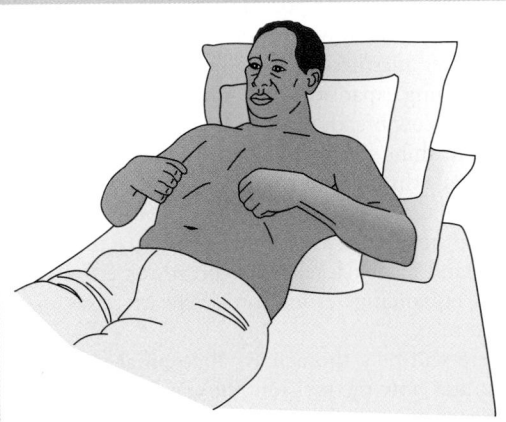

Diaphragmatic breathing

3. Breathe out gently and fully as the ribs sink down and inward toward midline.
4. Then take a deep breath through your nose and mouth, letting the abdomen rise as the lungs fill with air.
5. Hold this breath for a count of five.
6. Exhale and let out *all* the air through your nose and mouth.
7. Repeat this exercise 15 times with a short rest after each group of five.
8. Practice this twice a day preoperatively.

Coughing
1. Lean forward slightly from a sitting position in bed, interlace your fingers together, and place your hands across the incisional site to act as a splintlike support when coughing.

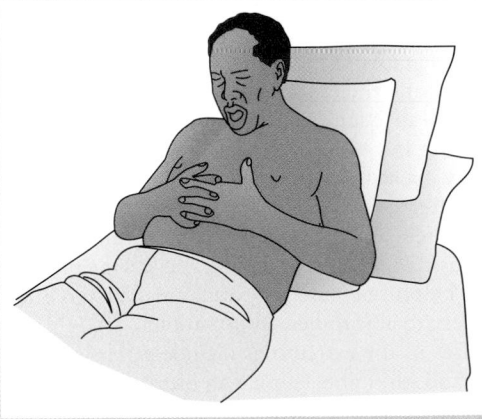

Splinting when coughing

2. Breathe with the diaphragm as described under "Diaphragmatic Breathing."
3. With your mouth slightly open, breathe in fully.
4. "Hack" out sharply for three short breaths.
5. Then, keeping your mouth open, take in a quick deep breath and immediately give a strong cough once or twice. This helps clear secretions from your chest. It may cause some discomfort but will not harm your incision.

Leg Exercises
1. Lie in a semi-Fowler's position and perform the following simple exercises to improve circulation.
2. Bend your knee and raise your foot—hold it a few seconds, then extend the leg and lower it to the bed.

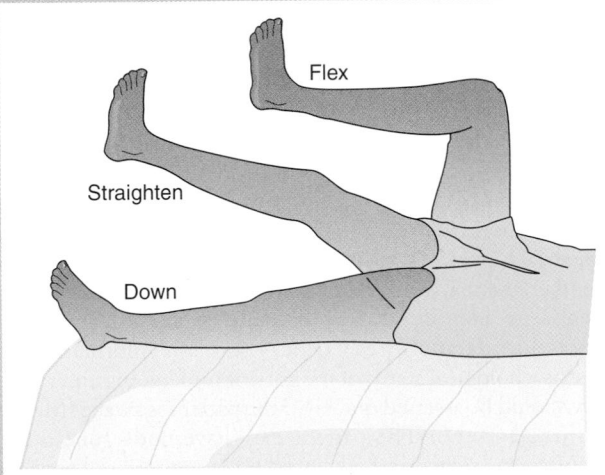

Leg exercises

3. Do this five times with one leg, then repeat with the other leg.
4. Then trace circles with the feet by bending them down, in toward each other, up, and then out.
5. Repeat these movements five times.

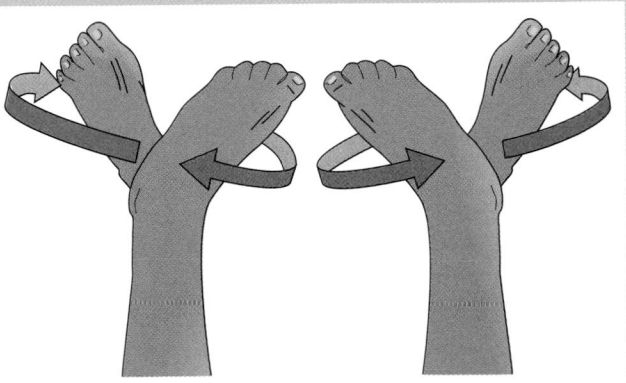

Foot exercises

Turning to the Side
1. Turn on your side with the uppermost leg flexed most and supported on a pillow.
2. Grasp the side rail as an aid to maneuver to the side.
3. Practice diaphragmatic breathing and coughing while on your side.

Getting Out of Bed
1. Turn on your side.
2. Push yourself up with one hand as you swing your legs out of bed.

the patient is assisted and reminded to perform these exercises. Later, the patient is encouraged to do them independently. Muscle tone is maintained so that ambulation will be easier.

The nurse should remember to use proper body mechanics and to instruct the patient to do the same. Whenever the patient is positioned, his or her body needs to be properly aligned.

Pain Management

An assessment should include a determination between acute and chronic pain so that the patient may differentiate postoperative pain from a chronic condition. It is at this point that a pain scale should be introduced and its use explained to the patient. Chapter 13 contains several examples of pain scales.

Postoperatively, medications are administered to relieve pain and maintain comfort without increasing the risk for inadequate air exchange. The patient is instructed to take the medication as frequently as prescribed during the initial postoperative period for pain relief. Anticipated methods of administration of analgesic agents for inpatients include patient-controlled analgesia (PCA), epidural catheter bolus or infusion, or patient-controlled epidural analgesia (PCEA). A patient who is expected to go home would receive oral analgesic agents. These are discussed with the patient before surgery, and the patient's interest and willingness to use those methods are assessed. The patient is instructed in use of a pain intensity rating scale to promote effective postoperative pain management.

Cognitive Coping Strategies

Cognitive strategies may be useful for relieving tension, overcoming anxiety, decreasing fear, and achieving relaxation. Examples of such strategies include the following:

- Imagery—The patient concentrates on a pleasant experience or restful scene.
- Distraction—The patient thinks of an enjoyable story or recites a favorite poem or song.
- Optimistic self-recitation—The patient recites optimistic thoughts ("I know all will go well").

Instruction for Ambulatory Surgical Patients

Preoperative education for the same-day or ambulatory surgical patient comprises all the material presented earlier in this chapter as well as collaborative planning with the patient and family for discharge and follow-up home care. The major difference in outpatient preoperative education is the teaching environment (Quinn, 1999).

Preoperative teaching content may be presented in a group meeting, on a videotape, during night classes, at preadmission testing, or by telephone in conjunction with the preoperative interview. In addition to answering questions and describing what to expect, the nurse tells the patient when and where to report, what to bring (insurance card, list of medications and allergies), what to leave at home (jewelry, watch, medications, contact lenses), and what to wear (loose-fitting, comfortable clothes; flat shoes). The nurse in the surgeon's office may initiate teaching before the perioperative telephone contact.

The last preoperative phone call is designed to remind the patient not to eat or drink as directed. A fasting period of 8 hours or more is recommended for a meal that includes fried or fatty foods or meat (Crenshaw, Winslow & Jacobson, 1999). The anesthesiologist or anesthetist may restrict foods and fluids for

longer periods of time depending on the patient's fluid status, age, and pulmonary status and the nature of the surgical procedure.

The purpose of withholding food before surgery is to prevent aspiration. Aspiration occurs when food or fluid is regurgitated from the stomach and enters the pulmonary system. Such inhaled material, which is a foreign substance, is irritating and causes an inflammatory reaction that interferes with adequate air exchange. Aspiration is a serious problem, and mortality is high (60% to 70%). If the patient is assessed as being at high risk for aspiration, the anesthesiologist or anesthetist prescribes more stringent food and fluid restrictions. Fluids may be administered intravenously

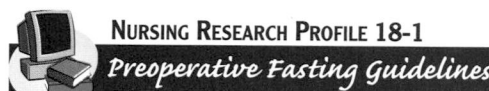

NURSING RESEARCH PROFILE 18-1
Preoperative Fasting Guidelines

Crenshaw, J., & Winslow, E. (2002). Preoperative fasting: Old habits die hard. *American Journal of Nursing, 102*(5), 36–44.

Purpose
In 1999 the American Society of Anesthesiologists (ASA) made the "NPO after Midnight" rule obsolete with revised practice guidelines that support much more liberal preoperative fasting in healthy adults. This study sought to determine if these guidelines had changed preoperative fasting practices.

Study Sample and Design
This was a descriptive study conducted in a 935-bed medical center in the United States. The center did not have a fasting policy. A convenience sample of 155 patients were interviewed about their preoperative fasting, comparing instructed, actual, and ASA-recommended fasting durations for liquids and solids. A semi-structured interview was used by trained staff nurses to collect the data. Subjects were all over 18 years old, admitted to the hospital from home for an elective, nonobstetric or nongastrointestinal surgery. All were in stable condition, had been without an IV infusion for more than 4 hours prior to surgery, were admitted to a noncritical care unit after surgery, and consented to participate. The patients all spoke and understood English; 87% were Caucasian, 7% were African American, and 9.6% were Hispanic, Asian, or of other ethnic origin.

Findings
The patients interviewed fasted from liquids and solids for an average of 12 to 14 hours, with some patients fasting for as long as 20 hours from liquids and 37 hours from solid foods. Ninety-seven percent of the 155 patients fasted from liquids for more than 6 hours. Actual fasting durations were found (using paired t-tests) to be significantly longer than both the instructed fasting durations (mean 10 hours) and the ASA recommendations. Most patients (91%) were instructed to maintain NPO status after midnight. A nurse participated in the preoperative fasting instruction with 63% of the patients. Almost half of the patients rated thirst and worry at a 5 on a 0-to-10 scale.

Nursing Implications
Nurses are an important part of the surgical team and are involved in preoperative fasting instruction with the majority of patients. Therefore, they share the responsibility for recommending excessively long and unnecessary fasting for patients and for patients' lack of understanding of instructions demonstrated in this study. Clear and specific instructions must be given to patients about fasting time for liquids and solids. The rationale for the fasting should also be clearly explained. Patients should be warned that they will feel thirsty and should be taught strategies (as permitted) for coping with thirst, such as brushing teeth, rinsing the mouth, and chewing gum.

in some patients to ensure an adequate fluid volume when oral fluids are restricted.

PREOPERATIVE PSYCHOSOCIAL INTERVENTIONS

Reducing Preoperative Anxiety

Cognitive strategies useful for reducing anxiety were addressed previously in this chapter. In addition to these strategies, music therapy is an easy-to-administer, inexpensive, noninvasive intervention that can reduce anxiety in the perioperative patient. The patient should be allowed to choose his or her own music and be provided with quiet uninterrupted listening time (White, 2000).

The general preoperative teaching addressed earlier in this section will also help decrease anxiety in many patients. Knowing ahead of time about the possible need for a ventilator, drainage tubes, or other types of equipment will help decrease anxiety in the postoperative period.

Decreasing Fear

During the preoperative assessment the nurse should assist the patient to identify coping strategies that he or she has previously used to decrease fear. The patient benefits from knowing when family and friends will be able to visit after surgery and that a spiritual advisor will be available if desired. Research suggests that hypnosis may be a useful strategy for reducing fear and overcoming the anxiety associated with surgery (Hernandez & Tatarunis, 2000).

Respecting Cultural, Spiritual, and Religious Beliefs

Psychosocial interventions include identifying and showing respect for cultural, spiritual, and religious beliefs. In some cultures, for example, individuals are stoic in regard to pain, whereas others are more expressive. These responses should be recognized as normal for those patients and families and respected by perioperative personnel. When patients decline blood transfusions for religious reasons (Jehovah's Witnesses), this information needs to be clearly identified in the preoperative period, documented, and communicated to the appropriate personnel.

GENERAL PREOPERATIVE NURSING INTERVENTIONS

Managing Nutrition and Fluids

The major purpose of withholding food and fluid before surgery is to prevent aspiration. However, studies demonstrate that in patients who do not have a compromised airway or coexisting diseases or disorders that affect gastric emptying or fluid volume (eg, pregnancy, obesity, diabetes, gastroesophageal reflux, enteral tube feeding, ileus or bowel obstruction), lengthy restriction of fluid and food is unnecessary (Crenshaw & Winslow, 2002; Pandit, Loberg & Pandit, 2000). Until recently, fluid and food were restricted preoperatively overnight and often longer. However, recent review of this practice by the American Society of Anesthesiologists has resulted in new recommendations for persons undergoing elective surgery who are otherwise healthy (ASA Task Force on Preoperative Fasting, 1999). The recommendations depend on the age of the patient and type of food eaten. For ex-

ample, adults are advised to fast for 8 hours after eating fatty food and 4 hours after ingesting milk products (Crenshaw, Winslow & Jacobson, 1999; Crenshaw & Winslow, 2002). Most patients are currently allowed clear liquids up to 2 hours before an elective procedure (Crenshaw & Winslow, 2002).

Preparing the Bowel for Surgery

Enemas are not commonly ordered preoperatively unless the patient is undergoing abdominal or pelvic surgery. In this case, a cleansing enema or laxative may be prescribed the evening before surgery and may be repeated the morning of surgery. The goals of this preparation are to allow satisfactory visualization of the surgical site and to prevent trauma to the intestine or contamination of the peritoneum by feces. Unless the condition of the patient presents some contraindication, the toilet or bedside commode, rather than the bedpan, is used for evacuating the enema if the patient is hospitalized during this time. Additionally, antibiotics may be prescribed to reduce intestinal flora.

Preparing the Skin

The goal of preoperative skin preparation is to decrease bacteria without injuring the skin. If the surgery is not performed as an emergency, the patient may be instructed to use a soap containing a detergent-germicide to cleanse the skin area for several days before surgery to reduce the number of skin organisms; this preparation may be carried out at home.

Generally, hair is not removed preoperatively unless the hair at or around the incision site is likely to interfere with the operation. If hair must be removed, electric clippers are used for safe hair removal immediately before the operation.

IMMEDIATE PREOPERATIVE NURSING INTERVENTIONS

The patient changes into a hospital gown that is left untied and open in the back. The patient with long hair may braid it, remove hairpins, and cover the head completely with a disposable paper cap.

The mouth is inspected, and dentures or plates are removed. If left in the mouth, these items could easily fall to the back of the throat during induction of anesthesia and cause respiratory obstruction.

Jewelry is not worn to the operating room; wedding rings and jewelry of body piercings should be removed to prevent injury (Fogg, 2001). If a patient objects to removing a ring, some institutions allow the ring to be securely fastened to the finger with tape. All articles of value, including assistive devices, dentures, glasses, and prosthetic devices, are given to family members or are labeled clearly with the patient's name and stored in a safe place according to the institution's policy.

All patients (except those with urologic disorders) should void immediately before going to the operating room to promote continence during low abdominal surgery and to make abdominal organs more accessible. Urinary catheterization is performed in the operating room as necessary.

Administering Preanesthetic Medication

The use of preanesthetic medication is minimal with ambulatory or outpatient surgery. If prescribed, it is usually administered in the preoperative holding area. If a preanesthetic medication is administered, the patient is kept in bed with the side rails raised because the medication can cause lightheadedness or drowsiness. During this time, the nurse observes the patient for any untoward reaction to the medications. The immediate surroundings are kept quiet to promote relaxation.

Often, surgery is delayed or operating room schedules are changed, and it becomes impossible to request that a medication be given at a specific time. In these situations, the preoperative medication is prescribed "on call from operating room." The nurse can have the medication ready to give and administer it as soon as a call is received from the operating room staff. It usually takes 15 to 20 minutes to prepare the patient for the operating room. If the nurse gives the medication before attending to the other details of preoperative preparation, the patient will have at least partial benefit from the preoperative medication and will have a smoother anesthetic and operative course.

Maintaining the Preoperative Record

A preoperative checklist contains critical elements that need to be checked preoperatively (Meeker & Rothrock, 1999). An example is shown in Figure 18-3. The completed chart accompanies the patient to the operating room with the surgical consent form attached, along with all laboratory reports and nurses' records. Any unusual last-minute observations that may have a bearing on anesthesia or surgery are noted at the front of the chart in a prominent place.

Transporting the Patient to the Presurgical Area

The patient is transferred to the holding area or presurgical suite in a bed or on a stretcher about 30 to 60 minutes before the anesthetic is to be given. The stretcher should be as comfortable as possible, with a sufficient number of blankets to prevent

1. Patient's name: _____ Date: _____ Height: _____ Weight: _____
   Identification band present: _____
2. Informed consent signed: _____ Special permits signed: _____
3. Surgical site: _____ (Ex: Sterilization)
4. History & physical examination report present: _____ Date: _____
5. Laboratory records present: _____
   CBC: _____ Hgb: _____ Urinalysis: _____ Hct: _____

6. Item	Present	Removed
a. Natural teeth		
Dentures; upper, lower, partial		
Bridge, fixed; crown		
b. Contact lenses		
c. Other prostheses—type: _____		
d. Jewelry:		
Wedding band (taped/tied)`		
Rings		
Earrings: pierced, clip-on		
Neck chains		
Any other body piercings		
e. Make-up		
Nail polish		
7. Clothing		
a. Clean patient gown		
b. Cap		
c. Sanitary pad, etc.		

8. Family instructed where to wait? _____
9. Valuables secured? _____
10. Blood available? _____ Ordered? _____ Where? _____
11. Preanesthetic medication given: _____
    Type _____ Time
12. Voided: _____ Amount: _____ Time: _____ Catheter: _____
    Mouth care given: _____
13. Vital signs: Temperature: _____ Pulse: _____ Resp: _____ Blood Pressure: _____
14. Special problems/precautions: (Allergies, deafness, *etc.*): _____
15. Area of skin preparation: _____
16. _____ Date: _____ Time: _____
    Signature: Nurse releasing patient

FIGURE 18-3 Preoperative checklist.

chilling in air-conditioned rooms. A small head pillow is usually provided.

The patient is taken to the preoperative holding area, greeted by name, and positioned comfortably on the stretcher or bed. The surrounding area should be kept quiet if the preoperative medication is to have maximal effect. Unpleasant sounds or conversation should be avoided because a sedated patient who overhears them might misinterpret them.

Patient safety in the preoperative area is a priority. Using a process to verify patient identification, the surgical procedure, and the surgical site maximizes patient safety and allows for early identification and intervention if any discrepancies are identified (Brown, Riippa & Shaneberger, 2001).

> **NURSING ALERT** It is important for someone to be with the preoperative patient at all times. Someone must be present to provide reassurance as well as to ensure safety. Facial expression, or the warm grasp of a hand can communicate reassurance nonverbally.

Attending to Family Needs

Most hospitals and ambulatory surgery centers have a waiting room where the family and significant others can wait while the patient is undergoing surgery. This room may be equipped with comfortable chairs, television, telephones, and facilities for light refreshment. Volunteers may remain with the family, offer them coffee, and keep them informed of the patient's progress. After surgery, the surgeon may meet the family in the waiting room and discuss the outcome.

The family and significant others should never judge the seriousness of an operation by the length of time the patient is in the operating room. A patient may be in surgery much longer than the actual operating time for several reasons:

- Patients are routinely transported well in advance of the actual operating time.
- The anesthesiologist or anesthetist often makes additional preparations that may take 30 to 60 minutes.
- The surgeon may take longer than expected with the preceding case, which delays the start of the next surgical procedure.

After surgery, the patient is taken to the PACU to ensure safe emergence from anesthesia.

Family members and significant others waiting to see the patient after surgery should be informed that the patient may have certain equipment or devices (eg, intravenous lines, indwelling urinary catheter, nasogastric tube, oxygen lines, monitoring equipment, and blood transfusion lines) in place when he or she returns from surgery. When the patient returns to the room, the nurse provides explanations regarding the frequent postoperative observations that will be made. However, it is the responsibility of the surgeon, not the nurse, to relay the surgical findings and the prognosis, even when the findings are favorable.

NURSING PROCESS: CARE OF THE PATIENT IN THE PREOPERATIVE PERIOD

Preoperative assessment of the surgical patient involves evaluating the elements addressed in the previous section on the factors that affect the patient undergoing surgery. A variety of patient problems or nursing diagnoses can be anticipated or identified on the basis of the assessment data.

Assessment

During the preoperative phase of care, nursing assessment usually addresses the following parameters:

- Physical condition, including respiratory, cardiac, and other major body systems as discussed earlier in this chapter
- Results of blood tests, x-ray studies, and other diagnostic tests
- Nutritional and fluid status
- Medication use, as previously described
- Psychological preparedness for surgery (anxiety, fear, spiritual and cultural beliefs)
- Special considerations, including the ambulatory surgery patient, gerontologic considerations, obesity, the patient with a disability, or the patient undergoing emergency surgery, as discussed earlier in this chapter

Diagnosis

NURSING DIAGNOSES

Based on the assessment data, major preoperative nursing diagnoses of the surgical patient may include the following:

- Anxiety related to the surgical experience (anesthesia, pain) and the outcome of surgery
- Fear related to perceived threat of the surgical procedure and separation from support system
- Knowledge deficit of preoperative procedures and protocols and postoperative expectations

COLLABORATIVE PROBLEMS/ POTENTIAL COMPLICATIONS

Failure to identify and communicate pertinent preoperative risk factors may lead to complications.

Planning and Goals

The major goals for the preoperative surgical patient may include relief of preoperative anxiety, decreased fear, increased knowledge of perioperative expectations, and absence of preoperative complications.

Nursing Interventions

REDUCING PREOPERATIVE ANXIETY

Specific nursing interventions are discussed in detail under psychosocial interventions and preoperative teaching in the previous sections.

DECREASING FEAR

Nursing management is discussed under psychosocial interventions in the previous section.

PROVIDING PATIENT EDUCATION

Specific nursing interventions pertaining to preoperative patient education are discussed in detail in earlier sections of this chapter.

MONITORING AND MANAGING POTENTIAL COMPLICATIONS

Nursing interventions to prevent preoperative complications include identification and documentation of factors that affect patients preparing to undergo surgery (discussed earlier in this chapter).

Evaluation

EXPECTED PATIENT OUTCOMES

Expected patient outcomes may include:

1. Reports relief of anxiety
   a. Discusses with anesthesiologist or anesthetist concerns related to types of anesthesia and induction
   b. Verbalizes an understanding of the preanesthetic medication and general anesthesia
   c. Discusses last-minute concerns with nurse or physician
   d. Discusses financial concerns with social worker, when appropriate
   e. Requests visit with member of clergy when appropriate
   f. Relaxes quietly after being visited by health care team members
2. Reports that fear is decreased
   a. Discusses fears with health care professionals
   b. Verbalizes an understanding of the location of family members or significant others during procedure
3. Voices understanding of surgical intervention
   a. Participates in preoperative preparation
   b. Demonstrates and describes exercises he or she is expected to perform postoperatively
   c. Reviews information about postoperative care
   d. Accepts preanesthetic medication, if prescribed
   e. Remains in bed once premedicated
   f. Relaxes during transportation to operating room or unit
   g. States rationale for use of side rails
   h. Discusses postoperative expectations
4. Shows no evidence of preoperative complications.

Critical Thinking Exercises

1. During the preoperative assessment of a man scheduled for hand surgery in an ambulatory setting, you think that the patient's responses indicate that he does not understand the procedure and that he has not made plans for postoperative care. What further assessment and teaching is indicated? What nursing interventions are warranted?

2. A patient with a long history of the use of several herbal supplements is scheduled for major surgery. What effect would this information have on your preoperative care of this patient?

3. Two patients are admitted to the same-day surgery unit for bilateral knee replacements. One patient is a 30-year-old who ambulates with crutches and the other is a 75-year-old who lives alone. How would your assessments, preoperative teaching, and preparation differ for these two patients?

REFERENCES AND SELECTED READINGS

Books

American Society of PeriAnesthesia Nurses. (2000). *Standards of perianesthesia nursing practice.* Thorofare, NJ: ASPAN.

Beyea, S. (Ed.). (2000). *Perioperative nursing data set: The perioperative nursing vocabulary.* Denver: AORN, Inc.

Dudek, S. G. (Ed.). (2001). *Nutrition essentials for nursing practice.* Philadelphia: Lippincott Williams & Wilkins.

Economou, S. G., & Economou, T. S. (1999). *Instructions for surgery patients.* Philadelphia: W. B. Saunders.

Fitzpatrick, J. J. (1998). *Encyclopedia of nursing research.* New York: Springer.

Fortunato, N. H. (2000). *Berry & Kohn's operating room technique.* St. Louis: Mosby, Inc.

Karch, A. (Ed.). (2002). *Nursing drug guide.* Philadelphia: Lippincott Williams & Wilkins.

Kuhn, M. (1999). *Complementary therapies for health care providers.* Philadelphia: Lippincott Williams & Wilkins.

Litwack, K. (Ed.). (1999). *Core curriculum for perianesthesia nursing practice.* Philadelphia: W. B. Saunders.

Meeker, M. H., & Rothrock, J. C. (Eds.). (1999). *Alexander's care of the patient in surgery.* St. Louis: Mosby Year Book.

Merli, G., & Weitz, H. (Eds.). (1998). *Medical management of the surgical patient* (2nd ed.). Philadelphia: W. B. Saunders.

Miller, T. A. (Ed.). (1998). *Modern surgical care: Physiologic foundations and clinical applications.* St. Louis: Quality Medical.

National Institutes of Health, National Heart, Lung and Blood Institute, North American Association for the Study of Obesity. (2000). *The practical guide: Identification, evaluation, and treatment of overweight and obesity in adults.* NIH Publication Number 00-4084. Bethesda, MD.

Quinn, D. M. (Ed.). (1999). *Ambulatory surgical nursing core curriculum.* Philadelphia: W. B. Saunders.

Russell, R., Williams, N., & Bulstrode, C. (Eds.). (2000). *Bailey & Love's short practice of surgery* (23d ed.). New York: Oxford University Press Inc.

Journals

Ambulatory Surgery

Asterisks indicate nursing research articles.

Dunn, D. (1998). Preoperative assessment criteria and patient teaching for ambulatory surgery patients. *Journal of Perianesthesia Nursing, 13*(5), 274–291.

Hession, M. (1998). Factors influencing successful discharge after outpatient laparoscopic cholecystectomy. *Journal of Perianesthesia Nursing, 13*(1), 11–15.

Pandit, S., Loberg, K., & Pandit, U. (2000). Toast and tea before elective surgery? A national survey on current practice. *Anesthesia & Analgesia, 90*(6), 1348–1351.

Yellen, E., & Davis, G. (2001). Patient satisfaction in ambulatory surgery. *AORN Journal, 74*(4), 483–498.

Anesthesia and Surgery

American Society of Anesthesiologists Task Force on Preoperative Fasting (1999). Practice guidelines for preoperative fasting and the use of pharmacologic agents to reduce risk of pulmonary aspiration: Application to healthy patients undergoing elective procedures. *Anesthesiology, 90*(3), 896–905.

Booth, M. (1998). Clinical aspects of CRNA practice: Sedation and monitored anesthesia care. *Nursing Clinics of North America, 31*(3), 667–682.

Braunschweig, C., Gomez, S., & Sheean, P. (2000). Impact of declines in nutritional status on outcomes in adult patients hospitalized for more than 7 days. *Journal of the American Dietetic Association, 100*(11), 1316–1322.

*Crenshaw, J., Winslow, E., & Jacobson, A. (1999). Research for practice: New guidelines for preoperative fasting. *American Journal of Nursing, 99*(4), 49.

Iverson, R. (1999). Sedation and analgesia in ambulatory settings. *Plastic & Reconstructive Surgery, 104*(5), 1559–1564.

Mack, M. (2002). Minimally invasive and robotic surgery. *Journal of the American Medical Association, 285*(5), 568–572.

Perioperative Assessment

Ang-Lee, M., Moss, J., & Yuan, C. (2001). Herbal medicines and perioperative care. *Journal of the American Medical Association, 286*(2), 208–216.

Brown, B., Riippa, M., & Shaneberger, K. (2001). Promoting patient safety through preoperative patient verification. *AORN Journal, 74*(5), 690–694.

Brumly, C. (2000). Herbs and the perioperative patient. *AORN Journal, 72*(5), 783–804.

*Crenshaw, J., & Winslow, E. (2002). Preoperative fasting: Old habits die hard. *American Journal of Nursing, 102*(5), 36–44.

Fogg, D. (2002). Clinical issues: Patient jewelry. *AORN Journal, 74*(2), 249.

Hernandez, A., & Tatarunis, A. (2000). The use of pre-, intra-, and posthypnotic suggestion in anesthesia and surgery. *Clinical Forum for Nurse Anesthetists, 11*(4), 167–72.

King, M. (2000). Preoperative evaluation. *American Family Physician, 62*(2), 387–395.

Little, K. (2000). Screening for domestic violence. *Postgraduate Medicine, 108*(2), 135–141.

Lyons, T. (2002). Herbal medicines and possible anesthesia interactions. *AANA Journal, 70*(1), 47–51.

*McDonald, D., Freeland, M., Thomas, G., & Moore, J. (2001). Testing a preoperative pain management intervention for elders. *Research in Nursing & Health, 24,* 401–409.

Marshall, C., Benton, D., & Brazier, J. (2000). Elder abuse: Using clinical tools to identify clues of mistreatment. *Geriatrics, 55*(2), 42–53.

Miller, K., & Weed, P. (1998). The latex allergy triage or admission tool: An algorithm to identify which patients would benefit from latex precautions. *Journal of Emergency Nursing, 24*(2), 145–152.

Posel, N. (1998). Preoperative teaching in the preadmission clinic. *Journal of Nursing Staff Development, 14*(1), 52–56.

Smetana, G. W. (1999). Preoperative pulmonary evaluation. *New England Journal of Medicine, 340*(12), 937–944.

Shannon-Cain, J., Webster, S., & Cain, B. (2002). Prevalence of and reasons for preoperative tobacco use. *AANA Journal, 70*(1), 33–40.

Tappen, R., Muzic, J., & Kennedy, P. (2001). Preoperative assessment and discharge planning for older adults undergoing ambulatory surgery. *AORN Journal,* 464–470.

White, J. (2000). State of the science of music interventions. *Critical Care Nursing Clinics of North America, 12*(2), 219–225.

Whitney, J., & Parkman, S. (2002). Preoperative physical activity, anesthesia, and analgesia: Effects on early postoperative walking after total hip replacement. *Applied Nursing Research, 15*(1), 19–27.

Zambricki, C. (1998). Clinical aspects of the preanesthetic evaluation. *Nursing Clinics of North America, 31*(3), 607–621.

RESOURCES AND WEBSITES

American Academy of Ambulatory Care Nursing, East Holly Ave., Box 56, Pitman, NJ, 08071; (856) 256-2350; (800) AMB-NURS; http://www.aaacn.org.

American Society of PeriAnesthesia Nurses, 10 Melrose Ave., Suite 110, Cherry Hill, NJ 08003-3696; (877) 9696 (toll-free); fax (856) 616-9621; http://www.aspan.org.

Association of Perioperative Registered Nurses, Inc., 2170 S. Parker Rd., Suite 300, Denver, CO 80231; (856) 616-9600 or 9601; toll-free 1-877-737-9696; http://www.aorn.org.

Intraoperative Nursing Management

On completion of this chapter, the learner will be able to:

1. Describe the interdisciplinary approach to the care of the patient during surgery.
2. Describe the principles of surgical asepsis.
3. Describe various nursing roles as well as the role of the anesthesiologist or anesthetist in the intraoperative phase of care.
4. Identify adverse effects of surgery and anesthesia.
5. Identify the surgical risk factors related to age-specific populations and nursing interventions to reduce those risks.
6. Compare various types of anesthesia with regard to uses, advantages, disadvantages, and nursing responsibilities.
7. Identify the use of the nursing process for optimizing patient outcomes during the intraoperative period.

Anesthesia and surgery place the patient at risk for several complications or adverse events. Consciousness or full awareness, mobility, protective biologic functions, and personal control are totally or partially relinquished by the patient when entering the operating room. Staff from the departments of anesthesia, nursing, and surgery work collaboratively to implement professional standards of care, to control iatrogenic and individual risks, and to promote high-quality patient outcomes.

The Surgical Team

The surgical team consists of the patient, the anesthesiologist or anesthetist, the surgeon, the intraoperative nurses, and the surgical technologists. The anesthesiologist or nurse anesthetist administers the **anesthetic** agent and monitors the patient's physical status throughout the surgery. The surgeon and assistants scrub and perform the surgery. The individual in the scrub role, either a nurse or surgical technologist, provides sterile instruments and supplies to the surgeon during the procedure. The circulating nurse coordinates the care of the patient in the operating room. Care provided by the circulating nurse includes assisting with patient positioning, preparing the patient's skin for surgery, managing surgical specimens, and documenting intraoperative events.

THE PATIENT

As the patient enters the operating room, he or she may feel relaxed and prepared, or fearful and highly stressed. These feelings depend very much on the amount and timing of preoperative sedation and the patient's level of fear and anxiety. Fears about loss of control, the unknown, pain, death, changes in body structure or function, and disruption of lifestyle all may contribute to a generalized anxiety. These fears can increase the amount of anesthetic needed, the level of postoperative pain, and overall recovery time.

The patient is also subject to several risks. Infection, failure of the surgery to relieve symptoms, temporary or permanent complications related to the procedure or the anesthetic, and death are uncommon but potential outcomes of the surgical experience (Chart 19-1). In addition to fears and risks, the patient undergoing sedation and anesthesia temporarily loses both cognitive function and biologic self-protective mechanisms. Loss of pain sense, reflexes, and ability to communicate subjects the intraoperative patient to possible injury.

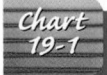

Chart 19-1 **Potential Adverse Effects of Surgery and Anesthesia**

Anesthesia and surgery disrupt all major body systems. Although most patients can compensate for surgical trauma and the effects of anesthesia, all patients are at risk during the operative procedure. These risks include the following:

- Cardiac dysrhythmia from electrolyte imbalance or adverse effect of anesthetic agents
- Myocardial depression, bradycardia, and circulatory collapse from toxic levels of local anesthetics
- Central nervous system agitation, seizures, and respiratory arrest from toxic levels of local anesthetics
- Oversedation or undersedation during moderate sedation
- Agitation or disorientation, especially in elderly patients
- Hypoxemia or hypercarbia from hypoventilation and inadequate respiratory support during anesthesia
- Laryngeal trauma, oral trauma, and broken teeth from difficult intubation
- Hypothermia from cool operating room temperatures, exposure of body cavities, and impaired thermoregulation secondary to anesthetic agents
- Hypotension from blood loss or adverse effect of anesthesia
- Infection
- Thrombosis from compression of blood vessels or stasis
- Malignant hyperthermia secondary to adverse effect of anesthesia
- Nerve damage, skin breakdown from prolonged or inappropriate positioning
- Electrical shock or burns
- Laser burns
- Drug toxicity, faulty equipment, and human error

 Gerontologic Considerations

Elderly patients face higher risks from anesthesia and surgery than younger adult patients (Polanczyk et al., 2001). Statistically, perioperative risk increases with each decade over 60 years, often because of the increased incidence of coexisting disease. Modifications tailored to the biologic changes of later life and the application of research findings for this population can reduce the risks.

Glossary

anesthesia: a state of narcosis, analgesia, relaxation, and loss of reflexes

anesthesiologist: physician trained to deliver anesthesia and to monitor the patient's condition during surgery

anesthetic: the substance, such as a chemical or gas, used to induce anesthesia

anesthetist: health care professional, such as a nurse anesthetist, who is trained to deliver anesthesia and to monitor the patient's condition during surgery

circulating nurse (or circulator): registered nurse who coordinates and documents patient care in the operating room

moderate sedation: use of sedation to depress the level of consciousness without altering the patient's ability to maintain a patent airway and to respond to physical stimuli and verbal commands

restricted zone: area in the operating room where scrub attire and surgical masks are required; includes operating room and sterile core areas

scrub role: registered nurse, licensed practical nurse, or surgical technologist who scrubs and dons sterile surgical attire, prepares instruments and supplies, and hands

instruments to the surgeon during the procedure

semirestricted zone: area in the operating room where scrub attire is required; may include areas where surgical instruments are processed

surgical asepsis: absence of microorganisms in the surgical environment to reduce the risk for infection

unrestricted zone: area in the operating room that interfaces with other departments; includes patient reception area and holding area

Biologic variations of particular importance include age-related cardiovascular and pulmonary changes (Townsend, 2002). The aging heart and blood vessels have decreased ability to respond to stress. Reduced cardiac output and limited cardiac reserve make the elderly patient vulnerable to changes in circulating volume and blood oxygen levels. Excessive or rapid administration of intravenous solutions may cause pulmonary edema. A sudden or prolonged drop in blood pressure may lead to cerebral ischemia, thrombosis, embolism, infarction, and anoxia. Reduced gas exchange can lead to cerebral hypoxia.

The elderly patient needs fewer anesthetics to produce anesthesia and eliminates the anesthetic agent over a longer time than a younger patient. As people age, the percentage of lean body tissue decreases and fatty tissue steadily increases (from age 20 years to 90 years). Anesthetic agents that have an affinity for fatty tissue concentrate in body fat and the brain (Dudek, 2001). Lower doses of anesthetic are appropriate for another reason. The older patient, particularly when malnourished, may have low plasma protein levels. With decreased plasma proteins, more of the anesthetic agent remains free or unbound, and the result is more potent action.

Also in elderly adults, body tissues made up predominantly of water and those with a rich blood supply, such as skeletal muscle, liver, and kidneys, shrink. Reduced liver size decreases the rate at which the liver can inactivate many anesthetics, whereas decreased kidney function slows elimination of waste products and anesthetics. Other factors affecting the elderly surgical patient in the intraoperative period include the following:

- Impaired ability to increase metabolic rate and impaired thermoregulatory mechanisms increase susceptibility to hypothermia.
- Bone loss (25% in women, 12% in men) necessitates careful manipulation and positioning during surgery.
- Reduced ability to adjust rapidly to emotional and physical stress influences surgical outcomes and requires meticulous observation of vital functions.

As expected, mortality is higher with emergency surgery (commonly required for traumatic injuries) than with elective surgery, making continuous and careful monitoring and prompt intervention especially important for older surgical patients (Phippen & Wells, 2000).

Nursing Care

Throughout surgery, nursing responsibilities include providing for the safety and well-being of the patient, coordinating the operating room personnel, and performing scrub and circulating activities. Because the patient's emotional state remains a concern, the care begun by preoperative nurses is continued by the intraoperative nursing staff, who provide the patient with information and realistic reassurance. The nurse supports coping strategies and reinforces the patient's ability to influence outcomes by encouraging his or her active participation in the plan of care.

In the role of patient advocate, intraoperative nurses monitor factors that can cause injury, such as patient position, equipment malfunction, and environmental hazards, and they protect patients' dignity and interests while they are anesthetized. Additional responsibilities include maintaining surgical standards of care, identifying existing patient risk factors, and assisting in modifying complicating factors to help reduce operative risk (Phippen & Wells, 2000).

THE CIRCULATING NURSE

The **circulating nurse** (also known as the **circulator**) must be a registered nurse. He or she manages the operating room and protects the patient's safety and health by monitoring the activities of the surgical team, checking the operating room conditions, and continually assessing the patient for signs of injury and implementing appropriate interventions. The main responsibilities include verifying consent, coordinating the team, and ensuring cleanliness, proper temperature, humidity, and lighting; the safe functioning of equipment; and the availability of supplies and materials. The circulating nurse monitors aseptic practices to avoid breaks in technique while coordinating the movement of related personnel (medical, radiography, and laboratory) as well as implementing fire safety precautions (Phippen & Wells, 2000). The circulating nurse monitors the patient and documents specific activities throughout the operation to ensure the patient's safety and well-being. Nursing activities directly relate to preventing complications and achieving optimal patient outcomes.

THE SCRUB ROLE

Activities of the **scrub role** include performing a surgical hand scrub; setting up the sterile tables; preparing sutures, ligatures, and special equipment (such as a laparoscope); and assisting the surgeon and the surgical assistants during the procedure by anticipating the instruments that will be required, such as sponges, drains, and other equipment (Phippen & Wells, 2000). As the surgical incision is closed, the scrub person and the circulator count all needles, sponges, and instruments to be sure they are accounted for and not retained as a foreign body in the patient. Tissue specimens obtained during surgery must also be labeled by the scrub person and sent to the laboratory by the circulator.

THE SURGEON

The surgeon performs the surgical procedure and heads the surgical team. He or she is a licensed physician (MD), osteopath (DO), oral surgeon (DDS or DMD), or podiatrist (DPM) who is specially trained and qualified. Qualifications may include certification by a specialty board, adherence to Joint Commission on Accreditation of Healthcare Organizations (JCAHO) standards, and adherence to hospital standards and admitting practices and procedures (Fortunato, 2000).

THE REGISTERED NURSE FIRST ASSISTANT

The registered nurse first assistant (RNFA) is another member of the operating room staff. Although the scope of practice of the RNFA depends on each state's nurse practice act, the RNFA practices under the direct supervision of the surgeon. RNFA responsibilities may include handling tissue, providing exposure at the operative field, suturing, and providing hemostasis. The entire process requires a thorough understanding of anatomy and physiology, tissue handling, and the principles of **surgical asepsis**. The competent RNFA needs to be aware of the objectives of the surgery, needs to have the knowledge and ability to anticipate needs and to work as a skilled member of a team, and needs to be able to handle any emergency situation in the operating room (Fortunato, 2000; Rothrock, 1999).

THE ANESTHESIOLOGIST AND ANESTHETIST

An **anesthesiologist** is a physician specifically trained in the art and science of anesthesiology. An **anesthetist** is a qualified health care professional who administers anesthetics. Most anesthetists are nurses who have graduated from an accredited nurse anesthesia program and have passed examinations sponsored by the American Association of Nurse Anesthetists to become a certified registered nurse anesthetist (CRNA). The anesthesiologist or anesthetist interviews and assesses the patient prior to surgery, selects the anesthesia, administers it, intubates the patient if necessary, manages any technical problems related to the administration of the anesthetic agent, and supervises the patient's condition throughout the surgical procedure. Before the patient enters the operating room, often at preadmission testing, the anesthesiologist or anesthetist visits the patient to provide information and answer questions. The type of anesthetic to be administered, previous reactions to anesthetics, and known anatomic abnormalities that would make airway management difficult are discussed. The anesthesiologist or anesthetist uses the American Society of Anesthesiologists (ASA) Physical Status Classification System to determine the patient's status (Chart 19-2).

When the patient arrives in the operating room, the anesthesiologist or anesthetist reassesses the patient's physical condition immediately prior to initiating anesthesia. The anesthetic is administered, and the patient's airway is maintained either through a laryngeal mask airway (LMA) or an endotracheal tube. During surgery, the anesthesiologist or anesthetist monitors the patient's blood pressure, pulse, and respirations as well as the electrocardiogram (ECG), blood oxygen saturation level, tidal volume, blood gas levels, blood pH, alveolar gas concentrations, and body temperature. Monitoring by electroencephalography is some-

times required. Levels of anesthetics in the body can also be determined; a mass spectrometer can provide instant readouts of critical concentration levels on display terminals. The device also assesses the patient's ability to breathe unassisted and indicates the need for mechanical assistance when ventilation is poor and the patient is not breathing well independently.

The Surgical Environment

The surgical environment is known for its stark appearance and cool temperature. The surgical suite is behind double doors, and access is limited to authorized personnel. External precautions include adhering to principles of surgical asepsis; strict control of the operating room (OR) environment is required, including traffic pattern restrictions. Policies governing this environment address such issues as the health of the staff; the cleanliness of the rooms; the sterility of equipment and surfaces; processes for scrubbing, gowning, and gloving; and OR attire.

To provide the best possible conditions for surgery, the OR is situated in a location that is central to all supporting services (eg, pathology, radiology, laboratory). The OR has special air filtration devices to screen out contaminating particles, dust, and pollutants. The temperature, humidity, and airflow patterns are controlled (Meeker et al., 1999).

Electrical hazards, emergency exit clearances, and storage of equipment and anesthetic gases are monitored periodically by official entities, such as state agencies and JCAHO. To help decrease microbes, the surgical area is divided into three zones: the **unrestricted zone**, where street clothes are allowed; the **semi-restricted zone**, where attire consists of scrub clothes and caps; and the **restricted zone**, where scrub clothes, shoe covers, caps, and masks are worn. The surgeons and other surgical team members wear additional sterile clothing and protective devices during the operation.

The Association of PeriOperative Registered Nurses, formerly known as the Association of Operating Room Nurses (and still abbreviated as AORN), recommends specific practices for those wearing surgical attire to promote a high level of cleanliness in a particular practice setting (AORN, 2002). OR attire includes close-fitting cotton dresses, pantsuits, jumpsuits, and gowns. Knitted cuffs on sleeves and pant legs prevent organisms shed from the perineum, legs, and arms from being released into the immediate surroundings. Shirts and waist drawstrings should be tucked inside the pants to prevent accidental contact with sterile areas and to contain skin shedding. Wet or soiled garments should be changed.

Masks are worn at all times in the restricted zone of the OR. High-filtration masks decrease the risk for postoperative wound infection by containing and filtering microorganisms from the oropharynx and nasopharynx. Masks should fit tightly, should cover the nose and mouth completely, and should not interfere with breathing, speech, or vision. Masks must be adjusted to prevent venting from the sides. Disposable masks have a filtration efficiency exceeding 95%. Masks are changed between patients and should not be worn outside the surgical department. The mask must be either on or off; it must not be allowed to hang around the neck.

Headgear should completely cover the hair (head and neckline, including beard) so that single strands of hair, bobby pins, clips, and particles of dandruff or dust do not fall on the sterile field.

Shoes should be comfortable and supportive. Shoes worn in from the outside must be covered with disposable shoe covers for protection from soiling. Shoe covers are worn one time only and are removed upon leaving the restricted area.

Chart 19-2	**American Society of Anesthesiologists Physical Status Classification System**

Anesthetists and anesthesiologists use the American Society of Anesthesiologists Physical (P) Status Classification System to describe the patient's general status and identify potential risks during surgery. There are five classes of physical status.

- **P 1.** A normally healthy patient
  Example: No systemic abnormality, localized infection without fever, benign tumor, hernia
- **P 2.** A patient with mild systemic disease
  Example: Well-controlled hypertension, well-controlled diabetes mellitus, chronic bronchitis, obesity, age over 80 yr
- **P 3.** A patient with severe systemic disease that is not incapacitating
  Example: Severe disease, compensated heart failure, myocardial infarction more than 6 mo ago, angina pectoris, severe dysrhythmia, cirrhosis, poorly controlled diabetes or hypertension, ileus
- **P 4.** A patient with an incapacitating systemic disease that is a constant threat to life
  Example: Severe heart failure, myocardial infarction less than 6 mo ago, severe respiratory failure, advanced liver or renal failure
- **P 5.** A moribund patient who is not expected to survive for 24 hours with or without operation
  Example: Unconscious patient with traumatic head injury and agonal cardiac rhythm

Barriers such as scrub attire and masks do not entirely protect the patient from microorganisms. Upper respiratory tract infections, sore throats, and skin infections in staff and patients are sources of pathogens and must be reported.

> **NURSING ALERT** Good health is essential for any person in the OR, and any perioperative team member with an infectious disease (eg, an upper respiratory tract infection or infected skin lesion) should not have direct patient contact. Until the infectious process has resolved, the perioperative team member should not work in the OR.

Because artificial fingernails harbor microorganisms and may cause nosocomial infections (Winslow & Jacobson, 2000), a ban on artificial nails by OR personnel is supported by the Centers for Disease Control and Prevention (CDC), AORN, and the Association of Professionals in Infection Control. Short, natural fingernails are encouraged (Winslow & Jacobson, 2000).

PRINCIPLES OF SURGICAL ASEPSIS

Surgical asepsis prevents the contamination of surgical wounds. The patient's natural skin flora or a previously existing infection may cause postoperative wound infection. Rigorous adherence to the principles of surgical asepsis by OR personnel is the foundation of preventing surgical site infections.

All surgical supplies, any instruments, needles, sutures, dressings, gloves, covers, and solutions that may come in contact with the surgical wound and exposed tissues, must be sterilized before use (Meeker & Rothrock, 1999; Townsend, 2002). Traditionally, the surgeon, surgical assistants, and nurses prepared themselves by scrubbing their hands and arms with antiseptic soap and water, but this traditional practice is being challenged by research investigating the optimal length of time to scrub and the best preparation to use (Larsen et al., 2001). (See Nursing Research Profile 19-1.)

Surgical team members wear long-sleeved sterile gowns and gloves. Head and hair are covered with a cap, and a mask is worn over the nose and mouth to minimize the possibility that bacteria from the upper respiratory tract will enter the wound. During surgery, the personnel who have scrubbed, gloved, and gowned touch only sterilized objects. Nonscrubbed personnel refrain from touching or contaminating anything sterile.

An area of the patient's skin considerably larger than that requiring exposure during the surgery is meticulously cleansed, and an antimicrobial agent is applied. If hair needs to be removed, it is done immediately prior to the procedure to minimize the risk of wound infection (Townsend, 2002). The remainder of the patient's body is covered with sterile drapes.

Environmental Controls

In addition to the protocols described previously, surgical asepsis requires meticulous cleaning and maintenance of the OR environment. Floors and horizontal surfaces are cleaned frequently with detergent, soap, and water, or a detergent germicide. Sterilizing equipment is inspected regularly to ensure optimal operation and performance.

All equipment that comes into direct contact with the patient must be sterile (Townsend, 2002). Sterilized linens, drapes, and solutions are used. Instruments are cleaned and sterilized in a unit near the operating room. Individually wrapped sterile items are used when additional individual items are needed.

Airborne bacteria are a concern. To decrease the amount of bacteria in the air, standard OR ventilation provides 15 air exchanges per hour (Meeker & Rothrock, 1999). Staff members shed skin scales, resulting in about 1,000 bacteria-carrying particles (or colony-forming units [CFUs]) per cubic foot per minute. With the standard air exchanges, air counts of bacteria are reduced to 50 to 150 CFUs per cubic foot per minute. The number of personnel and unnecessary physical movements may be restricted to minimize bacteria in the air and achieve an OR infection rate no greater than 3% to 5% in clean, infection-prone surgery.

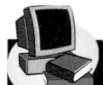

NURSING RESEARCH PROFILE 19-1

New Techniques for Surgical Hand Preparation

Larsen, E., Aiello, A., Heilman, J., Lyle, C., Cronquist, A., Stahl, J., & Dello-Latta, P. (2001). Comparison of different regimens for surgical hand preparation. *AORN Journal, 73*(2), 412–432.

Purpose
Staff members traditionally perform a lengthy regimen of scrubbing with an antiseptic agent before surgery, mostly due to concerns about reducing the risk for infection. The purpose of this study was to compare the traditional scrubbing technique in the operating room to a waterless hand preparation in terms of antimicrobial effectiveness, effect on skin condition, and time requirements.

Study Sample and Design
This was a 6-week, single-center, prospective clinical trial. Twenty surgical staff members used the waterless hand preparation for 3 weeks, had a 1-week hiatus, then used the traditional surgical scrub for 3 consecutive weeks. A reference group of five subjects was also included in the study, which was conducted at a 2,000-bed medical center in three operating suites. The participants were full-time surgical staff members who performed an average of at least 10 scrubs per week and ranged in age from 18 to 65 years of age. The three tools used to measure skin condition consisted of the visual scoring of skin, erythema grading scale, and the hand skin assessment. A total of 13 microbial skin counts were taken of each subject's hands during the study.

Findings
The waterless hand preparation was associated with less skin damage and lower microbial skin counts on days 5 and 19 compared to the traditional scrub. The researchers suggest that a lengthy scrub, as well as the use of a brush or sponge, appears to be counterproductive, causing skin damage and increased skin shedding. The waterless hand preparation protocol had shorter contact time (mean 80.7 seconds) compared to the traditional protocol (mean 145 seconds) and was preferred by the participants. They reported that it was easier, faster, milder on the hands, and conducive to donning gloves.

Nursing Implications
The waterless hand preparation performed better compared to the traditional surgical scrub, but nurses should keep in mind that this was a small study. The results of this study warrant evaluation of this new technique in a larger clinical trial before consideration for widespread implementation.

Some ORs have laminar airflow units. These units provide 400 to 500 air exchanges per hour. When used appropriately, laminar airflow units result in less than 10 CFUs per cubic foot per minute during surgery. The goal for a laminar flow-equipped OR is an infection rate under 1%. An OR equipped with this unit is frequently used for total joint replacement or organ transplant surgery.

Despite all these precautions, wound contamination may occur during surgery but may only become apparent days or weeks later in the form of an incisional infection or abscess. Constant surveillance and conscientious technique in carrying out aseptic practices is necessary to reduce the risk for contamination and infection.

Basic Guidelines for Maintaining Surgical Asepsis

All practitioners involved in the intraoperative phase have a responsibility to provide and maintain a safe environment. Adherence to aseptic practice is part of this responsibility. The eight basic principles of aseptic technique follow:

- All materials in contact with the surgical wound and used within the sterile field must be sterile. Sterile surfaces or articles may touch other sterile surfaces or articles and remain sterile; contact with unsterile objects at any point renders a sterile area contaminated.
- Gowns of the surgical team are considered sterile in front from the chest to the level of the sterile field. The sleeves are also considered sterile from 2 inches above the elbow to the stockinette cuff.
- Sterile drapes are used to create a sterile field. Only the top surface of a draped table is considered sterile. During draping of a table or patient, the sterile drape is held well above the surface to be covered and is positioned from front to back.
- Items should be dispensed to a sterile field by methods that preserve the sterility of the items and the integrity of the sterile field. After a sterile package is opened, the edges are considered unsterile. Sterile supplies, including solutions, are delivered to a sterile field or handed to a scrubbed person in such a way that the sterility of the object or fluid remains intact.
- The movements of the surgical team are from sterile to sterile areas and from unsterile to unsterile areas. Scrubbed persons and sterile items contact only sterile areas; circulating nurses and unsterile items contact only unsterile areas.
- Movement around a sterile field must not cause contamination of the field. Sterile areas must be kept in view during movement around the area. At least a 1-foot distance from the sterile field must be maintained to prevent inadvertent contamination.
- Whenever a sterile barrier is breached, the area must be considered contaminated. A tear or puncture of the drape permitting access to an unsterile surface underneath renders the area unsterile. Such a drape must be replaced.
- Every sterile field should be constantly monitored and maintained. Items of doubtful sterility are considered unsterile. Sterile fields should be prepared as close as possible to the time of use.

HEALTH HAZARDS ASSOCIATED WITH THE SURGICAL ENVIRONMENT

Safety issues in the OR include exposure to blood and body fluids, hazards associated with laser beams, and exposure to latex, radiation, and toxic agents. Internal monitoring of the OR includes the analysis of surface swipe samples and air samples for infectious and toxic agents. In addition, policies and procedures for minimizing exposure to body fluids and reducing the dangers associated with lasers and radiation have been established.

Laser Risks

The AORN has recommended practices for laser safety (AORN, 2002). While lasers are in use, warning signs should be clearly posted to alert personnel. Among the safety issues are the following: reducing the possibility of exposing the eyes and skin to laser beams, preventing inhalation of the laser plume (smoke and particulate matter), and protecting the patient and personnel from fire and electrical hazards. Because several types of lasers are available for clinical use, perioperative personnel should be familiar with the unique features, specific operation, and safety measures for each type of laser used in the practice setting (Townsend, 2002).

Nurses and other intraoperative personnel working with lasers must have a thorough eye examination before participating in procedures involving lasers. Special protective goggles, specific to the type of laser used in the procedure, are worn. There is controversy about the protection needed to avoid the laser plume and effects of its inhalation. Smoke evacuators are used in some procedures to remove the laser plume from the operative field. In recent years this technology has been applied to protect the surgical team from the hazards associated with the generalized smoke plume generated by standard electrocautery units.

Exposure to Blood and Body Fluids

Since the advent of the acquired immunodeficiency syndrome (AIDS) epidemic, OR attire has changed dramatically. Double gloving is routine, at least in trauma surgery where sharp bone fragments are present. In addition to the routine scrub suit and double gloves, some surgeons wear rubber boots, a waterproof apron, and sleeve protectors. Goggles, or a wrap-around face shield, are worn to protect against splashing when the surgical wound is irrigated or when bone drilling is performed. In hospitals where numerous total joint procedures are performed, a full bubble mask may be used. This mask provides full barrier protection from bone fragments and splashes. Safe ventilation is accomplished through an accompanying hood with a separate air-filtration system.

Latex Allergy

Both the AORN and the American Society of Perianesthesia Nurses (ASPAN) have recommended standards of care for the patient with latex allergy (AORN, 2002; ASPAN, 2000). These recommendations include early identification of the patient with a latex allergy, preparation of a latex allergy supply cart, and maintenance of latex allergy precautions throughout the perioperative period. Due to the increased number of patients with latex allergies, many latex-free products are now available. For safety, manufacturers and hospital material managers need to take responsibility for identifying the latex content in items used by patients and health care personnel. (see Chaps. 18 and 53 for assessment for latex allergy).

NURSING ALERT It is the responsibility of all nurses, and particularly perianesthesia and perioperative nurses, to be aware of latex allergies, necessary precautions, and products that are latex-free (Meeker & Rothrock, 1999). Hospital staff are also at risk for developing a latex allergy secondary to repeated exposure to latex products.

The Surgical Experience

During the surgical procedure, the patient will need sedation, anesthesia, or a combination of these.

SEDATION AND ANESTHESIA

Sedation and anesthesia have four levels: minimal sedation, moderate sedation, deep sedation, and anesthesia. Standards of care for each level have been set by JCAHO. A surgical procedure may also be performed using anesthetic agents that suspend sensation in parts of the body (local, regional, epidural, or spinal anesthesia).

For the patient, the anesthesia experience consists of having an intravenous line inserted, if it was not inserted earlier; receiving a sedating agent prior to induction with an anesthetic agent; losing consciousness; being intubated, if indicated; and then receiving a combination of anesthetic agents. Typically the experience is a smooth one and the patient has no recall of the events.

Minimal Sedation

The minimal sedation level is a drug-induced state during which the patient can respond normally to verbal commands. Cognitive function and coordination may be impaired, but ventilatory and cardiovascular functions are not affected (JCAHO, 2001; Patterson, 2000a, b).

Moderate Sedation

Moderate sedation is a form of anesthesia that may be produced intravenously. It is defined as a depressed level of consciousness that does not impair the patient's ability to maintain a patent airway and to respond appropriately to physical stimulation and verbal command. Its goal is a calm, tranquil, amnesic patient who, when sedation is combined with analgesic agents, is relatively pain-free during the procedure but able to maintain protective reflexes (JCAHO, 2001; Patterson, 2000a, b). Sedation can be administered by an anesthesiologist, anesthetist, other physician, or nurse. When administered by an anesthesiologist or anesthetist, moderate sedation is referred to as monitored anesthesia care. The medications permitted for use in moderate sedation vary with the credentials of the person administering the sedative. In addition, state departments of health are very specific about who may administer moderate sedation and about the training required for those individuals. These regulations vary greatly from state to state.

Midazolam (Versed) or diazepam (Valium) is used frequently for intravenous sedation. In some states, the physician must administer the first dose; a nurse with special training can administer subsequent doses. Other medications used include analgesic agents (eg, morphine, fentanyl) and reversal agonists, such as naloxone (Narcan). A nurse who is knowledgeable and skilled in detecting dysrhythmias, administering oxygen, and performing resuscitation must continuously monitor the patient who receives sedation. The patient receiving this form of anesthesia is never left alone and is closely monitored for respiratory, cardiovascular, and central nervous system depression using such methods as pulse oximetry, ECG, and frequent measurement of vital signs (Patterson, 2000a, b). The level of sedation is monitored by the patient's ability to maintain a patent airway and to respond to verbal commands.

Moderate sedation may be used alone or in combination with local, regional, or spinal anesthesia. Its use is increasing as more surgical procedures and diagnostic studies are performed in ambulatory and same-day settings with the expectation that the patient will be discharged home a few hours after the procedure.

Deep Sedation

Deep sedation is a drug-induced state during which a patient cannot be easily aroused but can respond purposefully after repeated stimulation (JCAHO, 2001). The difference between deep sedation and anesthesia is that the anesthetized patient is not arousable. Deep sedation and anesthesia are achieved when an anesthetic agent is inhaled or administered intravenously. Inhaled anesthetic agents include volatile liquid agents and gases (Aranda & Hanson, 2000; Townsend, 2002). Volatile liquid anesthetics produce anesthesia when their vapors are inhaled. Included in this group are halothane (Fluothane), enflurane (Ethrane), isoflurane (Forane), sevoflurane (Ultrane), and desflurane (Suprane). All are administered with oxygen, and usually with nitrous oxide as well.

Gas anesthetics are administered by inhalation and are always combined with oxygen. Nitrous oxide is the most commonly used gas anesthetic. When inhaled, the anesthetics enter the blood through the pulmonary capillaries and act on cerebral centers to produce loss of consciousness and sensation. When anesthetic administration is discontinued, the vapor or gas is eliminated through the lungs. Table 19-1 lists the advantages, disadvantages, and implications of the different volatile liquid and gas anesthetics.

Anesthesia

General anesthesia consists of four stages, each associated with specific clinical manifestations. When opioid agents (narcotics) and neuromuscular blockers (relaxants) are administered, several of the stages are absent. The anesthesia level consists of general anesthesia and spinal or major regional anesthesia but does not include local anesthesia (JCAHO, 2001). **Anesthesia** is a state of narcosis (severe central nervous system depression produced by pharmacologic agents), analgesia, relaxation, and reflex loss. Patients under general anesthesia are not arousable, even to painful stimuli. They lose the ability to maintain ventilatory function and require assistance in maintaining a patent airway. Cardiovascular function may be impaired as well (JCAHO, 2001).

STAGE I: BEGINNING ANESTHESIA

As the patient breathes in the anesthetic mixture, warmth, dizziness, and a feeling of detachment may be experienced. The patient may have a ringing, roaring, or buzzing in the ears and, though still conscious, may sense an inability to move the extremities easily. During this stage, noises are exaggerated; even low voices or minor sounds seem loud and unreal. For this reason, the nurse avoids making unnecessary noises or motions when anesthesia begins.

STAGE II: EXCITEMENT

The excitement stage, characterized variously by struggling, shouting, talking, singing, laughing, or crying, is often avoided if the anesthetic is administered smoothly and quickly. The pupils dilate, but contract if exposed to light; the pulse rate is rapid, and respirations may be irregular.

Because of the possibility of uncontrolled movements of the patient during this stage, the anesthesiologist or anesthetist must always be assisted by someone ready to help restrain the patient. A strap may be in place across the patient's thighs, and the hands may be secured to an armboard. The patient should not be touched except for purposes of restraint, but restraints should not be applied over the operative site. Manipulation increases circulation to the operative site and thereby increases the potential for bleeding.

Table 19-1 • Inhalation Anesthetic Agents

AGENT	ADMINISTRATION	ADVANTAGES	DISADVANTAGES	IMPLICATIONS/ CONSIDERATIONS
Volatile Liquids				
halothane (Fluothane)	Inhalation; special vaporizer	Not explosive or flammable Induction rapid and smooth Useful in almost every type of surgery Low incidence of postoperative nausea and vomiting	Requires skillful administration to prevent overdosage May cause liver damage May produce hypotension Requires special vaporizer for administration	In addition to observation of pulse and respiration postoperatively, blood pressure must be monitored frequently.
methoxyflurane (Penthrane)	Inhalation; special vaporizer	Nonflammable Seldom causes postoperative nausea and vomiting Analgesic action continues several hours after surgery Excellent muscle relaxation	Requires skillful administration Renal damage may occur. Unpleasant odor	Prolonged postoperative depressant action calls for careful observation by PACU personnel.
enflurane (Ethrane)	Inhalation	Rapid induction and recovery Potent analgesic Not explosive or flammable	Respiratory depression may develop rapidly, along with ECG abnormalities. Not compatible with epinephrine	Observe for possible respiratory depression. Administration with epinephrine may cause ventricular fibrillation.
isoflurane (Forane)	Inhalation	Rapid induction and recovery Muscle relaxants are markedly potentiated.	A profound respiratory depressant	Respirations must be monitored closely and supported when necessary.
sevoflurane (Ultrane)	Inhalation	Rapid induction and excretion; minimal side effects	Coughing and laryngospasm; trigger for malignant hyperthermia	Monitor for malignant hyperthermia.
desflurane (Suprane)	Inhalation	Rapid induction and emergence; rare organ toxicity	Respiratory irritation; trigger for malignant hyperthermia	Monitor for malignant hyperthermia, dysrhythmias.
Gases				
nitrous oxide (N_2O)	Inhalation (semiclosed method)	Induction and recovery rapid Nonflammable Useful with oxygen for short procedures Useful with other agents for all types of surgery	Poor relaxant Weak anesthetic May produce hypoxia	Most useful in conjunction with other agents with longer action Monitor for chest pain, hypertension, and stroke.

STAGE III: SURGICAL ANESTHESIA

Surgical anesthesia is reached by continued administration of the anesthetic vapor or gas. The patient is unconscious and lies quietly on the table. The pupils are small but contract when exposed to light. Respirations are regular, the pulse rate and volume are normal, and the skin is pink or slightly flushed. With proper administration of the anesthetic, this stage may be maintained for hours in one of several planes, ranging from light (1) to deep (4), depending on the depth of anesthesia needed.

STAGE IV: MEDULLARY DEPRESSION

This stage is reached when too much anesthesia has been administered. Respirations become shallow, the pulse is weak and thready, and the pupils become widely dilated and no longer contract when exposed to light. Cyanosis develops and, without prompt intervention, death rapidly follows. If this stage develops, the anesthetic is discontinued immediately and respiratory and circulatory support is initiated to prevent death. Stimulants,

although rarely used, may be administered; narcotic antagonists can be used if overdosage is due to opioids.

During smooth administration of an anesthetic, there is no sharp division between the first three stages, and there is no stage IV. The patient passes gradually from one stage to another, and it is only by close observation of the signs exhibited by the patient that an anesthesiologist or anesthetist can control the situation. The responses of the pupils, the blood pressure, and the respiratory and cardiac rates are probably the most reliable guides to the patient's condition.

METHODS OF ANESTHESIA ADMINISTRATION

Anesthetics produce anesthesia because they are delivered to the brain at a high partial pressure that enables them to cross the blood–brain barrier. Relatively large amounts of anesthetic must be administered during induction and the early maintenance phases because the anesthetic is recirculated and deposited in body tissues. As these sites become saturated, smaller amounts of the anesthetic agent are required to maintain anesthesia because equilibrium or near equilibrium has been achieved between brain, blood, and other tissues.

Anything that diminishes peripheral blood flow, such as vasoconstriction or shock, may reduce the amount of anesthetic required. Conversely, when peripheral blood flow is unusually high, as in the muscularly active or the apprehensive patient, induction is slower and greater quantities of anesthetic are required because the brain receives a smaller quantity of anesthetic.

Inhalation

Liquid anesthetics may be administered by mixing the vapors with oxygen or nitrous oxide–oxygen and then having the patient inhale the mixture (Townsend, 2002). The vapor is administered to the patient through a tube or a mask. The inhalation anesthetic may also be administered through a laryngeal mask (Fig. 19-1), a flexible tube with an inflatable silicone ring and cuff that can be inserted into the larynx (Fortunato, 2000). The endotracheal technique for administering anesthetics consists of introducing a soft rubber or plastic endotracheal tube into the trachea, usually by means of a laryngoscope. The endotracheal tube may be inserted through either the nose or mouth. When in place, the tube seals off the lungs from the esophagus so that if the patient vomits, stomach contents do not enter the lungs.

Intravenous

General anesthesia can also be produced by the intravenous injection of various substances, such as barbiturates, benzodiazepines, nonbarbiturate hypnotics, dissociative agents, and opioid agents (Aranda & Hanson, 2000; Townsend, 2002). These medications may be administered for induction (initiation) or maintenance of anesthesia. They are often used along with inhalation anesthetics but may be used alone. They can also be used to produce moderate sedation. Intravenous anesthetics are presented in Table 19-2.

An advantage of intravenous anesthesia is that the onset of anesthesia is pleasant; there is none of the buzzing, roaring, or dizziness known to follow administration of an inhalation anesthetic. For this reason, induction of anesthesia usually begins with an intravenous agent and is often preferred by patients who have experienced various methods. The duration of action is brief, and the patient awakens with little nausea or vomiting. Thiopental is usually the agent of choice, and it is often administered with other anesthetic agents in prolonged procedures.

Intravenous anesthetic agents are nonexplosive, they require little equipment, and they are easy to administer. The low incidence of postoperative nausea and vomiting makes the method useful in eye surgery because vomiting would increase intraocular pressure and endanger vision in the operated eye. Intravenous anesthesia is useful for short procedures but is used less often for the longer procedures of abdominal surgery. It is not indicated for children, who have small veins and require intubation because of their susceptibility to respiratory obstruction.

A disadvantage of an intravenous anesthetic such as thiopental is its powerful respiratory depressant effect. It must be administered by a skilled anesthesiologist or anesthetist and only when some method of oxygen administration is available immediately in case of difficulty. Sneezing, coughing, and laryngospasm are sometimes noted with its use.

Intravenous neuromuscular blockers (muscle relaxants) block the transmission of nerve impulses at the neuromuscular junction of skeletal muscles. Muscle relaxants are used to relax muscles in abdominal and thoracic surgery, relax eye muscles in certain types of eye surgery, facilitate endotracheal intubation, treat laryngospasm, and assist in mechanical ventilation.

Purified curare was the first widely used muscle relaxant; tubocurarine was isolated as the active ingredient. Succinylcholine was later introduced because it acts more rapidly than curare. Several other agents are also used (Table 19-3). The ideal muscle relaxant has the following characteristics:

- It is nondepolarizing (noncompetitive agent), with an onset and duration of action similar to succinylcholine but without its problems of bradycardia and cardiac dysrhythmias (Townsend, 2002).
- It has a duration of action between those of succinylcholine and pancuronium.
- It lacks cumulative and cardiovascular effects.
- It can be metabolized and does not depend on the kidneys for its elimination.

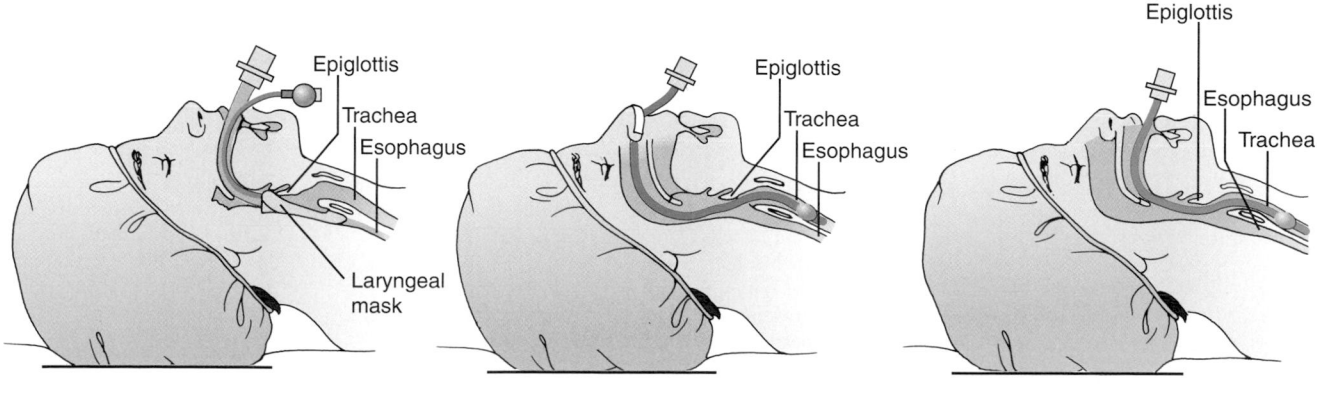

A. Laryngeal mask   B. Intranasal intubation   C. Oral intubation

FIGURE 19-1 Anesthetic delivery methods: (**A**) laryngeal mask, (**B**) nasal endotracheal catheter (in position), and (**C**) oral endotracheal intubation (tube is in position with cuff inflated).

Table 19-2 • Intravenous Anesthetic Agents

AGENT	ADMINISTRATION	ADVANTAGES	DISADVANTAGES	IMPLICATIONS/CONSIDERATIONS
Tranquilizers and Sedative–Hypnotics				
Benzodiazepines				
midazolam (Versed)	IV	Short acting; has antianxiety, sedative, amnesic, muscle relaxant effects	Increased sensitivity to its effects in chronic obstructive pulmonary disease patients	Monitor respiratory status closely.
diazepam (Valium)	IV Orally	Preoperative sedation Intraoperative tranquilization during regional anesthesia	Absorbed unpredictably when given IM	IV administration may produce thrombophlebitis (central vein is therefore preferred).
chlordiazepoxide (Librium)	IM	Production of hypnosis during anesthetic induction		
droperidol (Inapsine)	IM	Long duration of action	Weak antihistaminic action and α-adrenergic blocking action; inhibition of basic ganglionic dopaminergic pathways may lead to extrapyramidal rigidity resembling parkinsonism	Major tranquilizer Keep IV fluids and vasopressors available to treat hypotension.
lorazepam (Ativan)	IV	Long duration of action	Used with caution in patients with renal and liver impairment	Monitor laboratory values.
Opioids				
morphine (high doses)	IV	Not a myocardial depressant	Can depress arterial blood pressure by decreasing systemic vascular resistance Does not provide good amnesia Does not promote adequate muscular relaxation	Orthostatic hypotension may occur.
meperidine hydrochloride (Demerol)	IV Subcutaneously IM	Prompt onset Because of spasmolytic effect, it is drug of choice for surgery of bile duct, distal colon, and rectum; easily detoxified and excreted	May slow rate of respirations Adverse reactions: dizziness, nausea, and vomiting	In some patients, histamine may be released; treatment is diphenhydramine (Benadryl).

Neuroleptanalgesics

The term *neuroleptanalgesic* refers to the combination of a short-acting synthetic opioid agent (fentanyl) and a butyrophenone (droperidol). Patient becomes very drowsy; responds to voice command, although analgesia is profound. Of significance, the combination produces peripheral vasodilation followed by a decrease in arterial blood pressure. If administered rapidly, it may cause skeletal muscular rigidity and possibly respiratory impairment. These agents are also called narcotic agonist analgesics.

AGENT	ADMINISTRATION	ADVANTAGES	DISADVANTAGES	IMPLICATIONS/CONSIDERATIONS
fentanyl (Sublimaze)	IV Transdermally	75–100 times more potent than morphine and about 25% of duration of morphine (IV) Little effect on cardiovascular system	In very high dosage, an α-adrenergic blocking effect Respiratory depression	Short duration of action is due to its more rapid redistribution and more active metabolism by liver than other opioids.
sufentanil (Sufenta)	Injection	Onset extremely rapid		Duration is only about one third that of fentanyl.

Dissociative Agents

When under dissociative analgesia, the patient appears not to be asleep or anesthetized, but rather dissociated from the surroundings.

AGENT	ADMINISTRATION	ADVANTAGES	DISADVANTAGES	IMPLICATIONS/CONSIDERATIONS
ketamine (Ketalar; Ketaject)	IV IM	Rapid induction and short action; often used to supplement nitrous oxide Useful when hypotension may be hazardous; can be administered as analgesic or anesthetic	May cause elevated blood pressure and depressed respirations Patient may experience hallucinations. Vomiting and aspiration may occur.	Avoid verbal, visual, or tactile stimulation because this may trigger psychic aberration. Droperidol or diazepam (see below) may eliminate such psychic phenomena. Observe for signs of respiratory depression. Keep resuscitation equipment nearby.

(continued)

Table 19-2 • Intravenous Anesthetic Agents (Continued)

AGENT	ADMINISTRATION	ADVANTAGES	DISADVANTAGES	IMPLICATIONS/CONSIDERATIONS
Barbiturates				
thiopental sodium (Pentothal)	IV injection (or rectal)	Rapid induction Nonexplosive Requires little equipment Low incidence of post-operative nausea and vomiting	Powerful depressant of breathing Poor relaxant May produce coughing, sneezing, and laryngospasm Not useful for children because of small veins	Requires close observation because of potency and rapidity of drug action
methohexital sodium (Brevital)	IV	Rapid onset	Respiratory depression, involuntary muscle movement, seizures; may cause necrosis if IV infiltrates	Monitor respiratory status closely, monitor for seizure activity, ensure IV in vein.
Nonbarbiturate Hypnotics				
etomidate (Amidate)	IV	Few cardiovascular and respiratory effects; useful for frail patients	Transient adrenal suppression; involuntary muscle movements	
propofol (Diprivan)	IV	Rapid induction with minimal excitatory effects; may have antiemetic effect	Myocardial depression; hypotension; pain on injection	Monitor cardiac function and blood pressure closely; contraindicated in patients with allergy to eggs and soybean oil.

Regional Anesthesia

Regional anesthesia is a form of local anesthesia in which an anesthetic agent is injected around nerves so that the area supplied by these nerves is anesthetized. The effect depends on the type of nerve involved. Motor fibers are the largest fibers and have the thickest myelin sheath. Sympathetic fibers are the smallest and have a minimal covering. Sensory fibers are intermediate. Thus, a local anesthetic blocks motor nerves least readily and sympathetic nerves most readily. An anesthetic cannot be regarded as having worn off until all three systems (motor, sensory, and autonomic) are no longer affected.

The patient receiving spinal or local anesthesia is awake and aware of his or her surroundings unless medications are given to produce mild sedation or to relieve anxiety. The nurse must avoid careless conversation, unnecessary noise, and unpleasant odors; these may be noticed by the patient in the OR and may contribute to a negative view of the surgical experience. A quiet environment is therapeutic. The diagnosis must not be stated aloud if the patient is not to know it at this time.

Conduction Blocks and Spinal Anesthesia

There are many types of conduction blocks, depending on the nerve groups affected by the injection. Epidural anesthesia is achieved by injecting a local anesthetic into the spinal canal in the space surrounding the dura mater (Fig. 19-2). Epidural anesthesia also blocks sensory, motor, and autonomic functions, but it is differentiated from spinal anesthesia by the injection site and the amount of anesthetic used. Epidural doses are much higher because the epidural anesthetic does not make direct contact with the cord or nerve roots.

An advantage of epidural anesthesia is the absence of headache that occasionally results from subarachnoid injection. A dis-

advantage is the greater technical challenge of introducing the anesthetic into the epidural rather than the subarachnoid space. If inadvertent subarachnoid injection occurs during epidural anesthesia and the anesthetic travels toward the head, high spinal anesthesia can result; this can produce severe hypotension and respiratory depression and arrest. Treatment of these complications includes airway support, intravenous fluids, and use of vasopressors. Other types of nerve blocks include:

- Brachial plexus block, which produces anesthesia of the arm
- Paravertebral anesthesia, which produces anesthesia of the nerves supplying the chest, abdominal wall, and extremities
- Transsacral (caudal) block, which produces anesthesia of the perineum and, occasionally, the lower abdomen

Spinal anesthesia is a type of extensive conduction nerve block that is produced when a local anesthetic is introduced into the subarachnoid space at the lumbar level, usually between L4 and L5 (see Fig. 19-2). It produces anesthesia of the lower extremities, perineum, and lower abdomen. For the lumbar puncture procedure, the patient usually lies on the side in a knee–chest position. Sterile technique is used as a spinal puncture is made and the medication is injected through the needle. As soon as the injection has been made, the patient is positioned on his or her back. If a relatively high level of block is sought, the head and shoulders are lowered.

The spread of the anesthetic agent and the level of anesthesia depend on the amount of fluid injected, the speed with which it is injected, the positioning of the patient after the injection, and the specific gravity of the agent. If the specific gravity is greater than that of cerebrospinal fluid (CSF), the agent moves to the dependent position of the subarachnoid space. If the specific gravity is less than that of CSF, the anesthetic moves away from the dependent position. The anesthesiologist or anesthetist controls the spread of the agent. Generally, the agents used are procaine,

Table 19-3 • Neuromuscular Blocking Agents

MUSCLE RELAXANT	ACTION	ADVANTAGES	DISADVANTAGES	USES AND COMMENTS
Nondepolarizing Neuromuscular Blocking Agents				
tubocurarine chloride (Tubarine)	Peaks at 30–60 min	50%–70% excreted unchanged in 3–6 h	Histamine-like reaction Hypotension Increased airway resistance Skin erythema	Contraindicated with history of allergy, asthma
gallamine (Flaxedil)	20% as potent as curare Lasts 25% shorter time than curare Blocks vagal ganglia in heart	All excreted unchanged	Tachycardia	Used with cyclopropane or halothane
pancuronium bromide (Pavulon)	Similar to curare but 5 times more potent Duration: 60–85 min	Safe; stable Good muscle relaxant Reversible by neostigmine and atropine		Excellent for situations requiring complete relaxation Avoid with myasthenia gravis or renal disease. Avoid with patients sensitive to bromide.
vecuronium bromide (Norcuron)	Blocks depolarization	Facilitates endotracheal intubation; good muscle relaxant	Prolonged dose-related apnea	Related to Pavulon Well tolerated in patients with renal failure
Depolarizing Neuromuscular Blocking Agents				
These mimic the action of acetylcholine at the neuromuscular junction. Acetylcholine is discharged almost immediately on release, then repolarization of muscle takes place. When depolarizing neuromuscular blocking agents are used, skeletal muscle depolarizes.				
succinylcholine (Anectine; Sucostrin)	Onset is rapid: 1 min Duration: 4–8 min	Ideal for endotracheal intubation, fracture reduction; treatment of laryngospasm	Contraindicated in patients with low pseudo-cholinesterase On second IV injection, bradycardia and various dysrhythmias May cause fasciculations of the muscles and pain	Used to treat laryngospasm, status asthmaticus, and toxic reactions to local anesthetic drugs
decamethonium bromide (Syncurine)	Onset: 30–40 sec Duration: 15–20 min	Excreted unchanged by kidney	Some fasciculation of muscle: jaw masseter muscles; posterior calf muscles Difficult to reverse its action	Produces depolarization of end-plate region

tetracaine (Pontocaine), lidocaine (Xylocaine), and bupivacaine (Marcaine) (Table 19-4).

A few minutes after induction of a spinal anesthetic, anesthesia and paralysis affect the toes and perineum and then gradually the legs and abdomen. If the anesthetic reaches the upper thoracic and cervical spinal cord in high concentrations, a temporary partial or complete respiratory paralysis results. Paralysis of the respiratory muscles is managed by mechanical ventilation until the effects of the anesthetic on the respiratory nerves have worn off.

Nausea, vomiting, and pain may occur during surgery when spinal anesthesia is used. As a rule, these reactions result from manipulation of various structures, particularly those within the abdominal cavity. The simultaneous intravenous administration of a weak solution of thiopental and inhalation of nitrous oxide may prevent such reactions.

Headache may be an after-effect of spinal anesthesia. Several factors are involved in the incidence of headache: the size of the spinal needle used, the leakage of fluid from the subarachnoid space through the puncture site, and the patient's hydration status. Measures that increase cerebrospinal pressure are helpful in relieving headache. These include keeping the patient lying flat, quiet, and well hydrated.

In continuous spinal anesthesia, the tip of a plastic catheter remains in the subarachnoid space during the surgical procedure so that more anesthetics may be injected as needed. This technique allows greater control of the dosage, but there is greater potential for postanesthetic headache because of the large-gauge needle used.

Local Infiltration Anesthesia

Infiltration anesthesia is the injection of a solution containing the local anesthetic into the tissues at the planned incision site. Often it is combined with a local regional block by injecting the nerves immediately supplying the area. The advantages of local anesthesia are as follows:

- It is simple, economical, and nonexplosive.
- Equipment needed is minimal.
- Postoperative recovery is brief.
- Undesirable effects of general anesthesia are avoided.
- It is ideal for short and superficial surgical procedures.

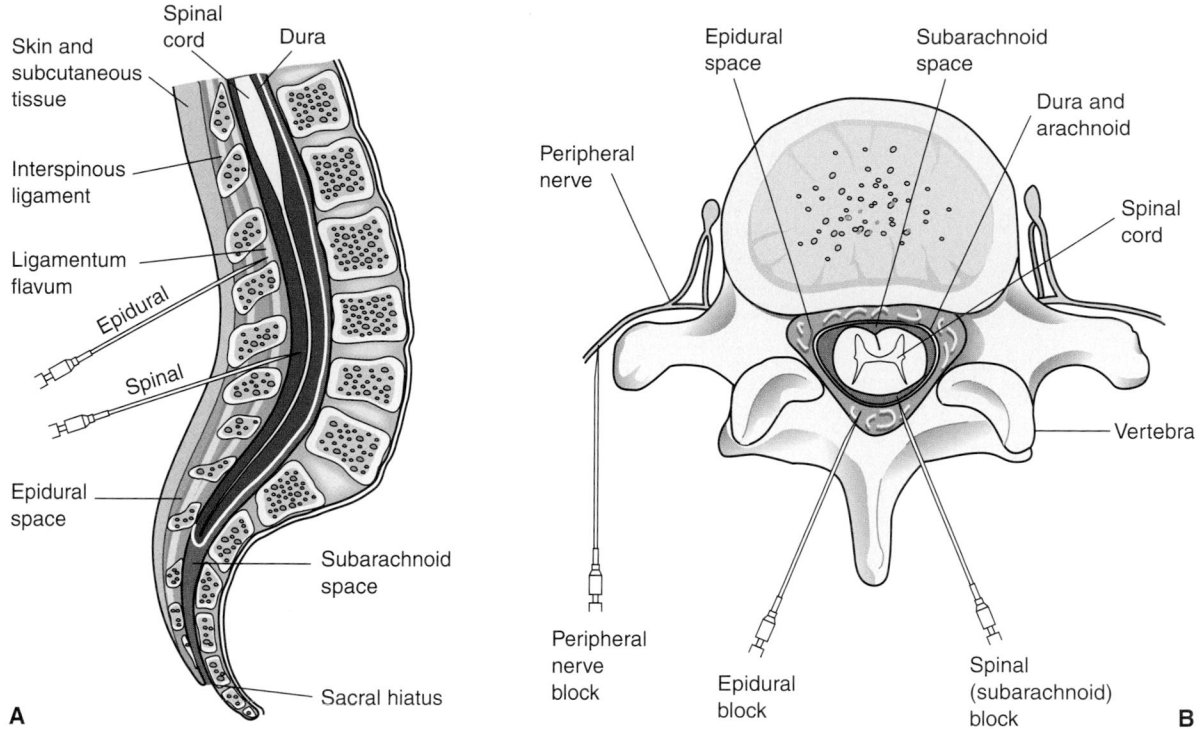

FIGURE 19-2 (**A**) Injection sites for spinal and epidural anesthesia. (**B**) Cross-section of injection sites for peripheral nerve, epidural, and spinal blocks.

Local anesthesia is often administered in combination with epinephrine. Epinephrine constricts blood vessels, which prevents rapid absorption of the anesthetic agent and thus prolongs its local action. Rapid absorption of the anesthetic agent into the bloodstream, which could cause seizures, is also prevented. Types of local anesthetic agents are listed in Table 19-5.

Local anesthesia is the anesthesia of choice in any surgical procedure in which it can be used. However, contraindications include high preoperative levels of anxiety, because surgery with local anesthesia may increase anxiety. A patient who requests general anesthesia rarely does well under local anesthesia. For some surgical procedures, local anesthesia is impractical because of the number of injections and the amount of anesthetic that would be required (breast reconstruction, for example).

The skin is prepared as for any surgical procedure, and a small-gauge needle is used to inject a modest amount of the anesthetic into the skin layers. This produces blanching or a wheal. Additional anesthetic is then injected in the skin until an area the length of the proposed incision is anesthetized. A larger, longer needle then is used to infiltrate deeper tissues with the anesthetic.

The action of the agent is almost immediate, so surgery may begin as soon as the injection is complete. Anesthesia lasts 45 minutes to 3 hours, depending on the anesthetic and the use of epinephrine.

Potential Intraoperative Complications

The surgical patient is subject to several risks. Potential intraoperative complications include nausea and vomiting, anaphylaxis, hypoxia, hypothermia, malignant hyperthermia, and disseminated intravascular coagulopathy.

NAUSEA AND VOMITING

Nausea and vomiting, or regurgitation, may affect patients during the intraoperative period. If gagging occurs, the patient is turned to the side, the head of the table is lowered, and a basin is provided to collect the vomitus. Suction is used to remove saliva and vomited gastric contents. There is no single way to prevent

AGENT	ADVANTAGES OF SPINAL ANESTHESIA (INCLUDES ALL AGENTS)	DISADVANTAGES OF SPINAL ANESTHESIA (INCLUDES ALL AGENTS)
procaine (Novocaine) tetracaine (Pontocaine) lidocaine (Xylocaine) bupivacaine (Marcaine)	Easily administered by a physician Inexpensive Minimum of equipment required Rapid onset Excellent muscular relaxation	Blood pressure may fall rapidly unless monitored carefully and treated with medications such as ephedrine. If the spinal anesthesia ascends to the chest, there may be respiratory distress. Occasionally, postoperative complications occur, such as headache or, rarely, meningitis or paralysis.

Table 19-4 • **Regional Anesthetic Agents**

Table 19-5 • **Local Anesthetic Agents**

AGENT	ADMINISTRATION	ADVANTAGES	DISADVANTAGES	IMPLICATIONS/ CONSIDERATIONS
lidocaine (Xylocaine) and mepivacaine (Carbocaine)	Topical or injection	Rapid Longer duration of action (compared with procaine) Free from local irritative effect	Occasional idiosyncrasy	Useful topically for cystoscopy Injected for use in dental work and surgery Observe for untoward reactions—drowsiness, depressed respiration.
bupivacaine (Marcaine)	Infiltration Peripheral nerve block Epidural	Duration is 2–3 times longer than lidocaine or mepivacaine	Use cautiously in patients with known drug allergies or sensitivities.	A period of analgesia persists after return of sensation; therefore, need for strong analgesics is reduced.
etidocaine (Duranest)	Infiltration Block			Greater potency and longer action than lidocaine
procaine (Novocaine)	Subcutaneously, intramuscularly, intravenously, or spinal	Low toxicity Inexpensive	Some idiosyncrasies Skin rash Poor stability	Observe for reaction: hypotension, bradycardia, weak pulse. Usually administered with epinephrine, causing vasoconstriction, thereby slowing absorption and prolonging nerve-deadening effect
tetracaine (Pontocaine)	Topical Infiltration Nerve block	Same as procaine	Same as procaine	More than 10 times as potent as procaine Usually administered with epinephrine

nausea and vomiting; an interdisciplinary approach involving the surgeon, anesthesiologist or anesthetist, and nurse is best (Meeker & Rothrock, 1999).

In some cases, the anesthesiologist administers antiemetics preoperatively or intraoperatively to counteract possible aspiration. If the patient aspirates vomitus, an asthma-like attack with severe bronchial spasms and wheezing is triggered. Pneumonitis and pulmonary edema can subsequently develop, leading to extreme hypoxia. Increasing medical attention is being paid to silent regurgitation of gastric contents, which occurs more frequently than previously realized. The importance of pH in the etiology of acid aspiration is being studied, as is the value of perioperative administration of a histamine-2 receptor antagonist, such as cimetidine (Tagamet), and similar medications (Meeker & Rothrock, 1999).

ANAPHYLAXIS

Any time a substance foreign to the patient is introduced, there is the potential for an anaphylactic reaction. Because medications are the most common cause of anaphylaxis, intraoperative nurses must be aware of the type and method of anesthesia used as well as the specific agents. An anaphylactic reaction can occur in response to many medications, latex, or other substances. The reaction may be immediate or delayed. Anaphylaxis is a life-threatening acute allergic reaction that causes vasodilation, hypotension, and bronchial constriction (Fortunato, 2000). See Chapters 15 and 53 for more details about the signs, symptoms, and treatment of anaphylaxis.

Fibrin sealants are used in a variety of surgical procedures, and cyanoacrylate tissue adhesives are used to close wounds without the use of sutures (Kassam et al., 2002; Vargas & Reger, 2000). These sealants have been implicated in allergic reactions and anaphylaxis. Although these reactions are rare, the nurse should be alert to the possibility and observe the patient for changes in vital signs and symptoms of anaphylaxis when these products are used.

HYPOXIA AND OTHER RESPIRATORY COMPLICATIONS

Inadequate ventilation, occlusion of the airway, inadvertent intubation of the esophagus, and hypoxia are significant potential problems of general anesthesia. Many factors can contribute to inadequate ventilation. Respiratory depression caused by anesthetic agents, aspiration of respiratory tract secretions or vomitus, and the patient's position on the operating table can compromise the exchange of gases. Anatomic variation can make the trachea difficult to visualize and result in the artificial airway being inserted into the esophagus rather than the trachea. In addition to these dangers, asphyxia caused by foreign bodies in the mouth, spasm of the vocal cords, relaxation of the tongue, or aspiration of vomitus, saliva, or blood can occur. Since brain damage from hypoxia occurs within minutes, vigilant assessment of the patient's oxygenation status is a primary function of the anesthesiologist or anesthetist and the circulating nurse. Peripheral perfusion is checked frequently, and pulse oximetry values are monitored continuously.

HYPOTHERMIA

During anesthesia, the patient's temperature may fall. Glucose metabolism is reduced, and as a result metabolic acidosis may develop. This condition is called hypothermia and is indicated by a core body temperature below normal (36.6°C [98.0°F] or lower). Inadvertent hypothermia may occur as a result of a low temperature in the OR, infusion of cold fluids, inhalation of cold gases, open body wounds or cavities, decreased muscle activity, advanced age, or the pharmaceutical agents used (eg, vasodilators, phenothiazines, general anesthetics). Hypothermia may also be intentionally induced in selected surgical procedures (such as cardiac surgeries requiring cardiopulmonary bypass) to reduce the patient's metabolic rate (Finkelmeier, 2000).

Preventing unintentional hypothermia is a major objective. If hypothermia occurs, the goal of intervention is to minimize or reverse the physiologic process. If hypothermia is intentional, the goal is safe return to normal body temperature. Environmental temperature in the OR can temporarily be set at 25° to 26.6°C (78° to 80°F). Intravenous and irrigating fluids are warmed to 37°C (98.6°F). Wet gowns and drapes are removed promptly and replaced with dry materials because wet linens promote heat loss. Whatever methods are used to rewarm the patient, warming must be accomplished gradually, not rapidly. Conscientious monitoring of core temperature, urinary output, ECG, blood pressure, arterial blood gas levels, and serum electrolyte levels is required.

MALIGNANT HYPERTHERMIA

Malignant hyperthermia is an inherited muscle disorder chemically induced by anesthetic agents (Fortunato-Phillips, 2000; Vermette, 1998). With the mortality rate exceeding 50%, identifying patients at risk for malignant hyperthermia is imperative. Susceptible people include those with strong and bulky muscles, a history of muscle cramps or muscle weakness and unexplained temperature elevation, and an unexplained death of a family member during surgery that was accompanied by a febrile response.

Pathophysiology

During anesthesia, potent agents such as inhalation anesthetics (halothane, enflurane) and muscle relaxants (succinylcholine), may trigger the symptoms of malignant hyperthermia (Fortunato-Phillips, 2000). Stress and some medications, such as sympathomimetics (epinephrine), theophylline, aminophylline, anticholinergics (atropine), and cardiac glycosides (digitalis), can induce or intensify such a reaction as well.

The pathophysiology is related to muscle cell activity. Muscle cells are composed of inner fluid (sarcoplasm) and an outer surrounding membrane. Calcium, an essential factor in muscle contraction, is normally stored in sacs in the sarcoplasm (Fortunato-Phillips, 2000). When nerve impulses stimulate the muscle, calcium is released, allowing contraction to occur. A pumping mechanism returns calcium to the sacs so that the muscle can relax. In malignant hyperthermia, this mechanism is disrupted. Calcium ions are not returned and they accumulate, causing clinical symptoms of hypermetabolism, which in turn increases muscle contraction (rigidity), hyperthermia, and damage to the central nervous system.

Clinical Manifestations

The initial symptoms of malignant hyperthermia are related to cardiovascular and musculoskeletal activity. Tachycardia (heart rate above 150 beats/min) is often the earliest sign. In addition to the tachycardia, sympathetic nervous stimulation leads to ventricular dysrhythmia, hypotension, decreased cardiac output, oliguria, and, later, cardiac arrest. With the abnormal transport of calcium, rigidity or tetanus-like movements occur, often in the jaw. The rise in temperature is actually a late sign that develops rapidly; body temperature can increase 1° to 2°C (2° to 4°F) every 5 minutes (Meeker & Rothrock, 1999). The temperature can reach or exceed 40°C (104°F) in a very short time (Fortunato-Phillips, 2000).

Medical Management

Recognizing symptoms early and discontinuing anesthesia promptly are imperative. Goals of treatment are to decrease metabolism, reverse metabolic and respiratory acidosis, correct dysrhythmias, decrease body temperature, provide oxygen and nutrition to tissues, and correct electrolyte imbalance. The Malignant Hyperthermia Association of North America (MHAUS) publishes a treatment protocol that should be posted in the OR or be readily available on a malignant hyperthermia cart.

Although malignant hyperthermia usually presents about 10 to 20 minutes after induction of anesthesia, it can also occur in the first 24 hours after surgery. As soon as the diagnosis is made, anesthesia and surgery are halted and the patient is hyperventilated with 100% oxygen. Dantrolene sodium, a skeletal muscle relaxant, and sodium bicarbonate are administered immediately (Fortunato-Phillips, 2000; Vermette, 1998). Continued monitoring of all parameters is necessary to evaluate the patient's status.

Nursing Management

Although malignant hyperthermia is uncommon, the nurse must identify patients at risk, recognize the signs and symptoms, have the appropriate medication and equipment available, and be knowledgeable about the protocol to follow (Fortunato-Phillips, 2000). This information may be lifesaving.

DISSEMINATED INTRAVASCULAR COAGULOPATHY

Disseminated intravascular coagulopathy is a life-threatening condition characterized by thrombus formation and depletion of select coagulation proteins (Dice, 2000). The exact cause is unknown, but predisposing factors include many conditions that may occur with emergency surgery, such as massive trauma, head injury, massive transfusion, liver or kidney involvement, embolic events, or shock. The signs and symptoms, nursing assessment, and treatment are discussed in Chapter 33.

NURSING PROCESS: THE PATIENT DURING SURGERY

The Perioperative Nursing Data Set (PNDS) is a helpful model used by nurses in the intraoperative phase of care (see Chap. 18, Fig. 18-1). Phenomena of concern to intraoperative nurses are nursing diagnoses, interventions, and outcomes that surgical patients and their families experience. Additional areas of concern include collaborative problems and expected goals.

Assessment

Nursing assessment of the intraoperative patient involves obtaining data from the patient and the patient's record to identify variables that can affect care and serve as guidelines for developing an individualized plan of patient care. The intraoperative nurse uses the focused preoperative nursing assessment documented on the patient record. This includes assessment of physiologic status (eg, health–illness level, level of consciousness), psychosocial status (eg, anxiety level, verbal communication problems, coping mechanisms), physical status (eg, surgical site, skin condition and effectiveness of preparation; immobile joints), and ethical concerns (Chart 19-3).

Diagnosis

NURSING DIAGNOSES
Based on the assessment data, some major nursing diagnoses may include the following:

- Anxiety related to expressed concerns due to surgery or OR environment
- Risk for perioperative positioning injury related to environmental conditions in the OR
- Risk for injury related to anesthesia and surgery
- Disturbed sensory perception (global) related to general anesthesia or sedation

COLLABORATIVE PROBLEMS/ POTENTIAL COMPLICATIONS
Based on the assessment data, potential complications may include the following:

- Nausea and vomiting
- Anaphylaxis
- Hypoxia
- Unintentional hypothermia
- Malignant hyperthermia
- Disseminated intravascular coagulopathy
- Infection

Chart 19-3 Ethics and Related Issues

To Resuscitate or Not?

Situation
Your hospital has developed a policy, authorized through the medical staff, that allows for patients to have a do-not-resuscitate order (DNR) in place during a surgical procedure. This policy follows the American Society of Anesthesiologists guidelines for DNR in the operating room. You are getting a patient ready for surgery and the anesthesiologist who will be administering the anesthetic writes an order for the DNR to be rescinded during surgery. The physician is refusing to talk to the patient concerning the DNR.

Problem
The patient believes his/her wishes will be followed with regard to resuscitation in the event of a cardiac arrest and the physician does not believe he can administer anesthesia if the DNR is in place.

Discussion
- What are the rights of the patient with regard to advance directives?
- What can you do to advocate for the patient?
- Should you contact the ethics committee of the hospital?
- How do you contact the ethics committee?

Planning and Goals

Goals for care of the patient during surgery include reducing anxiety, preventing positioning injuries, maintaining safety, maintaining the patient's dignity, and avoiding complications.

Nursing Interventions

REDUCING ANXIETY
The OR environment can seem cold, stark, and frightening to the patient, who may be feeling isolated and apprehensive. Introducing yourself, addressing the patient by name warmly and frequently, verifying details, providing explanations, and encouraging and answering questions provide a sense of professionalism and friendliness that can help the patient feel secure. When discussing what the patient can expect in surgery, the nurse uses common, basic communication skills, such as touch and eye contact, to reduce anxiety. Attention to physical comfort (warm blankets, position changes) helps the patient feel more comfortable. Telling the patient who else will be present in the OR, how long the procedure is expected to take, and other details helps the patient prepare for the experience and gain a sense of control.

PREVENTING INTRAOPERATIVE POSITIONING INJURY
The patient's position on the operating table depends on the surgical procedure to be performed as well as on his or her physical condition (Fig. 19-3). The potential for transient discomfort or even permanent injury is clear because many positions are awkward. Hyperextending joints, compressing arteries, or pressing on nerves and bony prominences usually results in discomfort simply because the position must be sustained for a long period (Meeker & Rothrock, 1999). Factors to consider include the following:

- The patient should be in as comfortable a position as possible, whether asleep or awake.
- The operative field must be adequately exposed.
- An awkward position, undue pressure on a body part, or use of stirrups or traction should not obstruct the vascular supply.
- Respiration should not be impeded by pressure of arms on the chest or by a gown that constricts the neck or chest.
- Nerves must be protected from undue pressure. Improper positioning of the arms, hands, legs, or feet may cause serious injury or paralysis. Shoulder braces must be well padded to prevent irreparable nerve injury, especially when the Trendelenburg position is necessary.
- Precautions for patient safety must be observed, particularly with thin, elderly, or obese patients, or those with a physical deformity (Curet, 2000).
- The patient needs gentle restraint before induction in case of excitement.

The usual position for surgery, called the dorsal recumbent position, is flat on the back. One arm is positioned at the side of the table, with the hand placed palm down; the other is carefully positioned on an armboard to facilitate intravenous infusion of fluids, blood, or medications. This position is used for most abdominal surgeries except for surgery of the gallbladder and pelvis (see Fig. 19-3A).

The Trendelenburg position usually is used for surgery on the lower abdomen and pelvis to obtain good exposure by displacing the intestines into the upper abdomen. In this position, the head and body are lowered. The patient is held in position by padded shoulder braces (see Fig. 19-3B).

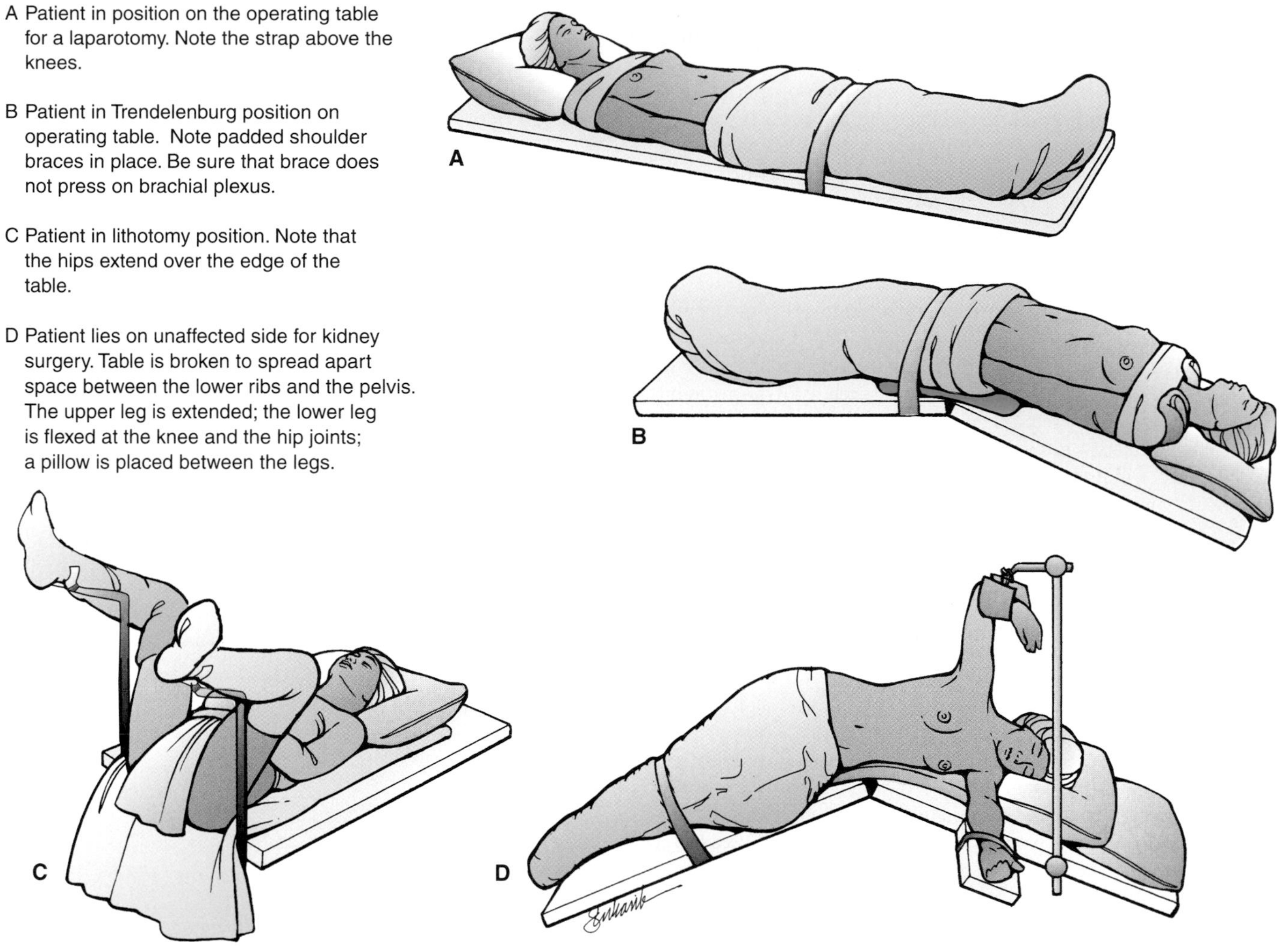

A Patient in position on the operating table for a laparotomy. Note the strap above the knees.

B Patient in Trendelenburg position on operating table. Note padded shoulder braces in place. Be sure that brace does not press on brachial plexus.

C Patient in lithotomy position. Note that the hips extend over the edge of the table.

D Patient lies on unaffected side for kidney surgery. Table is broken to spread apart space between the lower ribs and the pelvis. The upper leg is extended; the lower leg is flexed at the knee and the hip joints; a pillow is placed between the legs.

FIGURE 19-3 Positions on the operating table. Captions call attention to safety and comfort features. All surgical patients wear caps to cover the hair completely.

The lithotomy position is used for nearly all perineal, rectal, and vaginal surgical procedures (see Fig. 19-3C). The patient is positioned on the back with the legs and thighs flexed. The position is maintained by placing the feet in stirrups.

The Sims or lateral position is used for renal surgery. The patient is placed on the nonoperative side with an air pillow 12.5 to 15 cm (5 to 6 inches) thick under the loin, or on a table with a kidney or back lift (see Fig. 19-3D).

Other procedures, such as neurosurgery or abdominothoracic surgery, may require unique positioning and supplemental apparatus, depending on the operative approach.

PROTECTING THE PATIENT FROM INJURY

One way the nurse protects the patient from injury is by providing a safe environment. A variety of activities are used to address the diverse patient safety issues that arise in the OR. Verifying information, checking the chart for completeness, and maintaining surgical asepsis and an optimal environment are critical nursing responsibilities. Verifying that all required documentation is completed is one of the first functions of the intraoperative nurse. The patient is identified, and the planned surgical procedure and type of anesthesia are verified. It is important to review the patient's record for the following:

- Correct informed surgical consent, with patient's signature
- Completed records for health history and physical examination
- Results of diagnostic studies
- Allergies (including latex)

In addition to checking that all necessary patient data are complete, the perioperative nurse obtains the necessary equipment specific to the procedure. The need for nonroutine medications, blood components, instruments, and other equipment and supplies is assessed, and the readiness of the room, completeness of physical setup, and completeness of instrument, suture, and dressing setups are determined. Any aspects of the OR environment that may negatively affect the patient are identified. These include physical features, such as room temperature and humidity; electrical hazards; potential contaminants (dust, blood, and discharge on floor or surfaces, uncovered hair, faulty attire of personnel, jewelry worn by personnel); and unnecessary traffic. The circulating nurse also sets up and maintains suction equipment in working order, sets up invasive monitoring equipment, assists with insertion of vascular access and monitoring devices (arterial, Swan-Ganz, central venous pressure, intravenous lines), and initiates appropriate physical comfort measures for the patient.

Preventing physical injury includes using safety straps and bed rails and not leaving the sedated patient unattended. Transferring the patient from the stretcher to the OR table requires safe transferring practices. Other safety measures include properly positioning the grounding pad under the patient to prevent electrical burns and shock, removing excess povidone-iodine (Betadine) or other surgical germicide from the patient's skin, and promptly and completely draping exposed areas after the sterile field has been created to decrease the risk for hypothermia.

Nursing measures to prevent injury from excessive blood loss include blood conservation using equipment such a cell-saver (a device for recirculating the patient's own blood cells) or the administration of blood products (Finkelmeier, 2000). Few patients undergoing an elective procedure require blood transfusion, but those undergoing higher-risk procedures (such as orthopedic or cardiac surgeries) may require an intraoperative transfusion. The circulating nurse should anticipate this need, check that blood has been cross-matched and held in reserve, and be prepared to administer blood (Meeker & Rothrock, 1999).

SERVING AS PATIENT ADVOCATE

Because the patient undergoing general anesthesia or moderate sedation experiences temporary sensory/perceptual alteration or loss, he or she has an increased need for protection and advocacy. Patient advocacy in the OR entails maintaining the patient's physical and emotional comfort, privacy, rights, and dignity. Patients, whether conscious or not, should not be subjected to excess noise, inappropriate conversation, or, most of all, derogatory comments. As surprising as this sounds, banter in the OR occasionally includes jokes about the patient's physical appearance, job, personal history, and so forth. Cases have been reported in which seemingly deeply anesthetized patients recalled the entire surgical experience, including disparaging personal remarks made by OR personnel. As an advocate, the nurse never engages in this conversation and discourages others from doing so. Other advocacy activities include correcting for the clinical, dehumanizing aspects of being a surgical patient by making sure the patient is treated as a person, respecting cultural and spiritual values, providing physical privacy, and maintaining confidentiality.

MONITORING AND MANAGING POTENTIAL COMPLICATIONS

It is the responsibility of the surgeon and the anesthetist or anesthesiologist to monitor and manage complications. However, intraoperative nurses also play an important role. Being alert to and reporting changes in vital signs and symptoms of nausea and vomiting, anaphylaxis, hypoxia, hypothermia, malignant hyperthermia, or disseminated vascular coagulation and assisting with their management are important nursing functions (Dice, 2000; Fortunato-Phillips, 2000). Each of these complications was discussed earlier. Maintaining asepsis and preventing infection is the responsibility of all members of the surgical team.

Evaluation

EXPECTED PATIENT OUTCOMES

Expected patient outcomes may include:

1. Exhibits low level of anxiety
2. Remains free of perioperative positioning injury
3. Experiences no unexpected threats to safety
4. Has dignity preserved throughout OR experience

5. Is free of complications or experiences successful management of adverse effects of surgery and anesthesia

 Critical Thinking Exercises

1. A patient in the holding area awaiting surgery indicates that he had not received instructions not to take his usual medications (antihypertensive agent, diuretic, digoxin, potassium chloride, and insulin injection); as a result, he took them a few hours ago. What implications does this have for the patient's care and well-being while awaiting surgery, during surgery, and in the immediate postoperative period?

2. What are the differences in responsibility of the operating room nurse for care of patients who receive general anesthesia, conscious sedation, spinal anesthesia, and regional anesthesia?

3. While she is being transferred from the stretcher to the operating table, a female patient says she is very anxious about her surgery because of previous negative experiences. What assessment and interventions are indicated at this time?

REFERENCES AND SELECTED READINGS

Books

American Society of Perianesthesia Nurses. (2000). *Standards of perianesthesia nursing practice.* Thorofare, NJ: ASPAN.

AORN Standards, Recommended Practice, and Guidelines (2002). Denver: AORN, Inc.

Dudek, S. G. (2001). *Nutrition essentials for nursing practice.* Philadelphia: Lippincott Williams & Wilkins.

Finkelmeier, B. (2000). *Cardiothoracic surgical nursing* (2d ed.). Philadelphia: Lippincott Williams & Wilkins.

Fortunato, N. (2000). *Berry and Kohn's operating room technique* (9th ed.). St. Louis: Mosby, Inc.

Joint Commission on Accreditation of Healthcare Organizations (JCAHO) (2001). *Revisions to anesthesia care standards for comprehensive accreditation manual for ambulatory care.* Philadelphia: Lippincott Williams & Wilkins.

Litwack, K. (Ed.). (1999). *Core curriculum for perianesthesia nursing practice.* Philadelphia: WB Saunders.

Meeker, M. H., & Rothrock, J. C. (1999). *Alexander's care of the patient in surgery* (11th ed.). St. Louis: Mosby Year Book.

Perioperative Nursing Data Set: The perioperative nursing vocabulary. (2000). Denver: AORN, Inc.

Phippen, M., & Wells, M. (2000). *Patient care during operative and invasive procedures.* Philadelphia: WB Saunders.

Rothrock, J. (1999). *The RN first assistant: An expanded perioperative nursing role* (3rd ed.). Philadelphia: Lippincott.

Schwartz, S., & Shires, G. T. (1999). *Principles of surgery.* New York: McGraw-Hill.

Townsend, C. (2002). *Pocket companion to Sabiston textbook of surgery* (16th ed.). Philadelphia: WB Saunders.

Journals

Asterisks indicate nursing research articles.

Aranda, M., & Hanson, W. (2000). Anesthetics, sedatives, and paralytics: Understanding their use in the intensive care unit. *Surgical Clinics of North America, 80*(3), 933–947.

Curet, M. (2000). Special problems in laparoscopic surgery: Previous abdominal surgery, obesity, and pregnancy. *Surgical Clinics of North America, 80*(4), 1093–1110.

Dice, R. (2000). Intraoperative disseminated intravascular coagulopathy. *Critical Care Nursing Clinics of North America, 12*(2), 175–180.

Fortunato-Phillips, N. (2000). Malignant hyperthermia: Update 2000. *Critical Care Nursing Clinics of North America, 12*(2), 199–210.

Friberg, B. (1998). Ultraclean laminar airflow ORs. *AORN Journal, 67*(4), 841–851.

Kassam, A., Carrau, R., Horowitz, M., Snyderman, C., Hirsch, B., & Welch, W. (2002). The role of fibrin sealants in cranial-based surgery. *Clinical Update, 1280,* 1–36.

*Larsen, E., Aiello, A., Heilman, J., Lyle, C., Cronquist, A., Stahl, J., & Dello-Latta, P. (2001). Comparison of different regimens for surgical hand preparation. *AORN Journal, 73*(2), 412–432.

Patterson, C. (2000*a*). New rules impact sedation and anesthesia care, Part 1. *Nursing Management, 31*(5), 22.

Patterson, C. (2000*b*). New rules impact sedation and anesthesia care, Part 2. *Nursing Management, 31*(6), 16–17.

Polanczyk, C., Marcantonio, E., Goldman, L., et al. (2001). Impact of age on perioperative complications and length of stay in patients undergoing noncardiac surgery. *Annals of Internal Medicine, 134*(8), 637–643.

Vargas, G., & Reger, T. (2000). An alternative to sutures. *MedSurg Nursing, 9*(2), 83–85.

Vermette, E. (1998). Emergency! Malignant hyperthermia. *American Journal of Nursing, 98*(4), 45.

Williams, H., & Reeves, F. (1998). Anesthetic techniques and positioning: Implications for perioperative nurses. *Seminars in Perioperative Nursing, 7*(1), 14–20.

Winslow, E., & Jacobson, A. (2000). Can a fashion statement harm the patients? *American Journal of Nursing, 100*(9), 63–65.

RESOURCES AND WEBSITES

American Society of Anesthesiologists, 520 N. Northwest Highway, Park Ridge, IL, 60068; (847) 825-2286; http://www.asahq.org/practice.

American Society of PeriAnesthesia Nurses, 10 Melrose Ave., Suite 110, Cherry Hill, NJ 08003-3696; 877-9696 (toll-free); fax (856) 616-9621; http://www.aspan.org.

Association of PeriOperative Registered Nurses, Inc., 2170 S. Parker Rd., Suite 300, Denver, CO 80231; (800) 755-2676; http://www.aorn.org.

Malignant Hyperthermia Association of the United States (MHAUS), 39 East State Street, P.O. Box 1069, Sherburne, NY 13460; (607) 674-7901; http://www.mhaus.org.

Postoperative Nursing Management

On completion of this chapter, the learner will be able to:

1. Describe the responsibilities of the postanesthesia care unit nurse in the prevention of immediate postoperative complications.
2. Compare postoperative care of the ambulatory surgery patient and the hospitalized surgery patient.
3. Identify common postoperative problems and their management.
4. Describe the gerontologic considerations related to postoperative management of patients.
5. Describe variables that affect wound healing.
6. Demonstrate postoperative dressing techniques.
7. Identify assessment parameters appropriate for the early detection of postoperative complications.

The postoperative period extends from the time the patient leaves the operating room until the last follow-up visit with the surgeon. This period may be as short as 1 week or as long as several months. During the postoperative period, nursing care focuses on reestablishing the patient's physiologic equilibrium, alleviating pain, preventing complications, and teaching the patient self-care. Careful assessment and immediate intervention assist the patient in returning to optimal function quickly, safely, and as comfortably as possible. Ongoing care in the community through home care, clinic visits, office visits, or telephone follow-up facilitates an uncomplicated recovery.

The Postanesthesia Care Unit

The **postanesthesia care unit (PACU)**, also called the postanesthesia recovery room, is located adjacent to the operating rooms. Patients still under anesthesia or recovering from anesthesia are placed in this unit for easy access to experienced, highly skilled nurses, anesthesiologists or anesthetists, surgeons, advanced hemodynamic and pulmonary monitoring and support, special equipment, and medications (Litwack, 1999; Meeker & Rothrock, 1999).

The PACU is kept quiet, clean, and free of unnecessary equipment. This area is painted in soft, pleasing colors and has indirect lighting, a soundproof ceiling, equipment that controls or eliminates noise (eg, plastic emesis basins, rubber bumpers on beds and tables), and isolated but visible quarters for disruptive patients. The PACU should also be well ventilated. These features benefit the patient by helping to decrease anxiety and promote comfort. The PACU bed provides easy access to the patient, is safe and easily movable, can be readily placed in position to facilitate use of measures to counteract shock, and has features that facilitate care, such as intravenous (IV) poles, side rails, wheel brakes, and a chart storage rack.

PHASES OF POSTANESTHESIA CARE

Postanesthesia care in some hospitals and ambulatory surgical centers is divided into two phases (Litwack, 1999; Meeker & Rothrock, 1999). In the **phase I PACU**, used during the immediate recovery phase, intensive nursing care is provided. The **phase II PACU** is reserved for patients who require less frequent observation and less nursing care. In the phase II unit, the patient is prepared for discharge. Recliners rather than stretchers or beds are standard in many phase II units, which may also be referred to as step-down, sit-up, or progressive care units. Patients may remain in a phase II PACU unit for as long as 4 to 6 hours, depending on the type of surgery and any preexisting conditions of the patient. In facilities without separate phase I and phase II units, the patient remains in the PACU and may be discharged home directly from this unit.

Both phase I and phase II PACU nurses have special skills. The phase I PACU nurse provides frequent (every 15 minutes) monitoring of the patient's pulse, electrocardiogram, respiratory rate, blood pressure, and pulse oximeter value (blood oxygen level). In some cases, end-tidal carbon dioxide ($ETCO_2$) levels are monitored as well. The patient's airway may become obstructed because of the latent effects of recent anesthesia, and the PACU nurse must be prepared to assist in reintubation and in handling other emergencies that may occur. The nurse in the phase II PACU must possess strong clinical assessment and patient teaching skills.

ADMITTING THE PATIENT TO THE PACU

Transferring the postoperative patient from the operating room to the PACU is the responsibility of the anesthesiologist or anesthetist. During transport from the operating room to the PACU, the anesthesia provider remains at the head of the stretcher (to maintain the airway), and a surgical team member remains at the opposite end. Transporting the patient involves special consideration of the incision site, potential vascular changes, and exposure. The surgical incision is considered every time the postoperative patient is moved; many wounds are closed under considerable tension, and every effort is made to prevent further strain on the incision. The patient is positioned so that he or she is not lying on and obstructing drains or drainage tubes. Serious orthostatic hypotension may occur when a patient is moved from one position to another (eg, from a lithotomy position to a horizontal position or from a lateral to a supine position), so the patient must be moved slowly and carefully. As soon as the patient is placed on the stretcher or bed, the soiled gown is removed and replaced with a dry gown. The patient is covered with lightweight blankets and warmed. The side rails are raised to guard against falls.

The nurse who admits the patient to the PACU reviews the following information with the anesthesiologist or anesthetist:

- Medical diagnosis and type of surgery performed
- Pertinent past medical history and allergies
- Patient's age and general condition, airway patency, vital signs
- Anesthetics and other medications used during the procedure (eg, opioids and other analgesic agents, muscle relaxants, antibiotic agents)

Glossary

dehiscence: partial or complete separation of wound edges

evisceration: protrusion of abdominal organs through the surgical incision

first-intention healing: method of healing in which wound edges are surgically approximated and integumentary continuity is restored without granulation

Phase I PACU: area designated for care of surgical patients immediately after surgery and patients whose condition warrants close monitoring

Phase II PACU: area designated for care of surgical patients who have been transferred from a phase I PACU because their condition no longer requires the close monitoring provided in a phase I PACU

postanesthesia care unit (PACU): area where postoperative patients are monitored as they recover from anesthesia; formerly referred to as the recovery room or postanesthesia recovery room

second-intention healing: method of healing in which wound edges are not surgically approximated and integumentary continuity is restored by the process known as granulation

third-intention healing: method of healing in which surgical approximation of wound edges is delayed and integumentary continuity is restored by apposing areas of granulation

- Any problems that occurred in the operating room that might influence postoperative care (eg, extensive hemorrhage, shock, cardiac arrest)
- Pathology encountered (if malignancy is an issue during surgery, the nurse needs to know whether the patient and/or family have been informed)
- Fluid administered, estimated blood loss and replacement fluids
- Any tubing, drains, catheters, or other supportive aids
- Specific information about which the surgeon, anesthesiologist, or anesthetist wishes to be notified (eg, blood pressure or heart rate below or above a specified level)

NURSING MANAGEMENT IN THE PACU

The nursing management objectives for the patient in the PACU are to provide care until the patient has recovered from the effects of anesthesia (eg, until resumption of motor and sensory functions), is oriented, has stable vital signs, and shows no evidence of hemorrhage or other complications.

Assessing the Patient

Frequent, skilled assessments of the blood oxygen saturation level, pulse rate and regularity, depth and nature of respirations, skin color, level of consciousness, and ability to respond to commands are the cornerstones of nursing care in the PACU. The nurse performs a baseline assessment, then checks the surgical site for drainage or hemorrhage and makes sure that all drainage tubes and monitoring lines are connected and functioning.

After the initial assessment, vital signs are monitored and the patient's general physical status is assessed at least every 15 minutes. Patency of the airway and respiratory function are always evaluated first, followed by assessment of cardiovascular function, the condition of the surgical site, and function of the central nervous system. The nurse needs to be aware of any pertinent information from the patient's history that may be significant (eg, patient is hard of hearing, has a history of seizures, has diabetes, or is allergic to certain medications or to latex).

Maintaining a Patent Airway

The primary objective in the immediate postoperative period is to maintain pulmonary ventilation and thus prevent hypoxemia (reduced oxygen in the blood) and hypercapnia (excess carbon dioxide in the blood). Both can occur if the airway is obstructed and ventilation is reduced (hypoventilation). Besides checking the physician's orders for and administering supplemental oxygen, the nurse assesses respiratory rate and depth, ease of respirations, oxygen saturation, and breath sounds (Litwack, 1999; Meeker & Rothrock, 1999).

Patients who have experienced prolonged anesthesia usually are unconscious, with all muscles relaxed. This relaxation extends to the muscles of the pharynx. When the patient lies on his or her back, the lower jaw and the tongue fall backward and the air passages become obstructed (Fig. 20-1A). This is called hypopharyngeal obstruction. Signs of occlusion include choking, noisy and irregular respirations, decreased oxygen saturation scores, and within minutes a blue, dusky color (cyanosis) of the skin. Because movement of the thorax and the diaphragm does not necessarily indicate that the patient is breathing, the nurse needs to place the palm of the hand at the patient's nose and mouth to feel the exhaled breath.

> **NURSING ALERT** The treatment of hypopharyngeal obstruction involves tilting the head back and pushing forward on the angle of the lower jaw, as if to push the lower teeth in front of the upper teeth (Figs. 20-1**B, C**). This maneuver pulls the tongue forward and opens the air passages.

The anesthesiologist or anesthetist may leave a hard rubber or plastic airway in the patient's mouth (Fig. 20-2) to maintain a patent airway. Such a device should not be removed until signs such as gagging indicate that reflex action is returning. Alternatively, the patient may enter the PACU with an endotracheal tube still in place and may require continued mechanical ventilation. The nurse assists in initiating the use of the ventilator and in the weaning and extubation processes. Some patients, particularly those who have had extensive or lengthy surgical procedures, may be transferred from the operating room directly to the intensive care unit or may be transferred from the PACU to the intensive care unit while still intubated and on mechanical ventilation.

Respiratory difficulty can also result from excessive secretion of mucus or aspiration of vomitus. Turning the patient to one side allows the collected fluid to escape from the side of the mouth. If the teeth are clenched, the mouth may be opened manually but cautiously with a padded tongue depressor. The head of the bed is elevated 15 to 30 degrees unless contraindicated, and the patient is closely observed to maintain the airway as well as to minimize the risk of aspiration. If vomiting occurs, the patient is turned to the side to prevent aspiration and the vomitus is collected in the emesis basin. Mucus or vomitus obstructing the pharynx or the trachea is suctioned with a pharyngeal suction tip or a nasal catheter introduced into the nasopharynx or oropharynx. The catheter can be passed into the nasopharynx or oropharynx safely to a distance of 15 to 20 cm (6 to 8 inches). Caution is necessary in suctioning the throat of a patient who has had a tonsillectomy or other oral or laryngeal surgery because of risk for bleeding and discomfort.

Maintaining Cardiovascular Stability

To monitor cardiovascular stability, the nurse assesses the patient's mental status; vital signs; cardiac rhythm; skin temperature, color, and moisture; and urine output. Central venous pressure, pulmonary artery pressure, and arterial lines are monitored if the patient's condition requires such assessment. The nurse also assesses the patency of all IV lines. The primary cardiovascular complications seen in the PACU include hypotension and shock, hemorrhage, hypertension, and dysrhythmias.

HYPOTENSION AND SHOCK

Hypotension can result from blood loss, hypoventilation, position changes, pooling of blood in the extremities, or side effects of medications and anesthetics; the most common cause is loss of circulating volume through blood and plasma loss. If the amount of blood loss exceeds 500 mL (especially if the loss is rapid), replacement is usually indicated.

Shock, one of the most serious postoperative complications, can result from hypovolemia. Shock may be described as inadequate cellular oxygenation accompanied by the inability to excrete waste products of metabolism. Hypovolemic shock is characterized by a fall in venous pressure, a rise in peripheral resistance, and tachycardia. Neurogenic shock, a less common cause of shock in the surgical patient, occurs as a result of decreased arterial resistance caused by spinal anesthesia. It is characterized by a fall in blood

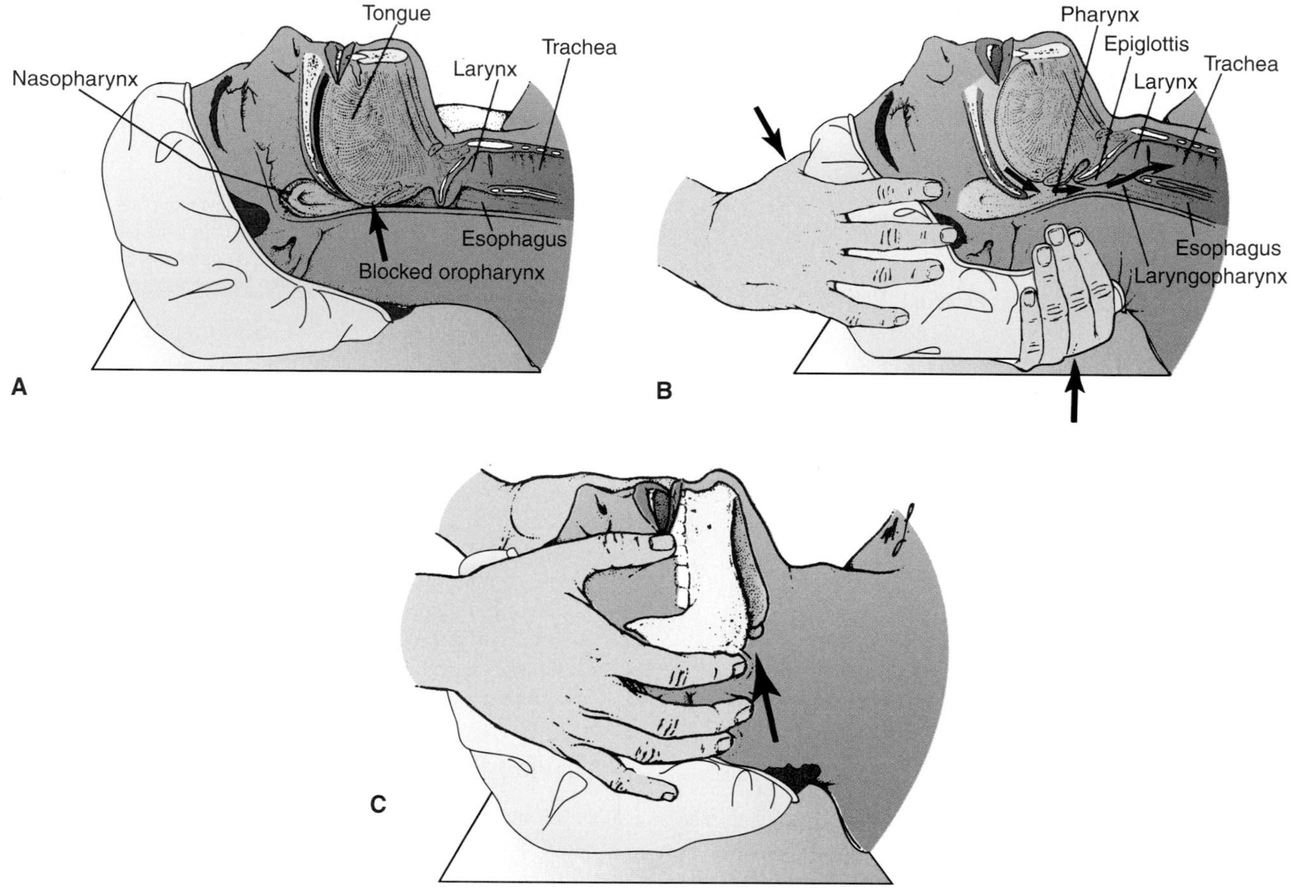

Tongue

Nasopharynx

Larynx

Trachea

Esophagus

Blocked oropharynx

A

Pharynx

Epiglottis

Larynx

Trachea

Esophagus

Laryngopharynx

B

C

FIGURE 20-1 (**A**) A hypopharyngeal obstruction occurs when neck flexion permits the chin to drop toward the chest; obstruction almost always occurs when the head is in the midposition. (**B**) Tilting the head back to stretch the anterior neck structure lifts the base of the tongue off the posterior pharyngeal wall. The direction of the arrows indicates the pressure of the hands. (**C**) Opening the mouth is necessary to correct valvelike obstruction of the nasal passage during expiration, which occurs in about 30% of unconscious patients. Open the patient's mouth (separate lips and teeth) and move the lower jaw forward so that the lower teeth are in front of the upper teeth. To regain backward tilt of the neck, lift with both hands at the ascending rami of the mandible.

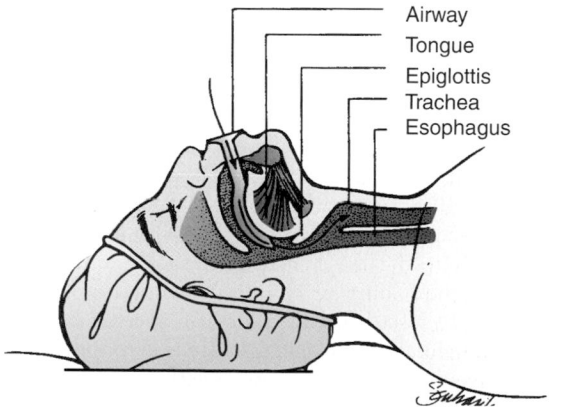

Airway

Tongue

Epiglottis

Trachea

Esophagus

FIGURE 20-2 Use of an airway to prevent respiratory difficulty after anesthesia. The airway passes over the base of the tongue and permits air to pass into the pharynx in the region of the epiglottis. Patients often leave the operating room with an airway in place. The airway should remain in place until the patient recovers sufficiently to breathe normally. As the patient regains consciousness, the airway usually causes irritation and should be removed.

pressure due to pooling of blood in dilated capacitance vessels (those with the ability to change volume capacity). Cardiogenic shock is unlikely in the surgical patient except if the patient has severe preexisting cardiac disease or experienced a myocardial infarction during surgery. See Chapter 15 for a detailed discussion of shock.

The classic signs of shock are:

- Pallor
- Cool, moist skin
- Rapid breathing
- Cyanosis of the lips, gums, and tongue
- Rapid, weak, thready pulse
- Decreasing pulse pressure
- Low blood pressure and concentrated urine

Hypovolemic shock can be avoided largely by the timely administration of IV fluids, blood, blood products, and medications that elevate blood pressure. Other factors may contribute to hemodynamic instability, and the PACU nurse implements multiple measures to manage these factors. Pain is controlled by making the patient as comfortable as possible and by using opioids judiciously. Exposure is avoided, and normothermia is maintained to prevent vasodilation.

Volume replacement is the primary intervention for shock. An infusion of lactated Ringer's solution or blood component therapy is initiated. Oxygen is administered by nasal cannula, facemask, or mechanical ventilation. Cardiotonic, vasodilator, and corticosteroid medications may be prescribed to improve cardiac function and reduce peripheral vascular resistance. The patient is kept warm while avoiding overheating to prevent cutaneous vessels from dilating and depriving vital organs of blood. The patient is placed flat in bed with the legs elevated. Respiratory and pulse rate, blood pressure, blood oxygen concentration, urinary output, level of consciousness, central venous pressure, pulmonary artery pressure, pulmonary capillary wedge pressure, and cardiac output are monitored to provide information on the patient's respiratory and cardiovascular status. Vital signs are monitored continuously until the patient's condition has stabilized.

HEMORRHAGE

Hemorrhage is an uncommon yet serious complication of surgery that can result in death (Finkelmeier, 2000). It can present insidiously or emergently at any time in the immediate postoperative period or up to several days after surgery (Table 20-1). When blood loss is extreme, the patient is apprehensive, restless, and thirsty; the skin is cold, moist, and pale. The pulse rate increases, the temperature falls, and respirations are rapid and deep, often of the gasping type spoken of as "air hunger." If hemorrhage progresses untreated, cardiac output decreases, arterial and venous blood pressure and hemoglobin level fall rapidly, the lips and the conjunctivae become pallid, spots appear before the eyes, a ringing is heard in the ears, and the patient grows weaker but remains conscious until near death.

Transfusing blood or blood products and determining the cause of hemorrhage are the initial therapeutic measures. The surgical site and incision should always be inspected for bleeding. If bleeding is evident, a sterile gauze pad and a pressure dressing are applied, and the site of the bleeding is elevated to heart level if possible. The patient is placed in the shock position (flat on back; legs elevated at a 20-degree angle; knees kept straight). If the source of bleeding is concealed, the patient may be taken back to the operating room for emergency exploration of the surgical site.

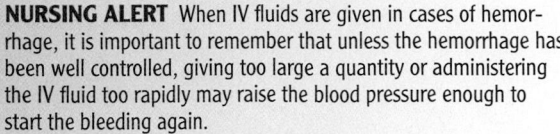

> **NURSING ALERT** When IV fluids are given in cases of hemorrhage, it is important to remember that unless the hemorrhage has been well controlled, giving too large a quantity or administering the IV fluid too rapidly may raise the blood pressure enough to start the bleeding again.

Special considerations must be given to patients who decline blood transfusions, such as Jehovah's Witnesses and those who identify specific requests on their advance directives or living will.

HYPERTENSION AND DYSRHYTHMIAS

Hypertension is common in the immediate postoperative period secondary to sympathetic nervous system stimulation from pain, hypoxia, or bladder distention. Dysrhythmias are associated with electrolyte imbalance, altered respiratory function, pain, hypothermia, stress, and anesthetic medications. Both conditions are managed by treating the underlying causes.

Relieving Pain and Anxiety

Opioid analgesics are administered judiciously and often intravenously in the PACU (Meeker & Rothrock, 1999). Intravenous opioids provide immediate relief and are short-acting, thus minimizing the potential for drug interactions or prolonged respiratory depression while anesthetics are still active in the patient's system. In addition to monitoring the patient's physiologic status and managing pain, the PACU nurse provides psychological support in an effort to relieve the patient's fears and concerns. The nurse checks the medical record for special needs and concerns of the patient. When the patient's condition permits, a close member of the family may visit in the PACU for a few moments. This often decreases the family's anxiety and makes the patient feel more secure.

Controlling Nausea and Vomiting

Nausea and vomiting are common problems in the PACU. The nurse should intervene at the patient's first report of nausea to control the problem rather than wait for it to progress to vomiting.

Many medications are available to control nausea and vomiting without oversedating the patient; they are commonly administered during surgery as well as in the PACU (Meeker & Rothrock, 1999). Intravenous or intramuscular administration of droperidol (Inapsine) is common, especially in the ambulatory setting. Other medications such as metoclopramide (Reglan), prochlorperazine (Compazine), and promethazine (Phenergan) are commonly prescribed (Karch, 2002; Meeker & Rothrock, 1999). Although it is costly, ondansetron (Zofran) is a frequently used, effective antiemetic with few side effects.

> **NURSING ALERT** At the slightest indication of nausea, the patient is turned completely to one side to promote mouth drainage and prevent aspiration of vomitus, which can cause asphyxiation and death.

Table 20-1 • **Classifications of Hemorrhage**

CLASSIFICATION	DEFINING CHARACTERISTIC
Time Frame	
Primary	Hemorrhage occurs at the time of surgery.
Intermediary	Hemorrhage occurs during the first few hours after surgery when the rise of blood pressure to its normal level dislodges insecure clots from untied vessels.
Secondary	Hemorrhage may occur some time after surgery if a ligature slips because a blood vessel was insecurely tied, became infected, or was eroded by a drainage tube.
Type of Vessel	
Capillary	Hemorrhage is characterized by a slow, general ooze.
Venous	Darkly colored blood bubbles out quickly.
Arterial	Blood is bright red and appears in spurts with each heartbeat.
Visibility	
Evident	Hemorrhage is on the surface and can be seen.
Concealed	Hemorrhage is in a body cavity and cannot be seen.

Gerontologic Considerations

The elderly patient, like all other patients, is transferred from the operating room table to the bed or stretcher slowly and gently. The effects of this action on blood pressure and ventilation are monitored. Special attention is given to keeping the patient warm because the elderly are more susceptible to hypothermia. The patient's position is changed frequently to stimulate respirations and to promote circulation and comfort.

Immediate postoperative care for the elderly patient is the same as that for any surgical patient, but additional support is given if there is impaired cardiovascular, pulmonary, or renal function. With invasive monitoring, it is possible to detect cardio-pulmonary deficits before signs and symptoms are apparent. The elderly patient has less physiologic reserve, and physiologic responses to stress are diminished or slowed. These changes reinforce the need for close monitoring and prompt treatment of hypotension, shock, and hemorrhage. Because of monitoring and improved individualized preoperative preparation, many older adults tolerate surgery well and have an uneventful recovery.

Postoperative confusion is common in older patients. The confusion is aggravated by social isolation, restraints, anesthetics and analgesics, and sensory deprivation. Reorienting the patient to the environment and using smaller amounts of sedatives, anesthetics, and analgesics may help prevent confusion. However, unrelieved pain, particularly pain at rest, may increase the risk for delirium and must be addressed (Lynch, Lazor, Gellis et al., 1998). Hypoxia can present as confusion and restlessness, as can blood loss and electrolyte imbalance. Excluding all other causes of confusion must precede the assumption that confusion is related to age, circumstances, and medications.

Determining Readiness for Discharge From the PACU

A patient remains in the PACU until he or she has fully recovered from the anesthetic agent (Meeker & Rothrock, 1999). Indicators of recovery include stable blood pressure, adequate respiratory function, adequate oxygen saturation level compared with baseline, and spontaneous movement or movement on command. Usually the following measures are used to determine the patient's readiness for discharge from the PACU:

- Stable vital signs
- Orientation to person, place, events, and time
- Uncompromised pulmonary function
- Pulse oximetry readings indicating adequate blood oxygen saturation
- Urine output at least 30 mL/h
- Nausea and vomiting absent or under control
- Minimal pain

Many hospitals use a scoring system (eg, Aldrete score) to determine the patient's general condition and readiness for transfer from the PACU (Quinn, 1999). Throughout the recovery period, the patient's physical signs are observed and evaluated by means of a scoring system based on a set of objective criteria. This evaluation guide, a modification of the Apgar scoring system used for evaluating newborns, allows a more objective assessment of the patient's condition in the PACU (Fig. 20-3). The patient is assessed at regular intervals (eg, every 15 or 30 minutes), and the score is totaled on the assessment record. Patients with a score lower than 7 must remain in the PACU until their condition improves or they are transferred to an intensive care area, depending on their preoperative baseline scores.

The patient is discharged from the phase I PACU by the anesthesiologist or anesthetist to the critical care unit, the medical-surgical unit, the phase II PACU, or home with a responsible family member (Quinn, 1999). Patients being discharged directly to home require verbal and written instructions and information about follow-up care.

Promoting Home and Community-Based Care

To ensure patient safety and recovery, expert patient teaching and discharge planning are necessary when a patient undergoes same-day or ambulatory surgery. Because anesthetics cloud memory for concurrent events, instructions should be given to both the patient and the adult who will be accompanying the patient home (Quinn, 1999).

TEACHING PATIENTS SELF-CARE

The patient and caregiver (eg, family member or friend) are informed about expected outcomes and immediate postoperative changes anticipated in the patient's capacity for self-care (Fox, 1998; Quinn, 1999). Written instructions about wound care, activity and dietary recommendations, medication, and follow-up visits to the same-day surgery unit or the surgeon are provided. Written instructions (designed to be copied and given to patients) about the postoperative care following many types of surgery are usually provided (Economou & Economou, 1999). The patient's caregiver at home is provided with verbal and written instructions about what to observe the patient for and about the actions to take if complications occur. Prescriptions are given to the patient. The nurse or surgeon's telephone number is provided, and the patient and caregiver are encouraged to call with questions and to schedule follow-up appointments (Chart 20-1).

Although recovery time varies depending on the type and extent of surgery and the patient's overall condition, instructions usually advise limited activity for 24 to 48 hours. During this time, the patient should not drive a vehicle, drink alcoholic beverages, or perform tasks that require energy or skill. Fluids may be consumed as desired, and smaller-than-normal amounts are eaten at mealtime. The patient is cautioned not to make important decisions at this time because the medications, anesthesia, and surgery may affect his or her decision-making ability.

CONTINUING CARE

Although most patients who undergo ambulatory surgery recover quickly and without complications, some patients require referral for home care. These may be elderly or frail patients, those who live alone, and patients with other health care problems that may interfere with self-care or resumption of usual activities. The home care nurse assesses the patient's physical status (eg, respiratory and cardiovascular status, adequacy of pain management, the surgical incision) and the patient's and family's ability to adhere to the recommendations given at the time of discharge. Previous teaching is reinforced as needed. The home care nurse may change surgical dressings, monitor the patency of a drainage system, or administer medications. The patient is assessed for any surgical complications. The patient and family are reminded about the importance of keeping follow-up appointments with the surgeon. Follow-up phone calls from the nurse or surgeon may also be used to assess the patient's progress and to answer any questions (Fox, 1998; Marley & Swanson, 2001).

Post Anesthesia Care Unit:
MODIFIED ALDRETE SCORE

Patient:

Room:

Date:

Final score:

Surgeon:

PACU nurse:

Area of Assessment	Point Score	Upon Admission	After		
			1 h	2 h	3 h
Muscle Activity:					
Moves spontaneously or on command:					
• Ability to move all extremities	2				
• Ability to move 2 extremities	1				
• Unable to control any extremity	0				
Respiration:					
• Ability to breathe deeply and cough	2				
• Limited respiratory effort (dyspnea or splinting)	1				
• No spontaneous effort	0				
Circulation:					
• BP ± 20% of preanesthetic level	2				
• BP ± 20%–49% of preanesthetic level	1				
• BP ± 50% of preanesthetic level	0				
Consciousness Level:					
• Fully awake	2				
• Arousable on calling	1				
• Not responding	0				
O₂ Saturation:					
• Able to maintain O₂ sat >92% on room air	2				
• Needs O₂ inhalation to maintain O₂ sat >90%	1				
• O₂ sat <90% even with O₂ supplement	0				
Totals:					

Required for discharge from Post Anesthesia Care Unit: 7–8 points

_____   _____

Time of release   Signature of nurse

FIGURE 20-3 Post anesthesia care unit record; Modified Aldrete Score. (O_2 sat = oxygen saturation.)

The Hospitalized Postoperative Patient

The patient admitted to the clinical unit for postoperative care has multiple needs. Seriously ill patients or those who have undergone major cardiovascular, pulmonary, or neurologic surgery are admitted to specialized intensive care units for close monitoring and advanced interventions and support. The care required by these patients in the immediate postoperative period is discussed in specific chapters. Postoperative care for the surgical patient returning to the general medical-surgical unit is discussed below.

Chart 20-1
Home Care Checklist • Discharge From Surgery

At the completion of the home care instruction, the patient or caregiver will be able to:	Patient	Caregiver
• Name the procedure that was performed and identify any permanent changes in anatomic structure or function.	✓	✓
• Describe ongoing postoperative therapeutic regimen, including medications, diet, activities to perform (such as walking and breathing exercises) and to avoid (such as driving a car or contact sports), adjuvant therapies, dressing changes and wound care, and any other treatments.	✓	✓
• Describe signs and symptoms of complications.	✓	✓
• State time and date of follow-up appointments.	✓	✓
• Identify interventions and strategies to use in adapting to any permanent changes in structure or function.	✓	✓
• Relate how to reach health care provider with questions or complications.	✓	✓
• State understanding of community resources and referrals (if any).	✓	✓
• Describe pertinent health promotion activities (eg, weight reduction, smoking cessation, stress management).	✓	✓

RECEIVING THE PATIENT IN THE CLINICAL UNIT

The patient's room is readied by assembling the necessary equipment and supplies: IV pole, drainage receptacle holder, emesis basin, tissues, disposable pads (Chux), blankets, and postoperative charting forms. When the call comes to the unit about the patient's transfer from the PACU, the need for any additional items that may be needed is communicated. The PACU nurse reports the baseline data about the patient's condition to the receiving nurse. The report includes demographic data, medical diagnosis, procedure performed, comorbid conditions, allergies, unexpected intraoperative events, estimated blood loss, the type and amount of fluids received, medications administered for pain, whether the patient has voided, and information that the patient and family have received about the patient's condition. Usually the surgeon speaks to the family after surgery and relates the general condition of the patient. The receiving nurse reviews the postoperative orders, admits the patient to the unit, performs an initial assessment, and attends to the patient's immediate needs (Chart 20-2).

NURSING MANAGEMENT AFTER SURGERY

During the first 24 hours after surgery, nursing care of the hospitalized patient on the general medical-surgical unit involves continuing to help the patient recover from the effects of anesthesia, frequently assessing the patient's physiologic status, monitoring for complications, managing pain, and implementing measures designed to achieve the long-range goals of independence with self-care, successful management of the therapeutic regimen, discharge to home, and full recovery. In the initial hours after admission to the clinical unit, adequate ventilation, hemodynamic stability, incisional pain, surgical site integrity, nausea and vomiting, neurologic status, and spontaneous voiding are primary concerns. The pulse rate, blood pressure, and respiration rate are recorded at least every 15 minutes for the first hour and every 30 minutes for the next 2 hours. Thereafter, they are measured less frequently if they remain stable. The temperature is monitored every 4 hours for the first 24 hours.

Patients usually begin to feel better several hours after surgery or after waking up the next morning. Although pain may still be intense, many patients feel more alert, less nauseous, and less anxious. They have begun their breathing and leg exercises, and many will have dangled their legs over the edge of the bed, stood, and ambulated a few feet or been assisted out of bed to the chair at least once. Many will have tolerated a light meal and had IV fluids discontinued. The focus of care shifts from intense physiologic management and symptomatic relief of the adverse effects of anesthesia to regaining independence with self-care and preparing for discharge. Despite these gains, the postoperative patient is still at risk for complications. Atelectasis, pneumonia, deep vein thrombosis, pulmonary embolism, constipation, paralytic ileus, and wound infection are ongoing threats for the postoperative patient (Fig. 20-4).

Chart 20-2 **Standard Postoperative Nursing Interventions**

Once the patient leaves the PACU and is admitted to the unit, immediate nursing interventions include the following:

- Assess breathing and administer supplemental oxygen, if prescribed.
- Monitor vital signs and note skin warmth, moisture, and color.
- Assess the surgical site and wound drainage systems.
- Assess level of consciousness, orientation, and ability to move extremities.
- Connect all drainage tubes to gravity or suction as indicated and monitor closed drainage systems.
- Assess pain level, pain characteristics (location, quality) and timing, type, and route of administration of last pain medication.
- Administer analgesics as prescribed and assess their effectiveness in relieving pain.
- Position patient to enhance comfort, safety, and lung expansion.
- Assess IV sites for patency and infusions for correct rate and solution.
- Assess urine output in closed drainage system or the patient's urge to void and bladder distention.
- Reinforce need to begin deep-breathing and leg exercises.
- Place call light, emesis basin, ice chips (if allowed), and bedpan or urinal within reach.
- Provide information to patient and family.

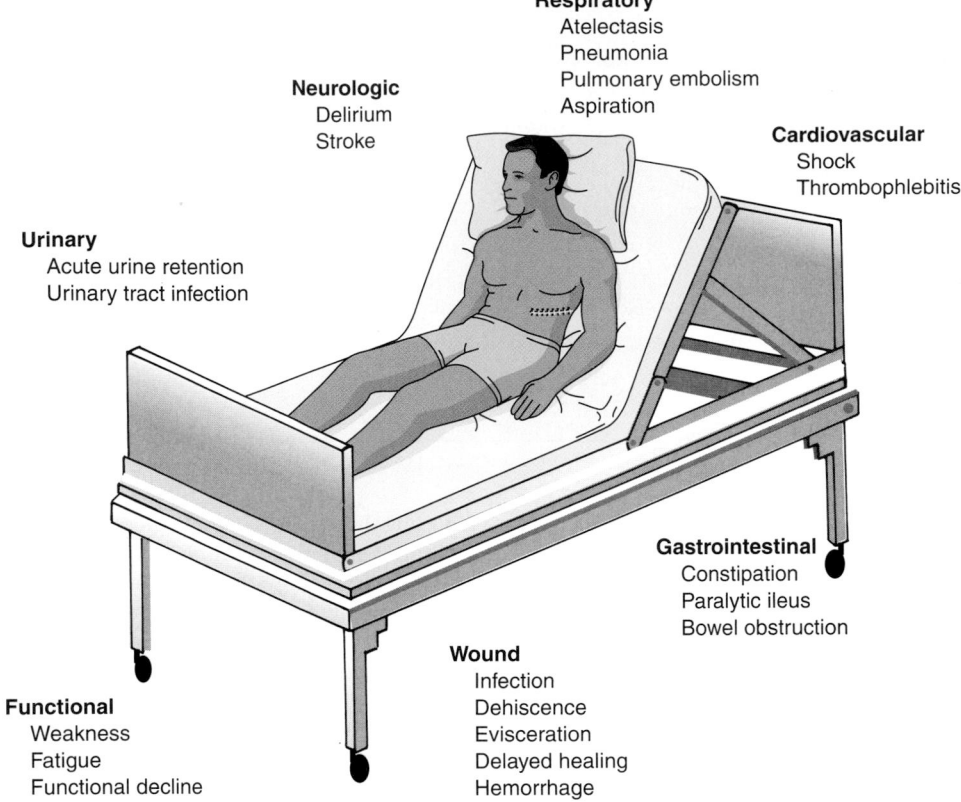

Respiratory
Atelectasis
Pneumonia
Pulmonary embolism
Aspiration

Neurologic
Delirium
Stroke

Cardiovascular
Shock
Thrombophlebitis

Urinary
Acute urine retention
Urinary tract infection

Gastrointestinal
Constipation
Paralytic ileus
Bowel obstruction

Wound
Infection
Dehiscence
Evisceration
Delayed healing
Hemorrhage
Hematoma

Functional
Weakness
Fatigue
Functional decline

FIGURE 20-4 The postoperative patient is subject to a number of potential complications.

NURSING PROCESS: THE HOSPITALIZED PATIENT RECOVERING FROM SURGERY

The Perioperative Nursing Data Set (PNDS) is a helpful model used by nurses in the postoperative phase of care (see Chap. 18, Fig. 18-1). Phenomena of concern to nurses on the clinical unit in the postoperative phase of care include nursing diagnoses, interventions, and outcomes for patients and their families. Additional areas of concern include collaborative problems and expected goals.

Assessment

Assessment of the hospitalized postoperative patient includes monitoring vital signs and completing a review of the systems upon arrival of the patient to the clinical unit and thereafter (see Chart 20-2).

Respiratory status is important because pulmonary complications are among the most frequent and serious problems encountered by the surgical patient. The nurse observes for airway patency and the quality of respirations, including depth, rate, and sound. Chest auscultation verifies that breath sounds are normal (or not normal) bilaterally, and the findings are documented as a baseline for later comparisons. Often, because of the effects of pain medications, respirations are slow. Shallow and rapid respirations may be due to pain, constricting dressings, gastric dilation, or obesity. Noisy breathing may be due to obstruction by secretions or the tongue.

The nurse assesses the patient's pain level using a verbal or visual analog scale and assesses the characteristics of the pain. The patient's appearance, pulse, respirations, blood pressure, skin color (adequate or cyanotic), and skin temperature (cold and clammy, warm and moist, or warm and dry) are clues to cardiovascular function. When the patient arrives in the clinical unit, the surgical site is observed for bleeding, type and integrity of dressing, and drains.

Also assessed when the patient arrives on the clinical unit are the patient's mental status and level of consciousness, speech, and orientation in comparison with preoperative baseline measures. Although a change in mental status or postoperative restlessness may be related to anxiety, pain, or medications, it may also be a symptom of oxygen deficit or hemorrhage. These serious causes must be investigated and excluded before other causes are pursued.

General discomfort resulting from lying in one position on the operating table, the surgeon's handling of tissues, the body's reaction to anesthesia, and anxiety are also common causes of restlessness. These discomforts may be relieved by administering the prescribed analgesics, changing the patient's position frequently, and assessing and alleviating the cause of anxiety. If tight, drainage-soaked bandages are causing discomfort, reinforcing or changing the dressing completely makes the patient more comfortable. The bladder is palpated for distention because urinary retention can also cause restlessness.

Diagnosis

NURSING DIAGNOSES

Based on the assessment data, major nursing diagnoses may include the following:

- Risk for ineffective airway clearance related to depressed respiratory function, pain, and bed rest

- Acute pain related to surgical incision
- Decreased cardiac output related to shock or hemorrhage
- Activity intolerance related to generalized weakness secondary to surgery
- Impaired skin integrity related to surgical incision and drains
- Risk for imbalanced body temperature related to surgical environment and anesthetic agents
- Risk for imbalanced nutrition, less than body requirements related to decreased intake and increased need for nutrients secondary to surgery
- Risk for constipation related to effects of medications, surgery, dietary change, and immobility
- Risk for urinary retention related to anesthetic agents
- Risk for injury related to surgical procedure or anesthetic agents
- Anxiety related to surgical procedure
- Risk for ineffective management of therapeutic regimen related to insufficient knowledge about wound care, dietary restrictions, activity recommendations, medications, follow-up care, or signs and symptoms of complications

COLLABORATIVE PROBLEMS/ POTENTIAL COMPLICATIONS

Based on the assessment data, potential complications may include the following:

- Deep vein thrombosis
- Hematoma
- Infection
- Wound dehiscence or evisceration

Planning and Goals

The major goals for the patient include optimal respiratory function, relief of pain, optimal cardiovascular function, increased activity tolerance, unimpaired wound healing, maintenance of body temperature, and maintenance of nutritional balance. Further goals include resumption of usual pattern of bowel and bladder elimination, identification of any perioperative positioning injury, acquisition of sufficient knowledge to manage self-care after discharge, and absence of complications.

Nursing Interventions

PREVENTING RESPIRATORY COMPLICATIONS

Respiratory depressive effects of opioid medications, decreased lung expansion secondary to pain, and decreased mobility combine to put the patient at risk for common respiratory complications, particularly atelectasis (incomplete expansion of the lung), pneumonia, and hypoxemia (Finkelmeier, 2000; Meeker & Rothrock, 1999). Atelectasis remains a risk for the patient who is not moving well or ambulating or who is not performing deep-breathing and coughing exercises or using an incentive spirometer. Signs and symptoms include decreased breath sounds over the affected area, crackles, and cough. Pneumonia is characterized by chills and fever, tachycardia, and tachypnea. Cough may or may not be present and may or may not be productive. Hypostatic pulmonary congestion, caused by a weakened cardiovascular system that permits stagnation of secretions at lung bases, may develop; it occurs most frequently in elderly patients who are not mobilized effectively. The symptoms are often vague, with perhaps a slight elevation of temperature, pulse, and respiratory rate

and a cough. Physical examination reveals dullness and crackles at the base of the lungs. If the condition progresses, the outcome may be fatal.

The types of hypoxemia that can affect postoperative patients are subacute and episodic. Subacute hypoxemia is a constant low level of oxygen saturation, although breathing appears normal. Episodic hypoxemia develops suddenly, and the patient may be at risk for cerebral dysfunction, myocardial ischemia, and cardiac arrest. Patients at risk for hypoxemia include those who have undergone major surgery (particularly abdominal), are obese, or have preexisting pulmonary problems. Hypoxemia can be detected by pulse oximetry, which measures blood oxygen saturation. Factors that may affect the accuracy of pulse oximetry readings include cold extremities, tremors, atrial fibrillation, acrylic nails, and black or blue nail polish (these colors interfere with the functioning of the pulse oximeter; other colors do not).

Preventive measures and timely recognition of signs and symptoms help avert pulmonary complications. Strategies to prevent respiratory complications include use of an incentive spirometer and deep-breathing and coughing exercises. Crackles indicate static pulmonary secretions that need to be mobilized by coughing and deep-breathing exercises. When a mucus plug obstructs one of the bronchi entirely, the pulmonary tissue beyond the plug collapses, and a massive atelectasis results.

To clear secretions and prevent pneumonia, the nurse encourages the patient to turn frequently and take deep breaths at least every 2 hours. Coughing is also encouraged to dislodge mucus plugs. These pulmonary exercises should begin as soon as the patient arrives on the clinical unit and continue until the patient is discharged. Even if he or she is not fully awake from anesthesia, the patient can be asked to take several deep breaths. This helps to expel residual anesthetic agents, mobilize secretions, and prevent alveolar collapse (atelectasis). Careful splinting of abdominal or thoracic incision sites helps the patient overcome the fear that the exertion of coughing might open the incision. Analgesic agents are administered to permit more effective coughing, and oxygen is administered as prescribed to prevent or relieve hypoxia. To encourage lung expansion, the patient is encouraged to yawn or take sustained maximal inspirations to create a negative intrathoracic pressure of −40 mm Hg and expand lung volume to total capacity. Chest physical therapy may be prescribed if indicated.

Coughing is contraindicated in patients who have head injuries or who have undergone intracranial surgery (because of the risk for increasing intracranial pressure), as well as in patients who have undergone eye surgery (risk for increasing intraocular pressure) or plastic surgery (risk for increasing tension on delicate tissues). In patients with an abdominal or thoracic incision, the nurse teaches the patient how to splint the incision while coughing.

Most postoperative patients, especially the elderly and those with an abdominal or thoracic incision, are given an incentive spirometer to use. In incentive spirometry, the patient performs sustained maximal inspirations and can see the results of these efforts as they register on the spirometer. Such feedback encourages the patient to continue to take deep breaths to maximize voluntary lung expansion. A target is established for each patient. The patient first exhales, then places the lips around the mouthpiece and slowly inhales, trying to drive the piston on the device to a marked goal. Using a spirometer has several advantages: it encourages the patient to participate actively in treatment; it ensures that the maneuver is physiologically appropriate and is repeated; and it is a cost-effective way of preventing complications. A common recommendation for use of the incentive spirometer is 10 deep breaths every hour while awake. Refer to Chapter 25 for additional discussion of incentive spirometry.

Early ambulation increases metabolism and pulmonary aeration and, in general, improves all body functions. The patient is encouraged to be out of bed as soon as possible (ie, on the day of surgery, or no later than the first postoperative day). This practice is especially valuable in preventing pulmonary complications in older patients.

RELIEVING PAIN

Most patients experience some pain after a surgical procedure (Meeker & Rothrock, 1999). Many factors (motivational, affective, cognitive, and emotional) influence the pain experience. Research findings have led to a better understanding of how perception, learning, personality, ethnic and cultural factors, and environment can affect anxiety, depression, and pain response (Schafheutle, Cantrill & Noyce, 2001; Watt-Watson, Stevens, Garfinkel et al., 2001). The degree and severity of postoperative pain and the patient's tolerance for pain depend on the incision site, the nature of the surgical procedure, the extent of surgical trauma, the type of anesthetic agent, and how the agent was administered. The preoperative preparation received by the patient (including information about what to expect as well as reassurance and psychological support) is a significant factor in decreasing anxiety, apprehension, and even the amount of postoperative pain.

The reasons for controlling pain are compelling. There is a well-known correlation between frequency of complications and localization of pain (Moline, 2001). Intense pain stimulates the stress response, which adversely affects the cardiac and immune systems. When pain impulses are transmitted, muscle tension increases, as does local vasoconstriction. The ischemia in the affected area causes further stimulation of pain receptors. When these noxious impulses travel centrally, sympathetic activity is compounded, which increases myocardial demand and oxygen consumption. Research has shown that cardiovascular insufficiency occurs three times more frequently, and the incidence of infection is five times greater, in people with poor postoperative pain control (Moline, 2001; Schafheutle et al., 2001; Watt-Watson et al., 2001). The hypothalamic stress response is also responsible for an increase in blood viscosity and platelet aggregation. This can lead to phlebothrombosis and pulmonary embolism.

Often the physician has prescribed different medications or dosages to cover various levels of pain. The nurse should discuss these options with the patient to determine the best medication. Then the nurse should assess the effectiveness of the medication periodically, beginning 30 minutes after administration or sooner if the medication is being delivered by patient-controlled analgesia.

Opioid Analgesics

About one third of patients report severe pain, one third moderate pain, and one third little or no pain. These statistics do not mean that the patients in the last group have no pain; rather, they appear to activate psychodynamic mechanisms that impair the registering of pain ("gate closing" theory and nociceptive transmission). See Chapter 13 for a more detailed discussion of pain and the factors influencing the pain experience.

Opioid analgesics are commonly prescribed for pain and immediate postoperative restlessness. A preventive approach rather than an "as needed" (PRN) approach, is more effective in relieving pain. With a preventive approach, the medication is administered at prescribed intervals rather than when the pain becomes severe or unbearable. Many patients (and some health

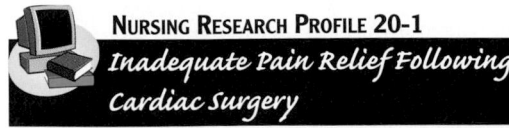

NURSING RESEARCH PROFILE 20-1
Inadequate Pain Relief Following Cardiac Surgery

Watt-Watson, J., Stevens, B., Garfinkel, P., Streiner, D., & Gallup, R. (2001). Relationships between nurses' pain knowledge and pain management outcomes for their postoperative cardiac patients. *Journal of Advanced Nursing, 36*(4), 535–545.

Purpose
Although studies have examined nurses' knowledge and perceived barriers to pain management, few studies have examined the relationship of nurses' knowledge and their actual implementation of pain management strategies. This Canadian study investigated the relationship between nursing pain knowledge and pain management outcomes for postoperative coronary artery bypass graft (CABG) patients.

Study Sample and Design
This was a descriptive, correlational, mixed between-within subjects design. A convenience sample of 94 nurses from four cardiovascular units in three university-affiliated hospitals were interviewed, along with 225 of their assigned patients. The nurses included 86 women and 8 men. The patients included 52 women and 173 men. Instruments used with the patients included the McGill Pain Questionnaire-Short Form (MPQ-SF), the present pain intensity (PPI) scale, and a visual analog scale (VAS); analgesic prescription and administration data were obtained by chart review. The Toronto Pain Management Inventory (TPMI) was used to measure pain knowledge in the nurses. The social desirability scale (SDS) was also used with the nurses.

Findings
The majority of patients reported moderate to severe pain during the previous 24 hours (86%) and at the time of interview while moving around (68%). The mean total score on the MPQ-SF, which has a range of possible scores from 0 to 45, was 11.8 ± 7. Chart review data indicated undermedication of patients for pain, with patients receiving only 47% of their prescribed analgesia. The nurses' scores on the TPMI indicated moderate pain knowledge, with the majority of nurses (53%) scoring 69% or less and only 15% scoring 75% or greater on the inventory. While hospital policy required documentation of pain as a fifth vital sign, charting of pain was minimal and high pain ratings did not result in an increase in analgesics administered.

Nursing Implications
Nurses caring for postoperative CABG patients need further education about pain management. Nurses also need to be aware that patients are undermedicated following CABG surgery and need to be more aware of patients' needs for medication, administer prescribed doses, and advocate for patients when pain medication is not prescribed.

care providers) are overly concerned with the risk of drug addiction in the postoperative patient. This risk, however, is negligible with the use of opioid medications for short-term pain control.

Patient-Controlled Analgesia

Given the negative impact of pain on recovery, nurses need to think "pain prevention" rather than sporadic pain control and should encourage the use of patient-controlled analgesia (PCA). Patients recover more quickly when adequate pain measures are used, and PCA permits patients to administer their own pain medication when needed (Quinn, 1999). The amount of medication delivered by the IV or epidural route and the time span during which the opioid medication is released are controlled by the PCA device. Self-administration promotes patient participation in care, eliminates delayed administration of pain medications, and maintains a therapeutic drug level.

Most patients are candidates for PCA. The two requirements for PCA are an understanding of the need to self-dose and the physical ability to self-dose. Upon sensing pain, the patient activates the medication-delivering pump with a hand-held button. PCA enables the patient to move, turn, cough, and take deep breaths with less pain, thus reducing postoperative pulmonary problems.

Epidural Infusions and Intrapleural Anesthesia

For thoracic, orthopedic, obstetric, and major abdominal surgery, certain opioid analgesics may be administered by epidural or intrathecal infusion. Epidural infusions produce a more profound analgesia. Epidural infusions are used with caution in chest procedures because the effect of the analgesic may ascend along the spinal cord and affect respiration. Intrapleural anesthesia involves the administration of local anesthetic by a catheter between the parietal and visceral pleura. It provides sensory anesthesia without affecting motor function to the intercostal muscles. This anesthesia allows more effective coughing and deep breathing in conditions such as cholecystectomy, renal surgery, and rib fractures in which pain in the thoracic region would interfere with these functions.

A local opioid or a combination anesthetic (opioid plus local anesthetic agent) is used in the epidural infusion. Other local anesthetic methods may be used to provide analgesia and anesthesia. Intrapleural anesthesia has fewer adverse effects than systemic or spinal opioids and a lower incidence of urinary retention, vomiting, and pruritus when compared with thoracic epidural opioids (Moline, 2001; Quinn, 1999).

Other Pain Relief Measures

For pain that is difficult to control, a subcutaneous pain management system may be used. This is a silicone catheter that is inserted at the affected area. The catheter is attached to a pump that delivers a continuous amount of local anesthetic at a specific amount determined and prescribed by the physician (Fig. 20-5).

Complete absence of pain in the area of the surgical incision may not occur for a few weeks, depending on the site and nature of surgery, but the intensity of postoperative pain gradually subsides on subsequent days. However, pain control continues to be an important concern for the patient and the nurse. Effective pain management allows the patient to participate in care, perform deep-breathing and leg exercises, and tolerate activity. As stated previously, poor pain control contributes to postoperative complications and increased length of stay. The nurse continues to assess the pain level, the effectiveness of pain medication, and factors that influence pain tolerance (eg, energy level, stress level, cultural background, meaning of pain to the patient). The nurse explains that taking pain medication before the pain becomes intense is more effective and offers pain medication at intervals rather than waiting for the patient to request medication. Nonpharmacologic pain relief measures, such as imagery, relaxation, massage, application of heat or cold (if prescribed), and distraction, can be used to supplement medications (Seers & Carroll, 1998). Changing the patient's position, using distraction, applying cool washcloths to the face, and rubbing the back with a soothing lotion may be useful in relieving general discomfort

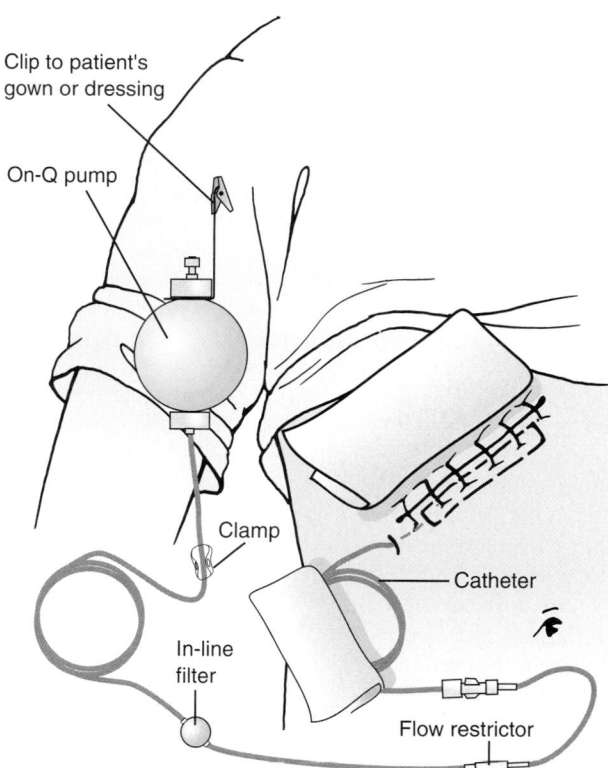

FIGURE 20-5 Subcutaneous pain management system comprises a pump, filter, and catheter that delivers a specific amount of prescribed local anesthetic at a rate determined by the physician. With permission from I-Flow Corporation, Lake Forest, CA.

temporarily and rendering medication more effective when it is administered.

PROMOTING CARDIAC OUTPUT

If signs and symptoms of shock or hemorrhage occur, treatment and nursing care are implemented as described in the discussion of care in the PACU.

> **NURSING ALERT** A systolic blood pressure of less than 90 mm Hg is usually considered reportable at once. However, the patient's preoperative or baseline blood pressure is used to make informed postoperative comparisons. A previously stable blood pressure that shows a downward trend of 5 mm Hg at each 15-minute reading should also be reported.

Although most patients do not hemorrhage or go into shock, changes in circulating volume, the stress of surgery, and the effects of medications and preoperative preparations all affect cardiovascular function. Intravenous fluid replacement is standard for up to 24 hours after surgery or until the patient is stable and tolerating oral fluids. Close monitoring is indicated to detect and correct conditions such as fluid volume deficit, altered tissue perfusion, and decreased cardiac output, all of which can increase the patient's discomfort, place him or her at risk for complications, and prolong the hospital stay. Some patients are at risk for fluid volume excess secondary to existing cardiovascular or renal disease, advanced age, or the release of adrenocorticotropic hormone and antidiuretic hormone as a result of the stress of surgery. Consequently, fluid replacement must be carefully managed, and intake and output records must be accurate.

Nursing management includes assessing the patency of the IV lines and ensuring that the appropriate fluids are administered at the prescribed rate. Intake and output, including emesis and output from wound drainage systems, are recorded separately and totaled to determine fluid balance. If the patient has an indwelling urinary catheter, hourly outputs are monitored and rates of less than 30 mL/h are reported; if the patient is voiding, an output of less than 240 mL per 8-hour shift is reported. Electrolyte levels and hemoglobin and hematocrit levels are monitored. Decreased hemoglobin and hematocrit levels can indicate blood loss or dilution of circulating volume by IV fluids. If dilution is contributing to the decreased levels, the hemoglobin and hematocrit rise as the stress response abates and fluids are mobilized and excreted.

Venous stasis from dehydration, immobility, and pressure on leg veins during surgery put the patient at risk for deep vein thrombosis. Leg exercises and frequent position changes are initiated early in the postoperative period to stimulate circulation. Patients should avoid positions that compromise venous return, such as raising the bed's knee gatch or placing a pillow under the knees, sitting for long periods, and dangling the legs with pressure at the back of the knees. Venous return is promoted by elastic compression stockings and early ambulation. Early ambulation has a significant effect on recovery and the prevention of complications and can begin, in many instances, the evening of surgery. Postoperative activity orders are checked before getting the patient out of bed. Sitting up at the edge of the bed for a few minutes may be all the patient can tolerate at first.

ENCOURAGING ACTIVITY

Most surgical patients are encouraged to be out of bed as soon as possible. Early ambulation reduces the incidence of postoperative complications, such as atelectasis, hypostatic pneumonia, gastrointestinal discomfort, and circulatory problems (Meeker & Rothrock, 1999). Ambulation increases ventilation and reduces the stasis of bronchial secretions in the lung. It also reduces postoperative abdominal distention by increasing gastrointestinal tract and abdominal wall tone and stimulating peristalsis. Thrombophlebitis or phlebothrombosis occurs less frequently because early ambulation prevents stasis of blood by increasing the rate of circulation in the extremities. Pain is often decreased when early ambulation is possible, and the hospital stay is shorter and less costly, a further advantage to the patient and the hospital.

Despite the advantages of early ambulation, patients may be reluctant to get up the evening of surgery. Reminding them of the importance of early mobility in preventing complications may help them overcome their fears. One concern when the patient is to get out of bed for the first time is orthostatic hypotension, also called postural hypotension. Orthostatic hypotension is an abnormal drop in blood pressure that occurs as the patient changes from a supine to a standing position. It is common after surgery because of changes in circulating volume and bed rest. Signs and symptoms include a 20-mm Hg decrease in systolic blood pressure or a 10-mm Hg decrease in diastolic blood pressure, weakness, dizziness, and fainting. Older adults are at increased risk for

orthostatic hypotension secondary to age-related changes in vascular tone. To detect orthostatic hypotension, the nurse assesses the patient's feelings of dizziness and his or her blood pressure first in the supine position, after the patient sits up, again after the patient stands, and 2 to 3 minutes later. Gradual position change gives the circulatory system time to adjust. If the patient becomes dizzy, he or she should be returned to the supine position, and getting out of bed should be delayed for several hours.

To assist the postoperative patient in getting out of bed for the first time after surgery, the nurse performs the following actions:

1. Help the patient to move gradually from the lying position to the sitting position until dizziness passes. This can be achieved by raising the head of the bed.
2. Position the patient completely upright (sitting) and turned so that both legs are hanging over the edge of the bed.
3. Assist the patient to stand beside the bed.

When accustomed to the upright position, the patient may start to walk. The nurse should be at the patient's side to give physical support and encouragement. Care must be taken not to tire the patient; the extent of the first few periods of ambulation varies with the type of surgical procedure and the patient's physical condition and age.

Whether or not the patient can ambulate early in the postoperative period, bed exercises are encouraged to improve circulation. Bed exercises consist of the following:

- Arm exercises (full range of motion, with specific attention to abduction and external rotation of the shoulder)
- Hand and finger exercises
- Foot exercises to prevent deep vein thrombosis, foot drop, and toe deformities and to aid in maintaining good circulation
- Leg flexion and leg-lifting exercises to prepare the patient for ambulation
- Abdominal and gluteal contraction exercises

Hampered by pain, dressings, IV lines, or drains, many patients cannot engage in activity without assistance. Prolonged inactivity may lead to pressure ulcers, deep vein thrombosis, atelectasis, or hypostatic pneumonia. Helping the patient increase his or her activity level on the first postoperative day is an important nursing function. One way to increase the patient's activity is to have the patient perform as much routine hygiene care as possible. Setting up the patient to bathe with a bedside wash basin or, if possible, assisting the patient to the bathroom to sit in a chair at the sink not only gets the patient moving but helps restore a sense of self-control and prepares the patient for discharge.

To be safely discharged to home, patients need to be able to ambulate a functional distance (length of the house or apartment), get in and out of bed unassisted, and be independent with toileting. Patients can be asked to perform as much as they can and then to call for assistance. The patient and the nurse can collaborate on a schedule for progressive activity that includes ambulating in the room and hallway and sitting out of bed in the chair. Assessing the patient's vital signs before, during, and after a scheduled activity helps the nurse and patient determine the rate of progression. By providing physical support, the nurse maintains the patient's safety; by communicating a positive attitude about the patient's ability to perform the activity, the nurse promotes the patient's confidence. The nurse should make sure the patient continues to perform bed exercises, wears pneumatic compression or thigh-high elastic compression stockings when in bed, and rests as needed.

PROMOTING WOUND HEALING

Ongoing assessment of the surgical site involves inspection for approximation of wound edges, integrity of sutures or staples, redness, discoloration, warmth, swelling, unusual tenderness, or drainage. The area around the wound should also be inspected for reactions to tape or trauma from tight bandages.

Nursing interventions to promote wound healing also include management of surgical drains and dressings. Wound drains are tubes exiting the peri-incisional area into either a portable wound suction device (closed) or into the dressings (open). The principle involved is to allow the escape of blood and serous fluids that can otherwise serve as a culture medium for bacteria. In portable wound suction, the use of gentle, constant suction enhances drainage of these fluids and collapses the skin flaps against the underlying tissue, thus removing "dead space." Types of wound drains include the Penrose, Hemovac, and Jackson-Pratt drains (Fig. 20-6). Output from wound drainage systems and all new drainage is recorded. The amount of bloody drainage on the surgical dressing is assessed frequently. Spots of drainage on the dressings are outlined with a pen, and the date and time of the outline are recorded on the dressing so that increased drainage can be easily seen. A certain amount of bloody drainage in a wound drainage system or on the dressing is expected, but excessive amounts should be reported to the surgeon. Increasing amounts of fresh blood on the dressing should be reported immediately. Some wounds are irrigated heavily before closure in the operating room, and open drains exiting the wound may be embedded in the dressings. These wounds may drain large amounts of blood-tinged fluid that saturate the dressing. The dressing can be reinforced with sterile gauze bandages; the time that they were reinforced should be documented. If drainage continues, the surgeon should be notified so that the dressing can be changed. Multiple similar drains are numbered or otherwise labeled (eg, left lower quadrant, left upper quadrant) so that output measurements can be reliably and consistently recorded.

Surgical wound healing occurs in three phases: the inflammatory, proliferative, and maturation phases (Table 20-2). Wounds also heal by different mechanisms, depending on the condition of the wound. These mechanisms include first-, second-, or third-intention wound healing (Meeker & Rothrock, 1999).

First-Intention Healing

Wounds made aseptically, with a minimum of tissue destruction, and properly closed heal with little tissue reaction by first intention (primary union) (Fig. 20-7). When wounds heal by **first-intention healing**, granulation tissue is not visible and scar formation is minimal. Postoperatively, many of these wounds are covered with a dry sterile dressing. If a cyanoacrylate tissue adhesive was used to close the incision without the use of sutures, a dressing is contraindicated (Vargas & Reger, 2000).

Second-Intention Healing

Second-intention healing (granulation) occurs in infected wounds (abscess) or in wounds in which the edges have not been approximated. When an abscess is incised, it collapses partly, but the dead and the dying cells forming its walls are still being released into the cavity. For this reason, drainage tubes or gauze packing are inserted into the abscess pocket to allow drainage to escape easily. Gradually, the necrotic material disintegrates and escapes, and the abscess cavity fills with a red, soft, sensitive tissue that bleeds easily. This tissue is composed of minute, thin-walled capillaries and buds that later form connective tissue. These buds, called granulations, enlarge until they fill the area left by the destroyed tissue (see Fig. 20-7). The cells surrounding the capillaries change their round shape to become long, thin, and intertwined to form a scar (cicatrix). Healing is complete when skin cells (epithelium) grow over these granulations. This method of repair is called healing by granulation, and it takes place whenever pus is formed or when loss of tissue has occurred for any reason. When the postoperative wound is allowed to heal by secondary intention, it is usually packed with saline-moistened sterile dressings and covered with a dry sterile dressing.

Third-Intention Healing

Third-intention healing (secondary suture) is used for deep wounds that have either not been sutured early or that break down and are resutured later, thus bringing together two apposing granulation surfaces. This results in a deeper and wider scar. These wounds are also packed postoperatively with moist gauze and covered with a dry sterile dressing.

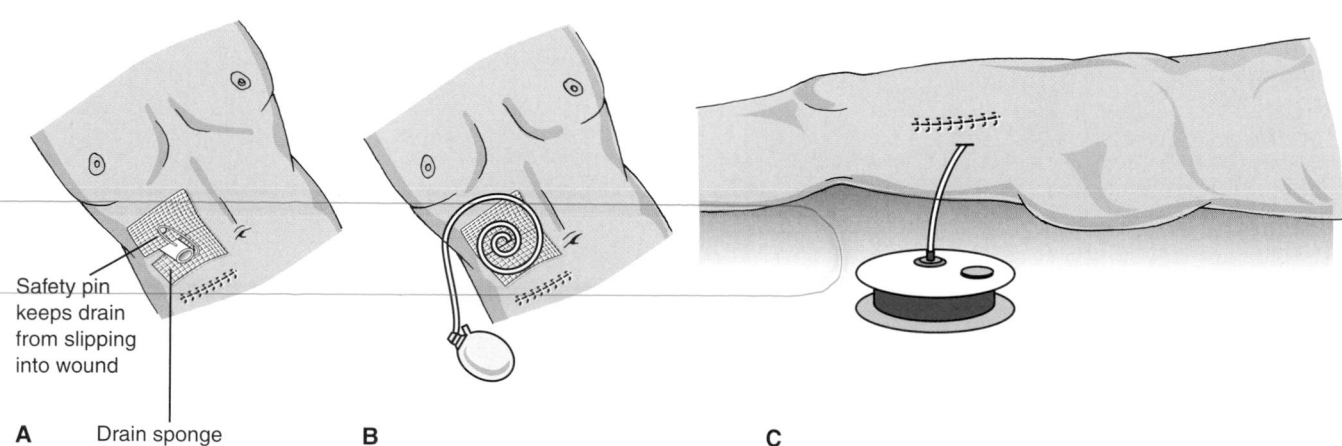

A Safety pin keeps drain from slipping into wound — Drain sponge **B** **C**

FIGURE 20-6 Types of surgical drains: (**A**) Penrose, (**B**) Jackson-Pratt, (**C**) Hemovac.

Table 20-2 • Phases of Wound Healing

PHASE	DURATION	EVENTS
Inflammatory (also called lag or exudative phase)	1–4 days	Blood clot forms Wound becomes edematous Debris of damaged tissue and blood clot are phagocytosed
Proliferative (also called fibroblastic or connective tissue phase)	5–20 days	Collagen produced Granulation tissue forms Wound tensile strength increases
Maturation (also called differentiation, resorptive, remodeling, or plateau phase)	21 days to months or even years	Fibroblasts leave wound Tensile strength increases Collagen fibers reorganize and tighten to reduce scar size

As a wound heals, many factors, such as adequate nutrition, cleanliness, rest, and position, determine how quickly healing occurs. These factors are influenced by nursing interventions. Specific nursing assessments and interventions that address these factors and help to promote wound healing are presented in Table 20-3. Other nursing interventions include assessment and care of the wound.

CHANGING THE DRESSING

While the first postoperative dressing is usually changed by a member of the surgical team, subsequent dressing changes in the immediate postoperative period are usually performed by the nurse. A dressing is applied to a wound for one or more of the following reasons: (1) to provide a proper environment for wound

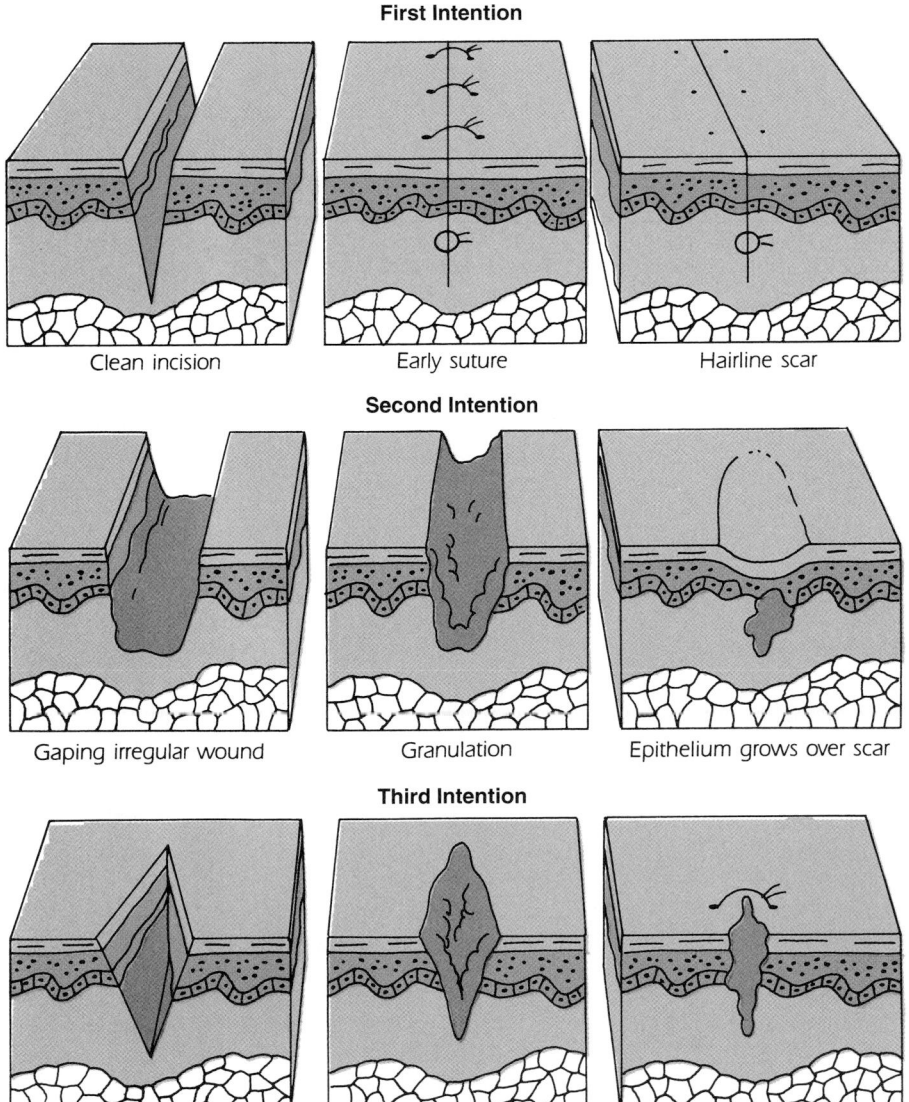

First Intention

Clean incision   Early suture   Hairline scar

Second Intention

Gaping irregular wound   Granulation   Epithelium grows over scar

Third Intention

Wound   Increased granulation   Late suturing with wide scar

FIGURE 20-7 Types of wound healing: first intention healing, second intention healing, and third intention healing.

Table 20-3 • Factors Affecting Wound Healing

FACTORS	RATIONALE	NURSING INTERVENTIONS
Age of patient	The older the patient, the less resilient the tissues.	Handle all tissues gently.
Handling of tissues	Rough handling causes injury and delayed healing.	Handle tissues carefully and evenly.
Hemorrhage	Accumulation of blood creates dead spaces as well as dead cells that must be removed. The area becomes a growth medium for organisms.	Monitor vital signs. Observe incision site for evidence of bleeding and infection.
Hypovolemia	Insufficient blood volume leads to vasoconstriction and reduced oxygen and nutrients available for wound healing.	Monitor for volume deficit (circulatory impairment). Correct by fluid replacement as prescribed.
Local factors		
Edema	Reduces blood supply by exerting increased interstitial pressure on vessels	Elevate part; apply cool compresses.
Inadequate dressing technique		
Too small	Permits bacterial invasion and contamination	Follow guidelines for proper dressing technique.
Too tight	Reduces blood supply carrying nutrients and oxygen	
Nutritional deficits	Protein-calorie depletion may occur. Insulin secretion may be inhibited, causing blood glucose to rise.	Correct deficits; this may require parenteral nutritional therapy. Monitor blood glucose levels. Administer vitamin supplements as prescribed.
Foreign bodies	Foreign bodies retard healing.	Keep wounds free of dressing threads, talcum, and powder from gloves.
Oxygen deficit (tissue oxygenation insufficient)	Insufficient oxygen may be due to inadequate lung and cardiovascular function as well as localized vasoconstriction.	Encourage deep breathing, turning, controlled coughing.
Drainage accumulation	Accumulated secretions hamper healing process.	Monitor closed drainage systems for proper functioning. Institute measures to remove accumulated secretions.
Medications		
Corticosteroids	May mask presence of infection by impairing normal inflammatory response	Be aware of action and effect of medications patient is receiving.
Anticoagulants	May cause hemorrhage	
Broad-spectrum and specific antibiotics	Effective if administered immediately before surgery for specific pathology or bacterial contamination. If administered after wound is closed, ineffective because of intravascular coagulation.	
Patient overactivity	Prevents approximation of wound edges. Resting favors healing.	Use measures to keep wound edges approximated: taping, bandaging, splints. Encourage rest.
Systemic disorders	These depress cell functions that directly affect wound healing.	Be familiar with the nature of the specific disorder.
Hemorrhagic shock		Administer prescribed treatment. Cultures may be indicated to determine appropriate antibiotic.
Acidosis		
Hypoxia		
Renal failure		
Hepatic disease		
Sepsis		
Immunosuppressed state	Patient is more vulnerable to bacterial and viral invasion; defense mechanisms are impaired.	Provide maximum protection to prevent infection. Restrict visitors with colds; institute mandatory hand hygiene by all staff.
Wound stressors	Produce tension on wounds, particularly of the torso.	Encourage frequent turning and ambulation and administer antiemetic medications as prescribed.
Vomiting		Assist patient in splinting incision.
Valsalva maneuver		
Heavy coughing		
Straining		

healing; (2) to absorb drainage; (3) to splint or immobilize the wound; (4) to protect the wound and new epithelial tissue from mechanical injury; (5) to protect the wound from bacterial contamination and from soiling by feces, vomitus, and urine; (6) to promote hemostasis, as in a pressure dressing; and (7) to provide mental and physical comfort for the patient.

The patient is told that the dressing is to be changed and that changing the dressing is a simple procedure associated with little discomfort. The dressing change is performed at a suitable time (eg, not at mealtimes or when visitors are present). Privacy is provided, and the patient is not unduly exposed. The nurse should avoid referring to the incision as a scar since the term may have negative connotations for the patient. Assurance is given that the incision will shrink as it heals and the redness will fade.

The nurse carries out hand hygiene before and after the dressing change and wears disposable gloves for the dressing change itself. The tape or adhesive portion of the dressing is removed by pulling it parallel with the skin surface and in the direction of hair growth, rather than at right angles. Alcohol wipes or nonirritating solvents aid in removing adhesive painlessly and quickly. The old dressing is removed and then deposited in a container designated for biomedical waste disposal. In accordance with standard precautions, dressings are never touched by ungloved hands because of the danger of transmitting pathogenic organisms.

If the patient is sensitive to adhesive tape, the dressing may be held in place with hypoallergenic tape. Many tapes are porous to permit ventilation and prevent skin maceration. The correct way to apply tape is to place the tape at the center of the dressing and then press the tape down on both sides, applying tension evenly away from the midline. The wrong method of applying tape— fixing one end of the tape to the skin and pulling it tight over the dressing—often wrinkles and pulls the skin in the process. The resulting continuous and forceful traction produces a shearing effect, causing the epidermal layer to slip sideways and become separated from the deeper dermal layers. Some wounds become edematous after having been dressed, causing considerable tension on the tape. If the tape is not flexible, the stretching bandage will also cause a shear injury to the skin. This can result in denuded areas or large blisters. An elastic adhesive bandage (Elastoplast, Microfoam-3M) may be used to hold dressings in place over mobile areas, such as the neck or the extremities, or where pressure is required.

While changing the dressing, the nurse has an opportunity to teach the patient how to care for the incision and change the dressings at home. The nurse observes for indicators of the patient's readiness to learn, such as looking at the incision, expressing interest, or assisting in the dressing change. Information on self-care activities and possible signs of infection are summarized in Chart 20-3.

MAINTAINING NORMAL BODY TEMPERATURE

The patient is still at risk for malignant hyperthermia and hypothermia in the postoperative period (Fortunato-Phillips, 2000). Efforts are made to identify malignant hyperthermia and to treat it early and promptly (Redmond, 2001). (See the discussion of malignant hyperthermia in Chap. 19.)

Patients who have been anesthetized are susceptible to chills and drafts. Attention to hypothermia management, begun in the intraoperative period, extends into the postoperative period to prevent significant nitrogen loss and catabolism. Signs of hypothermia are reported to the physician. The room is maintained at a comfortable temperature, and blankets are provided to prevent chilling. Treatment includes oxygen administration, adequate

---

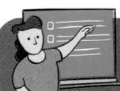

Chart 20-3 • **PATIENT EDUCATION**
Wound Care Instructions

Until Sutures Are Removed
1. Keep the wound dry and clean.
   - If there is no dressing, ask your nurse or physician if you can bathe or shower.
   - If a dressing or splint is in place, do not remove it unless it is wet or soiled.
   - If wet or soiled, change dressing yourself if you have been taught to do so; otherwise, call your nurse or physician for guidance.
   - If you have been taught, instruction might be as follows:
     Cleanse area *gently* with sterile normal saline once or twice daily.
     Cover with a sterile Telfa pad or gauze square large enough to cover wound.
     Apply hypoallergenic tape (Dermacel or paper). Adhesive is not recommended because it is difficult to remove without possible injury to the incisional site.
2. Immediately report any of these signs of infection:
   - Redness, marked swelling exceeding ½ inch (2.5 cm) from incision site; tenderness; or increased warmth around wound
   - Red streaks in skin near wound
   - Pus or discharge, foul odor
   - Chills or temperature higher than 37.7°C (100°F)
3. If soreness or pain causes discomfort, apply a dry cool pack (containing ice or cold water) or take prescribed

acetaminophen tablets (2) every 4–6 hours. Avoid using aspirin without direction or instruction because bleeding can occur with its use.
4. Swelling after surgery is common. To help reduce swelling, elevate the affected part to the level of the heart.
   - Hand or arm
     Sleep—elevate arm on pillow at side
     Sitting—place arm on pillow on adjacent table
     Standing—rest affected hand on opposite shoulder; support elbow with unaffected hand
   - Leg or foot
     Sitting—place a pillow on a facing chair; provide support underneath the knee
     Lying—place a pillow under affected leg

After Sutures Are Removed
Although the wound appears to be healed when sutures are removed, it is still tender and will continue to heal and strengthen for several weeks.
1. Follow recommendations of physician or nurse regarding extent of activity.
2. Keep suture line clean; do not rub vigorously; pat dry. Wound edges may look red and may be slightly raised. This is normal.
3. If the site continues to be red, thick, and painful to pressure after 8 weeks, consult the health care provider. (This may be due to excessive collagen formation and should be checked.)

hydration, and proper nutrition. The patient is also monitored for cardiac dysrhythmias. The risk for hypothermia is greater in the elderly and in patients who were in the cool operating room environment for a prolonged period.

MANAGING GASTROINTESTINAL FUNCTION AND RESUMING NUTRITION

Gastrointestinal discomfort (nausea, vomiting, hiccups) and resumption of oral intake are issues for both the patient and the nurse. Nausea and vomiting are common after anesthesia (Litwack, 1999; Meeker & Rothrock, 1999). They are more common in women, obese people (fat cells act as reservoirs for the anesthetic), patients prone to motion sickness, and patients who have undergone lengthy surgical procedures. Other causes of postoperative vomiting include an accumulation of fluid in the stomach, inflation of the stomach, and the ingestion of food and fluid before peristalsis resumes.

When vomiting is likely because of the nature of surgery, a nasogastric tube is inserted preoperatively and remains in place throughout the surgery and the immediate postoperative period. In addition, a nasogastric tube may be inserted when a patient who has food in the stomach requires emergency surgery.

Hiccups, produced by intermittent spasms of the diaphragm secondary to irritation of the phrenic nerve, can occur after surgery. The irritation may be direct, such as from stimulation of the nerve by a distended stomach, subdiaphragmatic abscess, or abdominal distention; indirect, such as from toxemia or uremia that stimulates the center; or reflexive, such as irritation from a drainage tube or obstruction of the intestines. Usually these occurrences are mild, transitory attacks that cease spontaneously. When hiccups persist, they may produce considerable distress and serious effects such as vomiting, exhaustion, and wound dehiscence. The physician may prescribe phenothiazine medications for severe, persistent hiccups.

Once nausea and vomiting have subsided and the patient is fully awake and alert, the sooner he or she can tolerate a usual diet, the more quickly normal gastrointestinal function will resume. Taking food by mouth stimulates digestive juices and promotes gastric function and intestinal peristalsis. The return to normal dietary intake should proceed at the pace set by the patient. Of course, the nature of surgery and the type of anesthesia directly affect the rate at which normal gastric activity resumes. Liquids are typically the first substances desired and tolerated by the patient after surgery. Water, fruit juices, and tea may be given in increasing amounts. Cool fluids are tolerated more easily than those that are ice cold or hot. Soft foods (gelatin, custard, milk, and creamed soups) are added gradually after clear fluids have been tolerated. As soon as the patient tolerates soft foods well, solid food may be given.

Assessment and management of gastrointestinal function are important after surgery because the gastrointestinal tract is subject to uncomfortable or potentially life-threatening complications. Any postoperative patient may suffer from distention. Postoperative distention of the abdomen results from the accumulation of gas in the intestinal tract. Manipulation of the abdominal organs during surgery may produce a loss of normal peristalsis for 24 to 48 hours, depending on the type and extent of surgery. Even though nothing is given by mouth, swallowed air and gastrointestinal secretions enter the stomach and the intestines; if not propelled by peristalsis, they collect in the intestines, producing distention and causing the patient to complain of fullness or pain in the abdomen. Most often, the gas collects in the colon.

Abdominal distention is further increased by immobility, anesthetic agents, and the use of opioid medications.

After major abdominal surgery, distention may be avoided by having the patient turn frequently, exercise, and ambulate as early as possible. This also alleviates distention produced by swallowing air, which is common in anxious patients. When postoperative distention is anticipated, a nasogastric tube may be inserted before surgery. The tube may remain in place until full peristaltic activity (indicated by the passage of flatus) has resumed. The nurse can determine when peristaltic bowel sounds return by listening to the abdomen with a stethoscope. Bowel sounds are documented so that diet progression can occur.

Paralytic ileus and intestinal obstruction are potential postoperative complications that occur more frequently in patients undergoing intestinal or abdominal surgery. Refer to Chapter 37 for discussion of treatment.

PROMOTING BOWEL FUNCTION

Constipation is common after surgery and can range from a minor irritation to a serious complication (Fox, 1998). Decreased mobility, decreased oral intake, and opioid analgesics contribute to difficulty having a bowel movement. In addition, irritation and trauma to the bowel during surgery may inhibit intestinal movement for several days. The combined effect of early ambulation, improved dietary intake, and a stool softener (if prescribed) promotes bowel elimination. Until the patient reports return of normal bowel function, the nurse should assess the abdomen for distention and the presence and frequency of bowel sounds. If the abdomen is not distended and bowel sounds are normal, and if the patient does not have a bowel movement by the second or third postoperative day, the physician should be notified so that a laxative can be given that evening.

MANAGING VOIDING

Urinary retention after surgery can occur for various reasons. Anesthetics, anticholinergic agents, and opioids interfere with the perception of bladder fullness and the urge to void and inhibit the ability to initiate voiding and completely empty the bladder. Abdominal, pelvic, and hip surgery may increase the likelihood of retention secondary to pain. Additionally, some patients find it difficult to use the bedpan or urinal in the recumbent position.

Bladder distention and the urge to void should be assessed on the patient's arrival on the unit and frequently thereafter. The patient is expected to void within 8 hours of surgery (this includes time spent in the PACU). If the patient has an urge to void and cannot, or if the bladder is distended and no urge is felt or the patient cannot void, catheterization is not delayed solely on the basis of the 8-hour time frame. All methods to encourage the patient to void should be tried (eg, letting water run, applying heat to the perineum). The bedpan should be warm; a cold bedpan causes discomfort and automatic tightening of muscles (including the urethral sphincter). When the patient cannot void on a bedpan, it may be permissible to use a commode rather than resorting to catheterization. Male patients are often permitted to sit up or stand beside the bed to use the urinal, but safeguards should be taken to prevent the patient from falling or fainting due to loss of coordination from medications or orthostatic hypotension. If the patient cannot void in the specified time frame, the patient is catheterized and the catheter removed after the bladder has emptied. Straight intermittent catheterization is preferred over indwelling catheterization because the risk for infection is increased with an indwelling catheter.

Even if the patient voids, the bladder may not necessarily be empty. The nurse notes the amount of urine voided and palpates the suprapubic area for distention or tenderness. A portable ultrasound device may also be used to assess residual volume. Intermittent catheterization continues every 4 to 6 hours until the patient can void spontaneously and the postvoid residual is less than 100 mL.

MAINTAINING A SAFE ENVIRONMENT

During the immediate postoperative period, the patient recovering from anesthesia should have all side rails up, and the bed should be in the low position. The nurse assesses the patient's level of consciousness and orientation and determines if the patient needs his or her eyeglasses or hearing aid, because impaired vision, inability to hear postoperative instructions, or inability to communicate verbally place the patient at risk for injury. All objects the patient may need should be within reach, especially the call bell. Any immediate postoperative orders concerning special positioning, equipment, or interventions should be implemented as soon as possible. The patient is instructed to ask for assistance with any activity. Although they are occasionally necessary for the disoriented patient, restraints should not be used if at all possible.

Any surgical procedure has the potential for injury due to disrupted neurovascular integrity resulting from prolonged awkward positioning in the operating room, manipulation of tissues, inadvertent severing of nerves, or tight bandages. Any orthopedic surgery or surgery involving the extremities carries a risk for peripheral nerve damage. Vascular surgeries, such as replacing sections of diseased peripheral arteries or inserting an arteriovenous graft, put the patient at risk for thrombus formation at the surgical site and subsequent ischemia of tissues distal to the thrombus. Assessment includes having the patient move the hand or foot distal to the surgical site through a full range of motion, assessing that all surfaces have intact sensation, and assessing peripheral pulses.

PROVIDING EMOTIONAL SUPPORT TO THE PATIENT AND FAMILY

Although patients and families are undoubtedly relieved that surgery is over, anxiety levels may remain high in the immediate postoperative period. Many factors contribute to this anxiety: pain, being in an unfamiliar environment, feeling unable to control one's circumstances, fear of the long-term effects of surgery, fear of complications, loss of ability to care for self, fatigue, spiritual distress, altered role responsibilities, ineffective coping, and altered body image are all potential reactions to the surgical experience. The nurse helps the patient and family work through their anxieties by providing reassurance and information and by spending time listening to and addressing their concerns. The nurse describes hospital routines and what to expect in the ensuing hours and days until discharge and explains the purpose of nursing assessments and interventions. Informing patients when they will be able to drink fluids or eat, when they will be getting out of bed, and when tubes and drains will be removed helps them gain a sense of control and participation in recovery and engages them in the plan of care. Acknowledging family members' concerns and accepting and encouraging their participation in the patient's care assists them in feeling they are helping their loved one. The nurse can manipulate the environment to enhance rest and relaxation by providing privacy, reducing noise, adjusting the lighting, providing enough seating for family members, and performing any other measures that will produce a supportive atmosphere.

MANAGING POTENTIAL COMPLICATIONS

Deep Vein Thrombosis

Deep vein thrombosis and other complications, such as pulmonary embolism, are serious potential complications of surgery (Chart 20-4). The stress response that is initiated as a result of surgery inhibits the fibrinolytic system, resulting in blood hypercoagulability. Dehydration, low cardiac output, blood pooling in the extremities, and bed rest add to the risk of thrombosis formation. Although all postoperative patients are at some risk, certain surgeries and patient populations carry a greater risk. The first symptom of deep vein thrombosis may be a pain or cramp in the calf. Although not present in all cases, calf pain elicited on ankle dorsiflexion (Homans' sign) suggests thrombosis (Fig. 20-8). Initial pain and tenderness may be followed by a painful swelling of the entire leg, often accompanied by a fever, chills, and diaphoresis.

Prophylactic treatment for postoperative patients at risk is common practice. Low-dose heparin may be prescribed and administered subcutaneously until the patient is ambulatory. Low-molecular-weight heparin and low-dose warfarin are other anticoagulants that may be used. External pneumatic compression and thigh-high elastic compression stockings can be used alone or in combination with low-dose heparin.

Chart 20-4

Risk Factors for Postoperative Complications

Patients at increased risk for postoperative complications (eg, deep vein thrombosis) and pulmonary problems include the following:

Deep Vein Thrombosis
- Orthopedic patients having hip surgery, knee reconstruction, and other lower extremity surgery
- Urologic patients having transurethral prostatectomy, and older patients having urologic surgery
- General surgical patients over 40 years of age, those who are obese, those with a malignancy, those who have had prior deep vein thrombosis or pulmonary embolism, or those undergoing extensive, complicated surgical procedures
- Gynecology (and obstetric) patients over 40 years of age with added risk factors (varicose veins, previous venous thrombosis, infection, malignancy, obesity)
- Neurosurgical patients, similar to other surgical high-risk groups (in patients with stroke, for instance, the risk of deep vein thrombosis in the paralyzed leg is as high as 75%)

Pulmonary Complications
- Type of surgery—greater incidence after all forms of abdominal surgery when compared with peripheral surgery
- Location of incision—the closer the incision to the diaphragm, the higher the incidence of pulmonary complications
- Preoperative respiratory problems
- Age—greater risk after age 40 than before age 40
- Sepsis
- Obesity—weight greater than 110% of ideal body weight
- Prolonged bed rest
- Duration of surgical procedure—more than 3 hours
- Aspiration
- Dehydration
- Malnutrition
- Hypotension and shock
- Immunosuppression

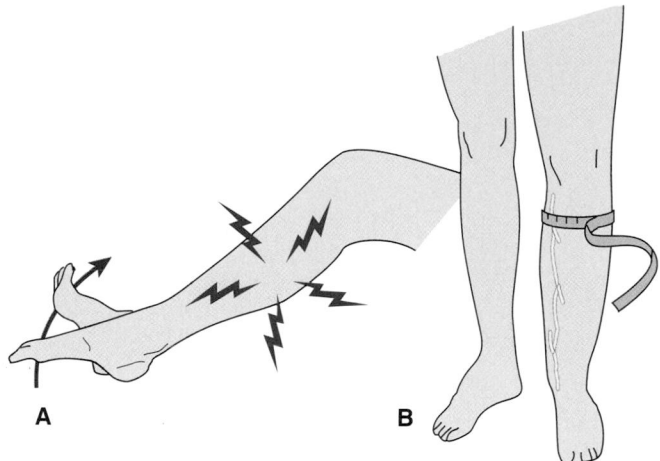

FIGURE 20-8 Assessment of signs and symptoms of deep vein thrombosis. (**A**) With the knee flexed, the patient may complain of pain in the calf on dorsiflexion of the foot (Homans' sign). This is a sign of early and subclinical thrombosis, which may or may not be present. Gentle compression reveals tenderness of the calf muscles (note arrow). (**B**) The affected leg may swell; veins are more prominent and may be palpated easily.

The benefits of early ambulation and hourly leg exercises in preventing deep vein thrombosis cannot be overemphasized, and these activities are recommended for all patients, regardless of their risk. It is important to avoid the use of blanket rolls, pillow rolls, or any form of elevation that can constrict vessels under the knees. Even prolonged "dangling" (having the patient sit on the edge of the bed with legs hanging over the side) can be dangerous and is not recommended in susceptible patients because pressure under the knees can impede circulation. Adequate hydration is also encouraged; the patient can be offered juices and water throughout the day to avoid dehydration. Refer to Chapter 30 for a complete discussion of deep vein thrombosis and to Chapter 23 for discussion of pulmonary embolus.

Hematoma

At times, concealed bleeding occurs beneath the skin at the surgical site. This hemorrhage usually stops spontaneously but results in clot (hematoma) formation within the wound. If the clot is small, it will be absorbed and need not be treated. When the clot is large, the wound usually bulges somewhat, and healing will be delayed unless the clot is removed. After several sutures are removed by the physician, the clot is evacuated and the wound is packed lightly with gauze. Healing occurs usually by granulation, or a secondary closure may be performed.

Infection (Wound Sepsis)

The creation of a surgical wound disrupts the integrity of the skin and its protective function. Exposure of deep body tissues to pathogens in the environment places the patient at risk for infection of the surgical site, a potentially life-threatening complication. Surgical site infection increases hospital length of stay, costs of care, and risk for further complications. In postoperative patients, surgical site infection is the most common nosocomial infection, with 67% of these infections occurring within the incision and 33% occurring in an organ or space around the surgical site (CDC, 1999). Recent research suggests that the administration of supplemental oxygen during colorectal resection and for 2 hours postoperatively reduces the incidence of postoperative infection (Greif, Ozan, Horn et al., 2000).

Multiple factors place the patient at risk for wound infection. One risk factor is the wound classification. Surgical wounds are classified according to the degree of contamination. Table 20-4 defines the terms used to describe surgical wounds and gives the expected rate of wound infection per category. Other risk factors

Table 20-4 • Wound Classification and Associated Surgical Site Infection Risk

SURGICAL CATEGORY	DETERMINANTS OF CATEGORY	EXPECTED RISK OF POSTSURGICAL INFECTION (%)
Clean	Nontraumatic site Uninfected site No inflammation No break in aseptic technique No entry into respiratory, alimentary, genitourinary, or oropharyngeal tracts	1–3
Clean-contaminated	Entry into respiratory, alimentary, genitourinary or oropharyngeal tracts without unusual contamination Appendectomy Minor break in aseptic technique Mechanical drainage	3–7
Contaminated	Open, newly experienced traumatic wounds Gross spillage from gastrointestinal tract Major break in aseptic technique Entry into genitourinary or biliary tract when urine or bile is infected	7–16
Dirty	Traumatic wound with delayed repair, devitalized tissue, foreign bodies, or fecal contamination Acute inflammation and purulent drainage encountered during procedure	16–29

include both patient-related factors and those associated with the surgical procedure. Patient-related factors include age, nutritional status, diabetes, smoking, obesity, remote infections, endogenous mucosal microorganisms, altered immune response, length of preoperative stay, and severity of illness (Bryant, 2000). Factors related to the surgical procedure include the method of preoperative skin preparation, surgical attire of the team, method of sterile draping, duration of surgery, antimicrobial prophylaxis, aseptic technique, factors related to surgical technique, drains or foreign material, operating room ventilation, and exogenous microorganisms. Efforts to prevent wound infection are directed at reducing these risks. Preoperative and intraoperative risks and interventions are discussed in Chapters 18 and 19. Although the conditions for surgical site infection and serious contamination of the wound occur in the preoperative and intraoperative time frames, postoperative care of the wound centers on assessing the wound, preventing contamination and infection before wound edges have sealed, and enhancing healing.

Wound infection may not present until at least postoperative day 5. Most patients are discharged before that time, and more than half of wound infections are diagnosed after discharge, highlighting the importance of patient education regarding wound care. Risk factors for wound sepsis include wound contamination, foreign body, faulty suturing technique, devitalized tissue, hematoma, debilitation, dehydration, malnutrition, anemia, advanced age, extreme obesity, shock, length of preoperative hospitalization, duration of surgical procedure, and associated disorders (eg, diabetes mellitus, immunosuppression). Signs and symptoms of wound infection include pulse rate and temperature elevation; an elevated white blood cell count; wound swelling, warmth, tenderness, or discharge; and incisional pain. Local signs may be absent if the infection is deep. *Staphylococcus aureus* accounts for many postoperative wound infections. Other infections may result from *Escherichia coli, Proteus vulgaris, Aerobacter aerogenes, Pseudomonas aeruginosa,* and other organisms. Although rare, beta-hemolytic streptococcal or clostridial infections can be rapid and deadly. If wound infection due to beta-hemolytic streptococcus or clostridium occurs, extreme care is needed to prevent spread of infection to others. Intensive medical and nursing care is essential if the patient is to survive.

When a wound infection is diagnosed in a surgical incision, the surgeon may remove one or more sutures or staples and, using aseptic precautions, separate the wound edges with a pair of blunt scissors or a hemostat. Once the incision is opened, a drain is inserted. If the infection is deep, an incision and drainage procedure may be necessary. Antimicrobial therapy and a wound care regimen are also initiated (Byrant, 2000).

Wound Dehiscence and Evisceration

Wound **dehiscence** (disruption of surgical incision or wound) and **evisceration** (protrusion of wound contents) are serious surgical complications (Fig. 20-9). Dehiscence and evisceration are especially serious when they involve abdominal incisions or wounds. These complications result from sutures giving way, from infection, and, more frequently, after marked distention or strenuous cough. They may also occur because of increasing age, poor nutritional status, and pulmonary or cardiovascular disease in patients undergoing abdominal surgery.

When the wound edges separate slowly, the intestines may protrude gradually or not at all, and the earliest sign may be a gush of bloody (serosanguineous) peritoneal fluid from the wound. When a wound ruptures suddenly, coils of intestine may push out of the abdomen. The patient may report that "something gave way."

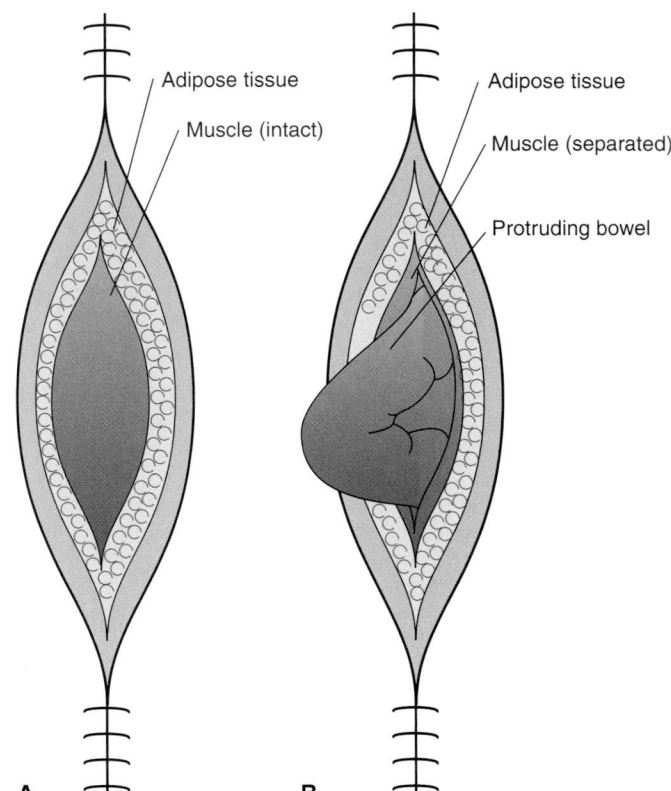

FIGURE 20-9 (**A**) Wound dehiscence; (**B**) wound evisceration.

thing gave way." The evisceration causes pain and can be associated with vomiting.

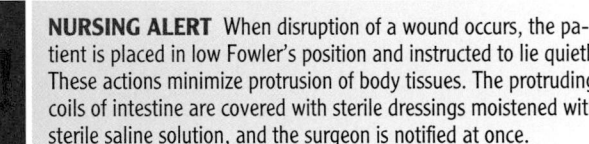

NURSING ALERT When disruption of a wound occurs, the patient is placed in low Fowler's position and instructed to lie quietly. These actions minimize protrusion of body tissues. The protruding coils of intestine are covered with sterile dressings moistened with sterile saline solution, and the surgeon is notified at once.

An abdominal binder, properly applied, is an excellent prophylactic measure against an evisceration and often is used along with the primary dressing, especially in patients with weak or pendulous abdominal walls or when rupture of a wound has occurred.

Gerontologic Considerations

Older adults recover more slowly, have a longer hospital stay, and are at greater risk for developing postoperative complications (Polanczyk et al., 2001). Delirium, pneumonia, decline in functional ability, exacerbation of comorbid conditions, pressure ulcers, decreased oral intake, gastrointestinal disturbance, and falls are all threats to recovery in the older adult. Expert nursing care can help the older adult avoid these complications or minimize their effects.

Postoperative delirium, characterized by confusion, perceptual and cognitive deficits, altered attention levels, disturbed sleep patterns, and impaired psychomotor skills, is a significant problem for older adults. Causes of delirium are multifactorial (Chart 20-5).

Chart 20-5

Causes of Postoperative Delirium

- Fluid and electrolyte imbalance
- Dehydration
- Hypoxia
- Hypercarbia
- Acid–base disturbance
- Infection (urinary tract, wound, respiratory)
- Medications (anticholinergics, benzodiazepines, central nervous system depressants)
- Unrelieved pain
- Blood loss
- Decreased cardiac output
- Cerebral hypoxia
- Heart failure
- Acute myocardial infarction
- Hypothermia or hyperthermia
- Unfamiliar surroundings and sensory deprivation
- Emergent surgery
- Alcohol withdrawal
- Urinary retention
- Fecal impaction

Skilled and frequent assessment of mental status and of all physiologic factors influencing mental status helps the nurse plan care, because in the elderly patient delirium may be the initial or only early indicator of infection, fluid and electrolyte imbalance, or deterioration of respiratory or hemodynamic status. Factors that determine if the patient is at risk for delirium include age, history of alcohol abuse, preoperative cognitive function, physical function, serum chemistries, and type of surgery.

Recognizing postoperative delirium and identifying and treating its underlying cause are the goals of care. Postoperative delirium is sometimes mistaken for preexisting dementia or is attributed to age. In addition to monitoring and managing identifiable causes, nurses can implement supportive interventions. Keeping the patient in a well-lit room and close to the nurses' station can help with sensory deprivation. At the same time, distracting and unfamiliar noises should be minimized. Because pain can contribute to postoperative delirium, the nurse collaborates with the physician or geriatric nurse specialist and the patient to achieve pain relief without oversedation (Lynch, Lazor, Gellis et al., 1998). The patient is reoriented as often as necessary, and staff should introduce themselves each time they come in contact with the patient. Engaging the patient in conversation and care activities and placing a clock and calender nearby may improve cognitive function. Physical activity should not be neglected while the patient is confused, because physical deterioration can worsen delirium and place the patient at increased risk for other complications. Restraints should be avoided because they can also worsen confusion. If possible, a family member or staff member is asked to sit with the patient instead. Haloperidol (Haldol) or lorazepam (Ativan) may be given during episodes of acute confusion, but these medications should be discontinued as soon as possible to avoid side effects.

Other problems confronting the older postoperative patient, such as pneumonia, altered bowel function, deep vein thrombosis, weakness, and functional decline, often can be prevented by early and progressive ambulation. Ambulation means walking, not just getting out of bed and sitting in a chair. Prolonged sitting positions that promote venous stasis in the lower extremities should be avoided. Assistance with ambulation may be required to keep the patient from bumping into objects and falling. A physical therapy referral may be indicated to promote safe, regular exercise for the older adult.

Urinary incontinence can be prevented by providing easy access to the call bell and the commode and by prompting voiding. Early ambulation and familiarity with the room help the patient to become self-sufficient sooner.

Optimal nutritional status is important for wound healing, return of normal bowel function, and fluid and electrolyte balance. The nurse and patient can consult with the dietitian to plan appealing, high-protein meals that provide sufficient fiber, calories, and vitamins. Nutritional supplements, such as Ensure or Sustacal, may be recommended. Multivitamins, iron, and vitamin C supplements aid in tissue healing, formation of new red blood cells, and overall nutritional status and are commonly prescribed postoperatively.

In addition to monitoring and managing the older adult's physiologic recovery, the nurse identifies and addresses psychosocial needs. The older adult may require more encouragement and support to resume activities, and the pace may be slower. Sensory deficits may require frequent repetition of instructions, and decreased physiologic reserve may necessitate frequent rest periods. The older adult may require extensive discharge planning to coordinate both professional and family care providers, and the nurse, social worker, or nurse case manager may institute the plan for continuing care.

PROMOTING HOME AND COMMUNITY-BASED CARE

Teaching Patients Self-Care

Patients have always required detailed discharge instructions to become proficient in special self-care needs after surgery; however, dramatically reduced hospital lengths of stay during the past decade have greatly increased the amount of information that should be provided while reducing the amount of time in which to provide it (Fox, 1998; Quinn, 1999). Although needs are specific to individual patients and the procedures they have undergone, general patient education needs for postoperative care have been identified (see Chart 20-1).

Continuing Care

Continuing care provided by community-based services is frequently necessary after surgery. Older patients, patients who live alone, patients without family support, and patients with preexisting disabilities are often in greatest need. Planning for discharge involves arranging for necessary services early in the acute care hospitalization. Wound care, drain management, catheter care, infusion therapy, and physical or occupational therapy are some of the needs addressed by community health care providers. The home care nurse coordinates these activities and services.

During home care visits, the nurse assesses the patient for postoperative complications; the nurse also assesses the surgical incision, respiratory and cardiovascular status, adequacy of pain management, fluid and nutritional status, and the patient's progress in returning to preoperative status. The nurse assesses the patient's and family's ability to manage dressing changes and drainage systems and other devices and to administer prescribed medications. The nurse may change dressings or catheters if needed. The nurse determines if any additional services are needed and assists the patient and family to arrange for them. Previous teaching is reinforced, and the patient is reminded to keep follow-up appointments. The patient and family are instructed about signs and symptoms to be reported to the surgeon. In addition, the nurse may provide information about how to obtain needed supplies and may suggest resources or support groups the patient may want to contact. In many settings, postoperative telephone calls are made to answer questions, assess recovery, and reassure patients and families.

Evaluation

EXPECTED PATIENT OUTCOMES

Expected patient outcomes may include:

1. Maintains optimal respiratory function
   a. Performs deep-breathing exercises
   b. Displays clear breath sounds
   c. Uses incentive spirometer as prescribed
   d. Splints incisional site when coughing to reduce pain
2. Indicates that pain is decreased in intensity
3. Exercises and ambulates as prescribed
   a. Alternates periods of rest and activity
   b. Progressively increases ambulation
   c. Resumes normal activities within prescribed time frame
   d. Performs activities related to self-care
4. Wound heals without complication
5. Maintains body temperature within normal limits
6. Resumes oral intake
   a. Reports absence of nausea and vomiting
   b. Takes at least 75% of usual diet
   c. Is free of abdominal distress and gas pains
   d. Exhibits normal bowel sounds
7. Reports resumption of usual bowel elimination pattern
8. Resumes usual voiding pattern
9. Is free of injury
10. Exhibits decreased anxiety
11. Acquires knowledge and skills necessary to manage therapeutic regimen
12. Experiences no complications

 Critical Thinking Exercises

1. Your patient has a history of esophageal cancer and is HIV positive. After undergoing ambulatory surgery to insert a gastric feeding tube, he is to be discharged to home. Indicate which assessment findings would indicate his readiness for discharge. Describe a teaching plan for the patient and his family. How would you modify the plan if the patient lives alone?

2. A patient who has undergone abdominal surgery reports severe pain and as a result is unable to cough and deep breathe. When you listen to the patient's lungs you hear crackles in the bases. Analyze these findings and indicate the interventions you would implement in this situation. How would your care differ if the patient has a musculoskeletal disorder that makes turning and ambulation difficult?

3. You are visiting a 72-year-old woman who had emergency surgery for a broken hip 3 weeks ago and has returned to her home, where she is living alone. How would you direct your assessment to identify the factors that might affect her recovery? How would you modify your assessment and nursing care plan because of her age?

REFERENCES AND SELECTED READINGS

Books

American Pain Society. (1999). *Principles of analgesic use in the treatment of acute pain and cancer pain.* Glenview, IL: Author.

American Society of Anesthesiologists. (1995). *ASA standards for postanesthesia care.* Park Ridge, IL: Author.

American Society of PeriAnesthesia Nurses. (2000). *Standards of perianesthesia nursing practice.* Thorofare, NJ: ASPAN.

Byrant, R. (2000). *Acute and chronic wounds* (2d ed.). St. Louis: Mosby.

Economou, S. G., & Economou, T. S. (1999). *Instructions for surgery patients.* Philadelphia: WB Saunders.

Ethicon Endo-Surgery, Inc. (2000). *Nursing quick reference card: On-Q Soaker catheter 6.5 pain management system.* Cincinnati, OH: Author.

Finkelmeier, B. (2000). *Cardiothoracic surgical nursing* (2d ed.). Philadelphia: Lippincott Williams & Wilkins.

Karch, A. (Ed.). (2002). *Nursing drug guide.* Philadelphia: Lippincott Williams & Wilkins.

Litwack, K. (1999). *Core curriculum for perianesthesia nursing practice.* Philadelphia: WB Saunders.

Meeker, M. H., & Rothrock, J. C. (1999). *Alexander's care of the patient in surgery.* St. Louis: Mosby Year Book.

Quinn, D. M. (Ed.). (1999). *Ambulatory surgical nursing core curriculum.* Philadelphia: WB Saunders.

Schwartz, S., & Shires, G. T. (1999). *Principles of surgery.* New York: McGraw-Hill.

Journals

Asterisks indicate nursing research articles.

Anesthesia care: New guidelines on postanesthesia care (2002). *OR Manager, 18*(1), 21.

Aldreta, J. A. (1998). Modifications to the postanesthesia score for use in ambulatory surgery. *Journal of Perianesthesia Nursing, 12*(3), 148–155.

Aranda, M., & Hanson, W. (2000). Anesthetics, sedatives, and paralytics: Understanding their use in the intensive care unit. *Surgical Clinics of North America, 80*(3), 933–947.

Bennet, J., Haas, R., & Wren, K. R. (2001). Opioid use during the perianesthesia period: Nursing implications. *Journal of Perianesthesia Nursing, 16*(4), 255–258.

Buckle, J. (1999). Aromatherapy in perianesthesia nursing. *Journal of Perianesthesia Nursing, 14*(6), 336–344.

Centers for Disease Control and Prevention (1999). Guideline for prevention of surgical site infections. *Infection Control and Hospital Epidemiology, 20*(4), 247–280.

Fortunato-Phillips, N. (2000). Malignant hyperthermia: Update 2000. *Critical Care Nursing Clinics of North America, 12*(2), 199–210.

Fox, V. J. (1998). Postoperative education that works. *AORN Journal, 67*(5), 1010, 1012–1017.

Goodwin, S. A. (1998). A review of preemptive analgesia. *Journal of Perianesthesia Nursing, 13*(2), 109–114.

Gordon, D. B. (1999). Pain management in the elderly. *Journal of Perianesthesia Nursing, 14*(6), 367–372.

Greif, R., Ozan, A., Horn, E., et al. (2000). Supplemental perioperative oxygen to reduce the incidence of surgical wound infection. *New England Journal of Medicine, 342*(3), 161–167.

Hession, M. C. (1998). Factors influencing successful discharge after outpatient laparoscopic cholecystectomy. *Journal of Perianesthesia Nursing, 13*(1), 11–15.

Hilbig, J. I., & Manning, J. (1999) Accountability and responsibility underpins successful pain management. *Journal of Perianesthesia Nursing, 14*(6), 390–392.

Jeran, L. (2001). Patient temperature: An introduction to the clinical guideline for the prevention of unplanned perioperative hypothermia. *Journal of Perianesthesia Nursing, 16*(5), 303–314.

Lynch, E. P., Lazor, M. A., Gellis, J. E., et al. (1998). The impact of postoperative pain in the development of postoperative delirium. *Anesthesia and Analgesia, 86,* 761–785.

Mamaril, M., & Hooper, V. (1998). Fast tracking versus bypassing phase I: rapid PACU progression. *Breathline, 17*(7), 12.

Marley, R. A., & Swanson, J. (2001). Patient care after discharge from the ambulatory surgical center. *Journal of Perianesthesia Nursing, 16*(6), 399–419.

Moline, B. M. (2001). Pain management in the ambulatory surgical population. *Journal of Perianesthesia Nursing, 16*(6), 388–398.

Polanczyk, C., Marcantonio, E., Goldman, L., et al. (2001). Impact of age on perioperative complications and length of stay in patients undergoing noncardiac surgery. *Annals of Internal Medicine, 134*(8), 637–643.

Redmond, M. C. (2001). Malignant hyperthermia: Perianesthesia recognition, treatment, and care. *Journal of Perianesthesia Nursing, 16*(4), 259–270.

Scales, B. (2001). CAMPing in the PACU: Using complementary and alternative medical practices in the PACU. *Journal of Perianesthesia Nursing, 16*(5), 325–334.

Schroeter, K. (1999). Pain management: Ethical issues for the perianesthesia nurse. *Journal of Perianesthesia Nursing, 14*(6), 393–397.

Schafheutle, E., Cantrill, J. & Noyce, P. (2001). Why is pain management suboptimal on surgical wards? *Journal of Advanced Nursing, 33*(6), 728–737.

Schwartz, L. B. (1998). Conventional and alternative therapies for acute deep vein thrombosis. *Journal of Care Management, 4,* 9–12, 32.

Seers, K., & Carroll, D. (1998). Relaxation techniques for acute pain management. *Journal of Advanced Nursing, 27*(3), 466–476.

Vargas, G., & Reger, T. (2000). An alternative to sutures. *Medsurg Nursing, 9*(2), 83–85.

Watkins, A. C., & White, P. F. (2001). Fast-tracking after ambulatory surgery. *Journal of Perianesthesia Nursing, 16*(6), 379–387.

*Watt-Watson, J., Stevens, B., Garfinkel, P., et al. (2001). Relationships between nurses' pain knowledge and pain management outcomes for their postoperative cardiac patients. *Journal of Advanced Nursing, 36*(4), 535–545.

RESOURCES AND WEBSITES

American Academy of Ambulatory Care Nursing, East Holly Ave., Box 56, Pitman, NJ, 08071; (856) 256-2350; (800) AMB-NURS; http://www.aaacn.org.

American Society of PeriAnesthesia Nurses, 10 Melrose Ave., Suite 110, Cherry Hill, NJ 08003-3696; (856) 616-9600 or 9601; toll-free 1-877-737-9696; fax (856) 616-9621; http://www.aspan.org.

Association of PeriOperative Registered Nurses, Inc., 2170 S. Parker Road, Suite 300, Denver, CO 80231; (800) 755-2676, (303) 755-6304; http://www.aorn.org.

Malignant Hyperthermia Association of the United States (MHAUS), 39 East State Street, P.O. Box 1069, Sherburne, NY 13460; (607) 674-7901; http://www.mhaus.org.

Unit 5

Gas Exchange and Respiratory Function

Applying Concepts from NANDA, NIC, and NOC

Mrs. Brant, age 73, is admitted to the hospital for LLL pneumonia. Her vital signs are: T: 100.6°; HR: 90 and regular; RR: 28; BP: 142/74. She has a weak cough, diminished breath sounds over the lower left lung field, and coarse rhonchi over the midtracheal area. She can expectorate some sputum, which is thick and grayish-green. She has a history of stroke. Secondary to the stroke she has impaired gag and cough reflexes and mild weakness of her left side. She is allowed food and fluids because she can swallow safely if she uses the chin-tuck maneuver. The concept map illustrates the relationships that exist among the nursing diagnoses, interventions, and outcomes for one of Mrs. Brant's clinical problems.

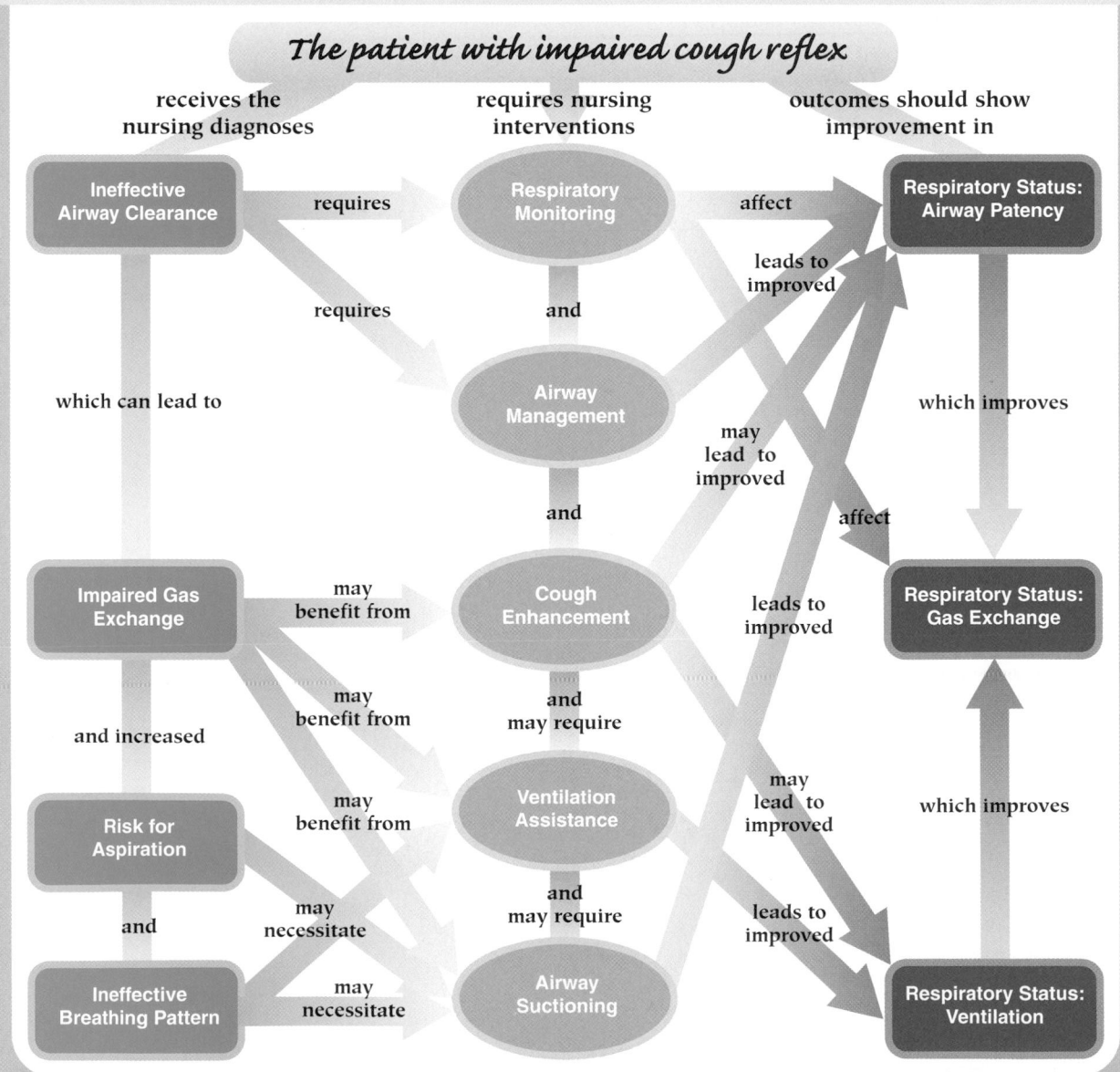

The patient with impaired cough reflex

receives the nursing diagnoses — requires nursing interventions — outcomes should show improvement in

Ineffective Airway Clearance — requires → Respiratory Monitoring — affect → Respiratory Status: Airway Patency

requires → and → leads to improved

which can lead to — Airway Management — which improves

may lead to improved — affect

Impaired Gas Exchange — may benefit from → Cough Enhancement — leads to improved — Respiratory Status: Gas Exchange

and increased — may benefit from — and may require

Risk for Aspiration — may benefit from → Ventilation Assistance — may lead to improved — which improves

and — may necessitate — and may require — leads to improved

Ineffective Breathing Pattern — may necessitate → Airway Suctioning — Respiratory Status: Ventilation

Nursing Classifications and Languages

NANDA
Nursing Diagnoses

Ineffective Airway Clearance—Inability to clear secretions or obstructions from the respiratory tract to maintain a clear airway

Impaired Gas Exchange—Excess or deficit in oxygenation and/or carbon dioxide elimination at the alveolar-capillary membrane

Risk for Aspiration—At risk for entry of gastrointestinal secretions, oropharyngeal secretions, solids or fluids into tracheo-bronchial passages

Ineffective Breathing Pattern—Inspiration and/or expiration that does not provide adequate ventilation

NIC
Nursing Interventions*

Respiratory Monitoring—Collection and analysis of patient data to ensure airway patency and adequate gas exchange

Airway Management—Facilitation of patency of air passages

Cough Enhancement—Promotion of deep inhalation by the patient with subsequent generation of high intrathoracic pressures and compression of underlying lung parenchyma for the forceful expulsion of air

Ventilation Assistance—Promotion of an optimal spontaneous breathing pattern that maximizes oxygen and carbon dioxide exchange in the lungs

Airway Suctioning—Removal of airway secretions by inserting a suction catheter into the patient's oral airway and/or trachea

NOC
Nursing Outcomes[†]

Return to functional baseline status, stabilization of, or improvement in

Respiratory Status: Airway Patency—Extent to which the tracheobronchial passages remain open; measured on a scale of extremely compromised to not compromised

Respiratory Status: Gas Exchange—The alveolar exchange of O_2 or CO_2 to maintain arterial blood gas concentrations; measured on a scale of extremely compromised to not compromised

Respiratory Status: Ventilation—Movement of air in and out of the lungs; measured on a scale of extremely compromised to not compromised

NANDA, North American Nursing Diagnosis Association; NIC, Nursing Interventions Classification; NOC, Nursing Outcomes Classification.

*Iowa Intervention Project © 2000. In McCloskey, J. C., & Bulechek, G. M. (2000). *Nursing interventions classification (NIC)* (3rd ed.). St. Louis: Mosby.

[†]Iowa Outcomes Project © 2000. In Johnson, M., Maas, M., & Moorhead, S. (2000). *Nursing outcomes classification (NOC)* (3rd ed.). St. Louis: Mosby.

Assessment of Respiratory Function

On completion of this chapter, the learner will be able to:

1. Describe the structures and functions of the upper and lower respiratory tracts.
2. Describe ventilation, perfusion, diffusion, shunting, and the relationship of pulmonary circulation to these processes.
3. Discriminate between normal and abnormal breath sounds.
4. Use assessment parameters appropriate for determining the characteristics and severity of the major symptoms of respiratory dysfunction.
5. Identify the nursing implications of the various procedures used for diagnostic evaluation of respiratory function.

Disorders of the respiratory system are common and are encountered by nurses in every setting from the community to the intensive care unit. To assess the respiratory system, the nurse must be skilled at differentiating normal assessment findings from abnormal ones. Good assessment skills must be developed and used when caring for patients with acute and chronic respiratory problems. In addition, an understanding of respiratory function and the significance of abnormal diagnostic test results is essential.

Anatomic and Physiologic Overview

The respiratory system is composed of the upper and lower respiratory tracts. Together, the two tracts are responsible for **ventilation** (movement of air in and out of the airways). The upper tract, known as the upper airway, warms and filters inspired air so that the lower respiratory tract (the lungs) can accomplish gas exchange. Gas exchange involves delivering oxygen to the tissues through the bloodstream and expelling waste gases, such as carbon dioxide, during expiration.

ANATOMY OF THE UPPER RESPIRATORY TRACT

Upper airway structures consist of the nose, sinuses and nasal passages, pharynx, tonsils and adenoids, larynx, and trachea.

Nose

The nose is composed of an external and an internal portion. The external portion protrudes from the face and is supported by the nasal bones and cartilage. The anterior nares (nostrils) are the external openings of the nasal cavities.

The internal portion of the nose is a hollow cavity separated into the right and left nasal cavities by a narrow vertical divider, the septum. Each nasal cavity is divided into three passageways by the projection of the turbinates (also called conchae) from the lateral walls. The nasal cavities are lined with highly vascular ciliated mucous membranes called the nasal mucosa. Mucus, secreted continuously by goblet cells, covers the surface of the nasal mucosa and is moved back to the nasopharynx by the action of the **cilia** (fine hairs).

The nose serves as a passageway for air to pass to and from the lungs. It filters impurities and humidifies and warms the air as it is inhaled. It is responsible for olfaction (smell) because the olfactory receptors are located in the nasal mucosa. This function diminishes with age.

Paranasal Sinuses

The paranasal sinuses include four pairs of bony cavities that are lined with nasal mucosa and ciliated pseudostratified columnar epithelium. These air spaces are connected by a series of ducts that drain into the nasal cavity. The sinuses are named by their location: frontal, ethmoidal, sphenoidal, and maxillary (Fig. 21-1). A prominent function of the sinuses is to serve as a resonating chamber in speech. The sinuses are a common site of infection.

Turbinate Bones (Conchae)

The turbinate bones are also called conchae (the name suggested by their shell-like appearance). Because of their curves, these bones increase the mucous membrane surface of the nasal passages and slightly obstruct the air flowing through them (Fig. 21-2).

Air entering the nostrils is deflected upward to the roof of the nose, and it follows a circuitous route before it reaches the nasopharynx. It comes into contact with a large surface of moist, warm mucous membrane that catches practically all the dust and organisms in the inhaled air. The air is moistened, warmed to body temperature, and brought into contact with sensitive nerves. Some of these nerves detect odors; others provoke sneezing to expel irritating dust.

Pharynx, Tonsils, and Adenoids

The pharynx, or throat, is a tubelike structure that connects the nasal and oral cavities to the larynx. It is divided into three regions: nasal, oral, and laryngeal. The nasopharynx is located posterior to the nose and above the soft palate. The oropharynx houses the faucial, or palatine, tonsils. The laryngopharynx extends from the hyoid bone to the cricoid cartilage. The epiglottis forms the entrance of the larynx.

The adenoids, or pharyngeal tonsils, are located in the roof of the nasopharynx. The tonsils, the adenoids, and other lymphoid tissue encircle the throat. These structures are important links in the chain of lymph nodes guarding the body from invasion by organisms entering the nose and the throat. The pharynx functions as a passageway for the respiratory and digestive tracts.

Larynx

The larynx, or voice organ, is a cartilaginous epithelium-lined structure that connects the pharynx and the trachea. The major function of the larynx is vocalization. It also protects the lower

Glossary

bronchoscopy: direct examination of larynx, trachea, and bronchi using an endoscope

cilia: short hairs that provide a constant whipping motion that serves to propel mucus and foreign substances away from the lung toward the larynx

crackles: soft, high-pitched, discontinuous popping sounds during inspiration caused by delayed reopening of the airways

diffusion: exchange of gas molecules from areas of high concentration to areas of low concentration

dyspnea: labored breathing or shortness of breath

hemoptysis: expectoration of blood from the respiratory tract

hypoxemia: decrease in arterial oxygen tension in the blood

hypoxia: decrease in oxygen supply to the tissues and cells

orthopnea: inability to breathe easily except in an upright position

physiologic dead space: portion of the tracheobronchial tree that does not participate in gas exchange

pulmonary perfusion: blood flow through the pulmonary vasculature

respiration: gas exchange between atmospheric air and the blood and between the blood and cells of the body

ventilation: movement of air in and out of airways

wheezes: continuous musical sounds associated with airway narrowing or partial obstruction

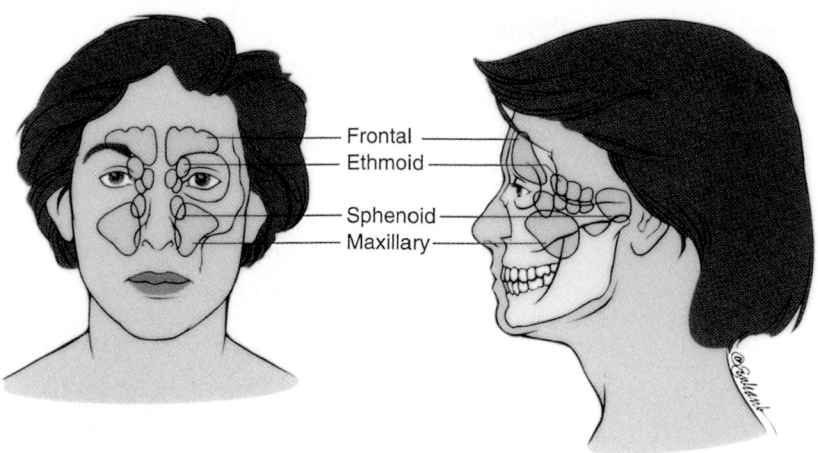

FIGURE 21-1 The paranasal sinuses.

airway from foreign substances and facilitates coughing. It is frequently referred to as the voice box and consists of the following:

- Epiglottis—a valve flap of cartilage that covers the opening to the larynx during swallowing
- Glottis—the opening between the vocal cords in the larynx
- Thyroid cartilage—the largest of the cartilage structures; part of it forms the Adam's apple
- Cricoid cartilage—the only complete cartilaginous ring in the larynx (located below the thyroid cartilage)
- Arytenoid cartilages—used in vocal cord movement with the thyroid cartilage

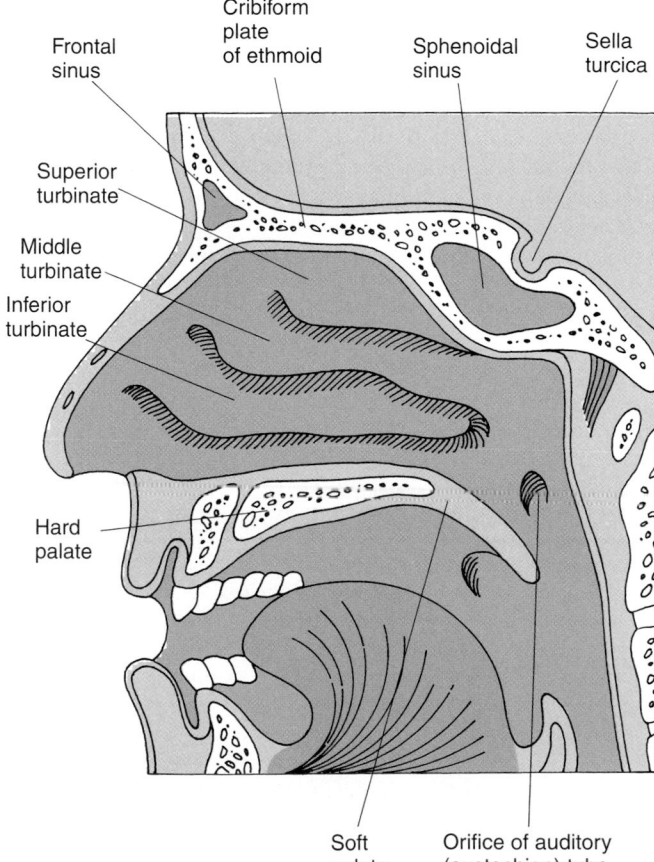

FIGURE 21-2 Cross-section of nasal cavity.

- Vocal cords—ligaments controlled by muscular movements that produce sounds; located in the lumen of the larynx

Trachea

The trachea, or windpipe, is composed of smooth muscle with C-shaped rings of cartilage at regular intervals. The cartilaginous rings are incomplete on the posterior surface and give firmness to the wall of the trachea, preventing it from collapsing. The trachea serves as the passage between the larynx and the bronchi.

ANATOMY OF THE LOWER RESPIRATORY TRACT: LUNGS

The lower respiratory tract consists of the lungs, which contain the bronchial and alveolar structures needed for gas exchange.

Lungs

The lungs are paired elastic structures enclosed in the thoracic cage, which is an airtight chamber with distensible walls (Fig. 21-3). Ventilation requires movement of the walls of the thoracic cage and of its floor, the diaphragm. The effect of these movements is alternately to increase and decrease the capacity of the chest. When the capacity of the chest is increased, air enters through the trachea (inspiration) because of the lowered pressure within and inflates the lungs. When the chest wall and diaphragm return to their previous positions (expiration), the lungs recoil and force the air out through the bronchi and trachea. The inspiratory phase of respiration normally requires energy; the expiratory phase is normally passive. Inspiration occurs during the first third of the respiratory cycle, expiration during the latter two thirds.

PLEURA

The lungs and wall of the thorax are lined with a serous membrane called the pleura. The visceral pleura covers the lungs; the parietal pleura lines the thorax. The visceral and parietal pleura and the small amount of pleural fluid between these two membranes serve to lubricate the thorax and lungs and permit smooth motion of the lungs within the thoracic cavity with each breath.

MEDIASTINUM

The mediastinum is in the middle of the thorax, between the pleural sacs that contain the two lungs. It extends from the sternum to the vertebral column and contains all the thoracic tissue outside the lungs.

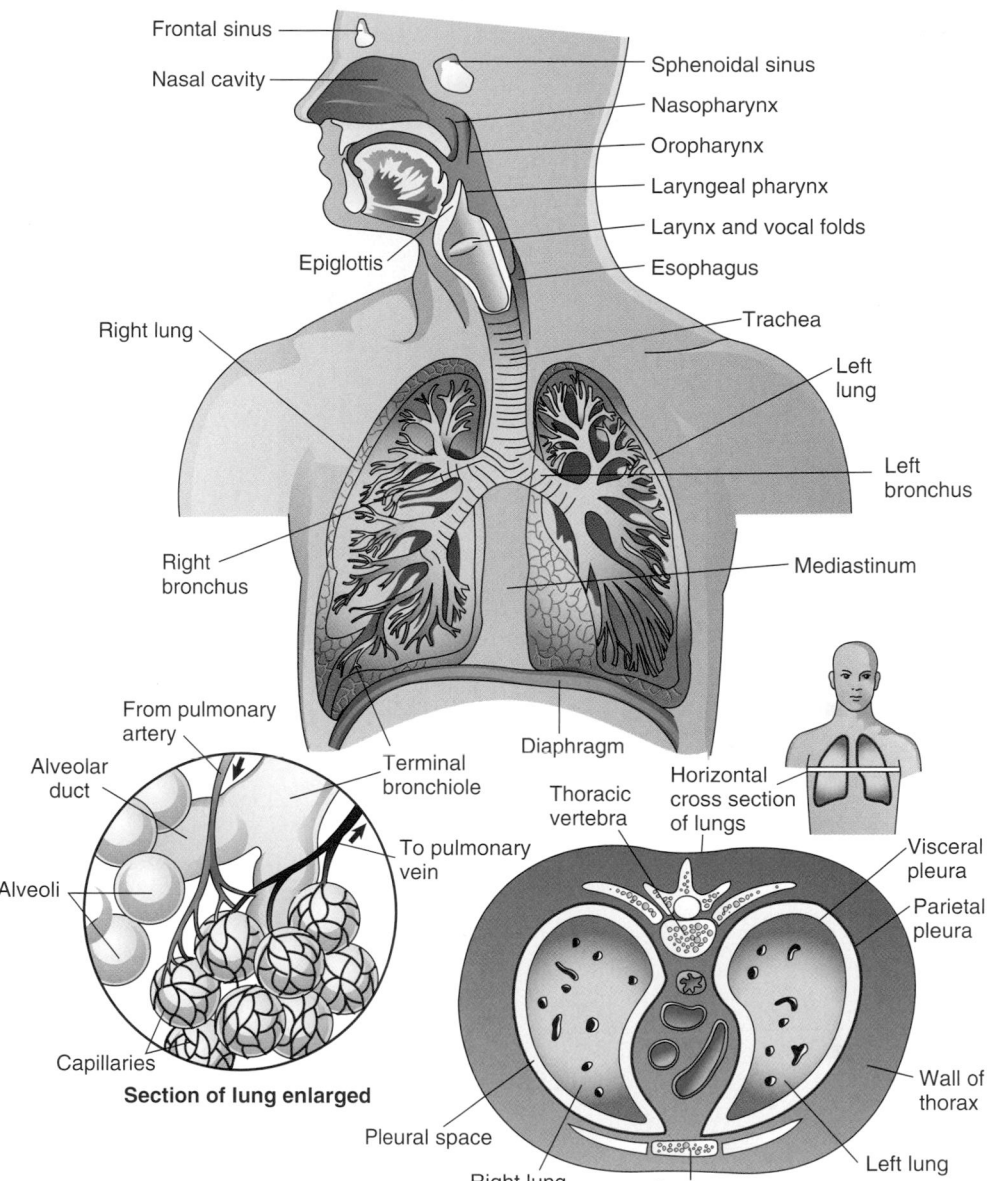

FIGURE 21-3 The respiratory system; upper respiratory structures and the structures of the thorax (*top*); alveoli and a horizontal cross section of the lungs (*bottom*).

LOBES

Each lung is divided into lobes. The left lung consists of an upper and lower lobe, whereas the right lung has an upper, middle, and lower lobe (Fig. 21-4). Each lobe is further subdivided into two to five segments separated by fissures, which are extensions of the pleura.

BRONCHI AND BRONCHIOLES

There are several divisions of the bronchi within each lobe of the lung. First are the lobar bronchi (three in the right lung and two in the left lung). Lobar bronchi divide into segmental bronchi (10 on the right and 8 on the left), which are the structures identified when choosing the most effective postural drainage position for a given patient. Segmental bronchi then divide into subsegmental bronchi. These bronchi are surrounded by connective tissue that contains arteries, lymphatics, and nerves.

The subsegmental bronchi then branch into bronchioles, which have no cartilage in their walls. Their patency depends entirely on the elastic recoil of the surrounding smooth muscle and

on the alveolar pressure. The bronchioles contain submucosal glands, which produce mucus that covers the inside lining of the airways. The bronchi and bronchioles are lined also with cells that have surfaces covered with cilia. These cilia create a constant whipping motion that propels mucus and foreign substances away from the lung toward the larynx.

The bronchioles then branch into terminal bronchioles, which do not have mucous glands or cilia. Terminal bronchioles then become respiratory bronchioles, which are considered to be the transitional passageways between the conducting airways and the gas exchange airways. Up to this point, the conducting airways contain about 150 mL of air in the tracheobronchial tree that does not participate in gas exchange. This is known as **physiologic dead space**. The respiratory bronchioles then lead into alveolar ducts and alveolar sacs and then alveoli. Oxygen and carbon dioxide exchange takes place in the alveoli.

ALVEOLI

The lung is made up of about 300 million alveoli, which are arranged in clusters of 15 to 20. These alveoli are so numerous

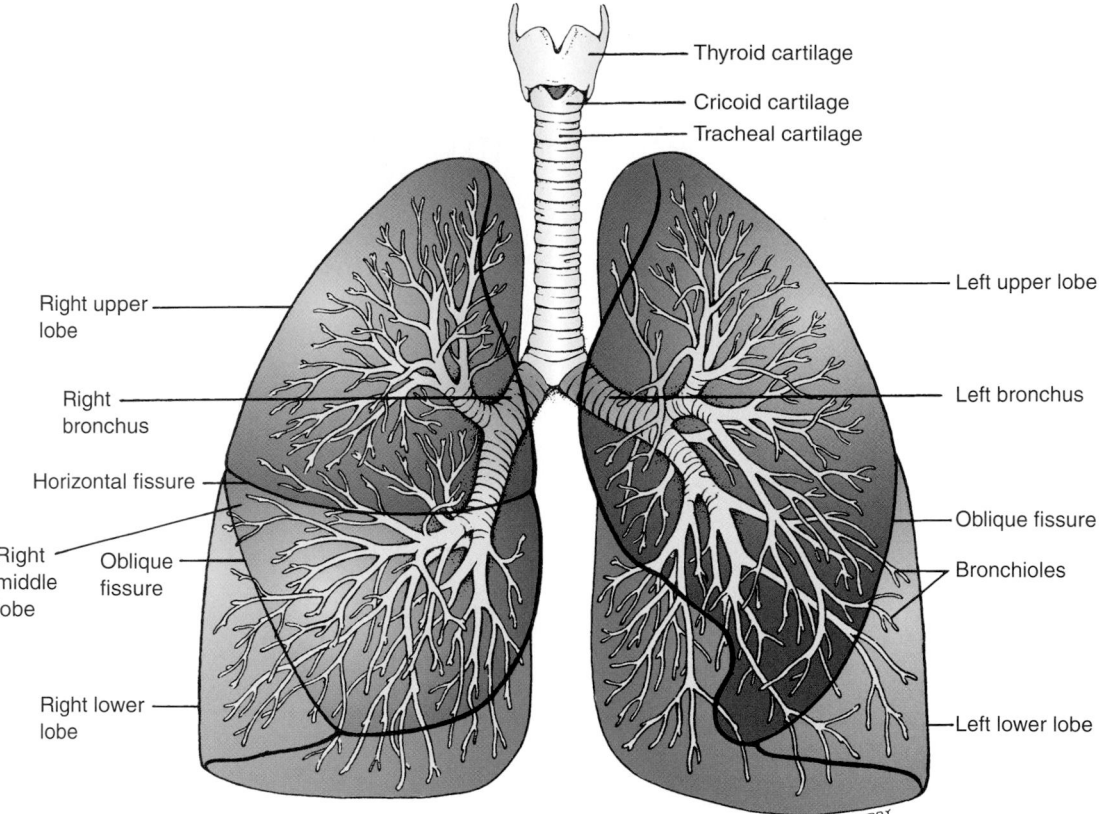

FIGURE 21-4 The lungs consist of five lobes. The right lung has three lobes (upper, middle, lower); the left has two (upper and lower). The lobes are further subdivided by fissures. The bronchial tree, another lung structure, inflates with air to fill the lobes.

that if their surfaces were united to form one sheet, it would cover 70 square meters—the size of a tennis court.

There are three types of alveolar cells. Type I alveolar cells are epithelial cells that form the alveolar walls. Type II alveolar cells are metabolically active. These cells secrete surfactant, a phospholipid that lines the inner surface and prevents alveolar collapse. Type III alveolar cell macrophages are large phagocytic cells that ingest foreign matter (eg, mucus, bacteria) and act as an important defense mechanism.

FUNCTION OF THE RESPIRATORY SYSTEM

The cells of the body derive the energy they need from the oxidation of carbohydrates, fats, and proteins. As with any type of combustion, this process requires oxygen. Certain vital tissues, such as those of the brain and the heart, cannot survive for long without a continuing supply of oxygen. However, as a result of oxidation in the body tissues, carbon dioxide is produced and must be removed from the cells to prevent the buildup of acid waste products. The respiratory system performs this function by facilitating life-sustaining processes such as oxygen transport, respiration and ventilation, and gas exchange.

Oxygen Transport

Oxygen is supplied to, and carbon dioxide is removed from, cells by way of the circulating blood. Cells are in close contact with capillaries, whose thin walls permit easy passage or exchange of oxygen and carbon dioxide. Oxygen diffuses from the capillary

through the capillary wall to the interstitial fluid. At this point, it diffuses through the membrane of tissue cells, where it is used by mitochondria for cellular respiration. The movement of carbon dioxide occurs by diffusion in the opposite direction—from cell to blood.

Respiration

After these tissue capillary exchanges, blood enters the systemic veins (where it is called venous blood) and travels to the pulmonary circulation. The oxygen concentration in blood within the capillaries of the lungs is lower than in the lungs' air sacs (alveoli). Because of this concentration gradient, oxygen diffuses from the alveoli to the blood. Carbon dioxide, which has a higher concentration in the blood than in the alveoli, diffuses from the blood into the alveoli. Movement of air in and out of the airways (ventilation) continually replenishes the oxygen and removes the carbon dioxide from the airways in the lung. This whole process of gas exchange between the atmospheric air and the blood and between the blood and cells of the body is called **respiration**.

Ventilation

During inspiration, air flows from the environment into the trachea, bronchi, bronchioles, and alveoli. During expiration, alveolar gas travels the same route in reverse.

Physical factors that govern air flow in and out of the lungs are collectively referred to as the mechanics of ventilation and include air pressure variances, resistance to air flow, and lung compliance.

AIR PRESSURE VARIANCES

Air flows from a region of higher pressure to a region of lower pressure. During inspiration, movement of the diaphragm and other muscles of respiration enlarges the thoracic cavity and thereby lowers the pressure inside the thorax to a level below that of atmospheric pressure. As a result, air is drawn through the trachea and bronchi into the alveoli.

During normal expiration, the diaphragm relaxes and the lungs recoil, resulting in a decrease in the size of the thoracic cavity. The alveolar pressure then exceeds atmospheric pressure, and air flows from the lungs into the atmosphere.

AIRWAY RESISTANCE

Resistance is determined chiefly by the radius or size of the airway through which the air is flowing. Any process that changes the bronchial diameter or width affects airway resistance and alters the rate of air flow for a given pressure gradient during respiration (Chart 21-1). With increased resistance, greater-than-normal respiratory effort is required by the patient to achieve normal levels of ventilation.

COMPLIANCE

The pressure gradient between the thoracic cavity and the atmosphere causes air to flow in and out of the lungs. When pressure changes are applied in the normal lung, there is a proportional change in the lung volume. A measure of the elasticity, expandability, and distensibility of the lungs and thoracic structures is called compliance. Factors that determine lung compliance are the surface tension of the alveoli (normally low with the presence of surfactant) and the connective tissue (ie, collagen and elastin) of the lungs.

Compliance is determined by examining the volume–pressure relationship in the lungs and the thorax. In normal compliance (1.0 L/cm H_2O), the lungs and thorax easily stretch and distend when pressure is applied. High or increased compliance occurs when the lungs have lost their elasticity and the thorax is overdistended (ie, in emphysema). When the lungs and thorax are "stiff," there is low or decreased compliance. Conditions associated with this include pneumothorax, hemothorax, pleural effusion, pulmonary edema, atelectasis, pulmonary fibrosis, and acute respiratory distress syndrome (ARDS), all of which are discussed in later chapters in this unit. Measurement of compliance is one method used to assess the progression and improvement in ARDS. Lungs with decreased compliance require greater-than-normal energy expenditure to achieve normal levels of ventilation. Compliance is usually measured under static conditions.

Lung Volumes and Capacities

Lung function, which reflects the mechanics of ventilation, is viewed in terms of lung volumes and lung capacities. Lung volumes are categorized as tidal volume, inspiratory reserve volume, expiratory reserve volume, and residual volume. Lung capacity is evaluated in terms of vital capacity, inspiratory capacity, functional residual capacity, and total lung capacity. These terms are described in Table 21-1.

Diffusion and Perfusion

Diffusion is the process by which oxygen and carbon dioxide are exchanged at the air–blood interface. The alveolar–capillary membrane is ideal for diffusion because of its large surface area and thin membrane. In the normal healthy adult, oxygen and carbon dioxide travel across the alveolar–capillary membrane without difficulty as a result of differences in gas concentrations in the alveoli and capillaries.

Pulmonary perfusion is the actual blood flow through the pulmonary circulation. The blood is pumped into the lungs by the right ventricle through the pulmonary artery. The pulmonary artery divides into the right and left branches to supply both lungs. These two branches divide further to supply all parts of each lung. Normally about 2% of the blood pumped by the right ventricle does not perfuse the alveolar capillaries. This shunted blood drains into the left side of the heart without participating in alveolar gas exchange.

The pulmonary circulation is considered a low-pressure system because the systolic blood pressure in the pulmonary artery is 20 to 30 mm Hg and the diastolic pressure is 5 to 15 mm Hg. Because of these low pressures, the pulmonary vasculature normally can vary its capacity to accommodate the blood flow it receives. When a person is in an upright position, however, the pulmonary artery pressure is not great enough to supply blood to the apex of the lung against the force of gravity. Thus, when a person is upright, the lung may be considered to be divided into three sections: an upper part with poor blood supply, a lower part with maximal blood supply, and a section in between the two with an intermediate supply of blood. When a person lying down turns to one side, more blood passes to the dependent lung.

Perfusion also is influenced by alveolar pressure. The pulmonary capillaries are sandwiched between adjacent alveoli. If the alveolar pressure is sufficiently high, the capillaries will be squeezed. Depending on the pressure, some capillaries completely collapse, whereas others narrow.

Pulmonary artery pressure, gravity, and alveolar pressure determine the patterns of perfusion. In lung disease these factors vary, and the perfusion of the lung may become very abnormal.

Ventilation and Perfusion Balance and Imbalance

Ventilation is the flow of gas in and out of the lungs, and perfusion is the filling of the pulmonary capillaries with blood. Adequate gas exchange depends on an adequate ventilation–perfusion ratio. In different areas of the lung, the ratio varies.

Alterations in perfusion may occur with a change in the pulmonary artery pressure, alveolar pressure, and gravity. Airway blockages, local changes in compliance, and gravity may alter ventilation.

A ventilation–perfusion $\dot{V}/\dot{Q}$ imbalance occurs from inadequate ventilation, inadequate perfusion, or both. There are four possible $\dot{V}/\dot{Q}$ states in the lung: normal $\dot{V}/\dot{Q}$ ratio, low $\dot{V}/\dot{Q}$ ratio

---

Chart 21-1 Causes of Increased Airway Resistance

Common phenomena that may alter bronchial diameter, which affects airway resistance, include:

- Contraction of bronchial smooth muscle—as in asthma
- Thickening of bronchial mucosa—as in chronic bronchitis
- Obstruction of the airway—by mucus, a tumor, or a foreign body
- Loss of lung elasticity—as in emphysema, which is characterized by connective tissue encircling the airways, thereby keeping them open during both inspiration and expiration

Table 21-1 • Lung Volumes and Lung Capacities

TERM	SYMBOL	DESCRIPTION	NORMAL VALUE*	SIGNIFICANCE
Lung Volumes				
Tidal volume	V_T or TV	The volume of air inhaled and exhaled with each breath	500 mL or 5–10 mL/kg	The tidal volume may not vary, even with severe disease.
Inspiratory reserve volume	IRV	The maximum volume of air that can be inhaled after a normal inhalation	3,000 mL	
Expiratory reserve volume	ERV	The maximum volume of air that can be exhaled forcibly after a normal exhalation	1,100 mL	Expiratory reserve volume is decreased with restrictive conditions, such as obesity, ascites, pregnancy.
Residual volume	RV	The volume of air remaining in the lungs after a maximum exhalation	1,200 mL	Residual volume may be increased with obstructive disease.
Lung Capacities				
Vital capacity	VC	The maximum volume of air exhaled from the point of maximum inspiration VC = TV + IRV + ERV	4,600 mL	A decrease in vital capacity may be found in neuromuscular disease, generalized fatigue, atelectasis, pulmonary edema, and COPD.
Inspiratory capacity	IC	The maximum volume of air inhaled after normal expiration IC = TV + IRV	3,500 mL	A decrease in inspiratory capacity may indicate restrictive disease.
Functional residual capacity	FRC	The volume of air remaining in the lungs after a normal expiration FRV = ERV + RV	2,300 mL	Functional residual capacity may be increased with COPD and decreased in ARDS.
Total lung capacity	TLC	The volume of air in the lungs after a maximum inspiration TLC = TV + IRV + ERV + RV	5,800 mL	Total lung capacity may be decreased with restrictive disease (atelectasis, pneumonia) and increased in COPD.

*Values for healthy men; women are 20%–25% less.

(shunt), high V̇/Q̇ ratio (dead space), and absence of ventilation and perfusion (silent unit) (Chart 21-2).

Ventilation and perfusion imbalance causes shunting of blood, resulting in **hypoxia** (low cellular oxygen level). Shunting appears to be the main cause of hypoxia after thoracic or abdominal surgery and most types of respiratory failure. Severe hypoxia results when the amount of shunting exceeds 20%. Supplemental oxygen may eliminate hypoxia, depending on the type of V̇/Q̇ imbalance.

Gas Exchange

The air we breathe is a gaseous mixture consisting mainly of nitrogen (78.62%) and oxygen (20.84%), with traces of carbon dioxide (0.04%), water vapor (0.05%), helium, and argon. The atmospheric pressure at sea level is about 760 mm Hg. Partial pressure is the pressure exerted by each type of gas in a mixture of gases. The partial pressure of a gas is proportional to the concentration of that gas in the mixture. The total pressure exerted by the gaseous mixture is equal to the sum of the partial pressures.

PARTIAL PRESSURE OF GASES
Based on these facts, the partial pressures of nitrogen and oxygen can be calculated. The partial pressure of nitrogen is 79% of 760 (0.79×760), or 600 mm Hg; that of oxygen is 21% of 760 (0.21×760), or 160 mm Hg. Chart 21-3 spells out terms and abbreviations related to partial pressure of gases.

Once the air enters the trachea, it becomes fully saturated with water vapor, which displaces some of the gases so that the air pressure within the lung remains equal to the air pressure outside (760 mm Hg). Water vapor exerts a pressure of 47 mm Hg when it fully saturates a mixture of gases at the body temperature of 37°C (98.6°F). Nitrogen and oxygen are responsible for the remaining 713 mm Hg (760 − 47) pressure. Once this mixture enters the alveoli, it is further diluted by carbon dioxide. In the alveoli, the water vapor continues to exert a pressure of 47 mm Hg. The remaining 713 mm Hg pressure is now exerted as follows: nitrogen, 569 mm Hg (74.9%); oxygen, 104 mm Hg (13.6%); and carbon dioxide, 40 mm Hg (5.3%).

PARTIAL PRESSURE IN GAS EXCHANGE
When a gas is exposed to a liquid, the gas dissolves in the liquid until an equilibrium is reached. The dissolved gas also exerts a partial pressure. At equilibrium, the partial pressure of the gas in the liquid is the same as the partial pressure of the gas in the gaseous mixture. Oxygenation of venous blood in the lung illustrates this point. In the lung, venous blood and alveolar oxygen are separated by a very thin alveolar membrane. Oxygen diffuses across this membrane to dissolve in the blood until the partial pressure of oxygen in the blood is the same as that in the alveoli (104 mm Hg). However, because carbon dioxide is a byproduct of oxidation in the cells, venous blood contains carbon dioxide at a higher partial pressure than that in the alveolar gas. In the lung, carbon dioxide diffuses out of venous blood into the alveolar gas. At equilibrium, the partial pressure of carbon dioxide in the blood and in alveolar gas is the same (40 mm Hg). The changes in partial pressure are shown in Figure 21-5.

EFFECTS OF PRESSURE ON OXYGEN TRANSPORT
Oxygen and carbon dioxide are transported simultaneously dissolved in blood or combined with some of the elements of blood. Oxygen is carried in the blood in two forms: first as physically dis-

Chart 21-2 Ventilation-Perfusion Ratios

Normal Ratio (A)
In the healthy lung, a given amount of blood passes an alveolus and is matched with an equal amount of gas (**A**). The ratio is 1:1 (ventilation matches perfusion).

Low Ventilation–Perfusion Ratio: Shunts (B)
Low ventilation–perfusion states may be called shunt-producing disorders. When perfusion exceeds ventilation, a shunt exists (**B**). Blood bypasses the alveoli without gas exchange occurring. This is seen with obstruction of the distal airways, such as with pneumonia, atelectasis, tumor, or a mucus plug.

High Ventilation–Perfusion Ratio: Dead Space (C)
When ventilation exceeds perfusion, dead space results (**C**). The alveoli do not have an adequate blood supply for gas exchange to occur. This is characteristic of a variety of disorders, including pulmonary emboli, pulmonary infarction, and cardiogenic shock.

Silent Unit (D)
In the absence of ventilation and perfusion or with limited ventilation and perfusion, a condition known as a silent unit occurs (**D**). This is seen with pneumothorax and severe acute respiratory distress syndrome.

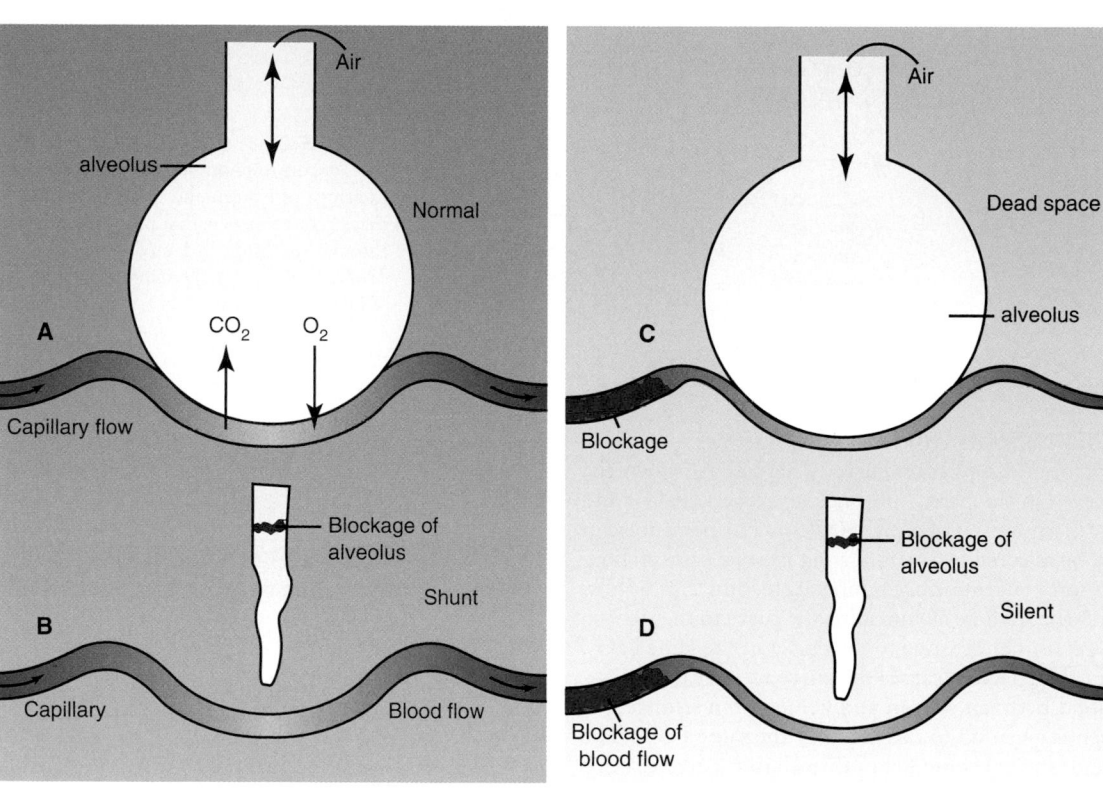

solved oxygen in the plasma, and second in combination with the hemoglobin of the red blood cells. Each 100 mL of normal arterial blood carries 0.3 mL of oxygen physically dissolved in the plasma and 20 mL of oxygen in combination with hemoglobin. Large amounts of oxygen can be transported in the blood because it combines easily with hemoglobin to form oxyhemoglobin:

$$O_2 + Hgb \leftrightarrow HgbO_2$$

The volume of oxygen physically dissolved in the plasma varies directly with the partial pressure of oxygen in the arteries (PaO_2). The higher the PaO_2, the greater the amount of oxygen dissolved. For example, at a PaO_2 of 10 mm Hg, 0.03 mL of oxygen is dissolved in 100 mL of plasma. At 20 mm Hg, twice this amount is dissolved in plasma, and at 100 mm Hg, 10 times this amount is dissolved. Therefore, the amount of dissolved oxygen is directly proportional to the partial pressure, regardless of how high the oxygen pressure rises.

The amount of oxygen that combines with hemoglobin also depends on PaO_2, but only up to a PaO_2 of about 150 mm Hg. When the PaO_2 is 150 mm Hg, hemoglobin is 100% saturated and will not combine with any additional oxygen. When hemoglobin is 100% saturated, 1 g of hemoglobin will combine with 1.34 mL of oxygen. Therefore, in a person with 14 g/dL of hemoglobin, each 100 mL of blood will contain about 19 mL of oxygen associated with hemoglobin. If the PaO_2 is less than 150 mm Hg, the percentage of hemoglobin saturated with oxygen is lower. For example, at a PaO_2 of 100 mm Hg (normal value), saturation is 97%; at a PaO_2 of 40 mm Hg, saturation is 70%.

Chart 21-3 Partial Pressure Abbreviations

P = pressure
PO_2 = partial pressure of oxygen
PCO_2 = partial pressure of carbon dioxide
PAO_2 = partial pressure of alveolar oxygen
$PACO_2$ = partial pressure of alveolar carbon dioxide
PaO_2 = partial pressure of arterial oxygen
$PaCO_2$ = partial pressure of arterial carbon dioxide
$P\bar{v}O_2$ = partial pressure of venous oxygen
$P\bar{v}CO_2$ = partial pressure of venous carbon dioxide
P_{50} = partial pressure of oxygen when the hemoglobin is 50% saturated

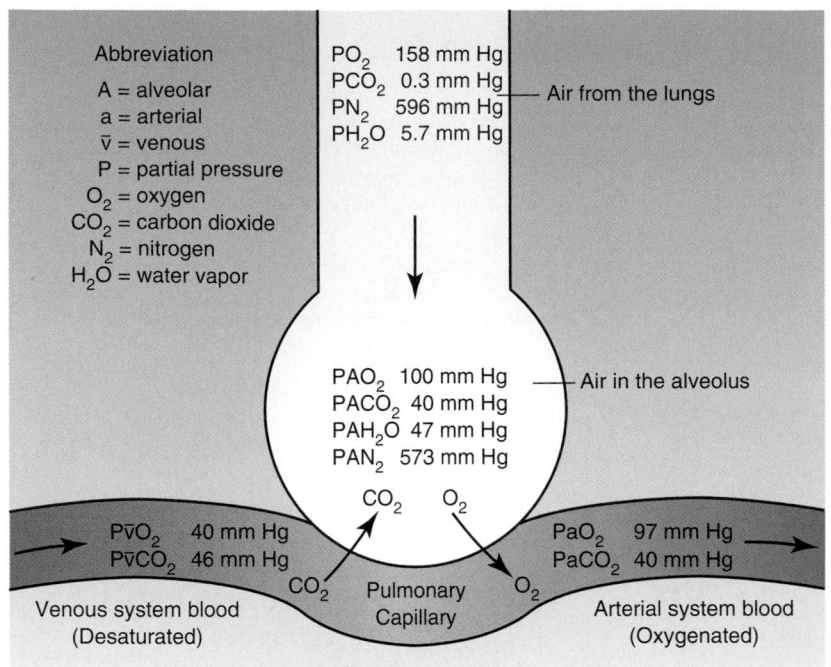

Abbreviation

A = alveolar
a = arterial
v̄ = venous
P = partial pressure
O_2 = oxygen
CO_2 = carbon dioxide
N_2 = nitrogen
H_2O = water vapor

PO_2 158 mm Hg
PCO_2 0.3 mm Hg
PN_2 596 mm Hg
PH_2O 5.7 mm Hg — Air from the lungs

PAO_2 100 mm Hg — Air in the alveolus
$PACO_2$ 40 mm Hg
PAH_2O 47 mm Hg
PAN_2 573 mm Hg

CO_2 O_2

PvO_2 40 mm Hg
$PvCO_2$ 46 mm Hg

PaO_2 97 mm Hg
$PaCO_2$ 40 mm Hg

CO_2 Pulmonary O_2
          Capillary

Venous system blood
(Desaturated)

Arterial system blood
(Oxygenated)

FIGURE 21-5 Changes occur in the partial pressure of gases during respiration. These values vary as a result of the exchange of oxygen and carbon dioxide and the changes that occur in their partial pressures as venous blood flows through the lungs. Adapted from Willis, M. C. (1996). *Medical terminology: The language of healthcare.* Baltimore: Williams & Wilkins.

OXYHEMOGLOBIN DISSOCIATION CURVE

The oxyhemoglobin dissociation curve (Chart 21-4) shows the relationship between the partial pressure of oxygen (PaO_2) and the percentage of saturation of oxygen (SaO_2). The percentage of saturation can be affected by the following factors: carbon dioxide, hydrogen ion concentration, temperature, and 2,3-diphosphoglycerate. A rise in these factors shifts the curve to the right so that more oxygen is then released to the tissues at the same PaO_2. A reduction in these factors causes the curve to shift to the left, making the bond between oxygen and hemoglobin stronger, so that less oxygen is given up to the tissues at the same PaO_2. The unusual shape of the oxyhemoglobin dissociation curve is a distinct advantage to the patient for two reasons:

1. If the arterial PO_2 decreases from 100 to 80 mm Hg as a result of lung disease or heart disease, the hemoglobin of the arterial blood remains almost maximally saturated (94%) and the tissues will not suffer from hypoxia.
2. When the arterial blood passes into tissue capillaries and is exposed to the tissue tension of oxygen (about 40 mm Hg), hemoglobin gives up large quantities of oxygen for use by the tissues.

Clinical Significance. The normal value of PaO_2 is 80 to 100 mm Hg (95% to 98% saturation). With this level of oxygenation, there is a 15% margin of excess oxygen available to the tissues. With a normal hemoglobin level of 15 mg/dL and a PaO_2 level of 40 mm Hg (oxygen saturation 75%), there is adequate oxygen available for the tissues but no reserve for physiologic stresses that increase tissue oxygen demand. When a serious incident occurs (eg, bronchospasm, aspiration, hypotension, or cardiac dysrhythmias) that reduces the intake of oxygen from the lungs, tissue hypoxia will result.

An important consideration in the transport of oxygen is cardiac output, which determines the amount of oxygen delivered to the body and which affects lung and tissue perfusion. If the cardiac output is normal (5 L/min), the amount of oxygen delivered to the

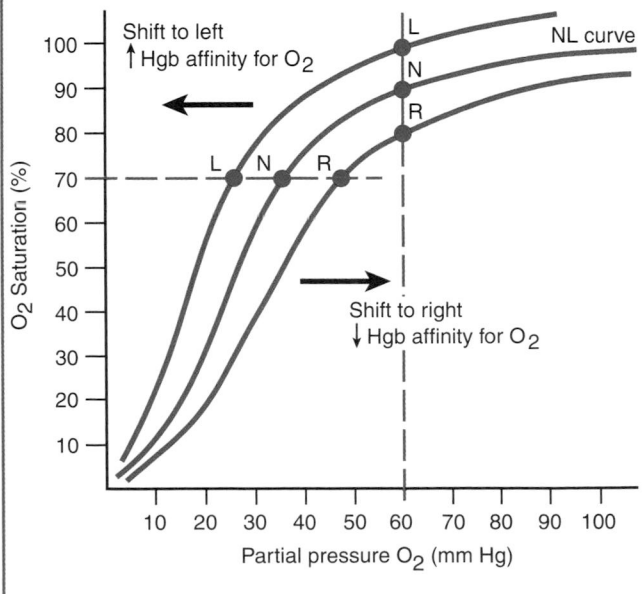

Chart 21-4 Oxyhemoglobin Dissociation Curve

The oxyhemoglobin dissociation curve is marked to show three oxygen levels:

1. Normal levels—PaO_2 above 70 mm Hg
2. Relatively safe levels—PaO_2 45 to 70 mm Hg
3. Dangerous levels—PaO_2 below 40 mm Hg

The normal (middle) curve (N) shows that 75% saturation occurs at a PaO_2 of 40 mm Hg. If the curve shifts to the right (R), the same saturation (75%) occurs at the higher PaO_2 of 57 mm Hg. If the curve shifts to the left (L), 75% saturation occurs at a PaO_2 of 25 mm Hg.

Shift to left
↑ Hgb affinity for O_2

NL curve

Shift to right
↓ Hgb affinity for O_2

O_2 Saturation (%)

Partial pressure O_2 (mm Hg)

body per minute is normal. If cardiac output falls, the amount of oxygen delivered to the tissues also falls. Under normal conditions, most of the oxygen delivered to the body is not used. In fact, only 250 mL of oxygen is used per minute. Under normal conditions, this is approximately 25% of available oxygen. The rest of the oxygen returns to the right side of the heart, and the PaO_2 of venous blood drops from 80 to 100 mm Hg to about 40 mm Hg.

Carbon Dioxide Transport

At the same time that oxygen diffuses from the blood into the tissues, carbon dioxide diffuses in the opposite direction (ie, from tissue cells to blood) and is transported to the lungs for excretion. The amount of carbon dioxide in transit is one of the major determinants of the acid–base balance of the body. Normally, only 6% of the venous carbon dioxide is removed, and enough remains in the arterial blood to exert a pressure of 40 mm Hg. Most of the carbon dioxide (90%) enters the red blood cells; the small portion (5%) that remains dissolved in the plasma (PCO_2) is the critical factor that determines carbon dioxide movement in or out of the blood.

In summary, the many processes involved in respiratory gas transport do not occur in intermittent stages; rather, they are rapid, simultaneous, and continuous.

Neurologic Control of Ventilation

Resting respiration is the result of cyclical excitation of the respiratory muscles by the phrenic nerve. The rhythm of breathing is controlled by respiratory centers in the brain. The inspiratory and expiratory centers in the medulla oblongata and pons control the rate and depth of ventilation to meet the body's metabolic demands.

The apneustic center in the lower pons stimulates the inspiratory medullary center to promote deep, prolonged inspirations. The pneumotaxic center in the upper pons is thought to control the pattern of respirations.

Several groups of receptor sites assist in the brain's control of respiratory function. The central chemoreceptors are located in the medulla and respond to chemical changes in the cerebrospinal fluid, which result from chemical changes in the blood. These receptors respond to an increase or decrease in the pH and convey a message to the lungs to change the depth and then the rate of ventilation to correct the imbalance. The peripheral chemoreceptors are located in the aortic arch and the carotid arteries and respond first to changes in PaO_2, then to $PaCO_2$ and pH. The Hering–Breuer reflex is activated by stretch receptors in the alveoli. When the lungs are distended, inspiration is inhibited; as a result, the lungs do not become overdistended. In addition, proprioceptors in the muscles and joints respond to body movements, such as exercise, causing an increase in ventilation. Thus, range-of-motion exercises in an immobile patient stimulate breathing. Baroreceptors, also located in the aortic and carotid bodies, respond to an increase or decrease in arterial blood pressure and cause reflex hypoventilation or hyperventilation.

Gerontologic Considerations

A gradual decline in respiratory function begins in early to middle adulthood and affects the structure and function of the respiratory system. The vital capacity of the lungs and respiratory muscle strength peak between ages 20 and 25 and decrease thereafter. With aging (40 years and older), changes occur in the alveoli that reduce the surface area available for the exchange of oxygen and carbon dioxide. At approximately age 50, the alveoli begin to lose elasticity. A decrease in vital capacity occurs with loss of chest wall mobility, thus restricting the tidal flow of air. The amount of respiratory dead space increases with age. These changes result in a decreased diffusion capacity for oxygen with age, producing lower oxygen levels in the arterial circulation. Elderly people have a decreased ability to move air rapidly in and out of the lungs. Gerontologic changes in the respiratory system are summarized in Table 21-2. Despite these changes, in the absence of chronic pulmonary disease, elderly people are able to carry out activities of daily living, but they may have decreased tolerance for and require additional rest after prolonged or vigorous activity.

Assessment

HEALTH HISTORY

The health history focuses on the physical and functional problems of the patient and the effect of these problems on his or her life. The reason the patient is seeking health care often is related to one of the following: **dyspnea** (shortness of breath), pain, accumulation of mucus, wheezing, **hemoptysis** (blood spit up from the respiratory tract), edema of the ankles and feet, cough, and general fatigue and weakness.

In addition to identifying the chief reason why the patient is seeking health care, the nurse tries to determine when the health problem or symptom started, how long it lasted, if it was relieved at any time, and how relief was obtained. The nurse collects information about precipitating factors, duration, severity, and associated factors or symptoms and also assesses for risk factors and genetic factors that may contribute to the patient's lung condition (Chart 21-5).

The nurse assesses the impact of signs and symptoms on the patient's ability to perform activities of daily living and to participate in usual work and family activities. In addition, psychosocial factors that may affect the patient are explored (Chart 21-6). These factors include anxiety, role changes, family relationships, financial problems, employment status, and the strategies the patient uses to cope with them.

Many respiratory diseases are chronic and progressively debilitating. Therefore, ongoing assessment of the patient's physical abilities, psychosocial supports, and quality of life is needed to plan appropriate interventions. It is important for the patient with a respiratory disorder to understand the condition and to be familiar with necessary self-care interventions. The nurse evaluates these factors over time and provides education as needed.

Signs and Symptoms

The major signs and symptoms of respiratory disease are dyspnea, cough, sputum production, chest pain, wheezing, clubbing of the fingers, hemoptysis, and cyanosis. These clinical manifestations are related to the duration and severity of the disease.

DYSPNEA

Dyspnea (difficult or labored breathing, shortness of breath) is a symptom common to many pulmonary and cardiac disorders, particularly when there is decreased lung compliance or increased airway resistance. The right ventricle of the heart will be affected ultimately by lung disease because it must pump blood through the lungs against greater resistance. It may also be associated with neurologic or neuromuscular disorders such as myasthenia gravis, Guillain-Barré syndrome, or muscular dystrophy.

Table 21-2 • **Age-Related Changes of the Respiratory System**

	STRUCTURAL CHANGES	FUNCTIONAL CHANGES	HISTORY AND PHYSICAL FINDINGS
Defense mechanisms (respiratory and nonrespiratory)	↓ Number of cilia and ↓ mucus ↓ Cough and gag reflex Loss of surface area of the capillary membrane Lack of a uniform or consistent ventilation and/or blood flow	↓ Protection against foreign particles ↓ Protection against aspiration ↓ Antibody response to antigens ↓ Response to hypoxia and hypercapnia (chemoreceptors)	↓ Cough reflex and mucus ↑ Infection rate History of respiratory infections, COPD, pneumonia. Risk factors: smoking, environmental exposure, TB exposure
Lung	↓ Size of airway ↑ Diameter of alveolar ducts ↑ Collagen of alveolar walls ↑ Thickness of alveolar membranes ↓ Elasticity of alveolar sacs	↑ Airway resistance ↑ Pulmonary compliance ↓ Expiratory flow rate ↓ Oxygen diffusion capacity ↑ Dead space Premature closure of airways ↑ Air trapping ↓ Expiratory flow rates Ventilation–perfusion mismatch ↓ Exercise capacity ↑ Anteroposterior (AP) diameter	Unchanged total lung capacity (TLC) ↑ Residual volume (RV) ↓ Inspiratory reserve volume (IRV) ↓ Expiratory reserve volume (ERV) ↓ Forced vital capacity (FVC) and vital capacity (VC) ↑ Functional residual capacity (FRC) ↓ PaO_2 ↑ CO_2
Chest wall and muscles	Calcification of intercostal cartilages Arthritis of costovertebral joints ↓ Continuity of diaphragm Osteoporotic changes ↓ Muscle mass Muscle atrophy	↑ Rigidity and stiffness of thoracic cage ↓ Respiratory muscle strength ↑ Work of breathing ↓ Capacity for exercise ↓ Peripheral chemosensitivity ↑ Risk for inspiratory muscle fatigue	Kyphosis, barrel chest Skeletal changes ↑ AP diameter Shortness of breath ↑ Abdominal and diaphragmatic breathing ↓ Maximum expiratory flow rates

Clinical Significance. In general, acute diseases of the lungs produce a more severe grade of dyspnea than do chronic diseases. Sudden dyspnea in a healthy person may indicate pneumothorax (air in the pleural cavity), acute respiratory obstruction, or ARDS. In immobilized patients, sudden dyspnea may denote pulmonary embolism. **Orthopnea** (inability to breathe easily except in an upright position) may be found in patients with heart disease and occasionally in patients with chronic obstructive pulmonary disease (COPD); dyspnea with an expiratory wheeze occurs with COPD. Noisy breathing may result from a narrowing of the airway or localized obstruction of a major bronchus by a tumor or foreign body. The presence of both inspiratory and expiratory wheezing usually signifies asthma if the patient does not have heart failure.

The circumstance that produces the dyspnea must be determined. Therefore, it is important to ask the patient the following questions:

- How much exertion triggers shortness of breath?
- Is there an associated cough?
- Is dyspnea related to other symptoms?
- Was the onset of shortness of breath sudden or gradual?

Chart 21-5
Risk Factors for Respiratory Disease

Smoking (the single most important contributor to lung disease)
Personal or family history of lung disease
Occupation
Allergens and environmental pollutants
Recreational exposure

- At what time of day or night does the dyspnea occur?
- Is the shortness of breath worse when the patient is flat in bed?
- Does the shortness of breath occur at rest? With exercise? Running? Climbing stairs?
- Is the shortness of breath worse while walking? If so, when walking how far? How fast?

Relief Measures. The management of dyspnea is aimed at identifying and correcting its cause. Relief of the symptom sometimes is achieved by placing the patient at rest with the head elevated (high Fowler's position) and, in severe cases, by administering oxygen.

COUGH

Cough results from irritation of the mucous membranes anywhere in the respiratory tract. The stimulus producing a cough may arise from an infectious process or from an airborne irritant, such as smoke, smog, dust, or a gas. The cough is the patient's chief protection against the accumulation of secretions in the bronchi and bronchioles.

Clinical Significance. Cough may indicate serious pulmonary disease. The nurse needs to evaluate the character of the cough—is it dry, hacking, brassy, wheezing, loose, or severe? A dry, irritative cough is characteristic of an upper respiratory tract infection of viral origin or may be a side effect of angiotensin-converting enzyme (ACE) inhibitor therapy. Laryngotracheitis causes an irritative, high-pitched cough. Tracheal lesions produce a brassy cough. A severe or changing cough may indicate bronchogenic carcinoma. Pleuritic chest pain accompanying coughing may indicate pleural or chest wall (musculoskeletal) involvement.

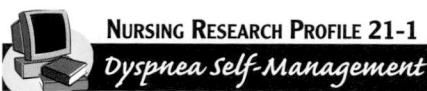

NURSING RESEARCH PROFILE 21-1
Dyspnea Self-Management

Nield, M. (2000). Dyspnea self-management in African Americans with chronic lung disease. *Heart & Lung, 29*(1), 50–55.

Purpose
The purpose of this qualitative analysis, part of a larger study of the relationship between dyspnea and respiratory muscle function in patients with chronic lung disease, was to explore dyspnea self-management in African Americans with COPD or chronic restrictive pulmonary disease resulting from sarcoidosis.

Study Sample and Design
A qualitative study approach was used with a convenience sample of 29 patients recruited from the pulmonary clinic at a large medical center in the midwestern United States. Fifteen of the subjects had COPD and 14 had sarcoidosis. All routinely experienced dyspnea. A semistructured interview guide was used to obtain data. The taped interviews were transcribed and content analysis was performed using open coding methods.

Findings
The investigators identified the following self-management themes from the data:
- Traditional medical care (formal health care and prescription medications)
- Self-care wisdom (learned insight regarding the impact of dyspnea on quality of life)
- Self-care action (specific strategies for dyspnea relief included exercise, environmental control, cognitive strategies, and controlled breathing, which refers to patient-initiated position and breathing to manage dyspnea). Patients with sarcoidosis used inhalation-focused breathing only, while patients with COPD used both inhalation- and exhalation-focused breathing.
- Self-care resources (internal or external assets that could be used for sustenance of the self-care actions such as spiritual and social support)

Nursing Implications
These findings mirror previous research; however, this study extends previous knowledge as it focused on African Americans exclusively. When working with patients with chronic respiratory disorders, nurses should assess all four aspects of dyspnea self-management, which reflect a holistic approach to care. Self-care actions should be encouraged and taught, and self-care resources facilitated. The breathing techniques used by patients with COPD and those with sarcoidosis should be considered during patient and family education. Further research is warranted to determine if the differences in the breathing techniques used by these two populations of patients are also found in a research study with a larger sample size.

The time of coughing is also noted. Coughing at night may herald the onset of left-sided heart failure or bronchial asthma. A cough in the morning with sputum production may indicate bronchitis. A cough that worsens when the patient is supine suggests postnasal drip (sinusitis). Coughing after food intake may indicate aspiration of material into the tracheobronchial tree. A cough of recent onset is usually from an acute infection.

SPUTUM PRODUCTION
A patient who coughs long enough almost invariably produces sputum. Violent coughing causes bronchial spasm, obstruction, and further irritation of the bronchi and may result in syncope (fainting). A severe, repeated, or uncontrolled cough that is nonproductive is exhausting and potentially harmful. Sputum pro-

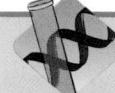

GENETICS IN NURSING PRACTICE—
Genetic Influences

Various conditions that affect gas exchange and respiratory function are influenced by genetic factors, including:
- Asthma
- Chronic obstructive pulmonary disease
- Cystic fibrosis
- Alpha-1 antitrypsin deficiency

NURSING ASSESSMENTS
FAMILY HISTORY ASSESSMENT
- Assess family history for other family members with histories of respiratory impairment.
- Assess family history for individuals with early-onset chronic pulmonary disease, family history of hepatic disease in infants (clinical symptoms of alpha-1 antitrypsin deficiency).
- Inquire about family history of genetic cystic fibrosis.

MANAGEMENT ISSUES SPECIFIC TO GENETICS
- Inquire whether DNA mutation or other genetic testing has been performed on affected family members.
- Refer for further genetic counseling and evaluation so that family members can discuss inheritance, risk to other family members, availability of genetic testing and gene-based interventions.
- Offer appropriate genetics information and resources.
- Assess patient's understanding of genetics information.
- Provide support to families with newly diagnosed genetic-related respiratory disorders.
- Participate in management and coordination of care of patients with genetic conditions, individuals predisposed to develop or pass on a genetic condition.

GENETIC RESOURCES FOR NURSES AND THEIR PATIENTS ON THE WEB
American Lung Association http://www.lungusa.org
Cystic Fibrosis Foundation http://www.cff.org
Genetic Alliance http://www.geneticalliance.org—a directory of support groups for patients and families with genetic conditions
Gene Clinics http://www.geneclinics.org—a listing of common genetic disorders with clinical summaries, genetic counseling and testing information
National Organization of Rare Disorders http://www.rarediseases.org—a directory of support groups and information for patients and families with rare genetic disorders
OMIM: Online Mendelian Inheritance in Man http://www.ncbi.nlm.nih.gov/omim/stats/html—a complete listing of inherited genetic conditions

---

duction is the reaction of the lungs to any constantly recurring irritant. It also may be associated with a nasal discharge.

Clinical Significance. A profuse amount of purulent sputum (thick and yellow, green, or rust-colored) or a change in color of the sputum probably indicates a bacterial infection. Thin, mucoid sputum frequently results from viral bronchitis. A gradual increase of sputum over time may indicate the presence of chronic bronchitis or bronchiectasis. Pink-tinged mucoid sputum suggests

Chart 21-6 • ASSESSMENT

Psychosocial Factors

Questions to consider when assessing psychosocial factors related to pulmonary disease and respiratory function include:

- What strategies does the patient use to cope with the signs and symptoms and challenges associated with pulmonary disease?
- Does the patient exhibit anxiety, anger, hostility, dependency, withdrawal, isolation, avoidance, noncompliance, acceptance, or denial?
- What support systems does the patient use to cope with the illness?
- Are resources (relatives, friends, or community groups) available? Do the patient and family use them effectively?

a lung tumor. Profuse, frothy, pink material, often welling up into the throat, may indicate pulmonary edema. Foul-smelling sputum and bad breath point to the presence of a lung abscess, bronchiectasis, or an infection caused by fusospirochetal or other anaerobic organisms.

Relief Measures. If the sputum is too thick for the patient to expectorate, it is necessary to decrease its viscosity by increasing its water content through adequate hydration (drinking water) and inhalation of aerosolized solutions, which may be delivered by any type of nebulizer. Strategies to assist the patient to cough productively are discussed later in this chapter.

Smoking is contraindicated with excessive sputum production because it interferes with ciliary action, increases bronchial secretions, causes inflammation and hyperplasia of the mucous membranes, and reduces production of surfactant. Thus, smoking impairs bronchial drainage. When the person stops smoking, sputum volume decreases and resistance to bronchial infections increases.

The patient's appetite may decrease because of the odor of the sputum or the taste it leaves in the mouth. The nurse encourages adequate oral hygiene and wise selection of food, measures that will stimulate appetite. In addition, the nurse encourages the patient and family to remove sputum cups, emesis basins, and soiled tissues before mealtime. Encouraging the patient to drink citrus juices at the beginning of the meal may increase the palatability of the rest of the meal because these juices cleanse the palate of the sputum taste.

CHEST PAIN

Chest pain or discomfort may be associated with pulmonary or cardiac disease. Chest pain associated with pulmonary conditions may be sharp, stabbing, and intermittent, or it may be dull, aching, and persistent. The pain usually is felt on the side where the pathologic process is located, but it may be referred elsewhere—for example, to the neck, back, or abdomen.

Clinical Significance. Chest pain may occur with pneumonia, pulmonary embolism with lung infarction, and pleurisy. It also may be a late symptom of bronchogenic carcinoma. In carcinoma the pain may be dull and persistent because the cancer has invaded the chest wall, mediastinum, or spine.

Lung disease does not always produce thoracic pain because the lungs and the visceral pleura lack sensory nerves and are insensitive to pain stimuli. However, the parietal pleura has a rich

supply of sensory nerves that are stimulated by inflammation and stretching of the membrane. Pleuritic pain from irritation of the parietal pleura is sharp and seems to "catch" on inspiration; patients often describe it as "like the stabbing of a knife." Patients are more comfortable when they lie on the affected side as this splints the chest wall, limits expansion and contraction of the lung, and reduces the friction between the injured or diseased pleurae on that side. Pain associated with cough may be reduced manually by splinting the rib cage.

The nurse assesses the quality, intensity, and radiation of pain and identifies and explores precipitating factors, along with their relationship to the patient's position. Also, it is important to assess the relationship of pain to the inspiratory and expiratory phases of respiration.

Relief Measures. Analgesic medications may be effective in relieving chest pain, but care must be taken not to depress the respiratory center or a productive cough, if present. Nonsteroidal anti-inflammatory drugs (NSAIDs) achieve this goal and thus are used for pleuritic pain. A regional anesthetic block may be performed to relieve extreme pain.

WHEEZING

Wheezing is often the major finding in a patient with bronchoconstriction or airway narrowing. It is heard with or without a stethoscope, depending on its location. Wheezing is a high-pitched, musical sound heard mainly on expiration.

Relief Measures. Oral or inhalant bronchodilator medications reverse wheezing in most instances.

CLUBBING OF THE FINGERS

Clubbing of the fingers is a sign of lung disease found in patients with chronic hypoxic conditions, chronic lung infections, and malignancies of the lung. This finding may be manifested initially as sponginess of the nailbed and loss of the nailbed angle (Fig. 21-6).

HEMOPTYSIS

Hemoptysis (expectoration of blood from the respiratory tract) is a symptom of both pulmonary and cardiac disorders. The onset of hemoptysis is usually sudden, and it may be intermittent or continuous. Signs, which vary from blood-stained sputum to a

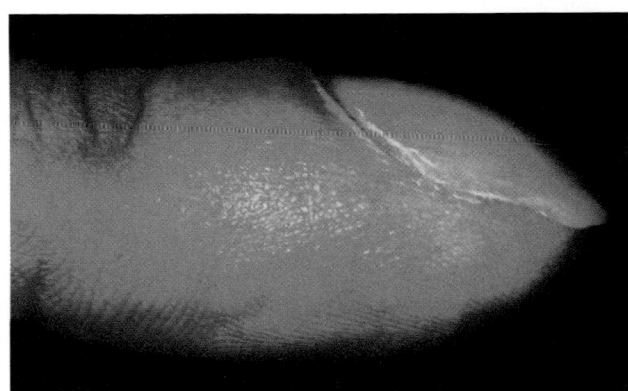

FIGURE 21-6 Clubbed finger. In clubbing, the distal phalanx of each finger is rounded and bulbous. The nail plate is more convex, and the angle between the plate and the proximal nail fold increases to 180 degrees or more. The proximal nail fold, when palpated, feels spongy or floating. Among the many causes are chronic hypoxia and lung cancer.

large, sudden hemorrhage, always merit investigation. The most common causes are:

- Pulmonary infection
- Carcinoma of the lung
- Abnormalities of the heart or blood vessels
- Pulmonary artery or vein abnormalities
- Pulmonary emboli and infarction

Diagnostic evaluation to determine the cause includes several studies: chest x-ray, chest angiography, and bronchoscopy. A careful history and physical examination are necessary to diagnose the underlying disease, irrespective of whether the bleeding involved a very small amount of blood in the sputum or a massive hemorrhage. The amount of blood produced is not always proportional to the seriousness of the cause.

First, it is important to determine the source of the bleeding—the gums, nasopharynx, lungs, or stomach. The nurse may be the only witness to the episode. When documenting the bleeding episode, the nurse considers the following points:

- Bloody sputum from the nose or the nasopharynx is usually preceded by considerable sniffing, with blood possibly appearing in the nose.
- Blood from the lung is usually bright red, frothy, and mixed with sputum. Initial symptoms include a tickling sensation in the throat, a salty taste, a burning or bubbling sensation in the chest, and perhaps chest pain, in which case the patient tends to splint the bleeding side. The term "hemoptysis" is reserved for the coughing up of blood arising from a pulmonary hemorrhage. This blood has an alkaline pH (greater than 7.0).
- If the hemorrhage is in the stomach, the blood is vomited (hematemesis) rather than coughed up. Blood that has been in contact with gastric juice is sometimes so dark that it is referred to as "coffee grounds." This blood has an acid pH (less than 7.0).

CYANOSIS

Cyanosis, a bluish coloring of the skin, is a very late indicator of hypoxia. The presence or absence of cyanosis is determined by the amount of unoxygenated hemoglobin in the blood. Cyanosis appears when there is 5 g/dL of unoxygenated hemoglobin. A patient with a hemoglobin level of 15 g/dL will not demonstrate cyanosis until 5 g/dL of that hemoglobin becomes unoxygenated, reducing the effective circulating hemoglobin to two thirds of the normal level. An anemic patient rarely manifests cyanosis, and a polycythemic patient may appear cyanotic even if adequately oxygenated. Therefore, cyanosis is *not* a reliable sign of hypoxia.

Assessment of cyanosis is affected by room lighting, the patient's skin color, and the distance of the blood vessels from the surface of the skin. In the presence of a pulmonary condition, central cyanosis is assessed by observing the color of the tongue and lips. This indicates a decrease in oxygen tension in the blood. Peripheral cyanosis results from decreased blood flow to a certain area of the body, as in vasoconstriction of the nailbeds or earlobes from exposure to cold, and does not necessarily indicate a central systemic problem.

PHYSICAL ASSESSMENT OF THE UPPER RESPIRATORY STRUCTURES

For a routine examination of the upper airway, only a simple light source, such as a penlight, is necessary. A more thorough examination requires the use of a nasal speculum.

Nose and Sinuses

The nurse inspects the external nose for lesions, asymmetry, or inflammation and then asks the patient to tilt the head backward. Gently pushing the tip of the nose upward, the nurse examines the internal structures of the nose, inspecting the mucosa for color, swelling, exudate, or bleeding. The nasal mucosa is normally redder than the oral mucosa, but it may appear swollen and hyperemic if the patient has a common cold. In allergic rhinitis, however, the mucosa appears pale and swollen.

Next the nurse inspects the septum for deviation, perforation, or bleeding. Most people have a slight degree of septal deviation, but actual displacement of the cartilage into either the right or left side of the nose may produce nasal obstruction. Such deviation usually causes no symptoms.

While the head is still tilted back, the nurse inspects the inferior and middle turbinates. In chronic rhinitis, nasal polyps may develop between the inferior and middle turbinates; they are distinguished by their gray appearance. Unlike the turbinates, they are gelatinous and freely movable.

Next the nurse may palpate the frontal and maxillary sinuses for tenderness (Fig. 21-7). Using the thumbs, the nurse applies gentle pressure in an upward fashion at the supraorbital ridges (frontal sinuses) and in the cheek area adjacent to the nose (maxillary sinuses). Tenderness in either area suggests inflammation. The frontal and maxillary sinuses can be inspected by transillumination (passing a strong light through a bony area, such as the sinuses, to inspect the cavity; Fig. 21-8). If the light fails to penetrate, the cavity is likely to contain fluid or pus.

Pharynx and Mouth

After the nasal inspection, the nurse may assess the mouth and pharynx, instructing the patient to open the mouth wide and take a deep breath. Usually this will flatten the posterior tongue and briefly allow a full view of the anterior and posterior pillars, tonsils, uvula, and posterior pharynx (Fig. 21-9). The nurse inspects these structures for color, symmetry, and evidence of exudate, ulceration, or enlargement. If a tongue blade is needed to depress the tongue to visualize the pharynx, it is pressed firmly beyond the midpoint of the tongue to avoid a gagging response.

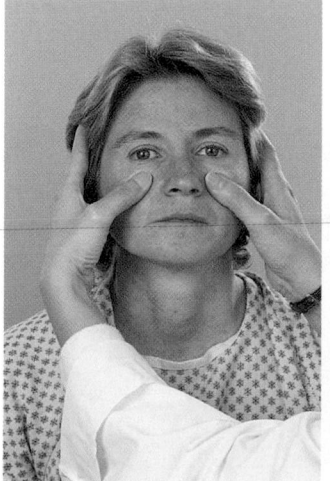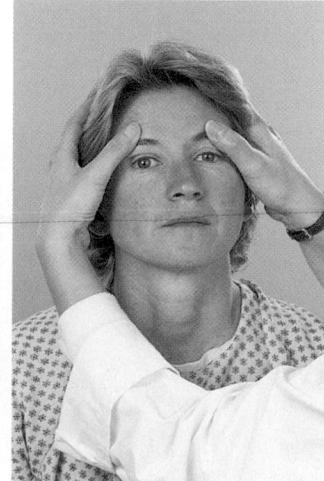

FIGURE 21-7 Technique for palpating the frontal sinuses at left and the maxillary sinuses at right. From Weber, J. & Kelley, J. (2003). *Health assessment in nursing* (2nd ed.). Philadelphia: Lippincott Williams & Wilkins.

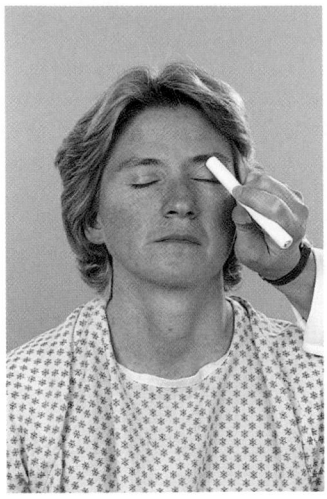 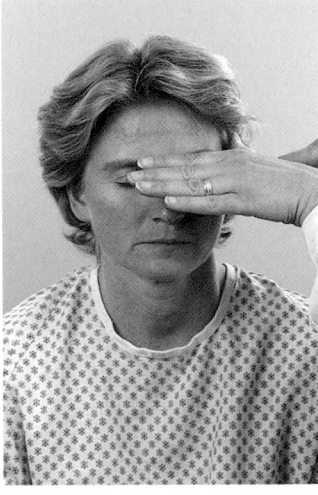

FIGURE 21-8 At left, the nurse positions the light source for transillumination of the frontal sinus. At right, the nurse shields the patient's brow and shines the light. In normal conditions (a darkened room), the light should shine through the tissues and appear as a reddish glow (above the nurse's hand) over the sinus. From Weber, J. & Kelley, J. (2003). *Health assessment in nursing* (2nd ed.). Philadelphia: Lippincott Williams & Wilkins.

Trachea

Next the position and mobility of the trachea are usually noted by direct palpation. This is performed by placing the thumb and index finger of one hand on either side of the trachea just above the sternal notch. The trachea is highly sensitive, and palpating too firmly may trigger a coughing or gagging response. The trachea is normally in the midline as it enters the thoracic inlet behind the sternum, but it may be deviated by masses in the neck or mediastinum. Pleural or pulmonary disorders, such as a pneumothorax, may also displace the trachea.

PHYSICAL ASSESSMENT OF THE LOWER RESPIRATORY STRUCTURES AND BREATHING

Thorax

Inspection of the thorax provides information about the musculoskeletal structure, the patient's nutritional status, and the respiratory system. The nurse observes the skin over the thorax for color and turgor and for evidence of loss of subcutaneous tissue. It is important to note asymmetry, if present. When findings are recorded or reported, anatomic landmarks are used as points of reference (Chart 21-7).

CHEST CONFIGURATION

Normally, the ratio of the anteroposterior diameter to the lateral diameter is 1 : 2. However, there are four main deformities of the chest associated with respiratory disease that alter this relationship: barrel chest, funnel chest (pectus excavatum), pigeon chest (pectus carinatum), and kyphoscoliosis.

Barrel Chest. Barrel chest occurs as a result of overinflation of the lungs. There is an increase in the anteroposterior diameter of the thorax. In a patient with emphysema, the ribs are more widely spaced and the intercostal spaces tend to bulge on expiration. The appearance of the patient with advanced emphysema is thus quite characteristic and often allows the observer to detect its presence easily, even from a distance.

Funnel Chest (Pectus Excavatum). Funnel chest occurs when there is a depression in the lower portion of the sternum. This may compress the heart and great vessels, resulting in murmurs. Funnel chest may occur with rickets or Marfan's syndrome.

Pigeon Chest (Pectus Carinatum). A pigeon chest occurs as a result of displacement of the sternum. There is an increase in the anteroposterior diameter. This may occur with rickets, Marfan's syndrome, or severe kyphoscoliosis.

Kyphoscoliosis. A kyphoscoliosis is characterized by elevation of the scapula and a corresponding S-shaped spine. This deformity limits lung expansion within the thorax. It may occur with osteoporosis and other skeletal disorders that affect the thorax.

BREATHING PATTERNS AND RESPIRATORY RATES

Observing the rate and depth of respiration is a simple but important aspect of assessment. The normal adult who is resting comfortably takes 12 to 18 breaths per minute. Except for occasional sighs, respirations are regular in depth and rhythm. This normal pattern is described as eupnea.

Bradypnea, also called slow breathing, is associated with increased intracranial pressure, brain injury, and drug overdose. Tachypnea, or rapid breathing, is commonly seen in patients with pneumonia, pulmonary edema, metabolic acidosis, septicemia,

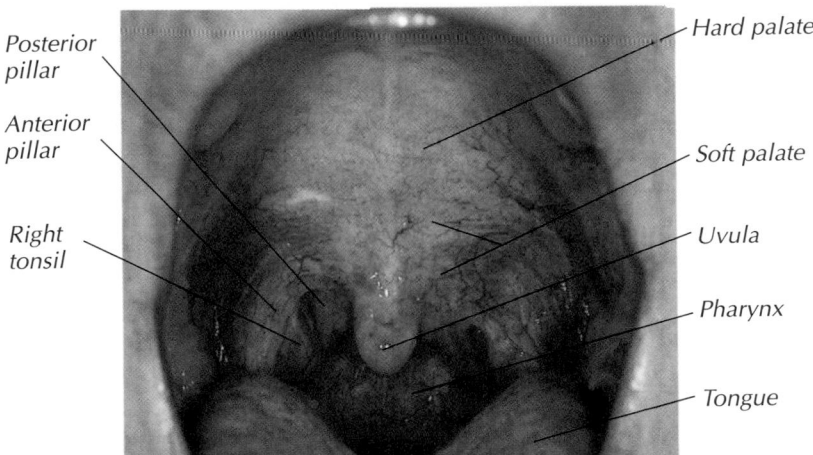

Posterior pillar
Anterior pillar
Right tonsil
Hard palate
Soft palate
Uvula
Pharynx
Tongue

FIGURE 21-9 The pharynx and other oral structures—pillars, tonsils, uvula, hard and soft palates, posterior pharynx, and tongue—are easily seen when the mouth is open.

Locating Thoracic Landmarks

With respect to the thorax, location is defined both horizontally and vertically. With respect to the lungs, location is defined by lobe.

Horizontal Reference Points

Horizontally, thoracic locations are identified according to their proximity to the rib or the intercostal space under the examiner's fingers. On the anterior surface, identification of a specific rib is facilitated by first locating the angle of Louis. This is where the manubrium joins the body of the sternum in the midline. The second rib joins the sternum at this prominent landmark.

Other ribs may be identified by counting down from the second rib. The intercostal spaces are referred to in terms of the rib immediately above the intercostal space; for example, the fifth intercostal space is directly below the fifth rib.

Locating ribs on the posterior surface of the thorax is more difficult. The first step is to identify the spinous process. This is accomplished by finding the seventh cervical vertebra (*vertebra prominens*), which is the most prominent spinous process. When the neck is slightly flexed, the seventh cervical spinous process stands out. Other vertebrae are then identified by counting downward.

Vertical Reference Points

Several imaginary lines are used as vertical referents or landmarks to identify the location of thoracic findings. The *midsternal line* passes through the center of the sternum. The *midclavicular line* is an imaginary line that descends from the middle of the clavicle. The *point of maximal impulse* of the heart normally lies along this line on the left thorax.

When the arm is abducted from the body at 90°, imaginary vertical lines may be drawn from the anterior axillary fold, from the middle of the axilla, and from the posterior axillary fold. These lines are called, respectively, the *anterior axillary line*, the *midaxillary line*, and the *posterior axillary line*. A line drawn vertically through the superior and inferior poles of the scapula is called the *scapular line*, and a line drawn down the center of the vertebral column is called the *vertebral line*. Using these landmarks, for example, the examiner communicates findings by referring to an area of dullness extending from the vertebral to the scapular line between the seventh and tenth ribs on the right.

Lobes of the Lungs

The lobes of the lung may be mapped on the surface of the chest wall in the following manner. The line between the upper and lower lobes on the left begins at the fourth thoracic spinous process posteriorly, proceeds around to cross the fifth rib in the midaxillary line, and meets the sixth rib at the sternum. This line on the right divides the right middle lobe from the right lower lobe. The line dividing the right upper lobe from the middle lobe is an incomplete one that begins at the fifth rib in the midaxillary line, where it intersects the line between the upper and lower lobes and traverses horizontally to the sternum. Thus, the upper lobes are dominant on the anterior surface of the thorax and the lower lobes are dominant on the posterior surface. There is no presentation of the middle lobe on the posterior surface of the chest.

Anterior thorax

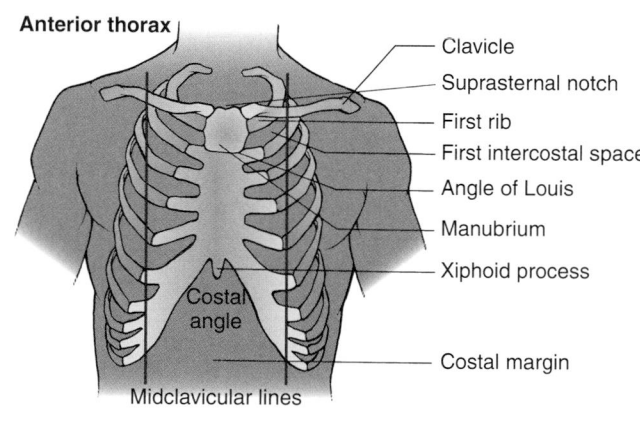

- Clavicle
- Suprasternal notch
- First rib
- First intercostal space
- Angle of Louis
- Manubrium
- Xiphoid process
- Costal angle
- Costal margin
- Midclavicular lines

Posterior thorax

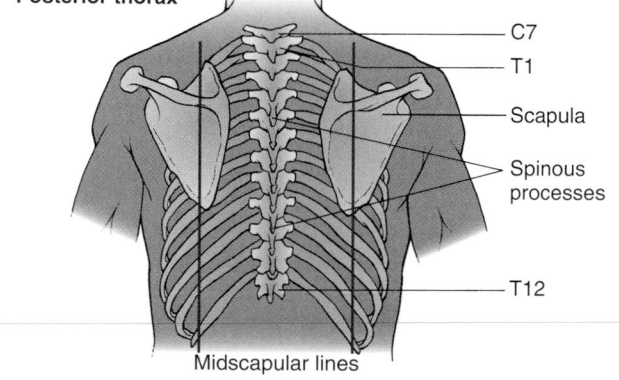

- C7
- T1
- Scapula
- Spinous processes
- T12
- Midscapular lines

Anterior view

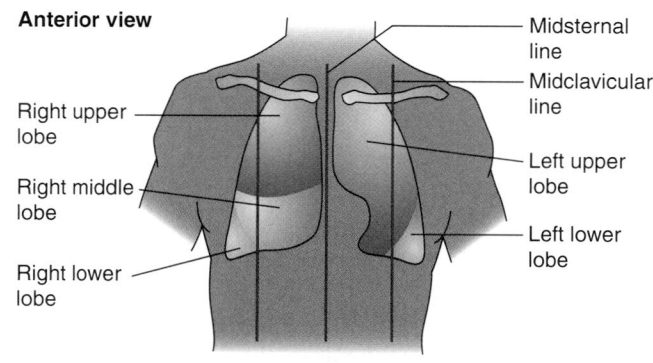

- Midsternal line
- Midclavicular line
- Right upper lobe
- Right middle lobe
- Right lower lobe
- Left upper lobe
- Left lower lobe

Lateral view

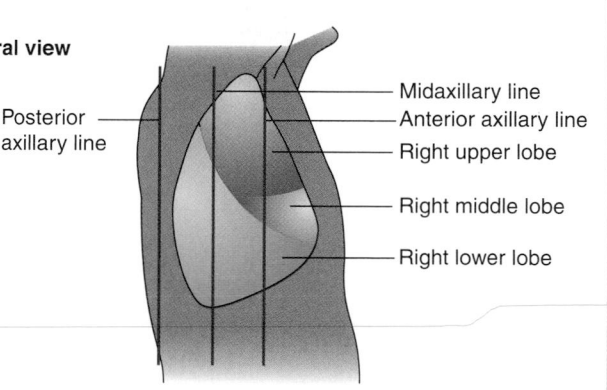

- Posterior axillary line
- Midaxillary line
- Anterior axillary line
- Right upper lobe
- Right middle lobe
- Right lower lobe

severe pain, and rib fracture. Shallow, irregular breathing is referred to as hypoventilation.

An increase in depth of respirations is called hyperpnea. An increase in both rate and depth that results in a lowered arterial PCO_2 level is referred to as hyperventilation. With rapid breathing, inspiration and expiration are nearly equal in duration. Hyperventilation that is marked by an increase in rate and depth, associated with severe acidosis of diabetic or renal origin, is called Kussmaul's respiration.

Apnea describes varying periods of cessation of breathing. If sustained, apnea is life-threatening.

Cheyne-Stokes respiration is characterized by alternating episodes of apnea (cessation of breathing) and periods of deep breathing. Deep respirations become increasingly shallow, followed by apnea that may last approximately 20 seconds. The cycle repeats after each apneic period. The duration of the period of apnea may vary and may progressively lengthen; therefore, it is timed and reported. Cheyne-Stokes respiration is usually associated with heart failure and damage to the respiratory center (drug-induced, tumor, trauma).

Biot's respirations, or cluster breathing, are cycles of breaths that vary in depth and have varying periods of apnea. Biot's respirations are seen with some central nervous system disorders.

Certain patterns of respiration are characteristic of specific disease states. Respiratory rhythms and their deviation from normal are important observations that the nurse reports and documents. The rate and depth of different patterns of respiration are presented in Figure 21-10.

In thin people, it is quite normal to note a slight retraction of the intercostal spaces during quiet breathing. Bulging during expiration implies obstruction of expiratory airflow, as in emphysema. Marked retraction on inspiration, particularly if asymmetric, implies blockage of a branch of the respiratory tree. Asymmetric bulging of the intercostal spaces, on one side or the other, is created by an increase in pressure within the hemithorax. This may be a result of air trapped under pressure within the pleural cavity where it does not normally appear (pneumothorax) or the pressure of fluid within the pleural space (pleural effusion).

Thoracic Palpation

The nurse palpates the thorax for tenderness, masses, lesions, respiratory excursion, and vocal fremitus. If the patient has reported an area of pain or if lesions are apparent, the nurse performs direct palpation with the fingertips (for skin lesions and subcutaneous masses) or with the ball of the hand (for deeper masses or generalized flank or rib discomfort).

RESPIRATORY EXCURSION

Respiratory excursion is an estimation of thoracic expansion and may disclose significant information about thoracic movement during breathing. The nurse assesses the patient for range and symmetry of excursion. The patient is instructed to inhale deeply while the movement of the nurse's thumbs (placed along the costal margin on the anterior chest wall) during inspiration and expiration is observed. This movement is normally symmetric.

Posterior assessment is performed by placing the thumbs adjacent to the spinal column at the level of the tenth rib (Fig. 21-11). The hands lightly grasp the lateral rib cage. Sliding the thumbs medially about 2.5 cm (1 inch) raises a small skinfold between the thumbs. The patient is instructed to take a full inspiration and to exhale fully. The nurse observes for normal flattening of the skinfold and feels the symmetric movement of the thorax.

	Definition	Graphic Representation
Eupnea	Normal, breathing at 12-18 breaths/minute	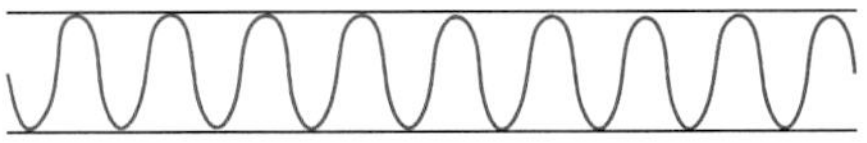
Bradypnea	Slower than normal rate (< 10 breaths/minute), with normal depth and regular rhythm	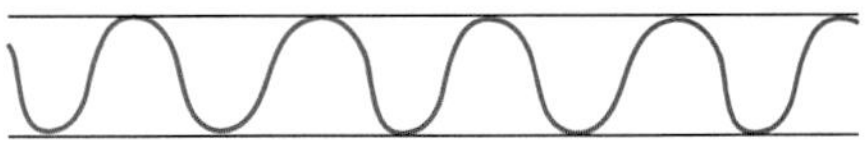
Tachypnea	Rapid, shallow breathing > 24 breaths/minute	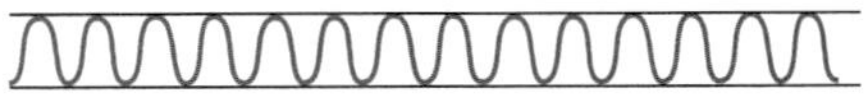
Hypoventilation	Shallow, irregular breathing	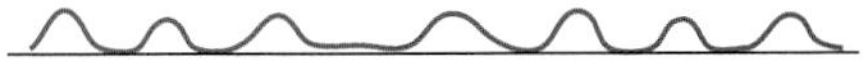
Hyperventilation	Increased rate and depth of breathing (called Kussmaul's respiration if caused by diabetic ketoacidosis)	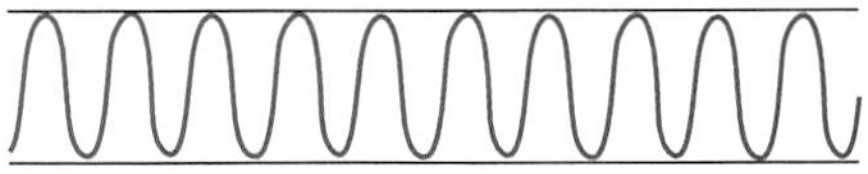
Apnea	Period of cessation of breathing. Time duration varies; apnea may occur briefly during other breathing disorders, such as with sleep apnea. Life threatening if sustained.	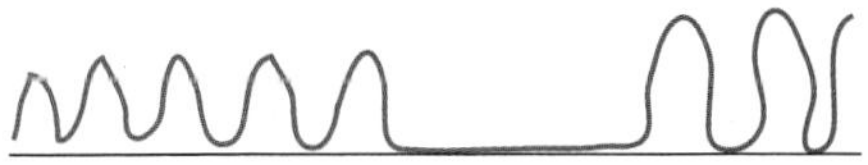
Cheyne-Stokes	Regular cycle where the rate and depth of breathing increase, then decrease until apnea (usually about 20 seconds) occurs.	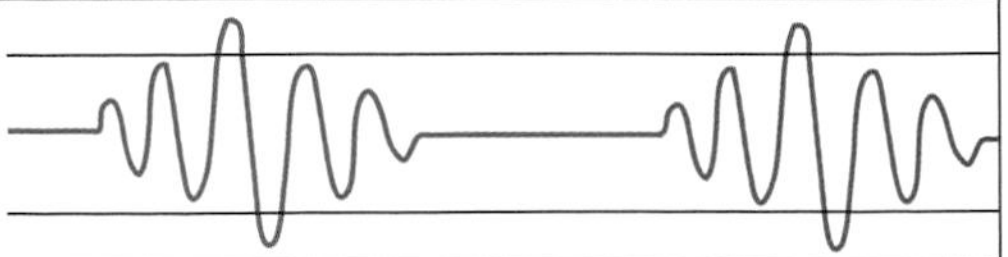
Biot's respiration	Periods of normal breathing (3-4 breaths) followed by a varying period of apnea (usually 10 seconds to 1 minute).	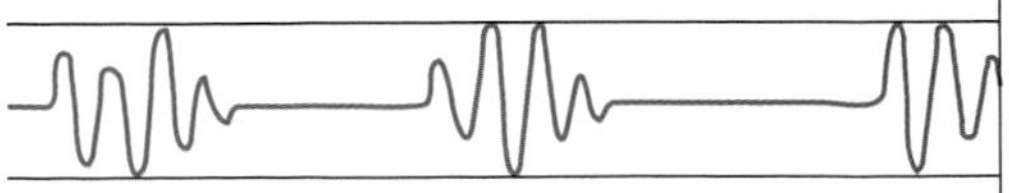

FIGURE 21-10 Graphic representation of different rates and depths of respiration.

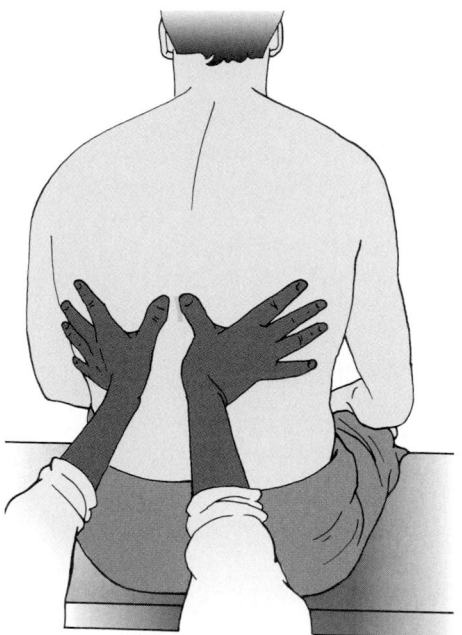

FIGURE 21-11 Method for assessing posterior respiratory excursion. Place both hands posteriorly at the level of T9 or T10. Slide hands medially to pinch a small amount of skin between your thumbs. Observe for symmetry.

Decreased chest excursion may be due to chronic fibrotic disease. Asymmetric excursion may be due to splinting secondary to pleurisy, fractured ribs, trauma, or unilateral bronchial obstruction.

TACTILE FREMITUS

Sound generated by the larynx travels distally along the bronchial tree to set the chest wall in resonant motion. This is especially true of consonant sounds. The detection of the resulting vibration on the chest wall by touch is called tactile fremitus.

Normal fremitus is widely varied. It is influenced by the thickness of the chest wall, especially if that thickness is muscular. However, the increase in subcutaneous tissue associated with obesity may also affect fremitus. Lower-pitched sounds travel better through the normal lung and produce greater vibration of the chest wall. Thus, fremitus is more pronounced in men than in women because of the deeper male voice. Normally, fremitus is most pronounced where the large bronchi are closest to the chest wall and least palpable over the distant lung fields. Therefore, it is most palpable in the upper thorax, anteriorly and posteriorly.

The patient is asked to repeat "ninety-nine" or "one, two, three," or "eee, eee, eee" as the nurse's hands move down the patient's thorax. The vibrations are detected with the palmar surfaces of the fingers and hands, or the ulnar aspect of the extended hands, on the thorax. The hand or hands are moved in sequence down the thorax. Corresponding areas of the thorax are compared (Fig. 21-12). Bony areas are not tested.

Air does not conduct sound well but a solid substance such as tissue does, provided that it has elasticity and is not compressed. Thus, an increase in solid tissue per unit volume of lung will enhance fremitus; an increase in air per unit volume of lung will impede sound. Patients with emphysema, which results in the rupture of alveoli and trapping of air, exhibit almost no tactile fremitus. A patient with consolidation of a lobe of the lung from pneumonia will have increased tactile fremitus over that lobe. Air in the pleural space will not conduct sound.

Thoracic Percussion

Percussion sets the chest wall and underlying structures in motion, producing audible and tactile vibrations. The nurse uses percussion to determine whether underlying tissues are filled with air, fluid, or solid material. Percussion also is used to estimate the size and location of certain structures within the thorax (eg, diaphragm, heart, liver).

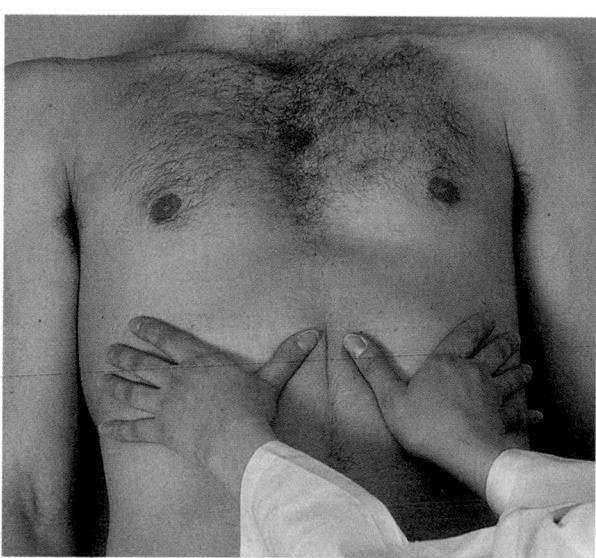
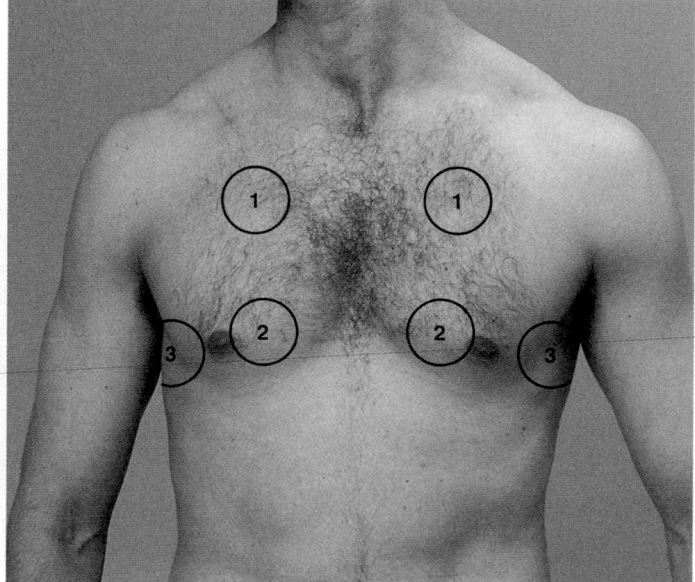

FIGURE 21-12 When palpating for tactile fremitus (*left*), the nurse places the ball or ulnar surface of the hands on the chest area being assessed. The palpation sequence is at right. From Bickley L. S. (2003). *Bates' guide to physical examination and history taking* (8th ed.). Philadelphia: Lippincott Williams & Wilkins.

Percussion usually begins with the posterior thorax. Ideally, the patient is in a sitting position with the head flexed forward and the arms crossed on the lap. This position separates the scapulae widely and exposes more lung area for assessment. The nurse percusses across each shoulder top, locating the 5-cm width of resonance overlying the lung apices (Fig. 21-13). Then the nurse proceeds down the posterior thorax, percussing symmetric areas at 5- to 6-cm (2- to 2.5-inch) intervals. The middle finger is positioned parallel to the ribs in the intercostal space; the finger is placed firmly against the chest wall before striking it with the middle finger of the opposite hand. Bony structures (scapulae or ribs) are not percussed.

Percussion over the anterior chest is performed with the patient in an upright position with shoulders arched backward and arms at the side. The nurse begins in the supraclavicular area and proceeds downward, from one intercostal space to the next. In the female patient, it may be necessary to displace the breasts for an adequate examination. Dullness noted to the left of the sternum between the third and fifth intercostal spaces is a normal finding because it is the location of the heart. Similarly, there is a normal span of liver dullness in the right thorax from the fifth intercostal space to the right costal margin at the midclavicular line.

The anterior and lateral thorax is examined with the patient in a supine position. If the patient cannot sit up, percussion of the posterior thorax is performed with the patient positioned on the side.

Dullness over the lung occurs when air-filled lung tissue is replaced by fluid or solid tissue. Table 21-3 reviews percussion sounds and their characteristics.

DIAPHRAGMATIC EXCURSION

The normal resonance of the lung stops at the diaphragm. The position of the diaphragm is different during inspiration than during expiration.

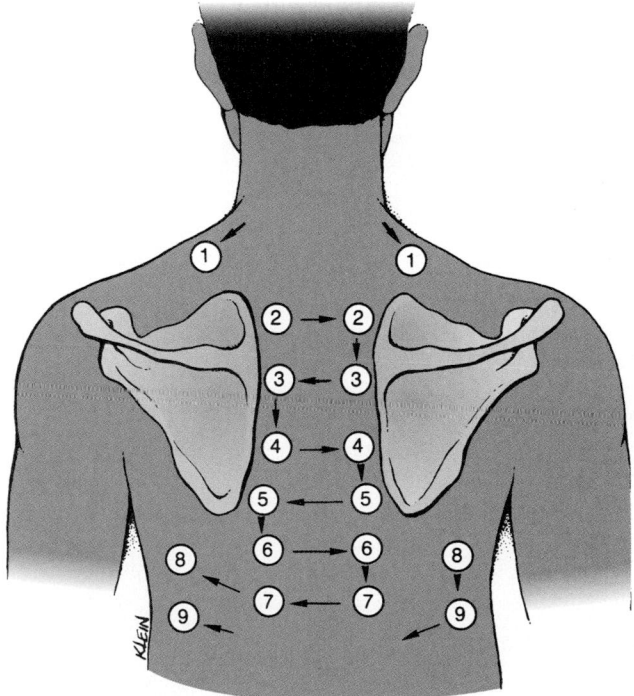

FIGURE 21-13 Percussion of the posterior thorax. With the patient in a sitting position, symmetric areas of the lungs are percussed at 5-cm intervals. This progression starts at the apex of each lung and concludes with percussion of each lateral chest wall.

To assess the position and motion of the diaphragm, the nurse instructs the patient to take a deep breath and hold it while the maximal descent of the diaphragm is percussed. The point at which the percussion note at the midscapular line changes from resonance to dullness is marked with a pen. The patient is then instructed to exhale fully and hold it while the nurse again percusses downward to the dullness of the diaphragm. This point is also marked. The distance between the two markings indicates the range of motion of the diaphragm.

Maximal excursion of the diaphragm may be as much as 8 to 10 cm (3 to 4 inches) in healthy, tall young men, but for most people it is usually 5 to 7 cm (2 to 2.75 inches). Normally, the diaphragm is about 2 cm (0.75 inches) higher on the right because of the position of the heart and the liver above and below the left and right segments of the diaphragm, respectively. Decreased diaphragmatic excursion may occur with pleural effusion and emphysema. An increase in intra-abdominal pressure, as in pregnancy or ascites, may account for a diaphragm that is positioned high in the thorax.

Thoracic Auscultation

Auscultation is useful in assessing the flow of air through the bronchial tree and in evaluating the presence of fluid or solid obstruction in the lung structures. The nurse auscultates for normal breath sounds, adventitious sounds, and voice sounds.

Examination includes auscultation of the anterior, posterior, and lateral thorax and is performed as follows. The nurse places the diaphragm of the stethoscope firmly against the chest wall as the patient breathes slowly and deeply through the mouth. Corresponding areas of the chest are auscultated in a systematic fashion from the apices to the bases and along midaxillary lines. The sequence of auscultation and the positioning of the patient are similar to those used for percussion. It often is necessary to listen to two full inspirations and expirations at each anatomic location for valid interpretation of the sound heard. Repeated deep breaths may result in symptoms of hyperventilation (eg, light-headedness); this is avoided by having the patient rest and breathe normally periodically during the examination.

BREATH SOUNDS

Normal breath sounds are distinguished by their location over a specific area of the lung and are identified as vesicular, bronchovesicular, and bronchial (tubular) breath sounds (Table 21-4).

The location, quality, and intensity of breath sounds are determined during auscultation. When airflow is decreased by bronchial obstruction (atelectasis) or when fluid (pleural effusion) or tissue (obesity) separates the air passages from the stethoscope, breath sounds are diminished or absent. For example, the breath sounds of the patient with emphysema are faint or often completely inaudible. When heard, the expiratory phase is prolonged. Bronchial and bronchovesicular sounds that are audible anywhere except over the main bronchus in the lungs signify pathology, usually indicating consolidation in the lung (eg, pneumonia, heart failure). This finding requires further evaluation.

ADVENTITIOUS SOUNDS

An abnormal condition that affects the bronchial tree and alveoli may produce adventitious (additional) sounds. Adventitious sounds are divided into two categories: discrete, noncontinuous sounds (crackles) and continuous musical sounds (wheezes). The duration of the sound is the important distinction to make in identifying the sound as noncontinuous or continuous. Pleural friction rubs are specific examples of crackles (Table 21-5).

Table 21-3 • Characteristics of Percussion Sounds

SOUND	RELATIVE INTENSITY	RELATIVE PITCH	RELATIVE DURATION	LOCATION EXAMPLE	EXAMPLES
Flatness	Soft	High	Short	Thigh	Large pleural effusion
Dullness	Medium	Medium	Medium	Liver	Lobar pneumonia
Resonance	Loud	Low	Long	Normal lung	Simple chronic bronchitis
Hyperresonance	Very loud	Lower	Longer	None normally	Emphysema, pneumothorax
Tympany	Loud	High*	*	Gastric air bubble or puffed-out cheek	Large pneumothorax

*Distinguished mainly by its musical timbre

Crackles (formerly referred to as rales) are discrete, noncontinuous sounds that result from delayed reopening of deflated airways. Crackles may or may not be cleared by coughing. Crackles reflect underlying inflammation or congestion and are often present in such conditions as pneumonia, bronchitis, heart failure, bronchiectasis, and pulmonary fibrosis.

Friction rubs result from inflammation of the pleural surfaces that induces a crackling, grating sound usually heard in inspiration and expiration. The sound can be enhanced by applying pressure to the chest wall with the diaphragm of the stethoscope. The sound is imitated by rubbing the thumb and index finger together near the ear. A friction rub is best heard over the lower lateral anterior surface of the thorax.

Wheezes are associated with bronchial wall oscillation and changes in airway diameter. Wheezes are commonly heard in patients with asthma, chronic bronchitis, and bronchiectasis.

VOICE SOUNDS
The sound heard through the stethoscope as the patient speaks is known as vocal resonance. The vibrations produced in the larynx are transmitted to the chest wall as they pass through the bronchi and alveolar tissue. During the process, the sounds are diminished in intensity and altered so that syllables are not distinguishable. Voice sounds are usually assessed by having the patient repeat "ninety-nine" or "eee" while the nurse listens with the stethoscope in corresponding areas of the chest from the apices to the bases.

Bronchophony describes vocal resonance that is more intense and clearer than normal. Egophony describes voice sounds that are distorted. It is best appreciated by having the patient repeat the letter E. The distortion produced by consolidation transforms the sound into a clearly heard A rather than E. Bronchophony and egophony have precisely the same significance as bronchial breathing with an increase in tactile fremitus. When an abnormality is detected, it should be evident using more than one assessment method. A change in tactile fremitus is more subtle and can be missed, but bronchial breathing and bronchophony can be noted loudly and clearly.

Whispered pectoriloquy is a very subtle finding, heard only in the presence of rather dense consolidation of the lungs. Transmission of high-frequency components of sound is so enhanced by the consolidated tissue that even whispered words are heard, a circumstance not noted in normal physiology. The significance is the same as that of bronchophony.

Table 21-4 • Breath Sounds

	DURATION OF SOUNDS	INTENSITY OF EXPIRATORY SOUND	PITCH OF EXPIRATORY SOUND	LOCATIONS WHERE HEARD NORMALLY
Vesicular*	Inspiratory sounds last longer than expiratory ones.	Soft	Relatively low	Entire lung field except over the upper sternum and between the scapulae
Broncho-vesicular	Inspiratory and expiratory sounds are about equal.	Intermediate	Intermediate	Often in the 1st and 2nd interspaces anteriorly and between the scapulae (over the main bronchus)
Bronchial	Expiratory sounds last longer than inspiratory ones.	Loud	Relatively high	Over the manubrium, if heard at all
Tracheal	Inspiratory and expiratory sounds are about equal.	Very loud	Relatively high	Over the trachea in the neck

*The thickness of the bars indicates intensity of breath sounds; the steeper their incline, the higher the pitch of the sounds.

Table 21-5 • Abnormal (Adventitious) Breath Sounds

BREATH SOUND	DESCRIPTION	ETIOLOGY
Crackles		
Crackles in general	Soft, high-pitched, discontinuous popping sounds that occur during inspiration	Secondary to fluid in the airways or alveoli or to opening of collapsed alveoli
Coarse crackles	Discontinuous popping sounds heard in early inspiration; harsh, moist sound originating in the large bronchi	Associated with obstructive pulmonary disease
Fine crackles	Discontinuous popping sounds heard in late inspiration; sounds like hair rubbing together; originates in the alveoli	Associated with interstitial pneumonia, restrictive pulmonary disease (eg, fibrosis). Fine crackles in early inspiration are associated with bronchitis or pneumonia.
Wheezes		
Sonorous wheezes (rhonchi)	Deep, low-pitched rumbling sounds heard primarily during expiration; caused by air moving through narrowed tracheobronchial passages	Secretions or tumor
Sibilant wheezes	Continuous, musical, high-pitched, whistle-like sounds heard during inspiration and expiration caused by air passing through narrowed or partially obstructed airways; may clear with coughing	Bronchospasm, asthma, and buildup of secretions
Friction rubs		
Pleural friction rub	Harsh, crackling sound, like two pieces of leather being rubbed together. Heard during inspiration alone or during both inspiration and expiration. May subside when patient holds breath. Coughing will not clear sound.	Secondary to inflammation and loss of lubricating pleural fluid

The physical findings for the most common respiratory diseases are summarized in Table 21-6.

PHYSICAL ASSESSMENT OF BREATHING ABILITY IN THE ACUTELY ILL PATIENT

Tests of the patient's breathing ability are easily performed at the bedside by measuring the respiratory rate (see the previous section "Breathing Patterns and Respiratory Rates"), tidal volume, minute ventilation, vital capacity, inspiratory force, and compliance. These tests are particularly important for patients at risk for developing pulmonary complications, including those who have undergone chest or abdominal surgery, have had prolonged anesthesia, have preexisting pulmonary disease, or are elderly. These tests are also used routinely for mechanically ventilated patients.

Patients whose chest expansion is limited by external restrictions such as obesity or abdominal distention and who cannot breathe deeply because of postoperative pain or sedation will inhale and exhale a low volume of air (referred to as low tidal volumes). Prolonged hypoventilation at low tidal volumes can produce alveolar collapse or atelectasis. The amount of air remaining in the lungs after a normal expiration (functional residual capacity) falls, the ability of the lungs to expand (compliance) is reduced, and the patient must breathe faster to maintain the same degree of tissue oxygenation. These events can be exaggerated in patients who have preexisting pulmonary diseases and in elderly patients whose airways are less compliant, because the small airways may collapse during expiration.

NURSING ALERT One should not rely only on visual inspection of the rate and depth of a patient's respiratory excursions to determine the adequacy of ventilation. Respiratory excursions may appear normal or exaggerated due to an increased work of breathing, but the patient may actually be moving only enough air to ventilate the dead space. If there is any question regarding adequacy of ventilation, auscultation and/or pulse oximetry should be used for additional assessment of respiratory status.

Tidal Volume

The volume of each breath is referred to as the tidal volume (see Table 21-1 to review lung capacities and volumes). A spirometer is an instrument that can be used at the bedside to measure volumes. If the patient is breathing through an endotracheal tube or tracheostomy, the spirometer is directly attached to it and the exhaled volume is obtained from the reading on the gauge. In other patients, the spirometer is attached to a facemask or a mouthpiece positioned so that it is airtight, and the exhaled volume is measured.

The tidal volume may vary from breath to breath. To make the measurement reliable, it is important to measure the volumes of several breaths and to note the range of tidal volumes, together with the average tidal volume.

Minute Ventilation

Respiratory rates and tidal volume alone are unreliable indicators of adequate ventilation because both can vary widely from breath to breath. Together, however, the tidal volume and respiratory

Table 21-6 • Assessment Findings in Common Respiratory Problems

PROBLEM	TACTILE FREMITUS	PERCUSSION	AUSCULTATION
Consolidation (eg, pneumonia)	Increased	Dull	Bronchial breath sounds, crackles, bronchophony, egophony, whispered pectoriloquy
Bronchitis	Normal	Resonant	Normal to decreased breath sounds, wheezes
Emphysema	Decreased	Hyperresonant	Decreased intensity of breath sounds, usually with prolonged expiration
Asthma (severe attack)	Normal to decreased	Resonant to hyperresonant	Wheezes
Pulmonary edema	Normal	Resonant	Crackles at lung bases, possibly wheezes
Pleural effusion	Absent	Dull to flat	Decreased to absent breath sounds, bronchial breath sounds and bronchophony, egophony, and whispered pectoriloquy above the effusion over the area of compressed lung
Pneumothorax	Decreased	Hyperresonant	Absent breath sounds
Atelectasis	Absent	Flat	Decreased to absent breath sounds

rate are important because the minute ventilation, which is useful in detecting respiratory failure, can be determined from them. Minute ventilation is the volume of air expired per minute. It is equal to the product of the tidal volume and the respiratory rate or frequency. In practice, the minute ventilation is not calculated but is measured directly using a spirometer.

Minute ventilation may be decreased by a variety of conditions that result in hypoventilation. When the minute ventilation falls, alveolar ventilation in the lungs also decreases, and the $PaCO_2$ increases. Risk factors for hypoventilation are listed in Chart 21-8.

Vital Capacity

Vital capacity is measured by having the patient take in a maximal breath and exhale fully through a spirometer. The normal value depends on the patient's age, gender, body build, and weight.

> **NURSING ALERT** Most patients can generate a vital capacity twice the volume they normally breathe in and out (tidal volume). If the vital capacity is less than 10 mL/kg, the patient will be unable to sustain spontaneous ventilation and will require respiratory assistance.

When the vital capacity is exhaled at a maximal flow rate, the forced vital capacity is measured. Most patients can exhale at least 80% of their vital capacity in 1 second (forced expiratory volume in 1 second, or FEV_1) and almost all of it in 3 seconds (FEV_3). A reduction in FEV_1 suggests abnormal pulmonary air flow. If the patient's FEV_1 and forced vital capacity are proportionately reduced, maximal lung expansion is restricted in some way. If the reduction in FEV_1 greatly exceeds the reduction in forced vital capacity, the patient may have some degree of airway obstruction.

Inspiratory Force

Inspiratory force evaluates the effort the patient is making during inspiration. It does not require patient cooperation and thus is

useful in the unconscious patient. The equipment needed for this measurement includes a manometer that measures negative pressure and adapters that are connected to an anesthesia mask or a cuffed endotracheal tube. The manometer is attached and the airway is completely occluded for 10 to 20 seconds while the inspiratory efforts of the patient are registered on the manometer. The normal inspiratory pressure is about 100 cm H_2O. If the negative pressure registered after 15 seconds of occluding the airway is less than about 25 cm H_2O, mechanical ventilation is usually required because the patient lacks sufficient muscle strength for deep breathing or effective coughing.

Diagnostic Evaluation

A wide range of diagnostic studies, described on the following pages, may be performed in patients with respiratory conditions.

PULMONARY FUNCTION TESTS

Pulmonary function tests (PFTs) are routinely used in patients with chronic respiratory disorders. They are performed to assess respiratory function and to determine the extent of dysfunction. Such tests include measurements of lung volumes, ventilatory

> **Chart 21-8**
> ### Risk Factors for Hypoventilation
>
> - Limited neurologic impulses transmitted from the brain to the respiratory muscles, as in spinal cord trauma, cerebrovascular accidents, tumors, myasthenia gravis, Guillain-Barré syndrome, polio, and drug overdose
> - Depressed respiratory centers in the medulla, as with anesthesia and drug overdose
> - Limited thoracic movement (kyphoscoliosis), limited lung movement (pleural effusion, pneumothorax), or reduced functional lung tissue (chronic pulmonary diseases, severe pulmonary edema)

function, and the mechanics of breathing, diffusion, and gas exchange (Table 21-7).

PFTs are useful in following the course of a patient with an established respiratory disease and assessing the response to therapy. They are useful as screening tests in potentially hazardous industries, such as coal mining and those that involve exposure to asbestos and other noxious fumes, dusts, or gases. They are useful for screening patients scheduled for thoracic and upper abdominal surgery, and symptomatic patients with a history suggesting high risk.

PFTs generally are performed by a technician using a spirometer that has a volume-collecting device attached to a recorder that demonstrates volume and time simultaneously. A number of tests are carried out because no single measurement provides a complete picture of pulmonary function. The most frequently used PFTs are described in Table 21-7. Technology is available that allows for more complex assessment of pulmonary function. Methods include exercise tidal flow-volume loops, negative expiratory pressure, nitric oxide, and forced oscillation. These assessment methods allow for detailed evaluation of expiratory flow limitations and airway inflammation (Johnson, Beck, Zeballos & Weisman, 1999).

PFT results are interpreted on the basis of the degree of deviation from normal, taking into consideration the patient's height, weight, age, and gender. Because there is a wide range of normal values, PFTs may not detect early localized changes. The patient with respiratory symptoms (dyspnea, wheezing, cough, sputum production) usually undergoes a complete diagnostic evaluation, even though the results of PFTs are "normal." Trends of results provide information about disease progression as well as the patient's response to therapy.

Patients with respiratory disorders may be taught how to measure their peak flow rate (reflects maximal expiratory flow) at home using a spirometer. This allows them to monitor the progress of therapy, to alter medications and other interventions as needed based on caregiver guidelines, or to notify the health care provider if there is inadequate response to their own interventions. Home care teaching instructions are described in Chapter 24, which discusses asthma.

ARTERIAL BLOOD GAS STUDIES

Measurements of blood pH and of arterial oxygen and carbon dioxide tensions are obtained when managing patients with respiratory problems and in adjusting oxygen therapy as needed. The arterial oxygen tension (PaO_2) indicates the degree of oxygenation of the blood, and the arterial carbon dioxide tension ($PaCO_2$) indicates the adequacy of alveolar ventilation. Arterial blood gas studies aid in assessing the ability of the lungs to provide adequate oxygen and remove carbon dioxide and the ability of the kidneys to reabsorb or excrete bicarbonate ions to maintain normal body pH. Serial blood gas analysis also is a sensitive indicator of whether the lung has been damaged after chest trauma. Arterial blood gas levels are obtained through an arterial puncture at the radial, brachial, or femoral artery or through an indwelling arterial catheter. Arterial blood gas levels are discussed in detail in Chapter 14.

PULSE OXIMETRY

Pulse oximetry is a noninvasive method of continuously monitoring the oxygen saturation of hemoglobin (SpO_2 or SaO_2). Although pulse oximetry does not replace arterial blood gas measurement, it is an effective tool to monitor for subtle or sudden changes in oxygen saturation. It is used in all settings where oxygen saturation monitoring is needed, such as the home, clinics, ambulatory surgical settings, and hospitals.

A probe or sensor is attached to the fingertip (Fig. 21-14), forehead, earlobe, or bridge of the nose. The sensor detects changes in oxygen saturation levels by monitoring light signals generated by the oximeter and reflected by blood pulsing through the tissue at the probe. Normal SpO_2 values are 95% to 100%. Values less than 85% indicate that the tissues are not receiving enough oxygen, and the patient needs further evaluation. SpO_2 values obtained by pulse oximetry are unreliable in cardiac arrest and shock, when dyes (ie, methylene blue) or vasoconstrictor medications have been used, or when the patient has severe anemia or a high carbon monoxide level.

Table 21-7 • Pulmonary Function Tests

TERM USED	SYMBOL	DESCRIPTION	REMARKS
Forced vital capacity	FVC	Vital capacity performed with a maximally forced expiratory effort	Forced vital capacity is often reduced in COPD because of air trapping.
Forced expiratory volume (qualified by subscript indicating the time intervals in seconds)	FEV_t, usually FEV_1	Volume of air exhaled in the specified time during the performance of forced vital capacity; FEV_1 is volume exhaled in 1 second	A valuable clue to the severity of the expiratory airway obstruction
Ratio of timed forced expiratory volume to forced vital capacity	$FEV_t/FVC\%$, usually $FEV_1/FVC\%$	FEV_t expressed as a percentage of the forced vital capacity	Another way of expressing the presence or absence of airway obstruction
Forced expiratory flow	$FEF_{200-1200}$	Mean forced expiratory flow between 200 and 1,200 mL of the FVC	An indicator of large airway obstruction
Forced midexpiratory flow	$FEF_{25\%-75\%}$	Mean forced expiratory flow during the middle half of the FVC	Slowed in small airway obstruction
Forced end expiratory flow	$FEF_{75\%-85\%}$	Mean forced expiratory flow during the terminal portion of the FVC	Slowed in obstruction of smallest airways
Maximal voluntary ventilation	MVV	Volume of air expired in a specified period (12 seconds) during repetitive maximal effort	An important factor in exercise tolerance

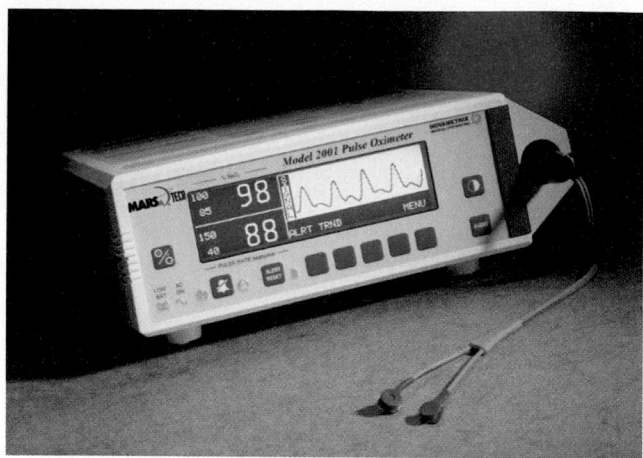

FIGURE 21-14 Measuring blood oxygenation with pulse oximetry reduces the need for invasive procedures, such as drawing blood for analysis of oxygen levels. After the pulse oximeter sensor slips easily over a patient's finger, the oxygen saturation level appears on the monitor. The oximeter is portable and ideal for home use. Courtesy Novametrix Medical Systems, Inc.

CULTURES

Throat cultures may be performed to identify organisms responsible for pharyngitis. Throat culture may also assist in identifying organisms responsible for infection of the lower respiratory tract. Nasal swabs also may be performed for the same purpose.

SPUTUM STUDIES

Sputum is obtained for analysis to identify pathogenic organisms and to determine whether malignant cells are present. It also may be used to assess for hypersensitivity states (in which there is an increase in eosinophils). Periodic sputum examinations may be necessary for patients receiving antibiotics, corticosteroids, and immunosuppressive medications for prolonged periods because these agents are associated with opportunistic infections. In general, sputum cultures are used in diagnosis, for drug sensitivity testing, and to guide treatment.

Expectoration is the usual method for collecting a sputum specimen. The patient is instructed to clear the nose and throat and rinse the mouth to decrease contamination of the sputum. After taking a few deep breaths, the patient coughs (rather than spits), using the diaphragm, and expectorates into a sterile container.

If the sputum cannot be raised spontaneously, the patient often can be induced to cough deeply by breathing an irritating aerosol of supersaturated saline, propylene glycol, or some other agent delivered with an ultrasonic nebulizer. Other methods of collecting sputum specimens include endotracheal aspiration, bronchoscopic removal, bronchial brushing, transtracheal aspiration, and gastric aspiration—usually for tuberculosis organisms (see Chap. 23). Generally, the deepest specimens (those from the base of the lungs) are obtained in the early morning after they have accumulated overnight.

The specimen is delivered to the laboratory within 2 hours by the patient or nurse. Allowing the specimen to stand for several hours in a warm room results in the overgrowth of contaminant organisms and may make it difficult to identify the organisms (especially *Mycobacterium tuberculosis*). The home care nurse may assist patients who need help obtaining the sample or who cannot deliver the specimen to the laboratory in a timely fashion.

IMAGING STUDIES

Imaging studies, including x-rays, computed tomography (CT) scans, magnetic resonance imaging (MRI), contrast studies, and radioisotope diagnostic scans may be part of any diagnostic workup, ranging from a determination of the extent of infection in sinusitis to tumor growth in cancer.

Chest X-Ray

Normal pulmonary tissue is radiolucent; therefore, densities produced by fluid, tumors, foreign bodies, and other pathologic conditions can be detected by x-ray examination. A chest x-ray may reveal an extensive pathologic process in the lungs in the absence of symptoms. The routine chest x-ray consists of two views—the posteroanterior projection and the lateral projection. Chest x-rays are usually taken after full inspiration (a deep breath) because the lungs are best visualized when they are well aerated. Also, the diaphragm is at its lowest level and the largest expanse of lung is visible. If taken on expiration, x-ray films may accentuate an otherwise unnoticed pneumothorax or obstruction of a major artery.

Computed Tomography

CT is an imaging method in which the lungs are scanned in successive layers by a narrow-beam x-ray. The images produced provide a cross-sectional view of the chest. Whereas a chest x-ray shows major contrast between body densities, such as bones, soft tissues, and air, CT scans can distinguish fine tissue density. CT may be used to define pulmonary nodules and small tumors adjacent to pleural surfaces that are not visible on routine chest x-ray, and to demonstrate mediastinal abnormalities and hilar adenopathy, which are difficult to visualize with other techniques. Contrast agents are useful when evaluating the mediastinum and its contents.

Magnetic Resonance Imaging

MRIs are similar to CT scans except that magnetic fields and radiofrequency signals are used instead of a narrow-beam x-ray. MRIs yield a much more detailed diagnostic image than CT scans. MRI is used to characterize pulmonary nodules, stage bronchogenic carcinoma (assessment of chest wall invasion), and evaluate inflammatory activity in interstitial lung disease, acute pulmonary embolism, and chronic thrombolytic pulmonary hypertension (Kauczor & Kreitner, 2000).

Fluoroscopic Studies

Fluoroscopy is used to assist with invasive procedures, such as a chest needle biopsy or transbronchial biopsy, performed to identify lesions. It also may be used to study the movement of the chest wall, mediastinum, heart, and diaphragm, to detect diaphragm paralysis, and to locate lung masses.

Pulmonary Angiography

Pulmonary angiography is most commonly used to investigate thromboembolic disease of the lungs, such as pulmonary emboli and congenital abnormalities of the pulmonary vascular tree. It involves the rapid injection of a radiopaque agent into the vasculature of the lungs for radiographic study of the pulmonary vessels.

It can be performed by injecting the radiopaque agent into a vein in one or both arms (simultaneously) or into the femoral vein, with a needle or catheter. The agent also can be injected into a catheter that has been inserted in the main pulmonary artery or its branches or into the great veins proximal to the pulmonary artery.

Radioisotope Diagnostic Procedures (Lung Scans)

Several types of lung scans—ventilation-perfusion scan, gallium scan, and positron emission tomography—are used to detect normal lung functioning, pulmonary vascular supply, and gas exchange.

A ventilation-perfusion lung scan is first performed by injecting a radioactive agent into a peripheral vein and then obtaining a scan of the chest to detect radiation. The isotope particles pass through the right side of the heart and are distributed into the lungs in amounts proportional to the regional blood flow, making it possible to trace and measure blood perfusion through the lung. This procedure is used clinically to measure the integrity of the pulmonary vessels relative to blood flow and to evaluate blood flow abnormalities, as seen in pulmonary emboli. The imaging time is 20 to 40 minutes, during which the patient will lie under the camera with a mask fitted over the nose and mouth. This is followed by the ventilation component of the scan. The patient takes a deep breath of a mixture of oxygen and radioactive gas, which diffuses throughout the lungs. A scan is performed to detect ventilation abnormalities in patients who have regional differences in ventilation. It may be helpful in the diagnosis of bronchitis, asthma, inflammatory fibrosis, pneumonia, emphysema, and lung cancer. Ventilation without perfusion is seen with pulmonary emboli.

A gallium scan is a radioisotope lung scan used to detect inflammatory conditions, abscesses, adhesions, and the presence, location, and size of tumors. It is used to stage bronchogenic cancer and record tumor regression after chemotherapy or radiation. Gallium is injected intravenously, and scans are taken at 6, 24, and/or 48 hours to evaluate gallium uptake by the pulmonary tissues.

Positron emission tomography (PET) is a radioisotope study with advanced diagnostic capabilities. It is used to evaluate lung nodules for malignancy. PET scans can detect and display metabolic changes in tissue, distinguish normal tissue from tissues that are diseased (such as in cancer), differentiate viable from dead or dying tissue, show regional blood flow, and determine the distribution and fate of medications in the body (Shuster, 1998). PET scans are more accurate in detecting malignancies than CT scans (Coleman, 1999; Graeber, Gupta & Murray, 1999) and have equivalent accuracy in detecting malignant nodules when compared to invasive procedures such as thoracoscopy (Lowe, Fletcher, Gobar et al., 1998).

ENDOSCOPIC PROCEDURES

Bronchoscopy

Bronchoscopy is the direct inspection and examination of the larynx, trachea, and bronchi through either a flexible fiberoptic bronchoscope or a rigid bronchoscope. The fiberoptic scope is used more frequently in current practice.

The purposes of diagnostic bronchoscopy are: (1) to examine tissues or collect secretions, (2) to determine the location and extent of the pathologic process and to obtain a tissue sample for diagnosis (by biting or cutting forceps, curettage, or brush biopsy), (3) to determine if a tumor can be resected surgically, and (4) to diagnose bleeding sites (source of hemoptysis).

Therapeutic bronchoscopy is used to: (1) remove foreign bodies from the tracheobronchial tree, (2) remove secretions obstructing the tracheobronchial tree when the patient cannot clear them, (3) treat postoperative atelectasis, and (4) destroy and excise lesions.

The fiberoptic bronchoscope is a thin, flexible bronchoscope that can be directed into the segmental bronchi (Fig. 21-15). Because of its small size, its flexibility, and its excellent optical system, it allows increased visualization of the peripheral airways and is ideal for diagnosing pulmonary lesions. Fiberoptic bronchoscopy allows biopsy of previously inaccessible tumors and can be performed at the bedside. It also can be performed through endotracheal or tracheostomy tubes of patients on ventilators. Cytologic examinations can be performed without surgical intervention.

The rigid bronchoscope is a hollow metal tube with a light at its end. It is used mainly for removing foreign substances, investigating the source of massive hemoptysis, or performing endobronchial surgical procedures. Rigid bronchoscopy is performed in the operating room, not at the bedside.

Possible complications of bronchoscopy include a reaction to the local anesthetic, infection, aspiration, bronchospasm, **hypoxemia** (low blood oxygen level), pneumothorax, bleeding, and perforation.

NURSING INTERVENTIONS

Before the procedure, a signed consent form is obtained from the patient, and food and fluids are withheld for 6 hours before the test to reduce the risk of aspiration when the cough reflex is blocked by anesthesia. The nurse explains the procedure to the patient to reduce fear and decrease anxiety and administers preoperative medications (usually atropine and a sedative or opioid) as prescribed to inhibit vagal stimulation (thereby guarding against bradycardia, dysrhythmias, and hypotension), suppress the cough reflex, sedate the patient, and relieve anxiety.

 NURSING ALERT Sedation given to patients with respiratory insufficiency may precipitate respiratory arrest.

The patient must remove dentures and other oral prostheses. The examination is usually performed under local anesthesia, but general anesthesia may be needed for rigid bronchoscopy. A topical anesthetic such as lidocaine (Xylocaine) may be sprayed on the pharynx or dropped on the epiglottis and vocal cords and into the trachea to suppress the cough reflex and minimize discomfort. Sedatives or opioids are administered intravenously as prescribed to provide moderate sedation.

After the procedure, it is important that the patient takes nothing by mouth until the cough reflex returns, because the preoperative sedation and local anesthesia impair the protective laryngeal reflex and swallowing for several hours. Once the patient demonstrates a cough reflex, the nurse may offer ice chips and eventually fluids. The nurse assesses for confusion and lethargy in the elderly, which may be due to the large doses of lidocaine given during the procedure. The nurse also monitors the patient's res-

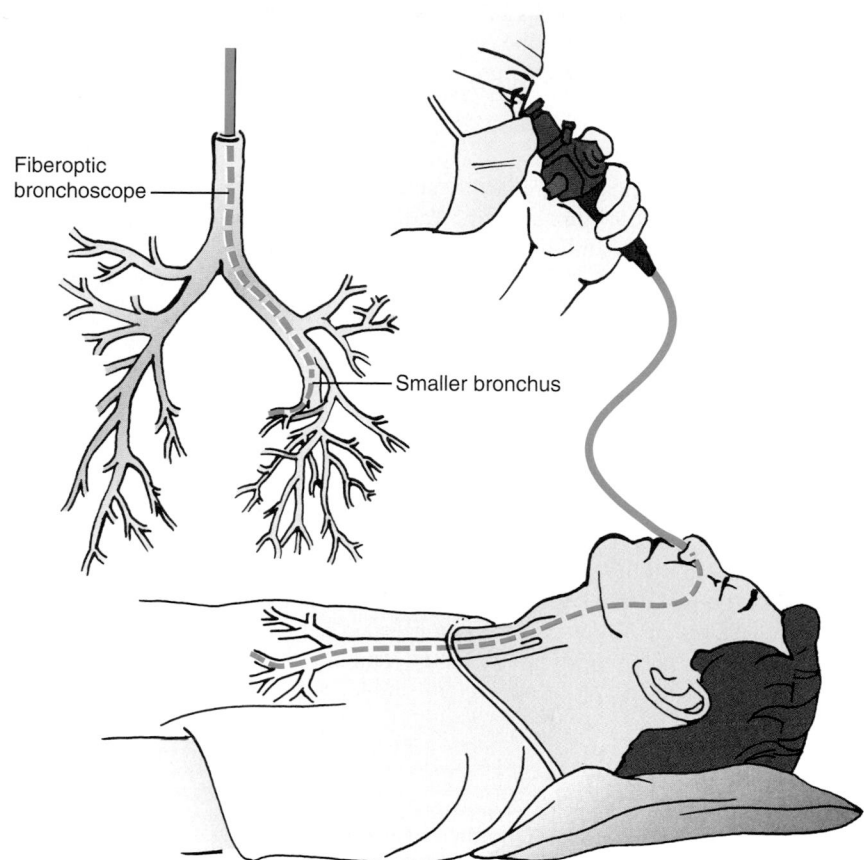

FIGURE 21-15 Endoscopic bronchoscopy permits visualization of bronchial structures. The bronchoscope is advanced into bronchial structures orally. Bronchoscopy permits the clinician not only to diagnose but also to treat various lung problems.

piratory status and observes for hypoxia, hypotension, tachycardia, dysrhythmias, hemoptysis, and dyspnea. Any abnormality is reported promptly. The patient is not discharged from the recovery area until adequate cough reflex and respiratory status are present. The nurse instructs the patient and family caregivers to report any shortness of breath or bleeding immediately.

Thoracoscopy

Thoracoscopy is a diagnostic procedure in which the pleural cavity is examined with an endoscope (Fig. 21-16). Small incisions are made into the pleural cavity in an intercostal space; the location of the incision depends on the clinical and diagnostic findings. After any fluid present in the pleural cavity is aspirated, the fiberoptic mediastinoscope is inserted into the pleural cavity, and its surface is inspected through the instrument. After the procedure, a chest tube may be inserted, and the pleural cavity is drained by negative-pressure water-seal drainage.

Thoracoscopy is primarily indicated in the diagnostic evaluation of pleural effusions, pleural disease, and tumor staging. Biopsies of the lesions can be performed under visualization for diagnosis.

Thoracoscopic procedures have expanded with the availability of video monitoring, which permits improved visualization of the lung. Such procedures also have been used with the carbon dioxide laser in the removal of pulmonary blebs and bullae and in the treatment of spontaneous pneumothorax. Lasers have also

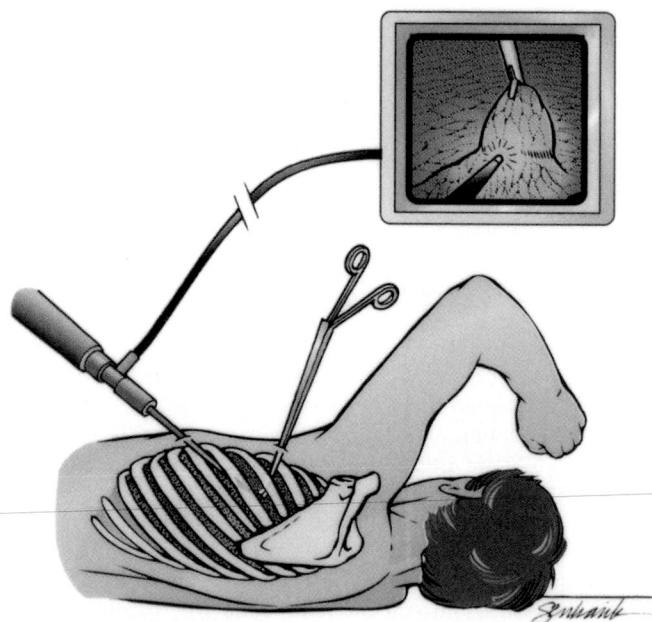

FIGURE 21-16 Endoscopic thoracoscopy. Like bronchoscopy, thoracoscopy uses fiberoptic instruments and video cameras for visualizing thoracic structures. Unlike bronchoscopy, thoracoscopy usually requires the surgeon to make a small incision before inserting the endoscope. A combined diagnostic–treatment procedure, thoracoscopy includes excising tissue for biopsy.

been used in the excision of peripheral pulmonary nodules. Although the laser does not replace the need for thoracotomy in the treatment of some lung cancers, its use continues to expand because it is less invasive.

NURSING INTERVENTIONS

Follow-up care in the health care facility and at home involves monitoring the patient for shortness of breath (which might indicate a pneumothorax), and minor activity restrictions, which vary depending on the intensity of the procedure. If a chest tube is in place, monitoring the chest drainage system and chest tube insertion site is essential (see Chap. 25).

THORACENTESIS

A thin layer of pleural fluid normally remains in the pleural space. An accumulation of pleural fluid may occur with some disorders. A sample of this fluid can be obtained by thoracentesis (aspiration of pleural fluid for diagnostic or therapeutic purposes). It is important to position the patient as shown in Chart 21-9.

A needle biopsy of the pleura may be performed at the same time. Studies of pleural fluid include Gram's stain culture and sensitivity, acid-fast staining and culture, differential cell count, cytology, pH, specific gravity, total protein, and lactic dehydrogenase.

BIOPSY

Biopsy, the excision of a small amount of tissue, may be performed to permit examination of cells from the pharynx, larynx, and nasal passages. Local, topical, or general anesthesia may be administered, depending on the site and the procedure (see also "Lung Biopsy Procedures" below).

Pleural Biopsy

Pleural biopsy is accomplished by needle biopsy of the pleura or by pleuroscopy, a visual exploration through a fiberoptic bronchoscope inserted into the pleural space. Pleural biopsy is performed when there is pleural exudate of undetermined origin and when there is a need to culture or stain the tissue to identify tuberculosis or fungi.

Lung Biopsy Procedures

When the chest x-ray findings are inconclusive or show pulmonary density (indicating an infiltrate or lesion), biopsy may be performed to obtain lung tissue for examination to identify the nature of the lesion. There are several nonsurgical lung biopsy techniques that are used because they yield accurate information with low morbidity: (1) transcatheter bronchial brushing, (2) transbronchial lung biopsy, or (3) percutaneous (through-the-skin) needle biopsy.

In transcatheter bronchial brushing, a fiberoptic bronchoscope is introduced into the bronchus under fluoroscopy. A small brush attached to the end of a flexible wire is inserted through the bronchoscope. Under direct visualization, the area under suspicion is brushed back and forth, causing cells to slough off and adhere to the brush. The catheter port of the bronchoscope may be used to irrigate the lung tissue with saline solution to secure material for additional studies. The brush is removed from the bronchoscope and a microscopic slide is made. The brush may be cut off and sent to the pathology laboratory for analysis.

This procedure is useful for cytologic evaluations of lung lesions and for the identification of pathogenic organisms (*Nocardia, Aspergillus, Pneumocystis carinii,* and other pathogens). It is especially useful in the immunologically compromised patient.

A transbronchial lung biopsy uses biting or cutting forceps introduced by a fiberoptic bronchoscope. A biopsy is indicated when a lung lesion is suspected and the results of routine sputum samples and bronchoscopic washings are negative.

Another method of bronchial brushing involves the introduction of the catheter through the transcricothyroid membrane by needle puncture. After this procedure, the patient is instructed to hold a finger or thumb over the puncture site while coughing to prevent air from leaking into the surrounding tissues.

Percutaneous needle biopsy may be accomplished with a cutting needle or by aspiration with a spinal-type needle that provides a tissue specimen for histologic study. Analgesia may be administered before the procedure. The skin over the biopsy site is cleansed and anesthetized and a small incision is made. The biopsy needle is inserted through the incision into the pleura with the patient holding the breath in mid-expiration. Using fluoroscopic monitoring, the surgeon guides the needle into the periphery of the lesion and obtains a tissue sample from the mass. Possible complications include pneumothorax, pulmonary hemorrhage, and empyema.

NURSING INTERVENTIONS

After the procedure, recovery and home care are similar to those for bronchoscopy and thoracoscopy. Nursing care involves monitoring the patient for shortness of breath, bleeding, and infection. In preparation for discharge, the patient and/or family is instructed to report pain, shortness of breath, visible bleeding, or redness of the biopsy site or pus to the health care provider immediately. Patients who have undergone biopsy are often anxious because of the need for the biopsy and the potential findings; the nurse must consider this in providing postbiopsy care and teaching.

Lymph Node Biopsy

The scalene lymph nodes are enmeshed in the deep cervical pad of fat overlying the scalenus anterior muscle. They drain the lungs and mediastinum and may show histologic changes from intrathoracic disease. When these nodes are palpable on physical examination, a scalene node biopsy may be performed. A biopsy of these nodes may be performed to detect lymph node spread of pulmonary disease and to establish a diagnosis or prognosis in such diseases as Hodgkin's disease, sarcoidosis, fungal disease, tuberculosis, and carcinoma.

Mediastinoscopy is the endoscopic examination of the mediastinum for exploration and biopsy of mediastinal lymph nodes that drain the lungs; this examination does not require a thoracotomy. Biopsy is usually performed through a suprasternal incision. Mediastinoscopy is carried out to detect mediastinal involvement of pulmonary malignancy and to obtain tissue for diagnostic studies of other conditions (eg, sarcoidosis).

An anterior mediastinotomy is thought to provide better exposure and diagnostic possibilities than a mediastinoscopy. An incision is made in the area of the second or third costal cartilage. The mediastinum is explored and biopsies are performed on any lymph nodes found. Chest tube drainage is required after the procedure. Mediastinotomy is particularly valuable to determine whether a pulmonary lesion is resectable.

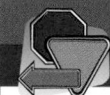

Chart 21-9

GUIDELINES FOR Assisting the Patient Undergoing Thoracentesis

A thoracentesis (aspiration of fluid or air from the pleural space) is performed on patients with various clinical problems. A diagnostic or therapeutic procedure, thoracentesis may be used for:
- Removal of fluid and air from the pleural cavity
- Aspiration of pleural fluid for analysis
- Pleural biopsy
- Instillation of medication into the pleural space

The responsibilities of the nurse and rationale for the nursing actions are summarized below.

NURSING ACTIVITIES	RATIONALE
1. Ascertain in advance that a chest x-ray has been ordered and completed and the consent form has been signed.	1. Posteroanterior and lateral chest x-ray films are used to localize fluid and air in the pleural cavity and to aid in determining the puncture site. When fluid is loculated (isolated in a pocket of pleural fluid), ultrasound scans are performed to help select the best site for needle aspiration.
2. Assess the patient for allergy to the local anesthetic to be used. Administer sedation if prescribed.	2. If the patient is allergic to the initially prescribed anesthetic, assessment findings provide an opportunity to use a safer anesthetic.
3. Inform the patient about the nature of the procedure and: a. The importance of remaining immobile b. Pressure sensations to be experienced c. That minimal discomfort is anticipated after the procedure	3. An explanation helps to orient the patient to the procedure, assists the patient to mobilize resources, and provides an opportunity to ask questions and verbalize anxiety.
4. Position the patient comfortably with adequate supports. If possible, place the patient upright or in one of the following positions: a. Sitting on the edge of the bed with the feet supported and arms and head on a padded over-the-bed table	4. The upright position facilitates the removal of fluid that usually localizes at the base of the chest. A position of comfort helps the patient to relax.

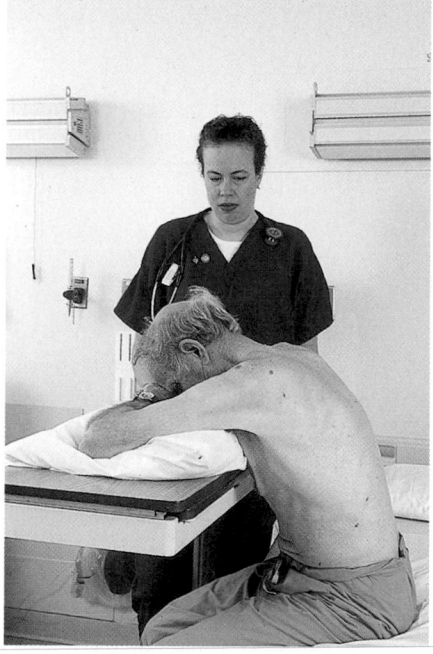

Patient positioned for thoracentesis.

b. Straddling a chair with arms and head resting on the back of the chair

c. Lying on the unaffected side with the bed elevated 30 degrees to 45 degrees if unable to assume a sitting position

5. Support and reassure the patient during the procedure.
   a. Prepare the patient for the cold sensation of skin germicide solution and for a pressure sensation from infiltration of local anesthetic agent.
   b. Encourage the patient to refrain from coughing.

5. Sudden and unexpected movement, such as coughing, by the patient can traumatize the visceral pleura and lung.

(continued)

Chart 21-9

GUIDELINES FOR Assisting the Patient Undergoing Thoracentesis (Continued)

NURSING ACTIVITIES	RATIONALE
6. Expose the entire chest. The site for aspiration is visualized by chest x-ray film and percussion. If fluid is in the pleural cavity, the thoracentesis site is determined by the chest x-ray, ultrasound scanning, and physical findings, with attention to the site of maximal dullness on percussion.	6. If air is in the pleural cavity, the thoracentesis site is usually in the second or third intercostal space in the midclavicular line because air rises in the thorax.
7. The procedure is performed under aseptic conditions. After the skin is cleansed, the physician uses a small-caliber needle to inject a local anesthetic slowly into the intercostal space.	7. An intradermal wheal is raised slowly; rapid injection causes pain. The parietal pleura is very sensitive and should be well infiltrated with anesthetic before the physician passes the thoracentesis needle through it.

8. The physician advances the thoracentesis needle with the syringe attached. When the pleural space is reached, suction may be applied with the syringe.
  a. A 20-mL syringe with a three-way stopcock is attached to the needle (one end of the adapter is attached to the needle and the other to the tubing leading to a receptacle that receives the fluid being aspirated).
  b. If a considerable quantity of fluid is removed, the needle is held in place on the chest wall with a small hemostat.
	
	a. When a large quantity of fluid is withdrawn, a three-way stopcock serves to keep air from entering the pleural cavity.
	
	b. The hemostat steadies the needle on the chest wall. Sudden pleuritic chest pain or shoulder pain may indicate that the needle point is irritating the visceral or the diaphragmatic pleura.

9. After the needle is withdrawn, pressure is applied over the puncture site and a small, sterile dressing is fixed in place.	9. Pressure helps to stop bleeding and the dressing protects the site.
10. Advise the patient that he or she will be on bed rest and a chest x-ray will be obtained after thoracentesis.	10. A chest x-ray verifies that there is no pneumothorax.
11. Record the total amount of fluid withdrawn from the procedure and document the nature of the fluid, its color, and its viscosity. If indicated, prepare samples of fluid for laboratory evaluation. A specimen container with formalin may be needed for a pleural biopsy.	11. The fluid may be clear, serous, bloody, purulent, etc.
12. Monitor the patient at intervals for increasing respiratory rate; asymmetry in respiratory movement; faintness; vertigo; tightness in chest; uncontrollable cough; blood-tinged, frothy mucus; a rapid pulse; and signs of hypoxemia.	12. Pneumothorax, tension pneumothorax, subcutaneous emphysema, or pyrogenic infection are complications of a thoracentesis. Pulmonary edema or cardiac distress can occur after a sudden shift in mediastinal contents when large amounts of fluid are aspirated.

NURSING INTERVENTIONS

Postprocedure care focuses on providing adequate oxygenation, monitoring for bleeding, and providing pain relief. The patient may be discharged a few hours after the chest drainage system is removed. The nurse should instruct the patient and family about monitoring for changes in respiratory status, taking into consideration the impact of anxiety about the potential findings of the biopsy on their ability to remember those instructions.

Critical Thinking Exercises

1. After a transbronchial lung biopsy, your patient reports shortness of breath and appears anxious. He is coughing up blood-tinged sputum. Based on your knowledge of the risks associated with lung biopsy, how would you focus your assessment? What physical and psychological nursing interventions would be appropriate for the patient at this time?

2. Your patient is scheduled for a video-assisted thoracoscopy. Describe the postprocedure nursing care and teaching for a patient undergoing this procedure. Identify the specific assessment parameters that are indicated.

3. Your patient has had a thoracentesis to remove pleural fluid for laboratory analysis and to relieve shortness of breath. What assessment should be carried out following the procedure? What teaching is warranted for the patient and family if she is to be discharged an hour after the procedure? How would you modify your instructions to the patient if she lives alone?

4. Your frail, elderly patient has a diagnosis of long-standing cardiac disease and is scheduled for PFTs prior to surgery to repair her cardiac valves. What specific explanations about the tests would you provide to the patient? What problems would you monitor for following the PFT?

REFERENCES AND SELECTED READINGS

Books

Bickley, L. S. (2003). *Bates' guide to physical examination and history taking* (8th ed.). Philadelphia: Lippincott Williams & Wilkins.

Blair, K. A. (1999). The aging pulmonary system. In M. Stanley & P. G. Bear (Eds.), *Gerontological nursing* (2d ed.). Philadelphia: F. A. Davis.

Levitzky, M. G. (1999). *Pulmonary physiology* (4th ed.). New York: McGraw Hill.

Sole, M. L., & Byers, J. F. (2001). Ventilatory assistance. In M. L. Sole, J. C. Hartshorn, & M. L. Lamborn (Eds.), *Introduction to critical care nursing* (3rd ed.). Philadelphia: W. B. Saunders.

West, J. B. (2000). *Respiratory physiology: The essentials.* Philadelphia: Lippincott Williams & Wilkins.

West, J. B. (2001). *Pulmonary physiology and pathophysiology: An integrated, case-based approach.* Philadelphia: Lippincott Williams & Wilkins.

Wilkins, R. L., Sheldon, R. L., & Knider, S. J. (2000). *Clinical assessment in respiratory care* (4th ed.). St. Louis: Mosby-Year Book.

Journals

Asterisks indicate nursing research articles.

Boyle, A. H., & Waters, H. F. (2000). Issues in respiratory nursing: Focus on prevention: recommendations of the National Lung Health Education Program. *Heart & Lung, 29*(6), 446–449.

Camhi, S. L., & Enright, P. L. (2000). How to assess pulmonary function in older persons. *Journal of Respiratory Diseases, 21*(6), 395–399.

Coleman, R. E. (1999). PET in lung cancer. *Journal of Nuclear Medicine, 40*(5), 814–820.

Graeber, G. M., Gupta, N. C., & Murray, G. F. (1999). Positron emission tomographic imaging with fluorodeoxyglucose is efficacious in evaluating malignant pulmonary disease. *Journal of Thoracic and Cardiovascular Surgery, 117*(4), 719–727.

Horne, C., & Derrico, D. (1999). Mastering ABGs. The art of arterial blood gas measurement. *American Journal of Nursing, 99*(8), 26–32.

Janssens, J. P., de Muralt, B., & Titelion, V. (2000). Management of dyspnea in severe chronic obstructive pulmonary disease. *Journal of Pain and Symptom Management, 19*(5), 378–392.

Johnson, B. D., Beck, K. C., Zeballos, R. J., & Weisman, I. M. (1999). Advances in pulmonary laboratory testing. *Chest, 116*(5), 1377–1387.

Kauczor, H. U., & Kreitner, K. E. (2000). Contrast-enhanced MRI of the lung. *European Journal of Radiology, 34*(3), 196–207.

Lowe, V. J., Fletcher, J. W., Gobar, L., Lawson, M., et al. (1998). Prospective investigation of positron emission tomography in lung nodules. *Journal of Clinical Oncology, 16*(3), 1075–1084.

Martin, B., Llewellyn, J., Faut-Callahan, M., & Meyer, P. (2000). The use of telemetric oximetry in the clinical setting. *MedSurg Nursing, 9*(2), 71–76.

*Nield, M. (2000). Dyspnea self-management in African Americans with chronic lung disease. *Heart & Lung, 29*(1), 50–55.

Salzman, S. (1999). Pulmonary function testing: Tips on how to interpret the results. *Journal of Respiratory Diseases, 20*(12), 809–812.

Shortall, S. P., & Perkins, L. A. (1999). Interpreting the ins and outs of pulmonary function tests. *Nursing, 29*(12), 41–47.

Shuster, D. P. (1998). The evaluation of lung function with PET. *Seminars in Nuclear Medicine, 28*(4), 341–351.

Wong, F. W. H. (1999). A new approach to ABG interpretation. *American Journal of Nursing, 99*(8), 34–36.

RESOURCES AND WEBSITES

American Lung Association, 1740 Broadway, New York, NY 10019; (212) 315-8700; 1-800-LUNG USA; http://www.lungusa.org.

American Association for Respiratory Care, 11030 Ables Lane, Dallas, TX 75229; (972) 243-2272; http://www.aarc.org.

National Heart, Lung, and Blood Institute/National Institutes of Health, Rockville Pike, Bldg. 31, Bethesda, MD 20892; (301) 496-5166; http://www.nhlbi.nih.gov/nhlbi/index.htm.

National Lung Health Education Program: http://www.nlhep.org. Has easy-to-read teaching resources for patients.

Management of Patients With Upper Respiratory Tract Disorders

On completion of this chapter, the learner will be able to:

1. Describe nursing management of patients with upper airway disorders.
2. Compare and contrast the upper respiratory tract infections with regard to cause, incidence, clinical manifestations, management, and the significance of preventive health care.
3. Use the nursing process as a framework for care of patients with upper airway infection.
4. Describe nursing management of the patient with epistaxis.
5. Use the nursing process as a framework for care of patients undergoing laryngectomy.

$\mathcal{M}$any upper airway disorders are relatively minor, and their effects are limited to mild and temporary discomfort and inconvenience for the patient. However, other upper airway disorders are acute, severe, and life-threatening and may require permanent alterations in breathing and speaking. Thus, the nurse must have good assessment skills, an understanding of the wide variety of disorders that may affect the upper airway, and an awareness of the impact of these alterations on patients.

Because many of the disorders are treated outside the hospital or at home by patients themselves, patient teaching is an important aspect of nursing care. When caring for patients with acute, life-threatening disorders, the nurse needs highly developed assessment and clinical management skills, along with a focus on rehabilitation needs.

Upper Airway Infections

Upper airway infections are common conditions that affect most people on occasion. Some infections are acute, with symptoms that last several days; others are chronic, with symptoms that last a long time or recur. Patients with these conditions seldom require hospitalization. However, nurses working in community settings or long-term care facilities may encounter patients who have these infections. Thus, it is important for the nurse to recognize the signs and symptoms and to provide appropriate care.

RHINITIS

Rhinitis is a group of disorders characterized by inflammation and irritation of the mucous membranes of the nose. It may be classified as nonallergic or allergic. It is estimated that 10% to 15% of the population of the United States has allergic rhinitis (Middleton et al., 1998). Rhinitis may be an acute or chronic condition.

Pathophysiology

Nonallergic rhinitis may be caused by a variety of factors, including environmental factors such as changes in temperature or humidity, odors, or foods; infection; age; systemic disease; drugs (cocaine) or prescribed medications; or the presence of a foreign body. Drug-induced rhinitis is associated with use of antihypertensive agents and oral contraceptives and chronic use of nasal decongestants. Rhinitis also may be a manifestation of an allergy (see Chap. 53), in which case it is referred to as allergic rhinitis. Figure 22-1 shows the pathological processes involved in rhinitis and sinusitis.

Clinical Manifestations

The signs and symptoms of rhinitis include **rhinorrhea** (excessive nasal drainage, runny nose), nasal congestion, nasal discharge (purulent with bacterial rhinitis), nasal itchiness, and sneezing. Headache may occur, particularly if sinusitis is also present.

Medical Management

The management of rhinitis depends on the cause, which may be identified in the history and physical examination. The examiner asks the patient about recent symptoms as well as possible exposure to allergens in the home, environment, or workplace. If viral rhinitis is the cause, medications are given to relieve the symptoms. In allergic rhinitis, tests may be performed to identify possible allergens. Depending on the severity of the allergy, desensitizing immunizations and corticosteroids may be required (see Chap. 53 for more details). If symptoms suggest a bacterial infection, an antimicrobial agent will be used (see "Medical Management of Sinusitis").

PHARMACOLOGIC THERAPY

Medication therapy for allergic and nonallergic rhinitis focuses on symptom relief. Antihistamines are administered for sneezing, itching, and rhinorrhea. Oral decongestant agents are used for nasal obstruction. In addition, intranasal corticosteroids may be used for severe congestion, and ophthalmic agents are used to relieve irritation, itching, and redness of the eyes.

Nursing Management

TEACHING PATIENTS SELF-CARE

The nurse instructs the patient with allergic rhinitis to avoid or reduce exposure to allergens and irritants, such as dusts, molds, animals, fumes, odors, powders, sprays, and tobacco smoke. The patient is instructed about the importance of controlling the environment at home and work. Saline nasal or aerosol sprays may be helpful in soothing mucous membranes, softening crusted secretions, and removing irritants. The nurse instructs the patient in the proper use of and technique for administrating nasal medications. To achieve maximal relief, the patient is instructed to blow the nose before applying any medication into the nasal cavity. In the case of infectious rhinitis, the nurse reviews with the patient hand hygiene technique as a measure to prevent transmission of organisms. The nurse teaches methods to treat symptoms of the viral rhinitis. In the elderly and other high-risk populations, the nurse reviews the value of receiving a vaccination

Glossary

alaryngeal communication: alternative modes of speaking that do not involve the normal larynx; used by patients whose larynx has been surgically removed

aphonia: impaired ability to use one's voice due to disease or injury to the larynx

apnea: cessation of breathing

dysphagia: difficulties in swallowing

epistaxis: hemorrhage from the nose due to rupture of tiny, distended vessels in the mucous membrane of any area of the nose

herpes simplex: cold sore (cutaneous viral infection with painful vesicles and erosions on the tongue, palate, gingival, buccal membranes, or lips)

laryngitis: inflammation of the larynx; may be due to voice abuse, exposure to irritants, or infectious organisms

laryngectomy: removal of all or part of the larynx and surrounding structures

pharyngitis: inflammation of the throat; usually viral or bacterial in origin

rhinitis: inflammation of the mucous membranes of the nose; may be infectious, allergic, or inflammatory in origin

rhinorrhea: drainage of a large amount of fluid from the nose

sinusitis: inflammation of the sinuses; may be acute or chronic; may be viral, bacterial, or fungal in origin

submucous resection: surgical procedure to correct nasal obstruction due to deviated septum; also called septoplasty

tonsillitis: inflammation of the tonsils, usually due to an acute infection

xerostomia: dryness of the mouth from a variety of causes

Physiology/Pathophysiology

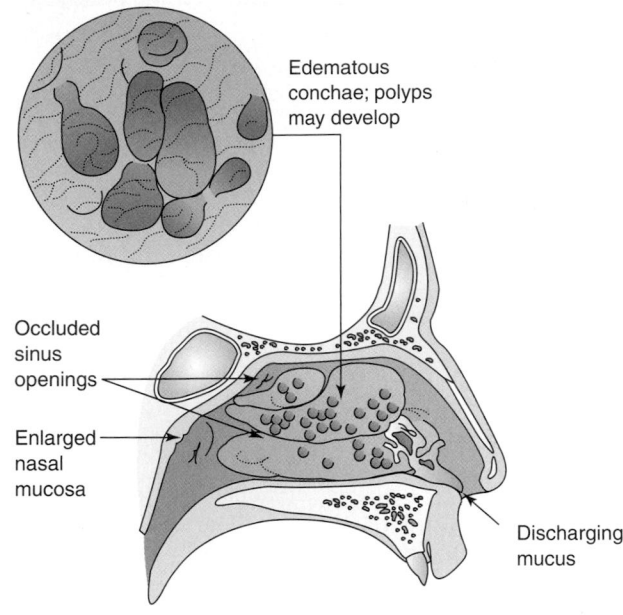

A. Rhinitis

Edematous conchae; polyps may develop

Occluded sinus openings

Enlarged nasal mucosa

Discharging mucus

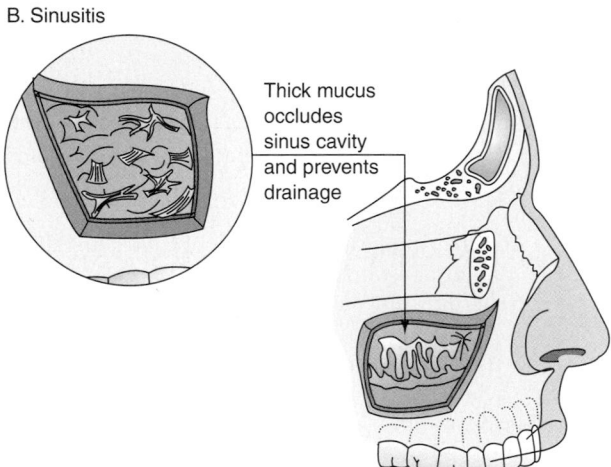

B. Sinusitis

Thick mucus occludes sinus cavity and prevents drainage

FIGURE 22-1 Pathophysiologic processes in rhinitis and sinusitis. Although pathophysiologic processes are similar in rhinitis and sinusitis, they affect different structures. In rhinitis (**A**), the mucous membranes lining the nasal passages become inflamed, congested, and edematous. The swollen nasal conchae block the sinus openings, and mucus is discharged from the nostrils. Sinusitis (**B**) is also marked by inflammation and congestion, with thickened mucous secretions filling the sinus cavities and occluding the openings.

in the fall in order to achieve immunity prior to the beginning of the "flu season."

VIRAL RHINITIS (COMMON COLD)

The term "common cold" often is used when referring to an upper respiratory tract infection that is self-limited and caused by a virus (viral rhinitis). Nasal congestion, rhinorrhea, sneezing, sore throat, and general malaise characterize it. Specifically, the term "cold" refers to an afebrile, infectious, acute inflammation

of the mucous membranes of the nasal cavity. More broadly, the term refers to an acute upper respiratory tract infection, whereas terms such as "rhinitis," "pharyngitis," and "laryngitis" distinguish the sites of the symptoms. It can also be used when the causative virus is influenza ("the flu"). Colds are highly contagious because virus is shed for about 2 days before the symptoms appear and during the first part of the symptomatic phase. It is estimated that adults in the United States average two to four colds each year. The common cold is the most common cause of absenteeism from work and school (Mandell, Bennett, & Dolin, 2000).

The six viruses known to produce the signs and symptoms of the viral rhinitis are rhinovirus, parainfluenza virus, coronavirus, respiratory syncytial virus (RSV), influenza virus, and adenovirus. Each virus may have multiple strains. For example, there are over 100 strains of rhinovirus, which accounts for 50% of all colds. The incidence of viral rhinitis follows a specific pattern during the year, depending on the causative agent (Fig. 22-2). Even though viral rhinitis can occur at any time of the year, three waves account for the epidemics in the United States:

- In September, just after the opening of school
- In late January
- Toward the end of April

Immunity after recovery is variable and depends on many factors, including a person's natural host resistance and the specific virus that caused the cold.

Clinical Manifestations

Signs and symptoms of viral rhinitis are nasal congestion, runny nose, sneezing, nasal discharge, nasal itchiness, tearing watery eyes, "scratchy" or sore throat, general malaise, low-grade fever, chills,

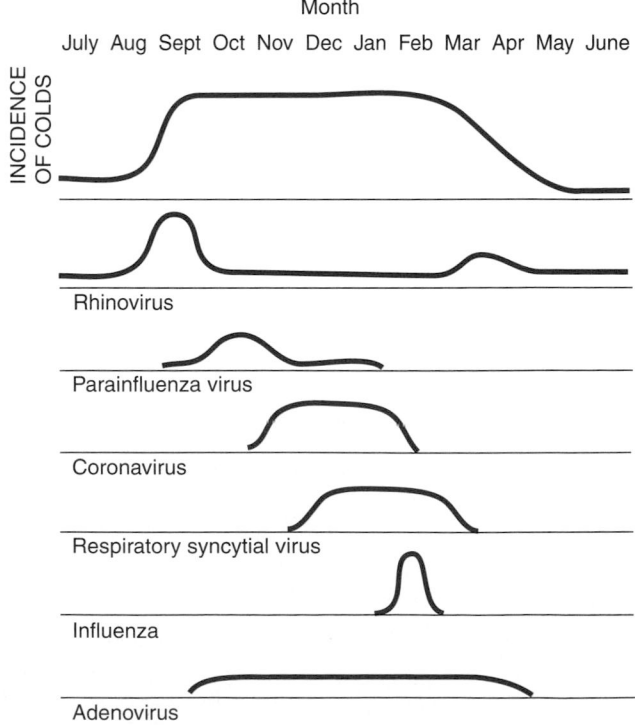

Month

July Aug Sept Oct Nov Dec Jan Feb Mar Apr May June

INCIDENCE OF COLDS

Rhinovirus

Parainfluenza virus

Coronavirus

Respiratory syncytial virus

Influenza

Adenovirus

FIGURE 22-2 Schematic diagram incidence of viral rhinitis (common cold) in the United States and the frequency of the causative agents. Redrawn from Goldman, L. & Bennett, J. C. (eds.) (2000) *Cecil textbook of medicine* (21st ed., Vol. 2). Philadelphia: W. B. Saunders, p. 1791.

and often headache and muscle aches. As the illness progresses, cough usually appears. In some people, viral rhinitis exacerbates the **herpes simplex**, commonly called a cold sore (Chart 22-1).

The symptoms last from 1 to 2 weeks. If there is significant fever or more severe systemic respiratory symptoms, it is no longer viral rhinitis but one of the other acute upper respiratory tract infections. Allergic conditions can also affect the nose, mimicking the symptoms of a cold.

Medical Management

There is no specific treatment for the common cold or influenza. Management consists of symptomatic therapy. Some measures include providing adequate fluid intake, encouraging rest, preventing chilling, increasing intake of vitamin C, and using expectorants as needed. Warm salt-water gargles soothe the sore throat and nonsteroidal anti-inflammatory agents (NSAIDs) such as aspirin or ibuprofen relieve the aches, pains, and fever in adults. Antihistamines are used to relieve sneezing, rhinorrhea, and nasal congestion. Topical (nasal) decongestant agents may re-

lieve nasal congestion; however, if they are overused they may create a rebound congestion that may be worse than the original symptoms. Some research suggests that zinc lozenges may reduce the duration of cold symptoms if taken within the first 24 hours of onset (Prasad, Fitzgerald, & Bao, 2000). Amantadine (Symmetrel) or rimantadine (Flumadine) may be prescribed prophylactically to decrease the signs and symptoms as well. Antimicrobial agents (antibiotics) should not be used because they do not affect the virus or reduce the incidence of bacterial complications.

Nursing Management

TEACHING PATIENTS SELF-CARE
Most viruses can be transmitted in several ways: direct contact with infected secretions; inhalation of large particles that land on a mucosal surface from coughing or sneezing; or inhalation of small particles (aerosol) that may be suspended in the air for up to an hour. It is important to teach the patient how to break the chain of infection. Hand washing remains the most effective measure to prevent transmission of organisms. The nurse teaches methods to treat symptoms of the common cold and preventive measures (Chart 22-2).

ACUTE SINUSITIS

The sinuses, mucus-lined cavities filled with air that drain normally into the nose, are involved in a high proportion of upper respiratory tract infections. If their openings into the nasal passages are clear, the infections resolve promptly. However, if their drainage is obstructed by a deviated septum or by hypertrophied turbinates, spurs, or nasal polyps or tumors, sinus infection may persist as a smoldering secondary infection or progress to an acute suppurative process (causing purulent discharge). **Sinusitis** affects over 14% of the population and accounts for billions of dollars in direct health care costs (Tierney, McPhee, & Papadakis, 2001). Some individuals are more prone to sinusitis because of their occupations. For example, continuous exposure to environmental hazards such as paint, sawdust, and chemicals may result in chronic inflammation of the nasal passages.

Pathophysiology

Acute sinusitis is an infection of the paranasal sinuses. It frequently develops as a result of an upper respiratory infection, such as an unresolved viral or bacterial infection, or an exacerbation of allergic rhinitis. Nasal congestion, caused by inflammation, edema, and transudation of fluid, leads to obstruction of the sinus cavities (see Fig. 22-1). This provides an excellent medium for bacterial growth. Bacterial organisms account for more than 60% of the cases of acute sinusitis, namely *Streptococcus pneumoniae,* *Haemophilus influenzae,* and *Moraxella catarrhalis* (Murray & Nadel, 2001). Dental infections also have been associated with acute sinusitis.

Clinical Manifestations

Symptoms of acute sinusitis may include facial pain or pressure over the affected sinus area, nasal obstruction, fatigue, purulent nasal discharge, fever, headache, ear pain and fullness, dental pain, cough, a decreased sense of smell, sore throat, eyelid edema, or facial congestion or fullness. Acute sinusitis can be difficult to differentiate from an upper respiratory infection or allergic rhinitis.

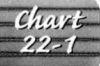

| *Chart* 22-1 | **Colds and Cold Sores (Herpes Simplex Virus)** |

The herpes simplex virus (HSV-1) produces the familiar *herpes labialis,* commonly called a cold sore or fever blister. In the past, this painful blisterlike lip sore was thought to be caused by a cold or a fever. Even now that scientists recognize the origin of herpes labialis, the condition is still referred to as a cold sore. The herpes virus infection remains latent in cells of the lips or nose and is activated by stress, sunlight, and febrile illnesses from the common cold to streptococcal pneumonia, meningococcal meningitis, and even malaria.

The incubation period is 2 to 12 days. The virus is transmitted primarily by direct contact with infected secretions. The virus may also be transmitted from an asymptomatic person. Small vesicles, single or clustered, may erupt on the lips, inside the mouth, including the tongue, soft and hard palate, gums, buccal mucosa, and the pharynx. These soon rupture, forming sore shallow ulcers that increase in number. The gums may bleed and feel painful.

The herpes virus may subside spontaneously in 10 to 14 days. If it does not, acyclovir, an antiviral agent, may be administered orally or topically to minimize the symptoms and the duration or length of the flare-up. Analgesics, such as acetaminophen (Tylenol) with codeine or aspirin with codeine, are helpful in relieving pain and discomfort. Topical anesthetics, such as lidocaine (Xylocaine) or dyclonine (Dyclone), and over-the-counter preparations, such as Herpecin-L, may relieve oral pain. Applications of drying lotions or liquids may help to dry the lesions.

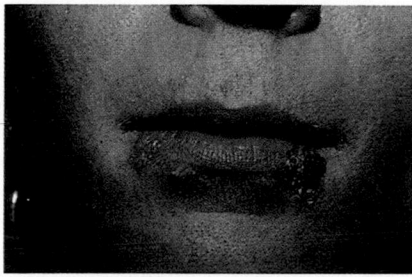

With permission from Goodheart, H. P. (1999). *Photoguide of common skin disorders: Diagnosis and management.* Baltimore: Lippincott Williams & Wilkins.

Chart 22-2
Home Care Checklist • **Preventing and Managing Upper Respiratory Infections**

At the completion of the home care instruction, the patient or caregiver will be able to:	Patient	Caregiver
Prevention		
• Identify strategies to prevent infection and, if infected, to prevent spread of infection to others	✓	✓
Perform hand hygiene often		
Use disposable tissues		
Avoid crowds during the flu season		
Avoid individuals with colds or respiratory infections		
Obtain influenza vaccination, if recommended (especially if elderly or diagnosed with a chronic illness)		
• Practice good health habits	✓	✓
Eat a nutritious diet		
Get plenty of rest and sleep		
Avoid or reduce stress when possible		
Exercise appropriately		
Avoid smoking or second-hand smoke and excessive intake of alcohol		
Increase humidity in house, especially during winter		
Practice adequate oral hygiene		
• Avoid allergens, if allergies are associated with upper respiratory infections	✓	
Prevention and Management		
• Identify strategies to control the environment	✓	✓
Adequately humidify (avoid overhumidifying) living quarters		
Place a dehumidifier in the basement, if appropriate		
Provide central ventilation fans, air conditioning with microstatic air filters		
Reduce irritants (dust, chemical, tobacco smoke) when possible		
Limit exposure to animals and house pets, particularly in the bedroom		
Management		
• Describe strategies to relieve symptoms of upper respiratory infection	✓	✓
Gargle with salt water		
Increase fluid intake, particularly of hot liquids		
Provide warm, moist air by shower or humidifier to relieve swollen mucous membranes		
Avoid irritants (dust, chemicals, tobacco smoke) when possible		
• Recognize signs and symptoms of infection and state when to contact a health care provider	✓	✓
Upper respiratory infection symptoms persisting longer than 7 to 10 days		
Extreme red throat or white patches on the back of the throat		
Discolored drainage or foul-smelling nasal discharge		
Prolonged fever of 100.5°F (38°C) >2 days		
Shortness of breath, wheezing		
Swollen lymph nodes		
Severe pain or tenderness around the eyes or persistent pain in sinus areas		
Severe headache		

Assessment and Diagnostic Findings

A careful history and physical examination are performed. The head and neck, particularly the nose, ears, teeth, sinuses, pharynx, and chest, are examined. There may be tenderness to palpation over the infected sinus area. The sinuses are percussed using the index finger, tapping lightly to determine if the patient experiences pain. The affected area is also transilluminated; with sinusitis, there is a decrease in the transmission of light (see Chap. 21, Fig. 21-8). Sinus x-rays may be performed to detect sinus opacity, mucosal thickening, bone destruction, and air–fluid levels. Computed tomography scanning of the sinuses is the most effective diagnostic tool. It is also used to rule out other local or systemic disorders, such as tumor, fistula, and allergy.

Complications

Acute sinusitis, if left untreated, may lead to severe and occasionally life-threatening complications such as meningitis, brain abscess, ischemic infarction, and osteomyelitis. Other complica-

tions of sinusitis, although uncommon, include severe orbital cellulitis, subperiosteal abscess, and cavernous sinus thrombosis.

Medical Management

The goals of treatment of acute sinusitis are to treat the infection, shrink the nasal mucosa, and relieve pain. There is a growing concern over the inappropriate use of antibiotics for viral upper respiratory infections; such overuse has resulted in antibiotics being less effective (more resistant) in treating bacterial infections such as sinusitis. As a result, careful consideration is given to the potential pathogen before antimicrobial agents are prescribed.

The antimicrobial agents of choice for a bacterial infection vary in clinical practice. First-line antibiotics include amoxicillin (Amoxil), trimethoprim/sulfamethoxazole (Bactrim, Septra), and erythromycin. Second-line antibiotics include cephalosporins such as cefuroxime axetil (Ceftin), cefpodoxime (Vantin), and cefprozil (Cefzil) and amoxicillin clavulanate (Augmentin). Newer and more expensive antibiotics with a broader spectrum include macrolides, azithromycin (Zithromax), and clarithromycin (Biaxin). Quinolones such as ciprofloxacin (Cipro), levofloxacin (Levaquin) (used with severe penicillin allergy), and sparfloxacin (Zagam) have also been used. The course of treatment is usually 10 to 14 days. A recent report found little difference in clinical outcomes between first-line and second-line antibiotics; however, costs were greater when newer second-line antibiotics were used (Piccirillo, Mager, Frisse et al., 2001).

Use of oral and topical decongestant agents may decrease mucosal swelling of nasal polyps, thereby improving drainage of the sinuses. Heated mist and saline irrigation also may be effective for opening blocked passages. Decongestant agents such as pseudoephedrine (Sudafed, Dimetapp) have proven effective because of their vasoconstrictive properties. Topical decongestant agents such as oxymetazoline (Afrin) may be used for up to 72 hours. It is important to administer them with the patient's head tilted back to promote maximal dispersion of the medication. Guaifenesin (Robitussin, Anti-Tuss), a mucolytic agent, may also be effective in reducing nasal congestion.

In 2000, the U.S. Food and Drug Administration issued a public health advisory concerning phenylpropanolamine, which previously had been commonly used in oral decongestants and diet pills. The voluntary recall of products containing this ingredient was based on a study linking its use with hemorrhagic stroke in women. Men may also be at risk (Kernan et al., 2000).

Antihistamines such as diphenhydramine (Benadryl), cetirizine (Zyrtec), and fexofenadine (Allegra) may be used if an allergic component is suspected. If the patient continues to have symptoms after 7 to 10 days, the sinuses may need to be irrigated and hospitalization may be required.

Nursing Management

TEACHING PATIENTS SELF-CARE

Patient teaching is an important aspect of nursing care for the patient with acute sinusitis. The nurse instructs the patient about methods to promote drainage such as inhaling steam (steam bath, hot shower, and facial sauna), increasing fluid intake, and applying local heat (hot wet packs). The nurse also informs the patient about the side effects of nasal sprays and about rebound congestion. In the case of rebound congestion, the body's receptors, which have become dependent on the decongestant sprays to keep the nasal passages open, close and congestion results after the spray is discontinued.

The nurse stresses the importance of following the recommended antibiotic regimen, because a consistent blood level of the medication is critical to treat the infection. The nurse teaches the patient the early signs of a sinus infection and recommends preventive measures such as following healthy practices and avoiding contact with people who have upper respiratory infections (see Chart 22-2).

The nurse should explain to the patient that fever, severe headache, and nuchal rigidity are signs of potential complications. If fever persists despite antibiotic therapy, the patient should seek additional care.

CHRONIC SINUSITIS

Chronic sinusitis is an inflammation of the sinuses that persists for more than 3 weeks in an adult and 2 weeks in a child. It is estimated that 32 million people a year develop chronic sinusitis.

Pathophysiology

A narrowing or obstruction in the ostia of the frontal, maxillary, and anterior ethmoid sinuses usually causes chronic sinusitis, preventing adequate drainage to the nasal passages. This combined area is known as the osteomeatal complex. Blockage that persists for greater than 3 weeks in an adult may occur because of infection, allergy, or structural abnormalities. This results in stagnant secretions, an ideal medium for infection. The organisms that cause chronic sinusitis are the same as those implicated in acute sinusitis. Immunocompromised patients, however, are at increased risk for developing fungal sinusitis. *Aspergillus fumigatus* is the most common organism associated with fungal sinusitis.

Clinical Manifestations

Clinical manifestations of chronic sinusitis include impaired mucociliary clearance and ventilation, cough (because the thick discharge constantly drips backward into the nasopharynx), chronic hoarseness, chronic headaches in the periorbital area, and facial pain. These symptoms are generally most pronounced on awakening in the morning. Fatigue and nasal stuffiness are also common. In addition, some patients experience a decrease in smell and taste and a fullness in the ears.

Assessment and Diagnostic Findings

A careful history and diagnostic assessment, including a computed tomography scan of the sinuses or magnetic resonance imaging (if fungal sinusitis is suspected), are performed to rule out other local or systemic disorders, such as tumor, fistula, and allergy. Nasal endoscopy may be indicated to rule out underlying diseases such as tumors and sinus mycetomas (fungus balls). The fungus ball is usually a brown or greenish-black material with the consistency of peanut butter or cottage cheese.

Complications

Complications of chronic sinusitis, although uncommon, include severe orbital cellulitis, subperiosteal abscess, cavernous sinus thrombosis, meningitis, encephalitis, and ischemic infarction.

Medical Management

Medical management of chronic sinusitis is almost the same as for acute sinusitis. The antimicrobial agents of choice include amoxicillin clavulanate (Augmentin) or ampicillin (Ampicin). Clarithromycin (Biaxin) and third-generation cephalosporins such as cefuroxime axetil (Ceftin), cefpodoxime (Vantin), and cefprozil (Cefzil) have also been effective. Levofloxacin (Levaquin), a quinolone, may also be used. The course of treatment may be 3 to 4 weeks. Decongestant agents, antihistamines, saline sprays, and heated mist may also provide some symptom relief.

SURGICAL MANAGEMENT

When standard medical therapy fails, surgery, usually endoscopic, may be indicated to correct structural deformities that obstruct the ostia (openings) of the sinus. Excising and cauterizing nasal polyps, correcting a deviated septum, incising and draining the sinuses, aerating the sinuses, and removing tumors are some of the specific procedures performed. When sinusitis is caused by a fungal infection, surgery is required to excise the fungus ball and necrotic tissue and drain the sinuses. Oral and topical corticosteroids are usually prescribed. Antimicrobial agents are administered before and after surgery. Some patients with severe chronic sinusitis obtain relief only by moving to a dry climate.

Nursing Management

Because the patient usually performs care measures for sinusitis at home, nursing management consists mainly of patient teaching.

TEACHING PATIENTS SELF-CARE

The nurse teaches the patient how to promote sinus drainage by increasing the environmental humidity (steam bath, hot shower, and facial sauna), increasing fluid intake, and applying local heat (hot wet packs). The nurse also instructs the patient about the importance of following the medication regimen. Instructions on the early signs of a sinus infection are provided and preventive measures are reviewed.

ACUTE PHARYNGITIS

Acute **pharyngitis** is an inflammation or infection in the throat, usually causing symptoms of a sore throat.

Pathophysiology

Most cases of acute pharyngitis are caused by viral infection. When group A beta-hemolytic streptococcus, the most common bacterial organism, causes acute pharyngitis, the condition is known as strep throat (Bisno, 2001). The body responds by triggering an inflammatory response in the pharynx. This results in pain, fever, vasodilation, edema, and tissue damage, manifested by redness and swelling in the tonsillar pillars, uvula, and soft palate. A creamy exudate may be present in the tonsillar pillars (Fig. 22-3).

Uncomplicated viral infections usually subside promptly, within 3 to 10 days after the onset. However, pharyngitis caused by more virulent bacteria such as group A beta-hemolytic streptococci is a more severe illness. If left untreated, the complications can be severe and life-threatening. Complications include sinusitis, otitis media, peritonsillar abscess, mastoiditis, and cervical adenitis. In rare cases the infection may lead to bacteremia, pneumonia, meningitis, rheumatic fever, or nephritis.

Clinical Manifestations

The signs and symptoms of acute pharyngitis include a fiery-red pharyngeal membrane and tonsils, lymphoid follicles that are swollen and flecked with white-purple exudate, and enlarged and tender cervical lymph nodes and no cough. Fever, malaise, and sore throat also may be present.

Assessment and Diagnostic Findings

Rapid screening tests for streptococcal antigens such as the latex agglutination (LA) antigen test and solid-phase enzyme immunoassays (ELISA), optical immunoassay (OIA), streptolysin titers, and throat cultures are used to determine the causative organism, after which appropriate therapy is prescribed. Nasal swabs and blood cultures may also be necessary to identify the organism (Corneli, 2001).

Medical Management

Viral pharyngitis is treated with supportive measures since antibiotics will have no effect on the organism. Bacterial pharyngitis is treated with a variety of antimicrobial agents.

PHARMACOLOGIC THERAPY

If a bacterial cause is suggested or demonstrated, penicillin is usually the treatment of choice. For patients who are allergic to penicillin or have organisms that are resistant to erythromycin (one fifth of group A beta-hemolytic streptococci and most *S. aureus* organisms are resistant to penicillin and erythromycin), cephalosporins and macrolides (clarithromycin and azithromycin) may be used. Antibiotics are administered for at least 10 days to eradicate the infection from the oropharynx.

Severe sore throats can also be relieved by analgesic medications, as prescribed. For example, aspirin or acetaminophen (Tylenol) can be taken at 3- to 6-hour intervals; if required, acetaminophen with codeine can be taken three or four times daily. Antitussive medication, in the form of codeine, dextromethorphan (Robitussin DM), or hydrocodone bitartrate (Hycodan), may be required to control the persistent and painful cough that often accompanies acute pharyngitis.

NUTRITIONAL THERAPY

A liquid or soft diet is provided during the acute stage of the disease, depending on the patient's appetite and the degree of discomfort that occurs with swallowing. Occasionally, the throat is so sore that liquids cannot be taken in adequate amounts by mouth. In severe situations, fluids are administered intravenously. Otherwise, the patient is encouraged to drink as much fluid as possible (at least 2 to 3 L per day).

Nursing Management

The nurse instructs the patient to stay in bed during the febrile stage of illness and to rest frequently once up and about. Used tissues should be disposed of properly to prevent the spread of infection. It is important to examine the skin once or twice daily for

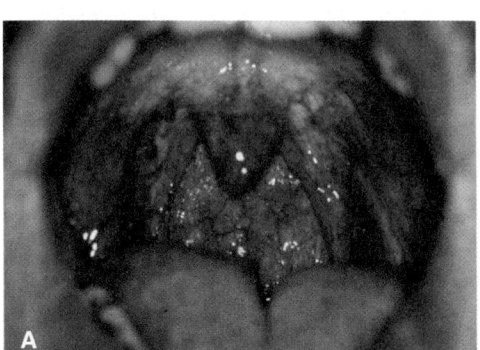
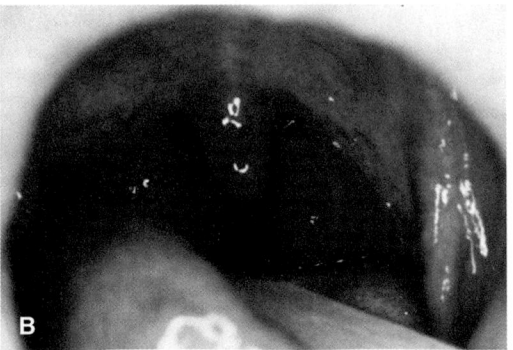

FIGURE 22-3 Pharyngitis—inflammation without exudate. (**A**) Redness and vascularity of the pillars and uvula are mild to moderate. (**B**) Redness is diffuse and intense. Each patient would probably complain of a sore throat. From Bickley, L. S. (2003). *Bates' guide to physical examination and history taking* (8th ed.). Philadelphia: Lippincott Williams & Wilkins.

possible rash, because acute pharyngitis may precede some other communicable diseases (ie, rubella).

Warm saline gargles or irrigations are used depending on the severity of the lesion and the degree of pain. The benefits of this treatment depend on the degree of heat that is applied. The nurse teaches the patient about the recommended temperature of the solution: high enough to be effective and as warm as the patient can tolerate, usually 105°F to 110°F (40.6°C to 43.3°C). Irrigating the throat properly is an effective means of reducing spasm in the pharyngeal muscles and relieving soreness of the throat. Unless the purpose of the procedure and its technique are understood clearly by the patient and family, the results may be less than satisfactory.

An ice collar also can relieve severe sore throats. Mouth care may add greatly to the patient's comfort and prevent the development of fissures (cracking) of the lips and oral inflammation when bacterial infection is present. The nurse instructs the patient to resume activity gradually. A full course of antibiotic therapy is indicated in patients with group A beta-hemolytic streptococcal infection in view of the possible development of complications such as nephritis and rheumatic fever, which may have their onset 2 or 3 weeks after the pharyngitis has subsided. The nurse instructs the patient and family about the importance of taking the full course of therapy and informs them about the symptoms to watch for that may indicate complications.

CHRONIC PHARYNGITIS

Chronic pharyngitis is a persistent inflammation of the pharynx. It is common in adults who work or live in dusty surroundings, use their voice to excess, suffer from chronic cough, and habitually use alcohol and tobacco.

Three types of chronic pharyngitis are recognized:

- Hypertrophic: characterized by general thickening and congestion of the pharyngeal mucous membrane
- Atrophic: probably a late stage of the first type (the membrane is thin, whitish, glistening, and at times wrinkled)
- Chronic granular ("clergyman's sore throat"): characterized by numerous swollen lymph follicles on the pharyngeal wall

Clinical Manifestations

Patients with chronic pharyngitis complain of a constant sense of irritation or fullness in the throat, mucus that collects in the throat and can be expelled by coughing, and difficulty swallowing.

Medical Management

Treatment of chronic pharyngitis is based on relieving symptoms, avoiding exposure to irritants, and correcting any upper respiratory, pulmonary, or cardiac condition that might be responsible for a chronic cough.

Nasal congestion may be relieved by short-term use of nasal sprays or medications containing ephedrine sulfate (Kondon's Nasal) or phenylephrine hydrochloride (Neo-Synephrine). If there is a history of allergy, one of the antihistamine decongestant medications, such as Drixoral or Dimetapp, is taken orally every 4 to 6 hours. Aspirin or acetaminophen is recommended for its anti-inflammatory and analgesic properties.

Nursing Management

TEACHING PATIENTS SELF-CARE

To prevent the infection from spreading, the nurse instructs the patient to avoid contact with others until the fever subsides. Alcohol, tobacco, second-hand smoke, and exposure to cold are avoided, as are environmental or occupational pollutants if possible. The patient may minimize exposure to pollutants by wearing a disposable facemask. The nurse encourages the patient to drink plenty of fluids. Gargling with warm saline solutions may relieve throat discomfort. Lozenges will keep the throat moistened.

TONSILLITIS AND ADENOIDITIS

The tonsils are composed of lymphatic tissue and are situated on each side of the oropharynx. The faucial or palatine tonsils and lingual tonsils are located behind the pillars of fauces and tongue, respectively. They frequently serve as the site of acute infection (**tonsillitis**). Chronic tonsillitis is less common and may be mistaken for other disorders such as allergy, asthma, and sinusitis.

The adenoids or pharyngeal tonsils consist of lymphatic tissue near the center of the posterior wall of the nasopharynx. Infection of the adenoids frequently accompanies acute tonsillitis. Group A beta-streptococcus is the most common organism associated with tonsillitis and adenoiditis.

Clinical Manifestations

The symptoms of tonsillitis include sore throat, fever, snoring, and difficulty swallowing. Enlarged adenoids may cause mouth-breathing, earache, draining ears, frequent head colds, bronchitis, foul-smelling breath, voice impairment, and noisy respiration. Unusually enlarged adenoids fill the space behind the posterior nares, making it difficult for the air to travel from the nose to the throat and resulting in a nasal obstruction. Infection can extend to the middle ears by way of the auditory (eustachian) tubes and may result in acute otitis media, which can lead to spontaneous rupture of the eardrums and further extension of the infection into the mastoid cells, causing acute mastoiditis. The infection also may reside in the middle ear as a chronic, low-grade, smoldering process that eventually may cause permanent deafness.

Assessment and Diagnostic Findings

A thorough physical examination is performed and a careful history is obtained to rule out related or systemic conditions. The tonsillar site is cultured to determine the presence of bacterial infection. In adenoiditis, if recurrent episodes of suppurative otitis media result in hearing loss, the patient should be given a comprehensive audiometric examination (see Chap. 59).

Medical Management

Tonsillectomy is usually performed for recurrent tonsillitis when medical treatment is unsuccessful and there is severe hypertrophy, asymmetry, or peritonsillar abscess that occludes the pharynx, making swallowing difficult and endangering the airway (particularly during sleep). Enlargement of the tonsils is rarely an indication for their removal; most children normally have large tonsils, which decrease in size with age. Despite the continuing debate over the effectiveness of many tonsillectomies, the operation is still a common surgical procedure in the United States.

Tonsillectomy or adenoidectomy is indicated only if the patient has had any of the following problems: repeated bouts of tonsillitis; hypertrophy of the tonsils and adenoids that could cause obstruction and obstructive sleep apnea; repeated attacks of purulent otitis media; suspected hearing loss due to serous otitis media that has occurred in association with enlarged tonsils and adenoids; and some other conditions, such as an exacerbation of asthma or rheumatic fever. Appropriate antibiotic therapy is initiated for patients undergoing tonsillectomy or adenoidectomy. The most common antimicrobial agent is oral penicillin, which is taken for 7 days. Amoxicillin and erythromycin are alternatives.

Nursing Management

PROVIDING POSTOPERATIVE CARE

Continuous nursing observation is required in the immediate postoperative and recovery period because of the significant risk of hemorrhage. In the immediate postoperative period, the most comfortable position is prone with the head turned to the side to allow drainage from the mouth and pharynx. The nurse must not remove the oral airway until the patient's gag and swallowing reflexes have returned. The nurse applies an ice collar to the neck, and a basin and tissues are provided for the expectoration of blood and mucus.

Bleeding may be bright red if the patient expectorates blood before swallowing it. Often, however, the patient swallows the blood, which immediately becomes brown because of the action of the acidic gastric juice.

Hemorrhage is a potential complication after a tonsillectomy and adenoidectomy. If the patient vomits large amounts of dark blood or bright-red blood at frequent intervals, or if the pulse rate and temperature rise and the patient is restless, the nurse notifies the surgeon immediately. The nurse should have the following items ready for examination of the surgical site for bleeding: a light, a mirror, gauze, curved hemostats, and a waste basin.

Occasionally, suture or ligation of the bleeding vessel is required. In such cases, the patient is taken to the operating room and given general anesthesia. After ligation, continuous nursing observation and postoperative care are required, as in the initial postoperative period.

If there is no bleeding, water and ice chips may be given to the patient as soon as desired. The patient is instructed to refrain from too much talking and coughing because these activities can produce throat pain.

TEACHING PATIENTS SELF-CARE

Tonsillectomy and adenoidectomy usually do not require hospitalization and are performed as outpatient surgery with a short length of stay. Because the patient will be sent home soon after surgery, the patient and family must understand the signs and symptoms of hemorrhage. Hemorrhage usually occurs in the first 12 to 24 hours. The patient is instructed to report frank red bleeding to the physician.

Alkaline mouthwashes and warm saline solutions are useful in coping with the thick mucus and halitosis that may be present after surgery. It is important to explain to the patient that a sore throat, stiff neck, and vomiting may occur in the first 24 hours. A liquid or semiliquid diet is given for several days. Sherbet and gelatin are acceptable foods. The patient should avoid spicy, hot, acidic, or rough foods. Milk and milk products (ice cream and yogurt) may be restricted because they may make removal of mucus more difficult.

The nurse explains to the patient that halitosis and some minor ear pain may occur for the first few days. The nurse instructs the patient to avoid vigorous tooth brushing or gargling, since these actions could cause bleeding.

PERITONSILLAR ABSCESS

A peritonsillar abscess is a collection of purulent exudate between the tonsillar capsule and the surrounding tissues, including the soft palate. It is believed to develop after an acute tonsillar infection, which progresses to a local cellulitis and abscess.

Clinical Manifestations

The usual symptoms of an infection are present, together with such local symptoms as a raspy voice, odynophagia (a severe sensation of burning, squeezing pain while swallowing), **dysphagia** (difficulty swallowing), otalgia (pain in the ear), and drooling. An examination shows marked swelling of the soft palate, often occluding almost half of the opening from the mouth into the pharynx, unilateral tonsillar hypertrophy, and dehydration.

Assessment and Diagnostic Findings

Aspiration of purulent material (pus) by needle aspiration is required to make the appropriate diagnosis. The aspirated material is sent for culture and Gram's stain. A CTscan is performed when it is not possible to aspirate the abscess.

Medical Management

Antibiotics (usually penicillin) are extremely effective in controlling the infection in peritonsillar abscess. If antibiotics are prescribed early in the course of the disease, the abscess may resolve without needing to be incised.

SURGICAL MANAGEMENT

If treatment is delayed, the abscess is evacuated as soon as possible. The mucous membrane over the swelling is first sprayed with a topical anesthetic and then injected with a local anesthetic. Single or repeated needle aspirations are performed to decompress the abscess. The abscess may also be incised and drained. These procedures are performed best with the patient in the sitting position to make it easier to expectorate the pus and blood that accumulate in the pharynx. Almost immediate relief is experienced. Approximately 30% of patients with peritonsillar abscess have indications for tonsillectomy (Tierney et al., 2001).

Nursing Management

Considerable relief may be obtained by the use of topical anesthetic agents and throat irrigations or the frequent use of mouthwashes or gargles, using saline or alkaline solutions at a temperature of 105°F to 110°F (40.6°C to 43.3°C). The nurse instructs the patient to gargle at intervals of 1 or 2 hours for 24 to 36 hours. Liquids that are cool or at room temperature are usually well tolerated.

LARYNGITIS

Laryngitis, an inflammation of the larynx, often occurs as a result of voice abuse or exposure to dust, chemicals, smoke, and other pollutants, or as part of an upper respiratory tract infection.

It also may be caused by isolated infection involving only the vocal cords.

The cause of infection is almost always a virus. Bacterial invasion may be secondary. Laryngitis is usually associated with allergic rhinitis or pharyngitis. The onset of infection may be associated with exposure to sudden temperature changes, dietary deficiencies, malnutrition, and an immunosuppressed state. Laryngitis is common in the winter and is easily transmitted.

Clinical Manifestations

Signs of acute laryngitis include hoarseness or **aphonia** (complete loss of voice) and severe cough. Chronic laryngitis is marked by persistent hoarseness. Laryngitis may be a complication of upper respiratory infections.

Medical Management

Management of acute laryngitis includes resting the voice, avoiding smoking, resting, and inhaling cool steam or an aerosol. If the laryngitis is part of a more extensive respiratory infection due to a bacterial organism or if it is severe, appropriate antibacterial therapy is instituted. The majority of patients recover with conservative treatment; however, laryngitis tends to be more severe in elderly patients and may be complicated by pneumonia.

For chronic laryngitis, the treatment includes resting the voice, eliminating any primary respiratory tract infection, eliminating smoking, and avoiding second-hand smoke. Topical corticosteroids, such as beclomethasone dipropionate (Vanceril) inhalation, may also be used. These preparations have no systemic or long-lasting effects and may reduce local inflammatory reactions.

Nursing Management

The nurse instructs the patient to rest the voice and to maintain a well-humidified environment. If laryngeal secretions are present during acute episodes, expectorant agents are suggested, along with a daily fluid intake of 3 L to thin secretions.

NURSING PROCESS: THE PATIENT WITH UPPER AIRWAY INFECTION

Assessment

A health history may reveal signs and symptoms of headache, sore throat, pain around the eyes and on either side of the nose, difficulty in swallowing, cough, hoarseness, fever, stuffiness, and generalized discomfort and fatigue. Determining when the symptoms began, what precipitated them, what if anything relieves them, and what aggravates them is part of the assessment. It also is important to determine any history of allergy or the existence of a concomitant illness.

Inspection may reveal swelling, lesions, or asymmetry of the nose as well as bleeding or discharge. The nurse inspects the nasal mucosa for abnormal findings such as increased redness, swelling, or exudate, and nasal polyps, which may develop in chronic rhinitis.

The nurse palpates the frontal and maxillary sinuses for tenderness, which suggests inflammation, and then inspects the throat by having the patient open the mouth wide and take a deep breath. The tonsils and pharynx are inspected for abnormal findings such as redness, asymmetry, or evidence of drainage, ulceration, or enlargement.

Next the nurse palpates the trachea to determine the midline position in the neck and to detect any masses or deformities. The neck lymph nodes also are palpated for associated enlargement and tenderness.

Diagnosis

NURSING DIAGNOSES

Based on the assessment data, the patient's major nursing diagnoses may include the following:

- Ineffective airway clearance related to excessive mucus production secondary to retained secretions and inflammation
- Acute pain related to upper airway irritation secondary to an infection
- Impaired verbal communication related to physiologic changes and upper airway irritation secondary to infection or swelling
- Deficient fluid volume related to increased fluid loss secondary to diaphoresis associated with a fever
- Deficient knowledge regarding prevention of upper respiratory infections, treatment regimen, surgical procedure, or postoperative care

COLLABORATIVE PROBLEMS/ POTENTIAL COMPLICATIONS

Based on assessment data, potential complications may include:

- Sepsis
- Meningitis
- Peritonsillar abscess
- Otitis media
- Sinusitis

Planning and Goals

The major goals for the patient may include maintenance of a patent airway, relief of pain, maintenance of effective means of communication, normal hydration, knowledge of how to prevent upper airway infections, and absence of complications.

Nursing Interventions

MAINTAINING A PATENT AIRWAY

An accumulation of secretions can block the airway in patients with an upper airway infection. As a result, changes in the respiratory pattern occur, and the work of breathing required to get beyond the blockage increases. The nurse can implement several measures to loosen thick secretions or to keep the secretions moist so that they can be easily expectorated. Increasing fluid intake helps thin the mucus. Use of room vaporizers or steam inhalation also loosens secretions and reduces inflammation of the mucous membranes. To enhance drainage from the sinuses, the nurse instructs the patient about the best position to assume; this depends on the location of the infection or inflammation. For example, drainage for sinusitis or rhinitis is achieved in the upright position. In some conditions, topical or systemic medications, when prescribed, help to relieve nasal or throat congestion.

PROMOTING COMFORT

Upper respiratory tract infections usually produce localized discomfort. In sinusitis, pain may occur in the area of the sinuses or may produce a general headache. In pharyngitis, laryngitis, or tonsillitis, a sore throat occurs. The nurse encourages the patient to take analgesics, such as acetaminophen with codeine, as prescribed, which will help relieve this discomfort. Other helpful measures include topical anesthetic agents for symptomatic relief of herpes simplex blisters (see Chart 22-1) and sore throats, hot packs to relieve the congestion of sinusitis and promote drainage, and warm water gargles or irrigations to relieve the pain of a sore throat. The nurse encourages rest to relieve the generalized discomfort and fever that accompany many upper airway conditions (especially rhinitis, pharyngitis, and laryngitis). The nurse instructs the patient in general hygiene techniques to prevent the spread of infection. For postoperative care following tonsillectomy and adenoidectomy, an ice collar may reduce swelling and decrease bleeding.

PROMOTING COMMUNICATION

Upper airway infections may result in hoarseness or loss of speech. The nurse instructs the patient to refrain from speaking as much as possible and to communicate in writing instead, if possible. Additional strain on the vocal cords may delay full return of the voice.

ENCOURAGING FLUID INTAKE

In upper airway infections, the work of breathing and the respiratory rate increase as inflammation and secretions develop. This, in turn, may increase insensible fluid loss. Fever further increases the metabolic rate, diaphoresis, and fluid loss.

Sore throat, malaise, and fever may interfere with a patient's willingness to eat. The nurse encourages the patient to drink 2 to 3 L of fluid per day during the acute stage of airway infection, unless contraindicated, to thin secretions and promote drainage. Liquids (hot or cold) may be soothing, depending on the illness.

PROMOTING HOME AND COMMUNITY-BASED CARE

Teaching Patients Self-Care

Prevention of most upper airway infections is difficult because of the many potential causes. However, most upper respiratory infections are transmitted by hand-to-hand contact. Therefore, it is important to teach the patient and family how to minimize the spread of infection to others. Other preventive strategies are identified in Chart 22-2. The nurse advises the patient to avoid exposure to others at risk for serious illness if respiratory infection is transmitted. Those at risk include elderly adults, immunosuppressed people, and those with chronic health problems.

The nurse teaches patients and their families strategies to relieve symptoms of upper respiratory infections. These include increasing the humidity level, encouraging adequate fluid intake, getting adequate rest, using warm water gargles or irrigations and topical anesthetic agents to relieve sore throat, and applying hot packs to relieve congestion. The nurse reinforces the need to complete the treatment regimen, particularly when antibiotics are prescribed.

Continuing Care

Referral for home care is rare. However, it may be indicated for the person whose health status was compromised before the onset of the respiratory infection and for those who cannot manage self-care without assistance. In such circumstances, the home care nurse assesses the patient's respiratory status and progress in recovery. The nurse may advise elderly patients and those who would be at increased risk from a respiratory infection to consider an annual influenza vaccine. A follow-up appointment with the primary care provider may be indicated for patients with compromised health status to ensure that the respiratory infection has resolved.

MONITORING AND MANAGING POTENTIAL COMPLICATIONS

While major complications of upper respiratory infections are rare, the nurse must be aware of them and assess the patient for them. Because most patients with upper respiratory infections are managed at home, patients and their families must be instructed to monitor for signs and symptoms and to seek immediate medical care if the patient's condition does not improve or if the patient's physical status appears to be worsening.

Sepsis and meningitis may occur in patients with compromised immune status or in those with an overwhelming bacterial infection. The patient with an upper respiratory infection and family members are instructed to seek medical care if the patient's condition fails to improve within several days of the onset of symptoms, if unusual symptoms develop, or if the patient's condition deteriorates. They are instructed about signs and symptoms that require further attention: persistent or high fever, increasing shortness of breath, confusion, and increasing weakness and malaise. The patient with sepsis requires expert care to treat the infection, stabilize vital signs, and prevent or treat septicemia and shock. Deterioration of the patient's condition necessitates intensive care measures (eg, hemodynamic monitoring and administration of vasoactive medications, intravenous fluids, nutritional support, corticosteroids) to monitor the patient's status and to support the patient's vital signs. High doses of antibiotics may be administered to treat the causative organism. The nurse's role is to monitor the patient's vital signs, hemodynamic status, and laboratory values, administer needed treatment, alleviate the patient's physical discomfort, and provide explanations, teaching, and emotional support to the patient and family.

Peritonsillar abscess may develop following an acute infection of the tonsils. The patient requires treatment to drain the abscess and receives antibiotics for infection and topical anesthetic agents and throat irrigations to relieve pain and sore throat. Follow-up is necessary to ensure that the abscess resolves; tonsillectomy may be required. The nurse assists the patient in administering throat irrigations and instructs the patient and family about the importance of adhering to the prescribed treatment regimen and recommended follow-up appointments.

Otitis media and sinusitis may develop with upper respiratory infection. The patient and family are instructed about the signs and symptoms of otitis media and sinusitis and about the importance of follow-up with the primary health care practitioner to ensure adequate evaluation and treatment of these conditions.

Evaluation

EXPECTED PATIENT OUTCOMES

Expected patient outcomes may include:

1. Maintains a patent airway by managing secretions
   a. Reports decreased congestion
   b. Assumes best position to facilitate drainage of secretions
2. Reports feeling more comfortable
   a. Uses comfort measures: analgesics, hot packs, gargles, rest
   b. Demonstrates adequate oral hygiene
3. Demonstrates ability to communicate needs, wants, level of comfort

4. Maintains adequate fluid intake
5. Identifies strategies to prevent upper airway infections and allergic reactions
   a. Demonstrates hand hygiene technique
   b. Identifies the value of the influenza vaccine
6. Demonstrates an adequate level of knowledge and performs self-care adequately
7. Becomes free of signs and symptoms of infection
   a. Exhibits normal vital signs (temperature, pulse, respiratory rate)
   b. Absence of purulent drainage
   c. Free of pain in ears, sinuses, and throat

Obstruction and Trauma of the Upper Respiratory Airway

OBSTRUCTION DURING SLEEP

A variety of respiratory disorders are associated with sleep, the most common being sleep apnea syndrome. Sleep apnea syndrome is defined as cessation of breathing (**apnea**) during sleep.

Pathophysiology

Sleep apnea is classified into three types:

- Obstructive—lack of air flow due to pharyngeal occlusion
- Central—simultaneous cessation of both air flow and respiratory movements
- Mixed—a combination of central and obstructive apnea within one apneic episode

The most common type of sleep apnea syndrome, obstructive sleep apnea, will be presented here.

Clinical Manifestations

It is estimated that 12 million Americans have sleep apnea (National Institute of Health, 2000). It is more prevalent in men, especially those who are older and overweight. Cigarette smoking is a risk factor. Obstructive sleep apnea is defined as frequent and loud snoring and breathing cessation for 10 seconds or more for five episodes per hour or more, followed by awakening abruptly with a loud snort as the blood oxygen level drops. Patients with sleep apnea may experience anywhere from five apneic episodes per hour to several hundred per night. Other symptoms include excessive daytime sleepiness, morning headache, sore throat, intellectual deterioration, personality changes, behavioral disorders, enuresis, impotence, obesity, and complaints by the partner that the patient snores loudly or is unusually restless during sleep (Chart 22-3).

The obstruction may be caused by mechanical factors such as a reduced diameter of the upper airway or dynamic changes in the upper airway during sleep. The activity of the tonic dilator muscles of the upper airway is reduced during sleep. These sleep-related changes may predispose the patient to increased upper airway collapse with the small amounts of negative pressure generated during inspiration. Obstructive sleep apnea may be associated with obesity and with other conditions that reduce pharyngeal muscle tone (eg, neuromuscular disease, sedative/hypnotic medications, acute ingestion of alcohol). The diagnosis of sleep apnea is made based on clinical features plus polysomnographic findings (sleep test), in which the cardiopulmonary status of the patient is monitored during an episode of sleep.

Chart 22-3 • ASSESSMENT

Obstructive Sleep Apnea

Clinical features of obstructive sleep apnea include:
Excessive daytime sleepiness
Frequent nocturnal awakening
Insomnia
Loud snoring
Morning headaches
Intellectual deterioration
Personality changes, irritability
Impotence
Systemic hypertension
Dysrhythmias
Pulmonary hypertension, cor pulmonale
Polycythemia
Enuresis

The effects of obstructive sleep apnea can seriously tax the heart and lungs. Repetitive apneic events result in hypoxia and hypercapnia, which triggers a sympathetic response. As a consequence, patients have a high prevalence of hypertension and an increased risk of myocardial infarction and stroke. In patients with underlying cardiovascular disease, the nocturnal hypoxemia may predispose to dysrhythmias.

Medical Management

Patients usually seek medical treatment because their partners express concern or because they experience excessive sleepiness at inappropriate times or settings (eg, while driving a car). A variety of treatments are used. In mild cases, the patient is advised to avoid alcohol and medications that depress the upper airway and to lose weight. In more severe cases involving hypoxemia with severe CO_2 retention (hypercapnia), the treatment includes continuous positive airway pressure or bilevel positive airway pressure therapy with supplemental oxygen via nasal cannula. These treatment methods are described in Chapter 25.

Surgical procedures (eg, uvulopalatopharyngoplasty) may be performed to correct the obstruction. As a last resort, a tracheostomy is performed to bypass the obstruction if the potential for respiratory failure or life-threatening dysrhythmias exists. The tracheostomy is unplugged only during sleep. Although this is an effective treatment, it is used in a limited number of patients because of its associated physical disfigurement (Murray & Nadel, 2001).

PHARMACOLOGIC THERAPY

Treatment of central sleep apnea also includes medication. Protriptyline (Triptil) given at bedtime is thought to increase the respiratory drive and improve upper airway muscle tone. Medroxyprogesterone acetate (Provera) and acetazolamide (Diamox) have been recommended for sleep apnea associated with chronic alveolar hypoventilation, but their benefits have not been well established. Administration of low-flow nasal oxygen at night can help relieve hypoxemia in some patients but has little effect on the frequency or severity of apnea.

Nursing Management

The patient with obstructive sleep apnea may not recognize the potential consequences of the disorder. Therefore, the nurse explains the disorder in language that is understandable to the patient and relates symptoms (daytime sleepiness) to the underlying disorder. The nurse also instructs the patient and family about treatments, including the correct and safe use of oxygen, if prescribed.

EPISTAXIS (NOSEBLEED)

A hemorrhage from the nose, referred to as **epistaxis**, is caused by the rupture of tiny, distended vessels in the mucous membrane of any area of the nose. Rarely does epistaxis originate in the densely vascular tissue over the turbinates. Most commonly, the site is the anterior septum, where three major blood vessels enter the nasal cavity: (1) the anterior ethmoidal artery on the forward part of the roof (Kesselbach's plexus), (2) the sphenopalatine artery in the posterosuperior region, and (3) the internal maxillary branches (the plexus of veins located at the back of the lateral wall under the inferior turbinate).

There are a variety of causes associated with epistaxis, including trauma, infection, inhalation of illicit drugs, cardiovascular diseases, blood dyscrasias, nasal tumors, low humidity, a foreign body in the nose, and a deviated nasal septum. Additionally, vigorous nose blowing and nose picking have been associated with epistaxis.

Medical Management

Management of epistaxis depends on the location of the bleeding site. A nasal speculum or headlight may be used to determine the site of bleeding in the nasal cavity. Most nosebleeds originate from the anterior portion of the nose. Initial treatment may include applying direct pressure. The patient sits upright with the head tilted forward to prevent swallowing and aspiration of blood and is directed to pinch the soft outer portion of the nose against the midline septum for 5 or 10 minutes continuously. If this measure is unsuccessful, additional treatment is indicated. In anterior nosebleeds, the area may be treated with a silver nitrate applicator and Gelfoam, or by electrocautery. Topical vasoconstrictors,

such as adrenaline (1 : 1,000), cocaine (0.5%), and phenylephrine may be prescribed.

If bleeding is occurring from the posterior regions, cotton pledgets soaked in a vasoconstricting solution may be inserted into the nose to reduce the blood flow and improve the examiner's view of the bleeding site. Alternatively, a cotton tampon may be used to try to stop the bleeding. Suction may be used to remove excess blood and clots from the field of inspection. The search for the bleeding site should shift from the anteroinferior quadrant to the anterosuperior, then to the posterosuperior, and finally to the posteroinferior area. The field is kept clear by using suction and by shifting the cotton tampon. Only about 60% of the total nasal cavity can actually be seen, however.

When the origin of the bleeding cannot be identified, the nose may be packed with gauze impregnated with petrolatum jelly or antibiotic ointment; a topical anesthetic spray and decongestant agent may be used prior to inserting the gauze packing, or a balloon-inflated catheter may be used (Fig. 22-4). The packing may remain in place for 48 hours or up to 5 or 6 days if necessary to control bleeding. Antibiotics may be prescribed because of the risk of iatrogenic sinusitis and toxic shock syndrome.

Nursing Management

The nurse monitors the vital signs, assists in the control of bleeding, and provides tissues and an emesis basin to allow the patient to expectorate any excess blood. It is not uncommon for patients to be anxious in response to a nosebleed. Blood loss on clothing and handkerchiefs can be frightening, and the nasal examination and treatment are uncomfortable. Assuring the patient in a calm, efficient manner that bleeding can be controlled can help reduce anxiety.

TEACHING PATIENTS SELF-CARE
Discharge teaching includes reviewing ways to prevent epistaxis: avoiding forceful nose blowing, straining, high altitudes, and

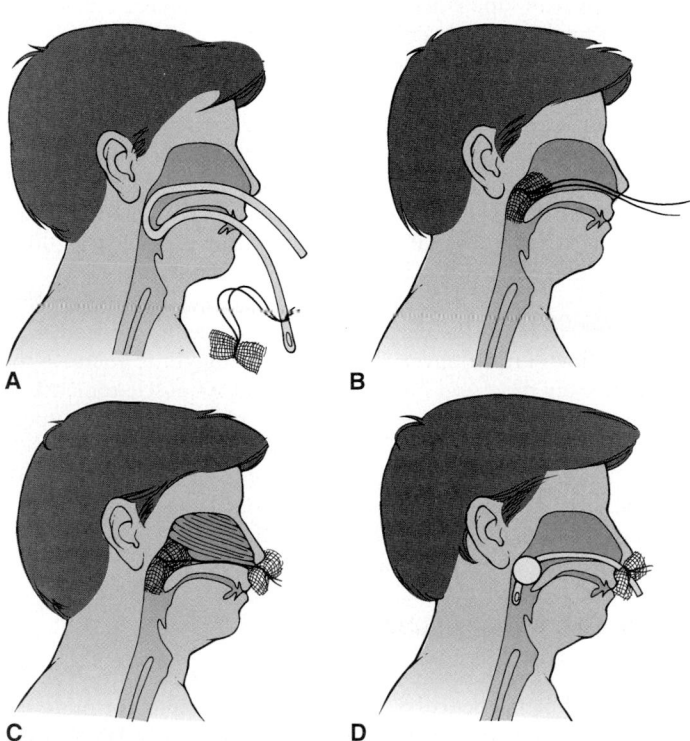

A   **B**

C   **D**

FIGURE 22-4 Packing to control bleeding from the posterior nose. (**A**) Catheter is inserted and packing is attached. (**B**) Packing is drawn into position as the catheter is removed. (**C**) Strip is tied over a bolster to hold the packing in place with an anterior pack installed "accordion pleat" style. (**D**) Alternative method, using a balloon catheter instead of gauze packing.

nasal trauma (including nose picking). Adequate humidification may prevent drying of the nasal passages. The nurse instructs the patient how to apply direct pressure to the nose with the thumb and the index finger for 15 minutes in the case of a recurrent nosebleed. If recurrent bleeding cannot be stopped, the patient is instructed to seek additional medical attention.

NASAL OBSTRUCTION

The passage of air through the nostrils is frequently obstructed by a deviation of the nasal septum, hypertrophy of the turbinate bones, or the pressure of nasal polyps, which are grapelike swellings that arise from the mucous membrane of the sinuses, especially the ethmoids. This obstruction also may lead to a condition of chronic infection of the nose and result in frequent episodes of nasopharyngitis. Frequently, the infection extends to the sinuses of the nose. When sinusitis develops and the drainage from these cavities is obstructed by deformity or swelling within the nose, pain is experienced in the region of the affected sinus.

Medical Management

The treatment of nasal obstruction requires the removal of the obstruction, followed by measures to overcome whatever chronic infection exists. In many patients an underlying allergy requires treatment. At times endoscopic surgery is necessary to drain the nasal sinuses. The specific procedure performed depends on the type of nasal obstruction found. Usually, surgery is performed under local anesthesia.

If a deviation of the septum is the cause of the obstruction, the surgeon makes an incision into the mucous membrane and, after raising it from the bone, removes the deviated bone and cartilage with bone forceps. The mucosa then is allowed to fall back in place and is held there by tight packing. Generally, the packing is soaked in liquid petrolatum so that it can be removed easily in 24 to 36 hours. This operation is called a **submucous resection** or septoplasty.

Nasal polyps are removed by clipping them at their base with a wire snare. Hypertrophied turbinates may be treated by applying an astringent agent to shrink them.

Nursing Management

Most of these procedures are performed on an outpatient basis. If the patient is hospitalized, the nurse elevates the head of the bed to promote drainage and to help alleviate discomfort from edema. Frequent oral hygiene is encouraged to overcome dryness caused by breathing through the mouth.

FRACTURES OF THE NOSE

The location of the nose makes it susceptible to injury by a wide variety of causes. In fact, nasal fractures are more common than those of any other bone in the body. Fractures of the nose usually result from a direct assault. As a rule, no serious consequences result, but the deformity that may follow often gives rise to obstruction of the nasal air passages and to facial disfigurement.

Clinical Manifestations

The signs and symptoms of a nasal fracture are bleeding from the nose externally and internally into the pharynx, swelling of the soft tissues adjacent to the nose, and deformity.

Assessment and Diagnostic Findings

The nose is examined internally to rule out the possibility that the injury may be complicated by a fracture of the nasal septum and a submucosal septal hematoma. Because of the swelling and bleeding that occur with a nasal fracture, an accurate diagnosis can be made only after the swelling subsides.

Clear fluid draining from either nostril suggests a fracture of the cribriform plate with leakage of cerebrospinal fluid. Because cerebrospinal fluid contains glucose, it can readily be differentiated from nasal mucus by means of a dipstick (Dextrostix). Usually, careful inspection or palpation will disclose any deviations of the bone or disruptions of the nasal cartilages. An x-ray may reveal displacement of the fractured bones and may help rule out extension of the fracture into the skull.

Medical Management

As a rule, bleeding is controlled with the use of cold compresses. The nose is assessed for symmetry either before swelling has occurred or after it has subsided. The patient is referred to a specialist, usually 3 to 5 days after the injury, to evaluate the need to realign the bones. Nasal fractures are surgically reduced 7 to 10 days after the injury.

Nursing Management

The nurse instructs the patient to apply ice packs to the nose for 20 minutes four times each day to decrease swelling. The patient who experiences bleeding from the nose (epistaxis) because of injury or for unexplained reasons is usually frightened and anxious. The packing inserted to stop the bleeding may be uncomfortable and unpleasant, and obstruction of the nasal passages by the packing forces the patient to breathe through the mouth. This in turn causes the oral mucous membranes to become dry. Mouth rinses will help to moisten the mucous membranes and to reduce the odor and taste of dried blood in the oropharynx and nasopharynx.

LARYNGEAL OBSTRUCTION

Edema of the larynx is a serious, often fatal, condition. The larynx is a stiff box that will not stretch. It contains a narrow space between the vocal cords (glottis) through which air must pass. Swelling of the laryngeal mucous membranes, therefore, may close off the opening tightly, leading to suffocation. Edema of the glottis occurs rarely in patients with acute laryngitis, occasionally in patients with urticaria, and more frequently in patients with severe inflammations of the throat, as in scarlet fever. It is an occasional cause of death in severe anaphylaxis (angioneurotic edema).

Foreign bodies frequently are aspirated into the pharynx, the larynx, or the trachea and cause a twofold problem. First, they obstruct the air passages and cause difficulty in breathing, which may lead to asphyxia; later, they may be drawn farther down, entering the bronchi or a bronchial branch and causing symptoms of irritation, such as a croupy cough, expectoration of blood or mucus, or labored breathing. The physical signs and x-ray findings confirm the diagnosis.

Medical Management

When the obstruction is caused by edema resulting from an allergic reaction, treatment includes administering subcutaneous epinephrine or a corticosteroid (see Chap. 53) and applying an ice pack to the neck. In emergencies caused by obstruction by a foreign body, when signs of asphyxia are apparent, immediate treatment is necessary. Frequently, if the foreign body has lodged in the pharynx and can be visualized, the finger can dislodge it.

If the obstruction is in the larynx or the trachea, the nurse or other rescuer tries the subdiaphragmatic abdominal thrust maneuver (Chart 22-4). If all efforts are unsuccessful, an immediate tracheotomy is necessary (see Chap. 25 for further discussion).

Cancer of the Larynx

Cancer of the larynx is a malignant tumor in the larynx (voice box). It is potentially curable if detected early. It represents less than 1% of all cancers and occurs about four times more frequently in men than in women, and most commonly in persons 50 to 70 years of age. The incidence of laryngeal cancer continues to decline, but the incidence in women versus men continues to increase. Each year in the United States, approximately 9,000 new cases are discovered, and 3,700 persons with cancer of the larynx will die (American Cancer Society, 2002).

Carcinogens that have been associated with the development of laryngeal cancer include tobacco (smoke, smokeless) and alcohol and their combined effects, exposure to asbestos, mustard gas, wood dust, cement dust, tar products, leather, and metals. Other contributing factors include straining the voice, chronic laryngitis, nutritional deficiencies (riboflavin), and family predisposition (Chart 22-5).

A malignant growth may occur in three different areas of the larynx: the glottic area (vocal cords), supraglottic area (area above the glottis or vocal cords, including epiglottis and false cords), and subglottis (area below the glottis or vocal cords to the cricoid). Two thirds of laryngeal cancers are in the glottic area. Supraglottic cancers account for approximately one third of the cases, subglottic tumors for less than 1%. Glottic tumors seldom spread if found early because of the limited lymph vessels found in the vocal cords (Lenhard, Osteen, & Gansler, 2001).

Chart 22-5
Risk Factors for Laryngeal Cancer

Carcinogens
Tobacco (smoke, smokeless)
Combined effects of alcohol and tobacco
Asbestos
Second-hand smoke
Paint fumes
Wood dust
Cement dust
Chemicals
Tar products
Mustard gas
Leather and metals

Other Factors
Straining the voice
Chronic laryngitis
Nutritional deficiencies (riboflavin)
History of alcohol abuse
Familial predisposition
Age (higher incidence after 60 years of age)
Gender (more common in men)
Race (more prevalent in African Americans)
Weakened immune system

Clinical Manifestations

Hoarseness of more than 2 weeks' duration is noted early in the patient with cancer in the glottic area because the tumor impedes the action of the vocal cords during speech. The voice may sound harsh, raspy, and lower in pitch. Affected voice sounds are not early signs of subglottic or supraglottic cancer. The patient may complain of a cough or sore throat that does not go away and pain and burning in the throat, especially when consuming hot liquids or citrus juices. A lump may be felt in the neck. Later symptoms include dysphagia, dyspnea (difficulty breathing), unilateral nasal

Chart 22-4   Performing the Abdominal Thrust Maneuver

To assist a patient or other person who is choking on a foreign object, the nurse performs the abdominal thrust maneuver (sometimes called the Heimlich maneuver) according to guidelines set forth by the American Heart Association. (*Note:* Hands crossed at the neck is the universal sign for choking.)

1. Stand behind the person who is choking.
2. Place both arms around the person's waist.
3. Make a fist with one hand with the thumb outside the fist.
4. Place thumb side of fist against the person's abdomen above the navel and below the xiphoid process.
5. Grasp fist with other hand.
6. Quickly and forcefully exert pressure against the person's diaphragm, pressing upward with quick, firm thrusts.
7. Apply thrusts 6 to 10 times until the obstruction is cleared.
8. The pressure from the thrusts should lift the diaphragm, force air into the lungs, and create an artificial cough powerful enough to expel the aspirated object.

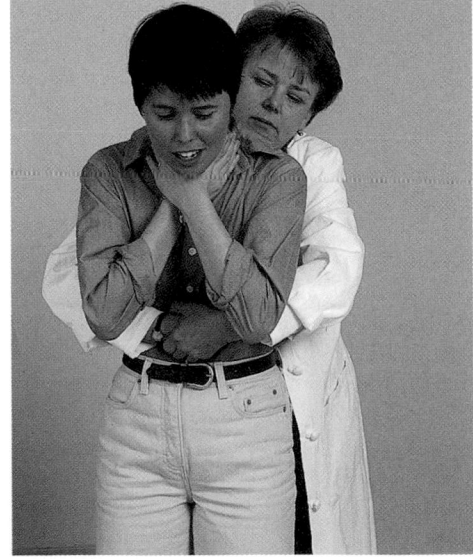

obstruction or discharge, persistent hoarseness, persistent ulceration, and foul breath. Cervical lymph adenopathy, unplanned weight loss, a general debilitated state, and pain radiating to the ear may occur with metastasis.

Assessment and Diagnostic Findings

An initial assessment includes a complete history and physical examination of the head and neck. This will include assessment of risk factors, family history, and any underlying medical conditions. An indirect laryngoscopy, using a flexible endoscope, is initially performed in the otolaryngologist's office to visually evaluate the pharynx, larynx, and possible tumor. Mobility of the vocal cords is assessed; if normal movement is limited, the growth may affect muscle, other tissue, and even the airway. The lymph nodes of the neck and the thyroid gland are palpated to determine spread of the malignancy (Haskell, 2001).

If a tumor of the larynx is suspected on an initial examination, a direct laryngoscopic examination is scheduled. This examination is done under local or general anesthesia and allows evaluation of all areas of the larynx. Samples of the suspicious tissue are obtained for histologic evaluation. The tumor may involve any of the three areas of the larynx and may vary in appearance.

Squamous cell carcinoma accounts for over 90% of the cases of laryngeal carcinoma (Haskell, 2001). The staging of the tumor serves as a framework for the therapeutic regimen. The TNM classification system, developed by the American Joint Committee on Cancer (AJCC) (Chart 22-6), is the accepted method used to classify head and neck tumors. The classification of the tumor determines the suggested treatment modalities. Because many of

---

Chart 22-6 — Staging System for Cancer of Larynx: Tumor-Node-Metastasis (TNM) System

Primary Tumor (T)

TX: Primary tumor cannot be assessed
T0: No evidence of primary tumor
Tis: Carcinoma in situ

Supraglottis

T1: Tumor limited to one subsite of supraglottis with normal vocal cord mobility
T2: Tumor invades mucosa of more than one adjacent subsite of supraglottis or glottis or region outside the supraglottis (eg, mucosa of base of tongue, vallecula, medial wall of pyriform sinus) without fixation of the larynx
T3: Tumor limited to larynx with vocal cord fixation and/or invades any of the following: postcricoid area, pre-epiglottic tissues, paraglottic space, and/or minor thyroid cartilage erosion (eg, inner cortex)
T4a: Tumor invades through the thyroid cartilage, and/or invades tissues beyond the larynx (eg, trachea, soft tissues of neck including deep extrinsic muscle of the tongue, strap muscles, thyroid, or esophagus)
T4b: Tumor invades prevertebral space, encases carotid artery, or invades mediastinal structures

Glottis

T1: Tumor limited to vocal cord(s) (may involve anterior or posterior commissure) with normal mobility
T1a: Tumor limited to one vocal cord
T1b: Tumor involves both vocal cords
T2: Tumor extends to supraglottis and/or subglottis, and/or with impaired vocal cord mobility
T3: Tumor limited to the larynx with vocal cord fixation and/or invades paraglottic space, and or minor thyroid cartilage erosion (eg, inner cortex)
T4a: Tumor invades through the thyroid cartilage and/or invades tissues beyond the larynx (eg, trachea, soft tissues of neck including deep extrinsic muscle of the tongue, strap muscles, thyroid, or esophagus)
T4b: Tumor invades prevertebral space, encases carotid artery, or invades mediastinal structures

Subglottis

T1: Tumor limited to the subglottis
T2: Tumor extends to vocal cord(s) with normal or impaired mobility
T3: Tumor limited to larynx with vocal cord fixation

T4a: Tumor invades cricoid or thyroid cartilage and/or invades tissues beyond the larynx (eg, trachea, soft tissues of neck including deep extrinsic muscles of the tongue, strap muscles, thyroid, or esophagus)
T4b: Tumor invades prevertebral space, encases carotid artery, or invades mediastinal structures

Regional Lymph Nodes (N)

NX: Regional lymph nodes cannot be assessed
N0: No regional lymph node metastasis
N1: Metastasis in single ipsilateral lymph node, 3 cm or less in greatest dimension
N2: Metastasis in single ipsilateral lymph node, more than 3 cm but not more than 6 cm in greatest dimension, or in multiple ipsilateral lymph nodes, none more than 6 cm in greatest dimension, or in bilateral or contralateral lymph nodes, none more than 6 cm in greatest dimension
   N2a: Metastasis in a single ipsilateral lymph node more than 3 cm but not more than 6 cm in greatest dimension
   N2b: Metastasis in multiple ipsilateral lymph nodes, none more than 6 cm in greatest dimension
   N2c: Metastasis in bilateral or contralateral lymph nodes, none more than 6 cm in greatest dimension
N3: Metastasis in a lymph node more than 6 cm in greatest dimension

Distant Metastasis (M)

MX: Distant metastasis cannot be assessed
M0: No distant metastasis
M1: Distant metastasis

Stage Grouping

Stage	T	N	M
Stage 0	Tis	N0	M0
Stage I	T1	N0	M0
Stage II	T2	N0	M0
Stage III	T3	N0	M0
	T1	N1	M0
	T2	N1	M0
	T3	N1	M0
Stage IV A	T4a	N0	M0
	T4a	N1	M0
	Any T	N2	M0
Stage IV B	Any T	N3	M0
Stage IV C	Any T	Any N	M1

Used with the permission of the American Joint Committee on Cancer (AJCC), Chicago, Illinois. The original source for this material is the *AJCC Cancer Staging Manual, Sixth Edition* (2002) published by Springer-Verlag, New York, www.springer-ny.com.

these lesions are submucosal, biopsy may require that an incision be made using microlaryngeal techniques or using a CO_2 laser to transect the mucosa and reach the tumor.

Computed tomography and magnetic resonance imaging (MRI) are used to assess regional adenopathy and soft tissue and to help stage and determine the extent of a tumor. MRI is also helpful in post-treatment follow-up in order to detect a recurrence. Positron emission tomography (PET scan) may also be used to detect recurrence of a laryngeal tumor after treatment.

Medical Management

Treatment of laryngeal cancer depends on the staging of the tumor, which includes the location, size, and histology of the tumor and the presence and extent of cervical lymph node involvement. Treatment options include surgery, radiation therapy, and chemotherapy. The prognosis depends on a variety of factors: tumor stage, the patient's gender and age, and pathologic features of the tumor, including the grade and depth of infiltration. The treatment plan also depends on whether this is an initial diagnosis or a recurrence. Small glottic tumors, stage I and II, with no infiltration to the lymph nodes are associated with a 75% to 95% survival rate. Patients with stage III and IV or advanced tumors have a 50% to 60% survival rate and have a 50% chance of recurrence and a 30% chance of metastasis. The highest risk of laryngeal cancer recurrence is in the first 2 to 3 years. Recurrence after 5 years is rare and is usually due to a new primary malignancy (Lenhard et al., 2001) (Chart 22-7).

Surgery and radiation therapy are both effective methods in the early stages of cancer of the larynx. Chemotherapy traditionally has been used for recurrence or metastatic disease. It has also been used more recently in conjunction with either radiation

therapy to avoid a total laryngectomy or preoperatively to shrink a tumor before surgery. A complete dental examination is performed to rule out any oral disease. Any dental problems are resolved, if possible, prior to surgery. If surgery is to be performed, a multidisciplinary team evaluates the needs of the patient and family to develop a successful plan of care (Forastiere et al., 2001).

SURGICAL MANAGEMENT

Recent advances in surgical techniques for treating laryngeal cancer may minimize the ensuing cosmetic and functional deficits. Depending on the location and staging of the tumor, four different types of **laryngectomy** (surgical removal of part or all of the larynx and surrounding structures) are considered:

- Partial laryngectomy
- Supraglottic laryngectomy
- Hemilaryngectomy
- Total laryngectomy

Some microlaryngeal surgery can be performed endoscopically. The CO_2 laser can be used for the treatment of many laryngeal tumors, with the exception of large vascular tumors.

Partial Laryngectomy. A partial laryngectomy (laryngofissure–thyrotomy) is recommended in the early stages of cancer in the glottic area when only one vocal cord is involved. The surgery is associated with a very high cure rate. It may also be performed for a recurrence when high-dose radiation has failed. A portion of the larynx is removed, along with one vocal cord and the tumor; all other structures remain. The airway remains intact and the patient is expected to have no difficulty swallowing. The voice quality may change or the patient may be hoarse.

Supraglottic Laryngectomy. A supraglottic laryngectomy is indicated in the management of early (stage I) supraglottic and stage II lesions. The hyoid bone, glottis, and false cords are removed. The true vocal cords, cricoid cartilage, and trachea remain intact. During surgery, a radical neck dissection is performed on the involved side. A tracheostomy tube (see Chap. 25) is left in the trachea until the glottic airway is established. It is usually removed after a few days and the stoma is allowed to close. Nutrition is provided through a nasogastric tube until there is healing, followed by a semisolid diet. Postoperatively, the patient may experience some difficulty swallowing for the first 2 weeks. Aspiration is a potential complication since the patient must learn a new method of swallowing (supraglottic swallowing). The chief advantage of this surgical procedure is that it preserves the voice, even though the quality of the voice may change. Speech therapy is required before and after surgery. The major problem is the high risk for recurrence of the cancer; therefore, patients are selected carefully.

Hemilaryngectomy. A hemilaryngectomy is performed when the tumor extends beyond the vocal cord but is less than 1 cm in size and is limited to the subglottic area. It may be used in stage I glottic lesions. In this procedure, the thyroid cartilage of the larynx is split in the midline of the neck and the portion of the vocal cord (one true cord and one false cord) is removed with the tumor. The arytenoid cartilage and half of the thyroid are removed. The patient will have a tracheostomy tube and nasogastric tube in place for 10 to 14 days following surgery. The patient is at risk for aspiration postoperatively. Some change may occur in the voice quality. The voice may be rough, raspy, and hoarse and have limited projection. The airway and swallowing remain intact.

Chart 22-7 • Ethics and Related Issues

Situation
A 68-year-old attorney was diagnosed with cancer of the larynx 8 years ago. He was treated successfully with radiation therapy, resulting in an altered voice quality. Recently, he has complained of shortness of breath and difficulty swallowing. In the past few months, he also has noticed a marked change in his voice and physical condition, which he attributed to "winter colds."

After a complete physical exam and an extensive diagnostic workup and biopsy, it is determined that the cancer has recurred at a new primary site. His health care provider recommends surgery (a total laryngectomy) and chemotherapy as the best options. The patient states that he is not willing to "lose my voice and my livelihood" but instead will "take my chances." He has also expressed concern about his quality of life after surgery. His family has approached you about trying to convince him to have surgery.

Dilemma
The patient's right to refuse treatment conflicts with the family's wishes and recommendation from his health care provider.

Discussion
1. Is the patient making a decision based upon all pertinent information concerning his health status, treatment, options, risk/benefits, and long-term prognosis?
2. What arguments can be made to support the patient's decision to forego treatment?
3. What arguments can be made to question the patient's decision to forego treatment?

Total Laryngectomy. A total laryngectomy is performed in the most advanced stage IV laryngeal cancer, when the tumor extends beyond the vocal cords, or for recurrent or persistent cancer following radiation therapy. In a total laryngectomy, the laryngeal structures are removed, including the hyoid bone, epiglottis, cricoid cartilage, and two or three rings of the trachea. The tongue, pharyngeal walls, and trachea are preserved. A total laryngectomy will result in permanent loss of the voice and a change in the airway.

Many surgeons recommend that a radical neck dissection be performed on the same side as the lesion even if no lymph nodes are palpable because metastasis to the cervical lymph nodes is common. Surgery is more difficult when the lesion involves the midline structures or both vocal cords. With or without neck dissection, a total laryngectomy requires a permanent tracheal stoma because the larynx that provides the protective sphincter is no longer present. The tracheal stoma prevents the aspiration of food and fluid into the lower respiratory tract. The patient will have no voice but will have normal swallowing. A total laryngectomy changes the manner in which airflow is used for breathing and speaking, as depicted in Figure 22-5. Complications that may occur include a salivary leak, wound infection from the development of a pharyngocutaneous fistula, stomal stenosis, and dysphagia secondary to pharyngeal and cervical esophageal stricture.

RADIATION THERAPY

The goal of radiation therapy is to eradicate the cancer and preserve the function of the larynx. The decision to use radiation therapy is based on several factors, including the staging of the tumor (usually used for stage I and stage II tumors as a standard treatment option) and the patient's overall health status, lifestyle (including occupation), and personal preference. Excellent results have been achieved with radiation therapy in patients with early-stage (I and II) glottic tumors when only one vocal cord is involved and there is normal mobility (ie, moves with phonation) and in small supraglottic lesions. One of the benefits of radiation therapy is that patients retain a near-normal voice. A few may develop chondritis (inflammation of the cartilage) or stenosis; a small number may later require laryngectomy.

Radiation therapy may also be used preoperatively to reduce the tumor size. Radiation therapy is combined with surgery in advanced (stages III and IV) laryngeal cancer as adjunctive therapy to surgery or chemotherapy, and as a palliative measure. A variety of clinical trials have combined chemotherapy and radiation therapy in the treatment of advanced laryngeal tumors. Early studies suggest that combined modality therapy may improve the tumor's response to radiation therapy. Radiation therapy combined with chemotherapy may be an alternative to a total laryngectomy.

The complications from radiation therapy are a result of external radiation to the head and neck area, which may also include the parotid gland responsible for mucus production. The symptoms may include acute mucositis, ulceration of the mucous membranes, pain, **xerostomia** (dry mouth), loss of taste, dysphasia, fatigue, and skin reactions. Later complications may include laryngeal necrosis, edema, and fibrosis.

SPEECH THERAPY

The loss or alteration of speech is discussed with the patient and family before surgery, and the speech therapist conducts a preoperative evaluation. During this time, the nurse should inform the patient and family about methods of communication that will be available in the immediate postoperative period. These include

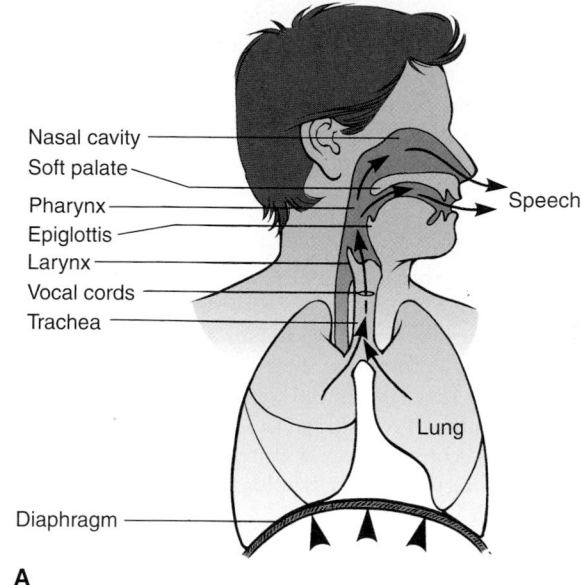

A

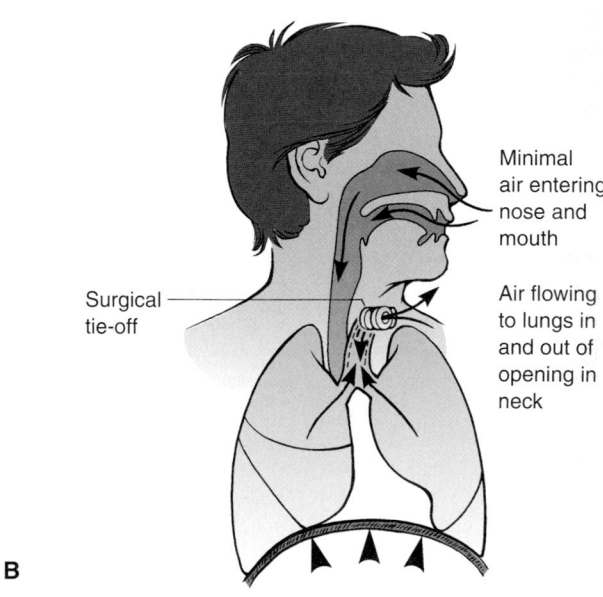

B

FIGURE 22-5 Total laryngectomy produces a change in airflow for breathing and speaking. (**A**) Normal airflow. (**B**) Airflow after total laryngectomy.

writing, lip speaking, and communication or word boards. A system of communication is established with the patient, family, nurse, and physician and implemented consistently after surgery.

A postoperative communication plan is also developed. The three most common techniques of **alaryngeal communication** are esophageal speech, artificial larynx (electrolarynx), and tracheoesophageal puncture. Training in these techniques begins once medical clearance is obtained from the physician.

Esophageal Speech. Esophageal speech was the primary method of alaryngeal speech taught to patients until the 1980s. The patient needs the ability to compress air into the esophagus and expel it, setting off a vibration of the pharyngeal esophageal segment. The technique can be taught once the patient begins oral feedings, approximately 1 week after surgery. First, the patient learns to belch and is reminded to do so an hour after eating. Then the technique is practiced repeatedly. Later, this conscious belching action is transformed into simple explosions of air from the esophagus for speech purposes. Thereafter, the speech therapist works with the patient in an attempt to make speech intelligible and as close to normal as possible. Because it takes a long time to become proficient, the success rate is low.

Electric Larynx. If esophageal speech is not successful, or until the patient masters the technique, an electric larynx may be used for communication. This battery-powered apparatus projects sound into the oral cavity. When the mouth forms words (articulated), the sounds from the electric larynx become audible words. The voice that is produced sounds mechanical, and some words may be difficult to distinguish. The advantage is that the patient is able to communicate with relative ease while working to become proficient at either esophageal or tracheoesophageal puncture speech.

Tracheoesophageal Puncture. The third technique of alaryngeal speech is tracheoesophageal puncture (Fig. 22-6). This technique is the most widely used because the speech associated with it most resembles normal speech (the sound produced is a combination of esophageal speech and voice), and it is easily learned. A valve is placed in the tracheal stoma to divert air into the esophagus and out of the mouth. Once the puncture is surgically created and has healed, a voice prosthesis (Blom–Singer) is fitted over the puncture site. To prevent airway obstruction, the prosthesis is removed and cleaned when mucus builds up. A speech therapist teaches the patient how to produce sounds. Moving the tongue and lips to form the sound into words produces speech as before. Tracheoesophageal speech is successful in 80% to 90% of patients (DeLisa & Gans, 1998).

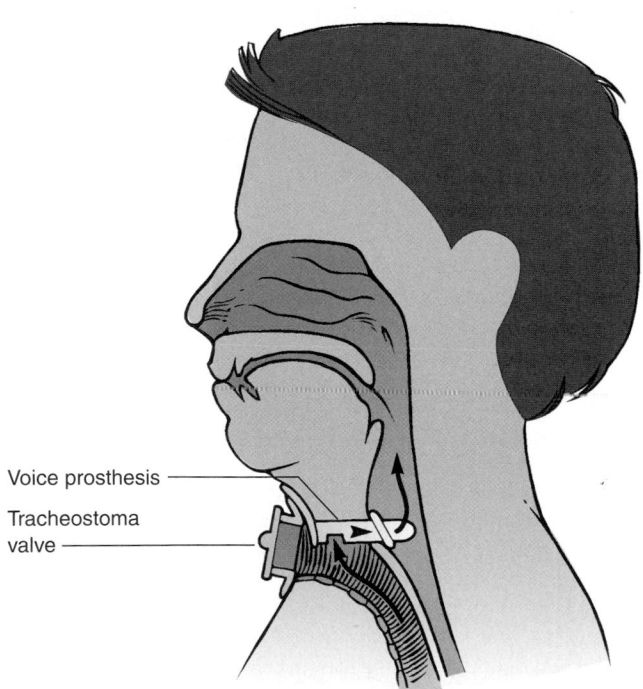

Voice prosthesis
Tracheostoma valve

FIGURE 22-6 Schematic representation of tracheoesophageal puncture speech (TEP). Air travels from the lung through a puncture in the posterior wall of the trachea into the esophagus and out the mouth. A voice prosthesis is fitted over the puncture site.

NURSING PROCESS: THE PATIENT UNDERGOING LARYNGECTOMY

Assessment

The nurse assesses the patient for the following symptoms: hoarseness, sore throat, dyspnea, dysphagia, or pain and burning in the throat. The neck is palpated for swelling.

If treatment includes surgery, the nurse must know the nature of the surgery to plan appropriate care. If the patient is expected to have no voice, a preoperative evaluation by the speech therapist is indicated. The patient's ability to hear, see, read, and write is assessed. Visual impairment and functional illiteracy may create additional problems with communication and require creative approaches to ensure that the patient is able to communicate any needs.

In addition, the nurse determines the psychological readiness of the patient and family. The idea of cancer is terrifying to most people. Fear is compounded by the possibility of permanently losing one's voice and, in some cases, of having some degree of disfigurement. The nurse evaluates the patient's and family's coping methods to support them effectively both preoperatively and postoperatively.

Diagnosis

NURSING DIAGNOSES

Based on all the assessment data, major nursing diagnoses may include the following:

- Deficient knowledge about the surgical procedure and postoperative course
- Anxiety and depression related to the diagnosis of cancer and impending surgery
- Ineffective airway clearance related to excess mucus production secondary to surgical alterations in the airway
- Impaired verbal communication related to anatomic deficit secondary to removal of the larynx and to edema
- Imbalanced nutrition: less than body requirements, related to inability to ingest food secondary to swallowing difficulties
- Disturbed body image and low self-esteem secondary to major neck surgery, change in the structure and function of the larynx
- Self-care deficit related to pain, weakness, fatigue, musculoskeletal impairment related to surgical procedure and postoperative course

COLLABORATIVE PROBLEMS/ POTENTIAL COMPLICATIONS

Based on assessment data, potential complications that may develop include:

- Respiratory distress (hypoxia, airway obstruction, tracheal edema)
- Hemorrhage
- Infection
- Wound breakdown

Planning and Goals

The major goals for the patient may include attainment of an adequate level of knowledge, reduction in anxiety, maintenance of a patent airway (patient is able to handle own secretions), effective use of alternative means of communication, attainment of optimal levels of nutrition and hydration, improvement in body image and self-esteem, improved self-care management, and absence of complications.

Nursing Interventions

TEACHING THE PATIENT PREOPERATIVELY

The diagnosis of laryngeal cancer is associated with misconceptions and fears. Many people assume that loss of speech and disfigurement are inevitable with this condition. Once the physician explains the diagnosis to the patient, the nurse clarifies any misconceptions by identifying the location of the larynx, its function, the nature of the surgical procedure, and its effect on speech. Informational materials (written and audiovisual) about the surgery are given to the patient and family for review and reinforcement.

If a complete laryngectomy is planned, the patient should know that the natural voice will be lost, but that special training can provide a means for communicating. However, the ability to sing, laugh, or whistle will be lost. Until this training is initiated, the patient needs to know that communication will be possible by using the call light or special communication board and by writing. The nurse answers questions about the nature of the surgery and reinforces the physician's explanation that the patient will lose the ability to vocalize, but that a rehabilitation program is available. The multidisciplinary team conducts an initial assessment of the patient and family. The team might include the nurse, physician, respiratory therapist, speech therapist, clinical nurse specialist, social worker, dietitian, and home care nurse.

Next, the nurse reviews equipment and treatments for postoperative care with the patient and family, teaches important coughing and deep-breathing exercises, and assists the patient to perform a return demonstration. The nurse clarifies the patient's role in the postoperative and rehabilitation periods.

REDUCING ANXIETY AND DEPRESSION

Because surgery of the larynx is performed most commonly for a malignant tumor, the patient may have many questions: Will the surgeon be able to remove all of the tumor? Is it cancer? Will I die? Will I choke? Will I suffocate? Will I ever speak again? What will I look like? The psychological preparation of the patient is as important as the physical preparation.

Any patient undergoing surgery may have many fears. In laryngeal surgery, these fears may relate to the diagnosis of cancer and may be compounded by the possibility of permanent loss of the voice and disfigurement. The nurse provides the patient and family with opportunities to ask questions, verbalize feelings, and discuss perceptions. It is important to address any questions and misconceptions the patient and family have. During the preoperative or postoperative period, a visit from someone who has had a laryngectomy may reassure the patient that people are available to help and that rehabilitation is possible.

MAINTAINING A PATENT AIRWAY

The nurse promotes a patent airway by positioning the patient in the semi-Fowler's or Fowler's position after recovery from anesthesia. Observing the patient for restlessness, labored breathing, apprehension, and increased pulse rate helps the nurse identify possible respiratory or circulatory problems. Medications that depress respiration, particularly opioids, should be used cautiously. As with other surgical patients, the nurse encourages the laryngectomy patient to turn, cough, and take deep breaths. If necessary, suctioning may be performed to remove secretions. The

nurse also encourages and assists the patient with early ambulation to prevent atelectasis and pneumonia.

If a total laryngectomy was performed, a laryngectomy tube will most likely be in place. (In some instances a laryngectomy tube is not used; in others it is used temporarily, and in many it is used permanently.) The laryngectomy tube, which is shorter than a tracheostomy tube but has a larger diameter, is the patient's only airway. The care of this tube is the same as for a tracheostomy tube (see Chap. 25). The nurse cleans the stoma daily with saline solution or another prescribed solution. If a non–oil-based antibiotic ointment is prescribed, the nurse applies it around the stoma and suture line. If crusting appears around the stoma, the nurse removes the crusts with sterile tweezers and applies additional ointment.

Wound drains may be in place to assist in removal of fluid and air from the surgical site. Suction also may be used, but cautiously, to avoid trauma to the surgical site and incision. The nurse observes, measures, and records drainage. When drainage is less than 50 to 60 mL/day, the physician usually removes the drains.

Frequently, the patient coughs up large amounts of mucus through this opening. Because air passes directly into the trachea without being warmed and moistened by the upper respiratory mucosa, the tracheobronchial tree compensates by secreting excessive amounts of mucus. Therefore, the patient will have frequent coughing episodes and may develop a brassy-sounding, mucus-producing cough. The nurse should reassure the patient that these problems will diminish in time as the tracheobronchial mucosa adapts to the altered physiology.

After the patient coughs, the tracheostomy opening must be wiped clean and clear of mucus. A simple gauze dressing, washcloth, or even paper towel (because of its size and absorbency) worn below the tracheostomy may serve as a barrier to protect the clothing from the copious mucus that the patient may expel initially.

One of the most important factors in decreasing cough, mucus production, and crusting around the stoma is adequate humidification of the environment. Mechanical humidifiers and aerosol generators (nebulizers) increase the humidity and are important for the patient's comfort.

The laryngectomy tube may be removed when the stoma is well healed, within 3 to 6 weeks after surgery. The nurse can teach the patient how to clean and change the tube (see Chap. 25) and remove secretions.

PROMOTING ALTERNATIVE COMMUNICATION METHODS

Understanding the patient's postoperative needs is critical. Alternative means of communication are established and used consistently by all personnel who come in contact with the patient—for example, a call bell or hand bell may be placed within easy reach of the patient. Because a Magic Slate often is used for communication, the nurse should document which hand the patient uses for writing so that the opposite arm can be used for intravenous infusions. (The nurse should discard any old notes used for communication to ensure the patient's privacy.) If the patient cannot write, a picture-word-phrase board or hand signals can be used. Preoperatively, the nurse reviews the system of communication to be used postoperatively with the patient.

Because it is very time-consuming to have to write everything or communicate through gestures, the inability to speak can be very frustrating. The patient may become impatient and angry when not understood. In such cases, other staff members need to be alert to the problem and also recognize that the patient will be unable to use the intercom system.

The return of communication is generally the ultimate goal in the rehabilitation of the laryngectomy patient. The nurse works with the patient, speech therapist, and family to encourage use of alternative communication methods.

PROMOTING ADEQUATE NUTRITION

Postoperatively, the patient may not be permitted to eat or drink for 10 to 14 days. Alternative sources of nutrition and hydration include intravenous fluids, enteral feedings through a nasogastric tube, and parenteral nutrition.

Once the patient is ready to start oral feedings, the nurse explains that thick liquids will be used first because they are easy to swallow. The nurse instructs the patient to avoid sweet foods, which increase salivation and suppress the appetite. Solid foods are introduced as tolerated. The nurse instructs the patient to rinse the mouth with warm water or mouthwash and to brush the teeth frequently.

The patient can expect to have a diminished sense of taste and smell for a period of time after surgery. Inhaled air passes directly into the trachea, bypassing the nose and the olfactory end organs. Because taste and smell are so closely connected, taste sensations are altered. In time, however, the patient usually accommodates to this problem and olfactory sensation adapts, often with return of interest in eating. The nurse observes the patient for any difficulty swallowing, particularly when eating resumes, and reports its occurrence to the physician.

PROMOTING POSITIVE BODY IMAGE AND SELF-ESTEEM

Disfiguring surgery and an altered communication pattern are a threat to a patient's body image and self-esteem. The reaction of family members and friends is a major concern for the patient. The nurse encourages the patient to express any feelings about the changes brought about by surgery, particularly those related to fear, anger, depression, and isolation.

A positive approach is important when caring for the patient. Promoting self-care activities is part of this approach. It is important for the patient and family to begin participating in self-care activities as soon as possible. The nurse needs to be a good listener and a support to the family, especially when explaining the tubes, dressings, and drains that are in place postoperatively. Referral to a support group, such as Lost Chord or New Voice clubs (through the International Association of Laryngectomees) and I Can Cope (through the American Cancer Society), may help the patient and family deal with the changes in their lives. Groups such as Lost Chord and New Voice promote and support the rehabilitation of people who have had a laryngectomy by providing an opportunity for exchanging ideas and sharing information.

MONITORING AND MANAGING POTENTIAL COMPLICATIONS

The immediate potential complications after laryngectomy include respiratory distress and hypoxia, hemorrhage, infection, and wound breakdown.

Respiratory Distress and Hypoxia

The nurse monitors the patient for signs and symptoms of respiratory distress and hypoxia, particularly restlessness, irritation, agitation, confusion, tachypnea, use of accessory muscles, and decreased oxygen saturation on pulse oximetry (SpO_2). Any change in the respiratory status requires immediate intervention. Obstruction needs to be ruled out immediately by suctioning and having the patient cough and breathe deeply. Hypoxia and airway obstruction, if not immediately treated, are life-threatening.

The nurse contacts the physician immediately if nursing measures do not improve the patient's respiratory status.

Hemorrhage

Bleeding at the surgical site from the drains or with tracheal suctioning may signal the occurrence of hemorrhage. The nurse should notify the surgeon of any active bleeding immediately. Bleeding may occur at a variety of sites, including the surgical site, drains, or trachea. Rupture of the carotid artery is especially dangerous. Should this occur, the nurse should apply direct pressure over the artery, summon assistance, and provide emotional support to the patient until the vessel can be ligated. It is important to monitor vital signs for changes, particularly increased pulse rate, decreased blood pressure, and rapid deep respirations. Cold, clammy, pale skin may indicate active bleeding.

Infection

The nurse observes for postoperative infection. Early signs of infection include an increase in temperature and pulse, a change in the type of wound drainage, or increased areas of redness or tenderness at the surgical site. Other signs include purulent drainage, odor, and increased wound drainage. The nurse reports any significant change to the surgeon.

Wound Breakdown

Wound breakdown due to infection, poor wound healing, or development of a fistula or as a result of radiation therapy or tumor growth can create a life-threatening emergency. The carotid artery, which is close to the stoma, may rupture from erosion if the wound does not heal properly. The nurse observes the stoma area for wound breakdown, hematoma, and bleeding and reports any significant changes to the surgeon. If wound breakdown occurs, the patient must be monitored carefully and identified as being at high risk for carotid hemorrhage.

PROMOTING HOME AND COMMUNITY-BASED CARE

Teaching Patients Self-Care

The nurse has an important role in the recovery and rehabilitation of the laryngectomy patient. In an effort to facilitate the patient's ability to manage self-care, discharge instruction begins as soon as the patient is able to participate. Nursing care and patient teaching in the hospital, outpatient setting, and rehabilitation or long-term care facility must take into consideration the many emotions, physical changes, and lifestyle changes experienced by the patient. In preparing the patient to go home, the nurse assesses the patient's readiness to learn and the level of knowledge about self-care management. The nurse also reassures the patient and family that most self-care management strategies can be mastered. The patient will need to learn a variety of self-care behaviors, including tracheostomy and stoma care, wound care, and oral hygiene. In addition, the nurse instructs the patient about the need for safe hygiene and recreational activities.

Tracheostomy and Stoma Care. The nurse provides specific instructions to the patient and family about what to expect from the tracheostomy and its management. The nurse teaches the patient and family caregiver to perform suctioning and emergency measures and tracheostomy and stoma care. The nurse stresses the importance of humidification at home and instructs the family to set up a humidification system before the patient returns home. In addition, the nurse cautions the patient and family that air-conditioned air may be too cool or too dry, and thus too irritating, for the patient with a new laryngectomy. (See Chap. 25 for details about tracheostomy care.)

Hygiene and Safety Measures. The nurse instructs the patient and family about safety precautions needed because of the structural changes resulting from the surgery. Special precautions are needed in the shower to prevent water from entering the stoma. Wearing a loose-fitting plastic bib over the tracheostomy or simply holding the hand over the opening is effective. Swimming is not recommended, however, because people with a laryngectomy can drown without getting their face wet. Barbers and beauticians need to be alerted so that hair sprays, loose hair, and powder do not get near the stoma, because they can block or irritate the trachea and possibly cause infection. These self-care points are summarized in Chart 22-8.

Recreation and exercise are important, and all but very strenuous exercise can be enjoyed safely. Avoidance of strenuous exercise and fatigue is important because, when tired, the patient has more difficulty speaking, which can be discouraging. Additional safety points to address include the need for the patient to wear or carry medical identification, such as a bracelet or card, to alert medical personnel to the special requirements for resuscitation should this need arise. When resuscitation is needed, direct mouth-to-stoma ventilation should be performed. For home emergency situations, prerecorded emergency messages for police, the fire department, or other rescue services can be kept near the phone to be used quickly.

The nurse instructs and encourages the patient to perform oral care on a regular basis to prevent halitosis and infection. If the patient is receiving radiation therapy, there will be a decrease in saliva, and synthetic saliva may be required. The nurse instructs the patient to drink water or sugar-free liquids throughout the day and to use a humidifier at home. Brushing the teeth or dentures and rinsing the mouth several times a day will assist in maintaining proper oral hygiene.

Continuing Care

Referral for home care is an important aspect of postoperative care for the patient who has had a laryngectomy and will assist the patient and family in the transition to the home. The home care nurse assesses the patient's general health status and the ability of the patient and family to care for the stoma and tracheostomy.

The nurse assesses the surgical incisions, nutritional and respiratory status, and adequacy of pain management. The nurse assesses not only for signs and symptoms of complications but also for the patient's and family's knowledge of which signs and symptoms to report to the physician. During the home visit, the nurse identifies and addresses other learning needs of the patient and family, such as adaptation to physical, lifestyle, and functional changes. It is important to assess the patient's psychological status as well. The home care nurse reinforces previous teaching and provides reassurance and support to the patient and family as needed.

The nurse encourages the person who has had a laryngectomy to have regular physical examinations and to seek advice concerning any problems related to recovery and rehabilitation. The patient is also reminded to participate in health promotion activities and health screening and about the importance of keeping scheduled appointments with the physician, speech therapist, and other health care providers.

Evaluation

EXPECTED PATIENT OUTCOMES

Expected patient outcomes may include:

1. Acquires an adequate level of knowledge, verbalizing an understanding of the surgical procedure and performing self-care adequately
2. Demonstrates less anxiety and depression
   a. Expresses a sense of hope
   b. Is aware of available community organizations and agencies such as the Lost Chord or New Voice groups
   c. Participates in support group, such as I Can Cope
3. Maintains a clear airway and handles own secretions; also demonstrates practical, safe, and correct technique for cleaning and changing the laryngectomy tube
4. Acquires effective communication techniques
   a. Uses assistive devices and strategies for communication (Magic Slate, call bell, picture board, sign language, lip reading, computer aids)
   b. Follows the recommendations of the speech therapist

Chart 22-8

Home Care Checklist • The Patient With a Laryngectomy

At the completion of the home care instruction, the patient or caregiver will be able to:	Patient	Caregiver
• Demonstrate methods to clear the airway and handle secretions	✓	✓
• Explain the rationale for maintaining adequate humidification with a humidifier or nebulizer	✓	✓
• Demonstrate how to clean the skin around the stoma and how to use ointments and tweezers to remove encrustations	✓	✓
• State the rationale for wearing a loose-fitting protective cloth at the stoma	✓	✓
• Discuss the need to avoid cold air from air conditioning and the environment to prevent irritation of the airway	✓	✓
• Demonstrate safe technique in changing the laryngectomy tube	✓	✓
• Identify the signs and symptoms of wound infection and state what to do about them	✓	✓
• Describe safety or emergency measures to implement in case of breathing difficulty or bleeding	✓	✓
• State the rationale for wearing or carrying special medical identification and ways to obtain help in an emergency	✓	✓
• Explain the importance of covering the stoma when showering or bathing	✓	✓
• Identify fluid and caloric needs	✓	✓
• Describe mouth care and discuss its importance	✓	✓
• Demonstrate alternative communication methods	✓	✓
• Identify support groups and agency resources	✓	✓
• State the need for regular check-ups and reporting of any problems immediately	✓	✓

5. Maintains balanced nutrition and adequate fluid intake
6. Exhibits improved body image, self-esteem, and self-concept
   a. Expresses feelings and concerns
   b. Participates in self-care and decision making
   c. Accepts information about support group
7. Exhibits no complications
   a. Vital signs (blood pressure, temperature, pulse, respiratory rate) normal
   b. No redness, tenderness, or purulent drainage at surgical site
   c. Demonstrates a patent airway and appropriate respirations
   d. No bleeding from surgical site and minimal bleeding from drains
   e. No wound breakdown
8. Adheres to rehabilitation and home care program
   a. Practices recommended speech therapy
   b. Demonstrates proper methods for caring for stoma and laryngectomy tube (if present)
   c. Verbalizes understanding of symptoms that require medical attention
   d. States safety measures to take in emergencies
   e. Performs oral hygiene as prescribed

Critical Thinking Exercises

1. A 36-year-old teacher is diagnosed with acute sinusitis. She has been self-medicating with over-the-counter medications for the past 2 weeks with no relief. What assessment and treatment should the nurse anticipate? What teaching and management strategies would you discuss with the patient? What is the rationale for your approach?

2. Your 68-year-old patient is scheduled for total laryngectomy for treatment of laryngeal cancer. What information would you provide to the patient about managing changes in breathing and speech that are expected in the immediate postoperative period and in the long term? What information would you provide to the patient's family?

3. You are making the first home visit to a patient who has just been discharged from the hospital following treatment for pneumonia and a 60-lb weight loss. He had a laryngectomy 8 months ago to treat laryngeal cancer. What will be the focus of your initial home visit? What aspects of assessment and nursing management are key at this point in caring for this patient? How would you assist this patient and his family to plan his care for the next month? Next 6 months?

4. Your patient, age 36, has been admitted to the emergency department with profuse epistaxis following a car crash. He tells you that he has hemophilia and is HIV-positive as a result of repeated use of clotting factors. What are the initial measures you would use to stop the bleeding? What other options are available if the bleeding does not stop within a reasonable period? How will his HIV status and the diagnosis of hemophilia affect your plan of care for him?

REFERENCES AND SELECTED READINGS

Books

American Cancer Society. (2002). *Cancer facts and figures.* Atlanta: American Cancer Society Inc.

Bast, R. C., Kufe, D. W., Pollock, R. E., et al. (Eds.) (2000). *Holland & Frei cancer medicine* (5th ed.) Hamilton: B.C. Decker, Inc.

DeLisa, J. A., & Gans, B. M. (1998). *Rehabilitation medicine principles and practice* (3d ed.). Philadelphia: Lippincott-Raven.

Goldman, L., & Bennett, J. C. (Eds.) (2000). *Cecil textbook of medicine* (21st ed.). Philadelphia: W. B. Saunders.

Green, E., et al. (Eds.) (2002). *AJCC cancer staging manual* (6th ed.). New York: Springer-Verlag.

Haskell, C. M. (2001) *Cancer treatment* (5th ed.). Philadelphia: W. B. Saunders.

Lenhard, R. E., Osteen, R. T., & Gansler, T. (2001) *The American Cancer Society's clinical oncology* (1st ed.). Atlanta: American Cancer Society Inc.

Mandell, G. L., Bennett, J. E., & Dolin, R (Eds.) (2000). *Principles and practice of infectious diseases* (5th ed.). Philadelphia: Churchill Livingstone.

McKenry, L. M., & Salerno, E. (2001). *Mosby's principles in nursing* (21st ed.). St. Louis: Mosby.

Middleton, E., Ellis, E. F., Yunginger, J. W., et al. (1998). *Allergy: principles and practice* (Vol. II, 5th ed.). St. Louis: Mosby.

Murray, J. F., & Nadel, J. A. (2001). *Textbook of respiratory medicine* (Vols. 1 & 2, 3d ed.). Philadelphia: W. B. Saunders.

Peckenpaugh, N. J., & Poleman, C. M. (1999). *Nutrition essentials and diet therapy* (8th ed.). Philadelphia: W. B. Saunders.

Tierney, L. M., McPhee, S. J., & Papadakis, M. A. (2001). *Current medical diagnosis and treatment 2001* (40th ed.). New York: Lange Medical Books/McGraw Hill.

Tintinalli, J. E., Kelen, G. D., & Stapczynski, J. S. (2000). *Emergency medicine: A comprehensive study guide* (5th ed.). New York: McGraw-Hill.

Townsend, C. M. (Ed.) (2001). *Sabiston textbook of surgery* (16th ed.). Philadelphia: W. B. Saunders.

Yarbro, C. H., Goodman, M., Frogge, M. H., & Groenwald, S. L. I. (Eds.) (2000). *Cancer nursing: Principles and practice* (5th ed.). Boston: Jones & Bartlett.

Journals

Asterisks indicate nursing research articles.

General

Casale, T. B., Condemi, J., LaForce, C., et al. (2001). Effect of omalizumab on symptoms of seasonal allergic rhinitis: A randomized controlled trial. *Journal of the American Medical Association, 286*(23), 2956–2967.

Chan, E., & Welsh, C. H. (1998). Geriatric respiratory medicine. *Chest, 114*(6), 1704–1733.

Upper Respiratory Infections

Bisno, A. L. (2001) Primary care: Acute pharyngitis. *New England Journal of Medicine, 344*(3), 205–211.

Cifu, A., & Levinson, W. (2000) Influenza. *Journal of the American Medical Association, 284*(22), 2847–2849.

Cooper, R. J., Hoffman, J. R., Bartlett, J. G., et al. (June 2001). Centers for Disease Control and Prevention. Principles of appropriate antibiotic use for acute pharyngitis in adults: background. *Annals of Emergency Medicine. 37*(6), 711–719.

Corneli, H. (2001). Rapid strep tests in the emergency department: An evidence-based approach. *Pediatric Emergency Care, 17*(4), 272–278.

Ebell, M. H., Smith, M. A., Barry, H. C., Ives, K., & Carey, M. (2000). Does this patient have strep throat? *Journal of the American Medical Association, 284*(22), 2912–2918.

Hall, C. B. (2001). Respiratory syncytial virus and parainfluenza virus. *New England Journal of Medicine, 344*(25), 1917–1928.

Hickner, J. M. (2001). Acute rhinosinusitis: A diagnostic and therapeutic challenge. *Journal of Family Practice, 50*(1), 38–40.

Hickner, J. M., Bartlett, J. G., Besser, R. E., et al. (2001). American Academy of Family Physicians/American Society of Internal Medicine. Centers for Disease Control Infectious Diseases Society of America. Principles of appropriate antibiotic use for acute rhinosinusitis in adults: background. *Annals of Internal Medicine, 134*(6), 498–505.

Kearney, K. (2001). Emergency: Epiglottis. *American Journal of Nursing, 101*(8), 37–38.

Kernan, W. N., Viscoli, C. M., Brass, L. M., et al. (2000). Phenylpropanolamine and the risk of hemorrhagic stroke. *New England Journal of Medicine, 343*(25), 1826–1832.

Luna, B., Drew, R. H., & Perfect, J. R. (2000). Agents for the treatment of invasive fungal infections. *Otolaryngologic Clinics of North America, 33*(4), 277–299.

Mattila, P. (2001). Causes of tonsillar disease and frequency of tonsillectomy operations. *Archives of Otolaryngology- Head & Neck Surgery, 127*(1), 37–44.

Piccirillo, J. F., Mager, D. E., Frisse, M. E., Brophy, R. H. & Goggin, A. (2001). Impact of first-line vs. second-line antibiotics for the treatment of acute uncomplicated sinusitis. *Journal of the American Medical Association, 286*(15), 1849–1856.

Prasad, A. S., Fitzgerald, J. T., Bao, B., et al. (2000). Duration of symptoms and plasma cytokine levels in patients with the common cold treated with zinc acetate: A randomized, double-blind, placebo-controlled trial. *Annals of Internal Medicine, 133*(4), 245–252.

Sly, M. (1999). Changing prevalence of allergic rhinitis and asthma. *Annals of Allergy, Asthma, & Immunology, 82*(3), 233–252.

Snow, V., Mottur-Pilson, C., Hickner, J. M., et al. (2001). Principles of appropriate antibiotic use for acute sinusitis in adults. *Annals of Internal Medicine, 134*(6), 495–497.

Stephenson, K. (2000). Acute and chronic pharyngitis across the lifespan. *Lippincott's Primary Care Practice. Ear, Nose, and Throat Problems, 4*(5), 471–489.

Stone, S., Gonzales, R., Maselli, J., & Lowenstein, S. R. (2000). Antibiotic prescribing for patients with colds, upper respiratory tract infections, and bronchitis: A national study of hospital-based emergency departments. *Annals of Emergency Medicine. 36*(4), 320–327.

Youngs, R. (2000) Sinusitis in adults. *Current Opinion in Pulmonary Medicine, 6*(3), 217–220.

Obstruction and Trauma of the Airway

Boehlecke, B. A. (2000). Epidemiology and pathogenesis of sleep-disordered breathing. *Current Opinion in Pulmonary Medicine, 6*(6), 471–478.

Flemons, W. W. (2002). Clinical practice. Obstructive sleep apnea. *New England Journal of Medicine, 347*(7), 498–504.

Goldberg, R. (2000). Treatment of obstructive sleep apnea, other than with continuous positive airway pressure. *Current Opinion in Pulmonary Medicine, 6*(6), 496–500.

Harding, S. M. (2000). Complications and consequences of obstructive sleep apnea. *Current Opinion in Pulmonary Medicine, 6*(6), 485–489.

Krieger, A. C. & Redeker, N. S. (2002) Obstructive sleep apnea syndrome: its relationship with hypertension. *Journal of Cardiovascular Nursing, 17*(1), 1–11.

Krishna, P., & Lee, D. (2001). Post-tonsillectomy bleeding: A meta-analysis. *Laryngoscope, 111*(8), 1358–1361.

Liu, J., Anderson, K. E., Willging, J. P., et al. (2001). Post-tonsillectomy hemorrhage: What is it and what should be recorded? *Archives of Otolaryngology—Head & Neck Surgery, 127*(10), 1271–1275.

Marchiondo, K. (2000). Pickwickian syndrome: The challenge of severe sleep apnea. *MedSurg Nursing, 9*(4), 183–188.

Narkiewicz, K., Kato, M., Phillips, B. G., et al. (1999). Nocturnal continuous positive airway pressure decreases daytime sympathetic traffic in obstructive sleep apnea. *Circulation, 100*(23), 2332–2335.

National Institutions of Health. (2000). NHLBI study shows association between sleep apnea and hypertension (Press release, 4-11-00). http://www.nhlbi.nih.gov/about/ncsdr.

Nieto, F. J., Young, T. B., Lind, B. K., et al. (2000). Association of sleep-disordered breathing, sleep apnea, and hypertension in a large community-based study. Sleep Heart Health Study. *Journal of the American Medical Association, 283*(14), 1829–1836.

Parker, K. P. & Dunbar, S. B. (2002). Sleep and heart failure. *Journal of Cardiovascular Nursing, 17*(1), 12–29.

Peppard, P. E., Young, T., Palta, M., et al. (2000). Longitudinal study of moderate weight change and sleep-disordered breathing. *Journal of the American Medical Association, 284*(23), 3015–3021.

Redeker, N. S. (2002). Why is sleep relevant to cardiovascular disease? *Journal of Cardiovascular Nursing, 17*(1), v–ix.

Cancer of the Larynx

Bauer, A. M. (2001). Current trends in surgical management of head and neck carcinomas. *Nursing Clinics of North America, 36*(3), 501–506.

*Dropkin, M. J. (2001). Anxiety, coping strategies and coping behaviors in patients undergoing head and neck cancer surgery. *Cancer Nursing, 24*(2), 143–148.

Finizia, C., & Bergman, B. (2001). Health-related quality of life in patients with laryngeal cancer: A post-treatment comparison of different modes of communication. *Laryngoscope, 111*(5), 918–923.

Forastiere, A., Koch, W., Trotti, A., & Sidransky, D. (2001). Head and neck cancer. *New England Journal of Medicine, 345*(26), 1890–1900.

Friedman, M., Landsberg, R., Pryor, S., et al. (2001). The occurrence of sleep-disordered breathing among patients with head and neck cancer. *Laryngoscope, 111*(11), 1917–1919.

*Hemsley, B. (2001). Nursing the patient with severe communication impairment. *Journal of Advanced Nursing, 35*(6), 827–835.

Koch, W. (2001). A fail-safe technique for endoscopic tracheoesophageal puncture. *Laryngoscope, 111*(9), 1663–1665.

*Major, M. S., Bumpous, J. M., Flynn, M. B., & Schill, K. (2001). Quality of life after treatment for advanced laryngeal and hypopharyngeal cancer. *Laryngoscope, 111*(8), 1379–1382.

Owen, C., et al. (2001). The psychosocial impact of head and neck cancer. *Clinical Otolaryngology & Allied Sciences, 26*(5), 351–356.

Rose, P., & Yates, P. (2001). Quality of life experienced by patients receiving radiation treatment for cancers of the head and neck. *Cancer Nursing, 24*(4), 255–263.

Serra, A. (2000). Tracheostomy care. *Nursing Standard, 14*(42), 45–55.

Tamura, E. (2001). Clinical assessment of intralaryngeal ultrasonography. *Laryngoscope, 111*(10), 767–770.

Weinstein, G. S., El-Sawy, M. M., Ruiz, C., et al. (2001). Laryngeal preservation with supracricoid partial laryngectomy results in improved quality of life when compared with total laryngectomy. *Laryngoscope, 111*(12), 191–199.

RESOURCES AND WEBSITES

American Cancer Society, 1599 Clifton Rd., NE, Atlanta, GA 30329-4251; (404) 320-3333; (800) ACS-2345; http://www.cancer.org.

American Lung Association, 1740 Broadway, New York, NY 10019-4374; (212) 315-8700; http://www.lungusa.org.

American Sleep Apnea Association, 1424 K Street, NW, Suite 302, Washington, DC 20005; 202-293-3650; http://www.sleepapnea.org.

International Association of Laryngectomees, 7400 N. Shadeland Ave., Suite 100, Indianapolis, IN 46250; (317) 570-4568; http://www.larynxlink.com.

National Cancer Institute (NCI), Bldg. 31, 31 Center Drive, MSC 2580, Bethesda, MD 20892-2580; http://cancernet.nci.nih.gov.

National Institute of Allergy and Infectious Disease, Building 31, 31 Center Drive MSC 2520, Bethesda, MD 20892-2520; http://www.niaid.nih.gov.

National Heart, Lung, and Blood Institute (NHBLI), National Institutes of Health, Bldg. 31, Rm. 4A21, Bethesda, MD 20892; 301-592-8573 800-575-9355; http://www.nhlbi.nih.gov.

National Sleep Foundation, 1522 K Street NW, Suite 500, Washington, DC 20005; 202-437-3471; Fax: 202-347-3472; http://www.sleepfoundation.org.

Voice Center at Eastern Virginia Medical School, Norfolk, VA 23507; http://www.voice-center.com.

Management of Patients With Chest and Lower Respiratory Tract Disorders

LEARNING OBJECTIVES

On completion of this chapter, the learner will be able to:

1. Identify patients at risk for atelectasis and nursing interventions related to its prevention and management.

2. Compare the various pulmonary infections with regard to causes, clinical manifestations, nursing management, complications, and prevention.

3. Use the nursing process as a framework for care of the patient with pneumonia.

4. Relate pleurisy, pleural effusion, and empyema to pulmonary infection.

5. Describe smoking and air pollution as causes of pulmonary disease.

6. Relate the therapeutic management techniques of acute respiratory distress syndrome to the underlying pathophysiology of the syndrome.

7. Describe risk factors for and measures appropriate for prevention and management of pulmonary embolism.

8. Describe preventive measures appropriate for controlling and eliminating the problem of occupational lung disease.

9. Discuss the modes of therapy and related nursing management for patients with lung cancer.

10. Describe the complications of chest trauma and their clinical manifestations and nursing management.

11. Describe nursing measures to prevent aspiration.

*C*onditions affecting the lower respiratory tract range from acute problems to long-term chronic disorders. Many of these disorders are serious and often life-threatening. The patient with a lower respiratory tract disorder requires care from nurses with astute assessment and clinical management skills as well as an understanding of the impact of the disorder on the patient's quality of life and ability to carry out usual activities of daily living. Patient and family teaching is an important nursing intervention in the management of all lower respiratory tract disorders.

Atelectasis

Atelectasis refers to closure or collapse of alveoli and often is described in relation to x-ray findings and clinical signs and symptoms. Atelectasis may be acute or chronic and may cover a broad range of pathophysiologic changes, from microatelectasis (which is not detectable on chest x-ray) to macroatelectasis with loss of segmental, lobar, or overall lung volume. The most commonly described atelectasis is acute atelectasis, which occurs frequently in the postoperative setting or in people who are immobilized and have a shallow, monotonous breathing pattern. Excess secretions or mucus plugs may also cause obstruction of airflow and result in atelectasis in an area of the lung. Atelectasis also is observed in patients with a chronic airway obstruction that impedes or blocks air flow to an area of the lung (eg, obstructive atelectasis in the patient with lung cancer that is invading or compressing the airways). This type of atelectasis is more insidious and slower in onset.

Pathophysiology

Atelectasis may occur in the adult as a result of reduced alveolar ventilation or any type of blockage that impedes the passage of air to and from the alveoli that normally receive air through the bronchi and network of airways. The trapped alveolar air becomes absorbed into the bloodstream, but outside air cannot replace the absorbed air because of the blockage. As a result, the isolated portion of the lung becomes airless and the alveoli collapse. This may occur with altered breathing patterns, retained secretions, pain, alterations in small airway function, prolonged supine positioning, increased abdominal pressure, reduced lung volumes due to musculoskeletal or neurologic disorders, restrictive defects, and specific surgical procedures (eg, upper abdominal, thoracic, or open heart surgery). Persistent low lung volumes, secretions or a mass obstructing or impeding airflow, and compression of lung tissue may all cause collapse or obstruction of the airways, which leads to atelectasis.

The postoperative patient is at high risk for atelectasis because of the numerous respiratory changes that may occur. A monotonous low tidal breathing pattern may cause airway closure and alveolar collapse. This results from the effects of anesthesia or analgesic agents, supine positioning, splinting of the chest wall because of pain, and abdominal distention. The postoperative patient may also have secretion retention, airway obstruction, and an impaired cough reflex or may be reluctant to cough because of pain. Figure 23-1 shows the pathogenic mechanisms and consequences of acute atelectasis in the postoperative patient.

Atelectasis resulting from bronchial obstruction by secretions may occur in patients with impaired cough mechanisms (eg, postoperative, musculoskeletal or neurologic disorders) or in debilitated, bedridden patients. Atelectasis may also result from excessive pressure on the lung tissue, which restricts normal lung expansion on inspiration. Such pressure may be produced by fluid accumulating within the pleural space (**pleural effusion**), air in the pleural space (**pneumothorax**), or blood in the pleural space (**hemothorax**). The **pleural space** is the area between the parietal and the visceral pleurae. Pressure may also be produced

Glossary

acute respiratory distress syndrome (ARDS): nonspecific pulmonary response to a variety of pulmonary and nonpulmonary insults to the lung; characterized by interstitial infiltrates, alveolar hemorrhage, atelectasis, decreased compliance, and refractory hypoxemia

asbestosis: diffuse lung fibrosis resulting from exposure to asbestos fibers

atelectasis: collapse or airless condition of the alveoli caused by hypoventilation, obstruction to the airways, or compression

central cyanosis: bluish discoloration of the skin or mucous membranes due to hemoglobin carrying reduced amounts of oxygen

consolidation: lung tissue that has become more solid in nature due to collapse of alveoli or infectious process (pneumonia)

cor pulmonale: "heart of the lungs"; enlargement of the right ventricle from hypertrophy or dilation or as a secondary response to disorders that affect the lungs

empyema: accumulation of purulent material in the pleural space

fine-needle aspiration: insertion of a needle through the chest wall to obtain cells of a mass or tumor; usually performed under fluoroscopy or chest CT guidance

hemoptysis: the coughing up of blood from the lower respiratory tract

hemothorax: partial or complete collapse of the lung due to blood accumulating in the pleural space; may occur after surgery or trauma

induration: an abnormally hard lesion or reaction, as in a positive tuberculin skin test

nosocomial: pertaining to or originating from a hospitalization; not present at the time of hospital admission

open lung biopsy: biopsy of lung tissue performed through a limited thoracotomy incision

orthopnea: shortness of breath when reclining or in the supine position

pleural effusion: abnormal accumulation of fluid in the pleural space

pleural friction rub: localized grating or creaking sound caused by the rubbing together of inflamed parietal and visceral pleurae

pleural space: the area between the parietal and visceral pleurae; a potential space

pneumothorax: partial or complete collapse of the lung due to positive pressure in the pleural space

pulmonary edema: increase in the amount of extravascular fluid in the lung

pulmonary embolism: obstruction of the pulmonary vasculature with an embolus; embolus may be due to blood clot, air bubbles, or fat droplets

purulent: consisting of, containing, or discharging pus

restrictive lung disease: disease of the lung that causes a decrease in lung volumes

tension pneumothorax: pneumothorax characterized by increasing positive pressure in the pleural space with each breath; this is an emergency situation and the positive pressure needs to be decompressed or released immediately

thoracentesis: insertion of a needle into the pleural space to remove fluid that has accumulated and decrease pressure on the lung tissue; may also be used diagnostically to identify potential causes of a pleural effusion

transbronchial: through the bronchial wall, as in a transbronchial lung biopsy

ventilation–perfusion ratio: the ratio between ventilation and perfusion in the lung; matching of ventilation to perfusion optimizes gas exchange

Physiology/Pathophysiology

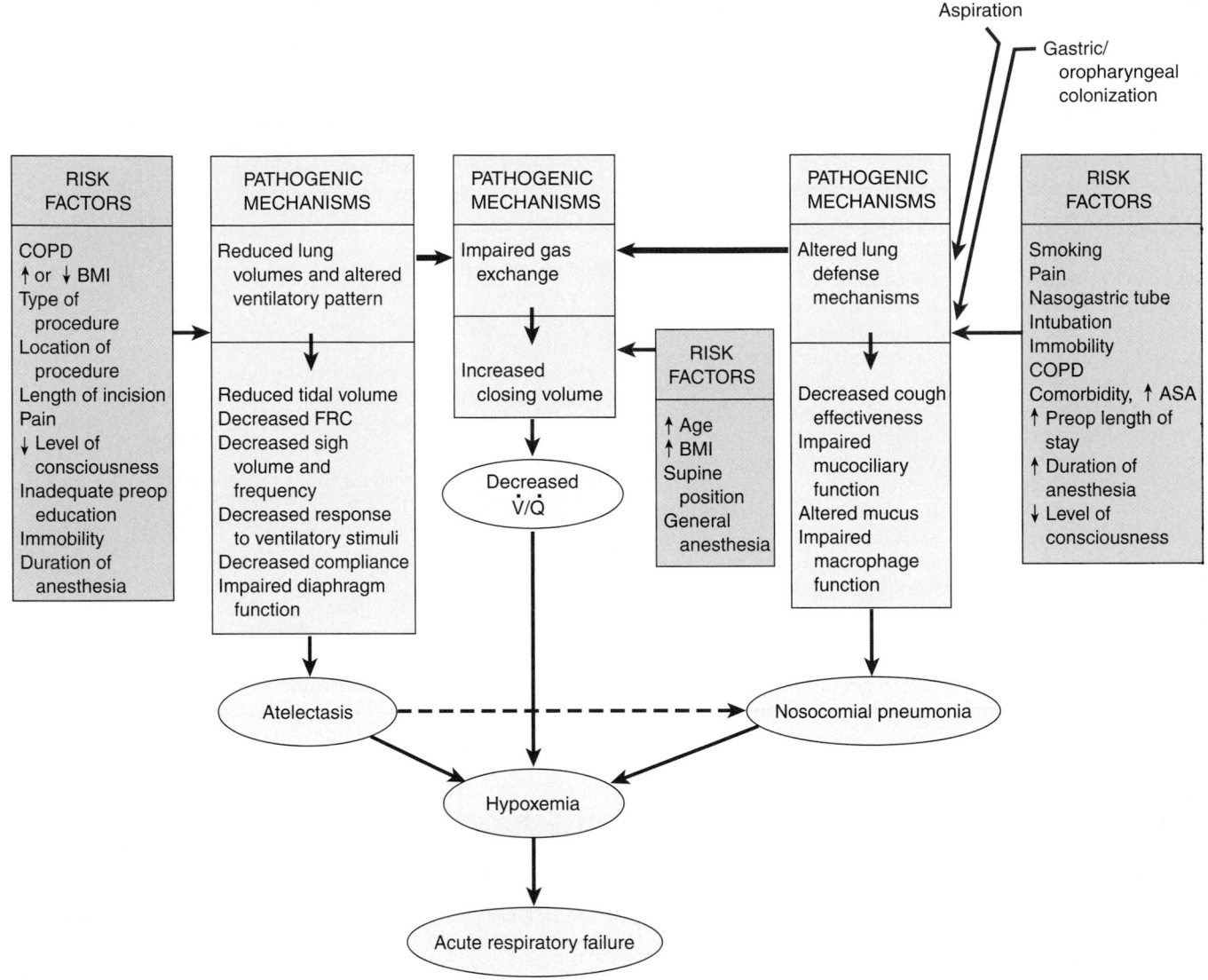

FIGURE 23-1 Relationship of risk factors, pathogenic mechanisms, and consequences of acute atelectasis in the post-operative patient. COPD, chronic obstructive pulmonary disease; BMI, body mass index; FRC, functional residual capacity; diaphragm fx, diaphragm function; ASA, American Society of Anesthesiology physical status; V̇/Q̇, ventilation-perfusion ratio. From the work of Jo Ann Brooks-Brunn, DNS, RN, FAAN, FCCP, Indiana University Medical Center, Indianapolis.

by a pericardium distended with fluid (pericardial effusion), tumor growth within the thorax, or an elevated diaphragm.

Clinical Manifestations

The development of atelectasis usually is insidious. Signs and symptoms include cough, sputum production, and low-grade fever. Fever is universally cited as a clinical sign of atelectasis, but there are few data to support this. Most likely the fever that accompanies atelectasis is due to infection or inflammation distal to the obstructed airway.

In acute atelectasis involving a large amount of lung tissue (lobar atelectasis), marked respiratory distress may be observed. In addition to the above signs and symptoms, dyspnea, tachycar-

dia, tachypnea, pleural pain, and **central cyanosis** (a bluish skin hue that is a late sign of hypoxemia) may be anticipated. The patient characteristically has difficulty breathing in the supine position and is anxious. Signs and symptoms of chronic atelectasis are similar to those of acute atelectasis. Because the alveolar collapse is chronic, infection may occur distal to the obstruction. Thus, the signs and symptoms of a pulmonary infection also may be present.

Assessment and Diagnostic Findings

Decreased breath sounds and crackles are heard over the affected area. In addition, chest x-ray findings may reveal patchy infiltrates or consolidated areas. In the patient who is confined to bed, atelectasis is usually diagnosed by chest x-ray or identified by physical assessment in the dependent, posterior, basilar areas of the lungs. Depending on the degree of hypoxemia, pulse oximetry (SpO$_2$) may demonstrate a low saturation of hemoglobin with oxygen (less than 90%) or a lower-than-normal partial pressure of arterial oxygen (PaO$_2$).

Prevention

Nursing measures to prevent atelectasis include frequent turning, early mobilization, and strategies to expand the lungs and to manage secretions. Deep-breathing maneuvers (at least every 2 hours) assist in preventing and treating atelectasis. The performance of these maneuvers requires a patient who is alert and cooperative. Patient education and reinforcement are key to the success of these interventions. The use of incentive spirometry or voluntary deep breathing enhances lung expansion, decreases the potential for airway closure, and may generate a cough. Secretion management techniques may include directed cough, suctioning, aerosol nebulizer treatments followed by chest physical therapy (postural drainage and chest percussion), or bronchoscopy. In some settings, a metered-dose inhaler (MDI) is used to dispense a bronchodilator rather than an aerosol nebulizer treatment. Chart 23-1 summarizes measures to prevent atelectasis.

Management

The goal in treating the patient with atelectasis is to improve ventilation and remove secretions. The strategies to prevent atelectasis, which include frequent turning, early ambulation, lung volume expansion maneuvers (eg, deep-breathing exercises, incentive spirometry), and coughing also serve as the first-line measures to minimize or treat atelectasis by improving ventilation. In patients who do not respond to first-line measures or who cannot perform deep-breathing exercises, other treatments such as positive expiratory pressure or PEP therapy (a simple mask and one-way valve system that provides varying amounts of expiratory resistance [usually 5 to 15 cm H$_2$O]), continuous or intermittent positive pressure-breathing (IPPB), or bronchoscopy may be used. Although IPPB may be used in some settings, few data support its use in the postoperative setting (Duffy & Farley, 1993). Before initiating more complex, costly, and labor-intensive therapies, the nurse should ask several questions:

- Has the patient been given an adequate trial of deep-breathing exercises?

- Has the patient received adequate education, supervision, and coaching to carry out the deep-breathing exercises?
- Have other factors been evaluated that may impair ventilation or prohibit a good patient effort (eg, lack of turning, mobilization; excessive pain; excessive sedation)?

If the cause of atelectasis is bronchial obstruction from secretions, the secretions must be removed by coughing or suctioning to permit air to re-enter that portion of the lung. Chest physical therapy (chest percussion and postural drainage) may also be used to mobilize secretions. Nebulizer treatments with a bronchodilator medication or sodium bicarbonate may be used to assist the patient in the expectoration of secretions. If respiratory care measures fail to remove the obstruction, a bronchoscopy is performed. Severe or massive atelectasis may lead to acute respiratory failure, especially in a patient with underlying lung disease. Endotracheal intubation and mechanical ventilation may be necessary. Prompt treatment reduces the risk for acute respiratory failure or pneumonia.

If atelectasis has resulted from compression of lung tissue, the goal is to decrease the compression. With a large pleural effusion that is compressing lung tissue and causing alveolar collapse, treatment may include **thoracentesis**, removal of the fluid by needle aspiration, or insertion of a chest tube. The measures to increase lung expansion described above also are used.

Management of chronic atelectasis focuses on removing the cause of the obstruction of the airways or the compression of the lung tissue. For example, bronchoscopy may be used to open an airway obstructed by lung cancer or a nonmalignant lesion, and the procedure may involve cryotherapy or laser therapy. The goal is to reopen the airways and provide ventilation to the collapsed area. In some cases, surgical management may be indicated.

Respiratory Infections

ACUTE TRACHEOBRONCHITIS

Acute tracheobronchitis, an acute inflammation of the mucous membranes of the trachea and the bronchial tree, often follows infection of the upper respiratory tract. A patient with a viral infection has decreased resistance and can readily develop a secondary bacterial infection. Thus, adequate treatment of upper respiratory tract infection is one of the major factors in the prevention of acute bronchitis. Aside from infection, inhalation of physical and chemical irritants, gases, and other air contaminants can also cause acute bronchial irritation.

Pathophysiology

In acute tracheobronchitis, the inflamed mucosa of the bronchi produces mucopurulent sputum, often in response to *Streptococcus pneumoniae, Haemophilus influenzae,* and *Mycoplasma pneumoniae.* In addition, a fungal infection (eg, *Aspergillus* tracheobronchitis) may also cause tracheobronchitis. A sputum culture is essential to identify the specific causative organism.

Clinical Manifestations

Initially, the patient has a dry, irritating cough and expectorates a scanty amount of mucoid sputum. The patient complains of sternal soreness from coughing and has fever or chills and night sweats, headache, and general malaise. As the infection progresses, the patient may be short of breath, have noisy inspiration and expiration (inspiratory stridor and expiratory wheeze), and

---

Chart 23-1   Preventing Atelectasis

- Change patient's position frequently, especially from supine to upright position, to promote ventilation and prevent secretions from accumulating.
- Encourage early mobilization from bed to chair followed by early ambulation.
- Encourage appropriate deep breathing and coughing to mobilize secretions and prevent them from accumulating.
- Teach/reinforce appropriate technique for incentive spirometry.
- Administer prescribed opioids and sedatives judiciously to prevent respiratory depression.
- Perform postural drainage and chest percussion, if indicated.
- Institute suctioning to remove tracheobronchial secretions, if indicated.

produce **purulent** (pus-filled) sputum. With severe tracheobronchitis, blood-streaked secretions may be expectorated as a result of the irritation of the mucosa of the airways.

Medical Management

Antibiotic treatment may be indicated depending on the symptoms, sputum purulence, and results of the sputum culture. Antihistamines are usually not prescribed because they may cause excessive drying and make secretions more difficult to expectorate. Expectorants may be prescribed, although their efficacy is questionable. Fluid intake is increased to thin the viscous and tenacious secretions. Copious, purulent secretions that cannot be cleared by coughing place the patient at risk for increasing airway obstruction and the development of a more severe lower respiratory tract infection, such as pneumonia. Suctioning and bronchoscopy may be needed to remove secretions. Rarely, endotracheal intubation may be required in cases of acute tracheobronchitis leading to acute respiratory failure. This may be necessary for patients who are severely debilitated or who have coexisting diseases that also impair the respiratory system.

In most cases, treatment of tracheobronchitis is largely symptomatic. The patient is advised to rest. Increasing the vapor pressure (moisture content) in the air will reduce irritation. Cool vapor therapy or steam inhalations may help relieve laryngeal and tracheal irritation. Moist heat to the chest may relieve the soreness and pain. Mild analgesics or antipyretics may be indicated.

Nursing Management

Acute tracheobronchitis is frequently treated in the home setting. A primary nursing function is to encourage bronchial hygiene, such as increasing fluid intake and directed coughing to remove secretions. The nurse should encourage and assist the patient to sit up frequently to cough effectively and to prevent retention of mucopurulent sputum. If the patient is treated with antibiotics for an underlying infection, it is important to emphasize the need to complete the full course of antibiotics prescribed. Fatigue is a consequence of tracheobronchitis; therefore, the nurse must caution the patient against overexertion, which can induce a relapse or exacerbation of the infection.

PNEUMONIA

Pneumonia is an inflammation of the lung parenchyma that is caused by a microbial agent. "Pneumonitis" is a more general term that describes an inflammatory process in the lung tissue that may predispose a patient to or place a patient at risk for microbial invasion. Pneumonia is the most common cause of death from infectious diseases in the United States. It is the seventh leading cause of death in the United States for all ages and both genders, resulting in almost 70,000 deaths per year. In persons 65 years of age and older, it is the fifth leading cause of death (National Center for Health Statistics, 2000; Minino & Smith, 2001). It is treated extensively on both an inpatient and outpatient basis.

Bacteria commonly enter the lower airway but do not cause pneumonia in the presence of an intact host defense mechanism. When pneumonia does occur, it is caused by various microorganisms, including bacteria, mycobacteria, chlamydiae, mycoplasma, fungi, parasites, and viruses. Several systems are used to classify pneumonias. Classically, pneumonia has been categorized into one of four categories: bacterial or typical, atypical, anaerobic/cavitary, and opportunistic. However, there is overlap in the microorganisms thought to be responsible for typical and atypical pneu-

monias. A more widely used classification scheme categorizes the major pneumonias as community-acquired pneumonia, hospital-acquired pneumonia, pneumonia in the immunocompromised host, and aspiration pneumonia (Table 23-1). There is overlap in how specific pneumonias are classified because they may occur in differing settings.

Community-acquired pneumonia (CAP) occurs either in the community setting or within the first 48 hours of hospitalization or institutionalization. The need for hospitalization for CAP depends on the severity of the pneumonia. The agents that most frequently cause CAP requiring hospitalization are *S. pneumoniae, H. influenzae, Legionella, Pseudomonas aeruginosa,* and other gram-negative rods. The specific etiologic agent of CAP is identified in about 50% of the cases. The absence of a responsible caregiver in the home may be another indication for hospitalization. More than 5.5 million people develop CAP and as many as 1.1 million require hospitalization each year (Centers for Disease Control and Prevention [CDC], 1997; Marston, Plouffe, File et al., 1997).

Pneumonia caused by *S. pneumoniae* (pneumococcus) is the most common CAP in people younger than 60 without comorbidity and in those older than 60 with comorbidity. It is most prevalent during the winter and spring, when upper respiratory tract infections are most frequent. *S. pneumoniae* is a gram-positive, capsulated, nonmotile coccus that resides naturally in the upper respiratory tract. The organism colonizes the upper respiratory tract and can cause the following types of illnesses: disseminated invasive infections, pneumonia and other lower respiratory tract infections, and upper respiratory tract infections, including otitis media and sinusitis (CDC, 1998). It may occur as a lobar or bronchopneumonic form in patients of any age and may follow a recent respiratory illness.

Mycoplasma pneumonia, another type of CAP, occurs most often in older children and young adults and is spread by infected respiratory droplets through person-to-person contact. Patients can be tested for mycoplasma antibodies. The inflammatory infiltrate is primarily interstitial rather than alveolar. It spreads throughout the entire respiratory tract, including the bronchioles, and has the characteristics of a bronchopneumonia. Earache and bullous myringitis are common. Impaired ventilation and diffusion may occur.

H. influenzae is another cause of CAP. It frequently affects elderly people or those with comorbid illnesses (eg, chronic obstructive pulmonary disease [COPD], alcoholism, diabetes mellitus). The presentation of this pneumonia is indistinguishable from that of other forms of bacterial CAP. The presentation may be subacute, with cough or low-grade fever for weeks before diagnosis. Chest x-rays may reveal multilobar, patchy bronchopneumonia or areas of **consolidation** (tissue that solidifies as a result of collapsed alveoli or pneumonia).

Viruses are the most common cause of pneumonia in infants and children but are relatively uncommon causes of CAP in adults. The chief causes of viral pneumonia in the immunocompetent adult are influenza viruses types A and B, adenovirus, parainfluenza virus, coronavirus, and varicella-zoster virus. In immunocompromised adults, cytomegalovirus is the most common viral pathogen, followed by herpes simplex virus, adenovirus, and respiratory syncytial virus. The acute stage of a viral respiratory infection occurs within the ciliated cells of the airways. This is followed by infiltration of the tracheobronchial tree. With pneumonia, the inflammatory process extends into the alveolar area, resulting in edema and exudation. The clinical signs and symptoms of a viral pneumonia are often difficult to distinguish from those of a bacterial pneumonia.

(text continues on page 524)

Table 23-1 • **Commonly Encountered Pneumonias**

TYPE	ORGANISM RESPONSIBLE	EPIDEMIOLOGY	CLINICAL FEATURES	TREATMENT	COMMENTS
Community-Acquired Pneumonia					
Streptococcal pneumonia (pneumococcal)	*Streptococcus pneumoniae*	Highest occurrence in winter months. Incidence greatest in the elderly and in patients with COPD, heart failure, alcoholism, asplenia, following influenza. Leading infectious cause of illness worldwide among young children, persons with underlying chronic health conditions, and the elderly. Death occurs in 14% of hospitalized adults with invasive disease.	Abrupt onset, toxic appearance, pleuritic chest pain. Usually involves one or more lobes. Lobar infiltrate common on chest x-ray or bronchopneumonia pattern. Bacteremia in 15% to 25% of all patients.	Penicillins Alternate antibiotic therapy, such as cefotaxime or ceftriaxone; antipseudomonal fluoroquinolones (levofloxacin, gatifloxacin, moxifloxacin).	Complications include shock, pleural effusion, superinfections, pericarditis, and otitis media.
Haemophilus influenzae	*Haemophilus influenzae*	Incidence greatest in alcoholics, the elderly, patients in chronic care facilities and nursing homes, patients with diabetes or COPD, and children <5 years old. Accounts for 5% to 20% of community-acquired pneumonias. Mortality rate: 30%.	Frequently insidious onset associated with upper respiratory tract infection 2 to 6 weeks before onset of illness. Fever, chills, productive cough. Usually involves one or more lobes. Bacteremia is common. Infiltrate, occasional bronchopneumonia pattern on chest x-ray.	Ampicillin, 3rd-generation cephalosporin, macrolides (azithromycin, clarithromycin), fluoroquinolones	Complications include lung abscess, pleural effusion, meningitis, arthritis, pericarditis, epiglottitis.
Legionnaires' disease	*Legionella pneumophila*	Highest occurrence in summer and fall. May cause disease sporadically or as part of an epidemic. Incidence greatest in middle-aged and older men, smokers, and patients with chronic diseases, those receiving immunosuppressive therapy, or those in close proximity to excavation sites. Accounts for 15% of community-acquired pneumonias. Mortality rate: 15% to 50%.	Flulike symptoms. High fevers, mental confusion, headache, pleuritic pain, myalgias, dyspnea, productive cough, hemoptysis, leukocytosis. Bronchopneumonia, unilateral or bilateral disease, lobar consolidation.	Erythromycin +/− rifampin (in severely compromised patient) or clarithromycin, or a macrolide (azithromycin), or a fluoroquinolone (ofloxacin, levofloxacin, sparfloxacin).	Complications include hypotension, shock, and acute renal failure.

(continued)

Table 23-1 • **Commonly Encountered Pneumonias** (Continued)

TYPE	ORGANISM RESPONSIBLE	EPIDEMIOLOGY	CLINICAL FEATURES	TREATMENT	COMMENTS
Mycoplasma pneumoniae	*Mycoplasma pneumoniae*	Increase in fall and winter. Responsible for epidemics of respiratory illness. Most common type of atypical pneumonia. Accounts for 20% of community-acquired pneumonias. More common in children and young adults. Mortality rate: <0.1%.	Onset is usually insidious. Patients not usually as ill as in other pneumonias. Sore throat, nasal congestion, ear pain, headache, low-grade fever, pleuritic pain, myalgias, diarrhea, erythematous rash, pharyngitis. Interstitial infiltrates on chest x-ray.	Erythromycin; macrolide, fluoroquinolone or tetracycline.	Complications include aseptic meningitis, meningo-encephalitis, transverse myelitis, cranial nerve palsies, pericarditis, myocarditis.
Viral pneumonia	Influenza viruses types A, B adenovirus, parainfluenza, cytomegalovirus, coronavirus	Incidence greatest in winter months. Epidemics occur every 2 to 3 years. Most common causative organisms in adults. Other organisms in children (eg, cytomegalovirus and respiratory syncytial virus). Accounts for 20% of community-acquired pneumonias.	Patchy infiltrate, small pleural effusion on chest x-ray. In majority of patients, influenza begins as an acute upper respiratory infection; others have bronchitis, pleurisy, etc., and still others develop gastrointestinal symptoms.	Amantadine; rimantadine; oseltamivir phosphate, ribavirin aerosol. Treated symptomatically. Does not respond to treatment with currently available antimicrobials.	Complications include a super-imposed bacterial infection, bronchopneumonia.
Chlamydial pneumonia (TWAR agent)	*C. pneumoniae*	Reported mainly in college students, military recruits, and the elderly. May be a common cause of community-acquired pneumonia or observed in combination with other pathogens. Mortality rate is low as the majority of cases are relatively mild. The elderly with coexistent infections, comorbidities, and re-infections may require hospitalization.	Hoarseness, fever, chills, pharyngitis, rhinitis, nonproductive cough, myalgias, arthralgias. Single infiltrate on chest x-ray; pleural effusion possible.	Tetracycline, erythromycin, macrolide, quinolone.	Complications include reinfection and acute respiratory failure.

(continued)

Table 23-1 • **Commonly Encountered Pneumonias** (Continued)

TYPE	ORGANISM RESPONSIBLE	EPIDEMIOLOGY	CLINICAL FEATURES	TREATMENT	COMMENTS
Hospital-Acquired Pneumonia					
Pseudomonas pneumonia	*Pseudomonas aeruginosa*	Incidence greatest in those with pre-existing lung disease, cancer (particularly leukemia); those with homograft transplants, burns; debilitated persons; and patients receiving anti-microbial therapy and treatments such as tracheostomy, suctioning, and in postoperative settings. Almost always of nosocomial origin. Accounts for 15% of hospital-acquired pneumonias. Mortality rate: 40% to 60%.	Diffuse consolidation on chest x-ray. Toxic appearance: fever, chills, productive cough, relative bradycardia, leukocytosis.	Aminoglycoside and anti-pseudomonal agents (ticarcillin, piperacillin, mezlocillin, ceftazidine).	Complications include lung cavitation. Has capacity to invade blood vessels, causing hemorrhage and lung infarction. Usually requires hospitalization.
Staphylococcal pneumonia	*Staphylococcus aureus*	Incidence greatest in immunocompromised patients, IV drug users, and as a complication of epidemic influenza. Commonly nosocomial in origin. Accounts for 10% to 30% of hospital-acquired pneumonias. Mortality rate: 25% to 60%.	Severe hypoxemia, cyanosis, necrotizing infection. Bacteremia is common.	Nafcillin/oxacillin +/− rifampin or gentamicin; methicillin-resistant: vancomycin +/− rifampin or gentamicin.	Complications include pleural effusion/pneumothorax, lung abscess, empyema, meningitis, endocarditis. Frequently requires hospitalization. Treatment must be vigorous and prolonged because disease tends to destroy lung tissue.
Klebsiella pneumonia	*Klebsiella pneumoniae* (Friedlander's bacillus-encapsulated gram-negative aerobic bacillus)	Incidence greatest in the elderly; alcoholics; patients with chronic disease, such as diabetes, heart failure, COPD; patients in chronic care facilities and nursing homes. Accounts for 2% to 5% of community-acquired and 10% to 30% of hospital-acquired pneumonias. Mortality rate: 40% to 50%.	Tissue necrosis occurs rapidly. Toxic appearance: fever, cough, sputum production, bronchopneumonia, lung abscess. Lobar consolidation, bronchopneumonia pattern on chest x-ray.	Third-generation cephalosporins (cefotaxime, ceftriaxone) plus aminoglycoside, antipseudomonal penicillin, monobactam (aztreonam), or quinolone.	Complications include multiple lung abscesses with cyst formation, empyema, pericarditis, pleural effusion. May be fulminating, progressing to fatal outcome.

(continued)

Table 23-1 • **Commonly Encountered Pneumonias** (Continued)

TYPE	ORGANISM RESPONSIBLE	EPIDEMIOLOGY	CLINICAL FEATURES	TREATMENT	COMMENTS
Pneumonia in Immunocompromised Host					
Pneumocystis carinii pneumonia (PCP)	*Pneumocystis carinii*	Incidence greatest in patients with AIDS and patients receiving immuno-suppressive therapy for cancer, organ transplants, and other disorders. Frequently seen with cyto-megalovirus infection. Mortality rate 15% to 20% in hospitalized and fatal if not treated.	Pulmonary infil-trates on chest x-ray. Nonpro-ductive cough, fever, dyspnea.	Trimethoprim/sulfa-methoxazole (TMP-SMZ), dapsone-trimethoprim, pentamidine, primequine plus clindamycin.	Complications in-clude respiratory failure.
Fungal pneumonia	*Aspergillus fumigatus*	Incidence greatest in immunocompro-mised and neutro-penic patients. Mortality rate: 15% to 20%.	Cough, hemoptysis, infiltrates, fungus ball on chest x-ray.	Flucytosine with amphotericin B in non-neutropenic patients, ampho-tericin B, itra-conazole, ketoconazole. Lobectomy for fungus ball.	Complications in-clude dissemina-tion to brain, myocardium, and/or thyroid gland.
Tuberculosis	*Mycobacterium tuberculosis*	Incidence increased in indigent, immi-grant, and prison populations, peo-ple with AIDS, and the homeless. Mortality rate <1% (depending on comorbidity)	Weight loss, fever, night sweats, cough, sputum production, he-moptysis, non-specific infiltrate (lower lobe), hilar node enlargement, pleural effusion on chest x-ray.	Rifampin, strepto-mycin, etham-butol, INH (isoniazid), pyrazinamide	Complications in-clude reinfection and acute respira-tory infection.

+/− = may add depending upon situation

Hospital-acquired pneumonia (HAP), also known as **nosoco-mial** pneumonia, is defined as the onset of pneumonia symptoms more than 48 hours after admission to the hospital. HAP ac-counts for approximately 15% of hospital-acquired infections but is the most lethal nosocomial infection. It is estimated to occur in 0.5% to 1% of all hospitalized patients and in 15% to 20% of intensive care patients. Ventilator-associated pneumonia can be considered a type of nosocomial pneumonia that is associated with endotracheal intubation and mechanical ventilation.

The common organisms responsible for HAP include the pathogens *Enterobacter* species, *Escherichia coli*, *Klebsiella* species, *Proteus*, *Serratia marcescens*, *P. aeruginosa*, and methicillin-sensitive or methicillin-resistant *Staphylococcus aureus*. These respiratory infections occur when at least one of three conditions exists: host defenses are impaired, an inoculum of organisms reaches the pa-tient's lower respiratory tract and overwhelms the host's defenses, or a highly virulent organism is present. Certain illnesses may pre-dispose a patient to HAP because of impaired host defenses. Examples include severe acute or chronic illness, a variety of co-morbid conditions, coma, malnutrition, prolonged hospitalization, hypotension, and metabolic disorders. The hospitalized patient is also exposed to potential bacteria from other sources (eg, respira-

tory therapy devices and equipment, transmission of pathogens by the hands of health care personnel). Numerous intervention-related factors also may play a role in the development of HAP (eg, therapeutic agents leading to central nervous system depres-sion with decreased ventilation, impaired removal of secretions, or potential aspiration; prolonged or complicated thoraco-abdominal procedures, which may impair mucociliary function and cellular host defenses; endotracheal intubation; prolonged or inappropriate use of antibiotics; use of nasogastric tubes). In addi-tion, immunocompromised patients are at particular risk. HAP is associated with a high mortality rate, in part because of the vir-ulence of the organisms, their resistance to antibiotics, and the patient's underlying disorder.

Dominant pathogens for HAP are gram-negative bacilli (*P. aeruginosa* and *Enterobacteriaceae/Klebsiella* species, *Enter-obacter, Proteus, Serratia*) and *S. aureus*. Pseudomonal pneumo-nia occurs in patients who are debilitated, those with altered mental status, and those with prolonged intubation or with tra-cheostomies. Staphylococcal pneumonia can occur through in-halation of the organism or spread through the hematogenous route. It is often accompanied by bacteremia and positive blood cultures. Although responsible for less than 10% of cases of CAP, staphylococcal pneumonia may be responsible for more than 30% of cases of HAP. Its mortality rate is high. Specific strains of staphylococci are resistant to all available antimicrobials except vancomycin. These strains of *S. aureus* are referred to as methicillin-resistant *S. aureus* (MRSA). Overuse and misuse of antimicrobial agents are major risk factors for the emergence of these resistant pathogens. Because MRSA is highly virulent, steps must be taken to prevent the spread of this organism. The patient with MRSA should be isolated in a private room, and contact precautions (gown, mask, glove, and antibacterial soap) are used. The number of people in contact with the patient should be minimized, and appropriate precautions must be taken when transporting the patient within or between facilities.

The usual presentation of an HAP is a new pulmonary infiltrate on chest x-ray combined with evidence of infection such as fever, respiratory symptoms, purulent sputum, and/or leukocytosis. Pneumonias from *Klebsiella* or other gram-negative organisms (*E. coli, Proteus, Serratia*) are characterized by destruction of lung structure and alveolar walls, consolidation, and bacteremia. Elderly patients and those with alcoholism, chronic lung disease, or diabetes are at particular risk. A sudden onset of cough is a common presentation, and blood-tinged sputum may be present. In the debilitated or dehydrated patient, sputum production may be minimal or absent. Pleural effusions, high fevers, and tachycardia are often observed. Even with treatment, the mortality rate remains high.

Pneumonia in the immunocompromised host is seen with greater frequency because immunocompromised hosts represent a growing portion of the patient population. Examples of pneumonia in the immunocompromised host are *Pneumocystis carinii* pneumonia (PCP), fungal pneumonias, and mycobacterium tuberculosis. These types of pneumonia may also occur in the immunocompetent person and in different settings, but these are less common. Immunocompromised states occur with the use of corticosteroids or other immunosuppressive agents, chemotherapy, nutritional depletion, use of broad-spectrum antimicrobial agents, AIDS, genetic immune disorders, and long-term advanced life-support technology (mechanical ventilation). Patients with compromised immune systems commonly acquire pneumonia from organisms of low virulence. In addition, increasing numbers of patients with impaired defenses develop HAP from gram-negative bacilli (*Klebsiella, Pseudomonas, E. coli, Enterobacteriaceae, Proteus, Serratia*).

Pneumonia in the compromised host may be caused by the organisms also observed in CAP or HAP (*S. pneumoniae, S. aureus, H. influenzae, P. aeruginosa, M. tuberculosis*). PCP is rarely observed in the immunocompetent host and is often an initial AIDS-defining complication. Whether the patient is immunocompromised or immunocompetent, the clinical presentation of pneumonia is similar. PCP has a subtle onset with progressive dyspnea, fever, and a nonproductive cough.

Aspiration pneumonia refers to the pulmonary consequences resulting from the entry of endogenous or exogenous substances into the lower airway. The most common form of aspiration pneumonia is bacterial infection from aspiration of bacteria that normally reside in the upper airways. Aspiration pneumonia may occur in the community or hospital setting; common pathogens are *S. pneumoniae, H. influenzae,* and *S. aureus*. Other substances may be aspirated into the lung, such as gastric contents, exogenous chemical contents, or irritating gases. This type of aspiration or ingestion may impair the lung defenses, cause inflammatory changes, and lead to bacterial growth and a resulting pneumonia. (Aspiration is described in more detail at the end of this chapter.)

Pathophysiology

Upper airway characteristics normally prevent potentially infectious particles from reaching the normally sterile lower respiratory tract. Thus, patients with pneumonia caused by infectious agents often have an acute or chronic underlying disease that impairs host defenses. Pneumonia arises from normally present flora in a patient whose resistance has been altered, or it results from aspiration of flora present in the oropharynx. It may also result from bloodborne organisms that enter the pulmonary circulation and are trapped in the pulmonary capillary bed, becoming a potential source of pneumonia.

Pneumonia often affects both ventilation and diffusion. An inflammatory reaction can occur in the alveoli, producing an exudate that interferes with the diffusion of oxygen and carbon dioxide. White blood cells, mostly neutrophils, also migrate into the alveoli and fill the normally air-containing spaces. Areas of the lung are not adequately ventilated because of secretions and mucosal edema that cause partial occlusion of the bronchi or alveoli, with a resultant decrease in alveolar oxygen tension. Bronchospasm may also occur in patients with reactive airway disease. Because of hypoventilation, a ventilation–perfusion mismatch occurs in the affected area of the lung. Venous blood entering the pulmonary circulation passes through the underventilated area and exits to the left side of the heart poorly oxygenated. The mixing of oxygenated and unoxygenated or poorly oxygenated blood eventually results in arterial hypoxemia.

If a substantial portion of one or more lobes is involved, the disease is referred to as "lobar pneumonia." The term "bronchopneumonia" is used to describe pneumonia that is distributed in a patchy fashion, having originated in one or more localized areas within the bronchi and extending to the adjacent surrounding lung parenchyma. Bronchopneumonia is more common than lobar pneumonia (Fig. 23-2).

Risk Factors

Being knowledgeable about the factors and circumstances that commonly predispose a person to pneumonia will aid in identifying patients at high risk for this disorder (Chart 23-2).

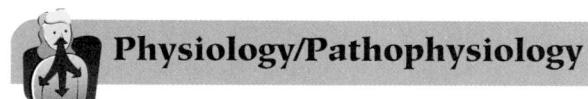

Physiology/Pathophysiology

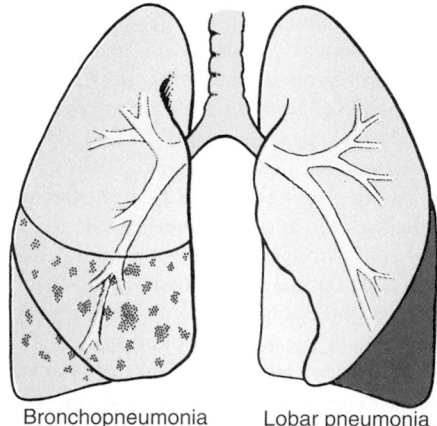

Bronchopneumonia   Lobar pneumonia

FIGURE 23-2 Distribution of lung involvement in bronchial and lobar pneumonia. In bronchopneumonia (*left*), patchy areas of consolidation occur. In lobar pneumonia (*right*), an entire lobe is consolidated.

Chart 23-2
Risk Factors for Pneumonia

Risk Factor	Preventive Measure
Conditions that produce mucus or bronchial obstruction and interfere with normal lung drainage (eg, cancer, cigarette smoking, COPD)	Promote coughing and expectoration of secretions. Encourage smoking cessation.
Immunosuppressed patients and those with a low neutrophil count (neutropenic)	Initiate special precautions against infection.
Smoking; cigarette smoke disrupts both mucociliary and macrophage activity	Encourage smoking cessation.
Prolonged immobility and shallow breathing pattern	Reposition frequently and promote lung expansion exercises and coughing. Initiate suctioning and chest physical therapy if indicated.
Depressed cough reflex (due to medications, a debilitated state, or weak respiratory muscles); aspiration of foreign material into the lungs during a period of unconsciousness (head injury, anesthesia, depressed level of consciousness), or abnormal swallowing mechanism	Reposition frequently to prevent aspiration and administer medications judiciously, particularly those that increase risk for aspiration. Perform suctioning and chest physical therapy if indicated.
Nothing-by-mouth (NPO) status; placement of nasogastric, orogastric, or endotracheal tube	Promote frequent oral hygiene. Minimize risk for aspiration by checking placement of tube and proper positioning of patient.
Antibiotic therapy (in very ill people, the oropharynx is likely to be colonized by gram-negative bacteria)	
Alcohol intoxication (because alcohol suppresses the body's reflexes, may be associated with aspiration, and decreases white cell mobilization and tracheobronchial ciliary motion)	Encourage reduced or moderate alcohol intake (in case of alcohol stupor, position patient to prevent aspiration).
General anesthetic, sedative, or opioid preparations that promote respiratory depression, which causes a shallow breathing pattern and predisposes to the pooling of bronchial secretions and potential development of pneumonia	Observe the respiratory rate and depth during recovery from general anesthesia and before giving medications. If respiratory depression is apparent, withhold the medication and contact the physician.
Advanced age, because of possible depressed cough and glottic reflexes and nutritional depletion	Promote frequent turning, early ambulation and mobilization, effective coughing, breathing exercises, and nutritious diet.
Respiratory therapy with improperly cleaned equipment	Make sure that respiratory equipment is cleaned properly; participate in continuous quality improvement monitoring with the respiratory care department.

Increasing numbers of patients who have compromised defenses against infections are susceptible to pneumonia. Some types of pneumonia, such as those caused by viral infections, occur in previously healthy people and often follow a viral illness.

Pneumonia is common with certain underlying disorders such as heart failure, diabetes, alcoholism, COPD, and AIDS. Certain diseases also have been associated with specific pathogens. For example, staphylococcal pneumonia has been noted after epidemics of influenza, and patients with COPD are at increased risk for developing pneumonia caused by pneumococci or *H. influenzae*. In addition, cystic fibrosis is associated with respiratory infection caused by pseudomonal and staphylococcal organisms, and PCP has been associated with AIDS. Pneumonias occurring in hospitalized patients often involve organisms not usually found in CAP, including enteric gram-negative bacilli and *S. aureus*.

The CDC has identified three specific strategies for preventing HAP: (1) staff education and infection surveillance, (2) interruption of transmission of microorganisms through person-to-person transmission and equipment transmission, and (3) modification of host risk of infection (CDC, 1997). Providing anticipatory and preventive care is an important nursing measure.

To reduce or prevent serious complications of CAP in high-risk groups, vaccination against pneumococcal infection is advised for the following:

- People 65 years of age or older
- Immunocompetent people who are at increased risk for illness and death associated with pneumococcal disease because of chronic illness (eg, cardiovascular, pulmonary, diabetes mellitus, chronic liver disease)
- People with functional or anatomic asplenia
- People living in environments or social settings in which the risk of disease is high
- Immunocompromised people at high risk for infection (CDC, 1998)

The vaccine provides specific prevention against pneumococcal pneumonia and other infections caused by this organism (otitis media, other upper respiratory tract infections). Vaccines should be avoided in the first trimester of pregnancy.

Clinical Manifestations

Pneumonia varies in its signs and symptoms depending on the organism and the patient's underlying disease. However, regardless of the type of pneumonia (CAP, HAP, immunocompromised host, aspiration), a specific type of pneumonia cannot be diagnosed by clinical manifestations alone. For example, the patient with streptococcal (pneumococcal) pneumonia usually has a sudden onset of shaking chills, rapidly rising fever (38.5° to 40.5°C [101° to 105°F]), and pleuritic chest pain that is aggravated by deep breathing and coughing. The patient is severely ill, with marked tachypnea (25 to 45 breaths/min), accompanied by other signs of respiratory distress (eg, shortness of breath, use of accessory muscles in respiration). The pulse is rapid and bounding, and it usually increases about 10 beats/min for every degree of temperature (Celsius) elevation. A relative bradycardia for the amount of fever may suggest viral infection, mycoplasma infection, or infection with a *Legionella* organism.

Some patients exhibit an upper respiratory tract infection (nasal congestion, sore throat), and the onset of symptoms of pneumonia is gradual and nonspecific. The predominant symptoms may be headache, low-grade fever, pleuritic pain, myalgia, rash, and pharyngitis. After a few days, mucoid or mucopurulent sputum is expectorated. In severe pneumonia, the cheeks are flushed and the lips and nailbeds demonstrate central cyanosis (a late sign of poor oxygenation [hypoxemia]).

Typically, the patient has **orthopnea** (shortness of breath when reclining); he or she prefers to be propped up in bed leaning forward (orthopneic position), trying to achieve adequate gas exchange without coughing or breathing deeply. Appetite is poor, and the patient is diaphoretic and tires easily. Sputum is often purulent; this is not a reliable indicator of the etiologic agent. Rusty, blood-tinged sputum may be expectorated with streptococcal (pneumococcal), staphylococcal, and *Klebsiella* pneumonia.

Signs and symptoms of pneumonia may also depend on underlying conditions. Differing signs occur in patients with other conditions, such as cancer, or in those who are undergoing treatment with immunosuppressants, which lower the resistance to infection. Such patients have fever, crackles, and physical findings that indicate consolidation of lung tissue, including increased tactile fremitus (vocal vibration detected on palpation), percussion dullness, bronchial breath sounds, egophony (when auscultated, the spoken "E" becomes a loud, nasal-sounding "A"), and whispered pectoriloquy (whispered sounds are easily auscultated through the chest wall). These changes occur because sound is transmitted better through solid or dense tissue (consolidation) than through normal air-filled tissue; these sounds are described in Chapter 21.

Purulent sputum or slight changes in respiratory symptoms may be the only sign of pneumonia in patients with COPD. It may be difficult to determine whether an increase in symptoms is an exacerbation of the underlying disease process or an additional infectious process.

Assessment and Diagnostic Findings

The diagnosis of pneumonia is made by history (particularly of a recent respiratory tract infection), physical examination, chest x-ray studies, blood culture (bloodstream invasion, called bacteremia, occurs frequently), and sputum examination. The sputum sample is obtained by having the patient: (1) rinse the mouth with water to minimize contamination by normal oral flora, (2) breathe deeply several times, (3) cough deeply, and (4) expectorate the raised sputum into a sterile container.

More invasive procedures may be used to collect specimens. Sputum may be obtained by nasotracheal or orotracheal suctioning with a sputum trap or by fiberoptic bronchoscopy (see Chap. 21). Bronchoscopy is often used in patients with acute severe infection, patients with chronic or refractory infection, or immunocompromised patients when a diagnosis cannot be made from an expectorated or induced specimen.

Medical Management

The treatment of pneumonia includes administration of the appropriate antibiotic as determined by the results of the Gram stain. However, an etiologic agent is not identified in 50% of CAP cases and empiric therapy must be initiated. Therapy for CAP is continuing to evolve. Guidelines exist to guide antibiotic choice; however, the resistance patterns, prevalence of etiologic

agents, patient risk factors, and costs and availability of newer antibiotic agents must all be taken into consideration.

Several organizations have published guidelines for the medical management of CAP (Bartlett et al., 2000; American Thoracic Society, 2001). Recommendations are classified by existing risk factors, setting (inpatient vs. outpatient treatment), or specific pathogens. Examples of risk factors that may increase the risk of infection with certain types of pathogens appear in Chart 23-3.

Recommendations for treatment of outpatients with CAP who have no cardiopulmonary disease or other modifying factors include a macrolide (erythromycin, azithromycin [Zithromax], or clarithromycin [Biaxin]), doxycycline (Vibramycin), or a fluoroquinolone (eg, gatifloxacin [Tequin], levofloxacin [Levaquin]) with enhanced activity against *S. pneumoniae* (Bartlett et al., 2000; American Thoracic Society, 2001). Erythromycin should be avoided in areas where *H. influenzae* and *S. aureus* are more prevalent (Kenreigh & Wagner, 2000; Lynch, 2000). For those outpatients who have cardiopulmonary disease or other modifying factors, treatment should include a beta-lactam (oral cefpodoxime [Vantin], cefuroxime [Zinacef, Ceftin], high-dose amoxicillin or amoxicillin/clavulanate [Augmentin, Clavulin]) plus a macrolide or doxycycline. Also, a beta-lactam plus an antipneumococcal fluoroquinolone can be used (American Thoracic Society, 2001). These are guidelines; treatment for individual patients may be modified.

For patients with CAP who are hospitalized and do not have cardiopulmonary disease or modifying factors, management consists of intravenous azithromycin (Zithromax) or monotherapy with an antipneumococcal fluoroquinolone. For inpatients with cardiopulmonary disease or modifying factors, the treatment involves an intravenous beta-lactam plus an intravenous or oral macrolide or doxycycline. An intravenous antipneumococcal fluoroquinolone may also be used alone (American Thoracic Society, 2001). For acutely ill patients admitted to the intensive care unit, management includes an intravenous beta-lactam plus either an intravenous macrolide or fluoroquinolone. For patients

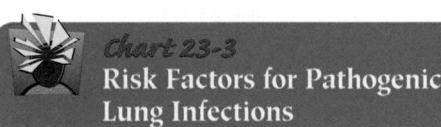

Chart 23-3
Risk Factors for Pathogenic Lung Infections

Risk Factors for Infection with Penicillin-Resistant and Drug-Resistant Pneumococci
- Age over 65 years
- Alcoholism
- Beta-lactam therapy (eg, cephalosporins) in past 3 months
- Immunosuppressive disorders
- Multiple medical comorbidities
- Exposure to a child in a day care facility

Risk Factors for Infection with Enteric Gram-Negative Bacteria
- Nursing home residency
- Underlying cardiopulmonary disease
- Multiple medical comorbidities
- Recent antibiotic therapy

Risk Factors for Infection with *Pseudomonas aeruginosa*
- Structural lung disease (eg, bronchiectasis)
- Corticosteroid therapy
- Broad-spectrum antibiotic therapy (more than 7 days in the past month)
- Malnutrition

(American Thoracic Society, 2001)

at high risk for *P. aeruginosa,* more select antipseudomonal antibiotics are administered intravenously.

If specific pathogens have been identified for the CAP, more specific agents may be utilized. Mycoplasma pneumonia is treated with doxycycline or a macrolide. PCP responds best to pentamidine and trimethoprim–sulfamethoxazole (TMP-SMZ). Amantadine and rimantadine are effective with influenza A and have been shown to reduce the duration of fever and other systemic complications when administered within 24 to 48 hours of the onset of an uncomplicated influenza infection. These medications also reduce the duration and quantity of virus shedding in the respiratory secretions. They are most effective when used in combination with influenza vaccine. Ganciclovir is used to treat cytomegalovirus in the non-AIDS patient; cytomegalovirus immunoglobulin may also be used.

HAP has a different etiology from CAP. In suspected HAP or nosocomial pneumonia, empirical treatment is usually initiated with a broad-spectrum intravenous antibiotic and may be monotherapy or combination therapy. In patients who are mildly to moderately ill with a low risk of *Pseudomonas,* the following antibiotics may be used: second-generation cephalosporins (eg, cefuroxime [Ceftin, Zinacef] or cefamandole [Mandol]), nonpseudomonal third-generation cephalosporins (ceftriaxone [Rocephin], cefotaxime [Claforan], ampicillin-sulbactam [Unasyn]), or fluoroquinolones (eg, ciprofloxacin [Cipro], levofloxacin [Levaquin]). For combination therapy, any of the above may be used with an aminoglycoside.

For patients at high risk for *Pseudomonas* infection, an antipseudomonal penicillin plus an aminoglycoside (amikacin [Amikin], gentamicin) or beta-lactamase inhibitor (ampicillin/sulbactam [Unasyn], ticarcillin/clavulanate [Timentin]) may be used. Other types of combination therapy may also be used depending upon the individual characteristics of the patient.

Of concern is the rampant rise in respiratory pathogens that are resistant to available antibiotics. Examples include vancomycin-resistant enterococcus (VRE) and drug-resistant *S. pneumoniae* (McGeer & Low, 2000). There is a tendency for clinicians to aggressively use antibiotics inappropriately or to use broad-spectrum agents when narrow-spectrum agents are more appropriate. Mechanisms to monitor and minimize the inappropriate use of antibiotics are in place. Education of clinicians to use evidence-based guidelines in the treatment of respiratory infection is important. Monitoring and surveillance of susceptibility patterns for pathogens are also important.

Therapy with parenteral agents usually is changed to oral antimicrobial agents when there is evidence of a clinical response and the patient is able to tolerate oral medications. The recommended duration of treatment for pneumococcal pneumonia is 72 hours after the patient becomes afebrile. Most other forms of pneumonia caused by bacterial pathogens are treated for 1 to 2 weeks after the patient becomes afebrile. Atypical pneumonia is usually treated for 10 to 21 days (Bartlett, Dowell, Mandell et al., 2000).

Treatment of viral pneumonia is primarily supportive. Antibiotics are ineffective in viral upper respiratory infections and pneumonia and may be associated with adverse effects. Treatment of viral infections with antibiotics is a major reason for the overuse of these medications in the United States. Antibiotics are indicated with a viral respiratory infection *only* when a secondary bacterial pneumonia, bronchitis, or sinusitis is present. Hydration is a necessary part of therapy because fever and tachypnea may result in insensible fluid losses. Antipyretics may be used to treat headache and fever; antitussive medications may be used for the associated cough. Warm, moist inhalations are helpful in relieving bronchial

irritation. Antihistamines may provide benefit with reduced sneezing and rhinorrhea. Nasal decongestants may also be used to treat symptoms and improve sleep; however, excessive use may cause rebound nasal congestion. Treatment of viral pneumonia (with the exception of antimicrobial therapy) is the same as that for bacterial pneumonia. The patient is placed on bed rest until the infection shows signs of clearing. If hospitalized, the patient is observed carefully until the clinical condition improves.

If hypoxemia develops, oxygen is administered. Pulse oximetry or arterial blood gas analysis is performed to determine the need for oxygen and to evaluate the effectiveness of the therapy. A high concentration of oxygen is contraindicated in patients with COPD because it may worsen alveolar ventilation by decreasing the patient's ventilatory drive, leading to further respiratory decompensation. Respiratory support measures include high oxygen concentrations (fraction of inspired oxygen [FiO_2]), endotracheal intubation, and mechanical ventilation. Different modes of mechanical ventilation may be required; see Chapter 25.

Figure 23-3 provides an algorithm for patients with suspected CAP.

Gerontologic Considerations

Pneumonia in the elderly patient may occur as a primary problem or as a complication of a chronic disease process. Pulmonary infections in the elderly frequently are difficult to treat and have a higher mortality rate than in younger patients. General deterioration, weakness, abdominal symptoms, anorexia, confusion, tachycardia, and tachypnea may signal the onset of pneumonia. The diagnosis of pneumonia may be missed because the classic symptoms of cough, chest pain, sputum production, and fever may be absent or masked in the elderly patient. Also, the presence of some signs may be misleading. Abnormal breath sounds, for example, may be due to microatelectasis that occurs in the aged as a result of decreased mobility, decreased lung volumes, and other respiratory function changes. Because chronic heart failure is often seen in the elderly, chest x-rays may be obtained to assist in differentiating it from pneumonia as the cause of clinical signs and symptoms.

Supportive treatment includes hydration (with caution and frequent assessment because of the risk of fluid overload in the elderly), supplemental oxygen therapy, assistance with deep breathing, coughing, frequent position changes, and early ambulation. All of these are particularly important in the care of the elderly patient with pneumonia. To reduce or prevent serious complications of pneumonia in the elderly, vaccination against pneumococcal and influenza infections is recommended.

Complications

SHOCK AND RESPIRATORY FAILURE

Severe complications of pneumonia include hypotension and shock and respiratory failure (especially with gram-negative bacterial disease in elderly patients). These complications are encountered chiefly in patients who have received no specific treatment or inadequate or delayed treatment. These complications are also encountered when the infecting organism is resistant to therapy and when a comorbid disease complicates the pneumonia.

If the patient is seriously ill, aggressive therapy may include hemodynamic and ventilatory support to combat peripheral collapse, maintain arterial blood pressure, and provide adequate oxygenation. A vasopressor agent may be administered intravenously by continuous infusion and at a rate adjusted in accordance with

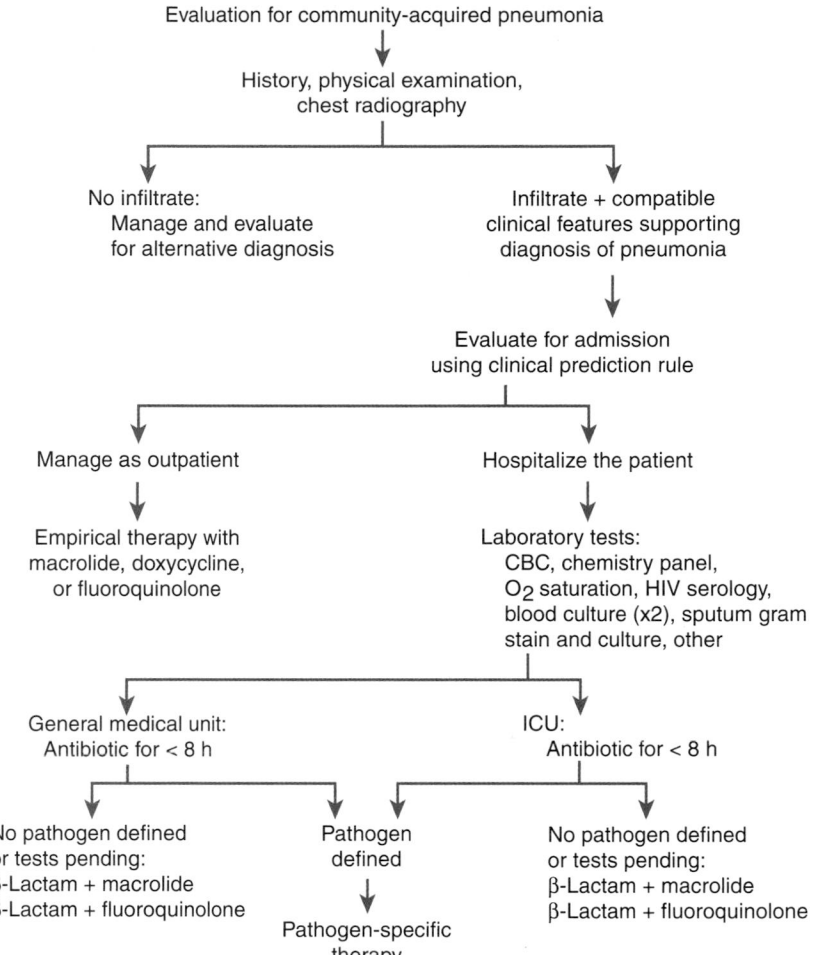

FIGURE 23-3 Treatment algorithm for patient with suspected CAP. From Bartlett, J. G. et al. (2000). Practice guidelines for the management of community-acquired pneumonia in adults. *Clinical Infectious Diseases, 31* (2), 347–382.

the pressure response. Corticosteroids may be administered parenterally to combat shock and toxicity in patients who are extremely ill with pneumonia and in apparent danger of dying of the infection. Patients may require endotracheal intubation and mechanical ventilation. Congestive heart failure, cardiac dysrhythmias, pericarditis, and myocarditis also are complications of pneumonia that may lead to shock.

ATELECTASIS AND PLEURAL EFFUSION

Atelectasis (from obstruction of a bronchus by accumulated secretions) may occur at any stage of acute pneumonia. Parapneumonic pleural effusions occur in at least 40% of bacterial pneumonias. A parapneumonic effusion is any pleural effusion associated with bacterial pneumonia, lung abscess, or bronchiectasis. After the pleural effusion is detected on a chest x-ray, a thoracentesis may be performed to remove the fluid. The fluid is sent to the laboratory for analysis. There are three stages of parapneumonic pleural effusions based on pathogenesis: uncomplicated, complicated, and thoracic empyema. An **empyema** occurs when thick, purulent fluid accumulates within the pleural space, often with fibrin development and a loculated (walled-off) area where the infection is located. (Empyema is discussed in greater detail in the section Pleural Conditions, below.) A chest tube may be inserted to treat pleural infection by establishing proper drainage of the empyema. Sterilization of the empyema cavity requires 4 to 6 weeks of antibiotics. Sometimes surgical management is required.

SUPERINFECTION

Superinfection may occur with the administration of very large doses of antibiotics, such as penicillin, or with combinations of antibiotics. Superinfection may also occur in the patient who has been receiving numerous courses and types of antibiotics. In such cases, bacteria may become resistant to the antibiotic therapy. If the patient improves and the fever diminishes after initial antibiotic therapy, but subsequently there is a rise in temperature with increasing cough and evidence that the pneumonia has spread, a superinfection is likely. Antibiotics are changed appropriately or discontinued entirely in some cases.

NURSING PROCESS: THE PATIENT WITH PNEUMONIA

Assessment

Nursing assessment is critical in detecting pneumonia. A fever, chills, or night sweats in a patient who also has respiratory symptoms should alert the nurse to the possibility of bacterial pneumonia. A respiratory assessment will further identify the clinical manifestations of pneumonia: pleuritic-type pain, fatigue, tachypnea, use of accessory muscles for breathing, bradycardia or relative bradycardia, coughing, and purulent sputum. It is important to identify the severity, location, and cause of the chest pain, along with any medications or procedures that provide relief. The nurse should monitor the following:

- Changes in temperature and pulse
- Amount, odor, and color of secretions
- Frequency and severity of cough
- Degree of tachypnea or shortness of breath
- Changes in physical assessment findings (primarily assessed by inspecting and auscultating the chest)
- Changes in the chest x-ray findings

In addition, it is important to assess the elderly patient for unusual behavior, altered mental status, dehydration, excessive fatigue, and concomitant heart failure.

Diagnosis

NURSING DIAGNOSES

Based on the assessment data, the patient's major nursing diagnoses may include:

- Ineffective airway clearance related to copious tracheobronchial secretions
- Activity intolerance related to impaired respiratory function
- Risk for deficient fluid volume related to fever and dyspnea
- Imbalanced nutrition: less than body requirements
- Deficient knowledge about the treatment regimen and preventive health measures

COLLABORATIVE PROBLEMS/ POTENTIAL COMPLICATIONS

Based on the assessment data, collaborative problems or potential complications that may occur include:

- Continuing symptoms after initiation of therapy
- Shock
- Respiratory failure
- Atelectasis
- Pleural effusion
- Confusion
- Superinfection

Planning and Goals

The major goals for the patient may include improved airway patency, rest to conserve energy, maintenance of proper fluid volume, maintenance of adequate nutrition, an understanding of the treatment protocol and preventive measures, and absence of complications.

Nursing Interventions

IMPROVING AIRWAY PATENCY

Removing secretions is important because retained secretions interfere with gas exchange and may slow recovery. The nurse encourages hydration (2 to 3 L/day) because adequate hydration thins and loosens pulmonary secretions. Humidification may be used to loosen secretions and improve ventilation. A high-humidity facemask (using either compressed air or oxygen) delivers warm, humidified air to the tracheobronchial tree, helps to liquefy secretions, and relieves tracheobronchial irritation. Coughing can be initiated either voluntarily or by reflex. Lung expansion maneuvers, such as deep breathing with an incentive spirometer, may induce a cough. A directed cough may be necessary to improve airway patency. The nurse encourages the patient to perform an effective, directed cough, which includes correct positioning, a deep inspiratory maneuver, glottic closure, contraction of the expiratory muscles against the closed glottis, sudden glottic opening, and an explosive expiration. In some cases, the nurse may assist the patient by placing both hands on the patient's lower rib cage (anteriorly or posteriorly) to focus the patient on a slow deep breath, and then manually assisting the patient by applying external pressure during the expiratory phase.

Chest physiotherapy (percussion and postural drainage) is important in loosening and mobilizing secretions (see Chap. 25). Indications for chest physiotherapy include sputum retention not responsive to spontaneous or directed cough, a history of pulmonary problems previously treated with chest physiotherapy, continued evidence of retained secretions (decreased or abnormal breath sounds, change in vital signs), abnormal chest x-ray findings consistent with atelectasis or infiltrates, or deterioration in oxygenation. The patient is placed in the proper position to drain the involved lung segments, and then the chest is percussed and vibrated either manually or with a mechanical percussor.

After each position change, the nurse encourages the patient to breathe deeply and cough. If the patient is too weak to cough effectively, the nurse may need to remove the mucus by nasotracheal suctioning (see Chap. 25). It may take time for secretions to mobilize and move into the central airways for expectoration. Thus, it is important for the nurse to monitor the patient for cough and sputum production after the completion of chest physiotherapy.

The nurse administers and titrates oxygen therapy as prescribed. The effectiveness of oxygen therapy is monitored by improvement in clinical signs and symptoms, and adequate oxygenation values measured by pulse oximetry or arterial blood gas analysis.

PROMOTING REST AND CONSERVING ENERGY

The nurse encourages the debilitated patient to rest and avoid overexertion and possible exacerbation of symptoms. The patient should assume a comfortable position to promote rest and breathing (eg, semi-Fowler's) and should change positions frequently to enhance secretion clearance and ventilation/perfusion in the lungs. It is important to instruct outpatients not to overexert themselves and to engage in only moderate activity during the initial phases of treatment.

PROMOTING FLUID INTAKE

The respiratory rate of a patient with pneumonia increases because of the increased workload imposed by labored breathing and fever. An increased respiratory rate leads to an increase in insensible fluid loss during exhalation and can lead to dehydration. Therefore, it is important to encourage increased fluid intake (at least 2 L/day), unless contraindicated.

MAINTAINING NUTRITION

Patients with shortness of breath and fatigue often have a decreased appetite and will take only fluids. Fluids with electrolytes (commercially available drinks, such as Gatorade) may help provide fluid, calories, and electrolytes. Other nutritionally enriched drinks or shakes may be helpful. In addition, fluids and nutrients may be administered intravenously if necessary.

PROMOTING THE PATIENT'S KNOWLEDGE

The patient and family are instructed about the cause of pneumonia, management of symptoms of pneumonia, and the need for follow-up (discussed later). The patient also needs information about factors (both patient risk factors and external factors) that may have contributed to developing pneumonia and strategies to promote recovery and to prevent recurrence. If hospitalized for treatment, the patient is instructed about the purpose and importance of management strategies that have been implemented and about the importance of adhering to them during and after the hospital stay. Explanations need to be given simply and in language that the patient can understand. If possible, written instructions and information should be provided. Because of the severity of symptoms, the patient may require that instructions and explanations be repeated several times.

MONITORING AND MANAGING POTENTIAL COMPLICATIONS

Continuing Symptoms After Initiation of Therapy

Patients usually begin to respond to treatment within 24 to 48 hours after antibiotic therapy is initiated. The patient is observed for response to antibiotic therapy. The patient is monitored for changes in physical status (deterioration of condition or resolution of symptoms) and for persistent recurrent fever, which may be due to medication allergy (signaled possibly by a rash); medication resistance or slow response (greater than 48 hours) of the susceptible organism to therapy; superinfection; pleural effusion; or pneumonia caused by an unusual organism, such as *P. carinii* or *Aspergillus fumigatus*. Failure of the pneumonia to resolve or persistence of symptoms despite changes on the chest x-ray raises the suspicion of other underlying disorders, such as lung cancer. As described earlier, lung cancers may invade or compress airways, causing an obstructive atelectasis that may lead to a pneumonia.

In addition to monitoring for continuing symptoms of pneumonia, the nurse also monitors for other complications, such as shock and multisystem failure, atelectasis, pleural effusion, and superinfection, which may develop during the first few days of antibiotic treatment.

Shock and Respiratory Failure

The nurse assesses for signs and symptoms of shock and respiratory failure by evaluating the patient's vital signs, pulse oximetry values, and hemodynamic monitoring parameters. The nurse reports signs of deteriorating patient status and assists in administering intravenous fluids and medications prescribed to combat shock. Intubation and mechanical ventilation may be required if respiratory failure occurs. Shock is described in detail in Chapter 15, and care of the patient receiving mechanical ventilation is described in Chapter 25.

Atelectasis and Pleural Effusion

The patient is assessed for atelectasis, and preventive measures are initiated to prevent its development. If pleural effusion develops and thoracentesis is performed to remove fluid, the nurse assists in the procedure and explains it to the patient. After thoracentesis, the nurse monitors the patient for pneumothorax or recurrence of pleural effusion. If a chest tube needs to be inserted, the nurse monitors the patient's respiratory status (see Chap. 25 for more information on care of the patient with a chest tube).

Superinfection

The patient is monitored for manifestations of superinfection (ie, minimal improvement in signs and symptoms, rise in temperature with increasing cough, increasing fremitus and adventitious breath sounds on auscultation of the lungs). These signs are re-

ported, and the nurse assists in implementing therapy to treat superinfection.

Confusion

The patient with pneumonia is assessed for confusion and other more subtle changes in cognitive status. Confusion and changes in cognitive status resulting from pneumonia are poor prognostic signs. Confusion may be related to hypoxemia, fever, dehydration, sleep deprivation, or developing sepsis. The patient's underlying comorbid conditions may also play a part in the development of confusion. Addressing the underlying factors and ensuring the patient's safety are important nursing interventions.

PROMOTING HOME AND COMMUNITY-BASED CARE

Teaching Patients Self-Care

Depending on the severity of the pneumonia, treatment may occur in the hospital or in the outpatient setting. Patient education is crucial regardless of the setting, and the proper administration of antibiotics is important. In some instances, the patient may be initially treated with intravenous antibiotics as an inpatient and then be discharged to continue the intravenous antibiotics in the home setting. It is important that a seamless system of care be maintained for the patient from hospital to home; this includes communication between the nurses caring for this patient in both settings. In addition, if oral antibiotics are prescribed, it is important to teach the patient about their proper administration and potential side effects.

After the fever subsides, the patient may gradually increase activities. Fatigue and weakness may be prolonged after pneumonia, especially in the elderly. The nurse encourages breathing exercises to promote secretion clearance and volume expansion. It is important to instruct the patient to return to the clinic or caregiver's office for a follow-up chest x-ray and physical examination. Often improvement in chest x-ray findings lags behind improvement in clinical signs and symptoms.

The nurse encourages the patient to stop smoking. Smoking inhibits tracheobronchial ciliary action, which is the first line of defense of the lower respiratory tract. Smoking also irritates the mucous cells of the bronchi and inhibits the function of alveolar macrophage (scavenger) cells. The patient is instructed to avoid stress, fatigue, sudden changes in temperature, and excessive alcohol intake, all of which lower resistance to pneumonia. The nurse reviews with the patient the principles of adequate nutrition and rest, because one episode of pneumonia may make the patient susceptible to recurring respiratory tract infections.

Continuing Care

Patients who are severely debilitated or who cannot care for themselves may require referral for home care. During home visits, the nurse assesses the patient's physical status, monitors for complications, assesses the home environment, and reinforces previous teaching. The nurse evaluates the patient's adherence to the therapeutic regimen (ie, taking medications as prescribed, performing breathing exercises, consuming adequate fluid and dietary intake, and avoiding smoking, alcohol, and excessive activity). The nurse stresses to the patient and family the importance of monitoring for complications. The nurse encourages the patient to obtain an influenza vaccine at the prescribed times, because influenza increases susceptibility to secondary bacterial pneumonia, especially that caused by staphylococci, *H. influenzae*, and *S. pneumoniae*. The nurse also encourages the patient to seek medical advice about receiving the vaccine (Pneumovax) against *S. pneumoniae*.

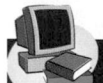

NURSING RESEARCH PROFILE 23-1

Tobacco-Related Nursing Interventions

Sarna, L. P., Brown, J. K., Lillington, L., Rose, M., Wewers, M. E., & Brecht, M. (2000). Tobacco interventions by oncology nurses in clinical practice. *Cancer, 89*(4), 881–889.

Purpose

Smoking remains a major cause of death in all populations in the U.S. The purpose of this study was to describe the frequency of interventions related to the use of tobacco used by oncology nurses, using the Agency for Health Care Policy and Research (AHCPR) guidelines as a framework.

Study Sample and Design

This was a descriptive study; a self-report questionnaire was mailed to a random sample of 4,000 members of the Oncology Nursing Society. The response rate was 38%, with 1,508 completed questionnaires available for analysis. Subjects were asked to identify those interventions related to tobacco use that they used in their clinical practice.

Findings

The majority of respondents were female (98%), with an average age of 44 years. The educational background of respondents was varied, with 39% with baccalaureate preparation, 41% with associate or diploma education, and 20% with master's or doctoral level education. Sixty-two percent of the respondents reported their position as staff nurse. Overall, the sample was characterized as experienced nurses, with average number of years in nursing at 18 ± 9.4 years

and as an oncology nurse for 11.5 ± 5.5 years. Thirty percent of the sample were ex-smokers, while 7% were active smokers. The results demonstrated that most respondents (86%) encountered smokers in their clinical practice on a weekly basis, but only 10% had any knowledge of the AHCPR guidelines for smoking cessation. Sixty-four percent of the respondents assessed and documented smoking status in their clinical patients and 38% assessed readiness to quit. However, fewer nurses reported providing interventions for smoking cessation. The most frequent barriers cited included perceived lack of patient motivation (74%), time (52%), and skills to provide a cessation intervention (53%).

Nursing Implications

Nurses have frequent contacts with active smokers in the inpatient and outpatient setting and could have a tremendous impact on smoking prevention and cessation. Even in this sample of oncology nurses, few provided smoking cessation interventions on a regular basis. Nurses need a heightened awareness of the importance of smoking cessation and the potential impact they may have on this growing problem. It is imperative that students and practicing nurses receive improved education regarding smoking cessation techniques and use of evidence-based guidelines like those of the AHCPR.

Evaluation

EXPECTED PATIENT OUTCOMES

Expected patient outcomes may include:

1. Demonstrates improved airway patency, as evidenced by adequate oxygenation by pulse oximetry or arterial blood gas analysis, normal temperature, normal breath sounds, and effective coughing
2. Rests and conserves energy by limiting activities and remaining in bed while symptomatic and slowly increasing activities
3. Maintains adequate hydration, as evidenced by an adequate fluid intake and urine output and normal skin turgor
4. Consumes adequate dietary intake, as evidenced by maintenance or increase in body weight without excess fluid gain
5. States explanation for management strategies
6. Complies with management strategies
7. Exhibits no complications
   a. Has normal vital signs, pulse oximetry, and arterial blood gas measurements
   b. Reports productive cough that diminishes over time
   c. Has absence of signs or symptoms of shock, respiratory failure, or pleural effusion
   d. Remains oriented and aware of surroundings
   e. Maintains or increases weight
8. Complies with treatment protocol and prevention strategies

PULMONARY TUBERCULOSIS

Tuberculosis (TB) is an infectious disease that primarily affects the lung parenchyma. It also may be transmitted to other parts of the body, including the meninges, kidneys, bones, and lymph nodes. The primary infectious agent, *Mycobacterium tuberculosis*,

is an acid-fast aerobic rod that grows slowly and is sensitive to heat and ultraviolet light. *Mycobacterium bovis* and *Mycobacterium avium* have rarely been associated with the development of a TB infection.

TB is a worldwide public health problem, and the mortality and morbidity rates continue to rise. *M. tuberculosis* infects an estimated one third of the world's population and remains the leading cause of death from infectious disease in the world. It is the leading cause of death among HIV-positive people (World Health Organization, 2000). TB is closely associated with poverty, malnutrition, overcrowding, substandard housing, and inadequate health care.

In 1952, anti-TB medications were introduced, and the rate of reported cases of TB in the United States declined an average of 6% each year between 1953 and 1985. It was thought that by the early part of the 21st century, TB might be eliminated in the United States. However, since 1985 the trend has reversed and the number of cases has increased. This change has been attributed to several factors, including increased immigration, the HIV epidemic, the emergence of multidrug-resistant strains of TB, increased homelessness, decreased interest and detection by health care providers, and inadequate funding of the U.S. public health system (Small & Fujiwara, 2001).

Transmission and Risk Factors

TB spreads from person to person by airborne transmission. An infected person releases droplet nuclei (generally particles 1 to 5 micrometers in diameter) through talking, coughing, sneezing, laughing, or singing. Larger droplets settle; smaller droplets remain suspended in the air and are inhaled by the susceptible person. Risk factors for TB are listed in Chart 23-4. Chart 23-5 summarizes the CDC's recommendations for prevention of TB transmission in health care settings.

Chart 23-4

Risk Factors for Tuberculosis

- Close contact with someone who has active TB. Inhalation of airborne nuclei from an infected person is proportional to the amount of time spent in the same air space, the proximity of the person, and the degree of ventilation.
- Immunocompromised status (eg, those with HIV infection, cancer, transplanted organs, and prolonged high-dose corticosteroid therapy)
- Substance abuse (IV or injection drug users and alcoholics)
- Any person without adequate health care (the homeless; impoverished; minorities, particularly children under age 15 years and young adults between ages 15 and 44 yrs)
- Preexisting medical conditions or special treatment (eg, diabetes, chronic renal failure, malnourishment, selected malignancies, he-

modialysis, transplanted organ, gastrectomy, or jejunoileal bypass)
- Immigration from countries with a high prevalence of TB (southeastern Asia, Africa, Latin America, Caribbean)
- Institutionalization (eg, long-term care facilities, psychiatric institutions, prisons)
- Living in overcrowded, substandard housing
- Being a health care worker performing high-risk activities: administration of aerosolized pentamidine and other medications, sputum induction procedures, bronchoscopy, suctioning, coughing procedures, caring for the immunosuppressed patient, home care with the high-risk population, and administering anesthesia and related procedures (eg, intubation, suctioning)

Pathophysiology

A susceptible person inhales mycobacterium bacilli and becomes infected. The bacteria are transmitted through the airways to the alveoli, where they are deposited and begin to multiply. The bacilli also are transported via the lymph system and bloodstream to other parts of the body (kidneys, bones, cerebral cortex) and other areas of the lungs (upper lobes). The body's immune system responds by initiating an inflammatory reaction. Phagocytes (neutrophils and macrophages) engulf many of the bacteria, and TB-specific lymphocytes lyse (destroy) the bacilli and normal tissue. This tissue reaction results in the accumulation of exudate in the alveoli, causing bronchopneumonia. The initial infection usually occurs 2 to 10 weeks after exposure.

Granulomas, new tissue masses of live and dead bacilli, are surrounded by macrophages, which form a protective wall around the granulomas. Granulomas are then transformed to a fibrous tissue mass, the central portion of which is called a Ghon tubercle. The material (bacteria and macrophages) becomes necrotic, forming a cheesy mass. This mass may become calcified and form a col-

lagenous scar. At this point, the bacteria become dormant, and there is no further progression of active disease.

After initial exposure and infection, the person may develop active disease because of a compromised or inadequate immune system response. Active disease also may occur with reinfection and activation of dormant bacteria. In this case, the Ghon tubercle ulcerates, releasing the cheesy material into the bronchi. The bacteria then become airborne, resulting in further spread of the disease. Then the ulcerated tubercle heals and forms scar tissue. This causes the infected lung to become more inflamed, resulting in further development of bronchopneumonia and tubercle formation.

Unless the process is arrested, it spreads slowly downward to the hilum of the lungs and later extends to adjacent lobes. The process may be prolonged and characterized by long remissions when the disease is arrested, only to be followed by periods of renewed activity. Approximately 10% of people who are initially infected develop active disease. Some people develop reactivation TB (also called adult-type TB). This type of TB results from a breakdown of the host defenses. It most commonly occurs within

Chart 23-5

CDC Recommendations for Preventing Transmission of Tuberculosis in Health Care Settings

1. Early identification and treatment of persons with active TB
   a. Maintain a high index of suspicion for TB to identify cases rapidly.
   b. Promptly initiate effective multidrug anti-TB therapy based on clinical and drug-resistance surveillance data.
2. Prevention of spread of infectious droplet nuclei by source control methods and by reduction of microbial contamination of indoor air
   a. Initiate acid-fast bacilli (AFB) isolation precautions immediately for all patients who are suspected or confirmed to have active TB and who may be infectious. AFB isolation precautions include use of a private room with negative pressure in relation to surrounding areas and a minimum of six air exchanges per hour. Air from the room should be exhausted directly to the outside. Use of ultraviolet lamps and/or high-efficiency particulate air filters to supplement ventilation may be considered.
   b. Persons entering the AFB isolation room should use disposable particulate respirators that fit snugly around the face.
   c. Continue AFB isolation precautions until there is clinical evidence of reduced infectiousness (ie, cough has substantially de-

creased, and the number of organisms on sequential sputum smears is decreasing). If drug resistance is suspected or confirmed, continue AFB precautions until the sputum smear is negative for AFB.
   d. Use special precautions during cough-inducing procedures.
3. Surveillance for TB transmission
   a. Maintain surveillance for TB infection among health care workers (HCWs) by routine, periodic tuberculin skin testing. Recommend appropriate preventive therapy for HCWs when indicated.
   b. Maintain surveillance for TB cases among patients and HCWs.
   c. Promptly initiate contact investigation procedures among HCWs, patients, and visitors exposed to an untreated, or ineffectively treated, infectious TB patient for whom appropriate AFB procedures are not in place. Recommend appropriate therapy or preventive therapy for contacts with disease or TB infection without current disease. Therapeutic regimens should be chosen based on the clinical history and local drug-resistance surveillance data.

the lungs, usually in the apical or posterior segments of the upper lobes, or the superior segments of the lower lobes.

Clinical Manifestations

The signs and symptoms of pulmonary TB are insidious. Most patients have a low-grade fever, cough, night sweats, fatigue, and weight loss. The cough may be nonproductive, or mucopurulent sputum may be expectorated. Hemoptysis also may occur. Both the systemic and pulmonary symptoms are usually chronic and may have been present for weeks to months. The elderly usually present with less pronounced symptoms than do younger patients. Extrapulmonary disease occurs in up to 16% of cases in the United States. In patients with AIDS, extrapulmonary disease is more prevalent and may occur in up to 70% of cases (Niederman & Sarosi, 2000; Small & Fujiwara, 2001).

Assessment and Diagnostic Findings

A complete history, physical examination, tuberculin skin test, chest x-ray, acid-fast bacillus smear, and sputum culture are used to diagnose TB. If the person is infected with TB, the chest x-ray usually reveals lesions in the upper lobes and the acid-fast bacillus smear contains mycobacterium.

TUBERCULIN SKIN TEST

The Mantoux test is used to determine if a person has been infected with the TB bacillus. The Mantoux test is a standardized procedure and should be performed only by those trained in its administration and reading. Tubercle bacillus extract (tuberculin), purified protein derivative (PPD), is injected into the intradermal layer of the inner aspect of the forearm, approximately 4 inches below the elbow (Fig. 23-4). Intermediate-strength (5 TU) PPD in a tuberculin syringe with a half-inch 26- or 27-gauge nee-

dle is used. The needle, with the bevel facing up, is inserted beneath the skin. Then 0.1 mL of PPD is injected, creating an elevation in the skin, a wheal or bleb. The site, antigen name, strength, lot number, date, and time of the test are recorded. The test result is read 48 to 72 hours after injection. Tests read after 72 hours tend to underestimate the true size of **induration** (hardening). A delayed localized reaction indicates that the person is sensitive to tuberculin.

A reaction occurs when both induration and erythema (redness) are noted. After the area is inspected for induration, it is lightly palpated across the injection site, from the area of normal skin to the margins of the induration. The diameter of the induration (not erythema) is measured in millimeters at its widest part (see Fig. 23-4), and the size of the induration is documented. Erythema without induration is not considered significant.

Interpretation of Results. The size of the induration determines the significance of the reaction. A reaction of 0 to 4 mm is considered not significant; a reaction of 5 mm or greater may be significant in individuals who are considered at risk. An induration of 10 mm or greater is usually considered significant in individuals who have normal or mildly impaired immunity. A significant reaction indicates that a patient has been exposed to *M. tuberculosis* recently or in the past or has been vaccinated with bacille Calmette-Guerin (BCG) vaccine. The BCG vaccine is given to produce a greater resistance to developing TB. It is effective in up to 76% of those who receive it. The vaccine is used in Europe and Latin America but not routinely in the United States.

A reaction of 5 mm or greater is defined as positive for patients who are HIV-positive or have HIV risk factors and are of unknown HIV status, those who are close contacts with an active case, and those who have chest x-ray results consistent with tuberculosis.

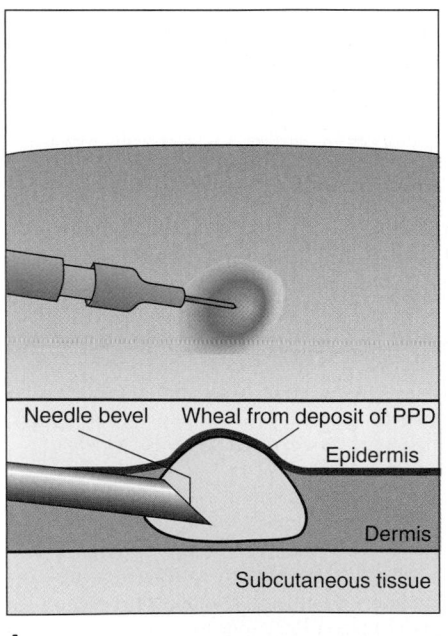

Needle bevel   Wheal from deposit of PPD
Epidermis
Dermis
Subcutaneous tissue

A

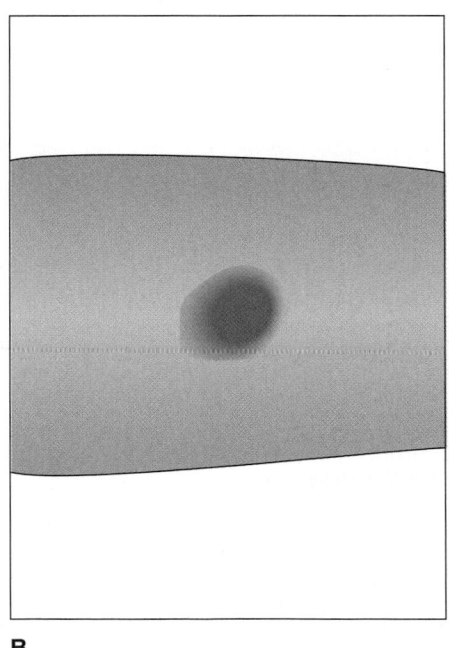

B

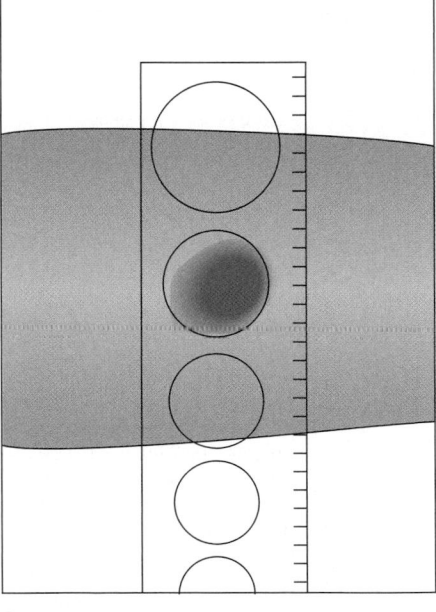

C

FIGURE 23-4 The Mantoux test for tuberculosis. (**A**) Correct technique for inserting the needle involves depositing the PPD subcutaneously with the needle bevel facing upward. (**B**) The reaction to the Mantoux test usually consists of a wheal, a hivelike, firm welt. (**C**) To determine the extent of the reaction, the wheal is measured using a commercially prepared gauge. A wheal measuring 5 mm or more is considered significant.

A significant (positive) reaction does not necessarily mean that active disease is present in the body. Most (more than 90%) people who are tuberculin-significant reactors do not develop clinical TB. However, all significant reactors are candidates for active TB. In general, the more intense the reaction, the greater the likelihood of an active infection.

A nonsignificant (negative) skin test does not exclude TB infection or disease because patients who are immunosuppressed cannot develop an immune response adequate to produce a positive skin test. This is referred to as anergy.

The accuracy of the skin test depends on the skill of the person interpreting the test reaction. One study (Kendig, Kirkpatrick, Carter et al., 1998) revealed that health care professionals tend to underestimate the size of induration: only 7% of a sample of 107 health care providers charted the correct size of induration.

CLASSIFICATION OF TB

Data from the history, physical examination, skin test, chest x-ray, and microbiologic studies are used to classify TB into one of five classes. A classification scheme provides public health officials with a systematic way to monitor epidemiology and treatment of the disease (American Thoracic Society, 2000).

- Class 0: no exposure; no infection
- Class 1: exposure; no evidence of infection
- Class 2: latent infection; no disease (eg, positive PPD reaction but no clinical evidence of active TB)
- Class 3: disease; clinically active
- Class 4: disease; not clinically active
- Class 5: suspected disease; diagnosis pending

 Gerontologic Considerations

TB may have atypical manifestations in elderly patients, whose symptoms may include unusual behavior and altered mental status, fever, anorexia, and weight loss. Many elderly patients may have no reaction (loss of immunologic memory) or delayed reactivity for up to a week (recall phenomenon). A second skin test is performed in 1 to 2 weeks.

Medical Management

Pulmonary TB is treated primarily with chemotherapeutic agents (antituberculosis agents) for 6 to 12 months. A prolonged treatment duration is necessary to ensure eradication of the organisms and to prevent relapse. A worldwide concern and challenge in TB therapy is the continuing (since the 1950s) and increasing resistance of *M. tuberculosis* to TB medications. Several types of drug resistance must be considered when planning effective therapy:

- Primary drug resistance: resistance to one of the first-line antituberculosis agents in a person who has not had previous treatment
- Secondary or acquired drug resistance: resistance to one or more antituberculosis agents in a patient undergoing therapy
- Multidrug resistance: resistance to two agents, isoniazid (INH) and rifampin. The populations at highest risk for multidrug resistance are those who are HIV-positive, institutionalized, or homeless.

The increasing prevalence of drug resistance points out the need to begin TB treatment with four or more medications, to ensure completion of therapy, and to develop and evaluate new anti-TB medications.

PHARMACOLOGIC THERAPY

In current TB therapy, five first-line medications are used (Table 23-2): INH, rifampin, pyrazinamide, and either streptomycin or ethambutol.

Combination medications, such as INH and rifampin (Rifamate) or INH, pyrazinamide and rifampin and medications administered twice a week (eg, rifapentine) are available to help improve patient adherence. Capreomycin, ethionamide, para-aminosalicylate sodium, and cycloserine are second-line medications. Additional potentially effective medications include other aminoglycosides, quinolones, rifabutin, clofazimine, and combinations of medications.

Recommended treatment guidelines for newly diagnosed cases of pulmonary TB (CDC, 2000) consist of a multiple-medication regimen of INH, rifampin, pyrazinamide, and either streptomycin or ethambutol. This initial intensive-treatment regimen is usually administered daily for 8 weeks. If cultures demonstrate that the organism is sensitive to the medications before the 8 weeks of therapy have been completed, either ethambutol or streptomycin can be discontinued. After 8 weeks of this medication regimen, pyrazinamide can be discontinued and INH and rifampin are administered for an additional 4 months. The medication regimen, however, may continue for 12 months. A person is considered noninfectious after 2 to 3 weeks of continuous medication therapy. Vitamin B (pyridoxine) is usually administered with INH to prevent INH-associated peripheral neuropathy (see Table 23-2).

INH also may be used as a prophylactic (preventive) measure for those at risk for significant disease, including:

- Household family members of patients with active disease
- HIV-infected patients with a PPD test reaction of 5 mm of induration or more
- Patients with fibrotic lesions detected on a chest x-ray, suggestive of old TB, and a PPD reaction of 5 mm of induration or more
- Patients whose current PPD test results show a change from former test results, suggesting recent exposure to TB and possible infection (also called skin test converters)
- Drug (intravenous or injectable) users with PPD test results of 10 mm of induration or more
- Patients with high-risk comorbid conditions with a PPD result of 10 mm of induration or more

Other candidates for preventive INH therapy are those age 35 years or younger with PPD test results of 10 mm of induration or more and one of the following criteria:

- Foreign-born individuals from countries with a high prevalence of TB
- High-risk, medically underserved populations
- Institutionalized patients

Prophylactic INH treatment involves taking daily doses for 6 to 12 months. Liver enzyme, blood urea nitrogen, and creatinine levels are monitored monthly. Sputum culture results are monitored for acid-fast bacillus to evaluate the effectiveness of treatment and the patient's compliance with therapy.

In 1998, the federal Advisory Council for the Elimination of Tuberculosis published recommendations for the development of TB vaccines. The recommendations include a focus on a "postinfection vaccine" to prevent people infected with TB from developing active disease (CDC, 1998). To date, this vaccine has

Table 23-2 • **First-Line Antitubercular Medications**

COMMONLY USED AGENTS	ADULT DAILY DOSAGE*	MOST COMMON SIDE EFFECTS	DRUG INTERACTIONS†	REMARKS*
isoniazid (INH)	5 mg/kg (300 mg maximum daily)	Peripheral neuritis, hepatic enzyme elevation, hepatitis, hypersensitivity	Phenytoin— synergistic Antabuse Alcohol	Bactericidal. Pyridoxine as prophylaxis for neuritis. Monitor AST (SGOT) and ALT (SGPT).
rifampin (Rifadin)	10 mg/kg (600 mg maximum daily)	Hepatitis, febrile reaction, purpura (rare), nausea, vomiting	Rifampin increases metabolism of oral contraceptives, quinidine, corticosteroids, coumarin derivatives and methadone, digoxin, oral hypoglycemics; PAS may interfere with absorption of rifampin.	Bactericidal. Orange urine and other body secretions. Discoloring of contact lenses. Monitor AST (SGOT) and ALT (SGPT).
rifabutin (Mycobutin)	5 mg/kg (300 mg maximum daily)			
streptomycin	15 mg/kg (1 g maximum daily)*	8th cranial nerve damage (may lead to deafness), nephrotoxicity	Neuromuscular blocking agents; may be potentiated to cause prolonged paralysis	Bactericidal in alkaline pH. Use with caution in elderly or in those with renal disease. Monitor vestibular function, audiograms, BUN and creatinine.
pyrazinamide	15 to 30 mg/kg (2.0 g maximum daily)*	Hyperuricemia, hepatotoxicity, skin rash, arthralgias, GI distress		Bactericidal. Monitor uric acid, AST (SGOT), ALT (SGPT).
ethambutol (Myambutol)	15 to 25 mg/kg (no maximum daily dose, but base on lean body wt)*	Optic neuritis (may lead to blindness; very rare at 15 mg/kg), skin rash		Bacteriostatic. Use with caution with renal disease or when eye testing is not feasible. Monitor visual acuity, color discrimination.‡
Combinations: INH + rifampin (eg, Rifamate)	150-mg & 300-mg caps (2 caps daily)			

*Check product labeling for detailed information on dose, contraindications, drug interaction, adverse reactions, and monitoring.
†Refer to current literature, particularly on rifampin, because it increases hepatic microenzymes and therefore interacts with many drugs.
‡Initial examination should be performed at start of treatment.

not become clinically available. In 2000, recommendations were released regarding the treatment of latent TB infection (American Thoracic Society and CDC, 2000). Isoniazid (INH) for 6 to 12 months has been the mainstay of treatment for latent TB infection. However, this long duration of treatment has been limited due to poor adherence and concerns of toxicity. The American Thoracic Society and CDC released newer guidelines in the 2000 document, which focused on treating a latent infection over a shorter period of time. The CDC released case reports of liver injury associated with the 2-month rifampin-pyrazinamide (RIF-PZA) dosing regimen in August 2001 (MMWR, 2001). This prompted a review and changes to the 2000 guidelines. In summary, a 2-month RIF-PZA treatment regimen for latent TB infection should be used with caution, especially in patients who are concurrently taking medications for liver disease or those with a history of alcoholism. For patients not infected with HIV, 9 months of daily INH remains the preferred treatment, and 4 months of daily RIF is an acceptable alternative. No more than

a 2-week supply of RIF-PZA should be dispensed at any one time to facilitate periodic clinical assessments. Lastly, serum aminotransferase and bilirubin should be measured at baseline and at 2, 4, and 6 weeks of treatment in patients taking RIF-PZA (MMWR, 2001).

NURSING PROCESS: THE PATIENT WITH TUBERCULOSIS

Assessment

The nurse performs a complete history and physical examination. Clinical manifestations of fever, anorexia, weight loss, night sweats, fatigue, cough, and sputum production prompt a more thorough assessment of respiratory function—for example, assessing the lungs for consolidation by evaluating breath sounds (diminished, bronchial sounds, crackles), fremitus, egophony, and dullness on percussion. Enlarged, painful lymph nodes may be palpated as well. The nurse also assesses the patient's living arrangements, perceptions and understanding of TB and its treatment, and readiness to learn.

Nursing Diagnoses

Based on the assessment data, the nursing diagnoses may include:

- Ineffective airway clearance related to copious tracheobronchial secretions
- Deficient knowledge about treatment regimen and preventive health measures and related ineffective individual management of the therapeutic regimen (noncompliance)
- Activity intolerance related to fatigue, altered nutritional status, and fever

Collaborative Problems/ Potential Complications

Based on the assessment data, collaborative problems or potential complications that may occur include:

- Malnutrition
- Adverse side effects of medication therapy: hepatitis, neurologic changes (deafness or neuritis), skin rash, gastrointestinal upset
- Multidrug resistance
- Spread of TB infection (miliary TB)

Planning and Goals

The major goals for the patient include maintenance of a patent airway, increased knowledge about the disease and treatment regimen and adherence to the medication regimen, increased activity tolerance, and absence of complications.

Nursing Interventions

PROMOTING AIRWAY CLEARANCE

Copious secretions obstruct the airways in many patients with TB and interfere with adequate gas exchange. Increasing fluid intake promotes systemic hydration and serves as an effective expectorant. The nurse instructs the patient about correct positioning to facilitate airway drainage (postural drainage); this is described in Chapter 25.

ADVOCATING ADHERENCE TO TREATMENT REGIMEN

The multiple-medication regimen that a patient must follow can be quite complex. Understanding the medications, schedule, and side effects is important. The patient must understand that TB is a communicable disease and that taking medications is the most effective means of preventing transmission. The major reason treatment fails is that patients do not take their medications regularly and for the prescribed duration. The nurse carefully instructs the patient about important hygiene measures, including mouth care, covering the mouth and nose when coughing and sneezing, proper disposal of tissues, and hand hygiene.

PROMOTING ACTIVITY AND ADEQUATE NUTRITION

Patients with TB are often debilitated from a prolonged chronic illness and impaired nutritional status. The nurse plans a progressive activity schedule that focuses on increasing activity tolerance and muscle strength. Anorexia, weight loss, and malnutrition are common in patients with TB. The patient's willingness to eat may be altered by fatigue from excessive coughing, sputum production, chest pain, generalized debilitated state, or cost, if the person has few resources. A nutritional plan that allows for small, frequent meals may be required. Liquid nutritional supplements may assist in meeting basic caloric requirements.

MONITORING AND MANAGING POTENTIAL COMPLICATIONS

Malnutrition

This may be a consequence of the patient's lifestyle, lack of knowledge about adequate nutrition and its role in health maintenance, lack of resources, fatigue, or lack of appetite because of coughing and mucus production. To counter the effects of these factors, the nurse collaborates with the dietitian, physician, social worker, family, and patient to identify strategies to ensure an adequate nutritional intake and availability of nutritious food. Identifying facilities (eg, shelters, soup kitchens, Meals on Wheels, and other community resources) that provide meals in the patient's neighborhood may increase the likelihood that the patient with limited resources and energy will have access to a more nutritious intake. High-calorie nutritional supplements may be suggested as a strategy for increasing dietary intake using food products normally found in the home. Purchasing food supplements may be beyond the patient's budget, but a dietitian can help develop recipes to increase caloric intake despite minimal resources.

Side Effects of Medication Therapy

It is important to assess medication side effects because they are often a reason the patient fails to adhere to the prescribed medication regimen. Efforts are made to reduce the side effects to increase the patient's willingness to take the medications as prescribed.

The nurse instructs the patient to take the medication either on an empty stomach or at least 1 hour before meals, because food interferes with medication absorption (although taking medications on an empty stomach frequently results in gastrointestinal upset). Patients taking INH should avoid foods containing tyramine and histamine (tuna, aged cheese, red wine, soy sauce, yeast extracts). Eating these types of foods while taking INH may result in headache, flushing, hypotension, light-headedness, palpitations, and diaphoresis.

In addition, rifampin can increase the metabolism of other medications, making them less effective. These medications include beta-blockers, oral anticoagulants such as warfarin (Coumadin), digoxin, quinidine, corticosteroids, oral hypoglycemic agents, oral contraceptives, theophylline, and verapamil. This issue should be discussed with the physician and pharmacist so that medication dosages can be adjusted accordingly. The nurse informs the patient that rifampin may discolor contact lenses, so the patient may want to wear eyeglasses during treatment. The nurse monitors for other side effects of anti-TB medications, including hepatitis, neurologic changes (hearing loss, neuritis), and rash. Liver enzyme, blood urea nitrogen, and serum creatinine levels are monitored to detect medication-related changes in liver and kidney function. Sputum culture results are monitored for acid-fast bacillus to evaluate the effectiveness of the treatment regimen and adherence to therapy.

Multidrug Resistance

The nurse carefully monitors vital signs and observes for spikes in temperature or changes in the clinical status. The nurse reports any change in the patient's respiratory status to the primary health care provider. The nurse instructs the patient about the risk of drug resistance if the medication regimen is not strictly and continuously followed.

Spread of TB Infection

Spread of TB infection to nonpulmonary sites of the body is known as miliary TB. It is the result of invasion of the bloodstream by the tubercle bacillus (Ghon tubercle). Usually it results from late reactivation of a dormant infection in the lung or elsewhere. The origin of the bacilli that enter the bloodstream is either a chronic focus that has ulcerated into a blood vessel or multitudes of miliary tubercles lining the inner surface of the thoracic duct. The organisms migrate from these foci into the bloodstream, are carried throughout the body, and disseminate throughout all tissues, with tiny miliary tubercles developing in the lungs, spleen, liver, kidneys, meninges, and other organs.

The clinical course of miliary TB may vary from an acute, rapidly progressive infection with high fever to an indolent process with low-grade fever, anemia, and debilitation. At first, there may be no localizing signs except an enlarged spleen and a reduced number of leukocytes. Within a few weeks, however, the chest x-ray reveals small densities scattered diffusely throughout both lung fields; these are the miliary tubercles, which gradually grow.

The possibility of TB in nonpulmonary sites in the body requires careful monitoring for this very serious form of the infection. The nurse monitors vital signs and observes for spikes in temperature as well as changes in renal and cognitive function. Few physical signs may be elicited on physical examination of the chest, but at this stage the patient has a severe cough and dyspnea. Treatment of miliary TB is the same as for pulmonary TB.

PROMOTING HOME AND COMMUNITY-BASED CARE

Teaching Patients Self-Care

The nurse plays a vital role in caring for the patient with TB and the family, which includes assessing the patient's ability to continue therapy at home. The nurse instructs the patient and family about infection control procedures, such as proper disposal of tissues, covering the mouth during coughing, and hand hygiene. Assessment of the patient's adherence to the medication regimen is imperative because of the risk of developing resistant strains of TB if the regimen is not followed faithfully. In some cases, when the patient's ability to comply with the medication regimen is in question, referral to an outpatient clinic for daily medication administration may be required. This is referred to as directly observed therapy (DOT).

Continuing Care

The nurse evaluates the patient's environment, including home or workplace and social setting, to identify other people who may have been in contact with the patient during the infectious stage. It is important to arrange follow-up screening for any contacts of the infected person. Nurses who have contact with the patient in home, shelter, hospital, clinic, or work settings assess the patient's physical and psychological status and ability to adhere to the prescribed treatment. The nurse assesses the patient for adverse effects of medications and adherence to the therapeutic regimen (eg, taking medications as prescribed, practicing safe hygiene, consuming a nutritious and adequate diet, and participating in an appropriate level of activity). The nurse reinforces previous teaching and emphasizes the importance of keeping scheduled appointments with the primary health care provider. In addition, the patient is reminded of the importance of other health promotion activities and recommended health screening.

Evaluation

EXPECTED PATIENT OUTCOMES

Expected patient outcomes may include:

1. Maintains a patent airway by managing secretions with hydration, humidification, coughing, and postural drainage
2. Demonstrates an adequate level of knowledge
   a. Lists medications by name and the correct schedule for taking them
   b. Names expected side effects of medications
   c. Identifies how and when to contact health care provider
3. Adheres to treatment regimen by taking medications as prescribed and reporting for follow-up screening
4. Participates in preventive measures
   a. Disposes of used tissues properly
   b. Encourages people who are close contacts to report for testing
   c. Adheres to hand hygiene recommendations
5. Maintains activity schedule
6. Exhibits no complications
   a. Maintains adequate weight or gains weight if indicated
   b. Exhibits normal results of tests of liver and kidney function
7. Takes steps to minimize side effects of medications
   a. Takes supplemental vitamins (vitamin B), as prescribed, to minimize peripheral neuropathy
   b. Avoids use of alcohol
   c. Avoids foods containing tyramine and histamine
   d. Has regular physical examinations and blood tests to evaluate liver and kidney function, neuropathy, hearing and visual acuity

LUNG ABSCESS

A lung abscess is a localized necrotic lesion of the lung parenchyma containing purulent material that collapses and forms a cavity. It is generally caused by aspiration of anaerobic bacteria. By definition, the chest x-ray will demonstrate a cavity of at least 2 cm. Patients who have impaired cough reflexes and cannot close the glottis, or those with swallowing difficulties, are at risk for aspirating foreign material and developing a lung abscess. Other at-risk patients include those with central nervous system disorders (seizure, stroke), drug addiction, alcoholism, esophageal disease, or compromised immune function, those without teeth, as well as patients receiving nasogastric tube feedings and those with an altered state of consciousness from anesthesia.

Pathophysiology

Most lung abscesses are a complication of bacterial pneumonia or are caused by aspiration of oral anaerobes into the lung. Abscesses also may occur secondary to mechanical or functional obstruction of the bronchi by a tumor, foreign body, or bronchial stenosis, or from necrotizing pneumonias, TB, pulmonary embolism, or chest trauma.

Most abscesses are found in areas of the lung that may be affected by aspiration. The site of the lung abscess is related to gravity and is determined by the patient's position. For patients who are confined to bed, the posterior segment of an upper lobe and the superior segment of the lower lobe are the most common areas in which lung abscess occurs. However, atypical presentations may occur, depending on the position of the patient when the aspiration occurred.

Initially, the cavity in the lung may or may not extend directly into a bronchus. Eventually the abscess becomes surrounded, or encapsulated, by a wall of fibrous tissue. The necrotic process may extend until it reaches the lumen of a bronchus or the pleural space and establishes communication with the respiratory tract, the pleural cavity, or both. If the bronchus is involved, the purulent contents are expectorated continuously in the form of sputum. If the pleura is involved, an empyema results. A communication or connection between the bronchus and pleura is known as a bronchopleural fistula.

The organisms frequently associated with lung abscesses are *S. aureus, Klebsiella,* and other gram-negative species. Anaerobic organisms, however, may also be present. The organism varies depending on the underlying predisposing factors.

Clinical Manifestations

The clinical manifestations of a lung abscess may vary from a mild productive cough to acute illness. Most patients have a fever and a productive cough with moderate to copious amounts of foul-smelling, often bloody, sputum. Leukocytosis may be present. Pleurisy or dull chest pain, dyspnea, weakness, anorexia, and weight loss are common. Fever and cough may develop insidiously and may have been present for several weeks before diagnosis.

Assessment and Diagnostic Findings

Physical examination of the chest may reveal dullness on percussion and decreased or absent breath sounds with an intermittent **pleural friction rub** (grating or rubbing sound) on auscultation. Crackles may be present. Confirmation of the diagnosis is made by chest x-ray, sputum culture, and in some cases fiberoptic bronchoscopy. The chest x-ray reveals an infiltrate with an air–fluid level. A computed tomography (CT) scan of the chest may be required to provide more detailed pictures of different cross-sectional areas of the lung.

Prevention

The following measures will reduce the risk of lung abscess:

- Appropriate antibiotic therapy before any dental procedures in patients who must have teeth extracted while their gums and teeth are infected
- Adequate dental and oral hygiene, because anaerobic bacteria play a role in the pathogenesis of lung abscess
- Appropriate antimicrobial therapy for patients with pneumonia

Medical Management

The findings of the history, physical examination, chest x-ray, and sputum culture indicate the type of organism and the treatment required. Adequate drainage of the lung abscess may be achieved through postural drainage and chest physiotherapy. The patient should be assessed for an adequate cough. A few patients need a percutaneous chest catheter placed for long-term drainage of the abscess. Therapeutic use of bronchoscopy to drain an abscess is uncommon. A diet high in protein and calories is necessary because

chronic infection is associated with a catabolic state, necessitating increased intake of calories and protein to facilitate healing. Surgical intervention is rare, but pulmonary resection (lobectomy) is performed when there is massive **hemoptysis** (coughing up of blood) or little or no response to medical management.

PHARMACOLOGIC THERAPY

Intravenous antimicrobial therapy depends on the results of the sputum culture and sensitivity and is administered for an extended period. Penicillin G or clindamycin (Cleocin) is the medication of choice, followed by penicillin with metronidazole. Large intravenous doses are generally required because the antibiotic must penetrate the necrotic tissue and the fluid in the abscess. The intravenous dose is continued until there is evidence of symptom improvement.

Long-term therapy with oral antibiotics replaces intravenous therapy after the patient shows signs of improvement (usually 3 to 5 days). Improvement is demonstrated by normal temperature, decreased white blood cell count, and improvement on the chest x-ray (resolution of surrounding infiltrate, reduction in cavity size, absence of fluid). Oral administration of antibiotic therapy is continued for an additional 4 to 8 weeks. If treatment stops too soon, a relapse may occur.

Nursing Management

The nurse administers antibiotics and intravenous therapies as prescribed and monitors for adverse effects. Chest physiotherapy is initiated as prescribed to facilitate drainage of the abscess. The nurse teaches the patient to perform deep-breathing and coughing exercises to help expand the lungs. To ensure proper nutritional intake, the nurse encourages a diet high in protein and calories. The nurse also offers emotional support because the abscess may take a long time to resolve.

PROMOTING HOME AND COMMUNITY-BASED CARE

Teaching Patients Self-Care. The patient who has had surgery may return home before the wound closes entirely or with a drain or tube in place. Thus, the patient or a caregiver needs instruction on how to change the dressings to prevent skin excoriation and odor, how to monitor for signs and symptoms of infection, and how to care for and maintain the drain or tube. The nurse instructs the patient to perform deep-breathing and coughing exercises every 2 hours during the day and shows a caregiver how to perform chest percussion and postural drainage to facilitate expectoration of lung secretions.

Continuing Care. Referral for home care may be required by some patients whose condition requires therapy at home. During visits to the patient at home, the nurse assesses the patient's physical condition, nutritional status, and home environment as well as the patient's and family's ability to carry out the therapeutic regimen. Patient teaching is reinforced during home visits, and nutrition counseling is provided with the goal of attaining and maintaining an optimal state of nutrition. To prevent a relapse, the nurse emphasizes the importance of completing the antibiotic regimen and of following the suggestions for rest and appropriate activity. If intravenous antibiotic therapy is to continue at home, the services of a home care nurse may be arranged to initiate intravenous therapy and to evaluate its administration by the patient or family. Although most outpatient intravenous therapy is administered in the home setting, a patient may visit a nearby clinic or physician's office for this treatment. In some cases the patient with lung abscess may have ignored his or her health. Therefore, it is important to use this opportunity to address health promotion strategies and health screening with the patient.

Pleural Conditions

Pleural conditions are disorders that involve the membranes covering the lungs (visceral pleura) and the surface of the chest wall (parietal pleura) or disorders affecting the pleural space.

PLEURISY

Pathophysiology

Pleurisy (pleuritis) refers to inflammation of both layers of the pleurae (parietal and visceral). Pleurisy may develop in conjunction with pneumonia or an upper respiratory tract infection, TB, or collagen disease; after trauma to the chest, pulmonary infarction, or pulmonary embolism; in patients with primary and metastatic cancer; and after thoracotomy. The parietal pleura has nerve endings; the visceral pleura does not. When the inflamed pleural membranes rub together during respiration (intensified on inspiration), the result is severe, sharp, knifelike pain.

Clinical Manifestations

The key characteristic of pleuritic pain is its relationship to respiratory movement. Taking a deep breath, coughing, or sneezing worsens the pain. Pleuritic pain is restricted in distribution rather than diffuse; it usually occurs only on one side. The pain may become minimal or absent when the breath is held, or it may be localized or radiate to the shoulder or abdomen. Later, as pleural fluid develops, the pain decreases.

Assessment and Diagnostic Findings

In the early period, when little fluid has accumulated, a pleural friction rub can be heard with the stethoscope, only to disappear later as more fluid accumulates and separates the inflamed pleural surfaces. Diagnostic tests may include chest x-rays, sputum examinations, thoracentesis to obtain a specimen of pleural fluid for examination, and less commonly a pleural biopsy.

Medical Management

The objectives of treatment are to discover the underlying condition causing the pleurisy and to relieve the pain. As the underlying disease (pneumonia, infection) is treated, the pleuritic inflammation usually resolves. At the same time, it is necessary to monitor for signs and symptoms of pleural effusion, such as shortness of breath, pain, assumption of a position that decreases pain, and decreased chest wall excursion.

Prescribed analgesics and topical applications of heat or cold provide symptomatic relief. Indomethacin (Indocin), a nonsteroidal anti-inflammatory drug (NSAID), may provide pain relief while allowing the patient to take deep breaths and cough more effectively. If the pain is severe, an intercostal nerve block may be required.

Nursing Management

Because the patient has considerable pain on inspiration, the nurse can offer suggestions to enhance comfort, such as turning frequently onto the affected side to splint the chest wall and reduce the stretching of the pleurae. The nurse also can teach the patient to use the hands or a pillow to splint the rib cage while coughing.

PLEURAL EFFUSION

Pleural effusion, a collection of fluid in the pleural space, is rarely a primary disease process but is usually secondary to other diseases. Normally, the pleural space contains a small amount of fluid (5 to 15 mL), which acts as a lubricant that allows the pleural surfaces to move without friction (Fig. 23-5). Pleural effusion may be a complication of heart failure, TB, pneumonia, pulmonary infections (particularly viral infections), nephrotic syndrome, connective tissue disease, pulmonary embolism, and neoplastic tumors. Bronchogenic carcinoma is the most common malignancy associated with a pleural effusion.

Pathophysiology

In certain disorders, fluid may accumulate in the pleural space to a point where it becomes clinically evident. This almost always has pathologic significance. The effusion can be composed of a relatively clear fluid, or it can be bloody or purulent. An effusion

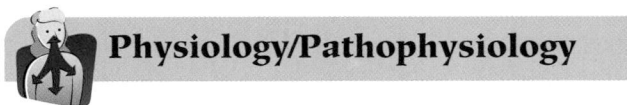

Physiology/Pathophysiology

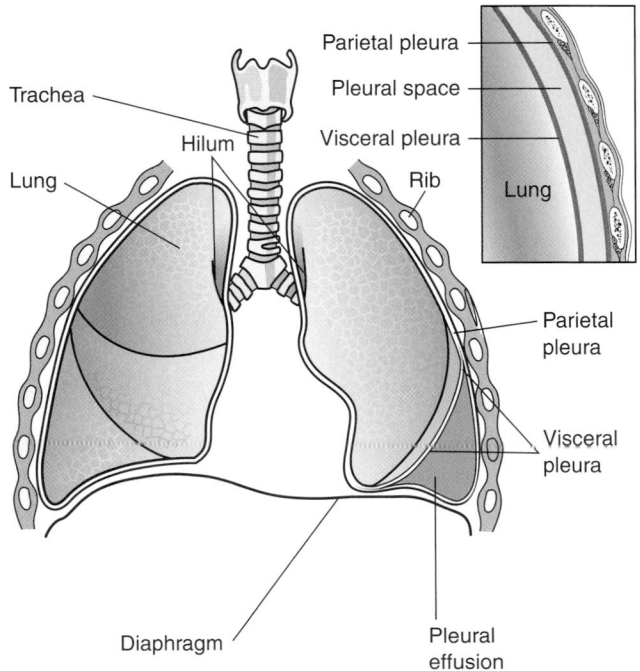

FIGURE 23-5 In pleural effusion, an abnormal volume of fluid collects in the pleural space, causing pain and shortness of breath. Pleural effusion is usually secondary to other disease processes.

of clear fluid may be a transudate or an exudate. A transudate (filtrates of plasma that move across intact capillary walls) occurs when factors influencing the formation and reabsorption of pleural fluid are altered, usually by imbalances in hydrostatic or oncotic pressures. The finding of a transudative effusion generally implies that the pleural membranes are not diseased. The most common cause of a transudative effusion is heart failure. An exudate (extravasation of fluid into tissues or a cavity) usually results from inflammation by bacterial products or tumors involving the pleural surfaces.

Clinical Manifestations

Usually the clinical manifestations are those caused by the underlying disease. Pneumonia causes fever, chills, and pleuritic chest pain, whereas a malignant effusion may result in dyspnea and coughing. The size of the effusion and the patient's underlying lung disease determine the severity of symptoms. A large pleural effusion causes shortness of breath. When a small to moderate pleural effusion is present, dyspnea may be absent or only minimal. The severity of the symptoms assessed depends on the time course of the development of the pleural effusion and the patient's underlying disease.

Assessment and Diagnostic Findings

Assessment of the area of the pleural effusion reveals decreased or absent breath sounds, decreased fremitus, and a dull, flat sound when percussed. In an extremely large pleural effusion, the assessment reveals a patient in acute respiratory distress. Tracheal deviation away from the affected side may also be noted.

Physical examination, chest x-ray, chest CT scan, and thoracentesis confirm the presence of fluid. In some instances, a lateral decubitus x-ray is obtained. For this x-ray, the patient lies on the affected side in a side-lying position. A pleural effusion can be diagnosed because this position allows for the "layering out" of the fluid, and an air–fluid line is visible.

Pleural fluid is analyzed by bacterial culture, Gram stain, acid-fast bacillus stain (for TB), red and white blood cell counts, chemistry studies (glucose, amylase, lactic dehydrogenase, protein), cytologic analysis for malignant cells, and pH. A pleural biopsy also may be performed.

Medical Management

The objectives of treatment are to discover the underlying cause, to prevent reaccumulation of fluid, and to relieve discomfort, dyspnea, and respiratory compromise. Specific treatment is directed at the underlying cause (eg, heart failure, pneumonia, lung cancer, cirrhosis). If the pleural fluid is an exudate, more extensive diagnostic procedures are performed to determine the cause. Treatment for the primary cause is then instituted.

Thoracentesis is performed to remove fluid, to obtain a specimen for analysis, and to relieve dyspnea and respiratory compromise (see Chap. 21). Thoracentesis may be performed under ultrasound guidance. Depending on the size of the pleural effusion, the patient may be treated by removing the fluid during the thoracentesis procedure or by inserting a chest tube connected to a water-seal drainage system or suction to evacuate the pleural space and re-expand the lung.

If the underlying cause is a malignancy, however, the effusion tends to recur within a few days or weeks. Repeated thoracente-

ses result in pain, depletion of protein and electrolytes, and sometimes pneumothorax. Once the pleural space is adequately drained, a chemical pleurodesis may be performed to obliterate the pleural space and prevent reaccumulation of fluid. Pleurodesis may be performed using a thoracoscopic approach or via a chest tube. Chemically irritating agents (eg., bleomycin or talc) are instilled in the pleural space. With the chest tube insertion approach, after the agent is instilled, the chest tube is clamped for 60 to 90 minutes and the patient is assisted to assume various positions to promote uniform distribution of the agent and to maximize its contact with the pleural surfaces. The tube is unclamped as prescribed, and chest drainage may be continued several days longer to prevent reaccumulation of fluid and to promote the formation of adhesions between the visceral and parietal pleurae.

Other treatments for malignant pleural effusions include surgical pleurectomy, insertion of a small catheter attached to a drainage bottle for outpatient management, or implantation of a pleuroperitoneal shunt. A pleuroperitoneal shunt consists of two catheters connected by a pump chamber containing two one-way valves. Fluid moves from the pleural space to the pump chamber and then to the peritoneal cavity. The patient manually pumps on the reservoir daily to move fluid from the pleural space to the peritoneal space (Taubert & Wright, 2000).

Nursing Management

The nurse's role in the care of the patient with a pleural effusion includes implementing the medical regimen. The nurse prepares and positions the patient for thoracentesis and offers support throughout the procedure. Pain management is a priority, and the nurse assists the patient to assume positions that are the least painful. However, frequent turning and ambulation are important to facilitate drainage. The nurse administers analgesics as prescribed and as needed.

If a chest tube drainage and water-seal system is used, the nurse is responsible for monitoring the system's function and recording the amount of drainage at prescribed intervals. Nursing care related to the underlying cause of the pleural effusion is specific to the underlying condition. Care of the patient with a chest tube is discussed in Chapter 25.

If the patient is to be managed as an outpatient with a pleural catheter for drainage, the nurse is responsible for educating the patient and family regarding management and care of the catheter and drainage system.

EMPYEMA

An empyema is an accumulation of thick, purulent fluid within the pleural space, often with fibrin development and a loculated (walled-off) area where infection is located. Most empyemas occur as complications of bacterial pneumonia or lung abscess. Other causes include penetrating chest trauma, hematogenous infection of the pleural space, nonbacterial infections, or iatrogenic causes (after thoracic surgery or thoracentesis).

Pathophysiology

At first the pleural fluid is thin, with a low leukocyte count, but it frequently progresses to a fibropurulent stage and, finally, to a stage where it encloses the lung within a thick exudative membrane (loculated empyema).

Clinical Manifestations

With an empyema, the patient is acutely ill and has signs and symptoms similar to those of an acute respiratory infection or pneumonia (fever, night sweats, pleural pain, cough, dyspnea, anorexia, weight loss). If the patient is immunocompromised, the symptoms may be more vague. If the patient has received antimicrobial therapy, the clinical manifestations may be less obvious.

Assessment and Diagnostic Findings

Chest auscultation demonstrates decreased or absent breath sounds over the affected area, and there is dullness on chest percussion as well as decreased fremitus. The diagnosis is established by a chest x-ray or chest CT scan. Usually a diagnostic thoracentesis is performed, often under ultrasound guidance.

Medical Management

The objectives of treatment are to drain the pleural cavity and to achieve full expansion of the lung. The fluid is drained and appropriate antibiotics, in large doses, are prescribed based on the causative organism. Sterilization of the empyema cavity requires 4 to 6 weeks of antibiotics. Drainage of the pleural fluid depends on the stage of the disease and is accomplished by one of the following methods:

- Needle aspiration (thoracentesis) with a thin percutaneous catheter, if the volume is small and the fluid not too purulent or thick
- Tube thoracostomy (chest drainage using a large-diameter intercostal tube attached to water-seal drainage [see Chap. 25]) with fibrinolytic agents instilled through the chest tube in patients with loculated or complicated pleural effusions
- Open chest drainage via thoracotomy, including potential rib resection, to remove the thickened pleura, pus, and debris and to remove the underlying diseased pulmonary tissue

With long-standing inflammation, an exudate can form over the lung, trapping it and interfering with its normal expansion. This exudate must be removed surgically (decortication). The drainage tube is left in place until the pus-filled space is obliterated completely. The complete obliteration of the pleural space is monitored by serial chest x-rays, and the patient should be informed that treatment may be long term. Patients are frequently discharged from the hospital with a chest tube in place, with instructions to monitor fluid drainage at home.

Nursing Management

Resolution of empyema is a prolonged process. The nurse helps the patient cope with the condition and instructs the patient in lung-expanding breathing exercises to restore normal respiratory function. The nurse also provides care specific to the method of drainage of the pleural fluid (eg, needle aspiration, closed chest drainage, or rib resection and drainage). When a patient is discharged to home with a drainage tube or system in place, the nurse instructs the patient and family on care of the drainage system and drain site, measurement and observation of drainage, signs and symptoms of infection, and how and when to contact the health care provider. (See Nursing Process: The Patient Undergoing Thoracic Surgery in Chapter 25.)

Pulmonary Edema

Pulmonary edema is defined as abnormal accumulation of fluid in the lung tissue and/or alveolar space. It is a severe, life-threatening condition.

Pathophysiology

Pulmonary edema most commonly occurs as a result of increased microvascular pressure from abnormal cardiac function. The backup of blood into the pulmonary vasculature resulting from inadequate left ventricular function causes an increased microvascular pressure, and fluid begins to leak into the interstitial space and the alveoli. Other causes of pulmonary edema are hypervolemia or a sudden increase in the intravascular pressure in the lung. One example of this is in the patient who has undergone pneumonectomy. When one lung has been removed, all the cardiac output then goes to the remaining lung. If the patient's fluid status is not monitored closely, pulmonary edema can quickly develop in the postoperative period as the patient's pulmonary vasculature attempts to adapt. This type of pulmonary edema is sometimes termed "flash" pulmonary edema. A second example is called re-expansion pulmonary edema. This may be due to a rapid reinflation of the lung after removal of air from a pneumothorax or evacuation of fluid from a large pleural effusion.

Clinical Manifestations

The patient has increasing respiratory distress, characterized by dyspnea, air hunger, and central cyanosis. The patient is usually very anxious and often agitated. As the fluid leaks into the alveoli and mixes with air, a foam or froth is formed. The patient coughs up or the nurse suctions out these foamy, frothy, and often blood-tinged secretions. The patient has acute respiratory distress and may become confused or stuporous.

Assessment and Diagnostic Findings

Auscultation reveals crackles in the lung bases (especially in the posterior bases) that rapidly progress toward the apices of the lungs. These crackles are due to the movement of air through the alveolar fluid. The chest x-ray reveals increased interstitial markings. The patient may be tachycardic, the pulse oximetry values begin to fall, and arterial blood gas analysis demonstrates increasing hypoxemia.

Medical Management

Management focuses on correcting the underlying disorder. If the pulmonary edema is cardiac in origin, then improvement in left ventricular function is the goal. Vasodilators, inotropic medications, afterload or preload agents, or contractility medications may be given. Additional cardiac measures (eg, intra-aortic balloon pump) may be indicated if the patient does not respond. If the problem is fluid overload, diuretics are given and the patient is placed on fluid restrictions. Oxygen is administered to correct the hypoxemia; in some circumstances, intubation and mechanical ventilation are necessary. The patient is extremely anxious, and morphine is administered to reduce anxiety and control pain.

Nursing Management

Nursing management of the patient with pulmonary edema includes assisting with administration of oxygen and intubation and mechanical ventilation if respiratory failure occurs. The nurse also administers medications (ie, morphine, vasodilators, inotropic medications, preload and afterload agents) as prescribed and monitors the patient's response. Nursing management in pulmonary edema is described in more detail in Chapter 30.

Acute Respiratory Failure

Respiratory failure is a sudden and life-threatening deterioration of the gas exchange function of the lung. It exists when the exchange of oxygen for carbon dioxide in the lungs cannot keep up with the rate of oxygen consumption and carbon dioxide production by the cells of the body.

Acute respiratory failure (ARF) is defined as a fall in arterial oxygen tension (PaO_2) to less than 50 mm Hg (hypoxemia) and a rise in arterial carbon dioxide tension ($PaCO_2$) to greater than 50 mm Hg (hypercapnia), with an arterial pH of less than 7.35. In ARF, the ventilation or perfusion mechanisms in the lung are impaired. Respiratory system mechanisms leading to ARF include:

- Alveolar hypoventilation
- Diffusion abnormalities
- Ventilation–perfusion mismatching
- Shunting

It is important to distinguish between ARF and chronic respiratory failure. Chronic respiratory failure is defined as a deterioration in the gas exchange function of the lung that has developed insidiously or has persisted for a long period after an episode of ARF. The absence of acute symptoms and the presence of a chronic respiratory acidosis suggest the chronicity of the respiratory failure. Two causes of chronic respiratory failure are COPD (discussed in Chap. 24) and neuromuscular diseases (discussed in Chap. 65). Patients with these disorders develop a tolerance to the gradually worsening hypoxemia and hypercapnia. However, a patient with chronic respiratory failure may develop ARF. This is seen in the COPD patient who develops an exacerbation or infection that causes additional deterioration of the gas exchange mechanism. The principles of management of acute versus chronic respiratory failure are different; the following discussion will be limited to ARF.

Pathophysiology

Common causes of ARF can be classified into four categories: decreased respiratory drive, dysfunction of the chest wall, dysfunction of the lung parenchyma, and other causes.

DECREASED RESPIRATORY DRIVE

Decreased respiratory drive may occur with severe brain injury, large lesions of the brain stem (multiple sclerosis), use of sedative medications, and metabolic disorders such as hypothyroidism. These disorders impair the normal response of chemoreceptors in the brain to normal respiratory stimulation.

DYSFUNCTION OF THE CHEST WALL

The impulses arising in the respiratory center travel through nerves that extend from the brain stem down the spinal cord to receptors in the muscles of respiration. Thus, any disease or disorder of the nerves, spinal cord, muscles, or neuromuscular junction involved in respiration seriously affects ventilation and may ultimately lead to ARF. These include musculoskeletal disorders (muscular dystrophy, polymyositis), neuromuscular junction disorders (myasthenia gravis, poliomyelitis), some peripheral nerve disorders, and spinal cord disorders (amyotrophic lateral sclerosis, Guillain-Barré syndrome, and cervical spinal cord injuries).

DYSFUNCTION OF LUNG PARENCHYMA

Pleural effusion, hemothorax, pneumothorax, and upper airway obstruction are conditions that interfere with ventilation by preventing expansion of the lung. These conditions, which may cause respiratory failure, usually are produced by an underlying lung disease, pleural disease, or trauma and injury. Other diseases and conditions of the lung that lead to ARF include pneumonia, status asthmaticus, lobar atelectasis, pulmonary embolism, and pulmonary edema.

OTHER CAUSES

In the postoperative period, especially after major thoracic or abdominal surgery, inadequate ventilation and respiratory failure may occur because of several factors. During this period, for example, ARF may be caused by the effects of anesthetic agents, analgesics, and sedatives, which may depress respiration as described earlier or enhance the effects of opioids and lead to hypoventilation. Pain may interfere with deep breathing and coughing. A mismatch of ventilation to perfusion is the usual cause of respiratory failure after major abdominal, cardiac, or thoracic surgery.

Clinical Manifestations

Early signs are those associated with impaired oxygenation and may include restlessness, fatigue, headache, dyspnea, air hunger, tachycardia, and increased blood pressure. As the hypoxemia progresses, more obvious signs may be present, including confusion, lethargy, tachycardia, tachypnea, central cyanosis, diaphoresis, and finally respiratory arrest. Physical findings are those of acute respiratory distress, including use of accessory muscles, decreased breath sounds if the patient cannot adequately ventilate, and other findings related specifically to the underlying disease process and cause of ARF.

Medical Management

The objectives of treatment are to correct the underlying cause and to restore adequate gas exchange in the lung. Intubation and mechanical ventilation may be required to maintain adequate ventilation and oxygenation while the underlying cause is corrected.

Nursing Management

Nursing management of the patient with ARF includes assisting with intubation and maintaining mechanical ventilation (described in Chap. 25). The nurse assesses the patient's respiratory status by monitoring the patient's level of response, arterial blood gases, pulse oximetry, and vital signs and assessing the respiratory system. The nurse implements strategies (eg, turning schedule, mouth care, skin care, range of motion of extremities) to prevent complications. The nurse also assesses the patient's understanding of the management strategies that are used and initiates some form of communication to enable the patient to express his or her needs to the health care team. Nursing care also addresses the problems that led to ARF. As the patient's status improves, the nurse assesses the patient's knowledge of the underlying disorder and provides teaching as appropriate to address the underlying disorder.

Acute Respiratory Distress Syndrome

Acute respiratory distress syndrome (ARDS; previously called adult respiratory distress syndrome) is a clinical syndrome characterized by a sudden and progressive pulmonary edema, increasing bilateral infiltrates on chest x-ray, hypoxemia refractory to oxygen supplementation, and reduced lung compliance. These signs occur in the absence of left-sided heart failure. Patients with ARDS usually require mechanical ventilation with a higher-than-normal airway pressure. A wide range of factors are associated with the development of ARDS (Chart 23-6), including direct injury to the lungs (eg, smoke inhalation) or indirect insult to the lungs (eg, shock). ARDS has been associated with a mortality rate as high as 50% to 60%. The major cause of death in ARDS is nonpulmonary multiple-system organ failure, often with sepsis.

Pathophysiology

ARDS occurs as a result of an inflammatory trigger that initiates the release of cellular and chemical mediators, causing injury to the alveolar capillary membrane. This results in leakage of fluid into the alveolar interstitial spaces and alterations in the capillary bed.

Severe ventilation–perfusion mismatching occurs in ARDS. Alveoli collapse because of the inflammatory infiltrate, blood, fluid, and surfactant dysfunction. Small airways are narrowed because of interstitial fluid and bronchial obstruction. The lung compliance becomes markedly decreased (stiff lungs), and the result is a characteristic decrease in functional residual capacity and severe hypoxemia. The blood returning to the lung for gas exchange is pumped through the nonventilated, nonfunctioning areas of the lung, causing a shunt to develop. This means that blood is interfacing with nonfunctioning alveoli and gas exchange is markedly impaired, resulting in severe, refractory hypoxemia. Figure 23-6 shows the sequence of pathophysiologic events leading to ARDS.

Chart 23-6

Etiologic Factors Related to ARDS

Aspiration (gastric secretions, drowning, hydrocarbons)
Drug ingestion and overdose
Hematologic disorders (disseminated intravascular coagulopathy [DIC], massive transfusions, cardiopulmonary bypass)
Prolonged inhalation of high concentrations of oxygen, smoke, or corrosive substances
Localized infection (bacterial, fungal, viral pneumonia)
Metabolic disorders (pancreatitis, uremia)
Shock (any cause)
Trauma (pulmonary contusion, multiple fractures, head injury)
Major surgery
Fat or air embolism
Systemic sepsis

Clinical Manifestations

Clinically, the acute phase of ARDS is marked by a rapid onset of severe dyspnea that usually occurs 12 to 48 hours after the initiating event. A characteristic feature is arterial hypoxemia that does not respond to supplemental oxygen. On chest x-ray, the findings are similar to those seen with cardiogenic pulmonary edema and present as bilateral infiltrates that quickly worsen. The acute lung injury then progresses to fibrosing alveolitis with persistent, severe hypoxemia. The patient also has increased alveolar dead space (ventilation to alveoli, but poor perfusion) and decreased pulmonary compliance ("stiff lungs," which are difficult to ventilate). Clinically, a patient is thought to be in the recovery phase if the hypoxemia gradually resolves, the chest x-ray improves, and the lungs become more compliant (Ware & Matthay, 2000).

Assessment and Diagnostic Findings

Intercostal retractions and crackles, as the fluid begins to leak into the alveolar interstitial space, are evident on physical examination. A diagnosis of ARDS may be made based on the following crite-

 **Physiology/Pathophysiology**

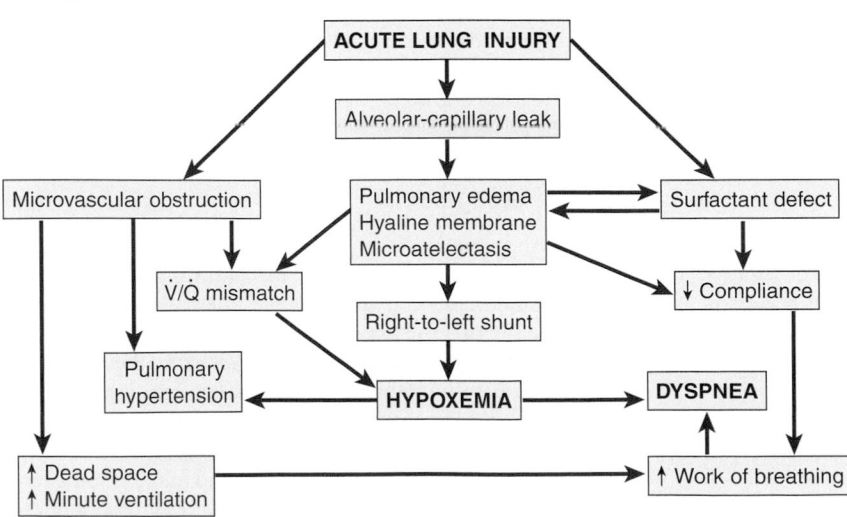

FIGURE 23-6 Pathogenesis and pathophysiology of acute respiratory distress syndrome. Adapted from Farzan, S. (1997). *A concise handbook of respiratory diseases* (4th ed.). Stamford, CT: Appleton & Lange.

ria: a history of systemic or pulmonary risk factors, acute onset of respiratory distress, bilateral pulmonary infiltrates, clinical absence of left-sided heart failure, and a ratio of partial pressure of oxygen of arterial blood to fraction of inspired oxygen (PaO_2/FiO_2) less than 200 mm Hg (severe refractory hypoxemia).

Medical Management

The primary focus in the management of ARDS includes identification and treatment of the underlying condition. Aggressive, supportive care must be provided to compensate for the severe respiratory dysfunction. This supportive therapy almost always includes intubation and mechanical ventilation. In addition, circulatory support, adequate fluid volume, and nutritional support are important. Supplemental oxygen is used as the patient begins the initial spiral of hypoxemia. As the hypoxemia progresses, intubation and mechanical ventilation are instituted. The concentration of oxygen and ventilator settings and modes are determined by the patient's status. This is monitored by arterial blood gas analysis, pulse oximetry, and bedside pulmonary function testing.

Positive end-expiratory pressure (PEEP) is a critical part of the treatment of ARDS. PEEP usually improves oxygenation, but it does not influence the natural history of the syndrome. Use of PEEP helps to increase functional residual capacity and reverse alveolar collapse by keeping the alveoli open, resulting in improved arterial oxygenation and a reduction in the severity of the ventilation–perfusion imbalance. By using PEEP, a lower FiO_2 may be required. The goal is a PaO_2 greater than 60 mm Hg or an oxygen saturation level of greater than 90% at the lowest possible FiO_2. PEEP and modes of mechanical ventilation are discussed in Chapter 25.

Systemic hypotension may occur in ARDS as a result of hypovolemia secondary to leakage of fluid into the interstitial spaces and depressed cardiac output from high levels of PEEP therapy. Hypovolemia must be carefully treated without causing further overload. Intravenous crystalloid solutions are administered, with careful monitoring of pulmonary status. Inotropic or vasopressor agents may be required. Pulmonary artery pressure catheters are used to monitor the patient's fluid status and the severe and progressive pulmonary hypertension sometimes observed in ARDS.

PHARMACOLOGIC THERAPY

Numerous pharmacologic treatments are under investigation to stop the cascade of events leading to ARDS. These include human recombinant interleukin-1 receptor antagonist, neutrophil inhibitors, pulmonary-specific vasodilators, surfactant replacement therapy, antisepsis agents, antioxidant therapy, and corticosteroids late in the course of ARDS (Ware & Matthay, 2000).

NUTRITIONAL THERAPY

Adequate nutritional support is vital in the treatment of ARDS. Patients with ARDS require 35 to 45 kcal/kg per day to meet caloric requirements. Enteral feeding is the first consideration; however, parenteral nutrition also may be required.

Nursing Management

GENERAL MEASURES

The patient with ARDS is critically ill and requires close monitoring because the condition could quickly change to a life-threatening situation. Most of the respiratory modalities discussed in Chapter 25 are used in this situation (oxygen administration, nebulizer therapy, chest physiotherapy, endotracheal intubation or tracheostomy, mechanical ventilation, suctioning, bronchoscopy). Frequent assessment of the patient's status is necessary to evaluate the effectiveness of treatment.

In addition to implementing the medical plan of care, the nurse considers other needs of the patient. Positioning is important. The nurse should turn the patient frequently to improve ventilation and perfusion in the lungs and enhance secretion drainage. However, the nurse must closely monitor the patient for deterioration in oxygenation with changes in position. Oxygenation in the ARDS patient is sometimes improved in the prone position and may be used in special circumstances; studies to assess the benefits and problems of such positioning are ongoing (Curley, 2000; Marion, 2001).

The patient is extremely anxious and agitated because of the increasing hypoxemia and dyspnea. The nurse should explain all procedures and provide care in a calm, reassuring manner. It is important to reduce the patient's anxiety because anxiety prevents rest and increases oxygen expenditure. Rest is essential to reduce oxygen consumption, thereby reducing oxygen needs.

VENTILATOR CONSIDERATIONS

If the patient is intubated and receiving mechanical ventilation with PEEP, several considerations must be addressed. PEEP, which causes increased end-expiratory pressure, is an unnatural pattern of breathing and feels strange to the patient. The patient may be anxious and "fight" the ventilator. Nursing assessment is important to assess for problems with ventilation that may be causing the anxiety reaction: tube blockage by kinking or retained secretions; other acute respiratory problems (eg, pneumothorax, pain); a sudden drop in the oxygen level; the patient's level of dyspnea; or ventilator malfunction. In some cases, sedation may be required to decrease the patient's oxygen consumption, allow the ventilator to provide full support of ventilation, and decrease the patient's anxiety. Possible sedatives are lorazepam (Ativan), midazolam (Versed), haloperidol (Haldol), propofol (Diprivan), and short-acting barbiturates.

If the PEEP level cannot be maintained despite the use of sedatives, neuromuscular blocking agents, such as pancuronium (Pavulon), vecuronium (Norcuron), atracurium (Tracrium), and rocuronium (Zemuron), may be given to paralyze the patient. This allows the patient to be ventilated more easily. With paralysis, the patient appears unconscious, loses motor function, and cannot breathe, talk, or blink independently. However, the patient retains sensation and is awake and able to hear. The nurse must reassure the patient that the paralysis is a result of the medication and is temporary. Paralysis should be used for the shortest possible time and never without adequate sedation.

Use of paralytic agents has many dangers and side effects. The nurse must be sure the patient does not become disconnected from the ventilator, because respiratory muscles are paralyzed and the patient will be apneic. Consequently, the nurse ensures that the patient is closely monitored at all times. All ventilator and patient alarms should be on at all times. Eye care is important as well because the patient cannot blink, increasing the risk of corneal abrasions. Neuromuscular blockers predispose patients to the development of deep venous thrombi, muscle atrophy, and skin breakdown. Nursing assessment is essential to minimize the complications related to neuromuscular blockade. The patient may have discomfort or pain but cannot communicate these sensations.

Analgesia is usually administered concurrently with neuromuscular blocking agents. The nurse must anticipate the patient's needs regarding pain and comfort. The nurse checks the patient's position to ensure it is comfortable and in normal alignment and talks to, and not about, the patient while in the patient's presence.

In addition, it is important for the nurse to describe the purpose and effects of the paralytic agents to the family. This experience can be very frightening to family members if they are unaware that these agents have been administered.

Pulmonary Hypertension

Pulmonary hypertension is a condition that is not clinically evident until late in its progression. Pulmonary hypertension exists when the systolic pulmonary artery pressure exceeds 30 mm Hg or the mean pulmonary artery pressure exceeds 25 mm Hg. These pressures cannot be measured indirectly as can systemic blood pressure; instead, they must be measured during right-sided heart catheterization. In the absence of these measurements, clinical recognition becomes the only indicator for the presence of pulmonary hypertension.

There are two forms of pulmonary hypertension: primary (or idiopathic) and secondary. Primary pulmonary hypertension is an uncommon disease in which the diagnosis is made by excluding all other possible causes. The exact cause is unknown, but there are several possible causes (Chart 23-7). The clinical presentation of primary pulmonary hypertension exists with no evidence of pulmonary and cardiac disease or pulmonary embolism. It occurs most often in women 20 to 40 years of age and is usually fatal within 5 years of diagnosis.

Chart 23-7 **Causes of Pulmonary Hypertension**

Primary or Idiopathic
    Altered immune mechanisms
    Silent pulmonary emboli
    Raynaud's phenomenon
    Oral contraceptive use
    Sickle cell disease
    Collagen diseases

Secondary
    Pulmonary vasoconstriction due to hypoxemia
        Chronic obstructive pulmonary disease
        Kyphoscoliosis
        Obesity
        Smoke inhalation
        High altitude
        Neuromuscular disorders
        Diffuse interstitial pneumonia
    Reduction of the pulmonary vascular bed (must impair 50% to 75% of the vascular bed)
        Pulmonary emboli
        Vasculitis
        Widespread interstitial lung disease (sarcoidosis, systemic sclerosis)
        Tumor emboli
    Primary cardiac disease
        Congenital (patent ductus arteriosus, atrial septal defect, ventricular septal defect)
        Acquired (rheumatic valvular disease, mitral stenosis, myxoma, left ventricular failure)

Secondary pulmonary hypertension is more common and results from existing cardiac or pulmonary disease. The prognosis depends on the severity of the underlying disorder and the changes in the pulmonary vascular bed. A common cause of secondary pulmonary hypertension is pulmonary artery constriction due to hypoxemia from COPD.

Pathophysiology

The underlying process of pulmonary hypertension varies, and multiple factors are often responsible. Normally, the pulmonary vascular bed can handle the blood volume delivered by the right ventricle. It has a low resistance to blood flow and compensates for increased blood volume by dilation of the vessels in the pulmonary circulation. However, if the pulmonary vascular bed is destroyed or obstructed, as in pulmonary hypertension, the ability to handle whatever flow or volume of blood it receives is impaired, and the increased blood flow then increases the pulmonary artery pressure. As the pulmonary arterial pressure increases, the pulmonary vascular resistance also increases. Both pulmonary artery constriction (as in hypoxemia or hypercapnia) and a reduction of the pulmonary vascular bed (which occurs with pulmonary emboli) result in an increase in pulmonary vascular resistance and pressure. This increased workload affects right ventricular function. The myocardium ultimately cannot meet the increasing demands imposed on it, leading to right ventricular hypertrophy (enlargement and dilation) and failure.

Clinical Manifestations

Dyspnea is the main symptom of pulmonary hypertension, occurring at first with exertion and eventually at rest. Substernal chest pain also is common, affecting 25% to 50% of patients. Other signs and symptoms include weakness, fatigue, syncope, occasional hemoptysis, and signs of right-sided heart failure (peripheral edema, ascites, distended neck veins, liver engorgement, crackles, heart murmur).

Assessment and Diagnostic Findings

A complete diagnostic evaluation includes a history, physical examination, chest x-ray, pulmonary function studies, electrocardiogram (ECG), echocardiogram, ventilation–perfusion scan, and cardiac catheterization. In some cases, a lung biopsy, performed by thoracotomy or thoracoscopy, may be needed to make a definite diagnosis. Cardiac catheterization of the right side of the heart reveals elevated pulmonary arterial pressure. An echocardiogram can assess the progression of the disease and rule out other conditions with similar signs and symptoms. The ECG reveals right ventricular hypertrophy, right axis deviation, and tall peaked P waves in inferior leads, tall anterior R waves, and ST-segment depression and/or T-wave inversion anteriorly. The PaO_2 also is decreased (hypoxemia). A ventilation–perfusion scan or pulmonary angiography detects defects in pulmonary vasculature, such as pulmonary emboli. Pulmonary function studies may be normal or show a slight decrease in vital capacity (VC) and lung compliance, with a mild decrease in the diffusing capacity.

Medical Management

The goal of treatment is to manage the underlying cardiac or pulmonary condition. Most patients with primary pulmonary hypertension do not have hypoxemia at rest but require supplemental oxygen with exercise. However, patients with severe right ventricular failure, decreased cardiac output, and progressive disease may have resting hypoxemia and require continuous oxygen supplementation. Appropriate oxygen therapy (see Chap. 25) reverses the vasoconstriction and reduces the pulmonary hypertension in a relatively short time.

In the presence of cor pulmonale, which is discussed in the section that follows, treatment should include fluid restriction, diuretics to decrease fluid accumulation, cardiac glycosides (eg, digitalis) in an attempt to improve cardiac function, calcium channel blockers for vasodilation, and rest. In primary pulmonary hypertension, vasodilators have been administered with variable success (eg, calcium channel blockers, intravenous prostacyclin). Prostacyclin (PGX [Flolan]) is one of the prostaglandins produced by the pulmonary endothelium. Intravenous prostacyclin (epoprostenol) helps to decrease pulmonary hypertension by reducing pulmonary vascular resistance and pressures and increasing cardiac output. Anticoagulants such as warfarin (Coumadin) have been given to patients because of chronic pulmonary emboli. Heart–lung transplantation has been successful in select patients with primary hypertension who have not been responsive to other therapies.

Nursing Management

The major nursing goal is to identify patients at high risk for pulmonary hypertension, such as those with COPD, pulmonary emboli, congenital heart disease, and mitral valve disease. The nurse also must be alert for signs and symptoms, administer oxygen therapy appropriately, and instruct patients and their families about the use of home oxygen supplementation.

Pulmonary Heart Disease (Cor Pulmonale)

Cor pulmonale is a condition in which the right ventricle of the heart enlarges (with or without right-sided heart failure) as a result of diseases that affect the structure or function of the lung or its vasculature. Any disease affecting the lungs and accompanied by hypoxemia may result in cor pulmonale. The most frequent cause is severe COPD (see Chap. 24), in which changes in the airway and retained secretions reduce alveolar ventilation. Other causes are conditions that restrict or compromise ventilatory function, leading to hypoxemia or acidosis (deformities of the thoracic cage, massive obesity), or conditions that reduce the pulmonary vascular bed (primary idiopathic pulmonary arterial hypertension, pulmonary embolus). Certain disorders of the nervous system, respiratory muscles, chest wall, and pulmonary arterial tree also may be responsible for cor pulmonale.

Pathophysiology

Pulmonary disease can produce physiologic changes that in time affect the heart and cause the right ventricle to enlarge and eventually fail. Any condition that deprives the lungs of oxygen can cause hypoxemia and hypercapnia, resulting in ventilatory insufficiency. Hypoxemia and hypercapnia cause pulmonary arterial vasoconstriction and possibly reduction of the pulmonary vascular bed, as in emphysema or pulmonary emboli. The result is increased resistance in the pulmonary circulatory system, with a subsequent rise in pulmonary blood pressure (pulmonary hypertension). A mean pulmonary arterial pressure of 45 mm Hg or more may occur in cor pulmonale. Right ventricular hypertrophy

may result, followed by right ventricular failure. In short, cor pulmonale results from pulmonary hypertension, which causes the right side of the heart to enlarge because of the increased work required to pump blood against high resistance through the pulmonary vascular system.

Clinical Manifestations

Symptoms of cor pulmonale are usually related to the underlying lung disease, such as COPD. With right ventricular failure, the patient may develop increasing edema of the feet and legs, distended neck veins, an enlarged palpable liver, pleural effusion, ascites, and a heart murmur. Headache, confusion, and somnolence may occur as a result of increased levels of carbon dioxide (hypercapnia). Patients often complain of increasing shortness of breath, wheezing, cough, and fatigue.

Medical Management

The objectives of treatment are to improve the patient's ventilation and to treat both the underlying lung disease and the manifestations of heart disease. Supplemental oxygen is administered to improve gas exchange and to reduce pulmonary arterial pressure and pulmonary vascular resistance. Improved oxygen transport relieves the pulmonary hypertension that is causing the cor pulmonale.

Better survival rates and greater reduction in pulmonary vascular resistance have been reported with continuous, 24-hour oxygen therapy for patients with severe hypoxemia. Substantial improvement may require 4 to 6 weeks of oxygen therapy, usually in the home. Periodic assessment of pulse oximetry and arterial blood gases is necessary to determine the adequacy of alveolar ventilation and to monitor the effectiveness of oxygen therapy.

Ventilation is further improved with chest physical therapy and bronchial hygiene maneuvers as indicated to remove accumulated secretions, and the administration of bronchodilators. Further measures depend on the patient's condition. If the patient is in respiratory failure, endotracheal intubation and mechanical ventilation may be necessary. If the patient is in heart failure, hypoxemia and hypercapnia must be relieved to improve cardiac function and output. Bed rest, sodium restriction, and diuretic therapy also are instituted judiciously to reduce peripheral edema (to lower pulmonary arterial pressure through a decrease in total blood volume) and the circulatory load on the right side of the heart. Digitalis may be prescribed to relieve pulmonary hypertension if the patient also has left ventricular failure, a supraventricular dysrhythmia, or right ventricular failure that does not respond to other therapy.

ECG monitoring may be indicated because of the high incidence of dysrhythmias in patients with cor pulmonale. Any pulmonary infection must be treated promptly to avoid further impaired gas exchange and exacerbations of hypoxemia and pulmonary heart disease. The prognosis depends on whether the pulmonary hypertension is reversible. (Management of acute respiratory failure was presented earlier in this chapter.)

Nursing Management

Nursing care of the patient with cor pulmonale addresses the underlying disorder leading to cor pulmonale as well as the problems related to pulmonary hyperventilation and right-sided cardiac failure. If intubation and mechanical ventilation are required to manage ARF, the nurse assists with the intubation procedure and maintains mechanical ventilation. The nurse assesses the patient's respiratory and cardiac status and administers medications as prescribed.

During the patient's hospital stay, the nurse instructs the patient about the importance of close monitoring (fluid retention, weight gain, edema) and adherence to the therapeutic regimen, especially the 24-hour use of oxygen. Factors that affect the patient's adherence to the treatment regimen are explored and addressed.

PROMOTING HOME AND COMMUNITY-BASED CARE

Teaching Patients Self-Care. Most of the care and monitoring of the patient with cor pulmonale is performed by the patient and family in the home because it is a chronic disorder. If supplemental oxygen is administered, the nurse instructs the patient and the family in its use. Nutrition counseling is warranted if the patient is on a sodium-restricted diet or is taking diuretics. The nurse teaches the family to monitor for signs and symptoms of right ventricular failure and about emergency interventions and when to call for assistance. Most importantly, the nurse urges the patient to stop smoking.

Continuing Care. A referral for home care may be warranted for the patient who cannot manage self-care or for the patient whose physical condition warrants close assessment. During the home visit, the home care nurse evaluates the patient's status and the patient's and family members' understanding of the therapeutic regimen and their adherence to it. If oxygen is used in the home, the nurse determines if it is being administered safely and as prescribed. It is important to assess the patient's progress in stopping smoking and to reinforce the importance of smoking cessation with the patient and family. The nurse identifies strategies to assist with smoking cessation and refers the patient and family to community support groups. In addition, the patient is reminded about the importance of other health promotion and screening practices.

Pulmonary Embolism

Pulmonary embolism (PE) refers to the obstruction of the pulmonary artery or one of its branches by a thrombus (or thrombi) that originates somewhere in the venous system or in the right side of the heart. Most commonly, PE is due to a blood clot or thrombus. However, there are other types of emboli: air, fat, amniotic fluid, and septic (from bacterial invasion of the thrombus). It is estimated that more than half a million people develop PE yearly, resulting in more than 50,000 deaths. PE is a common disorder and often is associated with trauma, surgery (orthopedic, major abdominal, pelvic, gynecologic), pregnancy, heart failure, age older than 50 years, hypercoagulable states, and prolonged immobility. It also may occur in an apparently healthy person. Risk factors for developing PE are identified in Chart 23-8.

Although most thrombi originate in the deep veins of the legs, other sites include the pelvic veins and the right atrium of the heart. A venous thrombosis can result from slowing of blood flow (stasis), secondary to damage to the blood vessel wall (particularly the endothelial lining) or changes in the blood coagulation mechanism. Atrial fibrillation is also a cause of pulmonary embolism. An enlarged right atrium in fibrillation causes blood to stagnate and form clots in this area. These clots are prone to travel into the pulmonary circulation.

Chart 23-8

Risk Factors for Pulmonary Embolus

Venous Stasis (slowing of blood flow in veins)
Prolonged immobilization (especially postoperative)
Prolonged periods of sitting/traveling
Varicose veins
Spinal cord injury

Hypercoagulability (due to release of tissue thromboplastin after injury/surgery)
Injury
Tumor (pancreatic, GI, GU, breast, lung)
Increased platelet count (polycythemia, splenectomy)

Venous Endothelial Disease
Thrombophlebitis
Vascular disease
Foreign bodies (IV/central venous catheters)

Certain Disease States (combination of stasis, coagulation alterations, and venous injury)
Heart disease (especially heart failure)
Trauma (especially fracture of hip, pelvis, vertebra, lower extremities)
Postoperative state/postpartum period
Diabetes mellitus
Chronic obstructive pulmonary disease

Other Predisposing Conditions
Advanced age
Obesity
Pregnancy
Oral contraceptive use
History of previous thrombophlebitis, pulmonary embolism
Constrictive clothing

Pathophysiology

When a thrombus completely or partially obstructs a pulmonary artery or its branches, the alveolar dead space is increased. The area, although continuing to be ventilated, receives little or no blood flow. Thus, gas exchange is impaired or absent in this area. In addition, various substances are released from the clot and surrounding area, causing regional blood vessels and bronchioles to constrict. This causes an increase in pulmonary vascular resistance. This reaction compounds the ventilation–perfusion imbalance.

The hemodynamic consequences are increased pulmonary vascular resistance from the regional vasoconstriction and reduced size of the pulmonary vascular bed. This results in an increase in pulmonary arterial pressure and, in turn, an increase in right ventricular work to maintain pulmonary blood flow. When the work requirements of the right ventricle exceed its capacity, right ventricular failure occurs, leading to a decrease in cardiac output followed by a decrease in systemic blood pressure and the development of shock.

Clinical Manifestations

The symptoms of PE depend on the size of the thrombus and the area of the pulmonary artery occluded by the thrombus; they may be nonspecific. Dyspnea is the most frequent symptom; tachypnea (very rapid respiratory rate) is the most frequent sign (Goldhaber, 1998). The duration and intensity of the dyspnea depend on the extent of embolization. Chest pain is common and is usually sudden and pleuritic. It may be substernal and mimic angina pectoris or a myocardial infarction. Other symptoms include anxiety, fever, tachycardia, apprehension, cough, diaphoresis, hemoptysis, and syncope.

A massive embolism is best defined by the degree of hemodynamic instability rather than the percentage of pulmonary vasculature occlusion. It is described as an occlusion of the outflow tract of the main pulmonary artery or the bifurcation of the pulmonary arteries that produces pronounced dyspnea, sudden substernal pain, rapid and weak pulse, shock, syncope, and sudden death. Multiple small emboli can lodge in the terminal pulmonary arterioles, producing multiple small infarctions of the lungs. A pulmonary infarction causes ischemic necrosis of an area of the lung and occurs in less than 10% of cases of PE (Arroliga, Matthay & Matthay, 2000). The clinical picture may mimic that of bronchopneumonia or heart failure. In atypical instances, the disease causes few signs and symptoms, whereas in other instances it mimics various other cardiopulmonary disorders.

Assessment and Diagnostic Findings

Death from PE commonly occurs within 1 hour of symptoms; thus, early recognition and diagnosis are priorities. Because the symptoms of PE can vary from few to severe, a diagnostic workup is performed to rule out other diseases. Deep venous thrombosis is closely associated with the development of PE. Typically, patients report sudden onset of pain and/or swelling and warmth of the proximal or distal extremity, skin discoloration, and superficial vein distention. The pain is usually relieved with elevation. The diagnostic workup includes a ventilation–perfusion scan, pulmonary angiography, chest x-ray, ECG, peripheral vascular studies, impedance plethysmography, and arterial blood gas analysis.

The chest x-ray is usually normal but may show infiltrates, atelectasis, elevation of the diaphragm on the affected side, or a pleural effusion. The chest x-ray is most helpful in excluding other possible causes. The ECG usually shows sinus tachycardia, PR-interval depression, and nonspecific T-wave changes. Peripheral vascular studies may include impedance plethysmography, Doppler ultrasonography, or venography (see Chap. 31). Test results confirm or exclude the diagnosis of PE. Arterial blood gas analysis may show hypoxemia and hypocapnia (from tachypnea); however, arterial blood gas measurements are normal in up to 20% of patients with PE.

A ventilation–perfusion scan is the test of choice in patients with suspected PE. The perfusion portion of the scan may indicate areas of diminished or absent blood flow and is the most useful test to rule out clinically important PE. A ventilation scan may show whether there is also a ventilation abnormality present. A normal perfusion scan rules out the diagnosis of PE. If there is a ventilation–perfusion mismatch, the probability of PE is high. Spiral CT of the chest may also assist in the diagnosis.

If lung scan results are not definitive, pulmonary angiography, considered the gold standard for the diagnosis of PE, can be used. This test is invasive and is performed in the interventional radiology department. A contrast agent is injected into the pulmonary arterial system, allowing visualization of obstructions to blood flow and abnormalities.

Prevention

For those at risk, the most effective approach to preventing PE is to prevent deep venous thrombosis. Active leg exercises to avoid venous stasis, early ambulation, and use of elastic compression stockings are general preventive measures. Additional strategies for prevention are listed in the checklist in Chart 23-9.

Chart 23-9

Home Care Checklist • Prevention of Recurrent Pulmonary Embolism

At the completion of the home care instruction, the patient or caregiver will be able to:	Patient	Caregiver
• Describe the underlying process leading to pulmonary embolism.	✓	✓
• Describe the need for continued anticoagulant therapy after the initial embolism.	✓	✓
• Name the anticoagulant prescribed and identify dosage and schedule of administration.	✓	✓
• Describe potential side effects of coagulation such as bruising and bleeding and identify ways to prevent bleeding.	✓	✓

Avoid the use of sharps (razors, knives, etc.) to prevent cuts; shave with an electric shaver.
    Use a toothbrush with soft bristles to prevent gum injury.
    Do not take aspirin or antihistamines while taking warfarin sodium (Coumadin).
    Always check with health care provider before taking any medicine, including over-the-counter medications.
    Avoid laxatives, because they may affect vitamin K absorption.
    Report the occurrence of dark, tarry stools to the health care provider immediately.
    Wear an identification bracelet or carry a medicine card stating that you are taking anticoagulants.		

• Describe strategies to prevent recurrent deep venous thrombosis and pulmonary emboli:	✓	✓

Continue to wear elastic pressure stockings (compression hose) as long as directed.
    Avoid sitting with legs crossed or sitting for prolonged periods of time.
    When traveling, change position regularly, walk occasionally, and do active exercises of moving the legs and ankles while sitting.
    Drink fluids, especially while traveling and in warm weather, to avoid hemoconcentration due to fluid deficit.		

• Describe the signs and symptoms of lower extremity circulatory compromise and potential deep venous thrombosis: calf or leg pain, swelling, pedal edema.	✓	✓
• Describe the signs and symptoms of pulmonary compromise related to recurrent pulmonary embolism.	✓	✓
• Describe how and when to contact the health care provider if symptoms of circulatory compromise or pulmonary compromise are identified.	✓	✓

Patients who are older than 40, whose hemostasis is adequate, and who are undergoing major elective abdominal or thoracic surgery may receive anticoagulant therapy. Low doses of heparin may be given before surgery to reduce the risk of postoperative deep venous thrombus and PE. Heparin should be administered subcutaneously 2 hours before surgery and continued every 8 to 12 hours until the patient is discharged. Low-dose heparin is thought to enhance the activity of antithrombin III, a major plasma inhibitor of clotting factor X. This regimen is not recommended for patients with an active thrombotic process or for those undergoing major orthopedic surgery, open prostatectomy, or surgery on the eye or brain. Low-molecular-weight heparin (eg, enoxaparin [Lovenox]) is an alternative therapy. It has a longer half-life, enhanced subcutaneous absorption, a reduced incidence of thrombocytopenia, and reduced interaction with platelets as compared to unfractionated heparin (Ansell, Hickey, Kleinschmidt et al., 2000).

The intermittent pneumatic leg compression device is useful in preventing thromboembolism. The device inflates a bag that intermittently compresses the leg from the calf to the thigh, thereby improving venous return. It may be applied before surgery and continued until the patient is ambulatory. The device is particularly useful for patients who are not candidates for anticoagulant therapy (Clagett, Anderson, Geerts et al., 1998).

Medical Management

Because PE is often a medical emergency, emergency management is of primary concern. After emergency measures have been taken and the patient's condition stabilizes, the treatment goal is to dissolve (lyse) the existing emboli and prevent new ones from forming. The treatment of PE may include a variety of modalities:

- General measures to improve respiratory and vascular status
- Anticoagulation therapy
- Thrombolytic therapy
- Surgical intervention

EMERGENCY MANAGEMENT

Massive PE is a life-threatening emergency. The immediate objective is to stabilize the cardiopulmonary system. A sudden rise in pulmonary resistance increases the work of the right ventricle, which can cause acute right-sided heart failure with cardiogenic shock. Most patients who die of massive PE do so in the first 1 to 2 hours after the embolic event. Emergency management consists of the following:

- Nasal oxygen is administered immediately to relieve hypoxemia, respiratory distress, and central cyanosis.
- Intravenous infusion lines are started to establish routes for medications or fluids that will be needed.
- A perfusion scan, hemodynamic measurements, and arterial blood gas determinations are performed. Spiral (helical) CT or pulmonary angiography may be performed. Spiral CT is more advanced and quicker than routine tomography. With spiral CT, the patient continuously moves as the x-ray tube rotates. With this type of CT, images can be reconstructed at select levels and locations for diagnostic purposes.
- Hypotension is treated by a slow infusion of dobutamine (Dobutrex) (which has a dilating effect on the pulmonary vessels and bronchi) or dopamine (Intropin).

- The ECG is monitored continuously for dysrhythmias and right ventricular failure, which may occur suddenly.
- Digitalis glycosides, intravenous diuretics, and antiarrhythmic agents are administered when appropriate.
- Blood is drawn for serum electrolytes, complete blood count, and hematocrit.
- If clinical assessment and arterial blood gas analysis indicate the need, the patient is intubated and placed on a mechanical ventilator.
- If the patient has suffered massive embolism and is hypotensive, an indwelling urinary catheter is inserted to monitor urinary output.
- Small doses of intravenous morphine or sedatives are administered to relieve the patient's anxiety, to alleviate chest discomfort, to improve tolerance of the endotracheal tube, and to ease adaptation to the mechanical ventilator.

GENERAL MANAGEMENT

Measures are initiated to improve the patient's respiratory and vascular status. Oxygen therapy is administered to correct the hypoxemia, relieve the pulmonary vascular vasoconstriction, and reduce the pulmonary hypertension. Using elastic compression stockings or intermittent pneumatic leg compression devices reduces venous stasis. These measures compress the superficial veins and increase the velocity of blood in the deep veins by redirecting the blood through the deep veins. Elevating the leg (above the level of the heart) also increases venous flow.

PHARMACOLOGIC THERAPY

Anticoagulation Therapy. Anticoagulant therapy (heparin, warfarin sodium) has traditionally been the primary method for managing acute deep vein thrombosis and PE (Goldhaber, 1998). Heparin is used to prevent recurrence of emboli but has no effect on emboli that are already present. It is administered as an intravenous bolus of 5,000 to 10,000 units, followed by a continuous infusion initiated at a dose of 18 U/kg per hour, not to exceed 1,600 U/hour in otherwise healthy patients (Goldhaber, 1998). The rate is reduced in patients with a high risk of bleeding. The goal is to keep the partial thromboplastin time 1.5 to 2.5 times normal (or 46 to 70 seconds). Heparin is usually administered for 5 to 7 days. Low-molecular-weight heparin (eg, enoxaparin [Lovenox]) may also be used.

Warfarin sodium (Coumadin) administration is begun within 24 hours after the start of heparin therapy because its onset of action is 4 to 5 days. Warfarin is usually continued for 3 to 6 months. The prothrombin time is maintained at 1.5 to 2.5 times normal (or an INR [international normalized ratio] of 2.0 to 3.0). Anticoagulation therapy is contraindicated in patients who are at risk for bleeding (eg, those with gastrointestinal conditions or with postoperative or postpartum bleeding).

Thrombolytic Therapy. Thrombolytic therapy (urokinase, streptokinase, alteplase, anistreplase, reteplase) also may be used in treating PE, particularly in patients who are severely compromised (eg, those who are hypotensive and have significant hypoxemia despite oxygen supplementation). Thrombolytic therapy resolves the thrombi or emboli more quickly and restores more normal hemodynamic functioning of the pulmonary circulation, thereby reducing pulmonary hypertension and improving perfusion, oxygenation, and cardiac output. Bleeding, however, is a significant side effect. Contraindications to thrombolytic therapy include a cerebrovascular accident within the past 2 months, other active intracranial processes, active bleeding, surgery within the past 10 days of the thrombotic event, recent labor and delivery, trauma, or severe hypertension. Consequently, thrombolytic agents are advocated only for PE affecting a significant area of blood flow to the lung and causing hemodynamic instability.

Before thrombolytic therapy is started, prothrombin time, partial thromboplastin time, hematocrit values, and platelet counts are obtained. Heparin is stopped prior to administration of a thrombolytic agent. During therapy, all but essential invasive procedures are avoided because of potential bleeding. If necessary, fresh whole blood, packed red cells, cryoprecipitate, or frozen plasma is administered to replace blood loss and reverse the bleeding tendency. After the thrombolytic infusion is completed (which varies in duration according to the agent used and the condition being treated), the patient is given anticoagulants.

SURGICAL MANAGEMENT

A surgical embolectomy is rarely performed but may be indicated if the patient has a massive PE or hemodynamic instability or if there are contraindications to thrombolytic therapy. Pulmonary embolectomy requires a thoracotomy with cardiopulmonary bypass technique. Transvenous catheter embolectomy is a technique in which a vacuum-cupped catheter is introduced transvenously into the affected pulmonary artery. Suction is applied to the end of the embolus and the embolus is aspirated into the cup. The surgeon maintains suction to hold the embolus within the cup, and the entire catheter is withdrawn through the right side of the heart and out the femoral vein. Catheters are available that pulverize the clot with high-velocity jets of normal saline solution (Goldhaber, 1998). An inferior caval filter is usually inserted at the time of surgery to protect against a recurrence.

Interrupting the inferior vena cava is another surgical technique used when PE recurs or when the patient is intolerant of anticoagulant therapy. This approach prevents dislodged thrombi from being swept into the lungs while allowing adequate blood flow. The preferred approach is the application of Teflon clips to the inferior vena cava to divide the lumen into small channels without occluding caval blood flow. Also, the use of transvenous devices that occlude or filter the blood through the inferior vena cava is a fairly safe way to prevent recurrent PE. One such technique involves inserting a filter (eg, Greenfield filter) through the internal jugular vein or common femoral vein (Fig. 23-7). This filter is advanced into the inferior vena cava, where it is opened. The perforated umbrella permits the passage of blood but prevents the passage of large thrombi. It is recommended that anticoagulation be continued in patients with a caval filter, if there are no contraindications to its use.

Nursing Management

MINIMIZING THE RISK OF PULMONARY EMBOLISM

A key role of the nurse is to identify patients at high risk for PE and to minimize the risk of PE in all patients. The nurse must have a high degree of suspicion for PE in any patient, but particularly in those with conditions predisposing to a slowing of venous return (see Chart 23-8).

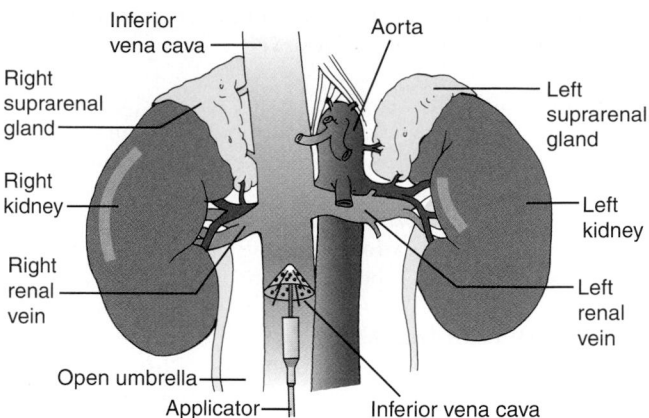

FIGURE 23-7 An umbrella filter is in place in the inferior vena cava to prevent pulmonary embolism. The filter (compressed within an applicator catheter) is inserted through an incision in the right internal jugular vein. The applicator is withdrawn when the filter fixes itself to the wall of the inferior vena cava after ejection from the applicator.

PREVENTING THROMBUS FORMATION

Preventing thrombus formation is a major nursing responsibility. The nurse encourages ambulation and active and passive leg exercises to prevent venous stasis in patients on bed rest. The nurse instructs the patient to move the legs in a "pumping" exercise so that the leg muscles can help increase venous flow. The nurse also advises the patient not to sit or lie in bed for prolonged periods, not to cross the legs, and not to wear constricting clothing. Legs should not be dangled or feet placed in a dependent position while the patient sits on the edge of the bed; instead, the patient's feet should rest on the floor or on a chair. In addition, intravenous catheters (for parenteral therapy or measurements of central venous pressure) should not be left in place for prolonged periods.

ASSESSING POTENTIAL FOR PULMONARY EMBOLISM

The nurse examines patients who are at risk for developing PE for a positive Homans' sign, which may or may not indicate impending thrombosis of the leg veins (see Chap. 31). To test for Homans' sign, the patient assumes a supine position, lifts the leg, and dorsiflexes the foot. The nurse asks the patient to report whether calf pain occurs during this maneuver. The occurrence of pain—a positive Homans' sign—may indicate deep venous thrombosis.

MONITORING THROMBOLYTIC THERAPY

The nurse is responsible for monitoring thrombolytic and anticoagulant therapy. Thrombolytic therapy (streptokinase, urokinase, tissue plasminogen activator) causes lysis of deep vein thrombi and pulmonary emboli, which helps dissolve the clots. During thrombolytic infusion, the patient remains on bed rest, vital signs are assessed every 2 hours, and invasive procedures are limited. Tests to determine prothrombin time or partial thromboplastin time are performed 3 to 4 hours after the thrombolytic infusion is started to confirm that the fibrinolytic systems have been activated. Because of the prolonged clotting time, only essential arterial punctures or venipunctures are performed, and manual pressure is applied to any puncture site for at least 30 minutes. Pulse oximetry is used to monitor changes in oxygenation. The nurse immediately discontinues the infusion if uncontrolled bleeding occurs.

See Chapter 31 for nursing management for the patient receiving anticoagulant or thrombolytic therapy.

MANAGING PAIN

Chest pain, if present, is usually pleuritic rather than cardiac in origin. A semi-Fowler's position provides a more comfortable position for breathing. However, it is important to continue to turn the patient frequently and reposition the patient to improve the **ventilation–perfusion ratio** in the lung. The nurse administers opioid analgesics as prescribed for severe pain.

MANAGING OXYGEN THERAPY

Careful attention is given to the proper use of oxygen. It is important to ensure that the patient understands the need for continuous oxygen therapy. The nurse assesses the patient frequently for signs of hypoxemia and monitors the pulse oximetry values to evaluate the effectiveness of the oxygen therapy. Deep breathing and incentive spirometry are indicated for all patients to minimize or prevent atelectasis and improve ventilation. Nebulizer therapy or percussion and postural drainage may be used for management of secretions.

RELIEVING ANXIETY

The nurse encourages the stabilized patient to talk about any fears or concerns related to this frightening episode, answers the patient's and family's questions concisely and accurately, explains the therapy, and describes how to recognize untoward effects early.

MONITORING FOR COMPLICATIONS

When caring for a patient who has had PE, the nurse must be alert for the potential complication of cardiogenic shock or right ventricular failure subsequent to the effect of PE on the cardiovascular system. Nursing activities for managing shock are found in Chapter 15.

PROVIDING POSTOPERATIVE NURSING CARE

After surgery, the nurse measures the patient's pulmonary arterial pressure and urinary output. The nurse assesses the insertion site of the arterial catheter for hematoma formation and infection. It is important to maintain the blood pressure at a level that supports perfusion of vital organs. To prevent peripheral venous stasis and edema of the lower extremities, the nurse elevates the foot of the bed and encourages isometric exercises, use of elastic compression stockings, and walking when the patient is permitted out of bed. Sitting is discouraged because hip flexion compresses the large veins in the legs.

PROMOTING HOME AND COMMUNITY-BASED CARE

Teaching Patients Self-Care. Before hospital discharge and at follow-up visits to the clinic or during home visits, the nurse instructs the patient about how to prevent recurrence and what signs and symptoms to report immediately. Patient instructions, as presented in Chart 23-9, are intended to help prevent recurrences and side effects of treatment.

Sarcoidosis

Sarcoidosis is a multisystem, granulomatous disease of unknown etiology. It may involve almost any organ or tissue but most commonly involves the lungs, lymph nodes, liver, spleen, central nervous system, skin, eyes, fingers, and parotid glands. The disease is not gender-specific, but some manifestations are more common in women. In the United States, the disease is 10 times more common in African Americans (40 cases per 100,000) than in Caucasians (5 cases per 100,000), and the disease usually begins in the third or fourth decade of life (American Thoracic Society, 1999).

Pathophysiology

Sarcoidosis is thought to be a hypersensitivity response to one or more agents (bacteria, fungi, virus, chemicals) in people with an inherited or acquired predisposition to the disorder. The hypersensitivity response results in granuloma formation due to the release of cytokines and other substances that promote replication of fibroblasts. In the lung, granuloma infiltration and fibrosis may occur, resulting in low lung compliance, impaired diffusing capacity, and reduced lung volumes (American Thoracic Society, 1999).

Clinical Manifestations

A hallmark of this disease is its insidious onset and lack of prominent clinical signs or symptoms. The clinical picture depends on the systems involved. With pulmonary involvement, signs and symptoms may include dyspnea, cough, hemoptysis, and congestion. Generalized symptoms include anorexia, fatigue, and weight loss. Other signs include uveitis, joint pain, fever, and granulomatous lesions of the skin, liver, spleen, kidney, and central nervous system. The granulomas may disappear or gradually convert to fibrous tissue. With multisystem involvement, the patient has fatigue, fever, anorexia, weight loss, and joint pain.

Assessment and Diagnostic Findings

Chest x-rays and CT scans are used to assess pulmonary adenopathy. The chest x-ray may show hilar adenopathy and disseminated miliary and nodular lesions in the lungs. A mediastinoscopy or **transbronchial** biopsy (in which a tissue specimen is obtained through the bronchial wall) may be used to confirm the diagnosis. In rare cases, an **open lung biopsy** is performed. Diagnosis is confirmed by a biopsy that shows noncaseating granulomas. Pulmonary function test results are abnormal if there is restriction of lung function (reduction in total lung capacity). Arterial blood gas measurements may be normal or may show reduced oxygen levels (hypoxemia) and increased carbon dioxide levels (hypercapnia).

Medical Management

Many patients undergo remission without specific treatment. Corticosteroid therapy may benefit some patients because of its anti-inflammatory effect, which relieves symptoms and improves organ function. It is useful for patients with ocular and myocardial involvement, skin involvement, extensive pulmonary disease that compromises pulmonary function, hepatic involvement, and hypercalcemia. Other cytotoxic and immunosuppressive agents have been used, but without the benefit of controlled clinical trials. There is no single test that monitors the progression or recurrence of sarcoidosis. Multiple tests are used to monitor the involved systems.

Occupational Lung Diseases: Pneumoconioses

Diseases of the lungs occur in numerous occupations as a result of exposure to organic and inorganic (mineral) dusts and noxious gases (fumes and aerosols). The effects of inhaling these materials depend on the composition of the substance, its concentration, its ability to initiate an immune response, its irritating properties, the duration of exposure, and the individual's response or susceptibility to the irritant. Smoking may compound the problem and may increase the risk of lung cancers in people exposed to the mineral asbestos. Key aspects of any assessment of patients with a potential occupational respiratory history include job and job activities, exposure levels, general hygiene, time frame of exposure, amount of respiratory protection used, and direct versus indirect exposures.

Pneumoconiosis refers to a nonneoplastic alteration of the lung resulting from inhalation of mineral or inorganic dust (eg, "dusty lung"). The most common pneumoconioses are silicosis, asbestosis, and coal workers' pneumoconiosis.

SILICOSIS

Silicosis is a chronic fibrotic pulmonary disease caused by inhalation of silica dust (crystalline silicon dioxide particles). Exposure to silica and silicates occurs in almost all mining, quarrying, and tunneling operations. Glass manufacturing, stone-cutting, the manufacture of abrasives and pottery, and foundry work are other occupations with exposure hazards. Finely ground silica, such as that found in soaps, polishes and filters, is extremely dangerous.

Pathophysiology

When the silica particles, which have fibrogenic properties, are inhaled, nodular lesions are produced throughout the lungs. With the passage of time and further exposure, the nodules enlarge and coalesce. Dense masses form in the upper portion of the lungs, resulting in the loss of pulmonary volume. **Restrictive lung disease** (inability of the lungs to expand fully) and obstructive lung disease from secondary emphysema result. Cavities can form as a result of superimposed TB. Exposure of 15 to 20 years is usually required before the onset of the disease and shortness of breath are manifested. Fibrotic destruction of pulmonary tissue can lead to emphysema, pulmonary hypertension, and cor pulmonale.

Clinical Manifestations

Patients with acute silicosis present with dyspnea, fever, cough, and weight loss and have a rapid progression of the disease. Symptoms are more severe in patients whose disease is complicated by progressive massive fibrosis. More commonly, this disease is a chronic problem with a long latency period. The patient may have slowly progressive symptoms indicative of hypoxemia, severe air-flow obstruction, and right-sided heart failure. Edema may occur because of the cardiac failure.

Medical Management

There is no specific treatment for silicosis, because the fibrotic process in the lung is irreversible. Supportive therapy is directed at managing complications and preventing infection. Testing is performed to rule out other lung diseases, such as TB, lung cancer, and sarcoidosis. If TB is present, it is aggressively treated. Additional therapy might include oxygen, diuretics, inhaled beta-adrenergic agonists, anticholinergics, and bronchodilator therapy.

ASBESTOSIS

Asbestosis is a disease characterized by diffuse pulmonary fibrosis from the inhalation of asbestos dust. Current laws restrict the use of asbestos, but many industries used it in the past. Therefore, exposure occurred, and may still occur, in numerous occupations, including asbestos mining and manufacturing, shipbuilding, demolition of structures containing asbestos, and roofing. Materials such as shingles, cement, vinyl asbestos tile, fireproof paint and clothing, brake linings, and filters all contained asbestos at one time, and many of these materials are still in existence. Additional diseases related to asbestos exposure include lung cancer, mesothelioma, and asbestos pleural effusion.

Pathophysiology

Inhaled asbestos fibers enter the alveoli, where they are surrounded by fibrous tissue. The fibrous tissue eventually obliterates the alveoli. Fibrous changes also affect the pleura, which thickens and develops plaque. The result of these physiologic changes is a restrictive lung disease, with a decrease in lung volume, diminished exchange of oxygen and carbon dioxide, and hypoxemia.

Clinical Manifestations

The onset of the disease is insidious, and the patient has progressive dyspnea, persistent, dry cough, mild to moderate chest pain, anorexia, weight loss, and malaise. Early physical findings include bibasilar fine, end-inspiratory crackles and in more advanced cases clubbing of the fingers. Cor pulmonale and respiratory failure occur as the disease progresses. A high proportion of workers who have been exposed to asbestos dust die of lung cancer, especially those who smoke or have a history of smoking. Malignant mesotheliomas may also occur. These are rare cancers of the pleura or peritoneum that are strongly associated with asbestos exposure.

Medical Management

There is no effective treatment for asbestosis as the lung damage is permanent and often progressive. Management is directed at controlling infection and treating the lung disease. When oxygen–carbon dioxide exchange becomes severely impaired, continuous oxygen therapy may help improve activity tolerance. The patient must be instructed to avoid additional exposure to asbestos and to stop smoking. A significant contributing cause to mortality in this population is the high incidence of lung carcinoma.

COAL WORKERS' PNEUMOCONIOSIS

Coal workers' pneumoconiosis ("black lung disease") includes a variety of respiratory diseases found in coal workers who have inhaled coal dust over the years. Coal miners are exposed to dusts that are mixtures of coal, kaolin, mica, and silica.

Pathophysiology

When coal dust is deposited in the alveoli and respiratory bronchioles, macrophages engulf the particles (by phagocytosis) and transport them to the terminal bronchioles, where they are removed by mucociliary action. In time, the clearance mechanisms cannot handle the excessive dust load, and the macrophages aggregate in the respiratory bronchioles and alveoli. Fibroblasts appear and a network of reticulin is laid down surrounding the dust-laden macrophages. The bronchioles and the alveoli become clogged with coal dust, dying macrophages, and fibroblasts. This leads to the formation of the coal macule, the primary lesion of the disorder. Macules appear as blackish dots on the lungs. Fibrotic lesions develop and, as the macules enlarge, the weakening bronchioles dilate, with subsequent development of a localized emphysema. The disease begins in the upper lobes of the lungs but may progress to the lower lobes.

Clinical Manifestations

The first signs are a chronic cough and sputum production, similar to the signs encountered in chronic bronchitis. As the disease progresses, the patient develops dyspnea and coughs up large amounts of sputum with varying amounts of black fluid (melanoptysis), particularly if the individual is a smoker. Eventually, cor pulmonale and respiratory failure result. The diagnosis may first be made based on chest x-ray findings and a history of exposure.

Medical Management

Preventing this disease is key because there is no effective treatment. Instead, treatment focuses on early diagnosis and management of complications. (See Chap. 24 for discussion of emphysema.)

Nursing Management

TEACHING ABOUT PREVENTION

The occupational health nurse serves as an employee advocate, making every effort to promote measures to reduce the exposure of workers to industrial products. Laws require that the work environment be ventilated properly to remove any noxious agent. Dust control can prevent many of the pneumoconioses. Dust control includes ventilation, spraying an area with water to control dust, and effective and frequent floor cleaning. Air samples need to be monitored. Toxic substances should be enclosed and placed in restricted areas. Workers must wear or use protective devices (facemasks, hoods, industrial respirators) to provide a safe air supply when a toxic element is present. Employees who are at risk should be carefully screened and followed. There is a risk of developing serious smoking-related illness (cancer) in industries in which there are unsafe levels of certain gases, dusts, fumes, fluids, and other toxic substances. Additionally, there is the potential for second-hand exposure. Asbestos and toxic dusts and substances may be transferred to others through the handling of clothing or shoes that have been exposed. Ongoing educational programs should be designed to teach workers to take responsibility for their own health and to stop smoking and receive an influenza vaccination.

The Right to Know law stipulates that employees must be informed about all hazardous and toxic substances in the workplace. Specifically, they must be educated about any hazardous or toxic substances they work with, what effects these substances can have on their health, and the measures they can take to protect themselves. The responsibility for implementing these controls inevitably falls on the federal or state government.

Chest Tumors

Tumors of the lung may be benign or malignant. A malignant chest tumor can be primary, arising within the lung, chest wall, or mediastinum, or it can be a metastasis from a primary tumor site elsewhere in the body. Metastatic lung tumors occur fre-

quently because the bloodstream transports cancer cells from primary cancers elsewhere in the body to the lungs.

LUNG CANCER (BRONCHOGENIC CARCINOMA)

Lung cancer is the number-one cancer killer among men and women in the United States, accounting for 31% of cancer deaths in men and 25% in women (American Cancer Society, 2002; Greenlee et al., 2001). For men, the incidence of lung cancer has remained relatively constant, but in women it continues to rise. Lung cancer affects primarily those in the sixth or seventh decade of life; less than 5% of patients are under the age of 40. In approximately 70% of lung cancer patients, the disease has spread to regional lymphatics and other sites by the time of diagnosis. As a result, the long-term survival rate for lung cancer patients is low. Evidence indicates that carcinoma tends to arise at sites of previous scarring (TB, fibrosis) in the lung. More than 85% of lung cancers are caused by the inhalation of carcinogenic chemicals, most commonly cigarette smoke (Schottenfeld, 2000).

Pathophysiology

Lung cancers arise from a single transformed epithelial cell in the tracheobronchial airways. A carcinogen (cigarette smoke, radon gas, other occupational and environmental agents) binds to a cell's DNA and damages it. This damage results in cellular changes, abnormal cell growth, and eventually a malignant cell. As the damaged DNA is passed on to daughter cells, the DNA undergoes further changes and becomes unstable. With the accumulation of genetic changes, the pulmonary epithelium undergoes malignant transformation from normal epithelium to eventual invasive carcinoma.

Squamous cell carcinoma is more centrally located and arises more commonly in the segmental and subsegmental bronchi in response to repetitive carcinogenic exposures. Adenocarcinoma is the most prevalent carcinoma of the lung for both men and women; it presents more peripherally as peripheral masses or nodules and often metastasizes. Large cell carcinoma (also called undifferentiated carcinoma) is a fast-growing tumor that tends to arise peripherally. Bronchioalveolar cell cancer arises from the terminal bronchus and alveoli and is usually slower growing as compared to other bronchogenic carcinomas. Lastly, small cell carcinomas arise primarily as a proximal lesion or lesions but may arise in any part of the tracheobronchial tree.

Classification and Staging

Non-small cell carcinoma represents 70% to 75% of tumors; small cell carcinoma represents 15% to 20% of tumors. For non-small cell carcinoma, the cell types include squamous cell carcinoma (30%), large cell carcinoma (10% to 16%), and adenocarcinoma (31% to 34%), including bronchioalveolar carcinoma (3% to 4%). Most small cell carcinomas arise in the major bronchi and spread by infiltration along the bronchial wall. Small cell cancers account for 20% to 25% of all bronchogenic cancers (Matthay, Tanoue & Carter, 2000).

In addition to cell type, lung cancers also are staged. The stage of the tumor refers to the size of the tumor, its location, whether lymph nodes are involved, and whether the cancer has spread (American Joint Committee on Cancer, 2002). Non-small cell lung cancer is staged as I to IV. Stage I is the earliest stage with the highest cure rates, while stage IV designates metastatic spread.

Small cell lung cancers are classified as limited or extensive. Diagnostic tools and further information on staging are described in Chapter 16.

Risk Factors

Various factors have been associated with the development of lung cancer, including tobacco smoke, second-hand (passive) smoke, environmental and occupational exposures, gender, genetics, and dietary deficits. Other factors that have been associated with lung cancer include genetic predisposition and other underlying respiratory diseases, such as COPD and TB.

TOBACCO SMOKE

Tobacco use is responsible for more than one of every six deaths in the United States from pulmonary and cardiovascular diseases. Smoking is the most important single preventable cause of death and disease in this country. More than 85% of lung cancers are attributable to inhalation of carcinogenic chemicals, such as cigarette smoke (American Cancer Society, 2002). Lung cancer is 10 times more common in cigarette smokers than nonsmokers. Risk is determined by the pack-year history (number of packs of cigarettes used each day, multiplied by the number of years smoked), the age of initiation of smoking, the depth of inhalation, and the tar and nicotine levels in the cigarettes smoked. The younger a person is when he or she starts smoking, the greater the risk of developing lung cancer. The risk of lung cancer decreases as the duration of smoking cessation increases.

SECOND-HAND SMOKE

Passive smoking has been identified as a possible cause of lung cancer in nonsmokers. In other words, people who are involuntarily exposed to tobacco smoke in a closed environment (home, car, building) are at increased risk for developing lung cancer as compared to unexposed nonsmokers. An average lifetime passive smoke exposure to a smoking spouse or partner increases a nonsmoker's risk of lung cancer by about 35% compared to the risk of 100% for a lifetime of active smoking (Matthay, Tanoue & Carter, 2000).

ENVIRONMENTAL AND OCCUPATIONAL EXPOSURE

Various carcinogens have been identified in the atmosphere, including motor vehicle emissions and pollutants from refineries and manufacturing plants. Evidence suggests that the incidence of lung cancer is greater in urban areas as a result of the buildup of pollutants and motor vehicle emissions.

Radon is a colorless, odorless gas found in soil and rocks. For many years it has been associated with uranium mines, but it is now known to seep into homes through ground rock. High levels of radon have been associated with the development of lung cancer, especially when combined with cigarette smoking. Homeowners are advised to have radon levels checked in their houses and to arrange for special venting if the levels are high.

Chronic exposure to industrial carcinogens, such as arsenic, asbestos, mustard gas, chromates, coke oven fumes, nickel, oil, and radiation, has been associated with the development of lung cancer. Laws have been passed to control exposure to such elements in the workplace.

GENETICS

Some familial predisposition to lung cancer seems apparent, because the incidence of lung cancer in close relatives of patients with lung cancer appears to be two to three times that of the general population regardless of smoking status.

DIETARY FACTORS

Prior research has demonstrated that smokers who eat a diet low in fruits and vegetables have an increased risk of developing lung cancer (Bast, Kufe, Pollock et al., 2000). The actual active agents in a diet rich in fruits and vegetables have yet to be determined. It has been hypothesized that carotenoids, particularly carotene or vitamin A, may be important. Several ongoing trials may help to determine if carotene supplementation has anticancer properties. Other nutrients, including vitamin E, selenium, vitamin C, fat, and retinoids, are also being evaluated regarding their protective role against lung cancer (Bast, Kufe, Pollock et al., 2000).

Clinical Manifestations

Often, lung cancer develops insidiously and is asymptomatic until late in its course. The signs and symptoms depend on the location and size of the tumor, the degree of obstruction, and the existence of metastases to regional or distant sites.

The most frequent symptom of lung cancer is cough or change in a chronic cough. People frequently ignore this symptom and attribute it to smoking or a respiratory infection. The cough starts as a dry, persistent cough, without sputum production. When obstruction of airways occurs, the cough may become productive due to infection.

 NURSING ALERT A cough that changes in character should arouse suspicion of lung cancer.

Wheezing is noted (occurs when a bronchus becomes partially obstructed by the tumor) in about 20% of patients with lung cancer. Patients also may report dyspnea. Hemoptysis or blood-tinged sputum may be expectorated. In some patients, a recurring fever occurs as an early symptom in response to a persistent infection in an area of pneumonitis distal to the tumor. In fact, cancer of the lung should be suspected in people with repeated unresolved upper respiratory tract infections. Chest or shoulder pain may indicate chest wall or pleural involvement by a tumor. Pain also is a late manifestation and may be related to metastasis to the bone.

If the tumor spreads to adjacent structures and regional lymph nodes, the patient may present with chest pain and tightness, hoarseness (involving the recurrent laryngeal nerve), dysphagia, head and neck edema, and symptoms of pleural or pericardial effusion. The most common sites of metastases are lymph nodes, bone, brain, contralateral lung, adrenal glands, and liver. Nonspecific symptoms of weakness, anorexia, and weight loss also may be diagnostic.

Assessment and Diagnostic Findings

If pulmonary symptoms occur in a heavy smoker, cancer of the lung is suspected. A chest x-ray is performed to search for pulmonary density, a solitary peripheral nodule (coin lesion), atelectasis, and infection. CT scans of the chest are used to identify small nodules not visualized on the chest x-ray and also to examine serially areas of the thoracic cage not clearly visible on the chest x-ray.

Sputum cytology is rarely used to make a diagnosis of lung cancer; however, fiberoptic bronchoscopy is more commonly used and provides a detailed study of the tracheobronchial tree and allows for brushings, washings, and biopsies of suspicious areas. For peripheral lesions not amenable to bronchoscopic biopsy, a transthoracic **fine-needle aspiration** may be performed under CT or fluoroscopic guidance to aspirate cells from a suspicious area. In some circumstances, an endoscopy with esophageal ultrasound (EUS) may be used to obtain a transesophageal biopsy of enlarged subcarinal lymph nodes that are not easily accessible by other means.

A variety of scans may be used to assess for metastasis of the cancer. These may include bone scans, abdominal scans, positron emission tomography (PET) scans, or liver ultrasound or scans. CT of the brain, magnetic resonance imaging (MRI), and other neurologic diagnostic procedures are used to detect central nervous system metastases. Mediastinoscopy or mediastinotomy may be used to obtain biopsy samples from lymph nodes in the mediastinum.

If surgery is a potential treatment, the patient is evaluated to determine whether the tumor is resectable and whether the physiologic impairment resulting from such surgery can be tolerated. Pulmonary function tests, arterial blood gas analysis, ventilation–perfusion scans, and exercise testing may all be used as part of the preoperative assessment (Knippel, 2001).

Medical Management

The objective of management is to provide a cure, if possible. Treatment depends on the cell type, the stage of the disease, and the physiologic status (particularly cardiac and pulmonary status) of the patient. In general, treatment may involve surgery, radiation therapy, or chemotherapy—or a combination of these. Newer and more specific therapies to modulate the immune system (gene therapy, therapy with defined tumor antigens) are under study and show promise in treating lung cancer.

SURGICAL MANAGEMENT

Surgical resection is the preferred method of treating patients with localized non-small cell tumors, no evidence of metastatic spread, and adequate cardiopulmonary function. If the patient's cardiovascular status, pulmonary function, and functional status are satisfactory, surgery is generally well tolerated. Coronary artery disease, pulmonary insufficiency, and other comorbidities, however, may contraindicate surgical intervention. The cure rate of surgical resection depends on the type and stage of the cancer. Surgery is primarily used for non-small cell carcinomas because small cell cancer of the lung grows rapidly and metastasizes early and extensively. Unfortunately, in many patients with bronchogenic cancer, the lesion is inoperable at the time of diagnosis.

Several different types of lung resections may be performed (Chart 23-10). The most common surgical procedure for a small, apparently curable tumor of the lung is lobectomy (removal of a lobe of the lung). In some cases, an entire lung may be removed (pneumonectomy) (see Chap. 25 for further details).

RADIATION THERAPY

Radiation therapy may cure a small percentage of patients. It is useful in controlling neoplasms that cannot be surgically resected but are responsive to radiation. Radiation also may be used to reduce the size of a tumor, to make an inoperable tumor operable, or to relieve the pressure of the tumor on vital structures. It can control symptoms of spinal cord metastasis and superior vena caval compression. Also, prophylactic brain irradiation is used in certain patients to treat microscopic metastases to the brain. Radiation may help relieve cough, chest pain, dyspnea, hemoptysis,

---

> ### *Chart 23-10* Types of Lung Resections
>
> - Lobectomy: a single lobe of lung is removed
> - Bilobectomy: two lobes of the lung are removed
> - Sleeve resection: cancerous lobe(s) is removed and a segment of the main bronchus is resected
> - Pneumonectomy: removal of entire lung
> - Segmentectomy: a segment of the lung is removed*
> - Wedge resection: removal of a small, pie-shaped area of the segment*
> - Chest wall resection with removal of cancerous lung tissue: for cancers that have invaded the chest wall
>
> ———————
> *Not recommended as curative resection for lung cancer.

---

and bone and liver pain. Relief of symptoms may last from a few weeks to many months and is important in improving the quality of the remaining period of life.

Radiation therapy usually is toxic to normal tissue within the radiation field, and this may lead to complications such as esophagitis, pneumonitis, and radiation lung fibrosis. These may impair ventilatory and diffusion capacity and significantly reduce pulmonary reserve. The patient's nutritional status, psychological outlook, fatigue level, and signs of anemia and infection are monitored throughout the treatment. See Chapter 16 for management of the patient receiving radiation therapy.

CHEMOTHERAPY

Chemotherapy is used to alter tumor growth patterns, to treat patients with distant metastases or small cell cancer of the lung, and as an adjunct to surgery or radiation therapy. Combinations of two or more medications may be more beneficial than single-dose regimens. A large number of medications are active against lung cancer. A variety of chemotherapeutic agents are used, including alkylating agents (ifosfamide), platinum analogues (cisplatin and carboplatin), taxanes (paclitaxel, docetaxel), vinca alkaloids (vinblastine and vindesine), doxorubicin, gemcitabine, vinorelbine, irinotecan (CPT-11), and etoposide (VP-16). The choice of agent depends on the growth of the tumor cell and the specific phase of the cell cycle that the medication affects. Numerous combinations of chemotherapy are undergoing investigation to identify the optimal regimen to treat differing types of lung cancer.

Chemotherapy may provide relief, especially of pain, but it does not usually cure the disease, nor does it often prolong life to any great degree. Chemotherapy is also accompanied by side effects. It is valuable in reducing pressure symptoms of lung cancer and in treating brain, spinal cord, and pericardial metastasis. See Chapter 16 for a discussion of chemotherapy for the patient with cancer.

PALLIATIVE THERAPY

Palliative therapy may include radiation therapy to shrink the tumor to provide pain relief, a variety of bronchoscopic interventions to open a narrowed bronchus or airway, and pain management and other comfort measures. Evaluation and referral for hospice care are important in planning for comfortable and dignified end-of-life care for the patient and family.

Treatment-Related Complications

A variety of complications may occur as a result of lung cancer treatments. Radiation therapy may result in diminished cardiopulmonary function and other complications, such as pulmonary fibrosis, pericarditis, myelitis, and cor pulmonale. Chemotherapy, particularly in combination with radiation therapy, can cause pneumonitis. Pulmonary toxicity is a potential side effect of chemotherapy. Surgical resection may result in respiratory failure, particularly when the cardiopulmonary system is compromised before surgery. Surgical complications and prolonged mechanical ventilation are potential outcomes.

Nursing Management

Nursing care of the patient with lung cancer is similar to that of other patients with cancer (see Chap. 16) and addresses the physiologic and psychological needs of the patient. The physiologic problems are primarily due to the respiratory manifestations of the disease. Nursing care includes strategies to ensure relief of pain and discomfort and to prevent complications.

MANAGING SYMPTOMS

The nurse instructs the patient and family about the potential side effects of the specific treatment and strategies to manage them. Strategies for managing such symptoms as dyspnea, fatigue, nausea and vomiting, and anorexia will assist the patient and family to cope with the therapeutic measures.

RELIEVING BREATHING PROBLEMS

Airway clearance techniques are key to maintaining airway patency through the removal of excess secretions. This may be accomplished through deep-breathing exercises, chest physiotherapy, directed cough, suctioning, and in some instances bronchoscopy. Bronchodilator medications may be prescribed to promote bronchial dilation. As the tumor enlarges or spreads, it may compress a bronchus or involve a large area of lung tissue, resulting in an impaired breathing pattern and poor gas exchange. At some stage of the disease, supplemental oxygen will probably be necessary.

Nursing measures focus on decreasing dyspnea by encouraging the patient to assume positions that promote lung expansion, breathing exercises for lung expansion and relaxation, and educating the patient on energy conservation and airway clearance techniques (Connolly & O'Neill, 1999). Many of the techniques used in pulmonary rehabilitation can be applied to the lung cancer patient. Depending on the severity of disease and the patient's wishes, a referral to a pulmonary rehabilitation program may be helpful in managing respiratory symptoms.

REDUCING FATIGUE

Fatigue is a devastating symptom that affects quality of life in the cancer patient. It is commonly experienced by the lung cancer patient and may be related to the disease itself, the cancer treatment and complications (eg, anemia), sleep disturbances, pain and discomfort, hypoxemia, poor nutrition, or the psychological ramifications of the disease (eg, anxiety, depression). The nurse is pivotal in thoroughly assessing the patient's level of fatigue, identifying potentially treatable causes, and validating with the patient that fatigue is indeed an important symptom. Educating the patient in energy conservation techniques or referring the patient to a physical therapy, occupational therapy, or pulmonary rehabilitation program may be helpful. In addition, guided exercise has been recently identified as a potential intervention for treating fatigue in cancer patients. This is an important area for research because few studies have been conducted, and only in select populations of cancer patients.

PROVIDING PSYCHOLOGICAL SUPPORT

Another important part of the nursing care of the patient with lung cancer is psychological support and identification of potential resources for the patient and family. Often, the nurse must help the patient and family deal with the poor prognosis and relatively rapid progression of this disease. The nurse must help the patient and family with informed decision making regarding the possible treatment options, methods to maintain the patient's quality of life during the course of this disease, and end-of-life treatment options.

TUMORS OF THE MEDIASTINUM

Tumors of the mediastinum include neurogenic tumors, tumors of the thymus, lymphomas, germ cell, cysts, and mesenchymal tumors. These tumors may be malignant or benign. These tumors are usually described in relation to location: anterior, middle, or posterior masses or tumors.

Clinical Manifestations

Nearly all the symptoms of mediastinal tumors result from the pressure of the mass against important intrathoracic organs. Symptoms may include cough, wheezing, dyspnea, anterior chest or neck pain, bulging of the chest wall, heart palpitations, angina, other circulatory disturbances, central cyanosis, superior vena caval syndrome (ie, swelling of the face, neck, and upper extremities), marked distention of the veins of the neck and the chest wall (evidence of the obstruction of large veins of the mediastinum by extravascular compression or intravascular invasion), and dysphagia and weight loss from pressure or invasion into the esophagus.

Assessment and Diagnostic Findings

Chest x-rays are the major method used initially to diagnose mediastinal tumors and cysts. CT scans are the gold standard for assessment of the mediastinum and surrounding structures. MRI may be used in some circumstances, as well as PET scans.

Medical Management

If the tumor is malignant and has infiltrated surrounding tissue, radiation therapy and/or chemotherapy are the therapeutic modalities used when complete surgical removal (discussed below) is not feasible.

SURGICAL MANAGEMENT

Many mediastinal tumors are benign and operable. The location of the tumor (anterior, middle, or posterior compartments) in the mediastinum dictates the type of incision. The common incision used is a median sternotomy; however, a thoracotomy may be used, depending on the location of the tumor. Additional approaches may include a bilateral anterior thoracotomy (clamshell incision) or video-assisted thoracoscopic surgery (see Chap. 25). The care is the same as for any patient undergoing thoracic surgery. The major complications include hemorrhage, injury to the phrenic or recurrent laryngeal nerve, and infection.

Chest Trauma

Approximately 60% of all multisystem trauma victims have some type of chest or thoracic trauma (Owens, Chaudry, Eggerstedt & Smith, 2000). Chest trauma is classified as either blunt or penetrating. Blunt chest trauma results from sudden compression or positive pressure inflicted to the chest wall. Motor vehicle crashes (trauma due to steering wheel, seat belt), falls, and bicycle crashes (trauma due to handlebars) are the most common causes of blunt chest trauma. Penetrating trauma occurs when a foreign object penetrates the chest wall. The most common causes of penetrating chest trauma include gunshot wounds and stabbings.

BLUNT TRAUMA

Although blunt chest trauma is more common, it is often difficult to identify the extent of the damage because the symptoms may be generalized and vague. In addition, patients may not seek immediate medical attention, which may complicate the problem.

Pathophysiology

Injuries to the chest are often life-threatening and result in one or more of the following pathologic mechanisms:

- Hypoxemia from disruption of the airway; injury to the lung parenchyma, rib cage, and respiratory musculature; massive hemorrhage; collapsed lung; and pneumothorax
- Hypovolemia from massive fluid loss from the great vessels, cardiac rupture, or hemothorax
- Cardiac failure from cardiac tamponade, cardiac contusion, or increased intrathoracic pressure

These mechanisms frequently result in impaired ventilation and perfusion leading to ARF, hypovolemic shock, and death.

Assessment and Diagnostic Findings

Time is critical in treating chest trauma. Therefore, it is essential to assess the patient immediately to determine the following:

- When the injury occurred
- Mechanism of injury
- Level of responsiveness
- Specific injuries
- Estimated blood loss
- Recent drug or alcohol use
- Prehospital treatment

The initial assessment of thoracic injuries includes assessment of the patient for airway obstruction, tension pneumothorax, open pneumothorax, massive hemothorax, flail chest, and cardiac tamponade. These injuries are life-threatening and need immediate treatment. Secondary assessment would include simple pneumothorax, hemothorax, pulmonary contusion, traumatic aortic rupture, tracheobronchial disruption, esophageal perforation, traumatic diaphragmatic injury, and penetrating wounds to the mediastinum (Owens, Chaudry, Eggerstedt & Smith, 2000). Although listed as secondary, these injuries may be life-threatening as well depending upon the circumstances.

The physical examination includes inspection of the airway, thorax, neck veins, and breathing difficulty. Specifics include assessing the rate and depth of breathing for abnormalities, such as stridor, cyanosis, nasal flaring, use of accessory muscles, drooling, and overt trauma to the face, mouth, or neck. The chest should be assessed for symmetric movement, symmetry of breath sounds, open chest wounds, entrance or exit wounds, impaled objects, tracheal shift, distended neck veins, subcutaneous emphysema, and paradoxical chest wall motion. In addition, the chest wall should be assessed for bruising, petechiae, lacerations, and burns. The vital signs and skin color are assessed for signs of shock. The thorax is palpated for tenderness and crepitus; the position of the trachea is also assessed.

The initial diagnostic workup includes a chest x-ray, CT scan, complete blood count, clotting studies, type and cross-match, electrolytes, oxygen saturation, arterial blood gas analysis, and ECG. The patient is completely undressed to avoid missing additional injuries that can complicate care. Many patients with injuries involving the chest have associated head and abdominal injuries that require attention. Ongoing assessment is essential to monitor the patient's response to treatment and to detect early signs of clinical deterioration.

Medical Management

The goals of treatment are to evaluate the patient's condition and to initiate aggressive resuscitation. An airway is immediately established with oxygen support and, in some cases, intubation and ventilatory support. Re-establishing fluid volume and negative intrapleural pressure and draining intrapleural fluid and blood are essential.

The potential for massive blood loss and exsanguination with blunt or penetrating chest injuries is high because of injury to the great blood vessels. Many patients die at the scene or are in shock by the time help arrives. Agitation and irrational and combative behavior are signs of decreased oxygen delivery to the cerebral cortex. Strategies to restore and maintain cardiopulmonary function include ensuring an adequate airway and ventilation, stabilizing and re-establishing chest wall integrity, occluding any opening into the chest (open pneumothorax), and draining or removing any air or fluid from the thorax to relieve pneumothorax, hemothorax, or cardiac tamponade. Hypovolemia and low cardiac output must be corrected. Many of these treatment efforts, along with the control of hemorrhage, are usually carried out simultaneously at the scene of the injury or in the emergency department. Depending on the success of efforts to control the hemorrhage in the emergency department, the patient may be taken immediately to the operating room. Principles of management are essentially those pertaining to care of the postoperative thoracic patient (see Chap. 25).

Sternal and Rib Fractures

Sternal fractures are most common in motor vehicle crashes with a direct blow to the sternum via the steering wheel and are most common in women, patients over age 50, and those using shoulder restraints (Owens, Chaudry, Eggerstedt & Smith, 2000).

Rib fractures are the most common type of chest trauma, occurring in more than 60% of patients admitted with blunt chest injury. Most rib fractures are benign and are treated conservatively. Fractures of the first three ribs are rare but can result in a high mortality rate because they are associated with laceration of the subclavian artery or vein. The fifth through ninth ribs are the most common sites of fractures. Fractures of the lower ribs are associated with injury to the spleen and liver, which may be lacerated by fragmented sections of the rib.

CLINICAL MANIFESTATIONS

The patient with sternal fractures has anterior chest pain, overlying tenderness, ecchymosis, crepitus, swelling, and the potential of a chest wall deformity. For the patient with rib fractures, clinical manifestations are similar: severe pain, point tenderness, and muscle spasm over the area of the fracture, which is aggravated by coughing, deep breathing, and movement. The area around the fracture may be bruised. To reduce the pain, the patient splints the chest by breathing in a shallow manner and avoids sighs, deep breaths, coughing, and movement. This reluctance to move or breathe deeply results in diminished ventilation, collapse of unaerated alveoli (atelectasis), pneumonitis, and hypoxemia. Respiratory insufficiency and failure can be the outcomes of such a cycle.

ASSESSMENT AND DIAGNOSTIC FINDINGS

The patient with a sternal fracture must be closely evaluated for underlying cardiac injuries. A crackling, grating sound in the thorax (subcutaneous crepitus) may be detected with auscultation. The diagnostic workup may include a chest x-ray, rib films of a specific area, ECG, continuous pulse oximetry, and arterial blood gas analysis.

MEDICAL MANAGEMENT

Medical management of the patient with a sternal fracture is directed toward controlling pain, avoiding excessive activity, and treating any associated injuries. Surgical fixation is rarely necessary unless fragments are grossly displaced and pose a potential for further injury.

The goals of treatment for rib fractures are to control pain and to detect and treat the injury. Sedation is used to relieve pain and to allow deep breathing and coughing. Care must be taken to avoid oversedation and suppression of the respiratory drive. Alternative strategies to relieve pain include an intercostal nerve block and ice over the fracture site; a chest binder may decrease pain on movement. Usually the pain abates in 5 to 7 days, and discomfort can be controlled with epidural analgesia, patient-controlled analgesia, or nonopioid analgesia. Most rib fractures heal in 3 to 6 weeks. The patient is monitored closely for signs and symptoms of associated injuries.

Flail Chest

Flail chest is frequently a complication of blunt chest trauma from a steering wheel injury. It usually occurs when three or more adjacent ribs (multiple contiguous ribs) are fractured at two or more sites, resulting in free-floating rib segments. It may also re-

sult as a combination fracture of ribs and costal cartilages or sternum (Owens, Chaudry, Eggerstedt & Smith, 2000). As a result, the chest wall loses stability and there is subsequent respiratory impairment and usually severe respiratory distress.

PATHOPHYSIOLOGY

During inspiration, as the chest expands, the detached part of the rib segment (flail segment) moves in a paradoxical manner (pendelluft movement) in that it is pulled inward during inspiration, reducing the amount of air that can be drawn into the lungs. On expiration, because the intrathoracic pressure exceeds atmospheric pressure, the flail segment bulges outward, impairing the patient's ability to exhale. The mediastinum then shifts back to the affected side (Fig. 23-8). This paradoxical action results in increased dead space, a reduction in alveolar ventilation, and decreased compliance. Retained airway secretions and atelectasis frequently accompany flail chest. The patient has hypoxemia, and if gas exchange is greatly compromised, respiratory acidosis develops as a result of CO_2 retention. Hypotension, inadequate tissue perfusion, and metabolic acidosis often follow as the paradoxical motion of the mediastinum decreases cardiac output.

MEDICAL MANAGEMENT

As with rib fracture, treatment of flail chest is usually supportive. Management includes providing ventilatory support, clearing secretions from the lungs, and controlling pain. The specific management depends on the degree of respiratory dysfunction. If only a small segment of the chest is involved, the objectives are to clear the airway through positioning, coughing, deep breathing, and suctioning to aid in the expansion of the lung, and to relieve pain by intercostal nerve blocks, high thoracic epidural blocks, or cautious use of intravenous opioids.

For mild to moderate flail chest injuries, the underlying pulmonary contusion is treated by monitoring fluid intake and appropriate fluid replacement, while at the same time relieving chest pain. Pulmonary physiotherapy focusing on lung volume expansion and secretion management techniques are performed. The patient is closely monitored for further respiratory compromise.

When a severe flail chest injury is encountered, endotracheal intubation and mechanical ventilation are required to provide internal pneumatic stabilization of the flail chest and to correct abnormalities in gas exchange. This helps to treat the underlying

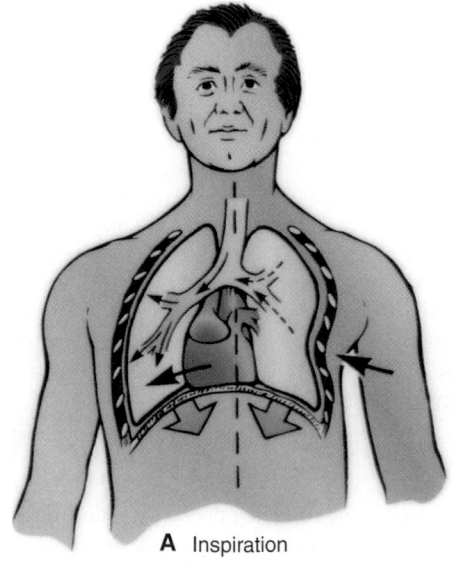
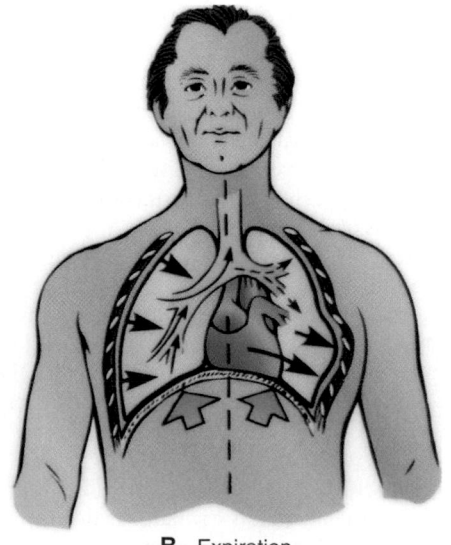

FIGURE 23-8 Flail chest is caused by a free-floating segment of rib cage resulting from multiple rib fractures. (**A**) Paradoxical movement on inspiration occurs when the flail rib segment is sucked inward and the mediastinal structures shift to the unaffected side. The amount of air drawn into the affected lung is reduced. (**B**) On expiration, the flail segment bulges outward and the mediastinal structures shift back to the affected side.

A Inspiration

B Expiration

pulmonary contusion, serves to stabilize the thoracic cage to allow the fractures to heal, and improves alveolar ventilation and intrathoracic volume by decreasing the work of breathing. This treatment modality requires endotracheal intubation and ventilator support. Differing modes of ventilation are used depending on the patient's underlying disease and specific needs.

In rare circumstances, surgery may be required to more quickly stabilize the flail segment. This may be used in the patient who is difficult to ventilate or the high-risk patient with underlying lung disease who may be difficult to wean from mechanical ventilation.

Regardless of the type of treatment, the patient is carefully monitored by serial chest x-rays, arterial blood gas analysis, pulse oximetry, and bedside pulmonary function monitoring. Pain management is key to successful treatment. Patient-controlled analgesia, intercostal nerve blocks, epidural analgesia, and intrapleural administration of opioids may be used to control thoracic pain.

Pulmonary Contusion

Pulmonary contusion is observed in about 20% of adult patients with multiple traumatic injuries and in a higher percentage of children due to increased compliance of the chest wall. It is defined as damage to the lung tissues resulting in hemorrhage and localized edema. It is associated with chest trauma when there is rapid compression and decompression to the chest wall (ie, blunt trauma). It may not be evident initially on examination but will develop in the posttraumatic period.

PATHOPHYSIOLOGY
The primary pathologic defect is an abnormal accumulation of fluid in the interstitial and intra-alveolar spaces. It is thought that injury to the lung parenchyma and its capillary network results in a leakage of serum protein and plasma. The leaking serum protein exerts an osmotic pressure that enhances loss of fluid from the capillaries. Blood, edema, and cellular debris (from cellular response to injury) enter the lung and accumulate in the bronchioles and alveolar surface, where they interfere with gas exchange. An increase in pulmonary vascular resistance and pulmonary artery pressure occurs. The patient has hypoxemia and carbon dioxide retention. Occasionally, a contused lung occurs on the other side of the point of body impact; this is called a contrecoup contusion.

CLINICAL MANIFESTATIONS
Pulmonary contusion may be mild, moderate, or severe. The clinical manifestations vary from tachypnea, tachycardia, pleuritic chest pain, hypoxemia, and blood-tinged secretions to more severe tachypnea, tachycardia, crackles, frank bleeding, severe hypoxemia, and respiratory acidosis. Changes in sensorium, including increased agitation or combative irrational behavior, may be signs of hypoxemia.

In addition, the patient with moderate pulmonary contusion has a large amount of mucus, serum, and frank blood in the tracheobronchial tree; the patient often has a constant cough but cannot clear the secretions. A patient with severe pulmonary contusion has the signs and symptoms of ARDS; these may include central cyanosis, agitation, combativeness, and productive cough with frothy, bloody secretions.

ASSESSMENT AND DIAGNOSTIC FINDINGS
The efficiency of gas exchange is determined by pulse oximetry and arterial blood gas measurements. Pulse oximetry is also used to measure oxygen saturation continuously. The chest x-ray may show pulmonary infiltration. The initial chest x-ray may show no changes; in fact, changes may not appear for 1 or 2 days after the injury.

MEDICAL MANAGEMENT
Treatment priorities include maintaining the airway, providing adequate oxygenation, and controlling pain. In mild pulmonary contusion, adequate hydration via intravenous fluids and oral intake is important to mobilize secretions. However, fluid intake must be closely monitored to avoid hypervolemia. Volume expansion techniques, postural drainage, physiotherapy including coughing, and endotracheal suctioning are used to remove the secretions. Pain is managed by intercostal nerve blocks or by opioids via patient-controlled analgesia or other methods. Usually, antimicrobial therapy is administered because the damaged lung is susceptible to infection. Supplemental oxygen is usually given by mask or cannula for 24 to 36 hours.

The patient with moderate pulmonary contusion may require bronchoscopy to remove secretions; intubation and mechanical ventilation with PEEP may also be necessary to maintain the pressure and keep the lungs inflated. Diuretics may be given to reduce edema. A nasogastric tube is inserted to relieve gastrointestinal distention.

The patient with severe contusion may develop respiratory failure and may require aggressive treatment with endotracheal intubation and ventilatory support, diuretics, and fluid restriction. Colloids and crystalloid solutions may be used to treat hypovolemia.

Antimicrobial medications may be prescribed for the treatment of pulmonary infection. This is a common complication of pulmonary contusion (especially pneumonia in the contused segment), because the fluid and blood that extravasates into the alveolar and interstitial spaces serve as an excellent culture medium.

PENETRATING TRAUMA: GUNSHOT AND STAB WOUNDS

Gunshot and stab wounds are the most common types of penetrating chest trauma. They are classified according to their velocity. Stab wounds are generally considered of low velocity because the weapon destroys a small area around the wound. Knives and switchblades cause most stab wounds. The appearance of the external wound may be very deceptive, because pneumothorax, hemothorax, lung contusion, and cardiac tamponade, along with severe and continuing hemorrhage, can occur from any small wound, even one caused by a small-diameter instrument such as an ice pick.

Gunshot wounds to the chest may be classified as of low, medium, or high velocity. The factors that determine the velocity and resulting extent of damage include the distance from which the gun was fired, the caliber of the gun, and construction and size of the bullet. A gunshot wound can produce a variety of pathophysiologic changes. A bullet can cause damage at the site of penetration and along its pathway. It also may ricochet off bony structures and damage the chest organs and great vessels. If the diaphragm is involved in either a gunshot wound or a stab wound, injury to the chest cavity must be considered.

Medical Management

The objective of immediate management is to restore and maintain cardiopulmonary function. After an adequate airway is ensured and ventilation is established, the patient is examined for shock and intrathoracic and intra-abdominal injuries. The patient is undressed completely so that additional injuries will not be missed. There is a high risk for associated intra-abdominal injuries with stab wounds below the level of the fifth anterior intercostal space. Death can result from exsanguinating hemorrhage or intra-abdominal sepsis.

After the status of the peripheral pulses is assessed, a large-bore intravenous line is inserted. The diagnostic workup includes a chest x-ray, chemistry profile, arterial blood gas analysis, pulse oximetry, and ECG. Blood typing and cross-matching are done in case blood transfusion is required. An indwelling catheter is inserted to monitor urinary output. A nasogastric tube is inserted to prevent aspiration, minimize leakage of abdominal contents, and decompress the gastrointestinal tract.

Shock is treated simultaneously with colloid solutions, crystalloids, or blood, as indicated by the patient's condition. Chest x-rays are obtained, and other diagnostic procedures are carried out as dictated by the needs of the patient (eg, CT scans of chest or abdomen, flat plate x-ray of the abdomen, abdominal tap to check for bleeding).

A chest tube is inserted into the pleural space in most patients with penetrating wounds of the chest to achieve rapid and continuing re-expansion of the lungs. The insertion of the chest tube frequently results in a complete evacuation of the blood and air. The chest tube also allows early recognition of continuing intrathoracic bleeding, which would make surgical exploration necessary. If the patient has a penetrating wound of the heart and great vessels, the esophagus, or the tracheobronchial tree, surgical intervention is required.

PNEUMOTHORAX

Pneumothorax occurs when the parietal or visceral pleura is breached and the pleural space is exposed to positive atmospheric pressure. Normally the pressure in the pleural space is negative or subatmospheric compared to atmospheric pressure; this negative pressure is required to maintain lung inflation. When either pleura is breached, air enters the pleural space, and the lung or a portion of it collapses. Types of pneumothorax include simple, traumatic, and tension pneumothorax.

Simple Pneumothorax

A simple, or spontaneous, pneumothorax occurs when air enters the pleural space through a breach of either the parietal or visceral pleura. Most commonly this occurs as air enters the pleural space through the rupture of a bleb or a bronchopleural fistula. A spontaneous pneumothorax may occur in an apparently healthy person in the absence of trauma due to rupture of an air-filled bleb, or blister, on the surface of the lung, allowing air from the airways to enter the pleural cavity. It may be associated with diffuse interstitial lung disease and severe emphysema.

Traumatic Pneumothorax

Traumatic pneumothorax occurs when air escapes from a laceration in the lung itself and enters the pleural space or enters the pleural space through a wound in the chest wall. It can occur with blunt trauma (eg, rib fractures) or penetrating chest trauma. It may also occur from abdominal trauma (eg, stab wounds or gunshot wounds to the abdomen) and from diaphragmatic tears. Traumatic pneumothorax may occur with invasive thoracic procedures (ie, thoracentesis, transbronchial lung biopsy, insertion

of a subclavian line) in which the pleura is inadvertently punctured, or with barotrauma from mechanical ventilation.

Traumatic pneumothorax resulting from major injury to the chest is often accompanied by hemothorax (collection of blood in the pleural space resulting from torn intercostal vessels, lacerations of the great vessels, and lacerations of the lungs). Often both blood and air are found in the chest cavity (hemopneumothorax) after major trauma. Chest surgery can cause what is classified as a traumatic pneumothorax as a result of the entry into the pleural space and the accumulation of air and fluid in the pleural space.

Open pneumothorax is one form of traumatic pneumothorax. It occurs when a wound in the chest wall is large enough to allow air to pass freely in and out of the thoracic cavity with each attempted respiration. Because the rush of air through the hole in the chest wall produces a sucking sound, such injuries are termed sucking chest wounds. In such patients, not only does the lung collapse, but the structures of the mediastinum (heart and great vessels) also shift toward the uninjured side with each inspiration and in the opposite direction with expiration. This is termed mediastinal flutter or swing, and it produces serious circulatory problems.

Clinical Manifestations

The signs and symptoms associated with pneumothorax depend on its size and cause. Pain is usually sudden and may be pleuritic. The patient may have only minimal respiratory distress with slight chest discomfort and tachypnea with a small simple or uncomplicated pneumothorax. If the pneumothorax is large and the lung collapses totally, acute respiratory distress occurs. The patient is anxious, has dyspnea and air hunger, has increased use of the accessory muscles, and may develop central cyanosis from severe hypoxemia. Severe chest pain may occur, accompanied by tachypnea, decreased movement of the affected side of the thorax, a tympanic sound on percussion of the chest wall, and decreased or absent breath sounds and tactile fremitus on the affected side.

Medical Management

Medical management of pneumothorax depends on its cause and severity. The goal of treatment is to evacuate the air or blood from the pleural space. A small chest tube (28 French) is inserted near the second intercostal space; this space is used because it is the thinnest part of the chest wall, minimizes the danger of contacting the thoracic nerve, and leaves a less visible scar. If the patient also has a hemothorax, a large-diameter chest tube (32 French or greater) is inserted, usually in the fourth or fifth intercostal space at the midaxillary line. The tube is directed posteriorly to drain the fluid and air. Once the chest tube or tubes are inserted and suction is applied (usually to 20 mm Hg suction), effective decompression of the pleural cavity (drainage of blood or air) occurs.

If an excessive amount of blood enters the chest tube in a relatively short period, an autotransfusion may be needed. This technique involves taking the patient's own blood that has been drained from the chest, filtering it, and then transfusing it back into the patient's vascular system.

 NURSING ALERT Traumatic open pneumothorax calls for emergency interventions. Stopping the flow of air through the opening in the chest wall is a life-saving measure.

In such an emergency, anything may be used that is large enough to fill the chest wound—a towel, a handkerchief, or the heel of the hand. If conscious, the patient is instructed to inhale and strain against a closed glottis. This action assists in re-expanding the lung and ejecting the air from the thorax. In the hospital, the opening is plugged by sealing it with gauze impregnated with petrolatum. A pressure dressing is applied. Usually, a chest tube connected to water-seal drainage is inserted to permit air and fluid to drain. Antibiotics usually are prescribed to combat infection from contamination.

The severity of open pneumothorax depends on the amount and rate of thoracic bleeding and the amount of air in the pleural space. The pleural cavity can be decompressed by needle aspiration (thoracentesis) or chest tube drainage of the blood or air. The lung is then able to re-expand and resume the function of gas exchange. As a rule of thumb, the chest wall is opened surgically (thoracotomy) when more than 1,500 mL of blood is aspirated initially by thoracentesis (or is the initial chest tube output) or when chest tube output continues at greater than 200 mL/hour. The urgency with which the blood must be removed is determined by the respiratory compromise. An emergency thoracotomy may also be performed in the emergency department if there is suggested cardiovascular injury secondary to chest or penetrating trauma.

Tension Pneumothorax

A **tension pneumothorax** occurs when air is drawn into the pleural space from a lacerated lung or through a small hole in the chest wall. It may be a complication of other types of pneumothorax. In contrast to open pneumothorax, the air that enters the chest cavity with each inspiration is trapped; it cannot be expelled during expiration through the air passages or the hole in the chest wall. In effect, a one-way valve or ball valve mechanism occurs where air enters the pleural space but cannot escape. With each breath, tension (positive pressure) is increased within the affected pleural space. This causes the lung to collapse and the heart, the great vessels, and the trachea to shift toward the unaffected side of the chest (mediastinal shift). Both respiration and circulatory function are compromised because of the increased intrathoracic pressure. The increased intrathoracic pressure decreases venous return to the heart, causing decreased cardiac output and impairment of peripheral circulation. In extreme cases, the pulse may be undetectable—this is known as pulseless electrical activity.

CLINICAL MANIFESTATIONS
The clinical picture is one of air hunger, agitation, increasing hypoxemia, central cyanosis, hypotension, tachycardia, and profuse diaphoresis. A comparison of open and tension pneumothorax is shown in Figure 23-9.

 NURSING ALERT Relief of tension pneumothorax is considered an emergency measure.

MEDICAL MANAGEMENT
If a tension pneumothorax is suspected, the patient should immediately be given a high concentration of supplemental oxygen to treat the hypoxemia, and pulse oximetry should be used to monitor oxygen saturation.

In an emergency situation, gas tension pneumothorax can be decompressed or quickly converted to a simple pneumothorax by inserting a large-bore needle (14-gauge) at the second intercostal

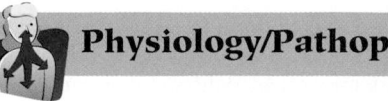 **Physiology/Pathophysiology**

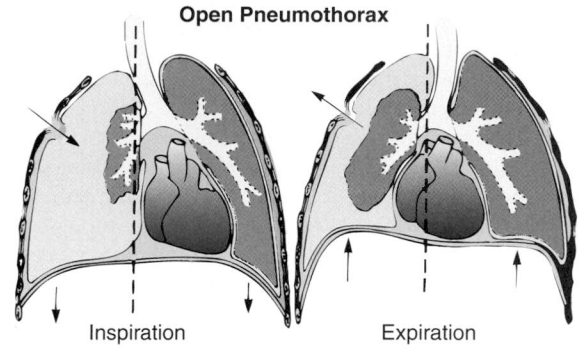

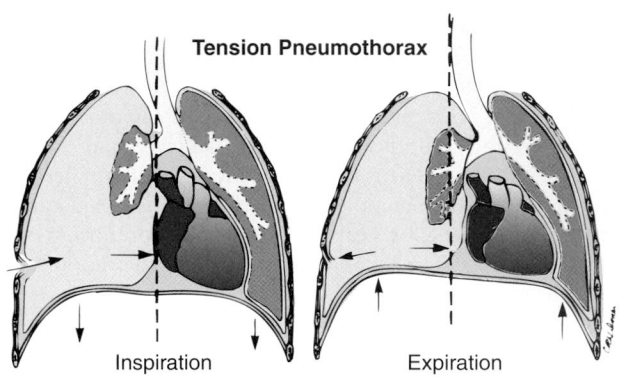

FIGURE 23-9 Open pneumothorax (*top*) and tension pneumothorax (*bottom*). In open pneumothorax, air enters the chest during inspiration and exits during expiration. A slight shift of the affected lung may occur because of a decrease in pressure as air moves out of the chest. In tension pneumothorax, air enters but cannot leave the chest. As the pressure increases, the heart and great vessels are compressed and the mediastinal structures are shifted toward the opposite side of the chest. The trachea is pushed from its normal midline position toward the opposite side of the chest, and the unaffected lung is compressed.

space, midclavicular line on the affected side. This relieves the pressure and vents the positive pressure to the external environment. A chest tube is then inserted and connected to suction to remove the remaining air and fluid, re-establish the negative pressure, and re-expand the lung. If the lung re-expands and air leakage from the lung parenchyma stops, further drainage may be unnecessary. If a prolonged air leak continues despite chest tube drainage to underwater seal, surgery may be necessary to close the leak.

CARDIAC TAMPONADE

Cardiac tamponade is the compression of the heart as a result of fluid within the pericardial sac. It usually is caused by blunt or penetrating trauma to the chest. A penetrating wound of the heart is associated with a high mortality rate. Cardiac tamponade also may follow diagnostic cardiac catheterization, angiographic procedures, and pacemaker insertion, which can produce perforations of the heart and great vessels. Pericardial effusion with fluid compressing the heart also may develop from metastases to the pericardium from malignant tumors of the breast, lung, and mediastinum and may occur with lymphomas and leukemias, renal failure, TB, and high-dose radiation to the chest. Cardiac tamponade is discussed in detail in Chapter 30.

SUBCUTANEOUS EMPHYSEMA

No matter what kind of chest trauma the patient has, when the lung or the air passages are injured, air may enter the tissue planes and pass for some distance under the skin (eg, neck, chest). The tissues give a crackling sensation when palpated, and the subcutaneous air produces an alarming appearance as the face, neck, body, and scrotum become misshapen by subcutaneous air. Fortunately, subcutaneous emphysema is of itself usually not a serious complication. The subcutaneous air is spontaneously absorbed if the underlying air leak is treated or stops spontaneously. In severe cases in which there is widespread subcutaneous emphysema, a tracheostomy is indicated if airway patency is threatened.

Aspiration

Aspiration of stomach contents into the lungs is a serious complication that may cause pneumonia and result in the following clinical picture: tachycardia, dyspnea, central cyanosis, hypertension, hypotension, and finally death. It can occur when the protective airway reflexes are decreased or absent from a variety of factors (Chart 23-11).

> **NURSING ALERT** When a nonfunctioning nasogastric tube allows the gastric contents to accumulate in the stomach, a condition known as silent aspiration may result. Silent aspiration often occurs unobserved and may be more common than suspected. If untreated, massive inhalation of gastric contents develops in a period of several hours.

Pathophysiology

The primary factors responsible for death and complications after aspiration of gastric contents are the volume and character of the aspirated gastric contents. For example, a small, localized aspiration from regurgitation can cause pneumonia and acute respiratory distress; a massive aspiration is usually fatal.

A full stomach contains solid particles of food. If these are aspirated, the problem then becomes one of mechanical blockage of the airways and secondary infection. During periods of fasting, the stomach contains acidic gastric juice, which, if aspirated, may be very destructive to the alveoli and capillaries. Fecal contamination (more likely seen in intestinal obstruction) increases the

Chart 23-11
Risk Factors for Aspiration

Seizure activity
Decreased level of consciousness from trauma, drug or alcohol
    intoxication, excessive sedation, or general anesthesia
Nausea and vomiting in the patient with a decreased level of
    consciousness
Stroke
Swallowing disorders
Cardiac arrest
Silent aspiration

likelihood of death because the endotoxins produced by intestinal organisms may be absorbed systemically, or the thick proteinaceous material found in the intestinal contents may obstruct the airway, leading to atelectasis and secondary bacterial invasion.

Aspiration pneumonitis may develop from aspiration of substances with a pH of less than 2.5 and a volume of gastric aspirate greater than 0.3 mL per kilogram of body weight (20 to 25 mL in adults) (Marik, 2001). Aspiration of gastric contents causes a chemical burn of the tracheobronchial tree and pulmonary parenchyma (Marik, 2001). An inflammatory response occurs. This results in the destruction of alveolar–capillary endothelial cells, with a consequent outpouring of protein-rich fluids into the interstitial and intra-alveolar spaces. As a result, surfactant is lost, which in turn causes the airways to close and the alveoli to collapse. Finally, the impaired exchange of oxygen and carbon dioxide causes respiratory failure.

Aspiration pneumonia develops following inhalation of colonized oropharyngeal material. The pathologic process involves an acute inflammatory response to bacteria and bacterial products. Most commonly, the bacteriologic findings include gram-positive cocci, gram-negative rods, and occasionally anaerobic bacteria (Marik, 2001).

Prevention

Prevention is the primary goal when caring for patients at risk for aspiration.

COMPENSATING FOR ABSENT REFLEXES

Aspiration is likely to occur if the patient cannot adequately coordinate protective glottic, laryngeal, and cough reflexes. This hazard is increased if the patient has a distended abdomen, is in a supine position, has the upper extremities immobilized by intravenous infusions or hand restraints, receives local anesthetics to the oropharyngeal or laryngeal area for diagnostic procedures, has been sedated, or has had long-term intubation.

When vomiting, a person can normally protect the airway by sitting up or turning on the side and coordinating breathing, coughing, gag, and glottic reflexes. If these reflexes are active, an oral airway should not be inserted. If an airway is in place, it should be pulled out the moment the patient gags so as not to stimulate the pharyngeal gag reflex and promote vomiting and aspiration. Suctioning of oral secretions with a catheter should be performed with minimal pharyngeal stimulation.

ASSESSING FEEDING TUBE PLACEMENT

Even when the patient is intubated, aspiration may occur even with a nasogastric tube in place. This aspiration may result in nosocomial pneumonia. Assessment of tube placement is key to prevent aspiration. The best method for determining tube placement is via an x-ray. There are other nonradiologic methods that have been studied. Observation of the aspirate and testing of its pH are the most reliable. Gastric fluid may be grassy green, brown, clear, or colorless. An aspirate from the lungs may be off-white or tan mucus. Pleural fluid is watery and usually straw-colored (Metheny & Titler, 2001). Gastric pH values are typically lower or more acidic that that of the intestinal or respiratory tract. Gastric pH is usually between 1 and 5, while intestinal or respiratory pH is 7 or higher (Metheny & Titler, 2001). There are differences in assessing tube placement with continuous versus intermittent feedings. For intermittent feedings with small-bore tubes, observation of aspirated contents and pH evaluation should be performed. For continuous feedings, the pH method

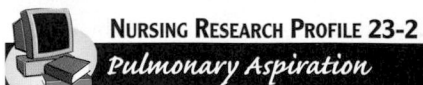

NURSING RESEARCH PROFILE 23-2
Pulmonary Aspiration

Elpern, E. H., Okonek, M. B., Bacon, M., Gerstung, C., & Skrzynski, M. (2000). Effect of the Passy-Muir tracheostomy speaking valve on pulmonary aspiration in adults. *Heart Lung, 29*(4), 287–293.

Purpose
The purpose of this study was to investigate the frequency of aspiration in adults with tracheostomies and to investigate the effect of the Passy-Muir speaking valve on aspiration occurrences.

Study Sample and Design
Fifteen subjects were included in this study. Inclusion criteria were that there was a tracheostomy in place and the patient was scheduled for a videofluoroscopic swallowing examination. During the swallowing examination, six presentations of thin liquids were recorded: three with and three without the Passy-Muir tracheostomy speaking valve applied.

Findings
Seven of the 15 subjects (47%) aspirated material on one or more presentations of the thin liquid. Five subjects aspirated without the valve and two subjects aspirated with and without the valve. No subjects aspirated only when the valve was applied. Aspiration occurred less frequently with the Passy-Muir tracheostomy speaking valve on than with it off.

Nursing Implications
Aspiration is a common problem that can lead to severe pulmonary complications. Potential complications of aspiration include obstruction, inflammation (pneumonitis), and infection (aspiration pneumonia). Nursing assessment and knowledge of risk factors are key in evaluating patients at risk for potential aspiration problems and preventing this complication.

---

is not clinically useful due to the infused formula (Metheny & Titler, 2001).

The patient who is receiving continuous or timed-interval tube feedings must be positioned properly. The patient receiving a continuous infusion is given small volumes under low pressure in an upright position, which helps to prevent aspiration. Patients receiving tube feedings at timed intervals are maintained in an upright position during the feeding and for a minimum of 30 minutes afterward to allow the stomach to empty partially. Tube feedings must be given only when it is certain that the feeding tube is positioned correctly in the stomach. Many patients today receive enteral feeding directly into the duodenum through a small-bore flexible feeding tube or surgically implanted tube. Feedings are given slowly and regulated by a feeding pump. Correct placement is confirmed by chest x-ray.

IDENTIFYING DELAYED STOMACH EMPTYING
A full stomach may cause aspiration because of increased intragastric or extragastric pressure. The following clinical situations cause a delayed emptying time of the stomach and may contribute to aspiration: intestinal obstruction; increased gastric secretions in gastroesophageal reflex disease; increased gastric secretions during anxiety, stress, or pain; or abdominal distention because of ileus, ascites, peritonitis, use of opioids and sedatives, severe illness, or vaginal delivery.

When a feeding tube is present, contents are aspirated, usually every 4 hours, to determine the amount of the last feeding left in the stomach (residual volume). If more than 50 mL is aspirated, there may be a problem with delayed emptying, and the next

feeding should be delayed or the continuous feeding stopped for a period of time.

MANAGING EFFECTS OF PROLONGED INTUBATION
Prolonged endotracheal intubation or tracheostomy can depress the laryngeal and glottic reflexes because of disuse. Patients with prolonged tracheostomies are encouraged to phonate and exercise their laryngeal muscles. For patients who have had long-term intubation or tracheostomies, it may be helpful to have a rehabilitation therapist experienced in speech and swallowing disorders work with the patient to assess the swallowing reflex.

Critical Thinking Exercises

1. Your patient, a 44-year-old unemployed man who lives with his 80-year-old mother, has recently been diagnosed with active TB. He has been started on treatment and given specific instructions about his medications. What strategies would you initiate to be sure that he takes his medications correctly? What strategies would you use to ensure that his mother is not infected? How would your care differ if the patient lived alone or were homeless?

2. You are working on a surgical unit. Your patient is a 67-year-old woman who has had surgery to repair a fractured hip that occurred following a fall associated with heavy alcohol use. She has been a heavy smoker for over 35 years and is reluctant to move in bed because of pain. What are the potential postoperative pulmonary complications? What assessment criteria would you use to assess her respiratory status? What interventions would you implement to prevent pulmonary complications in this patient? What changes, if any, would you implement if she had a history of deep vein thrombosis?

3. Your patient has experienced blunt chest trauma following a motor vehicle crash. A chest tube has been inserted to treat a pneumothorax. The chest drainage system has drained 400 mL of light-red fluid during the first 6 hours following the tube's insertion. The patient is unable to recall how he was injured or what has happened to him over the last 24 hours. The patient is experiencing pain requiring opioids and is asking that the chest tube be removed to enable him to walk to the bathroom. What additional information would you obtain through assessment and what actions would you take? How would you explain to the patient and his family the purpose of the chest tubes? How would you modify your explanation and teaching if he has little understanding of English?

REFERENCES AND SELECTED READINGS
Books
American Cancer Society. (2002). *Cancer facts and figures.* Atlanta: American Cancer Society.

American Joint Committee on Cancer (AJCC). (2002). *Cancer staging manual* (6th ed.). New York: Springer-Verlag.

Ansell, J. E., Hickey, A. D., Kleinschmidt, K. C., Merli, G. J., Tillman, D. J., & Yusen, R. D. (2000). *Advancing the treatment of deep venous thrombosis and pulmonary embolism.* Cincinnati: Sci-Health Communications.

Arroliga, A. C., Matthay, M. A., & Matthay, R. A. (2000). Pulmonary thromboembolism and other pulmonary vascular diseases. In R. George, R. Light, M. Matthay, & R. Matthay (eds.), *Chest medicine: Essentials of pulmonary and critical care medicine* (4th ed., pp 233–261). Philadelphia: Lippincott Williams & Wilkins.

Bartlett, J. G. (1999). *Management of respiratory tract infections* (2d ed). Philadelphia: Lippincott Williams & Wilkins.

Bast, R. C., Kufe, D. W., Pollock, R. E. et al. (eds.) (2000). *Cancer medicine* (5th ed.). Hamilton, Ontario: B. C. Decker, Inc.

Centers for Disease Control and Prevention (2000). *TB elimination: Now is the time.* National Center for HIV, STD and TB Prevention.

Cherniack, N. S., Homma, I., & Altose, M. (1999). *Rehabilitation of the patient with respiratory disease.* New York: McGraw-Hill.

Davis, G. S. (1999). *Medical management of pulmonary diseases.* New York: Marcel Dekker, Inc.

Duffy, S. Q., & Farley, D. E. (1993). *Intermittent positive pressure breathing: Old technologies rarely die* (AHCPR Publication No. 94-0001). Division of Provider Studies Research Note 18, Agency for Health Care Policy and Research, Rockville, MD: Public Health Service.

Farzan, S. (1997). *A concise handbook of respiratory diseases.* Stamford, CT: Appleton & Lange.

Matthay, R. A., Tanoue, L. T., & Carter, D. C. (2000). Lung neoplasms. In R. George, R. Light, M. Matthay, & R. Matthay (eds.), *Chest medicine: essentials of pulmonary and critical care medicine* (4th ed., pp 346–376). Philadelphia: Lippincott Williams & Wilkins.

Niederman, M. S., & Sarosi, G. A. (2000). Respiratory tract infections. In R. George, R. Light, M. Matthay, & R. Matthay (eds.), *Chest medicine: Essentials of pulmonary and critical care medicine* (4th ed., pp 377–429). Philadelphia: Lippincott Williams & Wilkins.

Nield, M. J. (ed.). Committee on Regulating Occupational Exposure to Tuberculosis (2000). *Tuberculosis in the workplace.* Division of Health Promotion and Disease Prevention, National Academy of Sciences, Institute of Medicine.

Owens, M. W., Chaudry, M. S., Eggerstedt, J. M., & Smith, L. M. (2000). Thoracic trauma, surgery and perioperative management. In R. George, R. Light, M. Matthay, & R. Matthay (eds.), *Chest medicine: Essentials of pulmonary and critical care medicine* (4th ed., pp 592–619). Philadelphia: Lippincott Williams & Wilkins.

Respiratory Nursing Society and American Nurses Association. (1994). *Standards and scope of respiratory nursing practice/Joint Standards Task Force for Respiratory Nursing Practice.* Washington, DC: Author.

Schottenfeld, D. (2000). Etiology and epidemiology of lung cancer. In H. I. Pass, J. B. Mitchell, D. H. Johnson, & J. D. Minna (eds). *Lung cancer: Principles and practice* (2d ed., pp 367–388). Philadelphia: Lippincott Williams & Wilkins.

Tanoue, L. T., & Elias, J. A. (1998). Systemic sarcoidosis. In G. L. Baum, J. D. Crapo, B. R. Celli, & J. B. Karlinsky (eds.), *Textbook of pulmonary disease* (pp 407–430). Philadelphia: Lippincott-Raven.

Velmahos, G. C., Kern, J., Chan, L., et al. (2000). *Prevention of venous thromboembolism after injury.* Evidence Report/Technology Assessment No. 22 (Prepared by Southern California Evidence-based Practice Center/RAND under Contract no. 290-97-0001). AHRQ Publication No. 01-E004. Rockville, MD: Agency for Healthcare Research and Quality.

Wilcox, W. (1998). *Public health sourcebook* (vol. 34, p 49). Detroit: Omnigraphics.

Winningham, M. L., & Barton-Burke, M. (2000). *Fatigue in cancer: A multidimensional approach.* Boston: Jones and Bartlett Publishers.

World Health Organization. (2000). *Global tuberculosis control: WHO report.* Geneva, Switzerland: Author.

Journals

Asterisks indicate nursing research articles.
General
American Thoracic Society. (1999). Statement on sarcoidosis. *American Journal of Respiratory and Critical Care Medicine, 160*(2), 736–755.

American Thoracic Society and European Respiratory Society. (2000). Idiopathic pulmonary fibrosis: diagnosis and treatment. International consensus statement. *American Journal of Respiratory and Critical Care Medicine, 161*(2), 646–664.

Bryce, J. C. (1995). Aspiration: causes, consequences, and prevention. *ORL Head and Neck Nursing, 13*(2), 14–19.

Centers for Disease Control and Prevention (1997). Premature deaths, monthly mortality and monthly physician contacts: United States. *MMWR Morbidity and Mortality Weekly Report, 46*(24), 556–561.

Clagett, G. P., Anderson, F. A. Jr., Geerts, W., et al. (1998). Prevention of venous thromboembolism. *Chest, 114*(5), 531S-560S.

Dalen, J. E., Hirsh, J., & Guyatt, G. H. (2001). Sixth ACCP consensus conference on antithrombotic therapy. *Chest, 119*(1), supplement, 1S-370S.

Elpern, E. H. (1997). Pulmonary aspiration in hospitalized adults. *Nutrition in Clinical Practice, 12*(1), 5–13.

*Elpern, E. H., Okonek, M. B., Bacon, M., et al. (2000). Effect of the Passy-Muir tracheostomy speaking valve on pulmonary aspiration in adults. *Heart Lung, 29*(4), 287–293.

Goldhaber, S. Z. (1998). Medical progress: Pulmonary embolism. *New England Journal of Medicine, 339*(2), 93–104.

Lomotan, J. R., George, S. S., & Brandsetter, R. D. (1997). Aspiration pneumonia: Strategies for early recognition and prevention. *Postgraduate Medicine, 102*(2), 225–231.

Marik, P. E. (2001). Aspiration pneumonitis and aspiration pneumonia. *New England Journal of Medicine, 344*(9), 665–671.

Metheny, N. A., & Titler, M. G. (2001). Assessing placement of feeding tubes. *American Journal of Nursing, 101*(5), 36–45.

Seijo, L. M., & Sterman, D. H. (2001). Interventional pulmonology. *New England Journal of Medicine, 344*(10), 740–749.

Taubert, J., & Wright, S. (2000). Malignant pleural effusion: nursing interventions using an indwelling pleural catheter with intermittent drainage. *Nursing Interventions in Oncology, 12,* 2–7.

Acute Respiratory Failure and ARDS
Acute Respiratory Distress Syndrome Network. (2000). Ventilation with lower tidal volumes as compared with traditional tidal volumes for acute lung injury and the acute respiratory distress syndrome. *New England Journal of Medicine, 342*(18), 1301–1308.

Bernard, G. R., Artigas, A., Brigham, K. L., et al. (1994). Report of the American-European consensus conference on acute respiratory distress syndrome: Definitions, mechanisms, relevant outcomes, and clinical trial coordination. *American Journal of Critical Care Medicine, 9*(1), 72–81.

Brower, R. G., Ware, L. B., Berthiaume, Y., & Matthay, M. A. (2001). Treatment of ARDS. *Chest, 120*(4), 1347–1367.

Curley, M. A. (2000). Prone positioning of patients with acute respiratory distress syndrome: a systematic review. *American Journal of Critical Care, 9*(4), 295–296.

Davidson, T. A., Caldwell, E. S., Curtis, J. R., et al. (1999). Reduced quality of life in survivors of acute respiratory distress syndrome compared with critically ill control patients. *Journal of the American Medical Association, 281*(4), 354–360.

Marion, B. S. (2001). A turn for the better: 'Prone Positioning' of patients with ARDS. *American Journal of Nursing, 101*(5), 26–34.

Thompson, B. T., Hayden, D., Matthay, M. A., et al. (2001). Clinicians' approaches to mechanical ventilation in acute lung injury and ARDS. *Chest, 120*(5), 1622–1627.

Ware, L. B., & Matthay, M. A. (2000). The acute respiratory distress syndrome. *New England Journal of Medicine, 342*(18), 1334–1349.

Lung Cancer
Alpha-Tocopherol Beta-Carotene Cancer Prevention Study Group. (1994). The effect of vitamin E and beta-carotene on the incidence of lung cancer and other cancers in male smokers. *New England Journal of Medicine, 330,* 1029–1035.

American Thoracic Society. (2000). Management of malignant pleural effusions. *American Journal of Respiratory and Critical Care Medicine, 162*(5), 1987–2001.

*Brown, J. K., & Radke, K. J. (1998). Nutritional assessment, intervention, and evaluation of weight loss in patients with non-small-cell lung cancer. *Oncology Nursing Forum, 25*(3), 547–554.

*Connolly, M., & O'Neill, J. (1999). Teaching a research-based approach to the management of breathlessness in patients with lung cancer. *European Journal of Cancer Care, 8*(1), 30–36.

Greenlee, R. T., Hill-Harmon, M. B., Murray, T., & Thun, M. (2001). Cancer statistics 2001. *CA: A Cancer Journal for Clinicians, 51*(1), 15–36.

Hennekens, C., Buring, J., & Manson, J. (1996). Lack of effect of long-term supplementations with beta carotene on the incidence of malignant neoplasms and cardiovascular disease. *New England Journal of Medicine, 334*, 1145–1149.

Knippel, S. L. (2001). Surgical therapies for lung carcinomas. *Nursing Clinics of North America, 36*(3), 517–525.

Mountain, C. F. (1997). Revisions in the international system for staging lung cancer. *Chest, 111*(6), 1710–1717.

*Rice, V. H. (1999). Nursing intervention and smoking cessation: a meta-analysis. *Heart Lung, 28*(6), 438–454.

*Sarna, L. P., Brown, J. K., Lillington, L., et al. (2000). Tobacco interventions by oncology nurses in clinical practice. *Cancer, 89*(4), 881–889.

Taubert, J. (2001). Management of malignant pleural effusion. *Nursing Clinics of North America, 36*(4), 665–683.

Yeatman, T. J. (2000). Nutritional support for the surgical oncology patient. *Cancer Control, 7*(6), 563–565.

Pulmonary Infections

American Thoracic Society. (2001). Guidelines for the management of adults with community-acquired pneumonia. *American Journal of Respiratory and Critical Care Medicine, 163*(7), 1730–1754.

American Thoracic Society. (1995). Hospital-acquired pneumonia in adults: Diagnosis, assessment of severity, initial antimicrobial therapy, and preventive strategies. A consensus statement. *American Journal of Critical Care Medicine, 153*(5), 1711–1725.

Bartlett, J. G., Dowell, S. F., Mandell, L. A., File, T. M., Musher, D. M., & Fine, M. J. (2000). Practice guidelines for the management of community-acquired pneumonia in adults. *Clinical Infectious Diseases, 31*(2), 347–382.

*Brooks-Brunn, J. A. (1997). Predictors of postoperative pulmonary complications following abdominal surgery. *Chest, 111*(3), 564–571.

Brooks, J. A. (2001). Postoperative nosocomial pneumonia: nurse-sensitive interventions. *AACN Clinical Issues, 12*(2), 305–323.

Centers for Disease Control and Prevention. (1997). Guidelines for prevention of nosocomial pneumonia. *MMWR Morbidity and Mortality Weekly Report, 46*:RR1, 1–79.

Centers for Disease Control and Prevention. (1998). Influenza and pneumococcal vaccination levels among adults aged >65 years—United States. *MMWR Morbidity and Mortality Weekly Report, 47*, 797–802.

Centers for Disease Control and Prevention. (2000a). Prevention and control of influenza: recommendations of the Advisory Committee on Immunization Practices (ACIP). *MMWR Morbidity and Mortality Weekly Report, 49*(RR03), 1–38.

Centers for Disease Control and Prevention. (2000b). Influenza, pneumococcal, and tetanus toxoid vaccination of adults—United States, 1993–1997. *MMWR Morbidity and Mortality Weekly Report, 49*(SS09), 39–62.

Colice, G. L., Curtis, A., Deslauriers, J., et al. (2000). Medical and surgical treatment of parapneumonic effusions: an evidence-based guideline. *Chest, 18*(4), 1158–1171.

Fine, M. J., Auble, T. E., Yealy, D. M., et al. (1997). A prediction rule to identify low-risk patients with community-acquired pneumonia. *New England Journal of Medicine, 336*(4), 243–250.

Fine, M. J., Smith, M. A., Carson, C. A., et al. (1996). Prognosis and outcomes of patients with community-acquired pneumonia: a meta-analysis. *Journal of the American Medical Association, 75*(2), 134–141.

Goodwin, R. S. (1996). Prevention of aspiration pneumonia: A research-based protocol. *Dimensions of Critical Care Nursing, 15*(2), 58–74.

Gross, T. J., & Hunninghake, G. W. (2001). Idiopathic pulmonary fibrosis. *New England Journal of Medicine, 345*(7), 517–525.

Kenreigh, C. A., & Wagner, L. T. (2000). Treatment of CAP: optimizing formulary decisions. http://www.medscape.com.

Kollef, M. H. (1999). The prevention of ventilator-associated pneumonia. *New England Journal of Medicine, 340*(8), 627–634.

Lynch, J. P. (2000). Treating community-acquired pneumonia. *Journal of Respiratory Diseases, 23*(10), 602–608.

Marston, B. J., Plouffe, J. F., File, T. M., et al. (1997). Incidence of community-acquired pneumonia requiring hospitalizations: Results of a population-based active surveillance study in Ohio. *Archives of Internal Medicine, 157*(15), 1709–1718.

McGeer, A. J., & Low, D. E. (2000). Vancomycin-resistant enterococci. *Seminars in Respiratory Infections, 15*(4), 261–263.

McIntosh, K. (2002). Community-acquired pneumonia in children. *New England Journal of Medicine, 346*(6), 429–437.

Minino, A. M., & Smith, B. L. (2001). Deaths: preliminary data for 2000. *National Vital Statistics Reports, 49*(12), 1–40.

National Center for Health Statistics (2000). *United States Mortality Public Use Data Tape 1998,* Centers for Disease Control and Prevention.

Smith-Sims, K. (2001). Hospital-acquired pneumonia. *American Journal of Nursing, 101*(1), 24AA–24EE.

Tasota, F. J., Fisher, E. M., Coulson, C. F., & Hoffman, L. A. (1998). Protecting ICU patients from nosocomial infections: Practical measures for favorable outcomes. *Critical Care Nurse, 18*(1), 54–67.

Zimmer, J. G., & Hall, W. J. (1997). Nursing home-acquired pneumonia: Avoiding the hospital. *Journal of the American Geriatrics Society, 45*(3), 380–381.

Trauma

Collins, J. (2000). Chest wall trauma. *Journal of Thoracic Imaging, 15*(2), 112–119.

Flynn, M. B., & Bonini, S. (1999) Blunt chest trauma: Case report. *Critical Care Nurse, 19*(5), 68–77.

Karlet, M. C. (1997). Update for nurse anesthetists: Thoracic trauma. *American Association of Nurse Anesthetists Journal, 65*(1), 73–80.

Pape, H. C., Remmers, D., Rice, J., Ebisch, M., Krettek, C., & Tscherne, H. (2000). Appraisal of early evaluation of blunt chest trauma: Development of a standardized scoring system for initial clinical decision making. *Journal of Trauma-Injury Infection & Critical Care, 49*(3), 496–504.

Tuberculosis

American Thoracic Society. (2000). Diagnostic standards and classification of tuberculosis in adults and children. *American Journal of Respiratory and Critical Care Medicine, 161*(4), 1376–1395.

American Thoracic Society and Centers for Disease Control and Prevention. (2000). Targeted tuberculin testing and treatment of latent infection. *American Journal of Respiratory and Critical Care Medicine, 161*(4), S221–S247.

American Thoracic Society and Centers for Disease Control and Prevention. (2001). Fatal and severe liver injuries associated with rifampin and pyrazinamide for latent tuberculosis infection and revisions in American Thoracic Society/CDC Recommendations—United States 2001. *MMWR Morbidity Mortality Weekly Report, 50*(34), 733–735.

Centers for Disease Control and Prevention. (1995). Essential components of a tuberculosis prevention and control program: recommendations of the Advisory Council for the Elimination of Tuberculosis. *MMWR Morbidity and Mortality Weekly Report, 44*(RR-11), 1–16.

Centers for Disease Control and Prevention. (1995). Screening for tuberculosis and tuberculosis infection in high-risk populations: recommendations of the Advisory Council for the Elimination of Tuberculosis. *MMWR Morbidity and Mortality Weekly Report, 44*(RR-11), 18–34.

Centers for Disease Control and Prevention. (1998). Development of new vaccines for tuberculosis. *MMWR Morbidity and Mortality Weekly Report, 47*(RR13), 1–6.

Centers for Disease Control and Prevention. (1998). Tuberculosis morbidity, United States. *MMWR Morbidity and Mortality Weekly Report, 47*(13), 253–257.

Centers for Disease Control and Prevention. (2000). *Core curriculum on tuberculosis: What the clinician should know* (4th ed.). Atlanta: Author.

Horsburgh, C. R., Feldman, S., & Ridzon, R. (2000) Practice guidelines for the treatment of tuberculosis. *Clinical Infectious Diseases, 31*(3), 633–639.

Kendig, E. L., Kirkpatrick, B. V., Carter, W. H., Hill, F. A., Caldwell, K., & Entwistle, M. (1998). Underreading of the tuberculin skin test reaction. *Chest, 113*(5), 1175–1177.

Small, P. M., & Fujiwara, P. I. (2001). Management of tuberculosis in the United States. *New England Journal of Medicine, 345*(3), 189–200.

RESOURCES AND WEBSITES

Agency for Healthcare Quality and Research, 2101 E. Jefferson St., Suite 501, Rockville, MD 20852; 1-301-594-1364; http://www.ahrq.org.

American Association for Respiratory Care, 1720 Regal Row, Dallas, TX 75235; 1-214-630-3540; http://www.aarc.org.

American Cancer Society, 1599 Clifton Road NE, Atlanta, GA 30329; 1-888-ACS-5552; http://www.cancer.org.

American College of Chest Physicians, 3300 Dundee Road, Northbrook, IL 60062; 1-847-498-1400; http://www.chest.org.

American Lung Association, 1740 Broadway, New York, NY 10019-4374; 1-212-315-8700; http://www.lungusa.org.

American Thoracic Society, 1740 Broadway, New York, NY 10019; 1-212-315-8700; http://www.thoracic.org.

Centers for Disease Control and Prevention, 1600 Clifton Road, NE, Atlanta, GA 30333; http://www.cdc.gov.

National Heart, Lung and Blood Institute, National Institutes of Health, 900 Rockville Pike, Bldg. 31, Bethesda, MD 20892; 1-301-496-5166; http://www.nhlbi.nih.gov.

National Cancer Institute, National Institutes of Health, 31 Center Drive MSC 2580, Bldg. 31, Room 10A16, Bethesda, MD 20892; 1-800-4-CANCER (Cancer Information Services); http://www.nci.nih.gov.

Respiratory Nursing Society, c/o NYSNA, 11 Cornell Road, Latham, NY 12110; 1-518-782-9400 × 286; http://www.respiratorynursingsociety.org.

U.S. Department of Labor, Occupational Safety and Health Administration (OSHA), Directorate of Technical Support, 200 Constitution Avenue, NW, Washington, DC 20210; 1-202-219-7047; http://www.osha.gov.

Management of Patients With Chronic Obstructive Pulmonary Disease

On completion of this chapter, the learner will be able to:

1. Describe the pathophysiology of chronic obstructive pulmonary disease (COPD).
2. Discuss the major risk factors for developing COPD and nursing interventions to minimize or prevent these risk factors.
3. Use the nursing process as a framework for care of the patient with COPD.
4. Develop a teaching plan for patients with COPD.
5. Describe the pathophysiology of asthma.
6. Discuss the medications used in asthma management.
7. Describe asthma self-management strategies.
8. Describe the pathophysiology of cystic fibrosis.

Chronic obstructive pulmonary disease (COPD) is a leading cause of morbidity and mortality in the United States. Nurses are involved with COPD patients across the spectrum of care, from outpatient and home care to critical care and the hospice setting. Patients with COPD or asthma need care from nurses who not only have astute assessment and clinical management skills, but who also understand how these disorders can affect patients' quality of life. Patient and family teaching is an important nursing intervention to enhance self-management of COPD, asthma, and cystic fibrosis.

Chronic Obstructive Pulmonary Disease

Chronic obstructive pulmonary disease (COPD) is a disease state characterized by airflow limitation that is not fully reversible. This newest definition of COPD, provided by the Global Initiative for Chronic Obstructive Lung Disease, provides a broad description that better explains this disorder and its signs and symptoms (National Institutes of Health [NIH], 2001). While previous definitions have included emphysema and chronic bronchitis under the umbrella classification of COPD, this was often confusing because most patients with COPD present with overlapping signs and symptoms of these two distinct disease processes.

COPD may include diseases that cause airflow obstruction (eg, emphysema, chronic bronchitis) or a combination of these disorders. Other diseases such as cystic fibrosis, bronchiectasis, and asthma were previously classified as types of chronic obstructive lung disease. However, asthma is now considered a separate disorder and is classified as an abnormal airway condition characterized primarily by reversible inflammation. COPD can coexist with asthma. Both of these diseases have the same major symptoms; however, symptoms are generally more variable in asthma than in COPD. This chapter discusses COPD as a disease and briefly describes chronic bronchitis and emphysema as distinct disease states, providing a foundation for understanding the pathophysiology of COPD. Bronchiectasis, asthma, and cystic fibrosis are discussed separately.

COPD is the fifth leading cause of death in the United States for all ages and both genders; fifth for men and fourth for women (National Center for Health Statistics [NCHS], 2000). In 1998, more than 12,000 persons died of COPD. This represents a rise in the mortality rate for this disorder at a time when death rates from other serious illnesses, such as heart disease and cerebral vascular disease, were declining. Approximately 16 million people in the United States have some form of COPD; it is responsible for over 13.4 million office visits per year and is the third most frequent justification for home care services (NCHS, 2000; National Heart, Lung and Blood Institute [NHLBI], 1998). People with COPD commonly become symptomatic during the middle adult years, and the incidence of COPD increases with age. Although certain aspects of lung function normally decrease with age (eg, vital capacity and forced expiratory volume in 1 second [FEV_1]), COPD accentuates and accelerates these physiologic changes.

Pathophysiology

In COPD, the airflow limitation is both progressive and associated with an abnormal inflammatory response of the lungs to noxious particles or gases. The inflammatory response occurs throughout the airways, parenchyma, and pulmonary vasculature (NIH, 2001). Because of the chronic inflammation and the body's attempts to repair it, narrowing occurs in the small peripheral airways. Over time, this injury-and-repair process causes scar tissue formation and narrowing of the airway lumen. Airflow obstruction may also be due to parenchymal destruction as seen with emphysema, a disease of the alveoli or gas exchange units.

In addition to inflammation, processes relating to imbalances of proteinases and antiproteinases in the lung may be responsible for airflow limitation. When activated by chronic inflammation, proteinases and other substances may be released, damaging the parenchyma of the lung. The parenchymal changes may also be consequences of inflammation, environmental, or genetic factors (eg, alpha$_1$ antitrypsin deficiency).

Early in the course of COPD, the inflammatory response causes pulmonary vasculature changes that are characterized by thickening of the vessel wall. These changes may occur as a result of exposure to cigarette smoke or use of tobacco products or as a result of the release of inflammatory mediators (NIH, 2001).

Chronic Bronchitis

Chronic **bronchitis**, a disease of the airways, is defined as the presence of cough and sputum production for at least 3 months in each of 2 consecutive years. In many cases, smoke or other environmental pollutants irritate the airways, resulting in hypersecretion

Glossary

air trapping: incomplete emptying of alveoli during expiration due to loss of lung tissue elasticity (emphysema), bronchospasm (asthma), or airway obstruction

alpha$_1$ antitrypsin deficiency: genetic disorder resulting from deficiency of alpha$_1$ antitrypsin, a protective agent for the lung; increases patient's risk for developing panacinar emphysema even in the absence of smoking

asthma: a disease with multiple precipitating mechanisms resulting in a common clinical outcome of reversible airflow obstruction; no longer considered a category of COPD

bronchiectasis: chronic dilation of a bronchus or bronchi; the dilated airways become saccular and are a medium for chronic infection. Is no longer considered a category of COPD.

bronchitis: a disease of the airways defined as the presence of cough and sputum production for at least a combined total of 3 months in each of 2 consecutive years; is a category of COPD

chronic obstructive pulmonary disease: disease state characterized by airflow limitation that is not fully reversible; sometimes referred to as chronic airway obstruction or chronic obstructive lung disease

emphysema: a disease of the airways characterized by destruction of the walls of overdistended alveoli; is a category of COPD

metered-dose inhaler (MDI): patient-activated medication canister that provides aerosolized medication that the patient inhales into the lungs

polycythemia: increase in the red blood cell concentration in the blood; in COPD, the body attempts to improve oxygen carrying capacity by producing increasing amounts of red blood cells

spirometry: pulmonary function tests that measure specific lung volumes (eg, FEV_1, FVC) and rates ($FEF_{25-75\%}$); may be measured before and after bronchodilator administration

of mucus and inflammation. This constant irritation causes the mucus-secreting glands and goblet cells to increase in number, ciliary function is reduced, and more mucus is produced. The bronchial walls become thickened, the bronchial lumen is narrowed, and mucus may plug the airway (Fig. 24-1). Alveoli adjacent to the bronchioles may become damaged and fibrosed, resulting in altered function of the alveolar macrophages. This is significant because the macrophages play an important role in destroying foreign particles, including bacteria. As a result, the patient becomes more susceptible to respiratory infection. A wide range of viral, bacterial, and mycoplasmal infections can produce acute episodes of bronchitis. Exacerbations of chronic bronchitis are most likely to occur during the winter.

Emphysema

In **emphysema**, impaired gas exchange (oxygen, carbon dioxide) results from destruction of the walls of overdistended alveoli. "Emphysema" is a pathological term that describes an abnormal distention of the air spaces beyond the terminal bronchioles, with destruction of the walls of the alveoli. It is the end stage of a process that has progressed slowly for many years. As the walls of the alveoli are destroyed (a process accelerated by recurrent infections), the alveolar surface area in direct contact with the pulmonary capillaries continually decreases, causing an increase in dead space (lung area where no gas exchange can occur) and impaired oxygen diffusion, which leads to hypoxemia. In the later stages of the disease, carbon dioxide elimination is impaired, resulting in increased carbon dioxide tension in arterial blood (hypercapnia) and causing respiratory acidosis. As the alveolar walls continue to break down, the pulmonary capillary bed is reduced. Consequently, pulmonary blood flow is increased, forcing the right ventricle to maintain a higher blood pressure in the pulmonary artery. Hypoxemia may further increase pulmonary artery pressure. Thus, right-sided heart failure (cor pulmonale) is one of the complications of emphysema. Congestion, dependent edema, distended neck veins, or pain in the region of the liver suggests the development of cardiac failure.

There are two main types of emphysema, based on the changes taking place in the lung: panlobular (panacinar) and centrilobular (centroacinar) (Fig. 24-2). Both types may occur in the same pa-

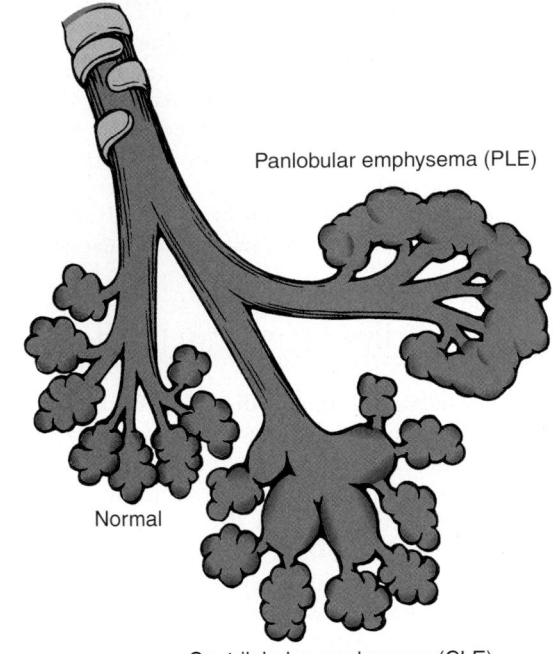

FIGURE 24-2 Changes in alveolar structure in centrilobular and panlobular emphysema. In panlobular emphysema, the bronchioles, alveolar ducts, and alveoli are destroyed and the air spaces within the lobule are enlarged. In centrilobular emphysema, the pathologic changes occur in the lobule, while the peripheral portions of the acinus are preserved.

tient. In the panlobular (panacinar) type, there is destruction of the respiratory bronchiole, alveolar duct, and alveoli. All air spaces within the lobule are essentially enlarged, but there is little inflammatory disease. The patient with this type of emphysema typically has a hyperinflated (hyperexpanded) chest (barrel chest on physical examination), marked dyspnea on exertion, and weight loss. To move air into and out of the lungs, negative pressure is required during inspiration, and an adequate level of positive pressure must be attained and maintained during expiration. The resting position is one of inflation. Instead of being an involuntary passive act, expiration becomes active and requires mus-

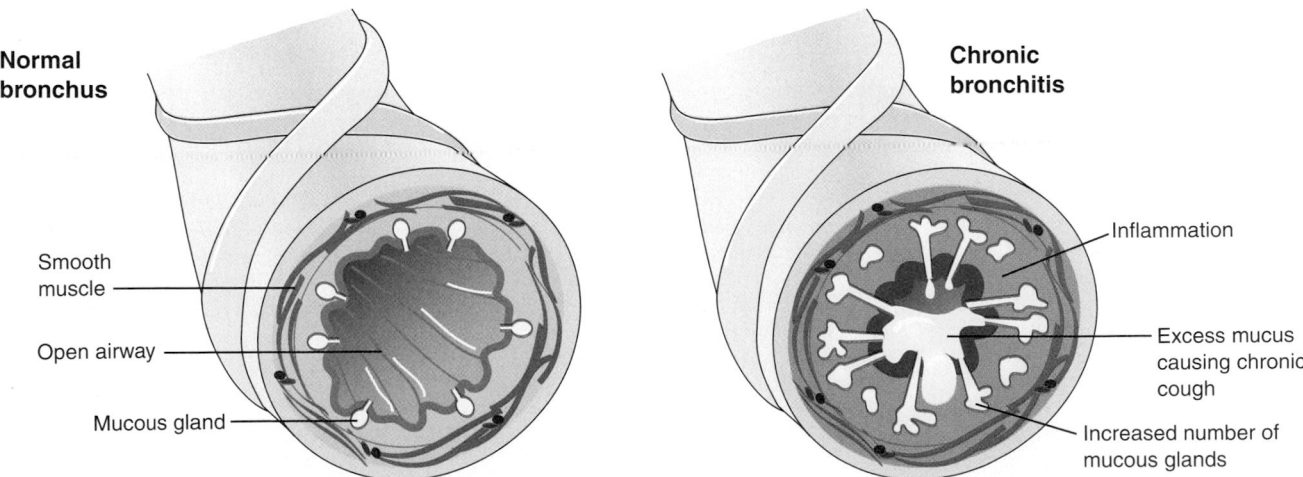

FIGURE 24-1 Pathophysiology of chronic bronchitis as compared to a normal bronchus. The bronchus in chronic bronchitis is narrowed and has impaired air flow due to multiple mechanisms: inflammation, excess mucus production, and potential smooth muscle constriction (bronchospasm).

cular effort. The patient becomes increasingly short of breath, the chest becomes rigid, and the ribs are fixed at their joints.

In the centrilobular (centroacinar) form, pathologic changes take place mainly in the center of the secondary lobule, preserving the peripheral portions of the acinus. Frequently, there is a derangement of ventilation–perfusion ratios, producing chronic hypoxemia, hypercapnia (increased CO_2 in the arterial blood), **polycythemia,** and episodes of right-sided heart failure. This leads to central cyanosis, peripheral edema, and respiratory failure. The patient may receive diuretic therapy for edema.

Risk Factors

Risk factors for COPD include environmental exposures and host factors (Chart 24-1). The most important risk factor for COPD is cigarette smoking. Pipe, cigar, and other types of tobacco smoking are also risk factors. In addition, passive smoking contributes to respiratory symptoms and COPD (NIH, 2001). Smoking depresses the activity of scavenger cells and affects the respiratory tract's ciliary cleansing mechanism, which keeps breathing passages free of inhaled irritants, bacteria, and other foreign matter. When smoking damages this cleansing mechanism, airflow is obstructed and air becomes trapped behind the obstruction. The alveoli greatly distend, diminishing lung capacity. Smoking also irritates the goblet cells and mucus glands, causing an increased accumulation of mucus, which in turn produces more irritation, infection, and damage to the lung. In addition, carbon monoxide (a byproduct of smoking) combines with hemoglobin to form carboxyhemoglobin. Hemoglobin that is bound by carboxyhemoglobin cannot carry oxygen efficiently.

Smoking is not the only risk factor for COPD. Other factors include prolonged and intense exposure to occupational dusts and chemicals, indoor air pollution, and outdoor air pollution, which adds to the total burden of inhaled particles on the lung (NIH, 2001).

A host risk factor for COPD is a deficiency of alpha$_1$ antitrypsin, an enzyme inhibitor that protects the lung parenchyma from injury. This deficiency predisposes young patients to rapid development of lobular emphysema even in the absence of smoking. **Alpha$_1$ antitrypsin deficiency** is one of the most common genetically linked lethal diseases among Caucasians and affects approximately one in every 3,000 Americans or approximately 80,000 to 100,000 cases (George, San Pedro & Stoller, 2000). The genetically susceptible person is sensitive to environmental factors (smoking, air pollution, infectious agents, allergens) and in time develops chronic obstructive symptoms. Carriers of this genetic defect must be identified so that they can modify environmental risk factors to delay or prevent overt symptoms of disease. Genetic counseling should also be offered. Alpha-protease inhibitor replacement therapy, which slows the progression of the disease, is available for patients with this genetic defect and for those with severe disease. This intermittent infusion therapy is costly and is required on an ongoing basis.

Clinical Manifestations

COPD is characterized by three primary symptoms: cough, sputum production, and dyspnea on exertion (NIH, 2001). These symptoms often worsen over time. Chronic cough and sputum production often precede the development of airflow limitation by many years. However, not all individuals with cough and sputum production will develop COPD. Dyspnea may be severe and often interferes with the patient's activities. Weight loss is common because dyspnea interferes with eating, and the work of breathing is energy-depleting. Often the patient cannot participate in even mild exercise because of dyspnea; as COPD progresses, dyspnea occurs even at rest. As the work of breathing increases over time, the accessory muscles are recruited in an effort to breathe. The patient with COPD is at risk for respiratory insufficiency and respiratory infections, which in turn increase the risk for acute and chronic respiratory failure.

In COPD patients with a primary emphysematous component, chronic hyperinflation leads to the "barrel chest" thorax configuration. This results from fixation of the ribs in the inspiratory position (due to hyperinflation) and from loss of lung elasticity (Fig. 24-3). Retraction of the supraclavicular fossae occurs on inspiration, causing the shoulders to heave upward (Fig. 24-4). In advanced emphysema, the abdominal muscles also contract on inspiration.

Assessment and Diagnostic Findings

The nurse should obtain a thorough health history for a patient with known or potential COPD. Chart 24-2 lists the key factors to assess. Pulmonary function studies are used to help confirm the diagnosis of COPD, determine disease severity, and follow disease progression. **Spirometry** is used to evaluate airflow obstruction, which is determined by the ratio of FEV_1 (volume of air that the patient can forcibly exhale in 1 second) to forced vital capacity (FVC). Spirometric results are expressed as an absolute volume and as percent-predicted using appropriate normal values for gender, age, and height. With obstruction, the patient either has difficulty exhaling or cannot forcibly exhale air from the lungs, reducing the FEV_1. Obstructive lung disease is defined as a FEV_1/FVC ratio of less than 70%.

In addition, bronchodilator reversibility testing may be performed to rule out the diagnosis of asthma and to guide initial treatment. With this type of testing, spirometry is first obtained, then the patient is given an inhaled bronchodilator per a protocol, and finally spirometry is repeated. The patient demonstrates a degree of reversibility if the pulmonary function values improve after administration of the bronchodilator.

Arterial blood gas measurements may also be obtained to assess baseline oxygenation and gas exchange. In addition, a chest x-ray may be obtained to exclude alternative diagnoses. Lastly, alpha$_1$ antitrypsin deficiency screening may be performed for patients under age 45 or for those with a strong family history of COPD.

The severity of COPD is classified into four stages (Table 24-1) (National Institutes of Health, 2001). Factors that determine the clinical course and survival of patients with COPD include history

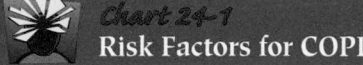

Chart 24-1
Risk Factors for COPD

Exposure to tobacco smoke accounts for an estimated 80% to 90% of COPD cases (Rennard, 1998)
Passive smoking
Occupational exposure
Ambient air pollution
Genetic abnormalities, including a deficiency of alpha$_1$-antitrypsin, an enzyme inhibitor that normally counteracts the destruction of lung tissue by certain other enzymes

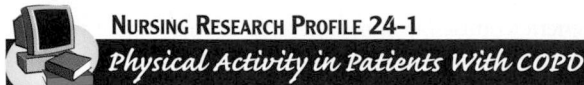

NURSING RESEARCH PROFILE 24-1
Physical Activity in Patients With COPD

Belza, B., Steele, B. G., Hunziker, J., Lakshminaryan, S., Holt, L., & Buchner, D. M. (2001). Correlates of physical activity in chronic obstructive pulmonary disease. *Nursing Research, 50*(4), 195–202.

Purpose

For patients with chronic obstructive pulmonary disease (COPD), physical activity is an important part of their quality of life. Yet little is known about the contributions of psychological and physiologic variables to physical activity in this population. The purpose of this study was to determine the relationships among differing functional performance measures (physical activity, functional capacity, symptom experience, and health-related quality of life) in this population.

Study Sample and Design

This cross-sectional, descriptive study evaluated 63 outpatients with COPD prior to entry into a pulmonary rehabilitation program. The sample was predominantly male (60 men and 3 women) with a mean age of 65.4 ± 8.0 years. None of the participants had been hospitalized in the past 2 months for a respiratory problem, and none was engaged in a formalized exercise program. Functional performance was measured by physical activity (evaluated by an accelerometer and self-report). Functional capacity was measured by three measures of impairment (pulmonary function tests [FEV_1], 6-minute walk test, and

a self-efficacy questionnaire for walking). The symptom experiences of dyspnea and fatigue as well as health-related quality of life were measured by widely used reliable and valid questionnaires.

Findings

Sixty-nine subjects were initially enrolled in the study but six were withdrawn due to missing data. Daily physical activity as measured by the accelerometer was strongly associated with the maximal distance walked in the 6-minute walk test, the level of airway obstruction as measured by pulmonary function tests, walking self-efficacy, and physical health status. Physical activity was not correlated with the subjects' self-report of functional status. The 6-minute walk test was the only predictor of physical activity in this sample.

Nursing Implications

Functional performance status is an important multidimensional outcome measure for both nursing and medicine. This study demonstrates that the multiple measures of functional performance status, which are frequently used in clinical practice and research, may differ in their relationship to the actual physical activity level of the patient.

---

of cigarette smoking, passive smoking exposure, age, rate of decline of FEV_1, hypoxemia, pulmonary artery pressure, resting heart rate, weight loss, and reversibility of airflow obstruction (George, San Pedro & Stoller, 2000).

In diagnosing COPD, several differential diagnoses must be ruled out. The primary differential diagnosis is asthma. Key characteristics of asthma include onset often early in life, variation in daily symptoms and day-to-day occurrence or timing of symptoms, family history of asthma, and a largely reversible airflow obstruction. It may be difficult to differentiate between a patient with COPD and one with chronic asthma. A key part of differentiation is the patient history, as well as the patient's respon-

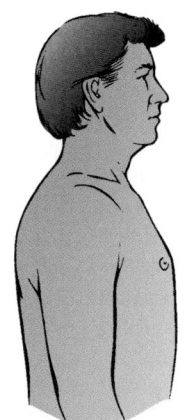

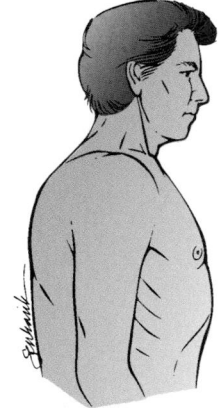

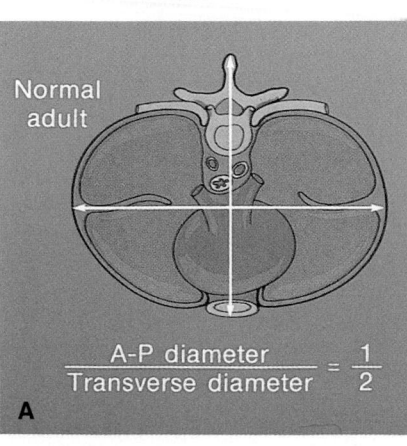

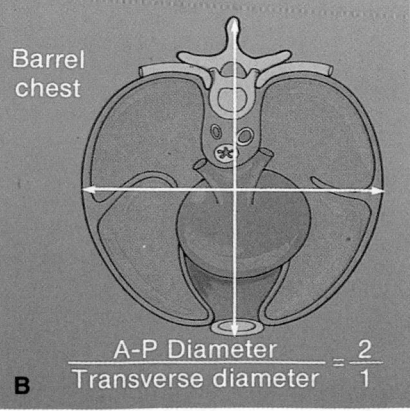

FIGURE 24-3 Characteristics of normal chest wall and chest wall in emphysema. The normal chest wall and its cross section are illustrated on the left (**A**). The barrel-shaped chest of emphysema and its cross section are illustrated on the right (**B**).

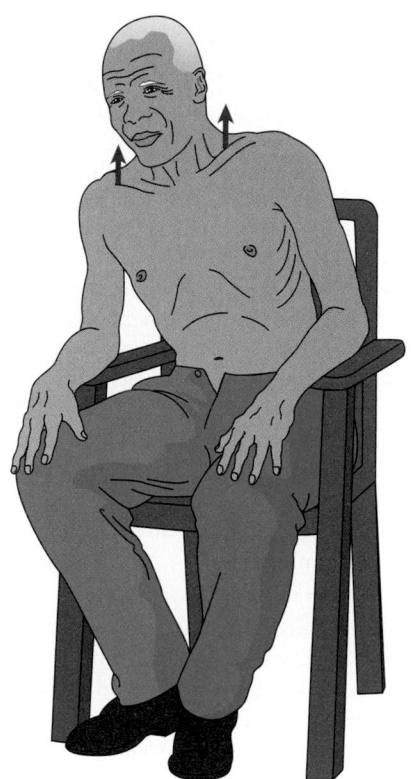

FIGURE 24-4 Typical posture of person with COPD—primarily emphysema. The person tends to lean forward and uses the accessory muscles of respiration to breathe, forcing the shoulder girdle upward and causing the supraclavicular fossae to retract on inspiration.

siveness to bronchodilators. Other diseases that must be considered in the differential diagnosis include heart failure, bronchiectasis, and tuberculosis (NIH, 2001).

Complications

Respiratory insufficiency and failure are major life-threatening complications of COPD. The acuity of the onset and the severity of respiratory failure depend on the patient's baseline pulmonary function, pulse oximetry or arterial blood gas values, comorbid conditions, and the severity of other complications of COPD. Respiratory insufficiency and failure may be chronic

---

Table 24-1 • Stages of COPD

STAGE	CHARACTERISTICS
0	Normal spirometry Chronic symptoms of cough, sputum production
I (mild COPD)	$FEV_1/FVC < 70\%$ $FEV_1 \geq 80\%$ predicted May or may not have chronic symptoms of cough, sputum production
II (moderate COPD)	$FEV_1/FVC < 70\%$ FEV_1 between 30% and 80% predicted May or may not have chronic symptoms of cough, sputum production
III (severe COPD)	$FEV_1/FVC < 70\%$ $FEV_1 < 30\%$ predicted or $FEV_1 < 50\%$ predicted plus respiratory failure or clinical signs of right heart failure

National Institutes of Health (2001). *Global initiative for chronic obstructive lung disease: Global strategy for the diagnosis, management, and prevention of chronic obstructive pulmonary disease.* U.S. Department of Health and Human Services, NIH Publication Number 2701B.

(with severe COPD) or acute (with severe bronchospasm or pneumonia in the patient with severe COPD). Acute respiratory insufficiency and failure may necessitate ventilatory support until other acute complications, such as infection, can be treated. Management of the patient requiring ventilatory support is discussed in Chapter 25. Other complications of COPD include pneumonia, atelectasis, pneumothorax, and cor pulmonale.

Medical Management

RISK REDUCTION

Smoking cessation is the single most effective intervention to prevent COPD or slow its progression (NIH, 2001). Recent surveys indicate that 25% of all American adults smoke (USPHS, 2000). Nurses play a key role in promoting smoking cessation and educating patients about ways to do so. Patients diagnosed with COPD who continue to smoke must be encouraged and assisted to quit. Factors associated with continued smoking vary among patients and may include the strength of nicotine addiction, continued exposure to smoking-associated stimuli (at work or in social settings), stress, depression, and habit. Continued smoking is also more prevalent among those with low incomes, a low level of education, and psychosocial problems (Pohl, 2000).

Because there are multiple factors associated with continued smoking, successful cessation often requires multiple strategies. The health care provider should promote cessation by explaining the risks of smoking and personalizing the "at-risk" message to the patient. After giving a strong warning about smoking, the health care provider should work with the patient to set a definite "quit date." Referral to a smoking cessation program may be helpful. Follow-up within 3 to 5 days after the quit date to review progress and to address any problems is associated with an increased rate of success; this should be repeated as needed. Continued reinforcement with telephone calls or clinic visits is extremely beneficial. Relapses should be analyzed, and the patient and health care provider should jointly identify possible solutions to prevent future backsliding. It is important to emphasize successes rather

---

Chart 24-2 • ASSESSMENT

Key Factors to Assess in the COPD Patient's Health History

Exposure to risk factors—types, intensity, duration
Past medical history—respiratory diseases/problems, including asthma, allergy, sinusitis, nasal polyps, history of respiratory infections
Family history of COPD or other chronic respiratory diseases
Pattern of symptom development
History of exacerbations or previous hospitalizations for respiratory problems
Presence of comorbidities
Appropriateness of current medical treatments
Impact of the disease on quality of life
Available social and family support for patient
Potential for reducing risk factors (eg, smoking cessation)

than failures. First-line pharmacotherapies that reliably increase long-term smoking abstinence rates are bupropion SR (Zyban, Wellbutrin), nicotine gum, nicotine inhaler, nicotine nasal spray, or nicotine patches. Second-line pharmacotherapies include clonidine (Catapres) and nortriptyline (Aventyl) (USPHS, 2000).

Smoking cessation can begin in a variety of health care settings—outpatient clinic, pulmonary rehabilitation, community, hospital, and the patient's home. Regardless of the setting, the nurse has the opportunity to teach the patient about the risks of smoking and the benefits of smoking cessation. A variety of materials, resources, and programs are available to assist with this effort (eg, Agency for Healthcare Research and Quality [formerly Agency for Healthcare Policy and Research], United States Public Health Service, Centers for Disease Control and Prevention, National Cancer Institute, American Lung Association, American Cancer Society).

PHARMACOLOGIC THERAPY

Bronchodilators. Bronchodilators relieve bronchospasm and reduce airway obstruction by allowing increased oxygen distribution throughout the lungs and improving alveolar ventilation. These medications, which are central in the management of COPD (NIH, 2001), are delivered through a metered-dose inhaler, by nebulization, or via the oral route in pill or liquid form. Bronchodilators are often administered regularly throughout the day as well as on an as-needed basis. They may also be used prophylactically to prevent breathlessness by having the patient use them before an activity, such as eating or walking.

A **metered-dose inhaler** (MDI) is a pressurized device containing an aerosolized powder of medication. A precise amount of medication is released with each activation of the canister (Dhand, 2000). Patients need to be instructed on the correct use

of the device. A spacer (holding chamber) may also be used to enhance deposition of the medication in the lung and help the patient coordinate activation of the MDI with inspiration. Spacers come in several designs, but all are attached to the MDI and have a mouthpiece on the opposite end (Fig. 24-5). Once the canister is activated, the spacer holds the aerosol in the chamber until the patient inhales (Dhand, 2000). The patient should take a slow, 3- to 5-second inhalation immediately following activation of the MDI (Expert Panel Report II, 1997).

Several classes of bronchodilators are used: beta-adrenergic agonists, anticholinergic agents, and methylxanthines. These medications may be used in combination to optimize the bronchodilation effect. Some of these medications are short-acting; others are long-acting. Long-acting bronchodilators are more convenient for patient use. Examples of medications in these differing classes are shown in Table 24-2. Nebulized medications (nebulization of medication via an air compressor) may also be effective in patients who cannot use an MDI properly or who prefer this method of administration.

Corticosteroids. Inhaled and systemic corticosteroids (oral or intravenous) may also be used in COPD but are used more frequently in asthma. Although it has been shown that corticosteroids do not slow the decline in lung function, these medications may improve symptoms. A short trial course of oral corticosteroids may be prescribed for patients with stage II or III COPD to see if pulmonary function improves and symptoms decrease. Inhaled corticosteroids via MDI may also be used. Examples of corticosteroids in the inhaled form are beclomethasone (Beclovent, Vanceril), budesonide (Pulmicort), flunisolide (AeroBid), fluticasone (Flovent), and triamcinolone (Azmacort).

Medication regimens used to manage COPD are based on disease severity. For stage I or mild COPD, a short-acting bron-

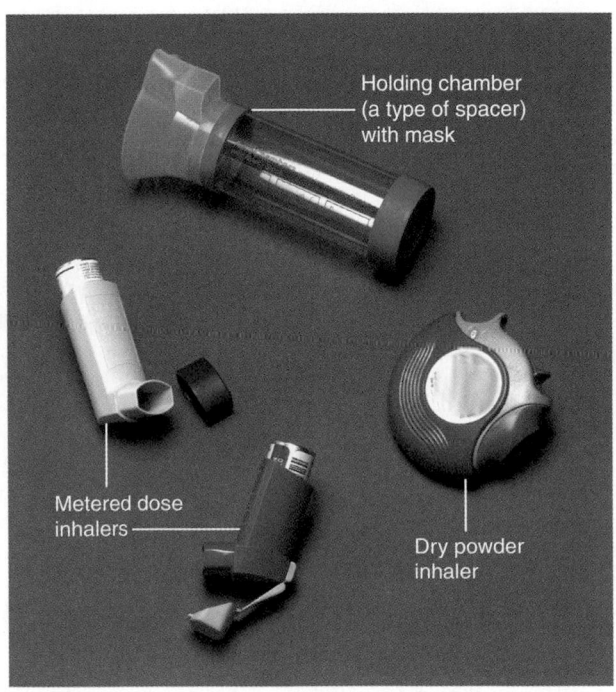

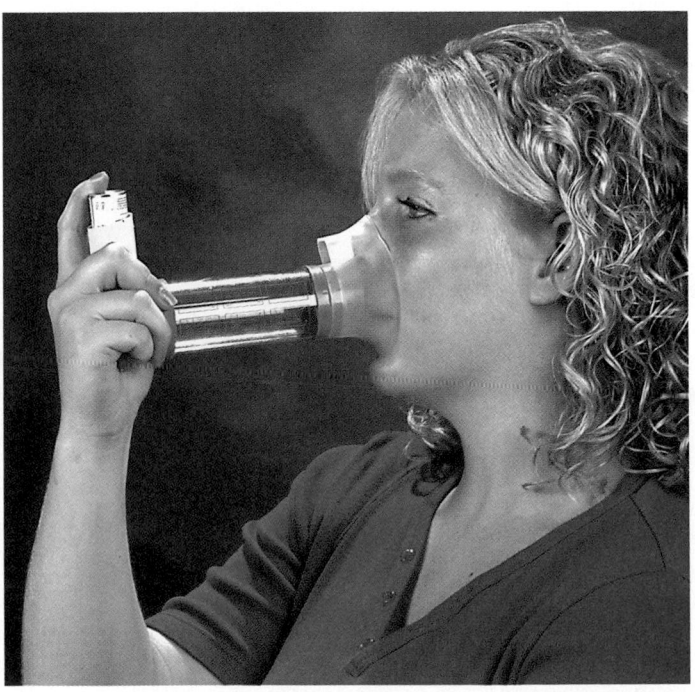

A   **B**

FIGURE 24-5 (**A**) Examples of metered dose inhalers and spacers. (**B**) A metered dose inhaler and spacer in use.

Table 24-2 • Types of Bronchodilator Medications

CLASS/DRUG	METHOD OF ADMINISTRATION			DURATION OF ACTION
	Metered-Dose Inhaler	Nebulizer	Oral	
Beta-Adrenergic Agonist Agents				
Albuterol (Proventil, Ventolin, Volmax)	X	X	X	Short
Bitolerol (Tornate)	X	X		Medium
Levalbuterol (Xopenax)		X		Medium
Metaproterenol (Alupent)	X	X	X	Short
Pirbuterol (Maxair)	X			Short
Salbutamol (Asmavent)	X	X	X	Short
Salmeterol (Serevent)	X			Long
Terbutaline (Brethaire)			X	Short
Anticholinergic Agents				
Ipratropium bromide (Atrovent)	X	X		Short
Oxitropium bromide (Oxivent)	X			Medium
Methylxanthines				
Aminophylline (Phyllocontin)			X	Variable
Theophylline (Slo-bid, Theo-Dur)			X	Variable

Short-acting: 4–6 hours
Medium-acting: 6–9 hours
Long-acting: 12+ hours

chodilator may be prescribed. For stage II or moderate COPD, one or more bronchodilators may be prescribed along with inhaled corticosteroids, if symptoms are significant. For stage III or severe COPD, medication therapy includes regular treatment with one or more bronchodilators and inhaled corticosteroids (NIH, 2001).

Other Medications. Patients should receive a yearly influenza vaccine and the pneumococcal vaccine every 5 to 7 years as preventive measures. In most healthy adults, pneumococcal vaccine titers persist for 5 or more years (George, San Pedro & Stoller, 2000). Other pharmacologic treatments that may be used in COPD include alpha$_1$ antitrypsin augmentation therapy, antibiotic agents, mucolytic agents, and antitussive agents.

MANAGEMENT OF EXACERBATION

An exacerbation of COPD is difficult to diagnose, but signs and symptoms may include increased dyspnea, increased sputum production and purulence, respiratory failure, changes in mental status, or worsening blood gas abnormalities. Primary causes for an acute exacerbation include tracheobronchial infection and air pollution (NIH, 2001). Secondary causes are pneumonia; pulmonary embolism; pneumothorax; rib fractures or chest trauma; inappropriate use of sedative, opioid, or beta-blocking agents; and right- or left-sided heart failure. First, the primary cause of the exacerbation is identified, and then specific treatment is administered. Optimization of bronchodilator medications is the first-line therapy and involves identifying the best medication or combinations of medications taken on a regular schedule for that patient. Depending on the signs and symptoms, corticosteroids, antibiotic agents, oxygen therapy, and intensive respiratory interventions may also be used. Indications for hospitalization of a patient with an acute exacerbation of COPD include severe dyspnea that does not respond adequately to initial therapy, confu-

sion or lethargy, respiratory muscle fatigue, paradoxical chest wall movement, peripheral edema, worsening or new onset of central cyanosis, persistent or worsening hypoxemia, and/or need for noninvasive or invasive assisted mechanical ventilation (Celli, Snider, Heffner et al., 1995; NIH, 2001).

OXYGEN THERAPY

Oxygen therapy can be administered as long-term continuous therapy, during exercise, or to prevent acute dyspnea. Long-term oxygen therapy has been shown to improve the patient's quality of life and survival (NIH, 2001). For patients with an arterial oxygen pressure (PaO$_2$) of 55 mm Hg or less on room air, maintaining a constant and adequate oxygen saturation (>90%) is associated with significantly reduced mortality and improved quality of life. Indications for oxygen supplementation include a PaO$_2$ of 55 mm Hg or less or evidence of tissue hypoxia and organ damage such as cor pulmonale, secondary polycythemia, edema from right heart failure, or impaired mental status. In patients with exercise-induced hypoxemia, oxygen supplementation during exercise can improve performance. Patients who are hypoxemic while awake are likely to be so during sleep. Therefore, nighttime oxygen therapy is recommended as well, and the prescription for oxygen therapy is for continuous, 24-hour use. Intermittent oxygen therapy is indicated for those who desaturate only during exercise or sleep.

NURSING ALERT Because hypoxemia stimulates respiration in the patient with severe COPD, increasing the oxygen flow to a high rate may greatly raise the patient's blood oxygen level. At the same time, this will suppress the respiratory drive, causing increased retention of carbon dioxide and CO$_2$ narcosis. The nurse should closely monitor the patient's respiratory response to oxygen administration via physical assessment, pulse oximetry, and/or arterial blood gases.

NURSING RESEARCH PROFILE 24-2

Oxygen Administration and Dyspnea Management in Patients With AAT Deficiency

Knebel, A. R., Bentz, E., & Barnes, P. (2000). Dyspnea management in alpha-1 antitrypsin deficiency: Effect of oxygen administration. *Nursing Research, 49*(6), 333–338.

Purpose

Limitations in activity due to dyspnea are common in persons with emphysema, including patients with alpha$_1$ antitrypsin (AAT) deficiency. The purpose of this study was to examine whether short-term oxygen administration decreased dyspnea and improved exercise tolerance in nonhypoxemic patients with emphysema caused by AAT deficiency.

Study Sample and Design

Thirty-one Caucasian subjects participated in a double-blind, crossover study. The subjects' mean age was 47 ± 7 years; 62% were male and 38% were female. Twenty-four percent had used oxygen supplementation at some point during their illness. Oxygen saturation, 6-minute walk distance, and end-of-walk dyspnea were measured during three practice walks and during walks with nasal cannula administration of oxygen (intervention) and compressed air (control).

Findings

Researchers found significant differences in subjects' oxygen saturation during walks with oxygen vs. walks with compressed air ($p = 0.0001$),

with oxygen saturation higher with oxygen supplementation than with compressed air. There was no difference in subjects' walk distance and severity of self-reported dyspnea between oxygen and compressed air use. However, some gender differences were noted. Men showed no benefit from oxygen supplementation while walking, but women experienced less dyspnea, which corresponded with an increased walking distance.

Nursing Implications

The findings demonstrated that oxygen supplementation did not significantly improve the sensation of dyspnea or the distance walked in 6 minutes in the total sample of patients with AAT deficiency. However, there were trends in gender differences in relation to dyspnea levels and distance walked while receiving the intervention (oxygen supplementation). Future studies should examine subjects with differing levels of room air hypoxemia and explore potential gender differences in exercise performance with oxygen supplementation. Nurses should be aware that patients may respond differently to oxygen supplementation depending upon the underlying disease process, level of hypoxemia, and gender.

SURGICAL MANAGEMENT

Bullectomy. A bullectomy is a surgical option for select patients with bullous emphysema. Bullae are enlarged airspaces that do not contribute to ventilation but occupy space in the thorax; these areas may be surgically excised. Many times these bullae compress areas of the lung that do have adequate gas exchange. Bullectomy may help reduce dyspnea and improve lung function. It can be done thoracoscopically (with a video-assisted thoracoscope) or via a limited thoracotomy incision (see Chap. 25).

Lung Volume Reduction Surgery. Treatment options for patients with end-stage COPD (stage III) with a primary emphysematous component are limited, although lung volume reduction surgery is an option for a specific subset of patients. This subset includes patients with homogenous disease or disease that is focused in one area and not widespread throughout the lungs. Lung volume reduction surgery involves the removal of a portion of the diseased lung parenchyma. This allows the functional tissue to expand, resulting in improved elastic recoil of the lung and improved chest wall and diaphragmatic mechanics. This type of surgery does not cure the disease, but it may decrease dyspnea, improve lung function, and improve the patient's overall quality of life. Careful selection of patients for this procedure is essential to decrease the morbidity and mortality. The long-term outcomes of this surgery are unknown.

The National Emphysema Treatment Trial (NETT) is a large, multicenter randomized clinical trial that began in 1997 and is ongoing. It is attempting to answer many questions regarding the risks and benefits of lung volume reduction surgery in the treatment of severe emphysema. All patients in this trial receive a 6- to 10-week pulmonary rehabilitation program and comprehensive medical management. Following completion of pulmonary rehabilitation, patients are randomized to continue medical management or undergo lung volume reduction surgery. The results

of this trial will help to determine the role of lung volume reduction surgery for patients with severe emphysema (NIH, 2001). It is expected that 2,500 patients will be entered into the study.

Lung Transplantation. Lung transplantation is a viable alternative for definitive surgical treatment of end-stage emphysema. It has been shown to improve quality of life and functional capacity (NIH, 2001). Specific criteria exist for referral for lung transplantation; however, organs are in short supply and many patients die while waiting for a transplant.

PULMONARY REHABILITATION

Pulmonary rehabilitation for patients with COPD is well established and widely accepted as a means to alleviate symptoms and optimize functional status. In both randomized and nonrandomized clinical trials, pulmonary rehabilitation has been shown to improve exercise tolerance, reduce dyspnea, and increase health-related quality of life (Rochester, 2000). The primary goal of rehabilitation is to restore patients to the highest level of independent function possible and to improve their quality of life. A successful rehabilitation program is individualized for each patient, is multidisciplinary, and attends to both the physiologic and emotional needs of the patient. Most pulmonary rehabilitation programs include educational, psychosocial, behavioral, and physical components. Breathing exercises and retraining and exercise programs are used to improve functional status, and the patient is taught methods to alleviate symptoms.

Pulmonary rehabilitation may be used therapeutically in other diseases besides COPD, including asthma, cystic fibrosis, lung cancer, interstitial lung disease, thoracic surgery, and lung transplantation. It may be conducted in the inpatient, outpatient, or home setting; the lengths of programs vary. Selection of a program depends upon the patient's physical, functional, and psychosocial status; insurance coverage; changing health care trends; availability of programs; and patient preference (Rochester, 2000).

Nursing Management

The nurse plays a key role in identifying potential candidates for pulmonary rehabilitation and in facilitating and reinforcing the material learned in the rehabilitation program. Not all patients have access to a formal rehabilitation program. However, the nurse can be instrumental in teaching the patient and family as well as facilitating specific services for the patient (eg, respiratory therapy education, physical therapy for exercise and breathing re-training, occupational therapy for conserving energy during activities of daily living, and nutritional counseling). In addition, numerous educational materials are available to assist the nurse in teaching patients with COPD. Potential resources include the American Lung Association, the American Association of Cardiovascular and Pulmonary Rehabilitation, the American Thoracic Society, the American College of Chest Physicians, and the American Association for Respiratory Therapy.

PATIENT EDUCATION

Patient education is a major component of pulmonary rehabilitation and includes a broad variety of topics. Depending on the length and setting of the program, topics may include normal anatomy and physiology of the lung, pathophysiology and changes with COPD, medications and home oxygen therapy, nutrition, respiratory therapy treatments, symptom alleviation, smoking cessation, sexuality and COPD, coping with chronic disease, communicating with the health care team, and planning for the future (advance directives, living wills, informed decision making about health care alternatives).

Breathing Exercises. The breathing pattern of most people with COPD is shallow, rapid, and inefficient; the more severe the disease, the more inefficient the breathing pattern. With practice, this type of upper chest breathing can be changed to diaphragmatic breathing, which reduces the respiratory rate, increases alveolar ventilation, and sometimes helps expel as much air as possible during expiration (see Chap. 25 for technique). Pursed-lip breathing helps to slow expiration, prevents collapse of small airways, and helps the patient to control the rate and depth of respiration. It also promotes relaxation, enabling the patient to gain control of dyspnea and reduce feelings of panic.

Inspiratory Muscle Training. Once the patient masters diaphragmatic breathing, a program of inspiratory muscle training may be prescribed to help strengthen the muscles used in breathing. This program requires that the patient breathe against resistance for 10 to 15 minutes every day. As the resistance is gradually increased, the muscles become better conditioned. Conditioning of the respiratory muscles takes time, and the patient is instructed to continue practicing at home (Larson, Covey, Wirtz et al., 1999; NIH, 2001).

Activity Pacing. A patient with COPD has decreased exercise tolerance during specific periods of the day. This is especially true on arising in the morning, because bronchial secretions collect in the lungs during the night while the person is lying down. The patient may have difficulty bathing or dressing. Activities requiring the arms to be supported above the level of the thorax may produce fatigue or respiratory distress but may be tolerated better after the patient has been up and moving around for an hour or more. Working with the nurse, the patient can reduce these limitations by planning self-care activities and determining the best time for bathing, dressing, and daily activities.

Self-Care Activities. As gas exchange, airway clearance, and the breathing pattern improve, the patient is encouraged to assume increasing participation in self-care activities. The patient is taught to coordinate diaphragmatic breathing with activities such as walking, bathing, bending, or climbing stairs. The patient should bathe, dress, and take short walks, resting as needed to avoid fatigue and excessive dyspnea. Fluids should always be readily available, and the patient should begin to drink fluids without having to be reminded. If postural drainage is to be done at home, the nurse instructs and supervises the patient before discharge or in the outpatient setting.

Physical Conditioning. Physical conditioning techniques include breathing exercises and general exercises intended to conserve energy and increase pulmonary ventilation. There is a close relationship between physical fitness and respiratory fitness. Graded exercises and physical conditioning programs using treadmills, stationary bicycles, and measured level walks can improve symptoms and increase work capacity and exercise tolerance. Any physical activity that can be done regularly is helpful. Lightweight portable oxygen systems are available for ambulatory patients who require oxygen therapy during physical activity.

Oxygen Therapy. Oxygen supplied to the home comes in compressed gas, liquid, or concentrator systems. Portable oxygen systems allow the patient to exercise, work, and travel. To help the patient adhere to the oxygen prescription, the nurse explains the proper flow rate and required number of hours for oxygen use as well as the dangers of arbitrary changes in flow rates or duration of therapy. The nurse cautions the patient that smoking with or near oxygen is extremely dangerous. The nurse also reassures the patient that oxygen is not "addictive" and explains the need for regular evaluations of blood oxygenation by pulse oximetry or arterial blood gas analysis.

Nutritional Therapy. Nutritional assessment and counseling are important aspects in the rehabilitation process for the patient with COPD. Approximately 25% of patients with COPD are undernourished (NIH, 2001; Ferreira, Brooks, Lacasse & Goldstein, 2001). A thorough assessment of caloric needs and counseling about meal planning and supplementation are part of the rehabilitation process.

Coping Measures. Any factor that interferes with normal breathing quite naturally induces anxiety, depression, and changes in behavior. Many patients find the slightest exertion exhausting. Constant shortness of breath and fatigue may make the patient irritable and apprehensive to the point of panic. Restricted activity (and reversal of family roles due to loss of employment), the frustration of having to work to breathe, and the realization that the disease is prolonged and unrelenting may cause the patient to react with anger, depression, and demanding behavior. Sexual function may be compromised, which also diminishes self-esteem. In addition, the nurse needs to provide education and support to the spouse/significant other and family because the caregiver role in end-stage COPD can be difficult.

NURSING PROCESS: THE PATIENT WITH COPD

Assessment

Assessment involves obtaining information about current symptoms as well as previous disease manifestations. Chart 24-3 lists sample questions that may be used to obtain a clear history of the disease process. In addition to the history, the nurse also reviews the results of available diagnostic tests.

Diagnosis

NURSING DIAGNOSES

Based on the assessment data, the patient's major nursing diagnoses may include the following:

- Impaired gas exchange and airway clearance due to chronic inhalation of toxins
- Impaired gas exchange related to ventilation–perfusion inequality

Chart 24-3 • ASSESSMENT

Chronic Obstructive Pulmonary Disease

Health History
- How long has the patient had respiratory difficulty?
- Does exertion increase the dyspnea? What type of exertion?
- What are limits of the patient's tolerance for exercise?
- At what times during the day does the patient complain most of fatigue and shortness of breath?
- Which eating and sleeping habits have been affected?
- What does the patient know about the disease and his or her condition?
- What is the patient's smoking history (primary and secondary)?
- Is there occupational exposure to smoke or other pollutants?
- What are the triggering events (exertion, strong odors, dust, exposure to animals, etc.)?

Inspection and Examination Findings
- What position does the patient assume during the interview?
- What are the pulse and the respiratory rates?
- What is the character of respirations? Even and without effort? Other?
- Can the patient complete a sentence without having to take a breath?
- Does the patient contract the abdominal muscles during inspiration?
- Does the patient use accessory muscles of the shoulders and neck when breathing?
- Does the patient take a long time to exhale (prolonged expiration)?
- Is central cyanosis evident?
- Are the patient's neck veins engorged?
- Does the patient have peripheral edema?
- Is the patient coughing?
- What is the color, amount, and consistency of the sputum?
- Is clubbing of the fingers present?
- What types of breath sounds (ie, clear, diminished or distant, crackles, wheezes) are heard? Describe and document findings and locations.
- What is the status of the patient's sensorium?
- Is there short-term or long-term memory impairment?
- Is there increasing stupor?
- Is the patient apprehensive?

- Ineffective airway clearance related to bronchoconstriction, increased mucus production, ineffective cough, bronchopulmonary infection, and other complications
- Ineffective breathing pattern related to shortness of breath, mucus, bronchoconstriction, and airway irritants
- Activity intolerance due to fatigue, ineffective breathing patterns, and hypoxemia
- Deficient knowledge of self-care strategies to be performed at home.
- Ineffective coping related to reduced socialization, anxiety, depression, lower activity level, and the inability to work

COLLABORATIVE PROBLEMS/POTENTIAL COMPLICATIONS

Based on the assessment data, potential complications that may develop include:

- Respiratory insufficiency or failure
- Atelectasis
- Pulmonary infection
- Pneumonia
- Pneumothorax
- Pulmonary hypertension

Planning and Goals

The major goals for the patient may include smoking cessation, improved gas exchange, airway clearance, improved breathing pattern, improved activity tolerance, maximal self-management, improved coping ability, adherence to the therapeutic program and home care, and absence of complications.

Nursing Interventions

PROMOTING SMOKING CESSATION

Because smoking has such a detrimental effect on the lungs, the nurse must discuss smoking cessation strategies with patients. Although patients may believe that it is too late to reverse the damage from years of smoking and that smoking cessation is futile, they should be informed that continuing to smoke impairs the mechanisms that clear the airways and keep them free of irritants. The nurse should educate the patient regarding the hazards of smoking and cessation strategies and provide resources regarding smoking cessation, counseling, and formalized programs available in the community.

IMPROVING GAS EXCHANGE

Bronchospasm, which occurs in many pulmonary diseases, reduces the caliber of the small bronchi and may cause dyspnea, static secretions, and infection. Bronchospasm can sometimes be detected when wheezing or diminished breath sounds are heard on auscultation with a stethoscope. Increased mucus production, along with decreased mucociliary action, contributes to further reduction in the caliber of the bronchi and results in decreased airflow and decreased gas exchange. This is further aggravated by the loss of lung elasticity that occurs with COPD (NIH, 2001).

These changes in the airway require that the nurse monitor the patient for dyspnea and hypoxemia. If bronchodilators or corticosteroids are prescribed, the nurse must administer the medications properly and be alert for potential side effects. The relief of bronchospasm is confirmed by measuring improvement in expiratory flow rates and volumes (the force of expiration, how long it takes to exhale, and the amount of air exhaled) and assessing whether the patient has less dyspnea.

ACHIEVING AIRWAY CLEARANCE

Diminishing the quantity and viscosity of sputum can clear the airway and improve pulmonary ventilation and gas exchange. All pulmonary irritants should be eliminated or reduced, particularly cigarette smoking, which is the most persistent source of pulmonary irritation. The nurse instructs the patient in directed or controlled coughing, which is more effective and reduces the fatigue associated with undirected forceful coughing. Directed coughing consists of a slow, maximal inspiration followed by breath-holding for several seconds and then two or three coughs. "Huff" coughing may also be effective. The technique consists of one or two forced exhalations ("huffs") from low to medium lung volumes with the glottis open.

Chest physiotherapy with postural drainage, intermittent positive-pressure breathing, increased fluid intake, and bland aerosol mists (with normal saline solution or water) may be useful for some patients with COPD. The use of these measures must be based on the patient's response and tolerance.

IMPROVING BREATHING PATTERNS

Ineffective breathing patterns and shortness of breath are due to the ineffective respiratory mechanics of the chest wall and lung resulting from **air trapping**, ineffective diaphragmatic movement, airway obstruction, the metabolic cost of breathing, and stress. Inspiratory muscle training and breathing retraining may help to improve breathing patterns. Training in diaphragmatic breathing reduces the respiratory rate, increases alveolar ventilation, and sometimes helps expel as much air as possible during expiration. Pursed-lip breathing helps to slow expiration, prevents collapse of small airways, and helps the patient to control the rate and depth of respiration. It also promotes relaxation, which enables the patient to gain control of dyspnea and reduce feelings of panic.

IMPROVING ACTIVITY TOLERANCE

Patients with COPD experience progressive activity and exercise intolerance. Education is focused on rehabilitative therapies to promote independence in executing activities of daily living. These may include pacing activities throughout the day or using supportive devices to decrease energy expenditure. The nurse evaluates the patient's activity tolerance and limitations and teaching strategies to promote independent activities of daily living. Also, the patient may be a candidate for exercise training to strengthen the muscles of the upper and lower extremities and improve exercise tolerance and endurance. Other health care professionals (rehabilitation therapy, occupational therapy, physical therapy) may be consulted as additional resources.

ENHANCING SELF-CARE STRATEGIES

In addition to a pulmonary rehabilitation program, the nurse helps the patient manage self-care by emphasizing the importance of setting realistic goals, avoiding temperature extremes, and modifying lifestyle (particularly stopping smoking) as applicable.

Setting Realistic Goals

A major area of teaching is the importance of setting and accepting realistic short-term and long-range goals. If the patient is severely disabled, the objectives of treatment are to preserve current pulmonary function and relieve symptoms as much as possible. If the disease is mild, the objectives are to increase exercise tolerance and prevent further loss of pulmonary function. It is important to plan and share the goals and expectations of treatment with the patient. The patient and those providing care need patience to achieve these goals.

Avoiding Temperature Extremes

The nurse instructs the patient to avoid extremes of heat and cold. Heat increases the body temperature, thereby raising oxygen requirements; cold tends to promote bronchospasm. Air pollutants such as fumes, smoke, dust, and even talcum, lint, and aerosol sprays may initiate bronchospasm. High altitudes aggravate hypoxemia.

Modifying Lifestyle

Patients with COPD should adopt a lifestyle of moderate activity, ideally in a climate with minimal shifts in temperature and humidity. As much as possible, the patient should avoid emotional disturbances and stressful situations that might trigger a coughing episode. The medication regimen for patients with COPD can be quite complex; patients receiving aerosol medications by an MDI may be particularly challenged. It is crucial to review this material and to have the patient perform a return demonstration before discharge, during follow-up visits to the caregiver's office or clinic, and during home visits (Chart 24-4).

Smoking cessation goes hand in hand with lifestyle changes, and reinforcement of the patient's efforts is a key nursing activity. Smoking cessation is the single most important therapeutic intervention for patients with COPD. There are many strategies, including prevention, cessation with or without oral or topical patch medications, and behavior modification techniques.

ENHANCING INDIVIDUAL COPING STRATEGIES

COPD and its progression promote a cycle of physical, social, and psychological consequences, all which are interrelated. Patients experience depression, altered mood states, social isolation, and altered functional status. The nurse is key to identifying this cycle and promoting interventions for improved physical functioning, psychological and emotional stability, and social support. Following the initial assessment of the patient, the nurse may provide referrals to health care professionals in these specific areas.

MONITORING AND MANAGING POTENTIAL COMPLICATIONS

The nurse caring for the patient with COPD must assess for various complications, such as life-threatening respiratory insufficiency and failure and respiratory infection and atelectasis, which may increase the patient's risk for respiratory failure. The nurse also monitors for cognitive changes (personality and behavioral changes, memory impairment), increasing dyspnea, tachypnea, and tachycardia, which may indicate increasing hypoxemia and impending respiratory failure.

The nurse monitors pulse oximetry values to assess the patient's need for oxygen and administers supplemental oxygen as prescribed. The nurse also instructs the patient about signs and symptoms of respiratory infection that may worsen hypoxemia and reports changes in the patient's physical and cognitive status to the physician. Other activities require assisting with the management of developing complications, with possible intubation and mechanical ventilation (see Chap. 25).

Bronchopulmonary infections must be controlled to diminish inflammatory edema and to permit recovery of normal ciliary action. Minor respiratory infections that are of no consequence to the person with normal lungs can be life-threatening to the person with COPD. The cough associated with bronchial infection introduces a vicious cycle with further trauma and damage to the lungs, progression of symptoms, increased bronchospasm, and increased susceptibility to bronchial infection. Infection compromises lung

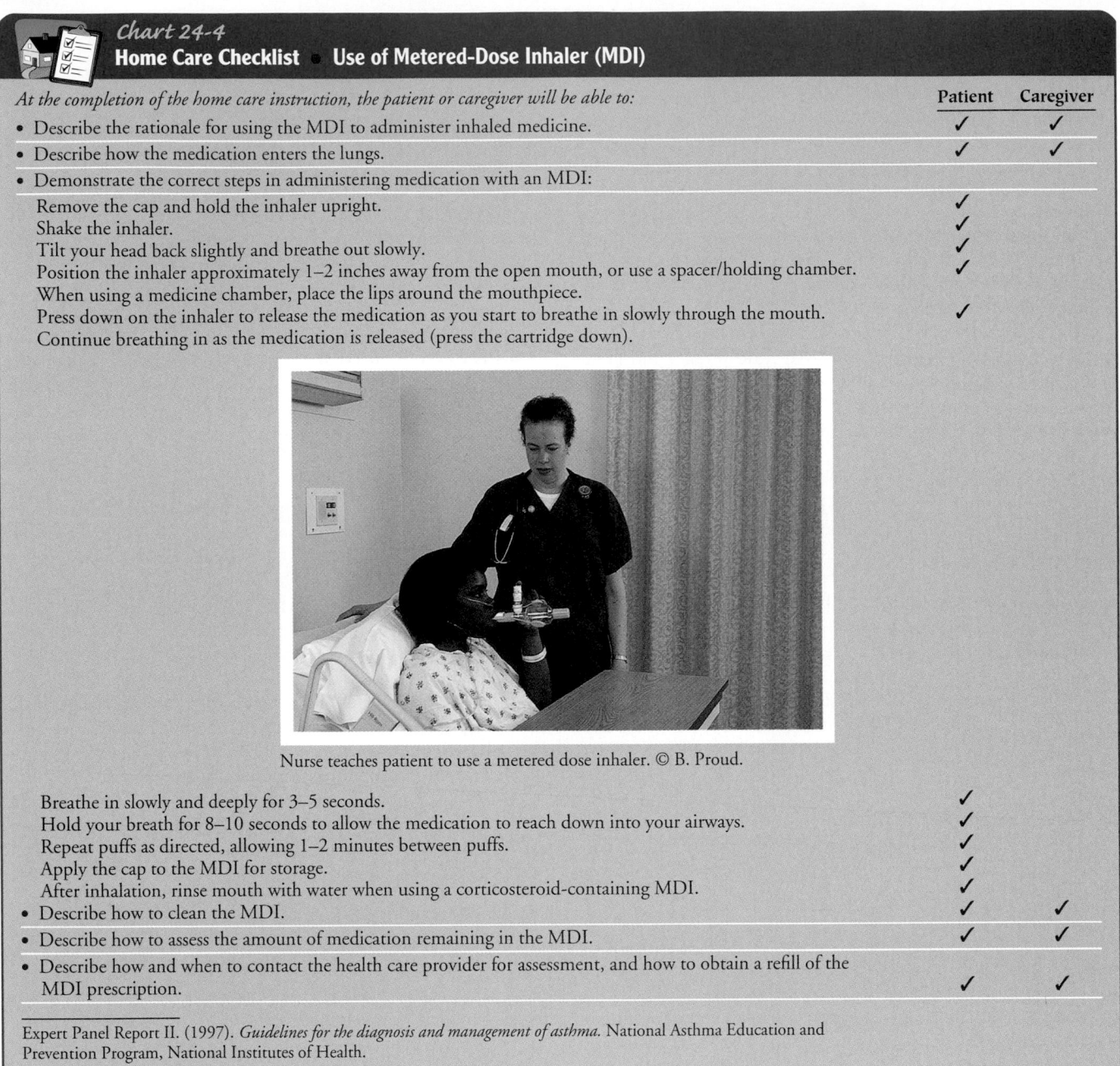

Chart 24-4

Home Care Checklist ● **Use of Metered-Dose Inhaler (MDI)**

At the completion of the home care instruction, the patient or caregiver will be able to:	Patient	Caregiver
● Describe the rationale for using the MDI to administer inhaled medicine.	✓	✓
● Describe how the medication enters the lungs.	✓	✓
● Demonstrate the correct steps in administering medication with an MDI:		
Remove the cap and hold the inhaler upright.	✓	
Shake the inhaler.	✓	
Tilt your head back slightly and breathe out slowly.	✓	
Position the inhaler approximately 1–2 inches away from the open mouth, or use a spacer/holding chamber.	✓	
When using a medicine chamber, place the lips around the mouthpiece.		
Press down on the inhaler to release the medication as you start to breathe in slowly through the mouth.	✓	
Continue breathing in as the medication is released (press the cartridge down).		

Nurse teaches patient to use a metered dose inhaler. © B. Proud.

	Patient	Caregiver
Breathe in slowly and deeply for 3–5 seconds.	✓	
Hold your breath for 8–10 seconds to allow the medication to reach down into your airways.	✓	
Repeat puffs as directed, allowing 1–2 minutes between puffs.	✓	
Apply the cap to the MDI for storage.	✓	
After inhalation, rinse mouth with water when using a corticosteroid-containing MDI.	✓	
● Describe how to clean the MDI.	✓	✓
● Describe how to assess the amount of medication remaining in the MDI.	✓	✓
● Describe how and when to contact the health care provider for assessment, and how to obtain a refill of the MDI prescription.	✓	✓

Expert Panel Report II. (1997). *Guidelines for the diagnosis and management of asthma.* National Asthma Education and Prevention Program, National Institutes of Health.

function and is a common cause of respiratory failure in patients with COPD.

In COPD, infection may be accompanied by subtle changes. The nurse instructs the patient to report any signs of infection, such as a fever or change in sputum color, character, consistency, or amount. Any worsening of symptoms (increased tightness of the chest, increased dyspnea and fatigue) also suggests infection and must be reported. Viral infections are hazardous to these patients because they are often followed by infections caused by bacterial organisms, such as *Streptococcus pneumoniae* and *Haemophilus influenzae.*

The nurse should encourage patients with COPD to be immunized against influenza and *S. pneumoniae* because these patients are prone to respiratory infection. It is important to caution patients to avoid going outdoors if the pollen count is high or if there is significant air pollution because of the risk of bron-

chospasm. The patient also should avoid exposure to high outdoor temperatures with high humidity.

Pneumothorax is a potential complication of COPD. Patients with severe emphysematous changes can develop large bullae, which may rupture and cause a pneumothorax. The development of a pneumothorax may be spontaneous or related to an activity such as severe coughing or large intrathoracic pressure changes. If the patient develops a rapid onset of shortness of breath, the nurse should quickly evaluate the patient for a potential pneumothorax by assessing the symmetry of chest movement, differences in breath sounds, and pulse oximetry. A pneumothorax is a life-threatening event in the patient with COPD who has minimal pulmonary reserve.

Over time, pulmonary hypertension may occur as a result of chronic hypoxemia. The pulmonary arteries respond to hypoxemia by constriction, thus leading to pulmonary hypertension.

The complication may be prevented by maintaining adequate oxygenation through an adequate hemoglobin level, improved ventilation/perfusion of the lungs, or continuous administration of supplemental oxygen (if needed).

PROMOTING HOME AND COMMUNITY-BASED CARE

Teaching Patients Self-Care

Teaching is essential throughout the course of COPD and should be part of the nursing care given to every patient with COPD. Patients' and family members' knowledge and comfort level with their knowledge should be assessed and considered when providing instructions about self-management strategies. In addition to the aspects of patient education previously described, patients and family members must become familiar with the medications that are prescribed and knowledgeable about potential side effects. Patients and family members need to learn the early signs and symptoms of infection and other complications so that they seek appropriate health care promptly.

Continuing Care

Referral for home care is important to enable the nurse to assess the patient's home environment and physical and psychological status, to evaluate the patient's adherence to the prescribed regimen, and to assess the patient's ability to cope with changes in lifestyle and physical status. The nurse assesses the patient's and family's understanding of the complications and side effects of medications. The home care visit provides an opportunity to reinforce the information and activities learned in the inpatient or outpatient pulmonary rehabilitation program and to have the patient and family demonstrate correct administration of medications and oxygen, if indicated, and performance of exercises. If the patient does not have access to a formal pulmonary rehabilitation program, it is important for the nurse to provide the education and breathing retraining necessary to optimize the patient's functional status.

The nurse may direct patients to community resources such as pulmonary rehabilitation programs and smoking cessation programs to help improve their ability to cope with their chronic condition and the therapeutic regimen and to give them a sense of worth, hope, and well-being. In addition, the nurse reminds the patient and family about the importance of participating in general health promotion activities and health screening.

Evaluation

EXPECTED PATIENT OUTCOMES

Expected patient outcomes may include:

1. Demonstrates knowledge of hazards of smoking
   a. Verbalizes willingness/interest to quit smoking
   b. Verbalizes information about smoking, risks of continuing, benefits of quitting, and techniques to optimize cessation efforts
2. Demonstrates improved gas exchange
   a. Shows no signs of restlessness, confusion, or agitation
   b. Has stable pulse oximetry or arterial blood gas values (but not necessarily normal values due to chronic changes in the gas exchange ability of the lungs)
3. Achieves maximal airway clearance
   a. Stops smoking
   b. Avoids noxious substances and extremes of temperature
   c. Maintains adequate hydration
   d. If indicated, performs postural drainage correctly

   e. Knows signs of early infection and is aware of how and when to report them if they occur
   f. Performs controlled coughing without experiencing excessive fatigue
4. Improves breathing pattern
   a. Practices and uses pursed-lip and diaphragmatic breathing
   b. Shows signs of decreased respiratory effort (decreased respiratory rate, less dyspnea)
5. Demonstrates knowledge of strategies to improve activity tolerance and maintain maximum level of self-care
   a. Performs self-care activities within tolerance range
   b. Paces self to avoid fatigue and dyspnea
   c. Uses controlled breathing while performing activities
   d. Uses devices to assist with activity tolerance and decrease energy expenditure
6. Demonstrates knowledge of self-care strategies
   a. Participates in determining the therapeutic program
   b. Understands the rationale for activities and medications
   c. Follows the medication plan
   d. Uses bronchodilators and oxygen therapy as prescribed
   e. Stops smoking
   f. Maintains acceptable activity level
7. Uses effective coping mechanisms for dealing with consequences of disease
   a. Uses self-care strategies to lessen stress associated with disease
   b. Verbalizes resources available to deal with psychological burden of disease
   c. Participates in pulmonary rehabilitation, if appropriate
8. Uses community resources and home-based care
   a. Verbalizes knowledge of community resources (eg, smoking cessation, hospital/community-based support groups)
   b. Participates in pulmonary rehabilitation, if appropriate
9. Avoids or reduces complications
   a. Has no evidence of respiratory failure or insufficiency
   b. Maintains adequate pulse oximetry and arterial blood gas values
   c. Shows no signs or symptoms of infection, pneumothorax, or pulmonary hypertension

For more information, see Plan of Nursing Care: Care of the Patient With COPD.

Bronchiectasis

Bronchiectasis is a chronic, irreversible dilation of the bronchi and bronchioles. Under the new definition of COPD, it is considered a separate disease process from COPD (NIH, 2001). Bronchiectasis may be caused by a variety of conditions, including:

- Airway obstruction
- Diffuse airway injury
- Pulmonary infections and obstruction of the bronchus or complications of long-term pulmonary infections
- Genetic disorders such as cystic fibrosis
- Abnormal host defense (eg, ciliary dyskinesia or humoral immunodeficiency)
- Idiopathic causes

(text continues on page 586)

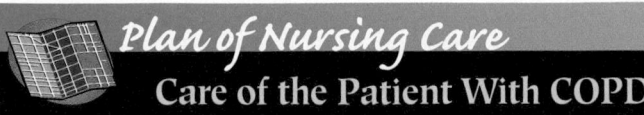

Plan of Nursing Care
Care of the Patient With COPD

Nursing Interventions	Rationale	Expected Outcomes

Nursing Diagnosis: Impaired gas exchange and airway clearance due to chronic inhalation of toxins
Goal: Improvement in gas exchange

Nursing Interventions	Rationale	Expected Outcomes

1. Evaluate current smoking status, educate regarding smoking cessation, and facilitate efforts to quit.
  a. Evaluate current smoking habits of patient and family.
  b. Educate regarding hazards of smoking and relationship to COPD.
  c. Evaluate previous smoking cessation attempts.
  d. Provide educational materials.
  e. Refer to a smoking cessation program or resource.
2. Evaluate current exposure to occupational exposures and indoor/outdoor pollution.
  a. Evaluate current exposures to occupational toxins, indoor and outdoor air pollution (eg, smog, toxic fumes, chemicals).
  b. Emphasize primary prevention to occupational exposures. This is best achieved by elimination or reduction of exposures in the workplace.
  c. Educate regarding types of indoor and outdoor air pollution (eg, biomass fuel burned for cooking and heating in poorly ventilated buildings, outdoor air pollution).
  d. Advise patient to monitor public announcements regarding air quality.
	1. Smoking causes permanent damage to the lung and diminishes the lungs' protective mechanisms. Airflow is obstructed, secretions are increased, and lung capacity is reduced. Continued smoking increases morbidity and mortality in COPD and is also a risk factor for lung cancer.
	
	2. Chronic inhalation of both indoor and outdoor toxins causes damage to the airways and impairs gas exchange.
		• Identifies the hazards of cigarette smoking
		• Enrolls in smoking cessation program
		• Reports success in stopping smoking
		• Identifies resources for smoking cessation
		• Verbalizes types of inhaled toxins
		• Minimizes or eliminates exposures
		• Monitors public announcements regarding air quality and minimizes or eliminates exposures during episodes of severe pollution

Nursing Diagnosis: Impaired gas exchange related to ventilation–perfusion inequality
Goal: Improvement in gas exchange

Nursing Interventions	Rationale	Expected Outcomes

1. Administer bronchodilators as prescribed:
  a. Inhalation is the preferred route.
  b. Observe for side effects: tachycardia, dysrhythmias, central nervous system excitation, nausea, and vomiting.
  c. Assess for correct technique of metered-dose inhaler (MDI) administration.
2. Evaluate effectiveness of nebulizer or MDI treatments.
  a. Assess for decreased shortness of breath, decreased wheezing or crackles, loosened secretions, decreased anxiety.
  b. Ensure that treatment is given before meals to avoid nausea and to reduce fatigue that accompanies eating.
3. Instruct and encourage patient in diaphragmatic breathing and effective coughing.
	1. Bronchodilators dilate the airways. The medication dosage is carefully adjusted for each patient, in accordance with clinical response.
	
	2. Combining medication with aerosolized bronchodilators is typically used to control bronchoconstriction in an acute exacerbation. Generally, however, the MDI with spacer is the preferred route (less cost and time to treatment).
	
	3. These techniques improve ventilation by opening airways to facilitate clearing the airways of sputum. Gas exchange is improved and fatigue is minimized.
		• Verbalizes need for bronchodilators and for taking as prescribed
		• Evidences minimal side effects; heart rate near normal, absence of dysrhythmias, normal mentation
		• Reports a decrease in dyspnea
		• Shows an improved expiratory flow rate
		• Uses and cleans respiratory therapy equipment as applicable
		• Demonstrates diaphragmatic breathing and coughing
		• Uses oxygen equipment appropriately when indicated
		• Evidences improved arterial blood gases or pulse oximetry
		• Demonstrates correct technique for use of MDI

(continued)

Plan of Nursing Care

Care of the Patient With COPD (Continued)

Nursing Interventions	Rationale	Expected Outcomes

4. Administer oxygen by the method prescribed.
  a. Explain rationale and importance to patient.
  b. Evaluate effectiveness; observe for signs of hypoxemia. Notify physician if restlessness, anxiety, somnolence, cyanosis, or tachycardia is present.
  c. Analyze arterial blood gases and compare with baseline values. When arterial puncture is performed and a blood sample is obtained, hold puncture site for 5 minutes to prevent arterial bleeding and development of ecchymoses.
  d. Initiate pulse oximetry to monitor oxygen saturation.
  e. Explain that no smoking is permitted by patient or visitors while oxygen is in use.
	4. Oxygen will correct the hypoxemia. Careful observation of the liter flow or the percentage administered and its effect on the patient is important. If the patient has chronic CO_2 retention, excessive oxygen could suppress the hypoxic drive and respirations. These patients generally need low-flow oxygen rates of 1 to 2 L/min. Periodic arterial blood gases and pulse oximetry help to evaluate adequacy of oxygenation. Smoking may render pulse oximetry inaccurate because the carbon monoxide from cigarette smoke also saturates hemoglobin.	

Nursing Diagnosis: Ineffective airway clearance related to bronchoconstriction, increased mucus production, ineffective cough, bronchopulmonary infection, and other complications

Goal: Achievement of airway clearance

1. Adequately hydrate the patient.	1. Systemic hydration keeps secretions moist and easier to expectorate. Fluids must be given with caution if right- or left-sided heart failure is present.	• Verbalizes need to drink fluids • Demonstrates diaphragmatic breathing and coughing • Performs postural drainage correctly • Coughing is minimized • Does not smoke • Verbalizes that pollens, fumes, gases, dusts, and extremes of temperature and humidity are irritants to be avoided • Identifies signs of early infection • Is free of infection (no fever, no change in sputum, lessening of dyspnea) • Verbalizes need to notify health care provider at the earliest sign of infection • Verbalizes need to stay away from crowds or people with colds in flu season • Discusses flu and pneumonia vaccines with clinician to help prevent infection
2. Teach and encourage the use of diaphragmatic breathing and coughing techniques.	2. These techniques help to improve ventilation and mobilize secretions without causing breathlessness and fatigue.	
3. Assist in administering nebulizer or MDI.	3. This ensures adequate delivery of medication to the airways.	
4. If indicated, perform postural drainage with percussion and vibration in the morning and at night as prescribed.	4. Uses gravity to help raise secretions so they can be more easily expectorated or suctioned.	
5. Instruct patient to avoid bronchial irritants such as cigarette smoke, aerosols, extremes of temperature, and fumes.	5. Bronchial irritants cause bronchoconstriction and increased mucus production, which then interferes with airway clearance.	

6. Teach early signs of infection that are to be reported to the clinician immediately:
  a. Increased sputum production
  b. Change in color of sputum
  c. Increased thickness of sputum
  d. Increased shortness of breath, tightness in chest, or fatigue
  e. Increased coughing
  f. Fever or chills
	6. Minor respiratory infections that are of no consequence to the person with normal lungs can produce fatal disturbances in the lungs of the person with emphysema. Early recognition is crucial.	

7. Administer antibiotics as prescribed.	7. Antibiotics may be prescribed to prevent or treat infection.	
8. Encourage patient to be immunized against influenza and *Streptococcus pneumoniae*.	8. People with respiratory conditions are prone to respiratory infections and are encouraged to be immunized.	

(continued)

Plan of Nursing Care
Care of the Patient With COPD (Continued)

Nursing Interventions	Rationale	Expected Outcomes
Nursing Diagnosis: Ineffective breathing pattern related to shortness of breath, mucus, bronchoconstriction, and airway irritants **Goal:** Improvement in breathing pattern		
1. Teach patient diaphragmatic and pursed-lip breathing.	1. Helps patient prolong expiration time and decreases air trapping. With these techniques, patient will breathe more efficiently and effectively.	• Practices pursed-lip and diaphragmatic breathing and uses them when short of breath and with activity • Shows signs of decreased respiratory effort and paces activities • Uses inspiratory muscle trainer as prescribed
2. Encourage alternating activity with rest periods. Allow patient to make some decisions (bath, shaving) about care based on tolerance level.	2. Pacing activities permits patient to perform activities without excessive distress.	
3. Encourage use of an inspiratory muscle trainer if prescribed.	3. Strengthens and conditions the respiratory muscles.	
Nursing Diagnosis: Self-care deficits related to fatigue secondary to increased work of breathing and insufficient ventilation and oxygenation **Goal:** Independence in self-care activities		
1. Teach patient to coordinate diaphragmatic breathing with activity (eg, walking, bending).	1. This will allow the patient to be more active and to avoid excessive fatigue or dyspnea during activity.	• Uses controlled breathing while bathing, bending, and walking • Paces activities of daily living to alternate with rest periods to reduce fatigue and dyspnea
2. Encourage patient to begin to bathe self, dress self, walk, and drink fluids. Discuss energy conservation measures.	2. As condition resolves, patient will be able to do more but needs to be encouraged to avoid increasing dependence.	• Describes energy conservation strategies • Performs same self-care activities as before • Performs postural drainage correctly
3. Teach postural drainage if appropriate.	3. Encourages patient to become involved in own care. Prepares patient to manage at home.	
Nursing Diagnosis: Activity intolerance due to fatigue, hypoxemia, and ineffective breathing patterns **Goal:** Improvement in activity tolerance		

1. Support patient in establishing a regular regimen of exercise using treadmill and exercycle, walking, or other appropriate exercises, such as mall walking.
  a. Assess the patient's current level of functioning and develop exercise plan based on baseline functional status.
  b. Suggest consultation with a physical therapist or pulmonary rehabilitation program to determine an exercise program specific to the patient's capability. Have portable oxygen unit available if oxygen is prescribed for exercise.
	1. Muscles that are deconditioned consume more oxygen and place an additional burden on the lungs. Through regular, graded exercise, these muscle groups become more conditioned, and the patient can do more without getting as short of breath. Graded exercise breaks the cycle of debilitation.	• Performs activities with less shortness of breath
		• Verbalizes need to exercise daily and demonstrates an exercise plan to be carried out at home
		• Walks and gradually increases walking time and distance to improve physical condition
		• Exercises both upper and lower body muscle groups

Nursing Diagnosis: Ineffective coping related to reduced socialization, anxiety, depression, lower activity level, and the inability to work **Goal:** Attainment of an optimal level of coping		
1. Help the patient develop realistic goals.	1. Developing realistic goals will promote a sense of hope and accomplishment rather than defeat and hopelessness.	• Expresses interest in the future • Participates in the discharge plan • Discusses activities or methods that can be performed to ease shortness of breath
2. Encourage activity to level of symptom tolerance.	2. Activity reduces tension and decreases degree of dyspnea as patient becomes conditioned.	• Uses relaxation techniques appropriately • Expresses interest in a pulmonary rehabilitation program

(continued)

Plan of Nursing Care

Care of the Patient With COPD (*Continued*)

Nursing Interventions	Rationale	Expected Outcomes
3. Teach relaxation technique or provide a relaxation tape for patient. 4. Enroll patient in pulmonary rehabilitation program where available.	3. Relaxation reduces stress, anxiety, and dyspnea and helps patient to cope with disability. 4. Pulmonary rehabilitation programs have been shown to promote a subjective improvement in a patient's status and self-esteem as well as increased exercise tolerance and decreased hospitalizations.	

Nursing Diagnosis: Deficient knowledge about self-management to be performed at home.
Goal: Adherence to therapeutic program and home care

Nursing Interventions	Rationale	Expected Outcomes

1. Help patient understand short- and long-term goals.
  a. Teach the patient about disease, medications, procedures, and how and when to seek help.
  b. Refer patient to pulmonary rehabilitation.
2. Give strong message to stop smoking. Discuss smoking cessation strategies. Provide information about resource groups (eg, SmokEnders, American Cancer Society, American Lung Association).
	1. Patient needs to be a partner in developing the plan of care and needs to know what to expect. Teaching about the condition is one of the most important aspects of care; it will prepare the patient to live and cope with the condition and improve quality of life.
	2. Smoking causes permanent damage to the lung and diminishes the lungs' protective mechanisms. Air flow is obstructed and lung capacity is reduced. Smoking increases morbidity and mortality and is also a risk factor for lung cancer.
		• Understands disease and what affects it
		• Verbalizes the need to preserve existing lung function by adhering to the prescribed program
		• Understands purposes and proper administration of medications
		• Stops smoking or enrolls in a smoking cessation program
		• Identifies when and whom to call for assistance

Collaborative Problem: Atelectasis
Goal: Absence of atelectasis on x-ray and physical examination

Nursing Interventions	Rationale	Expected Outcomes
1. Monitor respiratory status, including rate and pattern of respirations, breath sounds, signs and symptoms of respiratory distress, and pulse oximetry. 2. Instruct in and encourage diaphragmatic breathing and effective coughing techniques. 3. Promote use of lung expansion techniques (eg, deep-breathing exercises, incentive spirometry) as prescribed.	1. A change in respiratory status, including tachypnea, dyspnea, and diminished or absent breath sounds, may indicate atelectasis. 2. These techniques improve ventilation and lung expansion and ideally improve gas exchange. 3. Deep-breathing exercises and incentive spirometry promote maximal lung expansion.	• Normal (baseline for patient) respiratory rate and pattern • Normal breath sounds for patient • Demonstrates diaphragmatic breathing and effective coughing • Performs deep-breathing exercises, incentive spirometry as prescribed • Pulse oximetry is ≥ 90%

Collaborative Problem: Pneumothorax
Goal: Absence of signs and symptoms of pneumothorax

Nursing Interventions	Rationale	Expected Outcomes
1. Monitor respiratory status, including rate and pattern of respirations, symmetry of chest wall movement, breath sounds, signs and symptoms of respiratory distress, and pulse oximetry. 2. Assess pulse. 3. Assess for chest pain and precipitating factors. 4. Palpate for tracheal deviation/shift away from the affected side.	1. Dyspnea, tachypnea, tachycardia, acute pleuritic chest pain, tracheal deviation away from the affected side, absence of breath sounds on the affected side, and decreased tactile fremitus may indicate pneumothorax. 2. Tachycardia is associated with pneumothorax and anxiety. 3. Pain may accompany pneumothorax. 4. Early detection of pneumothorax and prompt intervention will prevent other serious complications.	• Normal respiratory rate and pattern for patient • Normal breath sounds bilaterally • Normal pulse for patient • Normal tactile fremitus • Absence of pain • Tracheal position is midline • Pulse oximetry ≥ 90% • Maintains normal oxygen saturation and arterial blood gas measurements for patient • Exhibits no hypoxemia and hypercapnia (or returns to baseline values)

(continued)

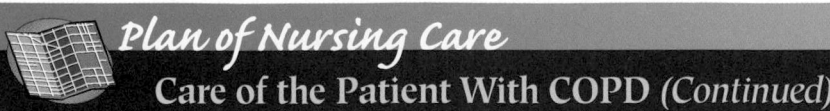

Plan of Nursing Care
Care of the Patient With COPD (Continued)

Nursing Interventions	Rationale	Expected Outcomes
5. Monitor pulse oximetry and if indicated arterial blood gases.	5. Recognition of a deterioration in respiratory function will prevent serious complications.	• Absence of pain • Symmetric chest wall movement • Lung is reexpanded on chest x-ray • Breath sounds are heard on the affected side
6. Administer supplemental oxygen therapy, as indicated.	6. Oxygen will correct hypoxemia; administer it with caution.	
7. Administer analgesics, as indicated, for chest pain.	7. Pain interferes with deep breathing, resulting in a decrease in lung expansion.	
8. Assist with chest tube insertion and use pleural drainage system, as prescribed.	8. Removal of air from the pleural space will reexpand the lung.	

Collaborative Problem: Respiratory failure
Goal: Absence of signs and symptoms of respiratory failure; no evidence of respiratory failure on laboratory tests

1. Monitor respiratory status, including rate and pattern of respirations, breath sounds, and signs and symptoms of acute respiratory distress.	1. Early recognition of a deterioration in respiratory function will avert further complications, such as respiratory failure, severe hypoxemia, and hypercapnia.	• Normal respiratory rate and pattern for patient with no acute distress • Recognizes symptoms of hypoxemia and hypercapnia • Maintains normal arterial blood gases/pulse oximetry or returns to baseline values
2. Monitor pulse oximetry and arterial blood gases.	2. Recognition of changes in oxygenation and acid–base balance will guide in correcting and preventing complications.	
3. Administer supplemental oxygen and initiate mechanisms for mechanical ventilation, as prescribed.	3. Acute respiratory failure is a medical emergency. Hypoxemia is a hallmark sign. Administration of oxygen therapy and mechanical ventilation (if indicated) are critical to survival.	

Collaborative Problem: Pulmonary hypertension
Goal: Absence of evidence of pulmonary hypertension on physical examination or laboratory tests

1. Monitor respiratory status, including rate and pattern of respirations, breath sounds, pulse oximetry, and signs and symptoms of acute respiratory distress.	1. Dyspnea is the primary symptom of pulmonary hypertension. Other symptoms include fatigue, angina, near syncope, edema, and palpitations.	• Normal respiratory rate and pattern for patient • Exhibits no signs and symptoms of right-sided failure • Maintains baseline pulse oximetry values and arterial blood gases
2. Assess for signs and symptoms of right-sided heart failure, including peripheral edema, ascites, distended neck veins, crackles, and heart murmur.	2. Right-sided heart failure is a common clinical manifestation of pulmonary hypertension due to increased right ventricular workload.	
3. Administer oxygen therapy, as prescribed.	3. Continuous oxygen therapy is a major component of management of pulmonary hypertension by preventing hypoxemia and thereby reducing pulmonary vascular constriction (resistance) secondary to hypoxemia.	

A person may be predisposed to bronchiectasis as a result of recurrent respiratory infections in early childhood, measles, influenza, tuberculosis, and immunodeficiency disorders.

Pathophysiology

The inflammatory process associated with pulmonary infections damages the bronchial wall, causing a loss of its supporting structure and resulting in thick sputum that ultimately obstructs the bronchi. The walls become permanently distended and distorted, impairing mucociliary clearance. The inflammation and infection extend to the peribronchial tissues; in the case of saccular bronchiectasis, each dilated tube virtually amounts to a lung abscess, the exudate of which drains freely through the bronchus. Bronchiectasis is usually localized, affecting a segment or lobe of a lung, most frequently the lower lobes.

The retention of secretions and subsequent obstruction ultimately cause the alveoli distal to the obstruction to collapse (atelectasis). Inflammatory scarring or fibrosis replaces functioning lung tissue. In time the patient develops respiratory insufficiency with reduced vital capacity, decreased ventilation, and an increased ratio of residual volume to total lung capacity. There is impairment in the matching of ventilation to perfusion (ventilation–perfusion imbalance) and hypoxemia.

Clinical Manifestations

Characteristic symptoms of bronchiectasis include chronic cough and the production of purulent sputum in copious amounts. Many patients with this disease have hemoptysis. Clubbing of the fingers also is common because of respiratory insufficiency. The patient usually has repeated episodes of pulmonary infection. Even with modern treatment approaches, the average age at death is approximately 55 years.

Assessment and Diagnostic Findings

Bronchiectasis is not readily diagnosed because the symptoms can be mistaken for those of simple chronic bronchitis. A definite sign is offered by the prolonged history of productive cough, with sputum consistently negative for tubercle bacilli. The diagnosis is established by a computed tomography (CT) scan, which demonstrates either the presence or absence of bronchial dilation.

Medical Management

Treatment objectives are to promote bronchial drainage to clear excessive secretions from the affected portion of the lungs and to prevent or control infection. Postural drainage is part of all treatment plans because draining the bronchiectatic areas by gravity reduces the amount of secretions and the degree of infection. Sometimes mucopurulent sputum must be removed by bronchoscopy. Chest physiotherapy, including percussion and postural drainage, is important in secretion management.

Smoking cessation is important because smoking impairs bronchial drainage by paralyzing ciliary action, increasing bronchial secretions, and causing inflammation of the mucous membranes, resulting in hyperplasia of the mucous glands. Infection is controlled with antimicrobial therapy based on the results of sensitivity studies on organisms cultured from sputum. A year-round regimen of antibiotic agents may be prescribed, with different types of antibiotics at intervals. Some clinicians prescribe antibiotic agents throughout the winter or when acute upper respiratory tract infections occur. Patients should be vaccinated against influenza and pneumococcal pneumonia. Bronchodilators, which may be prescribed for patients who also have reactive airway disease, may also assist with secretion management.

Surgical intervention, although used infrequently, may be indicated for the patient who continues to expectorate large amounts of sputum and has repeated bouts of pneumonia and hemoptysis despite adhering to the treatment regimen. However, the disease must involve only one or two areas of the lung that can be removed without producing respiratory insufficiency. The goals of surgical treatment are to conserve normal pulmonary tissue and to avoid infectious complications. Diseased tissue is removed, provided that the postoperative lung function will be adequate. It may be necessary to remove a segment of a lobe (segmental resection), a lobe (lobectomy), or rarely an entire lung (pneumonectomy). (See Chart 25-16 for further information.) Segmental resection is the removal of an anatomic subdivision of a pulmonary lobe. The chief advantage is that only diseased tissue is removed and healthy lung tissue is conserved.

The surgery is preceded by a period of careful preparation. The objective is to obtain a dry (free of infection) tracheobronchial tree to prevent complications (atelectasis, pneumonia, bronchopleural fistula, and empyema). This is accomplished by postural drainage or, depending on the location, by direct suction through a bronchoscope. A course of antibacterial therapy may be prescribed. After surgery, the care is the same as for any patient undergoing chest surgery (see Chap. 25).

Nursing Management

Nursing management of the patient with bronchiectasis focuses on alleviating symptoms and assisting the patient to clear pulmonary secretions. Smoking and other factors that increase the production of mucus and hamper its removal are targeted in patient teaching. The patient and family are taught to perform postural drainage and to avoid exposure to others with upper respiratory and other infections. If the patient experiences fatigue and dyspnea, strategies to conserve energy while maintaining as active a lifestyle as possible are discussed. The patient needs to become knowledgeable about early signs of respiratory infection and the progression of the disorder so that appropriate treatment can be implemented promptly. Because the presence of a large amount of mucus may decrease the patient's appetite and result in an inadequate dietary intake, the patient's nutritional status is assessed and strategies are implemented to ensure an adequate diet.

Asthma

Asthma is a chronic inflammatory disease of the airways that causes airway hyperresponsiveness, mucosal edema, and mucus production. This inflammation ultimately leads to recurrent episodes of asthma symptoms: cough, chest tightness, wheezing, and dyspnea (Fig. 24-6). Estimates show that nearly 17 million Americans have asthma, and more than 5,000 die from this disease annually (Centers for Disease Control and Prevention [CDC], 1998; CDC, 1999; NCHS, 2001). In 1998, asthma accounted for over 13.9 million outpatient visits to physician offices or hospital clinics and over 2.0 million emergency room visits (NCHS, 2001).

Asthma differs from the other obstructive lung diseases in that it is largely reversible, either spontaneously or with treatment. Patients with asthma may experience symptom-free periods alternating with acute exacerbations, which last from minutes to hours or days. Asthma can occur at any age and is the most common chronic disease of childhood. Despite increased knowledge regarding the pathology of asthma and the development of better medications and management plans, the death rate from asthma continues to increase. For most patients it is a disruptive disease, affecting school and work attendance, occupational choices, physical activity, and general quality of life.

Allergy is the strongest predisposing factor for asthma. Chronic exposure to airway irritants or allergens also increases the risk for developing asthma. Common allergens can be seasonal (eg, grass, tree, and weed pollens) or perennial (eg, mold, dust, roaches, or animal dander). Common triggers for asthma symptoms and exacerbations in patients with asthma include airway irritants (eg, air pollutants, cold, heat, weather changes, strong odors or perfumes, smoke), exercise, stress or emotional upsets, sinusitis with postnasal drip, medications, viral respiratory tract infections, and gastroesophageal reflux. Most people who have asthma are sensitive to a variety of triggers. A patient's asthma condition will change depending upon the environment, activities, management practices, and other factors (NHLBI, 1998).

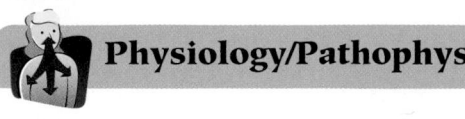

Physiology/Pathophysiology

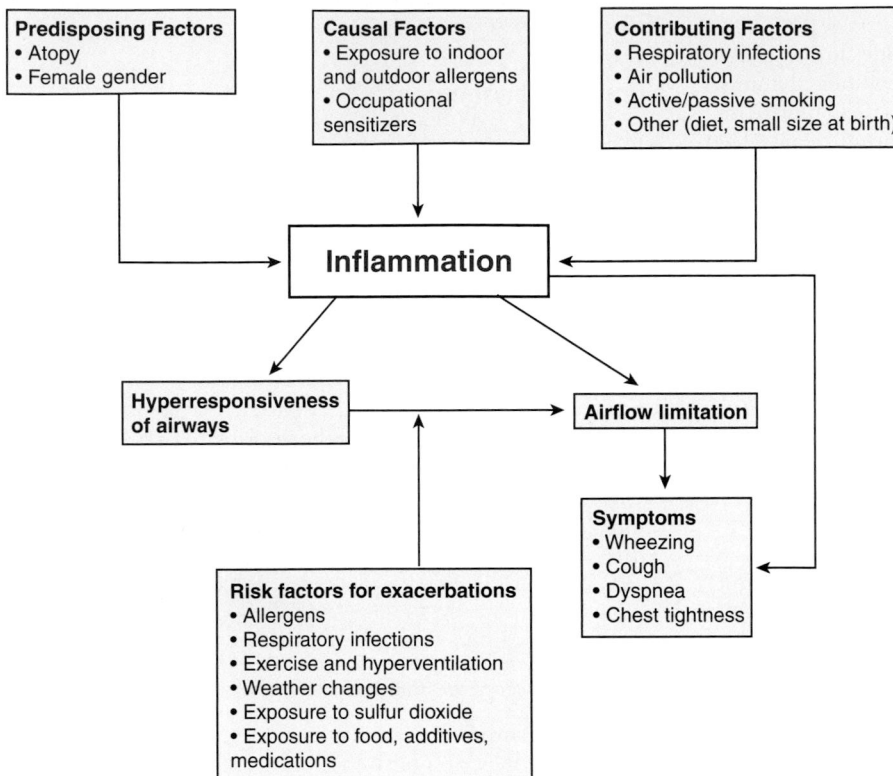

Predisposing Factors
• Atopy
• Female gender

Causal Factors
• Exposure to indoor and outdoor allergens
• Occupational sensitizers

Contributing Factors
• Respiratory infections
• Air pollution
• Active/passive smoking
• Other (diet, small size at birth)

Inflammation

Hyperresponsiveness of airways

Airflow limitation

Symptoms
• Wheezing
• Cough
• Dyspnea
• Chest tightness

Risk factors for exacerbations
• Allergens
• Respiratory infections
• Exercise and hyperventilation
• Weather changes
• Exposure to sulfur dioxide
• Exposure to food, additives, medications

FIGURE 24-6 Pathophysiology of asthma. Adapted from materials developed for the Global Initiative for Asthma (GINA): Global Strategy for Asthma Management and Prevention, National Institutes of Health–National Heart, Lung, and Blood Institute, revised 2002.

Pathophysiology

The underlying pathology in asthma is reversible and diffuse airway inflammation. The inflammation leads to obstruction from the following: swelling of the membranes that line the airways (mucosal edema), reducing the airway diameter; contraction of the bronchial smooth muscle that encircles the airways (bronchospasm), causing further narrowing; and increased mucus production, which diminishes airway size and may entirely plug the bronchi.

The bronchial muscles and mucus glands enlarge; thick, tenacious sputum is produced; and the alveoli hyperinflate. Some patients may have airway subbasement membrane fibrosis. This is called airway "remodeling" and occurs in response to chronic inflammation. The fibrotic changes in the airway lead to airway narrowing and potentially irreversible airflow limitation (NIH, 2001; NHLBI, 1998).

Cells that play a key role in the inflammation of asthma are mast cells, neutrophils, eosinophils, and lymphocytes. Mast cells, when activated, release several chemicals called mediators. These chemicals, which include histamine, bradykinin, prostaglandins, and leukotrienes, perpetuate the inflammatory response, causing increased blood flow, vasoconstriction, fluid leak from the vasculature, attraction of white blood cells to the area, and bronchoconstriction (NHLBI, 1998). Regulation of these chemicals is the aim of much of the current research regarding pharmacologic therapy for asthma.

Further, alpha- and beta₂-adrenergic receptors of the sympathetic nervous system are located in the bronchi. When the alpha-adrenergic receptors are stimulated, bronchoconstriction occurs; when the beta₂-adrenergic receptors are stimulated, bronchodila-

tion results. The balance between alpha and beta₂ receptors is controlled primarily by cyclic adenosine monophosphate (cAMP). Alpha-adrenergic receptor stimulation results in a decrease in cAMP, which leads to an increase of chemical mediators released by the mast cells and bronchoconstriction. Beta₂-receptor stimulation results in increased levels of cAMP, which inhibits the release of chemical mediators and causes bronchodilation (NHLBI, 1998).

Clinical Manifestations

The three most common symptoms of asthma are cough, dyspnea, and wheezing. In some instances, cough may be the only symptom. Asthma attacks often occur at night or early in the morning, possibly due to circadian variations that influence airway receptor thresholds.

An asthma exacerbation may begin abruptly but most frequently is preceded by increasing symptoms over the previous few days. There is cough, with or without mucus production. At times the mucus is so tightly wedged in the narrowed airway that the patient cannot cough it up. There may be generalized wheezing (the sound of airflow through narrowed airways), first on expiration and then possibly during inspiration as well. Generalized chest tightness and dyspnea occur. Expiration requires effort and becomes prolonged. As the exacerbation progresses, diaphoresis, tachycardia, and a widened pulse pressure may occur along with hypoxemia and central cyanosis (a late sign of poor oxygenation). Although life-threatening and severe hypoxemia can occur in asthma, it is relatively uncommon. The hypoxemia is secondary to a ventilation–perfusion mismatch and readily responds to supplemental oxygenation.

Symptoms of exercise-induced asthma include maximal symptoms during exercise, absence of nocturnal symptoms, and sometimes only a description of a "choking" sensation during exercise.

Asthma is categorized according to symptoms and objective measures of airflow obstruction (Table 24-3) (Expert Panel Report II, 1997).

Assessment and Diagnostic Findings

A complete family, environmental, and occupational history is essential. To establish the diagnosis, the clinician must determine that periodic symptoms of airflow obstruction are present, airflow is at least partially reversible, and other etiologies have been excluded. A positive family history and environmental factors, including seasonal changes, high pollen counts, mold, climate changes (particularly cold air), and air pollution, are primarily associated with asthma. In addition, asthma is associated with a variety of occupation-related chemicals and compounds, including metal salts, wood and vegetable dust, medications (eg, aspirin, antibiotics, piperazine, cimetidine), industrial chemicals and plastics, biologic enzymes (eg, laundry detergents), animal and insect dusts, sera, and secretions. Comorbid conditions that may accompany asthma include gastroesophageal reflux, drug-induced asthma, and allergic bronchopulmonary aspergillosis. Other possible allergic reactions that may accompany asthma include eczema, rashes, and temporary edema.

During acute episodes, sputum and blood tests may disclose eosinophilia (elevated levels of eosinophils). Serum levels of immunoglobulin E may be elevated if allergy is present. Arterial blood gas analysis and pulse oximetry reveal hypoxemia during acute attacks. Initially, hypocapnia and respiratory alkalosis are present. As the condition worsens and the patient becomes more fatigued, the $PaCO_2$ may rise. A normal $PaCO_2$ value may be a signal of impending respiratory failure. Because CO_2 is 20 times more diffusible than oxygen, it is rare for $PaCO_2$ to be normal or elevated in a person who is breathing very rapidly. During an exacerbation, the FEV_1 and FVC are markedly decreased but improve with bronchodilator administration (demonstrating reversibility). Pulmonary function is usually normal between exacerbations.

The occurrence of a severe, continuous reaction is referred to as status asthmaticus and is considered life-threatening (see below).

Prevention

Patients with recurrent asthma should undergo tests to identify the substances that precipitate the symptoms. Possible causes are dust, dust mites, roaches, certain types of cloth, pets, horses, detergents, soaps, certain foods, molds, and pollens. If the attacks are seasonal, pollens can be strongly suspected. The patient is instructed to avoid the causative agents whenever possible.

Knowledge is the key to quality asthma care. Although national guidelines are available for the care of the asthma patient, unfortunately health care providers may not follow them. Failure to follow the guidelines in the following areas has been noted: lack of treatment of patients who have symptoms more than 2 days per week with a regular medication schedule, lack of patient-specific advice on improving the environment and an explanation about the importance of doing so, lack of encouragement for patients to monitor their peak flow measurements with a diary, and lack of written, up-to-date educational materials (Plaut, 2001).

A 1998 survey by a group called "Asthma in America" found that 11% of physicians were unaware of the national asthma guidelines. Only 35% of patients with asthma who were surveyed reported having pulmonary function testing in the past year.

While 83% of physicians reported prescribing peak flow meter monitoring, only 62% of patients had ever heard of a peak flow meter (Rickard & Stempel, 1999). All health care providers caring for asthma patients need to be aware of the national guidelines and use them (Expert Panel Report II, 1997).

Complications

Complications of asthma may include status asthmaticus, respiratory failure, pneumonia, and atelectasis. Airway obstruction, particularly during acute asthmatic episodes, often results in hypoxemia, requiring the administration of oxygen and the monitoring of pulse oximetry and arterial blood gases. Fluids are administered because people with asthma are frequently dehydrated from diaphoresis and insensible fluid loss with hyperventilation.

Medical Management

Immediate intervention is necessary because the continuing and progressive dyspnea leads to increased anxiety, aggravating the situation.

PHARMACOLOGIC THERAPY

Two general classes of asthma medications are long-acting medications to achieve and maintain control of persistent asthma and quick-relief medications for immediate treatment of asthma symptoms and exacerbations (Table 24-4). Because the underlying pathology of asthma is inflammation, control of persistent asthma is accomplished primarily with regular use of anti-inflammatory medications. These medications have systemic side effects when used long term. The route of choice for administration of these medications is the MDI because it allows for topical administration. Critical to the success of inhaled therapy is the proper use of the MDI (see Chart 24-4). If the patient has difficulty with this procedure, the use of a spacer device is indicated. Table 24-3 presents a stepwise approach for managing asthma (Expert Panel Report II, 1997). Information on use of the MDI and spacer device is given in the previous section on COPD.

Long-Acting Control Medications. Corticosteroids are the most potent and effective anti-inflammatory medications currently available. They are broadly effective in alleviating symptoms, improving airway function, and decreasing peak flow variability. Initially, the inhaled form is used. A spacer should be used with inhaled corticosteroids and the patient should rinse the mouth after administration to prevent thrush, a common complication of inhaled corticosteroid use. A systemic preparation may be used to gain rapid control of the disease; to manage severe, persistent asthma; to treat moderate to severe exacerbations; to accelerate recovery; and to prevent recurrence (Dhand, 2000).

Cromolyn sodium (Intal) and nedocromil (Tilade) are mild to moderate anti-inflammatory agents that are used more commonly in children. They are also effective on a prophylactic basis to prevent exercise-induced asthma or in unavoidable exposure to known triggers. These medications are contraindicated in acute asthma exacerbations.

Long-acting beta$_2$-adrenergic agonists are used with anti-inflammatory medications to control asthma symptoms, particularly those that occur during the night. These agents are also effective for preventing exercise-induced asthma. Long-acting beta$_2$-adrenergic agonists are not indicated for immediate relief of symptoms.

(text continues on page 592)

Table 24-3 • Stepwise Approach for Managing Asthma in Adults and Children Over 5 Years Old

Goals of Asthma Treatment
- Prevent chronic and troublesome symptoms (eg, coughing or breathlessness in the night, in the early morning, or after exertion)
- Maintain near-normal pulmonary function
- Maintain normal activity levels (including exercise and other physical activity)

- Prevent recurrent exacerbations of asthma and minimize the need for emergency department visits or hospitalizations
- Provide optimal pharmacotherapy with minimal or no adverse effects
- Meet patients' and families' expectation of and satisfaction with asthma care

	SYMPTOMS**	NIGHTTIME SYMPTOMS	LUNG FUNCTION	LONG-TERM CONTROL	QUICK RELIEF	EDUCATION
STEP 4 Severe Persistent*	• Continual symptoms • Limited physical activity • Frequent exacerbations	Frequent	• FEV_1 or PEF ≤60% predicted • PEF variability >30%	Daily medications: • Anti-inflammatory: inhaled corticosteroid (high dose) AND • Long-acting bronchodilator: either long-acting inhaled beta₂-agonist, sustained-release theophylline, or long-acting beta₂-agonist tablets AND • Corticosteroid tablets or syrup long term (2 mg/kg/day, generally do not exceed 60 mg per day).	• Short-acting bronchodilator: inhaled beta₂-agonists as needed for symptoms. • Intensity of treatment will depend on severity of exacerbation. • Use of short-acting inhaled beta₂-agonists on a daily basis, or increasing use, indicates the need for additional long-term control therapy.	Steps 2 and 3 actions plus: • Refer to individual education/counseling
STEP 3 Moderate Persistent	• Daily symptoms • Daily use of inhaled short-acting beta₂-agonist • Exacerbations affect activity • Exacerbations ≥2 times a week; may last days	>1 time a week	• FEV_1 or PEF 60% to 80% predicted • PEF variability >30%	Daily medication: • Either – Anti-inflammatory: inhaled corticosteroid (medium dose) OR – Inhaled corticosteroid (low–medium dose) and add a long-acting bronchodilator, especially for nighttime symptoms; either long-acting inhaled beta₂-agonist, sustained-release theophylline, or long-acting beta₂-agonist tablets. • If needed – Anti-inflammatory: inhaled corticosteroids (medium–high dose) AND – Long-acting bronchodilator, especially for nighttime symptoms; either long-acting inhaled beta₂-agonist, sustained-release theophylline, or long-acting beta₂-agonist tablets.	• Short-acting bronchodilator: inhaled beta₂-agonists as needed for symptoms. • Intensity of treatment will depend on severity of exacerbation. • Use of short-acting inhaled beta₂-agonists on a daily basis, or increasing use, indicates the need for additional long-term control therapy.	Step 1 actions plus: • Teach self-monitoring • Refer to group education if available • Review and update self-management plan
STEP 2 Mild Persistent	• Symptoms >2 times a week but <1 time a day • Exacerbations may affect activity	>2 times a month	• FEV_1 or PEF ≥80% predicted • PEF variability 20%–30%	Daily medication: • Anti-inflammatory: either inhaled corticosteroid (low doses) or cromolyn or nedocromil (children usually begin with a trial of cromolyn or nedocromil).	• Short-acting bronchodilator: inhaled beta₂-agonists as needed for symptoms. • Intensity of treatment will depend on severity of exacerbation.	Step 1 actions plus: • Teach self-monitoring • Refer to group education if available

(continued)

Table 24-3 • **Stepwise Approach for Managing Asthma in Adults and Children Over 5 Years Old** (Continued)

	SYMPTOMS**	NIGHTTIME SYMPTOMS	LUNG FUNCTION	LONG-TERM CONTROL	QUICK RELIEF	EDUCATION
				• Sustained-release theophylline to serum concentration of 5–15 µg/mL is an alternative. Zafirlukast or zileuton may also be considered for patients ≥12 years of age, although their position in therapy is not fully established.	• Use of short-acting inhaled beta₂-agonists on a daily basis, or increasing use, indicates the need for additional long-term-control therapy.	• Review and update self-management plan
STEP 1 Mild Intermittent	• Symptoms ≤2 times a week • Asymptomatic and normal PEF between exacerbations • Exacerbations brief (from a few hours to a few days); intensity may vary	≤2 times a month	• FEV₁ or PEF ≥80% predicted • PEF variability <20%	• No daily medication needed.	• Short-acting bronchodilator: inhaled beta₂-agonists as needed for symptoms. • Intensity of treatment will depend on severity of exacerbation. • Use of short-acting inhaled beta₂-agonists more than 2 times a week may indicate the need to initiate long-term control therapy.	• Teach basic facts about asthma • Teach inhaler/spacer/holding chamber technique • Discuss roles of medications • Develop self-management plan • Develop action plan for when and how to take rescue actions • Discuss appropriate environmental control measures to avoid exposure to known allergens and irritants

↓*Step Down*
Review treatment every 1 to 6 months; a gradual stepwise reduction in treatment may be possible.

Notes:
• The stepwise approach presents general guidelines to assist clinical decision making; it is not intended to be a specific prescription. Asthma is highly variable; clinicians should tailor specific medication plans to the needs and circumstances of individual patients.
• Gain control as quickly as possible; then decrease treatment to the least medication necessary to maintain control. Gaining control may be accomplished either by starting treatment at the step most appropriate to the initial severity of the condition or by starting at a higher level of therapy (eg, a course of systemic corticosteroids or higher dose of inhaled corticosteroids).

↑ *Step Up*
If control is not maintained, consider step up. First, review patient medication technique, adherence, and environmental control (avoidance of allergens or other factors that contribute to asthma severity).
• A rescue course of systemic corticosteroid may be needed at any time and at any step.
• Some patients with intermittent asthma experience severe and life-threatening exacerbations separated by long periods of normal lung function and no symptoms. This may be especially common with exacerbations provoked by respiratory infections. A short course of systemic corticosteroids is recommended.
• At each step, patients should control their environment to avoid or control factors that make their asthma worse (eg, allergens, irritants); this requires specific diagnosis and education.

PEF, peak expiratory flow
*The presence of one of the features of severity is sufficient to place a patient in that category. An individual should be assigned to the most severe grade in which any feature occurs. The characteristics noted in this table are general and may overlap because asthma is highly variable. Furthermore, an individual's classification may change over time.
**Patients at any level of severity can have mild, moderate, or severe exacerbations. Some patients with intermittent asthma experience severe and life-threatening exacerbations separated by long periods of normal lung function and no symptoms.
Highlights of the Expert Panel Report 2. (1997). *Guidelines for the diagnosis and management of asthma.* National Institutes of Health, National Heart, Lung and Blood Institute, NIH Publication No 97-4051A, p. 29.

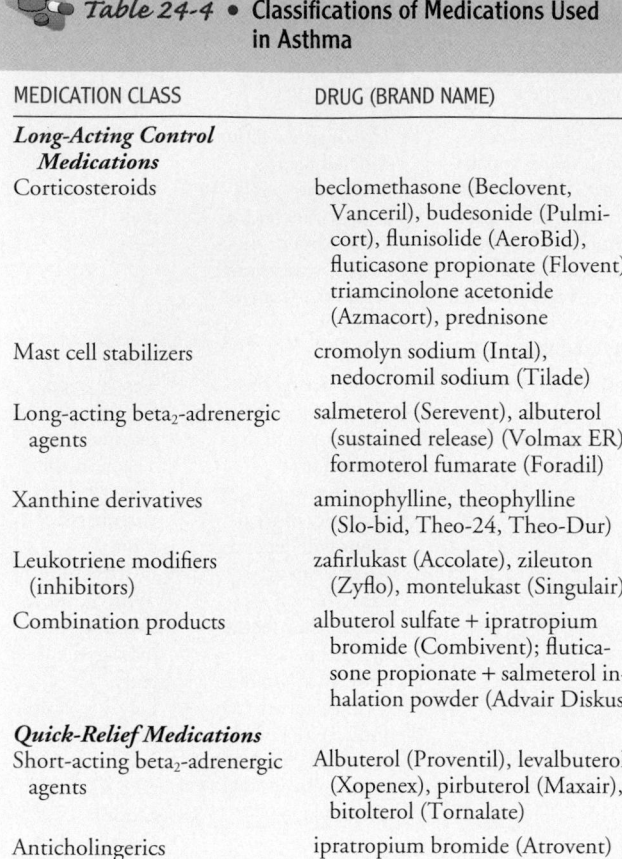

Table 24-4 • Classifications of Medications Used in Asthma

MEDICATION CLASS	DRUG (BRAND NAME)
Long-Acting Control Medications	
Corticosteroids	beclomethasone (Beclovent, Vanceril), budesonide (Pulmicort), flunisolide (AeroBid), fluticasone propionate (Flovent), triamcinolone acetonide (Azmacort), prednisone
Mast cell stabilizers	cromolyn sodium (Intal), nedocromil sodium (Tilade)
Long-acting beta$_2$-adrenergic agents	salmeterol (Serevent), albuterol (sustained release) (Volmax ER), formoterol fumarate (Foradil)
Xanthine derivatives	aminophylline, theophylline (Slo-bid, Theo-24, Theo-Dur)
Leukotriene modifiers (inhibitors)	zafirlukast (Accolate), zileuton (Zyflo), montelukast (Singulair)
Combination products	albuterol sulfate + ipratropium bromide (Combivent); fluticasone propionate + salmeterol inhalation powder (Advair Diskus)
Quick-Relief Medications	
Short-acting beta$_2$-adrenergic agents	Albuterol (Proventil), levalbuterol (Xopenex), pirbuterol (Maxair), bitolterol (Tornalate)
Anticholingerics	ipratropium bromide (Atrovent)

Expert Panel Report II. (1997). *Guidelines for the diagnosis and management of asthma.* National Asthma Education and Prevention Program, National Institutes of Health.

Methylxanthines (theophylline [Slo-bid, Theo-24, Theo-Dur]) are mild to moderate bronchodilators usually used in addition to inhaled corticosteroids, mainly for relief of nighttime asthma symptoms. There is some evidence that theophylline may have a mild anti-inflammatory effect (NHLBI, 1998).

Leukotriene modifiers (inhibitors) or antileukotrienes are a new class of medications. Leukotrienes are potent bronchoconstrictors that also dilate blood vessels and alter permeability. Leukotriene inhibitors act by either interfering with leukotriene synthesis or blocking the receptors where leukotrienes exert their action (Boushey, Fick, Lazarus & Martin, 2000). At this time, they may provide an alternative to inhaled corticosteroids for mild persistent asthma or may be added to a regimen of inhaled corticosteroids in more severe asthma to attain further control.

In addition, combination products are also available (eg, albuterol/ipratropium [Combivent]) and offer ease of use for the patient.

Quick-Relief Medications. Short-acting beta-adrenergic agonists are the medications of choice for relieving acute symptoms and preventing exercise-induced asthma. They have a rapid onset of action. Anticholinergics (eg, ipratropium bromide [Atrovent]) may bring added benefit in severe exacerbations, but they are used more frequently in COPD patients.

MANAGEMENT OF ASTHMA EXACERBATION

Asthma exacerbations are best managed by early treatment and education of the patient (Expert Panel Report II, 1997). Quick-acting beta-adrenergic medications are first used for prompt re-

lief of airflow obstruction. Systemic corticosteroids may be necessary to decrease airway inflammation in patients who fail to respond to inhaled beta-adrenergic medications. In some patients, oxygen supplementation may be required to relieve hypoxemia associated with a moderate to severe exacerbation (Expert Panel Report II, 1997). Also, response to treatment may be monitored by serial measurements of lung function.

A written action plan is the most useful tool for the patient (Fig. 24-7). This helps to guide the patient in self-management strategies regarding an exacerbation and also provides instructions regarding recognition of early warning signs of worsening asthma. Patient self-management and early recognition of problems lead to more efficient communication with health care providers regarding an asthma exacerbation (Expert Panel Report II, 1997).

PEAK FLOW MONITORING

Peak flow meters measure the highest airflow during a forced expiration (Fig. 24-8). Daily peak flow monitoring is recommended for all patients with moderate or severe asthma because it helps measure asthma severity and, when added to symptom monitoring, indicates the current degree of asthma control. The patient is instructed in the proper technique, particularly to give maximal effort. The "personal best" is determined after monitoring peak flows for 2 or 3 weeks after receiving optimal asthma therapy. The green (80% to 100% of personal best), yellow (60% to 80%), and red (less than 60%) zones are determined, and specific actions are delineated for each zone, enabling the patient to monitor and manipulate his or her own therapy after careful instruction (Expert Panel Report II, 1997). This reinforces compliance, independence, and self-efficacy (Reinke, 2000).

Nursing Management

The immediate nursing care of the patient with asthma depends on the severity of the symptoms. The patient may be treated successfully as an outpatient if asthma symptoms are relatively mild, or he or she may require hospitalization and intensive care for acute and severe asthma.

The patient and family are often frightened and anxious because of the patient's dyspnea. Thus, an important aspect of care is a calm approach. The nurse assesses the patient's respiratory status by monitoring the severity of symptoms, breath sounds, peak flow, pulse oximetry, and vital signs. The nurse obtains a history of allergic reactions to medications before administering medications and identifies the patient's current use of medications. The nurse administers medications as prescribed and monitors the patient's responses to those medications. Fluids may be administered if the patient is dehydrated, and antibiotic agents may be prescribed if the patient has an underlying respiratory infection. If the patient requires intubation because of acute respiratory failure, the nurse assists with the intubation procedure, continues close monitoring of the patient, and keeps the patient and family informed about procedures.

PROMOTING HOME AND COMMUNITY-BASED CARE

Teaching Patients Self-Care. A major challenge is to implement basic asthma management principles at the community level (Reinke, 2000). Key issues include education of health care providers, establishment of programs for asthma education (for patients and providers), use of outpatient follow-up care for patients, and a focus on chronic management versus acute episodic care. The nurse is pivotal to achieving all of these objectives.

ASTHMA ACTION PLAN FOR _____

Doctor's Name _____ Date _____

Doctor's Phone Number _____ Hospital/Emergency Room Phone Number _____

GREEN ZONE: Doing Well

- No cough, wheeze, chest tightness, or shortness of breath during the day or night
- Can do usual activities

And, if a peak flow meter is used,
Peak flow: more than _____
(80% or more of my best peak flow)

My best peak flow is: _____

Take These Long-Term-Control Medicines Each Day (include an anti-inflammatory)

Medicine	How much to take	When to take it

| Before exercise | ☐ | ☐ 2 or ☐ 4 puffs | 5 to 60 minutes before exercise |

YELLOW ZONE: Asthma Is Getting Worse

- Cough, wheeze, chest tightness, or shortness of breath, or
- Waking at night due to asthma, or
- Can do some, but not all, usual activities

-Or-

Peak flow: _____ to _____
(50% - 80% of my best peak flow)

FIRST Add: Quick-Relief Medicine – and keep taking your GREEN ZONE medicine

_____ ☐ 2 or ☐ 4 puffs, every 20 minutes for up to 1 hour
(short-acting beta₂-agonist) ☐ Nebulizer, once

SECOND If your symptoms (and peak flow, if used) return to GREEN ZONE after 1 hour of above treatment:

- ☐ Take the quick-relief medicine every 4 hours for 1 to 2 days.
- ☐ Double the dose of your inhaled steroid for _____ (7-10) days.

-Or-

If your symptoms (and peak flow, if used) do not return to GREEN ZONE after 1 hour of above treatment:

- ☐ Take: _____ ☐ 2 or ☐ 4 puffs or ☐ Nebulizer
  (short-acting beta₂-agonist)
- ☐ Add: _____ _____ mg. per day For _____ (3-10) days
  (oral steroid)
- ☐ Call the doctor ☐ before/ ☐ within _____ hours after taking the oral steroid.

RED ZONE: Medical Alert!

- Very short of breath, or
- Quick-relief medicines have not helped, or
- Cannot do usual activities, or
- Symptoms are same or get worse after 24 hours in Yellow Zone

-Or-

Peak flow: less than _____
(50% of my best peak flow)

Take this medicine:

☐ _____ ☐ 4 or ☐ 6 puffs or ☐ Nebulizer
(short-acting beta₂-agonist)

☐ _____ _____ mg.
(oral steroid)

Then call your doctor NOW. Go to the hospital or call for an ambulance if:

- You are still in the red zone after 15 minutes AND
- You have not reached your doctor.

DANGER SIGNS

- Trouble walking and talking due to shortness of breath
- Lips or fingernails are blue

■ Take ☐ 4 or ☐ 6 puffs of your quick-relief medicine AND
■ Go to the hospital or call for an ambulance (_____) NOW!

FIGURE 24-7 Asthma action plan. From *Facts about controlling asthma*, National Asthma Education and Prevention Program, National Heart, Lung, and Blood Institute. NIH Publication No. 97-2339.

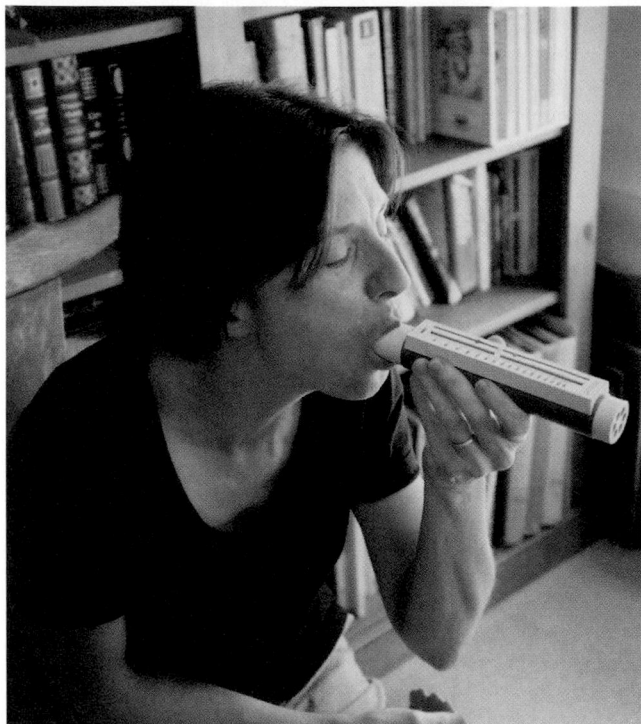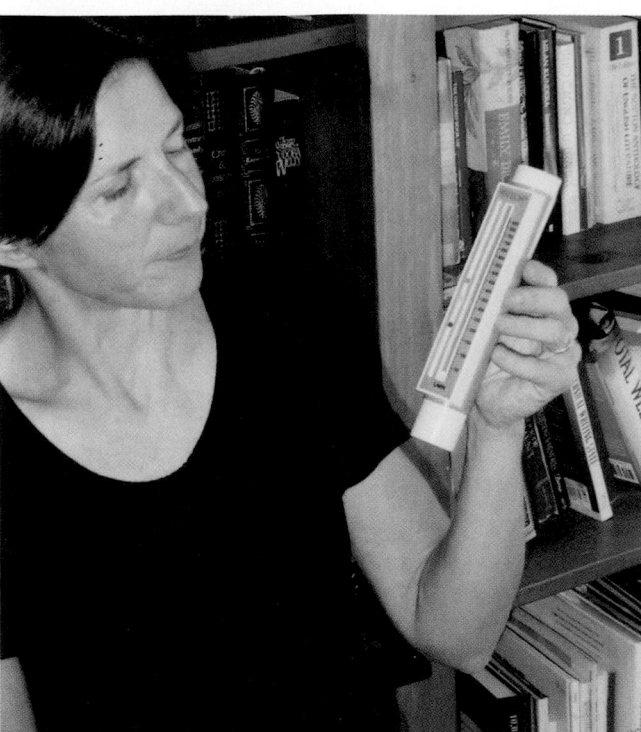

FIGURE 24-8 Peak flow meters measure the highest volume of air flow during a forced expiration (*left*). Volume is measured in color-coded zones (*right*): the green zone signifies 80% to 100% of personal best; yellow, 60% to 80%; and red, less than 60%. If peak flow falls below the red zone, the patient should take the appropriate actions prescribed by his or her health care provider.

Patient teaching is a critical component of care for the patient with asthma (Plaut, 2001). Multiple inhalers, different types of inhalers, antiallergy therapy, antireflux medications, and avoidance measures are all integral for long-term control. This complex therapy requires a patient–provider partnership to determine the desired outcomes and to formulate a plan to achieve those outcomes. The patient then carries out daily therapy as part of self-care management, with input and guidance by the health care provider. Before a partnership can be established, the patient needs to understand the following:

- The nature of asthma as a chronic inflammatory disease
- The definition of inflammation and bronchoconstriction
- The purpose and action of each medication
- Triggers to avoid, and how to do so
- Proper inhalation technique
- How to perform peak flow monitoring (Chart 24-5)
- How to implement an action plan
- When to seek assistance, and how to do so

An assortment of excellent educational materials is available from the Expert Panel Report II (1997) and the National Heart,

Chart 24-5
Home Care Checklist • Use of Peak Flow Meter

At the completion of the home care instruction, the patient or caregiver will be able to:	Patient	Caregiver
• Describe the rationale for using a peak flow meter in asthma management.	✓	✓
• Explain how peak flow monitoring is used along with symptoms to determine severity of asthma.	✓	✓
• Demonstrate steps for using the peak flow meter correctly:		
• Move the indicator to the bottom of the numbered scale.	✓	
• Stand up.	✓	
• Take a deep breath and fill the lungs completely.	✓	
• Place mouthpiece in mouth and close lips around mouthpiece (do not put tongue inside opening).	✓	
• Blow out hard and fast with a single blow.	✓	
• Record the number achieved on the indicator.	✓	
• Repeat steps 1–5 two more times and write the highest number in the asthma diary.	✓	
• Explain how to determine the "personal best" peak flow reading.	✓	✓
• Describe the significance of the color zones for peak flow monitoring.	✓	✓
• Demonstrate how to clean the peak flow meter.	✓	✓
• Discuss how and when to contact the health care provider about changes or decreases in peak flow values.	✓	✓

Lung and Blood Institute. The nurse should obtain current educational materials for the patient based on the patient's diagnosis, causative factors, educational level, and cultural factors.

Continuing Care. The nurse who has contact with the patient in the hospital, clinic, school, or office uses the opportunity to assess the patient's respiratory status and ability to manage self-care to prevent serious exacerbations. The nurse emphasizes adherence to the prescribed therapy, preventive measures, and the need to keep follow-up appointments with the primary health care provider. A home visit to assess the home environment for allergens may be indicated for the patient with recurrent exacerbations. The nurse refers the patient to community support groups. In addition, the nurse reminds the patient and family about the importance of health promotion strategies and recommended health screening.

STATUS ASTHMATICUS

Status asthmaticus is severe and persistent asthma that does not respond to conventional therapy. The attacks can last longer than 24 hours. Infection, anxiety, nebulizer abuse, dehydration, increased adrenergic blockage, and nonspecific irritants may contribute to these episodes. An acute episode may be precipitated by hypersensitivity to aspirin.

Pathophysiology

The basic characteristics of asthma (constriction of the bronchiolar smooth muscle, swelling of the bronchial mucosa, and thickened secretions) decrease the diameter of the bronchi and are apparent in status asthmaticus. A ventilation–perfusion abnormality results in hypoxemia and respiratory alkalosis initially, followed by respiratory acidosis. There is a reduced PaO_2 and an initial respiratory alkalosis, with a decreased $PaCO_2$ and an increased pH. As status asthmaticus worsens, the $PaCO_2$ increases and the pH falls, reflecting respiratory acidosis.

Clinical Manifestations

The clinical manifestations are the same as those seen in severe asthma: labored breathing, prolonged exhalation, engorged neck veins, and wheezing. However, the extent of wheezing does not indicate the severity of the attack. As the obstruction worsens, the wheezing may disappear, and this is frequently a sign of impending respiratory failure.

Assessment and Diagnostic Findings

Pulmonary function studies are the most accurate means of assessing acute airway obstruction. Arterial blood gas measurements are obtained if the patient cannot perform pulmonary function maneuvers because of severe obstruction or fatigue, or if the patient does not respond to treatment. Respiratory alkalosis (low $PaCO_2$) is the most common finding in patients with asthma. A rising $PaCO_2$ (to normal levels or levels indicating respiratory acidosis) frequently is a danger sign of impending respiratory failure.

Medical Management

In the emergency setting, the patient is treated initially with a short-acting beta-adrenergic agonist and corticosteroids. The patient usually requires supplemental oxygen and intravenous fluids for hydration. Oxygen therapy is initiated to treat dyspnea, central cyanosis, and hypoxemia. Humidified oxygen by either Venturi mask or nasal catheter is administered. The flow is based on pulse oximetry or arterial blood gas values. The PaO_2 is maintained at 65 to 85 mm Hg. Sedative medications are contraindicated. If there is no response to repeated treatments, hospitalization is required. Other criteria indicating the need for hospitalization include poor pulmonary function test results and deteriorating blood gas levels (respiratory acidosis), which may indicate that the patient is tiring and will require mechanical ventilation. Although most patients do not need mechanical ventilation, it is used for patients in respiratory failure, for those who tire and are too fatigued by the attempt to breathe, or for those whose conditions do not respond to initial treatment.

Death from asthma is associated with several risk factors, including the following:

- Past history of sudden and severe exacerbations
- Prior endotracheal intubation for asthma
- Prior admission to the intensive care unit for an asthma exacerbation
- Two or more hospitalizations for asthma within the past year
- Three or more emergency care visits for asthma in the past year
- Excessive use of short-acting beta-adrenergic inhalers (more than two canisters per month)
- Recent withdrawal from systemic corticosteroids
- Comorbidity of cardiovascular disease or COPD
- Psychiatric disease
- Low socioeconomic status
- Urban residence (Expert Panel Report II, 1997)

Nursing Management

The nurse constantly monitors the patient for the first 12 to 24 hours, or until status asthmaticus is under control. The nurse also assesses the patient's skin turgor to identify signs of dehydration. Fluid intake is essential to combat dehydration, to loosen secretions, and to facilitate expectoration. The nurse administers intravenous fluids as prescribed, up to 3 to 4 L/day, unless contraindicated. The patient's energy needs to be conserved, and the room should be quiet and free of respiratory irritants, including flowers, tobacco smoke, perfumes, or odors of cleaning agents. A nonallergenic pillow should be used.

Cystic Fibrosis

Cystic fibrosis (CF) is the most common fatal autosomal recessive disease among the Caucasian population. An individual must inherit a defective copy of the CF gene (one from each parent) to have CF. One in 31 Americans are unknowing symptom carriers of this gene (Katkin, 2002). The frequency of CF is 1 in 2,000 to 3,000 live births, and there are approximately 30,000 children and adults with this disease in the United States (Cystic Fibrosis Foundation, 2002). Although CF was once considered a fatal childhood disease, approximately 38% of people living with the disease are 18 years of age or older (Cystic Fibrosis Foundation, 2002). Cystic fibrosis is usually diagnosed in infancy or early childhood, but patients may be diagnosed later in life. For individuals diagnosed later in life, respiratory symptoms are frequently the major manifestation of the disease.

Pathophysiology

This disease is caused by mutations in the CF transmembrane conductance regulator protein, which is a chloride channel found in all exocrine tissues (Katkin, 2002). Chloride transport problems lead to thick, viscous secretions in the lungs, pancreas, liver, intestine, and reproductive tract as well as increased salt content in sweat gland secretions. In 1989, major breakthroughs were made in this disease with the identification of the CF gene. The ability to detect the common mutations of this gene allows for routine screening for this disease as well as the detection of carriers. Genetic counseling is an important part of health care for couples at risk.

Airflow obstruction is a key feature in the presentation of CF. This obstruction is due to bronchial plugging by purulent secretions, bronchial wall thickening due to inflammation, and, over time, airway destruction (Katkin, 2002). These chronic retained secretions in the airways set up an excellent reservoir for continued bronchial infections.

Clinical Manifestations

The pulmonary manifestations of this disease include a productive cough, wheezing, hyperinflation of the lung fields on chest x-ray, and pulmonary function test results consistent with obstructive airways disease (Katkin, 2002). Colonization of the airways with pathogenic bacteria usually occurs early in life. *Staphylococcus aureus* and *Haemophilus influenzae* are common organisms during early childhood. As the disease progresses, *Pseudomonas aeruginosa* is ultimately isolated from the sputum of most patients. Upper respiratory manifestations of the disease include sinusitis and nasal polyps.

Nonpulmonary clinical manifestations include gastrointestinal problems (eg, pancreatic insufficiency, recurrent abdominal pain, biliary cirrhosis, vitamin deficiencies, recurrent pancreatitis, weight loss), genitourinary problems (male and female infertility), and clubbing of the extremities. (See Chap. 40 for a discussion of pancreatitis.)

Assessment and Diagnostic Findings

Most of the time, the diagnosis of CF is made based on an elevated result of a sweat chloride concentration test, along with clinical signs and symptoms consistent with the disease. Repeated sweat chloride values of greater than 60 mEq/L distinguish most individuals with CF from those with other obstructive diseases. A molecular diagnosis may also be used in evaluating common genetic mutations of the CF gene.

Medical Management

Pulmonary problems remain the leading cause of morbidity and mortality in CF. Because chronic bacterial infection of the airways occurs in individuals with CF, control of infections is key in the treatment. Antibiotic medications are routinely prescribed for acute pulmonary exacerbations of the disease. Depending upon the severity of the exacerbation, aerosolized, oral, or intravenous antibiotic therapy may be used. Antibiotic agents are selected based upon the results of a sputum culture and sensitivity. Patients with CF have problems with bacteria that are resistant to multiple drugs and require multiple courses of antibiotic agents over long periods of time.

Bronchodilators are frequently administered to decrease airway obstruction. Differing pulmonary techniques are used to enhance secretion clearance. Examples include manual postural drainage and chest physical therapy, high-frequency chest wall oscillation, and other devices that assist in airway clearance (PEP masks [masks that generate positive expiratory pressure], "flutter devices" [devices that provide an oscillatory expiratory pressure pattern with positive expiratory pressure and assist with expectoration of secretions]).

Inhaled mucolytic agents such as dornase alfa (Pulmozyme) or N-acetylcysteine (Mucomyst) may also be used. These agents help to decrease the viscosity of the sputum and promote expectoration of secretions.

To decrease the inflammation and ongoing destruction of the airways, anti-inflammatory agents may also be used. These may include inhaled corticosteroids or systemic therapy. Other anti-inflammatory medications have also been studied in CF. Ibuprofen was studied in children with CF and some benefit was demonstrated, but there is little information on its use in young or older adults with CF (Katkin, 2002).

Supplemental oxygen is used to treat the progressive hypoxemia that occurs with CF. It helps to correct the hypoxemia and may minimize the complications seen with chronic hypoxemia (pulmonary hypertension).

Lung transplantation is an option for a small, select population of CF patients. A double lung transplant technique is used due to the chronically infected state of the lungs seen in end-stage CF. Because there is a long waiting list for lung transplant recipients, many patients die while awaiting a transplant.

Gene therapy is a promising approach to management, with many clinical trials underway. It is hoped that various methods of administering gene therapy will carry healthy genes to the damaged cells and correct defective CF cells. Efforts are underway to develop innovative methods of delivering therapy to the CF cells of the airways.

Nursing Management

Nursing care of the adult with CF includes assisting the patient to manage pulmonary symptoms and to prevent complications of CF. Specific nursing measures include strategies that promote removal of pulmonary secretions; chest physiotherapy, including postural drainage, chest percussion, and vibration, and breathing exercises are implemented and are taught to the patient and to the family when the patient is very young. The patient is reminded of the need to reduce risk factors associated with respiratory infections (eg, exposure to crowds and to persons with known infections). The patient is taught the early signs and symptoms of respiratory infection and disease progression that indicate the need to notify the primary health care provider.

The nurse emphasizes the importance of an adequate fluid and dietary intake to promote removal of secretions and to ensure an adequate nutritional status. Because CF is a life-long disorder, patients often have learned to modify their daily activities to accommodate their symptoms and treatment modalities. As the disease progresses, however, assessment of the home environment may be warranted to identify modifications required to address changes in the patient's needs, increasing dyspnea and fatigue, and nonpulmonary symptoms.

Although gene therapy and double lung transplantation are promising therapies for CF, they are limited in availability and largely experimental. As a result, the life expectancy of adults with CF is shortened. Therefore, end-of-life issues and concerns need to be addressed in patients when warranted. For the patient whose disease is progressing and who is developing increasing hypoxemia, preferences for end-of-life care should be discussed, documented, and honored (see Chap. 17). Patients and family members need support as they face a shortened life span and an uncertain future.

Critical Thinking Exercises

1. A 75-year-old woman with end-stage COPD was recently admitted to your unit from the emergency room. She cannot lie flat in bed, she is extremely short of breath, and she has decreased breath sounds throughout the chest and crackles in the posterior basilar areas. What is the pathophysiology associated with these findings? What medical and nursing interventions might be used to decrease or alleviate these signs/symptoms?

2. Your patient at an outpatient asthma clinic is a 35-year-old inner-city Mexican-American mother with asthma. Use of an MDI on a regular daily schedule has been repeatedly prescribed for her, but she reports that she does not use the MDI except as needed when extremely short of breath. Describe teaching techniques you might use to assess the patient's knowledge of the medication and provide education about the action of the MDI, frequency of use, and correct administration of the medication. What methods would you use to monitor use of the MDI and reinforce education?

3. As a nurse in your hospital's community outreach clinic, you are responsible for providing group education and counseling to patients with asthma. What areas would you address regarding triggers for asthma? How might you have patients assess their home environments?

4. Your 64-year-old patient has a history of bronchiectasis and heart failure following two myocardial infarctions. To promote removal of pulmonary secretions, his physician has prescribed chest physiotherapy and postural drainage. The patient reports that he is able to breathe easily only in a sitting position. Describe how you would modify chest physiotherapy and postural drainage given his statement that he cannot breathe in a supine or prone position.

5. Your 22-year-old patient is a college student with a history of cystic fibrosis; he has been admitted to your unit for intravenous antibiotic therapy. Describe what pulmonary rehabilitation techniques would be appropriate for his disease process, which are age-specific and consistent with his activity level.

REFERENCES AND SELECTED READINGS

Books

American Association of Cardiovascular & Pulmonary Rehabilitation. (1998). *Guidelines for pulmonary rehabilitation programs* (2nd ed.). Champaign, IL: Human Kinetics.

Cystic Fibrosis Foundation (2002). What is CF? http://www.cff.org (accessed June 13, 2002).

Cherniack, N. S., Homma, I., & Altose, M. (Eds.). (1999). *Rehabilitation of the patient with respiratory disease.* New York: McGraw-Hill.

Expert Panel Report II. (1997). *Guidelines for the diagnosis and management of asthma.* National Asthma Education and Prevention Program, National Institutes of Health.

FitzGerald, J. M. (2001). *Evidence-based asthma management.* Hamilton, Ontario: B. C. Decker.

George, R. B., San Pedro, G. S., & Stoller, J. K. (2000). Chronic obstructive pulmonary disease, bronchiectasis, and cystic fibrosis. In R. B. George, R. W. Light, M. A. Matthay & R. A. Matthay (Eds.), *Chest medicine: Essentials of pulmonary and critical care medicine* (4th ed.). Philadelphia: Lippincott Williams & Wilkins.

Hall, J. B. (2000). *Acute asthma: Assessment and management.* New York: McGraw-Hill, Health Professions Division.

Katkin, J. P. (2002). *Clinical manifestations and diagnosis of cystic fibrosis.* UpToDate, Vol. 10(1), Wellesley, MA.

Kavuru, M. S., & Wiedemann, H. P. (2000). Asthma. In R. B. George, R. W. Light, M. A. Matthay & R. A. Matthay (Eds.), *Chest medicine: Essentials of pulmonary and critical care medicine* (4th ed., pp. 133–173). Philadelphia: Lippincott Williams & Wilkins.

Lieberman, P., & Anderson, J. A. (Eds.). (2000). *Allergic diseases: Diagnosis and treatment.* Totowa, NJ: Humana.

National Center for Health Statistics. (2000). *US mortality public use data tape 1998.* Centers for Disease Control and Prevention, Hyattsville, MD.

National Center for Health Statistics. (2001). *New asthma estimates: Tracking prevalence, health care, and mortality.* Fact sheet released Oct. 5, 2001, Hyattsville, MD.

National Heart, Lung and Blood Institute (1998). *Morbidity and mortality: 1998 chart book on cardiovascular, lung and blood diseases.*

National Heart, Lung and Blood Institute (2000). *Morbidity and mortality: 2000 chart book on cardiovascular, lung and blood diseases.*

National Institutes of Health. (2001) *Global initiative for chronic obstructive lung disease: Global strategy for the diagnosis, management, and prevention of chronic obstructive pulmonary disease.* U.S. Department of Health and Human Services, NIH Publication Number 2701B.

O'Byrne, P. M. (2001). *Manual of asthma management* (2d ed.). London: W. B. Saunders.

Journals

Asterisks indicate nursing research articles.

General

ACCP/AACVPR Pulmonary Rehabilitation Guidelines Panel. (1997). Pulmonary rehabilitation: Joint ACCP/AACVPR evidence-based guidelines. *Chest, 112*(5), 1363–1396.

Adatsi, G. (1999). Health going up in smoke: How can you prevent it? *American Journal of Nursing, 99*(3), 63–69.

American Thoracic Society. (1999). Statement on pulmonary rehabilitation. *American Journal of Respiratory and Critical Care Medicine, 159*(5), 1666–1682.

Lacasse, Y., Guyatt, G., & Goldstein, R. (1997). The components of a respiratory rehabilitation program: A systematic overview. *Chest, 111*(4), 1977–2088.

*McEntee, D. J., & Badenhop, D. T. (2000). Quality of life comparisons: Gender and population differences in cardiopulmonary rehabilitation. *Heart Lung, 29*(5), 340–347.

Rochester, C. L. (2000). Which pulmonary rehabilitation program is best for your patient? *Journal of Respiratory Diseases, 21*(9), 539–546.

Asthma

Boushey, H. A., Fick, R. B., Lazarus, S., & Martin, A. (2000). *Anti-IgE: A unique approach to asthma management.* Gardiner-Caldwell SynerMed, Califon, NJ, 2–24.

Busse, W. W., & Lemanske, R. F. Jr. (2001). Advances in immunology: Asthma. *New England Journal of Medicine, 344*(5), 350–362.

Caprioti, T. (1999). Leukotriene antagonists offer a new mechanism for asthma control. *MedSurg Nursing, 8*(5), 318–322.

Centers for Disease Control and Prevention. (1998). Forecasted state-specific estimates of self-reported asthma prevalence: United States, 1998. *MMWR Morbidity and Mortality Weekly Report, 47*(47), 1022–1025.

Centers for Disease Control and Prevention. (1999). Asthma Prevention Program of the National Center for Environmental Health, At-A-Glance, 1999, 1–6.

Dhand, R. (2000). Aerosol therapy in asthma. *Current Opinion in Pulmonary Medicine, 6*(1), 59–70.

Drazen, J. M., Israel, E., & O'Byrne, P. M. (1999). Treatment of asthma with drugs modifying the leukotriene pathway. *New England Journal of Medicine, 340*(3), 197–206.

Janson, S. (1998). National Asthma Education and Prevention Program, Expert Panel Report II: Overview and application for primary care. *Lippincott's Primary Care Practice, 2*(6), 578–588.

McGann, E. (1999). Medication compliance in adults with asthma. *American Journal of Nursing, 99*(3), 45–46.

National Heart, Lung and Blood Institute. (1998). Asthma diagnosis and management. A continuing education module. http://www.nhlbi.nih.gov.

Naureckas, E. T., & Solway, J. (2001). Mild asthma. *New England Journal of Medicine, 345*(17), 1257–1262.

Owen, C. L. (1999). New directions in asthma management. *American Journal of Nursing, 99*(3), 26–33.

Plaut, T. F. (2001). Lack of knowledge leads to poor asthma care. *Advance for Managers of Respiratory Care, 10*(3), 38, 40–41.

Reinke, L. F. (2000). Asthma education: Creating a partnership. *Heart Lung, 29*(3), 225–236.

Rickard, K. A., & Stempel, D. A. (1999). Asthma survey demonstrates that the goals of the NHLBI have not been accomplished [abstract]. *Journal of Allergy and Clinical Immunology, 103*(1 Pt 2), S171.

*Schott-Baer, D., & Christensen, M. (1999). A pilot program to increase self-care of adult asthma patients. *MedSurg Nursing, 8*(3), 178–183.

Togger, D. A., & Brenner, P. S. (2001). Metered dose inhalers. *American Journal of Nursing, 101*(10), 26–32.

COPD

Barnes, P. J. (2000). Medical progress: Chronic obstructive pulmonary disease. *New England Journal of Medicine, 343*(4), 269–280.

*Belza, B., Steele, B. G., Hunziker, J., Lakshminaryan, S., Holt, L., & Buchner, D. M. (2001). Correlates of physical activity in chronic obstructive pulmonary disease. *Nursing Research, 50*(4), 195–202.

Boyle, A. H., & Waters, H. F. (2000). COPD: Focus on prevention. Recommendations of the National Lung Health Education Program. *Heart Lung, 29*(6), 446–449.

Celli, B. R., Snider, G. L, Heffner, J., et al. (1995). ATS standards for the diagnosis and care of patients with chronic obstructive pulmonary disease. *American Journal of Respiratory Critical Care Medicine, 152*(5), S77–S121.

Fiel, S. B. (2000). Bronchiectasis: The changing clinical scenario. *Journal of Respiratory Disease, 21*(11), 666–681.

Fein, A. (1998). Lung volume reduction surgery. *Chest, 113*(4), 277S–282S.

Ferreira, I., Brooks, D., Lacasse, Y., & Goldstein, R. (2001). Nutritional intervention in COPD: A systematic overview. *Chest, 119*(2), 353–363.

Garvey, C. (1998). COPD and exercise. *Lippincott's Primary Care Practice, 2*(6), 589–598.

*Knebel, A. R., Bentz, E., & Barnes, P. (2000). Dyspnea management in alpha-1 antitrypsin deficiency: Effect of oxygen administration. *Nursing Research, 49*(6), 333–338.

Larson, J. L., Covey, M. K., Wirtz, S. E., et al. (1999). Cycle ergometer and inspiratory muscle training in chronic obstructive pulmonary disease. *American Journal of Respiratory and Critical Care Medicine, 160*(2), 500–507.

*Meek, P. M. (2000). Influence of attention and judgment on perception of breathlessness in healthy individuals and patient with chronic obstructive pulmonary disease. *Nursing Research, 49*(1), 11–19.

National Institutes of Health. (2001). *NHLBI-funded emphysema study finds certain patients at high risk for death following lung surgery.* NIH news release, Aug. 14, 2001.

National Institutes of Health. (2001). National emphysema treatment trial (NETT), evaluation of lung volume reduction surgery for emphysema. June 20, 2001. http://www.nhlbi.nih.gov/health/prof/lung/nett/lvrsweb.htm.

National Emphysema Treatment Trial Research Group (2001). Patients at high risk of death after lung-volume-reduction surgery. *New England Journal of Medicine, 345*(18), 1075–1083.

*Nield, M. (2000). Dyspnea self-management in African-Americans with chronic lung disease. *Heart Lung, 29*(1), 50–55.

Pohl, J. M. (2000). Smoking cessation and low-income women: Theory, research, and interventions. *Nurse Practice Forum, 11*(2), 101–108.

Rennard, S. I. (1998). COPD: Overview of definitions, epidemiology, and factors influencing its development. *Chest, 113*(4, Suppl.), 235S–241S.

*Skilbeck, J., Mott, L., Smith, D., Page, H., & Clark, D. (1997). Research and development. Nursing care for people dying from chronic obstructive airway disease. *International Journal of Palliative Nursing, 3*(2), 100–106.

Stoller, J. K. (2002). Acute exacerbations of chronic obstructive pulmonary medicine. *New England Journal of Medicine, 346*(13), 988–994.

*Trudeau, M. E., & Solano-McGuire, S. M. (1999). Evaluating the quality of COPD care. *American Journal of Nursing, 99*(3), 47–50.

Truesdell, S. (2000). Helping patients with COPD manage episodes of acute shortness of breath. *MedSurg Nursing, 9*(4), 178–182.

United States Public Health Service. (2000). Treating tobacco use and dependence. Summary, June 2000. http://www.surgeongeneral.gov/tobacco.smokesum.htm.

*Wu, C-Y., Lee, Y-Y., Baig, K., & Wichaikhum O. (2001). Coping behaviors of individuals with chronic obstructive pulmonary disease. *MedSurg Nursing, 10*(6), 315–320.

RESOURCES AND WEBSITES

Agency for Healthcare Research and Quality, 2101 E. Jefferson St., Suite 501, Rockville, MD 20852; (301) 594-1364; http://www.ahrq.org.

American Academy of Allergy, Asthma, and Immunology, 611 E. Wells St., Milwaukee, WI 53202; (414) 272-6071; http://www.aaaai.org.

American Association of Cardiovascular and Pulmonary Rehabilitation, 7611 Elmwood Ave., Suite 201, Middleton, WI 53562, (608) 831-5122; http://www.aacvpr.org.

American Association for Respiratory Care, 1720 Regal Row, Dallas, TX 75235; (214) 630-3540; http://www.aarc.org.

American Cancer Society, 1599 Clifton Road NE, Atlanta, GA 30329-4251; (800) ACS-2345; http://www.cancer.org.

American College of Chest Physicians, 3300 Dundee Road, Northbrook, IL 60062; (847) 498-1400; http://www.chest.org.

American Lung Association, 1740 Broadway, New York, NY 10019-4374; (212) 315-8700; http://www.lungusa.org.

American Thoracic Society, 1740 Broadway, New York, NY 10019; (212) 315-8700; http://www.thoracic.org.

Centers for Disease Control and Prevention, 1600 Clifton Road, NE, Atlanta, GA 30333; http://www.cdc.gov.

Cystic Fibrosis Foundation, 6931 Arlington Road, Bethesda, MD 20814; (310) 951-4422 or (800) FIGHT CF; http://www.cff.org.

National Cancer Institute; (800) 4-Cancer or (301) 496-5585; http://www.cancer.gov or http://www.nci.nih.gov.

National Heart, Lung and Blood Institute, National Institutes of Health, 900 Rockville Pike, Bldg. 31, Bethesda, MD 20892; (301) 496-5166; http://www.nhlbi.nih.gov.

Respiratory Nursing Society, 11 Cornell Road, Latham, NY 12110; (518) 782-9400 x286l; e-mail: RNS@NYSNA.ORG.

U.S. Department of Health and Human Services, Department of Health and Human Services, 200 Independence Avenue, S.W., Washington DC 20201; (202) 619-0257; http://www.hhs.gov or http://www.healthfinder.gov.

Respiratory Care Modalities

On completion of this chapter, the learner will be able to:

1. Describe the nursing management for patients receiving oxygen therapy, intermittent positive-pressure breathing, mini-nebulizer therapy, incentive spirometry, chest physiotherapy, and breathing retraining.

2. Describe the patient education and home care considerations for patients receiving oxygen therapy.

3. Describe the nursing care for a patient with an endotracheal tube and for a patient with a tracheostomy.

4. Demonstrate the procedure of tracheal suctioning.

5. Use the nursing process as a framework for care of patients who are mechanically ventilated.

6. Describe the process of weaning the patient from mechanical ventilation.

7. Describe the significance of preoperative nursing assessment and patient teaching for the patient who is to have thoracic surgery.

8. Explain the principles of chest drainage and the nursing responsibilities related to the care of the patient with a chest drainage system.

9. Describe the patient education and home care considerations for patients who have had thoracic surgery.

*N*umerous treatment modalities are used when caring for patients with various respiratory conditions. The choice of modality is based on the oxygenation disorder and whether there is a problem with gas ventilation, diffusion, or both. Therapies range from simple and noninvasive modalities (oxygen and nebulizer therapy, chest physiotherapy, breathing retraining) to complex and highly invasive treatments (intubation, mechanical ventilation, surgery). Assessment and management of the patient with respiratory disorders are best accomplished when the approach is multidisciplinary and collaborative.

Noninvasive Respiratory Therapies

OXYGEN THERAPY

Oxygen therapy is the administration of oxygen at a concentration greater than that found in the environmental atmosphere. At sea level, the concentration of oxygen in room air is 21%. The goal of oxygen therapy is to provide adequate transport of oxygen in the blood while decreasing the work of breathing and reducing stress on the myocardium.

Oxygen transport to the tissues depends on factors such as cardiac output, arterial oxygen content, concentration of hemoglobin, and metabolic requirements. These factors must be kept in mind when oxygen therapy is considered. (Respiratory physiology and oxygen transport are discussed in Chap. 21.)

Indications

A change in the patient's respiratory rate or pattern may be one of the earliest indicators of the need for oxygen therapy. The change in respiratory rate or pattern may result from hypoxemia or hypoxia. **Hypoxemia** (a decrease in the arterial oxygen tension in the blood) is manifested by changes in mental status (progressing through impaired judgment, agitation, disorientation, confusion, lethargy, and coma), dyspnea, increase in blood pressure, changes in heart rate, dysrhythmias, central cyanosis (late sign), diaphoresis, and cool extremities. Hypoxemia usually leads to **hypoxia**, which is a decrease in oxygen supply to the tissues. Hypoxia, if severe enough, can be life-threatening.

The signs and symptoms signaling the need for oxygen may depend on how suddenly this need develops. With rapidly developing hypoxia, changes occur in the central nervous system because the higher neurologic centers are very sensitive to oxygen deprivation. The clinical picture may resemble that of alcohol intoxication, with the patient exhibiting lack of coordination and impaired judgment. Longstanding hypoxia (as seen in chronic obstructive pulmonary disease [COPD] and chronic heart failure) may produce fatigue, drowsiness, apathy, inattentiveness, and delayed reaction time. The need for oxygen is assessed by arterial blood gas analysis and pulse oximetry as well as by clinical evaluation. For more information about hypoxia, see Chart 25-1.

Cautions in Oxygen Therapy

As with other medications, the nurse administers oxygen with caution and carefully assesses its effects on each patient. Oxygen is a medication and except in emergency situations is administered only when prescribed by a physician.

In general, patients with respiratory conditions are given oxygen therapy only to raise the arterial oxygen pressure (PaO_2) back to the patient's normal baseline, which may vary from 60 to 95 mm Hg. In terms of the oxyhemoglobin dissociation curve (see Chap. 21),

---

Glossary

assist–control ventilation: mode of mechanical ventilation in which the patient's breathing pattern may trigger the ventilator to deliver a preset tidal volume; in the absence of spontaneous breathing, the machine delivers a controlled breath at a preset minimum rate and tidal volume

chest drainage system: use of a chest tube and closed drainage system to reexpand the lung and to remove excess air, fluid, and blood

chest percussion: manually cupping over the chest wall to mobilize secretions by mechanically dislodging viscous or adherent secretions in the lungs

chest physiotherapy (CPT): therapy used to remove bronchial secretions, improve ventilation, and increase the efficiency of the respiratory muscles. Types include postural drainage, chest percussion, and vibration.

controlled ventilation: mode of mechanical ventilation in which the ventilator completely controls the patient's ventilation according to preset tidal volumes and respiratory rate. Because of problems with synchrony, it is rarely used except in paralyzed or anesthetized patients.

endotracheal intubation: insertion of a breathing tube through the nose or mouth into the trachea

fraction of inspired oxygen (FiO$_2$): concentration of oxygen delivered (1.0 = 100% oxygen)

hypoxemia: decrease in arterial oxygen tension in the blood

hypoxia: decrease in oxygen supply to the tissues and cells

incentive spirometry: method of deep breathing that provides visual feedback to help the patient inhale deeply and slowly and achieve maximum lung inflation

mechanical ventilator: a positive- or negative-pressure breathing device that supports ventilation and oxygenation

pneumothorax: partial or complete collapse of the lung due to positive pressure in the pleural space

positive end-expiratory pressure (PEEP): positive pressure maintained by the ventilator at the end of exhalation (instead of a normal zero pressure) to increase functional residual capacity and open collapsed alveoli; improves oxygenation with lower FiO$_2$

postural drainage: positioning the patient to allow drainage from all the lobes of the lungs and airways

pressure support ventilation (PSV): mode of mechanical ventilation in which preset positive pressure is delivered with spontaneous breaths to decrease work of breathing

respiratory weaning: process of gradual, systematic withdrawal and/or removal of ventilator, breathing tube, and oxygen

synchronized intermittent mandatory ventilation (SIMV): mode of mechanical ventilation in which the ventilator allows the patient to breathe spontaneously while providing a preset number of breaths to ensure adequate ventilation; ventilated breaths are synchronized with spontaneous breathing

thoracotomy: surgical opening into the chest cavity

tracheotomy: surgical opening into the trachea

tracheostomy tube: indwelling tube inserted directly into the trachea to assist with ventilation

vibration: a type of massage administered by quickly tapping the chest with the fingertips or alternating the fingers in a rhythmic manner, or by using a mechanical device to assist in mobilizing lung secretions

Types of Hypoxia

Hypoxia can occur from either severe pulmonary disease (inadequate oxygen supply) or from extrapulmonary disease (inadequate oxygen delivery) affecting gas exchange at the cellular level. The four general types of hypoxia are hypoxemic hypoxia, circulatory hypoxia, anemic hypoxia, and histotoxic hypoxia.

Hypoxemic Hypoxia

Hypoxemic hypoxia is a decreased oxygen level in the blood resulting in decreased oxygen diffusion into the tissues. It may be caused by hypoventilation, high altitudes, ventilation–perfusion mismatch (as in pulmonary embolism), shunts in which the alveoli are collapsed and cannot provide oxygen to the blood (commonly caused by atelectasis), and pulmonary diffusion defects. It is corrected by increasing alveolar ventilation or providing supplemental oxygen.

Circulatory Hypoxia

Circulatory hypoxia is hypoxia resulting from inadequate capillary circulation. It may be caused by decreased cardiac output, local vascular obstruction, low-flow states such as shock, or cardiac arrest. Although tissue partial pressure of oxygen (PO_2) is reduced, arterial oxygen (PaO_2) remains normal. Circulatory hypoxia is corrected by identifying and treating the underlying cause.

Anemic Hypoxia

Anemic hypoxia is a result of decreased effective hemoglobin concentration, which causes a decrease in the oxygen-carrying capacity of the blood. It is rarely accompanied by hypoxemia. Carbon monoxide poisoning, because it reduces the oxygen-carrying capacity of hemoglobin, produces similar effects but is not strictly anemic hypoxia because hemoglobin levels may be normal.

Histotoxic Hypoxia

Histotoxic hypoxia occurs when a toxic substance, such as cyanide, interferes with the ability of tissues to use available oxygen.

---

the blood at these levels is 80% to 98% saturated with oxygen; higher inspired oxygen flow (FiO_2) values add no further significant amounts of oxygen to the red blood cells or plasma. Instead of helping, increased amounts of oxygen may produce toxic effects on the lungs and central nervous system or may depress ventilation (see discussion below).

It is important to observe for subtle indicators of inadequate oxygenation when oxygen is administered by any method. Therefore, the nurse assesses the patient frequently for confusion, restlessness progressing to lethargy, diaphoresis, pallor, tachycardia, tachypnea, and hypertension. Intermittent or continuous pulse oximetry is used to monitor oxygen levels.

OXYGEN TOXICITY

Oxygen toxicity may occur when too high a concentration of oxygen (greater than 50%) is administered for an extended period (longer than 48 hours). It is caused by overproduction of oxygen free radicals, which are byproducts of cell metabolism. If oxygen toxicity is untreated, these radicals can severely damage or kill cells. Antioxidants such as vitamin E, vitamin C, and beta-carotene may help defend against oxygen free radicals (Scanlan, Wilkins & Stoller, 1999). The dietitian can adjust the patient's diet so that it is rich in antioxidants; supplements are also available for patients who have a decreased appetite or who are unable to eat.

Signs and symptoms of oxygen toxicity include substernal discomfort, paresthesias, dyspnea, restlessness, fatigue, malaise, progressive respiratory difficulty, and alveolar infiltrates evident on chest x-rays.

Prevention of oxygen toxicity is achieved by using oxygen only as prescribed. If high concentrations of oxygen are necessary, it is important to minimize the duration of administration and reduce its concentration as soon as possible. Often, **positive end-expiratory pressure** (PEEP) or continuous positive airway pressure (CPAP) is used with oxygen therapy to reverse or prevent microatelectasis, thus allowing a lower percentage of oxygen to be used. The level of PEEP that allows the best oxygenation without hemodynamic compromise is known as "best PEEP."

SUPPRESSION OF VENTILATION

In patients with COPD, the stimulus for respiration is a decrease in blood oxygen rather than an elevation in carbon dioxide levels. Thus, administration of a high concentration of oxygen removes the respiratory drive that has been created largely by the patient's chronic low oxygen tension. The resulting decrease in alveolar ventilation can cause a progressive increase in arterial carbon dioxide pressure ($PaCO_2$), ultimately leading to the patient's death from carbon dioxide narcosis and acidosis. Oxygen-induced hypoventilation is prevented by administering oxygen at low flow rates (1 to 2 L/min).

OTHER COMPLICATIONS

Because oxygen supports combustion, there is always a danger of fire when it is used. It is important to post "no smoking" signs when oxygen is in use. Oxygen therapy equipment is also a potential source of bacterial cross-infection; thus, the nurse changes the tubing according to infection control policy and the type of oxygen delivery equipment.

Methods of Oxygen Administration

Oxygen is dispensed from a cylinder or a piped-in system. A reduction gauge is necessary to reduce the pressure to a working level, and a flow meter regulates the flow of oxygen in liters per minute. When oxygen is used at high flow rates, it should be moistened by passing it through a humidification system to prevent it from drying the mucous membranes of the respiratory tract.

The use of oxygen concentrators is another means of providing varying amounts of oxygen, especially in the home setting. These devices are relatively portable, easy to operate, and cost-effective. However, they require more maintenance than tank or liquid systems and probably cannot deliver oxygen flows in excess of 4 L, which provides an FiO_2 of about 36%.

Many different oxygen devices are used, and all deliver oxygen if they are used as prescribed and maintained correctly (Table 25-1). The amount of oxygen delivered is expressed as a percentage concentration (eg, 70%). The appropriate form of oxygen therapy is best determined by arterial blood gas levels, which indicate the patient's oxygenation status.

Oxygen delivery systems are classified as low-flow or high-flow delivery systems. Low-flow systems contribute partially to the inspired gas the patient breathes. This means the patient breathes some room air along with the oxygen. These systems do not provide a constant or known concentration of inspired oxygen. The amount of inspired oxygen changes as the patient's breathing changes. Examples of low-flow systems include nasal cannula, oropharyngeal catheter, simple mask, and partial-rebreather and non-rebreather masks. High-flow systems provide the total amount of inspired air. A specific percentage of oxygen is delivered independent of the patient's breathing. High-flow systems are indicated for patients who require a constant and precise amount of oxygen. Examples of such systems include transtracheal catheters, Venturi

Table 25-1 • **Oxygen Administration Devices**

DEVICE	SUGGESTED FLOW RATE (L/MIN)	O$_2$ PERCENTAGE SETTING	ADVANTAGES	DISADVANTAGES
Low-Flow Systems				
Cannula	1–2	23–30	Lightweight, comfortable, inexpensive, continuous use with meals and activity	Nasal mucosal drying, variable FiO$_2$
	3–5	30–40		
	6	42		
Oropharyngeal catheter	1–6	23–42	Inexpensive, does not require a tracheostomy	Nasal mucosa irritation; catheter should be changed frequently to alternate nostril
Mask, simple	6–8	40–60	Simple to use, inexpensive	Poor fitting, variable FiO$_2$, must remove to eat
Mask, partial rebreather	8–11	50–75	Moderate O$_2$ concentration	Warm, poorly fitting, must remove to eat
Mask, non-rebreather	12	80–100	High O$_2$ concentration	Poorly fitting
High-Flow Systems				
Transtracheal catheter	¼–4	60–100	More comfortable, concealed by clothing, less oxygen liters per minute needed than nasal cannula	Requires frequent and regular cleaning, requires surgical intervention
Mask, Venturi	4–6	24, 26, 28	Provides low levels of supplemental O$_2$	Must remove to eat
	6–8	30, 35, 40	Precise FiO$_2$, additional humidity available	
Mask, aerosol	8–10	30–100	Good humidity, accurate FiO$_2$	Uncomfortable for some
Tracheostomy collar	8–10	30–100	Good humidity, comfortable, fairly accurate FiO$_2$	
T-piece	8–10	30–100	Same as tracheostomy collar	Heavy with tubing
Face tent	8–10	30–100	Good humidity, fairly accurate FiO$_2$	Bulky and cumbersome

masks, aerosol masks, tracheostomy collars, T-piece, and face tents (Cairo & Philbeam, 1999; Scanlan, Wilkins & Stoller, 1999).

A nasal cannula is used when the patient requires a low to medium concentration of oxygen for which precise accuracy is not essential. This method is relatively simple and allows the patient to move about in bed, talk, cough, and eat without interrupting oxygen flow. Flow rates in excess of 6 to 8 L/min may lead to swallowing of air; this may cause irritation and drying of the nasal and pharyngeal mucosa.

The oropharyngeal catheter is rarely used but may be prescribed for short-term therapy to administer low to moderate concentrations of oxygen. The catheter should be changed every 8 hours, alternating nostrils to prevent infection and nasal irritation.

When oxygen is administered via cannula or catheter, the percentage of oxygen reaching the lungs varies with the depth and rate of respirations, particularly if the nasal mucosa is swollen or if the patient is a mouth breather.

Oxygen masks come in several forms. Each is used for different purposes (Fig. 25-1). *Simple masks* are used for low to moderate concentrations of oxygen. The body of the mask itself gathers and stores oxygen between breaths. The patient exhales directly through openings or ports in the body of the mask. If oxygen flow ceases, the patient can draw air in through these openings around the mask edges (Scanlan, Wilkins & Stoller, 1999). Although widely used, these masks cannot be used for controlled oxygen concentrations and must be adjusted for proper fit. They should not press too tightly against the skin, because this may cause a sense of claustrophobia and skin breakdown; adjustable elastic bands are provided to ensure comfort and security.

Partial-rebreathing masks have a reservoir bag that must remain inflated during both inspiration and expiration. The nurse

should adjust the liter flow to ensure that the bag does not collapse during inhalation. A higher concentration of oxygen can be delivered because both the mask and bag serve as reservoirs for oxygen. Oxygen enters the mask through small-bore tubing that connects at the junction of the mask and bag. As the patient inhales, gas is drawn from the mask, the bag, and potentially from room air through the exhalation ports. As the patient exhales, the first third of the exhalation fills the reservoir bag. This is mainly dead space and does not participate in gas exchange in the lungs. Therefore, it has a high oxygen concentration. The remainder of the exhaled gas is vented through the exhalation ports. The actual percentage of oxygen delivered is influenced by the patient's ventilatory pattern (Cairo & Philbeam, 1999).

Non-rebreathing masks are similar in design to partial-rebreathing masks except that they have two valves. The first valve is a one-way valve located between the reservoir bag and the base of the mask. The valve allows gas from the reservoir bag to enter the mask on inhalation and prevents gas in the mask from flowing back into the reservoir bag during exhalation. The second valve is a set of valves located at the exhalation ports. These one-way valves prevent room air from entering the mask during inhalation. They also allow the patient's exhaled gases to exit the mask on exhalation (Cairo & Pilbeam, 1999). As with the partial-rebreathing mask, it is important to adjust the liter flow so that the reservoir bag does not completely collapse on inspiration. In theory, if the non-rebreather mask fits the patient snugly and both side exhalation ports have one-way valves, it is possible for the patient to receive 100% oxygen, making the non-rebreather a high-flow oxygen system. However, because it is difficult to get an exact fit from the mask on every patient, and some non-rebreather masks have only one one-way exhalation valve, it is nearly impossible to ensure 100% oxygen delivery, making it a low-flow oxygen system.

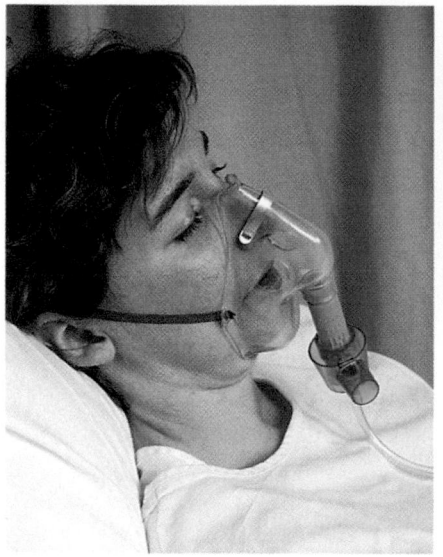
Venturi mask

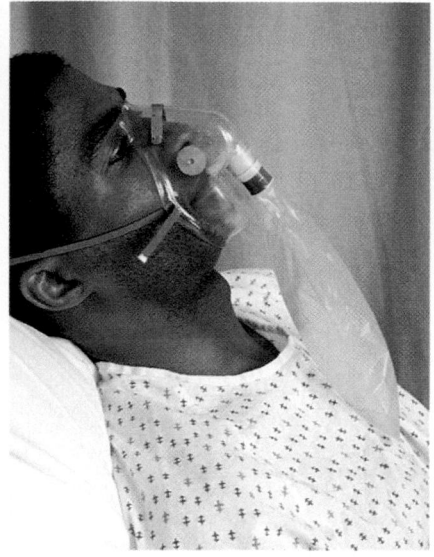
Nonrebreather mask

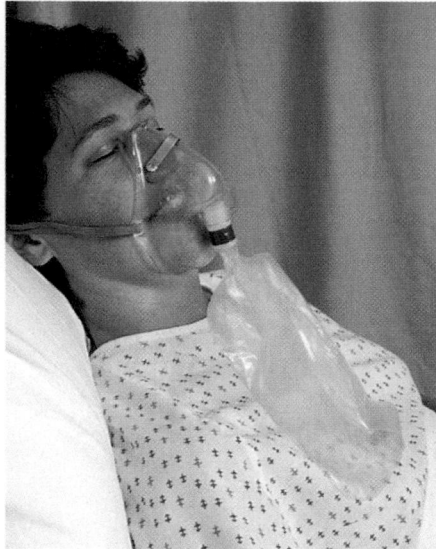
Partial rebreather mask

FIGURE 25-1 Types of oxygen masks used to deliver varying concentrations of oxygen. Photos © Ken Kaspar.

The *Venturi mask* is the most reliable and accurate method for delivering precise concentrations of oxygen through noninvasive means. The mask is constructed in a way that allows a constant flow of room air blended with a fixed flow of oxygen. It is used primarily for patients with COPD because it can provide low levels of supplemental oxygen, thus avoiding the risk of suppressing the hypoxic drive.

The Venturi mask employs the Bernoulli principle of air entrainment (trapping the air like a vacuum), which provides a high air flow with controlled oxygen enrichment. For each liter of oxygen that passes through a jet orifice, a fixed proportion of room air will be entrained. A precise volume of oxygen can be delivered by varying the size of the jet orifice and adjusting the flow of oxygen. Excess gas leaves the mask through the two exhalation ports, carrying with it the exhaled carbon dioxide. This method allows a constant oxygen concentration to be inhaled regardless of the depth or rate of respiration.

The mask should fit snugly enough to prevent oxygen from flowing into the patient's eyes. The nurse should check the patient's skin for irritation. It is necessary to remove the mask so that the patient can eat, drink, and take medications.

The *transtracheal oxygen catheter* is inserted directly into the trachea and is indicated for patients with chronic oxygen therapy needs. These catheters are more comfortable, less dependent on breathing patterns, and less obvious than other oxygen delivery methods. Because no oxygen is lost into the surrounding environment, the patient achieves adequate oxygenation at lower rates, making this method less expensive and more efficient.

The *T-piece* connects to the endotracheal tube and is useful in weaning patients from mechanical ventilation (Fig. 25-2).

Other oxygen devices include *aerosol masks, tracheostomy collars,* and *face tents,* all of which are used with aerosol devices (nebulizers) that can be adjusted for oxygen concentrations from 27% to 100% (0.27 to 1.00). If the gas mixture flow falls below patient demand, room air is pulled in, diluting the concentration. The aerosol mist must be available for the patient during the entire inspiratory phase.

Although most oxygen therapy is administered as continuous flow oxygen, new methods of oxygen conservation are coming into use. *Demand oxygen delivery systems* (DODS) interrupt the flow of oxygen during exhalation, when the oxygen flow is otherwise mostly wasted. Several versions of DODS are being researched for their effectiveness. Studies show that DODS models conserve oxygen and maintain oxygen saturations better than continuous-flow oxygen when the respiratory rate increases (Bliss, McCoy & Adams, 1999).

Hyperbaric oxygen therapy is the administration of oxygen at pressures greater than one atmosphere. As a result, the amount of oxygen dissolved in plasma is increased, which raises oxygen levels in the tissues. It is administered through a small (single patient use) or large (multiple patient use) cylinder chamber. During therapy, the patient is placed in the chamber. Hyperbaric oxygen therapy is used to treat conditions such as air embolism, carbon monoxide poisoning, gangrene, tissue necrosis, and hemorrhage. Other uses for this therapy include treatment for multiple sclerosis, diabetic foot ulcers, closed head trauma, and acute myocardial infarction. Research continues in the area of hyperbaric oxygen use because of potential side effects, including ear trauma, central nervous system disorders, and oxygen toxicity (Takezawa, 2000; Woodrow & Roe, 2000).

Gerontologic Considerations

The respiratory system changes throughout the aging process, and it is important for nurses to be aware of these changes when assessing patients who are receiving oxygen therapy. As the respiratory muscles weaken and the large bronchi and alveoli become enlarged, the available surface area of the lungs decreases, resulting in reduced ventilation and respiratory gas exchange. The number of functional cilia is also reduced, decreasing ciliary action and the cough reflex. As a result of osteoporosis and the calcification of the costal cartilages, chest wall compliance is decreased. Patients may display increased chest rigidity and respiratory rate and decreased PaO_2 and lung expansion. Nurses should be aware that the older adult is at risk for aspiration and infection related to these changes. In addition, patient education regarding adequate nutrition is essential, because appropriate dietary intake can help

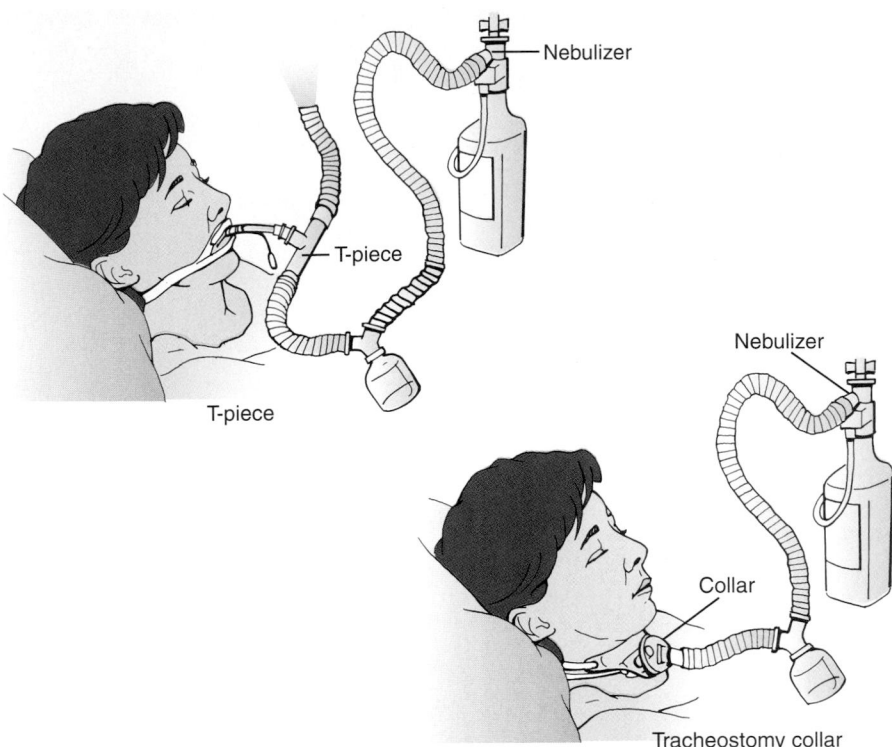

FIGURE 25-2 T-pieces and tracheostomy collars are devices used when weaning patients from mechanical ventilation.

to diminish the excess build-up of carbon dioxide and to maintain optimal respiratory functioning (Abraham, Bottrell, Fulmer & Mezey, 1999; Eliopoulos, 2001).

Nursing Management

PROMOTING HOME AND COMMUNITY-BASED CARE

Teaching Patients Self-Care. At times oxygen must be administered to the patient at home. The nurse instructs the patient or family in the methods for administering oxygen and informs the patient and family that oxygen is available in gas, liquid, and concentrated forms. The gas and liquid forms come in portable devices so that the patient can leave home while receiving oxygen therapy. Humidity must be provided while oxygen is used (except with portable devices) to counteract the dry, irritating effects of compressed oxygen on the airway (Chart 25-2).

Continuing Care. Home visits by a home health nurse or respiratory therapist may be arranged based on the patient's status and needs. It is important to assess the patient's home environment, the patient's physical and psychological status, and the need for further teaching. The nurse reinforces the teaching points on how to use oxygen safely and effectively, including fire safety tips because oxygen is flammable. To maintain a consistent quality of care and to maximize the patient's financial reimbursement for

---

Chart 25-2
Home Care Checklist • Oxygen Therapy

At the completion of the home care instruction, the patient or caregiver will be able to:	**Patient**	**Caregiver**
• State proper care of and administration of oxygen to patient		
State physician's prescription for oxygen and the manner in which it is to be used	✓	✓
Indicate when a humidifier should be used	✓	✓
Identify signs and symptoms indicating the need for change in oxygen therapy	✓	✓
Describe precautions and safety measures to be used when oxygen is in use	✓	✓
State how and when to place an order for more oxygen	✓	✓
Describe a diet that meets energy demands	✓	✓
• Maintain equipment properly		
Demonstrate correct adjustment of prescribed flow rate	✓	✓
Describe how to clean and when to replace oxygen tubing	✓	✓
Identify when a portable oxygen delivery device should be used	✓	✓
Demonstrate safe and appropriate use of portable oxygen delivery device	✓	✓
Identify causes of malfunction of equipment and when to call for replacement of equipment	✓	✓
Describe the importance of determining that all electrical outlets are working properly	✓	✓

home oxygen therapy, the nurse ensures that the physician's prescription includes the diagnosis, the prescribed oxygen flow, and conditions for use (eg, continuous use, nighttime use only). Because oxygen is a medication, the nurse reminds the patient receiving long-term oxygen therapy and family about the importance of keeping follow-up appointments with the physician. The patient is instructed to see the physician every 6 months or more often, if indicated. Blood gas measurements and laboratory tests are repeated annually, or more often if the patient's condition changes (Smith & Matti, 1999).

INTERMITTENT POSITIVE-PRESSURE BREATHING

Intermittent positive-pressure breathing (IPPB) is a form of assisted or controlled respiration produced by a ventilatory apparatus in which compressed gas is delivered under positive pressure into a person's airways until a preset pressure is reached. Passive exhalation is allowed through a valve. The specific pressure and volume amounts, along with the use of any nebulizing medications, are prescribed individually for patients. The nurse should encourage patients to relax and reassure them that the machine will automatically shut off airflow at the end of inspiration. The IPPB machine may be powered by electricity or gas and may be connected with a mouthpiece, mask, or tracheostomy adapter.

Indications

General indications for IPPB include difficulty in raising respiratory secretions, reduced vital capacity with ineffective deep breathing and coughing, or unsuccessful trials of simpler and less costly methods for loosening secretions, delivering aerosol, or expanding the lungs.

Complications

IPPB therapy is used rarely today because of its inherent hazards, which may include pneumothorax, mucosal drying, increased intracranial pressure, hemoptysis, gastric distention, vomiting with possible aspiration, psychological dependency (especially with long-term use, as in COPD patients), hyperventilation, excessive oxygen administration, and cardiovascular problems.

MINI-NEBULIZER THERAPY

The mini-nebulizer is a hand-held apparatus that disperses a moisturizing agent or medication, such as a bronchodilator or mucolytic agent, into microscopic particles and delivers it to the lungs as the patient inhales. The mini-nebulizer is usually air-driven by means of a compressor through connecting tubing. In some instances, the nebulizer is oxygen-driven rather than air-driven. To be effective, a visible mist must be available for the patient to inhale.

Indications

The indications for use of a mini-nebulizer are similar to the indications for IPPB, except that the patient must be able to generate a deep breath without the aid of the positive-pressure machine. Diaphragmatic breathing (Chart 25-3) is a helpful technique to prepare for proper use of the mini-nebulizer. Frequently,

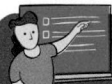

Chart 25-3 • PATIENT EDUCATION
Breathing Exercises

General Instructions
- Breathe slowly and rhythmically to exhale completely and empty the lungs completely.
- Inhale through the nose to filter, humidify, and warm the air before it enters the lungs.
- If you feel out of breath, breathe more slowly by prolonging the exhalation time.
- Keep the air moist with a humidifier.

Diaphragmatic Breathing
Goal: To use and strengthen the diaphragm during breathing
- Place one hand on the abdomen (just below the ribs) and the other hand on the middle of the chest to increase the awareness of the position of the diaphragm and its function in breathing.
- Breathe in slowly and deeply through the nose, letting the abdomen protrude as far as possible.
- Breathe out through pursed lips while tightening (contracting) the abdominal muscles.
- Press firmly inward and upward on the abdomen while breathing out.
- Repeat for 1 minute; follow with a rest period of 2 minutes.
- Gradually increase duration up to 5 minutes, several times a day (before meals and at bedtime).

Pursed-Lip Breathing
Goal: To prolong exhalation and increase airway pressure during expiration, thus reducing the amount of trapped air and the amount of airway resistance.
- Inhale through the nose while counting to 3—the amount of time needed to say "Smell a rose."
- Exhale slowly and evenly against pursed lips while tightening the abdominal muscles. (Pursing the lips increases intratracheal pressure; exhaling through the mouth offers less resistance to expired air.)
- Count to 7 while prolonging expiration through pursed lips—the length of time to say "Blow out the candle."
- While sitting in a chair:
  Fold arms over the abdomen.
  Inhale through the nose while counting to 3.
  Bend forward and exhale slowly through pursed lips while counting to 7.
- While walking:
  Inhale while walking two steps.
  Exhale through pursed lips while walking four or five steps.

mini-nebulizers are used for patients with COPD to dispense inhaled medications and are commonly used at home on a long-term basis.

Nursing Management

PROMOTING HOME AND COMMUNITY-BASED CARE

Teaching Patients Self-Care. The nurse instructs the patient to breathe through the mouth, taking slow, deep breaths, and then to hold the breath for a few seconds at the end of inspiration to increase intrapleural pressure and reopen collapsed alveoli, thereby increasing functional residual capacity. The nurse encourages the patient to cough and to monitor the effectiveness of the therapy. The nurse instructs the patient and family about the purpose of the treatment, equipment set-up, medication additive, and proper cleaning and storage of the equipment.

INCENTIVE SPIROMETRY (SUSTAINED MAXIMAL INSPIRATION)

Incentive spirometry is a method of deep breathing that provides visual feedback to help the patient inhale slowly and deeply to maximize lung inflation and prevent or reduce atelectasis. Ideally, the patient assumes a sitting or semi-Fowler's position to enhance diaphragmatic excursion (Chart 25-4). However, this procedure may be performed with the patient in any position.

Incentive spirometers may be one of two types: volume or flow. In the volume type, the tidal volume of the spirometer is set according to the manufacturer's instructions. The purpose of the device is to ensure that the volume of air inhaled is increased gradually as the patient takes deeper and deeper breaths. The patient takes a deep breath through the mouthpiece, pauses at peak lung inflation, and then relaxes and exhales. Taking several normal breaths before attempting another with the incentive spirometer helps avoid fatigue. The volume is periodically increased as tolerated.

A flow spirometer has the same purpose as a volume spirometer, but the volume is not preset. The spirometer contains a number of movable balls that are pushed up by the force of the breath and held suspended in the air while the patient inhales. The amount of air inhaled and the flow of the air are estimated by how long and how high the balls are suspended.

Indications

Incentive spirometry is used after surgery, especially thoracic and abdominal surgery, to promote the expansion of the alveoli and to prevent or treat atelectasis. As a preventive measure, incentive spirometry may be more effective than IPPB because it maximizes the amount of air inhaled while maintaining relatively low airway pressures.

Nursing Management

Nursing management of the patient using incentive spirometry includes placing the patient in the proper position, teaching the technique for using the incentive spirometer, setting realistic goals for the patient, and recording the results of the therapy.

CHEST PHYSIOTHERAPY

Chest physiotherapy (CPT) includes **postural drainage, chest percussion** and **vibration,** and breathing exercises/breathing retraining. In addition, teaching the patient effective coughing technique is an important part of chest physiotherapy. The goals of chest physiotherapy are to remove bronchial secretions, improve ventilation, and increase the efficiency of the respiratory muscles.

Postural Drainage (Segmented Bronchial Drainage)

Postural drainage uses specific positions that allow the force of gravity to assist in the removal of bronchial secretions. The secretions drain from the affected bronchioles into the bronchi and trachea and are removed by coughing or suctioning. Postural drainage is used to prevent or relieve bronchial obstruction caused by accumulation of secretions.

Because the patient usually sits in an upright position, secretions are likely to accumulate in the lower parts of the lungs. With postural drainage, different positions (Fig. 25-3) are used so that the force of gravity helps to move secretions from the smaller bronchial airways to the main bronchi and trachea. The secretions then are removed by coughing. The nurse should instruct the patient to inhale bronchodilators and mucolytic agents, if prescribed, before postural drainage because these medications improve bronchial tree drainage.

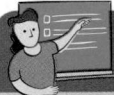 *Chart 25-4* • **PATIENT EDUCATION**
Assisting the Patient to Perform Incentive Spirometry

- Explain the reason and objective for the therapy: the inspired air helps to inflate the lungs. The ball or weight in the spirometer will rise in response to the intensity of the intake of air. The higher the ball rises, the deeper the breath.
- Assess the patient's level of pain and administer pain medication if prescribed.
- Position the patient in semi-Fowler's position or in an upright position (although any position is acceptable).
- Demonstrate how to use diaphragmatic breathing.
- Instruct the patient to place the mouthpiece of the spirometer firmly in the mouth, to breathe air in (inspire), and to hold the breath at the end of inspiration for about 3 seconds. The patient then exhales slowly.
- Encourage approximately 10 breaths per hour with the spirometer during waking hours.
- Set a reasonable volume and repetition goal (to provide encouragement and give the patient a sense of accomplishment).
- Encourage coughing during and after each session.
- Assist the patient to splint the incision when coughing postoperatively.
- Place the spirometer within easy reach of the patient.
- For the postoperative patient, begin the therapy immediately. (If the patient begins to hypoventilate, atelectasis can start to occur within an hour.)

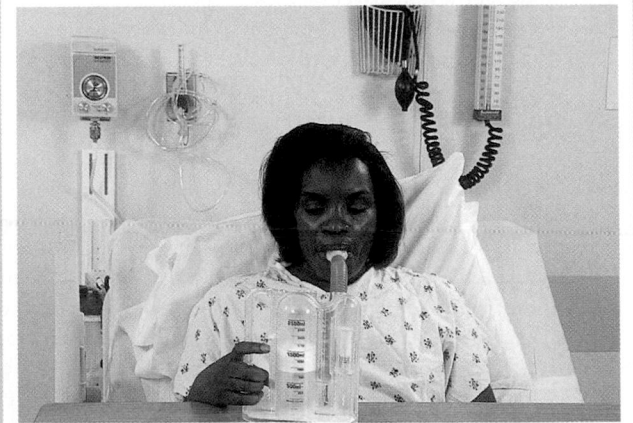

© B. Proud.

- Record how effectively the patient performs the therapy and the number of breaths achieved with the spirometer every 2 hours.

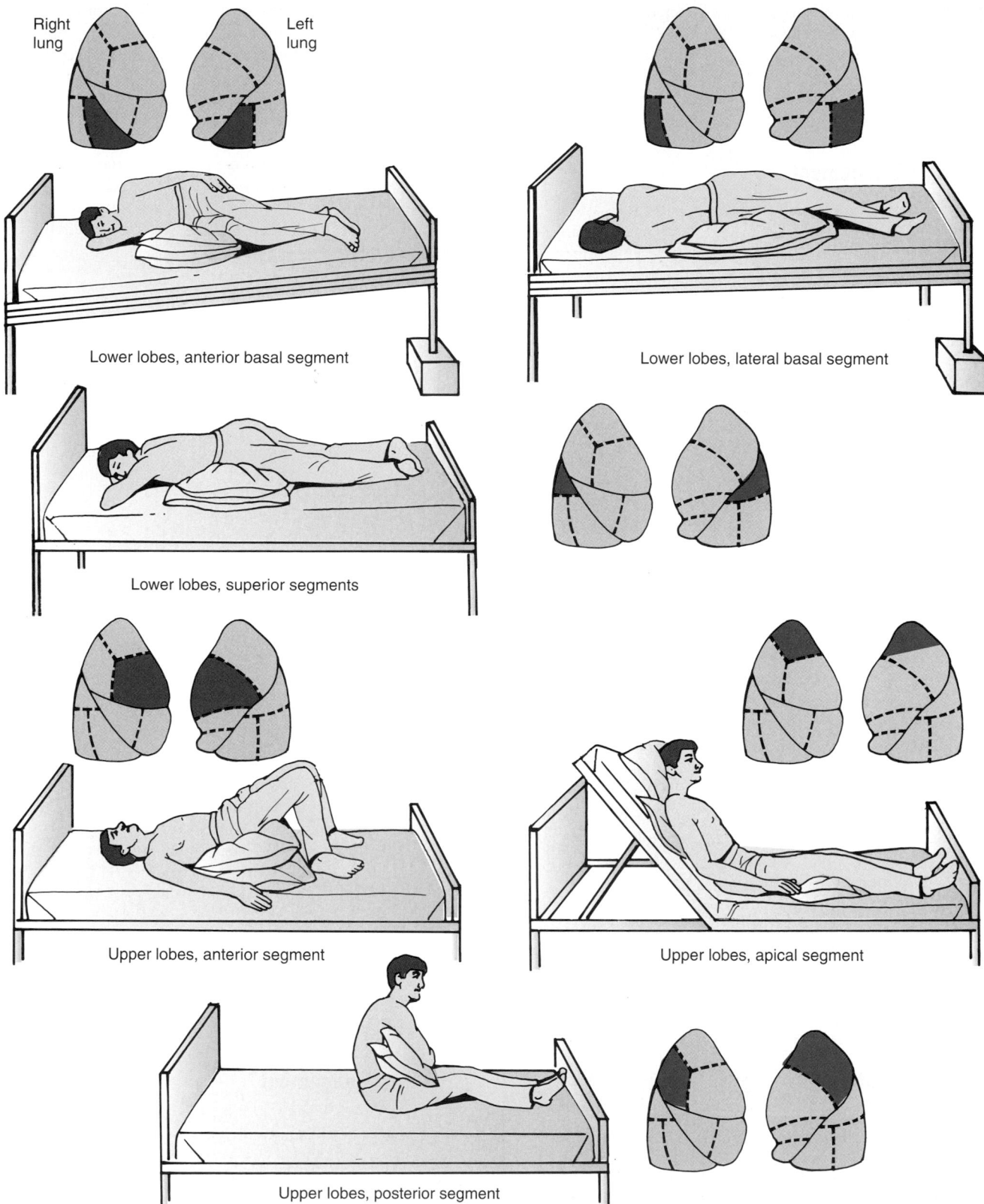

Right lung   Left lung

Lower lobes, anterior basal segment

Lower lobes, lateral basal segment

Lower lobes, superior segments

Upper lobes, anterior segment

Upper lobes, apical segment

Upper lobes, posterior segment

FIGURE 25-3 Postural drainage positions and the areas of lung drained by each position.

Postural drainage exercises can be directed at any of the segments of the lungs. The lower and middle lobe bronchi drain more effectively when the head is down; the upper lobe bronchi drain more effectively when the head is up. Frequently, five positions are used, one for drainage of each lobe: head down, prone, right and left lateral, and sitting upright.

Nursing Management

The nurse should be aware of the patient's diagnosis as well as the lung lobes or segments involved, the cardiac status, and any structural deformities of the chest wall and spine. Auscultating the chest before and after the procedure helps to identify the areas needing drainage and to assess the effectiveness of treatment. The nurse teaches family members who will be assisting the patient at home to evaluate breath sounds before and after treatment. The nurse explores strategies that will enable the patient to assume the indicated positions at home. This may require the creative use of objects readily available at home, such as pillows, cushions, or cardboard boxes.

Postural drainage is usually performed two to four times daily, before meals (to prevent nausea, vomiting, and aspiration) and at bedtime. Prescribed bronchodilators, water, or saline may be nebulized and inhaled before postural drainage to dilate the bronchioles, reduce bronchospasm, decrease the thickness of mucus and sputum, and combat edema of the bronchial walls. The recommended sequence of positioning is as follows: positions to drain the lower lobes first, then positions to drain the upper lobes.

The nurse makes the patient as comfortable as possible in each position and provides an emesis basin, sputum cup, and paper tissues. The nurse instructs the patient to remain in each position for 10 to 15 minutes and to breathe in slowly through the nose and then breathe out slowly through pursed lips to help keep the airways open so that secretions can drain while in each position. If a position cannot be tolerated, the nurse helps the patient to assume a modified position. When the patient changes position, the nurse explains how to cough and remove secretions (Chart 25-5).

If the patient cannot cough, the nurse may need to suction the secretions mechanically. It also may be necessary to use chest percussion and vibration to loosen bronchial secretions and mucus plugs that adhere to the bronchioles and bronchi and to propel sputum in the direction of gravity drainage (see "Chest Percussion and Vibration," below). If suctioning is required at home, the nurse instructs caregivers in safe suctioning technique and care of the suctioning equipment.

After the procedure, the nurse notes the amount, color, viscosity, and character of the expelled sputum. It is important to evaluate the patient's skin color and pulse the first few times the procedure is performed. It may be necessary to administer oxygen during postural drainage.

If the sputum is foul-smelling, it is important to perform postural drainage in a room away from other patients and/or family members and to use deodorizers unless contraindicated. Deodorizers delivered in aerosol sprays can cause bronchospasm and irritation to the patient with a respiratory disorder and should be used cautiously (Zang & Allender, 1999). After the procedure, the patient may find it refreshing to brush the teeth and use a mouthwash before resting.

Chest Percussion and Vibration

Thick secretions that are difficult to cough up may be loosened by tapping (percussing) and vibrating the chest. Chest percussion and vibration help to dislodge mucus adhering to the bronchioles and bronchi.

Percussion is carried out by cupping the hands and lightly striking the chest wall in a rhythmic fashion over the lung segment to be drained. The wrists are alternately flexed and extended so that the chest is cupped or clapped in a painless manner (Fig. 25-4). A soft cloth or towel may be placed over the segment of the chest that is being cupped to prevent skin irritation and redness from direct contact. Percussion, alternating with vibration, is performed for 3 to 5 minutes for each position. The patient uses diaphragmatic breathing during this procedure to promote relaxation (see "Breathing Retraining," below). As a precaution, percussion over chest drainage tubes, the sternum, spine, liver, kidneys, spleen, or breasts (in women) is avoided. Percussion is performed cautiously in the elderly because of their increased incidence of osteoporosis and risk of rib fracture.

Vibration is the technique of applying manual compression and tremor to the chest wall during the exhalation phase of respiration (see Fig. 25-4). This helps to increase the velocity of the air expired from the small airways, thus freeing the mucus. After three or four vibrations, the patient is encouraged to cough, using the abdominal muscles. (Contracting the abdominal muscles increases the effectiveness of the cough.)

A scheduled program of coughing and clearing sputum, together with hydration, reduces the amount of sputum in most patients. The number of times the percussion and vibration cycle is repeated depends on the patient's tolerance and clinical response. It is important to evaluate breath sounds before and after the procedures.

Nursing Management

When performing chest physiotherapy, the nurse ensures that the patient is comfortable, is not wearing restrictive clothing, and has not just eaten. The uppermost areas of the lung are treated first. The nurse gives medication for pain, as prescribed, before percussion and vibration and splints any incision and provides pillows for support as needed. The positions are varied, but focus is placed on the affected areas. On completion of the treatment, the nurse assists the patient to assume a comfortable position.

The nurse must stop treatment if any of the following occur: increased pain, increased shortness of breath, weakness, lightheadedness, or hemoptysis. Therapy is indicated until the patient has normal respirations, can mobilize secretions, and has normal breath sounds, and when the chest x-ray findings are normal.

Chart 25-5 Effective Coughing Technique

1. The patient assumes a sitting position and bends slightly forward. This upright position permits a stronger cough.
2. The patient's knees and hips are flexed to promote relaxation and reduce the strain on the abdominal muscles while coughing.
3. The patient inhales slowly through the nose and exhales through pursed lips several times.
4. The patient should cough twice during each exhalation while contracting (pulling in) the abdomen sharply with each cough.
5. The patient splints the incisional area, if any, with firm hand pressure or supports it with a pillow or rolled blanket while coughing (see Fig. 25-8). (The nurse can initially demonstrate this by using the patient's hands.)

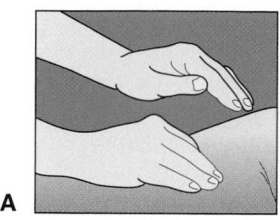
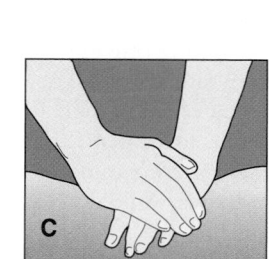
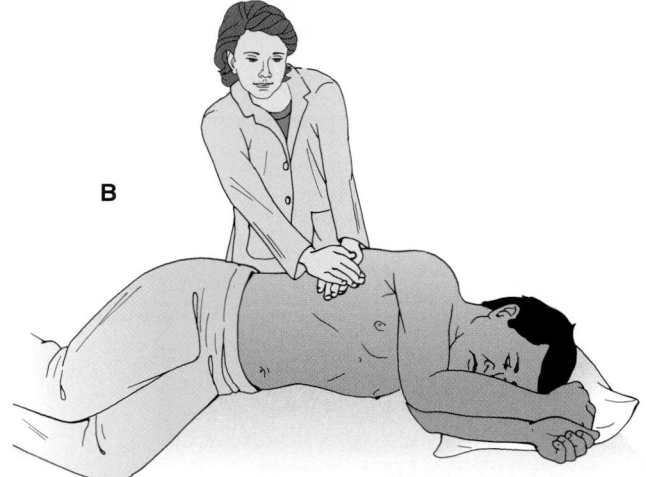

FIGURE 25-4 Percussion and vibration. (**A**) Proper hand position for percussion. (**B**) Proper technique for vibration. The wrists and elbows remain stiff; the vibrating motion is produced by the shoulder muscles. (**C**) Proper hand position for vibration.

PROMOTING HOME AND COMMUNITY-BASED CARE

Teaching Patients Self-Care. Chest physiotherapy is frequently indicated at home for patients with COPD, bronchiectasis, and cystic fibrosis. The techniques are the same as described above, but gravity drainage is achieved by placing the hips over a box, a stack of magazines, or pillows (unless a hospital bed is available). The nurse instructs the patient and family in the positions and techniques of percussion and vibration so that therapy can be continued in the home. In addition, the nurse instructs the patient to maintain an adequate fluid intake and air humidity to prevent secretions from becoming thick and tenacious. It also is important to teach the patient to recognize early signs of infection, such as fever and a change in the color or character of sputum. Resting 5 to 10 minutes in each postural drainage position before chest physiotherapy maximizes the amount of secretions obtained.

Continuing Care. Chest physical therapy may be carried out during visits by a home care nurse. The nurse also assesses the patient's physical status, understanding of the treatment plan, and compliance with recommended therapy, as well as the effectiveness of therapy. It is important to reinforce patient and family teaching during these visits. The nurse reports to the patient's physician any deterioration in the patient's physical status and inability to clear secretions.

Breathing Retraining

Breathing retraining consists of exercises and breathing practices designed to achieve more efficient and controlled ventilation and to decrease the work of breathing. Breathing retraining is especially indicated in patients with COPD and dyspnea. These exercises promote maximal alveolar inflation and muscle relaxation, relieve anxiety, eliminate ineffective, uncoordinated patterns of respiratory muscle activity, slow the respiratory rate, and decrease the work of breathing. Slow, relaxed, and rhythmic breathing also helps to control the anxiety that occurs with dyspnea. Specific breathing exercises include diaphragmatic and pursed-lip breathing (see Chart 25-3).

The goal of diaphragmatic breathing is to use and strengthen the diaphragm during breathing. Diaphragmatic breathing can become automatic with sufficient practice and concentration. Pursed-lip breathing, which improves oxygen transport, helps to induce a slow, deep breathing pattern and assists the patient to control breathing, even during periods of stress. This type of breathing helps prevent airway collapse secondary to loss of lung elasticity in emphysema. The goal of pursed-lip breathing is to train the muscles of expiration to prolong exhalation and increase airway pressure during expiration, thus lessening the amount of airway trapping and resistance. The nurse instructs the patient in diaphragmatic breathing and pursed-lip breathing, as described earlier in Chart 25-3. Breathing exercises may be practiced in several positions because air distribution and pulmonary circulation vary with the position of the chest. Many patients require additional oxygen, using a low-flow method, while performing breathing exercises. Emphysema-like changes in the lung occur as part of the natural aging process of the lung; therefore, breathing exercises are appropriate for all elderly patients who are hospitalized and elderly patients in any setting who are sedentary, even without primary lung disease.

Nursing Management

PROMOTING HOME AND COMMUNITY-BASED CARE

Teaching Patients Self-Care. The nurse instructs the patient to breathe slowly and rhythmically in a relaxed manner and to exhale completely to empty the lungs. The patient is instructed always to inhale through the nose because this filters, humidifies, and warms the air. If short of breath, the patient should concentrate on breathing slowly and rhythmically. To avoid initiating a cycle of increasing shortness of breath and panic, it is often helpful to instruct the patient to concentrate on prolonging the length of exhalation rather than merely slowing the rate of breathing. Minimizing the amount of dust or particles in the air and providing adequate humidification may also make it easier for the patient to breathe. Strategies to decrease dust or particles in the air include removing drapes or upholstered furniture, using air filters, and washing floors and dusting and vacuuming frequently.

The nurse instructs the patient that an adequate dietary intake promotes gas exchange and increases energy levels. It is important to provide adequate nutrition without overfeeding patients. Nurses should teach patients to consume small, frequent meals and snacks. Having ready-prepared meals and favorite foods available helps encourage nutrient consumption. Gas-producing foods such as beans, legumes, broccoli, cabbage, and Brussels sprouts should be avoided to prevent gastric distress. Because many of these patients lack the energy to eat, they should be taught to rest before and after meals to conserve energy (Lutz & Przytulski, 2001).

Airway Management

Adequate ventilation is dependent on free movement of air through the upper and lower airways. In many disorders, the airway becomes narrowed or blocked as a result of disease, bronchoconstriction (narrowing of airway by contraction of muscle fibers), a foreign body, or secretions. Maintaining a patent (open) airway is achieved through meticulous airway management, whether in an emergency situation such as airway obstruction or in long-term management, as in caring for a patient with an endotracheal or a tracheostomy tube.

EMERGENCY MANAGEMENT OF UPPER AIRWAY OBSTRUCTION

Upper airway obstruction has a variety of causes. Acute upper airway obstruction may be caused by food particles, vomitus, blood clots, or any other particle that enters and obstructs the larynx or trachea. It also may occur from enlargement of tissue in the wall of the airway, as in epiglottitis, laryngeal edema, laryngeal carcinoma, or peritonsillar abscess, or from thick secretions. Pressure on the walls of the airway, as occurs in retrosternal goiter, enlarged mediastinal lymph nodes, hematoma around the upper airway, and thoracic aneurysm, also may result in upper airway obstruction.

The patient with an altered level of consciousness from any cause is at risk for upper airway obstruction because of loss of the protective reflexes (cough and swallowing) and the tone of the pharyngeal muscles, causing the tongue to fall back and block the airway.

The nurse makes the following rapid observations to assess for signs and symptoms of upper airway obstruction:

- Inspection—Is the patient conscious? Is there any inspiratory effort? Does the chest rise symmetrically? Is there use or retraction of accessory muscles? What is the skin color? Are there any obvious signs of deformity or obstruction (trauma, food, teeth, vomitus)? Is the trachea midline?
- Palpation—Do both sides of the chest rise equally with inspiration? Are there any specific areas of tenderness, fracture, or subcutaneous emphysema (crepitus)?
- Auscultation—Is there any audible air movement, stridor (inspiratory sound), or wheezing (expiratory sound)? Are breath sounds present bilaterally in all lobes?

As soon as an upper airway obstruction is identified, the nurse takes emergency measures (Chart 25-6). (See "Guidelines for Managing a Foreign Body Airway Obstruction" in Chap. 71 for more details, or see Chap. 22.)

ENDOTRACHEAL INTUBATION

Endotracheal intubation involves passing an endotracheal tube through the mouth or nose into the trachea (Fig. 25-5). Intubation provides a patent airway when the patient is having respiratory distress that cannot be treated with simpler methods. It is the method of choice in emergency care. Endotracheal intubation is a means of providing an airway for patients who cannot maintain an adequate airway on their own (eg, comatose patients or pa-

tients with upper airway obstruction), for mechanical ventilation, and for suctioning secretions from the pulmonary tree.

An endotracheal tube usually is passed with the aid of a laryngoscope by specifically trained medical, nursing, or respiratory therapy personnel. (See "Guidelines for Inserting an Oropharyngeal Airway" in Chap. 71 for more details.) Once the tube is inserted, a cuff around the tube is inflated to prevent air from leaking around the outer part of the tube, to minimize the possibility of subsequent aspiration, and to prevent movement of the tube.

Nurses should be aware that complications could occur from pressure in the cuff on the tracheal wall. Cuff pressures should be checked with a calibrated aneroid manometer device every 8 to 12 hours to maintain cuff pressure between 20 and 25 mm Hg. High cuff pressure can cause tracheal bleeding, ischemia, and pressure necrosis, while low cuff pressure can increase the risk of aspiration pneumonia. Routine deflation of the cuff is not recommended due to the increased risk of aspiration and hypoxia. The cuff is deflated prior to removing the endotracheal tube (St. John, 1999b).

Tracheobronchial secretions are suctioned through the tube. Warmed, humidified oxygen should always be introduced through the tube, whether the patient is breathing spontaneously or is receiving ventilatory support. Endotracheal intubation may be used for no more than 3 weeks, by which time a tracheostomy must be considered to decrease irritation of and trauma to the tracheal lining, to reduce the incidence of vocal cord paralysis (secondary to laryngeal nerve damage), and to decrease the work of breathing. Chart 25-7 discusses the nursing care of the patient with an endotracheal tube.

There are several disadvantages of endotracheal and tracheostomy tubes. First, the tube causes discomfort. In addition, the cough reflex is depressed because closure of the glottis is hindered. Secretions tend to become thicker because the warming and humidifying effect of the upper respiratory tract has been bypassed. The swallowing reflexes, composed of the glottic, pharyngeal, and laryngeal reflexes, are depressed because of prolonged disuse and the mechanical trauma of the endotracheal or tracheostomy tube, which puts the patient at increased risk for aspiration. In addition, ulceration and stricture of the larynx or trachea may develop. Of great concern to the patient is the inability to talk and to communicate needs.

Unintentional or premature removal of the tube is a potentially life-threatening complication of endotracheal intubation. Removal of the tube is a frequent problem in intensive care units and occurs mainly during nursing care or by the patient. It is important for nurses to instruct patients and family members about the purpose of the tube and the dangers of removing it. Baseline and ongoing assessment of the patient and equipment ensures effective care. Providing comfort measures, including opioid analgesia and sedation, can improve the patient's tolerance of the endotracheal tube.

> **NURSING ALERT** Inadvertent removal of an endotracheal tube can cause laryngeal swelling, hypoxemia, bradycardia, hypotension, and even death. Measures must be taken to prevent premature or inadvertent removal.

To prevent tube removal by the patient, the nurse can use the following strategies: explain to the patient and family the purpose of the tube, distract the patient through one-to-one interaction with the nurse and family or with television, and maintain comfort measures. As a last resort, soft wrist restraints may be used, according to agency policy.

Chart 25-6 **Clearing an Upper Airway Obstruction**

Clearing the Airway

- Hyperextend the patient's neck by placing one hand on the forehead and placing the fingers of the other hand underneath the jaw and lifting upward and forward. This action pulls the tongue away from the back of the pharynx.

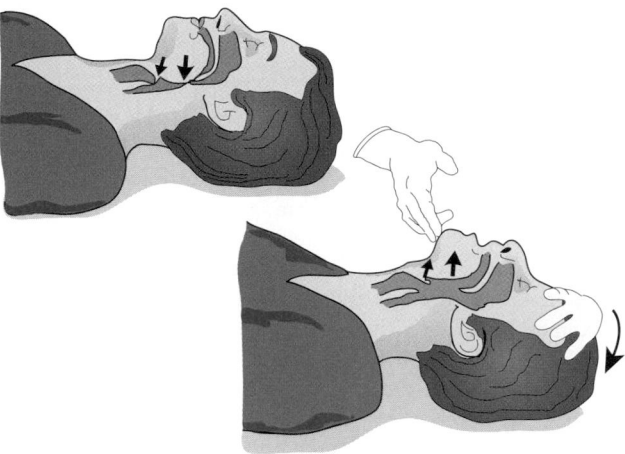

Opening the airway.

- Assess the patient by observing the chest and listening and feeling for the movement of air.
- Use a cross-finger technique to open the mouth and observe for obvious obstructions such as secretions, blood clots, or food particles.
- If no passage of air is detected, apply five quick sharp abdominal thrusts just below the xiphoid process to expel the obstruction (Heimlich maneuver). Repeat this procedure until the obstruction is expelled.
- After the obstruction is expelled, roll the patient as a unit onto the side for recovery.
- When the obstruction is relieved and the patient can breathe spontaneously but not cough, swallow, or gag, insert an oral or nasopharyngeal airway.

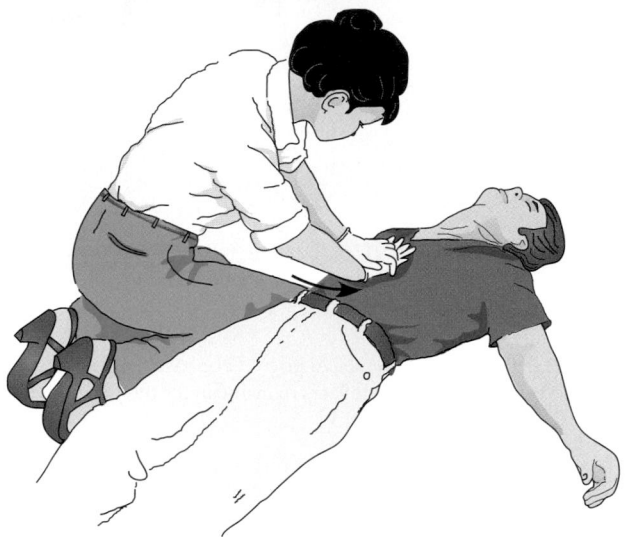

Abdominal thrust (Heimlich) maneuver administered to unconscious patient.

Bag and Mask Resuscitation

- Use a resuscitation bag and mask if assisted ventilation is required.
- Apply the mask to the patient's face and create a seal by pressing the thumb of the nondominant hand on the bridge of the nose and the index finger on the chin. Use the rest of the fingers on the hand and pull on the chin and the angle of the mandible to maintain the head in extension. Use the dominant hand to inflate the lungs by squeezing the bag to its full volume.

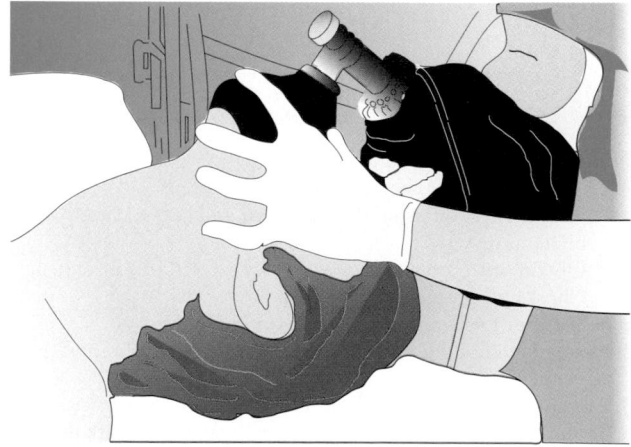

Resuscitation via bag and mask apparatus.

Studies have shown that the most effective way to prevent tube removal by the patient is through the use of soft wrist restraints (Happ, 2000). However, discretion and caution must always be used before applying any restraint. If the patient cannot move the arms and hands to the endotracheal tube, restraints would not be needed. If the patient is alert, oriented, able to follow directions, and cooperative to the point that it is highly unlikely that he or she will remove the endotracheal tube, restraints are not needed. On the other hand, if the nurse determines there is a risk that the patient may try to remove the tube, soft wrist restraints are appropriate with a physician's order (check agency policy). Close monitoring of the patient remains essential to ensure safety and prevent harm.

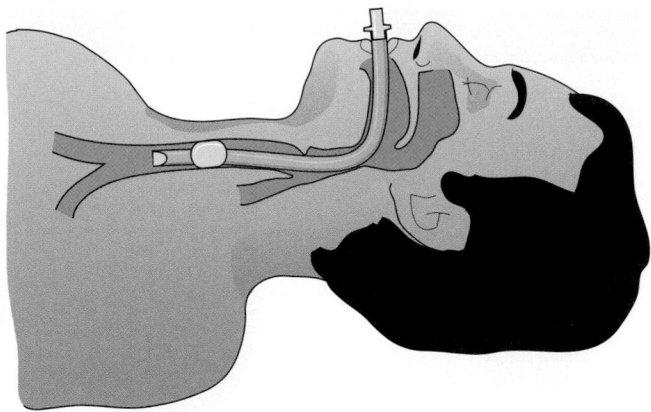

FIGURE 25-5 Endotracheal tube in place. Tube has been inserted using the oral route. The cuff has been inflated to maintain the tube's position and minimize the risk for aspiration.

TRACHEOSTOMY

A **tracheotomy** is a surgical procedure in which an opening is made into the trachea. The indwelling tube inserted into the trachea is called a **tracheostomy tube**. A tracheostomy may be either temporary or permanent.

A tracheostomy is used to bypass an upper airway obstruction, to allow removal of tracheobronchial secretions, to permit the long-term use of mechanical ventilation, to prevent aspiration of oral or gastric secretions in the unconscious or paralyzed patient (by closing off the trachea from the esophagus), and to replace an endotracheal tube. There are many disease processes and emergency conditions that make a tracheostomy necessary.

Procedure

The surgical procedure is usually performed in the operating room or in an intensive care unit, where the patient's ventilation can be well controlled and optimal aseptic technique can be maintained.

A surgical opening is made in the second and third tracheal rings. After the trachea is exposed, a cuffed tracheostomy tube of an appropriate size is inserted. The cuff is an inflatable attachment to the tracheostomy tube that is designed to occlude the space between the trachea walls and the tube to permit effective mechanical ventilation and to minimize the risk of aspiration.

The tracheostomy tube is held in place by tapes fastened around the patient's neck. Usually a square of sterile gauze is placed between the tube and the skin to absorb drainage and prevent infection.

Complications

Complications may occur early or late in the course of tracheostomy tube management. They may even occur years after the tube has been removed. Early complications include bleeding, pneumothorax, air embolism, aspiration, subcutaneous or mediastinal emphysema, recurrent laryngeal nerve damage, and posterior tracheal wall penetration. Long-term complications include airway obstruction from accumulation of secretions or protrusion of the cuff over the opening of the tube, infection, rupture of the innominate artery, dysphagia, tracheoesophageal fistula, tracheal dilation, and tracheal ischemia and necrosis. Tracheal stenosis may develop after the tube is removed. Chart 25-8 outlines measures nurses can take to prevent complications.

Postoperative Nursing Management

The patient requires continuous monitoring and assessment. The newly made opening must be kept patent by proper suctioning of secretions. After the vital signs are stable, the patient is placed in a semi-Fowler's position to facilitate ventilation, promote drainage, minimize edema, and prevent strain on the suture lines. Analgesia and sedative agents must be administered with caution because of the risk of suppressing the cough reflex.

Major objectives of nursing care are to alleviate the patient's apprehension and to provide an effective means of communica-

---

 Care of the Patient with an Endotracheal Tube

Immediately After Intubation
1. Check symmetry of chest expansion.
   - Auscultate breath sounds of anterior and lateral chest bilaterally.
   - Obtain order for chest x-ray to verify proper tube placement.
   - Check cuff pressure every 8–12 hours.
   - Monitor for signs and symptoms of aspiration.
2. Ensure high humidity; a visible mist should appear in the T-piece or ventilator tubing.
3. Administer oxygen concentration as prescribed by physician.
4. Secure the tube to the patient's face with tape, and mark the proximal end for position maintenance.
   - Cut proximal end of tube if it is longer than 7.5 cm (3 inches) to prevent kinking.
   - Insert an oral airway or mouth device to prevent the patient from biting and obstructing the tube.
5. Use sterile suction technique and airway care to prevent iatrogenic contamination and infection.
6. Continue to reposition patient every 2 hours and as needed to prevent atelectasis and to optimize lung expansion.
7. Provide oral hygiene and suction the oropharynx whenever necessary.

Extubation (Removal of Endotracheal Tube)
1. Explain procedure.
2. Have self-inflating bag and mask ready in case ventilatory assistance is required immediately after extubation.
3. Suction the tracheobronchial tree and oropharynx, remove tape, and then deflate the cuff.
4. Give oxygen for a few breaths, then insert a new, sterile suction catheter inside tube.
5. Have the patient inhale. At peak inspiration remove the tube, suctioning the airway through the tube as it is pulled out.
Note: In some hospitals this procedure can be performed by respiratory therapists; in others, by nurses. Check hospital policy.

Care of Patient Following Extubation
1. Give heated humidity and oxygen by face mask.
2. Monitor respiratory rate and quality of chest excursions. Note stridor, color change, and change in mental alertness or behavior.
3. Monitor the patient's oxygen level using a pulse oximeter.
4. Keep NPO or give only ice chips for next few hours.
5. Provide mouth care.
6. Teach patient how to perform coughing and deep-breathing exercises.

Chart 25-8 Preventing Complications Associated With Endotracheal and Tracheostomy Tubes

- Administer adequate warmed humidity.
- Maintain cuff around tube.
- Suction as needed per assessment findings.
- Maintain skin integrity. Change tape and dressing as needed or per protocol.
- Auscultate lung sounds.
- Monitor for signs and symptoms of infection, including temperature and white blood cell count.
- Administer prescribed oxygen and monitor oxygen saturation.
- Monitor for cyanosis.
- Maintain adequate hydration of the patient.
- Use sterile technique when suctioning and performing tracheostomy care.

tion. The nurse keeps paper and pencil or a Magic Slate and the call light within the patient's reach to ensure a means of communication. The care of the patient with a tracheostomy tube is summarized in Chart 25-9.

SUCTIONING THE TRACHEAL TUBE (TRACHEOSTOMY OR ENDOTRACHEAL TUBE)

When a tracheostomy or endotracheal tube is in place, it is usually necessary to suction the patient's secretions because of the decreased effectiveness of the cough mechanism. Tracheal suctioning is performed when adventitious breath sounds are detected or whenever secretions are obviously present. Unnecessary suctioning can initiate bronchospasm and cause mechanical trauma to the tracheal mucosa.

All equipment that comes into direct contact with the patient's lower airway must be sterile to prevent overwhelming pulmonary and systemic infections. The procedure for suctioning a tracheostomy is presented in Chart 25-10. In mechanically ventilated patients, an in-line suction catheter may be used to allow rapid suction when needed and to minimize cross-contamination of airborne pathogens. An in-line suction device allows the patient to be suctioned without being disconnected from the ventilator circuit.

MANAGING THE CUFF

As a general rule, the cuff on an endotracheal or tracheostomy tube should be inflated. The pressure within the cuff should be the lowest possible that allows delivery of adequate tidal volumes and prevents pulmonary aspiration. Usually the pressure is maintained at less than 25 cm H_2O to prevent injury and at more than 20 cm H_2O to prevent aspiration. Cuff pressure must be monitored at least every 8 hours by attaching a hand-held pressure gauge to the pilot balloon of the tube or by using the minimal leak volume or minimal occlusion volume technique. With long-term intubation, higher pressures may be needed to maintain an adequate seal.

PROMOTING HOME AND COMMUNITY-BASED CARE

Teaching Patients Self-Care. If the patient is at home with a tracheostomy, the nurse instructs the patient and family about its daily care as well as measures to take in an emergency. The nurse also makes sure the patient and family are aware of community contacts for education and support needs. It is important for the

nurse to teach the patient and family strategies to prevent infection when performing tracheostomy care (McConnell, 2000).

Mechanical Ventilation

Mechanical ventilation may be required for a variety of reasons, including the need to control the patient's respirations during surgery or during treatment of severe head injury, to oxygenate the blood when the patient's ventilatory efforts are inadequate, and to rest the respiratory muscles. Many patients placed on a ventilator can breathe spontaneously, but the effort needed to do so may be exhausting.

A mechanical ventilator is a positive- or negative-pressure breathing device that can maintain ventilation and oxygen delivery for a prolonged period. Caring for a patient on mechanical ventilation has become an integral part of nursing care in critical care or general medical-surgical units, extended care facilities, and the home. Nurses, physicians, and respiratory therapists must understand each patient's specific pulmonary needs and work together to set realistic goals. Positive patient outcomes depend on an understanding of the principles of mechanical ventilation and the patient's care needs as well as open communication among members of the health care team about the goals of therapy, weaning plans, and the patient's tolerance of changes in ventilator settings.

INDICATIONS FOR MECHANICAL VENTILATION

If a patient has a continuous decrease in oxygenation (PaO_2), an increase in arterial carbon dioxide levels ($PaCO_2$), and a persistent acidosis (decreased pH), mechanical ventilation may be necessary. Conditions such as thoracic or abdominal surgery, drug overdose, neuromuscular disorders, inhalation injury, COPD, multiple trauma, shock, multisystem failure, and coma all may lead to respiratory failure and the need for mechanical ventilation. The criteria for mechanical ventilation (Chart 25-11) guide the decision to place a patient on a ventilator. A patient with apnea that is not readily reversible also is a candidate for mechanical ventilation.

CLASSIFICATION OF VENTILATORS

Several types of mechanical ventilators exist; they are classified according to the manner in which they support ventilation. The two general categories are negative-pressure and positive-pressure ventilators. The most common category in use today is the positive-pressure ventilator.

Negative-Pressure Ventilators

Negative-pressure ventilators exert a negative pressure on the external chest. Decreasing the intrathoracic pressure during inspiration allows air to flow into the lung, filling its volume. Physiologically, this type of assisted ventilation is similar to spontaneous ventilation. It is used mainly in chronic respiratory failure associated with neuromuscular conditions, such as poliomyelitis, muscular dystrophy, amyotrophic lateral sclerosis, and myasthenia gravis. It is inappropriate for the unstable or complex patient or the patient whose condition requires frequent ventilatory changes. Negative-pressure ventilators are simple to use and do not require intubation of the airway; consequently, they are especially adaptable for home use.

Chart 25-9 | **Care of the Patient With a Tracheostomy Tube**

Nursing Intervention	Rationale
1. Gather the needed equipment, including sterile gloves, hydrogen peroxide, normal saline solution or sterile water, cotton-tipped applicators, dressing and twill tape (and the type of tube prescribed, if the tube is to be changed).	Everything needed to care for a tracheostomy should be readily on hand for the most effective care.
A cuffed tube (air injected into cuff) is required during mechanical ventilation. A low-pressure cuff is most commonly used.	A cuffed tube prevents air from leaking during positive-pressure ventilation and also prevents tracheal aspiration of gastric contents. An adequate seal is indicated by the disappearance of any air leakage from the mouth or tracheostomy or by the disappearance of the harsh, gurgling sound of air coming from the throat.
Patients requiring long-term use of a tracheostomy tube and who can breathe spontaneously commonly use an uncuffed, metal tube.	Low-pressure cuffs exert minimal pressure on the tracheal mucosa and thus reduce the danger of tracheal ulceration and stricture.
2. Provide patient and family instruction on the key points for tracheostomy care, beginning with how to inspect the tracheostomy dressing for moisture or drainage.	The tracheostomy dressing is changed as needed to keep the skin clean and dry. To prevent potential breakdown, moist or soiled dressings should not remain on the skin.
3. Perform hand hygiene.	Hand hygiene reduces bacteria on hands.
4. Explain procedure to patient and family as appropriate.	A patient with a tracheostomy is apprehensive and requires ongoing assurance and support.
5. Put on clean gloves; remove and discard the soiled dressing in a biohazard container.	Observing body substance isolation reduces cross-contamination from soiled dressings.
6. Prepare sterile supplies, including hydrogen peroxide, normal saline solution or sterile water, cotton-tipped applicators, dressing, and tape.	Having necessary supplies and equipment readily available allows the procedure to be completed efficiently.
7. Put on sterile gloves. (Some physicians approve clean technique for long-term tracheostomy patients in the home.)	Sterile equipment minimizes transmission of surface flora to the sterile respiratory tract. Clean technique may be used in the home because of decreased exposure to potential pathogens.
8. Cleanse the wound and the plate of the tracheostomy tube with sterile cotton-tipped applicators moistened with hydrogen peroxide. Rinse with sterile saline solution.	Hydrogen peroxide is effective in loosening crusted secretions. Rinsing prevents skin residue.
9. Soak inner cannula in peroxide and rinse with saline solution or replace with a new disposable inner cannula.	Soaking loosens and removes secretions from the inner lumen of the tracheostomy tube.
10. Remove soiled twill tape with clean tape, after the new tape is in place. Place clean twill tape in position to secure the tracheostomy tube by inserting one end of the tape through the side opening of the outer cannula. Take the tape around the back of the patient's neck and thread it through the opposite opening of the outer cannula. Bring both ends around so that they meet on one side of the neck. Tighten the tape until only two fingers can be comfortably inserted under it. Secure with a knot. For a new tracheostomy, two people should assist with tape changes.	This taping technique provides a double thickness of tape around the neck, which is needed because the tracheostomy tube can be dislodged by movement or by a forceful cough if left unsecured. A dislodged tracheostomy tube is difficult to reinsert, and respiratory distress may occur. Dislodgement of a new tracheostomy is a medical emergency.
11. Remove old tapes and discard in a biohazard container.	Tapes with old secretions may harbor bacteria.
12. Although some long-term tracheostomies with healed stomas may not require a dressing, other tracheostomies do. In such cases, use a sterile tracheostomy dressing, fitting it securely under the twill tapes and flange of tracheostomy tube so that the incision is covered, as shown below.	Healed tracheostomies with minimal secretions do not need a dressing. Dressings that will shred are not used around a tracheostomy because of the risk that pieces of material, lint, or thread may get into the tube, and eventually into the trachea, causing obstruction or abscess formation. Special dressings that do not have a tendency to shred are used.

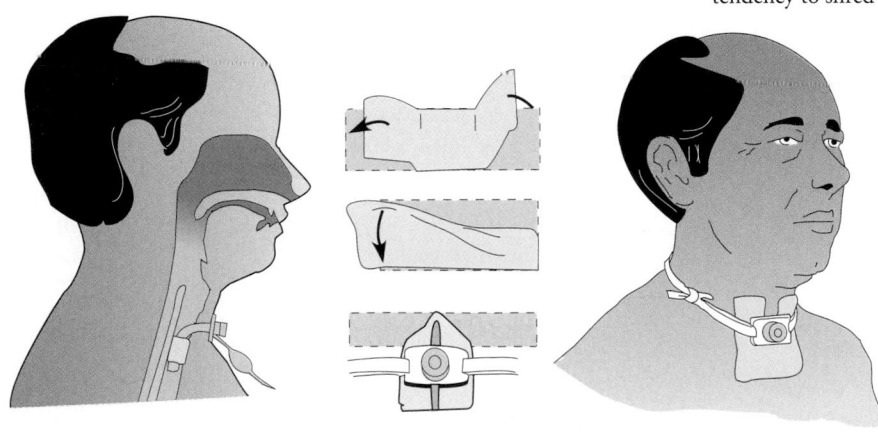

(**A**) The cuff of the tracheostomy tube fits smoothly and snugly in the trachea in a way that promotes circulation but seals off the escape of secretions and air surrounding the tube. (**B**) For a dressing change, a 4 × 4-inch gauze pad may be folded (cutting would promote shredding, placing the patient at risk for aspiration) around the tracheostomy tube and (**C**) stabilized by slipping the neck tape ties through the neck plate slots of the tracheostomy tube. The ties may be fastened to the side of the neck to eliminate the discomfort of lying on the knot.

A   B   C

Chart 25-10 **Performing Tracheal Suction**

Equipment
- Suction catheters
- Gloves
- Goggles for eye protection
- Basin for sterile normal saline solution for irrigation
- Manual resuscitation bag with supplemental oxygen
- Suction source

Procedure
1. Explain the procedure to the patient before beginning and offer reassurance during suctioning; the patient may be apprehensive about choking and about an inability to communicate.
2. Begin by carrying out hand hygiene.
3. Turn on suction source (pressure should not exceed 120 mm Hg).
4. Open suction catheter kit.
5. Fill basin with sterile normal saline solution.
6. Ventilate the patient with manual resuscitation bag and high-flow oxygen.
7. Put sterile glove on dominant hand.
8. Pick up suction catheter in gloved hand and connect to suction.
9. Hyperoxygenate the patient's lungs for several deep breaths. Instill normal saline solution into airway *only* if there are thick, tenacious secretions.
10. Insert suction catheter at least as far as the end of the tube without applying suction, just far enough to stimulate the cough reflex.
11. Apply suction while withdrawing and gently rotating the catheter 360° (no longer than 10 to 15 seconds, because hypoxia and dysrhythmias may develop, leading to cardiac arrest).
12. Reoxygenate and inflate the patient's lungs for several breaths.
13. Repeat previous three steps until the airway is clear.
14. Rinse catheter in basin with sterile normal saline solution between suction attempts if necessary.
15. Suction oropharyngeal cavity after completing tracheal suctioning.
16. Rinse suction tubing.
17. Discard catheter, gloves, and basin appropriately.

There are several types of negative-pressure ventilators: iron lung, body wrap, and chest cuirass.

IRON LUNG (DRINKER RESPIRATOR TANK)

The iron lung is a negative-pressure chamber used for ventilation. It was used extensively during polio epidemics in the past and currently is used by polio survivors and patients with other neuromuscular disorders.

BODY WRAP (PNEUMOWRAP) AND CHEST CUIRASS (TORTOISE SHELL)

Both of these portable devices require a rigid cage or shell to create a negative-pressure chamber around the thorax and abdomen.

Because of problems with proper fit and system leaks, these types of ventilators are used only with carefully selected patients.

Positive-Pressure Ventilators

Positive-pressure ventilators inflate the lungs by exerting positive pressure on the airway, similar to a bellows mechanism, forcing the alveoli to expand during inspiration. Expiration occurs passively. Endotracheal intubation or tracheostomy is necessary in most cases. These ventilators are widely used in the hospital setting and are increasingly used in the home for patients with primary lung disease. There are three types of positive-pressure ventilators, which are classified by the method of ending the inspiratory phase of respiration: pressure-cycled, time-cycled, and

---

NURSING RESEARCH PROFILE 25-1

The Effect of Normal Saline Instillation Before Suctioning on Oxygenation Status

Kinloch, D. (1999). Instillation of normal saline during endotracheal suctioning: effects on mixed venous oxygen saturation. *American Journal of Critical Care, 8*(4), 231–240.

Purpose

Although it has been suggested that instilling normal saline into an endotracheal tube before suctioning facilitates the removal of secretions, few studies have addressed this issue using in vivo measures of patients' oxygenation status. The purpose of this study was to determine if instillation of normal saline before endotracheal suctioning improves patients' oxygenation status.

Study Sample and Design

A descriptive, observational study design was used to investigate the effect of normal saline instillation (NSI) before endotracheal suctioning on mixed venous oxygen saturations. Thirty-five patients recovering from coronary artery bypass grafting were included in the study. The decision to instill normal saline into the endotracheal tube was made by the clinician caring for the patient. Patients were divided into NSI (n = 15) and non-NSI groups (n = 20). Patients in the NSI group received 5 mL of normal saline before endotracheal suctioning, and patients in the non-NSI group did not. A standardized suctioning protocol was used; other than NSI, suctioning procedures for both groups were identical. Baseline levels of mixed venous oxygenated

blood saturation ($S\bar{v}O_2$) levels were obtained through the use of a pulmonary artery catheter at 1-minute intervals for 5 minutes before the start of suctioning; the mean of these levels was considered the patient's baseline value. After suctioning, $S\bar{v}O_2$ levels were measured at 1-minute intervals until they returned to baseline levels.

Findings

The mean post-suctioning $S\bar{v}O_2$ level of the NSI group was significantly lower ($p = .007$) than that of the non-NSI group. Further, the NSI group took an average of 3.8 minutes longer to return to baseline $S\bar{v}O_2$ than the non-NSI group; this difference was statistically significant ($p = .05$).

Nursing Implications

The current standard of practice for nurses is to instill normal saline before suctioning, especially if the secretions are thick and tenacious. Although the findings of this study suggest that this practice should no longer be used, the issue needs further study with a larger sample and with randomization of patients to groups. The findings of this study are relevant to nurses caring for patients requiring endotracheal suctioning.

Chart 25-11

Indications for Mechanical Ventilation

$PaO_2 < 50$ mm Hg with $FiO_2 > 0.60$
$PaO_2 > 50$ mm Hg with pH < 7.25
Vital capacity $<$ 2 times tidal volume
Negative inspiratory force $<$ 25 cm H_2O
Respiratory rate $>$ 35/min

volume-cycled. Another type of positive-pressure ventilator used for selected patients is noninvasive positive-pressure ventilation.

PRESSURE-CYCLED VENTILATORS

The pressure-cycled ventilator ends inspiration when a preset pressure has been reached. In other words, the ventilator cycles on, delivers a flow of air until it reaches a predetermined pressure, then cycles off. Its major limitation is that the volume of air or oxygen can vary as the patient's airway resistance or compliance changes. As a result, the tidal volume delivered may be inconsistent, possibly compromising ventilation. Consequently, in adults, pressure-cycled ventilators are intended only for short-term use. The most common type is the IPPB machine (see previous discussion of IPPB).

TIME-CYCLED VENTILATORS

Time-cycled ventilators terminate or control inspiration after a preset time. The volume of air the patient receives is regulated by the length of inspiration and the flow rate of the air. Most ventilators have a rate control that determines the respiratory rate, but pure time-cycling is rarely used for adults. These ventilators are used in newborns and infants.

VOLUME-CYCLED VENTILATORS

Volume-cycled ventilators are by far the most commonly used positive-pressure ventilators today (Fig. 25-6). With this type of ventilator, the volume of air to be delivered with each inspiration is preset. Once this preset volume is delivered to the patient, the ventilator cycles off and exhalation occurs passively. From breath to breath, the volume of air delivered by the ventilator is relatively constant, ensuring consistent, adequate breaths despite varying airway pressures.

NONINVASIVE POSITIVE-PRESSURE VENTILATION

Positive-pressure ventilation can be given via facemasks that cover the nose and mouth, nasal masks, or other nasal devices. This eliminates the need for endotracheal intubation or tracheostomy and decreases the risk for nosocomial infections such as pneumonia. The most comfortable mode for the patient is pressure-controlled ventilation with pressure support. This eases the work of breathing and enhances gas exchange. The ventilator can be set with a minimum backup rate for patients with periods of apnea.

Patients are considered candidates for noninvasive ventilation if they have acute or chronic respiratory failure, acute pulmonary edema, COPD, or chronic heart failure with a sleep-related breathing disorder. The device also may be used at home to improve tissue oxygenation and to rest the respiratory muscles while the patient sleeps at night. It is contraindicated for those who have experienced respiratory arrest, serious dysrhythmias, cognitive impairment, or head or facial trauma. Noninvasive ventilation may also be used for patients at the end of life and those who do not want endotracheal intubation but may need short- or long-term ventilatory support (Scanlan, Wilkins & Stoller, 1999).

Bilevel positive airway pressure (bi-PAP) ventilation offers independent control of inspiratory and expiratory pressures while providing pressure support ventilation. It delivers two levels of

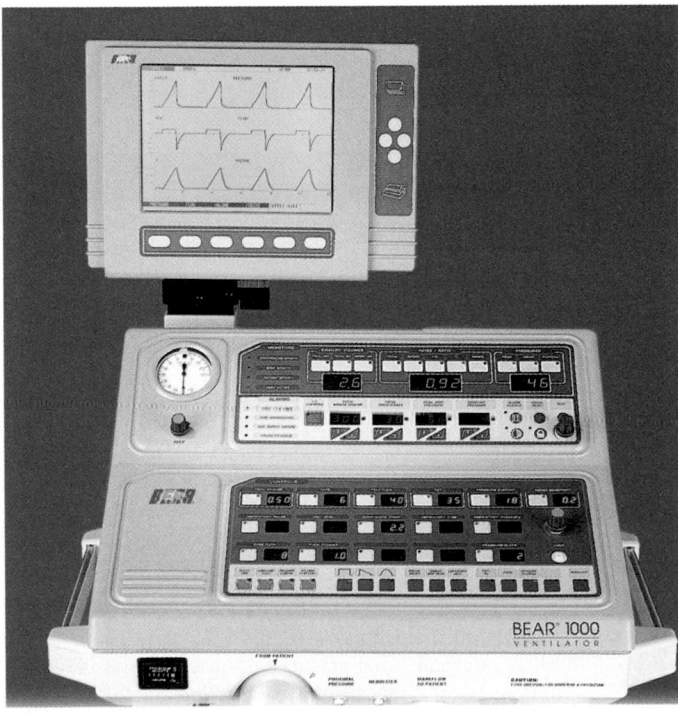

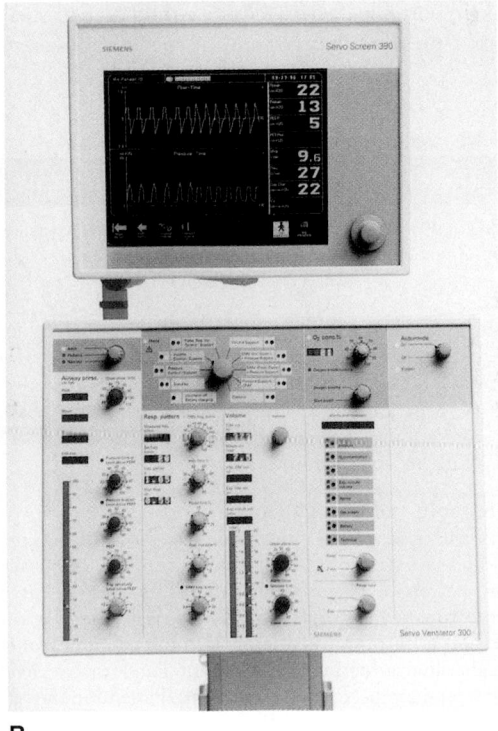

A **B**

FIGURE 25-6 Control panels of positive pressure ventilators in current use illustrate functions made possible by technologic advances. (**A**) Bear 1000 ventilator. Courtesy Bear Medical Systems. (**B**) Servo Ventilator 300 with Automode allows weaning to begin with the patient still intubated. Courtesy Siemens Medical Systems, Inc.

positive airway pressure provided via a nasal or oral mask, nasal pillow, or mouthpiece with a tight seal and a portable ventilator. Each inspiration can be initiated either by the patient or by the machine if it is programmed with a backup rate. The backup rate ensures that the patient will receive a set number of breaths per minute (Perkins & Shortall, 2000). Bi-PAP is most often used for patients who require ventilatory assistance at night, such as those with severe COPD or sleep apnea. Tolerance is variable; bi-PAP is usually most successful with highly motivated patients.

ADJUSTING THE VENTILATOR

The ventilator is adjusted so that the patient is comfortable and breathes "in sync" with the machine. Minimal alteration of the normal cardiovascular and pulmonary dynamics is desired. Modes of mechanical ventilation are described in Figure 25-7. If the volume ventilator is adjusted appropriately, the patient's arterial blood gas values will be satisfactory and there will be little or no cardiovascular compromise. Chart 25-12 discusses how to achieve adequate mechanical ventilation for each patient.

ASSESSING THE EQUIPMENT

The ventilator needs to be assessed to make sure that it is functioning properly and that the settings are appropriate. Even though the nurse is not primarily responsible for adjusting the settings on the ventilator or measuring ventilator parameters (usually the responsibility of the respiratory therapist), the nurse is responsible for the patient and therefore needs to evaluate how the ventilator affects the patient's overall status.

In monitoring the ventilator, the nurse should note the following:

- Type of ventilator (such as volume-cycled, pressure-cycled, negative-pressure)
- Controlling mode (such as **controlled ventilation, assist–control ventilation, synchronized intermittent mandatory ventilation**)
- Tidal volume and rate settings (tidal volume is usually 10 to 15 mL/kg; rate is usually 12 to 16/min)
- FiO_2 (**fraction of inspired oxygen**) setting

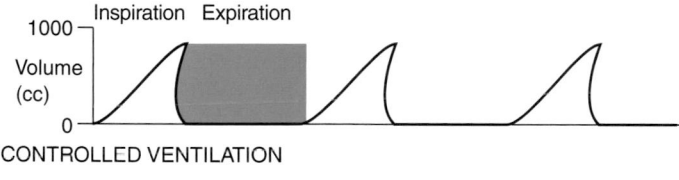

A CONTROLLED VENTILATION

A Flow in the controlled ventilation mode. A preset volume of gas is delivered to the patient under positive pressure while spontaneous patient respiratory effort is "locked out."

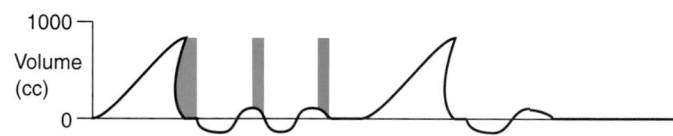

B ASSIST/CONTROLLED VENTILATION (A/C)

B Gas flow in the assist/control ventilation mode. In this mode, a preset volume of gas is delivered to the patient at a preset rate, but the patient may trigger a ventilator breath with negative inspiratory effort.

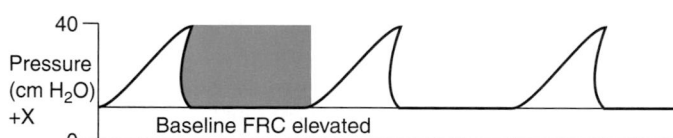

C SYNCHRONIZED INTERMITTENT MANDATORY VENTILATION (SIMV)

C Gas flow in the synchronized intermittent mandatory ventilation (SIMV) mode. A preset minimum number of breaths are synchronously delivered to the patient but the patient may also take spontaneous breaths of varying volumes. Note how inspiratory and expiratory pressures differ between spontaneous and ventilator breaths.

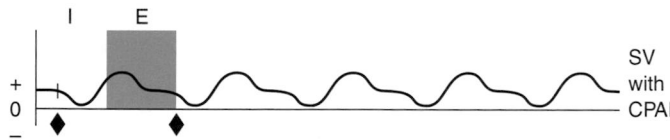

D POSITIVE END EXPIRATORY PRESSURE (PEEP)

D Airway pressure with varying levels of positive end-expiratory pressure (PEEP). Note that at end expiration, the airway is not allowed to return to zero. (FRC: functional residual capacity.)

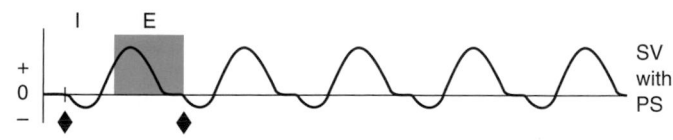

E CONTINUOUS POSITIVE AIRWAY PRESSURE (CPAP)

E Spontaneous ventilation with continous positive airway pressure (CPAP). This ventilatory adjunct is used only with spontaneous ventilation; the patient breathes spontaneously through the ventilator at an elevated baseline pressure throughout the breathing cycle.

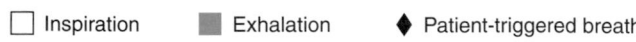

F PRESSURE SUPPORT (PS)

F Spontaneous ventilation with pressure support (PS). The patient breathes spontaneously with pressure assistance to each spontaneous inspiration.

☐ Inspiration   ▨ Exhalation   ◆ Patient-triggered breath

FIGURE 25-7 Modes of mechanical ventilation with air flow waveforms.

Chart 25-12 Initial Ventilator Settings

The following guide is an example of the steps involved in operating a mechanical ventilator. The nurse, in collaboration with the respiratory therapist, always reviews the manufacturer's instructions, which vary according to the equipment, before beginning mechanical ventilation.

1. Set the machine to deliver the tidal volume required (10 to 15 mL/kg).
2. Adjust the machine to deliver the lowest concentration of oxygen to maintain normal PaO_2 (80 to 100 mm Hg). This setting may be high initially but will gradually be reduced based on arterial blood gas results.
3. Record peak inspiratory pressure.
4. Set mode (assist–control or synchronized intermittent mandatory ventilation) and rate according to physician order. (See the glossary for definitions of modes of mechanical ventilation.) Set PEEP and pressure support if ordered.
5. Adjust sensitivity so that the patient can trigger the ventilator with a minimal effort (usually 2 mm Hg negative inspiratory force).
6. Record minute volume and measure carbon dioxide partial pressure (PCO_2), pH, and PO_2 after 20 minutes of continuous mechanical ventilation.
7. Adjust setting (FiO_2 and rate) according to results of arterial blood gas analysis to provide normal values or those set by the physician.
8. If the patient suddenly becomes confused or agitated or begins bucking the ventilator for some unexplained reason, assess for hypoxia and manually ventilate on 100% oxygen with a resuscitation bag.

- Inspiratory pressure reached and pressure limit (normal is 15 to 20 cm H_2O; this increases if there is increased airway resistance or decreased compliance)
- Sensitivity (a 2-cm H_2O inspiratory force should trigger the ventilator)
- Inspiratory-to-expiratory ratio (usually 1:3 [1 second of inspiration to 3 seconds of expiration] or 1:2)
- Minute volume (tidal volume × respiratory rate, usually 6 to 8 L/min)
- Sigh settings (usually 1.5 times the tidal volume and ranging from 1 to 3 per hour), if applicable
- Water in the tubing, disconnection or kinking of the tubing
- Humidification (humidifier filled with water) and temperature
- Alarms (turned on and functioning properly)
- PEEP and/or pressure support level, if applicable. PEEP is usually 5 to 15 cm H_2O

NURSING ALERT If the ventilator system malfunctions and the problem cannot be identified and corrected immediately, the nurse must ventilate the patient with a manual resuscitation bag until the problem is resolved.

PROBLEMS WITH MECHANICAL VENTILATION

Because of the seriousness of the patient's condition and the highly complex and technical nature of mechanical ventilation, a number of problems or complications can occur. Such situations fall into two categories: ventilator problems and patient problems. In either case, the patient must be supported while the problem is identified and corrected. Ventilator complications include cardiovascular compromise, pneumothorax, and pulmonary infection. These problems, their probable causes, and solutions are listed in Table 25-2.

BUCKING THE VENTILATOR

The patient is "in sync" with the ventilator when thoracic expansion coincides with the inspiratory phase of the machine and exhalation occurs passively. The patient is said to fight or buck the ventilator when out of phase with the machine. This is manifested when the patient attempts to breathe out during the ventilator's mechanical inspiratory phase or when there is jerky and increased abdominal muscle effort. The following factors contribute to this problem: anxiety, hypoxia, increased secretions, hypercapnia, inadequate minute volume, and pulmonary edema. These problems must be corrected before resorting to the use of paralyzing agents to reduce bucking; otherwise, the underlying problem is simply masked and the patient's condition will continue to deteriorate.

Muscle relaxants, tranquilizers, analgesic agents, and paralyzing agents are sometimes administered to patients receiving mechanical ventilation. Their purpose is ultimately to increase the patient–machine synchrony by decreasing the patient's anxiety, hyperventilation, or excessive muscle activity. The selection and dose of the appropriate medication are determined carefully and are based on the patient's requirements and the cause of his or her restlessness. Paralyzing agents are always used as a last resort, and always in conjunction with a sedative medication.

Nursing Management

PROMOTING HOME AND COMMUNITY-BASED CARE
Increasingly, patients are being cared for in extended care facilities or at home while on mechanical ventilators, with tracheostomy tubes, or on oxygen therapy. Patients receiving home ventilator care usually have chronic neuromuscular conditions or COPD.

Teaching Patients Self-Care. Caring for the patient with mechanical ventilator support at home can be accomplished successfully, but the family must be emotionally, educationally, and physically able to assume the role of primary caregiver. A home care team consisting of the nurse, physician, respiratory therapist, social service or home care agency, and equipment supplier is needed. The home is evaluated to determine if the electrical equipment needed can be operated safely. A summary of the basic assessment criteria needed for successful home care is presented in Chart 25-13.

Once the decision is made to initiate mechanical ventilation at home, the nurse prepares the patient and family for home care. It is important to teach them about the ventilator, suctioning, tracheostomy care, signs of pulmonary infection, cuff inflation and deflation, and assessment of vital signs. Teaching often begins in the hospital and continues at home. Nursing responsibilities include evaluating the patient's and family's understanding of the information presented.

The nurse teaches the family cardiopulmonary resuscitation, including mouth-to-tracheostomy tube (instead of mouth-to-mouth) breathing. The nurse also explains how to handle a power failure, which usually involves converting the ventilator from an electrical power source to a battery power source. Conversion is

Table 25-2 • **Troubleshooting Ventilator Problems**

PROBLEM	CAUSE	SOLUTION
Ventilator		
Increase in peak airway pressure	Coughing or plugged airway tube	Suction airway for secretions, empty condensation fluid from circuit.
	Patient "bucking" ventilator	Adjust sensitivity.
	Decreasing lung compliance	Manually ventilate patient.
		Assess for hypoxia or bronchospasm.
		Check arterial blood gas values.
		Sedate only if necessary.
	Tubing kinked	Check tubing; reposition patient; insert oral airway if necessary.
	Pneumothorax	Manually ventilate patient; notify physician.
	Atelectasis or bronchospasm	Clear secretions.
Decrease in pressure or loss of volume	Increase in compliance	None
	Leak in ventilator or tubing; cuff on tube/humidifier not tight	Check entire ventilator circuit for patency.
		Correct leak.
Patient		
Cardiovascular compromise	Decrease in venous return due to application of positive pressure to lungs	Assess for adequate volume status by measuring heart rate, blood pressure, central venous pressure, pulmonary capillary wedge pressure, and urine output. Notify physician if values are abnormal.
Barotrauma/pneumothorax	Application of positive pressure to lungs; high mean airway pressures lead to alveolar rupture	Notify physician. Prepare patient for chest tube insertion. Avoid high pressure settings for patients with COPD, ARDS, or history of pneumothorax.
Pulmonary infection	Bypass of normal defense mechanisms; frequent breaks in ventilator circuit; decreased mobility; impaired cough reflex	Use meticulous aseptic technique. Provide frequent mouth care. Optimize nutritional status.

Chart 25-13 • ASSESSMENT

Criteria for Successful Home Ventilator Care

The decision to proceed with home ventilation therapy is usually based on the following parameters.

Patient Criteria
• The patient has chronic underlying pulmonary abnormalities.
• The patient's clinical pulmonary status is stable.
• The patient is willing to go home on mechanical ventilation.

Home Criteria
• The home environment is conducive to care of the patient.
• The electrical facilities are adequate to operate all equipment safely.
• The home environment is controlled, without drafts in cold weather and with proper ventilation in warm weather.
• Space is available for cleaning and storing ventilator equipment.

Family Criteria
• Family members are competent, dependable, and willing to spend the time required for proper training with available professional support.
• Family members understand the diagnosis and prognosis.
• Family has sufficient financial and supportive resources.

automatic in most types of home ventilators and lasts approximately 1 hour. The nurse instructs the family on using a manual self-inflation bag should it be necessary. Some of the patient's and family's responsibilities are listed in Chart 25-14.

Continuing Care. A home care nurse monitors and evaluates how well the patient and family are adapting to providing care in the home. The nurse also assesses the adequacy of ventilation and oxygenation as well as airway patency. The nurse addresses any unique adaptation problems the patient may have and listens to the patient's and family's anxieties and frustrations, offering support and encouragement where possible. The home care nurse helps identify and contact community resources that may assist in home management of the patient with mechanical ventilation.

The technical aspects of the ventilator are managed by vendor follow-up. A respiratory therapist usually is assigned to the patient and makes frequent home visits to evaluate the patient and perform a maintenance check of the ventilator.

Transportation services are identified should the patient require transportation in an emergency. These arrangements must be made before an emergency arises.

Providing the opportunity for ventilator-dependent patients to return home to live with their families in familiar surroundings can be a positive experience. The ultimate goal of home ventilator therapy is to enhance the patient's quality of life, not simply to support or prolong life.

Chart 25-14
Home Care Checklist • Ventilator Care

At the completion of the home care instruction, the patient or caregiver will be able to:	Patient	Caregiver
• State proper care of patient on ventilator		
Observe physical signs such as color, secretions, breathing pattern, and state of consciousness.		✓
Perform physical care such as suctioning, postural drainage, and ambulation.		✓
Observe the tidal volume and pressure manometer regularly. Intervene when they are abnormal (ie, suction if airway pressure increases).		✓
Provide a communication method for the patient (eg, pad and pencil, electric larynx, talking tracheostomy).		✓
Monitor vital signs as directed.		✓
Indicate when feeling short of breath or in distress by a predetermined signal.	✓	
• Care for and maintain equipment properly		
Check the ventilator settings twice each day and whenever the patient is removed from the ventilator.		✓
Adjust the volume and pressure alarms if needed.		✓
Fill humidifier as needed and check its level three times a day.		✓
Empty water in tubing as needed.	✓	✓
Use a clean humidifier when circuitry is changed.		✓
Keep exterior of ventilator clean and free of any objects.		✓
Change external circuitry once a week or more often as indicated.		✓
Report malfunction or strange noises immediately	✓	✓

NURSING PROCESS: THE PATIENT ON A VENTILATOR

Assessment

The nurse has a vital role in assessing the patient's status and the functioning of the ventilator.

In assessing the patient, the nurse evaluates the patient's physiologic status and how he or she is coping with mechanical ventilation. Physical assessment includes systematic assessment of all body systems, with an in-depth focus on the respiratory system. Respiratory assessment includes vital signs, respiratory rate and pattern, breath sounds, evaluation of spontaneous ventilatory effort, and potential evidence of hypoxia. Increased adventitious breath sounds may indicate a need for suctioning. The nurse also evaluates the settings and functioning of the mechanical ventilator, as described previously.

Assessment also addresses the patient's neurologic status and effectiveness of coping with the need for assisted ventilation and the changes that accompany it. The nurse should assess the patient's comfort level and ability to communicate as well. Finally, weaning from mechanical ventilation requires adequate nutrition. Therefore, it is important to assess the function of the gastrointestinal system and nutritional status.

Diagnosis

NURSING DIAGNOSES

Based on the assessment data, the patient's major nursing diagnoses may include:

- Impaired gas exchange related to underlying illness, or ventilator setting adjustment during stabilization or weaning.
- Ineffective airway clearance related to increased mucus production associated with continuous positive-pressure mechanical ventilation
- Risk for trauma and infection related to endotracheal intubation or tracheostomy
- Impaired physical mobility related to ventilator dependency

- Impaired verbal communication related to endotracheal tube and attachment to ventilator
- Defensive coping and powerlessness related to ventilator dependency

COLLABORATIVE PROBLEMS/ POTENTIAL COMPLICATIONS

Based on assessment data, potential complications may include:

- Alterations in cardiac function
- Barotrauma (trauma to the alveoli) and pneumothorax
- Pulmonary infection
- Sepsis

Planning and Goals

The major goals for the patient may include achievement of optimal gas exchange, maintenance of a patent airway, absence of trauma or infection, attainment of optimal mobility, adjustment to nonverbal methods of communication, acquisition of successful coping measures, and absence of complications.

Nursing Interventions

Nursing care of the mechanically ventilated patient requires expert technical and interpersonal skills. Nursing interventions are similar regardless of the setting; however, the frequency of interventions and the stability of the patient vary from setting to setting. Nursing interventions for the mechanically ventilated patient are not uniquely different from other pulmonary patients, but astute nursing assessment and a therapeutic nurse–patient relationship are critical. The specific interventions used by the nurse are determined by the underlying disease process and the patient's response.

Two general nursing interventions important in the care of the mechanically ventilated patient are pulmonary auscultation and interpretation of arterial blood gas measurements. The nurse is often the first to note changes in physical assessment findings or significant trends in blood gases that signal the development of a serious problem (eg, pneumothorax, tube displacement, pulmonary embolus).

ENHANCING GAS EXCHANGE

The purpose of mechanical ventilation is to optimize gas exchange by maintaining alveolar ventilation and oxygen delivery. The alteration in gas exchange may be due to the underlying illness or to mechanical factors related to the adjustment of the machine to the patient. The health care team, including the nurse, physician, and respiratory therapist, continually assesses the patient for adequate gas exchange, signs and symptoms of hypoxia, and response to treatment. Thus, the nursing diagnosis impaired gas exchange is, by its complex nature, multidisciplinary and collaborative. The team members must share goals and information freely. All other goals directly or indirectly relate to this primary goal.

Nursing interventions to promote optimal gas exchange include judicious administration of analgesic agents to relieve pain without suppressing the respiratory drive and frequent repositioning to diminish the pulmonary effects of immobility. The nurse also monitors for adequate fluid balance by assessing for the presence of peripheral edema, calculating daily intake and output, and monitoring daily weights. The nurse administers medications prescribed to control the primary disease and monitors for their side effects.

PROMOTING EFFECTIVE AIRWAY CLEARANCE

Continuous positive-pressure ventilation increases the production of secretions regardless of the patient's underlying condition. The nurse assesses for the presence of secretions by lung auscultation at least every 2 to 4 hours. Measures to clear the airway of secretions include suctioning, chest physiotherapy, frequent position changes, and increased mobility as soon as possible. Frequency of suctioning should be determined by patient assessment. If excessive secretions are identified by inspection or auscultation techniques, suctioning should be performed. Sputum is not produced continuously or every 1 to 2 hours but as a response to a pathologic condition. Therefore, there is no rationale for routine suctioning of all patients every 1 to 2 hours. Although suctioning is used to aid in the clearance of secretions, it can damage the airway mucosa and impair cilia action (Scanlan, Wilkins & Stoller, 1999).

The sigh mechanism on the ventilator may be adjusted to deliver at least one to three sighs per hour at 1.5 times the tidal volume if the patient is on assist–control. Because of the risk of hyperventilation and trauma to pulmonary tissue from excess ventilator pressure (barotrauma, pneumothorax), this feature is not being used as frequently today. If the patient is on the synchronized intermittent mandatory ventilation (SIMV) mode, the mandatory ventilations act as sighs because they are of greater volume than the patient's spontaneous breaths. Periodic sighing prevents atelectasis and the further retention of secretions.

Humidification of the airway via the ventilator is maintained to help liquefy secretions so they are more easily removed. Bronchodilators are administered to dilate the bronchioles and are classified as adrenergic or anticholinergic. Adrenergic bronchodilators are mostly inhaled and work by stimulating the beta-receptor sites, mimicking the effects of epinephrine in the body. The desired effect is smooth muscle relaxation, thus dilating the constricted bronchial tubes. Medications include albuterol (Proventil, Ventolin), isoetharine (Bronkosol), isoproterenol (Isuprel), metaproterenol (Alupent, Metaprel), pirbuterol acetate (Maxair), salmeterol (Serevent), and terbutaline (Brethine, Brethaire, Bricanyl). Tachycardia, heart palpitations, and tremors are side effects that have been reported with use of these medications (Zang & Allender, 1999). Anticholinergic bronchodilators such as ipratropium (Atrovent) and ipratropium with albuterol (Combivent) produce airway relaxation by blocking cholinergic-induced bronchoconstriction. Patients receiving bronchodilator therapy of either type should be monitored for adverse effects including dizziness, nausea, decreased oxygen saturation, hypokalemia, increased heart rate, and urine retention. Mucolytic agents such as acetylcysteine (Mucomyst) are administered as prescribed to liquefy secretions so that they are more easily mobilized. Nursing management of patients receiving mucolytic therapy includes assessment for an adequate cough reflex, sputum characteristics, and improvement in incentive spirometry (McKenry & Salerno, 2001). Side effects include nausea, vomiting, bronchospasm, stomatitis (oral ulcers), urticaria, and runny nose (LeFever & Hayes, 2000).

PREVENTING TRAUMA AND INFECTION

Airway management must involve maintaining the endotracheal or tracheostomy tube. The nurse positions the ventilator tubing so that there is minimal pulling or distortion of the tube in the trachea; this reduces the risk of trauma to the trachea. Cuff pressure is monitored every 8 hours to maintain the pressure at less than 25 cm H_2O. The nurse evaluates for the presence of a cuff leak at the same time.

Patients with endotracheal intubation or a tracheostomy tube do not have the normal defenses of the upper airway. In addition, these patients frequently have multiple additional body system disturbances that lead to immunocompromise. Tracheostomy care is performed at least every 8 hours, and more frequently if needed, because of the increased risk of infection. The ventilator circuit and in-line suction tubing is replaced periodically, according to infection control guidelines, to decrease the risk of infection.

The nurse administers oral hygiene frequently because the oral cavity is a primary source of contamination of the lungs in the intubated and compromised patient. The presence of a nasogastric tube in the intubated patient can increase the risk for aspiration, leading to nosocomial pneumonia. The nurse positions the patient with the head elevated above the stomach as much as possible. Antiulcer medications such as sucralfate (Carafate) are given to maintain normal gastric pH; research has demonstrated a lower incidence of aspiration pneumonia when sucralfate is administered (Scanlan, Wilkins & Stoller, 1999).

PROMOTING OPTIMAL LEVEL OF MOBILITY

The patient's mobility is limited because he or she is connected to the ventilator. The nurse should assist a patient whose condition has become stable to get out of bed and to a chair as soon as possible. Mobility and muscle activity are beneficial because they stimulate respirations and improve morale. If the patient cannot get out of bed, the nurse encourages the patient to perform active range-of-motion exercises every 6 to 8 hours. If the patient cannot perform these exercises, the nurse performs passive range-of-motion exercises every 8 hours to prevent contractures and venous stasis.

PROMOTING OPTIMAL COMMUNICATION

It is important to develop alternative methods of communication for the patient on a ventilator. The nurse assesses the patient's communication abilities to evaluate for limitations. Questions to consider when assessing the ventilator-dependent patient's ability to communicate include the following:

- Is the patient conscious and able to communicate? Can the patient nod or shake the head?

- Is the patient's mouth unobstructed by the tube so that words can be mouthed?
- Is the patient's hand strong and available for writing? (For example, if the patient is right-handed, the intravenous line is placed in the left arm if possible so that the right hand is free.)

Once the patient's limitations are known, the nurse offers several appropriate communication approaches: lip reading (use single key words), pad and pencil or Magic Slate, communication board, gesturing, or electric larynx. Use of a "talking" or fenestrated tracheostomy tube may be suggested to the physician; this allows the patient to talk while on the ventilator. If indicated, the nurse should make sure that the patient's eyeglasses and hearing aid and a translator are available to enhance the patient's ability to communicate.

The patient must be assisted to find the most suitable communication method. Some methods may be frustrating to the patient, family, and nurse; these need to be identified and minimized. A speech therapist can assist in determining the most appropriate method.

PROMOTING COPING ABILITY

Dependence on a ventilator is frightening to both the patient and family and disrupts even the most stable families. Encouraging the family to verbalize their feelings about the ventilator, the patient's condition, and the environment in general is beneficial. Explaining procedures every time they are performed helps to reduce anxiety and familiarizes the patient with ventilator procedures. To restore a sense of control, the nurse encourages the patient to participate in decisions about care, schedules, and treatment when possible. The patient may become withdrawn or depressed while on mechanical ventilation, especially if its use is prolonged. To promote effective coping, the nurse informs the patient about progress when appropriate. It is important to provide diversions such as watching television, playing music, or taking a walk (if appropriate and possible). Stress reduction techniques (eg, a backrub, relaxation measures) help relieve tension and help the patient to deal with anxieties and fears about both the condition and the dependence on the ventilator.

MONITORING AND MANAGING POTENTIAL COMPLICATIONS

Alterations in Cardiac Function

Alterations in cardiac output may occur as a result of positive-pressure ventilation. The positive intrathoracic pressure during inspiration compresses the heart and great vessels, thereby reducing venous return and cardiac output. This is usually corrected during exhalation when the positive pressure is off. Patients may have decreased cardiac output and resultant decreased tissue perfusion and oxygenation.

To evaluate cardiac function, the nurse first looks for signs and symptoms of hypoxia (restlessness, apprehension, confusion, tachycardia, tachypnea, labored breathing, pallor progressing to cyanosis, diaphoresis, transient hypertension, and decreased urine output). If a pulmonary artery catheter is in place, cardiac output, cardiac index, and other hemodynamic values can be used to assess the patient's status.

Barotrauma and Pneumothorax

Excessive positive pressure may cause barotrauma, which results in a spontaneous pneumothorax. This may quickly develop into a tension pneumothorax, further compromising venous return, cardiac output, and blood pressure. The nurse should consider any sudden onset of changes in oxygen saturation or respiratory distress to be a life-threatening emergency requiring immediate action.

Pulmonary Infection

The patient is at high risk for infection, as described above. The nurse should report fever or a change in the color or odor of sputum to the physician for follow-up.

Evaluation

EXPECTED PATIENT OUTCOMES

Expected patient outcomes may include:

1. Exhibits adequate gas exchange, as evidenced by normal breath sounds, acceptable arterial blood gas levels, and vital signs
2. Demonstrates adequate ventilation with minimal mucus accumulation
3. Is free of injury or infection, as evidenced by normal temperature and white blood count
4. Is mobile within limits of ability
   a. Gets out of bed to chair, bears weight, or ambulates as soon as possible
   b. Performs range-of-motion exercises every 6 to 8 hours
5. Communicates effectively through written messages, gestures, or other communication strategies
6. Copes effectively
   a. Verbalizes fears and concerns about condition and equipment
   b. Participates in decision making when possible
   c. Uses stress reduction techniques when necessary
7. Absence of complications
   a. Absence of cardiac compromise, as evidenced by stable vital signs and adequate urine output
   b. Absence of pneumothorax, as evidenced by bilateral chest excursion, normal chest x-ray, and adequate oxygenation
   c. Absence of pulmonary infection, as evidenced by normal temperature, clear pulmonary secretions, and negative sputum cultures

WEANING THE PATIENT FROM THE VENTILATOR

Respiratory weaning, the process of withdrawing the patient from dependence on the ventilator, takes place in three stages: the patient is gradually removed from the ventilator, then from the tube, and finally from oxygen. Weaning from mechanical ventilation is performed at the earliest possible time consistent with patient safety. The decision must be made from a physiologic rather than from a mechanical viewpoint. A thorough understanding of the patient's clinical status is required in making this decision. Weaning is started when the patient is recovering from the acute stage of medical and surgical problems and when the cause of respiratory failure is sufficiently reversed.

Successful weaning involves collaboration among the physician, respiratory therapist, and nurse. Each health care provider must understand the scope and function of other team members in relation to patient weaning to conserve the patient's strength, use resources efficiently, and maximize successful outcomes.

NURSING RESEARCH PROFILE 25-2

Early Versus Late Tracheostomy Decannulation

Clini, E., Vitacca, M., Bianchi, L., Porta, R., & Ambrosino, N. (1999). Long-term tracheostomy in severe COPD patients weaned from mechanical ventilation. *Respiratory Care, 44*(4), 241–244.

Purpose

Patients with chronic obstructive pulmonary disease (COPD) who require mechanical ventilation for management of acute respiratory failure are at risk for relapse. It is not known if patients with spontaneous respirations would benefit from retaining a tracheostomy after discharge from the intensive care unit. This study was conducted to determine the effects of maintaining a tracheal cannula in spontaneously breathing patients following discharge.

Study Sample and Design

Investigators studied 20 patients with severe COPD who were undergoing weaning from mechanical ventilation. The researchers used a prospective, randomized, and controlled design to measure tracheal cannula use in two groups of patients: 10 patients had the tracheal cannula removed, and 10 did not. Breathing pattern, forced lung volumes, respiratory muscle strength, and arterial blood gases were evaluated in patients at hospital discharge and at 1, 3, and 6 months after discharge. Investigators measured breathing patterns and forced lung volumes with a portable spirometer and assessed respiratory muscle strength by measuring maximal inspiratory pressure. They also recorded number

of hospital days, mortality rate, and number of new exacerbations requiring antibiotics.

Results

No significant differences were found between the two groups with regard to breathing patterns, forced lung volumes, respiratory strength, or arterial blood gases. In both groups, 2 of the 10 patients (20%) died due to respiratory causes. During the follow-up period, exacerbations were significantly greater in the patients with tracheostomies than in those whose tracheostomies had been removed ($p < .005$).

Nursing Implications

The findings of this study suggest that retaining a chronic tracheostomy following weaning from mechanical ventilation in patients with COPD is associated with a higher frequency of adverse events, including exacerbations requiring treatment with antibiotics. Although there were no significant findings with regard to breathing pattern, forced lung volumes, respiratory muscle strength, and arterial blood gases, the patient population was small, thus necessitating further study. The results suggest that clinics should consider early decannulation in COPD patients weaned from mechanical ventilation.

Criteria for Weaning

Careful assessment is required to determine whether the patient is ready to be removed from mechanical ventilation. If the patient is stable and showing signs of improvement or reversal of the disease or condition that caused the need for mechanical ventilation, weaning indices should be assessed. These indices include:

- Vital capacity: the amount of air expired after maximum inspiration. Used to assess the patient's ability to take deep breaths. Vital capacity should be 10 to 15 mL/kg to meet the criteria for weaning.
- Maximum inspiratory pressure (MIP): used to assess the patient's respiratory muscle strength. It is also known as negative inspiratory pressure and should be at least −20 cm H_2O.
- Tidal volume: volume of air that is inhaled or exhaled from the lungs during an effortless breath. It is normally 7 to 9 mL/kg.
- Minute ventilation: equal to the respiratory rate multiplied by tidal volume. Normal is about 6 L/min.
- Rapid/shallow breathing index: used to assess the breathing pattern and is calculated by dividing the respiratory rate by tidal volume. Patients with indices below 100 breaths/min/L are more likely to be successful at weaning.

Other measurements used to assess readiness for weaning include a PaO_2 of greater than 60 mm Hg with an FiO_2 of less than 40%. Stable vital signs and arterial blood gases are also important predictors of successful weaning. Once readiness has been determined, the nurse records baseline measurements of weaning indices to monitor progress (Cull & Inwood, 1999).

Patient Preparation

To maximize the chances of success of weaning, the nurse must consider the patient as a whole, taking into account factors that impair the delivery of oxygen and elimination of carbon dioxide

as well as those that increase oxygen demand (sepsis, seizures, thyroid imbalances) or decrease the patient's overall strength (nutrition, neuromuscular disease). Adequate psychological preparation is necessary before and during the weaning process. Patients need to know what is expected of them during the procedure. They are often frightened by having to breathe on their own again and need reassurance that they are improving and are well enough to handle spontaneous breathing. The nurse explains what will happen during weaning and what role the patient will play in the procedure. The nurse emphasizes that someone will be with or near the patient at all times, and answers any questions simply and concisely. Proper preparation of the patient can reduce the weaning time.

Methods of Weaning

Considerable effort has been devoted to finding the best method of weaning from mechanical ventilation, but research has not established which method is best (Tasota & Dobbin, 2000). Success depends on the combination of adequate patient preparation, available equipment, and an interdisciplinary approach to solving patient problems (Chart 25-15). The most common weaning methods in use today are described below.

Assist–control may be used as the resting mode for patients undergoing weaning trials. This mode provides full ventilatory support by delivering a preset tidal volume and respiratory rate; if the patient takes a breath, the ventilator delivers the preset volume. The cycle does not adapt to the patient's spontaneous efforts. The nurse assesses patients being weaned on this mode for the following signs of distress: rapid shallow breathing, use of accessory muscles, reduced level of consciousness, increase in carbon dioxide levels, decrease in oxygen saturations, and tachycardia.

The patient on intermittent mandatory ventilation (IMV) can increase the respiratory rate, but each spontaneous breath receives only the tidal volume the patient generates. Mechanical breaths

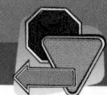

Chart 25-15

GUIDELINES FOR Care of the Patient Being Weaned From Mechanical Ventilation

NURSING INTERVENTIONS	RATIONALE
1. Assess patient for weaning criteria: Vital capacity—10 to 15 mL/kg Maximum inspiratory pressure (MIP) at least –20 cm H_2O Tidal volume—7 to 9 mL/kg Minute ventilation—6 L/min Rapid/shallow breathing index—below 100 breaths/minute/L PaO_2 greater than 60 mm Hg with FiO_2 less than 40%	1. Careful assessment of multiple weaning indices helps to determine readiness for weaning. When the criteria have been met, the patient's likelihood of successful weaning increases.
2. Monitor activity level, assess dietary intake, and monitor results of laboratory tests of nutritional status.	2. Reestablishing independent spontaneous ventilation can be physically exhausting. It is crucial that the patient have enough energy reserves to succeed. Providing periods of rest and recommended nutritional intake can increase the likelihood of successful weaning.
3. Assess the patient's and family's understanding of the weaning process and address any concerns about the process. Explain that the patient may feel short of breath initially and provide encouragement as needed. Reassure the patient that he or she will be attended closely and that if the weaning attempt is not successful, it can be tried again later.	3. The weaning process can be psychologically tiring; emotional support can help promote a sense of security. Explaining that weaning will be attempted again later helps reduce the sense of failure if the first attempts are unsuccessful.
4. Implement the weaning method prescribed: A/C, IMV, SIMV, PSV, PAV, CPAP, or T-piece.	4. The prescribed weaning method should reflect the patient's individualized criteria for weaning and weaning history. By having different methods to choose from, the physician can select the one that best fits the patient.
5. Monitor vital signs, pulse oximetry, ECG, and respiratory pattern constantly for the first 20 to 30 minutes and every 5 minutes after that until weaning is complete.	5. Monitoring the patient closely provides ongoing indications of success or failure.
6. Maintain a patent airway; monitor arterial blood gas levels and pulmonary function tests. Suction the airway as needed.	6. These values can be compared to baseline measurements to evaluate weaning. Suctioning helps to reduce the risk of aspiration and maintain the airway.
7. In collaboration with the physician, terminate the weaning process if adverse reactions occur. These include a heart rate increase of 20 beats/min, systolic blood pressure increase of 20 mm Hg, a decrease in oxygen saturation to less than 90%, respiratory rate less than 8 or greater than 20 breaths/minute, ventricular dysrhythmias, fatigue, panic, cyanosis, erratic or labored breathing, paradoxical chest movement.	7. These signs and symptoms indicate an unstable patient at risk for hypoxia and ventricular dysrhythmias. Continuing the weaning process can lead to cardiopulmonary arrest.
8. If the weaning process continues, measure tidal volume and minute ventilation every 20 to 30 minutes; compare with the patient's desired values, which have been determined in collaboration with the physician.	8. These values help to determine if weaning is successful and should be continued.
9. Assess for psychological dependence if the physiologic parameters indicate weaning is feasible and the patient still resists.	9. Psychological dependence is a common problem after mechanical ventilation. Possible causes include fear of dying and depression from chronic illness. It is important to address this issue before the next weaning attempt.

are delivered at preset intervals and a preselected tidal volume, regardless of the patient's efforts. IMV allows patients to use their own muscles of ventilation to help prevent muscle atrophy. IMV lowers mean airway pressure, which can assist in preventing barotrauma.

Synchronized intermittent mandatory ventilation (SIMV) delivers a preset tidal volume and number of breaths per minute. Between ventilator-delivered breaths, the patient can breathe spontaneously with no assistance from the ventilator on those extra breaths. As the patient's ability to breathe spontaneously increases, the preset number of ventilator breaths is decreased and the patient does more of the work of breathing. SIMV is indicated if the patient satisfies all the criteria for weaning but cannot sustain adequate spontaneous ventilation for long periods.

IMV and SIMV can be used to provide full or partial ventilatory support. Nursing interventions for both of these include

monitoring progress by recording respiratory rate, minute volume, spontaneous and machine-generated tidal volume, FiO_2, and arterial blood gas levels.

The **pressure support ventilation** (PSV) mode assists SIMV by applying a pressure plateau to the airway throughout the patient-triggered inspiration to decrease resistance by the tracheal tube and ventilator tubing. Pressure support is reduced gradually as the patient's strength increases. A SIMV backup rate may be added for extra support. The nurse must closely observe the patient's respiratory rate and tidal volumes on initiation of PSV. It may be necessary to adjust the pressure support to avoid tachypnea or large tidal volumes.

The proportional assist ventilation (PAV) mode of partial ventilatory support allows the ventilator to generate pressure in proportion to the patient's efforts. With every breath, the ventilator synchronizes with the patient's ventilatory efforts (Giannouli,

Webster, Roberts & Younes, 1999). Nursing assessment should include careful monitoring of the patient's respiratory rate, arterial blood gases, tidal volume, minute ventilation, and breathing pattern.

The continuous positive airway pressure (CPAP) mode allows the patient to breathe spontaneously, while applying positive pressure throughout the respiratory cycle to keep the alveoli open and promote oxygenation. Providing CPAP during spontaneous breathing also offers the advantage of an alarm system and may reduce patient anxiety if the patient has been taught that the machine is keeping track of breathing. It also maintains lung volumes and improves the patient's oxygenation status. CPAP is often used in conjunction with PSV. Nurses should carefully assess for tachypnea, tachycardia, reduced tidal volumes, decreasing oxygen saturations, and increasing carbon dioxide levels.

Weaning trials using a T-piece or tracheostomy mask (see Fig. 25-2) are normally conducted with the patient disconnected from the ventilator, receiving humidified oxygen only, and performing all work of breathing. Patients who do not have to overcome the resistance of the ventilator may find this mode more comfortable, or they may become anxious as they breathe with no support from the ventilator. During T-piece trials, the nurse monitors the patient closely and provides encouragement. This method of weaning is usually used when the patient is awake and alert, is breathing without difficulty, has good gag and cough reflexes, and is hemodynamically stable. During the weaning process, the patient is maintained on the same or a higher oxygen concentration than when on the ventilator. While on the T-piece, the patient should be observed for signs and symptoms of hypoxia, increasing respiratory muscle fatigue, or systemic fatigue. These include restlessness, increased respiratory rate greater than 35 breaths/min, use of accessory muscles, tachycardia with premature ventricular contractions, and paradoxical chest movement (asynchronous breathing, chest contraction during inspiration and expansion during expiration). Fatigue or exhaustion is initially manifested by an increased respiratory rate associated with a gradual reduction in tidal volume; later there is a slowing of the respiratory rate.

If the patient appears to be tolerating the T-piece trial, a second set of arterial blood gas measurements is drawn 20 minutes after the patient has been on spontaneous ventilation at a constant FiO_2 pressure support ventilation. (Alveolar–arterial equilibration takes 15 to 20 minutes to occur.)

Signs of exhaustion and hypoxia correlated with deterioration in the blood gas measurements indicate the need for ventilatory support. The patient is placed back on the ventilator each time signs of fatigue or deterioration develop.

If clinically stable, the patient usually can be extubated within 2 or 3 hours of weaning and allowed spontaneous ventilation by means of a mask with humidified oxygen. Patients who have had prolonged ventilatory assistance usually require more gradual weaning; it may take days or even weeks. They are weaned primarily during the day and placed back on the ventilator at night to rest.

Because patients respond in different manners to the various weaning methods, there is no definitive way to assess which method is best. With all of the methods, ongoing assessment of respiratory status is essential to monitor patient progress (Woodruff, 1999).

Successful weaning from the ventilator is supplemented by intensive pulmonary care. The following are continued:

- Oxygen therapy
- Arterial blood gas evaluation
- Pulse oximetry
- Bronchodilator therapy
- Chest physiotherapy
- Adequate nutrition, hydration, and humidification
- Incentive spirometry

These patients still have borderline pulmonary function and need vigorous supportive therapy before their respiratory status returns to a level that supports activities of daily living.

Weaning From the Tube

Weaning from the tube is considered when the patient can breathe spontaneously, maintain an adequate airway by effectively coughing up secretions, swallow, and move the jaw. If frequent suctioning is needed to clear secretions, tube weaning may be unsuccessful (Ecklund, 1999). Secretion clearance and aspiration risks are assessed to determine if active pharyngeal and laryngeal reflexes are intact.

Once the patient can clear secretions adequately, a trial period of mouth breathing or nose breathing is conducted. This can be accomplished by several methods. The first method requires changing to a smaller size tube to increase the resistance to airflow and simultaneously plugging the tracheostomy tube (deflating the cuff). The smaller tube is sometimes replaced by a cuffless tracheostomy tube, which allows the tube to be plugged at lengthening intervals to monitor patient progress. A second method involves changing to a fenestrated tube (a tube with an opening or window in its bend). This permits air to flow around and through the tube to the upper airway and enables talking. A third method involves switching to a smaller tracheostomy button (stoma button). A tracheostomy button is a plastic tube approximately 1 inch long that helps to keep the windpipe open after the larger tracheostomy tube has been removed. Finally, when the patient demonstrates the ability to maintain a patent airway without a tracheostomy tube, the tube can be removed. An occlusive dressing is placed over the stoma, which usually heals anywhere from several days to many weeks (Ecklund, 1999).

Weaning From Oxygen

The patient who has been successfully weaned from the ventilator, cuff, and tube and has adequate respiratory function is then weaned from oxygen. The FiO_2 is gradually reduced until the PaO_2 is in the range of 70 to 100 mm Hg while the patient is breathing room air. If the PaO_2 is less than 70 mm Hg on room air, supplemental oxygen is recommended. The Centers for Medicare and Medicaid Services, formerly the Health Care Financing Administration (HCFA), requires that the patient's PaO_2 on room air be less than 55 mm Hg for the patient to be eligible for financial reimbursement for in-home oxygen.

Nutrition

Success in weaning the long-term ventilator-dependent patient requires early and aggressive but judicious nutritional support. The respiratory muscles (diaphragm and especially intercostals) become weak or atrophied after just a few days of mechanical ventilation, especially if nutrition is inadequate. Fat kilocalories produce less carbon dioxide than carbohydrate kilocalories. For this reason, a high-fat diet may assist patients with respiratory failure who are being weaned from mechanical ventilation. Research is being conducted on the role of fatty acids in lung disease (Schwartz,

2000). A high-fat diet may provide as much as 50% of the total daily kilocalories. Adequate protein intake is important in increasing respiratory muscle strength. Protein intake should be approximately 25% of total daily kilocalories, or 1.2 to 1.5 g/kg/day. Because a high-carbohydrate diet can lead to increased carbon dioxide production and retention, total carbohydrate intake should not exceed 25% of total daily kilocalories, or 2 g/kg/day in patients being weaned from mechanical ventilation. Care must be taken not to overfeed patients because excessive intake can raise the demand for oxygen and the production of carbon dioxide. Total daily kilocalories should be closely monitored (Lutz & Przytulski, 2001).

Soon after the patient is admitted, a consultation with a dietitian or nutrition support team should be arranged to plan the best form of nutritional replacement. Adequate nutrition may decrease the duration of mechanical ventilation and prevent other complications, especially sepsis. Sepsis can occur if bacteria enter the bloodstream and release toxins that, in turn, cause vasodilation and hypotension, fever, tachycardia, increased respiratory rate, and coma. Aggressive treatment of sepsis is essential to reverse this threat to survival and to promote weaning from the ventilator when the patient's condition improves. Optimal nutritional intake is an essential part of the treatment of sepsis.

The Patient Undergoing Thoracic Surgery

Assessment and management are particularly important in the patient undergoing thoracic surgery. Frequently, patients undergoing such surgery also have obstructive pulmonary disease with compromised breathing. Preoperative preparation and careful postoperative management are crucial for successful patient outcomes because these patients may have a narrow range between their physical tolerance for certain activities and their limitations, which, if exceeded, can lead to distress. Various types of thoracic surgical procedures are performed to relieve disease conditions such as lung abscesses, lung cancer, cysts, and benign tumors (Chart 25-16). An exploratory **thoracotomy** (creation of a surgical opening into the thoracic cavity) may be performed to diagnose lung or chest disease. A biopsy may be performed in this procedure with a small amount of lung tissue removed for analysis; the chest incision is then closed.

The objectives of preoperative care for the patient undergoing thoracic surgery are to ascertain the patient's functional reserve to determine if the patient can survive the surgery and to ensure that the patient is in optimal condition for surgery.

PREOPERATIVE MANAGEMENT

Assessment and Diagnostic Findings

The nurse performs chest auscultation to assess breath sounds in the different regions of the lungs (see Chap. 21). It is important to note if breath sounds are normal, indicating a free flow of air in and out of the lungs. (In the patient with emphysema, the breath sounds may be markedly decreased or even absent on auscultation.) The nurse notes crackles and wheezes and assesses for hyperresonance and decreased diaphragmatic motion. Unilateral diminished breath sounds and rhonchi can be the result of occlusion of the bronchi by mucus plugs. The nurse assesses for retained secretions during auscultation by asking the patient to cough. It is important to note any signs of rhonchi or wheezing.

The patient history and assessment should include the following questions:

- What signs and symptoms are present (cough, sputum expectorated [amount and color], hemoptysis, chest pain, dyspnea)?
- If there is a smoking history, how long has the patient smoked? Does the patient smoke currently? How many packs a day?
- What is the patient's cardiopulmonary tolerance while resting, eating, bathing, and walking?
- What is the patient's breathing pattern? How much exertion is required to produce dyspnea?
- Does the patient need to sleep in an upright position or with more than two pillows?
- What is the patient's physiologic status (eg, general appearance, mental alertness, behavior, nutritional status)?
- What other medical conditions exist (eg, allergies, cardiac disorders, diabetes)?

A number of tests are performed to determine the patient's preoperative status and to assess the patient's physical assets and limitations. Many patients are seen by their surgeons in the office, and many tests and examinations are performed on an outpatient basis. The decision to perform any pulmonary resection is based on the patient's cardiovascular status and pulmonary reserve. Pulmonary function studies (especially lung volume and vital capacity) are performed to determine whether the planned resection will leave sufficient functioning lung tissue. Arterial blood gas values are assessed to provide a more complete picture of the functional capacity of the lung. Exercise tolerance tests are useful to determine if the patient who is a candidate for pneumonectomy can tolerate removal of one of the lungs.

Preoperative studies are performed to provide a baseline for comparison during the postoperative period and to detect any unsuspected abnormalities. These studies may include a bronchoscopic examination (a lighted scope is inserted into the airways to examine the bronchi), chest x-ray, electrocardiogram (for arteriosclerotic heart disease, conduction defects), nutritional assessment, determination of blood urea nitrogen and serum creatinine (renal function), glucose tolerance or blood glucose (diabetes), assessment of serum electrolytes and protein levels, blood volume determinations, and complete blood cell count.

PREOPERATIVE NURSING MANAGEMENT

Improving Airway Clearance

The underlying lung condition often is associated with increased respiratory secretions. Before surgery, the airway is cleared of secretions to reduce the possibility of postoperative atelectasis or infection. Risk factors for postoperative atelectasis and pneumonia are listed in Chart 25-17. Strategies to reduce the risk for atelectasis and infection include humidification, postural drainage, and chest percussion after bronchodilators are administered, if prescribed. The nurse estimates the volume of sputum if the patient expectorates large amounts of secretions. Such measurements are carried out to determine if and when the amount decreases. Antibiotics are administered as prescribed for infection, which may be causing the excessive secretions.

Chart 25-16 **Thoracic Surgeries and Procedures**

Pneumonectomy

The removal of an entire lung (pneumonectomy) is performed chiefly for cancer when the lesion cannot be removed by a less extensive procedure. It also may be performed for lung abscesses, bronchiectasis, or extensive unilateral tuberculosis. The removal of the right lung is more dangerous than the removal of the left, because the right lung has a larger vascular bed and its removal imposes a greater physiologic burden.

A posterolateral or anterolateral thoracotomy incision is made, sometimes with resection of a rib. The pulmonary artery and the pulmonary veins are ligated and severed. The main bronchus is divided and the lung removed. The bronchial stump is stapled, and usually no drains are used because the accumulation of fluid in the empty hemithorax prevents mediastinal shift.

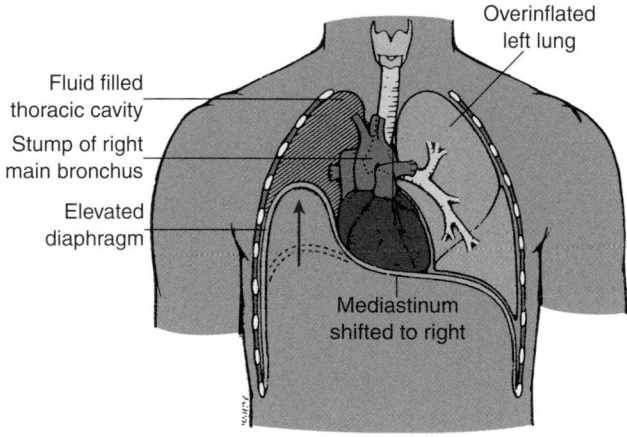

Pneumonectomy

Lobectomy

When the pathology is limited to one area of a lung, a lobectomy (removal of a lobe of a lung) is performed. Lobectomy, which is more common than pneumonectomy, may be carried out for bronchogenic carcinoma, giant emphysematous blebs or bullae, benign tumors, metastatic malignant tumors, bronchiectasis, and fungus infections.

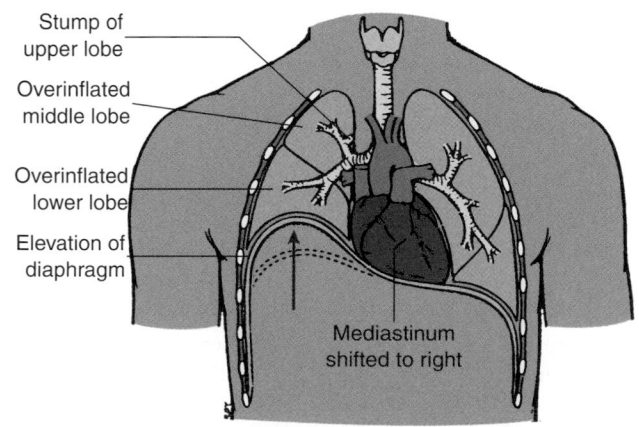

Lobectomy

The surgeon makes a thoracotomy incision: its exact location depends on the lobe to be resected. When the pleural space is entered, the involved lung collapses and the lobar vessels and the bronchus are ligated and divided. After the lobe is removed, the remaining lobes of the lung are reexpanded. Usually, two chest catheters are inserted for drainage. The upper tube is for air removal; the lower one is for fluid drainage. Sometimes, only one catheter is needed. The chest tube is connected to a chest drainage apparatus for several days.

Segmentectomy (Segmental Resection)

Some lesions are located in only one segment of the lung. Bronchopulmonary segments are subdivisions of the lung that function as individual units. They are held together by delicate connective tissue. Disease processes may be limited to a single segment. Care is used to preserve as much healthy and functional lung tissue as possible, especially in patients who already have limited cardiopulmonary reserve. Single segments can be removed from any lobe; the right middle lobe, which has only two small segments, invariably is removed entirely. On the left side, corresponding to a middle lobe, is a "lingular" segment of the upper lobe. This can be removed as a single segment or by lingulectomy. This segment frequently is involved in bronchiectasis.

Wedge Resection

A wedge resection of a small, well-circumscribed lesion may be performed without regard for the location of the intersegmental planes. The pleural cavity usually is drained because of the possibility of an air or blood leak. This procedure is performed for diagnostic lung biopsy and for the excision of small peripheral nodules.

Bronchoplastic or Sleeve Resection

Bronchoplastic resection is a procedure in which only one lobar bronchus, together with a part of the right or left bronchus, is excised. The distal bronchus is reanastomosed to the proximal bronchus or trachea.

Lung Volume Reduction

Lung volume reduction is a surgical procedure involving the removal of 20% to 30% of a patient's lung through a midsternal incision or video thoracoscopy. The diseased lung tissue is identified on a lung perfusion scan. Although some patients with chronic obstructive pulmonary disease have reported an improvement in the quality of their lives for at least 6 months to 1 year after the surgery, results have generally been disappointing. Research is ongoing to examine the benefits of lung volume reduction surgery using video thoracoscopy (Baker & Flynn, 1999; National Institutes of Health, 2001).

Video Thoracoscopy

A video thoracoscopy is an endoscopic procedure that allows the surgeon to look into the thorax without making a large incision. The procedure is performed to obtain specimens of tissue for biopsy, to treat recurrent spontaneous pneumothorax, and to diagnose either pleural effusions or pleural masses. Thoracoscopy has also been found to be an effective diagnostic and therapeutic alternative for the treatment of mediastinal disorders (Cirino et al., 2000). Some advantages of video thoracoscopy include rapid diagnosis and treatment of some conditions, a decrease in postoperative complications, and a shortened hospital stay (see Chap. 21).

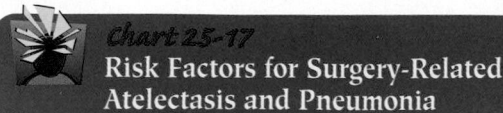

Chart 25-17

Risk Factors for Surgery-Related Atelectasis and Pneumonia

Preoperative Risk Factors
Increased age
Obesity
Poor nutritional status
Smoking history
Abnormal pulmonary function tests
Preexisting lung disease
Emergency surgery
History of aspiration
Comorbid states
Preexisting disability

Intraoperative Risk Factors
Thoracic incision
Prolonged anesthesia

Postoperative Risk Factors
Immobilization
Supine position
Decreased level of consciousness
Inadequate pain management
Prolonged intubation/mechanical ventilation
Presence of nasogastric tube
Inadequate preoperative education

Teaching the Patient

Increasingly, patients are admitted on the day of surgery, which does not provide much time for the acute care nurse to talk with the patient. Nurses in all settings must take an active role in educating the patient and relieving anxiety. The nurse informs the patient what to expect, from administration of anesthesia to thoracotomy and the likely use of chest tubes and a drainage system in the postoperative period. The patient is also informed about the usual postoperative administration of oxygen to facilitate breathing, and the possible use of a ventilator. It is essential to explain the importance of frequent turning to promote drainage of lung secretions. Instruction in the use of incentive spirometry begins before surgery to familiarize the patient with its correct use. The nurse should teach diaphragmatic and pursed-lip breathing, and the patient should begin practicing these techniques (see Chart 25-3, "Breathing Exercises," and Chart 25-4, "Assisting the Patient to Perform Incentive Spirometry").

Because a coughing schedule will be necessary in the postoperative period to promote the clearance or removal of secretions, the nurse instructs the patient in the technique of coughing and warns the patient that the coughing routine may be uncomfortable. The nurse teaches the patient to splint the incision with the hands, a pillow, or a folded towel (see Chart 25-5).

Another technique, "huffing," may be helpful for the patient with diminished expiratory flow rates or for the patient who refuses to cough because of severe pain. Huffing is the expulsion of air through an open glottis. This type of forced expiration technique (FET) stimulates pulmonary expansion and assists in alveolar inflation. The nurse instructs the patient as follows:

- Take a deep diaphragmatic breath and exhale forcefully against your hand in a quick, distinct pant, or huff.
- Practice doing small huffs and progress to one strong huff during exhalation.

Patients should be informed preoperatively that blood and other fluids may be administered, oxygen will be administered, and vital signs will be checked often for several hours after surgery. If a chest tube is needed, the patient should be informed that it will drain the fluid and air that normally accumulate after chest surgery. The patient and family are informed that the patient may be admitted to the intensive care unit for 1 to 2 days after surgery, that the patient may experience pain at the incision site, and that medication is available to relieve pain and discomfort (Finkelmeier, 2000).

Relieving Anxiety

The nurse listens to the patient to evaluate his or her feelings about the illness and proposed treatment. The nurse also determines the patient's motivation to return to normal or baseline function. The patient may reveal significant concerns: fear of hemorrhage because of bloody sputum, fear of discomfort from a chronic cough and chest pain, fear of ventilator dependence, or fear of death because of dyspnea and the underlying disease (eg, tumor).

The nurse helps the patient to overcome these fears and to cope with the stress of surgery by correcting any misconceptions, supporting the patient's decision to undergo surgery, reassuring the patient that the incision will "hold," and dealing honestly with questions about pain and discomfort and their treatment. The management and control of pain begin before surgery, when the nurse informs the patient that many postoperative problems can be overcome by following certain routines related to deep breathing, coughing, turning, and moving. If patient-controlled analgesia or epidural analgesia is to be used after surgery, the nurse instructs the patient in its use.

POSTOPERATIVE MANAGEMENT

After surgery the vital signs are checked frequently. Oxygen is administered by a mechanical ventilator, nasal cannula, or mask for as long as necessary. A reduction in lung capacity requires a period of physiologic adjustment, and fluids may be given at a low hourly rate to prevent fluid overload and pulmonary edema. When the patient is conscious and the vital signs have stabilized, the head of the bed may be elevated 30 to 45 degrees. Careful positioning of the patient is important. Following pneumonectomy, a patient is usually turned every hour from the back to the operative side and should not be completely turned to the unoperated side. This allows the fluid left in the space to consolidate and prevents the remaining lung and the heart from shifting (mediastinal shift) toward the operative side. The patient with a lobectomy may be turned to either side, and a patient with a segmental resection usually is not turned onto the operative side unless the surgeon prescribes this position (Finkelmeier, 2000).

Medication for pain is needed for several days after surgery. Because coughing can be painful, patients should be taught to splint the chest. Exercises are resumed early in the postoperative period to facilitate lung ventilation. The nurse assesses for signs of complications, including cyanosis, dyspnea, and acute chest pain. These may indicate atelectasis and should be reported immediately. Increased temperature or white blood cell count may indicate an infection, and pallor and increased pulse may indicate internal hemorrhage. Dressings should be assessed for fresh bleeding.

Mechanical Ventilation

Depending on the nature of the surgery, the patient's underlying condition, the intraoperative course, and the depth of anesthesia, the patient may require mechanical ventilation after surgery. The physician is responsible for determining the ventilator settings and modes, as well as determining the overall method and pace of weaning. However, the physician, nurse, and respiratory therapist work together closely to assess the patient's tolerance and weaning progress. Early extubation from mechanical ventilation can also lead to earlier removal of arterial lines (Zevola & Maier, 1999).

Chest Drainage

A crucial intervention for improving gas exchange and breathing in the postoperative period is the proper management of chest drainage and the **chest drainage system**. After thoracic surgery, chest tubes and a closed drainage system are used to re-expand the involved lung and to remove excess air, fluid, and blood. Chest

drainage systems also are used in treatment of spontaneous pneumothorax and trauma resulting in pneumothorax. Table 25-3 describes and compares the main features of these systems. Management of chest drainage systems is explained in Chart 25-18. Prevention of cardiopulmonary complications following thoracic surgery is discussed in Chart 25-19.

The normal breathing mechanism operates on the principle of negative pressure; that is, the pressure in the chest cavity normally is lower than the pressure of the atmosphere, causing air to move into the lungs during inspiration. Whenever the chest is opened, there is a loss of negative pressure, which can result in the collapse of the lung. The collection of air, fluid, or other substances in the chest can compromise cardiopulmonary function and can also cause the lung to collapse. Pathologic substances that collect in the pleural space include fibrin, or clotted blood; liquids (serous fluids, blood, pus, chyle); and gases (air from the lung, tracheobronchial tree, or esophagus).

Chest tubes may be inserted to drain fluid or air from any of the three compartments of the thorax (the right and left pleural spaces and the mediastinum). The pleural space, located between the visceral and parietal pleura, normally contains 20 mL or less of fluid, which helps to lubricate the visceral and parietal pleura. Surgical incision of the chest wall almost always causes some degree of pneumothorax (air accumulating in the pleural space) or hemothorax (build-up of serous fluid or blood in the pleural space). Air and fluid collect in the pleural space, restricting lung expansion and reducing gas exchange. Placement of a chest tube in the pleural space restores the negative intrathoracic pressure needed for lung re-expansion following surgery or trauma.

Table 25-3 • Comparison of Chest Drainage Systems

TYPES OF CHEST DRAINAGE SYSTEMS	DESCRIPTION	COMMENTS
Traditional Water Seal Also referred to as wet suction	Has 3 chambers: a collection chamber, water seal chamber (middle chamber), and wet suction control chamber	Requires that sterile fluid be instilled into water seal and suction chambers Has positive- and negative-pressure release valves Intermittent bubbling indicates that the system is functioning properly Additional suction can be added by connecting system to a suction source
Dry Suction Water Seal Also referred to as dry suction	Has 3 chambers: a collection chamber, water seal chamber (middle chamber), and wet suction control chamber	Requires that sterile fluid be instilled in water seal chamber at 2-cm level No need to fill suction chamber with fluid Suction pressure is set with a regulator Has positive- and negative-pressure release valves Has an indicator to signify that the suction pressure is adequate Quieter than traditional water seal systems
Dry Suction Also referred to as one-way valve system	Has a one-way mechanical value that allows air to leave the chest and prevents air from moving back into the chest	No need to fill suction chamber with fluid; thus, can be set up quickly in an emergency Works even if knocked over, making it ideal for patients who are ambulatory

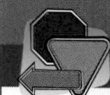

Chart 25-18

GUIDELINES FOR Managing Chest Drainage Systems

NURSING INTERVENTIONS	RATIONALE
1. If using a chest drainage system with a water seal, fill the water seal chamber with sterile water to the level specified by the manufacturer.	Water seal drainage allows air and fluid to escape into a drainage chamber. The water acts as a seal and keeps the air from being drawn back into the pleural space.
2. When using suction in chest drainage systems with a water seal, fill the suction control chamber with sterile water to the 20-cm level or as prescribed. In systems without a water seal, set the regulator dial at the appropriate suction level.	The water level regulator dial setting determines the degree of suction applied.
3. Attach the drainage catheter exiting the thoracic cavity to the tubing coming from the collection chamber. Tape securely with adhesive tape.	In chest drainage units, the system is closed. The only connection is the one to the patient's catheter.
4. If suction is used, connect the suction control chamber tubing to the suction unit. If using a wet suction system, turn on the suction unit and increase pressure until slow but steady bubbling appears in the suction control chamber. If using a chest drainage system with a dry suction control chamber, turn the regulator dial to 20 cm H_2O.	With a wet suction system, the degree of suction is determined by the amount of water in the suction control chamber and is not dependent on the rate of bubbling or the pressure gauge setting on the suction unit. With a dry suction control chamber, the regulator dial replaces the water.

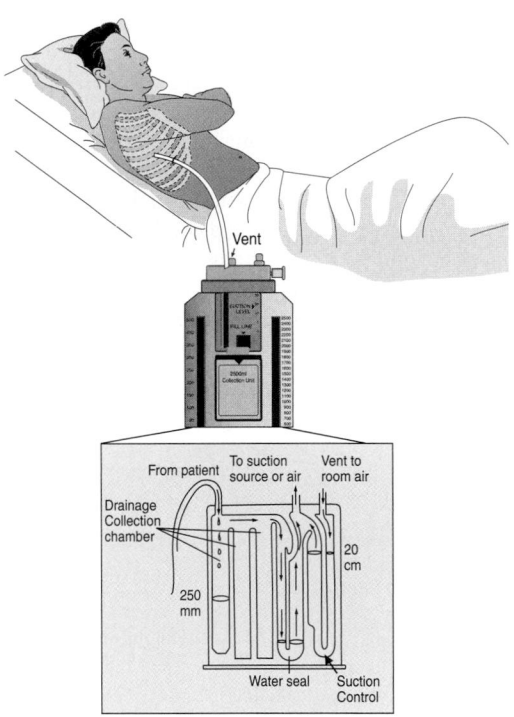

Example of a disposable chest drainage system.

5. Mark the drainage from the collection chamber with tape on the outside of the drainage unit. Mark hourly/daily increments (date and time) at the drainage level.	This marking shows the amount of fluid loss and how fast fluid is collecting in the drainage chamber. It serves as a basis for determining the need for blood replacement, if the fluid is blood. Visibly bloody drainage will appear in the chamber in the immediate postoperative period but should gradually becomes serous. If the patient is bleeding as heavily as 100 mL every 15 minutes, check the drainage every few minutes. A reoperation or autotransfusion may be needed. The transfusion of blood collected in the drainage chamber must be reinfused within 4 to 6 hours. Usually, however, drainage decreases progressively in the first 24 hours.
6. Ensure that the drainage tubing does not kink, loop, or interfere with the patient's movements.	Kinking, looping, or pressure on the drainage tubing can produce back-pressure, which may force fluid back into the pleural space or impede its drainage.
7. Encourage the patient to assume a comfortable position with good body alignment. With the lateral position, make sure that the patient's body does not compress the tubing. The patient should be turned and repositioned every 1.5 to 2 hours. Provide adequate analgesia.	Frequent position changes promote drainage, and good body alignment helps prevent postural deformities and contractures. Proper positioning also helps breathing and promotes better air exchange. Analgesics may be needed to promote comfort.

(continued)

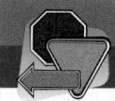

Chart 25-18

GUIDELINES FOR Managing Chest Drainage Systems (Continued)

NURSING INTERVENTIONS	RATIONALE
8. Assist the patient with range-of-motion exercises for the affected arm and shoulder several times daily. Provide adequate analgesia.	Exercise helps to prevent ankylosis of the shoulder and to reduce postoperative pain and discomfort. Analgesics may be needed to relieve pain.
9. Gently "milk" the tubing in the direction of the drainage chamber as needed.	"Milking" prevents the tubing from becoming obstructed by clots and fibrin. Constant attention to maintaining the patency of the tube facilitates prompt expansion of the lung and minimizes complications.
10. Make sure there is fluctuation ("tidaling") of the fluid level in the water seal chamber (in wet systems), or check the air leak indicator for leaks (in dry systems with a one-way valve). *Note:* Fluid fluctuations in the water seal chamber or air leak indicator area will stop when: • The lung has reexpanded • The tubing is obstructed by blood clots, fibrin, or kinks • A loop of tubing hangs below the rest of the tubing • Suction motor or wall suction is not working properly	Fluctuation of the water level in the water seal shows effective connection between the pleural cavity and the drainage chamber and indicates that the drainage system remains patent. Fluctuation is also a gauge of intrapleural pressure in systems with a water seal (wet and dry, but not with the one-way valve). An air leak indicator shows changes in intrathoracic pressure in dry systems with a one-way valve. Bubbles will appear if a leak is present. The air leak indicator takes the place of fluid fluctuations in the water seal chamber.
11. With a dry system, assess for the presence of the indicator (bellows or float device) when setting the regulator dial to the desired level of suction.	The indicator shows that the vacuum is adequate to maintain the desired level of suction.
12. Observe for air leaks in the drainage system; they are indicated by constant bubbling in the water seal chamber, or by the air leak indicator in dry systems with a one-way valve. Also assess the chest tube system for correctable external leaks. Notify the physician immediately of excessive bubbling in the water seal chamber not due to external leaks.	Leaking and trapping of air in the pleural space can result in tension pneumothorax.
13. When turning down the dry suction, depress the manual high-negativity vent, and assess for a rise in the water level of the water seal chamber.	A rise in the water level of the water seal chamber indicates high negative pressure in the system that could lead to increased intrathoracic pressure.
14. Observe and immediately report rapid and shallow breathing, cyanosis, pressure in the chest, subcutaneous emphysema, symptoms of hemorrhage, or significant changes in vital signs.	Many clinical conditions can cause these signs and symptoms, including tension pneumothorax, mediastinal shift, hemorrhage, severe incisional pain, pulmonary embolus, and cardiac tamponade. Surgical intervention may be necessary.
15. Encourage the patient to breathe deeply and cough at frequent intervals. Provide adequate analgesia. If needed, request an order for patient-controlled analgesia. Also teach the patient how to perform incentive spirometry.	Deep breathing and coughing help to raise the intrapleural pressure, which promotes drainage of accumulated fluid in the pleural space. Deep breathing and coughing also promote removal of secretions from the tracheobronchial tree, which in turn promotes lung expansion and prevents atelectasis (alveolar collapse).
16. If the patient is lying on a stretcher and must be transported to another area, place the drainage system below the chest level. If the tubing disconnects, cut off the contaminated tips of the chest tube and tubing, insert a sterile connector in the cut ends, and reattach to the drainage system. Do *not* clamp the chest tube during transport.	The drainage apparatus must be kept at a level lower than the patient's chest to prevent fluid from flowing backward into the pleural space. Clamping can result in a tension pneumothorax.
17. When assisting in the chest tube's removal, instruct the patient to perform a gentle Valsalva maneuver or to breathe quietly. The chest tube is then clamped and quickly removed. Simultaneously, a small bandage is applied and made airtight with petrolatum gauze covered by a 4 × 4-inch gauze pad and thoroughly covered and sealed with nonporous tape.	The chest tube is removed as directed when the lung is reexpanded (usually 24 hours to several days), depending on the cause of the pneumothorax. During tube removal, the chief priorities are preventing air from entering the pleural cavity as the tube is withdrawn and preventing infection.

The mediastinal space is an extrapleural space that lies between the right and left thoracic cavities. Mediastinal chest tubes promote the removal of blood or other fluid from around the heart (Finkelmeier, 2000). Accumulating fluid can stop the heart from beating if it is not drained. A mediastinal tube can be inserted either anteriorly or posteriorly to the heart to drain blood after surgery or trauma. Without a tube, compression of the heart could occur, leading to death (Carroll, 2000).

There are two types of chest tubes: small-bore and large-bore catheters. Small-bore catheters (7F to 12F) have a one-way valve apparatus to prevent air from moving back into the patient. They can be inserted through a small skin incision. Large-bore catheters, which range in size up to 40F, are usually connected to a chest drainage system to collect any pleural fluid and monitor for air leaks (Scanlan, Wilkins & Stoller, 1999). After the chest tube is positioned, it is sutured to the skin and connected to a drainage apparatus to remove the residual air and fluid from the pleural or mediastinal space. This results in the re-expansion of remaining lung tissue.

CHEST DRAINAGE SYSTEMS

Chest drainage systems have a suction source, a collection chamber for pleural drainage, and a mechanism to prevent air from reentering the chest with inhalation. Various types of

Chart 25-19 **Preventing Postoperative Cardiopulmonary Complications After Thoracic Surgery**

Patient Management
- Auscultate lung sounds and assess for rate, rhythm, and depth.
- Monitor oxygenation with pulse oximetry.
- Monitor electrocardiogram for rate and rhythm changes.
- Assess capillary refill, skin color, and status of the surgical dressing.
- Encourage and assist the patient to turn, cough, and take deep breaths.

Chest Drainage Management
- Verify that all connection tubes are patent and connected securely.
- Assess that the water seal is intact when using a wet suction system and assess the regulator dial in dry suction systems.
- Monitor characteristics of drainage including color, amount, and consistency. Assess for significant increases or decreases in drainage output.
- Note fluctuations in the water seal chamber for wet suction systems and the air leak indicator for dry suction systems.
- Keep system below the patient's chest level.
- Assess suction control chamber for bubbling in wet suction systems.
- Keep suction at level ordered.
- Maintain appropriate fluid in water seal for wet suction systems.
- Keep air vent open when suction is off.

chest drainage systems are available for use in removal of air and fluid from the pleural space and re-expansion of the lungs. Chest drainage systems come with either wet (water seal) or dry suction control. In wet suction systems, the amount of suction is determined by the amount of water instilled in the suction chamber. The amount of bubbling in the suction chamber indicates how strong the suction is. Wet systems use a water seal to prevent air from moving back into the chest on inspiration. Dry systems use a one-way valve and a suction control dial in place of the water needed with wet or water seal system. Both systems can operate by gravity drainage, without a suction source.

Water Seal Chest Drainage Systems. The traditional water seal chest drainage system (or wet suction) has three chambers: a collection chamber, a water seal chamber, and a wet suction control chamber. The collection chamber acts as a reservoir for fluid draining from the chest tube. It is graduated to permit easy measurement of drainage. Suction may be added to create negative pressure and promote drainage of fluid and removal of air. The suction control chamber regulates the amount of negative pressure applied to the chest. The amount of suction is determined by the water level. It is generally set at 20-cm water; adding more fluid results in more suction. After the suction is turned on, bubbling appears in the suction chamber. A positive-pressure valve is located at the top of the suction chamber that automatically opens with increases in positive pressure within the system. Air will automatically be released through a positive-pressure relief valve if the suction tubing is inadvertently clamped or kinked.

The water seal chamber has a one-way valve or water seal that prevents air from moving back into the chest when the patient in-

hales. There will be an increase in the water level with inspiration and a return to the baseline level during exhalation; this is referred to as tidaling. Intermittent bubbling in the water seal chamber is normal, but continuous bubbling can indicate an air leak. Bubbling and tidaling do not occur when the tube is placed in the mediastinal space; however, fluid may pulsate with the patient's heartbeat. If the chest tube is connected to gravity drainage only, suction is not used. The pressure is equal to the water seal only. Two-chamber chest drainage systems (water seal chamber and collection chamber) are available for use with patients who need only gravity drainage.

The water level in the water seal chamber reflects the negative pressure present in the intrathoracic cavity. A rise in the water level indicates negative pressure in the pleural or mediastinal space. Excessive negative pressure can cause trauma to tissue (Bar-El, Ross, Kablawi & Egenburg, 2001). Most chest drainage systems have an automatic means to prevent excessive negative pressure. By pressing and holding a manual high-negativity vent (usually located on the top of the chest drainage system) until the water level in the water seal chamber returns to the 2-cm mark, excessive negative pressure is avoided, preventing damage to tissue.

> **NURSING ALERT** When the wall vacuum is turned off, the drainage system must be open to the atmosphere so that intrapleural air can escape from the system. This can be done by detaching the tubing from the suction port to provide a vent.

> **NURSING ALERT** If the chest tube and drainage system become disconnected, air can enter the pleural space, producing a pneumothorax. To prevent pneumothorax if the chest tube is inadvertently disconnected from the drainage system, a temporary water seal can be established by immersing the chest tube's open end in a bottle of sterile water.

Dry Suction Water Seal Systems. Dry suction water seal systems, also referred to as dry suction, have a collection chamber for drainage, a water seal chamber, and a dry suction control chamber. The water seal chamber is filled with water to the 2-cm level. Bubbling in this area can indicate an air leak. The dry suction control chamber contains a regulator dial that conveniently regulates vacuum to the chest drain. Water is not needed for suction as it is in the wet system. Without the bubbling in the suction chamber, the machine is quieter.

Once the tube is connected to the suction source, the regulator dial allows the desired level of suction to be dialed in; the suction is increased until an indicator appears. The indicator has the same function as the bubbling in the traditional water seal system; that is, it indicates that the vacuum is adequate to maintain the desired level of suction. Some drainage systems use a bellows (a chamber that can be expanded or contracted) or an orange-colored float device as an indicator of when the suction control regulator is set.

When the water in the water seal rises above the 2-cm level, intrathoracic pressure increases. Dry suction water seal systems have a manual high-negativity vent located on top of the drain. Pressing the manual high-negativity vent until the indicator appears (either a float device or bellows) and the water level in the water seal returns to the desired level, intrathoracic pressure is decreased.

> **NURSING ALERT** The manual vent should not be used to lower the water level in the water seal when the patient is on gravity drainage (no suction) because intrathoracic pressure is equal to the pressure in the water seal.

Dry Suction with a One-Way Valve System. A third type of chest drainage system is dry suction with a one-way mechanical valve. This system has a collection chamber, a one-way mechanical valve, and a dry suction control chamber. The valve acts in the same way as a water seal and permits air to leave the chest but prevents it from moving back into the pleural space. This model lacks a water seal chamber and therefore has the advantage of a system that operates without water. For example, it can be set up quickly in emergency situations, and the dry control drain will still work even if it is knocked over. If the wet suction drain is knocked over, the water seal could be lost. This makes the dry suction systems useful for the patient who is ambulating or being transported. However, without the water seal chamber, there is no way to tell by inspection if the pressure in the chest has changed. An air leak indicator is present so that the system can be checked for air leaks. If an air leak is suspected, 30 mL of water are injected into the air leak indicator. Bubbles will appear if a leak is present (Carroll, 2000).

NURSING PROCESS: THE PATIENT UNDERGOING THORACIC SURGERY

Postoperative Assessment

The nurse monitors the heart rate and rhythm by auscultation and electrocardiography because episodes of major dysrhythmias are common after thoracic and cardiac surgery. In the immediate postoperative period, an arterial line may be maintained to allow frequent monitoring of arterial blood gases, serum electrolytes, hemoglobin and hematocrit values, and arterial pressure. Central venous pressure may be monitored to detect early signs of fluid volume disturbances. Central venous pressure monitoring devices are being used less frequently and for shorter periods of time than in the past. Early extubation from mechanical ventilation can also lead to earlier removal of arterial lines (Zevola & Maier, 1999). Another important component of postoperative assessment is to note the results of the preoperative evaluation of the patient's lung reserve by pulmonary function testing. A preoperative FEV_1 of more than 2 L or more than 70% of predicted value indicates a good lung reserve. Patients who have a postoperative predicted FEV_1 of less than 40% of predicted value have a higher incidence of morbidity and mortality (Scanlan, Wilkins & Stoller, 1999). This results in decreased tidal volumes, placing the patient at risk for respiratory failure.

Diagnosis

NURSING DIAGNOSES

Based on the assessment data, the patient's major postoperative nursing diagnoses may include:

- Impaired gas exchange related to lung impairment and surgery
- Ineffective airway clearance related to lung impairment, anesthesia, and pain
- Acute pain related to incision, drainage tubes, and the surgical procedure
- Impaired physical mobility of the upper extremities related to thoracic surgery
- Risk for imbalanced fluid volume related to the surgical procedure
- Imbalanced nutrition, less than body requirements related to dyspnea and anorexia
- Deficient knowledge about self-care procedures at home

COLLABORATIVE PROBLEMS/ POTENTIAL COMPLICATIONS

Based on assessment data, potential complications may include:

- Respiratory distress
- Dysrhythmias
- Atelectasis, pneumothorax, and bronchopleural fistula
- Blood loss and hemorrhage
- Pulmonary edema

Planning and Goals

The major goals for the patient may include improvement of gas exchange and breathing, improvement of airway clearance, relief of pain and discomfort, increased arm and shoulder mobility, maintenance of adequate fluid volume and nutritional status, understanding of self-care procedures, and absence of complications.

Nursing Interventions

IMPROVING GAS EXCHANGE AND BREATHING

Gas exchange is determined by evaluating oxygenation and ventilation. In the immediate postoperative period, this is achieved by measuring vital signs (blood pressure, pulse, and respirations) at least every 15 minutes for the first 1 to 2 hours, then less frequently as the patient's condition stabilizes.

Pulse oximetry is used for continuous monitoring of the adequacy of oxygenation. It is important to draw blood for arterial blood gas measurements early in the postoperative period to establish a baseline to assess the adequacy of oxygenation and ventilation and the possible retention of CO_2. The frequency with which postoperative arterial blood gases are measured depends on whether the patient is mechanically ventilated or exhibits signs of respiratory distress; these measurements can help determine appropriate therapy. It also is common practice for patients to have an arterial line in place to obtain blood for blood gas measurements and to monitor blood pressure closely. Hemodynamic monitoring may be used to assess hemodynamic stability.

Breathing techniques, such as diaphragmatic and pursed-lip breathing, that were taught before surgery should be performed by the patient every 2 hours to expand the alveoli and prevent atelectasis. Another technique to improve ventilation is sustained maximal inspiration therapy or incentive spirometry. This technique promotes lung inflation, improves the cough mechanism, and allows early assessment of acute pulmonary changes. (See Charts 25-3 and 25-4 for more information.)

Positioning also improves breathing. When the patient is oriented and blood pressure is stabilized, the head of the bed is elevated 30 to 40 degrees during the immediate postoperative period. This facilitates ventilation, promotes chest drainage from the lower chest tube, and helps residual air to rise in the upper portion of the pleural space, where it can be removed through the upper chest tube.

The nurse should consult with the surgeon about patient positioning. There is controversy regarding the best side-lying position. In general, the patient should be positioned from back to side frequently and moved from horizontal to semi-upright position as soon as tolerated. Most commonly, the patient is instructed to lie on the operative side. However, the patient with unilateral lung pathology may not be able to turn well onto that side because of pain. In addition, positioning the patient with the "good lung" (the nonoperated lung) down allows a better match of ventilation and perfusion and therefore may actually improve oxygenation. The patient's position is changed from horizontal to semi-upright as soon as possible, because remaining in one position tends to promote the retention of secretions in the dependent portion of the lungs. After a pneumonectomy, the operated side should be dependent so that fluid in the pleural space remains below the level of the bronchial stump, and the other lung can fully expand.

The procedure for turning the patient is as follows:

- Instruct the patient to bend the knees and use the feet to push.
- Have the patient shift hips and shoulders to the opposite side of the bed while pushing with the feet.
- Bring the patient's arm over the chest, pointing it in the direction toward which the patient is being turned. Have the patient grasp the side rail with the hand.
- Turn the patient in log-roll fashion to prevent twisting at the waist and pain from possible pulling on the incision.

IMPROVING AIRWAY CLEARANCE

Retained secretions are a threat to the thoracotomy patient after surgery. Trauma to the tracheobronchial tree during surgery, diminished lung ventilation, and diminished cough reflex all result in the accumulation of excessive secretions. If the secretions are retained, airway obstruction occurs. This, in turn, causes the air in the alveoli distal to the obstruction to become absorbed and the affected portion of the lung to collapse. Atelectasis, pneumonia, and respiratory failure may result.

Several techniques are used to maintain a patent airway. First, secretions are suctioned from the tracheobronchial tree before the endotracheal tube is discontinued. Secretions continue to be removed by suctioning until the patient can cough up secretions effectively. Nasotracheal suctioning may be needed to stimulate a deep cough and aspirate secretions that the patient cannot cough up. However, it should be used only after other methods to raise secretions have been unsuccessful (Chart 25-20).

Coughing technique is another measure used in maintaining a patent airway. The patient is encouraged to cough effectively; ineffective coughing results in exhaustion and retention of secretions (see Chart 25-5). To be effective, the cough must be low-pitched, deep, and controlled. Because it is difficult to cough in a supine position, the patient is helped to a sitting position on the edge of the bed, with the feet resting on a chair. The patient should cough at least every hour during the first 24 hours and when necessary thereafter. If audible crackles are present, it may be necessary to use chest percussion with the cough routine until the lungs are clear. Aerosol therapy is helpful in humidifying and mobilizing secretions so that they can easily be cleared with coughing. To minimize incisional pain during coughing, the nurse supports the incision or encourages the patient to do so (Fig. 25-8).

After helping the patient to cough, the nurse should listen to both lungs, anteriorly and posteriorly, to determine whether there are any changes in breath sounds. Diminished breath sounds may indicate collapsed or hypoventilated alveoli.

Chart 25-20 — **Performing Nasotracheal Suction**

Sterile Technique to Be Used

1. Explain procedure to the patient.
2. Medicate patient for pain if necessary.
3. Place the patient in a sitting or semi-Fowler's position. Make sure the patient's head is not flexed forward. Remove excess pillows if necessary.
4. Oxygenate the patient several minutes before initiating the suctioning procedure. Have oxygen source ready nearby during procedure.
5. Put on sterile gloves.
6. Lubricate catheter with water-soluble gel.
7. Gently pass catheter through the patient's nose to the pharynx. If it is difficult to pass the catheter, and repeated suctioning is expected, a soft rubber nasal trumpet may be placed nasopharyngeally to provide easier catheter passage. Check the position of the tip of the catheter by asking the patient to open the mouth and inspecting it; the tip of the catheter should be in the lower pharynx.
8. Instruct the patient to take a deep breath or stick out the tongue. This action opens the epiglottis and promotes downward movement of the catheter.
9. Advance the catheter into the trachea only during inspiration. Listen for cough or for passage of air through the catheter.
10. Attach the catheter to suction apparatus. Apply intermittent suction while slowly withdrawing the catheter. Do not let suction exceed 120 mm Hg.
11. Do not suction for longer than 10 to 15 seconds, as dysrhythmias, bradycardia, or cardiac arrest may occur in patients with borderline oxygenation.
12. If additional suctioning is needed, withdraw the catheter to the back of the pharynx. Reassure patient and oxygenate for several minutes before resuming suctioning.

Chest physiotherapy is the final technique for maintaining a patent airway. If a patient is identified as being at high risk for developing postoperative pulmonary complications, then chest physiotherapy is started immediately (perhaps even before surgery). The techniques of postural drainage, vibration, and percussion help to loosen and mobilize the secretions so that they can be coughed up or suctioned.

RELIEVING PAIN AND DISCOMFORT

Pain after a thoracotomy may be severe, depending on the type of incision and the patient's reaction to and ability to cope with pain. Deep inspiration is very painful after thoracotomy. Pain can lead to postoperative complications if it reduces the patient's ability to breathe deeply and cough, and if it further limits chest excursions so that ventilation becomes ineffective.

Immediately after the surgical procedure and before the incision is closed, the surgeon may perform a nerve block with a long-acting local anesthetic such as bupivacaine (Marcaine, Sensorcaine). Bupivacaine is titrated to relieve postoperative pain while allowing the patient to cooperate in deep breathing, coughing, and mobilization. However, it is important to avoid depressing the respiratory system with excessive analgesia: the patient should not be so sedated as to be unable to cough. There is controversy about the effectiveness of injections of local anesthetic for pain relief after thoracotomy surgery. Research has shown that bupivacaine was no

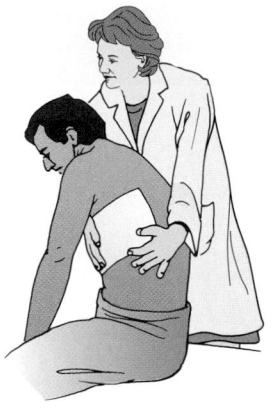

A The nurse's hands should support the chest incision anteriorly and posteriorly. The patient is instructed to take several deep breaths, inhale, and then cough forcibly.

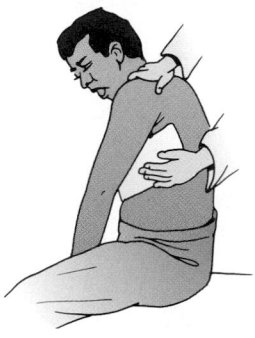

B With one hand, the nurse exerts downward pressure on the shoulder of the affected side while firmly supporting the area beneath the wound with the other hand. The patient is instructed to take several deep breaths, inhale, and then cough forcibly.

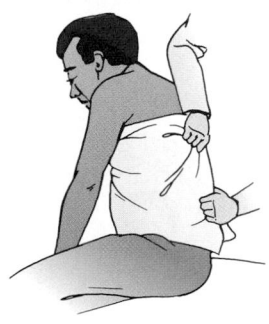

C The nurse can wrap a towel or sheet around the patient's chest and hold the ends together, pulling slightly as the patient coughs, and releasing during deep breaths.

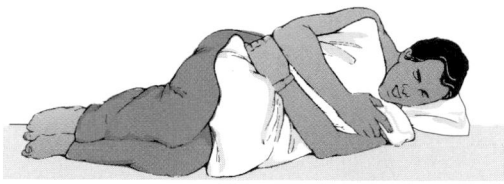

FIGURE 25-8 Techniques for supporting incision while a patient recovering from thoracic surgery coughs.

D The patient can be taught to hold a pillow firmly against the incision while coughing. This can be done while lying down or sitting in an upright position.

more effective than saline injections in treating postoperative thoracotomy pain (Silomon et al., 2000).

Lidocaine and prilocaine are local anesthetic agents used to treat pain at the site of the chest tube insertion. These medications are administered as topical transdermal analgesics that penetrate the skin. Lidocaine and prilocaine have also been found to be effective when used together. EMLA cream, which is a mixture of the two medications, has been found to be effective in treating pain from chest tube removal, and recent studies found it to be more effective than intravenous morphine (Valenzuela & Rosen, 1999).

Because of the need to maximize patient comfort without depressing the respiratory drive, patient-controlled analgesia (PCA) is often used. Opioid analgesic agents such as morphine are commonly used. PCA, administered through an intravenous pump or an epidural catheter, allows the patient to control the frequency and total dosage. Preset limits on the pump avoid overdosage. With proper instruction, these methods are well tolerated and allow earlier mobilization and cooperation with the treatment regimen. (See Chap. 13 for a more extensive discussion of PCA and pain management.)

> **NURSING ALERT** It is important not to confuse the restlessness of hypoxia with the restlessness caused by pain. Dyspnea, restlessness, increasing respiratory rate, increasing blood pressure, and tachycardia are warning signs of impending respiratory insufficiency. Pulse oximetry is used to monitor oxygenation and to differentiate causes of restlessness.

PROMOTING MOBILITY AND SHOULDER EXERCISES

Because large shoulder girdle muscles are transected during a thoracotomy, the arm and shoulder must be mobilized by full range of motion of the shoulder. As soon as physiologically possible, usually within 8 to 12 hours, the patient is helped to get out of bed. Although this may be painful initially, the earlier the patient moves, the sooner the pain will subside. In addition to getting out of bed, the patient begins arm and shoulder exercises to restore movement and prevent painful stiffening of the affected arm and shoulder (Chart 25-21).

MAINTAINING FLUID VOLUME AND NUTRITION

Intravenous Therapy

During the surgical procedure or immediately after, the patient may receive a transfusion of blood products, followed by a continuous intravenous infusion. Because a reduction in lung capacity often occurs following thoracic surgery, a period of physiologic adjustment is needed. Fluids should be administered at a low hourly rate and titrated (as prescribed) to prevent overloading the vascular system and precipitating pulmonary edema. The nurse performs careful respiratory and cardiovascular assessments, as well as intake and output, vital signs, and assessment of jugular vein distention. The nurse should also monitor the infusion site for signs of infiltration, including swelling, tenderness, and redness.

Diet

It is not unusual for patients undergoing thoracotomy to have poor nutritional status before surgery because of dyspnea, sputum production, and poor appetite. Therefore, it is especially important

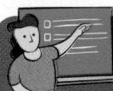

Chart 25-21 • PATIENT EDUCATION
Performing Arm and Shoulder Exercises

Arm and shoulder exercises are performed after thoracic surgery to restore movement, prevent painful stiffening of the shoulder, and improve muscle power.

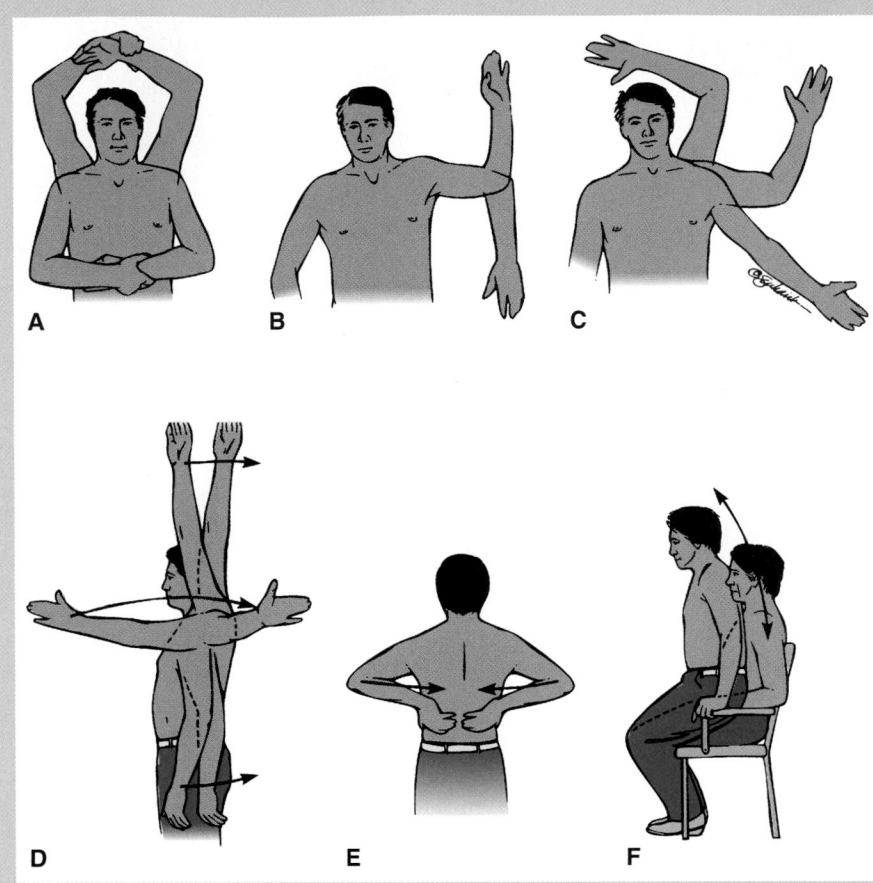

(**A**) Hold hand of the affected side with the other hand, palms facing in. Raise the arms forward, upward, and then overhead, while taking a deep breath. Exhale while lowering the arms. Repeat five times. (**B**) Raise arm sideward, upward, and downward in a waving motion. (**C**) Place arm at side. Raise arm sideward, upward, and over the head. Repeat five times. These exercises can also be performed while lying in bed. (**D**) Extend the arm up and back, out to the side and back, down at the side and back. (**E**) Place hands in small of back. Push elbows as far back as possible. (**F**) Sit erect in an armchair; place the hands on the arms of the chair directly opposite the sides of the body. Press down on hands, consciously pulling the abdomen in and stretching up from the waist. Inhale while raising the body until the elbows are extended completely. Hold this position a moment, and begin exhaling while lowering the body slowly to the original position.

that adequate nutrition be provided. A liquid diet is provided as soon as bowel sounds return; the patient is progressed to a full diet as soon as possible. Small, frequent meals are better tolerated and are crucial to the recovery and maintenance of lung function.

MONITORING AND MANAGING POTENTIAL COMPLICATIONS

Complications after thoracic surgery are always a possibility and must be identified and managed early. In addition, the nurse monitors the patient at regular intervals for signs of respiratory distress or developing respiratory failure, dysrhythmias, bronchopleural fistula, hemorrhage and shock, atelectasis, and pulmonary infection.

Respiratory distress is treated by identifying and eliminating its cause while providing supplemental oxygen. If the patient progresses to respiratory failure, intubation and mechanical ventilation are necessary, eventually requiring weaning.

Dysrhythmias are often related to the effects of hypoxia or the surgical procedure. They are treated with antiarrhythmic medication and supportive therapy (see Chap. 27). Pulmonary infec-

tions or effusion, often preceded by atelectasis, may occur a few days into the postoperative course.

Pneumothorax may occur following thoracic surgery if there is an air leak from the surgical site to the pleural cavity or from the pleural cavity to the environment. Failure of the chest drainage system will prevent return of negative pressure in the pleural cavity and result in pneumothorax. In the postoperative patient pneumothorax is often accompanied by hemothorax. The nurse maintains the chest drainage system and monitors the patient for signs and symptoms of pneumothorax: increasing shortness of breath, tachycardia, increased respiratory rate, and increasing respiratory distress.

Bronchopleural fistula is a serious but rare complication preventing the return of negative intrathoracic pressure and lung reexpansion. Depending on its severity, it is treated with closed chest drainage, mechanical ventilation, and possibly talc pleurodesis (described in Chap. 23).

Hemorrhage and shock are managed by treating the underlying cause, whether by reoperation or by administration of blood products or fluids. Pulmonary edema from overinfusion of intravenous fluids is a significant danger. The early symptoms are dyspnea, crackles, bubbling sounds in the chest, tachycardia, and pink, frothy sputum. This constitutes an emergency and must be reported and treated immediately.

PROMOTING HOME AND COMMUNITY-BASED CARE

Teaching Patients Self-Care

The nurse instructs the patient and family about postoperative care that will be continued at home. The nurse explains signs and symptoms that should be reported to the physician. These include:

- Change in respiratory status: increasing shortness of breath, fever, increased restlessness or other changes in mental or cognitive status, increased respiratory rate, change in respiratory pattern, change in amount or color of sputum
- Bleeding or other drainage from the surgical incision or chest tube exit sites
- Increased chest pain

In addition, respiratory care and other treatment modalities (oxygen, incentive spirometer, chest physiotherapy, and oral, inhaled, or intravenous medications) may be continued at home. Therefore, the nurse needs to instruct the patient and family in their correct and safe use.

The nurse emphasizes the importance of progressively increased activity. The nurse instructs the patient to ambulate within limits and explains that return of strength is likely to be very gradual. Another important aspect of patient teaching addresses shoulder exercises. It is important to instruct the patient to do these exercises five times daily. Additional patient teaching is described in Chart 25-22.

Continuing Care

Depending on the patient's physical status and the availability of family assistance, a home care referral may be indicated. The home care nurse assesses the patient's recovery from surgery, with special attention to respiratory status, the surgical incision, chest drainage, pain control, ambulation, and nutritional status. The patient's use of respiratory modalities should be assessed to ensure they are being used correctly and safely. In addition, the nurse assesses the patient's compliance with the postoperative treatment plan and identifies acute or late postoperative complications.

The recovery process may be longer than the patient had expected, and providing support to the patient is an important task for the home care nurse. Because of shorter hospital stays, attending follow-up physician appointments is essential. The nurse teaches the patient about the importance of keeping follow-up appointments and completing laboratory tests as prescribed to assist the physician in evaluating recovery. The home care nurse provides continuous encouragement and education to the patient and family during the process. As recovery progresses, the nurse also reminds the patient and family about the importance of participating in health promotion activities and recommended health screening.

Evaluation

EXPECTED PATIENT OUTCOMES

Expected patient outcomes may include:

1. Demonstrates improved gas exchange, as reflected in arterial blood gas measurements, breathing exercises, and use of incentive spirometry
2. Shows improved airway clearance, as evidenced by deep, controlled coughing and clear breath sounds or decreased presence of adventitious sounds
3. Has decreased pain and discomfort by splinting incision during coughing and increasing activity level
4. Shows improved mobility of shoulder and arm; demonstrates arm and shoulder exercises to relieve stiffening
5. Maintains adequate fluid intake and maintains nutrition for healing
6. Exhibits less anxiety by using appropriate coping skills, and demonstrates a basic understanding of technology used in care
7. Adheres to therapeutic program and home care
8. Is free of complications, as evidenced by normal vital signs and temperature, improved arterial blood gas measurements, clear lung sounds, and adequate respiratory function

For a detailed plan of nursing care for the patient who has had a thoracotomy, see the Plan of Nursing Care.

Chart 25-22
Home Care Checklist • The Patient With a Thoracotomy

At the completion of the home care instruction, the patient or caregiver will be able to:	Patient	Caregiver
• Use local heat and oral analgesia to relieve intercostal pain.	✓	✓
• Alternate walking and other activities with frequent rest periods, expecting weakness and fatigue for the first 3 weeks.	✓	✓
• Perform breathing exercises several times daily for the first few weeks at home.	✓	
• Avoid lifting more than 20 pounds until complete healing has taken place; the chest muscles and incision may be weaker than normal for 3 to 6 months after surgery.	✓	
• Walk at a moderate pace, gradually and persistently extending walking time and distance.	✓	
• Immediately stop any activity that causes undue fatigue, increased shortness of breath, or chest pain.	✓	
• Avoid bronchial irritants (smoke, fumes, air pollution, aerosol sprays).	✓	✓
• Avoid others with known colds or lung infections.	✓	✓
• Obtain an annual influenza vaccine and discuss vaccination against pneumonia with the physician.	✓	
• Report for follow-up care by the surgeon or clinic as necessary.	✓	✓
• Stop smoking, if applicable.	✓	✓

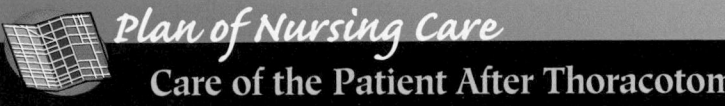

Plan of Nursing Care
Care of the Patient After Thoracotomy

Nursing Interventions	Rationale	Expected Patient Outcomes

Nursing Diagnosis: Impaired gas exchange related to lung impairment and surgery
Goal: Improvement of gas exchange and breathing

Nursing Interventions	Rationale	Expected Patient Outcomes
1. Monitor pulmonary status as directed and as needed: a. Auscultate breath sounds. b. Check rate, depth, and pattern of respirations. c. Assess blood gases for signs of hypoxemia or CO_2 retention. d. Evaluate patient's color for cyanosis.	1. Changes in pulmonary status indicate improvement or onset of complications.	• Lungs are clear on auscultation • Respiratory rate is within acceptable range with no episodes of dyspnea • Vital signs are stable • Dysrhythmias are not present or are under control • Demonstrates deep, controlled, effective breathing to allow maximal lung expansion • Uses incentive spirometer every 2 hours while awake • Demonstrates deep, effective coughing technique • Lungs are expanded to capacity (evidenced by chest x-ray)
2. Monitor and record blood pressure, apical pulse, and temperature every 2–4 hours, central venous pressure (if indicated) every 2 hours.	2. Aid in evaluating effect of surgery on cardiac status.	
3. Monitor continuous electrocardiogram for pattern and dysrhythmias.	3. Dysrhythmias (especially atrial fibrillation and atrial flutter) are more frequently seen after thoracic surgery. A patient with total pneumonectomy is especially prone to cardiac irregularity.	
4. Elevate head of bed 30–40 degrees when patient is oriented and hemodynamic status is stable.	4. Maximum lung excursion is achieved when patient is as close to upright as possible.	
5. Encourage deep-breathing exercises (see section on Breathing Retraining) and effective use of incentive spirometer (sustained maximal inspiration).	5. Helps to achieve maximal lung inflation and to open closed airways.	
6. Encourage and promote an effective cough routine to be performed every 1–2 hours during first 24 hours.	6. Coughing is necessary to remove retained secretions.	
7. Assess and monitor the chest drainage system:* a. Assess for leaks and patency as needed. b. Monitor amount and character of drainage and document every 2 hours. Notify physician if drainage is 150 mL/h or greater. c. See Chart 25-18 for summary of nurse's role in management of chest drainage systems.	7. System is used to eliminate any residual air or fluid after thoracotomy.	

Nursing Diagnosis: Ineffective airway clearance related to lung impairment, anesthesia, and pain
Goal: Improvement of airway clearance and achievement of a patent airway

Nursing Interventions	Rationale	Expected Patient Outcomes
1. Maintain an open airway.	1. Provides for adequate ventilation and gas exchange	• Airway is patent • Coughs effectively • Splints incision while coughing • Sputum is clear or colorless • Lungs are clear on auscultation
2. Perform endotracheal suctioning until patient can raise secretions effectively.	2. Endotracheal secretions are present in excessive amounts in post-thoracotomy patients due to trauma to the tracheobronchial tree during surgery, diminished lung ventilation, and cough reflex.	
3. Assess and medicate for pain. Encourage deep-breathing and coughing exercises. Help splint incision during coughing.	3. Helps to achieve maximal lung inflation and to open closed airways. Coughing is painful; incision needs to be supported.	

---

*A patient with a pneumonectomy usually does not have water seal chest drainage because it is desirable that the pleural space fill with an effusion, which eventually obliterates this space. Some surgeons do use a modified water seal system.

(continued)

Plan of Nursing Care
Care of the Patient After Thoracotomy *(Continued)*

Nursing Interventions	Rationale	Expected Patient Outcomes
4. Monitor amount, viscosity, color, and odor of sputum. Notify physician if sputum is excessive or contains bright-red blood.	4. Changes in sputum suggest presence of infection or change in pulmonary status. Colorless sputum is not unusual; opacification or coloring of sputum may indicate dehydration or infection.	
5. Administer humidification and mini-nebulizer therapy as prescribed.	5. Secretions must be moistened and thinned if they are to be raised from the chest with the least amount of effort.	
6. Perform postural drainage, percussion, and vibration as prescribed. Do not percuss or vibrate directly over operative site.	6. Chest physiotherapy uses gravity to help remove secretions from the lung.	
7. Auscultate both sides of chest to determine changes in breath sounds.	7. Indications for tracheal suctioning are determined by chest auscultation.	

Nursing Diagnosis: Acute pain related to incision, drainage tubes, and the surgical procedure
Goal: Relief of pain and discomfort

1. Evaluate location, character, quality, and severity of pain. Administer analgesic medication as prescribed and as needed. Observe for respiratory effect of opioid. Is patient too somnolent to cough? Are respirations depressed?	1. Pain limits chest excursions and thereby decreases ventilation.	• Asks for pain medication, but verbalizes that he or she expects some discomfort while deep breathing and coughing • Verbalizes that he or she is comfortable and not in acute distress • No signs of incisional infection evident

2. Maintain care postoperatively in positioning the thoracotomy patient:
  a. Place patient in semi-Fowler's position.
  b. Patients with limited respiratory reserve may not be able to turn on unoperated side.
  c. Assist or turn patient every 2 hours.
	2. The patient who is comfortable and free of pain will be less likely to splint the chest while breathing. A semi-Fowler's position permits residual air in the pleural space to rise to upper portion of pleural space and be removed via the upper chest catheter.	

3. Assess incision area every 8 hours for redness, heat, induration, swelling, separation, and drainage.	3. These signs indicate possible infection.	
4. Request order for patient-controlled analgesia pump if appropriate for patient.	4. Allowing patient control over frequency and dose improves comfort and compliance with treatment regimen.	

Nursing Diagnosis: Anxiety related to outcomes of surgery, pain, technology
Goal: Reduction of anxiety to a manageable level

1. Explain all procedures in understandable language.	1. Explaining what can be expected in understandable terms decreases anxiety and increases cooperation.	• States that anxiety is at a manageable level • Participates with health care team in treatment regimen • Uses appropriate coping skills (verbalization, pain relief strategies, use of support systems such as family, clergy) • Demonstrates basic understanding of technology used in care
2. Assess for pain and medicate, especially before potentially painful procedures.	2. Premedication before painful procedures or activities improves comfort and minimizes undue anxiety.	
3. Silence all *unnecessary* alarms on technology (monitors, ventilators).	3. *Unnecessary* alarms increase the risk of sensory overload and may increase anxiety.	
4. Encourage and support patient while increasing activity level.	4. Positive reinforcement improves patient motivation and independence.	
5. Mobilize resources (family, clergy, social worker) to help patient cope with outcomes of surgery (diagnosis, change in functional abilities).	5. A multidisciplinary approach promotes the patient's strengths and coping mechanisms.	

(continued)

Nursing Interventions	Rationale	Expected Patient Outcomes

Nursing Diagnosis: Impaired physical mobility of the upper extremities related to thoracic surgery
Goal: Increased mobility of the affected shoulder and arm

1. Assist patient with normal range of motion and function of shoulder and trunk: a. Teach breathing exercises to mobilize thorax. b. Encourage skeletal exercises to promote abduction and mobilization of shoulder (see Chart 25-21). c. Assist out of bed to chair as soon as pulmonary and circulatory systems are stable (usually by evening of surgery). 2. Encourage progressive activities according to level of fatigue.	1. Necessary to regain normal mobility of arm and shoulder and to speed recovery and minimize discomfort 2. Increases patient's use of affected shoulder and arm	• Demonstrates arm and shoulder exercises and verbalizes intent to perform them on discharge • Regains previous range of motion in shoulder and arm

Nursing Diagnosis: Risk for imbalanced fluid volume related to the surgical procedure
Goal: Maintenance of adequate fluid volume

1. Monitor and record hourly intake and output. Urine output should be at least 30 mL/h after surgery. 2. Administer blood component therapy and parenteral fluids and/or diuretics as prescribed to restore and maintain fluid volume.	1. Fluid management may be altered before, during, and after surgery, and patient's response to and need for fluid management must be assessed. 2. Pulmonary edema due to transfusion or fluid overload is an ever-present threat; after pneumonectomy, the pulmonary vascular system has been greatly reduced.	• Patient is adequately hydrated, as evidenced by: • Urine output greater than 30 mL/h • Vital signs stable, heart rate, and central venous pressure approaching normal • No excessive peripheral edema

Nursing Diagnosis: Deficient knowledge of home care procedures
Goal: Increased ability to carry out care procedures at home

1. Encourage patient to practice arm and shoulder exercises five times daily at home. 2. Instruct patient to practice assuming a functionally erect position in front of a full-length mirror. 3. Instruct patient in following aspects of home care: a. Relieve intercostal pain by local heat or oral analgesia. b. Alternate activities with frequent rest periods. c. Practice breathing exercises at home. d. Avoid heavy lifting until complete healing has occurred. e. Avoid undue fatigue, increased shortness of breath, or chest pain. f. Avoid bronchial irritants. g. Prevent colds or lung infection. h. Get annual influenza vaccine. i. Keep follow-up appointment with physician. j. Stop smoking.	1. Exercise accelerates recovery of muscle function and reduces long-term pain and discomfort. 2. Practice will help restore normal posture. 3. Knowing what to expect facilitates recovery. a. Some soreness may persist for several weeks. b. Weakness and fatigue are common for the first 3 weeks or longer. c. Effective breathing is necessary to prevent splinting of affected side, which may lead to atelectasis. d. Chest muscles and incision may be weaker than normal for 3–6 months. e. Undue stress may prolong the healing process. f. The lung is more susceptible to irritants. g. The lung is more susceptible to infection during the recovery phase. h. Vaccination helps prevent flu. i. This allows timely follow-up assessment. j. Smoking will slow healing process by decreasing oxygen delivery to tissues and make lung susceptible to infection and other complications.	• Demonstrates arm and shoulder exercises • Verbalizes need to try to assume an erect posture • Verbalizes the importance of relieving discomfort, alternating walking and rest, performing breathing exercises, avoiding heavy lifting, avoiding undue fatigue, avoiding bronchial irritants, preventing colds or lung infections, getting flu vaccine, keeping follow-up visits, and stopping smoking

Critical Thinking Exercises

1. Oxygen therapy is required for the following patients: a 45-year-old patient who has undergone a right lower lobe lobectomy and needs short-term, low-flow oxygen; a 62-year-old patient with severe COPD admitted to the hospital for the fourth time in the past year; and a 74-year-old patient with dyspnea secondary to advanced lung cancer. Describe the explanations and safety precautions indicated for each of these patients and their families.

2. Your patient has just returned from the operating room after chest surgery with an endotracheal tube, a chest tube, and two intravenous lines and cardiac monitoring in place. Identify the priorities of assessment and interventions for this patient.

3. Your patient, who underwent a thoracotomy less than 24 hours ago, has a chest tube in place on the right side. Identify the actions that are indicated for each of the following situations and state the rationale for your actions:
    a. Output in chest drainage chamber of 500 mL of serous drainage in the last 8 hours
    b. Continuous bubbling in the water seal chamber
    c. Patient reports chest pain and dyspnea; absence of breath sounds on the right side of the thorax

4. A patient is being discharged home on oxygen therapy for the first time. The physician's prescription is for 2 L of oxygen via nasal cannula. Write a teaching plan for home oxygen therapy to be discussed with the patient before discharge from the hospital.

5. A patient who had a chest tube inserted 8 hours ago becomes confused and disconnects the chest tube from the drainage system. What immediate actions are indicated in this situation? What nursing assessments and interventions are needed once the immediate situation has been corrected?

REFERENCES AND SELECTED READINGS

Books

Abraham, I., Bottrell, M., Fulmer, T., & Mezey, M. (1999). *Geriatric nursing protocols for best practice.* New York: Springer.

Cairo, J., & Pilbeam, S. (1999). *Respiratory care equipment.* St. Louis: Mosby.

Clinical practice guidelines. (2000). Dallas, Texas: American Association for Respiratory Care.

Doenges, M. E., & Moorhouse, F. (2000). *Nurse's pocket guide. Diagnoses, interventions, and rationales.* Philadelphia: F. A. Davis.

Dudek, S. G. (2001). *Nutrition essentials for nursing practice.* Philadelphia: Lippincott.

Eliopoulos, C. (2001). *Gerontological nursing.* Philadelphia: Lippincott Williams & Wilkins.

Finkelmeier, B. (2000). *Cardiothoracic-surgical nursing.* Philadelphia: Lippincott Williams & Wilkins.

Hill, N. S. (2000). *Long-term mechanical ventilation.* New York: Marcel Dekker, Inc.

Hurford, W. E. (2000). *Airway management.* Philadelphia: Lippincott Williams & Wilkins.

Kacmarek, R. M. (2000). *Advanced respiratory care.* Philadelphia: Lippincott Williams & Wilkins.

LeFever, J., & Hayes, E. (2000). *Pharmacology: A nursing process approach.* Philadelphia: W. B. Saunders.

Lutz, C., & Przytulski, K. (2001). *Nutrition and diet therapy.* Philadelphia: F. A. Davis.

MacIntyre, N. R., & Branson, R. D. (2001). *Mechanical ventilation.* Philadelphia: W. B. Saunders.

McKenry, L., & Salerno, E. (2001). *Pharmacology in nursing.* St. Louis: Mosby.

Mishoe, S. C., & Welch, A. (2001). *Critical thinking in respiratory care: A problem-based learning approach.* New York: McGraw-Hill, Medical Publishing Division.

Ochroch, E. A., & Deutschman, C. S. (2000). *Managing the airway in the critically ill patient.* Philadelphia: W. B. Saunders.

Scanlan, C., Wilkins, R., & Stoller, J. (1999). *Fundamentals of respiratory care.* St. Louis: Mosby.

Wilkins, R. L., Krider, S. J., & Sheldon, R. L. (2000). *Clinical assessment in respiratory care.* St. Louis: Mosby.

Woodrow, P., & Roe, J. (2000). *Intensive care nursing: A framework for practice.* New York: Routledge.

Zang, S., & Allender, J. (1999). *Home care of the elderly.* Philadelphia: Lippincott Williams & Wilkins.

Journals

Asterisks indicate nursing research articles.

Avery, S. (2000). Insertion and management of chest drains. *Nursing Times, 96*(37), 1–6.

Baker, S., & Flynn, M. B. (1999). New hope for patients with emphysema: Lung volume reduction surgery. *Heart and Lung, 28*(6), 455–458.

Bar-El, Y., Ross, A., Kablawi, A., & Egenburg, S. (2001). Potentially dangerous negative intrapleural pressures generated by ordinary pleural drainage systems. *Chest, 119*(2), 511–514.

Blackwood, B. (1999). Normal saline instillation with endotracheal suctioning: Primum non nocere (first do no harm). *Journal of Advanced Nursing, 29*(4), 928–934.

Bliss, P., McCoy, R., & Adams, A. (1999). A bench study of comparison of demand oxygen delivery systems and continuous flow oxygen. *Respiratory Care, 44*(8), 925–929.

*Byers, J. F., & Sole, M. L. (2000). Analysis of factors related to the development of ventilator associated pneumonia: Use of existing databases. *American Journal of Critical Care, 9*(5), 344–351.

Carroll, P. (2000). Exploring chest drain options. *RN, 63*(10), 50–58.

Cirino, L., Campos, J., Fernandez, A., Samano, M., Fernandez, P., Filomeno, L. & Jatene, F. (2000). Diagnosis and treatment of mediastinal tumors by thoracoscopy. *Chest, 117*(6), 1787–1792.

Clini, E., Vitacca, M. D., Bianchi, L., Porta, R., & Ambrosino, N. (1999). Long-term tracheostomy in severe COPD patients weaned from mechanical ventilation. *Respiratory Care, 44*(4), 241–244.

Creechan, T. (2000). Combining mechanical ventilation with hospice care in the home: death with dignity. *Critical Care Nurse, 20*(3), 49–53.

Cull, C. (1999). Weaning patients from mechanical ventilation. *Professional Nurse, 14*(8), 535–538.

Cull, C., & Inwood, H. (1999). Extubation in ICU: Enhancing the nursing role. *Professional Nurse, 14*(9), 535–538.

Day, T. (2000). Tracheal suctioning: When, why, and how? *Nursing Times, 96*(20), 13–15.

Doherty, M. J., & Greenstone, M. A. (2000). Noninvasive ventilation in acute exacerbations of chronic obstructive pulmonary disease. *Care of the Critically Ill, 116*(4), 126–130.

Estaban, A., Anzueto, A., Frutos, F., et al. (2002). Characteristics and outcomes in adult patients receiving mechanical ventilation. A 28-day international study. *Journal of the American Medical Association, 287*(3), 345–355.

Ecklund, M. (1999). Successful outcomes for the ventilator-dependent patient. *Critical Care Nursing Clinics of North America, 11*(2), 249–260.

Ferreira, M. M., Brooks, D., Lacasse, Y., & Goldstein, R. S. (2000). Nutritional support for individuals with COPD: A meta-analysis. *Chest, 117*(3), 672–678.

Giannouli, E., Webster, K., Roberts, D., & Younes, M. (1999). Response of ventilator-dependent patients to different levels of pressure support and proportional assist. *American Journal of Respiratory and Critical Care Medicine, 159*(6), 1716–1725.

Goodfellow, L. T., & Jones, M. (2002). Bronchial hygiene therapy. *American Journal of Nursing, 102*(1), 37–43.

Hanneman, S. K. (1999). Protocols for practice: Applying research at the bedside. Weaning from short-term mechanical ventilation. *Critical Care Nurse, 19*(5), 86–89.

Hanneman, S. K. (1999). Weaning from short-term mechanical ventilation. *Critical Care Nurse, 19*(5), 86–89.

Happ, M. B. (2000). Preventing treatment interference: The nurse's role in maintaining technologic devices. *Heart & Lung, 29*(1), 60–69.

Kacmarek, R. M. (2000). Delivery systems for long-term oxygen therapy. State-of-the-art conference on long-term oxygen therapy. *Respiratory Care, 45*(1), 84–94.

*Kinloch, D. (1999). Instillation of normal saline during endotracheal suctioning: Effects on mixed venous oxygen saturation. *American Journal of Critical Care, 8*(4), 231–240.

Kruger, M., & Sandler, A. (1999). Post-thoracotomy pain control. *Current Opinion of Anaesthesiology, 12*(1), 55–58.

Manaligod, J. M., Bendel-Stenzel, E. M., Meyers, P. A., et al. (2000). Variations in end-expiratory pressure during partial liquid ventilation. *Chest, 117*(1), 184–190.

*Mazolewski, P., Turner, J., Baker, M., Kurtz, T., & Little, A. (1999). The impact of nutritional status on the outcome of lung volume reduction surgery. *Chest, 116*(3), 693–696.

McConnell, E. A. (2000). Do's and don'ts. Suctioning a tracheostomy. *Nursing, 30*(1), 79–80.

National Institutes of Health (2001). *National emphysema treatment trial (NETT): Evaluation of lung volume reduction surgery for emphysema.* June 20, 2001. http://www.nhlbi.nih.gov/health/prof/lung/nett/lvrsweb.htm

Perkins, L., & Shortall, S. P. (2000). Ventilation without intubation. *RN, 63*(1), 34–39.

*Powers, J., & Bennett, S. J. (1999). Measurement of dyspnea in patients treated with mechanical ventilation. *American Journal of Critical Care, 8*(4), 254–261.

Roviaro, G., Varoli, F., Nucca, O., Vergani, C., & Maciocco, M. (2000). Videothorascopic approach to primary mediastinal pathology. *Chest, 117*(4), 1179–1183.

Schwartz, J. (2000). Role of polyunsaturated fatty acids in lung disease. *American Journal of Clinical Nutrition, 71*(1), 393–396.

Sclafani, J. C. (1999). Clinical perspectives. Home oxygen for adults: selection of appropriate oxygen delivery system. *AARC Times, 23*(9), 51–54.

Seijo, L. M., & Sterman, D. H. (2001). Interventional pulmonology. *New England Journal of Medicine, 344*(10), 740–749.

Serra, A. (2000). Tracheostomy care. *Nursing Standard, 14*(42), 45–55.

Silomon, M., Claus, T., Hower, H., Biedler, A., Larsen, R., & Molter, G. (2000). Interpleural analgesia does not influence post-thoracotomy pain. *Anesthesia and Analgesia, 91*(1), 44–50.

Smith, L., & McDougall, C. (1999). Removal of chest drains. *Nursing Times, 95*(12), 24–30.

Smith, T., & Matti, A. M. (1999). Respiratory care. Air apparent long-term oxygen therapy. *Nursing Times, 95*(41), 34–38.

*Steuer, J. D., Stone, K. S., Nickel, J., & Steinfeld, Y. (2000). Methodologic issues associated with secretion weight as a dependent variable in research using closed-system suction catheters. *Nursing Research, 49*(5), 295–299.

St. John, R. (1999a). Advances in artificial airway management. *Critical Care Nursing Clinics of North America, 11*(1), 7–17.

St. John, R. E. (1999b). Protocols for practice: applying research at the bedside. Airway management. *Critical Care Nurse, 19*(4), 79–83.

Tasota, F. J., & Dobbin, K. (2000). Weaning your patient from mechanical ventilation. *Nursing, 30*(10), 41–47.

Takezawa, J. (2000). Hyperbaric oxygen therapy. *Critical Care Alert, 8*(8), 88–93.

Tamburri, L. M. (2000). Care of the patient with a tracheostomy. *Orthopaedic Nursing, 19*(2), 49–60.

Tobin, M. J. (2001). Advances in mechanical ventilation. *New England Journal of Medicine, 344*(26), 1986–1996.

Tonelli, M. R. (1999). Withdrawing mechanical ventilation: Conflicts and consensus. *Respiratory Care, 44*(11), 1383–1387.

Truesdell, S. (2000). Helping patients with COPD manage episodes of acute shortness of breath. *MedSurg Nursing, 9*(4), 178–182.

Valenzuela, R., & Rosen, D. (1999). Topical lidocaine-prilocaine cream (EMLA) for thoracostomy tube removal. *Anesthesia and Analgesia, 88*(1), 1107–1108.

Wilmoth, D. (1999). New strategies for mechanical ventilation: Lung protective ventilation. *Critical Care Nursing Clinics of North America, 11*(4), 447–454.

Woodruff, D. W. (1999). How to ward off complications of mechanical ventilation. *Nursing, 29*(11), 34–39.

Zevola, D. R., & Maier, B. (1999). Improving the care of cardiothoracic surgery patients through advanced nursing skills. *Critical Care Nurse, 19*(1), 34–36.

RESOURCES AND WEBSITES

American Association for Respiratory Care, 11030 Ables Lane, Dallas, TX 75229; (972) 243-2272; http://www.aarc.org.

American Lung Association, 1740 Broadway, New York, NY 10019; (212) 315-8700, (800) LUNG-USA; http://www.lungusa.org.

American Thoracic Society, 1740 Broadway, New York, NY 10019; (212) 315-8700; http://www.thoracic.org.

National Heart, Lung and Blood Institute, National Institutes of Health, 9000 Rockville Pike, Bldg 31, Rm 5A52, Bethesda, MD 20892; (301) 496-5166 or (301) 496-4236; http://www.nhlbi.nih.gov.

Cardiovascular, Circulatory, and Hematologic Function

Applying Concepts from NANDA, NIC, and NOC

Mr. Arno, age 57, has a history of peripheral arterial occlusive disease (2 years), hypertension, hypercholesterolemia, Type 2 diabetes, and smoking. He eats low-fat foods and cut back on smoking to half a pack a day. His home-monitored blood glucose levels range from 180 to 215 mg/dL. Because he has severe calf pain after walking, he now walks only two blocks a day: one block from home and one block back. He now receives medical treatment for a nonhealing ulcer on the plantar aspect of his left foot. The concept map illustrates the relationships that exist among the nursing diagnoses, interventions, and outcomes for one of Mr. Arno's clinical problems.

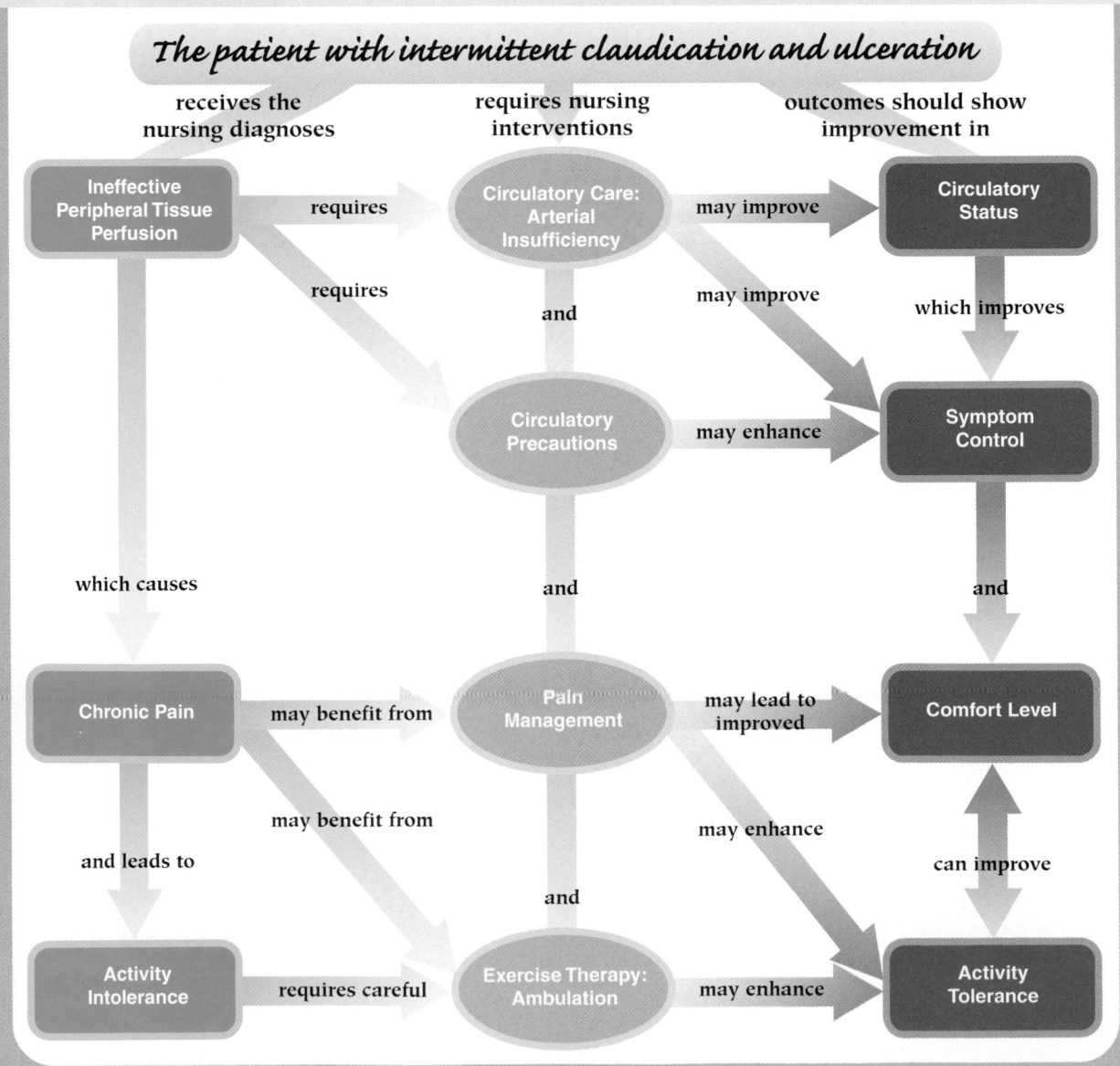

The patient with intermittent claudication and ulceration

Nursing Classifications and Languages

NANDA
Nursing Diagnoses

Ineffective Tissue Perfusion—Decrease in oxygen resulting in the failure to nourish tissues at the capillary level

Chronic Pain—Unpleasant sensory and emotional experience arising from actual or potential tissue damage or described in terms of such damage; sudden or slow onset of any intensity from mild to severe, constant or recurring without an anticipated or predictable end and a duration of greater than 6 months

Activity Intolerance—Insufficient physiological or psychological energy to endure or complete required or desired daily activities

NIC
Nursing Interventions*

Circulatory Care: Arterial Insufficiency—Promotion of arterial circulation

Circulatory Precautions—Protection of localized area with limited perfusion

Pain Management—Alleviation of pain or reduction in pain to a level of comfort that is acceptable to the patient

Exercise Therapy: Ambulation—Promotion and assistance with walking to maintain or restore autonomic and voluntary body functions during treatment and recovery from illness or injury

NOC
Nursing Outcomes†

Return to functional baseline status, stabilization of, or improvement in

Circulatory Status—Extent to which blood flows unobstructed, unidirectionally, and at an appropriate pressure through large vessels of the systemic and pulmonary circuits

Symptom Control—Personal actions to minimize perceived adverse changes in physical and emotional functioning

Comfort Level—Extent of physical and psychological ease

Activity Tolerance—Responses to energy-consuming body movements involved in required or desired daily activities

NANDA, North American Nursing Diagnosis Association; NIC, Nursing Interventions Classification; NOC, Nursing Outcomes Classification

*Iowa Intervention Project © 2000. In McCloskey, J. C., & Bulechek, G. M. (2000). *Nursing interventions classification (NIC)* (3rd ed.). St. Louis: Mosby.

†Iowa Outcomes Project © 2000. In Johnson, M., Maas, M., & Moorhead, S. (2000). *Nursing outcomes classification (NOC)* (3rd ed.). St. Louis: Mosby.

Assessment of Cardiovascular Function

LEARNING OBJECTIVES

On completion of this chapter, the learner will be able to:

1. Explain cardiac physiology in relation to cardiac anatomy and the conduction system of the heart.

2. Incorporate assessment of functional health patterns and cardiac risk factors into the health history and physical assessment of the patient with cardiac conditions.

3. Identify the clinical significance and related nursing implications of the various tests and procedures used for diagnostic assessment of cardiac function.

4. Compare central venous pressure monitoring, pulmonary artery pressure monitoring, and systemic intra-arterial monitoring with regard to clinical usefulness and significance, possible complications, and nursing responsibilities.

Throughout the continuum of care, whether in a home, hospital, or rehabilitation setting, all patients with cardiovascular disease (disorders of the heart and major blood vessels; CVD) require similar assessments. Key components of the cardiovascular assessment include obtaining a health history, performing a physical assessment, and monitoring a variety of laboratory and diagnostic test results. An accurate and timely assessment of cardiovascular function provides the data necessary to identify nursing diagnoses, formulate a plan of care, and evaluate the response of the patient to the care provided. Essential to the development of these assessment skills is an understanding of the structure and function of the heart in health and in disease.

Anatomic and Physiologic Overview

The heart is a hollow, muscular organ located in the center of the thorax, where it occupies the space between the lungs (mediastinum) and rests on the diaphragm. It weighs approximately 300 g (10.6 oz), although heart weight and size are influenced by age, gender, body weight, extent of physical exercise and conditioning, and heart disease. The heart pumps blood to the tissues, supplying them with oxygen and other nutrients.

The pumping action of the heart is accomplished by the rhythmic contraction and relaxation of its muscular wall. During **systole** (contraction of the muscle), the chambers of the heart become smaller as the blood is ejected. During **diastole** (relaxation of the muscle), the heart chambers fill with blood in preparation for the subsequent ejection. A normal resting adult heart beats approximately 60 to 80 times per minute. Each ventricle ejects approximately 70 mL of blood per beat and has an output of approximately 5 L per minute.

ANATOMY OF THE HEART

The heart is composed of three layers (Fig. 26-1). The inner layer, or endocardium, consists of endothelial tissue and lines the inside of the heart and valves. The middle layer, or myocardium, is made up of muscle fibers and is responsible for the pumping action. The exterior layer of the heart is called the epicardium.

The heart is encased in a thin, fibrous sac called the pericardium, which is composed of two layers. Adhering to the epicardium is the visceral pericardium. Enveloping the visceral pericardium is the parietal pericardium, a tough fibrous tissue that attaches to the great vessels, diaphragm, sternum, and vertebral column and supports the heart in the mediastinum. The space between these two layers (pericardial space) is filled with about 30 mL of fluid, which lubricates the surface of the heart and reduces friction during systole.

Heart Chambers

The four chambers of the heart constitute the right- and left-sided pumping systems. The right side of the heart, made up of the right atrium and right ventricle, distributes venous blood (deoxygenated blood) to the lungs via the pulmonary artery (pulmonary circulation) for oxygenation. The right atrium receives blood returning from the superior vena cava (head, neck, and upper extremities), inferior vena cava (trunk and lower extremities), and coronary sinus (coronary circulation). The left

Glossary

afterload: the amount of resistance to ejection of blood from the ventricle

apical impulse (also called point of maximum impulse [PMI]): impulse normally palpated at the fifth intercostal space, left midclavicular line; caused by contraction of the left ventricle

baroreceptors: nerve fibers located in the aortic arch and carotid arteries that are responsible for reflex control of the blood pressure

cardiac catheterization: an invasive procedure used to measure cardiac chamber pressures and assess patency of the coronary arteries

cardiac conduction system: specialized heart cells strategically located throughout the heart that are responsible for methodically generating and coordinating the transmission of electrical impulses to the myocardial cells

cardiac output: amount of blood pumped by each ventricle in liters per minute; normal cardiac output is 5 L per minute in the resting adult heart

cardiac stress test: a test used to evaluate the functioning of the heart during a period of increased oxygen demand

contractility: ability of the cardiac muscle to shorten in response to an electrical impulse

depolarization: electrical activation of a cell caused by the influx of sodium into the cell while potassium exits the cell

diastole: period of ventricular relaxation resulting in ventricular filling

ejection fraction: percentage of the end-diastolic blood volume ejected from the ventricle with each heartbeat

hemodynamic monitoring: use of monitoring devices to measure cardiovascular function

hypertension: blood pressure greater than 140/90 mm Hg

hypotension: a decrease in blood pressure to less than 100/60 mm Hg

international normalized ratio (INR): a standard method for reporting prothrombin levels, eliminating the variation in test results from laboratory to laboratory

murmurs: sounds created by abnormal, turbulent flow of blood in the heart

myocardial ischemia: condition in which heart muscle cells receive less oxygen than needed

myocardium: muscle layer of the heart responsible for the pumping action of the heart

normal heart sounds: sounds produced when the valves close; normal heart sounds are S_1 (atrioventricular valves) and S_2 (semilunar valves)

postural (orthostatic) hypotension: a significant drop in blood pressure (usually 10 mm Hg systolic or more) after an upright posture is assumed

preload: degree of stretch of the cardiac muscle fibers at the end of diastole

pulmonary vascular resistance: resistance to right ventricle ejection of blood

radioisotopes: unstable atoms that emit small amounts of energy in the form of gamma rays; used in cardiac nuclear medicine studies

repolarization: return of the cell to resting state, caused by reentry of potassium into the cell while sodium exits the cell

sinoatrial (SA) node: primary pacemaker of the heart, located in the right atrium

stroke volume: amount of blood ejected from the ventricle per heartbeat; normal stroke volume is 70 mL in the resting heart

systemic vascular resistance: resistance to left ventricle ejection

systole: period of ventricular contraction resulting in ejection of blood from the ventricles into the pulmonary artery and aorta

telemetry: the process of continuous electrocardiographic monitoring by the transmission of radiowaves from a battery-operated transmitter worn by the patient

venodilating agent: medication causing dilation of veins

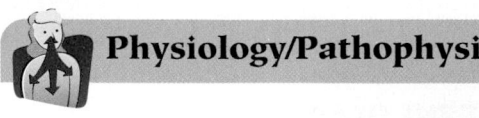

Physiology/Pathophysiology

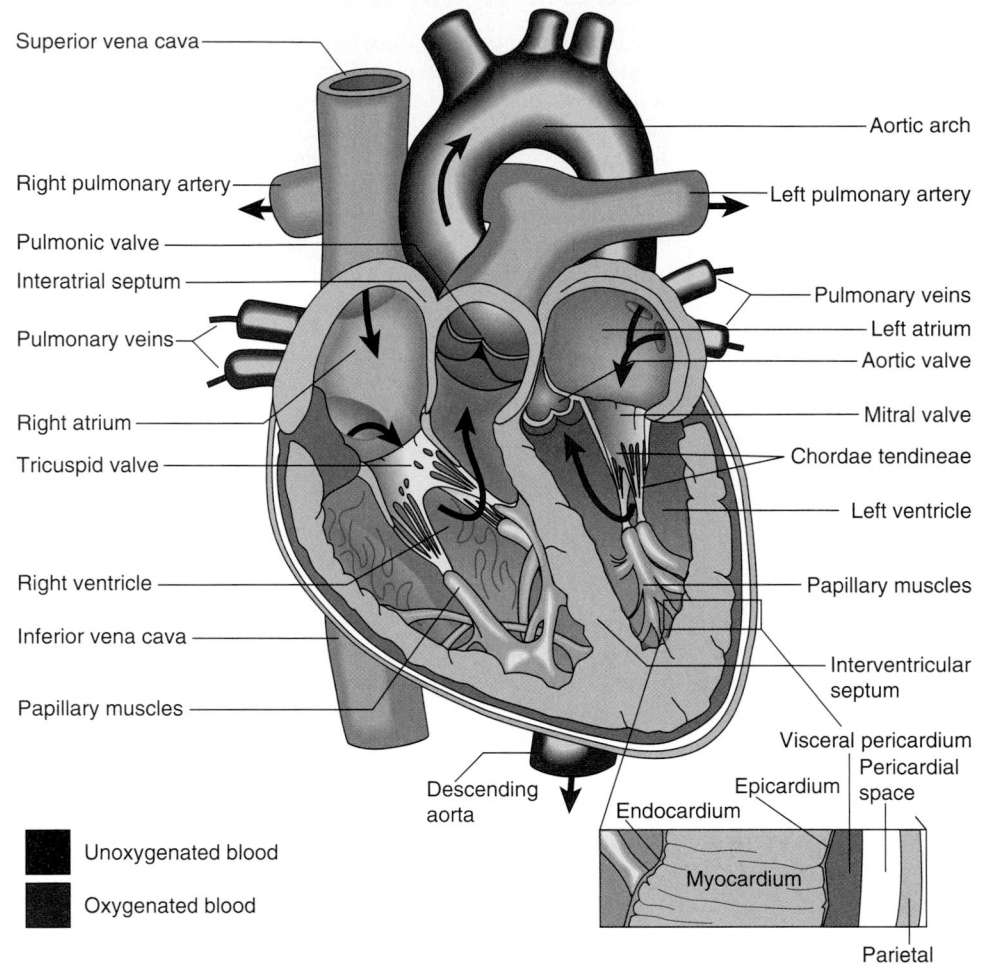

FIGURE 26-1 Structure of the heart. Arrows show course of blood flow through the heart chambers.

Labels (left side, top to bottom): Superior vena cava · Right pulmonary artery · Pulmonic valve · Interatrial septum · Pulmonary veins · Right atrium · Tricuspid valve · Right ventricle · Inferior vena cava · Papillary muscles · Descending aorta

Labels (right side, top to bottom): Aortic arch · Left pulmonary artery · Pulmonary veins · Left atrium · Aortic valve · Mitral valve · Chordae tendineae · Left ventricle · Papillary muscles · Interventricular septum · Visceral pericardium · Pericardial space · Epicardium · Endocardium · Myocardium · Parietal pericardium

Legend: Unoxygenated blood · Oxygenated blood

side of the heart, composed of the left atrium and left ventricle, distributes oxygenated blood to the remainder of the body via the aorta (systemic circulation). The left atrium receives oxygenated blood from the pulmonary circulation via the pulmonary veins. The relationships of the four heart chambers are shown in Figure 26-1.

The varying thicknesses of the atrial and ventricular walls relate to the workload required by each chamber. The atria are thin-walled because blood returning to these chambers generates low pressures. In contrast, the ventricular walls are thicker because they generate greater pressures during systole. The right ventricle contracts against low pulmonary vascular pressure and has thinner walls than the left ventricle. The left ventricle, with walls two-and-a-half times more muscular than those of the right ventricle, contracts against high systemic pressure.

Because the heart lies in a rotated position within the chest cavity, the right ventricle lies anteriorly (just beneath the sternum) and the left ventricle is situated posteriorly. The left ventricle is responsible for the apex beat or the point of maximum impulse (PMI), which is normally palpable in the left midclavicular line of the chest wall at the fifth intercostal space.

Heart Valves

The four valves in the heart permit blood to flow in only one direction. The valves, which are composed of thin leaflets of fibrous tissue, open and close in response to the movement of blood and pressure changes within the chambers. There are two types of valves: atrioventricular and semilunar.

ATRIOVENTRICULAR VALVES

The valves that separate the atria from the ventricles are termed atrioventricular valves. The tricuspid valve, so named because it is composed of three cusps or leaflets, separates the right atrium from the right ventricle. The mitral, or bicuspid (two cusps) valve, lies between the left atrium and the left ventricle (see Fig. 26-1).

Normally, when the ventricles contract, ventricular pressure rises, closing the atrioventricular valve leaflets. Two additional structures, the papillary muscles and the chordae tendineae, maintain valve closure. The papillary muscles, located on the sides of the ventricular walls, are connected to the valve leaflets by thin fibrous bands called chordae tendineae. During systole, contraction of the papillary muscles causes the chordae tendineae to become taut, keeping the valve leaflets approximated and closed.

SEMILUNAR VALVES

The two semilunar valves are composed of three half-moon-like leaflets. The valve between the right ventricle and the pulmonary artery is called the pulmonic valve; the valve between the left ventricle and the aorta is called the aortic valve.

Coronary Arteries

The left and right coronary arteries and their branches (Fig. 26-2) supply arterial blood to the heart. These arteries originate from the aorta just above the aortic valve leaflets. The heart has large metabolic requirements, extracting approximately 70% to 80% of the oxygen delivered (other organs consume, on average, 25%). Unlike other arteries, the coronary arteries are perfused during diastole. An increase in heart rate shortens diastole and can decrease myocardial perfusion. Patients, particularly those with coronary artery disease (CAD), can develop **myocardial ischemia** (inadequate oxygen supply) when the heart rate accelerates.

The left coronary artery has three branches. The artery from the point of origin to the first major branch is called the left main coronary artery. Two bifurcations arise off the left main coronary artery. These are the left anterior descending artery, which courses down the anterior wall of the heart, and the circumflex artery, which circles around to the lateral left wall of the heart.

The right side of the heart is supplied by the right coronary artery, which progresses around to the bottom or inferior wall of the heart. The posterior wall of the heart receives its blood supply by an additional branch from the right coronary artery called the posterior descending artery.

Superficial to the coronary arteries are the coronary veins. Venous blood from these veins returns to the heart primarily through the coronary sinus, which is located posteriorly in the right atrium.

Cardiac Muscle

The myocardium is composed of specialized muscle tissue. Microscopically, myocardial muscle resembles striated (skeletal) muscle, which is under conscious control. Functionally, however, myocardial muscle resembles smooth muscle because its contraction is involuntary. The myocardial muscle fibers are arranged in an interconnected manner (called a syncytium) that allows for coordinated myocardial contraction and relaxation. The sequential pattern of contraction and relaxation of individual muscle fibers ensures the rhythmic behavior of the myocardium as a whole and enables it to function as an effective pump.

FUNCTION OF THE HEART: CONDUCTION SYSTEM

The specialized heart cells of the **cardiac conduction system** methodically generate and coordinate the transmission of electrical impulses to the myocardial cells. The result is sequential atrioventricular contraction, which provides for the most effective flow of blood, thereby optimizing cardiac output. Three physiologic characteristics of the cardiac conduction cells account for this coordination:

Automaticity: ability to initiate an electrical impulse
Excitability: ability to respond to an electrical impulse
Conductivity: ability to transmit an electrical impulse from one cell to another

The **sinoatrial (SA) node**, referred to as the primary pacemaker of the heart, is located at the junction of the superior vena cava and the right atrium (Fig. 26-3). The SA node in a normal resting heart has an inherent firing rate of 60 to 100 impulses per minute, but the rate can change in response to the metabolic demands of the body.

The electrical impulses initiated by the SA node are conducted along the myocardial cells of the atria via specialized tracts called internodal pathways. The impulses cause electrical stimulation

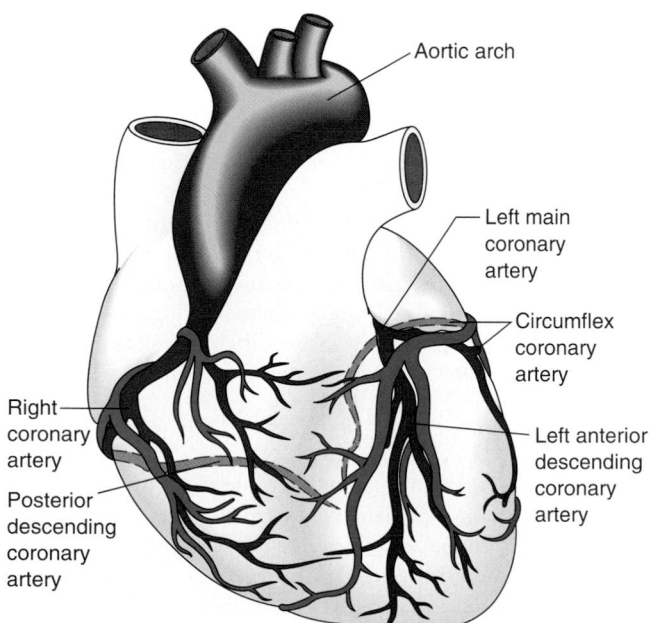

FIGURE 26-2 Coronary arteries (*red vessels*) arise from the aorta and encircle the heart. Coronary veins are shown in blue.

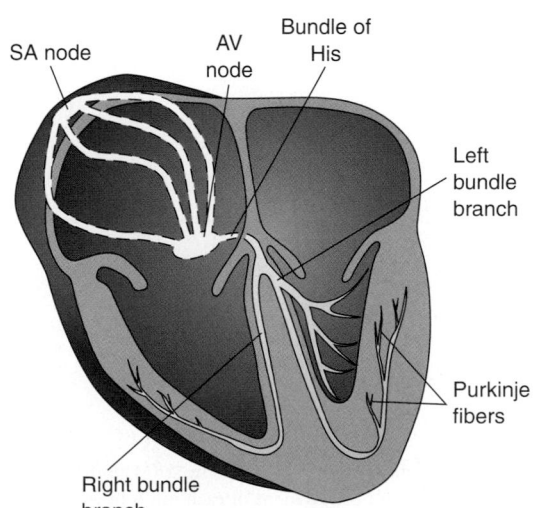

FIGURE 26-3 The cardiac conduction system. AV, atrioventricular; SA, sinoatrial.

and subsequent contraction of the atria. The impulses are then conducted to the atrioventricular (AV) node. The AV node (located in the right atrial wall near the tricuspid valve) consists of another group of specialized muscle cells similar to those of the SA node. The AV node coordinates the incoming electrical impulses from the atria and, after a slight delay (allowing the atria time to contract and complete ventricular filling), relays the impulse to the ventricles. This impulse is then conducted through a bundle of specialized conduction cells (bundle of His) that travel in the septum separating the left and right ventricles. The bundle of His divides into the right bundle branch (conducting impulses to the right ventricle) and the left bundle branch (conducting impulses to the left ventricle). To transmit impulses to the largest chamber of the heart, the left bundle branch bifurcates into the left anterior and left posterior bundle branches. Impulses travel through the bundle branches to reach the terminal point in the conduction system, called the Purkinje fibers. This is the point at which the myocardial cells are stimulated, causing ventricular contraction.

The heart rate is determined by the myocardial cells with the fastest inherent firing rate. Under normal circumstances, the SA node has the highest inherent rate, the AV node has the second-highest inherent rate (40 to 60 impulses per minute), and the ventricular pacemaker sites have the lowest inherent rate (30 to 40 impulses per minute). If the SA node malfunctions, the AV node generally takes over the pacemaker function of the heart at its inherently lower rate. Should both the SA and the AV nodes fail in their pacemaker function, a pacemaker site in the ventricle will fire at its inherent bradycardic rate of 30 to 40 impulses per minute.

Physiology of Cardiac Conduction

Cardiac electrical activity is the result of the movement of ions (charged particles such as sodium, potassium, and calcium) across the cell membrane. The electrical changes recorded within a single cell result in what is known as the cardiac action potential (Fig. 26-4).

In the resting state, cardiac muscle cells are polarized, which means an electrical difference exists between the negatively charged inside and the positively charged outside of the cell membrane.

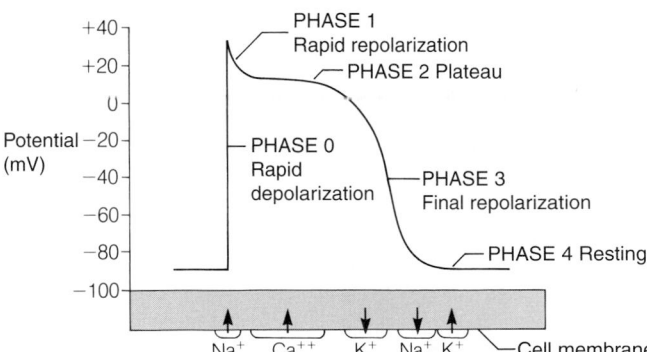

FIGURE 26-4 Cardiac action potential. The arrows indicate the approximate time and direction of movement of each ion influencing membrane potential. Ca^{++} movement out of the cell is not well defined but is thought to occur during Phase 4.

As soon as an electrical impulse is initiated, cell membrane permeability changes and sodium moves rapidly into the cell, while potassium exits the cell. This ionic exchange begins **depolarization** (electrical activation of the cell), converting the internal charge of the cell to a positive one (see Fig. 26-4). Contraction of the myocardium follows depolarization. The interaction between changes in membrane voltage and muscle contraction is called electromechanical coupling. As one cardiac muscle cell is depolarized, it acts as a stimulus to its neighboring cell, causing it to depolarize. Sufficient depolarization of a single specialized conduction system cell results in depolarization and contraction of the entire myocardium. **Repolarization** (return of the cell to its resting state) occurs as the cell returns to its baseline or resting state; this corresponds to relaxation of myocardial muscle.

After the rapid influx of sodium into the cell during depolarization, the permeability of the cell membrane to calcium is changed. Calcium enters the cell and is released from intracellular calcium stores. The increase in calcium, which occurs during the plateau phase of repolarization, is much slower than that of sodium and continues for a longer period.

Cardiac muscle, unlike skeletal or smooth muscle, has a prolonged refractory period during which it cannot be restimulated to contract. There are two phases of the refractory period, referred to as the absolute refractory period and the relative refractory period. The absolute refractory period is the time during which the heart cannot be restimulated to contract regardless of the strength of the electrical stimulus. This period corresponds with depolarization and the early part of repolarization. During the latter part of repolarization, however, if the electrical stimulus is stronger than normal, the myocardium can be stimulated to contract. This short period at the end of repolarization is called the relative refractory period.

Refractoriness protects the heart from sustained contraction (tetany), which would result in sudden cardiac death. Normal electromechanical coupling and contraction of the heart depend on the composition of the interstitial fluid surrounding the heart muscle cells. In turn, the composition of this fluid is influenced by the composition of the blood. A change in serum calcium concentration may alter the contraction of the heart muscle fibers. A change in serum potassium concentration is also important, because potassium affects the normal electrical voltage of the cell.

Cardiac Hemodynamics

An important determinant of blood flow in the cardiovascular system is the principle that fluid flows from a region of higher pressure to one of lower pressure. The pressures responsible for blood flow in the normal circulation are generated during systole and diastole. Figure 26-5 depicts the pressure differences in the great vessels and in the four chambers of the heart during systole and diastole.

CARDIAC CYCLE

Beginning with systole, the pressure inside the ventricles rapidly rises, forcing the atrioventricular valves to close. As a result, blood ceases to flow from the atria into the ventricles and regurgitation (backflow) of blood into the atria is prevented. The rapid rise of pressure inside the right and left ventricles forces the pulmonic and aortic valves to open, and blood is ejected into the pulmonary artery and aorta, respectively. The exit of blood is at first rapid;

Physiology/Pathophysiology

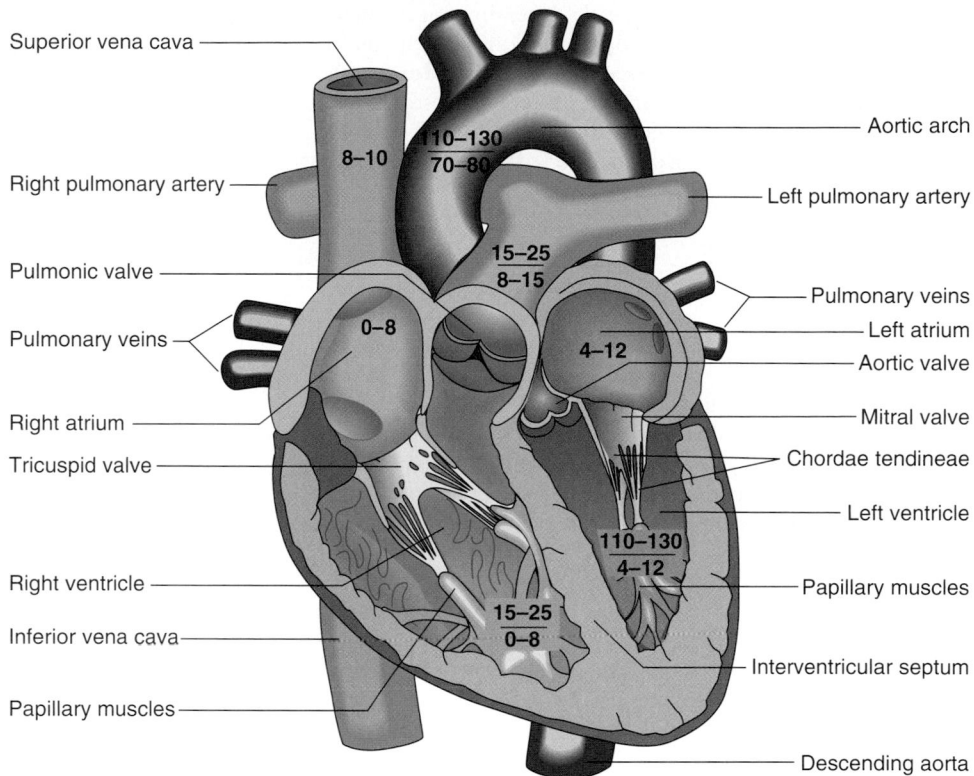

Superior vena cava

Aortic arch

Right pulmonary artery

Left pulmonary artery

Pulmonic valve

Pulmonary veins

Pulmonary veins

Left atrium

Aortic valve

Right atrium

Mitral valve

Tricuspid valve

Chordae tendineae

Left ventricle

Right ventricle

Papillary muscles

Inferior vena cava

Interventricular septum

Papillary muscles

Descending aorta

8–10

$\frac{110–130}{70–80}$

$\frac{15–25}{8–15}$

0–8

4–12

$\frac{110–130}{4–12}$

$\frac{15–25}{0–8}$

FIGURE 26-5 Great vessel and chamber pressures. Pressures are identified in millimeters of mercury (mm Hg) as mean pressure or systolic over diastolic pressure.

then, as the pressure in each ventricle and its corresponding artery equalizes, the flow of blood gradually decreases. At the end of systole, pressure within the right and left ventricles rapidly decreases. This lowers pulmonary artery and aortic pressure, causing closure of the semilunar valves. These events mark the onset of diastole.

During diastole, when the ventricles are relaxed and the atrioventricular valves are open, blood returning from the veins flows into the atria and then into the ventricles. Toward the end of this diastolic period, the atrial muscles contract in response to an electrical impulse initiated by the SA node (atrial systole). The resultant contraction raises the pressure inside the atria, ejecting blood into the ventricles. Atrial systole augments ventricular blood volume by 15% to 25% and is sometimes referred to as the "atrial kick." At this point, ventricular systole begins in response to propagation of the electrical impulse that began in the SA node some milliseconds previously. The following section reviews the chamber pressures generated during systole and diastole.

Chamber Pressures. In the right side of the heart, the pressure generated during ventricular systole (15 to 25 mm Hg) exceeds the pulmonary artery diastolic pressure (8 to 15 mm Hg), and blood is ejected into the pulmonary circulation. During diastole, venous blood flows into the atrium because pressure in the superior and inferior vena cava (8 to 10 mm Hg) is higher than that in the atrium. Blood flows through the open tricuspid valve and

into the right ventricle until the two right chamber pressures equalize (0 to 8 mm Hg).

In the left side of the heart, similar events occur, although higher pressures are generated. As pressure mounts in the left ventricle during systole (110 to 130 mm Hg), resting aortic pressure (80 mm Hg) is exceeded and blood is ejected into the aorta. During left ventricular ejection, the resultant aortic pressure (110 to 130 mm Hg) forces blood progressively through the arteries. Forward blood flow into the aorta ceases as the ventricle relaxes and pressure drops. During diastole, oxygenated blood returning from the pulmonary circulation via the four pulmonary veins flows into the atrium, where pressure remains low. Blood readily flows into the left ventricle because ventricular pressure is also low. At the end of diastole, pressure in the atrium and ventricle equilibrates (4 to 12 mm Hg). Figure 26-5 depicts the systolic and diastolic pressures in the four chambers of the heart.

Pressure Measurement. Chamber pressures are measured with the use of special monitoring catheters and equipment. This technique is called hemodynamic monitoring. Nurses caring for critically ill patients must have a sophisticated working knowledge of normal chamber pressures and the hemodynamic changes that occur during serious illnesses. The data obtained from hemodynamic monitoring assist with the diagnosis and management of pathophysiologic conditions affecting critically ill patients. Hemodynamic monitoring is covered in more detail at the end of this chapter.

Cardiac Output

Cardiac output is the amount of blood pumped by each ventricle during a given period. The cardiac output in a resting adult is about 5 L per minute but varies greatly depending on the metabolic needs of the body. Cardiac output is computed by multiplying the stroke volume by the heart rate. **Stroke volume** is the amount of blood ejected per heartbeat. The average resting stroke volume is about 70 mL, and the heart rate is 60 to 80 beats per minute (bpm). Cardiac output can be affected by changes in either stroke volume or heart rate.

CONTROL OF HEART RATE

Cardiac output must be responsive to changes in the metabolic demands of the tissues. For example, during exercise the total cardiac output may increase fourfold, to 20 L per minute. This increase is normally accomplished by approximate doubling of both the heart rate and the stroke volume. Changes in heart rate are accomplished by reflex controls mediated by the autonomic nervous system, including its sympathetic and parasympathetic divisions. The parasympathetic impulses, which travel to the heart through the vagus nerve, can slow the cardiac rate, whereas sympathetic impulses increase it. These effects on heart rate result from action on the SA node, to either decrease or increase its inherent rate. The balance between these two reflex control systems normally determines the heart rate. The heart rate is stimulated also by an increased level of circulating catecholamines (secreted by the adrenal gland) and by excess thyroid hormone, which produces a catecholamine-like effect.

Heart rate is also affected by central nervous system and baroreceptor activity. **Baroreceptors** are specialized nerve cells located in the aortic arch and in both right and left internal carotid arteries (at the point of bifurcation from the common carotid arteries). The baroreceptors are sensitive to changes in blood pressure (BP). During elevations in BP (**hypertension**), these cells increase their rate of discharge, transmitting impulses to the medulla. This initiates parasympathetic activity and inhibits sympathetic response, lowering the heart rate and the BP. The opposite is true during **hypotension** (low BP). Hypotension results in less baroreceptor stimulation, which prompts a decrease in parasympathetic inhibitory activity in the SA node, allowing for enhanced sympathetic activity. The resultant vasoconstriction and increased heart rate elevate the BP.

CONTROL OF STROKE VOLUME

Stroke volume is primarily determined by three factors: preload, afterload, and contractility.

Preload is the term used to describe the degree of stretch of the cardiac muscle fibers at the end of diastole. The end of diastole is the period when filling volume in the ventricles is the highest and the degree of stretch on the muscle fibers is the greatest. The volume of blood within the ventricle at the end of diastole determines preload. Preload has a direct effect on stroke volume. As the volume of blood returning to the heart increases, muscle fiber stretch also increases (increased preload), resulting in stronger contraction and a greater stroke volume. This relationship, called the Frank-Starling law of the heart (or sometimes the Starling law of the heart), is maintained until the physiologic limit of the muscle is reached.

The Frank-Starling law is based on the fact that, within limits, the greater the initial length or stretch of the cardiac muscle cells (sarcomeres), the greater the degree of shortening that occurs. This result is caused by increased interaction between the thick and thin filaments within the cardiac muscle cells. Preload is decreased by a reduction in the volume of blood returning to the ventricles. Diuresis, **venodilating agents** (eg, nitrates), and loss of blood or body fluids from excessive diaphoresis, vomiting, or diarrhea reduce preload. Preload is increased by increasing the return of circulating blood volume to the ventricles. Controlling the loss of blood or body fluids and replacing fluids (ie, blood transfusions and intravenous fluid administration) are examples of ways to increase preload.

The second determinant of stroke volume is **afterload**, the amount of resistance to ejection of blood from the ventricle. The resistance of the systemic BP to left ventricular ejection is called **systemic vascular resistance**. The resistance of the pulmonary BP to right ventricular ejection is called **pulmonary vascular resistance**. There is an inverse relationship between afterload and stroke volume. For example, afterload is increased by arterial vasoconstriction, which leads to decreased stroke volume. The opposite is true with arterial vasodilation: afterload is reduced because there is less resistance to ejection, and stroke volume increases.

Contractility is a term used to denote the force generated by the contracting myocardium under any given condition. Contractility is enhanced by circulating catecholamines, sympathetic neuronal activity, and certain medications (eg, digoxin, intravenous dopamine or dobutamine). Increased contractility results in increased stroke volume. Contractility is depressed by hypoxemia, acidosis, and certain medications (eg, beta-adrenergic blocking agents such as atenolol [Tenormin]).

The heart can achieve a greatly increased stroke volume (eg, during exercise) by increasing preload (through increased venous return), increasing contractility (through sympathetic nervous system discharge), and decreasing afterload (through peripheral vasodilation with decreased aortic pressure).

The percentage of the end-diastolic volume that is ejected with each stroke is called the **ejection fraction**. With each stroke, about 42% (right ventricle) to 50% (left ventricle) or more of the end-diastolic volume is ejected by the normal heart. The ejection fraction can be used as an index of myocardial contractility: the ejection fraction decreases if contractility is depressed.

🍃 Gerontologic Considerations

Changes in cardiac structure and function are clearly observable in the older heart. To understand the changes specifically related to aging, it is helpful to distinguish the normal aging process from changes related to CVD. The anatomic and functional changes in the aging heart are listed in Table 26-1.

Studies show that the normal aging heart can produce adequate cardiac output under ordinary circumstances but may have a limited ability to respond to situations that cause physical or emotional stress. In an elderly person who is less active, the left ventricle may become smaller (atrophy) as a consequence of physical deconditioning. Aging also results in decreased elasticity and widening of the aorta, thickening and rigidity of the cardiac valves, and increased connective tissue in the SA and AV nodes and bundle branches.

These changes lead to decreased myocardial contractility, increased left ventricular ejection time (prolonged systole), and delayed conduction. Therefore, stressful physical and emotional conditions, especially those that occur suddenly, may have adverse effects on the aged person. The heart cannot respond to such conditions with an adequate rate increase and needs more time to return to a normal resting rate after even a minimal increase in heart rate. In some patients, the added stress may precipitate heart failure (HF).

Table 26-1 • **Age-Related Changes of the Cardiac System**

CARDIOVASCULAR SYSTEM	STRUCTURAL CHANGES	FUNCTIONAL CHANGES	HISTORY AND PHYSICAL FINDINGS
Atria	↑ Size of left atrium Thickening of the endocardium	↑ Atrial irritability	Irregular heart rhythm from atrial dysrhythmias
Left ventricle	Endocardial fibrosis Myocardial thickening (hypertrophy) Infiltration of fat into myocardium	Left ventricle stiff and less compliant Progressive decline in cardiac output ↑ Risk for ventricular dysrhythmias Prolonged systole	Fatigue ↓ Exercise tolerance Signs and symptoms of HF or ventricular dysrhythmias Point of maximal impulse palpated lateral to the midclavicular line ↓ Intensity S_1, S_2; split S_2 S_4 may be present
Valves	Thickening and rigidity of AV valves Calcification of aortic valve	Abnormal blood flow across valves during cardiac cycle	Murmurs may be present Thrill may be palpated if significant murmur is present
Conduction system	Connective tissue collects in SA node, AV node, and bundle branches ↓ Number SA node cells ↓ Number AV, bundle of His, right and left bundle branch cells	Slower SA node rate of impulse discharge Slowed conduction across AV node and ventricular conduction system	Bradycardia Heart block ECG changes consistent with slowed conduction (↑ PR interval, widened QRS complex)
Sympathetic nervous system	↓ Response to beta-adrenergic stimulation	↓ Adaptive response to exercise: contractility and heart rate slower to respond to exercise demands Heart rate takes more time to return to baseline	Fatigue Diminished exercise tolerance ↓ Ability to respond to stress
Aorta and arteries	Stiffening of vasculature ↓ Elasticity and widening of aorta Elongation of aorta, displacing the brachiocephalic artery upward	Left ventricular hypertrophy	Progressive increase in systolic BP; slight ↑ in diastolic BP Widening pulse pressure Pulsation visible above right clavicle
Baroreceptor response	↓ Sensitivity of baroreceptors in the carotid artery and aorta to transient episodes of hypertension and hypotension	Baroreceptors unable to regulate heart rate and vascular tone, causing slow response to postural changes in body position	Postural blood pressure changes and reports feeling dizzy, fainting when moving from lying to sitting or standing position

AV, atrioventricular; BP, blood pressure; CHF, congestive heart failure; ECG, electrocardiographic; SA, sinoatrial.

GENDER DIFFERENCES IN CARDIAC STRUCTURE AND FUNCTION

Compared with a man's heart, a woman's heart tends to be smaller. It weighs less and has smaller coronary arteries. These structural differences have significant implications. Because the coronary arteries of a woman are smaller, they occlude from atherosclerosis more easily, making procedures such as cardiac catheterization and angioplasty technically more difficult, with a higher incidence of postprocedure complications. In addition, the resting rate, stroke volume, and ejection fraction of a woman's heart are higher than those of a man's, and the conduction time of an electrical impulse coursing from the SA node through the AV node to the Purkinje fibers is briefer.

Another significant difference between the genders is the physiologic effects of estrogen on the cardiovascular system. Two important effects of estrogen, regulation of vasomotor tone and of response to vascular injury, may be the mechanisms that protect women against the development of atherosclerosis. An additional, potentially beneficial effect of estrogen is its action on the liver, which results in improved lipid profiles. On the other hand, less favorable effects of estrogen include an increase in coagulation proteins and a decrease in fibrinolytic protein, which enhance the risk of thrombus formation. Progesterone also has vascular effects, but its role in the development of CVD is unclear at this time. Beneficial effects of estrogen disappear after menopause, as evidenced by the increased incidence of CVD in this population. However, because of health risks associated with hormone replacement therapy, the American Heart Association does not recommend its use as a primary or secondary prevention intervention for CVD (Mosca et al., 2001; Roussouw et al., 2002).

Assessment

The severity of the patient's symptoms, the practice setting of the nurse, and the purpose of the assessment are factors that need to be considered when determining the frequency and extent of nursing assessment required. The assessment of the acutely ill cardiac patient will be different from that of a patient with stable or chronic cardiac conditions. For example, the assessment performed by an emergency department nurse caring for a patient who is experiencing an acute myocardial infarction (MI) must be very focused and must be performed rapidly. The nurse must assess the patient for complications associated with the MI, screen the patient for contraindications to coronary artery reperfusion strategies including thrombolytic therapy or primary percutaneous transluminal coronary angioplasty (PTCA), and evaluate the patient's response to medical and nursing interventions. For this patient, the health history, physical assessment, and important nursing interventions (eg, cardiac monitoring, administration of intravenous medications) are performed simultaneously.

HEALTH HISTORY AND CLINICAL MANIFESTATIONS

For the patient experiencing an acute MI, the nurse obtains the health history using a few specific questions about the onset and severity of chest discomfort, associated symptoms, current medications, and allergies. At the same time, the nurse observes the patient's general appearance and evaluates hemodynamic status (heart rate and rhythm, BP). Once the condition of the patient stabilizes, a more extensive history can be obtained.

With stable patients, a complete health history is obtained during the initial contact. Often, it is helpful to have the patient's spouse or partner available during the health history interview. Initially, demographic information regarding age, gender, and ethnic origin is obtained. The family history, as well as the physical examination, should include assessment for genetic abnormalities associated with cardiovascular disorders (see Genetics in Nursing Practice box). Height, current weight, and usual weight (if there has been a recent weight loss or gain) are established. During the interview, the nurse conveys sensitivity to the cultural background and religious practices of the patient. This removes barriers to communication that may result if the interview is based only on the nurse's personal frame of reference. Patients from different cultural and ethnic groups may have different ways of describing symptoms such as pain and may engage in different health practices before seeking formal medical attention.

NURSING RESEARCH PROFILE 26-1
Racial Differences in Coronary Artery Disease: Symptoms and Seeking Care

Richards, S. B., Funk, M., & Milner, K. A. (2000). Differences between blacks and whites with coronary heart disease in initial symptoms and delay in seeking care. *American Journal of Critical Care, 9*, 237–244.

Purpose

Mortality rates due to coronary artery disease (CAD) are higher in African American men (7%) and African American women (35%) than in their Caucasian counterparts. Recent findings suggest that African Americans may delay longer than Caucasians in seeking emergency care and commonly have atypical symptom presentation. The purpose of this study was to explore differences between African Americans and Caucasians in both manifestations of symptoms of CAD and delay in seeking treatment by answering the following research questions:

- Do African Americans and Caucasians differ in their manifestation of symptoms of CAD?
- Among patients with confirmed CAD, do African Americans and Caucasians differ in the elapsed time between the onset of symptoms and arrival at the emergency department?

Study Sample and Design

This study, part of a larger study investigating aspects of CAD presentation, is the first of its kind to use a prospective, observational design. One member of the team of nurse researchers unobtrusively observed patients in the emergency department as they described their symptoms to the clinician.

The sample consisted of African Americans and Caucasians drawn from a total of 545 patients who were recruited from the emergency department of an 810-bed university teaching hospital. Patients with one or more typical or atypical symptoms of CAD, who met age-specific inclusion criteria based on the Framingham Heart Study, were enrolled. Electrocardiographic and cardiac enzyme criteria were used to confirm the diagnosis of angina or myocardial infarction.

Findings

Of the 231 patients with CAD, 40 (17%) were African American and 191 (82.7%) were Caucasian. The majority of the patients were male (58%). Ages ranged from 31 to 91 years. There were statistically significant differences in age and cardiac risk factors between the groups of African Americans and Caucasians. The mean age was significantly younger in African Americans than in Caucasians. Caucasians were more likely than African Americans to have hyperlipidemia, and African Americans were more likely than Caucasians to have hypertension.

Among all patients, shortness of breath, not chest pain, was the most common symptom (39.8%). Next, in descending order, were substernal chest pain (34%) and arm pain (27.2%). Both research questions were answered affirmatively. African Americans were more likely than Caucasians to have atypical presentation of acute CAD symptoms. These patients, the majority of whom were female (62.5%), were about three times more likely than Caucasians to experience shortness of breath as the predominant symptom and two times more likely to complain of left-sided chest pain. African Americans were found to have a median delay time of 11 hours, while Caucasians delayed 5 hours. This difference was significant ($p = .05$), demonstrating a trend toward longer delays by African Americans compared with Caucasians. Nineteen people in this study delayed 72 hours or longer before seeking treatment.

Nursing Implications

Studies such as this one contribute to the growing body of evidence showing that there are racial differences in the presentation of acute CAD. Nurses and other health care professionals need to be aware that "atypical" symptoms of angina and myocardial infarction, such as shortness of breath or left-sided chest pain, are common, especially among African Americans. Any patient with shortness of breath or left-sided chest pain should be assessed for other symptoms of CAD. Nurses should consult with nurse practitioners or physicians regarding diagnostic studies for CAD for any patient experiencing one or both of these symptoms. Nurses can teach colleagues and the lay public about shortness of breath, left-sided chest pain, and other symptoms of CAD and instruct them on how to access the emergency medical system if any of these symptoms are experienced.

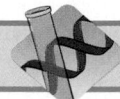

GENETICS IN NURSING PRACTICE—Cardiovascular Disorders

Several cardiovascular disorders are associated with genetic abnormalities. Some examples are:

- Familial hypercholesterolemia
- Hypertrophic cardiomyopathy
- Long QT syndrome (LQTS)
- Hereditary hemochromatosis
- Elevated homocystine levels

NURSING ASSESSMENTS

FAMILY HISTORY ASSESSMENT

- Assess all patients with cardiovascular symptoms for coronary artery disease, regardless of age (early-onset CAD occurs).
- Assess family history of sudden death in persons who may or may not have been diagnosed with coronary disease (especially of early onset).
- Ask about sudden death in a previously asymptomatic child, adolescent, or adult.
- Ask about other family members with biochemical or neuromuscular conditions (eg, hemochromatosis or muscular dystrophy).
- Assess whether DNA mutation or other genetic testing has been performed on an affected family member

ASSESSMENT

- Assess for signs and symptoms of hyperlipidemias (xanthomas, corneal arcus, abdominal pain of unexplained origin).
- Assess for muscular weakness.

MANAGEMENT ISSUES SPECIFIC TO GENETICS

- If indicated, refer for further genetic counseling and evaluation so that the family can discuss inheritance, risk to other family members, availability of genetic testing, and gene-based interventions
- Offer appropriate genetic information and resources (eg, Genetic Alliance website, American Heart Association, Muscular Dystrophy Association)
- Provide support to families newly diagnosed with genetic-related cardiovascular disease

GENETICS RESOURCES

Genetic Alliance—a directory of support groups for patients and families with genetic conditions; http://www.geneticalliance.org.

Gene Clinics—a listing of common genetic disorders with up-to-date clinical summaries, genetic counseling, and testing information; http://www.geneclinics.org.

National Organization of Rare Disorders—a directory of support groups and information for patients and families with rare genetic disorders; http://www.rarediseases.org.

OMIM: Online Mendelian Inheritance in Man—a complete listing of inherited genetic conditions; http://www.ncbi.nlm.nih.gov/omim/stats/html.

The baseline information derived from the history assists in identifying pertinent issues related to the patient's condition and educational and self-care needs. Once these problems are clearly identified, a plan of care is instituted. During subsequent contacts or visits with the patient, a more focused health history is performed to determine whether goals have been met, whether the plan needs to be modified, and whether new problems have developed. During the interview, the nurse asks questions to evaluate cardiac symptoms and health status.

Cardiac Signs and Symptoms

Patients with cardiovascular disorders commonly have one or more of the following signs and symptoms:

- Chest pain or discomfort (angina pectoris, MI, valvular heart disease)
- Shortness of breath or dyspnea (MI, left ventricular failure, HF)
- Edema and weight gain (right ventricular failure, HF)
- Palpitations (dysrhythmias resulting from myocardial ischemia, valvular heart disease, ventricular aneurysm, stress, electrolyte imbalance)
- Fatigue (earliest symptom associated with several cardiovascular disorders)

- Dizziness and syncope or loss of consciousness (postural hypotension, dysrhythmias, vasovagal effect, cerebrovascular disorders)

Not all chest discomfort is related to myocardial ischemia. When a patient has chest discomfort, questions should focus on differentiating a serious, life-threatening condition such as MI from conditions that are less serious or that would be treated differently (see Table 26-2).

The following points should be remembered when assessing patients with cardiac symptoms:

- Women are more likely to present with atypical symptoms of MI than are men.
- There is little correlation between the severity of the chest discomfort and the gravity of its cause. Elderly people and those with diabetes may not have pain with angina or MI because of neuropathies. Fatigue and shortness of breath may be the predominant symptoms in these patients.
- There is poor correlation between the location of chest discomfort and its source.
- The patient may have more than one clinical condition occurring simultaneously.
- In a patient with a history of CAD, the chest discomfort should be assumed to be secondary to ischemia until proven otherwise.

NURSING ALERT People experiencing myocardial ischemia can have a variety of symptoms. The typical symptom is angina presenting as pressure, fullness, squeezing pain, or discomfort in the center of the chest. This pain may radiate to the shoulders, neck, jaw, or arms. Angina can also have an atypical or uncommon presentation, referred to as anginal equivalent. It is characterized by shortness of breath, fatigue, weakness, or pain in other parts of the upper body, including the neck, shoulder, jaw, arm, back, or stomach. Angina patterns are usually predictable (eg, with activity). Rest or sublingual nitroglycerin relieves symptoms within a few minutes. A patient in the midst of an MI, however, can present with angina or its equivalent symptoms, which last longer than 15 minutes. Signs and symptoms associated with an MI include lightheadedness, fainting, diaphoresis, unexplained anxiety, nausea, and shortness of breath. Symptoms are unrelieved by rest or nitroglycerin.

HEALTH PERCEPTION AND MANAGEMENT

In an effort to determine how patients perceive their current health status. The nurse might ask some of the following questions:

> Do you have any health problems? If so, what do you think caused them?
>
> How has your health been recently? Have you noticed any changes from last year? from 5 years ago?
>
> Do you have a cardiologist or primary health care provider? How often do you go for checkups?
>
> Do you use tobacco or consume alcohol?
>
> What are your risk factors for heart disease? What do you do to stay healthy and take care of your heart?
>
> What prescription and over-the-counter medications are you taking? Do you take vitamins or herbal supplements?

Some patients may not be aware of their own medical diagnosis. For example, patients may not realize that their heart attack was caused by CAD. Patients who do not understand that their behaviors or diagnoses pose a threat to their health may be less motivated to make lifestyle changes or to manage their illness effectively. On the other hand, patients who perceive that their modifiable cardiovascular risk factors have contributed to their health conditions may be more likely to change these behaviors (Chart 26-1).

The patient's ability to recognize cardiac symptoms and to know what to do when they occur is essential for effective self-care

Chart 26-1
Risk Factors for Heart Disease

Nonmodifiable risk factors include the following:
Positive family history for premature coronary artery disease
Increasing age
Gender (men and postmenopausal women)
Race (higher incidence in African Americans than in Caucasians)

Modifiable risk factors include the following:
Hyperlipidemia
Hypertension
Cigarette smoking
Elevated blood glucose level (ie, diabetes mellitus)
Obesity
Physical inactivity
Type A personality characteristics, particularly hostility
Use of oral contraceptives

management. All too often, patients' new symptoms or symptoms of progressing cardiac dysfunction go unrecognized. This results in prolonged delays in seeking life-saving treatment. Major barriers to seeking prompt medical care include lack of knowledge about symptoms to expect with heart disease, attribution of symptoms to a benign source, psychological factors such as denial of symptom significance, and social factors, specifically feeling embarrassed about having symptoms (Zerwic, 1999).

An additional issue to consider is the patient's medication history, dosages, and schedules. Is the patient independent in taking medications? Are the medications taken as prescribed? Does the patient understand why the medication regimen is important? Are doses ever forgotten or skipped, or does the patient ever decide to stop taking a medication? An aspirin a day is a common nonprescription medication that improves patient outcomes after an MI. However, if patients are not aware of this benefit, they may be inclined to stop taking aspirin if they think it is a trivial medication. A careful medication history will often uncover common medication errors and causes for nonadherence to the medication regimen.

Table 26-2 summarizes the characteristics and patterns of the more common cardiac and noncardiac causes of chest pain. Table 26-3 identifies typical questions nurses use to assess cardiac signs and symptoms, as well as those used to determine the patient's ability to recognize and manage them. Some of the patient's responses may require further clarification and follow-up.

NUTRITION AND METABOLISM

Dietary modifications, exercise, weight loss, and careful monitoring are important strategies for managing three major cardiovascular risk factors: hyperlipidemia, hypertension, and hyperglycemia (diabetes mellitus). Diets that are restricted in sodium, fat, cholesterol, and/or calories are commonly prescribed. The nurse should obtain the following information:

- The patient's current height and weight (to determine body mass index), waist measurement (assessment for obesity), BP, and any laboratory test results such as blood glucose, glycosylated hemoglobin (diabetes), total blood cholesterol, high-density and low-density lipoprotein levels, and triglyceride levels (hyperlipidemia).
- How often the patient self-monitors BP, blood glucose, and weight as appropriate to the medical diagnoses.
- The patient's level of awareness regarding his or her target goals for each of the risk factors and any problems achieving or maintaining these goals.
- What the patient normally eats and drinks in a typical day and any food preferences (including cultural or ethnic preferences).
- Eating habits (canned or commercially prepared foods versus fresh foods, restaurant cooking versus home cooking, assessing for high sodium foods, dietary intake of fats).
- Who shops for groceries and prepares meals.

ELIMINATION

Typical bowel and bladder habits need to be identified. Nocturia (awakening at night to urinate) is common for patients with HF. Fluid collected in the dependent tissues (extremities) during the day redistributes into the circulatory system once the patient is recumbent at night. The increased circulatory volume is excreted by the kidneys (increased urine production). Patients need to be aware of their response to diuretic therapy and any changes in urination. This is vitally important for patients with HF. Patients may be taught to modify (titrate) their dose of diuretics based on urinary pattern, daily weight, and symptoms of dyspnea.

Table 26-2 • **Assessing Chest Pain**

	CHARACTER, LOCATION, AND RADIATION	DURATION	PRECIPITATING EVENTS	RELIEVING MEASURES
Angina Pectoris				
	Substernal or retrosternal pain spreading across chest; may radiate to inside of arm, neck, or jaw	5–15 min	Usually related to exertion, emotion, eating, cold	Rest, nitroglycerin, oxygen
Myocardial Infarction				
	Substernal pain or pain over precordium; may spread widely throughout chest. Pain in shoulders and hands may be present.	>15 min	Occurs spontaneously but may be sequela to unstable angina	Morphine sulfate, successful reperfusion of blocked coronary artery
Pericarditis				
	Sharp, severe substernal pain or pain to the left of sternum; may be felt in epigastrium and may be referred to neck, arms, and back	Intermittent	Sudden onset. Pain increases with inspiration, swallowing, coughing, and rotation of trunk.	Sitting upright, analgesia, anti-inflammatory medications

(continued)

Table 26-2 • Assessing Chest Pain (Continued)

	CHARACTER, LOCATION, AND RADIATION	DURATION	PRECIPITATING EVENTS	RELIEVING MEASURES
Pleuritic Pain	Pain arises from inferior portion of pleura; may be referred to costal margins or upper abdomen. Patient may be able to localize the pain.	30+ min	Often occurs spontaneously. Pain occurs or increases with inspiration.	Rest, time. Treatment of underlying cause, bronchodilators.
Esophageal Pain (Hiatal hernia, reflux esophagitis or spasm)	Substernal pain; may be projected around chest to shoulders.	5–60 min	Recumbency, cold liquids, exercise. May occur spontaneously.	Food, antacid. Nitroglycerin relieves spasm.
Anxiety	Pain over chest; may be variable. Does not radiate. Patient may complain of numbness and tingling of hands and mouth.	2–3 min	Stress, emotional tachypnea	Removal of stimulus, relaxation

To avoid straining, patients who become easily constipated need to establish a regular bowel regimen. When straining, the patient tends to bear down (the Valsalva maneuver), which momentarily increases pressure on the baroreceptors. This triggers a vagal response, causing the heart rate to slow down and resulting in syncope in some patients. For the same reason, straining during urination should be avoided. Because many cardiac medications can cause gastrointestinal side effects or bleeding, the nurse asks about bloating, diarrhea, constipation, stomach upset, heartburn, loss of appetite, nausea, and vomiting. Patients taking platelet-inhibiting medications such as aspirin and clopidogrel (Plavix); intravenous GP IIb/IIIa platelet aggregation inhibitors such as abciximab (ReoPro), eptifibatide (Integrilin), and tirofiban (Aggrastat); and anticoagulants such as low-molecular-weight heparin (ie, dalteparin [Fragmin]), enoxaparin (Lovenox), heparin, or warfarin (Coumadin) are screened for bloody urine or stools.

ACTIVITY AND EXERCISE

As the nurse assesses the patient's activity and exercise history, it is important to note that decreases in activity tolerance are typically gradual and may go unnoticed by the patient. Therefore, the nurse needs to determine whether there has been a change in the activity pattern during the last 6 to 12 months. The patient's subjective response to activity is an essential assessment parameter. New symptoms or a change in the usual angina or angina equivalent during activity is a significant finding. Fatigue, associated with low ejection fraction and certain medications (eg, beta-blockers), can result in activity intolerance. Patients with fatigue may benefit

Table 26-3 • **Asking Questions to Evaluate Cardiac Problems**

SYMPTOMS	ASSESSMENT QUESTIONS	ASSESSING PATIENT'S CAPACITY FOR SELF-MANAGEMENT
Chest pain, chest discomfort, angina pain	• Where is your pain (ask patient to point to location on chest) • What does the pain feel like? (pressure, heaviness, burning) • How severe is it on a scale of 0 to 10? • What causes the pain? (exertion, stress) • Does anything relieve it? (rest, nitroglycerin) • Does it spread to your arms, neck, jaw, shoulders, or back? • How long does the pain last? • Do you have any additional symptoms? (shortness of breath, palpitations, dizziness, sweating)	*Symptom Recognition* • If you have angina, what does it usually feel like? • If you have angina, how do your angina symptoms differ from the discomfort caused by your other medical conditions? (indigestion, GI disorders) • How do you think you would tell the difference between the symptoms of angina and a heart attack? • What were you doing when the pain started? *Symptom Management* • What did you do when the pain started? • How long did you wait before seeking medical attention (calling the doctor, coming to the emergency department, or calling the ambulance) *Use of Nitroglycerin* • Do you have a prescription for nitroglycerin (NTG) tablets or spray? • At the time of your chest pain, did you use your NTG? • How many tablets or sprays did you use and how frequently? • If you have NTG and did not take it with this angina episode, why do you think you did not take it? • When did you first open your NTG container? Where is it stored?
Shortness of breath, edema, weight gain	• When did you first notice feeling short of breath? • Do you have a cough? If yes, what do you cough up? • What makes you short of breath? Does anything make your breathing better or worse? • What activities are you no longer able to do because you are short of breath? • Do you ever wake up at night feeling short of breath? • What is your normal weight? • Have you had a recent weight gain? • Do you get up at night to urinate? Have you noticed an increase or decrease in the amount you usually urinate? • Have you noticed any weight gain or swelling in your feet, ankles, legs, or abdomen (sacrum if bedridden)? Do your shoes feel tight or clothes feel tight around your waist? • On how many pillows do you sleep, and has this changed recently? • Do you sleep in your bed, or do you breathe easier sleeping in a chair?	• Has anyone ever told you that you have heart failure? What does this mean to you? • Do you ever forget to take your diuretic medication (water pill) or other heart medicines or decide not to take them? If so, why do you think this happens? • What do you typically eat or drink? Who does the food shopping and meal preparation? • Are you on a sodium- or fluid-restricted diet? Have you been able to follow your special diet? • Do you have a scale to weigh yourself? How often do you weigh yourself? • What are important signs or symptoms to report to your doctor?
Palpitations	• Do you ever feel your heart racing, skipping beats, or pounding? • Do you ever feel lightheaded or dizzy? • Are there any other symptoms that occur at the same time? • How much caffeine do you consume? • Do you use tobacco (cigarettes, cigars, chew)? • Do you use any other stimulants, recreational drugs? • Do you use any nutritional supplements or herbs? • Have there been any changes in the amount of stress you experience?	• What did you do when your symptoms first occurred? • Is your primary health care provider aware of these symptoms? • Are you taking medication for this condition, and have you been taking it as directed?
Fatigue	• How would you describe your usual activity level? • What is your current activity level? • What were you able to do 1 month and 6 months ago? • What activities can you no longer do because of fatigue? • Do you feel rested when you wake up in the morning? • Can you rest during the day? • How often do you awaken at night, and for what reason?	• Have you spoken with your primary health care provider about decreases in your activity level? • Has anyone ever taught you energy conservation techniques? If so, are you able to use them?

(continued)

Table 26-3 • **Asking Questions to Evaluate Cardiac Problems** (Continued)

SYMPTOMS	ASSESSMENT QUESTIONS	ASSESSING PATIENT'S CAPACITY FOR SELF-MANAGEMENT
Dizziness, syncope (loss of consciousness)	• Do you ever feel dizzy or lightheaded? • Do you ever pass out or have fainting spells? • Does this happen when you move from a lying to a sitting or standing position? • Do you strain while having a bowel movement or when urinating? • Have you been urinating more than usual? • Have you decreased the amount of fluids you normally drink? • Do you have headaches?	• Have you ever been told you have high or low blood pressure? Has it been checked recently? • Are you taking any medications that can lower your blood pressure? • Before standing from a lying position, do you sit for a few minutes? Does that relieve the dizziness? • What are you using to prevent constipation?

from having their medications adjusted and learning energy conservation techniques.

Additional areas to ask about include possible architectural barriers and challenges in the home, and what the patient does for exercise. If the patient exercises, the nurse asks additional questions: What is the intensity, and how long and how often is exercise performed? Has the patient ever participated in a cardiac rehabilitation program? Functional levels are known to improve for almost all patients who participate in a cardiac rehabilitation program, and attendance is highly recommended (Smith et al., 2001). Patients with disabilities may require an individually tailored exercise program.

SLEEP AND REST

Clues to worsening cardiac disease, especially HF, can be revealed by sleep-related events. Determining where the patient sleeps or rests is important. Recent changes, such as sleeping upright in a chair instead of in bed, increasing the number of pillows used, awakening short of breath at night (paroxysmal nocturnal dyspnea [PND]), or awakening with angina (nocturnal angina), are all indicative of worsening HF.

COGNITION AND PERCEPTION

Evaluating cognitive ability helps to determine whether the patient has the mental capacity to manage safe and effective self-care. Is the patient's short-term memory intact? Is there any history of dementia? Is there evidence of depression or anxiety? Can the patient read? Can the patient read English? What is the patient's reading level? What is the patient's preferred learning style? What information does the patient perceive as important?

Providing the patient with written information can be a valuable part of patient education, but only if the patient can read and comprehend the information. Related assessments include possible hearing or visual impairments. If vision is impaired, patients with HF may not be able to weigh themselves independently nor keep records of weight, BP, pulse, or other data requested by the health care team.

SELF-PERCEPTION AND SELF-CONCEPT

Personality factors are associated with the development of and recovery from CAD. Most commonly cited is "type A behavior," which is characterized by competitive, hard-driving behaviors and a sense of time urgency. Although this behavior is not an independent risk factor for CAD, anger and hostility (personality traits common in people with "type A behavior") do affect the heart. People with these traits react to frustrating situations with an increase in BP, heart rate, and neuroendocrine responses. This

physiologic activation, called cardiac reactivity, is thought to trigger acute cardiovascular events (Woods et al., 1999).

During the health history, the nurse discovers how patients feel about themselves by asking questions such as: How would you describe yourself? Have you changed the way you feel about yourself since your heart attack or surgery? Do you find that you are easily angered or hostile? How do you feel right now? What helps to manage these feelings? To fully evaluate this health pattern, assistance from a psychiatric clinical nurse specialist, psychologist, or psychiatrist may be necessary.

ROLES AND RELATIONSHIPS

Determining the patient's social support systems is vitally important in today's health care environment. Hospital stays for cardiac illnesses have shortened. Many invasive diagnostic cardiac procedures, such as cardiac catheterization and percutaneous transluminal coronary angioplasty (PTCA) are performed as outpatient procedures. Patients are discharged back into the community with activity limitations, such as driving restrictions, and with greater nursing care and educational needs. These needs have significant implications for people who are independent under normal circumstances, and for people who are at higher risk for problems, such as older adults.

To assess support systems, the nurse needs to ask: Who is the primary caregiver? With whom does the patient live? Are there adequate services in place to provide a safe home environment? The nurse also assesses for any significant effects the cardiac illness has had on the patient's role in the family. Are there adequate finances and health insurance? The answers to these questions will assist the nurse in developing a plan to meet the patient's home care needs.

SEXUALITY AND REPRODUCTION

Although people recovering from cardiac illnesses or procedures are concerned about sexual activity, they are less likely to ask their nurse or other health care provider for information to help them resume their normal sex life. Lack of correct information and fear lead to reduced frequency and satisfaction with sexual activity. Therefore, nurses need to initiate this discussion with patients and not wait for them to bring it up in conversation. At first, inform the patient that it is common for people with similar heart problems to worry about resuming sexual activity. Then ask the patient to talk about his or her concerns.

The most commonly cited reasons for changes in sexual activity are fear of another heart attack or sudden death; untoward symptoms such as angina, dyspnea, or palpitations; and problems with impotence or depression. In men, impotence may develop as a side effect of cardiac medications (beta-adrenergic blocking agents) and may prompt patients to stop taking them. Other medications can be substituted, so patients should be encouraged to discuss this problem with their health care provider. Often, patients and their partners do not have adequate information about the physical demands related to sexual activity and ways in which these demands can be modified. The physiologic demands are greatest during orgasm, reaching 5 or 6 metabolic equivalents (METs). This level of activity is equivalent to walking 3 to 4 miles per hour on a treadmill. The METs expended before and after orgasm are considerably less, at 3.7 METs (Steinke, 2000). Having this information may make patients and their partners more comfortable with resuming sexual activity.

A reproductive history is necessary for women of childbearing age, particularly those with seriously compromised cardiac function. These women may be advised by their physicians not to become pregnant. The reproductive history includes information about previous pregnancies, plans for future pregnancies, oral contraceptive use (especially in women older than 35 years of age who are smokers), and use of hormone replacement therapy.

COPING AND STRESS TOLERANCE

It is important to determine the presence of psychosocial factors that adversely affect cardiac health. Anxiety, depression, and stress are known to influence both the development of and recovery from CAD. High levels of anxiety are associated with an increased incidence of CAD and increased in-hospital complication rates after MI. People with depression have an increased risk of MI and heart disease–related death, compared to people without depression. It is postulated that people who are depressed feel hopeless and are less motivated to make lifestyle changes and follow treatment plans, explaining the association between mortality and depression (Buselli & Stuart, 1999).

Stress initiates a variety of physiologic responses, including increases in the circulation of catecholamines and cortisol, and has been strongly linked to cardiovascular events. Therefore, patients need to be assessed for presence of negative and positive emotions, as well as sources of stress. This is achieved by asking questions about recent or ongoing stressors, previous coping styles and effectiveness, and the patient's perception of his or her current mood and coping ability. To adequately evaluate this health pattern, consultation with a psychiatric clinical nurse specialist, psychologist, or psychiatrist may be indicated.

PREVENTION STRATEGIES

Additional features of the health history include identification of risk factors and measures taken by the patient to prevent disease. The nurse's questions need to focus on the patient's health promotion practices. Epidemiologic studies show that certain conditions or behaviors (ie, risk factors) are associated with a greater incidence of coronary artery, peripheral vascular, and cerebrovascular disease. Risk factors are classified by the extent to which they can be modified by changing one's lifestyle or modifying personal behaviors.

Once a patient's risk factors are determined, the nurse assesses whether the patient has a plan for making necessary behavioral changes and whether assistance is needed to support these lifestyle changes. For example, tobacco use is the most common avoidable cause of CAD. The first step in treating this health risk is to identify patients who use tobacco products and those who have recently quit. Because 70% of smokers visit a health care facility each year, nurses have ample opportunities to assess patients for tobacco use. For those who use tobacco, it is imperative to ask whether they are willing to quit. Provide cessation advice, motivation to quit, and relapse prevention strategies, as outlined in a U.S. Public Health Service report (The Tobacco Use and Dependence Clinical Practice Guideline Update Panel, Staff, and Consortium Representatives, 2000), can be delivered. For patients who have obesity, hyperlipidemia, hypertension, and diabetes, the nurse determines any problems the patient may be having following the prescribed management plan (ie, diet, exercise, and medications). It may be necessary to clarify the patient's responsibilities, assist with finding additional resources, or make alternative plans for risk factor modification.

Comprehensive secondary prevention strategies (early diagnosis and prompt intervention to halt or slow the disease process and its consequences) aimed at reducing cardiovascular risk factors improve overall survival, improve quality of life, reduce the need for revascularization procedures (coronary artery bypass surgery and PTCA), and reduce the incidence of subsequent MIs. The overall benefits of secondary prevention also apply to other patient groups with atherosclerotic vascular disease, including patients with transient ischemic attacks, stroke, and peripheral vascular disease (the leading cause of disability and death in these patients being CAD). Despite these findings, only one third of eligible patients, over the long term, adhere to risk factor interventions. Patient compliance increases significantly with a team approach that includes long-term follow-up with office or clinic visits and telephone contact (Smith et al., 2001).

PHYSICAL ASSESSMENT

A physical examination is performed to confirm the data obtained in the health history. In addition to observing the patient's general appearance, a cardiac physical examination should include an evaluation of the following:

- Effectiveness of the heart as a pump
- Filling volumes and pressures
- Cardiac output
- Compensatory mechanisms

Indications that the heart is not contracting sufficiently or functioning effectively as a pump include reduced pulse pressure, cardiac enlargement, and murmurs and gallop rhythms (abnormal heart sounds).

The amount of blood filling the atria and ventricles and the resulting pressures (called filling volumes and pressures) are estimated by the degree of jugular vein distention and the presence or absence of congestion in the lungs, peripheral edema, and postural changes in BP that occur when the individual sits up or stands.

Cardiac output is reflected by cognition, heart rate, pulse pressure, color and texture of the skin, and urine output. Examples of compensatory mechanisms that help maintain cardiac output are increased filling volumes and elevated heart rate. Note that the findings on the physical examination are correlated with data obtained from diagnostic procedures, such as hemodynamic monitoring (discussed later).

The examination, which proceeds logically from head to toe, can be performed in about 10 minutes with practice and covers the following areas: (1) general appearance, (2) cognition, (3) skin, (4) BP, (5) arterial pulses, (6) jugular venous pulsations and pressures, (7) heart, (8) extremities, (9) lungs, and (10) abdomen.

General Appearance and Cognition

The nurse observes the patient's level of distress, level of consciousness, and thought processes as an indication of the heart's ability to propel oxygen to the brain (cerebral perfusion). The nurse also observes for evidence of anxiety, along with any effects emotional factors may have on cardiovascular status. The nurse attempts to put the anxious patient at ease throughout the examination.

Inspection of the Skin

Examination of the skin begins during the evaluation of the general appearance of the patient and continues throughout the assessment. It includes all body surfaces, starting with the head and finishing with the lower extremities. Skin color, temperature, and texture are assessed. The more common findings associated with cardiovascular disease are as follows.

- Pallor—a decrease in the color of the skin—is caused by lack of oxyhemoglobin. It is a result of anemia or decreased arterial perfusion. Pallor is best observed around the fingernails, lips, and oral mucosa. In patients with dark skin, the nurse observes the palms of the hands and soles of the feet.
- Peripheral cyanosis—a bluish tinge, most often of the nails and skin of the nose, lips, earlobes, and extremities—suggests decreased flow rate of blood to a particular area, which allows more time for the hemoglobin molecule to become desaturated. This may occur normally in peripheral vasoconstriction associated with a cold environment, in patients with anxiety, or in disease states such as HF.
- Central cyanosis—a bluish tinge observed in the tongue and buccal mucosa—denotes serious cardiac disorders (pulmonary edema and congenital heart disease) in which venous blood passes through the pulmonary circulation without being oxygenated.
- Xanthelasma—yellowish, slightly raised plaques in the skin—may be observed along the nasal portion of one or both eyelids and may indicate elevated cholesterol levels (hypercholesterolemia).
- Reduced skin turgor occurs with dehydration and aging.
- Temperature and moistness are controlled by the autonomic nervous system. Normally the skin is warm and dry. Under stress, the hands may become cool and moist. In cardiogenic shock, sympathetic nervous system stimulation causes vasoconstriction, and the skin becomes cold and clammy. During an acute MI, diaphoresis is common.
- Ecchymosis (bruise)—a purplish-blue color fading to green, yellow, or brown over time—is associated with blood outside of the blood vessels and is usually caused by trauma. Patients who are receiving anticoagulant therapy should be carefully observed for unexplained ecchymosis. In these patients, excessive bruising indicates prolonged clotting times (prothrombin or partial thromboplastin time) caused by an anticoagulant dosage that is too high.
- Wounds, scars, and tissue surrounding implanted devices should also be examined. Wounds are assessed for adequate healing, and any scars from previous surgeries are noted. The skin surrounding a pacemaker or implantable cardioverter defibrillator generator is examined for thinning, which could indicate erosion of the device through the skin.

Blood Pressure

Systemic arterial BP is the pressure exerted on the walls of the arteries during ventricular systole and diastole. It is affected by factors such as cardiac output, distention of the arteries, and the volume, velocity, and viscosity of the blood. BP usually is expressed as the ratio of the systolic pressure over the diastolic pressure, with normal adult values ranging from 100/60 to 140/90 mm Hg. The average normal BP usually cited is 120/80 mm Hg. An increase in BP above the upper normal range is called hypertension (see Chap. 32 for further definitions and management), whereas a decrease below the lower range is called hypotension.

BLOOD PRESSURE MEASUREMENT

BP can be measured with the use of invasive arterial monitoring systems (discussed later) or noninvasively by a sphygmomanometer and stethoscope or by an automated BP monitoring device. A detailed description of the procedure for obtaining BP can be found in nursing skills textbooks, and specific manufacturer's instructions review the proper use of the automated monitoring devices. Several important details must be observed to ensure that BP measurements are accurate; these are highlighted in Chart 26-2.

PULSE PRESSURE

The difference between the systolic and the diastolic pressures is called the pulse pressure. It is a reflection of stroke volume, ejection velocity, and systemic vascular resistance. Pulse pressure, which normally is 30 to 40 mm Hg, indicates how well the patient maintains cardiac output. The pulse pressure increases in conditions that elevate the stroke volume (anxiety, exercise, bradycardia), reduce systemic vascular resistance (fever), or reduce distensibility of the arteries (atherosclerosis, aging, hypertension). Decreased pulse pressure is an abnormal condition reflecting reduced stroke volume and ejection velocity (shock, HF, hypovolemia, mitral regurgitation) or obstruction to blood flow during systole (mitral or aortic

Chart 26-2   Ensuring Accurate Blood Pressure Measurement

- Cuff size must be appropriate for the patient. (The cuff size should have a bladder width at least 40% and length at least 80% of limb circumference.) The average adult cuff is 12 to 14 cm wide and 30 cm long. Using a cuff that is too small will give a high reading, whereas, too large a cuff results in a falsely low reading.
- Calibration of the sphygmomanometer should be performed routinely to ensure accuracy of blood pressure reading.
- Cuff is firmly wrapped around the arm, and cuff bladder is centered over the brachial artery.
- Patient's arm should be at heart level.
- Initial recordings are made on both arms, and subsequent measurements are taken on the arm with the higher pressure. Normally, in the absence of disease of the vasculature, there is a difference of no more than 5 mm Hg between arm pressures.
- Position of the patient and site of blood pressure measurement (eg, RA for right arm) are recorded.
- Palpation of the systolic pressure before auscultation helps to detect an auscultatory gap more readily.
- The patient is asked not to talk during blood pressure measurements. A significant increase in blood pressure and heart rate occurs when subjects are talking.

stenosis). A pulse pressure of less than 30 mm Hg signifies a serious reduction in cardiac output and requires further cardiovascular assessment.

POSTURAL BLOOD PRESSURE CHANGES

Postural (orthostatic) hypotension occurs when the BP drops significantly after the patient assumes an upright posture. It is usually accompanied by dizziness, lightheadedness, or syncope.

Although there are many causes of postural hypotension, the three most common causes in patients with cardiac problems are a reduced volume of fluid or blood in the circulatory system (intravascular volume depletion, dehydration), inadequate vasoconstrictor mechanisms, and insufficient autonomic effect on vascular constriction. Postural changes in BP and an appropriate history help health care providers differentiate among these causes. The following recommendations are important when assessing postural BP changes:

- Position the patient supine and flat (as symptoms permit) for 10 minutes before taking the initial BP and heart rate measurements.
- Check supine measurements before checking upright measurements.
- Do not remove the BP cuff between position changes, but check to see that it is still correctly placed.
- Assess postural BP changes with the patient sitting on the edge of the bed with feet dangling and, if appropriate, with the patient standing at the side of the bed.
- Wait 1 to 3 minutes after each postural change before measuring BP and heart rate.
- Be alert for any signs or symptoms of patient distress. If necessary, return the patient to a lying position before completing the test.
- Record both heart rate and BP and indicate the corresponding position (e.g., lying, sitting, standing) and any signs or symptoms that accompany the postural change.

Normal postural responses that occur when a person stands up or goes from a lying to a sitting position include (1) a heart rate increase of 5 to 20 bpm above the resting rate (to offset reduced stroke volume and maintain cardiac output); (2) an unchanged systolic pressure, or a slight decrease of up to 10 mm Hg; and (3) a slight increase of 5 mm Hg in diastolic pressure.

A decrease in the amount of blood or fluid in the circulatory system should be suspected after diuretic therapy or bleeding, when a postural change results in an increased heart rate and either a decrease in systolic pressure by 15 mm Hg or a drop in the diastolic pressure by 10 mm Hg. Vital signs alone do not differentiate between a decrease in intravascular volume and inadequate constriction of the blood vessels as a cause of postural hypotension. With intravascular volume depletion, the reflexes that maintain cardiac output (increased heart rate and peripheral vasoconstriction) function correctly; the heart rate increases, and the peripheral vessels constrict. However, because of lost volume, the BP falls. With inadequate vasoconstrictor mechanisms, the heart rate again responds appropriately, but because of diminished peripheral vasoconstriction the BP drops. The following is an example of a postural BP recording showing either intravascular volume depletion or inadequate vasoconstrictor mechanisms:

Lying down, BP 120/70, heart rate 70
Sitting, BP 100/55, heart rate 90
Standing, BP 98/52, heart rate 94

In autonomic insufficiency, the heart rate is unable to increase to completely compensate for the gravitational effects of an upright posture. Peripheral vasoconstriction may be absent or diminished. Autonomic insufficiency does not rule out a concurrent decrease in intravascular volume. The following is an example of autonomic insufficiency as demonstrated by postural BP changes:

Lying down, BP 150/90, heart rate 60
Sitting, BP 100/60, heart rate 60

Arterial Pulses

Factors to be evaluated in examining the pulse are rate, rhythm, quality, configuration of the pulse wave, and quality of the arterial vessel.

PULSE RATE

The normal pulse rate varies from a low of 50 bpm in healthy, athletic young adults to rates well in excess of 100 bpm after exercise or during times of excitement. Anxiety frequently raises the pulse rate during the physical examination. If the rate is higher than expected, it is appropriate to reassess it near the end of the physical examination, when the patient may be more relaxed.

PULSE RHYTHM

The rhythm of the pulse is as important to assess as the rate. Minor variations in regularity of the pulse are normal. The pulse rate, particularly in young people, increases during inhalation and slows during exhalation. This is called sinus arrhythmia.

For the initial cardiac examination, or if the pulse rhythm is irregular, the heart rate should be counted by auscultating the apical pulse for a full minute while simultaneously palpating the radial pulse.

Any discrepancy between contractions heard and pulses felt is noted. Disturbances of rhythm (dysrhythmias) often result in a pulse deficit, a difference between the apical rate (the heart rate heard at the apex of the heart) and the peripheral rate. Pulse deficits commonly occur with atrial fibrillation, atrial flutter, premature ventricular contractions, and varying degrees of heart block. See Chapter 27 for a detailed discussion of these dysrhythmias.

To understand the complexity of dysrhythmias that may be encountered during the examination, the nurse needs to have a sophisticated knowledge of cardiac electrophysiology, obtained through advanced education and training.

PULSE QUALITY

The quality, or amplitude, of the pulse can be described as absent, diminished, normal, or bounding. It should be assessed bilaterally. Scales can be used to rate the strength of the pulse. The following is an example of a 0-to-4 scale:

0	pulse not palpable or absent
+1	weak, thready pulse; difficult to palpate; obliterated with pressure
+2	diminished pulse; cannot be obliterated
+3	easy to palpate, full pulse; cannot be obliterated
+4	strong, bounding pulse; may be abnormal

The numerical classification is quite subjective; therefore, when documenting the pulse quality, it helps to specify a scale range (eg, "left radial +3/+4").

PULSE CONFIGURATION

The configuration (contour) of the pulse conveys important information. In patients with stenosis of the aortic valve, the valve opening is narrowed, reducing the amount of blood ejected into the aorta. The pulse pressure is narrow, and the pulse feels feeble. In aortic insufficiency, the aortic valve does not close completely, allowing blood to flow back or leak from the aorta into the left ventricle. The rise of the pulse wave is abrupt and strong, and its fall is precipitous—a "collapsing" or "water hammer" pulse. The true configuration of the pulse is best appreciated by palpating over the carotid artery rather than the distal radial artery, because the dramatic characteristics of the pulse wave may be distorted when the pulse is transmitted to smaller vessels.

EFFECT OF VESSEL QUALITY ON PULSE

The condition of the vessel wall also influences the pulse and is of concern, especially in older patients. Once rate and rhythm have been determined, the nurse assesses the quality of the vessel by palpating along the radial artery and comparing it with normal vessels. Does the vessel wall appear to be thickened? Is it tortuous?

To assess peripheral circulation, the nurse locates and evaluates all arterial pulses. Arterial pulses are palpated at points where the arteries are near the skin surface and are easily compressed against bones or firm musculature. Pulses are detected over the temporal, carotid, brachial, radial, femoral, popliteal, dorsalis pedis, and posterior tibial arteries. A reliable assessment of the pulses of the lower extremities depends on accurate identification of the location of the artery and careful palpation of the area. Light palpation is essential; firm finger pressure can easily obliterate the dorsalis pedis and posterior tibial pulses and confuse the examiner. In approximately 10% of patients, the dorsalis pedis pulses are not palpable. In such circumstances, both are usually absent together, and the posterior tibial arteries alone provide adequate blood supply to the feet. Arteries in the extremities are often palpated simultaneously to facilitate comparison of quality.

NURSING ALERT Do not palpate temporal or carotid arteries simultaneously, because it is possible to decrease the blood flow to the brain.

Jugular Venous Pulsations

An estimate of right-sided heart function can be made by observing the pulsations of the jugular veins of the neck. This provides a means of estimating central venous pressure, which reflects right atrial or right ventricular end-diastolic pressure (the pressure immediately preceding the contraction of the right ventricle).

Pulsations of the internal jugular veins are most commonly assessed. If they are difficult to see, pulsations of the external jugular veins may be noted. These veins are more superficial and are visible just above the clavicles, adjacent to the sternocleidomastoid muscles. The external jugular veins are frequently distended while the patient lies supine on the examining table or bed. As the patient's head is elevated, the distention of the veins disappears. The veins normally are not apparent if the head of the bed or examining table is elevated more than 30 degrees.

Obvious distention of the veins with the patient's head elevated 45 degrees to 90 degrees indicates an abnormal increase in the volume of the venous system. This is associated with right-sided HF, less commonly with obstruction of blood flow in the superior vena cava, and rarely with acute massive pulmonary embolism.

Heart Inspection and Palpation

The heart is examined indirectly by inspection, palpation, percussion, and auscultation of the chest wall. A systematic approach is the cornerstone of a thorough assessment. Examination of the chest wall is performed in the following six areas (Fig. 26-6):

1. *Aortic area*—second intercostal space to the right of the sternum. To determine the correct intercostal space, start at the angle of Louis by locating the bony ridge near the top of the sternum, at the junction of the body and the manubrium. From this angle, locate the second intercostal space by sliding one finger to the left or right of the sternum. Subsequent intercostal spaces are located from this reference point by palpating down the rib cage.
2. *Pulmonic area*—second intercostal space to the left of the sternum
3. *Erb's point*—third intercostal space to the left of the sternum
4. *Right ventricular or tricuspid area*—fourth and fifth intercostal spaces to the left of the sternum
5. *Left ventricular or apical area*—the PMI, location on the chest where heart contractions can be palpated
6. *Epigastric area*—below the xiphoid process

For most of the examination, the patient lies supine, with the head slightly elevated. The right-handed examiner is positioned at the right side of the patient and the left-handed examiner at the left side.

In a systematic fashion, each area of the precordium is inspected and then palpated. Oblique lighting is used to assist the examiner in identifying subtle pulsation. A normal impulse that is distinct and located over the apex of the heart is called the **apical impulse** (PMI). It may be observed in young people and in older people who are thin. The apical impulse is normally located and auscultated in the left fifth intercostal space in the midclavicular line (Fig. 26-7).

In many cases, the apical impulse is palpable and is normally felt as a light pulsation, 1 to 2 cm in diameter. It is felt at the onset of the first heart sound and lasts for only half of systole. (See the next section for a discussion of heart sounds.) The nurse uses the palm of the hand to locate the apical impulse initially and the fingerpads to assess its size and quality. A broad and forceful apical impulse is

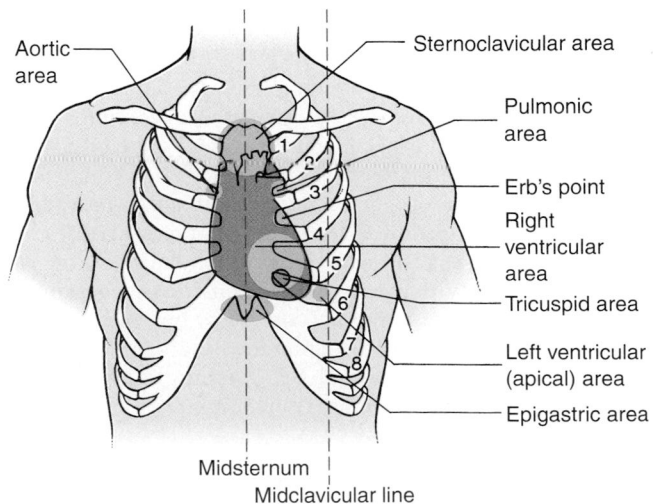

FIGURE 26-6 Areas of the precordium to be assessed when evaluating heart function. (Numerals identify ribs of adjacent intercostal spaces.)

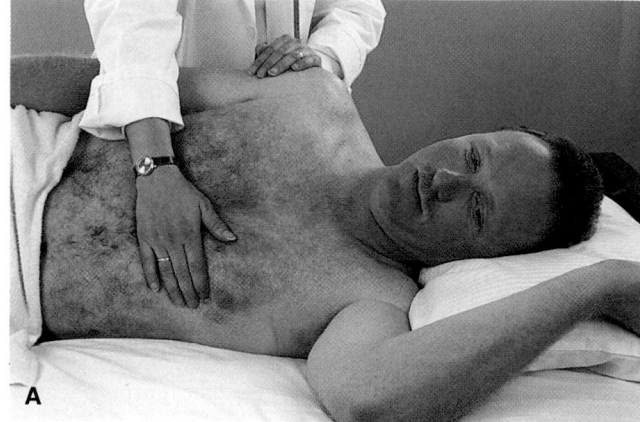

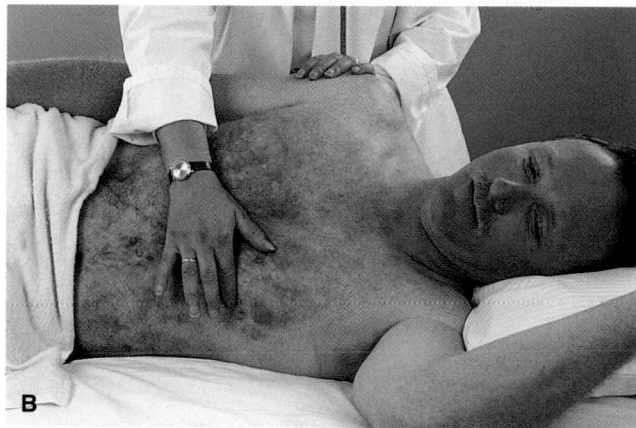

FIGURE 26-7 Locating (**A**) and palpating (**B**) the apical impulse (also called the point of maximal impulse, PMI). The apical impulse normally is located at the fifth intercostal space to the left of the sternum at the midclavicular line. The nurse locates the impulse with the palm of the hand and palpates with the fingerpads. © B. Proud in Weber, J. W., & Kelley, J. (2003). *Health assessment in nursing* (2nd ed.). Philadelphia: Lippincott Williams & Wilkins.

known as a left ventricular heave or lift. It is so named because it appears to lift the hand from the chest wall during palpation.

An apical impulse below the fifth intercostal space or lateral to the midclavicular line usually denotes left ventricular enlargement from left ventricular failure. Normally, the apical impulse is palpable in only one intercostal space; palpability in two or more adjacent intercostal spaces indicates left ventricular enlargement. If the apical impulse can be palpated in two distinctly separate areas and the pulsation movements are paradoxical (not simultaneous), a ventricular aneurysm should be suspected.

Abnormal, turbulent blood flow within the heart may be palpated with the palm of the hand as a purring sensation. This phenomenon is called a thrill and is associated with a loud murmur. A thrill is always indicative of significant pathology within the heart. Thrills also may be palpated over vessels when blood flow is significantly and substantially obstructed and over the carotid arteries if aortic stenosis is present or if the aortic valve is narrowed.

Chest Percussion

Normally, only the left border of the heart can be detected by percussion. It extends from the sternum to the midclavicular line in the third to fifth intercostal spaces. The right border lies under

the right margin of the sternum and is not detectable. Enlargement of the heart to either the left or right usually can be noted. In people with thick chests, obesity, or emphysema, the heart may lie so deep under the thoracic surface that not even its left border can be noted unless the heart is enlarged. In such cases, unless the nurse detects a displaced apical impulse and suspects cardiac enlargement, percussion is omitted.

Cardiac Auscultation

All areas identified in Figure 26-6, except the epigastric area, are auscultated. These include the aortic area, the pulmonary area, Erb's point, the tricuspid area, and the apical area. The actions of the four valves are uniquely reflected at specific locations on the chest wall. These locations do not correspond to the anatomic locations of the valves within the chest; rather, they reflect the patterns by which heart sounds radiate toward the chest wall. Sound in vessels through which blood is flowing is always reflected downstream. For example, the actions of the mitral valve are usually heard best in the fifth intercostal space at the midclavicular line. This is called the mitral valve area.

HEART SOUNDS

The **normal heart sounds**, S_1 and S_2, are produced primarily by the closing of the heart valves. The time between S_1 and S_2 corresponds to systole (Fig. 26-8). This is normally shorter than the time between S_2 and S_1 (diastole). As the heart rate increases, diastole shortens.

In normal physiology, the periods of systole and diastole are silent. Ventricular disease, however, can give rise to transient sounds in systole and diastole that are called gallops, snaps, or clicks. Significant narrowing of the valve orifices at times when they should be open, or residual gapping of valves at times when they should be closed, gives rise to prolonged sounds called murmurs.

S_1—First Heart Sound. Closure of the mitral and tricuspid valves creates the first heart sound (S_1), although vibration of the myocardial wall also may contribute to this sound. Although S_1 is heard over the entire precordium, it is heard best at the apex of the heart (apical area). Its intensity increases when the valve leaflets are made rigid by calcium in rheumatic heart disease and in any circumstance in which ventricular contraction occurs at a time when the valve is caught wide open. The latter circumstance occurs, for example, when a premature ventricular contraction interrupts the normal cardiac cycle. S_1 varies in intensity from beat to beat when atrial contraction is not synchronous with ventricular contraction. This is because the valve may be fully or partially closed on one beat and open on the subsequent one as a function of irregular atrial activity. S_1 is easily identifiable and serves as the point of reference for the remainder of the cardiac cycle.

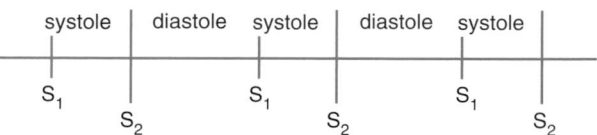

FIGURE 26-8 Normal heart sounds. The first heart sound (S_1) is produced by the closing of the mitral and tricuspid valves and is best heard at the apex of the heart (left ventricular or apical area). The second heart sound (S_2) is produced by the closing of the aortic and pulmonic valves and is loudest at the base of the heart. The time between S_1 and S_2 corresponds to systole. The time between S_2 and S_1 is diastole.

S₂—Second Heart Sound.

Closing of the aortic and pulmonic valves produces the second heart sound (S_2). Although these two valves close almost simultaneously, the pulmonic valve usually lags slightly behind. Therefore, under certain circumstances, the two components of the second sound may be heard separately (split S_2). The splitting is more likely to be accentuated on inspiration and to disappear on exhalation. (More blood is ejected from the right ventricle during inspiration than during exhalation.)

S_2 is heard loudest at the base of the heart. The aortic component of S_2 is heard clearly in both the aortic and pulmonic areas, and less clearly at the apex. The pulmonic component of S_2, if present, may be heard only over the pulmonic area. Therefore, one may hear a "single" S_2 in the aortic area and a split S_2 in the pulmonic area.

Gallop Sounds.

If the blood filling the ventricle is impeded during diastole, as occurs in certain disease states, then a temporary vibration may occur in diastole that is similar to, although usually softer than, S_1 and S_2. The heart sounds then come in triplets and have the acoustic effect of a galloping horse; they are called gallops. This may occur early in diastole, during the rapid-filling phase of the cardiac cycle, or later at the time of atrial contraction.

A gallop sound occurring during rapid ventricular filling is called a third heart sound (S_3); it represents a normal finding in children and young adults (Fig. 26-9A). Such a sound is heard in patients who have myocardial disease or in those who have HF and whose ventricles fail to eject all of their blood during systole. An S_3 gallop is heard best with the patient lying on the left side.

Gallop sounds heard during atrial contraction are called fourth heart sounds (S_4) (see Fig. 26-9B). An S_4 is often heard when the ventricle is enlarged or hypertrophied and therefore resistant to filling. Such a circumstance may be associated with CAD, hypertension, or stenosis of the aortic valve. On rare occasions, all four heart sounds are heard within a single cardiac cycle, giving rise to what is called a quadruple rhythm.

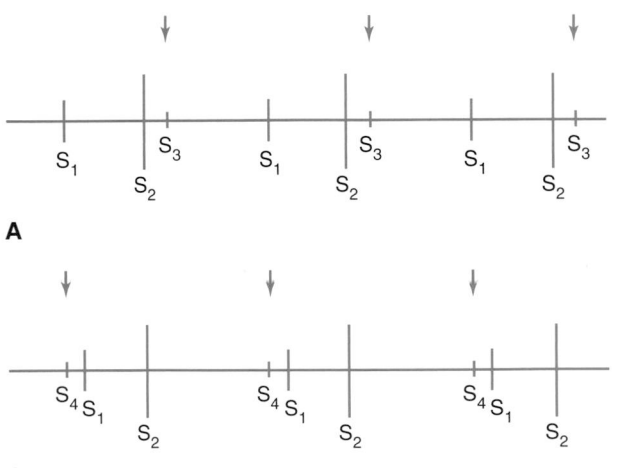

A

B

FIGURE 26-9 Gallops. (**A**) An S_3 gallop is heard immediately following the S_2 and occurs when the blood filling the ventricle is impeded during diastole, resulting in temporary vibrations. The heart sounds come in triplets and resemble the sound of a galloping horse. Myocardial disease and heart failure are associated with this sound. (**B**) An S_4 gallop is heard immediately preceding the S_1. The S_4 sound occurs during atrial contraction and is often heard when the ventricle is enlarged or hypertrophied. Associated conditions include coronary artery disease, hypertension, and stenosis of the aortic valve.

Gallop sounds are very low-frequency sounds and may be heard only with the bell of the stethoscope placed very lightly against the chest. They are heard best at the apex, although occasionally, when emanating from the right ventricle, they may be heard to the left of the sternum.

Snaps and Clicks.

Stenosis of the mitral valve resulting from rheumatic heart disease gives rise to an unusual sound very early in diastole that is high-pitched and is best heard along the left sternal border. The sound is caused by high pressure in the left atrium with abrupt displacement of a rigid mitral valve. The sound is called an opening snap. It occurs too long after S_2 to be mistaken for a split S_2 and too early in diastole to be mistaken for a gallop. It almost always is associated with the murmur of mitral stenosis and is specific to this disorder.

In a similar manner, stenosis of the aortic valve gives rise to a short, high-pitched sound immediately after S_1 that is called an ejection click. This is caused by very high pressure within the ventricle, displacing a rigid and calcified aortic valve.

Murmurs.

Murmurs are created by the turbulent flow of blood. The causes of the turbulence may be a critically narrowed valve, a malfunctioning valve that allows regurgitant blood flow, a congenital defect of the ventricular wall, a defect between the aorta and the pulmonary artery, or an increased flow of blood through a normal structure (eg, with fever, pregnancy, hyperthyroidism). Murmurs are characterized and consequently described by several characteristics, including timing in the cardiac cycle, location on the chest wall, intensity, pitch, quality, and pattern of radiation (Chart 26-3).

Friction Rub.

In pericarditis, a harsh, grating sound that can be heard in both systole and diastole is called a friction rub. It is caused by abrasion of the pericardial surfaces during the cardiac cycle. Because a friction rub may be confused with a murmur, care should be taken to identify the sound and to distinguish it from murmurs that may be heard in both systole and diastole. A pericardial friction rub can be heard best using the diaphragm of the stethoscope, with the patient sitting up and leaning forward.

AUSCULTATION PROCEDURE

During auscultation, the patient remains supine and the examining room is as quiet as possible. A stethoscope with a diaphragm and a bell is necessary for accurate auscultation of the heart.

Using the diaphragm of the stethoscope, the examiner starts at the apical area and progresses upward along the left sternal border to the pulmonic and aortic areas. If desired, the examiner may choose to begin the examination at the aortic and pulmonic areas and progress downward to the apex of the heart. Initially, S_1 is identified and evaluated with respect to its intensity and splitting. Next, S_2 is identified, and its intensity and any splitting are noted. After concentrating on S_1 and S_2, the examiner listens for extra sounds in systole and then in diastole.

Sometimes it helps to ask the following questions: Do I hear snapping or clicking sounds? Do I hear any high-pitched blowing sounds? Is this sound in systole, or diastole, or both? The examiner again proceeds to move the stethoscope to all of the designated areas of the precordium, listening carefully for these sounds. Finally, the patient is turned on the left side and the stethoscope is placed on the apical area, where an S_3, an S_4, and a mitral murmur are more readily detected.

Once an abnormality is heard, the entire chest surface is reexamined to determine the exact location of the sound and its

Chart 26-3 Characteristics of Heart Murmurs

Heart murmurs are described in terms of location, timing, intensity, pitch, quality, and radiation. These characteristics provide data about the location and nature of the cardiac abnormality.

Location

The location of the murmur (where it is detected on the chest wall) is crucial. Depending on the type of valvular disorder, a murmur can be heard only at the apex or more widely over the chest wall, or along the left sternal border between the third and fourth interspaces.

Timing

Timing of the murmur in the cardiac cycle is vital. The examiner first determines whether the murmur is occurring in systole or in diastole. Then, does it begin simultaneously with a heart sound, or is there some delay between the sound and the beginning of the murmur? Does the murmur continue to (or through) the second heart sound, or is there a delay between the end of the murmur and the second heart sound? Are diastolic murmurs (between the second and first heart sounds) continuous, or do they subside in mid- or late diastole?

Intensity

The intensity of murmurs is conventionally graded from I through VI. Sometimes, grade I murmurs are difficult to hear. However, a grade II cardiac murmur can be easily perceived by the experienced examiner. Murmurs of grades IV or louder are usually associated with thrills that may be palpated on the surface of the chest wall. A grade VI murmur can be heard with the stethoscope off the chest. A murmur may vary in intensity from its beginning to its conclusion. This is very characteristic of certain valvular disorders.

Pitch

The next important characteristic of a murmur is its pitch, which may be low, often heard only with the bell of the stethoscope placed lightly on the chest wall, or a very high-pitched murmur, heard best with the stethoscope's diaphragm. Other murmurs contain the full spectrum of sound frequency.

Quality

In addition to the intensity and pitch, the character of the sound. A murmur may be described as rumbling, blowing, whistling, harsh, or musical.

Radiation

The last feature of concern is radiation of the murmur. A murmur can radiate into the axilla, the carotid arteries in the neck, the left shoulder, or the back.

- Location of radiation of the sound away from where it is heard the loudest.

INTERPRETATION OF CARDIAC SOUNDS

Interpreting cardiac sounds requires detailed knowledge of cardiac physiology and the pathophysiology of cardiac diseases. There are different levels of performance at which the nurse may be expected to function. The first level is simply recognizing that what one is hearing is not normal—such as a third heart sound, a murmur in systole or diastole, a pericardial friction rub over the midsternum, or a second heart sound that is widely split. These findings are reported to the physician and acted on accordingly. This level of function is useful in screening. It is the kind of activity involved in performing physical examinations in schools on normal children or in performing routine physical examinations or screening examinations.

The second level involves recognizing patterns. The nurse correctly observes the findings and can recognize the constellation of sounds and the diagnostic significance of common ones.

At its most sophisticated level, cardiac diagnosis can be interpretive. Highly skilled nurses can differentiate among dysrhythmias and respond accordingly. They can determine the significance of the appearance and disappearance of gallops during the treatment of patients who have had MIs or who have HF. This is the role that the coronary care nurse and the cardiovascular advanced practice nurse assume. They function with a team of other health care professionals who have highly tuned skills of cardiovascular assessment and diagnosis.

Inspection of the Extremities

The hands, arms, legs, and feet are observed for skin and vascular changes. The most noteworthy changes include the following:

- Decreased capillary refill time indicates a slower peripheral flow rate from sluggish reperfusion and is often observed in patients with hypotension or HF. Capillary refill time provides the basis for estimating the rate of peripheral blood flow. To test capillary refill, briefly compress the nailbed so that it blanches, and then release the pressure. Normally, reperfusion occurs within 3 seconds, as evidenced by the return of color.
- Vascular changes from decreased arterial circulation include decrease in quality or loss of pulse, discomfort or pain, paresthesia, numbness, decrease in temperature, pallor, and loss of movement. During the first few hours after invasive cardiac procedures (eg, cardiac catheterization), affected extremities should be assessed for vascular changes frequently.
- Hematoma, or a localized collection of clotted blood in the tissue, may be observed in patients who have undergone invasive cardiac procedures such as cardiac catheterization, PTCA, or cardiac electrophysiology testing. Major blood vessels of the arms and legs are selected for catheter insertion. During these procedures, systemic anticoagulation with heparin is necessary, and minor or small hematomas may occur at the catheter puncture site. However, large hematomas are a serious complication that can compromise circulating blood volume and cardiac output, requiring blood transfusions. All patients who have undergone these procedures must have their puncture sites frequently observed until hemostasis is adequately achieved.
- Peripheral edema is fluid accumulation in dependent areas of the body (feet and legs, sacrum in the bedridden patient). Assess for pitting edema (a depression over an area of pres-

radiation. Also, the patient, who may be concerned about the prolonged examination, must be supported and reassured. The auscultatory findings, particularly murmurs, are documented by identifying the following characteristics:

- Location on chest wall.
- Timing of sound as either during systole or during diastole; described as early, middle, or late. (If heard throughout the systole, the sound is often referred to as pansystolic or holosystolic.)
- Intensity of the sound (I, very faint; II, quiet; III, moderately loud; IV, loud; V, very loud; or VI, heard with stethoscope removed from the chest).
- Pitch, described as high, medium, or low.
- Quality of the sound, commonly described as blowing, harsh, or musical.

sure) by pressing firmly for 5 seconds with the thumb over the dorsum of each foot, behind each medial malleolus, and over the shins. Pitting edema is graded as absent or as present on a scale from slight (1+ = 0 to 2 mm) to very marked (4+ = more than 8 mm). Peripheral edema is observed in patients with HF and in those with peripheral vascular diseases such as deep vein thrombosis or chronic venous insufficiency.

- Clubbing of the fingers and toes implies chronic hemoglobin desaturation, as in congenital heart disease.
- Lower extremity ulcers are observed in patients with arterial or venous insufficiency. Chapter 31 provides a complete description of differentiating characteristics.

Other Systems

LUNGS

The details of respiratory assessment are described in Chapter 21. Findings frequently exhibited by cardiac patients include the following:

Tachypnea: Rapid, shallow breathing may be noted in patients who have HF or pain, and in those who are extremely anxious.

Cheyne-Stokes respirations: Patients with severe left ventricular failure may exhibit Cheyne-Stokes breathing, a pattern of rapid respirations alternating with apnea. It is important to note the duration of the apnea.

Hemoptysis: Pink, frothy sputum is indicative of acute pulmonary edema.

Cough: A dry, hacking cough from irritation of small airways is common in patients with pulmonary congestion from HF.

Crackles: HF or atelectasis associated with bed rest, splinting from ischemic pain, or the effects of pain medications and sedatives often results in the development of crackles. Typically, crackles are first noted at the bases (because of gravity's effect on fluid accumulation and decreased ventilation of basilar tissue), but they may progress to all portions of the lung fields.

Wheezes: Compression of the small airways by interstitial pulmonary edema may cause wheezing. Beta-adrenergic blocking agents (beta-blockers), such as propranolol (Inderal), may precipitate airway narrowing, especially in patients with underlying pulmonary disease.

ABDOMEN

For the cardiac patient, two components of the abdominal examination are frequently performed.

Hepatojugular reflux: Liver engorgement occurs because of decreased venous return secondary to right ventricular failure. The liver is enlarged, firm, nontender, and smooth. The hepatojugular reflux may be demonstrated by pressing firmly over the right upper quadrant of the abdomen for 30 to 60 seconds and noting a rise of 1 cm or more in jugular venous pressure. This rise indicates an inability of the right side of the heart to accommodate increased volume.

Bladder distention: Urine output is an important indicator of cardiac function, especially when urine output is reduced. This may indicate inadequate renal perfusion or a less serious problem such as one caused by urinary retention. When the urine output is decreased, the patient needs to be assessed for a distended bladder or difficulty voiding. The bladder may be assessed with an ultrasound scanner or

the suprapubic area palpated for an oval mass and percussed for dullness, indicative of a full bladder.

 Gerontologic Considerations

When performing a cardiovascular examination on an elderly patient, the nurse may note such differences as more readily palpable peripheral pulses because of increased hardness of the arteries and a loss of adjacent connective tissue. Palpation of the precordium in the elderly is affected by the changes in the shape of the chest. For example, a cardiac impulse may not be palpable in patients with chronic obstructive pulmonary disease, because these patients usually have an increased anterior-posterior chest diameter. Kyphoscoliosis, a spinal deformity that occurs frequently in elderly patients, may dislocate the cardiac apex downward so that the diagnostic significance of palpating the apical impulse is obscured.

Systolic BP increases with age, but diastolic BP usually plateaus after 50 years. Medication therapy is usually initiated for high BP when consistent systolic readings of 160 mm Hg or diastolic readings of 95 mm Hg are observed. For the elderly patient, however, many factors are considered before initiating treatment. Orthostatic hypotension may reflect a decreasing sensitivity of postural reflexes, which must be considered when medication therapy is prescribed.

An S_4 is heard in about 90% of elderly patients; this is thought to be caused by decreased compliance of the left ventricle. The S_2 is usually split. At least 60% of elderly patients have murmurs, the most common being a soft systolic ejection murmur resulting from sclerotic changes of the aortic leaflets (see Table 26-1).

Diagnostic Evaluation

Diagnostic tests and procedures are used to confirm the data obtained by history and physical assessment. Some tests are easy to interpret, but others must be interpreted by expert clinicians. All tests should be explained to the patient. Some necessitate special preparation before they are performed and special monitoring by the nurse after the procedure.

LABORATORY TESTS

Laboratory tests may be performed for the following reasons:

- To assist in diagnosing an acute MI. (Angina pectoris, chest pain resulting from an insufficient supply of blood to the heart, cannot be confirmed by either blood or urine studies.)
- To identify abnormalities in the blood that affect the prognosis of a patient with a cardiac condition
- To assess the degree of inflammation
- To screen for risk factors associated with atherosclerotic coronary artery disease
- To determine baseline values before performing therapeutic interventions
- To monitor serum levels of medications
- To assess the effects of medications (e.g., the effects of diuretics on serum potassium levels)
- To screen generally for abnormalities

Because different laboratories use different equipment and different methods of measurements, normal test values may vary depending on the laboratory and the health care institution.

Cardiac Enzyme Analysis

Plasma cardiac enzyme analysis is part of a diagnostic profile that also includes the health history, symptoms, and electrocardiogram (ECG), associated with acute MI. Enzymes are released from injured cells when the cell membranes rupture. Most enzymes are nonspecific in relation to the particular organ that has been damaged. Certain isoenzymes, however, come only from myocardial cells and are released when the cells are damaged, such as by sustained hypoxia resulting in infarction or by trauma. The isoenzymes leak into the interstitial spaces of the myocardium and are carried into the general circulation by the lymphatic system and the coronary circulation, resulting in elevated serum enzyme concentrations.

Because different enzymes move into the blood at varying periods after MI, enzyme levels should be tested in relation to the time of onset of chest discomfort or other symptoms. Creatine kinase (CK) and its isoenzyme CK-MB are the most specific enzymes analyzed in acute MI, and they are the first enzyme levels to rise. Lactic dehydrogenase and its isoenzymes also are analyzed in patients who have delayed seeking medical attention, because these blood levels rise and peak in 2 to 3 days, much later than CK levels (see Table 28-5 in Chap. 28 for the time course of cardiac enzymes).

Myoglobin, an early marker of MI, is a heme protein with a small molecular weight. This allows it to be rapidly released from damaged myocardial tissue and accounts for its early rise, within 1 to 3 hours after the onset of an acute MI. Myoglobin peaks in 4 to 12 hours and returns to normal in 24 hours. Myoglobin is not used alone to diagnose MI, because elevations can also occur in patients with renal or musculoskeletal disease. However, negative results are helpful in ruling out an early diagnosis of MI.

Troponin I is measured in a laboratory test that has several advantages over traditional enzyme studies. Troponin I is a contractile protein found only in cardiac muscle. After myocardial injury, elevated serum troponin I concentrations can be detected within 3 to 4 hours; they peak in 4 to 24 hours and remain elevated for 1 to 3 weeks. These early and prolonged elevations make very early diagnosis of MI possible or allow for late diagnosis if the patient has delayed seeking treatment.

Blood Chemistry

LIPID PROFILE

Cholesterol, triglycerides, and lipoproteins are measured to evaluate a person's risk for developing atherosclerotic disease, especially if there is a family history of premature heart disease, or to diagnose a specific lipoprotein abnormality. Cholesterol and triglycerides are transported in the blood by combining with protein molecules to form lipoproteins. The lipoproteins are referred to as low-density lipoproteins (LDL) and high-density lipoproteins (HDL). The risk of CAD increases as the ratio of LDL to HDL or the ratio of total cholesterol (LDL + HDL) to HDL increases. Although cholesterol levels remain relatively constant over 24 hours, the blood specimen for the lipid profile should be obtained after a 12-hour fast.

CHOLESTEROL LEVELS

Cholesterol (normal level, less than 200 mg/dL) is a lipid required for hormone synthesis and cell membrane formation. It is found in large quantities in brain and nerve tissue. Two major sources of cholesterol are diet (animal products) and the liver, where cholesterol is synthesized. Elevated cholesterol levels are known to increase the risk for CAD. Factors that contribute to variations in cholesterol levels include age, gender, diet, exercise patterns, genetics, menopause, tobacco use, and stress levels.

LDLs (normal level, less than 130 mg/dL) are the primary transporters of cholesterol and triglycerides into the cell. One harmful effect of LDL is the deposition of these substances in the walls of arterial vessels. Elevated LDL levels are associated with a greater incidence of CAD. In people with known CAD or diabetes, the primary goal for lipid management is reduction of LDL levels to less than 100 mg/dL.

HDLs (normal range in men, 35 to 65 mg/dL; in women, 35 to 85 mg/dL) have a protective action. They transport cholesterol away from the tissue and cells of the arterial wall to the liver for excretion. Therefore, there is an inverse relationship between HDL levels and risk for CAD. Factors that lower HDL levels include smoking, diabetes, obesity, and physical inactivity. In patients with CAD, a secondary goal of lipid management is the increase of HDL levels to more than 40 mg/dL.

Triglycerides (normal range, 40 to 150 mg/dL), composed of free fatty acids and glycerol, are stored in the adipose tissue and are a source of energy. Triglyceride levels increase after meals and are affected by stress. Diabetes, alcohol use, and obesity can elevate triglyceride levels. These levels have a direct correlation with LDL and an inverse one with HDL.

SERUM ELECTROLYTE LEVELS

Sodium, potassium, and calcium are ions that are vital to cellular depolarization and repolarization. In addition, the serum sodium concentration reflects relative fluid balance. Generally, hyponatremia (low sodium level) indicates fluid excess, and hypernatremia (high sodium level) indicates fluid deficit.

Serum potassium is affected by renal function and may be decreased by diuretic agents that are used to treat HF. A decrease in potassium causes cardiac irritability and predisposes the patient receiving a digitalis preparation to digitalis toxicity and dysrhythmias. The effect of an elevated serum potassium concentration is myocardial depression and ventricular irritability. Both hypokalemia and hyperkalemia can lead to ventricular fibrillation or cardiac standstill. Calcium is necessary for blood coagulability and neuromuscular activity. Hypocalcemia and hypercalcemia can cause dysrhythmias.

Magnesium is integral to the absorption of calcium and the maintenance of potassium stores. It is required in the metabolism of adenosine triphosphate, playing a major role in protein synthesis, carbohydrate metabolism, and muscular contraction. Initial symptoms of hypermagnesemia are lethargy and decreased neuromuscular activity. On the ECG, hypomagnesemia lengthens the QT interval, predisposing the patient to life-threatening dysrhythmias.

BLOOD UREA NITROGEN LEVEL

Blood urea nitrogen (BUN) is an end product of protein metabolism and is excreted by the kidneys. In the patient with cardiac disease, an elevated BUN level may reflect reduced renal perfusion (from decreased cardiac output) or intravascular fluid volume deficit (from diuretic therapy or dehydration). The cause of elevated BUN is determined from the serum creatinine: high BUN and high creatinine reflect renal impairment, high BUN and normal creatinine reflect intravascular fluid volume deficit.

SERUM GLUCOSE LEVEL

The serum glucose level is important to monitor, because many patients with cardiac disease also have diabetes mellitus. In addition, the serum glucose level may be mildly elevated in stressful situations, when mobilization of endogenous epinephrine results in conversion of liver glycogen to glucose. Serum glucose levels are drawn in a fasting state. Glycosylated hemoglobin is an important measure to monitor in people with diabetes, because it reflects the blood glucose levels over 2 to 3 months. Hemoglobin A_{1C} is the common name for this test. The goal of diabetes management is to maintain the hemoglobin A_{1C} below 7% (normal range 4%–6%), reflecting consistent near-normal blood glucose levels. This is particularly important for primary and secondary prevention of CVD (Brundy et al., 2002; Smith et al., 2001).

Coagulation Studies

The formation of a thrombus is initiated by injury to a vessel wall or to the tissue. These events activate the coagulation cascade, a complex series of interactions among phospholipids, calcium, and various clotting factors that converts prothrombin to thrombin. The coagulation cascade has two pathways, the intrinsic pathway and the extrinsic pathway. Coagulation studies are routinely performed before invasive procedures, such as cardiac catheterization, electrophysiology testing, and coronary or cardiac surgery.

Partial thromboplastin time (PTT) and activated partial thromboplastin time (aPTT) measure the activity of the intrinsic pathway. The values of PTT and aPTT are used to assess the effects of heparin therapy. Patients receiving heparin have their PTT or aPTT levels maintained at 1.5 to 2.5 times their baseline values (reference range, 25 to 38 seconds). Prothrombin time (PT) measures the extrinsic pathway activity and is used to monitor the effects of therapeutic anticoagulation with warfarin (Coumadin). Laboratory results of PT also include the **International Normalized Ratio (INR)**. The INR provides a standard method for reporting PT levels, eliminating the variation of PT results from laboratory to laboratory. The INR, rather than the PT alone, is used to monitor patients receiving warfarin therapy. The INR is maintained between 2.0 and 3.0 for patients with deep vein thrombosis, pulmonary embolism, valvular heart disease, or atrial fibrillation, and between 2.5 and 3.5 for patients with mechanical prosthetic heart valve replacements.

Hematologic Studies

The complete blood cell count (CBC) identifies the total number of white and red blood cells, the platelet count, and the hemoglobin and hematocrit. The CBC is carefully monitored in patients with CVD. White blood cell counts are monitored in immunocompromised patients, including patients with transplanted hearts, and in situations where there is concern for infection (eg, after invasive procedures or surgery). The red blood cells carry hemoglobin, which transports oxygen to the cells. The hematocrit is a measure of the relative proportion of red blood cells and plasma. Low hemoglobin and hematocrit levels have serious consequences for patients with CAD, such as more frequent angina episodes. Platelets are the first line of protection against bleeding. Once activated by blood vessel wall injury or rupture of atherosclerotic plaque, platelets undergo chemical changes that form a thrombus. Patients are prescribed medications to inhibit platelet function, including aspirin, clopidogrel (Plavix), and intravenous GP IIb/IIIa inhibitors (abciximab [ReoPro], eptifibatide [Integrilin], tirofiban [Aggrastat]); therefore, it is essential to monitor for thrombocytopenia (low platelet counts). Chapter 33 provides an in-depth review of these laboratory tests and normal values.

CHEST X-RAY AND FLUOROSCOPY

A chest x-ray usually is obtained to determine the size, contour, and position of the heart. It reveals cardiac and pericardial calcifications and demonstrates physiologic alterations in the pulmonary circulation. It does not help diagnose acute MI but can help diagnose some complications (eg, HF). Correct placement of cardiac catheters, such as pacemakers and pulmonary artery catheters, is also confirmed by chest x-ray.

Fluoroscopy allows visualization of the heart on an x-ray screen. It shows cardiac and vascular pulsations and unusual cardiac contours. Fluoroscopy is useful for positioning intravenous pacing electrodes and for guiding catheter insertion during cardiac catheterization.

ELECTROCARDIOGRAPHY

The ECG is a diagnostic tool used in assessing the cardiovascular system. It is a graphic recording of the electrical activity of the heart; an ECG can be recorded with 12, 15, or 18 leads, showing the activity from those different reference points. The ECG is obtained by placing disposable electrodes in standard positions on the skin of the chest wall and extremities. The heart's electrical impulses are recorded as a tracing on special graph paper.

The standard 12-lead ECG is the most commonly used tool to diagnose dysrhythmias, conduction abnormalities, enlarged heart chambers, myocardial ischemia or infarction, high or low calcium and potassium levels, and effects of some medications. A 15-lead ECG adds 3 additional chest leads across the right precordium and is a valuable tool for the early diagnosis of right ventricular and posterior left ventricular infarction. The 18-lead ECG adds 3 posterior leads to the 15-lead ECG and is very useful for early detection of myocardial ischemia and injury (Wung & Drew, 1999). To enhance interpretation of the ECG, the patient's age, gender, BP, height, weight, symptoms, and medications (especially digitalis and antiarrhythmic agents) should be noted on the ECG requisition. The details of electrocardiography are covered in Chapter 27.

Continuous Electrocardiographic Monitoring

Continuous ECG monitoring is standard for patients who are at high risk for dysrhythmias. Two continuous ECG monitoring techniques are hardwire monitoring, found in critical care units and specialty step-down units, and telemetry, found in specialty step-down units and general nursing care units. Patients who are receiving continuous ECG monitoring need to be informed of its purpose and cautioned that this monitoring method will not detect symptoms such as dyspnea or chest pain. Therefore, patients need to be advised to report symptoms to the nurse whenever they occur.

HARDWIRE CARDIAC MONITORING

The patient's ECG can be continuously observed for dysrhythmias and conduction disorders on an oscilloscope at the bedside or at a central monitoring station by a hardwire monitoring system. This system is composed of three to five electrodes positioned on the patient's chest, a lead cable, and a bedside monitor. Hardwire monitoring systems vary in sophistication but in general can do the following:

- Monitor more than one lead simultaneously
- Monitor ST segments (ST-segment depression is a marker of myocardial ischemia; ST-segment elevation provides evidence of an evolving MI)

- Provide graded visual and audible alarms (based on priority, asystole would be highest)
- Computerize rhythm monitoring (dysrhythmias are interpreted and stored in memory)
- Print a rhythm strip
- Record a 12-lead ECG

Two leads commonly used for continuous monitoring are leads II and V1 or a modification of V1 (MCL1) (Fig. 26-10). Lead II provides the best visualization of atrial depolarization (represented by the P wave). Leads V1 and MCL1 best visualize the ventricle responsible for ectopic or abnormal ventricular beats.

TELEMETRY

In addition to hardwire monitoring systems, the ECG can be continuously observed by **telemetry**, the transmission of radio-waves from a battery-operated transmitter worn by the patient to a central bank of monitors. Although telemetry systems have the same capabilities as hardwire systems, they are wireless, allowing the patient to ambulate while being monitored. Following the guidelines for electrode placement will ensure good conduction and a clear picture of the patient's rhythm on the monitor:

- Clean the skin surface with soap and water and dry well (or as recommended by the manufacturer) before applying the electrodes. If the patient has much hair where the electrodes need to be placed, shave or clip the hair.
- Apply a small amount of benzoin to the skin if the patient is diaphoretic (sweaty) and the electrodes do not adhere well.
- Change the electrodes every 24 to 48 hours and examine the skin for irritation. Apply the electrodes to different locations each time they are changed.
- If the patient is sensitive to the electrodes, use hypoallergenic electrodes.

SIGNAL-AVERAGED ELECTROCARDIOGRAM

For some patients who are considered to be at high risk for sudden cardiac death, a signal-averaged ECG is performed. This high-resolution ECG assists in identifying the risk for life-threatening dysrhythmias and helps to determine the need for invasive diagnostic procedures. Signal averaging works by averaging about 150 to 300 QRS waveforms (QRS waveforms represent depolarization of the ventricle). The resulting averaged QRS complex is analyzed for certain characteristics that are likely to lead to lethal ventricular dysrhythmias. The recording is performed at the bedside and requires about 15 minutes.

CONTINUOUS AMBULATORY MONITORING

In ambulatory ECG monitoring, which may occur in the hospital but is more commonly prescribed for outpatients, one lead of the patient's ECG can be monitored by a Holter monitor. This monitor is a small tape recorder that continuously (for 10 to 24 hours) documents the heart's electrical activity on a magnetic tape. The tape recorder weighs approximately 2 pounds and can be carried over the shoulder or worn around the waist day and night to detect dysrhythmias or evidence of myocardial ischemia during activities of daily living. The patient keeps a diary of activity, noting the time of any symptoms, experiences, or unusual activities performed. The tape recording is then examined with a special scanner, analyzed, and interpreted. Evidence obtained in this way helps the physician diagnose dysrhythmias and myocardial ischemia and evaluate therapy, such as anti-arrhythmic and antianginal medications or pacemaker function.

TRANSTELEPHONIC MONITORING

Another method of evaluating the ECG of a patient at home is by transtelephonic monitoring. The patient attaches a specific lead system for transmitting the signals and places a telephone mouthpiece over the transmitter box; the ECG is recorded and evaluated at another location. This method is often used for diagnosing dysrhythmias and in follow-up evaluation of permanent cardiac pacemakers.

CARDIAC STRESS TESTING

Normally, the coronary arteries dilate to four times their usual diameter in response to increased metabolic demands for oxygen and nutrients. Coronary arteries with atherosclerosis, however, dilate much less, compromising blood flow to the myocardium and causing ischemia. Therefore, abnormalities in cardiovascular function are more likely to be detected during times of increased demand, or "stress." The **cardiac stress test** procedures—the exercise stress test, the pharmacologic stress test, and, more recently, the mental or emotional stress test—are noninvasive ways to evaluate the response of the cardiovascular system to stress. The stress

FIGURE 26-10 Two leads (views of the heart) commonly used for continuous monitoring. To monitor lead II, the negative electrode is placed on the right upper chest; the positive electrode is placed on the left lower chest. To monitor MCL1, the negative electrode is placed on the left upper chest; the positive electrode is placed in the V1 position. If three electrodes are used, the third electrode, which is the ground electrode, can be placed anywhere on the chest.

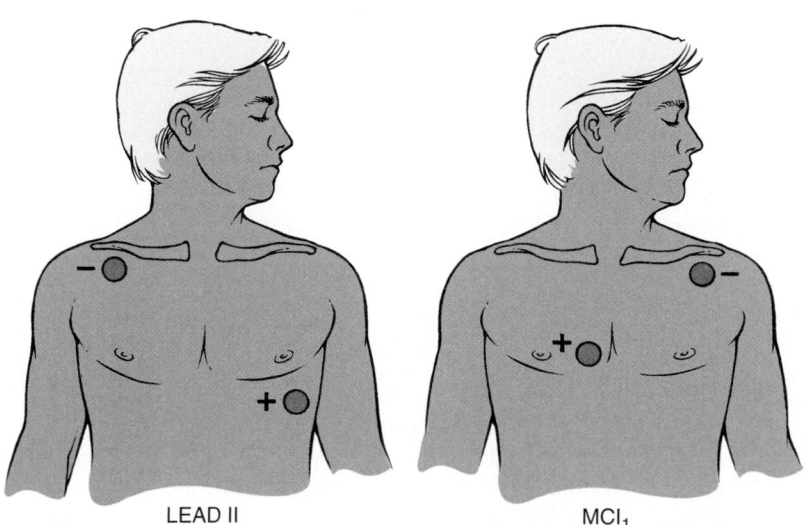

LEAD II   MCI₁

test helps determine the following: (1) CAD, (2) cause of chest pain, (3) functional capacity of the heart after an MI or heart surgery, (4) effectiveness of antianginal or antiarrhythmic medications, (5) dysrhythmias that occur during physical exercise, and (6) specific goals for a physical fitness program. Contraindications to stress testing include severe aortic stenosis, acute myocarditis or pericarditis, severe hypertension, suspected left main CAD, HF, and unstable angina. Because complications associated with stress testing can be life-threatening (MI, cardiac arrest, HF, and severe dysrhythmias), testing facilities must have staff and equipment ready to provide advanced cardiac life support.

Mental stress testing uses a mental arithmetic test or simulated public speech to determine whether an ischemic myocardial response occurs, similar to the response evoked by a conventional treadmill exercise test. Although its use for diagnostic purposes in patients with CAD is currently investigational, preliminary results indicate that the ischemic and hemodynamic measures obtained from mental stress testing may be useful in assessing the prognosis of patients with CHD who have had a positive exercise test (Krantz et al., 1999).

Stress testing is often combined with echocardiography or radionuclide imaging (discussed later). These techniques are performed during the resting state and immediately after stress.

Exercise Stress Testing

In an exercise stress test, the patient walks on a treadmill (most common) or pedals a stationary bicycle or arm crank. Exercise intensity progresses according to established protocols. The Bruce protocol, for example, is a common treadmill protocol in which the speed and grade of the treadmill are increased every 3 minutes. The goal of the test is to increase the heart rate to the "target heart rate." This is 80% to 90% of the maximum predicted heart rate and is based on the age and gender of the patient. During the test, the following are monitored: two or more ECG leads for heart rate, rhythm, and ischemic changes; BP; skin temperature; physical appearance; perceived exertion; and symptoms including chest pain, dyspnea, dizziness, leg cramping, and fatigue. The test is terminated when the target heart rate is achieved or when the patient experiences chest pain, extreme fatigue, a decrease in BP or pulse rate, serious dysrhythmias or ST segment changes on ECG, or other complications. When significant ECG abnormalities occur during the stress test (ST segment depressions), the test result is reported as positive and further diagnostic testing is required.

NURSING INTERVENTIONS

In preparation for the exercise stress test, the patient is instructed to fast for 4 hours before the test and to avoid stimulants such as tobacco and caffeine. Medications may be taken with sips of water. The physician may instruct patients not to take certain cardiac medications, such as beta-blockers, before the test. Clothes and sneakers or rubber-soled shoes suitable for exercising are to be worn. Women are advised to wear a bra that provides adequate support. The nurse describes the equipment used and the sensations and experiences that the patient may have during the test. The nurse explains the monitoring equipment used, the need to have an intravenous line placed, and the symptoms to report. The type of exercise is reviewed, and patients are asked to put forth their best exercise effort. If the test is to be performed with echocardiography or radionuclide imaging, this information is reviewed as well. After the test, patients are monitored for 10 to 15 minutes. Once stable, they may resume their usual activities.

Pharmacologic Stress Testing

Physically disabled or deconditioned patients will not be able to achieve their target heart rate by exercising on a treadmill or bicycle. Two vasodilating agents, dipyridamole (Persantin) and adenosine (Adenocard), administered intravenously, are used to mimic the effects of exercise by maximally dilating the coronary arteries. The effects of dipyridamole last about 15 to 30 minutes. The side effects are related to its vasodilating action and include chest discomfort, dizziness, headache, flushing, and nausea. Adenosine has similar side effects, although patients report these symptoms as more severe. A unique property of adenosine is that it has an extremely short half-life (less than 10 seconds), so any severe effects rapidly subside. Dipyridamole and adenosine are the agents of choice used in conjunction with radionuclide imaging techniques. Theophylline and other xanthines, such as caffeine, block the effects of dipyridamole and adenosine and must be avoided before either of these pharmacologic stress tests.

Dobutamine (Dobutrex) is another medication that may be used for patients who cannot exercise. Dobutamine, a synthetic sympathomimetic, increases heart rate, myocardial contractility, and BP, thereby increasing the metabolic demands of the heart. It is the agent of choice when echocardiography is used because of its effects on altering myocardial wall motion (due to enhanced contractility). In addition, dobutamine is used for patients who have bronchospasm or pulmonary disease and cannot tolerate having doses of theophylline withheld.

NURSING INTERVENTIONS

In preparation for the pharmacologic stress test, patients are instructed not to eat or drink anything for at least 4 hours before the test. This includes chocolate, caffeine, caffeine-free coffee, tea, carbonated beverages, or medications with caffeine (eg, Anacin, Darvon). If caffeine is ingested before a dipyridamole or adenosine stress test, the test will have to be rescheduled. Patients taking aminophylline or theophylline are instructed to stop taking these medications for 24 to 48 hours before the test (if tolerated). Oral doses of dipyridamole are to be withheld as well. Patients are informed about the transient sensations they may experience during infusion of the vasodilating agent, such as flushing or nausea, which will disappear quickly. The patient is instructed to report any other symptoms occurring during the test to the cardiologist or nurse. An explanation of echocardiography or radionuclide imaging is also provided as necessary. The stress test may take about 1 hour, or up to 3 hours if imaging is performed.

ECHOCARDIOGRAPHY

Echocardiography is a noninvasive ultrasound test that is used to examine the size, shape, and motion of cardiac structures. It is a particularly useful tool for diagnosing pericardial effusions, determining the etiology of heart murmurs, evaluating the function of prosthetic heart valves, determining chamber size, and evaluating ventricular wall motion. It involves transmission of high-frequency sound waves into the heart through the chest wall and recording of the return signals. The ultrasound is generated by a hand-held transducer applied to the front of the chest. The transducer picks up the echoes, converts them to electrical impulses, and transmits them to the echocardiography machine for display on an oscilloscope and recording on a videotape. An ECG is recorded simultaneously to assist with interpreting the echocardiogram.

M-mode (motion), the unidimensional mode that was first introduced, provides information about the cardiac structures and their motion. Two-dimensional or cross-sectional echocardiography (Fig. 26-11), an enhancement of the technique, creates a sophisticated, spatially correct image of the heart. Other techniques, such as Doppler and color flow imaging echocardiography, show the direction and velocity of the blood flow through the heart.

As previously mentioned, echocardiography may be performed with an exercise or pharmacologic stress test; resting and stress images are obtained. Myocardial ischemia from decreased perfusion during stress causes abnormalities in ventricular wall motion and is easily detected by echocardiography. A stress test using echocardiography is considered positive if abnormalities in ventricular wall motion are detected during stress but not during rest. These findings are highly suggestive of CAD and require further evaluation, such as a cardiac catheterization.

Transesophageal Echocardiography

A significant limitation of traditional echocardiography has been the poor quality of the images produced. Ultrasound loses its clarity as it passes through tissue, lung, and bone. Another echocardiographic technique involves threading a small transducer through the mouth and into the esophagus. This technique, called transesophageal echocardiography (TEE), provides clearer images because ultrasound waves are passing through less tissue. Pharmacologic stress testing using dobutamine and TEE can also be performed. The high-quality imaging obtained during TEE makes this technique an important adjunct to the technology available for detecting and evaluating the severity of CAD. Complications are uncommon during TEE, but if they do occur they are serious. These complications are caused by sedation and impaired swallowing from topical anesthesia (respiratory depression and aspiration) and by insertion and manipulation of the transducer into the esophagus and stomach (vasovagal response or esophageal perforation). The patient must be assessed before TEE for a history of dysphagia or radiation therapy to the chest that would increase the risk for complications.

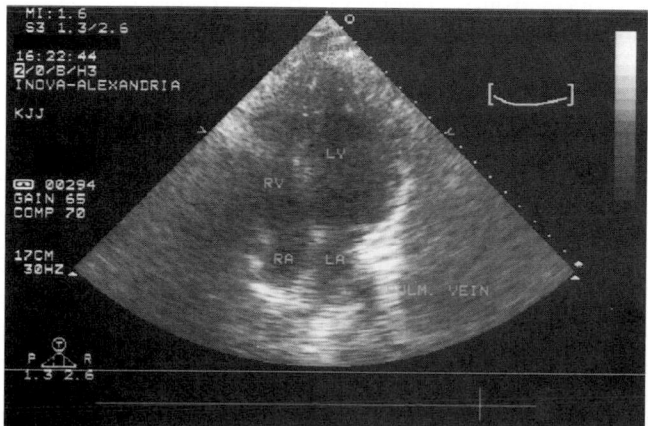

FIGURE 26-11 Two-dimensional echocardiogram, four-chamber view in a normal patient. The ventricles and atria are the dark areas outlined by the white. LA = left atrium, LV = left ventricle, RA = right atrium, RV = right ventricle. Courtesy of V. Bowles, RCS, CCT, Inova Alexandria Hospital, Alexandria, Virginia.

NURSING INTERVENTIONS

Before traditional echocardiography, the nurse informs the patient about the test, explaining that it is painless. Echocardiographic monitoring is performed while a transducer that emits the sound waves is moved about the chest. Gel applied to the skin helps transmit the sound waves. Periodically, the patient will have to turn onto the left side or hold a breath. The test takes about 30 to 45 minutes. If the patient is to undergo an exercise or pharmacologic stress test with echocardiography, information on stress testing is also reviewed.

In preparation for a TEE study, the following information is reviewed:

- The patient must fast for 6 hours before the study.
- An intravenous line is started for administering a sedative and any pharmacologic stress testing medications.
- The patient's throat is anesthetized before the probe is inserted.
- BP and the ECG are monitored throughout the study.
- The patient will be kept comfortable but not heavily sedated. The patient must be alert enough to follow instructions and to report symptoms such as chest pain.

After the study, monitoring continues for 30 to 60 minutes. The patient is to continue fasting for 4 hours. The patient may have a sore throat for the next 24 hours.

RADIONUCLIDE IMAGING

Radionuclide imaging studies involve the use of radioisotopes to evaluate coronary artery perfusion noninvasively, to detect myocardial ischemia and infarction, and to assess left ventricular function. **Radioisotopes** are atoms in an unstable form. Thallium 201 (Tl^{201}) and technetium 99m (Tc^{99m}) are two of the most common radioisotopes used in cardiac nuclear medicine studies. As they decay, they give off small amounts of energy in the form of gamma rays. When they are injected intravenously into the bloodstream, the energy emitted by the radioisotope can be detected by a gamma scintillation camera positioned over the body. Planar imaging, used with thallium, is a technique that provides a one-dimensional view of the heart from three locations. A relatively new technique called single photon emission computed tomography (SPECT) provides three-dimensional images. With SPECT, the patient is positioned supine with arms raised above the head, while the camera moves around the patient's chest in a 180- to 360-degree arc to identify the areas of decreased myocardial perfusion more precisely.

Myocardial Perfusion Imaging

The radioisotope Tl^{201} is used to assess myocardial perfusion. It resembles potassium and readily crosses into the cells of healthy myocardium. It is taken up more slowly and in smaller amounts by myocardial cells that are ischemic from decreased blood flow. However, thallium will not cross into the necrotic tissue that results from an MI.

Often, thallium is used with stress testing to assess changes in myocardial perfusion immediately after exercise (or after injection of one of the agents used in stress testing) and at rest. One or two minutes before the end of the stress test, a dose of Tl^{201} is injected into the intravenous line, allowing the radioisotope to be distributed into the myocardium. Images are taken immediately. Areas that do not show thallium uptake are noted as defects and indicate areas of either infarction or stress-induced myocardial ischemia. The resting images, taken 3 hours later, help to differentiate infarction from ischemia. Infarcted tissue is unable to take up thallium regardless of when the scan is taken; the defect remains the same size. This is called a fixed defect, indicating that there is no perfusion in that area of the myocardium. Ischemic myocardium, on the other hand, recovers in a few hours. Once perfusion is restored, thallium crosses into the myocardial cells, and the area of defect on the resting images is either smaller or completely reversed. These reversible defects constitute positive stress test findings. Usually, cardiac catheterization is recommended after a positive test result to determine whether angioplasty or coronary artery bypass graft surgery is needed.

Another radioisotope used for cardiac imaging is Tc^{99m}. Technetium can be combined with various chemical compounds, giving it an affinity for different types of cells. For example, Tc^{99m} sestamibi (Cardiolite) is distributed to myocardial cells in proportion to their amount of perfusion, making this tracer excellent for assessing perfusion to the myocardium. The procedure for cardiac imaging using Tc^{99m} sestamibi with stress testing is similar to the one using thallium, with two differences. Patients receiving Tc^{99m} sestamibi can have their resting images recorded before or after the exercise images. Timing of the images is not important because the half-life of Tc^{99m} is short, and Tc^{99m} needs to be injected before each scan. Also, SPECT imaging with Tc^{99m} sestamibi provides high-quality images.

NURSING INTERVENTIONS

The patient undergoing nuclear imaging techniques with stress testing should be prepared for the type of stressor to be used (exercise or drug) and the type of imaging technique (planar or SPECT). The patient may be concerned about receiving a radioactive substance and needs to be reassured that these tracers are safe, the radiation exposure being similar to that of other diagnostic x-ray studies. No postprocedure radiation precautions are necessary.

When providing teaching for patients undergoing SPECT, the nurse should instruct them that their arms will need to be positioned over their head for about 20 to 30 minutes. If they are physically unable to do this, thallium with planar imaging can be used.

Test of Ventricular Function and Wall Motion

Equilibrium radionuclide angiocardiography (ERNA), also known as multiple-gated acquisition (MUGA) scanning, is a common noninvasive technique that uses a conventional scintillation camera interfaced with a computer to record images of the heart during several hundred heartbeats. The computer processes the data and allows for sequential viewing of the functioning heart. The sequential images are analyzed to evaluate left ventricular function, wall motion, and ejection fraction. MUGA scanning can also be used to assess the differences in left ventricular function during rest and exercise.

The patient is reassured that there is no known radiation danger and is instructed to remain motionless during the scan.

Computed Tomography

Computed tomography (CT), also called computerized axial tomographic (CAT) scanning or electron-beam computed tomography (EBCT), uses x-rays to provide cross-sectional images of the chest, including the heart and great vessels. These techniques are used to evaluate cardiac masses and diseases of the aorta and pericardium.

EBCT, also known as the Ultrafast CT, is an especially fast x-ray scanning technique that results in much faster image acquisition with a higher degree of resolution than traditional x-ray or CT scanning provides (Woods et al., 1999). It is used to evaluate bypass graft patency, congenital heart lesions, left and right ventricular muscle mass, chamber volumes, cardiac output, and ejection fraction. For people without previous MI, PTCA, or coronary artery bypass surgery, the EBCT is used to determine the amount of calcium deposits in the coronary arteries and underlying atherosclerosis. From this scan, a calcium score is derived that predicts the incidence of cardiac events, such as MI or the need for a revascularization procedure within the next 1 to 2 years.

The EBCT is not widely used, but it does show great promise for early detection of CAD that is not yet clinically significant and that would not be identified by traditional testing methods, such as the exercise stress test.

NURSING INTERVENTIONS

Patient preparation is the primary role of the nurse for these tests. The nurse should instruct the patient that he will be positioned on a table during the scan while the scanner rotates around him. The procedure is noninvasive and painless. However, to obtain adequate images, the patient must lie perfectly still during the scanning process. An intravenous access line is necessary if contrast enhancement is to be used.

Positron Emission Tomography

Positron emission tomography (PET) is a noninvasive scanning method that was used in the past primarily to study neurologic dysfunction. More recently, and with increasing frequency, PET has been used to diagnose cardiac dysfunction. PET provides more specific information about myocardial perfusion and viability than does TEE or thallium scanning. For cardiac patients, including those without symptoms, PET helps in planning treatment (eg, coronary artery bypass surgery, angioplasty). PET also helps evaluate the patency of native and previously grafted vessels and the collateral circulation.

During a PET scan, radioisotopes are administered by injection; one compound is used to determine blood flow in the myocardium, and another shows the metabolic function. The PET camera provides detailed three-dimensional images of the distributed compounds. The viability of the myocardium is determined by comparing the extent of glucose metabolism in the myocardium to the degree of blood flow. For example, ischemic but viable tissue would show decreased blood flow and elevated metabolism. For a patient with this finding, revascularization through surgery or angioplasty would be likely to improve heart function. Restrictions of food intake before the test vary among institutions, but, because PET evaluates glucose metabolism, the patient's blood glucose level should be in the normal range. Although PET equipment is costly, it is increasingly valued and available.

NURSING INTERVENTIONS

Nurses involved in PET and other scanning procedures may instruct the patient to refrain from using tobacco and ingesting caffeine for 4 hours before the procedure. They should also reassure the patient that radiation exposure is at safe and acceptable levels, similar to those of other diagnostic x-ray studies.

Magnetic Resonance Imaging

Magnetic resonance imaging (MRI) is a noninvasive, painless technique that is used to examine both the physiologic and anatomic properties of the heart. MRI uses a powerful magnetic field and computer-generated pictures to image the heart and great vessels. It is valuable in diagnosing diseases of the aorta, heart muscle, and pericardium, as well as congenital heart lesions. The application of this technique to the evaluation of coronary artery anatomy, cardiac blood flow, and myocardial viability in conjunction with pharmacologic stress testing is being investigated.

NURSING INTERVENTIONS

Because of the strong magnetic field used during MRI, diagnostic centers where these procedures are performed carefully screen patients for contraindications. Standardized questionnaires are commonly used to determine whether the patient has a pacemaker, metal plates, prosthetic joints, or other metallic implants that can become dislodged if exposed to MRI. During an MRI, the patient is positioned supine on a table that is placed into an enclosed imager or tube that contains the magnetic field. People who are claustrophobic may need to receive a mild sedative before undergoing an MRI. As the MRI is performed, there is an intermittent clanking or thumping sound from the magnetic coils that can be annoying to the patient, so patients are offered headsets to listen to music. The scanner is equipped with a microphone so that the patient can communicate with the staff. During the scanning, the patient is instructed to remain still and not move.

 **NURSING ALERT** No metal can be in the MRI room because metal objects can become dangerous projectiles; this includes such items as clipboards, paperclips, oxygen tanks, and monitors.

CARDIAC CATHETERIZATION

Cardiac catheterization is an invasive diagnostic procedure in which radiopaque arterial and venous catheters are introduced into selected blood vessels of the right and left sides of the heart. Catheter advancement is guided by fluoroscopy. Most commonly, the catheters are inserted percutaneously through the blood vessels, or via a cutdown procedure if the patient has poor vascular access. Pressures and oxygen saturations in the four heart chambers are measured. Cardiac catheterization is used to diagnose CAD, assess coronary artery patency, and determine the extent of atherosclerosis based on the percentage of coronary artery obstruction. These results determine whether revascularization procedures including PTCA or coronary artery bypass surgery may be of benefit to the patient (see Chap. 28).

During cardiac catheterization, the patient has an intravenous line in place for the administration of sedatives, fluids, heparin, and other medications. Noninvasive hemodynamic monitoring that includes BP and multiple ECG tracings is necessary to continuously observe for dysrhythmias or hemodynamic instability. The myocardium can become ischemic and trigger dysrhythmias as catheters are positioned in the coronary arteries or during injection of contrast agents. Resuscitation equipment must be readily available during the procedure. Staff must be prepared to provide advanced cardiac life support measures as necessary.

Radiopaque contrast agents are used to visualize the coronary arteries; some contrast agents contain iodine. The patient is assessed before the procedure for previous reactions to contrast agents or allergies to iodine-containing substances (eg, seafood). If the patient has a suspected or known allergy to the substance, antihistamines or methylprednisolone (Solu-Medrol) may be administered before the procedure. In addition, the following blood tests are performed to identify abnormalities that may complicate recovery: BUN and creatinine levels, INR or PT, aPTT, hematocrit and hemoglobin values, platelet count, and electrolyte levels.

Diagnostic cardiac catheterizations are commonly performed on an outpatient basis and require 2 to 6 hours of bed rest before ambulation. For most patients, bed rest for 6 hours compared to 2 hours has no advantage with regard to groin bleeding complications (Logemann et al., 1999). However, variations in time to ambulation are most often related to the size of the catheter used during the procedure, the anticoagulation status of the patient, other patient variables (eg, advanced age, obesity, bleeding disorder), the method used for hemostasis of the arterial puncture site after the procedure, and institutional policies. The use of smaller (4 or 6 Fr) catheters, which are more amenable to shorter recovery times, is common in diagnostic cardiac catheterizations. There are several methods available to achieve arterial hemostasis after catheter removal, including manual pressure, mechanical compression devices such as the FemoStop (placed over puncture site for 30 minutes), and percutaneously deployed devices. The latter devices are positioned at the femoral arterial puncture site after completion of the procedure. They deploy collagen (VasoSeal), sutures (Perclose, Techstar), or a combination of both (Angio-Seal). Major benefits of these devices include reliable, immediate hemostasis and shorter time on bed rest without a significant increase in bleeding or other complications (Baim et al., 2000). A number of factors determine which hemostatic methods are used and are based on the physician's preference, the patient's condition, cost, and institutional availability of the equipment.

Patients hospitalized for angina or acute MI may also require cardiac catheterization. After the procedure, these patients usually return to their hospital rooms for recovery. In some cardiac catheterization laboratories, an angioplasty may be performed immediately after the catheterization if indicated.

ANGIOGRAPHY

Cardiac catheterization is usually performed with angiography, a technique of injecting a contrast agent into the vascular system to outline the heart and blood vessels. When a particular heart chamber or blood vessel is singled out for study, the procedure is known as selective angiography. Angiography makes use of cineangiograms, a series of rapidly changing films on an intensified fluoroscopic screen that record the passage of the contrast agent through the vascular site or sites. The recorded information allows for comparison of data over time. Common sites for selective angiography are the aorta, the coronary arteries, and the right and left sides of the heart.

Aortography

An aortogram is a form of angiography that outlines the lumen of the aorta and the major arteries arising from it. In thoracic aortography, a contrast agent is used to study the aortic arch and its major branches. The catheter may be introduced into the aorta using the translumbar or retrograde brachial or femoral artery approach.

Coronary Arteriography

In coronary arteriography, the catheter is introduced into the right or left brachial or femoral artery, then passed into the ascending aorta and manipulated into the appropriate coronary artery. Coronary arteriography is used to evaluate the degree of atherosclerosis and to guide the selection of treatment. It is also used to study suspected congenital anomalies of the coronary arteries.

Right Heart Catheterization

Right heart catheterization usually precedes left heart catheterization. It involves the passage of a catheter from an antecubital or femoral vein into the right atrium, right ventricle, pulmonary artery, and pulmonary arterioles. Pressures and oxygen saturations from each of these areas are obtained and recorded.

Although right heart catheterization is considered a relatively safe procedure, potential complications include cardiac dysrhythmias, venous spasm, infection of the insertion site, cardiac perforation, and, rarely, cardiac arrest.

Left Heart Catheterization

Left heart catheterization is performed to evaluate the patency of the coronary arteries and the function of the left ventricle and the mitral and aortic valves. Potential complications include dysrhythmias, MI, perforation of the heart or great vessels, and systemic embolization. Left heart catheterization is performed by retrograde catheterization of the left ventricle. In this approach, the physician usually inserts the catheter into the right brachial artery or a femoral artery and advances it into the aorta and left ventricle.

After the procedure, the catheter is carefully withdrawn and arterial hemostasis is achieved using manual pressure or other techniques previously described. If the physician performed an arterial or venous cutdown, the site is sutured and a sterile dressing is applied.

NURSING INTERVENTIONS

Nursing responsibilities before cardiac catheterization include the following:

- Instruct the patient to fast, usually for 8 to 12 hours, before the procedure. If catheterization is to be performed as an outpatient procedure, explain that a friend, family member, or other responsible person must transport the patient home.
- Prepare the patient for the expected duration of the procedure; indicate that it will involve lying on a hard table for less than 2 hours.
- Reassure the patient that mild sedatives or moderate sedation will be given intravenously.
- Prepare the patient to experience certain sensations during the catheterization. Knowing what to expect can help the patient cope with the experience. Explain that an occasional pounding sensation (palpitation) may be felt in the chest because of extrasystoles that almost always occur, particularly when the catheter tip touches the myocardium. The patient may be asked to cough and to breathe deeply, especially after the injection of contrast agent. Coughing may help to disrupt a dysrhythmia and to clear the contrast agent from the arteries. Breathing deeply and holding the breath helps to lower the diaphragm for better visualization of heart structures. The injection of a contrast agent into either side

of the heart may produce a flushed feeling throughout the body and a sensation similar to the need to void, which subsides in 1 minute or less.
- Encourage the patient to express fears and anxieties. Provide teaching and reassurance to reduce apprehension.

Nursing responsibilities after cardiac catheterization may include the following:

1. Observe the catheter access site for bleeding or hematoma formation, and assess the peripheral pulses in the affected extremity (dorsalis pedis and posterior tibial pulses in the lower extremity, radial pulse in the upper extremity) every 15 minutes for 1 hour, and then every 1 to 2 hours until the pulses are stable.
2. Evaluate temperature and color of the affected extremity and any patient complaints of pain, numbness, or tingling sensations to determine signs of arterial insufficiency. Report changes promptly.
3. Monitor for dysrhythmias by observing the cardiac monitor or by assessing the apical and peripheral pulses for changes in rate and rhythm. A vasovagal reaction, consisting of bradycardia, hypotension, and nausea, can be precipitated by a distended bladder or by discomfort during removal of the arterial catheter, especially if a femoral site has been used. Prompt intervention is critical; this includes raising the feet and legs above the head, administering intravenous fluids, and administering intravenous atropine.
4. Inform the patient that if the procedure is performed percutaneously through the femoral artery (and without the use of devices such as VasoSeal, Perclose, or Angio-Seal), the patient will remain on bed rest for 2 to 6 hours with the affected leg straight and the head elevated to 30 degrees (Logemann et al., 1999). For comfort, the patient may be turned from side to side with the affected extremity straight. If the cardiologist uses deployed devices, check local nursing care standards, but anticipate that the patient will have less restrictions on elevation of the head of the bed and will be allowed to ambulate in 2 hours or less (Baim et al., 2000). Analgesic medication is administered as prescribed for discomfort.
5. Instruct the patient to report chest pain and bleeding or sudden discomfort from the catheter insertion sites immediately.
6. Encourage fluids to increase urinary output and flush out the dye.
7. Ensure safety by instructing the patient to ask for help when getting out of bed the first time after the procedure, because orthostatic hypotension may occur and the patient may feel dizzy and lightheaded.

For patients being discharged from the hospital on the same day as the procedure, additional instructions are provided. They appear in Chart 26-4.

ELECTROPHYSIOLOGIC TESTING

The electrophysiology study (EPS) is an invasive procedure that plays a major role in the diagnosis and management of serious dysrhythmias and is used (1) to distinguish atrial from ventricular tachycardias when the determination cannot be made from the 12-lead ECG, (2) to evaluate how readily a life-threatening dysrhythmia (eg, ventricular tachycardia, ventricular fibrillation)

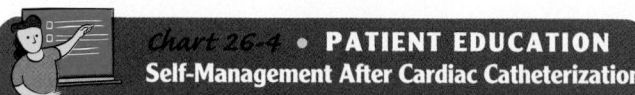

Chart 26-4 • PATIENT EDUCATION
Self-Management After Cardiac Catheterization

After discharge from the hospital for cardiac catheterization, guidelines for self-care include the following:

- For the next 24 hours, do not bend at the waist (to lift anything), strain, or lift heavy objects.
- Avoid tub baths, but shower as desired.
- Talk with your physician about when you may return to work, drive, or resume strenuous activities.
- Call your physician if any of the following occur: bleeding, swelling, new bruising or pain from your procedure puncture site, temperature of 101.5°F (38.6°C) or more.
- If test results show that you have coronary artery disease, talk with your physician about options for treatment, including cardiac rehabilitation programs in your community.
- Talk with your physician and nurse about lifestyle changes to reduce your risk for further or future heart problems, such as quitting smoking, lowering your cholesterol level, initiating dietary changes, beginning an exercise program, or losing weight.

can be induced, (3) to evaluate AV node function, (4) to evaluate the effectiveness of antiarrhythmic medications in suppressing the dysrhythmia, and (5) to determine the need for other therapeutic interventions, such as a pacemaker, implantable cardioverter defibrillator, or radiofrequency ablation (discussed in Chap. 27). EPS is indicated for patients with syncope and/or palpitations and for survivors of cardiac arrest from ventricular fibrillation (sudden cardiac death).

The initial study can take up to 4 hours. The patient receives moderate sedation. Catheters with recording and electrical stimulating (pacing) capabilities are inserted into the heart through the femoral and right subclavian veins to record electrical activity in the right and left atrium, bundle of His, and right ventricle. Fluoroscopy guides the positioning of these catheters. Baseline intracardiac recordings are obtained; programmed electrical stimulations of the atrium or ventricle are then administered in an attempt to induce the patient's dysrhythmia. If the dysrhythmia is induced, various antiarrhythmic medications are administered intravenously. The study is repeated after each medication to evaluate which medication or combination of medications is most effective in controlling the dysrhythmia.

After the study, the patient receives an equivalent oral antiarrhythmic agent, and subsequent studies may be necessary to evaluate the effectiveness of that medication. Results of the study may indicate the need for other therapeutic interventions, such as a pacemaker or implantable cardioverter defibrillator.

During EPS, lethal dysrhythmias may be induced; therefore, the procedure must be performed in a controlled environment with resuscitation equipment (eg, defibrillator) readily available. Possible complications include bleeding and hematoma from the catheter insertion sites, pneumothorax (air in the pleural cavity that may collapse portions of the lung), deep vein thrombosis, stroke, and sudden death.

Nursing Interventions

Patients receive nothing to eat or drink for 8 hours before the procedure. Antiarrhythmic medications are withheld for at least 24 hours before the initial study, and the patient's cardiac rate and rhythm are carefully monitored for dysrhythmias. Other medications may be taken with sips of water.

Thorough preparation before EPS will help to minimize patient anxiety. Ensure that the patient understands the reason for the study and is able to describe the common sensations and experiences expected during and after the study. Often the EPS laboratory has relaxation interventions available for patients, such as headsets with music. Also, the patient needs to be aware that the nurses in the EPS laboratory will be monitoring carefully for signs of discomfort and will offer intravenous medications to reduce discomfort or anxiety. Patients should be reminded to request these medications if necessary. Postprocedure interventions include careful monitoring for complications. The nurse takes vital signs, reviews tracings of continuous ECG monitoring, assesses the apical pulse, auscultates for pericardial friction rub (which indicates bleeding into the pericardial sac), and inspects the catheter insertion sites for bleeding or hematoma formation.

In addition, the nurse assists the patient to maintain bed rest with the affected extremity kept straight and the head of the bed elevated to 30 degrees for 4 to 6 hours. The frequency of assessments and the duration of bed rest may vary based on institutional policy and physician preference.

HEMODYNAMIC MONITORING

Critically ill patients require continuous assessment of their cardiovascular system to diagnose and manage their complex medical conditions. This is most commonly achieved by the use of direct pressure monitoring systems, often referred to as **hemodynamic monitoring**. Central venous pressure (CVP), pulmonary artery pressure, and intra-arterial BP monitoring are common forms of hemodynamic monitoring. Patients requiring hemodynamic monitoring are cared for in specialty critical care units. Some critical care step-down units also admit stable patients with CVP or intra-arterial BP monitoring. Noninvasive hemodynamic monitoring is used in some facilities.

To perform invasive monitoring, specialized equipment is necessary and includes the following:

- A CVP, pulmonary artery, or arterial catheter, which is introduced into the appropriate blood vessel or heart chamber
- A flush system composed of intravenous solution (which may include heparin), tubing, stopcocks, and a flush device, which provides for continuous and manual flushing of the system
- A pressure bag placed around the flush solution that is maintained at 300 mm Hg of pressure; the pressurized flush system delivers 3 to 5 mL of solution per hour through the catheter to prevent clotting and backflow of blood into the pressure monitoring system
- A transducer to convert the pressure coming from the artery or heart chamber into an electrical signal
- An amplifier or monitor, which increases the size of the electrical signal for display on an oscilloscope

Central Venous Pressure Monitoring

The CVP, the pressure in the vena cava or right atrium, is used to assess right ventricular function and venous blood return to the right side of the heart. The CVP can be continuously measured by connecting either a catheter positioned in the vena cava or the proximal port of a pulmonary artery catheter to a pressure monitoring system. The pulmonary artery catheter, described in greater detail later, is used for critically ill patients. Patients in general medical-surgical units who require CVP monitoring may have a single-lumen or multilumen catheter placed into the superior vena cava. Intermittent measurement of the CVP can then be obtained with the use of a water manometer.

Because the pressures in the right atrium and right ventricle are equal at the end of diastole (0 to 8 mm Hg), the CVP is also an indirect method of determining right ventricular filling pressure (preload). This makes the CVP a useful hemodynamic parameter to observe when managing an unstable patient's fluid volume status. CVP monitoring is most valuable when pressures are monitored over time and are correlated with the patient's clinical status. A rising pressure may be caused by hypervolemia or by a condition, such as HF, that results in a decrease in myocardial contractility. Pulmonary artery monitoring is preferred for the patient with HF. Decreased CVP indicates reduced right ventricular preload, most often caused by hypovolemia. This diagnosis can be substantiated when a rapid intravenous infusion causes the CVP to rise. (CVP monitoring is not clinically useful in a patient with HF in whom left ventricular failure precedes right ventricular failure, because in these patients an elevated CVP is a very late sign of HF.)

Before insertion of a CVP catheter, the site is prepared by shaving if necessary and by cleansing with an antiseptic solution. A local anesthetic may be used. The physician threads a single-lumen or multilumen catheter through the external jugular, antecubital, or femoral vein into the vena cava just above or within the right atrium.

NURSING INTERVENTIONS

Once the CVP catheter is inserted, it is secured and a dry, sterile dressing is applied. Catheter placement is confirmed by a chest x-ray, and the site is inspected daily for signs of infection. The dressing and pressure monitoring system or water manometer are changed according to hospital policy. In general, the dressing is to be kept dry and air occlusive. Dressing changes are performed with the use of sterile technique. CVP catheters can be used for infusing intravenous fluids, administering intravenous medications, and drawing blood specimens in addition to monitoring pressure.

To measure the CVP, the transducer (when a pressure monitoring system is used) or the zero mark on the manometer (when a water manometer is used) must be placed at a standard reference point, called the phlebostatic axis (Fig. 26-12). After locating this position, the nurse may make an ink mark on the

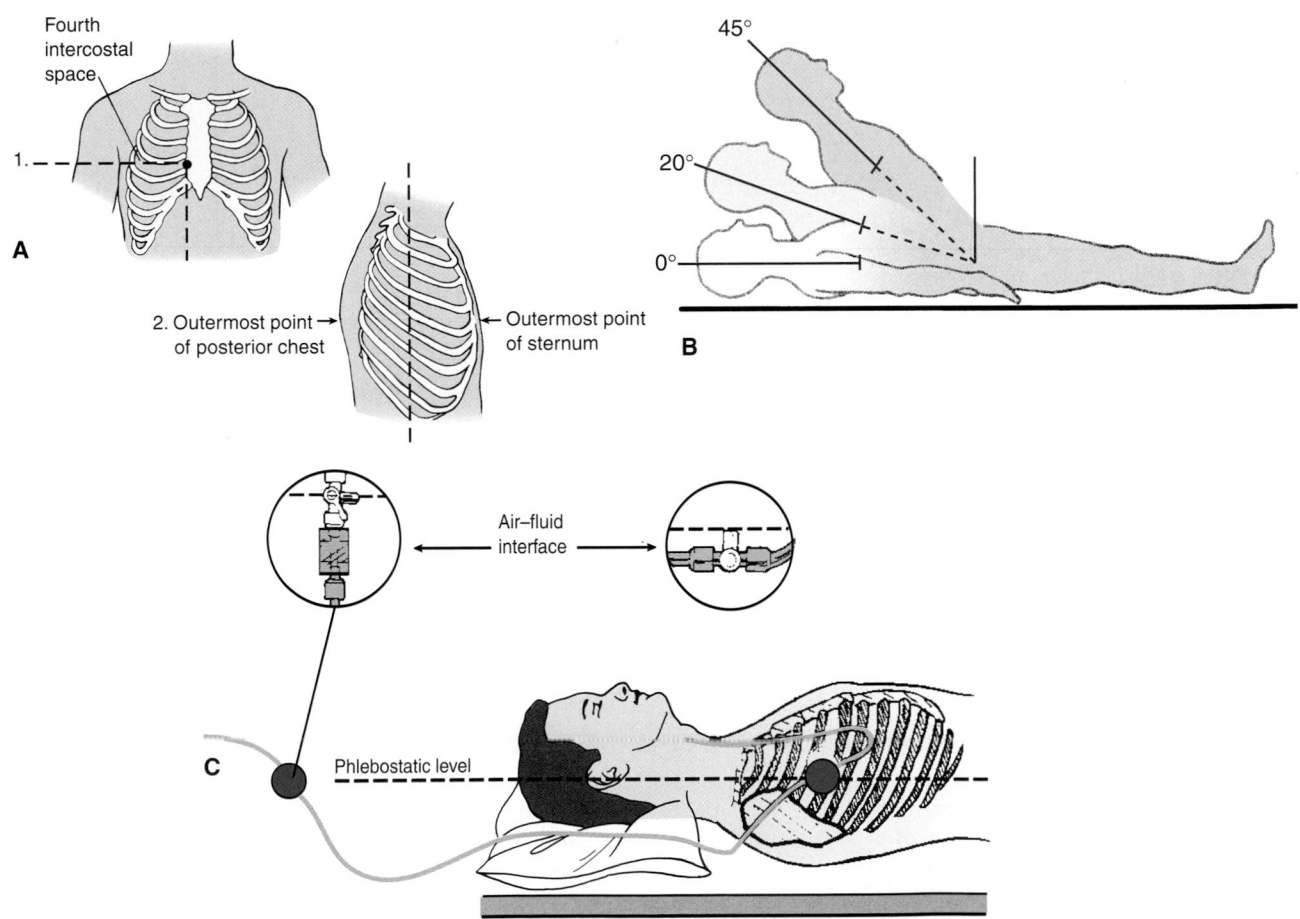

FIGURE 26-12 The phlebostatic axis and the phlebostatic level. **(A)** The phlebostatic axis is the crossing of two reference lines: (1) a line from the fourth intercostal space at the point where it joins the sternum, drawn out to the side of the body beneath the axilla; and (2) a line midway between the anterior and posterior surfaces of the chest. **(B)** The phlebostatic level is a horizontal line through the phlebostatic axis. The air–fluid interface of the stopcock of the transducer, or the zero mark on the manometer, must be level with this axis for accurate measurements. When moving from the flat to erect positions, the patient moves the chest and therefore the reference level; the phlebostatic level stays horizontal through the same reference point. **(C)** Two methods for referencing the pressure system to the phlebostatic axis. The system can be referenced by placing the air–fluid interface of either the in-line stopcock or stopcock on top of the transducer at the phlebostatic level.

patient's chest to indicate the location. If the phlebostatic axis is used, CVP can be measured correctly with the patient supine at any backrest position up to 45 degrees. The range for a normal CVP is 0 to 8 mm Hg with a pressure monitoring system or 3 to 8 cm H_2O with a water manometer system. The most common complications of CVP monitoring are infection and air embolism.

Pulmonary Artery Pressure Monitoring

Pulmonary artery pressure monitoring is an important tool used in critical care for assessing left ventricular function, diagnosing the etiology of shock, and evaluating the patient's response to medical interventions (eg, fluid administration, vasoactive medications). Pulmonary artery pressure monitoring is achieved by using a pulmonary artery catheter and pressure monitoring system. Catheters vary in their number of lumens and their types of measurement (eg, cardiac output, oxygen saturation) or pacing capabilities. All types require that a balloon-tipped, flow-directed catheter be inserted into a large vein (usually the subclavian, jugular, or femoral vein); the catheter is then passed into the vena cava and right atrium. In the right atrium, the balloon tip is inflated, and the catheter is carried rapidly by the flow of blood through the tricuspid valve, into the right ventricle, through the pulmonic valve, and into a branch of the pulmonary artery. When the catheter reaches a small pulmonary artery, the balloon is deflated and the catheter is secured with sutures. Fluoroscopy may be used during insertion to visualize the progression of the catheter through the heart chambers to the pulmonary artery. This procedure can be performed in the operating room or cardiac catheterization laboratory or at the bedside in the critical care unit. During insertion of the pulmonary artery catheter, the bedside monitor is observed for waveform and ECG changes as the catheter is moved

through the heart chambers on the right side and into the pulmonary artery.

After the catheter is correctly positioned, the following pressures can be measured: CVP or right atrial pressure, pulmonary artery systolic and diastolic pressures, mean pulmonary artery pressure, and pulmonary artery wedge pressure (Fig. 26-13). If a thermodilution catheter is used, the cardiac output can be measured and systemic vascular resistance and pulmonary vascular resistance can be calculated.

Normal pulmonary artery pressure is 25/9 mm Hg, with a mean pressure of 15 mm Hg (see Fig. 26-5 for normal ranges). When the balloon tip is inflated, usually with 1 mL of air, the catheter floats farther out into the pulmonary artery until it becomes wedged. This is an occlusive maneuver that impedes blood flow through that segment of the pulmonary artery. A pressure measurement, called pulmonary artery wedge pressure, is taken within seconds after wedging of the pulmonary artery catheter; then the balloon is immediately deflated and blood flow is restored. The nurse who obtains the wedge reading ensures that the catheter has returned to its normal position in the pulmonary artery by evaluating the pulmonary artery pressure waveform. The pulmonary artery diastolic reading and the wedge pressure reflect the pressure in the ventricle at end-diastole and are particularly important to monitor in critically ill patients, because they are used to evaluate left ventricular filling pressures (preload). At end-diastole, when the mitral valve is open, the wedge pressure is the same as the pressure in the left atrium and the left ventricle, unless the patient has mitral valve disease or pulmonary hypertension. Pulmonary capillary wedge pressure is a mean pressure and is normally 4.5 to 13 mm Hg. Critically ill patients usually require higher left ventricular filling pressures to optimize cardiac output. These patients may need to have their wedge pressure maintained as high as 18 mm Hg.

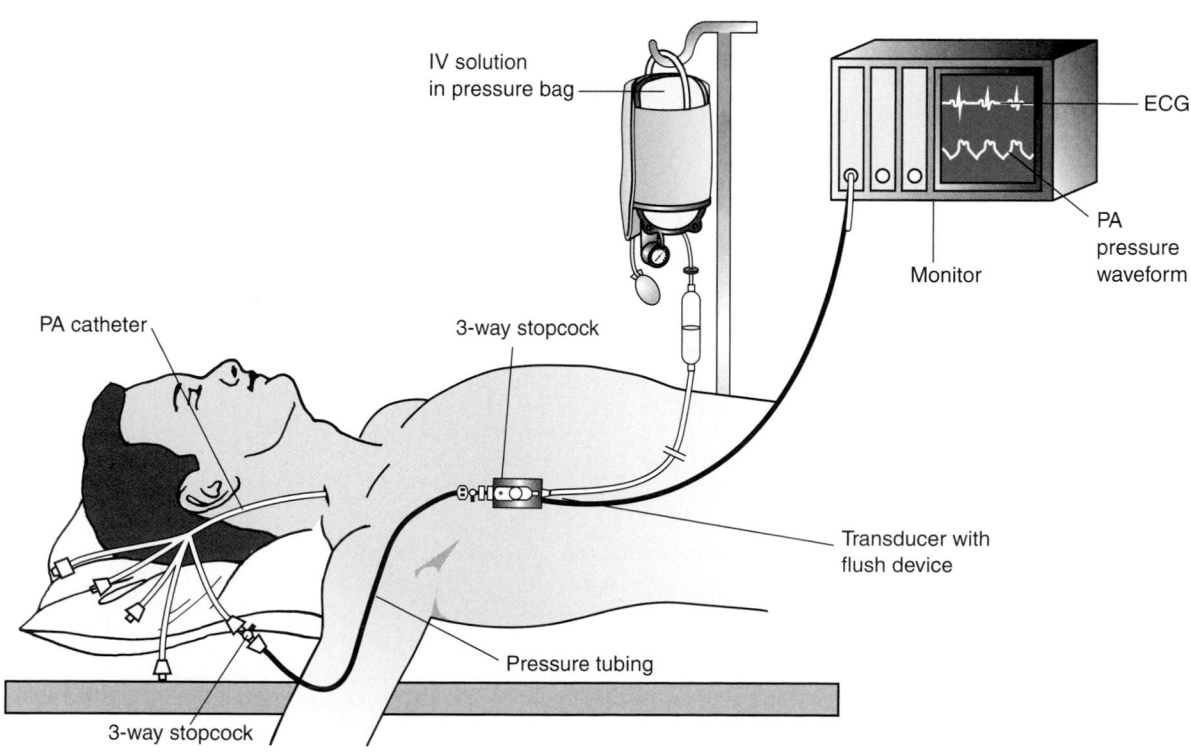

FIGURE 26-13 Example of a pulmonary artery (PA) pressure monitoring system. PA catheter is inserted into the internal jugular vein and advanced into the pulmonary artery.

NURSING INTERVENTIONS

Catheter site care is essentially the same as for a CVP catheter. As in measuring CVP, the transducer must be positioned at the phlebostatic axis to ensure accurate readings (see Fig. 26-12). Complications of pulmonary artery pressure monitoring include infection, pulmonary artery rupture, pulmonary thromboembolism, pulmonary infarction, catheter kinking, dysrhythmias, and air embolism.

Intra-arterial Blood Pressure Monitoring

Intra-arterial BP monitoring is used to obtain direct and continuous BP measurements in critically ill patients who have severe hypertension or hypotension (Fig. 26-14). Arterial catheters are also useful when arterial blood gas measurements and blood samples need to be obtained frequently.

Once an arterial site is selected (radial, brachial, femoral, or dorsalis pedis), collateral circulation to the area must be confirmed before the catheter is placed. This is a safety precaution to prevent compromised arterial perfusion to the area distal to the arterial catheter insertion site. If no collateral circulation exists and the cannulated artery became occluded, ischemia and infarction of the area distal to that artery could occur. Collateral circulation to the hand can be checked by the Allen test to evaluate the radial and ulnar arteries or by an ultrasonic Doppler test for any of the arteries. With the Allen test, the nurse compresses the radial and ulnar arteries simultaneously and asks the patient to make a fist, causing the hand to blanch. After the patient opens the fist, the nurse releases the pressure on the ulnar artery while maintaining pressure on the radial artery. The patient's hand will turn pink if the ulnar artery is patent.

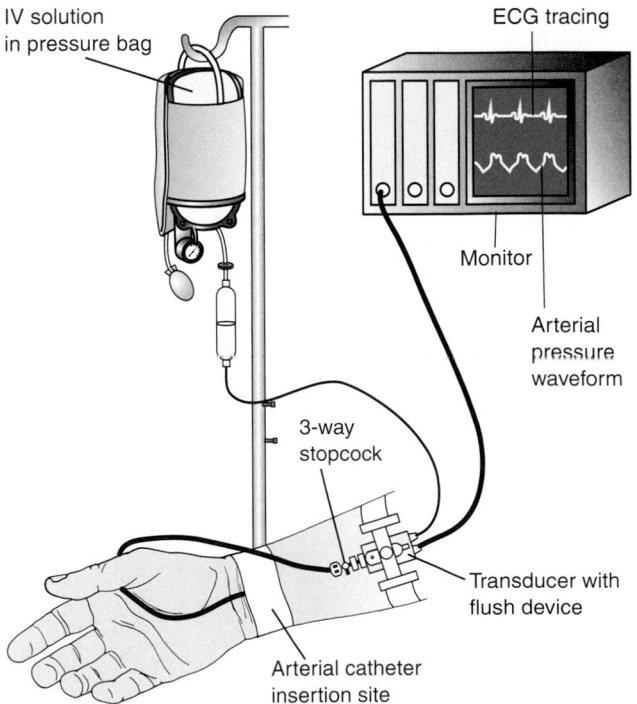

FIGURE 26-14 Example of an arterial pressure monitoring system. The arterial catheter is inserted into the radial artery. A three-way stopcock is used for drawing arterial blood samples.

NURSING INTERVENTIONS

Site preparation and care are the same as for CVP catheters. The catheter flush solution is the same as for pulmonary artery catheters. A transducer is attached, and pressures are measured in millimeters of mercury (mm Hg). Complications include local obstruction with distal ischemia, external hemorrhage, massive ecchymosis, dissection, air embolism, blood loss, pain, arteriospasm, and infection.

 Critical Thinking Exercises

1. You are caring for an elderly man who has had three hospital admissions in 6 months for HF. To plan for his discharge you need to fully understand what is causing these recurrent HF episodes. What medical and nursing history, physical examination, and laboratory data will you need to collect to help you understand the recurrent episodes of HF? What types of information are necessary to help you formulate his plan for discharge? With what other team members might you consult before completing this plan?

2. While working in a primary care clinic, you notice that many of the patients use tobacco products including cigarettes and chewing tobacco. What are the health risks of tobacco use? The clinic does not have a smoking cessation protocol. You want to help people become tobacco free but have little experience in providing cessation advice. What information and resources will you need to obtain to devise and implement a smoking cessation protocol?

3. While making a home visit, your patient, a 54-year-old African American woman with a history of hypertension, diabetes, and tobacco use, tells you she has had overwhelming fatigue and right scapular and shoulder pain going down into her arm for the last 10 hours. Describe your rapid chest pain assessment and management plan for this patient. Discuss the factors that may be contributing to her delay in seeking care for symptoms of acute MI. Compare and contrast symptoms of acute MI and factors contributing to delay in seeking care.

REFERENCES AND SELECTED READINGS

Books

American Heart Association. (2003). *Heart and stroke facts: 2002 statistical supplement.* Dallas, TX: Author.

Apple, S., & Lindsey, J. (1999). *Principles and practices of interventional cardiology.* Philadelphia: Lippincott Williams & Wilkins.

Bickley, L. S., & Szilagyi, P. G. (2003). *Bates' guide to physical examination* (8th ed.). Philadelphia: Lippincott Williams & Wilkins.

Braunwald, E., Libby, P., & Zipes, D. P. (Eds.). (2001). *Heart disease: A textbook of cardiovascular medicine* (6th ed.). Philadelphia: W. B. Saunders.

Chernecky, C., & Berger, B. (2001). *Laboratory tests and diagnostic procedures* (3rd ed.). Philadelphia: W. B. Saunders.

Darvic, G. (2002). *Handbook of hemodynamic monitoring.* Invasive and noninvasive clinical application (3rd ed.). Philadelphia: W. B. Saunders.

Fuller, J., & Schaller-Ayers, J. (2000). *Health assessment: A nursing approach* (3rd ed.). Philadelphia: Lippincott Williams & Wilkins.

Huff, J. (2001). *ECG workout: Exercises in arrhythmia interpretation* (4th ed.). Philadelphia: Lippincott Williams & Wilkins.

Jairath, N. (1999). *Coronary heart disease and risk factor management: A nursing perspective.* Philadelphia: W. B. Saunders.

Kern, M. (2003). *The interventional cardiac catheterization handbook* (2nd ed.). St. Louis: C. V. Mosby.

Maas, M. L., Buckwalter, K. C., Hardy, M. D., Tripp-Reimer, T., Titler, M. G., Specht, J. P., et al. (2001). *Nursing care of older adults: Diagnoses, outcomes, and interventions.* St. Louis: C. V. Mosby.

Miller, C. (1999). *Nursing care of older adults: Theory and practice* (3rd ed.). Philadelphia: Lippincott Williams & Wilkins.

Pohost, G. M., O'Rourke, R. A., Berman, D. S., & Shah, P. M. (2000). *Imaging in cardiovascular disease.* Philadelphia: Lippincott Williams & Wilkins.

Weber, J., & Kelley, J. (2003). *Health assessment in nursing* (2nd ed.). Philadelphia: Lippincott Williams & Wilkins.

Woods, S. L., Froelicher, E. S. S., & Motzer, S. U. (1999). *Cardiac nursing* (4th ed.). Philadelphia: Lippincott Williams & Wilkins.

Journals

Asterisks indicate nursing research articles.

Attin, M. (2001). Electrophysiology study: A comprehensive review. *American Journal of Critical Care, 10*(4), 260–273.

*Baim, D., Knopf, W., Hinohara, T., Schwarten, D. E., Schatz, R. A., Pinkerton, C. A., et al. (2000). Suture-mediated closure of the femoral access site after cardiac catheterization: Results of the suture to ambulate and discharge (STAND I and STAND II) trials. *American Journal of Cardiology, 85*(7), 864–869.

Beattie, S. (1999). Cut the risks for cardiac cath patients. *RN, 62*(1), 50–55.

*Bosworth, H., Feaganes, J., Vitaliano, P., Mark, D. B., & Siegler, I. C. (2001). Personality and coping with a common stressor: Cardiac catheterization. *Journal of Behavioral Medicine, 24*(1), 17–31.

*Botti, M., Williamson, B., & Steen, K. (2001). Coronary angiographic observations: Evidence-based or ritualistic practice? *Heart & Lung, 30*(2), 138–145.

Buselli, E. F., & Stuart, E. M. (1999). Influence of psychosocial factors and biopsychosocial interventions on outcomes after myocardial infarction. *J Cardiovasc Nurs, 13*(3), 60–72.

Chyun, D. (2001). Diabetes and coronary heart disease: A time for action. *Critical Care Nurse, 21*(1), 10–16.

Daleiden, A. M., & Schell, H. (2001). Setting a new gold standard: ST-segment monitoring provides early detection of myocardial ischemia. *American Journal of Nursing, 101,* (Suppl.), 4–8, 48–50.

Dracup, K., & Cannon, C. (1999). Combination treatment strategies for management of acute myocardial infarction: New directions with current therapies. *Critical Care Nurse, 19*(4), (Suppl.), 1–17.

Drew, B., & Krucoff, M. (1999). Multilead ST-segment monitoring in patients with acute coronary syndromes: A consensus statement for healthcare professionals. ST-segment monitoring practice guidelines international working group. *American Journal of Critical Care, 8*(6), 372–386.

Gibbar-Clements, T., Shirrell, D., Dooley, R., & Smiley, B. (2000). The challenge of warfarin therapy. *American Journal of Nursing, 100*(3), 38–40.

Grundy, S., Howard, B., Smith, S., Jr., Eckel, R., Redberg, R., & Bonow, R. O. (2002). Prevention Conference VI: Diabetes and cardiovascular disease executive summary: Conference proceeding for healthcare professionals from a special writing group of the American Heart Association. *Circulation, 105*(18), 2231–2239.

Hamel, W. (1999). Suppose a Perclose. *Progress in Cardiovascular Nursing, 14*(4), 136–142.

Hinkle, C., & Stegall, G. (2000). Ask the experts: Setting up 15 and 18 lead ECGs. *Critical Care Nurse, 20*(2), 125–126.

Jacobson, C. (2000). Optimum bedside cardiac monitoring. *Progress in Cardiovascular Nursing, 15*(4), 134–137.

*Krantz, D., Santiago, H., & Kop, W. (1999). Prognostic value of mental stress testing in coronary artery disease. *American Journal of Cardiology, 84*(11), 1292–1297.

*Logemann, T., Luetmer, P., Kaliebe, J., Olson, K., & Murdock, D. K. (1999). Two versus six hours of bed rest following left-sided cardiac catheterization and a meta-analysis of early ambulation trials. *American Journal of Cardiology, 84*(4), 486–488.

*Milner, K., Funk, M., Richards, S., Wilmes, R. M., Vaccarino, V., Krumholz, H. M., et al. (1999). Gender differences in symptom presentation associated with coronary heart disease. *American Journal of Cardiology, 84*(4), 396–399.

Mosca, L., Collins, P., Herrington, D., Mendelsohn, M. E., Pasternak, R. C., Robertson, R. M., et al. (2001). Hormone replacement therapy and cardiovascular disease: A statement for healthcare professionals from the American Heart Association. *Circulation, 104*(4), 499–503.

Mosca, L., Grungy, S. M., Judelson, D., King, K., Limacher, M., Oparil, S., et al. (1999). AHA/ACC scientific statement: Consensus panel statement. Guide to preventative cardiology for women. American Heart Association/American College of Cardiology. *Journal of the American College of Cardiology, 33*(6), 1751–1755.

*Mott, A. (1999). Psychologic preparation to decrease anxiety associated with cardiac catheterization. *Journal of Vascular Nursing, 17*(2), 41–49.

Pearson, T. A., Blair, S. W., Daniel, S. R., Eckel, R. H., Fair, J. M., Fortmann, S. P., et al. (2002). AHA guidelines for primary prevention of cardiovascular disease and stroke: 2002 update. Consensus panel guide to comprehensive risk reduction for adult patients without coronary or other atherosclerotic vascular diseases. *Circulation, 106*(3), 388–391.

*Richards, S., Funk, M., & Milner, K. (2000). Differences between blacks and whites with coronary heart disease in initial symptoms and delay in seeking care. *American Journal of Critical Care, 9*(4), 237–244.

Robertson, R. (2001). Women and cardiovascular disease: The risk of misperception and the need for action. *Circulation, 103*(19), 2318–2323.

*Roussouw, J. E., Anderson, G. L., Prentice, R. L., LaCroix, A. Z., Kooperberg, C., Stefanick, M. C., et al. (2002). Risk and benefits of estrogen plus progestin in healthy post menopausal women: Principle results from the Women's Health Initiative randomized controlled trial. *Journal of the American Medical Association, 288*(3), 321–333.

*Schickel, S., Adkisson, P., Miracle, V., Cronin, S. N. (1999). Achieving femoral artery hemostasis after cardiac catheterization: A comparison of methods. *American Journal of Critical Care, 8*(6), 406–415.

Siomko, A. J. (2000). Demystifying cardiac markers. *American Journal of Nursing, 100*(1), 36–41.

Smith, S. C. Jr., Blair, S. N., Bonow, R. O., Brass, L. M., Cerqueira, M. D., Dracup, K., et al. (2001). AHA/ACC guidelines for preventing heart attack and death in patients with atherosclerotic cardiovascular disease. *Circulation, 104*(13), 1577–1579.

Steinke, E. (2000). Sexual counseling: After myocardial infarction. *American Journal of Nursing, 100*(12), 38–44.

The Tobacco Use and Dependence Clinical Practice Guideline Update Panel, Staff, and Consortium Representatives. (2000). A clinical practice guideline for treating tobacco use and dependence: A U.S. Public Health Service Report. *Journal of the American Medical Association; 283*(24), 3244–3254.

*Then, K., Rankin, J., & Fofonoff, D. (2001). Atypical presentation of acute myocardial infarction in 3 age groups. *Heart & Lung, 30*(4), 285–293.

*Wung, S., & Drew, B. (1999). Comparison of 18-lead ECG and selected body surface potential mapping leads in determining maximally deviated ST lead and efficacy in detecting acute myocardial ischemia during coronary occlusion. *Journal of Electrophysiology, 32,* (Suppl.) 30–37.

Zerwic, J. (1999). Patient delay in seeking treatment for acute myocardial infarction symptoms. *Journal of Cardiovascular Nursing, 13*(3), 21–31.

RESOURCES AND WEBSITES

American Heart Association, 7272 Greenville Avenue, Dallas, TX 75231; 1-800-242-8721; http://www.americanheart.org.

New York Cardiac Center, 467 Sylvan Avenue, Englewood Cliffs, NJ 07632, 201-569-8180; http://nycardiaccenter.org.

Nurse-Beat: Cardiac Nursing Electronic Journal; http://www.nurse-beat.com.

Management of Patients With Dysrhythmias and Conduction Problems

On completion of this chapter, the learner will be able to:

1. Correlate the components of the normal ECG with physiologic events of the heart.

2. Define the ECG as a waveform that represents the cardiac electrical event in relation to the lead depicted (placement of electrodes).

3. Analyze elements of an ECG rhythm strip: ventricular and atrial rate, ventricular and atrial rhythm, QRS complex and shape, QRS duration, P wave and shape, PR interval, and P:QRS ratio.

4. Identify the ECG criteria, causes, and management of several dysrhythmias, including conduction disturbances.

5. Use the nursing process as a framework for care of patients with dysrhythmias.

6. Compare the different types of pacemakers, their uses, possible complications, and nursing implications.

7. Use the nursing process as a framework for care of patients with pacemakers.

8. Describe the key points of using a defibrillator.

9. Describe the purpose of an implantable cardioverter defibrillator (ICD), the types available, and the nursing implications.

10. Describe invasive methods to diagnose and treat recurrent dysrhythmias, and discuss the nursing implications.

Without a regular rate and rhythm, the heart may not perform efficiently as a pump to circulate oxygenated blood and other life-sustaining nutrients to all the body organs (including itself) and tissues. With an irregular or erratic rhythm, the heart is considered to be dysrhythmic (sometimes called arrhythmic). This has the potential to be a dangerous condition.

Dysrhythmias

Dysrhythmias are disorders of the formation or conduction (or both) of the electrical impulse within the heart. These disorders can cause disturbances of the heart rate, the heart rhythm, or both. Dysrhythmias may initially be evidenced by the hemodynamic effect they cause (eg, a change in conduction may change the pumping action of the heart and cause decreased blood pressure). Dysrhythmias are diagnosed by analyzing the electrocardiographic waveform. They are named according to the site of origin of the impulse and the mechanism of formation or conduction involved (Chart 27-1). For example, an impulse that originates in the sinoatrial (SA) node and that has a slow rate is called sinus bradycardia.

NORMAL ELECTRICAL CONDUCTION

The electrical impulse that stimulates and paces the cardiac muscle normally originates in the sinus node (SA node), an area located near the superior vena cava in the right atrium. Usually, the electrical impulse occurs at a rate ranging between 60 and 100 times a minute in the adult. The electrical impulse quickly travels from the sinus node through the atria to the atrioventricular (AV) node (Fig. 27-1). The electrical stimulation of the muscle cells of the atria causes them to contract. The structure of the AV node slows the electrical impulse, which allows time for the atria to contract and fill the ventricles with blood before the electrical impulse

---

Chart 27-1 **Identifying Dysrhythmias**

Sites of Origin
 Sinus (SA) node
 Atria
 Atrioventricular (AV) node or junction
 Ventricles

Mechanisms of Formation or Conduction
 Normal (idio) rhythm
 Bradycardia
 Tachycardia
 Dysrhythmia
 Flutter
 Fibrillation
 Premature complexes
 Blocks

---

travels very quickly through the bundle of His to the right and left bundle branches and the Purkinje fibers, located in the ventricular muscle. The electrical stimulation of the muscle cells of the ventricles, in turn, causes the mechanical contraction of the ventricles (systole). The cells repolarize and the ventricles then relax (diastole). The process from sinus node electrical impulse generation through ventricular repolarization completes the electromechanical circuit, and the cycle begins again.

Sinus rhythm promotes cardiovascular circulation. The electrical impulse causes (and, therefore, is followed by) the mechanical contraction of the heart muscle. The electrical stimulation is called **depolarization**; the mechanical contraction is called systole. Electrical relaxation is called **repolarization** and mechanical relaxation is called diastole. See Chapter 26 for a more complete explanation of cardiac function.

Glossary

ablation: purposeful destruction of heart muscle cells, usually in an attempt to control a dysrhythmia

antiarrhythmic: a medication that suppresses or prevents a dysrhythmia

automaticity: ability of the cardiac muscle to initiate an electrical impulse

cardioversion: electrical current administered in synchrony with the patient's own QRS to stop a dysrhythmia

conductivity: ability of the cardiac muscle to transmit electrical impulses

defibrillation: electrical current administered to stop a dysrhythmia, not synchronized with the patient's QRS complex

depolarization: process by which cardiac muscle cells change from a more negatively charged to a more positively charged intracellular state

dysrhythmia (also referred to as arrhythmia): disorder of the formation or conduction (or both) of the electrical impulse within the heart, altering the heart rate, heart rhythm, or both and potentially causing altered blood flow

implantable cardioverter defibrillator (ICD): a device implanted into the chest to treat dysrhythmias

inhibited: in reference to pacemakers, term used to describe the pacemaker withholding an impulse (not firing)

P wave: the part of an electrocardiogram (ECG) that reflects conduction of an electrical impulse through the atrium; atrial depolarization

paroxysmal: a dysrhythmia that has a sudden onset and/or termination and is usually of short duration

PR interval: the part of an ECG that reflects conduction of an electrical impulse from the sinoatrial (SA) node through the atrioventricular (AV) node

proarrhythmic: an agent (eg, a medication) that causes or exacerbates a dysrhythmia

QRS complex: the part of an ECG that reflects conduction of an electrical impulse through the ventricles; ventricular depolarization

QT interval: the part of an ECG that reflects the time from ventricular depolarization to repolarization

repolarization: process by which cardiac muscle cells return to a more negatively charged intracellular condition, their resting state

sinus rhythm: electrical activity of the heart initiated by the sinoatrial (SA) node

ST segment: the part of an ECG that reflects the end of ventricular depolarization (end of the QRS complex) through ventricular repolarization (end of the T wave)

supraventricular tachycardia (SVT): a rhythm that originates in the conduction system above the ventricles

T wave: the part of an ECG that reflects repolarization of the ventricles

triggered: in reference to pacemakers, term used to describe the release of an impulse in response to some stimulus

U wave: the part of an ECG that may reflect Purkinje fiber repolarization; usually seen when a patient's serum potassium level is low

ventricular tachycardia (VT): a rhythm that originates in the ventricles

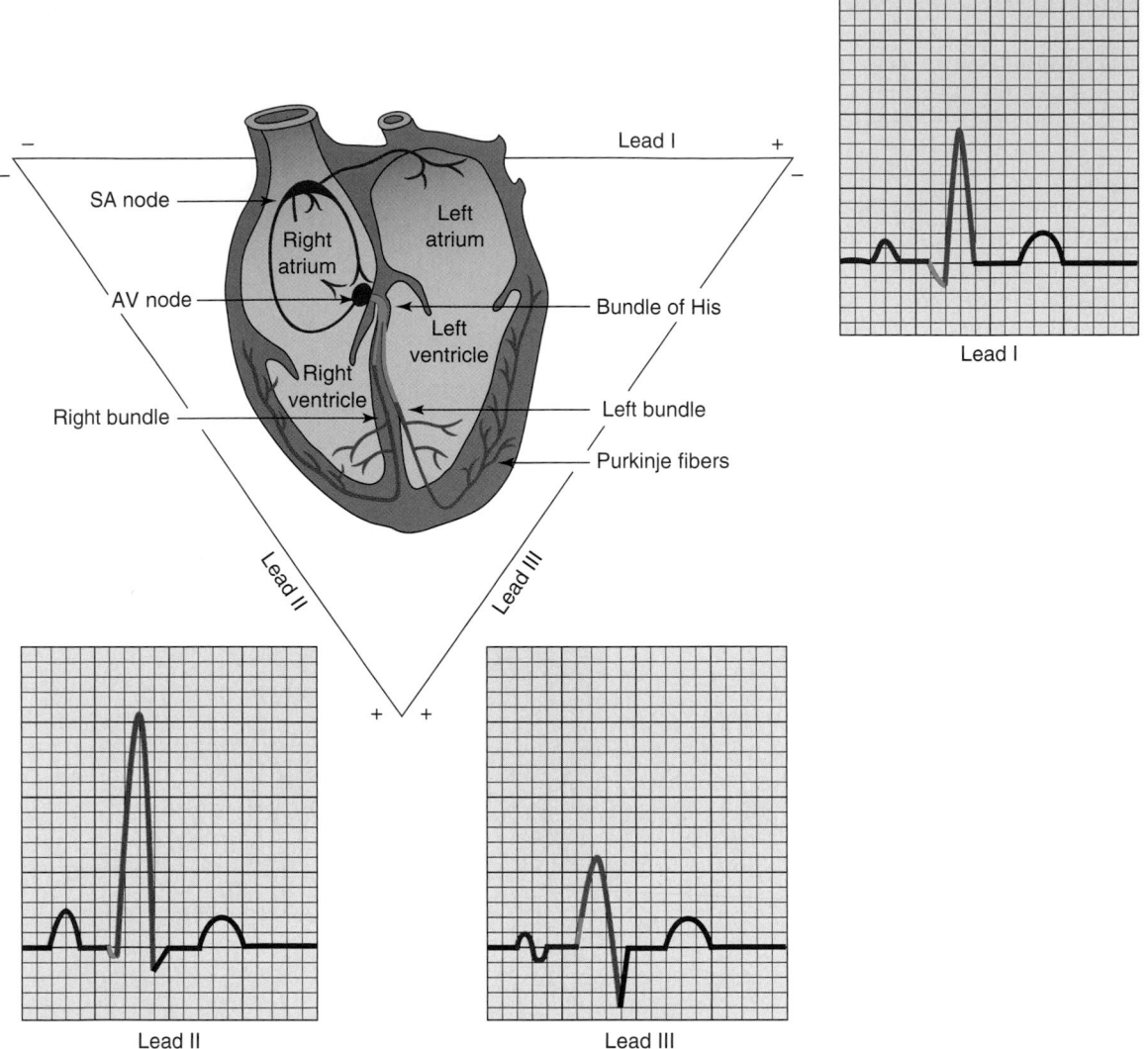

FIGURE 27-1 Relationship of electrocardiogram (ECG) complex, lead system, and electrical impulse. The heart conducts electrical activity, which the ECG measures and shows. The configurations of electrical activity displayed on the ECG vary depending on the lead (or view) of the ECG and on the rhythm of the heart. Therefore, the configuration of a normal rhythm tracing from lead I will differ from the configuration of a normal rhythm tracing from lead II, lead II will differ from lead III, and so on. The same is true for abnormal rhythms and cardiac disorders. To make an accurate assessment of the heart's electrical activity or to identify where, when, and what abnormalities occur, the ECG needs to be evaluated from every lead, not just from lead II. Here the different areas of electrical activity are identified by color.

Influences on Heart Rate and Contractility

The heart rate is influenced by the autonomic nervous system, which consists of sympathetic and parasympathetic fibers. Sympathetic nerve fibers (also referred to as adrenergic fibers) are attached to the heart and arteries as well as several other areas in the body. Stimulation of the sympathetic system increases heart rate (positive chronotropy), conduction through the AV node (positive dromotropy), and the force of myocardial contraction (positive inotropy). Sympathetic stimulation also constricts peripheral blood vessels, therefore increasing blood pressure. Parasympathetic nerve fibers are also attached to the heart and arteries. Parasympathetic stimulation reduces the heart rate (negative chronotropy), AV conduction (negative dromotropy), and the force of atrial myocardial contraction. The decreased sympathetic stimulation results in dilation of arteries, thereby lowering blood pressure.

Manipulation of the autonomic nervous system may increase or decrease the incidence of dysrhythmias. Increased sympathetic stimulation—caused, for example, by exercise, anxiety, fever, or administration of catecholamines (eg, dopamine [Intropin], aminophylline, dobutamine [Dobutrex])—may increase the incidence of dysrhythmias. Decreased sympathetic stimulation (eg, with rest, anxiety-reduction methods such as therapeutic communication or prayer, administration of beta-adrenergic blocking agents) may decrease the incidence of dysrhythmias.

INTERPRETATION OF THE ELECTROCARDIOGRAM

The electrical impulse that travels through the heart can be viewed by means of electrocardiography, the end product of which is an electrocardiogram (ECG). Each phase of the cardiac cycle is reflected by specific waveforms on the screen of a cardiac monitor or on a strip of ECG graph paper.

An ECG is obtained by slightly abrading the skin with a clean dry gauze pad and placing electrodes on the body at specific areas. Electrodes come in various shapes and sizes, but all have two components: (1) an adhesive substance that attaches to the skin to secure the electrode in place and (2) a substance that reduces the skin's electrical impedance and promotes detection of the electrical current.

The number and placement of the electrodes depend on the type of ECG needed. Most continuous monitors use two to five electrodes, usually placed on the limbs and the chest. These electrodes create an imaginary line, called a lead, that serves as a reference point from which the electrical activity is viewed. A lead is like an eye of a camera; it has a narrow peripheral field of vision, looking only at the electrical activity directly in front of it. Therefore, the ECG waveforms that appear on the paper or cardiac monitor represent the electrical current in relation to the lead (see Fig. 27-1). A change in the waveform can be caused by a change in the electrical current (where it originates or how it is conducted) or by a change in the lead.

Obtaining an Electrocardiogram

Electrodes are attached to cable wires, which are connected to one of the following:

- An ECG machine placed at the patient's side for an immediate recording (standard 12-lead ECG)
- A cardiac monitor at the patient's bedside for continuous reading; this kind of monitoring, usually called hardwire monitoring, is associated with intensive care units
- A small box that the patient carries and that continuously transmits the ECG information by radio waves to a central monitor located elsewhere (called telemetry)
- A small, lightweight tape recorder-like machine (called a Holter monitor) that the patient wears and that continuously records the ECG on a tape, which is later viewed and analyzed with a scanner

The placement of electrodes for continuous monitoring, telemetry, or Holter monitoring varies with the type of technology that is appropriate and available, the purpose of monitoring, and the standards of the institution. For a standard 12-lead ECG, 10 electrodes (six on the chest and four on the limbs) are placed on the body (Fig. 27-2). To prevent interference from the electrical activity of skeletal muscle, the limb electrodes are usually placed on areas that are not bony and that do not have significant movement. These limb electrodes provide the first six leads: leads I, II, III, aVR, aVL, and aVF. The six chest electrodes are attached to the chest at very specific areas. The chest electrodes provide the V or precordial leads, V_1 through V_6. To locate the fourth intercostal space and the placement of V_1, locate the sternal angle and then the sternal notch, which is about 1 or 2 inches below the sternal angle. When the fingers are moved to the patient's immediate right, the second rib can be palpated. The second intercostal space is the indentation felt just below the second rib.

Locating the specific intercostal space is critical for correct chest electrode placement. Errors in diagnosis can occur if electrodes are incorrectly placed. Sometimes, when the patient is in the hospital and needs to be monitored closely for ECG changes, the chest electrodes are left in place to ensure the same placement for follow-up ECGs.

A standard 12-lead ECG reflects the electrical activity primarily in the left ventricle. Placement of additional electrodes for

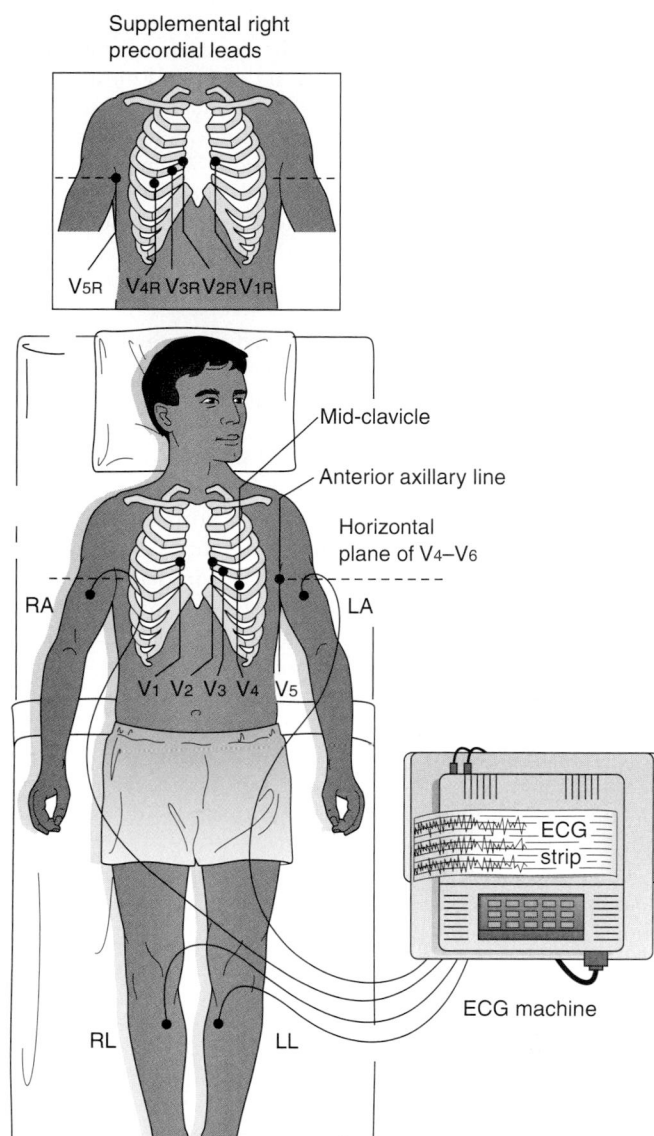

FIGURE 27-2 ECG electrode placement. The standard left precordial leads are V_1—4th intercostal space, right sternal border; V_2—4th intercostal space, left sternal border; V_3—diagonally between V_2 and V_4; V_4—5th intercostal space, left midclavicular line; V_5—same level as V_4, anterior axillary line; V_6 (not illustrated)—same level as V_4 and V_5, midaxillary line. The right precordial leads, placed across the right side of the chest, are the mirror opposite of the left leads. Adapted from Hosley, J. B., & Molle-Matthews, E. (1999). *Lippincott's pocket guide to medical assisting.* Philadelphia: Lippincott Williams & Wilkins.

other leads may be needed to obtain more complete information. For example, in patients with suspected right-sided heart damage, right-sided precordial leads are required to evaluate the right ventricle (see Fig. 27-2).

Analysis of the Electrocardiogram

The ECG waveform represents the function of the heart's conduction system, which normally initiates and conducts the electrical activity, in relation to the lead. When analyzed accurately, the ECG offers important information about the electrical activity of the heart. ECG waveforms are printed on graph paper that is divided by light and dark vertical and horizontal lines at standard intervals (Fig. 27-3). Time and rate are measured on the horizontal axis of the graph, and amplitude or voltage is measured on the vertical axis. When an ECG waveform moves toward the top of the paper, it is called a positive deflection. When it moves toward the bottom of the paper, it is called a negative deflection. When reviewing an ECG, each waveform should be examined and compared with the others.

WAVES, COMPLEXES, AND INTERVALS

The ECG is composed of waveforms (including the P wave, the QRS complex, the T wave, and possibly a U wave) and of segments or intervals (including the PR interval, the ST segment, and the QT interval) (see Fig. 27-3).

The **P wave** represents the electrical impulse starting in the sinus node and spreading through the atria. Therefore, the P wave represents atrial muscle depolarization. It is normally 2.5 mm or less in height and 0.11 second or less in duration.

The **QRS complex** represents ventricular muscle depolarization. Not all QRS complexes have all three waveforms. The first negative deflection after the P wave is the Q wave, which is normally less than 0.04 second in duration and less than 25% of the R wave amplitude; the first positive deflection after the P wave is the R wave; and the S wave is the first negative deflection after the R wave. When a wave is less than 5 mm in height, small letters (q, r, s) are used; when a wave is taller than 5 mm, capital letters (Q, R, S) are used. The QRS complex is normally less than 0.12 seconds in duration.

The **T wave** represents ventricular muscle repolarization (when the cells regain a negative charge; also called the resting state). It follows the QRS complex and is usually the same direction as the QRS complex.

The **U wave** is thought to represent repolarization of the Purkinje fibers, but it sometimes is seen in patients with hypokalemia (low potassium levels), hypertension, or heart disease. If present, the U wave follows the T wave and is usually smaller than the P wave. If tall, it may be mistaken for an extra P wave.

The **PR interval** is measured from the beginning of the P wave to the beginning of the QRS complex and represents the time needed for sinus node stimulation, atrial depolarization, and conduction through the AV node before ventricular depolarization. In adults, the PR interval normally ranges from 0.12 to 0.20 seconds in duration.

The **ST segment**, which represents early ventricular repolarization, lasts from the end of the QRS complex to the beginning of the T wave. The beginning of the ST segment is usually identified by a change in the thickness or angle of the terminal portion of the QRS complex. The end of the ST segment may be more difficult to identify because it merges into the T wave. The ST segment is normally isoelectric (see discussion of TP interval). It is analyzed to identify whether it is above or below the isoelectric line, which may be, among other signs and symptoms, a sign of cardiac ischemia (see Chap. 28).

The **QT interval**, which represents the total time for ventricular depolarization and repolarization, is measured from the beginning of the QRS complex to the end of the T wave. The QT interval varies with heart rate, gender, and age, and the measured interval needs to be corrected for these variables through a specific calculation. Several ECG interpretation books contain charts of these calculations. The QT interval is usually 0.32 to 0.40 seconds in duration if the heart rate is 65 to 95 beats per minute. If the QT interval becomes prolonged, the patient may be at risk for a lethal ventricular dysrhythmia called torsades de pointes.

The **TP interval** is measured from the end of the T wave to the beginning of the next P wave, an isoelectric period (see Fig 27-3).

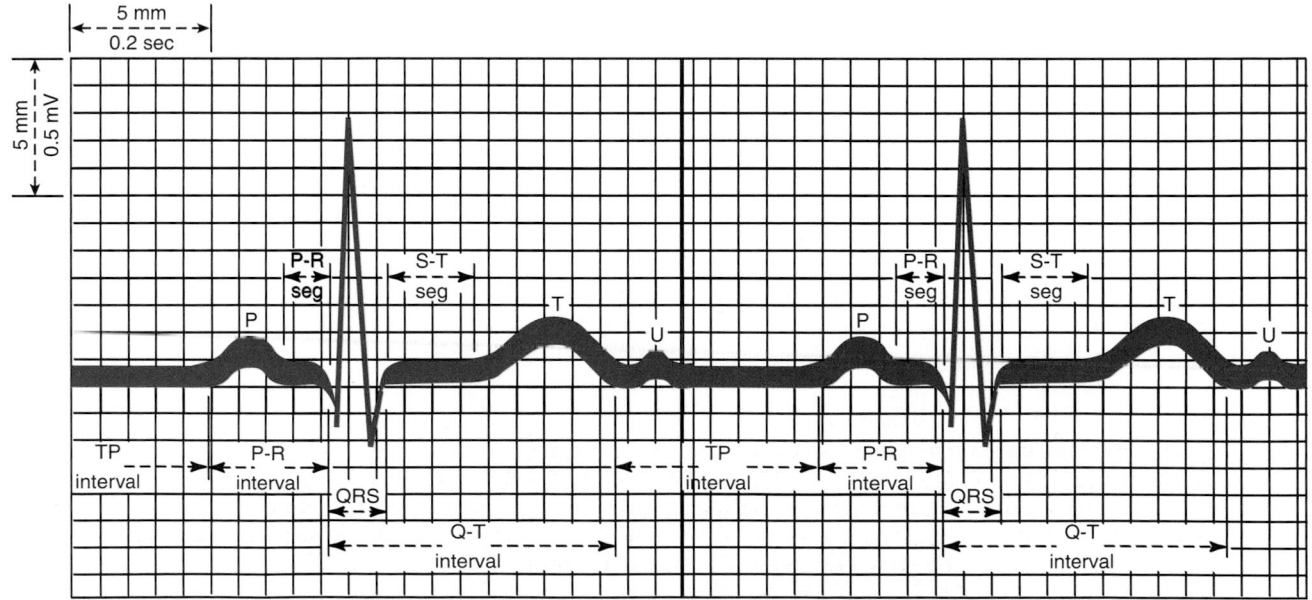

FIGURE 27-3 ECG graph and commonly measured components. Each small box represents 0.04 seconds on the horizontal axis and 1 mm or 0.1 millivolt on the vertical axis. The PR interval is measured from the beginning of the P wave to the beginning of the QRS complex; the QRS complex is measured from the beginning of the Q wave to the end of the S wave; the QT interval is measured from the beginning of the Q wave to the end of the T wave; and the TP interval is measured from the end of the T wave to the beginning of the next P wave.

When no electrical activity is detected, the line on the graph remains flat; this is called the isoelectric line. The ST segment is compared with the TP interval to detect changes from the line on the graph during the isoelectric period.

The **PP interval** is measured from the beginning of one P wave to the beginning of the next. The PP interval is used to determine atrial rhythm and atrial rate. The RR interval is measured from one QRS complex to the next QRS complex. The RR interval is used to determine ventricular rate and rhythm (Fig. 27-4).

DETERMINING VENTRICULAR HEART RATE FROM THE ELECTROCARDIOGRAM

Heart rate can be obtained from the ECG strip by several methods. A 1-minute strip contains 300 large boxes and 1500 small boxes. Therefore, an easy and accurate method of determining heart rate with a regular rhythm is to count the number of small boxes within an RR interval and divide 1500 by that number. If, for example, there are 10 small boxes between two R waves, the heart rate is 1500 ÷ 10, or 150; if there are 25 small boxes, the heart rate is 1500 ÷ 25, or 60 (see Fig. 27-4A).

An alternative but less accurate method for estimating heart rate, which is usually used when the rhythm is irregular, is to count the number of RR intervals in 6 seconds and multiply that number by 10. The top of the ECG paper is usually marked at 3-second intervals, which is 15 large boxes horizontally (see Fig. 27-4B). The RR intervals are counted, rather than QRS complexes, because a computed heart rate based on the latter might be inaccurately high.

The same methods may be used for determining atrial rate, using the PP interval instead of the RR interval.

DETERMINING HEART RHYTHM FROM THE ELECTROCARDIOGRAM

The rhythm is often identified at the same time the rate is determined. The RR interval is used to determine ventricular rhythm and the PP interval to determine atrial rhythm. If the intervals are the same or nearly the same throughout the strip, the rhythm is called regular. If the intervals are different, the rhythm is called irregular.

ANALYZING THE ELECTROCARDIOGRAM RHYTHM STRIP

The ECG must be analyzed in a systematic manner to determine the patient's cardiac rhythm and to detect dysrhythmias and conduction disorders, as well as evidence of myocardial ischemia, injury, and infarction. Chart 27-2 is an example of a method that can be used to analyze the patient's rhythm.

Once the rhythm has been analyzed, the findings are compared with and matched to the ECG criteria for dysrhythmias to determine a diagnosis. It is important for the nurse to assess the patient to determine the physiologic effect of the dysrhythmia and to identify possible causes. Treatment of dysrhythmias is based on the etiology and the effect of the dysrhythmia, not on its presence alone.

Normal Sinus Rhythm

Normal sinus rhythm occurs when the electrical impulse starts at a regular rate and rhythm in the sinus node and travels through the normal conduction pathway. The following are the ECG criteria for normal sinus rhythm (Fig. 27-5):

Ventricular and atrial rate: 60 to 100 in the adult
Ventricular and atrial rhythm: Regular
QRS shape and duration: Usually normal, but may be regularly abnormal
P wave: Normal and consistent shape; always in front of the QRS
PR interval: Consistent interval between 0.12 and 0.20 seconds
P: QRS ratio: 1 : 1

Types of Dysrhythmias

Dysrhythmias include sinus node, atrial, junctional, and ventricular dysrhythmias and their various subcategories.

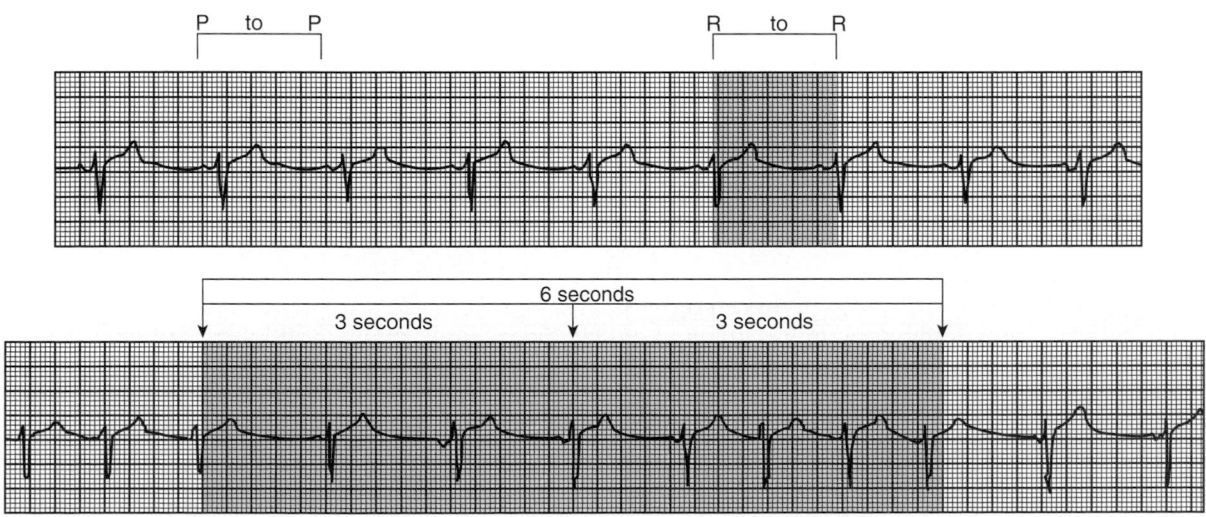

FIGURE 27-4 (**A**) Heart rate determination for a regular rhythm: 1500 divided by the number of small boxes between two R waves (there are 25 in this example) equals the ventricular heart rate. The heart rate in this example is 60. (**B**) Heart rate determination if the rhythm is irregular. There are approximately seven RR intervals in 6 seconds. Seven times 10 equals 70. The heart rate is 70.

Chart 27-2 Interpreting Dysrhythmias: Systematic Analysis of the Electrocardiogram

When examining an ECG rhythm strip to learn more about a patient's dysrhythmia, the nurse conducts the following assessment:
1. Determine the ventricular rate.
2. Determine the ventricular rhythm.
3. Determine QRS duration.
4. Determine whether the QRS duration is consistent throughout the strip. If not, identify other duration.
5. Identify QRS shape; if not consistent, then identify other shapes.
6. Identify P waves; is there a P in front of every QRS?
7. Identify P-wave shape; identify whether it is consistent or not.
8. Determine the atrial rate.
9. Determine the atrial rhythm.
10. Determine each PR interval.
11. Determine if the PR intervals are consistent, irregular but with a pattern to the irregularity, or just irregular.
12. Determine how many P waves for each QRS (P:QRS ratio).

In many cases, the nurse may use a checklist and document the findings next to the appropriate ECG criterion.

SINUS NODE DYSRHYTHMIAS

Sinus Bradycardia. Sinus bradycardia occurs when the sinus node creates an impulse at a slower-than-normal rate. Causes include lower metabolic needs (eg, sleep, athletic training, hypothermia, hypothyroidism), vagal stimulation (eg, from vomiting, suctioning, severe pain, extreme emotions), medications (eg, calcium channel blockers, amiodarone, beta-blockers), increased intracranial pressure, and myocardial infarction (MI), especially of the inferior wall. The following are characteristics of sinus bradycardia (Fig. 27-6):

Ventricular and atrial rate: Less than 60 in the adult
Ventricular and atrial rhythm: Regular
QRS shape and duration: Usually normal, but may be regularly abnormal
P wave: Normal and consistent shape; always in front of the QRS
PR interval: Consistent interval between 0.12 and 0.20 seconds
P:QRS ratio: 1:1

All characteristics of sinus bradycardia are the same as those of normal sinus rhythm, except for the rate. The patient is assessed to determine the hemodynamic effect and the possible cause of the dysrhythmia. If the decrease in heart rate results from stimulation of the vagus nerve, such as with bearing down during defecation or vomiting, attempts are made to prevent further vagal

stimulation. If the bradycardia is from a medication such as a beta-blocker, the medication may be withheld. If the slow heart rate causes significant hemodynamic changes, resulting in shortness of breath, decreased level of consciousness, angina, hypotension, ST-segment changes, or premature ventricular complexes, treatment is directed toward increasing the heart rate.

Atropine, 0.5 to 1.0 mg given rapidly as an intravenous (IV) bolus, is the medication of choice in treating sinus bradycardia. It blocks vagal stimulation, thus allowing a normal rate to occur. Rarely, catecholamines and emergency transcutaneous pacing also may be implemented.

Sinus Tachycardia. Sinus tachycardia occurs when the sinus node creates an impulse at a faster-than-normal rate. It may be caused by acute blood loss, anemia, shock, hypervolemia, hypovolemia, congestive heart failure, pain, hypermetabolic states, fever, exercise, anxiety, or sympathomimetic medications. The ECG criteria for sinus tachycardia follow (Fig. 27-7):

Ventricular and atrial rate: Greater than 100 in the adult
Ventricular and atrial rhythm: Regular
QRS shape and duration: Usually normal, but may be regularly abnormal
P wave: Normal and consistent shape; always in front of the QRS, but may be buried in the preceding T wave
PR interval: Consistent interval between 0.12 and 0.20 seconds
P:QRS ratio: 1:1

All aspects of sinus tachycardia are the same as those of normal sinus rhythm, except for the rate. As the heart rate increases, the diastolic filling time decreases, possibly resulting in reduced cardiac output and subsequent symptoms of syncope and low blood pressure. If the rapid rate persists and the heart cannot compensate for the decreased ventricular filling, the patient may develop acute pulmonary edema.

Treatment of sinus tachycardia is usually directed at abolishing its cause. Calcium channel blockers and beta-blockers (Table 27-1) may be used to reduce the heart rate quickly.

Sinus Arrhythmia. Sinus arrhythmia occurs when the sinus node creates an impulse at an irregular rhythm; the rate usually increases with inspiration and decreases with expiration. Nonrespiratory causes include heart disease and valvular disease, but these are rarely seen. The ECG criteria for sinus arrhythmia follow (Fig. 27-8):

Ventricular and atrial rate: 60 to 100 in the adult
Ventricular and atrial rhythm: Irregular
QRS shape and duration: Usually normal, but may be regularly abnormal

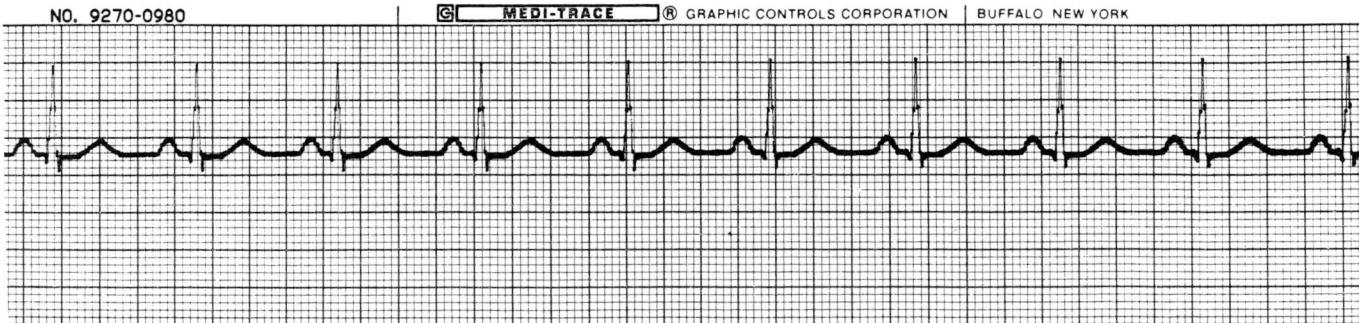

NO. 9270-0980   MEDI-TRACE ® GRAPHIC CONTROLS CORPORATION | BUFFALO NEW YORK

FIGURE 27-5 Normal sinus rhythm in lead II.

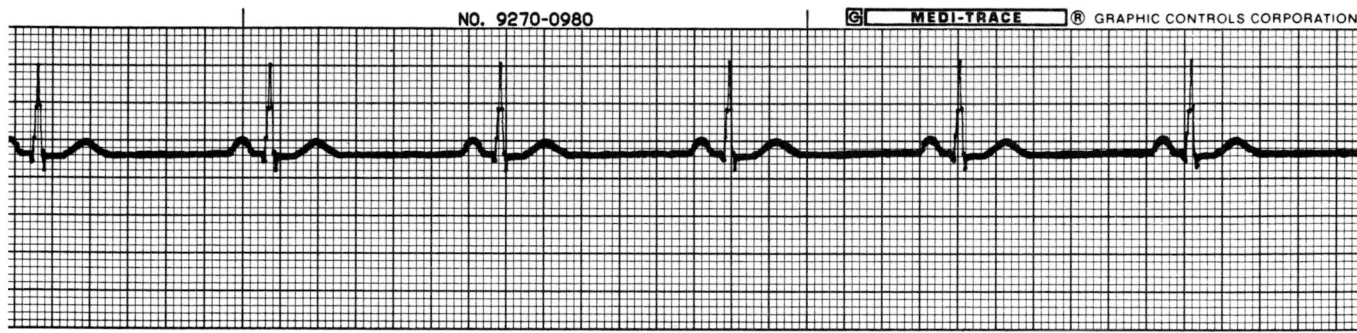

FIGURE 27-6 Sinus bradycardia in lead II.

P wave: Normal and consistent shape; always in front of the QRS
PR interval: Consistent interval between 0.12 and 0.20 seconds
P: QRS ratio: 1 : 1

Sinus arrhythmia does not cause any significant hemodynamic effect and usually is not treated.

ATRIAL DYSRHYTHMIAS

Premature Atrial Complex. A premature atrial complex (PAC) is a single ECG complex that occurs when an electrical impulse starts in the atrium before the next normal impulse of the sinus node. The PAC may be caused by caffeine, alcohol, nicotine, stretched atrial myocardium (as in hypervolemia), anxiety, hypokalemia (low potassium level), hypermetabolic states, or atrial ischemia, injury, or infarction. PACs are often seen with sinus tachycardia. PACs have the following characteristics (Fig. 27-9):

Ventricular and atrial rate: Depends on the underlying rhythm (eg, sinus tachycardia)
Ventricular and atrial rhythm: Irregular due to early P waves, creating a PP interval that is shorter than the others. This is sometimes followed by a longer-than-normal PP interval, but one that is less than twice the normal PP interval. This type of interval is called a noncompensatory pause.
QRS shape and duration: The QRS that follows the early P wave is usually normal, but it may be abnormal (aberrantly conducted PAC). It may even be absent (blocked PAC).
P wave: An early and different P wave may be seen or may be hidden in the T wave; other P waves in the strip are consistent.
PR interval: The early P wave has a shorter-than-normal PR interval, but still between 0.12 and 0.20 seconds.
P: QRS ratio: usually 1 : 1

PACs are common in normal hearts. The patient may say, "My heart skipped a beat." A pulse deficit (a difference between the apical and radial pulse rate) may exist.

If PACs are infrequent, no treatment is necessary. If they are frequent (more than 6 per minute), this may herald a worsening disease state or the onset of more serious dysrhythmias, such as atrial fibrillation. Treatment is directed toward the cause.

Atrial Flutter. Atrial flutter occurs in the atrium and creates impulses at an atrial rate between 250 and 400 times per minute. Because the atrial rate is faster than the AV node can conduct, not all atrial impulses are conducted into the ventricle, causing a therapeutic block at the AV node. This is an important feature of this dysrhythmia. If all atrial impulses were conducted to the ventricle, the ventricular rate would also be 250 to 400, which would result in ventricular fibrillation, a life-threatening dysrhythmia. Causes are similar to that of atrial fibrillation. Atrial flutter is characterized by the following (Fig. 27-10):

Ventricular and atrial rate: Atrial rate ranges between 250 and 400; ventricular rate usually ranges between 75 and 150.
Ventricular and atrial rhythm: The atrial rhythm is regular; the ventricular rhythm is usually regular but may be irregular because of a change in the AV conduction.
QRS shape and duration: Usually normal, but may be abnormal or may be absent
P wave: Saw-toothed shape. These waves are referred to as F waves.
PR interval: Multiple F waves may make it difficult to determine the PR interval.
P: QRS ratio: 2 : 1, 3 : 1, or 4 : 1

Atrial flutter can cause serious signs and symptoms, such as chest pain, shortness of breath, and low blood pressure. If the

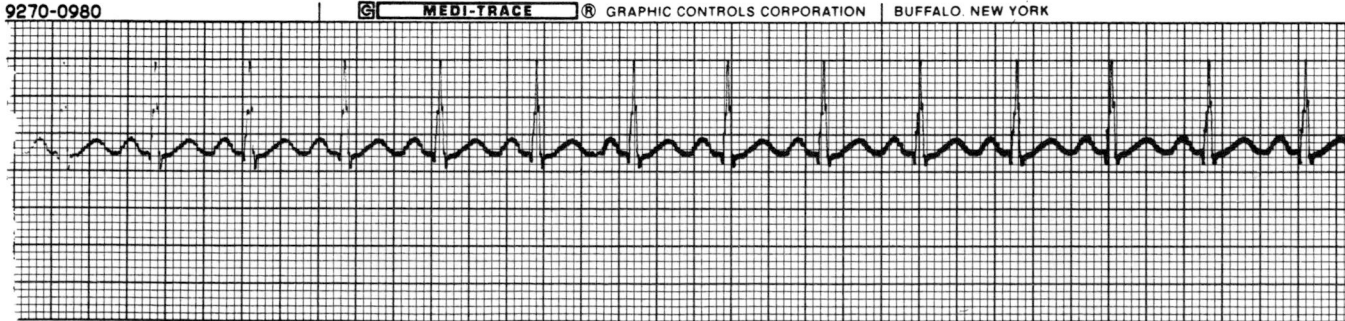

FIGURE 27-7 Sinus tachycardia in lead II.

Table 27-1 • Summary of Antiarrhythmic Medications*

CLASS	ACTION	DRUGS: GENERIC (TRADE) NAMES	SIDE EFFECTS	NURSING INTERVENTIONS
1A	Moderate depression of depolarization; prolongs repolarization Treats and prevents atrial and ventricular dysrhythmias	quinidine (Quinaglute, Quinalan, Quinora, Quinidex, Cardioquin) procainamide (Pronestyl) disopyramide (Norpace)	Decreased cardiac contractility Prolonged QRS, QT Proarrhythmic Hypotension with IV administration Lupus-like syndrome with Pronestyl Anticholinergic effects: dry mouth, decreased urine output	Observe for HF Monitor BP with IV administration Monitor QRS duration for increase >50% from baseline Monitor for prolonged QT Monitor N-acetyl procainamide (NAPA) laboratory values during procainamide therapy
1B	Minimal depression of depolarization; shortened repolarization Treats ventricular dysrhythmias	lidocaine (Xylocaine) mexiletine (Mexitil) tocainide (Tonocard)	CNS changes (eg, confusion, lethargy)	Discuss with physician decreasing the dose in elderly patients and patients with cardiac/liver dysfunction
1C	Marked depression of depolarization; little effect on repolarization Treats atrial and ventricular dysrhythmias	flecainide (Tambocor) propafenone (Rhythmol)	Proarrhythmic HF Bradycardia AV blocks	Discuss patient's left ventricular function with physician
II	Decreases automaticity and conduction Treats atrial and ventricular dysrhythmias	acebutolol (Sectral) atenolol (Tenormin) esmolol (Brevibloc) labetalol (Normodyne) metoprolol (Lopressor, Toprol) nadolol (Corgard) propranolol (Betachron E-R, Inderal) sotalol (Betapace; also has class III actions)	Bradycardia, AV block Decreased contractility Bronchospasm Hypotension with IV administration Masks hypoglycemia and thyrotoxicosis CNS disturbances	Monitor heart rate, PR interval, signs and symptoms of HF Monitor blood glucose level in patients with type 2 diabetes mellitus
III	Prolongs repolarization Primarily treats and prevents ventricular dysrhythmias; may also be used to treat atrial dysrhythmias	amiodarone (Cordarone, Pacerone) dofetilide (Tikosyn) ibutilide (Corvert)	Pulmonary toxicity (amiodarone) Corneal microdeposits (amiodarone) Photosensitivity (amiodarone) Hypotension with IV administration Polymorphic ventricular dysrhythmias Nausea and vomiting See beta-blockers (sotalol)	Make sure patient is sent for baseline pulmonary function tests (amiodarone) Closely monitor patient
IV	Blocks calcium channel Treats atrial dysrhythmias	verapamil (Calan, Isoptin, Verlan) diltiazem (Cardizem, Dilacor, Tiazac)	Bradycardia, AV blocks Hypotension with IV administration HF, peripheral edema	Monitor heart rate, PR interval Monitor blood pressure closely with IV administration Monitor for signs and symptoms of HF

*Based on Vaughn-Williams classification.
AV, atrioventricular; BP, blood pressure; CNS, central nervous system; HF, heart failure; IV, intravenous.

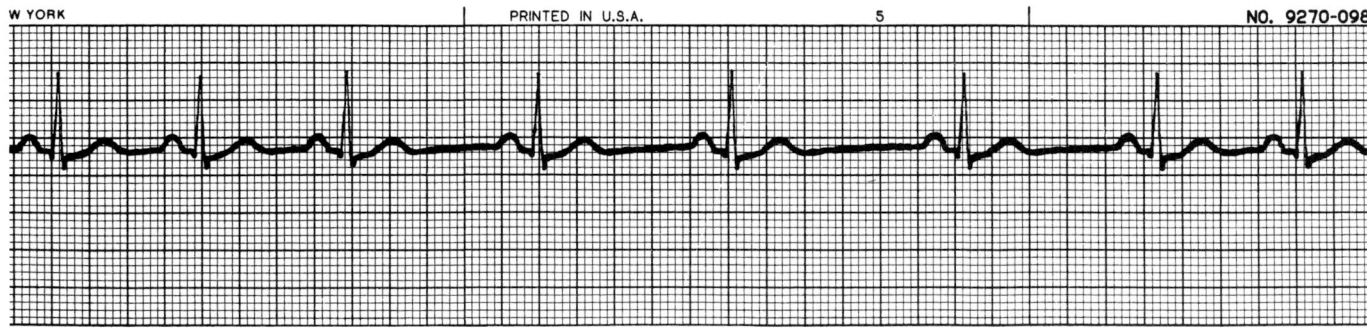

FIGURE 27-8 Sinus arrhythmia in lead II.

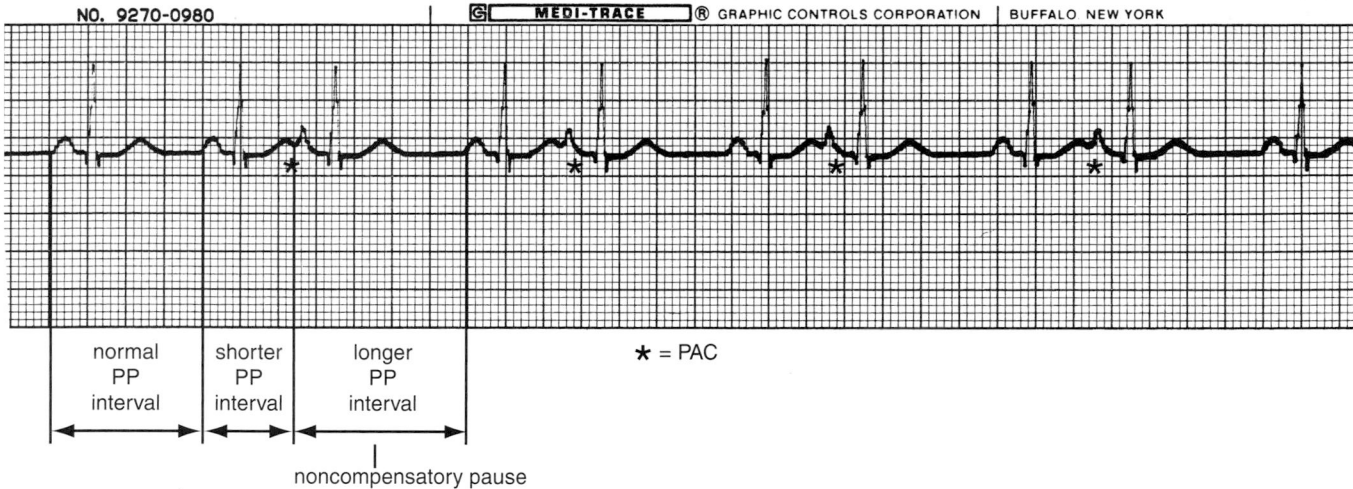

normal
PP
interval

shorter
PP
interval

longer
PP
interval

★ = PAC

noncompensatory pause

FIGURE 27-9 Premature atrial complexes (PACs) in lead II. Note pause following PAC that is longer than the normal PP interval, but shorter than twice the normal PP interval.

patient is unstable, electrical cardioversion (discussed later) is usually indicated. If the patient is stable, diltiazem (eg, Cardizem), verapamil (eg, Calan, Isoptin), beta-blockers, or digitalis may be administered intravenously to slow the ventricular rate. These medications can slow conduction through the AV node. Flecainide (Tambocor), ibutilide (Corvert), dofetilide (Tikosyn), quinidine (eg, Cardioquin, Quinaglute), disopyramide (Norpace), or amiodarone (Cordarone, Pacerone) may be given to promote conversion to sinus rhythm (see Table 27-1). If medication therapy is unsuccessful, electrical cardioversion is often successful. Once conversion has occurred, quinidine, disopyramide, flecainide, propafenone (Rhythmol), amiodarone, or sotalol (Betapace) may be given to maintain sinus rhythm (see Table 27-1).

Atrial Fibrillation. Atrial fibrillation causes a rapid, disorganized, and uncoordinated twitching of atrial musculature. It is the most common dysrhythmia that causes patients to seek medical attention. It may start and stop suddenly. Atrial fibrillation may occur for a very short time (**paroxysmal**), or it may be chronic. Atrial fibrillation is usually associated with advanced age, valvular heart disease, coronary artery disease, hypertension, cardiomyopathy, hyperthyroidism, pulmonary disease, acute moderate to heavy ingestion of alcohol ("holiday heart" syndrome), or the aftermath of open heart surgery. Sometimes it occurs in people without any underlying pathophysiology (termed lone atrial fibrillation). Atrial fibrillation is characterized by the following (Fig. 27-11):

Ventricular and atrial rate: Atrial rate is 300 to 600. Ventricular rate is usually 120 to 200 in untreated atrial fibrillation
Ventricular and atrial rhythm: Highly irregular
QRS shape and duration: Usually normal, but may be abnormal
P wave: No discernible P waves; irregular undulating waves are seen and are referred to as fibrillatory or f waves
PR interval: Cannot be measured
P: QRS ratio: many : 1

A rapid ventricular response reduces the time for ventricular filling, resulting in a smaller stroke volume. Because this rhythm causes the atria and ventricles to contract at different times, the atrial kick (the last part of diastole and ventricular filling, which accounts for 25% to 30% of the cardiac output) is also lost. This leads to symptoms of irregular palpitations, fatigue, and malaise. There is usually a pulse deficit, a numerical difference between apical and radial pulse rates. The shorter time in diastole reduces the time available for coronary artery perfusion, thereby increasing the risk for myocardial ischemia. The erratic atrial contraction promotes the formation of a thrombus within the atria, increasing the risk for an embolic event. There is a two- to five-fold increase in the risk of stroke (brain attack).

Treatment of atrial fibrillation depends on its cause and duration and the patient's symptoms, age, and comorbidities. In many patients, atrial fibrillation converts to sinus rhythm within 24 hours and without treatment. Both stable and unstable atrial fibrillation

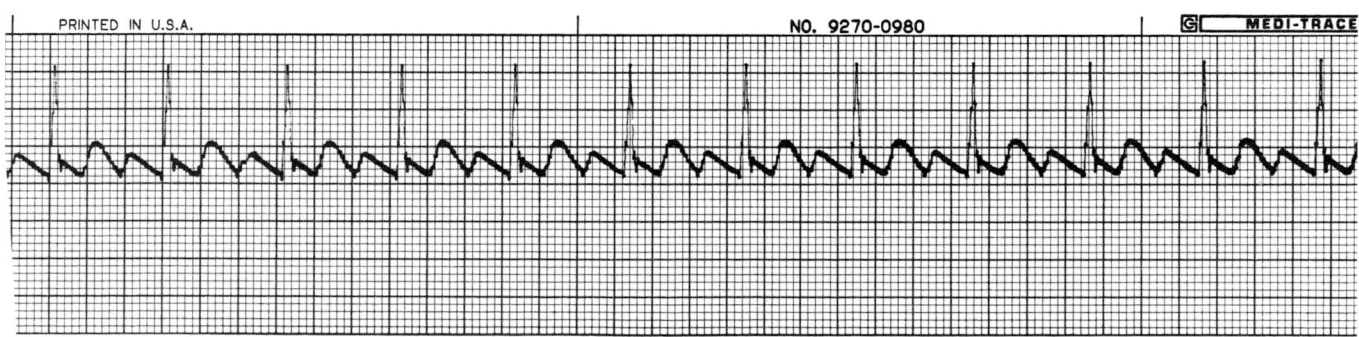

FIGURE 27-10 Atrial flutter in lead II.

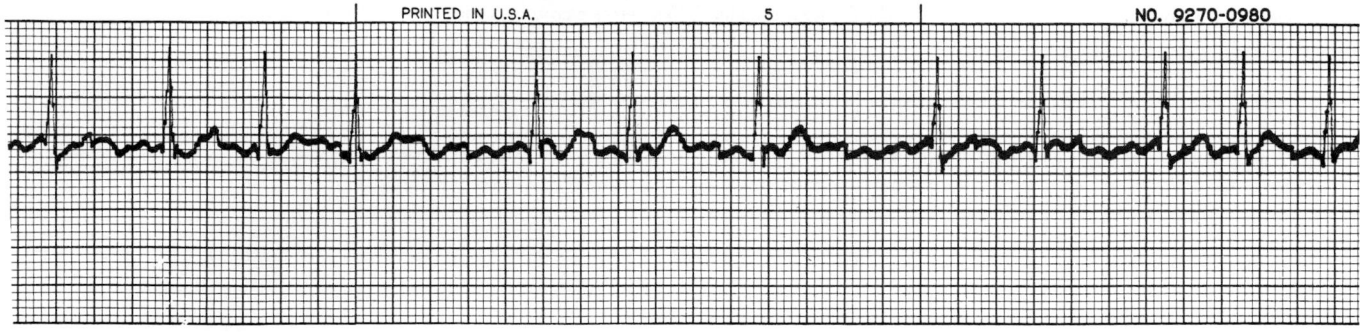

FIGURE 27-11 Atrial fibrillation in lead II.

of short duration are treated the same as stable and unstable atrial flutter. Cardioversion may be indicated for atrial fibrillation that has been present for less than 48 hours, a condition termed acute-onset atrial fibrillation. Cardioversion of atrial fibrillation that has lasted longer than 48 hours should be avoided unless the patient has received anticoagulants, due to the high risk for embolization of atrial thrombi.

For atrial fibrillation of acute onset, the medications quinidine, ibutilide, flecainide, dofetilide, propafenone, procainamide (Pronestyl), disopyramide, or amiodarone (see Table 27-1) may be given to achieve conversion to sinus rhythm (McNamara et al., 2001). Intravenous adenosine (Adenocard, Adenoscan) has also been used for conversion, as well as to assist in the diagnosis. To prevent recurrence and to maintain sinus rhythm, quinidine, disopyramide, flecainide, propafenone, sotalol, or amiodarone may be prescribed. Calcium-channel blockers [diltiazem (Cardizem, Dilacor, Tiazac) and verapamil (Calan, Isoptin, Verelan)] and beta blockers (see Table 27-1) are effective in controlling the ventricular rate in atrial fibrillation, especially during exercise (McNamara, et al., 2001). Use of digoxin is recommended to control the ventricular rate in those patients with poor cardiac function (ejection fraction less than 40%) (Hauptman & Kelly, 1999). In addition, warfarin is indicated if the patient is at higher risk for a stroke (ie, is elderly or has hypertension, heart failure, or a history of stroke). Aspirin may be substituted for warfarin for those with contraindications to warfarin and those who are at lower risk of stroke. The choice of antithrombotic medication can be guided by transesophageal echocardiography. Pacemaker implantation or surgery is sometimes indicated for patients who are unresponsive to medications.

JUNCTIONAL DYSRHYTHMIAS

Premature Junctional Complex. A premature junctional complex is an impulse that starts in the AV nodal area before the next normal sinus impulse reaches the AV node. Premature junctional complexes are less common than PACs. Causes of premature junctional complex include digitalis toxicity, congestive heart failure, and coronary artery disease. The ECG criteria for premature junctional complex are the same as for PACs, except for the P wave and the PR interval. The P wave may be absent, may follow the QRS, or may occur before the QRS but with a PR interval of less than 0.12 seconds. Premature junctional complexes rarely produce significant symptoms. Treatment for frequent premature junctional complexes is the same as for frequent PACs.

Junctional Rhythm. Junctional or idionodal rhythm occurs when the AV node, instead of the sinus node, becomes the pacemaker of the heart. When the sinus node slows (eg, from increased vagal tone) or when the impulse cannot be conducted through the AV node (eg, because of complete heart block), the AV node automatically discharges an impulse. The following are the ECG criteria for junctional rhythm not caused by complete heart block (Fig. 27-12):

Ventricular and atrial rate: Ventricular rate 40 to 60; atrial rate also 40 to 60 if P waves are discernible
Ventricular and atrial rhythm: Regular
QRS shape and duration: Usually normal, but may be abnormal
P wave: May be absent, after the QRS complex, or before the QRS; may be inverted, especially in lead II

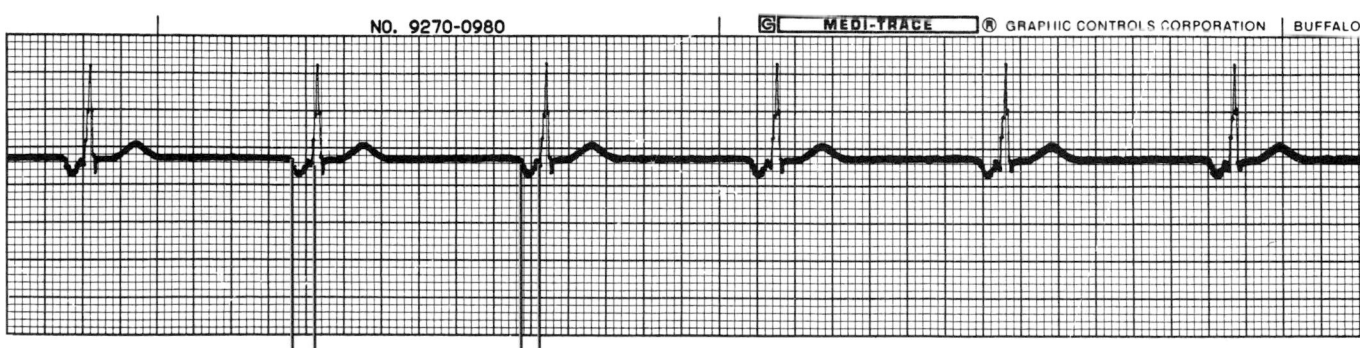

FIGURE 27-12 Junctional rhythm in lead II; note short PR intervals.

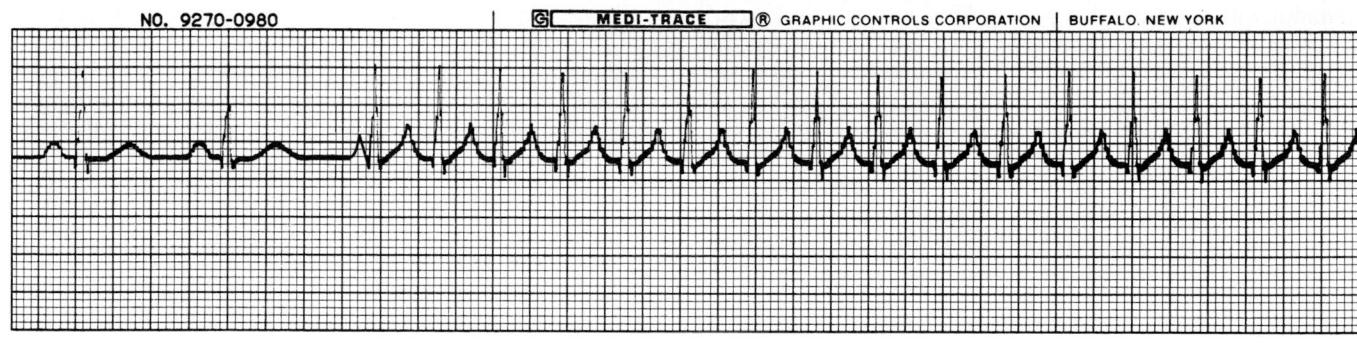

NO. 9270-0980 | MEDI-TRACE ® GRAPHIC CONTROLS CORPORATION | BUFFALO, NEW YORK

FIGURE 27-13 AV nodal reentry tachycardia in lead II.

PR interval: If P wave is in front of the QRS, PR interval is less than 0.12 second.
P: QRS ratio: 1:1 or 0:1

Junctional rhythm may produce signs and symptoms of reduced cardiac output. If so, the treatment is the same as for sinus bradycardia. Emergency pacing may be needed.

Atrioventricular Nodal Reentry Tachycardia.

AV nodal reentry tachycardia occurs when an impulse is conducted to an area in the AV node that causes the impulse to be rerouted back into the same area over and over again at a very fast rate. Each time the impulse is conducted through this area, it is also conducted down into the ventricles, causing a fast ventricular rate. AV nodal reentry tachycardia that has an abrupt onset and an abrupt cessation with a QRS of normal duration had been called paroxysmal atrial tachycardia (PAT). Factors associated with the development of AV nodal reentry tachycardia include caffeine, nicotine, hypoxemia, and stress. Underlying pathologies include coronary artery disease and cardiomyopathy. The ECG criteria are as follows (Fig. 27-13):

Ventricular and atrial rate: Atrial rate usually ranges between 150 to 250; ventricular rate usually ranges between 75 to 250
Ventricular and atrial rhythm: Regular; sudden onset and termination of the tachycardia
QRS shape and duration: Usually normal, but may be abnormal
P wave: Usually very difficult to discern
PR interval: If P wave is in front of the QRS, PR interval is less than 0.12 seconds
P: QRS ratio: 1:1, 2:1

The clinical symptoms vary with the rate and duration of the tachycardia and the patient's underlying condition. The tachycardia usually is of short duration, resulting only in palpitations. A fast rate may also reduce cardiac output, resulting in significant signs and symptoms such as restlessness, chest pain, shortness of breath, pallor, hypotension, and loss of consciousness.

Treatment is aimed at breaking the reentry of the impulse. Vagal maneuvers, such as carotid sinus massage (Fig. 27-14), gag reflex, breath holding, and immersing the face in ice water, increase parasympathetic stimulation, causing slower conduction through the AV node and blocking the reentry of the rerouted impulse. Some patients have learned to use some of these methods to terminate the episode on their own. Because of the risk of a cerebral embolic event, carotid sinus massage is contraindicated in patients with carotid bruits. If the vagal maneuvers are ineffective, the patient may then receive a bolus of adenosine, verapamil, or diltiazem. Cardioversion is the treatment of choice if the patient is unstable or does not respond to the medications.

If P waves cannot be identified, the rhythm may be called **supraventricular tachycardia (SVT)**, which indicates only that it is not **ventricular tachycardia (VT)**. SVT could be atrial fibrillation, atrial flutter, or AV nodal reentry tachycardia, among others. Vagal maneuvers and adenosine are used to slow conduction in the AV node to allow visualization of the P waves.

VENTRICULAR DYSRHYTHMIAS

Premature Ventricular Complex.

Premature ventricular complex (PVC) is an impulse that starts in a ventricle and is conducted through the ventricles before the next normal sinus impulse. PVCs can occur in healthy people, especially with the use of caffeine, nicotine, or alcohol. They are also caused by cardiac ischemia or infarction, increased workload on the heart (eg, exercise, fever, hypervolemia, heart failure, tachycardia), digitalis toxicity, hypoxia, acidosis, or electrolyte imbalances, especially hypokalemia.

In the absence of disease, PVCs are not serious. In the patient with an acute MI, PVCs may indicate the need for more aggressive therapy. PVCs may indicate the possibility of ensuing VT. However, PVCs that are (1) more frequent than 6 per minute,

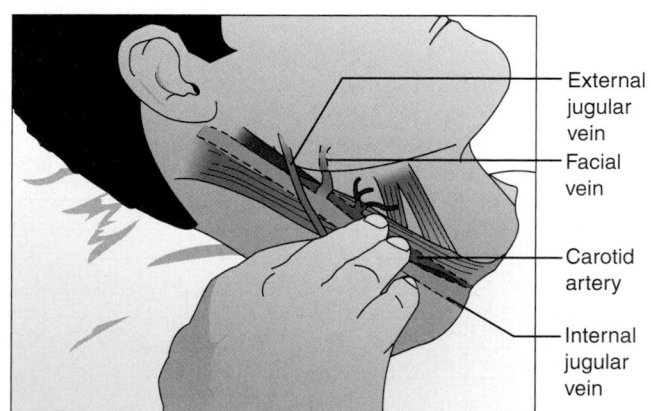

External jugular vein

Facial vein

Carotid artery

Internal jugular vein

FIGURE 27-14 Carotid sinus massage.

(2) multifocal or polymorphic (having different shapes), (3) occur two in a row (pair), and (4) occur on the T wave (the vulnerable period of ventricular depolarization) have not been found to be precursors of VT (Cardiac Arrhythmia Suppression Trial Investigators, 1989). These PVCs are no longer considered as warning or complex PVCs.

In a rhythm called bigeminy, every other complex is a PVC. Trigeminy is a rhythm in which every third complex is a PVC, and quadrigeminy is a rhythm in which every fourth complex is a PVC. PVCs have the following characteristics on the ECG (Fig. 27-15):

Ventricular and atrial rate: Depends on the underlying rhythm (eg, sinus rhythm)
Ventricular and atrial rhythm: Irregular due to early QRS, creating one RR interval that is shorter than the others. PP interval may be regular, indicating that the PVC did not depolarize the sinus node.
QRS shape and duration: Duration is 0.12 seconds or longer; shape is bizarre and abnormal
P wave: Visibility of P wave depends on the timing of the PVC; may be absent (hidden in the QRS or T wave) or in front of the QRS. If the P wave follows the QRS, the shape of the P wave may be different.
PR interval: If the P wave is in front of the QRS, the PR interval is less than 0.12 seconds.
P: QRS ratio: 0 : 1; 1 : 1

The patient may feel nothing or may say that the heart "skipped a beat." The effect of a PVC depends on its timing in the cardiac cycle and how much blood was in the ventricles when they contracted. Initial treatment is aimed at correcting the cause, if possible. Lidocaine (Xylocaine) is the medication most commonly used for immediate, short-term therapy (see Table 27-1). Long-term pharmacotherapy for only PVCs is not indicated.

Ventricular Tachycardia. Ventricular tachycardia (VT) is defined as three or more PVCs in a row, occurring at a rate exceeding 100 beats per minute. The causes are similar to those for PVC. VT is usually associated with coronary artery disease and may precede ventricular fibrillation. VT is an emergency because the patient is usually (although not always) unresponsive and pulseless. VT has the following characteristics (Fig. 27-16):

Ventricular and atrial rate: Ventricular rate is 100 to 200 beats per minute; atrial rate depends on the underlying rhythm (eg, sinus rhythm)
Ventricular and atrial rhythm: Usually regular; atrial rhythm may also be regular.
QRS shape and duration: Duration is 0.12 seconds or more; bizarre, abnormal shape

P wave: Very difficult to detect, so atrial rate and rhythm may be indeterminable
PR interval: Very irregular, if P waves seen.
P: QRS ratio: Difficult to determine, but if P waves are apparent, there are usually more QRS complexes than P waves.

The patient's tolerance or lack of tolerance for this rapid rhythm depends on the ventricular rate and underlying disease. If the patient is stable, continuing the assessment, especially obtaining a 12-lead ECG, may be the only action necessary. Cardioversion may be the treatment of choice, especially if the patient is unstable. Several factors determine the initial medication used for treatment, including the following: identifying the rhythm as monomorphic (having a consistent QRS shape and rate) or polymorphic (having varying QRS shapes and rates); determining the existence of a prolonged QT interval before the initiation of VT; and ascertaining the patient's heart function (normal or decreased). VT in a patient who is unconscious and without a pulse is treated in the same manner as ventricular fibrillation: immediate **defibrillation** is the action of choice.

Ventricular Fibrillation. Ventricular fibrillation is a rapid but disorganized ventricular rhythm that causes ineffective quivering of the ventricles. There is no atrial activity seen on the ECG. Causes of ventricular fibrillation are the same as for VT; it may also result from untreated or unsuccessfully treated VT. Other causes include electrical shock and Brugada syndrome, in which the patient (frequently of Asian descent) has a structurally normal heart, few or no risk factors for coronary artery disease, and a family history of sudden cardiac death. Ventricular fibrillation has the following characteristics (Fig. 27-17):

Ventricular rate: Greater than 300 per minute
Ventricular rhythm: Extremely irregular, without specific pattern
QRS shape and duration: Irregular, undulating waves without recognizable QRS complexes

This dysrhythmia is always characterized by the absence of an audible heartbeat, a palpable pulse, and respirations. Because there is no coordinated cardiac activity, cardiac arrest and death are imminent if ventricular fibrillation is not corrected. Treatment of choice is immediate defibrillation and activation of emergency services. The importance of defibrillation is evident in one of the recent changes in basic life support (American Heart Association, 2000): placing a call for emergency assistance and calling for a defibrillator takes precedence over initiating cardiopulmonary resuscitation in the adult victim. Also, application of an automatic external defibrillator (AED) is included in basic life support classes. After defibrillation, eradicating causes and administering vasoactive and **antiarrhythmic** medications alternating with defibril-

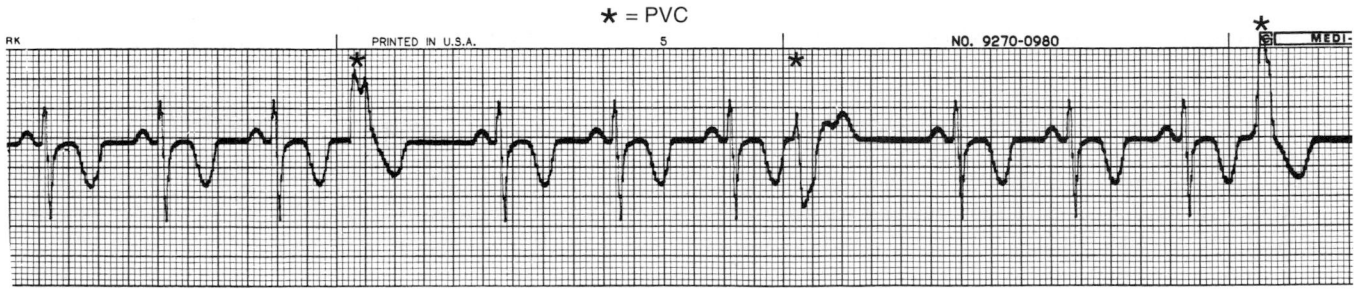

FIGURE 27-15 Multifocal PVCs in quadrigeminy in lead V$_1$. Note regular PP interval.

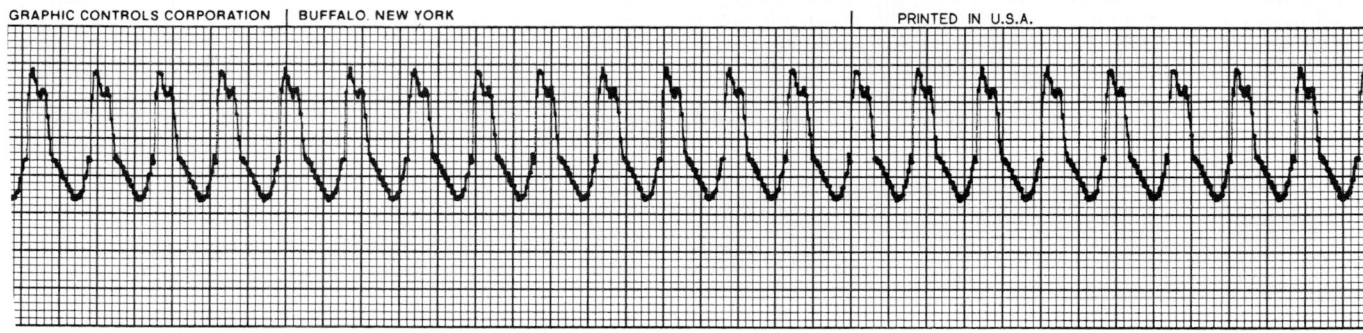

FIGURE 27-16 Ventricular tachycardia in lead V₁.

lation are treatments used to try to convert the rhythm to normal sinus rhythm.

Idioventricular Rhythm. Idioventricular rhythm, also called ventricular escape rhythm, occurs when the impulse starts in the conduction system below the AV node. When the sinus node fails to create an impulse (eg, from increased vagal tone), or when the impulse is created but cannot be conducted through the AV node (eg, due to complete AV block), the Purkinje fibers automatically discharge an impulse. The following are the ECG criteria when idioventricular rhythm is not caused by AV block (Fig. 27-18):

> *Ventricular rate:* Ranges between 20 and 40; if the rate exceeds 40, the rhythm is known as accelerated idioventricular rhythm (AIVR).
> *Ventricular rhythm:* Regular
> *QRS shape and duration:* Bizarre, abnormal shape; duration is 0.12 seconds or more

Idioventricular rhythm commonly causes the patient to lose consciousness and experience other signs and symptoms of reduced cardiac output. In such cases, the treatment is the same as for pulseless electrical activity if the patient is in cardiac arrest or for bradycardia if the patient is not in cardiac arrest. Interventions may include identifying the underlying cause, administering intravenous atropine and vasopressor medications, and initiating emergency transcutaneous pacing. In some cases, idioventricular rhythm may cause no symptoms of reduced cardiac output. However, bed rest is prescribed so as not to increase the cardiac workload.

Ventricular Asystole. Commonly called flatline, ventricular asystole (Fig. 27-19) is characterized by absent QRS complexes, although P waves may be apparent for a short duration in two different leads. There is no heartbeat, no palpable pulse, and no respiration. Without immediate treatment, ventricular asystole is fatal. Cardiopulmonary resuscitation and emergency services are necessary to keep the patient alive. The guidelines for advanced cardiac life support (American Heart Association, 2000) state that the key to successful treatment is rapid assessment to identify a possible cause, which may be hypoxia, acidosis, severe electrolyte imbalance, drug overdose, or hypothermia. Intubation and establishment of intravenous access are the first recommended actions. Transcutaneous pacing may be attempted. A bolus of intravenous epinephrine should be administered and repeated at 3- to 5-minute intervals, followed by 1-mg boluses of atropine at 3- to 5-minute intervals. Because of the poor prognosis associated with asystole, if the patient does not respond to these actions and others aimed at correcting underlying causes, resuscitation efforts are usually ended ("the code is called") unless special circumstances (eg, hypothermia) exist.

CONDUCTION ABNORMALITIES

When assessing the rhythm strip, the nurse takes care first to identify the underlying rhythm (eg, sinus rhythm, sinus arrhythmia). Then the PR interval is assessed for the possibility of an AV block. AV blocks occur when the conduction of the impulse through the AV nodal area is decreased or stopped. These blocks can be caused by medications (eg, digitalis, calcium channel blockers, beta-blockers), myocardial ischemia and infarction, valvular disorders, or myocarditis. If the AV block is caused by increased vagal tone (eg, suctioning, pressure above the eyes or on large vessels, anal stimulation), it is commonly accompanied by sinus bradycardia.

The clinical signs and symptoms of a heart block vary with the resulting ventricular rate and the severity of any underlying dis-

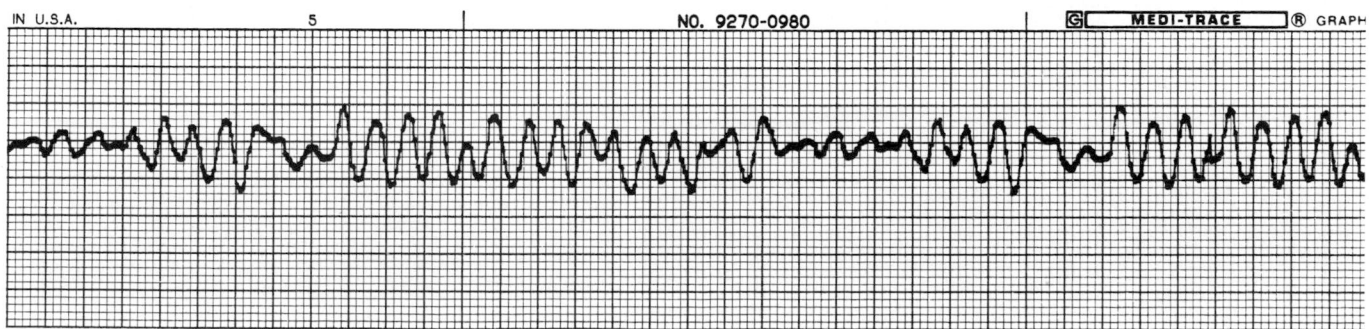

FIGURE 27-17 Ventricular fibrillation in lead II.

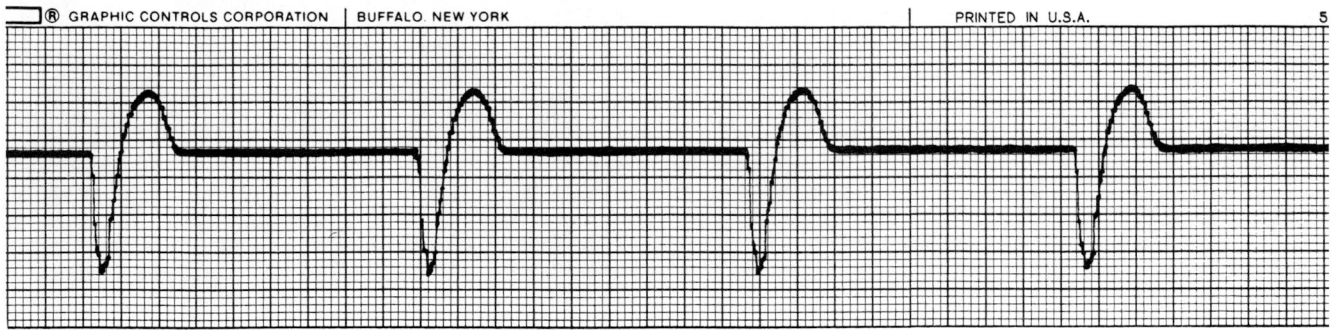

FIGURE 27-18 Idioventricular rhythm in lead V₁.

ease processes. Whereas first-degree AV block rarely causes any hemodynamic effect, the other blocks may result in decreased heart rate, causing a decrease in perfusion to vital organs, such as the brain, heart, kidneys, lungs, and skin. A patient with third-degree AV block caused by digitalis toxicity may be stable; another patient with the same rhythm caused by acute MI may be unstable. Health care providers must always keep in mind the need to treat the patient, not the rhythm. The treatment is based on the hemodynamic effect of the rhythm.

First-Degree Atrioventricular Block. First-degree heart block occurs when all the atrial impulses are conducted through the AV node into the ventricles at a rate slower than normal. This conduction disorder has the following characteristics (Fig. 27-20):

Ventricular and atrial rate: Depends on the underlying rhythm
Ventricular and atrial rhythm: Depends on the underlying rhythm
QRS shape and duration: Usually normal, but may be abnormal
P wave: In front of the QRS complex; shows sinus rhythm, regular shape
PR interval: Greater than 0.20 seconds; PR interval measurement is constant.
P: QRS ratio: 1:1

Second-Degree Atrioventricular Block, Type I. Second-degree, type I heart block occurs when all but one of the atrial impulses are conducted through the AV node into the ventricles. Each atrial impulse takes a longer time for conduction than the one before, until one impulse is fully blocked. Because the AV node is

not depolarized by the blocked atrial impulse, the AV node has time to fully repolarize, so that the next atrial impulse can be conducted within the shortest amount of time. Second-degree AV block, type I has the following characteristics (Fig. 27-21):

Ventricular and atrial rate: Depends on the underlying rhythm
Ventricular and atrial rhythm: The PP interval is regular if the patient has an underlying normal sinus rhythm; the RR interval characteristically reflects a pattern of change. Starting from the RR that is the longest, the RR interval gradually shortens until there is another long RR interval.
QRS shape and duration: Usually normal, but may be abnormal
P wave: In front of the QRS complex; shape depends on underlying rhythm
PR interval: PR interval becomes longer with each succeeding ECG complex until there is a P wave not followed by a QRS. The changes in the PR interval are repeated between each "dropped" QRS, creating a pattern in the irregular PR interval measurements.
P: QRS ratio: 3:2, 4:3, 5:4, and so forth

Second-Degree Atrioventricular Block, Type II. Second-degree, type II heart block occurs when only some of the atrial impulses are conducted through the AV node into the ventricles. Second-degree AV block, type II has the following characteristics (Fig. 27-22):

Ventricular and atrial rate: Depends on the underlying rhythm
Ventricular and atrial rhythm: The PP interval is regular if the patient has an underlying normal sinus rhythm. The RR

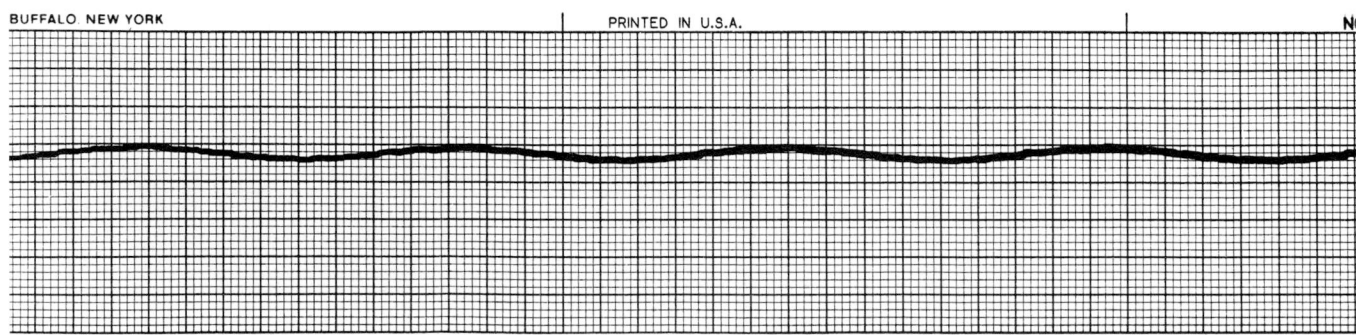

FIGURE 27-19 Asystole. (Always check two different leads to confirm rhythm.)

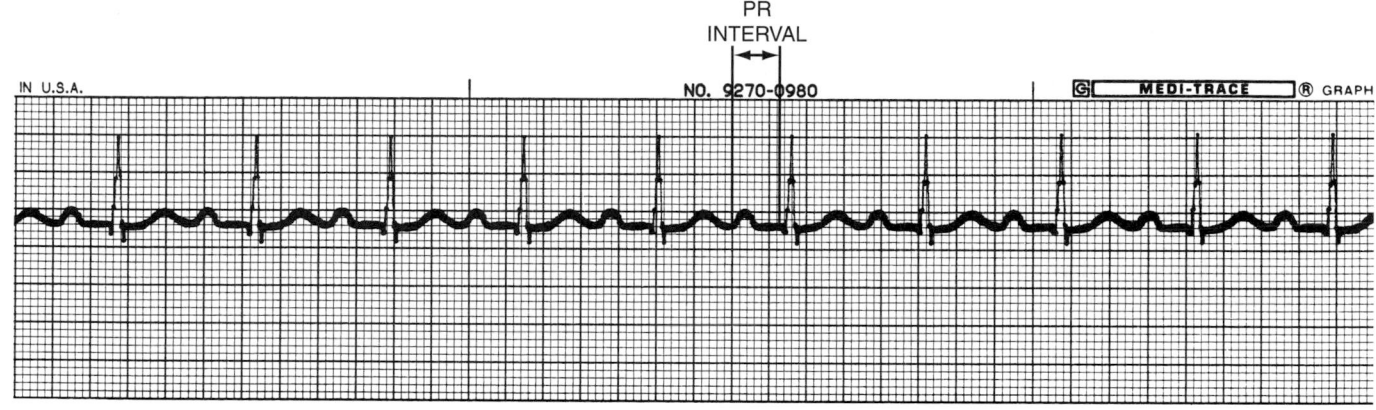

FIGURE 27-20 Sinus rhythm with first-degree AV block in lead II.

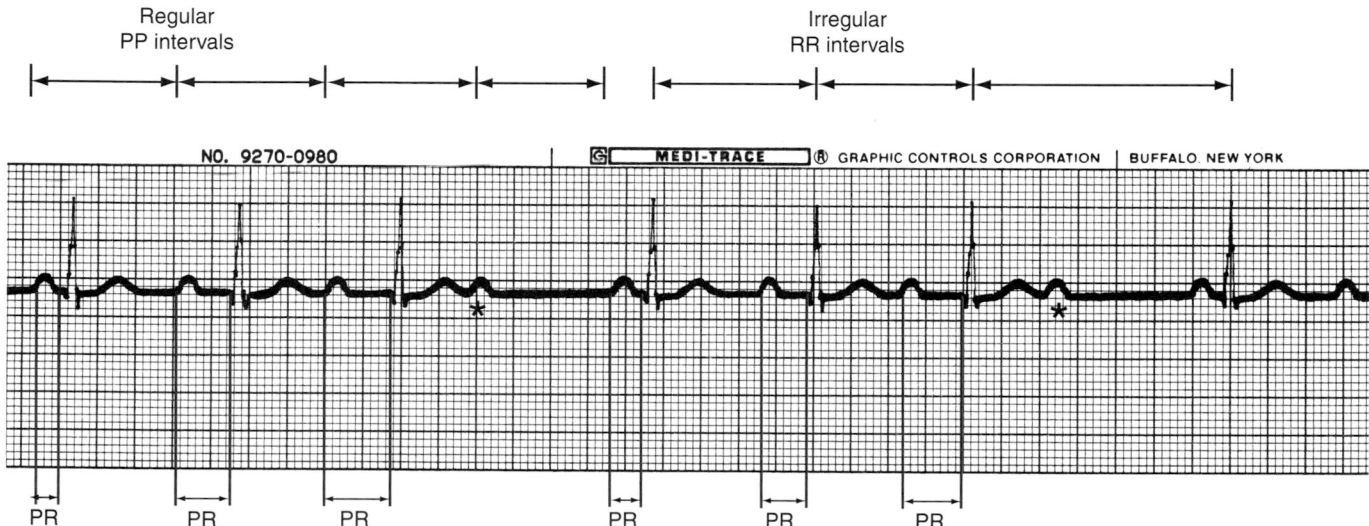

FIGURE 27-21 Sinus rhythm with second-degree AV block, type I in lead II. Note progressively longer PR durations until there is a nonconducted P wave, indicated by the asterisk (*).

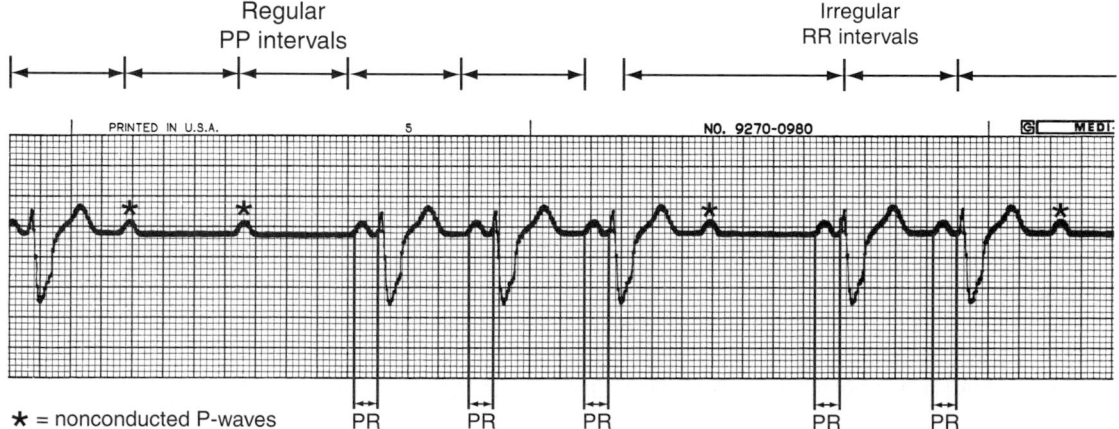

FIGURE 27-22 Sinus rhythm with second-degree AV block, type II in lead V₁; note constant PR interval.

interval is usually regular but may be irregular, depending on the P:QRS ratio.

QRS shape and duration: Usually abnormal, but may be normal
P wave: In front of the QRS complex; shape depends on underlying rhythm.
PR interval: PR interval is constant for those P waves just before QRS complexes.
P: QRS ratio: 2:1, 3:1, 4:1, 5:1, and so forth

Third-Degree Atrioventricular Block. Third-degree heart block occurs when no atrial impulse is conducted through the AV node into the ventricles. In third-degree heart block, two impulses stimulate the heart: one stimulates the ventricles (eg, junctional or ventricular escape rhythm), represented by the QRS complex, and one stimulates the atria (eg, sinus rhythm, atrial fibrillation), represented by the P wave. P waves may be seen, but the atrial electrical activity is not conducted down into the ventricles to cause the QRS complex, the ventricular electrical activity. This is called AV dissociation. Complete block (third-degree AV block) has the following characteristics (Fig. 27-23):

Ventricular and atrial rate: Depends on the escape and underlying atrial rhythm
Ventricular and atrial rhythm: The PP interval is regular and the RR interval is regular; however, the PP interval is not equal to the RR interval.
QRS shape and duration: Depends on the escape rhythm; in junctional escape, QRS shape and duration are usually normal, and in ventricular escape, QRS shape and duration are usually abnormal.
P wave: Depends on underlying rhythm
PR interval: Very irregular
P: QRS ratio: More P waves than QRS complexes

Based on the cause of the AV block and the stability of the patient, treatment is directed toward increasing the heart rate to maintain a normal cardiac output. If the patient is stable and has no symptoms, no treatment is indicated other than decreasing or eradicating the cause (eg, withholding the medication or treatment). If the patient is short of breath, complains of chest pain or lightheadedness, or has low blood pressure, an intravenous bolus of atropine is the initial treatment of choice. If the patient does not respond to atropine or has an acute MI, transcutaneous pacing should be started. A permanent pacemaker may be necessary if the block persists.

NURSING PROCESS: THE PATIENT WITH A DYSRHYTHMIA

Assessment

Major areas of assessment include possible causes of the dysrhythmia and the dysrhythmia's effect on the heart's ability to pump an adequate blood volume. When cardiac output is reduced, the amount of oxygen reaching the tissues and vital organs is diminished. This diminished oxygenation produces the signs and symptoms associated with dysrhythmias. If these signs and symptoms are severe or if they occur frequently, the patient may experience significant distress and disruption of daily life.

A health history is obtained to identify any previous occurrences of decreased cardiac output, such as syncope (fainting), lightheadedness, dizziness, fatigue, chest discomfort, and palpitations. Coexisting conditions that could be a possible cause of the dysrhythmia (eg, heart disease, chronic obstructive pulmonary disease) may also be identified. All medications, prescribed and over-the-counter (including herbs and nutritional supplements), are reviewed. Some medications (eg, digoxin) can cause dysrhythmias. A thorough psychosocial assessment is performed to identify the possible effects of the dysrhythmia and to determine whether anxiety is a significant contributing factor.

The nurse conducts a physical assessment to confirm the data obtained from the history and to observe for signs of diminished cardiac output during the dysrhythmic event, especially changes in level of consciousness. The nurse directs attention to the skin, which may be pale and cool. Signs of fluid retention, such as neck vein distention and crackles and wheezes auscultated in the lungs, may be detected. The rate and rhythm of apical and peripheral pulses are also assessed, and any pulse deficit is noted. The nurse auscultates for extra heart sounds (especially S_3 and S_4) and for heart murmurs, measures blood pressure, and determines pulse pressures. A declining pulse pressure indicates reduced cardiac output. Just one assessment may not disclose significant changes in cardiac output; therefore, the nurse compares multiple assessment findings over time, especially those that occur with and without the dysrhythmia.

Diagnosis

NURSING DIAGNOSES

Based on assessment data, major nursing diagnoses of the patient may include:

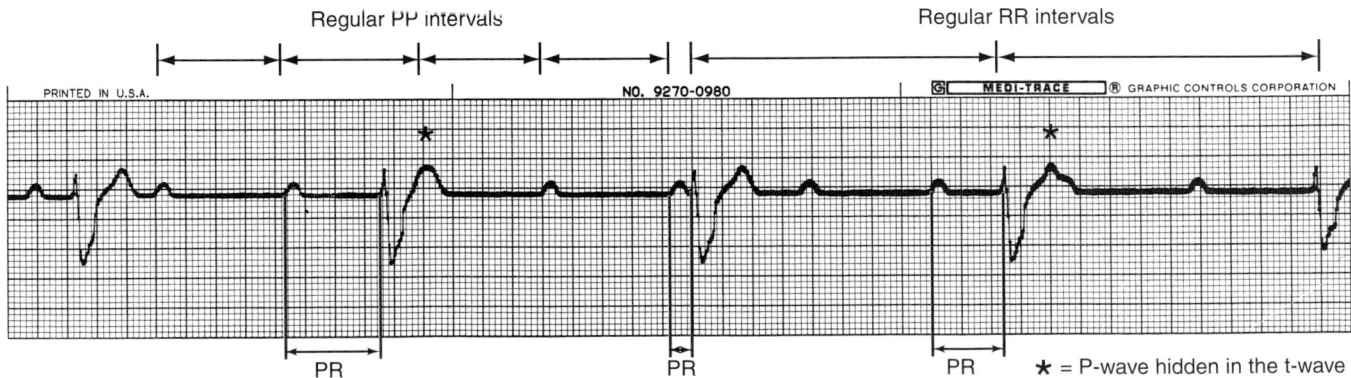

FIGURE 27-23 Sinus rhythm with third-degree AV block and idioventricular rhythm in lead V₁; note irregular PR intervals.

- Decreased cardiac output
- Anxiety related to fear of the unknown
- Deficient knowledge about the dysrhythmia and its treatment

COLLABORATIVE PROBLEMS/ POTENTIAL COMPLICATIONS

In addition to cardiac arrest, a potential complication that may develop over time is heart failure. Another potential complication, especially with atrial fibrillation, is a thromboembolic event. If the dysrhythmia necessitates treatment with medication, the beneficial and detrimental effects must be assessed.

Planning and Goals

The major goals for the patient may include eradicating or decreasing the incidence of the dysrhythmia (by decreasing contributory factors) to maintain cardiac output, minimizing anxiety, and acquiring knowledge about the dysrhythmia and its treatment.

Nursing Interventions

MONITORING AND MANAGING THE DYSRHYTHMIA

The nurse regularly evaluates blood pressure, pulse rate and rhythm, rate and depth of respirations, and breath sounds to determine the dysrhythmia's hemodynamic effect. The nurse also asks patients about episodes of lightheadedness, dizziness, or fainting as part of the ongoing assessment. If a patient with a dysrhythmia is hospitalized, the nurse may obtain a 12-lead ECG, continuously monitor the patient, and analyze rhythm strips to track the dysrhythmia.

Control of the incidence or the effect of the dysrhythmia, or both, is often achieved by the use of antiarrhythmic medications. The nurse assesses and observes for the beneficial and adverse effects of each of the medications. The nurse also manages medication administration carefully so that a constant serum blood level of the medication is maintained at all times.

In addition to medication, the nurse assesses for factors that contribute to the dysrhythmia (eg, caffeine, stress, nonadherence to the medication regimen) and assists the patient in developing a plan to make lifestyle changes that eliminate or reduce these factors.

MINIMIZING ANXIETY

When the patient experiences episodes of dysrhythmia, the nurse maintains a calm and reassuring attitude. This demeanor fosters a trusting relationship with the patient and assists in reducing anxiety (reducing the sympathetic response). Successes are emphasized with the patient to promote a sense of confidence in living with a dysrhythmia. For example, if a patient is experiencing episodes of dysrhythmia and a medication is administered that begins to reduce the incidence of the dysrhythmia, the nurse communicates that information to the patient. The nursing goal is to maximize the patient's control and to make the unknown less threatening.

PROMOTING HOME AND COMMUNITY-BASED CARE

Teaching Patients Self-Care

When teaching patients about dysrhythmias, the nurse presents the information in terms that are understandable and in a manner that is not frightening or threatening. The nurse explains the importance of maintaining therapeutic serum levels of anti-arrhythmic medications so that the patient understands why medications should be taken regularly each day. In addition, the relationship between a dysrhythmia and cardiac output is explained so that the patient understands the rationale for the medical regimen. If the patient has a potentially lethal dysrhythmia, it is also important to establish with the patient and family a plan of action to take in case of an emergency. This allows the patient and family to feel in control and prepared for possible events.

A referral for home care usually is not necessary for the patient with a dysrhythmia unless the patient is hemodynamically unstable and has significant symptoms of decreased cardiac output. Home care is also warranted if the patient has significant comorbidities, socioeconomic issues, or limited self-management skills that could potentiate the risk for nonadherence to the therapeutic regimen.

Evaluation

EXPECTED PATIENT OUTCOMES

Expected patient outcomes may include:

1. Maintains cardiac output
   a. Demonstrates heart rate, blood pressure, respiratory rate, and level of consciousness within normal ranges
   b. Demonstrates no or decreased episodes of dysrhythmia
2. Experiences reduced anxiety
   a. Expresses a positive attitude about living with the dysrhythmia
   b. Expresses confidence in ability to take appropriate actions in an emergency
3. Expresses understanding of the dysrhythmia and its treatment
   a. Explains the dysrhythmia and its effects
   b. Describes the medication regimen and its rationale
   c. Explains the need for therapeutic serum level of the medication
   d. Describes a plan to eradicate or limit factors that contribute to the occurrence of the dysrhythmia
   e. States actions to take in the event of an emergency

Adjunctive Modalities and Management

Dysrhythmia treatments depend on whether the disorder is acute or chronic as well as on the cause of the dysrhythmia and its actual or potential hemodynamic effects.

Acute dysrhythmias may be treated with medications or with external electrical therapy. Many antiarrhythmic medications are used to treat atrial and ventricular tachydysrhythmias. These medications are summarized in Table 27-1. The choice of medication depends on the specific dysrhythmia, presence of cardiac failure and other diseases, and the patient's response to previous treatment. The nurse is responsible for monitoring and documenting the patient's responses to the medication and for making sure that the patient has the knowledge and ability to manage the medication regimen.

If medications alone are ineffective in eradicating or decreasing the dysrhythmia, certain adjunctive mechanical therapies are available. The most common are pacemakers for bradycardias and tachycardias, elective cardioversion and defibrillation for acute tachydysrhythmia, and implantable devices for chronic tachydysrhythmia. Surgical treatments, although less common, are also available.

PACEMAKER THERAPY

A pacemaker is an electronic device that provides electrical stimuli to the heart muscle. Pacemakers are usually used when a patient has a slower-than-normal impulse formation or a conduction disturbance that causes symptoms. They may also be used to control some tachydysrhythmias that do not respond to medication therapy. Biventricular (both ventricles) pacing may be used to treat advanced heart failure that does not respond to medication therapy.

Pacemakers can be permanent or temporary. Permanent pacemakers are used most commonly for irreversible complete heart block. Temporary pacemakers are used (eg, after MI, after open heart surgery) to support patients until they improve or receive a permanent pacemaker.

Pacemaker Design and Types

Pacemakers consist of two components: an electronic pulse generator and pacemaker electrodes, which are located on leads or wires. The generator contains the circuitry and batteries that generate the rate (measured in beats per minute) and the strength (measured in milliamperes [mA]) of the electrical stimulus delivered to the heart. The pacemaker electrodes convey the heart's electrical activity through a lead to the generator; the generator's electrical response to the information received is then transmitted to the heart.

Leads can be threaded through a major vein into the right ventricle (endocardial leads), or they can be lightly sutured onto the outside of the heart and brought through the chest wall during open heart surgery (epicardial wires). The epicardial wires are always temporary and are removed by a gentle tug within a few days after surgery. The endocardial leads may be temporarily placed with catheters through the femoral, antecubital, brachial, or jugular vein (transvenous wires), usually guided by fluoroscopy. The endocardial and epicardial wires are connected to a temporary generator, which is about the size of a small paperback book. The energy source for a temporary generator is a common household battery; monitoring for pacemaker malfunctioning and battery failure is a nursing responsibility. This type of pacemaker therapy necessitates hospitalization of the patient.

The endocardial leads also may be placed permanently, usually through the external jugular vein, and connected to a permanent generator, which is usually implanted underneath the skin in a subcutaneous pocket in the pectoral region or below the clavicle (Fig. 27-24). Sometimes an abdominal site is selected. This procedure is usually performed in a cardiac catheterization laboratory with the patient receiving a local anesthetic. Permanent pacemaker generators are insulated to protect against body moisture and warmth. There are several different energy sources for permanent generators: mercury-zinc batteries (which last 3 to 4 years), lithium cell units (up to 10 years), and nuclear-powered sources such as plutonium 238 (up to 20 years). Some of the batteries are rechargeable. If the battery is not rechargeable and failure is impending, the old generator is removed and the new one is connected to the existing leads and reimplanted in the already existing subcutaneous pocket. This procedure is usually performed with the patient receiving a local anesthetic. Hospitalization of the patient is needed for implantation or battery replacement.

If a patient suddenly develops a bradycardia, emergency pacing may be started with transcutaneous pacing, which most defibrillators are now equipped to perform. AEDs are not able to do transcutaneous pacing (see later discussion). Large pacing ECG electrodes (sometimes the same conductive pads that are used for

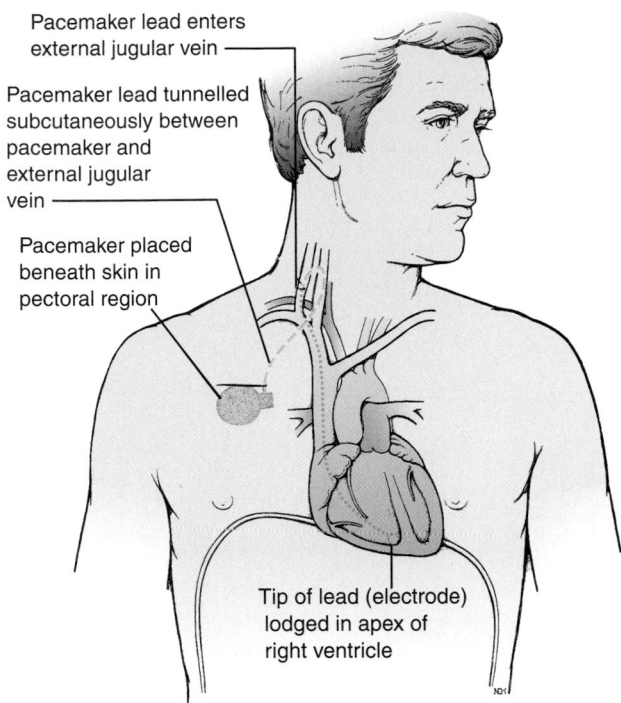

FIGURE 27-24 Implanted transvenous pacing lead (with electrode) and pacemaker generator.

cardioversion and defibrillation) are placed on the patient's chest and back. The electrodes are connected to the defibrillator, which is the temporary pacemaker generator (Fig. 27-25). Because the impulse must travel through the patient's skin and tissue before reaching the heart, transcutaneous pacing can cause significant discomfort and is intended to be used only in emergencies. This type of pacing necessitates hospitalization. If the patient is alert, the use of sedation and analgesia should be discussed with the physician.

Pacemaker Generator Functions

Because of the sophistication and wide use of pacemakers, a universal code has been adopted to provide a means of safe communication about their function. The coding is referred to as the NASPE-BPEG code because it is sanctioned by the North American Society of Pacing and Electrophysiology and the British Pacing and Electrophysiology Group. The complete code consists of five letters, but only the first three are commonly used.

The first letter of the code identifies the chamber or chambers being paced—that is, the chamber containing a pacing electrode. The letter characters for this code are A (atrium), V (ventricle), or D (dual, meaning both A and V).

The second letter describes the chamber or chambers being sensed by the pacemaker generator. Information from the electrode within the chamber is sent to the generator for interpretation and action by the generator. The possible letter characters are A (atrium), V (ventricle), D (dual), and O (indicating that the sensing function is turned off).

The third letter of the code describes the type of response by the pacemaker to what is sensed. The possible letter characters used to describe this response are I (**inhibited**), T (**triggered**), D (dual, inhibited and triggered), and O (none). Inhibited response means that the response of the pacemaker is controlled by the activity of the patient's heart; that is, the pacemaker will not func-

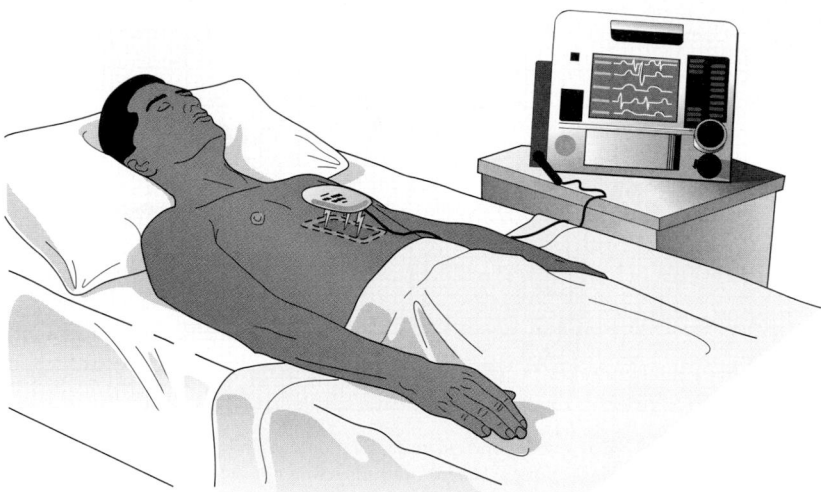

FIGURE 27-25 Transcutaneous pacemaker with electrode pads connected to the anterior and posterior chest walls.

tion when the patient's heart beats but will pace if no beat is sensed. In contrast, triggered response means that the pacemaker will provide a response (pace the heart) when it senses intrinsic heart activity.

The fourth and fifth letters are used only with permanent pacemaker generators. The fourth letter of the code is related to a permanent generator's ability to be programmed or reset. The possible letters are O (none), P (simple programmability), M (multiprogrammability; ability to change at least three factors, such as the rate at which pacing is initiated, the rate of pacing, and the amount of energy delivered), C (communicative or telemetry ability; information about the generator may be obtained [read or interrogated] with a hand-held device placed above the chest), and R (rate responsive capabilities; the ability of the pacemaker to change the rate from moment to moment based on parameters such as physical activity, acid-base changes, temperature, rate and depth of respirations, and oxygen saturation). A pacemaker with rate responsive ability will be capable of improving cardiac output during times of increased cardiac demand, such as with exercise.

The fifth letter of the code indicates that the permanent generator has antitachycardia and/or defibrillation capability. The possible letters are P (antitachycardia pacing), S (shock; defibrillation), D (dual—antitachycardia pacing and shock), and O (none). Antitachycardia pacing is used to terminate tachycardias caused by a conduction disturbance called reentry, which is repetitive restimulation of the heart by the same impulse. An impulse or series of impulses is delivered to the heart by the pacemaker at a fast rate to collide with and stop the heart's reentry conduction impulses, and therefore to stop the tachycardia.

An example of a NASPE-BPEG code is DVI:

D: Both the atrium and the ventricle have a pacing electrode in place.
V: The pacemaker is sensing the activity of the ventricle only.
I: The pacemaker's stimulating effect is inhibited by ventricular activity—in other words, it does not create an impulse when the patient's ventricle is active. The pacemaker paces the atrium and then the ventricle when no ventricular activity is sensed for a period of time (the time is individually programmed into the pacemaker for each patient).

The type of generator and its selected settings depend on the patient's dysrhythmia, underlying cardiac function, and age. A straight vertical line usually can be seen on the ECG when pacing is initiated. The line that represents pacing is called a pacemaker spike. The appropriate ECG complex should immediately follow the pacing spike; therefore, a P wave should follow an atrial pacing spike and a QRS complex should follow a ventricular pacing spike. Because the impulse starts in a different place than the patient's normal rhythm, the QRS complex or P wave that responds to pacing looks different from the patient's normal ECG complex. *Capture* is a term used to denote that the appropriate complex followed the pacing spike.

Pacemakers are generally set to sense and respond to intrinsic activity, which is called on-demand pacing (Fig. 27-26). If the pacemaker is set to pace but not to sense, it is called a fixed or asynchronous pacemaker (Fig. 27-27); this is written in code as AOO or VOO. The pacemaker will pace at a constant rate, independent of the patient's intrinsic rhythm. Because AOO pacing stimulates only the atrium, it may be used in a patient who has undergone open heart surgery and develops sinus bradycardia. AOO pacing ensures synchrony between atrial stimulation and ventricular stimulation (and therefore contraction), as long as the patient has no conduction disturbances in the AV node. VOO is rare because of the risk that the pacemaker may deliver an impulse during the vulnerable repolarization phase, leading to VT.

Complications of Pacemaker Use

Complications associated with pacemakers relate to their presence within the body, and improper functioning. The following complications may arise from a pacemaker:

- Local infection at the entry site of the leads for temporary pacing, or at the subcutaneous site for permanent generator placement
- Bleeding and hematoma at the lead entry sites for temporary pacing, or at the subcutaneous site for permanent generator placement
- Hemothorax from puncture of the subclavian vein or internal mammary artery
- Ventricular ectopy and tachycardia from irritation of the ventricular wall by the endocardial electrode
- Movement or dislocation of the lead placed transvenously (perforation of the myocardium)
- Phrenic nerve, diaphragmatic (hiccuping may be a sign of this), or skeletal muscle stimulation if the lead is dislocated or if the delivered energy (mA) is set high
- Rarely, cardiac tamponade from bleeding resulting from removal of epicardial wires used for temporary pacing

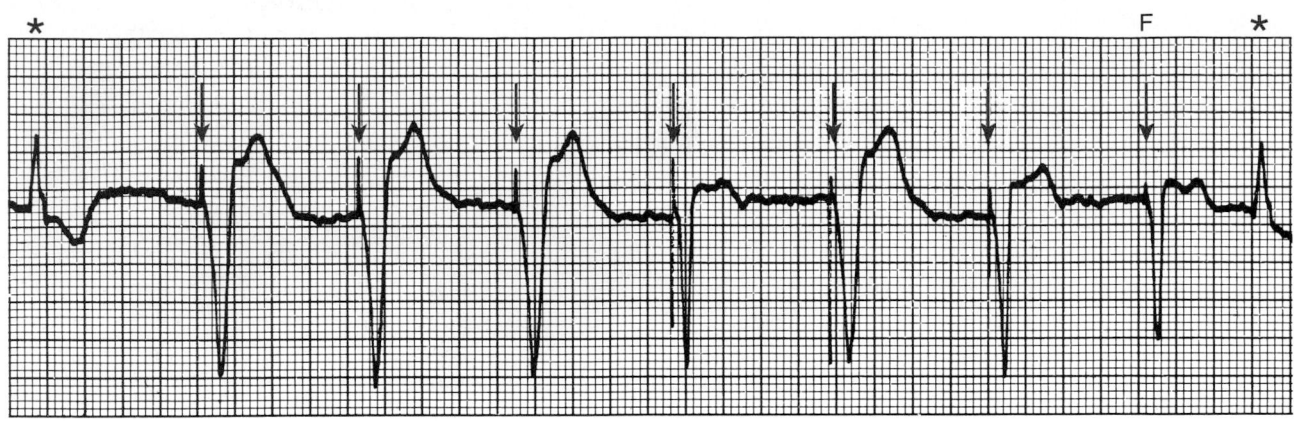

FIGURE 27-26 Pacing with appropriate sensing (on-demand pacing) in lead V_1. Arrows denote pacing spike. Asterisk (*) denotes intrinsic (patient's own) beats, therefore no pacing. F denotes a fusion beat, which is a combination of an intrinsic beat and a paced beat occurring at the same time.

In the initial hours after a temporary or permanent pacemaker is inserted, the most common complication is dislodgment of the pacing electrode. Minimizing patient activity can help to prevent this complication. If a temporary electrode is in place, the extremity through which the catheter has been advanced is immobilized. With a permanent pacemaker, the patient is instructed initially to restrict activity on the side of the implantation.

The ECG is monitored very carefully to detect pacemaker malfunction. Improper pacemaker function, which can arise from failure in one or more components of the pacing system, is outlined in Table 27-2. The following data should be noted on the patient's record: model of pacemaker, type of generator, date and time of insertion, location of pulse generator, stimulation threshold, pacer settings (eg, rate, energy output [mA], and duration between atrial and ventricular impulses [AV delay]). This information is important for identifying normal pacemaker function and diagnosing pacemaker malfunction.

A patient experiencing pacemaker malfunction may develop signs and symptoms of decreased cardiac output. The degree to which these symptoms become apparent depends on the severity of the malfunction, the patient's level of dependency on the pacemaker, and the patient's underlying condition. Pacemaker malfunction is diagnosed by analyzing the ECG. Manipulating the electrodes, changing the generator's settings, or replacing the pacemaker generator or leads (or both) may be necessary.

Inhibition of permanent pacemakers can occur with exposure to strong electromagnetic fields (electromagnetic interference). However, recent pacemaker technology allows patients to safely use most household electronic appliances and devices (eg, microwave ovens, electric tools) as long as they are not held close to the pacemaker generator. Gas-powered engines should be turned off before working on them. Objects that contain magnets (eg, the earpiece of a standard phone; large stereo speakers; magnet therapy products such as mattresses, jewelry, and wraps) should not be near the generator for longer than a few seconds. Patients are advised to use digital cellular phones on the side opposite the pacemaker generator. Large electromagnetic fields, such as those produced by magnetic resonance imaging (MRI), radio and TV transmitter towers and lines, transmission power lines (these are different from the distribution lines that bring electricity into a home), and electrical substations may cause electromagnetic interference. Patients should be cautioned to avoid such situations or to simply move farther away from the area if they experience dizziness or a feeling of rapid or irregular heartbeats (palpitations). Welding and use of a chain saw should be avoided. If such tools are used, precautionary steps such as limiting the welding current to a 60- to 130-ampere range or using electric rather than gasoline-powered chain saws are advised.

The metal of the pacemaker generator may trigger some store and airport security alarms, but these alarm systems will not interfere with the pacemaker function. However, the handheld screening devices used in airports may interfere with the pacemaker. Patients should be advised to request a hand search instead of the handheld screening device. Patients also should be instructed to wear or carry medical identification to alert personnel to the presence of the pacemaker.

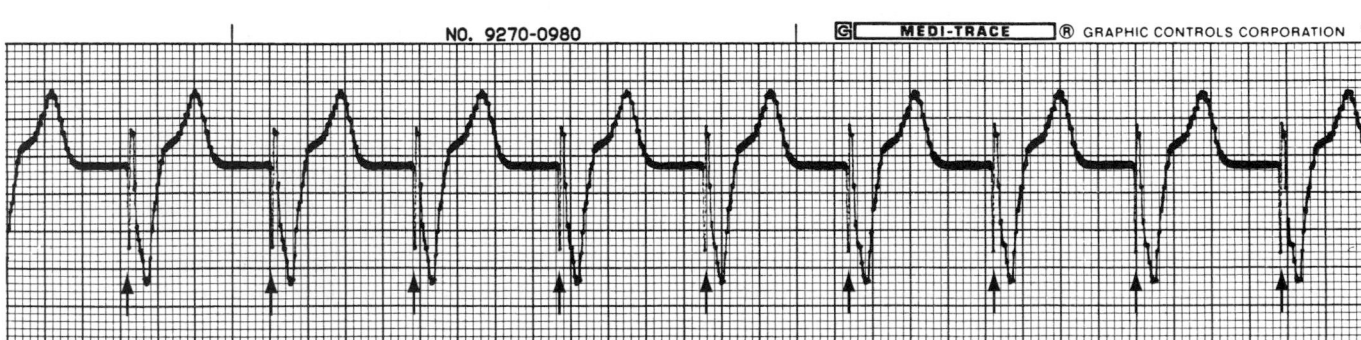

FIGURE 27-27 Fixed pacing or total loss of sensing pacing in lead V_1; arrows denote pacing spikes.

Table 27-2 • Assessing Pacemaker Malfunction

PROBLEM	POSSIBLE CAUSE	INTERVENTION
Loss of capture—complex does *not* follow pacing spike	Inadequate stimulus Catheter malposition Battery depletion Electronic insulation break	Check security of all connections; increase milliamperage. Reposition extremity; turn patient to left side. Change battery. Change generator.
Undersensing—pacing spike occurs at preset interval despite patient's intrinsic rhythm	Sensitivity too high Electrical interference (eg, by a magnet) Faulty generator	Decrease sensitivity. Eliminate interference. Replace generator.
Oversensing—loss of pacing artifact; pacing does *not* occur at preset interval despite lack of intrinsic rhythm	Sensitivity too low Electrical interference Battery depletion	Increase sensitivity. Eliminate interference. Change battery.
Loss of pacing—Total absence of pacing spikes	Battery depletion Loose or disconnected wires Perforation	Change battery. Check security of all connections. Obtain 12-lead ECG and portable chest x-ray. Assess for murmur. Call physician.
Change in pacing QRS shape	Septal perforation	Obtain 12-lead ECG and portable chest x-ray. Assess for murmur. Call physician.
Rhythmic diaphragmatic or chest wall twitching or hiccuping	Output too high Myocardial wall perforation	Decrease milliamperage. Turn pacer off. Call physician at once. Monitor closely for decreased cardiac output.

Pacemaker Surveillance

Pacemaker clinics have been established to monitor patients and to test pulse generators for impending pacemaker battery failure. Several other factors, such as lead fracture, muscle inhibition, and insulation disruption, are assessed depending on the type of pacemaker and the equipment available. If indicated, the pacemaker is turned off for a few seconds, using a magnet or a programmer, while the ECG is recorded to assess the patient's underlying cardiac rhythm.

Another follow-up method is transtelephonic transmission of the generator's pulse rate. Special equipment is used to transmit information about the patient's pacemaker over the telephone to a receiving system at a pacemaker clinic. The information is converted into tones, which equipment at the clinic converts to an electronic signal and records on an ECG strip. The pacemaker rate and other data concerning pacemaker function are obtained and evaluated by a cardiologist. This simplifies the diagnosis of a failing generator, reassures the patient, and improves management when the patient is physically remote from pacemaker testing facilities.

NURSING PROCESS:
THE PATIENT WITH A PACEMAKER

Assessment

After a temporary or a permanent pacemaker is inserted, the patient's heart rate and rhythm are monitored by ECG. The pacemaker's settings are noted and compared with the ECG recordings to assess pacemaker function. Pacemaker malfunction is detected by examining the pacemaker spike and its relationship to the surrounding ECG complexes (Fig. 27-28). In addition, cardiac output and hemodynamic stability are assessed to identify the patient's response to pacing and the adequacy of pacing. The ap-

pearance or increasing frequency of dysrhythmia is observed and reported to the physician.

The incision site where the pulse generator was implanted (or the entry site for the pacing electrode, if the pacemaker is a temporary transvenous pacemaker) is observed for bleeding, hematoma formation, or infection, which may be evidenced by swelling, unusual tenderness, unusual drainage, and increased heat. The patient may complain of continuous throbbing or pain. These symptoms are reported to the physician.

The patient with a temporary pacemaker is also assessed for electrical interference and the development of microshock. The nurse observes for potential sources of electrical hazards. All electrical equipment used in the vicinity of the patient should be grounded. Improperly grounded equipment can generate leakage of current capable of producing ventricular fibrillation. Exposed wires must be carefully covered with nonconductive material to prevent accidental ventricular fibrillation from stray currents. The nurse, working with a biomedical engineer or electrician, should make certain that the patient is in an electrically safe environment.

Patients, especially those receiving a permanent pacemaker, should be assessed for anxiety. In addition, for those receiving permanent pacemakers, the level of knowledge and learning needs of the patient and the family and the history of adherence to the therapeutic regimen should be identified.

Diagnosis

NURSING DIAGNOSES

Based on assessment data, major nursing diagnoses of the patient may include the following:

- Risk for infection related to pacemaker lead or generator insertion
- Risk for ineffective coping
- Deficient knowledge regarding self-care program

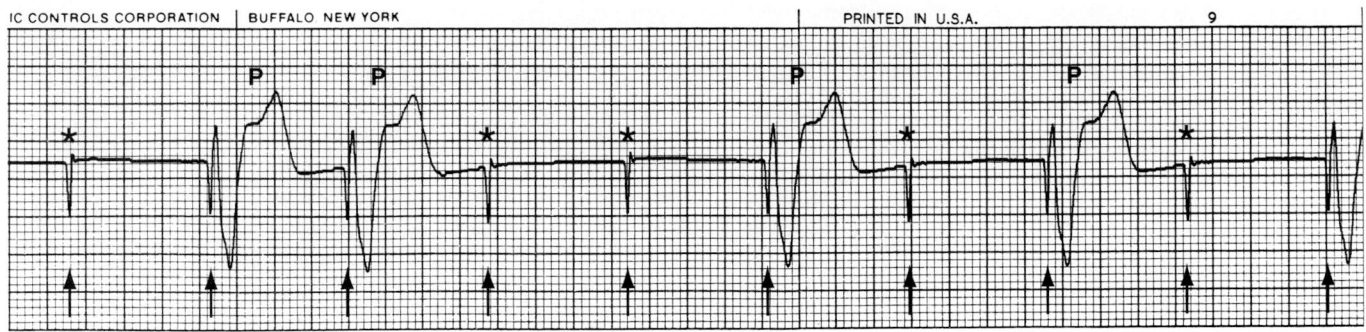

A

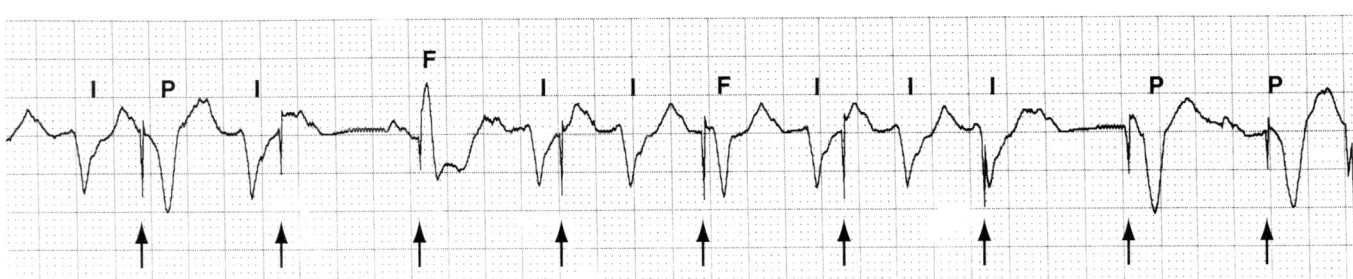

B

FIGURE 27-28 (**A**) Ventricular pacing with intermittent loss of capture (a pacing spike not followed by a QRS complex). (**B**) Ventricular pacing with loss of sensing (a pacing spike occurring at an inappropriate time). *Key:* ↑ = pacing spike; * = loss of capture; P = pacemaker-induced QRS complex; I = patient's intrinsic QRS complex; F = fusion (a QRS complex formed by a merging of the patient's intrinsic QRS complex and the pacemaker-induced QRS complex). Both in lead V₁.

COLLABORATIVE PROBLEMS/ POTENTIAL COMPLICATIONS

Based on the assessment findings, potential complications that may develop include decreased cardiac output related to pacemaker malfunction.

Planning and Goals

The major goals for the patient may include absence of infection, adherence to a self-care program, effective coping, and maintenance of pacemaker function.

Nursing Interventions

PREVENTING INFECTION

The nurse changes the dressing regularly and inspects the insertion site for redness, swelling, soreness, or any unusual drainage. An increase in temperature should be reported to the physician. Changes in wound appearance are also reported to the physician.

PROMOTING EFFECTIVE COPING

The patient treated with a pacemaker experiences not only lifestyle and physical changes but also emotional changes. At different times during the healing process, the patient may feel angry, depressed, fearful, anxious, or a combination of these emotions. Although each patient uses individual coping strategies (eg, humor, prayer, communication with a significant other) to manage emotional distress, some strategies may work better than others. Signs that may indicate ineffective coping include social isolation, increased or prolonged irritability or depression, and difficulty in relationships.

To promote effective coping strategies, the nurse must recognize the patient's emotional state and assist the patient to explore his or her feelings. The nurse may help the patient to identify per-

ceived changes (eg, loss of ability to participate in contact sports), the emotional response to the change (eg, anger), and how the patient responded to that emotion (eg, quickly became angry when talking with spouse). The nurse reassures the patient that the responses are normal, then assists the patient to identify realistic goals (eg, develop interest in another activity) and to develop a plan to attain those goals. The nurse may also teach the patient easy-to-use stress reduction techniques (eg, deep-breathing exercises) to facilitate coping. Education (Chart 27-3) may assist a patient to cope with changes that occur with pacemaker treatment.

PROMOTING HOME AND COMMUNITY-BASED CARE

Teaching Patients Self-Care

After pacemaker insertion, the patient's hospital stay may be less than 1 day, and follow-up in an outpatient clinic or office is common. The patient's anxiety and feelings of vulnerability may interfere with the ability to learn information provided. Nurses often need to include home caregivers in the teaching and provide printed materials for use by the patient and caregiver. Priorities for learning are established with the patient and caregiver. Teaching may include the importance of periodic pacemaker monitoring, promoting safety, avoiding infection, and sources of electromagnetic interference (see Chart 27-3).

Evaluation

EXPECTED PATIENT OUTCOMES

Expected patient outcomes may include:

1. Remains free of infection
   a. Has normal temperature
   b. Has white blood cell count within normal range (5,000 to 10,000/mm³)

Chart 27-3
Home Care Checklist • The Patient With a Pacemaker

At the completion of the home care instruction, the patient or caregiver will be able to:	Patient	Caregiver
Monitor pacemaker function.		
• Describe the importance of reporting to physician or pacemaker clinic periodically as prescribed, so that the pacemaker's rate and function can be monitored. This is especially important during the first month after implantation.	✓	
• Adhere to monitoring schedule as instructed after implantation.	✓	
• Check pulse daily. Report *immediately* any sudden slowing or increasing of the pulse rate. This may indicate pacemaker malfunction.	✓	✓
• Resume more frequent monitoring when battery depletion is anticipated. (The time for reimplantation depends on the type of battery in use.)	✓	
Promote safety and avoid infection.		
• Wear loose-fitting clothing around the area of the pacemaker.	✓	
• State the reason for the slight bulge over the pacemaker implant.	✓	✓
• Notify physician if the pacemaker area becomes red or painful.	✓	✓
• Avoid trauma to the area of the pacemaker generator.	✓	
• Study the manufacturer's instructions and become familiar with the pacemaker.	✓	✓
• Recognize that physical activity does not usually have to be curtailed, with the exception of contact sports.	✓	
• Carry medical identification indicating physician's name, type and model number of pacemaker, manufacturer's name, pacemaker rate, and hospital where pacemaker was inserted.	✓	
Electromagnetic interference: Describe the importance of the following:		
• Avoid large magnetic fields such as those surrounding magnetic resonance imaging, large motors, arc welding, electrical substations. Magnetic fields can deactivate the pacemaker.	✓	
• Some electrical and small motor devices, as well as cellular phones, may interfere with pacemaker function if placed very close to the generator. Avoid leaning directly over devices, or ensure that contact is brief; place cellular phone on opposite side of generator.	✓	✓
• Household items, such as microwave ovens, should not cause any concern.	✓	✓
• When going through security gates (eg, at airports, government buildings) show identification card and request hand search.	✓	✓
• Hospitalization may be necessary periodically to change battery or replace pacemaker unit.	✓	✓

c. Exhibits no redness or swelling of pacemaker insertion site
2. Adheres to a self-care program
   a. Responds appropriately when queried about the signs and symptoms of infection
   b. Identifies when to seek medical attention (as demonstrated in responses to signs and symptoms)
   c. Adheres to monitoring schedule
   d. Describes appropriate methods to avoid electromagnetic interference
3. Maintains pacemaker function (see Chart 27-3)
   a. Measures and records pulse rate at regular intervals
   b. Experiences no abrupt changes in pulse rate or rhythm

CARDIOVERSION AND DEFIBRILLATION

Cardioversion and defibrillation are treatments for tachydysrhythmias. They are used to deliver an electrical current to depolarize a critical mass of myocardial cells. When the cells repolarize, the sinus node is usually able to recapture its role as the heart's pacemaker. One major difference between cardioversion and defibrillation has to do with the timing of the delivery of electrical current. Another major difference concerns the circumstance: defibrillation is usually performed as an emergency treatment, whereas cardioversion is usually, but not always, a planned procedure.

Electrical current may be delivered through paddles or conductor pads. Both paddles may be placed on the front of the chest (Fig. 27-29), which is the standard paddle placement, or

one paddle may be placed on the front of the chest and the other connected to an adapter with a long handle and placed under the patient's back, which is called an anteroposterior placement (Fig. 27-30).

 NURSING ALERT When using paddles, apply the appropriate conductant between the paddles and the patient's skin. Do not substitute any other type of conductant, such as ultrasound gel.

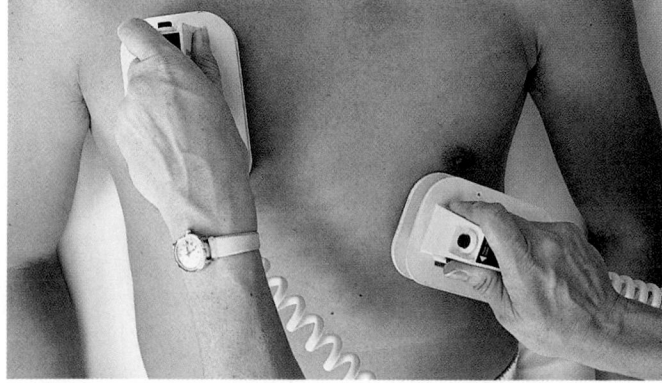
FIGURE 27-29 Standard paddle placement for defibrillation.

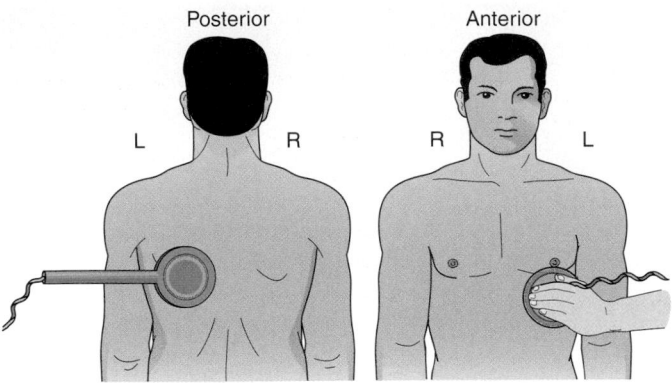

FIGURE 27-30 Anteroposterior paddle placement for defibrillation.

Instead of paddles, defibrillator multifunction conductor pads may be used (Fig. 27-31). The pads, which contain a conductive medium, are placed in the same position as the paddles. They are connected to the defibrillator and allow for hands-off defibrillation. This method reduces the risks of touching the patient during the procedure and increases electrical safety. AEDs use this type of delivery for the electrical current.

Whether using pads or paddles, the nurse must observe two safety measures. First, maintain good contact between the pads or paddles (with a conductive medium) and the patient's skin to prevent electrical current from leaking into the air (arcing) when the defibrillator is discharged. Second, ensure that no one is in contact with the patient or with anything that is touching the patient when the defibrillator is discharged, to minimize the chance that electrical current will be conducted to anyone other than the patient.

When performing defibrillation or cardioversion, the nurse should remember these key points:

- Use multifunction conductor pads or paddles with a conducting agent between the paddles and the skin (the conducting agent is available as a sheet, gel, or paste).
- Place paddles or pads so that they do not touch the patient's clothing or bed linen and are not near medication patches or direct oxygen flow.
- If cardioverting, ensure that the monitor leads are attached to the patient and that the defibrillator is in sync mode. If

defibrillating, ensure that the defibrillator is not in sync mode (most machines default to the "not-sync" mode).

- Do not charge the device until ready to shock; then keep thumbs and fingers off the discharge buttons until paddles or pads are on the chest and ready to deliver the electrical charge.
- Exert 20 to 25 pounds of pressure on the paddles to ensure good skin contact.
- Before pressing the discharge button, call "Clear!" three times: As "Clear" is called the first time, ensure that you are not touching the patient, bed or equipment; as "Clear" is called the second time, ensure that no one is touching the bed, the patient, or equipment, including the endotracheal tube or adjuncts; and as "Clear" is called the third time, perform a final visual check to ensure you and everyone else are clear of the patient and anything touching the patient.
- Record the delivered energy and the results (cardiac rhythm, pulse).
- After the event is complete, inspect the skin under the pads or paddles for burns; if any are detected, consult with the physician or a wound care nurse about treatment.

Cardioversion

Cardioversion involves the delivery of a "timed" electrical current to terminate a tachydysrhythmia. In cardioversion, the defibrillator is set to synchronize with the ECG on a cardiac monitor so that the electrical impulse discharges during ventricular depolarization (QRS complex). Because there may be a short delay until recognition of the QRS, the discharge buttons must be held down until the shock has been delivered. The synchronization prevents the discharge from occurring during the vulnerable period of repolarization (T wave), which could result in VT or ventricular fibrillation. When the synchronizer is on, no electrical current will be delivered if the defibrillator does not discern a QRS complex. Sometimes the lead and the electrodes must be changed for the monitor to recognize the patient's QRS complex.

If the cardioversion is elective, anticoagulation for a few weeks before cardioversion may be indicated. Digoxin is usually withheld for 48 hours before cardioversion to ensure the resumption of sinus rhythm with normal conduction. The patient is instructed not to eat or drink for at least 8 hours before the procedure. Gel-covered paddles or conductor pads are positioned front and back (anteroposteriorly) for cardioversion. Before cardio-

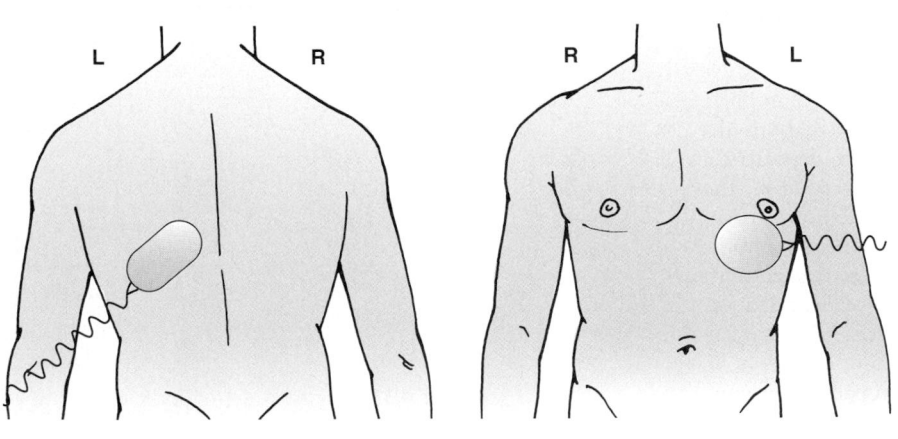

Back   Front

FIGURE 27-31 Multifunction pads for defibrillation.

version, the patient receives intravenous sedation as well as an analgesic medication or anesthesia. Respiration is then supported with supplemental oxygen delivered by a bag-mask-valve device with suction equipment readily available. Although patients rarely require intubation, equipment is nearby if it is needed. The amount of voltage used varies from 25 to 360 joules, depending on the defibrillator's technology and the type of dysrhythmia. If ventricular fibrillation occurs after cardioversion, the defibrillator is used to defibrillate the patient (sync mode is *not* used).

Indications of a successful response are conversion to sinus rhythm, adequate peripheral pulses, and adequate blood pressure. Because of the sedation, airway patency must be maintained and the patient's state of consciousness assessed. Vital signs and oxygen saturation are monitored and recorded until the patient is stable and recovered from sedation and the effects of analgesic medications or anesthesia. ECG monitoring is required during and after cardioversion.

Defibrillation

Defibrillation is used in emergency situations as the treatment of choice for ventricular fibrillation and pulseless VT. Defibrillation depolarizes a critical mass of myocardial cells at once; when they repolarize, the sinus node usually recaptures its role as the pacemaker. The electrical voltage required to defibrillate the heart is usually greater than that required for cardioversion. If three defibrillations of increasing voltage have been unsuccessful, cardiopulmonary resuscitation is initiated and advanced life support treatments are begun.

The use of epinephrine or vasopressin may make it easier to convert the dysrhythmia to a normal rhythm with defibrillation. These drugs may also increase cerebral and coronary artery blood flow. After the medication is administered and 1 minute of cardiopulmonary resuscitation is performed, defibrillation is again administered. Antiarrhythmic medications such as amiodarone (Cordarone, Pacerone), lidocaine (Xylocaine), magnesium, or procainamide (Pronestyl) are given if ventricular dysrhythmia persists (see Table 27-1). This treatment continues until a stable rhythm resumes or until it is determined that the patient cannot be revived.

IMPLANTABLE CARDIOVERTER DEFIBRILLATOR

The **implantable cardioverter defibrillator (ICD)** is a device that detects and terminates life-threatening episodes of VT or ventricular fibrillation in high-risk patients. Patients at high risk are those who have survived sudden cardiac death syndrome, usually caused by ventricular fibrillation, or have experienced symptomatic VT (syncope secondary to VT). In addition, an ICD may be indicated for patients who have survived an MI but are at high risk for cardiac arrest.

An ICD consists of a generator and at least one lead that can sense intrinsic electrical activity and deliver an electrical impulse. The device is usually implanted much like a pacemaker (Fig. 27-32). ICDs are designed to respond to two criteria: a rate that exceeds a predetermined level, and a change in the isoelectric line segments. When a dysrhythmia occurs, rate sensors take 5 to 10 seconds to sense the dysrhythmia. Then the device takes several seconds to charge and deliver the programmed charge through the lead to the heart. Battery life is about 5 years but varies depending on use of the ICD over time. The battery is checked during follow-up visits.

Antiarrhythmic medication usually is administered with this technology to minimize the occurrence of the tachydysrhythmia and to reduce the frequency of ICD discharge.

The first defibrillator, which was implanted in 1980 at Johns Hopkins University, simply defibrillated the heart. Today, however, several devices are available, and many are programmed for multiple treatments (Atlee & Bernstein, 2001). Each device offers a different delivery sequence, but all are capable of delivering high-energy (high-intensity) defibrillation to treat a tachycardia (atrial or ventricular). The device may deliver up to six shocks if necessary. Some ICDs can respond with antitachycardia pacing, in which the device delivers electrical impulses at a fast rate in an attempt to disrupt the tachycardia, by low-energy (low-intensity) cardioversion, by defibrillation, or all three (Atlee & Bernstein, 2001). Some also have pacemaker capability if the patient develops bradycardia, which sometimes occurs after treatment of the tachycardia. Usually the mode is VVI (V, paces the ventricle; V, senses ventricular activity; I, paces only if the ventricles do not depolarize) (Atlee & Bernstein, 2001). Some ICDs also deliver low-energy cardioversion, and some also treat atrial fibrillation (Bubien & Sanchez, 2001; Daoud et al., 2000). Which device is used and how it is programmed depends on the patient's dysrhythmia.

Complications are similar to those associated with pacemaker insertion. The primary complication associated with the ICD is surgery-related infection. There are a few complications associated with the technical aspects of the equipment, such as premature battery depletion and dislodged or fractured leads. Despite the possible complications, the consensus among clinicians is that the benefits of ICD therapy exceed the risks.

Nursing interventions for the patient with an ICD are provided throughout the preoperative, perioperative, and postoperative phases. In addition to providing the patient and family with explanations regarding implantation of the ICD in the preoperative phase, the nurse may need to manage acute episodes of life-threatening dysrhythmias. In the perioperative and postoperative phases, the nurse carefully observes the patient's responses to the ICD and provides the patient and family with further teaching as needed (White, 2000) (Chart 27-4). The nurse can also assist the patient and family in making lifestyle changes necessitated by the dysrhythmia and resulting ICD implantation (Dougherty, Benoliel, & Bellin, 2000).

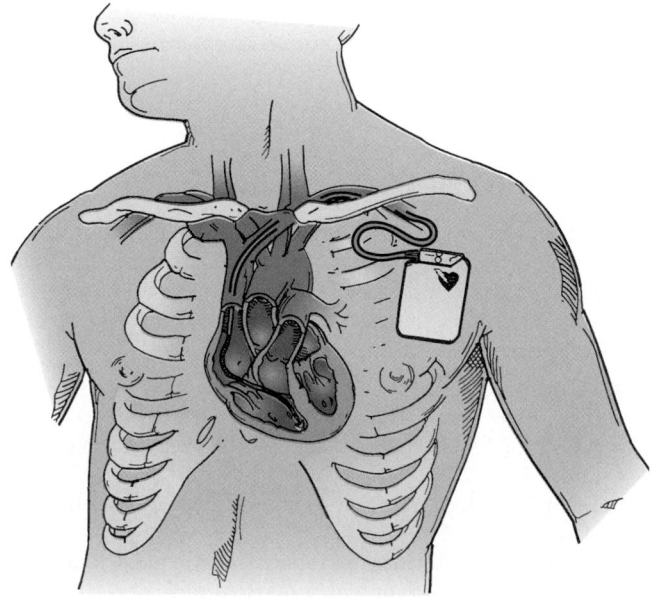

FIGURE 27-32 The implantable cardioverter defibrillator (ICD) consists of a generator and a sensing/pacing/defibrillating electrode.

Chart 27-4

Home Care Checklist • **The Patient With an ICD**

At the completion of the home care instruction, the patient or caregiver will be able to:	Patient	Caregiver
Avoid infection at the ICD insertion site.		
• Observe incision site daily for redness, swelling, and heat.	✓	✓
• Take temperature; report any increase.	✓	✓
• Avoid tight restrictive clothing that may cause friction over the insertion site.	✓	✓
Adhere to activity restrictions.		
• Movement of arm may continue to be restricted until incision heals if the ICD was implanted in pectoral region.	✓	
• Avoid heavy lifting.	✓	
• Discuss safety of activities (eg, driving) with physician.	✓	✓
• Avoid contact sports.	✓	
Electromagnetic interference: Understand the importance of the following:		
• Avoid large magnetic fields such as those created by magnetic resonance imaging, large motors, arc welding, electrical substations, and so forth. Magnetic fields may deactivate the ICD, negating any effect on a dysrhythmia.	✓	
• At security gates at airports, government buildings, or other secured areas, show identification card and request a hand search.	✓	
• Some electrical and small motor devices, as well as cellular phones, may interfere with the functioning of the ICD if placed very close to the ICD. Avoid leaning directly over devices, or ensure contact is of brief duration; place cellular phone on opposite side of ICD.	✓	
• Household appliances (eg, microwave ovens) should not cause any concern.	✓	✓
Promote safety.		
• Describe what to do if symptoms occur and notify physician if any discharges seem unusual.	✓	✓
• Maintain a log that records discharges. Record events that precipitate the sensation of shock. This provides important data for the physician to use in readjusting the medical regimen.	✓	✓
• Encourage family members to attend a CPR class.		✓
• Call 911 for emergency assistance if feeling of dizziness occurs.	✓	✓
• Wear medical identification (eg, Medic-Alert) that includes physician information.	✓	
• Avoid frightening family or friends with unexpected shocks, which will not harm them. Inform family and friends that in the event they are in contact with the patient when a shock is delivered, they may also feel the shock. It is especially important to warn sexual partners that this may occur.	✓	✓
• Discuss psychological responses to the ICD implantation, such as changes in self-image, depression due to loss of mobility secondary to driving restrictions, fear of shocks, increased anxiety, concerns that sexual activity may trigger the ICD, and changes in partner relationship.	✓	✓
Follow-up care		
• Adhere to appointments that are scheduled to test electronic performance of ICD. Remember to take log of discharges to review with physician.	✓	✓
• Attend an ICD support group within the area.	✓	

ELECTROPHYSIOLOGIC STUDIES

An electrophysiology (EP) study is used to evaluate and treat various dysrhythmias that have caused cardiac arrest or significant symptoms. It also is indicated for patients with symptoms that suggest a dysrhythmia that has gone undetected and undiagnosed by other methods. An EP study is used to

- Identify the impulse formation and propagation through the cardiac electrical conduction system
- Assess the function or dysfunction of the SA and AV nodal areas
- Identify the location (called mapping) and mechanism dysrhythmogenic foci
- Assess the effectiveness of antiarrhythmic medications and devices for the patient with a dysrhythmia
- Treat certain dysrhythmias through the destruction of the causative cells (**ablation**)

An EP procedure is a type of cardiac catheterization that is performed in a specially equipped cardiac catheterization laboratory. The patient is awake but lightly sedated. Usually a catheter with multiple electrodes is inserted through the femoral vein, threaded through the inferior vena cava, and advanced into the heart. The electrodes are positioned within the heart at specific locations—for instance, in the right atrium near the sinus node, in the coronary sinus, near the tricuspid valve, and at the apex of the right ventricle. The number and placement of electrodes depend on the type of study being conducted. These electrodes allow the electrical signal to be recorded from within the heart (intracardiogram).

The electrodes also allow the clinician to introduce a pacing stimulus to the intracardiac area at a precisely timed interval and rate, thereby stimulating the area (programmed stimulation). An area of the heart may be paced at a rate much faster than the normal rate of **automaticity**, the rate at which impulses are spontaneously formed (eg, in the sinus node). This allows the pacemaker to become an artificial focus of automaticity and to assume control (overdrive suppression). Then the pacemaker is stopped suddenly, and the time it takes for the sinus node to resume control is assessed. A prolonged time indicates dysfunction of the sinus node.

One of the main purposes of programmed stimulation is to assess the ability of the area surrounding the electrode to cause a reentry dysrhythmia. One or a series of premature impulses is delivered to an area in an attempt to cause the tachydysrhythmia. Because the precise location of the suspected area and the specific timing of the pacing needed are unknown, the electrophysiologist uses several different techniques to cause the dysrhythmia during the study. If the dysrhythmia can be reproduced by programmed stimulation, it is called inducible. Once a dysrhythmia is induced, a treatment plan is determined and implemented. If, on the follow-up EP study, the tachydysrhythmia cannot be induced, then the treatment is determined to be effective. Different medications may be administered and combined with electrical devices (pacemaker, ICD) to determine the most effective treatment to suppress the dysrhythmia.

Complications of an EP study are the same as those that can occur with cardiac catheterization. Because an artery is not always used, there is a lower incidence of vascular complications than with other catheterization procedures. Cardiac arrest may occur, but the incidence is low (less than 1%).

Patients who are to undergo an EP study may be anxious about the procedure and about its outcome. A detailed discussion involving the patient, the family, and the electrophysiologist usually occurs to ensure that the patient is able to give informed consent and to reduce anxiety about the procedure. Before the procedure, patients should receive instructions about the procedure and its usual duration, the environment where the procedure is performed, and what to expect. Although an EP study is not painful, it does cause discomfort and can be tiring. It may also cause feelings that were experienced when the dysrhythmia occurred in the past. In addition, patients also are taught what will be expected of them (eg, lying very still during the procedure, reporting symptoms or concerns).

Patients need to know that the dysrhythmia may occur during the procedure, but under very controlled circumstances. It often stops on its own; if it does not, treatment is given to restore the patient's normal rhythm. During the procedure, patients benefit from a calm, reassuring approach.

Postprocedural care includes restriction of activity to promote hemostasis at the insertion site. To identify any complications and to ensure healing, the patient's vital signs and the appearance of the insertion site are assessed frequently.

CARDIAC CONDUCTION SURGERY

Atrial tachycardias and ventricular tachycardias that do not respond to medications and are not suitable for antitachycardia pacing may be treated by methods other than medications and devices. Such methods include endocardial isolation, endocardial resection, and ablation. An ICD may be used with these surgical interventions.

Endocardial Isolation

Endocardial isolation involves making an incision into the endocardium that separates the area where the dysrhythmia originates from the surrounding endocardium. The edges of the incision are then sutured together. The incision and its resulting scar tissue prevent the dysrhythmia from affecting the whole heart.

Endocardial Resection

In endocardial resection, the origin of the dysrhythmia is identified, and that area of the endocardium is peeled away. No reconstruction or repair is necessary.

Catheter Ablation Therapy

Catheter ablation destroys specific cells that are the cause or central conduction method of a tachydysrhythmia. It is performed with or after an EP study. Usual indications for ablation are AV nodal reentry tachycardia, atrial fibrillation, or VT unresponsive to previous therapy (or for which the therapy produced significant side effects).

Ablation is also indicated to eliminate accessory AV pathways or bypass tracts that exist in the hearts of patients with preexcitation syndromes such as Wolff-Parkinson-White (WPW) syndrome. During normal embryonic development, all connections between the atrium and ventricles disappear, except for that between the AV node and the bundle of His. In some people, embryonic connections of normal heart muscle between the atrium and ventricles remain, providing an accessory pathway or a tract through which the electrical impulse can bypass the AV node. These pathways can be located in several different areas. If the patient develops atrial fibrillation, the impulse may be conducted into the ventricle at a rate of 300 times per minute or more, which can lead to ventricular fibrillation and sudden cardiac death. Preexcitation syndromes are identified by specific ECG findings. For example, in WPW syndrome there is a shortened PR interval, slurring (called a delta wave) of the initial QRS deflection, and prolonged QRS duration (Fig. 27-33).

Ablation may be accomplished by three different methods: radiofrequency ablation, cryoablation, or electrical ablation. The most often used method is radiofrequency, which involves placing a special catheter at or near the origin of the dysrhythmia. High-frequency, low-energy sound waves are passed through the catheter, causing thermal injury and cellular changes that result in localized destruction and scarring. The tissue damage is more specific to the dysrhythmic tissue, with less trauma to the surrounding cardiac tissue than occurs with cryoablation or electrical ablation.

Cryoablation involves placing a special probe, cooled to a temperature of −60°C (−76°F), on the endocardium at the site of the dysrhythmia's origin for 2 minutes. The tissue freezes and is later replaced by scar tissue, eliminating the origin of the dysrhythmia.

In electrical ablation, a catheter is placed at or near the origin of the dysrhythmia, and one to four shocks of 100 to 300 joules are administered through the catheter directly to the endocardium and surrounding tissue. The cardiac tissue burns and scars, thus eliminating the source of the dysrhythmia.

During the ablation procedure, defibrillation pads, an automatic blood pressure cuff, and a pulse oximeter are used on the patient, and an indwelling urinary catheter is inserted. The patient is given light sedation. An EP study is performed and attempts to induce the dysrhythmia are made. The ablation catheter is placed at the origin of the dysrhythmia, and the ablation procedure is performed. Multiple ablations may be necessary. Successful ablation is achieved when the dysrhythmia can no longer be induced. The patient is monitored for another 30 to 60 minutes and then retested to ensure that the dysrhythmia will not recur.

Postprocedural care is similar to that for an EP study, except that the patient is monitored more closely, depending on the time needed for recovery from sedation.

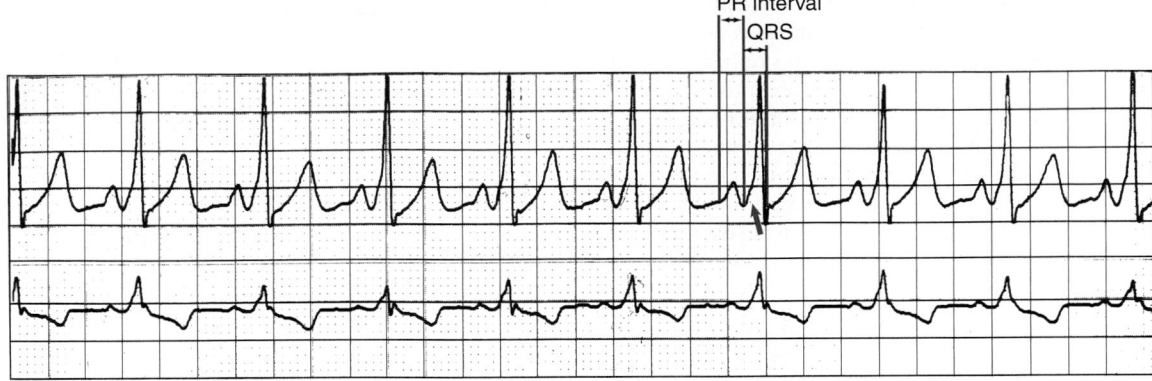

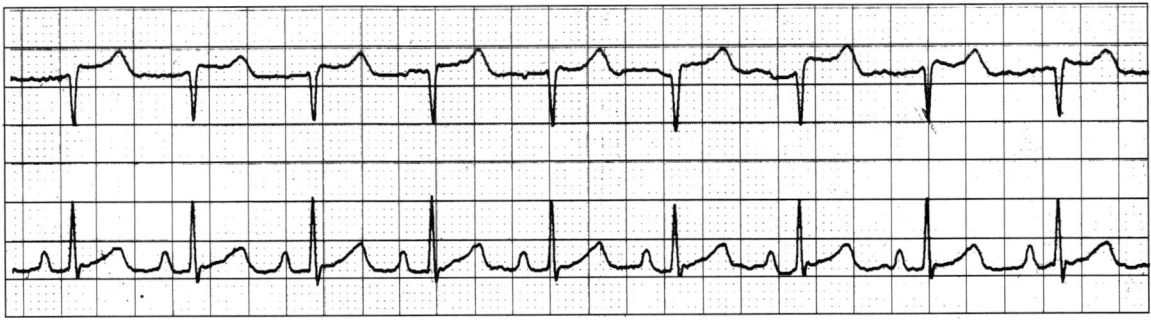

FIGURE 27-33 Wolff-Parkinson-White syndrome. (**A**) Sinus rhythm. Note the short PR interval, slurred initial upstroke of the QRS complex (delta wave, at the arrow), and prolonged QRS duration, upper lead II, lower lead V$_1$. (**B**) Rhythm strip of same patient following ablation, upper lead V$_1$, lower lead II. ECG strips courtesy of Linda Ardini and Catherine Berkmeyer, Inova Fairfax Hospital, Falls Church, VA.

Critical Thinking Exercises

1. You are caring for a 40 year-old male physician who had experienced a cardiac arrest at home, witnessed by his 9-year-old son and 15-year-old daughter. After having an ICD implanted, he appears sullen and withdrawn. On inquiry about how he feels, he replies, "I don't know if this device is a blessing or a punishment!" How would you respond? What other factors are important to assess? Discuss the impact that his children may have on his perception of the device. How would you alter your plan of care to address this patient's psychosocial concerns because he is a physician? How would the plan of care change if, instead of appearing sullen and withdrawn, he appeared irritable and confrontational?

2. Your patient is an active 80-year-old woman who has heart failure and chronic atrial fibrillation. She is taking an angiotensin-converting enzyme inhibitor, a beta-blocker, a diuretic, and digoxin. During your assessment, she tells you that she felt very dizzy this morning. How would you focus your assessment, and why? Identify some of the key assessment factors. What nursing interventions are needed? How would you modify your assessment and interventions if your patient also had chronic obstructive pulmonary disease and renal insufficiency?

REFERENCES AND SELECTED READINGS

Books and Pamphlets

Albert, J. S. (2001). *The AHA clinical cardiac consult.* Philadelphia: Lippincott Williams & Wilkins.

Braunwald, E., Zipes, D. P., & Libby, P. (2001). *Heart disease: A textbook of cardiovascular medicine* (6th ed.). Philadelphia: W. B. Saunders.

Conover, M. B. (1998). *Pocket guide to electrocardiology.* St. Louis: Mosby.

Ellenbogen, K. A., Kay, G. N, & Wilkoff, B. L. (Eds.). (2000). *Clinical cardiac pacing and defibrillation* (2nd ed.). Philadelphia: W. B. Saunders.

Fuster, V., Alexander R. W., & O'Rourke, R. A. (Eds.). (2001). *Hurst's the heart* (10th ed.). New York: McGraw-Hill.

Kinney, M., Brooks-Brunn, J. A., Molter, N., Dunbar, S. B., & Vitello-Ciccio, L. M. (Eds.). (1998). *AACN clinical reference for critical care nursing* (4th ed.). St. Louis: Mosby.

Management of new onset atrial fibrillation. Evidence Report/Technology Assessment: Number 12. AHRQ Publication No. 00-E007. (May 2000). Rockville, MD: Agency for Healthcare Research and Quality.

Marriott, H. J., & Conover, M. B. (1998). *Advanced concepts in arrhythmias.* St. Louis: Mosby.

McEvoy, G. K. (Ed.). (2001). *AHFS drug information 2001.* Bethesda, MD: American Society of Health System Pharmacists.

McNamara, R. L., Bass, E. B., Miller, M. R., Kim, N. L., Robinson, K. A., & Powe, N. R. (2001). *Management of new onset atrial fibrillation.* Evidence Report/Technology Assessment No. 12 (prepared by the Johns Hopkins University Evidence-Based Practice Center in Baltimore, MD, under Contract No. 290-97-0006). AHRQ Publication Number 01-E026. Rockville, MD: Agency for Healthcare Research and Quality.

Moses, H. W., Moulton, K. P., Miller, B. D., & Schneider, J. A. (2000). *A practical guide to cardiac pacing* (5th ed.). Philadelphia: Lippincott Williams & Wilkins.

Murphy, J. (Ed.). (2000). *Mayo Clinic cardiology review* (2nd ed.). Philadelphia: Lippincott Williams & Wilkins.

Singer, I. (2001). *Interventional electrophysiology.* Philadelphia: Lippincott.

Skidmore-Roth, L. (2002). *2002 Mosby's nursing drug reference.* St Louis: Mosby.

Wagner, G. S. (Ed.) (2001). *Marriott's practical electrocardiography* (10th ed.). Philadelphia: Lippincott Williams & Wilkins.

Journals

Asterisks indicate nursing research articles.

American College of Cardiology/American Heart Association Task Force on Practice Guidelines (Committee on Pacemaker Implantation). (1998). ACC/AHA Task Force Report. Guidelines for implantation of cardiac pacemakers and antiarrhythmia devices: Executive summary. *Circulation, 97*(13), 1325–1335.

American Heart Association, in collaboration with the International Liaison Committee on Resuscitation. (2000). Guidelines 2000 for cardiopulmonary resuscitation and emergency cardiovascular care: An international consensus on science. *Circulation, 102,* (8 Suppl.), I1–I384.

Aronow, W. S. (1999). Management of the older person with ventricular arrhythmias. *Journal of American Geriatrics Society, 47*(7), 886–895.

Asselin, M. E., & Cullen, H. A. (2001). What you need to know about the new ACLS guidelines: Find out about changes in algorithms and policies and how they'll affect your practice. *Nursing 2001, 31*(4), 48–50.

Atlee, J. L., & Bernstein, A. D. (2001). Cardiac rhythm management devices. Part I: Indications, device selection, and function. *Anesthesiology, 95*(5), 1265–1280.

Atkins, D. L., Dorian, P., Gonzalez, E. R., Gorgel, A. P., Kudenchuk, P. J., Luriek, K. G., Morley, P. T., Robertson, C., Samson, R. A., Silka, M. J., & Singh, B. N. (2001). Treatment of tachyarrhythmias: Proceedings of the International Guidelines 2000 Conference for Cardiopulmonary Resuscitation and Emergency Cardiovascular Care. *Annuals of Emergency Medicine, 37*(4), (Suppl.), S91–S109.

Bernstein, J. E. (1997). Recognizing when long QT intervals mean trouble. *Nursing 97, 27*(4), 32aa–32ff.

Boyle, J., & Rost, M. K. (2000). Present status of cardiac pacing: A nursing perspective. *Critical Care Nursing Quarterly, 23*(1), 1–19.

Brown, J., & Kellerman, A. L. (2000). The shocking truth about automated external defibrillators. *Journal of the American Medical Association, 284*(11), 1438–1441.

Bubien, R. S., & Sanchez, J. E. (2001). Atrial fibrillation: Treatment rationale and clinical utility of nonpharmacologic therapies. *AACN Clinical Issues: Advanced Practice Acute Critical Care 12*(1), 140–155.

The Cardiac Arrhythmia Suppression Trial Investigators. (1989). The Cardiac Arrhythmia Suppression Trial. *New England Journal of Medicine, 321*(25), 1754–1756.

Cannom, D. S. (2002). Implantable cardioverter defibrillator trials: What's new? *Current Opinion in Cardiology, 17*(1), 29–35.

Carroll, D. L., Hamilton, G. A., & McGovern, B. A. (1999). Changes in health status and quality of life and the impact of uncertainty in patients who survive life-threatening arrhythmia. *Heart & Lung, 28*(4), 251–260.

Daoud, E. G., Timmermans, C., Fellows, C., Hoyt, R., Lemery, R., Dawson, K., & Ayers, G. M. (2000). Initial clinical experience with ambulatory use of an implantable atrial defibrillator for conversion of atrial fibrillation. Metrix Investigators. *Circulation, 102*(12), 1407–1413.

Dickerson, S. S., Posluszny, M., & Kennedy, M. C. (2000). Help seeking in a support group for recipients of implantable cardioverter defibrillators and their support person. *Heart & Lung, 29*(2), 87–96.

Dougherty, C. M., Benoliel, J. Q., & Bellin, C. (2000). Domains of nursing intervention after sudden cardiac arrest and automatic internal cardioverter defibrillator implantation. *Heart & Lung, 29*(2), 79–86.

Drew, B. J., & Krucoff, M. W. (1999). Multilead ST-segment monitoring in patients with acute coronary syndromes: A consensus statement for healthcare professionals. *American Journal of Critical Care, 8*(6), 372–386.

Fenton, J. M. (2001). The clinician's approach to evaluating patients with dysrhythmias. *AACN Clinical Issues: Advanced Practice Acute Critical Care, 12*(1), 72–86.

Gilbert, C. J. (2001). Common supraventricular tachycardias: Mechanisms and management. *AACN Clinical Issues: Advanced Practice Acute Critical Care, 12*(1), 100–113, 170–172.

Gregoratos, G., Abrams, J., Epstein, A. E., Freedman, R. A., Hayes, D. L., Hlatky, M. A., Kerber, R. E., Naccarelli, G. V., Schoenfeld, M. H., Silka, M. J., Winters, S. L., Gibbons, R. J., Antman, E. M., Alpert, J. S., Gregoratos, G., Hiratzka, L. F., Faxon, D. P., Jacobs, A. K., Fuster, V., & Smith, S. C., Jr. ACC/AHA/NASPE 2002 guideline update for implantation of cardiac pacemakers and antiarrhythmia devices: Summary article. A report of the American College of Cardiology/American Heart Association Task Force on Practice Guidelines (ACC/AHA/NASPE Committee to Update the 1998 Pacemaker Guidelines). *Circulation, 106*(16), 2145–2161.

Hauptman, P. J., & Kelly, R. A. (1999). Digitalis. *Circulation, 99*(9), 1265–1270.

Kellen, J. C., Ettinger, A., Todd, L., Brezsnyak, M. L., Campion, J., McBride, R., Thomas, S., Corum, J., & Schron, E. (1996). The cardiac arrhythmia suppression trial: Implications for nursing practice. *American Journal of Critical Care, 5*(1), 19–25.

*Malm, D., Karlsson, J., & Fridlund, B. (1998). Quality of life in pacemaker patients from a nursing perspective. *Coronary Health Care, 2*(1), 17–27.

Mirowski M., Mower M. M., & Reid, P. R. (1980). The automatic implantable defibrillator. *American Heart Journal, 100,* (6 Part II), 1089–1092.

Ocampo, C. M. (2000). Living with an implantable cardioverter defibrillator: Impact on the patient, family and society. *Nursing Clinics of North America, 35*(4), 1019–1030.

Reynolds, J., & Apple, S. (2001). A systematic approach to pacemaker assessment. *AACN Clinical Issues: Advanced Practice Acute Critical Care, 12*(1), 14–26.

Shaffer, R. S. (2002). ICD therapy: The patient's perspective. *American Journal of Nursing, 102*(2), 46–49.

Thomas, S. A., Friedmann, E., & Kelley, F. J. (2001). Living with an implantable cardioverter-defibrillator: A review of the current literature related to psychosocial factors. *AACN Clinical Issues: Advanced Practice Acute Critical Care, 12*(1), 156–163.

*Tyndall, A., Nystrom, K. V., & Funk, M. (1997). Nausea and vomiting in patients undergoing radiofrequency catheter ablation. *American Journal of Critical Care, 6*(6), 437–444.

Wallace, C. J. (2001). Diagnosing and treating pacemaker syndrome. *Critical Care Nurse, 21*(1), 24–31, 35–37.

White, E. (2000). Patients with implantable cardioverter defibrillators: Transition to home. *Journal of Cardiovascular Nursing, 14*(3), 42–52.

Yager, M., Benson, J., & Kamajian, M. (2001). Brugada syndrome: A case study of aborted sudden cardiac death manifesting as seizures. *Critical Care Nurse, 21*(1), 38, 40, 42–46.

Zipes, D. P., & Wellens, H. J. (2000). What have we learned about cardiac arrhythmias? *Circulation, 102,* (20 Suppl. 4), IV52–IV57.

RESOURCES AND WEBSITES

American Association of Critical Care Nurses, 101 Columbia, Aliso Viejo, CA 92656-4109; 800-899-2226; http://www.aacn.org.

American College of Cardiology, 911 Old Georgetown Road, Bethesda, MD 20814; 800-253-4636; http://www.acc.org.

American Heart Association, National Center, 7272 Greenville Ave., Dallas, TX 75231; 1-800-242-8721; http://www.americanheart.org.

National Heart, Lung, Blood Institute, Health Information Center, National Institutes of Health, PO Box 30105, Bethesda, MD 20824; 301-592-8573; http://www.nhlbi.nih.gov.

National Institute on Aging, Building 31, Room 5C27, 31 Center Drive, MSC 2292, Bethesda, MD 20892; 301-496-1752; http://www.nih.gov/nia.

North American Society of Pacing and Electrophysiology, Six Strathmore Road, Natick, MA 01760-2499; 508-647-0100; http://www.naspe.org.

Management of Patients With Coronary Vascular Disorders

On completion of this chapter, the learner will be able to:

1. Describe the pathophysiology, clinical manifestations, and treatment of coronary atherosclerosis.

2. Describe the pathophysiology, clinical manifestations, and treatment of angina pectoris.

3. Use the nursing process as a framework for care of patients with angina pectoris.

4. Describe the pathophysiology, clinical manifestations, and treatment of myocardial infarction.

5. Use the nursing process as a framework for care of patients with myocardial infarction (acute coronary syndrome).

6. Describe the nursing care of a patient who has had an invasive interventional procedure for treatment of coronary artery disease.

7. Describe coronary artery revascularization procedures.

8. Describe the nursing care of the patient treated with cardiac surgery.

*I*n the past, identification and treatment of heart disease focused on white, middle-aged men. However, later studies showed that other segments of the population were also seriously affected by cardiac conditions. Cardiovascular disease is the leading cause of death in the United States for men and women of all racial and ethnic groups, and more women die of cardiovascular disease than all types of cancers combined (American Heart Association, 2001).

Coronary Artery Disease

Coronary artery disease (CAD) is the most prevalent type of cardiovascular disease. For this reason, it is important for nurses to become familiar with the various types of coronary artery conditions and the methods for assessing, preventing, and treating these disorders medically and surgically.

CORONARY ATHEROSCLEROSIS

The most common heart disease in the United States is **atherosclerosis**, which is an abnormal accumulation of lipid, or fatty, substances and fibrous tissue in the vessel wall. These substances create blockages or narrow the vessel in a way that reduces blood flow to the myocardium. Studies (Mehta et al., 1998) indicate that atherosclerosis involves a repetitious inflammatory response to artery wall injury and an alteration in the biophysical and biochemical properties of the arterial walls. An association between an infection (eg, gingivitis) and the later development of heart disease is being explored, as is the administration of antibiotics to prevent heart disease. Although authorities disagree about how atherosclerosis begins, they agree that atherosclerosis is a progressive disease that can be curtailed and, in some cases, reversed.

Pathophysiology

Atherosclerosis begins as fatty streaks, lipids that are deposited in the intima of the arterial wall. Although they are thought to be the precursors of atherosclerosis, fatty streaks are common, even in childhood. Moreover, not all develop into more advanced lesions. The reason why some fatty streaks continue to develop is unknown, although genetic and environmental factors are involved. The continued development of atherosclerosis involves an inflammatory response. T lymphocytes and monocytes (that become macrophages) infiltrate the area to ingest the lipids and then die; this causes smooth muscle cells within the vessel to proliferate and form a fibrous cap over the dead fatty core. These deposits, called **atheromas** or plaques, protrude into the lumen of the vessel, narrowing it and obstructing blood flow (Fig. 28-1). If the fibrous cap of the plaque is thick and the lipid pool remains relatively stable, it can resist the stress from blood flow and vessel movement. If the cap is thin, the lipid core may grow, causing it to rupture and hemorrhage into the plaque, allowing a thrombus to develop. The thrombus may obstruct blood flow, leading to sudden cardiac death or an acute **myocardial infarction (MI)**, which is the death of heart tissue.

The anatomic structure of the coronary arteries makes them particularly susceptible to the mechanisms of atherosclerosis. As Figure 28-2 shows, they twist and turn as they supply blood to the heart, creating sites susceptible to atheroma development. Although heart disease is most often caused by atherosclerosis of the coronary arteries, other phenomena decrease blood flow to the heart. Examples include vasospasm (sudden constriction or narrowing) of a coronary artery, myocardial trauma from internal or external forces, structural disease, congenital anomalies, decreased oxygen supply (eg, from acute blood loss, anemia, or low

Glossary

ACE inhibitor (ACE-I): abbreviation for medications that inhibit the angiotensin-converting enzyme

acute coronary syndrome (ACS): signs and symptoms that indicate unstable angina or acute myocardial infarction

angina pectoris: chest pain brought about by myocardial ischemia

atherosclerosis: abnormal accumulation of lipid deposits and fibrous tissue within arterial walls and lumen

atheroma: fibrous cap composed of smooth muscle cells that forms over lipid deposits within arterial vessels and that protrudes into the lumen of the vessel, narrowing the lumen and obstructing blood flow; also called plaque

collateral circulation: arteries that supply blood to tissue when the main arterial blood supply is partially or totally obstructed

contractility: ability of the cardiac muscle to shorten in response to an electrical impulse

coronary artery bypass graft (CABG): a surgical procedure in which a blood vessel from another part of the body is grafted onto the occluded coronary artery below the occlusion in such a way that blood flow bypasses the blockage

creatine kinase (CK): an enzyme found in human tissues; one of the three types of CK is specific to heart muscle and may be used as an indicator of heart muscle injury

high-density lipoprotein (HDL): a protein-bound lipid that transports cholesterol to the liver for excretion in the bile; composed of a higher proportion of protein to lipid than low-density lipoprotein; exerts a beneficial effect on the arterial wall

hormone replacement therapy (HRT): estrogen, progesterone, or both prescribed for postmenopausal or oophorectomized women

ischemia: insufficient tissue oxygenation

low-density lipoprotein (LDL): a protein-bound lipid that transports cholesterol to tissues in the body; composed of a lower proportion of protein to lipid than high-density lipoprotein; exerts a harmful effect on the arterial wall

myocardial infarction (MI): death of heart tissue caused by lack of oxygenated blood flow; if acute, abbreviated as AMI

percutaneous coronary intervention (PCI): an invasive procedure in which a catheter is placed in a coronary artery, and one of

several methods is employed to remove or reduce a blockage within the artery

percutaneous transluminal coronary angioplasty (PTCA): a type of percutaneous coronary intervention in which a balloon is inflated within a coronary artery to break an atheroma and open the vessel lumen, improving coronary artery blood flow

primary prevention: interventions taken to prevent the development of coronary artery disease

secondary prevention: interventions taken to prevent the advancement of existing coronary artery disease

streptokinase (SK): a thrombolytic agent

stent: a woven mesh that provides structural support to a coronary vessel, preventing its closure

sudden cardiac death: immediate cessation of effective heart activity

thrombolytic: an agent or process that breaks down blood clots

troponin: myocardial protein; measurement is used to indicate heart muscle injury

vasoconstrictor: an agent (usually a medication) that narrows the blood vessel lumen

vasodilator: an agent (usually a medication) that enlarges blood vessel lumen

Physiology/Pathophysiology

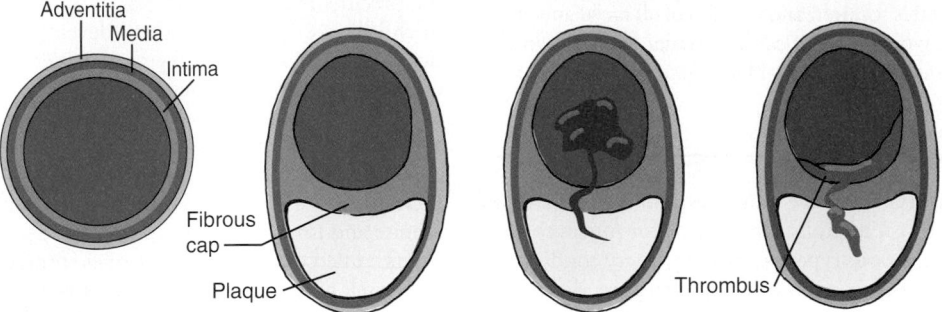

FIGURE 28-1 Atherosclerosis involves a normally patent artery (**A**) and an inflammatory response whereby smooth muscle cells proliferate within the blood vessel to form a fibrous cap (**B**). The proliferation results in deposits, called atheromas or plaques, which protrude into the lumen of the vessel, narrowing it and obstructing blood flow. If the cap ruptures and hemorrhages into the plaque (**C**), a thrombus (**D**) may develop and obstruct blood flow further.

blood pressure), and increased demand for oxygen (eg, from rapid heart rate, thyrotoxicosis, or ingestion of cocaine).

Clinical Manifestations

Coronary atherosclerosis produces symptoms and complications according to the location and degree of narrowing of the arterial lumen, thrombus formation, and obstruction of blood flow to the myocardium. This impediment to blood flow is usually progressive, causing an inadequate blood supply that deprives the muscle cells of oxygen needed for their survival. The condition is known as **ischemia**. **Angina pectoris** refers to chest pain that is brought about by myocardial ischemia. Angina pectoris usually is caused by significant coronary atherosclerosis. If the decrease in blood supply is great enough, of long enough duration, or both, irreversible damage and death of myocardial cells, or MI, may result. Over time, irreversibly damaged myocardium undergoes degener-

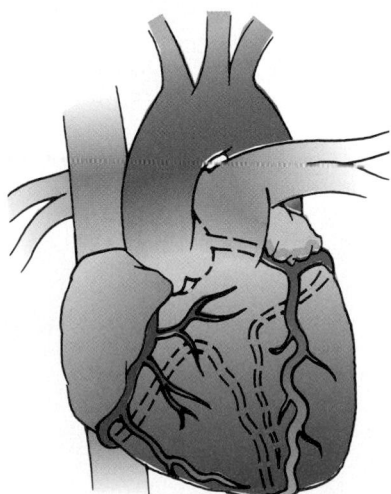

FIGURE 28-2 Angles of the coronary arteries. The many angles and curves of the coronary arteries contribute to the vessels' susceptibility to atheromatous plaques. Arteries shown as dashed lines supply the posterior wall of the heart.

ation and is replaced by scar tissue, causing various degrees of myocardial dysfunction. Significant myocardial damage may cause inadequate cardiac output, and the heart cannot support the body's needs for blood, which is called heart failure (HF). A decrease in blood supply from CAD may even cause the heart to stop abruptly, an event that is called **sudden cardiac death**.

The most common manifestation of myocardial ischemia is acute onset of chest pain. However, an epidemiologic study of the people in Framingham, Massachusetts, showed that nearly 15% of men and women who had MIs were totally asymptomatic (Kannel, 1986). Another study found that 33% of those diagnosed with MI did not present to the emergency room with chest pain (Canto et al., 2000; Ishihara et al., 2000). Those without chest pain tend to be older or women, or to have diabetes or a history of heart failure. Women have been found to have more atypical symptoms of myocardial ischemia (eg, shortness of breath, nausea, unusual fatigue) than men (Meischke et al., 1999). The incidence of prodromal angina (ie, angina a few hours to days before the MI) was found to be significantly lower in patients older than 70 years of age (Ishihara et al., 2000). Other clinical manifestations of CAD may be abnormalities signaled by changes on the electrocardiogram (ECG), high levels of cardiac enzymes, dysrhythmias, and sudden death.

Risk Factors

Epidemiologic studies point to several factors that increase the probability that heart disease will develop. Major risk factors include use of tobacco, hypertension, elevated blood lipid levels, family history of premature cardiovascular disease (first-degree relative with cardiovascular disease at age 55 or younger for men and at age 65 or younger for women) and age (>45 years for men; >55 years for women). The Third Report of the Expert Panel on Detection, Evaluation, and Treatment of High Blood Cholesterol in Adults (Adult Treatment Panel III [ATP III]; 2001) represents the updated clinical guidelines for cholesterol testing and management. ATP III addresses **primary prevention** (preventing the occurrence of CAD) and **secondary prevention** (preventing the progression of CAD).

ATP III is the standard for cholesterol management. ATP III continues to identify elevated **low-density lipoprotein (LDL)** cholesterol as the primary target of cholesterol-lowering therapy. Those at highest risk for having a cardiac event within 10 years are those with existing CAD or those with diabetes, peripheral arterial disease, abdominal aortic aneurysm, or carotid artery disease. The latter diseases are called CAD risk equivalents, because patients with these diseases have the same risk for a cardiac event as patients with CAD (Chart 28-1). The possibility of having a cardiac event within 10 years is also determined by points given to several factors, such as age, level of total cholesterol, level of LDL, level of **high-density lipoprotein (HDL)**, systolic blood pressure, and tobacco use. If the total points add up to more than 15 for men or 23 for women, the person has a greater than 20% risk for a cardiac event within 10 years. A composite of lipid and nonlipid risk factors of metabolic origin, called *metabolic syndrome,* is another risk factor for CAD. Metabolic syndrome includes abdominal obesity, an elevated triglyceride level, low HDL level, elevated blood pressure, and impaired function of insulin.

Measurement of other emerging risk factors, such as elevations of Lipoprotein(a) [Lp(a)], remnant lipoproteins, small LDL, fibrinogen, homocysteine, and impaired fasting plasma glucose (110–125 mg/dL), is optional and are not routinely recommended (ATP III, 2001). For example, the Homocysteine Studies Collaboration (2002) found that lower levels of homocysteine, an amino acid, were modestly associated with reduced risk of ischemic heart disease and stroke. The results of these retrospective studies suggest that homocysteine may promote atherosclerosis. A meta-analysis of prospective studies was done that showed a significant association between homocysteine levels and ischemic heart disease as well as between homocysteine and stroke (Wald, Law, & Morris, 2002). The authors recommend a daily intake of approximately 0.8 mg of folic acid to decrease blood homocysteine levels and reduce the risk of ischemic heart disease and CVA (brain attack, stroke). The American Heart Association has stated that until the results of large-scale randomized trials become available, routine testing of homocysteine concentrations cannot be justified (Malinow, Bostom, & Krauss, 1999).

Prevention

Four modifiable risk factors—cholesterol abnormalities, cigarette smoking (tobacco use), hypertension, and diabetes mellitus—have been cited as major risk factors for CAD and its consequent complications. As a result, they receive much attention in health promotion programs (Chart 28-2).

> ### Chart 28-1 Coronary Artery Disease Risk Equivalents
>
> Individuals at highest risk for a cardiac event within 10 years are those with existing coronary artery disease (CAD) and those with any of the following diseases, which are called CAD risk equivalents:
>
> * Diabetes
> * Peripheral arterial disease
> * Abdominal aortic aneurysm
> * Carotid artery disease
>
> From Expert Panel on Detection, Evaluation, and Treatment of High Blood Cholesterol in Adults. (2001). Executive summary of the third report of the National Cholesterol Education Program (NCEP) Expert Panel on Detection, Evaluation, and Treatment of High Blood Cholesterol in Adults (Adult Treatment Panel III). *Journal of the American Medical Association, 285*(19), 2486–2497.

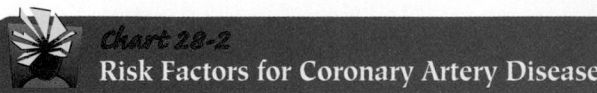

> ### Chart 28-2 Risk Factors for Coronary Artery Disease
>
> A modifiable risk factor is one over which individuals may exercise control, such as by changing a lifestyle or personal habit or by using medication. A nonmodifiable risk factor is a circumstance over which individuals have no control, such as age or heredity. A risk factor may operate independently or in tandem with other risk factors. The more risk factors individuals have, the greater the likelihood of coronary artery disease. Those at risk are advised to seek regular medical examinations and to engage in "heart-healthy" behavior (a deliberate effort to reduce the number and extent of risks).
>
> **Nonmodifiable Risk Factors**
> Family history of coronary heart disease
> Increasing age
> Gender (heart disease occurs three times more often in men than in premenopausal women)
> Race (higher incidence of heart disease in African Americans than in Caucasians)
>
> **Modifiable Risk Factors**
> High blood cholesterol level
> Cigarette smoking, tobacco use
> Hypertension
> Diabetes mellitus
> Lack of estrogen in women
> Physical inactivity
> Obesity

CONTROLLING CHOLESTEROL ABNORMALITIES

The association of a high blood cholesterol level with heart disease is well established and accepted. The metabolism of fats is important in understanding the development of heart disease.

Fats, which are insoluble in water, are encased in water-soluble lipoproteins to allow them to be transported within a circulatory system that is water-based. Four elements of fat metabolism—total cholesterol, LDL, HDL, and triglycerides—are primary factors affecting the development of heart disease (Fig. 28-3). Cholesterol and the lipoproteins are synthesized by the liver or ingested as part of the diet. All adults 20 years of age or older should have a fasting lipid profile (total cholesterol, LDL, HDL, and triglyceride) performed at least once every 5 years and more often if the profile is abnormal. Patients who have had an acute event (MI), percutaneous coronary intervention (PCI), or **coronary artery bypass graft (CABG)** require assessment of the LDL-cholesterol level within 60 to 365 days after the event (LDL levels may be low immediately after the acute event). Subsequently, lipids should be monitored every 6 weeks until the desired level is achieved and then every 4 to 6 months (Expert Panel on Detection, Evaluation, and Treatment of High Blood Cholesterol in Adults, 2001).

LDL exerts a harmful effect on the arterial wall and accelerates atherosclerosis. In contrast, HDL promotes the use of total cholesterol by transporting LDL to the liver, where it is biodegraded and then excreted. The desired goal is to have low LDL values and high HDL values. The desired level of LDL depends on the patient:

* Less than 160 mg/dL for patients with one or no risk factors
* Less than 130 mg/dL for patients with two or more risk factors
* Less than 100 mg/dL for patients with CAD or a CAD risk equivalent

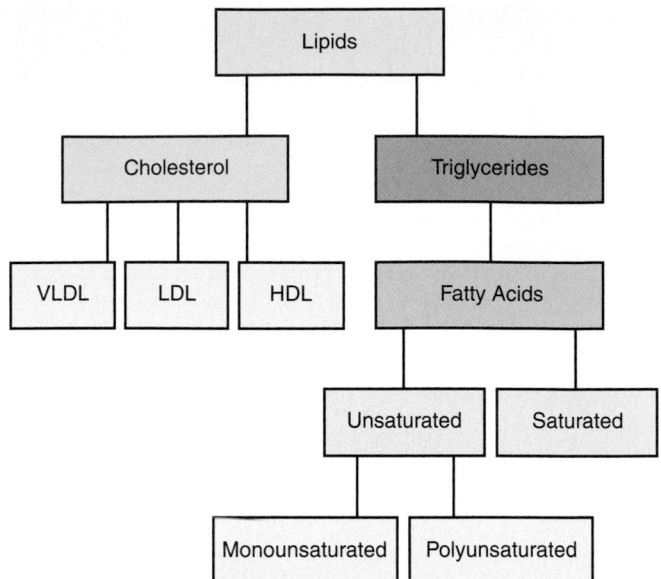

FIGURE 28-3 Types of lipids. Elevated levels of cholesterol, VLDL, LDL, and triglycerides, and low levels of HDL are risk factors for the development of atherosclerotic arterial disease, such as coronary artery disease. (VLDL, very low density lipoproteins; LDL, low density lipoproteins; HDL, high density lipoproteins.)

Serum cholesterol and LDL levels can usually be controlled by diet and physical activity. Depending on the patient's LDL level and risk of coronary heart disease, medication therapy may also be prescribed.

The level of HDL should exceed 40 mg/dL and should ideally be more than 60 mg/dL. A high HDL level is a strong negative risk factor (is protective) for heart disease.

Triglyceride is another fatty substance, made up of fatty acids, that is transported through the blood by a lipoprotein. Although an elevated triglyceride level (>200 mg/dL) may be genetic in origin, it also can be caused by obesity, physical inactiv-

ity, excessive alcohol intake, high-carbohydrate diets, diabetes mellitus, kidney disease, and certain medications, such as birth control pills, corticosteroids, and beta-adrenergic blockers when given in higher doses. Management of elevated triglyceride focuses on weight reduction and increased physical activity. Medications such as nicotinic acid and fibric acids (eg, fenofibrate [Tricor], clofibrate [Atromid-S]) may also be prescribed, especially if the triglyceride level is above 500 mg/dL (Expert Panel on Detection, Evaluation, and Treatment of High Blood Cholesterol in Adults, 2001).

Lipoprotein(a), or Lp(a), is a component of LDL and is attached to a special protein called apo(a). The level of Lp(a) is primarily determined by genetics. An elevated level of Lp(a) has been associated with a higher risk of CAD. However, clinical trials have not yet identified methods that lower the level of Lp(a) and have not demonstrated that lower levels of Lp(a) reduce the risk of CAD; therefore Lp(a) is not routinely monitored (Danesh, et al., 2000; Gibbons et al., 1999).

Dietary Measures. Table 28-1 provides recommendations of the Therapeutic Lifestyle Changes (TLC) diet (Expert Panel on Detection, Evaluation, and Treatment of High Blood Cholesterol in Adults, 2001). However, these recommendations may need to be adjusted to match the individual patient who has other nutritional needs, such as the requirements for pregnancy or diabetes. To assist in following the appropriate TLC diet, the patient should be referred to a registered dietitian. Other TLC recommendations are weight loss, cessation of tobacco use, and increased physical activity.

Soluble dietary fiber may also help lower cholesterol levels. Soluble fibers, which are found in fresh fruit, cereal grains, vegetables, and legumes, enhance the excretion of metabolized cholesterol. The ability of fiber to reduce serum cholesterol continues to be investigated. Intake of at least 20 to 30 grams of fiber each day is recommended (Expert Panel on Detection, Evaluation, and Treatment of High Blood Cholesterol in Adults, 2001).

Many resources are available to assist people who are attempting to control their cholesterol levels. The National Heart, Lung, and Blood Institute (NHLBI) and its National Cholesterol Education Program (NCEP), the American Heart Association, and the

Table 28-1 • **Nutrient Content of the Therapeutic Lifestyle Changes (TLC) Diet**

NUTRIENT	RECOMMENDED INTAKE
Total calories*	Balance intake and expenditure to maintain desirable weight
Total Fat	25%–35% of total calories
Saturated fat†	<7% of total calories
Polyunsaturated Fat	Up to 10% of total calories
Monounsaturated Fat	Up to 20% of total calories
Carbohydrate‡	50%–60% of total calories
Fiber	20–30 g/day
Protein	Approximately 15% of total calories
Cholesterol	<200 mg/day

*Daily energy expenditure should include at least moderate physical activity (contributing approximately 200 k/cal per day).
†Trans-fatty acids are formed from the processing (manufacturing, hydrogenation) of vegetable oils into a more solid form. The effects of trans-fatty acids are similar to saturated fats (ie, raising low-density lipoprotein and lowering high-density lipoprotein). Intake of trans-fatty acids should be kept low.
‡Carbohydrates should be derived predominately from foods rich in complex carbohydrates, including grains, especially whole grains, fruits, and vegetables.
From Expert Panel on Detection, Evaluation, and Treatment of High Blood Cholesterol in Adults. (2001). Executive summary of the third report of the National Cholesterol Education Program (NCEP) Expert Panel on Detection, Evaluation, and Treatment of High Blood Cholesterol in Adults (Adult Treatment Panel III). *Journal of the American Medical Association, 285*(19), 2486–2497.

American Diabetic Association, as well as CAD support groups and reliable Internet sources, are a few examples of the available resources. Cookbooks and recipes that include the nutritional breakdown of foods can be included as resources for patients. Dietary control has been made easier because food manufacturers are required to provide comprehensive nutritional data on product labels. The label information of interest to a person attempting to eat a heart-healthy diet is as follows:

- Serving size, expressed in household measures
- Amount of total fat per serving
- Amount of saturated fat per serving
- Amount of cholesterol per serving
- Amount of fiber per serving

Physical Activity. Regular, moderate physical activity increases HDL levels and reduces triglyceride levels. The goal for the average person is a total of 30 minutes of exercise, three to four times per week. The nurse helps patients set realistic goals for physical activity. For example, the inactive patient should start with activity that lasts 3 minutes, such as parking farther from a building to increase the walking time. For sustained activity, patients should begin with a 5-minute warm-up period to stretch and prepare the body for the exercise. They should end the exercise with a 5-minute cool-down period in which they gradually reduce the intensity of the activity to prevent a sudden decrease in cardiac output. Patients should be instructed to engage in an activity or variety of activities that interest them, to maintain motivation. They should also be taught to exercise to an intensity that does not preclude their ability to talk; if they cannot have a conversation, they should slow down or switch to a less intensive activity. When the weather is hot and humid, the patient should be advised to exercise during the early morning or indoors and wear loose-fitting clothing. When the weather is cold, the patient should be instructed to layer clothing and to wear a hat. The nurse can also advise the patient to avoid adverse weather conditions by participating in local community programs, such as those held at shopping malls. The nurse should inform patients to stop any activity if they develop chest pain, unusual shortness of breath, dizziness, lightheadedness, or nausea.

Medications. Medications (Table 28-2) are used in some instances to control cholesterol levels. If diet alone cannot normalize serum cholesterol levels, several medications have a synergistic effect with the prescribed diet. Lipid-lowering medications can reduce CAD mortality in patients with elevated lipid levels and in those with normal lipid levels. The lipid-lowering agents affect the different lipid components and are usually grouped into four types:

- 3-Hydroxy-3-methylglutaryl coenzyme A (HMG-CoA) reductase inhibitors or statins (eg, lovastatin [Mevacor], pravastatin [Pravachol], simvastatin [Zocor]; see Table 28-2) block cholesterol synthesis, lower LDL and triglyceride levels, and increase HDL levels. These medications are frequently the initial medication therapy for significantly elevated cholesterol and LDL levels. Because of their effect on the liver, results of hepatic function tests are monitored.
- Nicotinic acids (niacin [Niacor, Niaspan]; see Table 28-2) decrease lipoprotein synthesis, lower LDL and triglyceride levels, and increase HDL levels. The dose of niacin needs to be titrated weekly to achieve therapeutic dosage. Niacin is the medication most often used for minimally elevated cholesterol and LDL levels or as an adjunct to a statin when the lipid goal has not been achieved and the triglycerides are

elevated. Side effects include gastrointestinal upset, gout, and flushing. Because of its effect on the liver, hepatic function is monitored.
- Fibric acid or fibrates (eg, clofibrate [Atromid-S], fenofibrate [Ticor]; see Table 28-2) decrease the synthesis of cholesterol, reduce triglyceride levels, and increase HDL levels. Because they have the potential to increase LDLs, fibrates are the medications of choice for patients with triglyceride levels above 400 mg/dL. Because of the risk of myopathy and acute renal failure, fibrates should be used with caution in patients who are also taking a statin.
- Bile acid sequestrants or resins (eg, cholestyramine [LoCholest, Questran, Prevalite]; see Table 28-2) bind cholesterol in the intestine, increase its breakdown, and lower LDL levels with minimal effect on HDLs and no effect (or minimal increase) on triglyceride levels. These medications are more often used as adjunct therapy when statins alone have not been effective in controlling lipid levels and the triglyceride levels are less than 200 mg/dL. Significant side effects, such as gastric distention and constipation, can occur from using these medications.

Medication therapy is reserved for at-risk patients and is not regarded as a substitute for dietary modification. All of these medications have been shown to reduce major coronary events (Expert Panel on Detection, Evaluation, and Treatment of High Blood Cholesterol in Adults, 2001). Some of these may be used in combination to achieve synergistic effects. For example, LDL cholesterol can be lowered more effectively by adding a low dose of resin to a dose of niacin or statins, or both, than a maximum dose of an individual agent.

Patients with elevated cholesterol levels should be monitored for adherence to the medical plan, the effect of cholesterol-lowering medications, and the development of side effects from cholesterol-lowering medications. Lipid levels are obtained and adjustments made to the diet and medication every 6 weeks until the lipid goal or maximum dose is achieved and then every 6 months thereafter.

PROMOTING CESSATION OF TOBACCO USE

Cigarette smoking contributes to the development and severity of CAD in three ways. First, the inhalation of smoke increases the blood carbon monoxide level, causing hemoglobin, the oxygen-carrying component of blood, to combine more readily with carbon monoxide than with oxygen. A decreased amount of available oxygen may decrease the heart's ability to pump.

Second, the nicotinic acid in tobacco triggers the release of catecholamines, which raise the heart rate and blood pressure. Nicotinic acid can also cause the coronary arteries to constrict. Smokers have a tenfold increase in risk for sudden cardiac death. The increase in catecholamines may be a factor in the increased incidence of sudden cardiac death.

Third, use of tobacco causes a detrimental vascular response and increases platelet adhesion, leading to a higher probability of thrombus formation. A person with increased risk for heart disease is encouraged to stop tobacco use through any means possible: counseling, consistent motivation and reinforcement messages, support groups, and medications. Some people have found complementary therapies (eg, acupuncture, guided imagery, hypnosis) to be helpful. People who stop smoking reduce their risk of heart disease by 30% to 50% within the first year, and the risk continues to decline as long as they refrain from smoking.

Exposure to other smokers' smoke (passive or second-hand smoke) is believed to cause heart disease in nonsmokers. Oral contraceptive use by women who smoke is inadvisable because

Table 28-2 • Medications Affecting Lipoprotein Metabolism

MEDICATION AND DAILY DOSAGE	LIPID/LIPOPROTEIN EFFECTS	SIDE EFFECTS	CONTRAINDICATIONS
HMG-CoA Reductase Inhibitors (statins)			
Lovastatin (Mevacor) 20–80 mg	LDL ↓ 18–55%	Myopathy, increased liver enzyme levels	Absolute: active or chronic liver disease
Prevastatin (Pravachol) 20–40 mg	HDL ↑ 5–15% TG ↓ 7–30%		Relative: concomitant use of certain drugs*
Simvastatin (Zocor) 20–80 mg			
Fluvastatin (Lescol) 20–80 mg			
Atorvastatin calcium (Lipitor) 10–80 mg			
Nicotinic Acid			
Niacin (Niacor, Niaspan) Immediate-release nicotinic acid 1.5–3 g	LDL ↓ 5–25% HDL ↑ 15–35%	Flushing, hyperglycemia, hyperuricemia (or gout), upper gastrointestinal distress,	Absolute: chronic liver disease, severe gout Relative: diabetes, hyperuricemia, peptic
Extended-release nicotinic acid 1–2 g	TG ↓ 20–50%	hepatotoxicity	ulcer disease
Sustained-release nicotinic acid 1–2 g			
Fibric Acids			
Fenofibrate (Tricor) 200 mg	LDL ↓ 5–20% (may be increased in patients with high TG)	Dyspepsia, gallstones, myopathy, unexplained non-CHD deaths in World Health Organization study	Absolute: severe renal disease, severe hepatic disease
Clofibrate (Atromid-S) 1000 mg, b.i.d.	HDL ↑ 10–20% TG ↓ 20–50%		
Bile Acid Sequestrants			
Cholestyramine (LoCholest, Questran, Prevalite) 4–16 g	LDL ↓ 15–30% HDL ↑ 3–5% TG no change or	Gastrointestinal distress, constipation, decreased absorption of other drugs	Absolute: dysbetalipoproteinemia, TG >400 mg/dL
Colesevelam (Welchol) 2.6–3.8 g	increase		Relative: TG >200 mg/dL
Colestipol HCl (Colestid) 5–20 g			

HMG-CoA, 3-hydroxy-3-methylglutaryl coenzyme A; LDL, low-density lipoprotein; HDL, high-density lipoprotein; TG, triglycerides;
↓ decrease, ↑ increase; CHD, coronary heart disease
*Cyclosporine (Neoral, Sandimmune, SangCya); macrolide antibiotics (azithromycin [Zithromax], clarithromycin [Biaxin]; dirithromycin [Dynabac]; erythromycin [Aknemycin, E-mycin, Ery-Tab]; various antifungal agents and cytochrome P-450 inhibitors; fibrates; and niacin should be used with appropriate caution).
From Expert Panel on Detection, Evaluation, and Treatment of High Blood Cholesterol in Adults. (2001). Executive summary of the third report of the National Cholesterol Education Program (NCEP) Expert Panel on Detection, Evaluation, and Treatment of High Blood Cholesterol in Adults (Adult Treatment Panel III). *Journal of the American Medical Association, 285*(19), 2486–2497.

these medications significantly increase the risk of CAD and sudden cardiac death.

Cessation of tobacco use results in a lower rate of cardiac events. Patients should be advised to participate in an educational class, support group, or behavioral program. Use of medications such as the nicotine patch (Nicotrol, Nicoderm CQ, Habitrol) or bupropion (Zyban) may assist with stopping use of tobacco, but do have the same systemic effects: catecholamine release (increasing heart rate and blood pressure) and increased platelet adhesion. These medications should be used for the shortest time and at the lowest effective doses.

MANAGING HYPERTENSION

Hypertension is defined as blood pressure measurements that repeatedly exceed 140/90 mm Hg. Long-standing elevated blood pressure may result in increased stiffness of the vessel walls, leading to vessel injury and a resulting inflammatory response within the intima. Hypertension can also increase the work of the left ventricle, which must pump harder to eject blood into the arteries. Over time, the increased workload causes the heart to enlarge and thicken (ie, hypertrophy), a condition that may eventually lead to cardiac failure.

Early detection of high blood pressure and adherence to a therapeutic regimen can prevent the serious consequences associated with untreated elevated blood pressure. Hypertension is discussed in detail in Chapter 32.

CONTROLLING DIABETES MELLITUS

The relationship between diabetes mellitus and heart disease has been substantiated. For 65% to 75% of patients with diabetes, cardiovascular disease is listed as the cause of death (Braunwald et al., 2001; Grundy et al., 1999). Hyperglycemia fosters dyslipidemia, increased platelet aggregation, and altered red blood cell function, which can lead to thrombus formation. It has been suggested that these metabolic alterations impair endothelial cell–dependent vasodilation and smooth muscle function; treatment with insulin (eg, Humalog, Humulin, Novolin) and metformin (Glucophage) has demonstrated improvement in endothelial function: improved endothelial-dependent dilation (Gaenzer et al., 2002). Diabetes is considered equivalent to existing CAD in its risk of a cardiac event within 10 years (Expert Panel on Detection, Evaluation, and Treatment of High Blood Cholesterol in Adults, 2001). Diabetes is discussed in detail in Chapter 41.

Gender and Estrogen Level

Because heart disease had been considered to primarily affect white men, the disease was not as readily recognized and treated in women. However, in 1999 in the United States, 512,904 women died because of cardiovascular disease whereas 42,144 women died from breast cancer and 246,006 women died from any form of cancer (American Heart Association, 2002). Women tend to have a higher incidence of complications from CAD (American Heart Association, 2002). African-American women have a mortality rate nearly twice that of Caucasian women (Office for Social Environment and Health Research at West Virginia University, 2001). Women tend not to recognize the symptoms as early as men and to wait longer to report their symptoms and seek medical assistance (Meischke et al., 1999; Penque et al., 1998). In the past, women were less likely than men to be referred for coronary artery diagnostic procedures, to receive medical therapy (eg, **thrombolytic** therapy to break down the blood clots that cause acute MI, or nitroglycerin), and to be treated with invasive interventions, eg, angioplasty (Sheifer et al., 2000). It is anticipated that with better education of the general public and health care professionals, gender and racial differences will have less influence on the diagnosis, treatment, and incidence of complications of heart disease in the future.

In women younger than age 55, the incidence of CAD is significantly lower than in men. However, after age 55, the incidence in women is approximately equal to that in men. The age difference of the incidence of CAD in women may be related to estrogen. Although **hormone replacement therapy (HRT)** for menopausal women had been promoted as prevention for CAD, research studies do not support HRT as an effective means of CAD prevention (Hulley et al., 1998; Mosca, 2000). HRT has decreased postmenopausal symptoms and the risk for osteoporosis-related bone fractures, but HRT also has been associated with an increased risk for CAD, breast cancer, deep vein thrombosis, cerebrovascular accident (CVA, brain attack, stroke), and pulmonary embolism. The Women's Health Initiative (Gebbie, 2002) demonstrated that long-term HRT may have more risks than benefits, and that HRT should not be initiated or continued for primary prevention of CAD.

Behavior Patterns

Most clinicians believe that stress and certain behaviors contribute to the pathogenesis of CAD and a cardiac event, especially in women. Psychological and epidemiologic studies describe behaviors that characterize people who are prone to heart disease: excessive competitiveness, a sense of time urgency or impatience, aggressiveness, and hostility (Dembroski et al., 1989; Friedman

& Rosenman, 1959; Krantz et al., 2000). A person with these behaviors is classified as type A coronary-prone.

The type A coronary-prone classification may not be as significant as was once thought; evidence of its precise role remains inconclusive (Rozanski et al., 1999). To be on the safer side, however, such a person may be wise to alter behaviors and responses to triggering events and to reduce other risk factors. Nurses can assist these people by teaching them cognitive restructuring and relaxation techniques. Because people who are depressed have worse outcomes, these patients should be assessed for signs and symptoms of depression and, if diagnosed, appropriately treated.

ANGINA PECTORIS

Angina pectoris is a clinical syndrome usually characterized by episodes or paroxysms of pain or pressure in the anterior chest. The cause is usually insufficient coronary blood flow. The insufficient flow results in a decreased oxygen supply to meet an increased myocardial demand for oxygen in response to physical exertion or emotional stress. In other words, the need for oxygen exceeds the supply. The severity of angina is based on the precipitating activity and its effect on the activities of daily living (Table 28-3).

Pathophysiology

Angina is usually caused by atherosclerotic disease. Almost invariably, angina is associated with a significant obstruction of a major coronary artery. The characteristics of the various types of angina are listed in Chart 28-3. Identifying angina requires obtaining a thorough history. Effective treatment begins with reducing the demands placed on the heart and teaching the patient about the condition. Several factors are associated with typical anginal pain:

- Physical exertion, which can precipitate an attack by increasing myocardial oxygen demand
- Exposure to cold, which can cause vasoconstriction and an elevated blood pressure, with increased oxygen demand
- Eating a heavy meal, which increases the blood flow to the mesenteric area for digestion, thereby reducing the blood supply available to the heart muscle (In a severely compromised heart, shunting of blood for digestion can be sufficient to induce anginal pain.)
- Stress or any emotion-provoking situation, causing the release of adrenaline and increasing blood pressure, which may accelerate the heart rate and increase the myocardial workload

Table 28-3 • Canadian Cardiovascular Society Classification of Angina

CLASS	ACTIVITY EVOKING ANGINA	LIMITS TO ACTIVITY
I	Prolonged exertion	None
II	Walking >2 blocks	Slight
III	Walking <2 blocks	Marked
IV	Minimal or rest	Severe

Adapted from Campeau L. (1976). Grading of angina pectoris. *Circulation 54*, 522–523.

Chart 28-3   Types of Angina

- **Stable angina:** predictable and consistent pain that occurs on exertion and is relieved by rest
- **Unstable angina** (also called preinfarction angina or crescendo angina): symptoms occur more frequently and last longer than stable angina. The threshold for pain is lower, and pain may occur at rest.
- **Intractable or refractory angina:** severe incapacitating chest pain
- **Variant angina** (also called Prinzmetal's angina): pain at rest with reversible ST-segment elevation; thought to be caused by coronary artery vasospasm
- **Silent ischemia:** objective evidence of ischemia (such as electrocardiographic changes with a stress test), but patient reports no symptoms

Atypical angina is not associated with the listed factors. It may occur at rest.

Clinical Manifestations

Ischemia of the heart muscle may produce pain or other symptoms, varying in severity from a feeling of indigestion to a choking or heavy sensation in the upper chest that ranges from discomfort to agonizing pain accompanied by severe apprehension and a feeling of impending death. The pain is often felt deep in the chest behind the upper or middle third of the sternum (retrosternal area). Typically, the pain or discomfort is poorly localized and may radiate to the neck, jaw, shoulders, and inner aspects of the upper arms, usually the left arm. The patient often feels tightness or a heavy, choking, or strangling sensation that has a vise-like, insistent quality. The patient with diabetes mellitus may not have severe pain with angina because the neuropathy that accompanies diabetes can interfere with neuroreceptors, dulling the patient's perception of pain.

A feeling of weakness or numbness in the arms, wrists, and hands may accompany the pain, as may shortness of breath, pallor, diaphoresis, dizziness or lightheadedness, and nausea and vomiting. These symptoms may also appear alone and still represent myocardial ischemia. When these symptoms appear alone, they are called angina-like symptoms. Anxiety may accompany angina. An important characteristic of angina is that it abates or subsides with rest or nitroglycerin.

Gerontologic Considerations

The elderly person with angina may not exhibit the typical pain profile because of the diminished responses of neurotransmitters that occur in the aging process. Often, the presenting symptom in the elderly is dyspnea. If they do have pain, it is atypical pain that radiates to both arms rather than just the left arm. Sometimes, there are no symptoms ("silent" CAD), making recognition and diagnosis a clinical challenge. Elderly patients should be encouraged to recognize their chest pain–like symptom (eg, weakness) as an indication that they should rest or take prescribed medications. Noninvasive stress testing used to diagnose CAD may not be as useful in elderly patients because of other conditions (eg, peripheral vascular disease, arthritis, degenerative disk disease, physical disability, foot problems) that limit the patient's ability to exercise.

Assessment and Diagnostic Findings

The diagnosis of angina is often made by evaluating the clinical manifestations of ischemia and the patient's history. A 12-lead ECG and blood laboratory values help in making the diagnosis. The patient may undergo an exercise or pharmacologic stress test in which the heart is monitored by ECG, echocardiogram, or both. The patient may also be referred for an echocardiogram, nuclear scan, or invasive procedures (cardiac catheterization and coronary artery angiography).

CAD is believed to result from inflammation of the arterial endothelium. C-reactive protein (CRP) is a marker for inflammation of vascular endothelium. High blood levels of CRP have been associated with increased coronary artery calcification and risk of an acute cardiovascular event (eg, MI) in seemingly healthy individuals (Ridker et al., 2002; Wang et al., 2002). There is interest in using CRP blood levels as an additional risk factor for cardiovascular disease in clinical use and research, but the clinical value of CRP levels has not been fully established. The ability of CRP to predict cardiovascular disease when adjusted for other risk factors, how CRP levels can guide patient management, and if patient outcomes improve when using CRP levels must be established before CRP levels are used routinely for patient care (Mosca, 2002).

An elevated blood level of homocysteine, an amino acid, has also been proposed as an independent risk factor for cardiovascular disease. However, studies have not supported the relationship between mild to moderate elevations of homocysteine and atherosclerosis (Homocysteine Studies Collaboration, 2002). No study has yet shown that reducing homocysteine levels reduces the risk of CAD.

Medical Management

The objectives of the medical management of angina are to decrease the oxygen demand of the myocardium and to increase the oxygen supply. Medically, these objectives are met through pharmacologic therapy and control of risk factors.

Revascularization procedures to restore the blood supply to the myocardium include **percutaneous coronary interventional (PCI)** procedures (eg, **percutaneous transluminal coronary angioplasty [PTCA]**, intracoronary stents, and atherectomy), CABG, and percutaneous transluminal myocardial revascularization (PTMR).

PHARMACOLOGIC THERAPY

Among medications used to control angina are nitroglycerin, beta-adrenergic blocking agents, calcium channel blockers, and antiplatelet agents.

Nitroglycerin. Nitrates remain the mainstay for treatment of angina pectoris. A vasoactive agent, nitroglycerin (Nitrostat, Nitrol, Nitrobid IV) is administered to reduce myocardial oxygen consumption, which decreases ischemia and relieves pain. Nitroglycerin dilates primarily the veins and, in higher doses, also dilates the arteries. It helps to increase coronary blood flow by preventing vasospasm and increasing perfusion through the collateral vessels.

Dilation of the veins causes venous pooling of blood throughout the body. As a result, less blood returns to the heart, and filling pressure (preload) is reduced. If the patient is hypovolemic (does not have adequate circulating blood volume), the decrease in filling pressure can cause a significant decrease in cardiac output and blood pressure.

Nitrates in higher doses also relax the systemic arteriolar bed and lower blood pressure (decreased afterload). Nitrates may increase blood flow to diseased coronary arteries and through collateral coronary arteries, arteries that have been underused until the body recognizes poorly perfused areas. These effects decrease myocardial oxygen requirements and increase oxygen supply, bringing about a more favorable balance between supply and demand.

Nitroglycerin may be given by several routes: sublingual tablet or spray, topical agent, and intravenous administration. Sublingual nitroglycerin is generally placed under the tongue or in the cheek (buccal pouch) and alleviates the pain of ischemia within 3 minutes. Topical nitroglycerin is also fast acting and is a convenient way to administer the medication. Both routes are suitable for patients who self-administer the medication. Chart 28-4 provides more information.

A continuous or intermittent intravenous infusion of nitroglycerin may be administered to the hospitalized patient with recurring signs and symptoms of ischemia or after a revascularization procedure. The amount of nitroglycerin administered is based on the patient's symptoms while avoiding side effects such as hypotension. It usually is not given if the systolic blood pressure is 90 mm Hg or less. Generally, after the patient is symptom free, the nitroglycerin may be switched to a topical preparation within 24 hours.

Beta-Adrenergic Blocking Agents. Beta-blockers such as propranolol (Inderal), metoprolol (Lopressor, Toprol), and atenolol (Tenormin) appear to reduce myocardial oxygen consumption by blocking the beta-adrenergic sympathetic stimulation to the heart. The result is a reduction in heart rate, slowed conduction of an impulse through the heart, decreased blood pressure, and reduced myocardial **contractility** (force of contraction) that establishes a more favorable balance between myocardial oxygen needs (demands) and the amount of oxygen available (supply). This helps to control chest pain and delays the onset of ischemia during work or exercise. Beta-blockers reduce the incidence of recurrent angina, infarction, and cardiac mortality. The dose can be titrated to achieve a resting heart rate of 50 to 60 beats per minute.

Cardiac side effects and possible contraindications include hypotension, bradycardia, advanced atrioventricular block, and decompensated heart failure. If a beta-blocker is given intravenously for an acute cardiac event, the ECG, blood pressure, and heart rate are monitored closely after the medication has been administered. Because some beta-blockers also affect the beta-adrenergic receptors in the bronchioles, causing bronchoconstriction, they are contraindicated in patients with significant pulmonary constrictive diseases, such as asthma. Other side effects include worsening of hyperlipidemia, depression, fatigue, decreased libido, and masking of symptoms of hypoglycemia. Patients taking beta-blockers are cautioned not to stop taking them abruptly, because angina may worsen and MI may develop. Beta-blocker therapy needs to

---

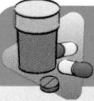

Chart 28-4 • PHARMACOLOGY
Self-Administration of Nitroglycerin

Most patients with angina pectoris must self-administer nitroglycerin on an as-needed basis. A key nursing role in such cases is educating patients about the medication and how to take it. Sublingual nitroglycerin comes in tablet and spray forms.

Teaching About Sublingual Nitroglycerin

- Instruct the patient to make sure the mouth is moist, the tongue is still, and saliva is not swallowed until the nitroglycerin tablet dissolves. If the pain is severe, the patient can crush the tablet between the teeth to hasten sublingual absorption.
- Advise the patient to carry the medication at all times as a precaution. However, because nitroglycerin is very unstable, it should be carried securely in its original container (eg, capped dark glass bottle); tablets should never be removed and stored in metal or plastic pillboxes.
- Explain that nitroglycerin is volatile and is inactivated by heat, moisture, air, light, and time. Instruct the patient to renew the nitroglycerin supply every 6 months.
- Inform the patient that the medication should be taken in anticipation of any activity that may produce pain. Because nitroglycerin increases tolerance for exercise and stress when taken prophylactically (ie, before angina-producing activity, such as exercise, stair-climbing, or sexual intercourse), it is best taken before pain develops.
- Recommend that the patient note how long it takes for the nitroglycerin to relieve the discomfort. Advise the patient that if pain persists after taking three sublingual tablets at 5-minute intervals, emergency medical services should be called.

- Discuss possible side effects of nitroglycerin, including flushing, throbbing headache, hypotension, and tachycardia.

Teaching About Topical Nitroglycerin
Nitroglycerin is also available in a lanolin-petrolatum base that is applied to the skin as a paste or a patch. Patients who use topical nitroglycerin need additional instruction.

- Advise the patient to read the instructions that accompany the product, because instructions vary according to the preparation. Also remind the patient to rotate the site of application to avoid skin irritation.
- Explain that the area of application needs to be an area that is well perfused for absorption to occur. Therefore, the medication should not be applied to areas with extensive body hair or scar tissue.
- Recommend that the patient protect clothing from the oil base in the paste.
- Explain that a long-term equally spaced dosing schedule of application of topical nitroglycerin is generally avoided to prevent tolerance (when the body does not respond as well to the same amount of medication). Most physicians prescribe application of topical nitroglycerin paste three or four times daily or every 6 hours (excluding the mid-night dose), and application of the nitroglycerin patch every morning and removed at 10 PM. This dosing regimen allows for a 6- to 8-hour nitrate-free period to prevent the body's development of tolerance.

be decreased gradually over several days before discontinuing it. Patients with diabetes who take beta-blockers are instructed to assess their blood glucose levels more often and to observe for signs and symptoms of hypoglycemia.

Calcium Channel Blocking Agents.

Calcium channel blockers (calcium ion antagonists) have different effects. Some decrease sinoatrial node automaticity and atrioventricular node conduction, resulting in a slower heart rate and a decrease in the strength of the heart muscle contraction (negative inotropic effect). These effects decrease the workload of the heart. Calcium channel blockers also relax the blood vessels, causing a decrease in blood pressure and an increase in coronary artery perfusion. Calcium channel blockers increase myocardial oxygen supply by dilating the smooth muscle wall of the coronary arterioles; they decrease myocardial oxygen demand by reducing systemic arterial pressure and the workload of the left ventricle.

The calcium channel blockers most commonly used are amlodipine (Norvasc), verapamil (Calan, Isoptin, Verelan), and diltiazem (Cardizem, Dilacor, Tiazac). They may be used by patients who cannot take beta-blockers, who develop significant side effects from beta-blockers or nitrates, or who still have pain despite beta-blocker and nitroglycerin therapy. Calcium channel blockers are used to prevent and treat vasospasm, which commonly occurs after an invasive interventional procedure. Use of short-acting nifedipine (Procardia) was found to be poorly tolerated and to increase the risk of MI in patients with hypertension and the risk of death in patients with **acute coronary syndrome** (Braunwald et al., 2000; Furberg et al., 1996; Ryan et al., 1999).

First-generation calcium channel blockers should be avoided or used with great caution in people with heart failure, because they decrease myocardial contractility. Amlodipine (Norvasc) and felodipine (Plendil) are the calcium channel blockers of choice for patients with heart failure. Hypotension may occur after the intravenous administration of any of the calcium channel blockers. Other side effects that may occur include atrioventricular blocks, bradycardia, constipation, and gastric distress.

Antiplatelet and Anticoagulant Medications.

Antiplatelet medications are administered to prevent platelet aggregation, which impedes blood flow.

Aspirin. Aspirin prevents platelet activation and reduces the incidence of MI and death in patients with CAD. A 160- to 325-mg dose of aspirin should be given to the patient with angina as soon as the diagnosis is made (eg, in the emergency room or physician's office) and then continued with 81 to 325 mg daily. Although it may be one of the most important medications in the treatment of CAD, aspirin may be overlooked because of its low cost and common use. Patients should be advised to continue aspirin even if concurrently taking nonsteroidal anti-inflammatory drugs (NSAIDs) or other analgesics. Because aspirin may cause gastrointestinal upset and bleeding, treatment of *Helicobacter pylori* and the use of H2-blockers (eg, cimetidine [Tagamet], famotidine [Mylanta AR, Pepcid], ranitidine [Zantac]) or misoprostol (Cytotec) should be considered to allow continued aspirin therapy.

Clopidogrel and Ticlopidine. Clopidogrel (Plavix) or ticlopidine (Ticlid) is given to patients who are allergic to aspirin or given in addition to aspirin in patients at high risk for MI. Unlike aspirin, these medications take a few days to achieve their antiplatelet effect. They also cause gastrointestinal upset, including nausea, vomiting, and diarrhea, and they decrease the neutrophil level.

Heparin. Unfractionated heparin prevents the formation of new blood clots. Use of heparin alone in treating patients with unstable angina reduces the occurrence of MI. If the patient's signs and symptoms indicate a significant risk for a cardiac event, the patient is hospitalized and may be given an intravenous bolus of heparin and started on a continuous infusion or given an intravenous bolus every 4 to 6 hours. The amount of heparin administered is based on the results of the activated partial thromboplastin time (aPTT). Heparin therapy is usually considered therapeutic when the aPTT is 1.5 to 2 times the normal aPTT value.

A subcutaneous injection of low-molecular-weight heparin (LMWH; enoxaparin [Lovenox] or dalteparin [Fragmin]) may be used instead of intravenous unfractionated heparin to treat patients with unstable angina or non–ST-segment elevation MIs. LMWH provides more effective and stable anticoagulation, potentially reducing the risk of rebound ischemic events, and it eliminates the need to monitor aPTT results (Cohen, 2001). LMWH may be beneficial before and during PCIs and for ST-segment elevation MIs.

Because unfractionated heparin and LMWH increase the risk of bleeding, the patient is monitored for signs and symptoms of external and internal bleeding, such as low blood pressure, an increased heart rate, and a decrease in serum hemoglobin and hematocrit values. The patient receiving heparin is placed on bleeding precautions, which include:

- Applying pressure to the site of any needle puncture for a longer time than usual
- Avoiding intramuscular injections
- Avoiding tissue injury and bruising from trauma or use of constrictive devices (eg, continuous use of an automatic blood pressure cuff)

A decrease in platelet count or skin lesions at heparin injection sites may indicate heparin-induced thrombocytopenia (HIT), an antibody-mediated reaction to heparin that may result in thrombosis (Hirsh et al., 2001). Patients who have received heparin within the past 3 months and those who have been receiving unfractionated heparin for 5 to 15 days are at high risk for HIT.

GPIIb/IIIa Agents. Intravenous GPIIb/IIIa agents (abciximab [ReoPro], tirofiban [Aggrastat], eptifibatide [Integrelin]) are indicated for hospitalized patients with unstable angina and as adjunct therapy for PCI. These agents prevent platelet aggregation by blocking the GPIIb/IIIa receptors on the platelet, preventing adhesion of fibrinogen and other factors that crosslink platelets to each other and thereby allow platelets to form a thrombus (clot). As with heparin, bleeding is the major side effect, and bleeding precautions should be initiated.

Oxygen Administration.

Oxygen therapy is usually initiated at the onset of chest pain in an attempt to increase the amount of oxygen delivered to the myocardium and to decrease pain. Oxygen inhaled directly increases the amount of oxygen in the blood. The therapeutic effectiveness of oxygen is determined by observing the rate and rhythm of respirations. Blood oxygen saturation is monitored by pulse oximetry; the normal oxygen saturation (SpO_2) level is greater than 93%. Studies are being conducted to assess the use of oxygen in patients without respiratory distress and its effect on outcome.

ALTERNATIVE THERAPIES

Researchers have reported significant improvement in the exercise endurance of patients with angina who were treated with acupuncture as well as with an intravenous infusion of a combination of ginseng (*Panax quinquefolium*), astragalus (*Astragalus membranaceus*), and angelica (*Angelica sinensis*) (Ballegaard et al., 1991; Reichter et al., 1991). Coenzyme Q10 was advocated for preventing the occurrence and progression of heart failure (Khatta et al., 2000). However, there have not been large, randomized, placebo-controlled studies that identify the direct beneficial effect from these therapies.

NURSING PROCESS:
THE PATIENT WITH ANGINA PECTORIS

Assessment

The nurse gathers information about the patient's symptoms and activities, especially those that precede and precipitate attacks of angina pectoris. Appropriate questions are identified in Table 28-4, using a PQRST format. Other helpful questions may be asked. How long does the angina usually last? Does nitroglycerin relieve the angina? If so, how many tablets or sprays are needed to achieve relief? How long does it takes for relief to occur?

The answers to these questions form a basis for designing a logical program of treatment and prevention. In addition to assessing angina pectoris or its equivalent, the nurse also assesses the patient's risk factors for CAD, the patient's response to angina, the patient's and family's understanding of the diagnosis, and adherence to the current treatment plan.

Diagnosis

NURSING DIAGNOSES
Based on the assessment data, major nursing diagnoses for the patient may include:

- Ineffective myocardial tissue perfusion secondary to CAD, as evidenced by chest pain or equivalent symptoms
- Anxiety related to fear of death
- Deficient knowledge about the underlying disease and methods for avoiding complications
- Noncompliance, ineffective management of therapeutic regimen related to failure to accept necessary lifestyle changes

COLLABORATIVE PROBLEMS/
POTENTIAL COMPLICATIONS
Potential complications that may develop include the following, which are discussed in the chapters indicated:

- Acute pulmonary edema (see Chap. 30)
- Congestive heart failure (see Chap. 30)
- Cardiogenic shock (see Chap. 30)
- Dysrhythmias and cardiac arrest (see Chaps. 27 and 30)
- MI (described later in this chapter)
- Myocardial rupture (see Chap. 30)
- Pericardial effusion and cardiac tamponade (see Chap. 30)

Planning and Goals

The major patient goals include immediate and appropriate treatment when angina occurs, prevention of angina, reduction of anxiety, awareness of the disease process and understanding of the prescribed care, adherence to the self-care program, and absence of complications.

Nursing Interventions

TREATING ANGINA

If the patient reports pain (or the individual's equivalent to pain), the nurse takes immediate action. When a patient experiences angina, the nurse should direct the patient to stop all activities and sit or rest in bed in a semi-Fowler position to reduce the oxygen requirements of the ischemic myocardium. The nurse assesses the patient's angina, asking questions to determine whether the angina is the same as the patient typically experiences. A difference may indicate a worsening of the disease or a different cause. The nurse then continues to assess the patient, measuring vital signs and observing for signs of respiratory distress. If the patient is in the hospital, a 12-lead ECG is usually obtained and scrutinized for ST-segment and T-wave changes. If the patient has been placed on cardiac monitoring with continuous ST-segment monitoring, the ST segment is assessed for changes.

Nitroglycerin is administered sublingually, and the patient's response is assessed (relief of chest pain and effect on blood pressure and heart rate). If the chest pain is unchanged or is lessened but still present, nitroglycerin administration is repeated up to three doses.

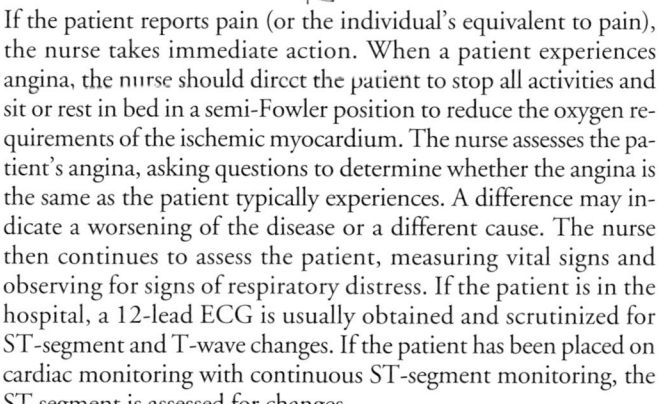

Table 28-4 • Assessment of Angina

ACRONYM	FACTORS ABOUT PAIN THAT NEED TO BE ASSESSED	ASSESSMENT QUESTIONS
P	Position/Location	"Where is the pain? Can you point to it?"
	Provocation	"What were you doing when the pain began?"
Q	Quality	"How would you describe the pain?"
		"Is it like the pain you had before?"
	Quantity	"Has the pain been constant?"
R	Radiation	"Can you feel the pain anywhere else?"
	Relief	"Did anything make the pain better?"
S	Severity	"How would you rate the pain on a 0–10 scale with 0 being no pain and 10 being the most amount of pain?" (or use visual analog scale or adjective rating scale)
	Symptoms	"Did you notice any other symptoms with the pain?"
T	Timing	"How long ago did the pain start?"

From Casey, P. E., Morrissey, A., & Nolan, E. M. (1998). Ischemic heart disease. In M. R. Kinney, B. S. Dunbar, J. A. Brooks-Brunn, et al. (Eds.), *AACN clinical reference for critical care nursing* (4th ed.) St. Louis: Mosby.

Each time, blood pressure, heart rate, and the ST segment (if the patient is on a monitor with ST segment monitoring capability) are assessed. The nurse administers oxygen therapy if the patient's respiratory rate is increased or the oxygen saturation level is decreased. Although there is no documentation of its effect on outcome, oxygen is usually administered at 2 L/min by nasal cannula, even without evidence of respiratory distress. If the pain is significant and continues after these interventions, the patient is usually transferred to a higher-acuity nursing unit.

REDUCING ANXIETY

Patients with angina often fear loss of their roles within society and the family. They may also be fearful that the pain may lead to an MI or death. Exploring the implications that the diagnosis has for the patient and providing information about the illness, its treatment, and methods of preventing its progression are important nursing interventions. Various stress reduction methods should be explored with the patient. For example, music therapy, in which patients are given the opportunity to listen to selected music through headphones for a predetermined duration, has been shown to reduce anxiety in patients who are in a coronary care unit and may serve as an adjunct to therapeutic communication (Chlan & Tracy, 1999; Evans, 2002). Addressing the spiritual needs of the patient and family may also assist in allaying anxieties and fears.

PREVENTING PAIN

The nurse reviews the assessment findings, identifies the level of activity that causes the patient's pain, and plans the patient's activities accordingly. If the patient has pain frequently or with minimal activity, the nurse alternates the patient's activities with rest periods. Balance of activity and rest is an important aspect of the educational plan for the patient and family.

PROMOTING HOME AND COMMUNITY-BASED CARE

Teaching Patients Self-Care. Learning about the modifiable risk factors that contribute to the continued development of CAD and resulting angina is essential. Exploring with the patient and family what they see as their priority in managing the disease and developing a plan based on their priorities can assist with patient adherence to the therapeutic regimen. It is important to explore with the patient methods to avoid, modify, or adapt the triggers for anginal pain. The teaching program for the patient with angina is designed so that the patient and family can explain the illness, identify the symptoms of myocardial ischemia, state the actions to take when symptoms develop, and discuss methods to prevent chest pain and the advancement of CAD. The goals of the educational program are to reduce the frequency and severity of anginal attacks, to delay the progress of the underlying disease, if possible, and to prevent any complications. The factors outlined in the accompanying checklist Chart 28-5 are important in educating the patient with angina pectoris.

The self-care program is prepared in collaboration with the patient and family or friends. Activities should be planned to minimize the occurrence of angina episodes. The patient needs to understand that any pain unrelieved within 15 minutes by the usual methods (see Chart 28-4) should be treated at the closest emergency center; the patient should call 911 for assistance.

Evaluation

EXPECTED PATIENT OUTCOMES

Expected patient outcomes may include:

1. Reports that pain is relieved promptly
   a. Recognizes symptoms
   b. Takes immediate action
   c. Seeks medical assistance if pain persists or changes in quality
2. Reports decreased anxiety
   a. Expresses acceptance of diagnosis
   b. Expresses control over choices within medical regimen
   c. Does not exhibit signs and symptoms that indicate a high level of anxiety
3. Understands ways to avoid complications and demonstrates freedom from complications
   a. Describes the process of angina

Chart 28-5

Home Care Checklist • Managing Angina Pectoris

At the completion of the home care instruction, the patient or caregiver will be able to:

	Patient	Caregiver
• Reduce the probability of an episode of anginal pain by balancing rest with activity:		
– Participate in a regular daily program of activities that do not produce chest discomfort, shortness of breath, or undue fatigue.	✓	
– Avoid exercises requiring sudden bursts of activity; avoid isometric exercise.	✓	
– State that temperature extremes (particularly cold) may induce anginal pain; therefore, avoid exercise in temperature extremes.	✓	
– Alternate activity with periods of rest.	✓	
– Use appropriate resources for support during emotionally stressful times (eg, counselor, nurse, clergy, physician).	✓	✓
• Avoid using medications or any over-the-counter substances (eg, diet pills, nasal decongestants) that can increase the heart rate and blood pressure without first discussing with a health care provider.	✓	✓
• Stop smoking and other use of tobacco, and avoid second-hand smoke (because smoking increases the heart rate, blood pressure, and blood carbon monoxide levels).	✓	✓
• Eat a diet low in saturated fat, high in fiber, and if indicated, lower in calories.	✓	✓
• Achieve and maintain normal blood pressure.	✓	
• Achieve and maintain normal blood glucose levels.	✓	
• Take medications, especially aspirin and beta-blockers, as prescribed.	✓	
• Carry nitroglycerin at all times; state when and how to use it; identify its side effects.	✓	✓

b. Explains reasons for measures to prevent complications
c. Exhibits normal ECG and cardiac enzyme levels
d. Experiences no signs and symptoms of acute MI
4. Adheres to self-care program
a. Takes medications as prescribed
b. Keeps health care appointments
c. Implements plan for reducing risk factors

MYOCARDIAL INFARCTION

Pathophysiology

MI refers to the process by which areas of myocardial cells in the heart are permanently destroyed. Like unstable angina, MI is usually caused by reduced blood flow in a coronary artery due to atherosclerosis and occlusion of an artery by an embolus or thrombus. Because unstable angina and acute MI are considered to be the same process but different points along a continuum, the term **acute coronary syndrome** (ACS) may be used for these diagnoses. Other causes of an MI include vasospasm (sudden constriction or narrowing) of a coronary artery; decreased oxygen supply (eg, from acute blood loss, anemia, or low blood pressure); and increased demand for oxygen (eg, from a rapid heart rate, thyrotoxicosis, or ingestion of cocaine). In each case, a profound imbalance exists between myocardial oxygen supply and demand.

Coronary occlusion, heart attack, and MI are terms used synonymously, but the preferred term is MI. The area of infarction takes time to develop. As the cells are deprived of oxygen, ischemia develops, cellular injury occurs, and over time, the lack of oxygen results in infarction, or the death of cells. The expression "time is muscle" reflects the urgency of appropriate treatment to improve patient outcomes. Each year in the United States, nearly 1 million people have acute MIs; one fourth of these people die of MI (American Heart Association, 2001; Ryan et al., 1999). One half of those who die never reach a hospital.

Various descriptions are used to further identify an MI: the location of the injury to the left ventricular wall (anterior, inferior, posterior, or lateral wall) or to the right ventricle and the point in time within the process of infarction (acute, evolving, or old).

The ECG usually identifies the location, and the ECG and patient history identify the timing. Regardless of the location of the infarction of cardiac muscle, the goal of medical therapy is to prevent or minimize myocardial tissue death and to prevent complications. The pathophysiology of heart disease and the risk factors involved are discussed earlier in this chapter.

Clinical Manifestations

Chest pain that occurs suddenly and continues despite rest and medication is the presenting symptom in most patients with an MI (Chart 28-6). One study showed that 2% of patients who eventually were diagnosed with an acute MI were incorrectly discharged and sent home from the emergency department (Pope et al., 2000). Most of these patients presented with atypical symptoms such as shortness of breath; they also tended to be female, younger than 55 years of age, of a minority group, and have normal ECGs. The Framingham Heart Study revealed that 50% of the men and 63% of the women who died suddenly of cardiovascular disease had no previous symptoms (Kannel, 1986). Patients may also be anxious and restless. They may have cool, pale, and moist skin. Their heart rate and respiratory rate may be faster than normal. These signs and symptoms, which are caused by stimulation of the sympathetic nervous system, may be present only for a short time or may not be present, or only some of them

---

Chart 28-6 • ASSESSMENT

Signs and Symptoms of an Acute Myocardial Infarction (MI) or Acute Coronary Syndrome (ACS)

Cardiovascular
Chest pain or discomfort, palpitations. Heart sounds may include S_3, S_4, and new onset of a murmur. Increased jugular venous distention may be seen if the MI has caused heart failure. Blood pressure may be elevated because of sympathetic stimulation or decreased because of decreased contractility, impending cardiogenic shock, or medications. Pulse deficit may indicate atrial fibrillation. In addition to ST-segment and T-wave changes, ECG may show tachycardia, bradycardia, and dysrhythmias.

Respiratory
Shortness of breath, dyspnea, tachypnea, and crackles if MI has caused pulmonary congestion. Pulmonary edema may be present.

Gastrointestinal
Nausea and vomiting.

Genitourinary
Decreased urinary output may indicate cardiogenic shock.

Skin
Cool, clammy, diaphoretic, and pale appearance due to sympathetic stimulation from loss of contractility may indicate cardiogenic shock. Dependent edema may also be present due to poor contractility.

Neurologic
Anxiety, restlessness, light-headedness may indicate increased sympathetic stimulation or a decrease in contractility and cerebral oxygenation. The same symptoms may also herald cardiogenic shock. Headache, visual disturbances, altered speech, altered motor function, and further changes in level of consciousness may indicate cerebral bleeding if patient is receiving thrombolytics.

Psychological
Fear with feeling of impending doom, or patient may deny that anything is wrong.

---

may occur. In many cases, the signs and symptoms of MI cannot be distinguished from those of unstable angina.

Assessment and Diagnostic Findings

Diagnosis of MI is generally based on the presenting symptoms, the ECG, and laboratory test results (eg, serial serum enzyme values). The prognosis depends on the severity of coronary artery obstruction and the extent of myocardial damage. Physical examination is always conducted, but the examination alone is insufficient to confirm the diagnosis.

PATIENT HISTORY

The patient history has two parts: the description of the presenting symptom (eg, pain) and the history of previous illnesses and family health history, particularly of heart disease. Previous history should also include information about the patient's risk factors for heart disease.

ELECTROCARDIOGRAM

The ECG provides information that assists in diagnosing acute MI. It should be obtained within 10 minutes from the time a patient reports pain or arrives in the emergency department. By monitoring the ECG over time, the location, evolution, and resolution of an MI can be identified and monitored.

The ECG changes that occur with an MI are seen in the leads that view the involved surface of the heart. The classic ECG changes are T-wave inversion, ST-segment elevation, and development of an abnormal Q wave (Fig. 28-4). Because infarction evolves over time, the ECG also changes over time. The first ECG signs of an acute MI are from myocardial ischemia and injury. Myocardial injury causes the T wave to become enlarged and symmetric. As the area of injury becomes ischemic, myocardial repolarization is altered and delayed, causing the T wave to invert. The ischemic region may remain depolarized while adjacent areas of the myocardium return to the resting state. Myocardial injury also causes ST-segment changes. The injured myocardial cells depolarize normally but repolarize more rapidly than normal cells, causing the ST segment to rise at least 1 mm above the isoelectric line (area between the T wave and the next P wave is used as the reference for the isoelectric line) when measured 0.08 seconds after the end of the QRS. If the myocardial injury is on the endocardial surface, the ST segment is depressed 1 mm or more for at least 0.08 seconds. The ST-segment depression is usually horizontal or has a downward slope (Wagner, 2001).

MI is classified as a Q-wave or non-Q-wave infarction. With Q-wave infarction, abnormal Q waves develop within 1 to 3 days because there is no depolarization current conducted from necrotic tissue (Wagner, 2001). The lead system then views the flow of current from other parts of the heart. An abnormal Q wave is 0.04 seconds or longer, 25% of the R-wave depth (provided the R wave exceeds a depth of 5 mm), or one that did not exist before the event (Wagner, 2001). An acute MI may cause a significant decrease in the height of the R wave. During an acute MI, injury and ischemic changes are also present. An abnormal Q wave may be present without ST-segment and T-wave changes, which indicates an old, not acute, MI. Patients with non-Q-wave MIs do not develop a Q wave on the ECG after the ST-segment and T-wave changes, but symptoms and cardiac enzyme analysis confirm the diagnosis of an MI.

During recovery from an MI, the ST segment often is the first to return to normal (1 to 6 weeks). The T wave becomes large and symmetric for 24 hours, and it then inverts within 1 to 3 days for 1 to 2 weeks. Q-wave alterations are usually permanent. An old Q-wave MI is usually indicated by an abnormal Q wave or decreased height of the R wave without ST-segment and T-wave changes.

ECHOCARDIOGRAM

The echocardiogram is used to evaluate ventricular function. It may be used to assist in diagnosing an MI, especially when the ECG is nondiagnostic. The echocardiogram can detect hypokinetic and akinetic wall motion and can determine the ejection fraction (see Chap. 26).

LABORATORY TESTS

Historically, laboratory tests used to diagnose an MI included **creatine kinase (CK)**, with evaluation of isoenzymes and lactic dehydrogenase (LDH) levels. Newer laboratory tests with faster results, resulting in earlier diagnosis, include myoglobin and troponin analysis. These tests are based on the release of cellular contents into the circulation when myocardial cells die. Table 28-5 shows the time courses of cardiac enzymes. An LDH test is now infrequently ordered because it is not useful in identifying cardiac events (Braunwald et al., 2000).

Creatine Kinase and Its Isoenzymes. There are three CK isoenzymes: CK-MM (skeletal muscle), CK-MB (heart muscle), and CK-BB (brain tissue). CK-MB is the cardiac-specific isoenzyme; CK-MB is found mainly in cardiac cells and therefore rises only when there has been damage to these cells. CK-MB assessed by mass assay is the most specific index for the diagnosis of acute MI (Braunwald et al., 2001). The level starts to increase within a few hours and peaks within 24 hours of an MI. If the area is reperfused (eg, due to thrombolytic therapy or PTCA), it peaks earlier.

Myoglobin. Myoglobin is a heme protein that helps to transport oxygen. Like CK-MB enzyme, myoglobin is found in cardiac and skeletal muscle. The myoglobin level starts to increase within 1 to 3 hours and peaks within 12 hours after the onset of symptoms.

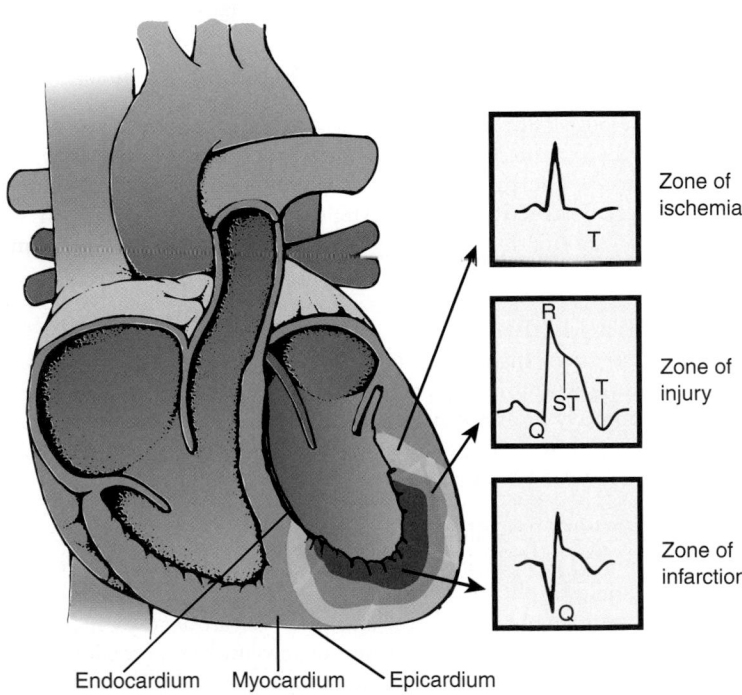

Endocardium   Myocardium   Epicardium

Zone of ischemia

Zone of injury

Zone of infarction

FIGURE 28-4 Effects of ischemia, injury, and infarction on ECG recording. Ischemia causes inversion of T wave because of altered repolarization. Cardiac muscle injury causes elevation of the ST segment and tall, symmetrical T waves. With Q-wave infarction, Q or QS waves develop because of the absence of depolarization current from the necrotic tissue and opposing currents from other parts of the heart.

Table 28-5 • **Serum Markers of Acute Myocardial Infarction**

SERUM TEST		EARLIEST INCREASE (HR)	TEST RUNNING TIME (MIN)	PEAK (HR)	RETURN TO NORMAL
Total CK		3–6	30–60	24–36	3 days
CK-MB:	isoenzyme	4–8	30–60	12–24	3–4 days
	mass assay	2–3	30–60	10–18	3–4 days
Myoglobin		1–3	30–60	4–12	12 hr
Troponin T or I		3–4	30–60	4–24	1–3 wk

Resource assistance by June Price, Laboratory Manager, Kaiser Permanente.

The test takes only a few minutes to run. An increase in myoglobin is not very specific in indicating an acute cardiac event; however, negative results are an excellent parameter for ruling out an acute MI. If the first myoglobin test results are negative, the test may be repeated 3 hours later. Another negative test result confirms that the patient did not have an MI.

Troponin. **Troponin**, a protein found in the myocardium, regulates the myocardial contractile process. There are three isomers of troponin (C, I, and T). Because of the smaller size of this protein and the increased specificity of the troponins I and T for cardiac muscle, these tests are used more frequently to identify myocardial injury (unstable angina or acute MI). The increase in the level of troponin in the serum starts and peaks at approximately the same time as CK-MB. However, it remains elevated for a longer period, often up to 3 weeks, and it therefore cannot be used to identify subsequent extension or expansion of an MI.

Medical Management

The goal of medical management is to minimize myocardial damage, preserve myocardial function, and prevent complications. These goals are achieved by reperfusing the area with the emergency use of thrombolytic medications or PTCA. Minimizing myocardial damage is also accomplished by reducing myocardial oxygen demand and increasing oxygen supply with medications, oxygen administration, and bed rest. The resolution of pain and ECG changes are the primary clinical indicators that demand and supply are in equilibrium; they may also indicate reperfusion. Visualization of blood flow through an open vessel in the catheterization laboratory is evidence of reperfusion.

PHARMACOLOGIC THERAPY

The patient with an acute MI receives the same medications as the patient with unstable angina, with the possible additions of thrombolytics, analgesics, and angiotensin-converting enzyme (ACE) inhibitors. Patients should receive a beta-blocker initially, throughout the hospitalization, and a prescription to continue its use after hospital discharge.

Thrombolytics. Thrombolytics are medications that are usually administered intravenously, although some may also be given directly into the coronary artery in the cardiac catheterization laboratory (Chart 28-7). The purpose of thrombolytics is to dissolve and lyse the thrombus in a coronary artery (thrombolysis), allowing blood to flow through the coronary artery again (reperfusion), minimizing the size of the infarction, and preserving ventricular function. Even though thrombolytics may dissolve the thrombus, they do not affect the underlying atherosclerotic lesion. The patient may be referred for a cardiac catheterization and other invasive interventions.

Thrombolytics dissolve all clots, not just the one in the coronary artery. They should not be used if the patient has formed a protective clot, such as after major surgery or hemorrhagic stroke. Because thrombolytics reduce the patient's ability to form a stabilizing clot, the patient is at risk for bleeding. Thrombolytics should not be used if the patient is bleeding or has a bleeding disorder. All patients who receive thrombolytic therapy are placed on bleeding precautions to minimize the risk for bleeding. This means minimizing the number of punctures for inserting intravenous lines, avoiding intramuscular injections, preventing tissue trauma, and applying pressure for longer than usual after any puncture.

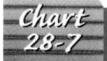 **Administration of Thrombolytic Therapy**

Indications
- Chest pain for longer than 20 minutes, unrelieved by nitroglycerin
- ST-segment elevation in at least two leads that face the same area of the heart
- Less than 24 hours from onset of pain

Absolute Contraindications
- Active bleeding
- Known bleeding disorder
- History of hemorrhagic stroke
- History of intracranial vessel malformation
- Recent major surgery or trauma
- Uncontrolled hypertension
- Pregnancy

Nursing Considerations
- Minimize the number of times the patient's skin is punctured.
- Avoid intramuscular injections.
- Draw blood for laboratory tests when starting the IV line.
- Start IV lines before thrombolytic therapy; designate one line to use for blood draws.
- Avoid continual use of noninvasive blood pressure cuff.
- Monitor for acute dysrhythmias, hypotension, and allergic reaction.
- Monitor for reperfusion: resolution of angina or acute ST-segment changes.
- Check for signs and symptoms of bleeding: decrease in hematocrit and hemoglobin values, decrease in blood pressure, increase in heart rate, oozing or bulging at invasive procedure sites, back pain, muscle weakness, changes in level of consciousness, complaints of headache
- Treat major bleeding by discontinuing thrombolytic therapy and any anticoagulants; apply direct pressure and notify the physician immediately.
- Treat minor bleeding by applying direct pressure if accessible and appropriate; continue to monitor.

To be effective, thrombolytics must be administered as early as possible after the onset of symptoms that indicate an acute MI. They are not given to patients with unstable angina. Hospitals monitor their ability to administer these medications within 30 minutes from the time the patient arrives in the emergency department. This is called *door-to-needle time* (Ryan et al., 1999). The thrombolytic agents used most often are **streptokinase** (Kabikinase, Streptase), alteplase (Activase), and reteplase (r-PA, TNKase). Anistreplase (Eminase) is another thrombolytic agent that may be used.

Streptokinase increases the amount of plasminogen activator, which then increases the amount of circulating and clot-bound plasmin. Because streptokinase is made from a bacterium, its use also entails a risk of an allergic reaction. Vasculitis has occurred up to 9 days after administration. Streptokinase is not used if the patient has been exposed to a recent *Streptococcus* infection or has received streptokinase in the past 6 to 12 months.

Alteplase is a type of tissue plasminogen activator (t-PA). In contrast to streptokinase, alteplase activates the plasminogen on the clot more than the circulating plasminogen. Because it does not decrease the clotting factors as much as streptokinase, unfractionated or low molecular weight heparin is used with t-PA to prevent another clot from forming at the same lesion site. Because t-PA is a naturally occurring enzyme, allergic reactions are minimized, but t-PA costs considerably more than streptokinase.

Reteplase is structurally very similar to alteplase and has similar effects. Anistreplase is similar to streptokinase and has similar effects.

Analgesics. The analgesic of choice for acute MI is morphine sulfate (Duramorph, Astramorph) administered in intravenous boluses. Morphine reduces pain and anxiety. It reduces preload, which decreases the workload of the heart. Morphine also relaxes bronchioles to enhance oxygenation. The cardiovascular response to morphine is monitored carefully, particularly the blood pressure, which can be lowered, and the respiratory rate, which can be depressed. Because morphine decreases sensation of pain, ST-segment monitoring may be a better indicator of subsequent ischemia than assessment of pain.

Angiotensin-Converting Enzyme Inhibitors (ACE-I). Angiotensin I is formed when the kidneys release renin in response to decreased blood flow. Angiotensin I is converted to angiotensin II by ACE, a substance found in the lumen of all blood vessels, especially the pulmonary vasculature. Angiotensin II causes the blood vessels to constrict and the kidneys to retain sodium and fluid while excreting potassium. These actions increase circulating fluid and raise the pressure against which the heart must pump, resulting in significantly increased cardiac workload. **ACE inhibitors (ACE-I)** prevent the conversion of angiotensin from I to II. In the absence of angiotensin II, the blood pressure decreases and the kidneys excrete sodium and fluid (diuresis), decreasing the oxygen demand of the heart. Use of ACE inhibitors in patients after MI decreases the mortality rate and prevents the onset of heart failure. It is important to ensure that the patient is not hypotensive, hyponatremic, hypovolemic, or hyperkalemic before ACE-I administration. Blood pressure, urine output, and serum sodium, potassium, and creatinine levels need to be monitored closely.

EMERGENT PERCUTANEOUS CORONARY INTERVENTION (PCI)

The patient in whom an acute MI is suspected may be referred for an immediate PCI. PCI may be used to open the occluded coronary artery in an acute MI and promote reperfusion to the area that has been deprived of oxygen. PCI treats the underlying atherosclerotic lesion. Because the duration of oxygen deprivation is directly related to the number of cells that die, the time from the patient's arrival in the emergency department to the time PCI is performed should be less than 60 minutes (time is muscle). This is frequently referred to as *door-to-balloon time* (Smith et al., 2001). To perform an emergent PCI within this short time, a cardiac catheterization laboratory and staff must be available.

Cardiac Rehabilitation

After the MI patient is free of symptoms, an active rehabilitation program is initiated. Cardiac rehabilitation is a program that targets risk reduction by means of education, individual and group support, and physical activity. Most insurance programs, including Medicare, cover the cost of a cardiac rehabilitation program. However, some studies indicate that only 8% to 39% of patients who are candidates for cardiac rehabilitation services typically participate in these programs (Wenger et al., 1995; Williams et al., 2002).

The goals of rehabilitation for the patient with an MI are to extend and improve the quality of life. The immediate objectives are to limit the effects and progression of atherosclerosis, return the patient to work and a pre-illness lifestyle, enhance the psychosocial and vocational status of the patient, and prevent another cardiac event. These objectives are accomplished by encouraging physical activity and physical conditioning, educating patient and family, and providing counseling and behavioral interventions.

Throughout all phases of rehabilitation, the goals of activity and exercise tolerance are achieved through gradual physical conditioning, aimed at improving cardiac efficiency over time. Cardiac efficiency is achieved when work and activities of daily living can be performed at a lower heart rate and lower blood pressure, thereby reducing the heart's oxygen requirements and reducing cardiac workload.

Physical conditioning is achieved gradually over time. It is not unusual for patients to "overdo it" in an attempt to achieve their goals too rapidly. Patients are observed for chest pain, dyspnea, weakness, fatigue, and palpitations and are instructed to stop exercise if any of the symptoms develop. In a monitored program, they are also monitored for an increase in heart rate above the target heart rate, an increase in systolic or diastolic blood pressure more than 20 mm Hg, a decrease in systolic blood pressure, onset or worsening of dysrhythmias, or ST-segment changes on the ECG.

The target heart rate in phase I is an increase of less than 10% from the resting heart rate, or 120 beats per minute. In phase II, the target heart rate is based on the results of the patient's stress test (usually 60% to 85% of the heart rate at which symptoms occurred), medications, and underlying condition. Oxygen saturation may also be assessed to ensure that it remains higher than 93%. If signs or symptoms occur, the patient is instructed to slow down or stop exercising. If the patient is exercising in an unmonitored program, he or she is cautioned to cease activity immediately if signs or symptoms occur and to seek appropriate medical attention. Table 28-6 identifies conditions in which an unmonitored home exercise program is not recommended.

Patients who are able to walk at 3 to 4 miles per hour are usually able to resume sexual activities. The nurse recommends that the patient be well rested and in a familiar setting; wait at least 1 hour after eating or drinking alcohol; and use a comfortable position. The patient is cautioned against anal sex. Sexual dysfunction or cardiac symptoms should be reported to the health care provider.

PHASES OF CARDIAC REHABILITATION

Cardiac rehabilitation occurs along the continuum of the disease and is typically categorized in three phases. Phase I may begin with the diagnosis of atherosclerosis, which may occur when the

Table 28-6 • Contraindications to Unsupervised Home Exercise

High-risk unstable angina (severe CAD)	Symptomatic severe aortic stenosis
Uncontrolled symptomatic dysrhythmia	Active pericarditis, myocarditis
Acute pulmonary embolism or infarction	High degree atrioventricular block
Acute aortic dissection	Resting diastolic BP > 110 mm Hg
Resting systolic BP > 200 mm Hg	Hypertrophic cardiomyopathy
Uncontrolled diabetes (BS > 400 mg/dL)	Active systemic illness or fever
Severe orthopedic problems	Orthostatic decrease in BP by ≥ 20 mm Hg
Uncompensated symptomatic HF	with symptoms

CAD, coronary artery disease; BS, blood sugar; BP, blood pressure; HF, heart failure; HR, heart rate.
Adapted from the American College of Cardiology Foundation and the American Heart Association (2002). *ACC/AHA 2002 Guideline Update for Exercise Testing: A report of the American College of Cardiology/American Heart Association Task Force on Practice Guidelines (Committee on Exercise Testing)*. Available at: http://www.acc.org/clinical/guidelines/exercise. Accessed December 3, 2002.

patient is admitted to the hospital for ACS (unstable angina, acute MI). It consists of low-level activities and initial education for the patient and family. Because of the brief hospital stay, mobilization occurs earlier, and patient teaching is prioritized to the essentials of self-care, rather than instituting behavioral changes for risk reduction. Priorities for in-hospital education include the signs and symptoms that indicate the need to call 911 (seek emergency assistance), the medication regimen, rest-activity balance, and follow-up appointments with the physician. The nurse needs to reassure the patient that, although CAD is a lifelong disease and must be treated as such, most patients can resume a normal life after an MI. This positive approach while in the hospital helps to motivate and teach the patient to continue the education and lifestyle changes that are usually needed after discharge. The amount of activity recommended at discharge depends on the age of the patient, his or her condition before the cardiac event, the extent of the disease, the course of the hospital stay, and the development of any complications.

Phase II occurs after the patient has been discharged. It usually lasts for 4 to 6 weeks but may last up to 6 months. This outpatient program consists of supervised, often ECG-monitored, exercise training that is individualized based on the results of an exercise stress test. Support and guidance related to the treatment of the disease and education and counseling related to lifestyle modification for risk factor reduction are a significant part of this phase. Short-term and long-range goals are collaboratively determined based on the patient's needs. At each session, the patient is assessed for the effectiveness of and adherence to the current medical plan. To prevent complications and another hospitalization, the cardiac rehabilitation staff alerts the referring physician to any problems. Outpatient cardiac rehabilitation programs are designed to encourage patients and families to support each other. Many programs offer support sessions for spouses and significant others while the patients exercise. The programs involve group educational sessions for both patients and families that are given by cardiologists, exercise physiologists, dietitians, nurses, and other health care professionals. These sessions may take place outside a traditional classroom setting. For instance, a dietitian may take a group of patients and their families to a grocery store to examine labels and meat selections or to a restaurant to discuss menu offerings for a "heart-healthy" diet.

Phase III focuses on maintaining cardiovascular stability and long-term conditioning. The patient is usually self-directed during this phase and does not require a supervised program, although it may be offered. The goals of each phase build on the accomplishments of the previous phase.

NURSING PROCESS: THE PATIENT WITH MYOCARDIAL INFARCTION

Assessment

One of the most important aspects of care of the patient with an MI is the assessment. It establishes the baseline for the patient so that any deviations may be identified, systematically identifies the patient's needs, and helps determine the priority of those needs. Systematic assessment includes a careful history, particularly as it relates to symptoms: chest pain or discomfort, difficulty breathing (dyspnea), palpitations, unusual fatigue, faintness (syncope), or sweating (diaphoresis). Each symptom must be evaluated with regard to time, duration, the factors that precipitate the symptom and relieve it, and comparison with previous symptoms. A precise and complete physical assessment is critical to detect complications and any change in patient status. Chart 28-6 identifies important assessments and possible findings.

Intravenous sites are examined frequently. At least one and possibly two intravenous lines are placed for any patient with ACS to ensure that access is available for administering emergency medications. Medications are administered intravenously to achieve rapid onset and to allow for timely adjustment. Intramuscular medications are avoided because of unpredictable absorption, delayed effect, and the risk of causing elevated serum enzyme levels by injuring muscle cells with an injection. After the patient's condition stabilizes, the intravenous line may be changed into a saline lock to maintain intravenous access.

Diagnosis

NURSING DIAGNOSES

Based on the clinical manifestations, history, and diagnostic assessment data, the patient's major nursing diagnoses may include:

- Ineffective cardiopulmonary tissue perfusion related to reduced coronary blood flow from coronary thrombus and atherosclerotic plaque
- Potential impaired gas exchange related to fluid overload from left ventricular dysfunction
- Potential altered peripheral tissue perfusion related to decreased cardiac output from left ventricular dysfunction
- Anxiety related to fear of death
- Deficient knowledge about post-MI self-care

COLLABORATIVE PROBLEMS/ POTENTIAL COMPLICATIONS

Based on the assessment data, potential complications that may develop include the following:

- Acute pulmonary edema (see Chap. 30)
- Heart failure (see Chap. 30)
- Cardiogenic shock (see Chap. 30)
- Dysrhythmias and cardiac arrest (see Chaps. 27 and 30)
- Pericardial effusion and cardiac tamponade (see Chap. 30)
- Myocardial rupture (see Chap. 30)

Planning and Goals

The major goals of the patient include relief of pain or ischemic signs and symptoms (eg, ST-segment changes), prevention of further myocardial damage, absence of respiratory dysfunction, maintenance or attainment of adequate tissue perfusion by decreasing the heart's workload, reduced anxiety, adherence to the self-care program, and absence or early recognition of complications. Care of the patient with an uncomplicated MI is summarized in the Plan of Nursing Care on pages 731–733.

Nursing Interventions

RELIEVING PAIN AND OTHER SIGNS AND SYMPTOMS OF ISCHEMIA

Balancing the cardiac oxygen supply with its oxygen demand (eg, as evidenced by the relief of chest pain) is the top priority for the patient with an acute MI. Although medication therapy is required to accomplish this goal, nursing interventions are also important. Collaboration among the patient, nurse, and physician is critical in assessing the patient's response to therapy and in altering the interventions accordingly.

The accepted method for relieving symptoms associated with MI is revascularization with thrombolytic therapy or emergent PCI for patients who present to the health care facility immediately and who have no major contraindications. These therapies are important because, in addition to relieving symptoms, they aid in minimizing or avoiding permanent injury to the myocardium. With or without revascularization, administration of aspirin, intravenous beta-blocker, and nitroglycerin is indicated. Use of a GPIIb/IIIa agent or heparin may also be indicated. The nurse administers morphine for relief of pain and other symptoms, anxiety, and reduction of preload.

Oxygen should be administered along with medication therapy to assist with relief of symptoms. Administration of oxygen even in low doses raises the circulating level of oxygen to reduce pain associated with low levels of myocardial oxygen. The route of administration, usually by nasal cannula, and the oxygen flow rate are documented. A flow rate of 2 to 4 L/min is usually adequate to maintain oxygen saturation levels of 96% to 100% if no other disease is present.

Vital signs are assessed frequently as long as the patient is experiencing pain and other signs or symptoms of acute ischemia. Physical rest in bed with the backrest elevated or in a cardiac chair helps to decrease chest discomfort and dyspnea. Elevation of the head is beneficial for the following reasons:

- Tidal volume improves because of reduced pressure from abdominal contents on the diaphragm and better lung expansion and gas exchange.
- Drainage of the upper lung lobes improves.
- Venous return to the heart (preload) decreases, which reduces the work of the heart.

IMPROVING RESPIRATORY FUNCTION

Regular and careful assessment of respiratory function can help the nurse detect early signs of pulmonary complications. Scrupulous attention to fluid volume status prevents overloading the heart and lungs. Encouraging the patient to breathe deeply and change position frequently helps keep fluid from pooling in the bases of the lungs.

PROMOTING ADEQUATE TISSUE PERFUSION

Limiting the patient to bed or chair rest during the initial phase of treatment is particularly helpful in reducing myocardial oxygen consumption ($m\dot{V}O_2$). This limitation should remain until the patient is pain-free and hemodynamically stable. Checking skin temperature and peripheral pulses frequently is important to ensure adequate tissue perfusion. Oxygen may be administered to enrich the supply of circulating oxygen.

REDUCING ANXIETY

Alleviating anxiety and fears is an important nursing function to reduce the sympathetic stress response. Decreased sympathetic stimulation decreases the workload of the heart, which may relieve pain and other signs and symptoms of ischemia.

Developing a trusting and caring relationship with the patient is critical in reducing anxiety. Providing information to the patient and family in an honest and supportive manner invites the patient to be a partner in care and greatly assists in developing a positive relationship. Ensuring a quiet environment, preventing interruptions that disturb sleep, using a caring and appropriate touch, teaching the patient the relaxation response, using humor and assisting the patient to laugh, and providing the appropriate prayer book and assisting the patient to pray if consistent with the patient's beliefs are other nursing interventions that can be used to reduce anxiety. Frequent opportunities are provided for the patient to privately share concerns and fears. An atmosphere of acceptance helps the patient to know that these concerns and fears are both realistic and normal. Music therapy, in which the patient listens to selected music for a predetermined duration and at a set time, has been found to be an effective method for reducing anxiety and managing stress (Chlan & Tracy, 1999; Evans, 2002). Pet therapy, in which animals are brought to the patient, appears to provide emotional support and reduce anxiety. Administrative and infectious control practitioners are usually involved in developing standards for the animals, animal handlers, and patients who are eligible for pet therapy.

MONITORING AND MANAGING POTENTIAL COMPLICATIONS

Complications that can occur after acute MI are caused by the damage that occurs to the myocardium and to the conduction system as a result of the reduced coronary blood flow. Because these complications can be lethal, close monitoring for and early identification of the signs and symptoms is critical (see Plan of Nursing Care, pp. 731–733).

The nurse monitors the patient closely for changes in cardiac rate and rhythm, heart sounds, blood pressure, chest pain, respiratory status, urinary output, skin color and temperature, sensorium, ECG changes, and laboratory values. Any changes in the patient's condition are reported promptly to the physician, and emergency measures are instituted when necessary.

PROMOTING HOME AND COMMUNITY-BASED CARE

Teaching Patients Self-Care

The most effective way to increase the probability the patient will implement a self-care regimen after discharge is to identify the

(text continues on page 733)

Plan of Nursing Care

Care of the Patient With an Uncomplicated Myocardial Infarction

Nursing Interventions	Rationale	Expected Outcomes

Nursing Diagnosis: Ineffective cardiopulmonary tissue perfusion related to reduced coronary blood flow
Goal: Relief of chest pain/discomfort

1. Initially assess, document, and report to the physician the following:

   a. The patient's description of chest discomfort, including location, intensity, radiation, duration, and factors that affect it. Other symptoms such as nausea, diaphoresis, or complaints of unusual fatigue.
   b. The effect of chest discomfort on cardiovascular perfusion—to the heart (eg, change in blood pressure, heart sounds), to the brain (eg, changes in LOC), to the kidneys (eg, decrease in urine output), and to the skin (eg, color, temperature).

2. Obtain a 12-lead ECG recording during the symptomatic event, as prescribed, to determine extension of infarction.
3. Administer oxygen as prescribed.

4. Administer medication therapy as prescribed and evaluate the patient's response continuously.

5. Ensure physical rest: use of the bedside commode with assistance; backrest elevated to promote comfort; diet as tolerated; arms supported during upper extremity activity; use of stool softener to prevent straining at stool. Provide a restful environment, and allay fears and anxiety by being supportive, calm, and competent. Individualized visitation, based on patient response.

1. These data assist in determining the cause and effect of the chest discomfort and provide a baseline with which post-therapy symptoms can be compared.
   a. There are many conditions associated with chest discomfort. There are characteristic clinical findings of ischemic pain and symptoms.

   b. MI decreases myocardial contractility and ventricular compliance and may produce dysrhythmias. Cardiac output is reduced, resulting in reduced blood pressure and decreased organ perfusion. The heart rate may increase as a compensatory mechanism to maintain cardiac output.

2. An ECG during symptoms may be useful in the diagnosis of an extension of MI.
3. Oxygen therapy may increase the oxygen supply to the myocardium if actual oxygen saturation is less than normal.
4. Medication therapy is the first line of defense in preserving myocardial tissue. The side effects of these medications can be hazardous and the patient's status must be assessed.
5. Physical rest reduces myocardial oxygen consumption. Fear and anxiety precipitate the stress response; this results in increased levels of endogenous catecholamines, which increase myocardial oxygen consumption. Also, with increased epinephrine, the pain threshold is decreased, and pain increases myocardial oxygen consumption.

- Reports beginning relief of chest discomfort and symptoms at once
- Appears comfortable and pain or symptom free:
  Is rested
  Respiratory rate, cardiac rate, and blood pressure return to prediscomfort level
  Skin warm and dry
- Adequate cardiac output as evidenced by:
  Heart rate and rhythm
  Blood pressure
  Mentation
  Urine output
  Serum BUN and creatinine
  Skin color, temperature, and moisture
- Is pain and symptom free

Nursing Diagnosis: Potential ineffective air exchange related to fluid overload
Goal: Absence of respiratory difficulties

1. Initially, every 4 hours, and with chest discomfort or symptoms, assess, document, and report to the physician abnormal heart sounds (particularly S_3 and S_4 gallops and the holosystolic murmur of left ventricular papillary muscle dysfunction), abnormal breath sounds (particularly crackles), and patient intolerance to specific activities.

1. These data are useful in diagnosing left ventricular failure. Diastolic filling sounds (S_3 and S_4 gallop) result from decreased left ventricular compliance associated with MI. Papillary muscle dysfunction (from infarction of the papillary muscle) can result in mitral regurgitation and a reduction in stroke volume, leading to left ventricular failure. The presence of crackles (usually at the lung bases) may indicate pulmonary

- No shortness of breath, dyspnea on exertion, orthopnea, or paroxysmal nocturnal dyspnea
- Respiratory rate less than 20 breaths/min with physical activity and 16 breaths/min with rest
- Skin color normal
- PaO_2 and $PaCO_2$ within normal range
- Heart rate less than 100 beats/min and greater than 60 beats/min, with blood pressure within patient's normal limits

(continued)

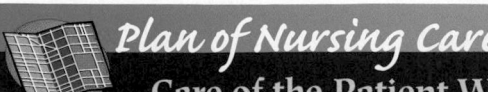

Plan of Nursing Care

Care of the Patient With an Uncomplicated Myocardial Infarction *(Continued)*

Nursing Interventions	Rationale	Expected Outcomes

	congestion from increased left heart pressures. The association of symptoms and activity can be used as a guide for activity prescription and a basis for patient teaching.	• Chest x-ray normal
		• Relief of chest discomfort
		• Appears comfortable:
		    Appears rested
		    Respiratory rate, cardiac rate, and blood pressure return to prediscomfort level
		    Skin warm and dry

2. Teach patient: a. To adhere to the diet prescribed (for example, explain low-sodium, low-calorie diet) b. To adhere to activity prescription	2. a. Low-sodium diet may reduce extra-cellular volume, thus reducing preload and afterload, and thus myocardial oxygen consumption. In the obese patient, weight reduction may decrease cardiac work and improve tidal volume. b. The activity prescription is determined individually to maintain the heart rate and blood pressure within safe limits.	

Nursing Diagnosis: Potential ineffective peripheral tissue perfusion related to decreased cardiac output
Goal: Maintenance/attainment of adequate tissue perfusion

Nursing Interventions	Rationale	Expected Outcomes

1. Initially, every 4 hours, and with chest discomfort, assess, document, and report to the physician the following:
a. Hypotension
b. Tachycardia and other dysrhythmia
c. Activity intolerance
d. Mentation changes (use family input)
e. Reduced urine output (less than 200 mL per 8 hours)
f. Cool, moist, cyanotic extremities
	1. These data are useful in determining a low cardiac output state. An ECG with pain may be useful in the diagnosis of an extension of myocardial ischemia, injury, and infarction, and of variant angina.	• Blood pressure within the patient's normal range
		• Ideally, normal sinus rhythm without dysrhythmia is maintained, or patient's baseline rhythm is maintained between 60 and 100 beats/min without further dysrhythmia.
		• No complaints of fatigue with prescribed activity
		• Remains fully alert and oriented and without cognitive or behavioral change
		• Appears comfortable
		    Appears rested
		    Respiratory rate, cardiac rate, and blood pressure return to prediscomfort level
		    Skin warm and dry
		• Urine output greater than 25 mL/hr
		• Extremities warm and dry with normal color

Nursing Diagnosis: Anxiety related to fear of death, change in health status
Goal: Reduction of anxiety

Nursing Interventions	Rationale	Expected Outcomes
1. Assess, document, and report to the physician the patient's and family's level of anxiety and coping mechanisms.	1. These data provide information about the psychological well-being and a baseline so that post-therapy symptoms can be compared. Causes of anxiety are variable and individual, and may include acute illness, hospitalization, pain, disruption of activities of daily living at home and at work, changes in role and self-image due to chronic illness, and lack of financial support. Because anxious family members can transmit anxiety to the patient, the nurse must also identify strategies to reduce the family's fear and anxiety.	• Reports less anxiety • Patient and family discuss their anxieties and fears about death • Patient and family appear less anxious • Appears restful, respiratory rate less than 16/min, heart rate less than 100/min without ectopic beats, blood pressure within patient's normal limits, skin warm and dry • Participates actively in a progressive rehabilitation program • Practices stress reduction techniques

(continued)

Plan of Nursing Care

Care of the Patient With an Uncomplicated Myocardial Infarction (*Continued*)

Nursing Interventions	Rationale	Expected Outcomes
2. Assess the need for spiritual counseling and refer as appropriate.	2. If a patient finds support in a religion, religious counseling may assist in reducing anxiety and fear.	

3. Allow patient (and family) to express anxiety and fear:
  a. By showing genuine interest and concern
  b. By facilitating communication (listening, reflecting, guiding)
  c. By answering questions
	3. Unresolved anxiety (the stress response) increases myocardial oxygen consumption.	

4. Use of flexible visiting hours allows the presence of a supportive family to assist in reducing the patient's level of anxiety.	4. The presence of supportive family members may reduce both patient's and family's anxiety.	
5. Encourage active participation in a cardiac rehabilitation program.	5. Prescribed cardiac rehabilitation may help to eliminate fear of death, reduce anxiety, and enhance feelings of well-being.	
6. Teach stress reduction techniques.	6. Stress reduction may help to reduce myocardial oxygen consumption and may enhance feelings of well-being.	

Nursing Diagnosis: Deficient knowledge about post-MI self-care
Goal: Adheres to the home health care program
      Chooses lifestyle consistent with heart-healthy recommendations.

(See Chart 28-8, Promoting Health After MI)

priorities as perceived by the patient, provide adequate education about heart-healthy living, and facilitate the patient's involvement in a cardiac rehabilitation program. Working with patients in developing plans to meet their specific needs further enhances the potential for an effective treatment plan (Chart 28-8).

Evaluation

EXPECTED PATIENT OUTCOMES

Expected patient outcomes may include the following:

1. Relief of angina
2. No signs of respiratory difficulties
3. Adequate tissue perfusion
4. Decreased anxiety
5. Adherence to a self-care program
6. Absence of complications

Invasive Coronary Artery Procedures

INVASIVE INTERVENTIONAL PROCEDURES

Angina pectoris may persist for many years in a stable form with brief attacks. However, unstable angina is a serious condition that can progress to MI or sudden cardiac death (ACS). Invasive interventional procedures to treat angina and CAD are PTCA, intracoronary stent implantation, atherectomy, brachytherapy, and transmyocardial laser revascularization. All of these procedures are classified as **percutaneous coronary interventions (PCIs)**.

Percutaneous Transluminal Coronary Angioplasty (PTCA)

PTCA may be used to treat patients who do not experience angina but are at high risk for a cardiac event as identified by noninvasive testing, with recurrent chest pain that is unresponsive to medical therapy, with a significant amount of myocardium at risk but are poor surgical candidates, or with an acute MI (as an alternate to thrombolysis and after thrombolysis) (Smith et al., 2001). The procedure is attempted when the cardiologist believes that PTCA can improve blood flow to the myocardium. PTCA alone is seldom attempted in the patient with occlusions of the left main coronary artery that do not demonstrate **collateral circulation** to the left anterior descending and circumflex arteries. The purpose of PTCA is to improve blood flow within a coronary artery by "cracking" the atheroma.

This invasive interventional procedure is carried out in the cardiac catheterization laboratory. The coronary arteries are examined by angiography, as they are during the diagnostic cardiac catheterization, and the location, extent, and calcification of the atheroma are verified. Hollow catheters, called sheaths, are inserted, usually in the femoral vein or artery (or both), providing a conduit for other catheters. After the presence of atheroma is verified, a balloon-tipped dilation catheter is passed through the sheath along a guide catheter and positioned over the lesion. The physician determines the catheter position by examining markers on the balloon that can be seen with fluoroscopy. When the catheter is properly positioned, the balloon is inflated with a radiopaque contrast agent (commonly called *dye*) to visualize the

Chart 28-8
Promoting Health After Myocardial Infarction and Other Acute Coronary Syndromes

To extend and improve the quality of life, a patient who has had an MI must learn to adjust his or her lifestyle to promote heart-healthy living. With this in mind, the nurse and patient develop a program to help the patient achieve desired outcomes.

Changing Lifestyle During Convalescence and Healing

Adaptation to a heart attack is an ongoing process and usually requires some modification of lifestyle. Some specific modifications include:

- Avoiding any activity that produces chest pain, extreme dyspnea, or undue fatigue
- Avoiding extremes of heat and cold and walking against the wind
- Losing weight, if indicated
- Stopping smoking and use of tobacco; avoiding second-hand smoke
- Using personal strengths to support lifestyle changes
- Developing heart-healthy eating patterns and avoiding large meals and hurrying while eating
- Modifying meals to align with the Therapeutic Lifestyle Changes (TLC) or the Dietary Approaches to Stopping Hypertension (DASH) diet
- Adhering to medical regimen, especially in taking medications
- Following recommendations that ensure blood pressure and blood glucose are in control
- Pursuing activities that relieve and reduce stress

Adopting an Activity Program

Additionally, the patient needs to undertake an *orderly* program of increasing activity and exercise for long-term rehabilitation as follows:

- Engaging in a regimen of physical conditioning with a gradual increase in activity duration and then a gradual increase in activity intensity
- Walking daily, increasing distance and time as prescribed
- Monitoring pulse rate during physical activity until the maximum level of activity is attained
- Avoiding activities that tense the muscles: isometric exercise, weight-lifting, any activity that requires sudden bursts of energy
- Avoiding physical exercise immediately after a meal
- Alternating activity with rest periods (some fatigue is normal and expected during convalescence)
- Participating in a daily program of exercise that develops into a program of regular exercise for a lifetime

Managing Symptoms

The patient must learn to recognize and take appropriate action for possible recurrences of symptoms as follows:

- Call 911 if chest pressure or pain (or anginal equivalent) is not relieved in 15 minutes by nitroglycerin
- Contacting the physician if any of the following occur: shortness of breath, fainting, slow or rapid heartbeat, swelling of feet and ankles

---

blood vessel and to provide a steady or oscillating pressure within the balloon. The balloon is inflated to a certain pressure for several seconds and then deflated. The pressure "cracks" and possibly compresses the atheroma (Fig. 28-5). The coronary artery's media and adventitia are also stretched.

Several inflations and several balloon sizes may be required to achieve the desired goal, usually defined as an improvement in blood flow and a residual stenosis of less than 20%. Other gauges of the success of a PTCA are an increase in the artery's lumen, a difference of less than 20 mm Hg in blood pressure from one side

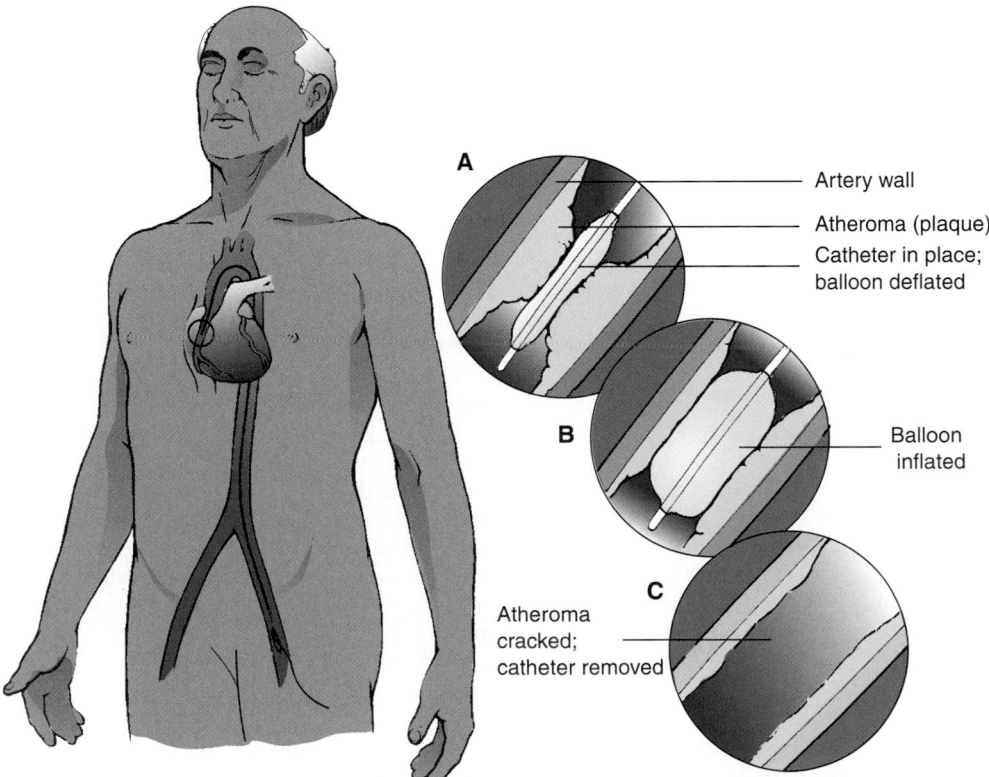

FIGURE 28-5 Percutaneous transluminal coronary angioplasty. (**A**) A balloon-tipped catheter is passed into the affected coronary artery and placed across the area of the atheroma (plaque). (**B**) The balloon is then rapidly inflated and deflated with controlled pressure. (**C**) After the atheroma is cracked, the catheter is removed, and blood flow improves.

of the lesion to the other, and no clinically obvious arterial trauma. Because the blood supply to the coronary artery decreases while the balloon is inflated, the patient may complain of chest pain (often called *stretch pain*), and the ECG may display significant ST-segment changes (Jeremias et al., 1998).

COMPLICATIONS

Possible complications during the PTCA procedure include dissection, perforation, abrupt closure, or vasospasm of the coronary artery, acute MI, acute dysrhythmias (eg, ventricular tachycardia), and cardiac arrest. These may require emergency surgical treatment. Complications after the procedure may include abrupt closure and vascular complications, such as bleeding at the insertion site, retroperitoneal bleeding, hematoma, pseudoaneurysm, arteriovenous fistula, or arterial thrombosis and distal embolization (Table 28-7).

POSTPROCEDURE CARE

Patient care is similar to that for a cardiac catheterization (see Chapter 26). Many patients are admitted to the hospital the day of the PTCA. Those with no complications go home the next day. During the PTCA, patients receive large amounts of heparin and are monitored closely for signs of bleeding. Most patients also receive intravenous nitroglycerin for a period after the procedure to prevent arterial spasm.

Hemostasis is usually achieved and sheaths are pulled immediately at the end of the procedure by using a vascular closure device (eg, Angio-Seal, VasoSeal, Duett, Syvek patch) or a device that sutures the vessels (Prostar, Perclose). Hemostasis after sheath removal may also be achieved by direct manual pressure, a mechanical compression device (eg, C-shaped clamp), or a pneumatic compression device (eg, FemStop).

The patient may return to the nursing unit with the large peripheral vascular access sheaths in place. The sheaths are removed after blood studies (eg, activated clotting time) indicate that the clotting time is within an acceptable range. This usually takes a few hours, depending on the amount of heparin given during the procedure. The patient must remain flat in bed and keep the affected leg straight until the sheaths are removed and then for a few hours after to maintain hemostasis. Because the immobility and bed rest usually cause the patient significant discomfort, treatment includes analgesics and sedation.

Several nursing interventions frequently used as part of the standard of care, such as applying a sandbag to the sheath insertion site, have not been shown to be effective in reducing the incidence of bleeding (Christensen et al., 1998; Juran et al., 1999). The method used to achieve hemostasis determines the length of time needed to achieve hemostasis, the duration of bed rest, and the risk of complications (Brachmann et al., 1998; Lehmann et al., 1999; Walker et al., 2001). Sheath removal and the application of pressure on the vessel insertion site may cause the heart rate to slow and the blood pressure to decrease (vasovagal response). An intravenous bolus of atropine is usually used to treat these side effects.

Some patients with unstable lesions and at high risk for abrupt vessel closure are restarted on heparin after sheath removal, or they receive an intravenous infusion of a GPIIb/IIIa inhibitor. These patients are monitored more closely and progressed more slowly.

After hemostasis is achieved, patients usually can be weaned from the intravenous medications, resume self-care, and ambulate unassisted within 1 to 12 hours of the procedure. The duration of immobilization depends on the size of the sheath inserted, the amount of anticoagulant administered, the method of hemostasis, the patient's underlying condition, and the physician's preference. The nurse teaches the patient to monitor the site for bleeding or development of a hard lump that is larger than a walnut. Most patients can return to their usual activities of daily living.

Table 28-7 • **Complications After Percutaneous Transluminal Coronary Angioplasty (PTCA)**

COMPLICATION	SIGNS AND SYMPTOMS	POSSIBLE CAUSES	NURSING ACTIONS
Bleeding or hematoma	Hard lump or bluish tinge at sheath insertion site	Coughing, vomiting, bending leg or hip, obesity, bladder distention, high blood pressure	Keep the head of the bed flat. Insert indwelling urinary catheter if needed Apply manual pressure at site of sheath insertion. Outline extent of hematoma with a marking pen. If bleeding does not stop, notify physician or nurse practitioner.
Lost or weakened pulse distal to sheath insertion site	Extremity cool, cyanotic, pale, or painful	Arterial thrombus or embolus	Notify physician or nurse practitioner. Anticipate surgery and anticoagulation or thrombolytic therapy.
Pseudoaneurysm and arteriovenous fistula	Pulsatile mass felt or bruit heard near sheath insertion site	Vessel trauma during procedure	Notify physician or nurse practitioner. Anticipate ultrasound-guided compression. Prepare patient for surgery to close fistula.
Retroperitoneal bleeding	Back or flank pain Low blood pressure Tachycardia Restlessness and agitation Decreased hemoglobin Decreased hematocrit	Arterial tear causing bleeding into flank area	Notify physician or nurse practitioner immediately. Stop any anticoagulation medication. Anticipate need for intravenous fluids and/or administration of blood.

Courtesy of Washington Adventist Hospital. Care of the interventional cardiology patient nursing protocol, based on communication from Amy Dukovic, Cardiac Interventional Nurse Practitioner.

Coronary Artery Stent

After PTCA, a portion of the plaque that was not removed may block the artery. The coronary artery may recoil (constrict) and the tissue remodels, increasing the risk for restenosis (Apple & Lindsay, 2000). A coronary artery stent is placed to overcome these risks. A **stent** is a woven mesh that provides structural support to a vessel at risk of acute closure. The stent is placed over the angioplasty balloon. When the balloon is inflated, the mesh expands and presses against the vessel wall, holding the artery open. The balloon is withdrawn, but the stent is left permanently in place within the artery (Fig. 28-6). Eventually, endothelium covers the stent and it is incorporated into the vessel wall. Because of the risk of thrombus formation in the stent, the patient receives antiplatelet medications (eg, clopidogrel [Plavix] therapy for 2 weeks and lifetime use of aspirin). Some stents have medication which may minimize the formation of thrombi or excessive scar tissue. It is estimated that 50% to 80% of all PCIs involve implanting at least one stent (Braunwald et al., 2001; Smith et al., 2001). Stents may be used in conjunction with PTCA or independently as a PCI. Use of stents without PTCA may decrease procedure time, use of the potentially nephrotoxic contrast agent, radiation exposure, and cost (Apple & Lindsay, 2000). Care of the patient after coronary artery stent placement is the same as for a patient after PTCA.

Atherectomy

Atherectomy is an invasive interventional procedure that involves the removal of the atheroma, or plaque, from a coronary artery (Smith et al., 2001). Directional (DCA) and transluminal extraction (TEC) coronary atherectomy procedures involve the use of a catheter that removes the lesion and its fragments. Rotational atherectomy uses a catheter with diamond chips impregnated on the tip (called a burr) that rotates like a dentist's drill at 130,000 to 180,000 rpm, pulverizing the lesion (Braunwald et al., 2001). Usually, several passes of these catheters are needed to achieve satisfactory results. Postprocedural patient care is the same as for a patient after PTCA.

Brachytherapy

PTCA and stent implantation cause a cellular reaction in the coronary artery that promotes proliferation of the intima of the artery, which also increases the possibility of arterial obstruction. Brachytherapy reduces the recurrence of obstruction, preventing vessel restenosis by inhibiting smooth muscle cell proliferation (Leon et al., 2001). Brachytherapy (from the Greek word, *brachys,* meaning *short*) involves the delivery of gamma or beta radiation by placing a radioisotope close to the lesion (Teirstein & Kuntz, 2001). The radioisotope may be delivered by a catheter or implanted with the stent. Long-term studies are needed to identify if the beneficial effects of radiation therapy are sustained and to determine the optimal dose and type of isotope to use for brachytherapy.

Transmyocardial Revascularization

Patients who have cardiac ischemia and who are not candidates for CABG may benefit from transmyocardial laser revascularization (TMR) (Burkhoff et al., 1999). The procedure may be performed percutaneously in the cardiac catheterization laboratory (percutaneous transmyocardial revascularization [PTMR]) or through a midsternal or thoracotomy incision in the operating room (Acorda et al., 2000). The tip of a fiberoptic catheter is held firmly against the ischemic area of the heart while a laser burns a channel into but not through the muscle. If the procedure is percutaneous, the catheter is positioned inside the ventricle. If the procedure is surgical, the catheter is positioned on the outer surface of the ventricle. Each procedure usually involves making 20 to 40 channels. It is thought that some blood flows into the channels, decreasing the ischemia directly. Within the next few days to months, the channels close as a result of the body's inflammatory process of healing a wound (Platek & Atzori, 1999). The long-term result is the formation of new blood vessels (angiogenesis) during the inflammatory process that follows the laser burns (Anderson, 2000; Braunwald et al., 2001; Fuster et al., 2001; Hayden, 1998; Platek, & Atzori, 1999). The new blood vessels provide enough blood to decrease the symptoms of cardiac ischemia. Nursing care before, during, and after the procedure depends on the approach: if the approach was percutaneous, the patient care is the same as following a PTCA; if the approach was surgical, the patient care is the same as following CABG.

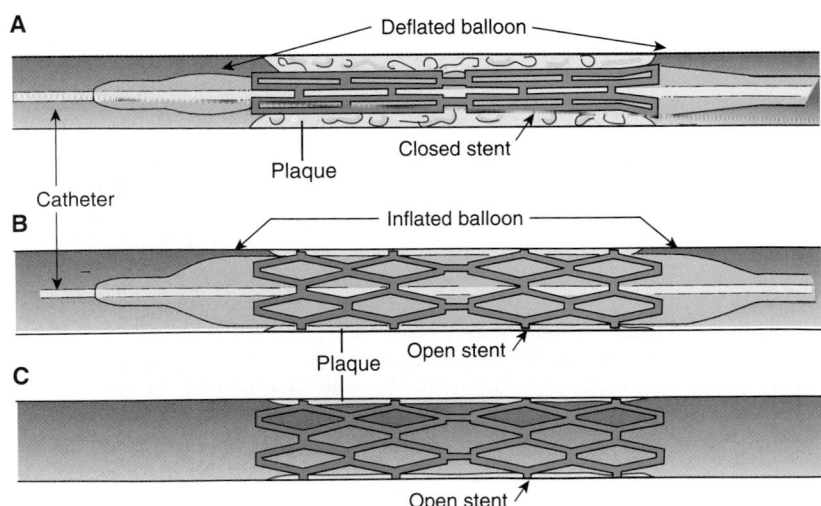

FIGURE 28-6 Intracoronary artery stent. (**A**) Stent closed, before balloon inflation. (**B**) Stent open, balloon inflated; stent will remain expanded after balloon is deflated and removed. (**C**) Stent open, balloon removed.

SURGICAL PROCEDURES

Coronary Artery Revascularization

Advances in diagnostics, medical management, surgical and anesthesia techniques, and cardiopulmonary bypass (CPB), as well as the care provided in critical care and surgical units, home care, and rehabilitation programs, have helped make surgery a viable treatment option for patients with cardiac disease. CAD has been treated by some form of myocardial revascularization since the 1960s; the most common CABG techniques have been performed for approximately 35 years. CABG is a surgical procedure in which a blood vessel from another part of the body is grafted to the occluded coronary artery so that blood can flow beyond the occlusion; it is also called a *bypass graft.*

Candidates for CABG are usually patients with the following conditions (Eagle et al., 1999):

- Angina that cannot be controlled by medical therapies
- Unstable angina
- A positive exercise tolerance test and lesions or blockage that cannot be treated by PCI
- A left main coronary artery lesion or blockage of more than 60%
- Blockage of two or three coronary arteries, one of which is the proximal left anterior descending artery
- Left ventricular dysfunction with blockages in two or more coronary arteries
- Complications from or unsuccessful PCIs

For a patient to be considered for CABG, the coronary arteries to be bypassed must have at least a 70% occlusion (60% if it is the left main coronary artery). If the lesion involves less than 70% of the artery, enough blood can flow through the blocked artery to prevent adequate blood flow through the bypass graft. As a result, the graft would clot, effectively negating the surgery.

The vessel most commonly used for CABG is the greater saphenous vein, followed by the lesser saphenous vein (Fig. 28-7). Cephalic and basilic veins are used also. The vein is removed from the leg (or arm) and grafted to the ascending aorta and to the coronary artery distal to the lesion. The saphenous veins are used in emergency CABG procedures because they can be obtained by one surgical team while another team performs the chest surgery. One side effect of using a large vein is edema, which may develop in the extremity from which it was taken. The degree of edema varies and may diminish over time. Approximately 5 to 10 years after CABG, symptomatic atherosclerotic changes develop in saphenous veins used for grafting. In arm veins, the same changes develop more quickly, approximately 3 to 6 years after the surgery.

The right and left internal mammary arteries and, occasionally, radial arteries are also used for CABG. Arterial grafts are preferred to vein grafts because they do not develop atherosclerotic changes as quickly and remain patent longer. In general, the surgeon leaves the proximal end of the mammary artery intact and detaches the distal end of the artery from the chest wall. This distal end of the artery is then grafted to the coronary artery distal to the occlusion. Disadvantages of using the internal mammary arteries are that they may not be long enough or wide enough for the bypass and ulnar nerve damage may result.

The gastroepiploic artery (located along the greater curvature of the stomach) may also be used, although it does not respond as well when used as a graft. It has a more extensive blood supply to its wall than the internal mammary arteries, making dissection from the stomach difficult and increasing the potential for injury

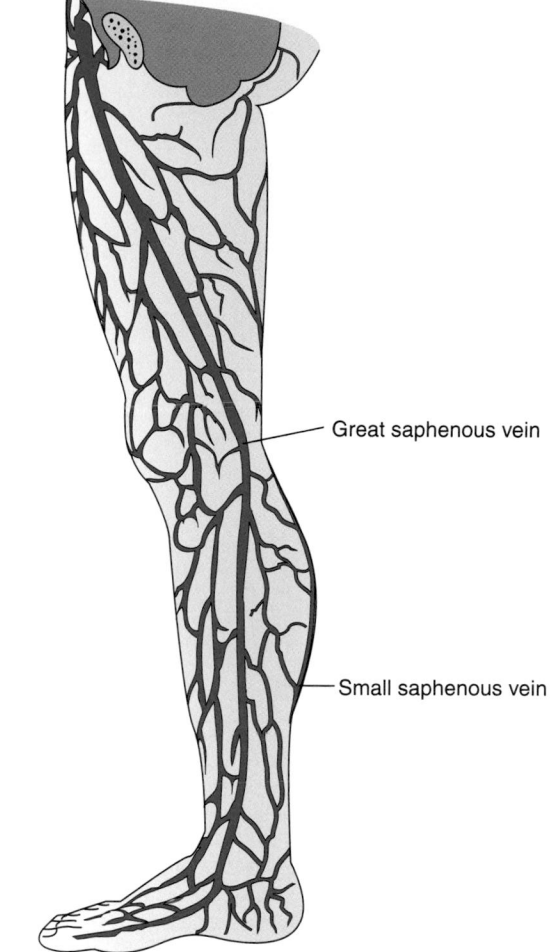

Great saphenous vein

Small saphenous vein

FIGURE 28-7 The greater and lesser saphenous veins are the vessels most commonly used in bypass graft procedures.

and ischemia of the graft. Use of the gastroepiploic artery requires the surgeon to extend the chest incision to the abdomen, thereby exposing the patient to the additional risks of an abdominal incision and infection at the surgical site from contamination by the gastrointestinal tract.

TRADITIONAL CORONARY ARTERY BYPASS GRAFT

The traditional CABG procedure is performed with the patient under general anesthesia. Usually, the surgeon makes a median sternotomy incision and connects the patient to the CPB machine. Next, a blood vessel from another part of the patient's body (eg, saphenous vein, left internal mammary artery) is grafted distal to the coronary artery lesion, bypassing the obstruction (Fig. 28-8). CPB is then discontinued and the incision is closed. The patient then is admitted to a critical care unit.

Cardiopulmonary Bypass (CPB). Many cardiac surgical procedures are possible because of CPB (ie, extracorporeal circulation). The procedure mechanically circulates and oxygenates blood for the body while bypassing the heart and lungs. CPB uses a heart-lung machine to maintain perfusion to other body organs and tissues while the surgeon works in a bloodless surgical field.

CPB, a common but complex technique, is accomplished by placing a cannula in the right atrium, vena cava, or femoral vein

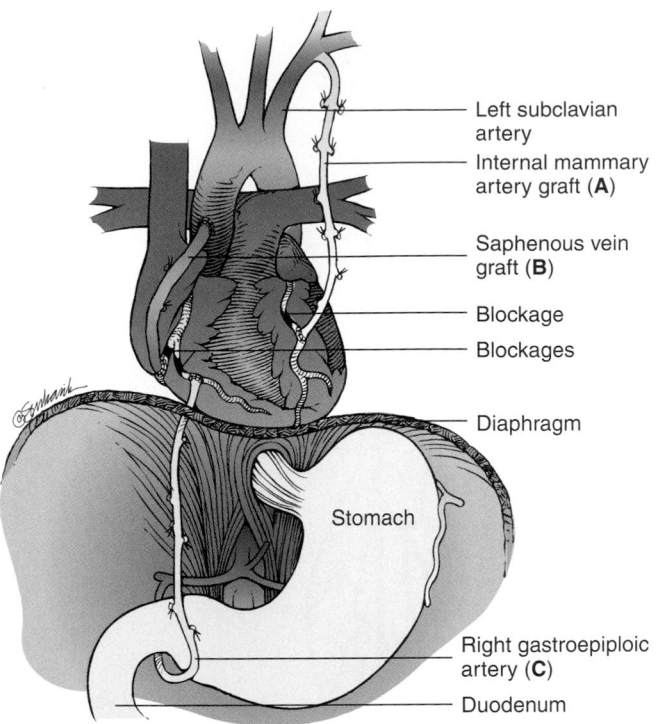

- Left subclavian artery
- Internal mammary artery graft (**A**)
- Saphenous vein graft (**B**)
- Blockage
- Blockages
- Diaphragm
- Stomach
- Right gastroepiploic artery (**C**)
- Duodenum

FIGURE 28-8 Three coronary artery bypass grafts. One or more procedures may be performed using various veins and arteries. (**A**) Left internal mammary artery, popular because of its functional longevity. (**B**) Saphenous vein, the most frequently constructed bypass. (**C**) Right gastroepiploic artery, rarely used because this artery has a more extensive blood supply to its wall (increasing the risk of bleeding and necrosis of the artery) and because of the risk of gastrointestinal tract contamination of the abdominal or mediastinal wound.

to withdraw blood from the body. The cannula is connected to tubing filled with an isotonic crystalloid solution (usually 5% dextrose in lactated Ringer's solution). Venous blood removed from the body by the cannula is filtered, oxygenated, cooled or warmed, and then returned to the body. The cannula used to return the oxygenated blood is usually inserted in the ascending aorta, but it may be inserted in the femoral artery (Fig. 28-9).

The patient receives heparin, an anticoagulant, to prevent thrombus formation and possible embolization that may occur when blood contacts the foreign surfaces of the CPB circuit and is pumped into the body by a mechanical pump (not the normal blood vessels and heart). After the patient is disconnected from the bypass machine, protamine sulfate is administered to reverse the effects of heparin.

During the procedure, hypothermia is maintained, usually 28°C to 32°C (82.4°F to 89.6°F). The blood is cooled during CPB and returned to the body. The cooled blood slows the body's basal metabolic rate, thereby decreasing its demand for oxygen. Cooled blood usually has a higher viscosity, but the crystalloid solution used to prime the bypass tubing dilutes the blood. When the surgical procedure is completed, the blood is rewarmed as it passes through the CPB circuit. Urine output, blood pressure, arterial blood gas measurements, electrolytes, coagulation studies, and the ECG are monitored to assess the patient's status during CPB.

MINIMALLY INVASIVE DIRECT CABG (MIDCAB)

For patients with single coronary artery blockages who cannot be treated by PTCA or with contraindications for CPB, an alternative to traditional CABG is minimally invasive direct CABG (MIDCAB). With the patient under general anesthesia, the surgeon makes one or more 2- to 4-inch (5- to 10-cm) incisions in

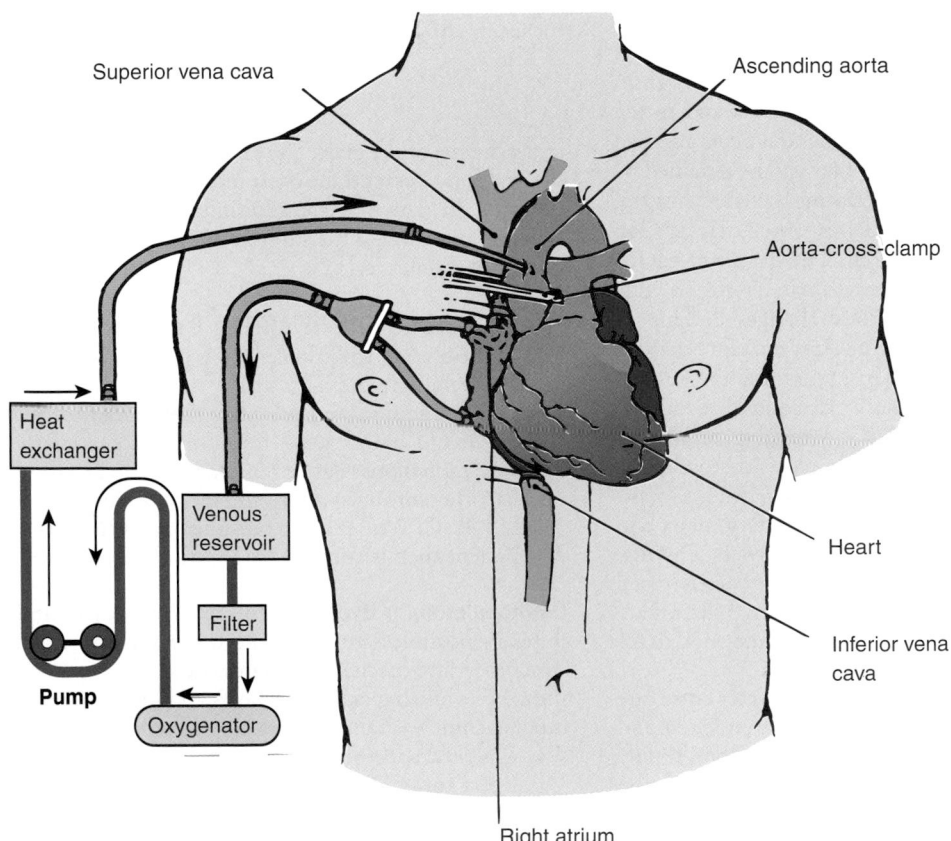

- Superior vena cava
- Ascending aorta
- Aorta-cross-clamp
- Heat exchanger
- Venous reservoir
- Filter
- **Pump**
- Oxygenator
- Heart
- Inferior vena cava
- Right atrium

FIGURE 28-9 The cardiopulmonary bypass system, in which cannulae are placed through the right atrium into the superior and inferior vena cavae to divert blood from the body and into the bypass system. The pump system creates a vacuum, pulling blood into the venous reservoir. The blood is cleared of air bubbles, clots, and particulates by the filter, and then is passed through the oxygenator, releasing carbon dioxide and obtaining oxygen. Next, the blood is pulled to the pump and pushed out to the heat exchanger, where its temperature is regulated. The blood is then returned to the body via the ascending aorta.

the chest wall for a left or right anterior thoracotomy or for a mid-sternal or midline upper laparotomy. The graft is prepared for the bypass (see previous graft selection description). The surgeon identifies the location of the coronary artery for the CAB, and a special instrument, a myocardial stabilizer, is put around the site. The stabilizer holds the graft site still for the surgeon while the heart continues to beat. Other techniques to minimize movement of the beating heart are to temporarily collapse the lung on the side of the chest where the surgery is being performed, decrease the respiratory rate and the volume of each breath, and give medications to cause bradycardia or up to 20 seconds of asystole.

Patients treated with MIDCAB may recover from anesthesia in the postanesthesia care unit (PACU) and then be admitted to a telemetry unit for 1 to 3 days. Nursing care is often directed toward routine postoperative pulmonary interventions (especially if a lung was collapsed during the MIDCAB) and incisional pain management (especially if a thoracotomy incision was made).

PORT ACCESS CORONARY ARTERY BYPASS GRAFT

Port access CABG is another alternative to traditional CABG. With the patient under general anesthesia, the surgeon makes three or more incisions (ports) to perform the CABG. One 0.5- to 1-inch (1.3- to 2.5-cm) incision in the groin provides access to a femoral artery and vein. The femoral artery is used for a multi-purpose catheter threaded retrograde through the aorta to the ascending aorta. The catheter is used to return blood from CPB to the patient, to occlude the aorta by inflating a balloon near the end of the catheter, to provide a cardioplegia solution to the coronary arteries, and to vent air from the aortic root during the surgical procedure. The femoral vein is used for a catheter threaded through the vena cava to the right atrium to drain blood from the patient for CPB. Another 0.5- to 1-inch (1.3- to 2.5-cm) incision in the neck provides access to the jugular vein for two catheters. One catheter is threaded into the pulmonary artery to remove air, fluid, and blood that may enter the right heart during surgery. The other catheter is threaded into the right atrium and the tip positioned in the coronary sinus for retrograde infusion of the cardioplegia solution. One or more thoracotomy incisions, usually 2 to 3.5 inches (5 to 9 cm) long, are made for insertion of the surgical instruments. One of the thoracotomy ports may be used for video-assisted imaging equipment.

CPB is begun when the equipment is in place through the groin, neck, and thoracotomy incisions. The balloon on the aortic catheter is inflated, and the cardioplegia solution is injected into the coronary arteries. Cardioplegia solution is a crystalloid and electrolyte liquid used to stop the heart and protect the myocardium during cardiac surgical procedures. One lung may be temporarily collapsed to assist with exposing the surgical site. The CABG is performed through a thoracotomy incision. When the CABG is complete, air is vented from the pulmonary artery and aorta. The balloon on the aortic catheter is deflated, and CPB is discontinued. The surgical instruments and the catheters are removed. The incisions are closed. The patient's postoperative care is similar to that after traditional CABG.

COMBINATION PERCUTANEOUS TRANSLUMINAL CORONARY ANGIOPLASTY AND CORONARY ARTERY BYPASS GRAFT

Patients who have blockages in the left anterior descending and at least one other coronary artery who are not candidates for traditional CABG or prefer less invasive procedures may be treated with both MIDCAB and PTCA. Because patients need their blood to be able to clot after MIDCAB, but require anticoagulation after PTCA, the sequence and timing of providing both treatments to the same patient are being investigated.

COMPLICATIONS

CABG may result in complications such as MI, dysrhythmias, and hemorrhage (see Table 28-2; these complications are discussed in depth in this chapter, in Chapter 27, and in Chapters 20 and 71). The patient's underlying heart disease remains, and angina, exercise intolerance, or other symptoms experienced before CABG may develop again. Medications required before surgery may need to be continued. Lifestyle modifications recommended before surgery remain important to treat the underlying CAD and for the continued viability of the newly implanted grafts (see Plan of Nursing Care, pp. 740–745).

NURSING PROCESS: THE PATIENT AWAITING CARDIAC SURGERY

The cardiac surgery patient has many of the same needs and requires the same perioperative care as other surgical patients (see Chaps. 18 through 20). The patient and family are experiencing a major life crisis. The association of the heart with life and death intensifies their emotional and psychological needs. Patients frequently are admitted the same day as the procedure. For these patients, the nurse must prioritize needs carefully; in the time allowed, the nurse focuses on the needs that have the highest priority.

Before surgery, physical and psychological assessments establish the baselines for future reference. The patient's understanding of the surgical procedure, informed consent, and adherence to treatment protocols are evaluated. Helping the patient to cope, understand the procedure, and maintain dignity are nursing responsibilities.

The preoperative phase of cardiac surgery begins before hospitalization. The nurse assesses the patient for other disorders, such as diabetes, hypertension, and respiratory, gastrointestinal, and hematologic diseases, and documents their treatment.

The nurse clarifies how the medication regimen is to be altered before surgery, such as tapering corticosteroids and digoxin, decreasing or discontinuing anticoagulants, and maintaining medications for treatment of blood pressure, angina, diabetes, and dysrhythmias. The nurse also clarifies the need to maintain activity patterns, a healthy diet, healthful sleep habits, and cessation of smoking to minimize the risks of surgery.

Assessment

Patients with nonacute heart disease may be admitted to the hospital the day of or the day before the surgery. Most of the preoperative evaluation is completed before the patient enters the hospital. Many surgeons' offices or hospitals mail an information packet to the patient's home.

A history and physical examination are performed by nursing and medical personnel. A chest x-ray, ECG, laboratory tests, blood typing and crossmatching, and autologous blood donation (patient's own blood) may also be performed. The health assessment focuses on obtaining baseline physiologic, psychological, and social information. The patient's and family's learning needs are identified and addressed as necessary. Of particular importance are the patient's usual functional level, coping mechanisms, and support systems. These are important because the support of the family or

(text continues on page 745)

Plan of Nursing Care
Care of the Patient After Cardiac Surgery

Nursing Interventions	Rationale	Expected Outcomes

Nursing Diagnosis: Decreased cardiac output related to blood loss and compromised myocardial function

Goal: Restoration of cardiac output to maintain/attain desired lifestyle

1. Monitor cardiovascular status. Serial readings of blood pressures (arterial, left atrial, pulmonary artery, pulmonary artery wedge pressure [PAWP], central venous pressure [CVP]), cardiac output/index, systemic and pulmonary vascular resistance, and cardiac rhythm and rate are obtained, recorded, and correlated with the patient's condition.	1. Effectiveness of cardiac output is determined by hemodynamic monitoring.	The following parameters are within the patient's normal ranges: • Arterial pressure • Left atrial pressures • PAWP • Pulmonary artery pressures • CVP • Heart sounds • Pulmonary and systemic vascular resistance • Cardiac output and cardiac index • Peripheral pulses • Cardiac rate and rhythm • Cardiac enzymes • Urine output • Skin and mucosal color • Skin temperature
a. Assess arterial blood pressure every 15 minutes until stable; then arterial or cuff blood pressure every 1–4 hours × 24 hours; then every 8–12 hours until hospital discharge; then every visit.	a. Blood pressure is one of the most important physiologic parameters to follow; vasoconstriction after cardiopulmonary bypass may make auscultatory blood pressure unobtainable.	
b. Auscultate for heart sounds and rhythm.	b. Auscultation provides evidence of cardiac tamponade (muffled distant heart sounds), pericarditis (precordial rub), dysrhythmias.	
c. Assess peripheral pulses (pedal, tibial, radial, carotid).	c. Presence or absence and quality of pulses provide data about cardiac output as well as obstructive lesions.	
d. Measure left atrial pressure, pulmonary artery diastolic (PAD) pressure, and PAWP to determine left ventricular end-diastolic volume and to assess cardiac output.	d. Rising pressures may indicate congestive heart failure or pulmonary edema.	
e. Monitor PAWP, PAD, left atrial pressure, and CVP to assess blood volume, vascular tone, and pumping effectiveness of the heart. *Remember: Trends are more important than isolated readings.* Mechanical ventilation may elevate CVP.	e. High PAWP, PAD, left atrial pressure, or CVP may result from hypervolemia, heart failure, cardiac tamponade. If blood pressure drop is due to low blood volume, PAWP, PAD, left atrial pressure, and CVP will show corresponding drop.	
f. Monitor ECG pattern for cardiac dysrhythmias (see Chap. 27 for discussion of dysrhythmias).	f. Dysrhythmias may occur with coronary ischemia, hypoxia, alterations in serum potassium, edema, bleeding, acid-base or electrolyte disturbances, digitalis toxicity, cardiac failure. ST-segment changes may indicate myocardial ischemia or coronary artery spasm. Pacemaker capture and anti-arrhythmic medication effects are used to maintain a heart rate and rhythm to support stable blood pressures.	
g. Assess cardiac enzyme test results when available.	g. Elevations may indicate myocardial infarction.	
h. Measure urine output every ½ hour to 1 hour at first, then with vital signs.	h. Urine output less than 25 mL/h indicates decreased renal perfusion and may reflect decreased cardiac output.	
i. Observe buccal mucosa, nailbeds, lips, earlobes, and extremities.	i. Duskiness and cyanosis may indicate decreased cardiac output.	
j. Assess skin; note temperature and color.	j. Cool moist skin indicates vasoconstriction and decreased cardiac output.	

(continued)

Nursing Interventions	Rationale	Expected Outcomes
2. Observe for persistent bleeding: steady, continuous drainage of blood; hypotension; low CVP; tachycardia. Prepare to administer blood products, IV solutions.	2. Bleeding can result from cardiac incision, tissue fragility, trauma to tissues, clotting defects.	• Less than 200 mL/hr of drainage through chest tubes during first 4 to 6 hours • Vital signs stable • Chest tube drainage expected amount • CVP and left atrial pressures within normal limits • Urinary output within normal limits • Skin color normal • Respirations unlabored, clear breath sounds • Pain limited to incision • ECG and isoenzymes negative for ischemic changes
3. Observe for cardiac tamponade: hypotension; rising PAWP, PAD, left atrial pressure, or CVP; muffled heart sounds; weak, thready pulse; jugular vein distention; decreasing urinary output. Check for diminished amount of blood in chest drainage collection system. Prepare for pericardiocentesis. Assess for pulsus paradoxus.	3. Cardiac tamponade results from bleeding into the pericardial sac or accumulation of fluid in the sac, which compresses the heart and prevents adequate filling of the ventricles. Decrease in chest drainage may indicate fluid is accumulating in the pericardial sac.	
4. Observe for cardiac failure: hypotension, rising PAWP, PAD, CVP, and left atrial pressure, tachycardia, restlessness, agitation, cyanosis, venous distention, dyspnea, moist crackles, ascites. Prepare to administer diuretics and digoxin.	4. Cardiac failure results from decreased pumping action of the heart; can cause deficient blood perfusion to vital organs.	
5. Observe for myocardial infarction: ST-segment elevations, T-wave changes, decreased cardiac output in the presence of normal circulating volume and filling pressures. Obtain serial ECGs and isoenzymes. Differentiate myocardial pain from incisional pain.	5. Symptoms may be masked by the patient's level of consciousness and pain medication.	

Nursing Diagnosis: Impaired gas exchange related to trauma of extensive chest surgery
Goal: Adequate gas exchange

Nursing Interventions	Rationale	Expected Outcomes
1. Maintain mechanical ventilation until the patient is able to breathe independently.	1. Ventilatory support may be used to decrease work of the heart, to maintain effective ventilation, and to provide an airway in the event of cardiac arrest.	• Airway patent • ABGs within normal range • Endotracheal tube correctly placed, as evidenced by x-ray • Breath sounds clear • Ventilator synchronous with respirations • Breath sounds clear after suctioning/FET • Nailbeds and mucous membranes pink • Mental acuity consistent with amount of sedatives and analgesics received • Oriented to person; able to respond yes and no appropriately
2. Monitor arterial blood gases, tidal volumes, peak inspiratory pressures, and extubation parameters.	2. ABGs and tidal volume indicate effectiveness of ventilator and changes that need to be made to improve gas exchange.	
3. Auscultate chest for breath sounds.	3. Crackles indicate pulmonary congestion; decreased or absent breath sounds may indicate pneumothorax or hemothorax.	
4. Sedate patient adequately, as prescribed, and monitor respiratory rate and depth if ventilations are not "controlled."	4. Sedation helps the patient to tolerate the endotracheal tube and to cope with ventilatory sensations; sedatives can depress respiratory rate and depth.	
5. Promote deep breathing, forced expiratory technique (FET, coughing), and turning. Encourage use of the incentive spirometer and compliance with breathing treatments. Teach incisional splinting with a "cough pillow" to decrease discomfort during deep breathing and FET (coughing).	5. Aids in keeping airway patent, preventing atelectasis, and facilitating lung expansion.	
6. Suction tracheobronchial secretions as needed, using strict aseptic technique.	6. Retention of secretions leads to hypoxia and possible cardiac arrest; retained secretions promote infection.	
7. Assist in weaning and endotracheal tube removal.	7. Decreased risk of pulmonary infections and enhanced ability of patient to communicate without an endotracheal tube.	

(continued)

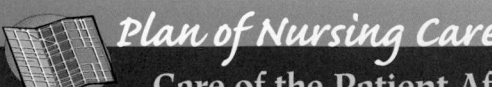

Plan of Nursing Care
Care of the Patient After Cardiac Surgery (Continued)

Nursing Interventions	Rationale	Expected Outcomes

Nursing Diagnosis: Risk for deficient fluid volume and electrolyte imbalance related to alterations in blood volume
Goal: Fluid and electrolyte balance

Nursing Interventions	Rationale	Expected Outcomes
1. Maintain fluid and electrolyte balance.	1. Adequate circulating blood volume is necessary for optimal cellular activity; metabolic acidosis and electrolyte imbalance can occur after use of cardiopulmonary bypass.	• Fluid intake and output balanced • Hemodynamic assessment parameters negative for fluid overload and dehydration • Normal blood pressure with position changes • Absence of dysrhythmia • Stable weight • Notify physician if weight gain of 2 lb or more in 1 day or 5 lb or more in 1 week. • Blood pH 7.35 to 7.45 • Serum potassium 3.5 to 5.0 mEq/L (3.5 to 5.0 mmol/L) • Serum magnesium 1.5 to 2.5 mEq/L (0.75 to 1.25 mmol/L) • Serum sodium 135 to 145 mEq/L (135 to 145 mmol/L) • Serum calcium 8.8 to 10.3 mg/100 mL (2.20 to 2.58 mmol/L)
a. Keep intake and output flow sheets; record urine volume every ½ hour to 4 hours while in critical care unit; then every 8 to 12 hours while hospitalized.	a. Provides a method to determine positive or negative fluid balance and fluid requirements.	
b. Assess the following parameters: pulmonary artery pressures, left atrial pressures, blood pressure, CVP, PAWP, weight, electrolyte levels, hematocrit, jugular venous pressure, tissue turgor, liver size, breath sounds, urinary output, and nasogastric tube drainage.	b. Provides information about state of hydration.	
c. Measure postoperative chest drainage (should not exceed 200 mL/hr for first 4 to 6 hours); cessation of drainage may indicate kinked or blocked chest tube. Ensure patency and integrity of the drainage system. Maintain autotransfusion system if in use.	c. Excessive blood loss from chest cavity can cause hypovolemia.	
d. Weigh daily once patient is ambulatory.	d. Indicator of fluid balance.	
2. Be alert to changes in serum electrolyte levels.	2. A specific concentration of electrolytes is necessary in both extracellular and intracellular body fluids to sustain life.	
a. Hypokalemia (low potassium) *Effects:* dysrhythmias, digitalis toxicity, metabolic alkalosis, weakened myocardium, cardiac arrest Observe for specific ECG changes. Administer IV potassium replacement as directed.	a. *Causes:* inadequate intake, diuretics, vomiting, excessive nasogastric drainage, stress from surgery	

b. Hyperkalemia (high potassium) *Effects:* mental confusion, restlessness, nausea, weakness, paresthesias of extremities
   Be prepared to administer an ion-exchange resin (sodium polystyrene sulfonate [Kayexalate]); IV sodium bicarbonate, or IV insulin and glucose.
	b. *Causes:* increased intake, hemolysis from cardiopulmonary bypass/mechanical assist devices, acidosis, renal insufficiency, tissue necrosis, adrenal cortical insufficiency.
	   The resin binds potassium and promotes intestinal excretion of it.
	   IV sodium bicarbonate drives potassium into the cells from extracellular fluid.
	   Insulin assists the cells with glucose absorption. The glucose provides the energy to activate the sodium–potassium pumps, which pull potassium into the cell while pumping sodium out.	

c. Hypomagnesemia (low magnesium) *Effects:* paresthesias, carpopedal spasm, muscle cramps, tetany, irritability, tremors, hyperexcitability, hyperreflexia, disorientation, depression, seizures, hypotension, dysrhythmias, prolonged PR and QT intervals, broad flat T waves.	c. *Causes:* decreased intake (chronic alcoholism, malnutrition, starvation), impaired absorption (malabsorption syndromes, excess intake of calcium) and increased excretion normal for 24 hours after major surgery, diuretic loss of intestinal fluids, diabetic ketoacidosis, primary aldosteronism, primary hyperparathyroidism.	

(continued)

Plan of Nursing Care
Care of the Patient After Cardiac Surgery (Continued)

Nursing Interventions	Rationale	Expected Outcomes
Be prepared to treat the cause. Magnesium supplements may be given (oral route preferred, extreme caution if IV).		
d. Hypermagnesemia (high magnesium) *Effects:* vasodilation, flushing, warm feeling, hypotension, loss of reflexes, slowing bowel function, drowsiness, respiratory depression, coma, apnea, cardiac arrest. Be prepared to treat cause; dialysis and calcium gluconate administration.	d. *Causes:* renal failure, excess intake of medications with magnesium (antacids, cathartics)	
e. Hyponatremia (low sodium) *Effects:* weakness, fatigue, confusion, seizures, coma Administer sodium or diuretics as prescribed.	e. *Causes:* reduction of total body sodium, or increased water intake causing dilution of sodium	
f. Hypocalcemia (low calcium) *Effects:* numbness and tingling in fingertips, toes, ears, nose; carpopedal spasm; muscle cramps; tetany Administer replacement therapy as prescribed.	f. *Causes:* alkalosis, multiple blood transfusions of citrated blood products	
g. Hypercalcemia (high calcium) *Effects:* dysrhythmias, digitalis toxicity, asystole Institute treatment as prescribed.	g. *Cause:* prolonged immobility	

Nursing Diagnosis: Disturbed sensory perception related to excessive environmental stimulation, sleep deprivation, electrolyte imbalance

Goal: Reduction of symptoms of sensory perceptual imbalance; prevention of postcardiotomy psychosis

1. Use measures to prevent postcardiotomy psychosis: a. Explain all procedures and the need for patient cooperation. b. Plan nursing care to provide for periods of uninterrupted sleep with patient's normal day–night pattern. c. Decrease sleep-preventing environmental stimuli as much as possible. d. Promote continuity of care from nurse to nurse. e. Orient to time and place frequently. Encourage family to visit at regular times. f. Assess for medications that may contribute to delirium. g. Teach relaxation techniques and diversions. h. Encourage self-care as much as tolerated to enhance self-control. Assess support systems and coping mechanisms 2. Observe for perceptual distortions, hallucinations, disorientation, and paranoid delusions.	1. Postcardiotomy psychosis may result from anxiety, sleep deprivation, increased sensory input, disorientation to night and day. Normally, sleep cycles are at least 50 min long. The first cycle may be as long as 90 to 120 min and then shorten during successive cycles. Sleep deprivation results when the sleep cycles are interrupted or there are not enough of them.	• Cooperates with procedures • Sleeps for long, uninterrupted intervals • Oriented to person, place, time • Experiences no perceptual distortions, hallucinations, disorientation, delusions

(continued)

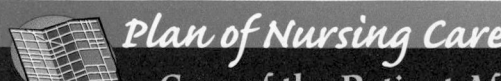

Plan of Nursing Care

Care of the Patient After Cardiac Surgery (*Continued*)

Nursing Interventions	Rationale	Expected Outcomes

Nursing Diagnosis: Acute pain related to surgical trauma and pleural irritation caused by chest tubes and/or internal mammary artery dissection
Goal: Relief of pain

1. Record nature, type, location, intensity, and duration of pain. 2. Assist patient to differentiate between surgical pain and anginal pain. 3. Encourage routine pain medication dosing for the first 24 to 72 hours and observe for side effects of lethargy, hypotension, tachycardia, respiratory depression.	1. Pain and anxiety increase pulse rate, oxygen consumption, and cardiac workload. 2. Anginal pain requires immediate treatment. 3. Analgesia promotes rest, decreases oxygen consumption caused by pain, and aids patient in performing deep-breathing and FET (coughing) exercises; pain medications is more effective when taken before pain is severe.	• States pain is decreasing in severity • Reports absence of pain • Restlessness decreased • Vital signs stable • Participates in deep-breathing and forced expiratory technique (FET, coughing) exercises • Verbalizes fewer complaints of pain each day • Positions self; participates in care activities • Gradually increases activity

Nursing Diagnosis: Ineffective renal tissue perfusion related to decreased cardiac output, hemolysis, or vasopressor drug therapy
Goal: Maintenance of adequate renal perfusion

1. Assess renal function: a. Measure urine output every ½ hour to 4 hours in critical care then every 8–12 hours until hospital discharge. b. Measure urine specific gravity. c. Monitor and report lab results: BUN, serum creatinine, urine and serum electrolytes. 2. Prepare to administer rapid-acting diuretics or inotropic drugs (eg, dopamine, dobutamine). 3. Prepare patient for dialysis or continuous renal replacement therapy if indicated.	1. Renal injury can be caused by deficient perfusion, hemolysis, low cardiac output, and use of vasopressor agents to increase blood pressure. a. Less than 25 mL/h indicates decreased renal function. b. Indicates kidneys' ability to concentrate urine in renal tubules. c. Indicate kidneys' ability to excrete waste products. 2. Promote renal function and increase cardiac output and renal blood flow. 3. Patients have the right to know what care is prescribed; provides patient with the opportunity to ask questions and prepare for the procedure.	• Urine output consistent with fluid intake; greater than 25 mL/hr • Urine specific gravity 1.015 to 1.025 • BUN, creatinine, electrolytes within normal limits

Nursing Diagnosis: Ineffective thermoregulation related to infection or postpericardiotomy syndrome
Goal: Maintenance of normal body temperature

1. Assess temperature every hour. 2. Use aseptic technique when changing dressings, suctioning endotracheal tube; maintain closed systems for all intravenous and arterial lines and for indwelling urinary catheter. 3. Observe for symptoms of postpericardiotomy syndrome: fever, malaise, pericardial effusion, pericardial friction rub, arthralgia. 4. Administer anti-inflammatory agents as directed.	1. Fever can indicate infectious process or postpericardiotomy syndrome. 2. Decreases risk of infection. 3. Occurs in 10% to 40% of patients after cardiac surgery. 4. Relieve symptoms of inflammation (eg, warm or flushed sensation, swelling, fullness, stiffness or aching sensation, and fatigue).	• Normal body temperature • Incisions are free of infection and are healing • Absence of symptoms of postpericardiotomy syndrome

(*continued*)

Plan of Nursing Care
Care of the Patient After Cardiac Surgery (Continued)

Nursing Interventions	Rationale	Expected Outcomes
Nursing Diagnosis: Deficient knowledge about self-care activities		
Goal: Ability to perform self-care activities		

Nursing Interventions	Rationale	Expected Outcomes

1. Develop teaching plan for patient and family. Provide specific instructions for the following:
  • Diet and daily weights
  • Activity progression
  • Exercise
  • Deep breathing, FET (coughing), lung expansion exercises
  • Temperature monitoring
  • Medication regimen
  • Pulse taking
  • CPR, if appropriate for the family to learn
  • Entry to the emergency medical system
  • Need for MedicAlert identification
	1. Each patient will have unique learning needs.	• Patient and family members explain and comply with all therapeutic regimen
		• Patient and family members identify lifestyle changes necessitated by therapeutic regimen
		• Has copy of discharge instructions (in the patient's primary language)
		• Makes follow-up phone calls
		• Keeps follow-up appointments

2. Provide verbal and written instructions; provide several teaching sessions for reinforcement and answering questions.	2. Repetition promotes learning by allowing for clarification of misinformation. After cardiac surgery, patients have short-term memory difficulty; information written in the patient's primary language is essential because it can be used as a resource after discharge. The less familiar or greater the amount of the content the patient and family need to learn, the more time it will take to learn.	
3. Involve family in all teaching sessions.	3. Family member responsible for home care is usually anxious and requires adequate time for learning.	
4. Provide information regarding follow-up phone call to surgeon, cardiologist, or liaison nurse; follow-up visit with surgeon.	4. Arrangements for phone contacts with health care personnel help to allay anxieties.	
5. Make appropriate referrals: home care agency, cardiac rehabilitation program, community support groups, Mended Hearts Club.	5. Learning and lifestyle changes continue after discharge from the hospital.	

significant others will affect the patient's postoperative course and rehabilitation. Discharge plans are influenced by the lifestyle demands of the home situation and the physical environment of the home.

HEALTH HISTORY
The preoperative history and health assessment should be thorough and well documented because they provide a basis for postoperative comparison. A systematic assessment of all systems is performed, with emphasis on cardiovascular functioning.

Functional status of the cardiovascular system is determined by reviewing the patient's symptoms, including past and present experiences with chest pain, hypertension, palpitations, cyanosis, breathing difficulty (dyspnea), leg pain that occurs with walking (intermittent claudication), orthopnea, paroxysmal nocturnal dyspnea, and peripheral edema. Because alterations in cardiac output can affect renal, respiratory, gastrointestinal, integumentary, hematologic, and neurologic functioning, a history of

these systems is also reviewed. The patient's history of major illnesses, previous surgeries, medication therapies, and use of drugs, alcohol, and tobacco is also obtained.

PHYSICAL ASSESSMENT
A complete physical examination is performed, with special emphasis on the following:

- General appearance and behavior
- Vital signs
- Nutritional and fluid status, weight, and height
- Inspection and palpation of the heart, noting the point of maximal impulse, abnormal pulsations, and thrills
- Auscultation of the heart, noting pulse rate, rhythm, and quality; S_3 and S_4, snaps, clicks, murmurs, and friction rub
- Jugular venous pressure
- Peripheral pulses
- Peripheral edema

PSYCHOSOCIAL ASSESSMENT

The psychosocial assessment and the assessment of the patient's and family's learning needs are as important as the physical examination. Anticipation of cardiac surgery is a source of great stress to the patient and family. They will be anxious and fearful and often have many unanswered questions. Their anxiety usually increases with the patient's admission to the hospital and the immediacy of surgery. An assessment of the level of anxiety is important. If it is low, it may indicate denial. If it is extremely high, it may interfere with the use of effective coping mechanisms and with preoperative teaching. Questions may be asked to obtain the following information:

- Meaning of the surgery to the patient and family
- Coping mechanisms that are being used
- Measures used in the past to deal with stress
- Anticipated changes in lifestyle
- Support systems in effect
- Fears regarding the present and the future
- Knowledge and understanding of the surgical procedure, postoperative course, and long-term rehabilitation

The nurse allows adequate time for the patient and family to express their fears. The fears most often expressed are fear of the unknown, fear of pain, fear of body image change, and fear of dying. During the assessment, the nurse determines how much the patient and family know about the impending surgery and the expected postoperative events. They are encouraged to ask questions and to indicate how much information they wish to receive. Some patients prefer not to have detailed information, whereas others want to know as much as possible. Patients are approached as unique individuals with their own specific learning needs, learning styles, and levels of understanding.

Patients requiring emergency heart surgery may have cardiac catheterization and surgery within several hours of admission. The nurse will have little opportunity to assess and meet their emotional and learning needs before surgery. As a result, patients will need extra help after surgery to adjust to the situation.

Diagnosis

NURSING DIAGNOSES

The nursing diagnoses for patients awaiting cardiac surgery vary according to each patient's cardiac disease and symptoms. Most patients have a nursing diagnosis of decreased cardiac output (see Cardiac Failure in Chap. 30). Preoperative nursing diagnoses for most patients may include:

- Fear related to the surgical procedure, its uncertain outcome, and the threat to well-being
- Deficient knowledge regarding the surgical procedure and the postoperative course

COLLABORATIVE PROBLEMS/POTENTIAL COMPLICATIONS

The stress of impending cardiac surgery may precipitate complications that require collaborative management with the physician. Based on the assessment data, potential complications that may develop include:

- Angina or anginal pain equivalent
- Severe anxiety requiring an anxiolytic (anxiety-reducing) medication
- Cardiac arrest

Planning and Goals

The major goals of the patient may include reducing fear, learning about the surgical procedure and postoperative course, and avoiding complications.

Nursing Interventions

During the preoperative phase of cardiac surgery, the nurse develops a plan of care that includes emotional support and teaching for the patient and family. Establishing rapport, answering questions, listening to fears and concerns, clarifying misconceptions, and providing information about what to expect are interventions the nurse uses to prepare the patient and family emotionally for the surgery and for the postoperative events.

REDUCING FEAR

The patient and family are provided time and opportunities to express their fears. If there is fear of the unknown, other surgical experiences that the patient has had can be compared with the impending surgery. It is often helpful to describe to the patient the sensations that are expected. If the patient has already had a cardiac catheterization, the similarities and differences between that procedure and the surgery may be compared. The patient is encouraged to talk about any concerns related to previous experiences.

A discussion of the patient's fears about pain is initiated. A comparison is made between the pain experienced with cardiac surgery and other pain experiences. The preoperative sedation, the anesthetic, and the postoperative pain medications are described. The nurse reassures the patient that the fear of pain is normal, that some pain will be experienced, that medication to relieve pain will be provided, and that the patient will be closely observed. The patient is encouraged to take pain medication before the pain becomes severe. Positioning and relaxation will make the pain more tolerable. Patients who have a fear of scarring from surgery are encouraged to discuss this concern, and misconceptions are corrected. It may be helpful to indicate that the health care team members will keep the patient informed about the healing process.

The patient and family are encouraged to talk about their fear of the patient dying. They should be reassured that this fear is normal. For those who only hint about this concern despite efforts to encourage them to talk about their fear, coaching may be helpful (eg, "Are you worrying about not making it through surgery? Most people who have heart surgery at least think about the possibility of dying."). After the fear is expressed, the patient and family can be helped to explore their feelings.

By alleviating undue anxiety and fear, preparing the patient emotionally for surgery decreases the chance of preoperative problems, promotes smooth anesthesia induction, and enhances the patient's involvement in care and recovery after surgery. Preparing the family for the events to come helps them to cope, be supportive to the patient, and participate in postoperative and rehabilitative care (Chart 28-9).

MONITORING AND MANAGING POTENTIAL COMPLICATIONS

Angina may occur because of increased stress and anxiety related to the forthcoming surgery. The patient who develops angina usually responds to normal angina therapy, most commonly nitroglycerin. Some patients require oxygen and intravenous nitroglycerin drips (see the Angina Pectoris section).

Chart 28-9 • Ethics and Related Issues

When Is Withholding or Withdrawing Life Support Discussed with Patients and Families?

Situation
Life support includes the use of intraaortic balloon pumps and ventricular assist devices, ventilators, vasoactive infusions, cardiopulmonary resuscitation, and antibiotics. Patients who receive these treatments include those who are acutely, chronically, and terminally ill. When dependent on life support, a patient may be unable to make decisions about his or her own care, and the patient's family may be asked to participate in decision making for the patient. At what point is the sensitive issue of withholding or withdrawing life support discussed?

Dilemma
A patient is unresponsive and utilizing life support in the critical care unit. The consulting cardiologist has written a progress note stating, "Patient is terminal. Further treatment is futile." The patient does not have a living will or a durable power of attorney for health care. The oldest child does not want the patient to suffer but states, "If there is any hope, I want everything done." The other child states that the patient "would not want to live like this."

Does the statement by the second child support the principle of autonomy? Does the statement by the oldest child provide precedence for the principles of sanctity of life, beneficence, or nonmaleficence? If you determined that the statement by the second child supported the principle of autonomy, should sanctity of life, beneficence, or nonmaleficence be used in decision making in this situation?

Discussion
What arguments would you offer to support the view that discussions about the extent of life-supporting treatments desired should occur before an individual experiences a life-threatening event?

What arguments would you offer to support the view that discussions about the extent of life-supporting treatment should occur only when certain circumstances arise?

For patients with extreme anxiety or fear and for whom emotional support and education are not successful, medication therapy may be helpful. The anxiolytic agents most commonly used before cardiac surgery are lorazepam (Ativan) and diazepam (Valium).

If cardiac arrest occurs in the preoperative period, advanced cardiac life support is provided (see Chap. 27).

PROMOTING HOME AND COMMUNITY-BASED CARE

Teaching Patients Self-Care
Patient and family teaching is based on assessed learning needs. Teaching usually includes information about hospitalization, surgery (eg, preoperative and postoperative care, length of surgery, pain and discomfort that can be expected, visiting hours, and procedures in the critical care unit), the recovery phase (eg, length of hospitalization, what to expect from home care and rehabilitation, when normal activities such as housework, shopping, and work can be resumed), and ongoing lifestyle habits. Any changes made in medical therapy and preoperative preparations need to be explained and reinforced.

The patient is informed that physical preparation usually involves several showers or scrubs with an antiseptic solution. A sedative may be prescribed the night before and the morning of

surgery. Most cardiac surgical teams use prophylactic antibiotic therapy, and the antibiotic therapy is initiated before surgery.

If no preadmission teaching has been done and the preoperative hospitalization period is very short, teaching the patient and family together may be most effective. Anxiety often increases with the admission process and impending surgery. Teaching the patient and family together capitalizes on their established support relationship. Teaching in this phase should be directed primarily by the patient's and family's questions. Too much detail may only increase anxiety.

The patient may be offered a tour of the critical care unit, the postanesthesia care unit, or both. (In some hospitals, the patient initially goes to the postanesthesia care unit.) The patient recovering from anesthesia may be reassured by having already seen the surroundings and having met someone from the unit. The patient and family are informed about the equipment, tubes, and lines that will be present after surgery and their purposes. They should know to expect monitors, several intravenous lines, chest tubes, and a urinary catheter. Explaining the purpose and the approximate time that these devices will be in place helps to reassure the patient. Most patients will remain intubated and on mechanical ventilation for 2 to 24 hours after surgery. They need to be aware that this prevents them from talking, and they should be reassured that the staff will be able to assist them with other means of communication.

The nurse takes care to answer the patient's questions about postoperative care and procedures. Deep breathing and huffing (or coughing), use of the incentive spirometer, and foot exercises are explained and practiced by the patient before surgery. The family's questions at this time usually focus on the length of the surgery, who will discuss the results of the procedure with them after surgery and when this may occur, where to wait during the surgery, the visiting procedures for the critical care unit, and how they can support the patient before surgery and in the critical care unit.

Evaluation

EXPECTED PATIENT OUTCOMES
Expected patient outcomes may include:

1. Demonstrates reduced fear
   a. Identifies fears
   b. Discusses fears with family
   c. Uses past experiences as a focus for comparison
   d. Expresses positive attitude about outcome of surgery
   e. Expresses confidence in measures to be used to relieve pain
2. Learns about the surgical procedure and postoperative course
   a. Identifies the purposes of the preoperative preparation procedure
   b. Tours the critical care unit, if desired
   c. Identifies limitations expected after surgery
   d. Discusses expected immediate postoperative environment (eg, tubes, machines, nursing surveillance)
   e. Demonstrates expected activities after surgery (eg, deep breathing, huffing [coughing], foot exercises)
3. Shows no evidence of complications
   a. Reports anginal pain is relieved with medications and rest
   b. Takes medications as prescribed

INTRAOPERATIVE NURSING MANAGEMENT

The perioperative nurse performs an assessment and prepares the patient for the operating room and recovery experience. Any changes in the patient's status and the need for changes in therapy are identified. Procedures are explained before they are performed, such as the application of electrodes and use of continuous monitoring, indwelling catheters, and an SpO_2 probe. Intravenous lines are inserted to administer fluids, medications, and blood products. The patient will receive general anesthesia, be intubated, and placed on mechanical ventilation. In addition to assisting with the surgical procedures, perioperative nurses are responsible for the comfort and safety of the patient. Some of the areas of intervention include positioning, skin care, wound care, and emotional support of the patient and family.

Before the chest incision is closed, chest tubes are positioned to evacuate air and drainage from the mediastinum and the thorax. Epicardial pacemaker electrodes are implanted on the surface of the right atrium and the right ventricle. These epicardial electrodes can be used to pace the heart and to monitor it for dysrhythmias through the atrial leads.

Possible intraoperative complications include dysrhythmias, hemorrhage, MI, CVA (stroke, brain attack), embolization, and organ failure from shock, embolus, or adverse drug reactions. Astute intraoperative patient assessment is critical in preventing these complications and for detecting symptoms and initiating prompt therapy.

NURSING PROCESS: THE PATIENT WHO HAS HAD CARDIAC SURGERY

Initial postoperative care focuses on achieving or maintaining hemodynamic stability and recovery from general anesthesia. Care may be provided in the postanesthesia care unit or intensive care unit. After hemodynamic stability and recovery from general anesthesia have been achieved, the patient is transferred to a surgical stepdown unit with telemetry. Care focuses on wound care, progressive activity, and nutrition. Education about medications and risk factor modification is emphasized (see Plan of Nursing Care: Care of the Patient After Cardiac Surgery). Discharge from the hospital usually occurs 3 to 5 days after CABG or 1 to 3 days after MIDCAB. Patients can expect fewer symptoms from CAD and an improved quality of life. CABG has been shown to increase the life span of high-risk patients—those with left main artery blockages, left ventricular dysfunction with multivessel blockages, three-vessel blockages with one being the left anterior descending artery, and diabetes (Eagle et al., 1999).

The immediate postoperative period for the patient who has undergone cardiac surgery presents many challenges to the health care team. All efforts are made to facilitate the transition from the operating room to the critical care unit or PACU with minimal risk. Specific information about the operation and important factors about postoperative management are communicated by the surgical team and anesthesia personnel to the critical care nurse, who then assumes responsibility for the patient's care. Figure 28-10 presents a graphic overview of the many aspects of postoperative care for the cardiac surgical patient.

Assessment

When the patient is admitted to the critical care unit or PACU and for at least every 12 hours thereafter, a complete assessment of all systems is performed to determine the postoperative status of the patient compared with the preoperative baseline and to identify anticipated changes since surgery. The following parameters are assessed:

Neurologic status: level of responsiveness, pupil size and reaction to light, reflexes, facial symmetry, movement of extremities, and hand grip strength

Cardiac status: heart rate and rhythm, heart sounds, arterial blood pressure, central venous pressure (CVP), pulmonary artery pressure, pulmonary artery wedge pressure (PAWP), left atrial pressure, waveforms from the invasive blood pressure lines, cardiac output or index, systemic and pulmonary vascular resistance, pulmonary artery oxygen saturation (SvO_2) if available, mediastinal chest tube drainage, and pacemaker status and function

Respiratory status: chest movement, breath sounds, ventilator settings (eg, rate, tidal volume, oxygen concentration, mode such as synchronized intermittent mandatory ventilation, positive end-expiratory pressure, pressure support), respiratory rate, ventilatory pressure, arterial oxygen saturation (SaO_2), percutaneous oxygen saturation (SpO_2), end-tidal CO_2, pleural chest tube drainage, arterial blood gases

Peripheral vascular status: peripheral pulses; color of skin, nailbeds, mucosa, lips, and earlobes; skin temperature; edema; condition of dressings and invasive lines

Renal function: urinary output; urine specific gravity and osmolality may be assessed

Fluid and electrolyte status: intake, output from all drainage tubes, all cardiac output parameters, and the following indications of electrolyte imbalance:

- *Hypokalemia:* digitalis toxicity, dysrhythmias, ECG changes (U wave, atrioventricular block, flat or inverted T waves)
- *Hyperkalemia:* mental confusion, restlessness, nausea, weakness, paresthesias of extremities, dysrhythmias, ECG changes (tall, peaked T waves; increased amplitude, widening QRS complex; prolonged QT interval)
- *Hypomagnesemia:* paresthesias, carpopedal spasm, muscle cramps, tetany, irritability, tremors, hyperexcitability, hyperreflexia, cardiac dysrhythmias, ECG changes (prolonged PR and QT intervals; broad, flat T waves), disorientation, depression, hypotension, seizures
- *Hypermagnesemia:* vasodilation, hypotension, hyporeflexia, slow gastrointestinal motility (hypoactive bowel sounds), lethargy, respiratory depression, coma, apnea, cardiac arrest
- *Hyponatremia:* weakness, fatigue, confusion, seizures, coma
- *Hypocalcemia:* paresthesias, carpopedal spasm, muscle cramps, tetany
- *Hypercalcemia:* digitalis toxicity, asystole

Pain: nature, type, location, duration (incisional pain must be differentiated from anginal pain); apprehension; response to analgesics

Some patients who have had a MIDCAB using a midsternal incision or an internal mammary artery CABG experience ulnar nerve paresthesia on the same side of the body as the graft. The paresthesia may be temporary or permanent. Patients who have had CABG using the gastroepiploic artery may experience an ileus for a longer period after surgery and have abdominal pain at the site of the incision and pain at the site of the chest incision.

Assessment also includes observing all equipment and tubes to determine whether they are functioning properly: endotracheal tube, ventilator, end-tidal CO_2 monitor, SpO_2 monitor, pul-

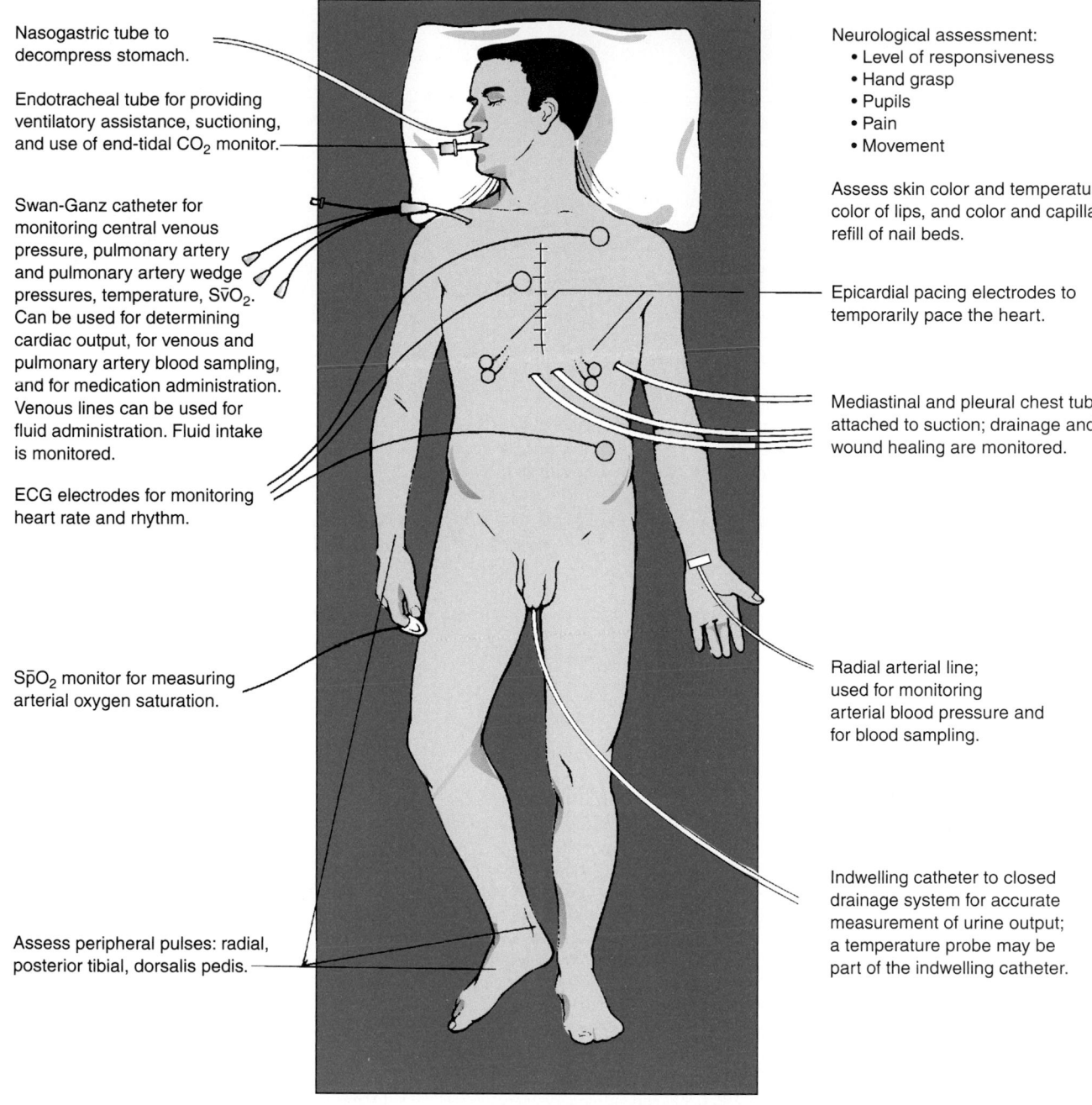

Nasogastric tube to decompress stomach.

Endotracheal tube for providing ventilatory assistance, suctioning, and use of end-tidal CO_2 monitor.

Swan-Ganz catheter for monitoring central venous pressure, pulmonary artery and pulmonary artery wedge pressures, temperature, $S\bar{v}O_2$. Can be used for determining cardiac output, for venous and pulmonary artery blood sampling, and for medication administration. Venous lines can be used for fluid administration. Fluid intake is monitored.

ECG electrodes for monitoring heart rate and rhythm.

$S\bar{p}O_2$ monitor for measuring arterial oxygen saturation.

Assess peripheral pulses: radial, posterior tibial, dorsalis pedis.

Neurological assessment:
• Level of responsiveness
• Hand grasp
• Pupils
• Pain
• Movement

Assess skin color and temperature, color of lips, and color and capillary refill of nail beds.

Epicardial pacing electrodes to temporarily pace the heart.

Mediastinal and pleural chest tubes attached to suction; drainage and wound healing are monitored.

Radial arterial line; used for monitoring arterial blood pressure and for blood sampling.

Indwelling catheter to closed drainage system for accurate measurement of urine output; a temperature probe may be part of the indwelling catheter.

FIGURE 28-10 Postoperative care of the cardiac surgical patient requires the nurse to be proficient in interpreting hemodynamics, correlating physical assessments with laboratory results, sequencing interventions, and evaluating progress toward desired outcomes.

monary artery catheter, $S\bar{v}O_2$ monitor, arterial and intravenous lines, intravenous infusion devices and tubing, cardiac monitor, pacemaker, chest tubes, and urinary drainage system.

As the patient regains consciousness and progresses through the postoperative period, the nurse expands the assessment to include parameters indicative of psychological and emotional status. The patient may exhibit behavior that reflects denial or depression or may experience postcardiotomy psychosis. Characteristic signs of psychosis include transient perceptual illusions, visual and auditory hallucinations, disorientation, and paranoid delusions.

The family's needs also should be assessed. The nurse ascertains how they are coping with the situation; determines their psychological, emotional, and spiritual needs; and finds out whether they are receiving adequate information about the patient's condition.

ASSESSING FOR COMPLICATIONS

The patient is continuously assessed for indications of impending complications (Table 28-8). The nurse and the surgeon function collaboratively to identify early signs and symptoms of complications and to institute measures to reverse their progression.

(text continues on page 754)

Table 28-8 • Potential Complications of Cardiac Surgery

COMPLICATION	DESCRIPTION	ASSESSMENT AND MANAGEMENT
Cardiac Complications (The patient may require interventions for more than one complication at a time. Collaboration among nurses, physicians, pharmacists, respiratory therapists, and dietitians is necessary to achieve the desired patient outcomes.)		
Decreased Cardiac Output		
Preload Alterations (the amount of myocardial muscle fiber stretch at the end of diastole)		
Hypovolemia (most common cause of decreased cardiac output after cardiac surgery)	• Blood loss (although some blood may be replaced to provide sufficient hemoglobin to carry oxygen to the tissues) • Surgical hypothermia (As the reduced body temperature rises after surgery, blood vessels dilate, and more volume is needed to fill the vessels.) • Intravenous fluid loss to the interstitial spaces because cardiopulmonary bypass makes capillary beds more permeable • Arterial hypotension with low pulmonary artery wedge pressure (PAWP) and low central venous pressures (CVP) often are seen with an increased heart rate.	• Fluid replacement may be prescribed. Replacement fluids include: colloid (albumin or protein), starch (hetastarch), packed red blood cells, or crystalloid solution (normal saline, lactated Ringer's solution).
Persistent bleeding	• Cardiopulmonary bypass procedure, which may cause platelet malfunction (blood clots abnormally) and hypothermia, which alters clotting mechanisms • Surgical trauma causing tissues and blood vessels to ooze bloody drainage • Anticoagulant (heparin) therapy	• Accurate measurement of wound bleeding and drainage tube blood is essential. Bloody drainage should not exceed 200 mL/h for the first 4 to 6 hours. Drainage should decrease and stop within a few days, while progressing from sanguineous to serosanguineous and serous drainage. • Protamine sulfate may be administered to neutralize unfractionated heparin; vitamin K and blood products may be used to treat hematologic deficiencies. • If bleeding persists, the patient may return to the operating room for corrective surgery.
Cardiac tamponade (may decrease preload to the heart by preventing available blood from entering the heart)	• Fluid accumulates in the pericardial sac, which compresses the heart, preventing blood from filling the ventricles. • Signs and symptoms include arterial hypotension, tachycardia, muffled heart sounds, decreasing urine output and equalizing of the PAWP, CVP, and pulmonary artery diastolic pressures. Additional signs and symptoms: arterial and pulmonary artery pressure waveforms demonstrating a pulsus paradoxus (decrease of more than 10 mm Hg during inspiration) and decreased chest tube drainage (suggesting that the drainage is trapped or clotted in the mediastinum).	• Equipment is checked to eliminate possible kinks or obstructions in the tubing. • Drainage system patency may be reestablished by milking the tubing (taking care not to strip the tubing, creating massive negative pressure within the chest, which may harm the surgical repair or trigger a dysrhythmia). • Chest x-ray may show a widening mediastinum. • Emergency medical management is required; may include pericardiocentesis or return to surgery.
Fluid overload	• High PAWP, CVP, and pulmonary artery diastolic pressures as well as crackles indicate fluid overload.	• Diuretics are usually prescribed and the rate of IV fluid administration is reduced. • Fluid restriction may be prescribed. Alternative treatments include continuous renal replacement therapy, dialysis, and phlebotomy.
Afterload Alterations (The force that the ventricle must overcome to move blood forward. Vascular resistance may be calculated to assess afterload and the effects of any vasoactive treatments. Alteration in the patient's body temperature is the most common cause of alterations in afterload after cardiac surgery.)		
Hypothermia	• Blood vessel constriction, which increases afterload. (Blood vessel dilation from fever or other hyperthermic condition decreases afterload.)	• Patient is rewarmed gradually, although vasodilators may be required if the resistance is too great to wait for rewarming. The patient may require volume support or vasopressors during a fever or severe vasodilation.
Hypertension	• Various causes. Some patients have a history of this condition and the nurse can anticipate the need for treatment postoperatively. Other patients experience transient hypertension.	• Vasodilators (nitroglycerin [Nitro-Bid], nitroprusside [Nipride, Nitropress]) may be used to treat hypertension. If patient had hypertension before surgery, the preoperative management regimen resumes as soon as possible.

(continued)

Table 28-8 • **Potential Complications of Cardiac Surgery** (Continued)

COMPLICATION	DESCRIPTION	ASSESSMENT AND MANAGEMENT
Heart Rate Alterations Tachydysrhythmias	• May or may not result from preload or afterload alterations	• Rhythms are assessed to establish that they are not the result of preload or afterload alterations. • If a tachydysrhythmia is the primary symptom, the heart rhythm is assessed and medications (eg, adenosine [Adenocard, Adenoscan], digoxin [Lanoxin], diltiazem [Cardizem], esmolol [Brevibloc], lidocaine [Xylocaine], procainamide [Procanbid, Pronestyl], propranolol [Inderal], quinidine [Cardioquin, Quinaglute, Quinidex], verapamil [Calan, Corvera, Isoptin, Verelan]) are prescribed. (Patients may be prescribed anti-arrhythmics before CABG to minimize the risk of postoperative tachydysrhythmias.) • Carotid massage may be performed by a physician to assist with diagnosing or treating the dysrhythmia. • Cardioversion and defibrillation are alternatives for symptomatic tachydysrhythmias.
Bradycardias	• Decreased heart rate	• Many postoperative patients will have temporary pacer wires that can be attached to a pulse generator (pacemaker) to stimulate the heart to beat faster. Less commonly, atropine, epinephrine or isoproterenol may be used to increase heart rate.
Dysrhythmias (may or may not affect cardiac output)	• Abnormal heart rates	• Treatment may include medication (Table 27-1), pacemakers (antibradycardiac, antitachycardiac), carotid massage, cardioversion, or defibrillation. Goal of treatment is to return the heart to a normal sinus rhythm. • For patients who cannot attain normal sinus rhythm, an alternate goal may be to establish a stable rhythm that produces a sufficient cardiac output.
Contractility Alterations Cardiac failure	• Possible when the heart fails as a pump and the chambers cannot adequately empty	• The nurse observes for and reports falling mean arterial pressure; rising PAWP, pulmonary artery diastolic pressure, and CVP; increasing tachycardia; restlessness and agitation; peripheral cyanosis; venous distention; labored respirations; and edema. • Medical management includes diuretics and digoxin.
Myocardial infarction (may occur intraoperatively or post-operatively)	• Portion of the cardiac muscle dies, therefore contractility decreases. Until the infarcted area becomes edematous, the ventricular wall moves paradoxically during contractions, further decreasing cardiac output. Symptoms may be masked by the postoperative surgical discomfort or the anesthesia–analgesia regimen.	• Careful assessment to determine the type of pain the patient is experiencing; MI suspected if the mean blood pressure is low with normal preload. The systemic vascular resistance (afterload) and heart rate may be elevated to compensate for poor contractility. • Serial ECGs and cardiac enzymes assist in making the diagnosis (alterations may be due to the surgical intervention). Analgesics are prescribed in small amounts while the patient's blood pressure and respiratory rate are monitored (because vasodilation secondary to analgesics or decreasing pain may occur and compound the hypotension). • Activity progression depends on the patient's activity tolerance.
Pulmonary Complications Impaired gas exchange	• During and after anesthesia, patients require mechanical assistance to breathe. • Potential for postperative atelectasis. • Endotracheal tubes stimulate production of mucus and chest incision pain may decrease the effectiveness of the forced expiratory technique (FET, cough).	• Pulmonary complications are often detected during assessment of breath sounds, oxygen saturation levels, and end-tidal CO_2 levels, and when monitoring peak pressure and exhaled tidal volumes on the ventilator. Arterial blood gas results and mixed venous saturations also are monitored when available.

(continued)

Table 28-8 • **Potential Complications of Cardiac Surgery** (Continued)

COMPLICATION	DESCRIPTION	ASSESSMENT AND MANAGEMENT
		• Extended periods of mechanical ventilation are often required while the complications are treated and until they are resolved. • In patients with hypoxia, ventricular stroke work index may be calculated to assist with assessment of contractility.
Fluid Volume Complications Hemorrhage	• Untoward and excessive bleeding may be life-threatening.	• Hemorrhage usually requires surgical intervention, and blood products are often administered. • Compression of a bleeding vessel is another treatment of hemorrhage. Lungs may be used to compress bleeding mediastinal blood vessels; lung volume and pressure are increased by adding PEEP to the ventilator settings of an intubated patient. The lungs slow or stop the bleeding by pushing in on the mediastinum and creating pressure on the bleeding vessels of the pericardium, coronary arteries, and bypass grafts.
Neurologic Complications Cerebrovascular accident (brain attack, stroke)	• Inability to follow simple command within 6 hours of recovery from anesthetic; different capabilities on right or left side of body	• Neurologically, most patients begin to recover from anesthesia in the operating room. • Patients who are elderly or who have renal or hepatic failure may take longer to recover. • Patient should be evaluated for CVA (brain attack, stroke) or air embolism.
Pain (see Chapter 13)		
Renal Failure and Electrolyte Imbalance Renal failure	• Usually acute and resolves within 3 months, but may become chronic and require ongoing dialysis	• May respond to diuretics or may require continuous renal replacement therapy (CRRT) or dialysis
Acute tubular necrosis	• Often results from hypoperfusion of the kidneys or from injury to the renal tubules by medications in the filtrate or from exacerbation of a preexisting condition	• Fluids, electrolytes, and urine output are monitored frequently.
Hypokalemia (low potassium level; normal level is 3.5 to 5.0 mEq/L [3.5 to 5.0 mmol/L])	• May be caused by inadequate intake, diuretics, vomiting, diarrhea, excessive nasogastric drainage without potassium replacement, and stress due to surgery (increased aldosterone secretion produces decreased potassium and increased sodium retention). • Signs and symptoms: digitalis toxicity, dysrhythmias, metabolic alkalosis, a weakened myocardium, and cardiac arrest • One specific ECG change is a U wave (a positive deflection after the T wave) that is more than 1 mm high. Additional signs are atrioventricular block, flat or inverted T waves, and low voltage.	• Must be detected and treated immediately • Patient must be observed carefully when serum potassium rises or falls outside the normal level • Some cardiac surgeons strive to maintain potassium level at 4.0 mEq/L (4.0 mmol/L) or higher to avoid dysrhythmias in the postoperative period. • When necessary, IV potassium replacement is prescribed.
Hyperkalemia (high potassium level)	• Hyperkalemia may be caused by increased intake, red blood cell hemolysis caused by cardiopulmonary bypass or mechanical assist devices, acidosis, renal insufficiency, tissue necrosis, and adrenal cortical insufficiency. • Signs and symptoms: mental confusion, restlessness, nausea, weakness, and paresthesias of the extremities. • ECG changes specific for hyperkalemia are tall peaked T waves, increased amplitude and widening of the QRS complex, and a prolonged QT interval.	• An ion exchange resin, sodium polystyrene sulfonate (Kayexalate), may be prescribed to bind the potassium in the gastrointestinal tract and decrease serum potassium. • Alternative treatments include IV sodium bicarbonate, IV insulin, and glucose to temporarily drive the potassium back into the cells from the extracellular fluid. • Hemodialysis or peritoneal dialysis may be used to reduce the potassium level.

(continued)

Table 28-8 • **Potential Complications of Cardiac Surgery** (Continued)

COMPLICATION	DESCRIPTION	ASSESSMENT AND MANAGEMENT
Hypomagnesemia (low magnesium level, <1.5 mEq/L (0.75 mmol/L), although symptoms usually develop with <1.0 mEq/L). Normal magnesium level ranges from 1.5–2.5 mEq/L (0.75–1.25 mmol/L)	• Can be caused by decreased intake, impaired absorption or increased excretion, and surgery, which causes the kidneys to excrete higher amounts of magnesium for 24 hours. Other causes may be decreased intake due to chronic alcoholism, malnutrition or starvation. Impaired absorption may be related to malabsorption syndromes (such as sprue, steatorrhea, or bowel resections) and excess intake of calcium. Increased excretion may result from diuretic use, loss of intestinal fluids (especially fistulas), diabetic ketoacidosis, primary aldosteronism, and primary hyperparathyroidism. Magnesium is important for the function of the neuromuscular system, so the signs and symptoms most often seen are neuromuscular. • Signs and symptoms: paresthesias, carpopedal spasm, muscle cramps, tetany, irritability, tremors, hyperexcitability, hyperreflexia, disorientation, depression, and seizures. Also, hypotension, dysrhythmias (atrial and ventricular), prolonged PR and QT intervals and broad flat T waves.	• Treatment is to correct the cause. If necessary, magnesium supplements may be given. The oral route is preferred to intramuscular injections, which are painful, and the IV route, which carries a significant risk for respiratory depression and hypotension. If the IV route is chosen for magnesium supplements, the nurse needs to assess the patient at least every 15 min for respiratory rate less than 16, hypotension, flushing, and diaphoresis. Loss of the patellar reflex may occur. If symptoms occur, the nurse slows or stops the infusion and notifies the physician.
Hypermagnesemia (high serum magnesium level, usually >3.0 Eq/L)	• Possibly caused by renal failure or intake of large amounts of medications with magnesium, such as some antacids and cathartics. • Signs and symptoms: vasodilation resulting in flushing, feeling warm, and hypotension. As the levels continue to rise, loss of reflexes, slowing bowel function, drowsiness, respiratory depression, coma, apnea and cardiac arrest may occur.	• Dialysis can be used to remove some magnesium but is not usually effective alone. Calcium gluconate is a temporary treatment until the cause can be identified and corrected.
Hypernatremia (high sodium level). and hyponatremia (low sodium level). Normal level is 135–145 mEq/L (135–145 mmol/L).	• Both may occur after cardiac surgery, but hyponatremia is more common. • Hyponatremia may result from reduced total body sodium or from increased water intake, which causes a dilution of body sodium. • Signs and symptoms of hyponatremia: weakness, fatigue, confusion, convulsions, and coma	• The patient must be observed for sodium values that vary from the normal ranges • When there is a true loss of sodium from the body, sodium replacement may be necessary. • Diuretics are prescribed when reduction in sodium is due to increased water intake.
Hypocalcemia (low calcium level). Normal level is 8.8–10.3 mg/100 mL (2.20–2.58 mmol/L).	• May result from alkalosis, which reduces the amount of calcium in the extracellular fluid, or from transfusions of large amounts of citrated blood products—packed red blood cells or whole blood. Citrate binds with calcium, reducing the amount of circulating ionized calcium. After 5–6 units of packed cells or whole blood from the blood bank, calcium binding may become a concern. • Signs and symptoms: numbness and tingling in the fingertips, toes, ears, and nose; carpopedal spasm; and muscle cramps and tetany	• Calcium level is monitored to determine if it is within normal limits. • Any symptoms of hypocalcemia are reported promptly so that calcium replacement can be instituted.
Hypercalcemia (high calcium level)	• Signs and symptoms: dysrhythmias that imitate those caused by digitalis toxicity (calcium can potentiate, or enhance, the action of digitalis)	• The nurse assesses the patient for signs of digitalis toxicity and reports these immediately so that the physician can institute treatment to prevent asystole and death.

(continued)

Table 28-8 • **Potential Complications of Cardiac Surgery** (Continued)

COMPLICATION	DESCRIPTION	ASSESSMENT AND MANAGEMENT
Other Complications		
Hepatic failure	• Most common in patients with cirrhosis, hepatitis, or prolonged right-sided heart failure	• Use of medications metabolized by the liver must be minimized. If hepatic failure cannot be reversed, death is inevitable. • Bilirubin, albumin, and amylase levels are monitored, and nutritional support must be provided.
Coagulopathies	• Result of hypothermia, blood component depletion, anticoagulation, or liver dysfunction	• Each patient must be carefully evaluated to determine the cause. Appropriate therapy is then provided.
Infection	• Cardiopulmonary bypass and anesthesia alter the patient's immune system. Many invasive devices are used to monitor and support the patient's recovery and may serve as a source of infection.	• The following must be monitored to detect signs of possible infection: body temperature, white blood cell counts and differential counts, incision and puncture sites, cardiac output and systemic vascular resistance, urine (clarity, color, and odor), bilateral breath sounds, sputum (color, odor, amount), as well as nasogastric secretions. • Antibiotic therapy may be expanded or modified as necessary. • Invasive devices must be discontinued as soon as they are no longer required. Institutional protocols for maintaining and replacing invasive lines and devices must be followed to minimize the patient's risk for infection.

Decreased Cardiac Output

A decrease in cardiac output is always a threat to the patient who has had cardiac surgery. It can have a variety of causes:

Preload alterations: too little or too much blood volume returning to the heart because of hypovolemia, persistent bleeding, cardiac tamponade, or fluid overload

Afterload alteration: hypertension and arterioles that are too constricted or too dilated because of alterations in body temperature or use of **vasoconstrictors** and **vasodilators**

Heart rate alterations: too fast, too slow, or dysrhythmias

Contractility alterations: cardiac failure, MI, electrolyte imbalances, hypoxia

Fluid Volume and Electrolyte Imbalance

The risk for fluid and electrolyte imbalance may occur after cardiac surgery. Nursing assessment for these complications includes monitoring of intake and output, weight, PAWP, left atrial pressure and CVP readings, hematocrit levels, distention of neck veins, edema, liver size, breath sounds (eg, fine crackles, wheezing), and electrolyte levels. Changes in serum electrolytes are reported promptly so that treatment can be instituted. Especially important are dangerously high or dangerously low levels of potassium, magnesium, sodium, and calcium.

Impaired Gas Exchange

Impaired gas exchange is another possible complication after cardiac surgery. All body tissues require an adequate supply of oxygen and nutrients for survival. To achieve this after surgery, an endotracheal tube with ventilator assistance may be used for 24 or more hours. The assisted ventilation is continued until the patient's blood gas measurements are acceptable and the patient demonstrates the ability to breathe independently. Patients who are stable after surgery may be extubated as early as 2 to 4 hours

after surgery, which reduces their anxiety regarding their limited ability to communicate.

The patient is continuously assessed for signs of impaired gas exchange: restlessness, anxiety, cyanosis of mucous membranes and peripheral tissues, tachycardia, and fighting the ventilator. Breath sounds are assessed often to detect fluid in the lungs and monitor lung expansion. Arterial blood gas values are monitored. Arterial blood gases, SpO_2, SaO_2, and end-tidal CO_2 are assessed for decreased oxygen and increased carbon dioxide.

Impaired Cerebral Circulation

Brain function depends on a continuous supply of oxygenated blood. The brain does not have the capacity to store oxygen and must rely on adequate continuous perfusion by the heart. It is important to observe the patient for any symptoms of hypoxia: restlessness, headache, confusion, dyspnea, hypotension, and cyanosis. An assessment of the patient's neurologic status includes level of consciousness, response to verbal commands and painful stimuli, pupil size and reaction to light, facial symmetry, movement of extremities, hand grip strength, presence of pedal and popliteal pulses, and temperature and color of extremities. Any indication of a changing status is documented, and abnormal findings are reported to the surgeon because they may signal the beginning of a complication. Hypoperfusion or microemboli may produce central nervous system injury after cardiac surgery.

Diagnosis

NURSING DIAGNOSES

Based on the assessment data and the type of surgical procedure performed, major nursing diagnoses of the patient may include:

• Decreased cardiac output related to blood loss, compromised myocardial function, and dysrhythmias

- Impaired gas exchange related to trauma of extensive chest surgery
- Risk for deficient fluid volume (and electrolyte imbalance) related to alteration in circulating blood volume
- Disturbed sensory perception (visual or auditory) related to excessive environmental stimuli (critical care environment, surgical experience), insufficient sleep, psychological stress, altered sensory integration, and electrolyte imbalances
- Acute pain related to surgical trauma and pleural irritation caused by chest tubes
- Ineffective tissue perfusion (renal, cerebral, cardiopulmonary, gastrointestinal, peripheral) related to decreased cardiac output, hemolysis, vasopressor drug therapy, venous stasis, embolization, underlying atherosclerotic disease, effects of vasopressors, or coagulation problems
- Ineffective thermoregulation related to infection or post-pericardiotomy syndrome
- Deficient knowledge about self-care activities

COLLABORATIVE PROBLEMS/POTENTIAL COMPLICATIONS

Based on the assessment data, potential complications that may develop include:

- Cardiac complications: heart failure, MI, stunned myocardium, dysrhythmias, tamponade, cardiac arrest
- Pulmonary complications: pulmonary edema, pulmonary emboli, pleural effusions, pneumothorax or hemothorax, respiratory failure, acute respiratory distress syndrome
- Hemorrhage
- Neurologic complications: CVA (brain attack, stroke), air emboli
- Renal failure, acute or chronic
- Electrolyte imbalances
- Hepatic failure
- Coagulopathies
- Infection, sepsis

Planning and Goals

The major goals for the patient include restoration of cardiac output, adequate gas exchange, maintenance of fluid and electrolyte balance, reduction of symptoms of sensory-perception alterations, relief of pain, maintenance of adequate tissue perfusion, maintenance of normal body temperature, learning self-care activities, and absence of complications.

Nursing Interventions

RESTORING CARDIAC OUTPUT

Nursing management of the patient involves continuously observing the patient's cardiac status and notifying the surgeon of any changes that indicate decreased cardiac output. The nurse and the surgeon then work collaboratively to correct the problem.

In evaluating the patient's cardiac status, the nurse primarily determines the effectiveness of cardiac output through clinical observations and routine measurements: serial readings of blood pressure, heart rate, CVP, arterial pressure, and left atrial or pulmonary artery pressure.

Renal function is related to cardiac function, as blood pressure and heart rate drive glomerular filtration; therefore, urinary output is measured and recorded. Urine output of less than 25 mL/hr may indicate a decrease in cardiac output. Urine specific gravity may also be assessed (normal: 1.010 to 1.025), as may urine osmolality. Inadequate fluid volume may be manifested by low urinary out-

put and high specific gravity, whereas overhydration is manifested by high urine output with low specific gravity.

The growth and function of body cells depend on adequate cardiac output to provide a continuous supply of oxygenated blood to meet the changing demands of the organs and body systems. Because the buccal mucosa, nailbeds, lips, and earlobes are sites with rich capillary beds, they should be observed for cyanosis or duskiness as possible signs of reduced heart action. Moist or dry skin may indicate vasodilation or vasoconstriction, respectively. Distention of the neck veins or of the dorsal surface of the hand raised to heart level may signal a changing demand or diminishing capacity of the heart. If cardiac output has fallen, the skin becomes cool, moist, and cyanotic or mottled.

Dysrhythmias, which may arise when poor perfusion of the heart exists, also serve as important indicators of cardiac function. The most common dysrhythmias encountered during the postoperative period are atrial fibrillation, bradycardias, tachycardias, and ectopic beats. Continuous observation of the cardiac monitor for various dysrhythmias is an essential part of patient care and management.

Any indications of decreased cardiac output are reported promptly to the physician. These assessment data and results of diagnostic tests are used by the physician to determine the cause of the problem. After a diagnosis has been made, the physician and the nurse work collaboratively to restore cardiac output and prevent further complications. When indicated, the physician prescribes blood components, fluids, digitalis or other antidysrhythmics, diuretics, vasodilators, or vasopressors. When additional surgery is necessary, the patient and family are prepared for the procedure.

PROMOTING ADEQUATE GAS EXCHANGE

To ensure adequate gas exchange, the nurse assesses and maintains the patency of the endotracheal tube. The patient is suctioned when wheezes, coarse crackles, or rhonchi are present. Suctioning may be performed with an in-line suction catheter; the nurse and respiratory therapist determine if the ventilator's fractional inspired oxygen (FIO_2) should be increased for three or more breaths before the patient is suctioned. Alternatively, 100% oxygen is delivered to the patient by a manual resuscitation bag (eg, Ambu-Bag) before and after suctioning to minimize the risk of hypoxia that can result from the suctioning procedure. Arterial blood gas determinations are compared with baseline data, and changes are reported to the physician promptly.

Because a patent airway is essential for oxygen and carbon dioxide exchange, the endotracheal tube must be secured to prevent it from slipping into the right mainstem bronchus and occluding the left bronchus. When the patient's condition stabilizes, body position is changed every 1 to 2 hours. Frequent changes of patient position provide for optimal pulmonary ventilation and perfusion by allowing the lungs to expand more fully. The nurse assesses breath sounds to detect crackles, wheezes, and fluid in the lungs.

The patient is usually weaned from the ventilator and extubated within 24 hours of CABG. Physical assessment and arterial blood gas results guide the process. Before being extubated, the patient should have cough and gag reflexes and stable vital signs; be able to lift the head off the bed or give firm hand grasps; have adequate vital capacity, negative inspiratory force, and minute volume appropriate for body size; and have acceptable arterial blood gas levels while breathing warmed humidified oxygen without the assistance of the ventilator.

Extubation has been performed within these parameters without any adverse effects on the patient's condition or prognosis.

During this time, the nurse assists with the weaning process and eventually with removal of the endotracheal tube. Deep breathing and forced expiration technique (FET, huffing) or coughing are encouraged at least every 1 to 2 hours after extubation to open the alveolar sacs and provide for increased perfusion. FET is the rapid exhalation of a deep breath using the diaphragm and abdominal muscles to force air out through an open mouth and glottis (the glottis is not held closed then suddenly opened, as in a cough). Patients may experience less pain with FET than coughing, which may increase the frequency with which a patient performs the exercises. The patient should be taught and assisted to splint the chest incision before and during FET or coughing to minimize discomfort.

MAINTAINING FLUID AND ELECTROLYTE BALANCE

To promote fluid and electrolyte balance, the nurse carefully assesses intake and output. Flow sheets are used to determine positive or negative fluid balance. All fluid intake is recorded, including intravenous, nasogastric tube, and oral fluids. All output is recorded, including urine, nasogastric drainage, and chest drainage.

Hemodynamic parameters (ie, blood pressure, pulmonary wedge and left atrial pressures, and CVP) are correlated with intake, output, and weight to determine the adequacy of hydration and cardiac output. Serum electrolytes are monitored, and the patient is observed for signs of potassium, magnesium, sodium, or calcium imbalance (ie, hypokalemia, hyperkalemia, hypomagnesemia, hyponatremia, or hypocalcemia).

Any indications of dehydration, fluid overload, or electrolyte imbalance are reported promptly, and the physician and nurse work collaboratively to restore fluid and electrolyte balance. The patient's response is monitored.

MINIMIZING SENSORY-PERCEPTION IMBALANCE

A large number of patients experience abnormal behaviors that occur with varying intensity and duration. In the early years of cardiac surgery, this phenomenon occurred more frequently than it does today. At that time, it was attributed to inadequate cerebral perfusion during surgery, microemboli, and the length of time that the patient remained on the CPB machine. Advances in surgical techniques have significantly decreased these factors. Today, when it occurs, it is thought to be caused by anxiety, sleep deprivation, increased sensory input, and disorientation to night and day when the patient loses track of time (Arrowsmith et al., 1999; Braunwald et al., 2001; Fuster et al., 2001). An important finding is that patients who do not or cannot express anxiety before surgery and those who are not able to sleep postoperatively are more prone to develop psychosis in the postoperative period. Psychosis may appear after a 2- to 5-day lucid interval.

Basic comfort measures used in conjunction with prescribed analgesics potentiate the effects of the analgesics and promote rest. The patient is assisted in changing positions every 1 to 2 hours and is positioned in such a way to avoid strain on incisions and chest tubes. Nursing care is scheduled as much as possible to provide undisturbed periods of rest. As the patient's condition stabilizes and the patient is disturbed less frequently for monitoring and therapeutic procedures, rest periods can be extended. As much uninterrupted sleep as possible is provided, especially during the patient's normal hours of sleep.

The nurse monitors the patient for signs of denial and provides an opportunity for emotional expression during the preoperative period. Careful explanations of all procedures and of the need for cooperation help to keep the patient oriented throughout the postoperative course. Continuity of care is desirable; a familiar face

and a nursing staff with a consistent approach promote the delivery of quality nursing care. A well-designed and individualized plan of nursing care can assist the nursing team in coordinating their efforts for the emotional well-being of the patient.

RELIEVING PAIN

Deep pain may not be reflected in the immediate area of injury but occur in a broader, more diffuse area. Patients who have had cardiac surgery experience pain caused by the interruption of intercostal nerves along the incision route and irritation of the pleura by the chest catheters. Incisional pain may also be experienced from peripheral vein or artery graft harvest sites.

It is essential to observe and listen to the patient for verbal and nonverbal clues about pain. The nurse accurately records the nature, type, location, and duration of the pain. (Chest incisional pain must be differentiated from anginal pain.) The patient is encouraged to use patient-controlled analgesia or accept medication as often as it is prescribed to reduce the amount of pain. Physical support of the incision during deep breathing and FET (or coughing) also helps to minimize pain. The patient should then be able to participate in respiratory exercises and to increase self-care progressively.

Pain produces tension, which may stimulate the central nervous system to release adrenaline, which results in constriction of the arterioles and increased heart rate. This can cause increased afterload and decreased cardiac output. Opioids alleviate anxiety and pain and induce sleep, which reduces the metabolic rate and oxygen demands. After the administration of opioids, any observations indicating relief of apprehension and pain are documented in the patient's record. The patient is observed for any respiratory depressant effects of the analgesic. If respiratory depression occurs, an opioid antagonist (eg, naloxone [Narcan]) is used to counteract the effect.

MAINTAINING ADEQUATE TISSUE PERFUSION

Peripheral pulses (eg, pedal, tibial, popliteal, femoral, radial, brachial) are routinely palpated to assess for arterial obstruction. If a pulse is absent in any extremity, the cause may be prior catheterization of that extremity. The newly identified absence of any pulse is immediately reported to the physician.

Thrombus formation and resulting embolus formation also can result from injury to the intima of the blood vessels, dislodging a clot from a damaged valve, loosening of mural thrombi, and coagulation problems. Air embolism may occur as a result of CPB or central venous cannulation. Symptoms of embolization vary according to site. The usual embolic sites are the lungs, coronary arteries, mesentery, spleen, extremities, kidneys, and brain. The patient is observed for:

- Chest pain and respiratory distress with pulmonary embolus or MI
- Midabdominal or midback pain
- Pain, cessation of pulses, blanching, numbness, or coldness in an extremity
- Decreased urine output
- One-sided weakness and pupillary changes, as occur in CVAs (brain attacks, strokes)

All such symptoms are promptly reported to the physician.

After surgery, the following measures are taken to prevent venous stasis, which can cause thrombus formation and subsequent embolization:

- Applying elastic compression stockings or elastic bandage wrap and pneumatic antiembolic stockings

- Discouraging crossing of legs
- Avoiding use of the knee gatch on the bed
- Omitting pillows in the popliteal space
- Instituting passive exercises followed by active exercises to promote circulation and prevent loss of muscle tone (patients need to ambulate as early as possible)

Inadequate renal perfusion can occur as a complication of cardiac surgery. One possible cause is low cardiac output. Trauma to blood cells during CPB can cause hemolysis of red blood cells, which then occlude the renal glomeruli. Use of vasopressor agents to increase blood pressure may constrict the renal arterioles and reduce blood flow to the kidneys.

Nursing management includes accurate measurement of urine output. An output of less than 25 mL/hr may indicate hypovolemia. Urine specific gravity can be monitored to determine the kidneys' ability to concentrate urine in the renal tubules. Rapid-acting diuretics or inotropic medications (eg, digoxin [Lanoxin], isoproterenol [Isuprel]) may be prescribed to increase cardiac output and renal blood flow. The nurse should be aware of the patient's blood urea nitrogen, serum creatinine, and urine and serum electrolyte levels. Abnormal levels are reported promptly because it may be necessary to adjust fluids and the dose or type of medication administered. If efforts to maintain renal perfusion are not effective, the patient may require dialysis or continuous renal replacement therapy (see Chap. 44).

MAINTAINING NORMAL BODY TEMPERATURE

Patients are usually hypothermic when admitted to the critical care unit from the cardiac surgical procedure. The patient must be gradually warmed to a normal temperature. This is accomplished partially by the patient's own basal metabolic processes and often with the assistance of warmed ventilator air, warm air or warm cotton blankets, or heat lamps. While the patient is hypothermic, the clotting process is less efficient, the heart is prone to dysrhythmias, and oxygen does not readily transfer from the hemoglobin to the tissues. Because anesthesia and hypothermia suppress the basal metabolism, oxygen supply usually meets the cellular demand.

After cardiac surgery, the patient is at risk for developing elevated body temperature caused by infection or postpericardiotomy syndrome. The resultant increase in metabolic rate increases tissue oxygen demands and increases cardiac workload. Measures are taken to prevent this sequence of events or to halt it as soon as it is recognized.

Sites of infection include the lungs, urinary tract, incisions, and intravascular catheters. Meticulous care is used to prevent contamination at the sites of catheter and tube insertions. Aseptic technique is used when changing dressings and when providing endotracheal tube and catheter care. Clearance of pulmonary secretions is accomplished by frequent repositioning of the patient, suctioning, and chest physical therapy, as well as teaching and encouraging the patient to breathe deeply and use FET (or cough). Closed systems are used to maintain all intravenous and arterial lines. All invasive equipment is discontinued as soon as possible after surgery.

Postpericardiotomy syndrome occurs in approximately 10% to 40% of patients who undergo cardiac surgery. Although the precise cause is unknown, a common factor appears to be trauma, with residual blood in the pericardial sac after surgery. The syndrome is characterized by fever, pericardial pain, pleural pain, dyspnea, pericardial effusion, pericardial friction rub, and arthralgia. There may be a combination of these signs and symptoms.

Leukocytosis occurs, along with elevation of the erythrocyte sedimentation rate. These symptoms frequently appear after the patient is discharged from the hospital.

The syndrome must be differentiated from other postoperative complications (eg, infection, incisional pain, MI, pulmonary embolus, bacterial endocarditis, pneumonia, atelectasis). Treatment depends on the severity of the symptoms. Bed rest and anti-inflammatory agents, such as salicylates and corticosteroids, produce a dramatic improvement in symptoms.

PROMOTING HOME AND COMMUNITY-BASED CARE

Teaching Patients Self-Care

Depending on the type of surgery and postoperative progress, the patient may be discharged from the hospital as early as 1 day after MIDCAB and 3 days after other surgery. Although the patient may be anxious to return home, the patient and family usually have apprehensions about this transition. The family members often express the fear that they are not capable of caring for the patient at home. They often are concerned that complications will occur that they are unprepared to handle.

The nurse helps the patient and family to set realistic, achievable goals. A teaching plan that meets the patient's individual needs is developed with the patient and family. This is done before admission and reviewed each shift through the hospitalization or with each home care and rehabilitation contact. Specific instructions are provided about incision care; signs and symptoms of infection; diet; activity progression and exercise; deep breathing, FET (or coughing), incentive spirometry; and smoking cessation; weight and temperature monitoring; the medication regimen; and follow-up visits with home care nurses, the rehabilitation personnel, the surgeon, and the cardiologist or internist.

Some patients may have difficulty learning and retaining information after cardiac surgery. Studies have documented that many patients have difficulties in cognitive function after cardiac surgery that do not occur after other types of major surgery (Arrowsmith et al., 1999; Roach et al., 1996). The patient may experience recent memory loss, short attention span, difficulty with simple math, poor handwriting, and visual disturbances. Patients with these difficulties often become frustrated when they try to resume normal activities and learn how to care for themselves at home. The patient and family are reassured that the difficulty is temporary and will subside, usually in 6 to 8 weeks. In the meantime, instructions are given to the patient at a much slower pace than normal, and a family member assumes responsibility for making sure that the prescribed regimen is followed. All information is provided in writing in the patient's primary language.

Continuing Care

Arrangements are made for a home care nurse to provide care when appropriate. Since the length of time that the patient remains in the hospital is relatively short, it is particularly important for the nurse to assess the patient's and family's ability to manage care in the home. The education plan is continued by the home care nurse. Vital signs and incisions are monitored, the patient is assessed for signs and symptoms of complications, and support for the patient and family is provided. Additional interventions may include dressing changes, intravenous antibiotic administration, diet counseling, and tobacco use cessation strategies. Patients and families need to know that cardiac surgery did not cure the patient's underlying heart disease. Lifestyle changes for risk factor reduction must be made, and medications taken preoperatively may be prescribed postoperatively.

NURSING RESEARCH PROFILE 28-1

Cardiac Surgery Patients' Transition From Hospital To Home

Weaver, L. A., & Doran, K. A. (2001). Telephone follow-up after cardiac surgery. *American Journal of Nursing, 101*(5), 24OO–24WW.

Purpose

Hospital length of stay (LOS) for patients after cardiac surgery may be 3 or 4 days. Formal patient/family education programs describing how to care for the patient at home are often provided during the hospitalization. These researchers identified that no health care professionals were contacting or seeing patients for 2 to 4 weeks after discharge from the hospital. The researchers implemented a telephone follow-up program. The purpose of the study was to evaluate the telephone follow-up program for patients who had undergone cardiac surgery.

Study Sample and Design

A convenience sample of heart surgery patients was selected, 46 of whom received usual care (control patients) and 44 of whom received usual care and postdischarge follow-up telephone calls (intervention patients). Patients in the intervention group were called by a cardiovascular stepdown unit registered nurse within 2 days after discharge, and then once a week for 1 month. At the end of this period, each participant was mailed a questionnaire to measure patient satisfaction, depression, recidivism, and complications. Patient satisfaction was measured with a modified four-question survey, the Continuity and Transition Dimensions, Picker Institute Survey. Depression was measured with a modified 15-question survey, the Geriatric Depression Scale. Recidivism was measured by the number of emergency department visits and hospital admissions during the 30 days after discharge from the hospital for cardiac surgery. Complications were self-reported by the participants.

Findings

Patient satisfaction in the intervention group was at least 10% higher than in the control group for three of four variables, but the results were not statistically significant. Twenty-two percent of the control group and 18% of the intervention group were readmitted or made emergency department visits during the first 30 days after discharge (recidivism); this difference in incidence was not statistically significant. There were no differences in the rate of depression or complications between the groups. The nurses who conducted the follow-up telephone program reported that they provided reassurance and support in each phone call. They provided reinforcement and clarification of postoperative education regarding leg swelling (31%), pain medication (23%), weight-taking and knowing when to call a health care provider (16%), and medication teaching (100%). The nurses also made referrals (to physicians, cardiac rehabilitation programs, dietitians, tobacco intervention programs [7%]) and coached patients with questions they wanted to ask their physicians (12%).

Nursing Implications

Telephone calls by step-down unit registered nurses to cardiac surgery patients after hospital discharge increase patient satisfaction (although not to statistical significance) and provide opportunities for reassurance and patient education. Development and use of scripts (algorithms, decision tree standards) may be helpful to the nurse making the telephone calls and facilitate consistency in the information provided to the patient. Script topics suggested by this study include incision care, leg swelling, fever, weight measurements and when to call a health care provider, pain management, medications (especially warfarin [Coumadin]), dysrhythmias, fluid status, constipation, nutrition, sleep, and depression.

Patient teaching does not end at the time of discharge from home health. The patient is encouraged to maintain telephone contact with the surgeon, cardiologist, and nurses. This provides the patient and family with reassurance that questions can be answered and problems can be resolved if they arise. Many hospitals provide family support sessions that help family members cope with their own stress related to the patient's home health care management. The patient is expected to have a follow-up visit with the surgeon.

Many patients and families benefit from supportive programs such as the postcardiac surgery rehabilitation programs offered by many medical centers. These programs provide exercise monitoring; instructions about diet and stress reduction; information about resuming exercise, work, driving, and sexual activity; assistance with tobacco use cessation; and support groups for patients and families. The American Heart Association sponsors the Mended Hearts Club, which provides information as well as an opportunity for families to share experiences.

Evaluation

EXPECTED PATIENT OUTCOMES

Expected patient outcomes may include:

1. Maintains adequate cardiac output
2. Maintains adequate gas exchange
3. Maintains fluid (and electrolyte) balance
4. Experiences decreased symptoms of sensory-perception disturbances
5. Experiences relief of pain
6. Maintains adequate tissue perfusion
7. Maintains normal body temperature
8. Performs self-care activities

A typical plan of postoperative nursing care and more-detailed expected outcomes for the cardiac surgery patient are presented in the Plan of Nursing Care, on pages 740–745.

Critical Thinking Exercises

1. You are caring for a patient who has undergone a PTCA with stent placement. The patient suddenly develops chest discomfort. In addition to the characteristics of the chest discomfort, identify the key factors that need to be assessed. Describe the actions that you would take and state why.

2. You are caring for a patient who is scheduled to have MIDCAB surgery. He appears quite anxious and states that he is afraid he will need to have traditional CABG surgery as discussed in obtaining informed consent. He states he does not want to have his "whole sternum cut open." His wife tends to minimize the significance of his concerns, commenting that, as the surgeon explained it, the possibility of having a traditional CABG is very small. How would you respond to this patient and his wife? How might your response differ if the wife shares her husband's concerns?

3. You are caring for a patient who underwent traditional CABG surgery 2 days ago and is progressing well. After ambulating in the corridor with his daughter, he returns to his room and notices that the dressing on his saphenous vein site is stained with bright red blood. His daughter is visibly upset. Explain what your first action will be and why. If your initial actions do not achieve the desired outcome, how would you proceed? How would you explain the episode to the daughter to help her understand the bleeding?

4. You are caring for two patients, both of whom were hospitalized for acute MI. One patient lives in his home with a supportive family, the other patient is homeless and living on the street. How does your plan of care and patient teaching differ for these patients?

REFERENCES AND SELECTED READINGS

Books

Agency for Health Care Policy and Research. (1994). *Unstable angina: Diagnosis and management.* Clinical Practice Guideline Number 10. AHCPR Publication No. 94-0602. Rockville, MD: Public Health Service, U.S. Department of Health and Human Services.

Albert, J. S. (2001). *The AHA clinical cardiac consult.* Philadelphia: Lippincott Williams & Wilkins.

American Heart Association (2001). *2001 Heart and Stroke Statistical Update.* Dallas, TX: American Heart Association.

Apple, S., & Lindsay, J. (2000). *Principles and practices of interventional cardiology.* Philadelphia: Lippincott Williams & Wilkins.

Bickley, L. S., & Szilagyi, P. G. (2003). *Bates's guide to physical examination and history taking* (8th ed.). Philadelphia: Lippincott Williams & Wilkins.

Braunwald, E., Zipes, D. P., & Libby, P. (Eds.). (2001). *Heart disease: A textbook of cardiovascular medicine* (6th ed.). Philadelphia: W. B. Saunders.

Carpenito, L. J. (2004). *Nursing diagnosis: Application to clinical practice* (10th ed.). Philadelphia: Lippincott Williams & Wilkins.

Effron, D. M. (Ed.). (1998). *Cardiopulmonary resuscitation: CPR* (4th ed.). Tulsa, OK: CPR Publishers, Inc.

Fuster, V., Alexander, R. W., O'Rourke, R. A., Roberts, R., King, S. B., III, & Wellens, H. J. J. (Eds.). (2001). *Hurst's the heart* (10th ed.). New York: McGraw-Hill.

Hudak, C. M., Gallo, B. M., & Morton, P. G. (1998). *Critical care nursing: A holistic approach* (7th ed.). Philadelphia: Lippincott-Raven.

Kuhn, M. A. (1999). *Complementary therapies for healthcare providers.* Philadelphia: Lippincott Williams & Wilkins.

McHale, D. J., & Carlson, K. K. (2001). *AACN procedure manual for critical care* (4th ed.). Philadelphia: W. B. Saunders.

Murphy, J. (Ed.). (2000). *Mayo Clinic cardiology review* (2nd ed.). Philadelphia: Lippincott Williams & Wilkins.

National Heart, Lung, Blood Institute, National High Blood Pressure Education Program. (1997). *The sixth report of the Joint Committee on Prevention, Detection, and Treatment of High Blood Pressure.* NIH Publication No. 98-4080. Bethesda, MD: National Institutes of Health.

North American Nursing Diagnosis Association. (2001). *Nursing diagnoses: Definitions and classification 2001–2002.* Philadelphia: North American Nursing Diagnosis Association.

Office for Social Environment and Health Research at West Virginia University. (2001). Women and heart disease: An atlas of racial and ethnic disparities in mortality (2nd ed.). Washington, DC: National Center for Chronic Disease Prevention and Health Promotion Centers for Disease Control and Prevention, U.S. Department of Health & Human Services.

Wagner, G. S. (2001). *Marriott's practical electrocardiography* (10th ed.). Philadelphia: Lippincott Williams & Wilkins.

Wenger, N. K., Froelicher, E. S., Smith, L. K., Ades, P. A., Berra, K., Blumenthal, J. A., et al. (1995). *Cardiac rehabilitation.* Clinical Practice Guideline Number 17. AHCPR Publication No. 96-0672. Rockville, MD: Public Health Service, Agency for Health Care Policy and Research and the National Heart, Lung, and Blood Institute.

Journals

Asterisks indicate nursing research articles.

Acorda, R., Kraus, T., & Casey, P. E. (2000). Advances in the surgical treatment of coronary artery disease. *Nursing Clinics of North America, 35*(4), 911–932.

American College of Cardiology Foundation and American Heart Association. (2002). ACC/AHA 2002 guideline update for exercise testing: A report of the American College of Cardiology/American Heart Association Task Force on Practice Guidelines (Committee on Exercise Testing). Available at: http://www.acc.org/clinical/guidelines/exercise. Accessed December 3, 2002.

American Heart Association. (2002). Women, heart disease and stroke statistics. Available at: http://www.americanheart.org/presenter.jhtml?identifier=4787. Accessed March 12, 2002.

Anderson, J. J. (2000). Transmyocardial laser revascularization. *Progress on Cardiovascular Nursing, 15*(3), 76–81.

Arrowsmith, J. E., Grocott, H. P., & Newman, M. F. (1999). Neurologic risk assessment, monitoring and outcome in cardiac surgery. *Journal of Cardiothoracic Vascular Anesthesia, 13*(6), 736–743.

Ballegaard, S., Meyer, C. N., & Trojaborg, W. (1991). Acupuncture in angina pectoris: Does acupuncture have a specific effect? *Journal of Internal Medicine, 229*(4), 357–362.

*Bengtson, A., Karlsson, T., & Herlitz, J. (2000). Differences between men and women on the waiting list for coronary revascularization. *Journal of Advanced Nursing, 31*(6), 1361–1367.

Brachmann, J., Ansah, M., Kosinski, E. J., & Schuler, G. C. (1998). Improved clinical effectiveness with a collagen vascular hemostasis device for shortened immobilization time following diagnostic angiography and percutaneous transluminal coronary angioplasty. *American Journal of Cardiology, 81*(12), 1502–1505.

Braunwald, E., Antman, E. M., Beasley, J. W., Califf, R., Cheitlin, M. D., Hochman, J. S., Jones, R. H, Kereiakes, D., Kupersmith, J., Levin, T. N., Pepine, C. J., Schaeffer, J. W., Smith, E. E., 3rd, Steward, D. E., Theroux, P., Alpert, J. S., Eagle, K. A., Faxon, D. P., Fuster, V., Gardner, T. J., Gregoratos, G., Russell, R. O., & Smith, S. C., Jr. (2000). ACC/AHA guidelines for the management of patients with unstable angina and non-ST-segment elevation MI: Executive summary and recommendations. A report of the American College of Cardiology/American Heart Association Task Force on Practice Guidelines (Committee on the Management of Patients with Unstable Angina). *Circulation, 102*(10), 1193–1209.

Burkhoff, D., Schmidt, S., Schulman, S. P., Myers, J., Resar, J., Becker, L. C., Weiss, J., & Jones, J. W. (1999). Transmyocardial laser revascularization compared with continued medical therapy for treatment of refractory angina pectoris: A prospective randomized trial. ATLANTIC (Angina Treatments: Lasers and Normal Therapies in Comparison) Investigators. *Lancet, 354*(9182), 885–890.

Buselli, E. F., & Stuart, E. M. (1999). Influence of psychosocial factors and biopsychosocial interventions on outcomes after myocardial infarction. *Journal of Cardiovascular Nursing, 13*(3), 60–72.

Canto, J. G., Shlipak, M. G., Rogers, W. J., Malmgren, J. A., Fraterick, P. D., Lambrew, C. T., Ornato, J. P., Barron, H. V., & Kiefe, C. I. (2000). Prevalence, clinical characteristics, and mortality among patients with myocardial infarction presenting without chest pain. *Journal of the American Medical Association, 283*(24), 3223–3229.

Casey, K., Bedker, D. L., & Roussel-McElmeel, P. L. (1998). Myocardial infarction: Review of clinical trials and treatment strategies. *Critical Care Nurse, 18*(2), 39–54.

Chlan, L., & Tracy, M. F. (1999). Music therapy in critical care: Indications and guidelines for intervention. *Critical Care Nurse, 19*(3), 35–41.

*Christensen, B. V., Manion, R. V., Iacarella, C. L., Meyer, S. M., Cartland, J. L., Bruhn-Ding, B. J., & Wilson, R. F. (1998). Vascular complications after angiography with and without the use of sandbags. *Nursing Research, 47*(1), 51–53.

Cohen, M. (2001). The role of low-molecular-weight heparin in the management of acute coronary syndromes. *Current Opinion in Cardiology, 16*(6), 384–389.

*Corrêa, C. G., & da Cruz, D. A. L. M. (2000). Pain: Clinical validation with postoperative heart surgery patients. *Nursing Diagnosis, 11*(1), 5–14.

Creek, D. J., Granger, B. B., & Prinkley-Briggs, L. A. (Eds.). (2000). Issues in acute cardiology. Continuing care in adult cardiology: Living with a cardiac diagnosis. *Nursing Clinics of North America, 35*(4), 833–1046.

Cucinelli, C. (2000). Minimally invasive coronary artery bypass surgery. *Critical Care Nursing Quarterly, 23*(1), 54–65.

Danesh, J., Collins, R., & Peto, R. (2000). Lipoprotein(a) and coronary heart disease: Meta-analysis of prospective studies. *Circulation, 102*(10), 1082–1085.

*Davies, N. (2000). Patients' and carers' perceptions of factors influencing recovery after cardiac surgery. *Journal of Advanced Nursing, 32*(2), 318–326.

Dembroski, T. M., MacDougall, J. M., Costa, P. T., & Grandits, G. A. (1989). Components of hostility as predictors of sudden death and myocardial infarction in the Multiple Risk Factor Intervention Trial. *Psychosomatic Medicine, 51*(5), 514–522.

*Dixon, T., Lim, L. L. Y., Powell, H., & Fisher, J. D. (2000). Psychosocial experiences of cardiac patients in early recovery: A community-based study. *Journal of Advanced Nursing, 31*(6), 1368–1375.

Doering, L. V. (1999). Pathophysiology of acute coronary syndromes leading to acute myocardial infarction. *Journal of Cardiovascular Nursing, 13*(3), 1–20.

Eagle, K. A., Guyton, R. A., Davidoff, R., Ewy, G. A., Fonger, J., Gardner, T. J., Gott, J. P., Herrmann, H. C., Marlow, R. A., Nugent, W. C., O'Connor, G. T., Orszulak, T. A., Rieselbach, R. E., Winters, W. L., Yusuf, S., Gibbons, R. J., Alpert, J. S., Eagle, K. A., Garson, A., Jr., Gregoratos, G., Russell, R. O., Smith, S. C., Jr. (1999). ACC/AHA guidelines for coronary artery bypass surgery: A report of the American College of Cardiology/American Heart Association Task Force on Practice Guidelines (Committee to Revise the 1991 Guidelines for Coronary Artery Bypass Graft Surgery). *Journal of the American College of Cardiology, 34*(4), 1262–1347.

Edgar, W. F., Ebersole, N., & Mayfield, M. G. (1999). MIDCAB. *American Journal of Nursing, 99*(7), 40–46.

*Elliott, D. (1994). The effects of music and muscle relaxation on patient anxiety in a coronary care unit. *Heart & Lung, 23*(1), 27–35.

Evans, D. (2002). The effectiveness of music as an intervention for hospital patients: A systematic review. *Journal of Advanced Nursing, 37*(1), 8–18.

Expert Panel on Detection, Evaluation, and Treatment of High Blood Cholesterol in Adults. (2001). Executive summary of the third report of the National Cholesterol Education Program (NCEP) Expert Panel on Detection, Evaluation, and Treatment of High Blood Cholesterol in Adults (Adult Treatment Panel III). *Journal of the American Medical Association, 285,* 2486–2497.

Expert Panel on Detection, Evaluation, and Treatment of High Blood Cholesterol in Adults. (2001). Third report of the National Cholesterol Education Program (NCEP) Expert Panel on detection, evaluation, and treatment of high blood cholesterol in adults (Adult Treatment Panel III): Full report. Available at: http://www.nhlbi.nih.gov/guidelines/cholesterol/atp3_rpt.htm. Accessed June 30, 2002.

Fair, J., & Fletcher, B. J. (Eds.). (2000). Abnormal lipids. *Journal of Cardiovascular Nursing, 14*(2), 1–103.

Friedman, M., & Rosenman, R. H. (1959). Association of specific overt behavior patterns with blood and cardiovascular findings: Blood cholesterol level, blood clotting time, incidence of arcus senilis and clinical coronary artery disease. *Journal of the American Medical Association, 169,* 1286–1297.

Furberg, C. D., Psaty, B. M., & Meyer, J. V. (1996). Nifedipine: Dose-related increase in mortality in patients with coronary heart disease. *Circulation, 92*(5), 1326–1331.

Gaenzer, H., Neumayr, G., Marschang, P., Sturm, W., Lechleitner, M., Föger, B., Kirchmair, R., & Patsch, J. (2002). Effect of insulin therapy on endothelium-dependent dilation in type 2 diabetes mellitus. *American Journal of Cardiology, 89*(4), 431–434.

Gebbie, A. (2002). Risks and benefits of estrogen plus progestin in healthy postmenopausal women: Principal results from the Women's Health Initiative Randomized Controlled Trial. Writing Group for the Women's Health Initiative Number 10 Investigators. *Journal of the American Medical Association, 288*(3), 321–333.

Gibbons, R. J., Chatterjee, K., Daley, J., Douglas, J. S., Fihn, S. D., Gardin, J. M., Grunwald, M. A., Levy, D., Lytle, B. W., O'Rourke, R. A., Schafer, W. P., Williams, S. V., Ritchie, J. L., Cheitlin, M. D., Eagle, K. A., Gardner, T. J., Garson, A., Jr., Russell, R. O., Ryan, T. J., & Smith, S. C., Jr. (1999). ACC/AHA/ACP-ASIM guidelines for the management of patients with chronic stable angina: A report of the American College of Cardiology/American Heart Association Task Force on Practice Guidelines (Committee on Management of Patients with Chronic Stable Angina). *Journal of the American College of Cardiology, 33*(7), 2092–2197.

Giuliano, K. K., Bloniasz, E., & Bell, J. (1999). Implementation of a pet visitation program in critical care. *Critical Care Nurse, 19*(3), 43–50.

Grady, D., Herrington, D., Bittner, V., Blumenthal, R., Davidson, M., Hlatky, M., Hsia, J., Hulley, S., Herd, A., Khan, S., Newby, L. K., Waters, D., Vittinghoff, E., Wenger, N., & HERS Research Group. (2002). Cardiovascular disease outcomes during 6.8 years of hormone therapy: Heart and Estrogen/Progestin Replacement Study follow-up (HERS II). *Journal of the American Medical Association, 288*(1), 49–57.

Greeland, P., Smith, S. C., Jr., & Grundy, S. M. (2001). Improving coronary heart disease risk assessment in asymptomatic people: Role of traditional risk factors and noninvasive cardiovascular tests. *Circulation, 104*(15), 1863–1867.

Grundy, S. M., Benjamin, I. J., Burke, G. L., Chait, A., Eckel, R. H., Howard, B. V., Mitch, W., Smith, S. C., Jr., & Sowers, J. R. (1999). Diabetes and cardiovascular disease: A statement for healthcare professionals from the American Heart Association. *Circulation, 100*(10), 1134–1146.

Harrison, H. (1999). Troponin I. *American Journal of Nursing, 99*(5), 24TT–26TT.

Hayden, A. M. (1998). Transmyocardial revascularization surgery. *Critical Care Nursing Quarterly, 21*(1), 48–57.

Hirsh, J., Anand, S. S., Halperin, J. L., & Fuster, V. (2001). Guide to anticoagulant therapy: Heparin. A statement for healthcare professionals from the American Heart Association. *Circulation, 103*(24), 2994–3018.

Homocysteine Studies Collaboration. (2002). Homocysteine and risk of ischemic heart disease and stroke: A meta-analysis. *Journal of the American Medical Association, 288*(16), 2015–2022.

Hulley, S., Grady, D., Bush, T., Furberg, C., Herrington, D., Riggs, B., & Vittinghoff, E. (1998). Randomized trial of estrogen plus progestin for secondary prevention of coronary heart disease in postmenopausal women. *Journal of the American Medical Association, 280*(7), 605–613.

*Hussey, L. C., Hynan, L., & Leeper, B. (2001). Risk factors for sternal wound infection in men versus women. *American Journal of Critical Care, 10*(2), 112–116.

Ishihara, M., Sato, H., Tateishi, H., Kawagoe, T., Shimatani, Y., Ueda, K., Noma, K., Yumoto, A., & Nishioka, K. (2000). Beneficial effect of prodromal angina pectoris is lost in elderly patients with acute myocardial infarction. *American Heart Journal, 139*(5), 881–888.

The Israeli SPRINT Study Group. (1988). Secondary Prevention Reinfarction Israeli Nifedipine Trial (SPRINT): A randomized intervention trial of nifedipine in patients with acute myocardial infarction. *European Heart Journal, 9*(4), 354–364.

Jeremias, A., Kutscher, S., Haude, M., Heinen, D., Holtmann, G., Senf, W., & Erbel, R. (1998). Nonischemic chest pain induced by coronary intervention: A prospective study comparing coronary angioplasty and stent implantation. *Circulation, 98*(24), 2656–2658.

*Juran, N. B., Rouse, C. L., Smith, D. D., O'Brien, M. A., DeLuca, S. A., & Sigmon, K. (1999). Nursing interventions to decrease bleeding at the femoral site after percutaneous coronary intervention. SANDBAG Nursing Coordinators: Standards of Angioplasty Nursing techniques to Diminish Bleeding Around the Groin. *American Journal of Critical Care, 8*(5), 303–313.

Kannel, W. B. (1986). Silent myocardial ischemia and infarction: Insights from the Framingham study. *Cardiology Clinics, 4*(4), 583–591.

Khatta, M., Alexander, B. S., Krichten, C. M., Fisher, M. L., Freudenberger, R., Robinson, S. W., & Gottlieb, S. S. (2000). The effect of coenzyme Q10 in patients with congestive heart failure. *Annals of Internal Medicine, 132*(8), 636–640.

*Knoll, S. M., & Johnson, J. L. (2000). Uncertainty and expectations: Taking care of a cardiac surgery patient at home. *Journal of Cardiovascular Nursing, 14*(3), 64–75.

Krantz, D. S., Sheps, D. S., Carney, R. M., & Natelson, B. H. (2000): Effects of mental stress in patients with coronary artery disease. *Journal of the American Medical Association, 283*(14), 1800–1802.

Lehmann, K. G., Heath-Lange, S. J., & Ferris, S. T. (1999). Randomized comparison of hemostasis techniques after invasive cardiovascular procedures. *American Heart Journal, 138*, (6 Part 1), 1118–1125.

Leon, M. B., Teirstein, P. S., Moses, J. W., Tripuraneni, P., Lansky, A. J., Jani, S., Wong, S. C., Fish, D., Ellis, S., Holmes, D. R., Kerieakes, D., & Kuntz, R. E. (2001). Localized intracoronary gamma-radiation therapy to inhibit the recurrence of restenosis after stenting. *New England Journal of Medicine, 344*(4), 250–256.

Livorsi-Moore, J., Gulanick, M., & Rosko, P. N. (1999). Port access: Another advance in cardiovascular surgery. *American Journal of Nursing, 99*(7), 52–55.

Malinow, M. R., Bostom, A. G., & Krauss, R. M. (1999). Homocyste(e)ine, diet, and cardiovascular diseases: A statement for healthcare professionals from the Nutrition Committee, American Heart Association. *Circulation, 99*(1), 178–182.

McErlean, E. S. (Ed.). (2000). Unstable angina. *Journal of Cardiovascular Nursing, 15*(1), 1–79.

Mehta, R. H., & Eagle, K. A. (2000). Missed diagnoses of acute coronary syndromes in the emergency room: Continued challenges. *New England Journal of Medicine, 342*(16), 1207–1210.

Mehta, J. L., Saldeen, T. G., & Rand, K. (1998). Interactive role of infection, inflammation and traditional risk factors in atherosclerosis and coronary artery disease. *Journal of the American College of Cardiology, 31*(6), 1217–1225.

*Meischke, H., Yasui, Y., Kuniyuki, A., Bowen, D. J., Andersen, R. F., Urban, N. (1999). How women label and respond to symptoms of acute myocardial infarction: Responses to hypothetical symptom scenarios. *Heart & Lung, 28*(4), 261–269.

Miller, K., & Grindel, C. G. (1999). Coronary artery bypass surgery in women and men: Preoperative profile and postoperative outcomes. *MedSurg Nursing, 8*(3), 167–172.

Morse, J. M. (2000). On comfort and comforting. *American Journal of Nursing, 100*(9), 34–38.

Mortality from coronary heart disease and acute myocardial infarction—United States, 1998. (2001). *Morbidity and Mortality Weekly Report, 50*(06), 90–93.

Mosca, L. (2002). C-reactive protein: To screen or not to screen? *New England Journal of Medicine, 347*(20), 1615–1617.

Mosca, L. (2000). The role of hormone replacement therapy in the prevention of postmenopausal heart disease. *Archive of Internal Medicine, 160*(15), 2263–2272.

Mueller, X. M., Tinguely, F., Tevaearai, H. T., Revelly, J. P., Chioléro, R., & von Segesser, L. K. (2000). Pain location, distribution, and intensity after cardiac surgery. *Chest, 118*(2), 391–396.

O'Hanlon, J. V., Jr. (2000). Minimally invasive saphenous vein harvesting. *Critical Care Nursing Quarterly, 23*(1), 42–46.

O'Rourke, R. A., Hochman, J. S., Cohen, M. C., Lucore, C. L., Popma, J. J., & Cannon, C. P. (2001). New approaches to diagnosis and management of unstable angina and non-ST segment elevation myocardial infarction. *Annals of Internal Medicine, 161*(5), 674–682.

*Penque, S., Halm, M., Smith, M., Deutsch, J., Van Roekel, M., McLaughline, L., Dzubay, S., Doll, N., & Beahrs, M. (1998). Women and coronary disease: relationship between descriptors of signs and symptoms and diagnostic and treatment course. *American Journal of Critical Care, 7*(3), 175–182.

Pepys, M. B., & Berger, A. (2001). The renaissance of C-reactive protein: It may be a marker not only of acute illness but also of future cardiovascular disease. *British Medical Journal, 322*(7277), 4–5.

*Plach, S. K., & Heidrich, S. M. (2001). Women's perceptions of their social roles after heart surgery and coronary angioplasty. *Heart & Lung, 30*(2), 117–127.

Platek, Y. M., & Atzori, M. (1999). PTMR. *American Journal of Nursing, 99*(7), 64–66.

Pope, J. H., Aufderheide, T. P., Ruthazer, R., Woolard, R. H., Feldman, J. A., & Beshansky, J. R., et al. (2000). Missed diagnoses of acute cardiac ischemia in the emergency department. *New England Journal of Medicine, 342*(16), 1163–1170.

Reichter, A., Herlitz, J., & Hjalmarson, A. (1991). Effect of acupuncture in patients with angina pectoris. *European Heart Journal, 2*(2), 175–178.

Ridker, P. M., Rifai, N., Rose, L., Burning, J. E., Cook, N. R. (2002). Comparison of C-reactive protein and low-density lipoprotein cholesterol levels in the prediction of first cardiovascular events. *New England Journal of Medicine, 347*(20), 1557–1565.

Ridker, P. M., Stampfer, M. J., & Rifai, N. (2001). Novel risk factors for systemic atherosclerosis: A comparison of C-reactive protein, fibrinogen, homocysteine, lipoprotein(a), and standard cholesterol screening as predictors of peripheral arterial disease. *Journal of the American Medical Association, 285*(19), 2481–2485.

Roach, G. W., Kanchuger, M., Mangano, C. M., Newman, M., Nussmeier, N., Wolman, R., Aggarwal, A., Marschall, K., Graham, S. H., & Ley, C. (1996). Adverse cerebral outcomes after coronary bypass surgery: Multicenter study of Perioperative Ischemia Research Group and the Ischemia Research and Education Foundation investigators. *New England Journal of Medicine, 335*(25), 1857–1863.

Rozanski, A., Blumenthal, J. A., & Kaplan, J. (1999). Impact of psychological factors on the pathogenesis of cardiovascular disease and implications for therapy. *Circulation, 99*(16), 2192–2217.

Ryan, T. J., Antman, E. M., Brooks, N. H., Califf, R. M., Hillis, L. D., Hiratzka, L. F., Rapaport, E., Riegel, B., Russell, R. O., Smith, E. E., 3rd, Weaver, W. D., Gibbons, R. J., Alpert, J. S., Eagle, K. A., Gardner, T. J., Garson, A., Jr., Gregoratos, G., Ryan, T. J., & Smith, S. C., Jr. (1999). 1999 Update: ACC/AHA guidelines for the management of patients with acute myocardial infarction. A report of the American College of Cardiology/American Heart Association Task Force on Practice Guidelines (Committee on Management of Acute Myocardial Infarction). *Journal of the American College of Cardiology, 34*(3), 890–911.

Scanlon, P. J., Faxon, D. P., Audet, A. M., Carabello, B., Dehmer, G. J., Eagle, K. A., Legako, R. D., Leon, D. F., Murray, J. A., Nissen, S. E., Pepine, C. J., Watson, R. M., Ritchie, J. L., Gibbons, R. J., Cheitlin, M. D., Gardner, T. J., Garson, A., Jr., Russell, R. O., Jr., Ryan, T. J., & Smith, S. C., Jr. (1999). ACC/AHA guidelines for coronary angiography. A report of the American College of Cardiology/American Heart Association Task Force on Practice Guidelines (Committee on Coronary Angiography). *Journal of the American College of Cardiology, 33*(6), 1756–1824.

Schouchoff, B., & Belhumeur, J. (2000). Radial artery: An alternative revascularization conduit. *Critical Care Nursing Quarterly, 23*(1), 28–34.

Sheifer, S. E., Escarce, J. J., & Schulman, K. A. (2000). Race and sex differences in the management of coronary artery disease. *American Heart Journal, 139*(5), 848–857.

*Skaggs, B. G., & Chrisopherson, B. (1999). Quality of life comparisons after coronary angioplasty and coronary artery bypass graft surgery. *Heart & Lung, 28*(6), 409–417.

Smith, S. C., Dove, J. T., Jacobs, A. K., Kennedy, J. W., Kereiakes, D., Kern, M. J., Kuntz, R. E., Popma, J. J., Schaff, H. V., Williams, D. O., Gibbons, R. J., Alpert, J. P., Eagle, K. A., Faxon, D. P., Fuster, V., Gardner, T. J., Gregoratos, G., Russell, R. O., Smith, S. C., Jr., American College of Cardiology, American Heart Association Task Force on Practice Guidelines, Committee to Revise the 1993 Guidelines for Percutaneous Transluminal Coronary Angioplasty. (2001). ACC/AHA Guidelines for percutaneous coronary intervention (revision of the 1993 PTCA Guidelines): Executive summary. A report of the American College of Cardiology/American Heart Association Task Force on Practice Guidelines (Committee to Revise the 1993 Guidelines for Percutaneous Transluminal Coronary Angioplasty). *Journal of the American College of Cardiology, 37*(8), 2215–2238.

Steinke, E. E. (2000). Sexual counseling after myocardial infarction. *American Journal of Nursing, 100*(12), 38–44.

Strong, J. P. (1999). Prevalence and extent of atherosclerosis in adolescents and young adults. *Journal of the American Medical Association, 281*(8), 727–735.

Teirstein, P. S., & Kuntz, R. E. (2001). New frontiers in interventional cardiology: intravascular radiation to prevent restenosis. *Circulation, 104*(21), 2620–2626.

*Tooth, L. R., McKenna, K. T., & Maas, F. (1999). Prediction of functional and psychological status after transluminal coronary angioplasty. *Heart & Lung, 28*(4), 276–283.

Wald, D. S., Law, M., & Morris, J. K. (2002). Homocysteine and cardiovascular disease: Evidence on causality from a meta-analysis. *British Medical Journal, 325*(7374), 1202–1206.

*Walker, S. B., Cleary, S., & Higgins, M. (2001). Comparison of the FemoStop device and manual pressure in reducing groin puncture site complications following coronary angioplasty and coronary stent placement. *International Journal of Nursing Practice, 7*(6), 366–375.

Wang, T. J., Larson, M. G., Levy, D., Benjamin, E. J., Kupka, M. J., Manning, W. J., Clouse, M. E., D'Agostino, R. B., Wilson, P. W.,

& O'Donnell, C. J. (2002). C-reactive protein is associated with subclinical epicardial coronary calcification in men and women: The Framingham Heart Study. *Circulation, 106*(10), 1189–1191.

*Weaver, L. A., & Doran, K. A. (2001). Telephone follow-up after cardiac surgery. *American Journal of Nursing, 101*(5), 24OO–24WW.

Williams, M. A., Fleg, J. L., Ades, P. A., Chaitman, B. R., Miller, N. H., Mohiuddin, S. M., Ockene, I. S., Taylor, C. B., Wenger, N. K., & American Heart Association Council on Clinical Cardiology Subcommittee on Exercise, Cardiac Rehabilitation, and Prevention. (2002). Secondary prevention of coronary heart disease in the elderly (with emphasis on patients ≥75 years of age): An American Heart Association scientific statement from the Council on Clinical Cardiology Subcommittee on Exercise, Cardiac Rehabilitation, and Prevention. *Circulation, 105*(14), 1735–1743.

Zalenski, R. J., Selker, H. P., Cannon, C. P., Farin, H. M., Gibler, W. B., Goldberg, R. J., Lambrew, C. T., Ornato, J. P., Rydman, R. J., & Steele, P. (2000). National Heart Attack Alert Program position paper: Chest pain centers and programs for the evaluation of acute cardiac ischemia. *Annals of Emergency Medicine, 35*(5), 462–471.

RESOURCES AND WEBSITES

American Dietetic Association, 216 W Jackson Blvd., Chicago, IL 60606-6995; 1-800-366-1644; http://www.eatright.org.

American Heart Association, 7320 Greenville Ave., Dallas, TX 75231; 1-800-AHA-USA1 (1-800-242-8721); http://www.americanheart.org.

Healthy People 2010; managed by the Office of Disease Prevention and Health Promotion, U.S. Department of Health and Human Services, 200 Independence Ave., SW, Washington, DC 20201; 1-800-877-696-6775; http://www.health.gov/healthypeople.

Heartmates, P.O. Box 16202, Minneapolis, MN 55416; 952-929-3331; http://www.heartmates.com.

National Heart, Lung, and Blood Institute, National Institutes of Health, Building 31, Room 5A52, Bethesda, MD 20892; 301-592-8593; http://www.nhlbi.nih.gov.

National Institute on Aging, Building 31, Room 5C27, 31 Center Drive, MSC 2292, Bethesda, MD 20892; http://www.nih.gov/nia.

Management of Patients With Structural, Infectious, and Inflammatory Cardiac Disorders

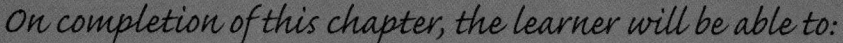

LEARNING OBJECTIVES ●

On completion of this chapter, the learner will be able to:

1. Define valvular disorders of the heart and describe the pathophysiology, clinical manifestations, and management of patients with mitral and aortic disorders.

2. Describe types of cardiac valve repair and replacement procedures used to treat valvular problems and the care needed by patients who undergo these procedures.

3. Describe the pathophysiology, clinical manifestations, and management of patients with cardiomyopathies.

4. Describe the pathophysiology, clinical manifestations, and management of patients with infections of the heart.

5. Describe the rationale for prophylactic antibiotic therapy for patients with mitral valve prolapse, valvular heart disease, rheumatic endocarditis, infective endocarditis, and myocarditis.

Structural disorders of the heart present many challenges for the patient, family, and health care team, as do the conduction and vascular disorders discussed in Chapters 27 and 28. Problems with the heart valves, holes in the intracardiac septum, cardiomyopathies, and infectious diseases of the heart muscle alter cardiac output. Treatments for these diagnoses may be noninvasive, such as medication therapy and activity and dietary modification. Invasive treatments, such as valve repair or replacement, septal repair, ventricular assist devices, total artificial hearts, cardiac transplantation, and other procedures may also be used. Nurses have an integral role in the care of patients with structural, infectious, and inflammatory cardiac conditions.

Acquired Valvular Disorders

The valves of the heart control the flow of blood through the heart into the pulmonary artery and aorta by opening and closing in response to the blood pressure changes as the heart contracts and relaxes through the cardiac cycle.

The atrioventricular valves separate the atria from the ventricles and include the **tricuspid valve**, which separates the right atrium from the right ventricle, and the **mitral valve**, which separates the left atrium from the left ventricle. The tricuspid valve has three leaflets; the mitral valve has two. Both valves have chordae tendineae that anchor the valve leaflets to the papillary muscles and ventricular wall.

The semilunar valves are located between the ventricles and their corresponding arteries. The **pulmonic valve** lies between the right ventricle and the pulmonary artery; the **aortic valve** lies between the left ventricle and the aorta. Figure 29-1 shows valves in the closed position.

When any of the heart valves do not close or open properly, blood flow is affected. When valves do not close completely, blood flows backward through the valve in a process called **regurgitation**. When valves do not open completely, a condition called **stenosis**, the flow of blood through the valve is reduced.

Disorders of the mitral valve fall into the following categories: mitral valve **prolapse** (ie, stretching of the valve leaflet into the atrium during systole), mitral regurgitation, and mitral stenosis. Disorders of the aortic valve are categorized as aortic regurgitation and aortic stenosis. These valvular disorders lead to various symptoms that, depending on their severity, may require surgical repair or replacement of the valve to correct the problem (Fig. 29-2). Tricuspid and pulmonic valve disorders also occur, usually with fewer symptoms and complications. Regurgitation and stenosis may occur at the same time in the same or different valves.

MITRAL VALVE PROLAPSE

Mitral valve prolapse, formerly known as mitral prolapse syndrome, is a deformity that usually produces no symptoms. Rarely, it progresses and can result in sudden death. Mitral valve prolapse occurs more frequently in women than in men. In recent years, this disorder has been diagnosed more frequently, probably as a result of improved diagnostic methods.

Pathophysiology

In mitral valve prolapse, a portion of a mitral valve leaflet balloons back into the atrium during systole. Rarely, the ballooning stretches the leaflet to the point that the valve does not remain closed during systole (ie, ventricular contraction). Blood then regurgitates from the left ventricle back into the left atrium (Braunwald et al., 2001).

Clinical Manifestations

Many people have a ballooned leaflet but no symptoms. Others have symptoms of fatigue, shortness of breath, light-headedness, dizziness, syncope, palpitations, chest pain, and anxiety (Braunwald et al., 2001; Freed et al., 1999; Fuster et al., 2001).

Fatigue may occur regardless of the person's activity level and amount of rest or sleep. Shortness of breath is not correlated with activity levels or pulmonary function. Atrial or ventricular dysrhythmias may produce the sensation of palpitations, but palpi-

Glossary

allograft: heart valve replacement made from a human heart valve (synonym: homograft)

annuloplasty: repair of a cardiac valve's outer ring

aortic valve: semilunar valve located between the left ventricle and the aorta

autograft: heart valve replacement made from the patient's own heart valve (ie, the pulmonic valve is excised and used as an aortic valve)

cardiomyopathy: disease of the heart muscle

chordoplasty: repair of the stringy, tendinous fibers that connect the free edges of the atrioventricular valve leaflets to the papillary muscles

commissurotomy: splitting or separating fused cardiac valve leaflets

heterograft: heart valve replacement made of tissue from an animal heart valve (synonym: xenograft)

heterotopic transplantation: procedure in which the recipient's heart remains in place and a donor heart is grafted to the right and anterior of it; the patient has two hearts

homograft: heart valve replacement made from a human heart valve (synonym: allograft)

leaflet repair: repair of a cardiac valve's movable "flaps" (leaflets)

mitral valve: atrioventricular valve located between the left atrium and left ventricle

orthotopic transplantation: the recipient's heart is removed, and a donor heart is grafted into the same site; the patient has one heart

prolapse (of a valve): stretching of an atrioventricular heart valve leaflet into the atrium during systole

pulmonic valve: semilunar valve located between the right ventricle and the pulmonary artery

regurgitation: backward flow of blood through a heart valve

stenosis: narrowing or obstruction of a cardiac valve's orifice

total artificial heart: mechanical device used to aid a failing heart, assisting the right and left ventricles

tricuspid valve: atrioventricular valve located between the right atrium and right ventricle

valve replacement: insertion of a device at the site of a malfunctioning heart valve to restore blood flow in one direction through the heart

valvuloplasty: repair of a stenosed or regurgitant cardiac valve by commissurotomy, annuloplasty, leaflet repair, or chordoplasty (or a combination of procedures)

ventricular assist device: mechanical device used to aid a failing right or left ventricle

xenograft: heart valve replacement made of tissue from an animal heart valve (synonym: heterograft)

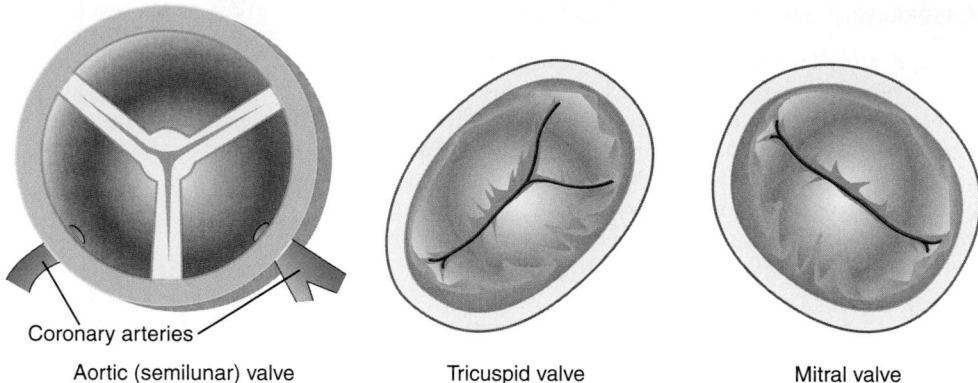

FIGURE 29-1 The valves of the heart (aortic or semilunar, tricuspid, and mitral) in closed position.

Coronary arteries
Aortic (semilunar) valve
Tricuspid valve
Mitral valve

tations have been reported while the heart has been beating normally. Another puzzling symptom is chest pain, which is often localized to the chest and may last for days.

Anxiety may be a response to the symptoms experienced by the patient; however, some patients report anxiety as the only symptom. Some clinicians speculate that the symptoms may be explained by dysautonomia, a dysfunction of the autonomic nervous system, although no consensus exists about the cause of the symptoms experienced by some patients with mitral valve prolapse.

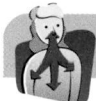 # Physiology/Pathophysiology

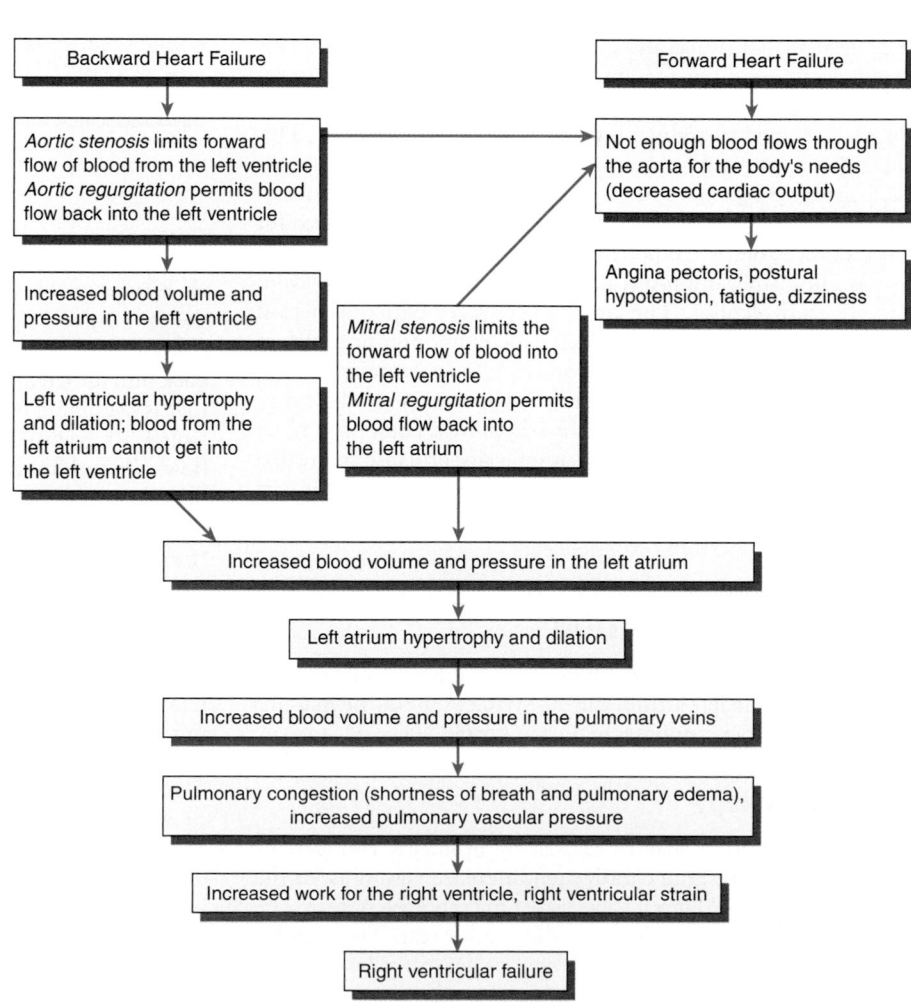

```
Backward Heart Failure                                    Forward Heart Failure

Aortic stenosis limits forward           ──────────→    Not enough blood flows through
flow of blood from the left ventricle                   the aorta for the body's needs
Aortic regurgitation permits blood                      (decreased cardiac output)
flow back into the left ventricle

Increased blood volume and                              Angina pectoris, postural
pressure in the left ventricle                          hypotension, fatigue, dizziness

Left ventricular hypertrophy          Mitral stenosis limits the
and dilation; blood from the          forward flow of blood into
left atrium cannot get into           the left ventricle
the left ventricle                    Mitral regurgitation permits
                                      blood flow back into
                                      the left atrium

         Increased blood volume and pressure in the left atrium

                Left atrium hypertrophy and dilation

         Increased blood volume and pressure in the pulmonary veins

      Pulmonary congestion (shortness of breath and pulmonary edema),
                    increased pulmonary vascular pressure

         Increased work for the right ventricle, right ventricular strain

                        Right ventricular failure
```

FIGURE 29-2 Pathophysiology: Left heart failure as a result of aortic and mitral valvular heart disease and the development of right ventricular failure.

Assessment and Diagnostic Findings

Often, the first and only sign of mitral valve prolapse is identified when a physical examination of the heart discloses an extra heart sound, referred to as a mitral click. The systolic click is an early sign that a valve leaflet is ballooning into the left atrium. In addition to the mitral click, a murmur of mitral regurgitation may be heard if progressive valve leaflet stretching and regurgitation have occurred. A small number of patients experience signs and symptoms of heart failure if mitral regurgitation exists.

Medical Management

Medical management is directed at controlling symptoms. If dysrhythmias are documented and cause symptoms, the patient is advised to eliminate caffeine and alcohol from the diet and to stop smoking; antiarrhythmic medications may be prescribed.

Chest pain that does not respond to nitrates may respond to calcium channel blockers or beta-blockers. Heart failure is treated the same as it would be for any other patient with heart failure (see Chap. 30). In advanced stages of disease, mitral valve repair or replacement may be necessary.

Nursing Management

The nurse educates patients about the diagnosis and the possibility that the condition is hereditary. Because most patients with mitral valve prolapse are asymptomatic, the nurse explains the need to inform the health care provider about any symptoms that may develop. The nurse also instructs patients about the need for prophylactic antibiotic therapy before undergoing invasive procedures (eg, dental work, genitourinary or gastrointestinal procedures) that may introduce infectious agents systemically. This therapy is prescribed for symptomatic patients and for asymptomatic patients who have both a systolic click and murmur or mitral regurgitation. If in doubt about risk factors and the need for antibiotics, patients should consult their physicians.

To minimize symptoms, the nurse teaches patients to avoid caffeine and alcohol. The nurse encourages patients to read product labels, particularly in over-the-counter products such as cough medicine, because these products may contain alcohol, caffeine, ephedrine, and epinephrine, which may produce dysrhythmias and other symptoms. Dysrhythmias, chest pain, heart failure, or other complications of mitral valve prolapse are treated as described in Chapter 30. The nurse also explores with patients possible diet, activity, sleep, and other lifestyle factors that may correlate with symptoms experienced.

MITRAL REGURGITATION

Mitral regurgitation involves blood flowing back from the left ventricle into the left atrium during systole. Often, the margins of the mitral valve cannot close during systole.

Pathophysiology

Mitral regurgitation may be caused by problems with one or more of the leaflets, the chordae tendineae, the annulus, or the papillary muscles. A mitral valve leaflet may shorten or tear. The chordae tendineae may elongate, shorten, or tear. The annulus may be stretched by heart enlargement or deformed by calcification. The papillary muscle may rupture, stretch, or be pulled out of position by changes in the ventricular wall (eg, scar from a

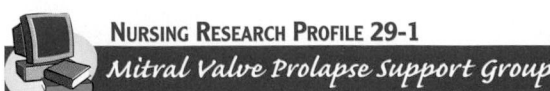

NURSING RESEARCH PROFILE 29-1
Mitral Valve Prolapse Support Group

Scordo, K. A. B. (2001). Factors associated with participating in a mitral valve prolapse support group. *Heart Lung, 30*(2), 128–137.

Purpose
The purpose of this study was to identify factors that influence a patient's attendance at mitral valve prolapse support groups.

Study Sample and Design
Questionnaires were used for this descriptive study of mitral valve support group leaders, current and former support group participants, and nonparticipants, all of whom had a diagnosis of mitral valve prolapse. A total of 376 questionnaires were analyzed.

Findings
People with mitral valve prolapse were more likely to participate in support groups if they were older than 50 years of age and participated in other self-help groups. The reason for attending was to obtain more information about mitral valve prolapse, information not usually available from family, friends, and physicians. No relationship was found between participation in a support group and patient gender, education level, marital status, age when first diagnosed, age when symptoms were first experienced, perceived social support, any symptoms experienced, or travel time or distance required to participate in the support group.

Nursing Implications
Nurses need to be aware that patients with mitral valve prolapse desire information about the condition, and not just at the time of diagnosis or development of symptoms. Nurses can provide education and facilitate support groups. Patients older than 50 years of age and those who participate in other self-help groups may be particularly interested in mitral valve prolapse support groups.

myocardial infarction or ventricular dilation). The papillary muscle may be unable to contract because of ischemia. Regardless of the cause, blood regurgitates back into the atrium during systole.

With each beat of the left ventricle, some of the blood is forced back into the left atrium. Because this blood is added to the blood that is beginning to flow in from the lungs, the left atrium must stretch. It eventually hypertrophies and dilates. The backward flow of blood from the ventricle diminishes the volume of blood flowing into the atrium from the lungs. As a result, the lungs become congested, eventually adding extra strain on the right ventricle. Mitral regurgitation ultimately involves the lungs and the right ventricle.

Clinical Manifestations

Chronic mitral regurgitation is often asymptomatic, but acute mitral regurgitation (eg, that resulting from a myocardial infarction) usually manifests as severe congestive heart failure. Dyspnea, fatigue, and weakness are the most common symptoms. Palpitations, shortness of breath on exertion, and cough from pulmonary congestion also occur.

Assessment and Diagnostic Findings

A systolic murmur is heard as a high-pitched, blowing sound at the apex. The pulse may be regular and of good volume, or it may be irregular as a result of extrasystolic beats or atrial fibrillation.

Echocardiography is used to diagnose and monitor the progression of mitral regurgitation.

Medical Management

Management of mitral regurgitation is the same as that for congestive heart failure. Surgical intervention consists of mitral valve replacement or valvuloplasty (ie, surgical repair of the heart valve).

MITRAL STENOSIS

Mitral stenosis is an obstruction of blood flowing from the left atrium into the left ventricle. It is most often caused by rheumatic endocarditis, which progressively thickens the mitral valve leaflets and chordae tendineae. The leaflets often fuse together. Eventually, the mitral valve orifice narrows and progressively obstructs blood flow into the ventricle.

Pathophysiology

Normally, the mitral valve opening is as wide as the diameter of three fingers. In cases of marked stenosis, the opening narrows to the width of a pencil. The left atrium has great difficulty moving blood into the ventricle because of the increased resistance of the narrowed orifice; it dilates (stretches) and hypertrophies (thickens) because of the increased blood volume it holds. Because there is no valve to protect the pulmonary veins from the backward flow of blood from the atrium, the pulmonary circulation becomes congested. As a result, the right ventricle must contract against an abnormally high pulmonary arterial pressure and is subjected to excessive strain. Eventually, the right ventricle fails.

Clinical Manifestations

The first symptom of mitral stenosis is often breathing difficulty (ie, dyspnea) on exertion as a result of pulmonary venous hypertension. Patients with mitral stenosis are likely to show progressive fatigue as a result of low cardiac output. They may expectorate blood (ie, hemoptysis), cough, and experience repeated respiratory infections.

Assessment and Diagnostic Findings

The pulse is weak and often irregular because of atrial fibrillation (caused by the strain on the atrium). A low-pitched, rumbling, diastolic murmur is heard at the apex. As a result of the increased blood volume and pressure, the atrium dilates, hypertrophies, and becomes electrically unstable, and the patient experiences atrial dysrhythmias. Echocardiography is used to diagnose mitral stenosis. Electrocardiography (ECG) and cardiac catheterization with angiography are used to determine the severity of the mitral stenosis.

Medical Management

Antibiotic prophylaxis therapy is instituted to prevent recurrence of infections. Congestive heart failure is treated as described in Chapter 30. Patients with mitral stenosis may benefit from anticoagulants to decrease the risk for developing atrial thrombus. They may also require treatment for anemia.

Surgical intervention consists of valvuloplasty, usually a commissurotomy to open or rupture the fused commissures of the mitral valve. Percutaneous transluminal valvuloplasty or mitral valve replacement may be performed.

AORTIC REGURGITATION

Aortic regurgitation is the flow of blood back into the left ventricle from the aorta during diastole. It may be caused by inflammatory lesions that deform the leaflets of the aortic valve, preventing them from completely closing the aortic valve orifice. This valvular defect also may result from endocarditis, congenital abnormalities, diseases such as syphilis, a dissecting aneurysm that causes dilation or tearing of the ascending aorta, or deterioration of an aortic valve replacement.

Pathophysiology

In aortic regurgitation, blood from the aorta returns to the left ventricle during diastole in addition to the blood normally delivered by the left atrium. The left ventricle dilates, trying to accommodate the increased volume of blood. It also hypertrophies, trying to increase muscle strength to expel more blood with above-normal force—raising systolic blood pressure. The arteries attempt to compensate for the higher pressures by reflex vasodilation; the peripheral arterioles relax, reducing peripheral resistance and diastolic blood pressure.

Clinical Manifestations

Aortic insufficiency develops without symptoms in most patients. Some patients are aware of a forceful heartbeat, especially in the head or neck. There may be marked arterial pulsations that are visible or palpable at the carotid or temporal arteries. This is a result of the increased force and volume of the blood ejected from the hypertrophied left ventricle. Exertional dyspnea and fatigue follow. Progressive signs and symptoms of left ventricular failure include breathing difficulties (eg, orthopnea, paroxysmal nocturnal dyspnea), especially at night.

Assessment and Diagnostic Findings

A diastolic murmur is heard as a high-pitched, blowing sound at the third or fourth intercostal space at the left sternal border. The pulse pressure (ie, difference between systolic and diastolic pressures) is considerably widened in patients with aortic regurgitation. One characteristic sign of the disease is the water-hammer pulse, in which the pulse strikes the palpating finger with a quick, sharp stroke and then suddenly collapses. Diagnosis may be confirmed by echocardiogram, radionuclide imaging, ECG, magnetic resonance imaging, and cardiac catheterization.

Medical Management

Before the patient undergoes invasive or dental procedures, antibiotic prophylaxis is needed to prevent endocarditis. Heart failure and dysrhythmias are treated as described in Chapters 27 and 30. Aortic valvuloplasty or valve replacement is the treatment of choice, preferably performed before left ventricular failure. Surgery is recommended for any patient with left ventricular hypertrophy, regardless of the presence or absence of symptoms.

AORTIC STENOSIS

Aortic valve stenosis is narrowing of the orifice between the left ventricle and the aorta. In adults, the stenosis may involve congenital leaflet malformations or an abnormal number of leaflets (ie, one or two rather than three), or it may result from rheumatic endocarditis or cusp calcification of unknown cause. The leaflets of the aortic valve may fuse.

Pathophysiology

There is progressive narrowing of the valve orifice, usually over a period of several years to several decades. The left ventricle overcomes the obstruction to circulation by contracting more slowly but with greater energy than normal, forcibly squeezing the blood through the very small orifice. The obstruction to left ventricular outflow increases pressure on the left ventricle, which results in thickening of the muscle wall. The heart muscle hypertrophies. When these compensatory mechanisms of the heart begin to fail, clinical signs and symptoms develop.

Clinical Manifestations

Many patients with aortic stenosis are asymptomatic. After symptoms develop, patients usually first have exertional dyspnea, caused by left ventricular failure. Other signs are dizziness and syncope because of reduced blood flow to the brain. Angina pectoris is a frequent symptom that results from the increased oxygen demands of the hypertrophied left ventricle, the decreased time in diastole for myocardial perfusion, and the decreased blood flow into the coronary arteries. Blood pressure can be low but is usually normal; there may be a low pulse pressure (30 mm Hg or less) because of diminished blood flow.

Assessment and Diagnostic Findings

On physical examination, a loud, rough systolic murmur may be heard over the aortic area. The sound to listen for is a systolic crescendo-decrescendo murmur, which may radiate into the carotid arteries and to the apex of the left ventricle. The murmur is low-pitched, rough, rasping, and vibrating. If the examiner rests a hand over the base of the heart, a vibration may be felt. The vibration is caused by turbulent blood flow across the narrowed valve orifice. Evidence of left ventricular hypertrophy may be seen on a 12-lead ECG and echocardiogram.

Echocardiography is used to diagnose and monitor the progression of aortic stenosis. After the stenosis progresses to the point that surgical intervention is considered, left-sided heart catheterization is necessary to measure the severity of the valvular abnormality and evaluate the coronary arteries. Pressure tracings are taken from the left ventricle and the base of the aorta. The systolic pressure in the left ventricle is considerably higher than that in the aorta during systole.

Medical Management

Antibiotic prophylaxis to prevent endocarditis is essential for anyone with aortic stenosis. After left ventricular failure or dysrhythmias occur, medications are prescribed. Definitive treatment for aortic stenosis is surgical replacement of the aortic valve. Patients who are symptomatic and are not surgical candidates may benefit from one- or two-balloon percutaneous valvuloplasty procedures.

VALVULAR HEART DISORDERS: NURSING MANAGEMENT

The nurse teaches all patients with valvular heart disease about the diagnosis, the progressive nature of valvular heart disease, and the treatment plan. The patient is taught to report any new symp-

toms or changes in symptoms to the health care provider. The nurse emphasizes the need for prophylactic antibiotic therapy before any invasive procedure (eg, dental work, genitourinary or gastrointestinal procedure) that may introduce infectious agents to the patient's bloodstream. The patient is taught that the infectious agent, usually a bacterium, is able to adhere to the diseased heart valve more readily than to a normal valve. Once attached to the valve, the infectious agent multiplies, resulting in endocarditis and further damage to the valve.

The patient's heart rate, blood pressure, and respiratory rate are measured and compared with previous data for any changes. Heart and lung sounds are auscultated and peripheral pulses palpated. The nurse assesses patients with valvular heart disease for signs and symptoms of heart failure: fatigue, dyspnea with exertion, an increase in coughing, hemoptysis, multiple respiratory infections, orthopnea, or paroxysmal nocturnal dyspnea (see Chap. 30). The nurse assesses for dysrhythmias by palpating the patient's pulse for strength and rhythm (ie, regular or irregular) and asks if the patient has experienced palpitations or felt forceful heartbeats (see Chap. 27). The nurse also assesses for dizziness, syncope, increased weakness, or angina pectoris (see Chap. 28).

The nurse collaborates with the patient to develop a medication schedule and teaches about the name, dosage, actions, side effects, and any drug-drug or drug-food interactions of the prescribed medications for heart failure, dysrhythmias, angina pectoris, or other symptoms. The nurse teaches the patient to weigh daily and report the gain of 2 pounds in 1 day or 5 pounds in 1 week to the health care provider. The nurse may assist the patient with planning activity and rest periods to achieve a lifestyle acceptable to the patient. If the patient is to have surgical valve replacement or valvuloplasty, the nurse teaches the patient about the procedure and anticipated recovery.

Valve Repair and Replacement Procedures

VALVULOPLASTY

The repair, rather than replacement, of a cardiac valve is referred to as **valvuloplasty**. The type of valvuloplasty depends on the cause and type of valve dysfunction. Repair may be made to the commissures between the leaflets in a procedure known as **commissurotomy**, to the annulus of the valve by annuloplasty, to the leaflets, or to the chordae by chordoplasty.

Most valvuloplasty procedures require general anesthesia and often require cardiopulmonary bypass. Some procedures, however, can be performed in the cardiac catheterization laboratory; these procedures do not always require general anesthesia or cardiopulmonary bypass. Percutaneous partial cardiopulmonary bypass is used in some cardiac catheterization laboratories. The cardiopulmonary bypass is achieved by inserting a large catheter (ie, cannula) into two peripheral blood vessels, usually a femoral vein and an artery. Blood is diverted from the body through the venous catheter to the cardiopulmonary bypass machine (see Chap. 28) and returned to the patient through the arterial catheter.

The patient is usually managed in a critical care unit for the first 24 to 72 hours after surgery. Care focuses on hemodynamic stabilization and recovery from anesthesia. Vital signs are assessed every 5 to 15 minutes and as needed until the patient recovers from anesthesia or sedation and then every 2 to 4 hours and as needed. Intravenous medications to increase or decrease blood pressure and to treat dysrhythmias or altered heart rates are administered, and their effects are monitored. The intravenous medications are gradually decreased until they are no longer required or the patient takes needed medication by another route (eg, oral, topical). Patient assessments are conducted every 1 to 4 hours and as needed, with particular attention to neurologic, respiratory, and cardiovascular assessments.

After the patient has recovered from anesthesia and sedation, is hemodynamically stable without intravenous medications, and assessments are stable, the patient is usually transferred to a telemetry or surgical unit for continued postsurgical care and teaching. The nurse provides wound care and patient teaching regarding diet, activity, medications, and self-care. Patients are discharged from the hospital in 1 to 7 days. In general, valves that have undergone valvuloplasty function longer than replacement valves, and the patients do not require continuous anticoagulation.

Commissurotomy

The most common valvuloplasty procedure is commissurotomy. Each valve has leaflets; the site where the leaflets meet is called the *commissure.* The leaflets may adhere to one another and close the commissure (ie, stenosis). Less commonly, the leaflets fuse in such a way that, in addition to stenosis, the leaflets are also prevented from closing completely, resulting in a backward flow of blood (ie, regurgitation). A commissurotomy is the procedure performed to separate the fused leaflets.

CLOSED COMMISSUROTOMY

Closed commissurotomies do not require cardiopulmonary bypass. The valve is not directly visualized. The patient receives a general anesthetic, a midsternal incision is made, a small hole is cut into the heart, and the surgeon's finger or a dilator is used to break open the commissure. This type of commissurotomy has been performed for mitral, aortic, tricuspid, and pulmonary valve disease.

Balloon Valvuloplasty. Balloon valvuloplasty (Fig. 29-3) is another type of closed commissurotomy beneficial for mitral valve stenosis in younger patients, for aortic valve stenosis in elderly patients, and for patients with complex medical conditions that place them at high risk for the complications of more extensive surgical procedures. Most commonly used for mitral and aortic valve stenosis, balloon valvuloplasty also has been used for tricuspid and pulmonic valve stenosis. The procedure is performed in the cardiac catheterization laboratory, and the patient may receive a local anesthetic. Patients remain in the hospital 24 to 48 hours after the procedure.

Mitral valvuloplasty is contraindicated for patients with left atrial or ventricular thrombus, severe aortic root dilation, significant mitral valve regurgitation, thoracolumbar scoliosis, rotation of the great vessels, and other cardiac conditions that require open heart surgery.

Mitral balloon valvuloplasty involves advancing one or two catheters into the right atrium, through the atrial septum into the left atrium, across the mitral valve into the left ventricle, and out into the aorta. A guide wire is placed through each catheter, and the original catheter is removed. A large balloon catheter is then placed over the guide wire and positioned with the balloon across the mitral valve. The balloon is then inflated with a dilute angiographic solution. When two balloons are used, they are inflated simultaneously. The advantage of two balloons is that they are each smaller than the one large balloon often used, making smaller atrial septal defects. As the balloons are inflated, they usually do not completely occlude the mitral valve, thereby permitting some forward flow of blood during the inflation period.

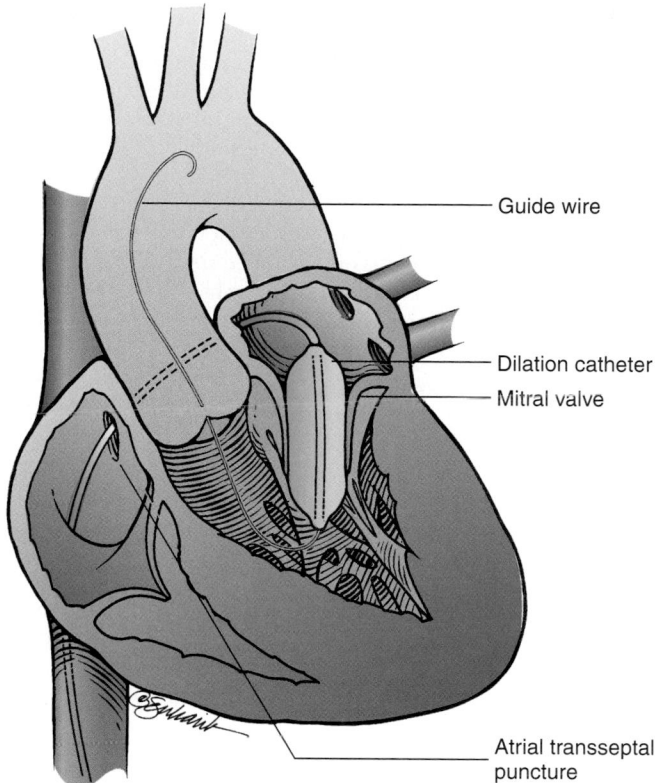

Guide wire

Dilation catheter
Mitral valve

Atrial transseptal puncture

FIGURE 29-3 Balloon valvuloplasty: cross-section of heart illustrating guide wire and dilation catheter placed through an atrial transseptal puncture and across the mitral valve. The guide wire is extended out from the aortic valve into the aorta for catheter support.

All patients have some degree of mitral regurgitation after the procedure. Other possible complications include bleeding from the catheter insertion sites, emboli resulting in complications such as strokes, and rarely, left-to-right atrial shunts through an atrial septal defect caused by the procedure.

Aortic balloon valvuloplasty also may be performed by passing the balloon or balloons through the atrial septum, but it is performed more commonly by introducing a catheter through the aorta, across the aortic valve, and into the left ventricle. The one-balloon or the two-balloon technique can be used for treating aortic stenosis. The aortic procedure is not as effective as the procedure for the mitral valve, and the rate of restenosis is nearly 50% in the first 12 to 15 months after the procedure (Braunwald et al., 2001). Possible complications include aortic regurgitation, emboli, ventricular perforation, rupture of the aortic valve annulus, ventricular dysrhythmias, mitral valve damage, and bleeding from the catheter insertion sites.

OPEN COMMISSUROTOMY

Open commissurotomies are performed with direct visualization of the valve. The patient is under general anesthesia, and a median sternotomy or left thoracic incision is made. Cardiopulmonary bypass is initiated, and an incision is made into the heart. A finger, scalpel, balloon, or dilator may be used to open the commissures. An added advantage of direct visualization of the valve is that thrombus may be identified and removed, calcifications can be seen, and if the valve has chordae or papillary muscles, they may be surgically repaired (chordoplasty is discussed later in this chapter).

Annuloplasty

Annuloplasty is the repair of the valve annulus (ie, junction of the valve leaflets and the muscular heart wall). General anesthesia and cardiopulmonary bypass are required for all annuloplasties. The procedure narrows the diameter of the valve's orifice and is useful for the treatment of valvular regurgitation.

There are two annuloplasty techniques. One technique uses an annuloplasty ring (Fig. 29-4). The leaflets of the valve are sutured to a ring, creating an annulus of the desired size. When the ring is in place, the tension created by the moving blood and contracting heart is borne by the ring rather than by the valve or a suture line, and progressive regurgitation is prevented by the repair. The other technique involves tacking the valve leaflets to the atrium with sutures or taking tucks to tighten the annulus. Because the valve's leaflets and the suture lines are subjected to the direct forces of the blood and heart muscle movement, the repair may degenerate more quickly than with the annuloplasty ring technique.

Leaflet Repair

Damage to cardiac valve leaflets may result from stretching, shortening, or tearing. **Leaflet repair** for elongated, ballooning, or other excess tissue leaflets is removal of the extra tissue. The elongated tissue may be folded over onto itself (ie, tucked) and sutured (ie, leaflet plication). A wedge of tissue may be cut from the middle of the leaflet and the gap sutured closed (ie., leaflet resection) (Fig. 29-5). Short leaflets are most often repaired by chordoplasty. After the short chordae are released, the leaflets often unfurl and can resume their normal function of closing the valve during systole. A piece of pericardium may also be sutured to extend the leaflet. A pericardial patch may be used to repair holes in the leaflets.

Chordoplasty

Chordoplasty is the repair of the chordae tendineae. The mitral valve is involved with chordoplasty (because it has the chordae tendineae); seldom is chordoplasty required for the tricuspid valve.

Regurgitation may be caused by stretched, torn, or shortened chordae tendineae. Stretched chordae tendineae can be shortened, torn ones can be reattached to the leaflet, and shortened ones can be elongated. Regurgitation may also be caused by stretched papillary muscles, which can be shortened.

VALVE REPLACEMENT

Prosthetic **valve replacement** began in the 1960s. When valvuloplasty or valve repair is not a viable alternative, such as when the annulus or leaflets of the valve are immobilized by calcifications, valve replacement is performed. General anesthesia and cardiopulmonary bypass are used for all valve replacements. Most procedures are performed through a median sternotomy (ie, incision through the sternum), although the mitral valve may be approached through a right thoracotomy incision.

After the valve is visualized, the leaflets and other valve structures, such as the chordae and papillary muscles, are removed. Some surgeons leave the posterior mitral valve leaflet, its chordae, and papillary muscles in place to help maintain the shape and function of the left ventricle after mitral valve replacement. Sutures are placed around the annulus and then into the valve prosthesis. The replacement valve is slid down the suture into position and tied into place (Fig. 29-6). The incision is closed, and the surgeon evaluates the function of the heart and the quality of the prosthetic repair. The patient is weaned from cardiopulmonary bypass, and surgery is completed.

Before surgery, the heart gradually adjusted to the pathology, but the surgery abruptly "corrects" the way blood flows through the heart. Complications unique to valve replacement are related to the sudden changes in intracardiac blood pressures. All prosthetic valve replacements create a degree of stenosis when they are implanted in the heart. Usually, the stenosis is mild and does not effect heart function. If valve replacement was for a stenotic valve, blood flow through the heart is often improved. The signs and symptoms of the backward heart failure resolve in a few hours or days. If valve replacement was for a regurgitant valve, it may take months for the chamber into which blood had been regurgitat-

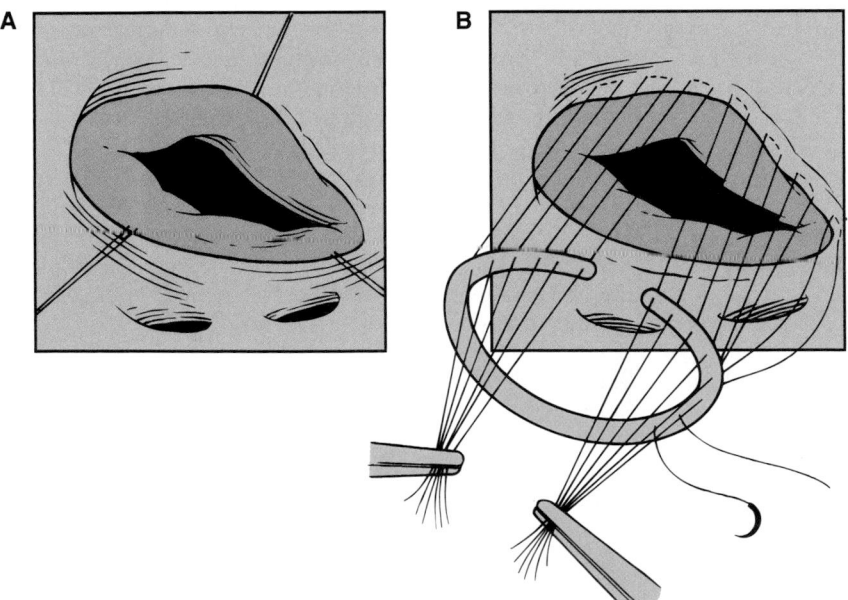
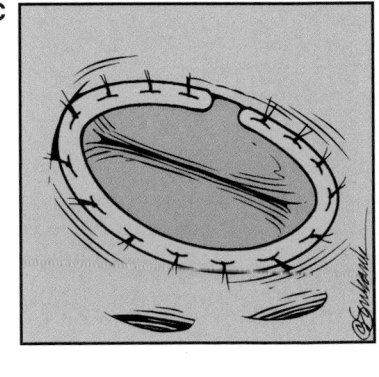

FIGURE 29-4 Annuloplasty ring insertion. (**A**) Mitral valve regurgitation; leaflets do not close. (**B**) Insertion of an annuloplasty ring. (**C**) Completed valvuloplasty; leaflets close.

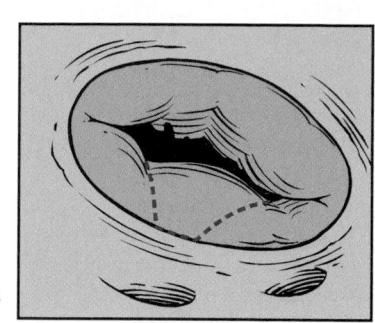
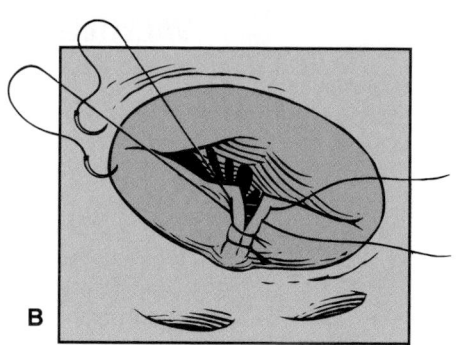
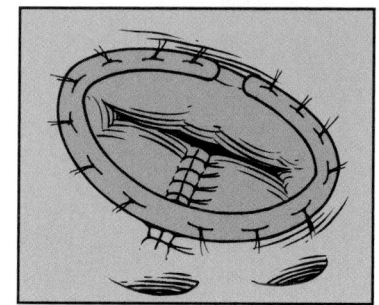

FIGURE 29-5 Valve leaflet resection and repair with a ring annuloplasty. (**A**) Mitral valve regurgitation; the section indicated by dashed lines is excised. (**B**) Approximation of edges and suturing. (**C**) Completed valvuloplasty, leaflet repair, and annuloplasty ring.

ing to achieve its optimal postoperative function. The signs and symptoms of heart failure resolve gradually as the heart function improves. The patient is at risk for many postoperative complications, such as bleeding, thromboembolism, infection, congestive heart failure, hypertension, dysrhythmias, hemolysis, and mechanical obstruction of the valve.

Types of Valve Prostheses

Two types of valve prostheses may be used: mechanical and tissue (ie, biologic) valves. Figure 29-7 shows mechanical and tissue valves.

MECHANICAL VALVES
The mechanical valves are of the ball-and-cage or disk design. Mechanical valves are thought to be more durable than tissue

prosthetic valves and often are used for younger patients. Mechanical valves are used if the patient has renal failure, hypercalcemia, endocarditis, or sepsis and requires valve replacement. The mechanical valves do not deteriorate or become infected as easily as the tissue valves used for patients with these conditions. Thromboemboli are significant complications associated with mechanical valves, and long-term anticoagulation with warfarin is required.

TISSUE OR BIOLOGIC VALVES
Tissue (ie, biologic) valves are of three types: xenografts, homografts, and autografts. Tissue valves are less likely to generate thromboemboli, and long-term anticoagulation is not required. Tissue valves are not as durable as mechanical valves and require replacement more frequently.

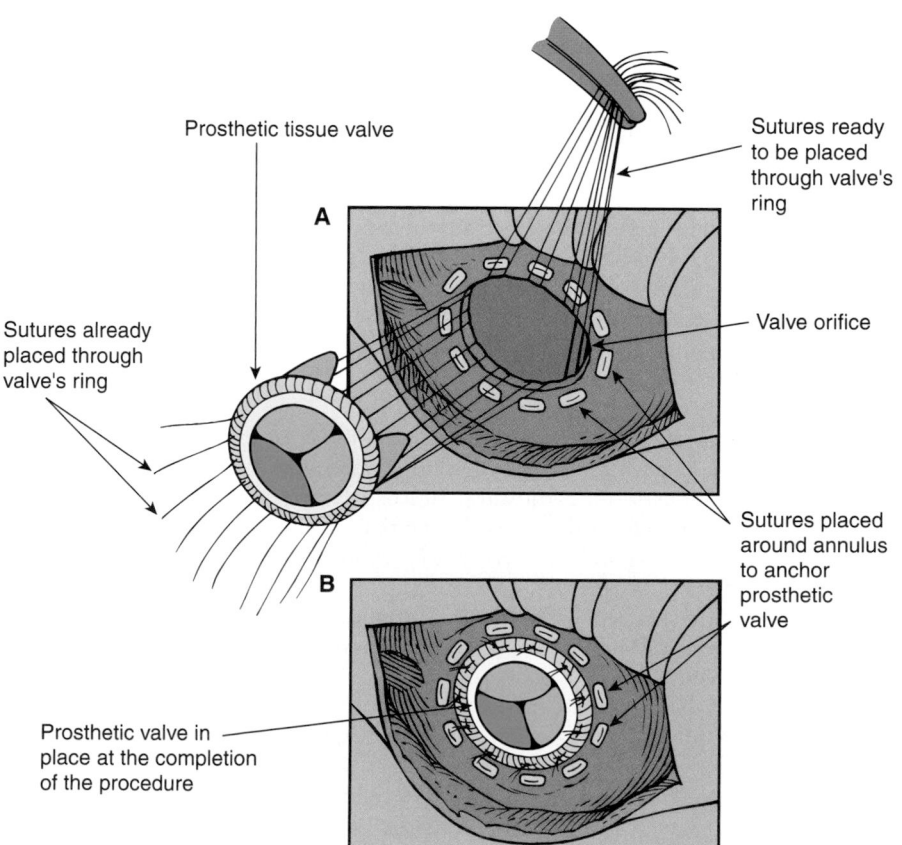

Prosthetic tissue valve

Sutures ready to be placed through valve's ring

Valve orifice

Sutures already placed through valve's ring

Sutures placed around annulus to anchor prosthetic valve

Prosthetic valve in place at the completion of the procedure

FIGURE 29-6 Valve replacement. (**A**) The native valve is excised and the prosthetic valve is sutured in place. (**B**) Once all sutures are placed through the ring, the surgeon slides the prosthetic valve down the sutures and into the natural orifice. The sutures are then tied off and trimmed.

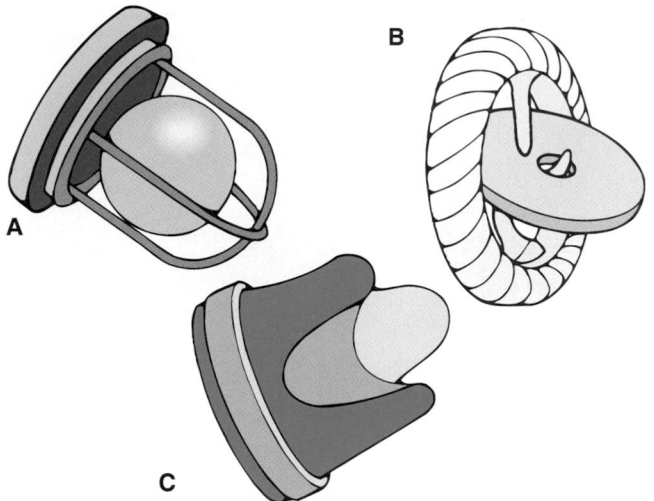

FIGURE 29-7 Common mechanical and tissue valve replacements. (**A**) Caged ball valve (Starr-Edwards, mechanical). (**B**) Tilting-disk valve (Medtronic-Hall, mechanical). (**C**) Porcine heterograft valve (Carpenter-Edwards, tissue).

Xenografts. **Xenografts** are tissue valves (eg, bioprostheses, **heterografts**); most are from pigs (porcine), but valves from cows (bovine) may also be used. Their viability is 7 to 10 years. They do not generate thrombi, thereby eliminating the need for long-term anticoagulation. They are used for women of childbearing age because the potential complications of long-term anticoagulation associated with menses, placental transfer to a fetus, and delivery of a child do not exist. Xenografts also are used for patients older than 70 years of age, patients with a history of peptic ulcer disease, and others who cannot tolerate long-term anticoagulation. Xenografts are used for all tricuspid valve replacements.

Homografts. **Homografts**, or **allografts** (ie, human valves), are obtained from cadaver tissue donations. The aortic valve and a portion of the aorta or the pulmonic valve and a portion of the pulmonary artery are harvested and stored cryogenically. Homografts are not always available and are very expensive. Homografts last for about 10 to 15 years, somewhat longer than xenografts. Homografts are not thrombogenic and are resistant to subacute bacterial endocarditis. They are used for aortic and pulmonic valve replacement.

Autografts. **Autografts** (ie, autologous valves) are obtained by excising the patient's own pulmonic valve and a portion of the pulmonary artery for use as the aortic valve. Anticoagulation is unnecessary because the valve is the patient's own tissue and is not thrombogenic. The autograft is an alternative for children (it may grow as the child grows), women of childbearing age, young adults, patients with a history of peptic ulcer disease, and those who cannot tolerate anticoagulation. Aortic valve autografts have remained viable for more than 20 years.

Most aortic valve autograft procedures are double valve-replacement procedures, because a homograft also is performed for pulmonic valve replacement. If pulmonary vascular pressures are normal, some surgeons elect not to replace the pulmonic valve. The patient can recover without a valve between the right ventricle and the pulmonary artery.

VALVULOPLASTY AND REPLACEMENT: NURSING MANAGEMENT

Patients who have had valvuloplasty or valve replacements are admitted to the intensive care unit; care focuses on recovery from anesthesia and hemodynamic stability. Vital signs are assessed every 5 to 15 minutes and as needed until the patient recovers from anesthesia or sedation and then assessed every 2 to 4 hours and as needed. Intravenous medications to increase or decrease blood pressure and to treat dysrhythmias or altered heart rates are administered and their effects monitored. The intravenous medications are gradually decreased until they are no longer required or the patient takes needed medication by another route (eg, oral, topical). Patient assessments are conducted every 1 to 4 hours and as needed, with particular attention to neurologic, respiratory, and cardiovascular systems. (See Plan of Nursing Care 28-2: Care of the Patient After Cardiac Surgery, in Chap. 28).

After the patient has recovered from anesthesia and sedation, is hemodynamically stable without intravenous medications, and assessment values are stable, the patient is usually transferred to a telemetry unit, typically within 24 to 72 hours after surgery. Nursing care continues as for most postoperative patients, including wound care and patient teaching regarding diet, activity, medications, and self-care.

The nurse educates the patient about long-term anticoagulant therapy, explaining the need for frequent follow-up appointments and blood laboratory studies, and provides teaching about any prescribed medication: the name of the medication, dosage, its actions, prescribed schedule, potential side effects, and any drug-drug or drug-food interactions. Patients with a mechanical valve prosthesis require education to prevent bacterial endocarditis with antibiotic prophylaxis, which is prescribed before all dental and surgical interventions. Patients are discharged from the hospital in 3 to 7 days. Home care and office or clinic nurses reinforce all new information and self-care instructions with the patient and family for 4 to 8 weeks after the procedure.

Septal Repair

The atrial or ventricular septum may have an abnormal opening between the right and left sides of the heart (ie, septal defect). Although most septal defects are congenital and are repaired during infancy or childhood, adults may not have undergone early repair or may develop septal defects as a result of myocardial infarctions or diagnostic and treatment procedures.

Repair of septal defects requires general anesthesia and cardiopulmonary bypass. The heart is opened, and a pericardial or synthetic (usually polyester or Dacron) patch is used to close the opening. Atrial septal defect repairs have low morbidity and mortality rates. When the mitral or tricuspid valve is involved, however, the procedure is more complicated because valve repair or replacement may be required and the heart failure may be more severe. Generally, ventricular septal repairs are uncomplicated, but the proximity of the defect to the intraventricular conduction system and the valves may make this repair more complex. (See Chapter 28, Plan of Nursing Care: Care of the Patient After Cardiac Surgery.)

Cardiomyopathies

Cardiomyopathy is a heart muscle disease associated with cardiac dysfunction. It is classified according to the structural and functional abnormalities of the heart muscle: dilated cardiomyopathy

(DCM), hypertrophic cardiomyopathy (HCM), restrictive or constrictive cardiomyopathy, arrhythmogenic right ventricular cardiomyopathy (ARVC), and unclassified cardiomyopathy (Richardson et al., 1996). *Ischemic cardiomyopathy* is a term frequently used to describe an enlarged heart caused by coronary artery disease, which is usually accompanied by heart failure (see Chap. 30). Regardless of the category and the cause, cardiomyopathy may lead to severe heart failure, lethal dysrhythmias, and death. Cardiomyopathy causes more than 27,000 deaths each year in the United States (American Heart Association, 2001). The mortality rate is highest for African Americans and the elderly (American Heart Association, 2001).

Pathophysiology

The pathophysiology of all cardiomyopathies is a series of progressive events that culminate in impaired cardiac output. Decreased stroke volume stimulates the sympathetic nervous system and the renin-angiotensin-aldosterone response, resulting in increased systemic vascular resistance and increased sodium and fluid retention, which places an increased workload on the heart. These alterations can lead to heart failure (see Chap. 30).

DILATED CARDIOMYOPATHY

DCM is the most common form of cardiomyopathy, with an incidence of 5 to 8 cases per 100,000 people per year and increasing (Braunwald et al., 2001). DCM occurs more often in men and African Americans, who also experience higher mortality rates (Braunwald et al., 2001). DCM is distinguished by significant dilation of the ventricles (Fig. 29-8) without significant concomitant hypertrophy (ie, increased muscle wall thickness) and systolic dysfunction. DCM was formerly named *congestive cardiomyopathy,* but DCM may exist without signs and symptoms of congestion.

Microscopic examination of the muscle tissue shows diminished contractile elements of the muscle fibers and diffuse necrosis of myocardial cells. The result is poor systolic function. These structural changes decrease the amount of blood ejected from the ventricle with systole, increasing the amount of blood remaining in the ventricle after contraction. Less blood is then able to enter the ventricle during diastole, increasing end-diastolic pressure and eventually increasing pulmonary pressures. Altered valve function can result from the enlarged stretched ventricle, usually resulting in regurgitation. Embolic events caused by ventricular and atrial thrombi as a result of the poor blood flow through the ventricle may also occur. More than 75 conditions and diseases may cause DCM, including pregnancy, heavy alcohol intake, and viral infection (eg, influenza). When the causative factor cannot be identified, the term used is *idiopathic DCM.* Idiopathic DCM accounts for approximately 25% of all heart failure cases (Braunwald et al., 2001). Early diagnosis and treatment can prevent or delay significant symptoms and sudden death from DCM. Echocardiography and ECG are used to diagnose DCM and should be conducted for all first-degree relatives (eg, parents, siblings, children) of patients with DCM (Braunwald et al., 2001).

HYPERTROPHIC CARDIOMYOPATHY

In HCM, the heart muscle increases in size and mass, especially along the septum (see Fig. 29-8). The increased thickness of the heart muscle reduces the size of the ventricular cavities and causes the ventricles to take a longer time to relax, making it more difficult for the ventricles to fill with blood during the first part of diastole and making them more dependent on atrial contraction for

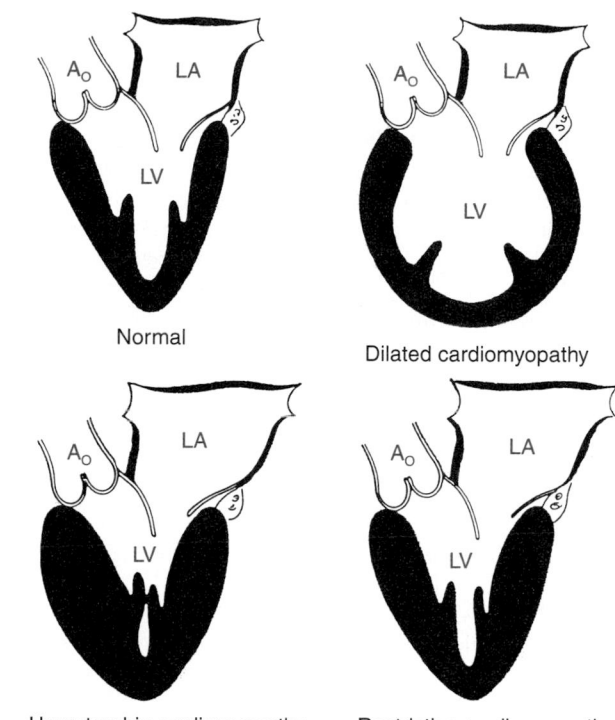

FIGURE 29-8 Cardiomyopathies that lead to congestive heart failure. A$_O$, aorta; LA, left atrium; LV, left ventricle. With permission from Braunwald, E., et al. (Eds.) (2001). *Heart disease: A textbook of cardiovascular medicine* (6th ed.). Philadelphia: W. B. Saunders.

filling. The increased septal size may misalign the papillary muscles so that the septum and mitral valve obstruct the flow of blood from the left ventricle into the aorta during ventricular contraction. Hence, HCM may be obstructive or nonobstructive. Because of the structural changes, HCM had also been called idiopathic hypertrophic subaortic stenosis (IHSS) or asymmetric septal hypertrophy (ASH). Structural changes may also result in a smaller than normal ventricular cavity and a higher velocity flow of blood out of the left ventricle into the aorta, which may be detected by echocardiography (Braunwald et al., 2001). HCM may cause significant diastolic dysfunction, but systolic function can be normal or high, resulting in a higher than normal ejection fraction.

Because HCM is a genetic disease, family members are observed closely for signs and symptoms indicating development of the disease (Fuster et al., 2001). HCM is rare, occurring in men, women, and children (often detected after puberty) (Oakley, 1997) with an estimated prevalence rate of 0.05% to 0.2% (Berul & Zevitz, 2002). It may also be idiopathic (ie, no cause can be found).

RESTRICTIVE CARDIOMYOPATHY

Restrictive cardiomyopathy (RCM) is characterized by diastolic dysfunction caused by rigid ventricular walls that impair ventricular stretch and diastolic filling (see Fig. 29-8). Systolic function is usually normal. Because RCM is the least common cardiomyopathy, representing approximately 5% of pediatric cardiomyopathies, its pathogenesis is the least understood (Shaddy, 2001). Restrictive cardiomyopathy can be associated with amyloidosis (in which amyloid, a protein substance, is deposited within the cells) and other such infiltrative diseases. However, the cause is unknown in most cases (ie, idiopathic).

ARRHYTHMOGENIC RIGHT VENTRICULAR CARDIOMYOPATHY

ARVC occurs when the myocardium of the right ventricle is progressively infiltrated and replaced by fibrous scar and adipose tissue. Initially, only localized areas of the right ventricle are affected, but as the disease progresses, the entire heart is affected. Eventually, the right ventricle dilates and develops poor contractility, right ventricular wall abnormalities, and dysrhythmias. The prevalence of ARVC is unknown because many cases are not recognized. ARVC should be suspected in patients with ventricular tachycardia originating in the right ventricle (ie, a left bundle branch block configuration on ECG) or sudden death, especially among previously symptom-free athletes (McRae et al., 2001). The disease may be genetic (ie, autosomal dominant) (Richardson et al., 1996). Family members should be screened for the disease with a 12-lead ECG, Holter monitor, and echocardiography.

UNCLASSIFIED CARDIOMYOPATHIES

Unclassified cardiomyopathies are different from or have characteristics of more than one of the previously described cardiomyopathies. Examples of unclassified cardiomyopathies include fibroelastosis, noncompacted myocardium, systolic dysfunction with minimal dilation, and mitochondrial involvement (Richardson et al., 1996).

Clinical Manifestations

The patient may have cardiomyopathy but remain stable and without symptoms for many years. As the disease progresses, so do symptoms. Frequently, dilated and restrictive cardiomyopathy are first diagnosed when the patient presents with signs and symptoms of heart failure (eg, dyspnea on exertion, fatigue). Patients with cardiomyopathy may also report paroxysmal nocturnal dyspnea, cough (especially with exertion), and orthopnea, which may lead to a misdiagnosis of bronchitis or pneumonia. Other symptoms include fluid retention, peripheral edema, and nausea, which is caused by poor perfusion of the gastrointestinal system. The patient may experience chest pain, palpitations, dizziness, nausea, and syncope with exertion. However, with HCM, cardiac arrest (ie, sudden cardiac death) may be the initial manifestation in young people, including athletes (Spirito et al., 2000).

Assessment and Diagnostic Findings

Physical examination in the early stage may reveal tachycardia and extra heart sounds. With disease progression, examination also reveals signs and symptoms of heart failure (eg, crackles on pulmonary auscultation, jugular vein distention, pitting edema of dependent body parts, enlarged liver).

Diagnosis is usually made from findings disclosed by the patient history and by ruling out other causes of heart failure, such as myocardial infarction. The echocardiogram is one of the most helpful diagnostic tools because the structure and function of the ventricles can be observed easily. ECG demonstrates dysrhythmias and changes consistent with left ventricular hypertrophy. The chest x-ray film reveals heart enlargement and possibly pulmonary congestion. Cardiac catheterization is sometimes used to rule out coronary artery disease as a causative factor. An endomyocardial biopsy may be performed to analyze myocardial tissue cells.

Medical Management

Medical management is directed toward determining and managing possible underlying or precipitating causes; correcting the heart failure with medications, a low-sodium diet, and an exercise-rest regimen (see Chap. 30); and controlling dysrhythmias with antiarrhythmic medications and possibly with an implanted electronic device, such as an implantable cardioverter-defibrillator (see Chap. 27). If patients exhibit signs and symptoms of congestion, their fluid intake may be limited to 2 liters each day. The person with HCM may also have to limit physical activity to avoid a life-threatening dysrhythmia. A pacemaker may be implanted to alter the electrical stimulation of the muscle and prevent the forceful hyperdynamic contractions that occur with HCM.

SURGICAL MANAGEMENT

When heart failure progresses and medical treatment is no longer effective, surgical intervention, including heart transplantation, is considered. However, because of the limited number of organ donors, many patients die waiting for transplantation. In some cases, a left ventricular assist device (LVAD) is implanted to support the failing heart until a suitable donor heart becomes available (mechanical assist devices and total artificial hearts are discussed later in this chapter).

Left Ventricular Outflow Tract Surgery. When a patient with HCM becomes symptomatic despite medical therapy and a difference in pressure of 50 mm Hg or more exists between the left ventricle and the aorta, surgery is considered. The most common procedure is a myectomy (sometimes referred to as a myotomy-myectomy), in which some of the heart tissue is excised. Septal tissue approximately 1 cm wide and deep is cut from the enlarged septum below the aortic valve. The length of septum removed depends on the degree of obstruction caused by the hypertrophied muscle.

Instead of a septal myectomy, the surgeon may open the left ventricular outflow tract to the aortic valve by removing the mitral valve, chordae, and papillary muscles. The mitral valve then is replaced with a low-profile disk valve. The space taken up by the mitral valve is substantially reduced by the prosthetic valve compared with the patient's own valve, chordae, and papillary muscles, allowing blood to move around the enlarged septum to the aortic valve in the area that the mitral valve once occupied. The primary complication of both procedures is dysrhythmia; additional complications are postoperative surgical complications such as pain, ineffective airway clearance, deep vein thrombosis, risk for infection, and delayed surgical recovery.

Heart Transplantation. The first human-to-human heart transplant was performed in 1967. Since then, transplant procedures, equipment, and medications have continued to improve. Since 1983, when cyclosporine became available, heart transplantation has become a therapeutic option for patients with end-stage heart disease. Cyclosporine (Neoral, Sandimmune, SangCya) is an immunosuppressant that greatly decreases the body's rejection of foreign proteins, such as transplanted organs. Unfortunately, cyclosporine also decreases the body's ability to resist infections, and a satisfactory balance must be achieved between suppressing rejection and avoiding infection.

Cardiomyopathy, ischemic heart disease, valvular disease, rejection of previously transplanted hearts, and congenital heart disease are the most common indications for transplantation (Becker & Petlin, 1999; Rourke et al., 1999). A typical candidate has severe symptoms uncontrolled by medical therapy, no other surgical options, and a prognosis of less than 12 months to live. A multidisciplinary team screens the candidate before recommending the transplantation procedure. The person's age, pulmonary status, other chronic health conditions, psychosocial status, family support, infections, history of other transplantations, compliance, and current health status are considered in the screening.

When a donor heart becomes available, a computer generates a list of potential recipients on the basis of ABO blood group compatibility, the sizes of the donor and the potential recipient, and the geographic locations of the donor and potential recipient; distance is a variable because postoperative function depends on the heart being implanted within 6 hours of harvest from the donor. Some patients are candidates for more than one organ transplant: heart-lung, heart-pancreas, heart-kidney, heart-liver.

Transplantation Techniques. Orthotopic transplantation is the most common surgical procedure for cardiac transplantation (Fig. 29-9). The recipient's heart is removed, and the donor heart is implanted at the vena cava and pulmonary veins. Some surgeons still prefer to remove the recipient's heart leaving a portion of the recipient's atria (with the vena cava and pulmonary veins) in place. The donor heart, which usually has been preserved in ice, is prepared for implant by cutting away a small section of the atria that corresponds with the sections of the recipient's heart that were left in place. The donor heart is implanted by suturing the donor atria to the residual atrial tissue of the recipient's heart. Both techniques then connect the recipient's pulmonary artery and aorta to those of the donor heart.

Heterotopic transplantation is less commonly performed (Fig. 29-10). The donor heart is placed to the right and slightly anterior to the recipient's heart; the recipient's heart is not removed. Initially, it was thought that the original heart might provide some protection for the patient in the event that the transplanted heart was rejected. Although the protective effect has not been proved, other reasons for retaining the original heart have been identified: a small donor heart or pulmonary hypertension (Becker & Petlin, 1999; Kadner et al., 2000).

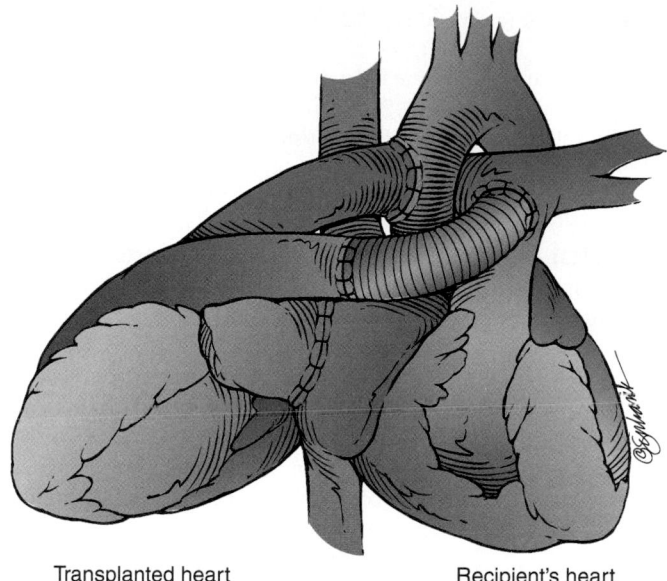

Transplanted heart   Recipient's heart

FIGURE 29-10 Heterotopic method of heart transplantation.

The transplanted heart has no nerve connections with the recipient's body (ie, denervated heart), and the sympathetic and vagus nerves do not affect the transplanted heart. The resting rate of the transplanted heart is approximately 70 to 90 beats per minute, but it increases gradually if catecholamines are in the circulation. Patients must gradually increase and decrease their exercise (ie, extended warm-up and cool-down periods), because 20 to 30 minutes may be required to achieve the desired heart rate. Atropine does not increase the heart rate of these patients.

Postoperative Course. Heart transplant patients are constantly balancing the risk of rejection with the risk of infection. They must comply with a complex regimen of diet, medications, activity, follow-up laboratory studies, biopsies (to diagnose rejection), and clinic visits. Most commonly, patients receive cyclosporine or tacrolimus (FK506, Prograf), azathioprine (Imuran) or mycophenolate mofetil (CellCept), and corticosteroids (ie, prednisone) to minimize rejection.

In addition to rejection and infection, complications may include accelerated atherosclerosis of the coronary arteries (ie, cardiac allograft vasculopathy [CAV] or accelerated graft atherosclerosis [AGA]). Although the cause is unknown, the disease is believed to be immunologically mediated (Augustine, 2000; Rourke et al., 1999). Hypertension may be experienced by patients taking cyclosporine or tacrolimus; the cause has not been identified. Osteoporosis frequently occurs as a side effect of the anti-rejection medications and pretransplantation dietary insufficiency and medications. Posttransplantation lymphoproliferative disease and cancer of the skin and lips are the most common malignancies after transplantation, possibly caused by immunosuppression. Weight gain, obesity, diabetes, dyslipidemias (eg, hypercholesterolemia), hypotension, renal failure, and central nervous system, respiratory, and gastrointestinal disturbances may be caused by the corticosteroids or other immunosuppressants. Other complications are immunosuppressant medication toxicities and responses to the psychosocial stresses imposed by organ transplantation. Patients may experience guilt that someone died for them to live, have anxiety about the new heart, experience depression or fear when rejection is identified, or have difficulty with family role changes before and after transplantation (Augustine, 2000; Becker &

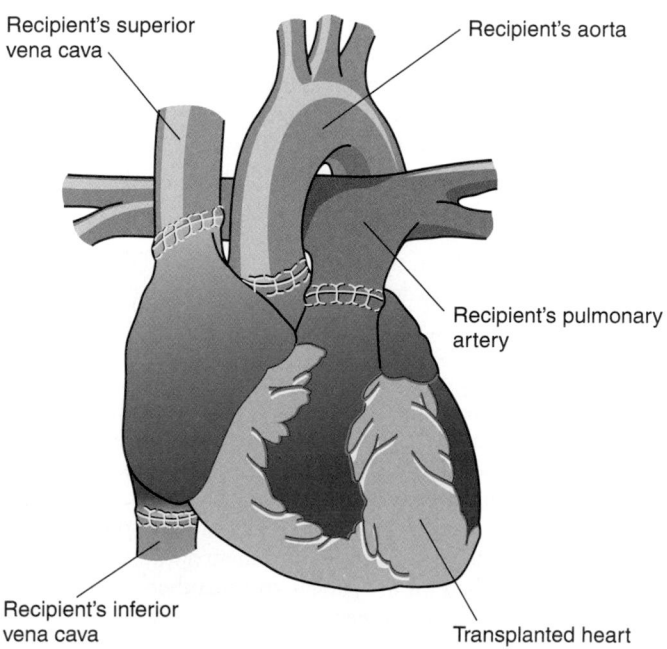

Recipient's superior vena cava

Recipient's aorta

Recipient's pulmonary artery

Recipient's inferior vena cava

Transplanted heart

FIGURE 29-9 Orthotopic method of heart transplantation.

Petlin, 1999; Braunwald et al., 2001; Fuster et al., 2001; Rourke et al., 1999).

The 1-year survival rate for patients with transplanted hearts is approximately 80% to 90%; the 5-year survival rate is approximately 60% to 70% (Augustine, 2000; Becker & Petlin, 1999; Braunwald et al., 2001; Fuster et al., 2001; Rourke et al., 1999).

Mechanical Assist Devices and Total Artificial Hearts. The use of cardiopulmonary bypass for cardiovascular surgery and the possibility of performing heart transplantation for end-stage cardiac disease have increased the need for mechanical assist devices. Patients who cannot be weaned from cardiopulmonary bypass or patients in cardiogenic shock may benefit from a period of mechanical heart assistance. The most commonly used device is the intra-aortic balloon pump (see Chap. 30). This pump decreases the work of the heart during contraction but does not perform the actual work of the heart.

Ventricular Assist Devices. More complex devices that actually perform some or all of the pumping function for the heart also are being used. These more sophisticated **ventricular assist devices** (VADs) (Fig. 29-11) can circulate as much blood per minute as the patient's heart, if not more. Each ventricular assist device is used to support one ventricle. Some ventricular assist devices can be combined with an oxygenator; the combination is called extracorporeal membrane oxygenation (ECMO). The oxygenator–ventricular assist device combination is used for the patient whose heart cannot pump adequate blood through the lungs or the body.

There are three basic types of devices: centrifugal, pneumatic, and electric or electromagnetic. Centrifugal VADs are external, nonpulsatile, cone-shaped devices with internal mechanisms that spin rapidly, creating a vortex (tornado-like action) that pulls blood from a large vein into the pump and then pushes it back into a large artery. Pneumatic VADs are external or implanted pulsatile devices with a flexible reservoir housed in a rigid exterior. The reservoir usually fills with blood drained from the patient's atrium or ventricle. The VAD then forces pressurized air into the rigid housing, compressing the reservoir and returning the blood to the patient's circulation, usually into the aorta. Electric or electromagnetic VADs are similar to the pneumatic VADs, but instead of pressurized air, one or more flat metal plates are pushed against the reservoir to return the blood to the patient's circulation.

Total Artificial Hearts. **Total artificial hearts** are designed to replace both ventricles. Some require the removal of the patient's heart to implant the total artificial heart; others do not. All of these devices are experimental. Although there has been some short-term success, the long-term results have been disappointing. Researchers hope to develop a device that can be permanently implanted and that will eliminate the need for donated human heart transplantation for the treatment of end-stage cardiac disease (Braunwald et al., 2001; Chillcott et al., 1998; Fuster et al., 2001; Rose et al., 1999; Schakenbach, 2001).

Most VADs and total artificial hearts are temporary treatments while the patient's own heart recovers or until a donor heart becomes available for transplantation (ie, "bridge to transplant"). Some devices are being investigated for permanent use. Bleeding disorders, hemorrhage, thrombus, emboli, hemolysis, infection, renal failure, right heart failure, multisystem failure, and mechanical failure are some of the complications of VADs and total artificial hearts (Braunwald et al., 2001; Duke & Perna, 1999; Schakenbach, 2001; Scherr et al., 1999). The nursing care for these patients focuses on assessing for and minimizing these complications and involves providing emotional support and education about the mechanical assist device.

NURSING PROCESS:
THE PATIENT WITH CARDIOMYOPATHY

Assessment

Nursing assessment for the patient with cardiomyopathy begins with a detailed history of the presenting signs and symptoms. The nurse identifies possible etiologic factors, such as heavy alcohol intake, recent illness or pregnancy, or history of the disease in immediate family members. If the patient complains of chest pain, a thorough review of the pain, including its precipitating factors, should be performed. The review of systems includes the presence of orthopnea, paroxysmal nocturnal dyspnea, and syncope or dyspnea with exertion. The number of pillows that are needed to sleep, usual weight, any weight change, and limitation to activities of daily living also are assessed. The New York Heart Association Classification for heart failure is determined. The patient's usual diet is evaluated to determine if alterations are needed to reduce sodium intake.

Because of the chronicity of cardiomyopathy, the nurse compiles a careful psychosocial history exploring the impact of the disease on the patient's role within the family and community. Identification of all perceived stressors helps the patient and the health care team to implement activities to relieve anxiety related to changes in health status. Very early on, the patient's support systems are identified, and members are involved in the patient's care and therapeutic regimen. The assessment addresses the effect the diagnosis has had on the patient and members of his or her support system and the patient's emotional status. Depression is not uncommon in patients with cardiomyopathy who have developed heart failure.

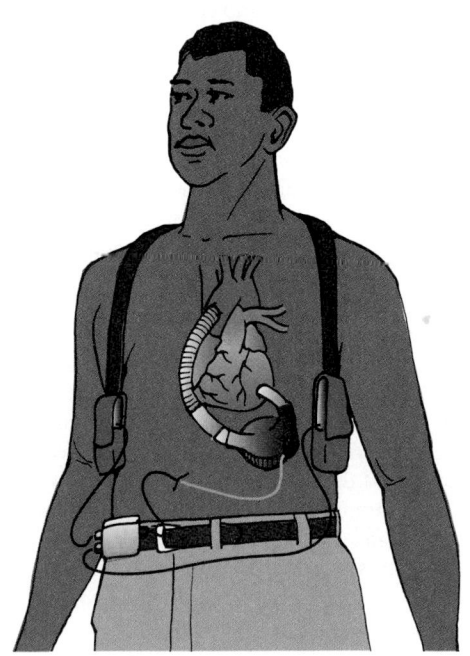

FIGURE 29-11 Left ventricular assist device.

The physical assessment focuses on signs and symptoms of congestive heart failure. The baseline assessment includes such key components as:

- Vital signs
- Calculation of pulse pressure and identification of pulsus paradoxus
- Current weight; determination of weight gain or loss
- Detection by palpation of the point of maximal impulse, often shifted to the left
- Cardiac auscultation for a systolic murmur and third and fourth heart sounds
- Pulmonary auscultation for crackles
- Measurement of jugular vein distention
- Identification of presence and severity of edema

Diagnosis

NURSING DIAGNOSES

Based on the assessment data, major nursing diagnoses for the patient may include:

- Decreased cardiac output related to structural disorders caused by cardiomyopathy or to dysrhythmia from the disease process and medical treatments
- Ineffective cardiopulmonary, cerebral, peripheral, and renal tissue perfusion related to decreased peripheral blood flow (resulting from decreased cardiac output)
- Impaired gas exchange related to pulmonary congestion caused by myocardial failure (decreased cardiac output)
- Activity intolerance related to decreased cardiac output or excessive fluid volume, or both
- Anxiety related to the change in health status and in role functioning
- Powerlessness related to disease process
- Noncompliance with medication and diet therapies

COLLABORATIVE PROBLEMS/ POTENTIAL COMPLICATIONS

Based on the assessment data, potential complications include:

- Congestive heart failure
- Ventricular dysrhythmias
- Atrial dysrhythmias
- Cardiac conduction defects
- Pulmonary or cerebral embolism
- Valvular dysfunction

These complications are discussed earlier in this chapter and in Chapters 27 and 30.

Planning and Goals

The major goals for the patient include improved or maintained cardiac output, increased activity tolerance, reduction of anxiety, adherence to the self-care program, increased sense of power with decision making, and absence of complications.

Nursing Interventions

IMPROVING CARDIAC OUTPUT

During a symptomatic episode, rest is indicated. Many patients with DCM find that sitting up with their legs down is more comfortable than lying down in a bed. This position is helpful in pooling venous blood in the periphery and reducing preload. As-

sessing the patient's oxygen saturation at rest and during activity may assist with determining a need for supplemental oxygen. Oxygen is usually given through nasal cannula when indicated.

Ensuring that medications are taken as prescribed is important to preserving adequate cardiac output. It is important to ensure that patients with HCM avoid diuretics and that patients with DCM avoid verapamil (Calan, Isoptin) to maintain contractility. The nurse may assist the patient with planning a schedule for taking medications and identifying methods to remember to follow it, such as associating the time to take a medication with an activity (eg, eating a meal, brushing teeth). Ensuring that the patient receives or chooses food selections that are appropriate for the low-sodium diet is also important. Determining the patient's weight every day and identifying any significant change is one way to monitor the patient's response to treatment. Assessing if the patient experiences shortness of breath after more or less activity than before treatment is another indication of the effect of treatment. Patients with low cardiac output may need assistance keeping warm and frequently changing position to stimulate circulation and reduce the possibility of skin breakdown.

INCREASING ACTIVITY TOLERANCE

The nurse plans the patient's activities so that they occur in cycles, alternating rest with activity periods. This benefits the patient's physiologic status, and it helps to teach the patient about the need for planned cycles of rest and activity. For example, after taking a bath or shower, the patient should plan to sit and read the paper or pay bills. Suggesting that patients sit while chopping vegetables, drying their hair, or shaving helps them to identify methods to balance rest with activity. The nurse can also make sure that the patient recognizes the symptoms that indicate the need for rest and the actions to take when the symptoms occur. Patients with HCM need to avoid strenuous activity and sports.

REDUCING ANXIETY

Spiritual, psychological, and emotional support may be indicated for the patient, family, and significant others. Interventions are directed toward eradicating or alleviating perceived stressors. The patient is provided with appropriate information about cardiomyopathy and self-management activities. An atmosphere in which the patient feels free to verbalize concerns is provided, as is assurance that these concerns are legitimate. If the patient is facing death or awaiting transplantation, time must be provided to discuss these issues. Providing the patient with realistic hope helps to reduce anxiety while the patient awaits a donor heart. Nurses help the patient, family, and significant others with anticipatory grieving. Accomplishing a goal, no matter how small, also promotes the patient's sense of well-being.

DECREASING THE SENSE OF POWERLESSNESS

Patients need to recognize that they go through a grieving process when given a diagnosis of cardiomyopathy. They are assisted in identifying the things in their life that they have lost (eg, foods that they have enjoyed eating but are high in sodium, ability to engage in constant active lifestyle, ability to play sports, ability to lift grandchildren). They also are assisted in identifying their emotional responses to the loss (eg, anger, depression). The nurse then assists patients in identifying the amount of control that they have in their lives, such as making food choices, managing their medications, and working with their provider to achieve the best possible outcomes. The use of patient tools that track behaviors with the resulting symptoms may be helpful. For example, a diary in which the patient records his or her food selections and weight may assist the patient with understanding the relationship between sodium intake and weight gain. Some patients are able to manage a self-titrating diuretic regimen, in which the patient is able to adjust the dose of diuretic to his or her symptoms.

PROMOTING HOME AND COMMUNITY-BASED CARE

Teaching Patients Self-Care. Teaching patients about the medication regimen, symptom monitoring, and symptom management is a key part of the plan of nursing care. The nurse is integral to the learning process as patients learn to balance their lifestyle and work while accomplishing their therapeutic activities. Helping patients cope with their disease status assists them in adjusting their lifestyles and implementing a self-care program at home.

Continuing Care. The nurse reinforces previous teaching and performs ongoing assessment of the patient's symptoms and progress. The nurse also assists the patient and family to adjust to lifestyle changes. Teaching patients to read nutritional labels, to maintain a record of daily weights and symptoms, and to organize daily activities to increase activity tolerance can be helpful. The patient's responses to diet and fluid restrictions and to the medication regimen are assessed, and explanations about symptoms that should be reported to the physician are emphasized. Because of the risk of dysrhythmia, the patient's family may be taught cardiopulmonary resuscitation. Women are often advised to avoid pregnancy; each case is assessed individually. The nurse assesses the psychosocial needs of the patient and family on an ongoing basis. There may be concerns and fears about the prognosis, changes in lifestyle, effects of medications, and the possibility of others in the family having the same condition that increase the patient's anxiety and interfere with effective coping strategies. Establishing trust is vital to the relationship with these chronically ill patients and their families. This is particularly significant when the nurse is involved with the patient and family in discussions about end-of-life decisions. Patients who have significant symptoms of heart failure or other complications of cardiomyopathy may need a home care referral.

Evaluation

EXPECTED PATIENT OUTCOMES
Expected patient outcomes may include:

1. Maintains or improves cardiac function
   a. Exhibits heart and respiratory rates within normal limits
   b. Reports decreased dyspnea and increased comfort; maintains or improves gas exchange
   c. Reports no weight gain
   d. Maintains or improves peripheral blood flow
2. Maintains or increases activity tolerance
   a. Carries out activities of daily living (eg, brushes teeth, feeds self)
   b. Reports increased tolerance to activity
3. Is less anxious
   a. Discusses prognosis freely
   b. Verbalizes fears and concerns
   c. Participates in support groups if appropriate
4. Decreases sense of powerlessness
   a. Identifies emotional response to diagnosis
   b. Discusses the control he or she has in life
5. Adheres to the self-care program
   a. Takes medications according to prescribed schedule

b. Modifies diet to accommodate sodium and fluid restrictions
c. Modifies lifestyle to accommodate recommended activity and rest behaviors
d. Identifies signs and symptoms to be reported to the health care professional

Cardiac Tumor and Trauma Surgery

TUMOR EXCISION

Tumors of the heart are rare; most (75% to 88%) are benign (Braunwald et al., 2001; Kamiya et al., 2001). Primary tumors occur in less than 1% of the population; metastatic tumors have been reported in 1.5% to 35% of oncology patients (Braunwald et al., 2001; Reynan, 1996; Shapiro, 2001). Tumors may be sites for thrombus formation and therefore create a risk of embolism. Dysrhythmias may occur as the myocardium or conduction system is affected.

Surgical excision is performed to prevent obstruction of a chamber or valve. Cardiopulmonary bypass is used, except for epicardial tumors, which can be excised without entering the heart and without stopping the heart from beating. The tumor location may necessitate valve replacement, myocardial patching, or pacemaker implantation. The nursing care is the same as that for patients undergoing other forms of cardiac surgery (see Chap. 28).

TRAUMA REPAIR

Patients who have sustained nonpenetrating (ie, blunt force) injury or penetrating injury (eg, gunshot wound, stabbing) causing cardiac trauma often do not survive to treatment (Flynn & Bonini, 1999; Thourani et al., 1999). Patients who do survive to treatment often require surgical treatment (Thourani et al., 1999; Wall et al., 1997). The repairs are typically to the valves or septum in blunt force injuries and to the ventricular and atrial walls in penetrating injuries. The wound is débrided and closed surgically when possible, but valve repair and replacement or patch grafts of the septum and atrial or ventricular walls may be required. The surgery is usually an emergency procedure, and the risk of complications from the injury and surgery is high. The nursing care is the same as that for patients undergoing other forms of cardiac surgery (See Chap. 28).

Infectious Diseases of the Heart

Among the most common infections of the heart are infective endocarditis, myocarditis, and pericarditis. The ideal management is prevention.

RHEUMATIC ENDOCARDITIS

Acute rheumatic fever, which occurs most often in school-age children, follows 0.3% to 3% of cases of group A beta-hemolytic streptococcal pharyngitis (Chin, 2001). Prompt treatment of strep throat with antibiotics can prevent the development of rheumatic fever (Chart 29-1). The *Streptococcus* is spread by direct contact with oral or respiratory secretions. Although the bacteria are the causative agents, malnutrition, overcrowding, and lower socioeconomic status may predispose individuals to rheumatic fever (Beers et al., 1999). The incidence of rheumatic fever in the United States and other developed countries is believed to have steadily decreased, but the exact incidence is difficult to deter-

Chart 29-1 • ASSESSMENT

Recognizing and Preventing Rheumatic Fever

Rheumatic fever is a preventable disease. Eradicating rheumatic fever would eliminate rheumatic heart disease. Penicillin therapy in patients with streptococcal infections can prevent almost all primary attacks of rheumatic fever. A throat culture is the only method by which an accurate diagnosis can be determined.

The signs and symptoms of streptococcal pharyngitis are the following:

- Fever (38.9° to 40°C [101° to 104°F])
- Chills
- Sore throat (sudden in onset)
- Diffuse redness of throat with exudate on oropharynx (may not appear until after the first day)
- Enlarged and tender lymph nodes
- Abdominal pain (more common in children)
- Acute sinusitis and acute otitis media (if due to streptococci)

mine because the infection may go unrecognized and patients may not seek treatment (Braunwald et al., 2001; Beers et al., 1999). As many as 39% of patients with rheumatic fever develop various degrees of rheumatic heart disease associated with valvular insufficiency, heart failure, and death (Chin, 2001). The disease also affects all bony joints, producing polyarthritis. The prevalence of rheumatic heart disease is difficult to determine because clinical diagnostic criteria are not standardized and autopsies are not routinely performed. Except for rare outbreaks, the prevalence of rheumatic heart disease in the United States is believed to be less than 0.05 cases per 1000 people (Chin, 2001). The number of U.S. citizens who die from rheumatic heart disease declined from approximately 15,000 in 1950 to about 4,000 in 2001 (AHA, 2001).

Pathophysiology

The heart damage and the joint lesions of rheumatic endocarditis are not infectious in the sense that these tissues are not invaded and directly damaged by destructive organisms; rather, they represent a sensitivity phenomenon or reaction occurring in response to hemolytic streptococci. Leukocytes accumulate in the affected tissues and form nodules, which eventually are replaced by scar tissue. The myocardium is certain to be involved in this inflammatory process; rheumatic myocarditis develops, which temporarily weakens the contractile power of the heart. The pericardium also is affected, and rheumatic pericarditis occurs during the acute illness. These myocardial and pericardial complications usually occur without serious sequelae. Rheumatic endocarditis, however, results in permanent and often crippling side effects.

Clinical Manifestations

Rheumatic endocarditis anatomically manifests first by tiny translucent vegetations or growths, which resemble pinhead-sized beads arranged in a row along the free margins of the valve flaps. These tiny beads look harmless enough and may disappear without injuring the valve leaflets. More often, however, they have serious effects. They are the starting point of a process that gradually thickens the leaflets, rendering them shorter and thicker than normal and preventing them from closing completely. The

result is leakage, a condition called *valvular regurgitation*. The most common site of valvular regurgitation is the mitral valve. In some patients, the inflamed margins of the valve leaflets become adherent, resulting in valvular stenosis, a narrowed or stenotic valvular orifice. Regurgitation and stenosis may occur in the same valve.

A few patients with rheumatic fever become critically ill with intractable heart failure, serious dysrhythmias, and pneumonia. These patients are treated in an intensive care unit. Most patients recover quickly. However, although the patient is free of symptoms, certain permanent residual effects remain that often lead to progressive valvular deformities. The extent of cardiac damage, or even its existence, might not have been apparent in clinical examinations during the acute phase of the disease. Eventually, however, the heart murmurs that are characteristic of valvular stenosis, regurgitation, or both become audible on auscultation and, in some patients, even detectable as thrills on palpation. Usually, the myocardium can compensate for these valvular defects very well for a time. As long as the myocardium can compensate, the patient remains in apparently good health. With continued valvular alterations, the myocardium is unable to compensate (see Fig. 29-2), as evidenced by signs and symptoms of heart failure, as described in Chapter 30.

Assessment and Diagnostic Findings

During assessment, the nurse should keep in mind that the symptoms depend on which side of the heart is involved. The mitral valve is most often affected, producing symptoms of left-sided heart failure: shortness of breath with crackles and wheezes in the lungs (see Chap. 30 for a discussion of left-sided versus right-sided failure). The severity of the symptoms depends on the size and location of the lesion. The systemic symptoms that are present are proportionate to the virulence of the invading organism. When a new murmur is detected in a patient with a systemic infection, infectious endocarditis should be suspected. The patient is also at risk for embolic phenomena of the lung (eg, recurrent pneumonia, pulmonary abscesses), kidney (eg, hematuria, renal failure), spleen (eg, left upper quadrant pain), heart (eg, myocardial infarction), brain (eg, stroke), or peripheral vessels.

Prevention

Rheumatic endocarditis is prevented through early and adequate treatment of streptococcal infections. A first-line approach in preventing initial attacks of rheumatic endocarditis is to recognize streptococcal infections, treat them adequately, and control epidemics in the community. Every nurse should be familiar with the signs and symptoms of streptococcal pharyngitis: high fever (38.9°C to 40°C [101°F to 104°F]), chills, sore throat, redness of the throat with exudate, enlarged lymph nodes, abdominal pain, and acute rhinitis.

NURSING ALERT A throat culture is the only method by which an accurate diagnosis of streptococcal infection of the throat can be made.

Medical Management

The objectives of medical management are to eradicate the causative organism and prevent additional complications, such as a thromboembolic event. Long-term antibiotic therapy is the recommended treatment, and penicillin administered parenterally remains the medication of choice.

The patient who has rheumatic endocarditis and whose valvular dysfunction is mild may require no further treatment. Nevertheless, the danger exists for recurrent attacks of acute rheumatic fever, bacterial endocarditis, embolism from vegetations or mural thrombi in the heart, and eventual cardiac failure.

Nursing Management

A key nursing role in rheumatic endocarditis is teaching patients about the disease, its treatment, and the preventive steps needed to avoid potential complications. After acute treatment with antibiotics, patients need to learn about the need to take prophylactic antibiotics before invasive procedures (see Prevention in the Infective Endocarditis section).

INFECTIVE ENDOCARDITIS

Infective endocarditis is an infection of the valves and endothelial surface of the heart. Endocarditis usually develops in people with cardiac structural defects (eg, valve disorders). Infective endocarditis is more common in older people, probably because of decreased immunologic response to infection and the metabolic alterations associated with aging. There is a high incidence of staphylococcal endocarditis among IV/injection drug users who most commonly have infections of the right heart valves (Bayer et al., 1998; Braunwald, 2001).

The incidence of infective endocarditis remained steady at about 4.2 cases per 100,000 patients in the years from 1950 to the mid-1980s (Braunwald et al., 2001). The incidence then increased, partially attributed to increased IV/injection drug abuse (Braunwald et al., 2001). In 1998, a total of 2212 deaths were attributed to infective endocarditis (American Heart Association, 2001). Invasive procedures, particularly those involving mucosal surfaces, can cause a bacteremia. The bacteremia rarely lasts for more than 15 minutes (Dajani et al., 1997). If a person has some anatomic cardiac defect, bacteremia can cause bacterial endocarditis (Dajani et al., 1997). The combination of the invasive procedure, the particular bacteria introduced into the bloodstream, and the cardiac defect may result in infective endocarditis.

Pathophysiology

Infective endocarditis is most often caused by direct invasion of the endocardium by a microbe (eg, streptococci, enterococci, pneumococci, staphylococci). The infection usually causes deformity of the valve leaflets, but it may affect other cardiac structures such as the chordae tendineae. Other causative microorganisms include fungi and rickettsiae. Patients at higher risk for infective endocarditis are those with prosthetic heart valves, a history of endocarditis, complex cyanotic congenital malformations, and systemic or pulmonary shunts or conduits that were surgically constructed (eg, saphenous vein grafts, internal mammary artery grafts). At high risk are patients with rheumatic heart disease or mitral valve prolapse and those who have prosthetic heart valves (Chart 29-2).

Hospital-acquired endocarditis occurs most often in patients with debilitating disease, those with indwelling catheters, and those receiving prolonged intravenous or antibiotic therapy. Patients receiving immunosuppressive medications or corticosteroids may develop fungal endocarditis.

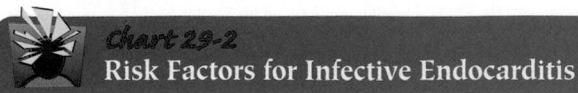

Chart 29-2

Risk Factors for Infective Endocarditis

High Risk
Prosthetic cardiac valves
History of bacterial endocarditis (even without heart disease)
Complex cyanotic congenital malformations
Surgically constructed systemic or pulmonary shunts or conduits

Moderate Risk
Mitral valve prolapse with valvular regurgitation or thickened leaflets
Hypertrophic cardiomyopathy
Acquired valvular dysfunction
Most congenital cardiac malformations (other than those listed above and surgical repair of atrial and ventricular septal defect, or patent ductus arteriosus)

A diagnosis of acute infective endocarditis is made when the onset of infection and resulting valvular destruction is rapid, occurring within days to weeks. The onset of infection may take 2 weeks to months, diagnosed as subacute infective endocarditis (Braunwald et al., 2001).

Clinical Manifestations

Usually, the onset of infective endocarditis is insidious. The signs and symptoms develop from the toxic effect of the infection, from destruction of the heart valves, and from embolization of fragments of vegetative growths on the heart. The occurrence of peripheral emboli is not experienced by patients with right heart valve infective endocarditis (Bayer et al., 1998; Braunwald, 2001). The patient exhibits signs and symptoms similar to those described in rheumatic endocarditis (see previous discussion).

Assessment and Diagnostic Findings

The general manifestations, which may be mistaken for influenza, include vague complaints of malaise, anorexia, weight loss, cough, and back and joint pain. Fever is intermittent and may be absent in patients who are receiving antibiotics or corticosteroids or in those who are elderly or have heart failure or renal failure. Splinter hemorrhages (ie, reddish-brown lines and streaks) may be seen under the fingernails and toenails, and petechiae may appear in the conjunctiva and mucous membranes. Small, painful nodules (Osler's nodes) may be present in the pads of fingers or toes. Hemorrhages with pale centers (Roth's spots) that may be seen in the fundi of the eyes are caused by emboli in the nerve fiber layer of the eye.

The cardiac manifestations include heart murmurs, which may be absent initially. Progressive changes in murmurs over time may be encountered and indicate valvular damage from vegetations or perforation of the valve or the chordae tendineae. Enlargement of the heart or evidence of heart failure is also found.

The central nervous system manifestations include headache, temporary or transient cerebral ischemia, and strokes, which may be caused by emboli to the cerebral arteries. Embolization may be a presenting symptom; it may occur at any time and may involve other organ systems. Embolic phenomena may occur, as discussed in the previous section on rheumatic endocarditis.

Although the described characteristics may indicate infective endocarditis, the signs and symptoms may indicate other diseases as well. A definitive diagnosis is made when a microorganism is found in two separate blood cultures, in a vegetation, or in an abscess. Three sets of blood cultures (with each set including one aerobic and one anaerobic culture) should be obtained before administration of any antimicrobial agents. Negative blood cultures do not totally rule out the diagnosis of infective endocarditis. An echocardiogram may assist in the diagnosis by demonstrating a moving mass on the valve, prosthetic valve, or supporting structures and by identification of vegetations, abscesses, new prosthetic valve dehiscence, or new regurgitation (Braunwald et al., 2001). An echocardiogram may also demonstrate the development of heart failure.

Prevention

Although rare, bacterial endocarditis may be life-threatening. A key strategy is primary prevention in high-risk patients (ie, those with rheumatic heart disease, mitral valve prolapse, or prosthetic heart valves). Antibiotic prophylaxis is recommended for high-risk patients immediately before and sometimes after the following procedures:

- Dental procedures that induce gingival or mucosal bleeding, including professional cleaning and placement of orthodontic bands (not brackets)
- Tonsillectomy or adenoidectomy
- Surgical procedures that involve intestinal or respiratory mucosa
- Bronchoscopy with a rigid bronchoscope
- Sclerotherapy for esophageal varices
- Esophageal dilation
- Gallbladder surgery
- Cystoscopy
- Urethral dilation
- Urethral catheterization if urinary tract infection is present
- Urinary tract surgery if urinary tract infection is present
- Prostatic surgery
- Incision and drainage of infected tissue
- Vaginal hysterectomy
- Vaginal delivery

The type of antibiotic used for prophylaxis varies with the type of procedure and the degree of risk. The patient is usually instructed to take 2 g of amoxicillin (Amoxil) 1 hour before dental, oral, respiratory, or esophageal procedures. If the patient is allergic to penicillin (eg, ampicillin [Omnipen, Polycillin], carbenicillin [Geocillin], cloxacillin [Cloxapen], methicillin [Staphcillin], nafcillin [Nafcil, Unipen], oxacillin [Prostaphlin, Bactocill], penicillin G [Bicillin, Permapen]), clindamycin (Cleocin), cephalexin (Keflex), cefadroxil (Duricef), azithromycin (Zithromax), or clarithromycin (Biaxin) may be used. Recommendations for gastrointestinal or genitourinary procedures are ampicillin and gentamicin (Garamycin) for high-risk patients, amoxicillin or ampicillin for moderate-risk patients, and substituting vancomycin (Vancocin) only for patients allergic to ampicillin or amoxicillin.

The severity of oral inflammation and infection is a significant factor in the incidence and degree of bacteremia. Poor dental hygiene can lead to bacteremia, particularly in the setting of a dental procedure. Regular personal and professional oral health care and rinsing with an antiseptic mouthwash for 30 seconds before dental procedures may assist in reducing the risk of bacteremia. Increased vigilance is also needed in patients with intravenous catheters. To minimize the risk of infection, nurses must ensure that meticulous hand hygiene, site preparation, and the use of

aseptic technique occur during the insertion and maintenance procedures (Schmid, 2000). All catheters are removed as soon as they are no longer needed or no longer function.

Complications

Even if the patient responds to the therapy, endocarditis can be destructive to the heart and other organs. Heart failure and cerebral vascular complications, such as stroke, may occur before, during, or after therapy. The development of heart failure, which may result from perforation of a valve leaflet, rupture of chordae, blood flow obstruction due to vegetations, or intracardiac shunts from dehiscence of prosthetic valves, indicates a poor prognosis with medical therapy alone and a higher surgical risk (Braunwald et al., 2001). Valvular stenosis or regurgitation, myocardial damage, and mycotic (fungal) aneurysms are potential heart complications. Many other organ complications can result from septic or nonseptic emboli, immunologic responses, abscess of the spleen, mycotic aneurysms, and hemodynamic deterioration.

Medical Management

The causative organism may be identified by serial blood cultures. The objective of treatment is to eradicate the invading organism through adequate doses of an appropriate antimicrobial agent.

PHARMACOLOGIC THERAPY
Antibiotic therapy is usually administered parenterally in a continuous intravenous infusion for 2 to 6 weeks. Parenteral therapy is administered in doses that achieve a high serum concentration and for a significant duration to ensure eradication of the dormant bacteria within the dense vegetations. This therapy is often delivered in the patient's home and is monitored by a home care nurse. Serum levels of the selected antibiotic are monitored. If the serum does not demonstrate bactericidal activity, increased dosages of the antibiotic are prescribed, or a different antibiotic is used. Numerous antimicrobial regimens are in use, but penicillin is usually the medication of choice. Blood cultures are taken periodically to monitor the effect of therapy. In fungal endocarditis, an antifungal agent, such as amphotericin B (Abelect, Amphocin, Fungizone), is the usual treatment.

The patient's temperature is monitored at regular intervals because the course of the fever is one indication of the effectiveness of treatment. However, febrile reactions also may occur as a result of medication. After adequate antimicrobial therapy is initiated, the infective organism usually disappears. The patient should begin to feel better, regain an appetite, and have less fatigue. During this time, patients require psychosocial support because, although they feel well, they may find themselves confined to the hospital or home with restrictive intravenous therapy.

SURGICAL MANAGEMENT
After the patient recovers from the infectious process, seriously damaged valves may need to be replaced. Surgical valve replacement greatly improves the prognosis for patients with severe symptoms from damaged heart valves. Aortic or mitral valve excision and replacement are required for patients who develop congestive heart failure despite adequate medical treatment, patients who have more than one serious systemic embolic episode, and patients with uncontrolled infection, recurrent infection, or fungal endocarditis. Many patients who have prosthetic valve endocarditis (ie, infected prostheses) require valve replacement.

Nursing Management

The nurse monitors the patient's temperature; the patient may have fever for weeks. Heart sounds are assessed; a new murmur may indicate involvement of the valve leaflets. The nurse monitors for signs and symptoms of systemic embolization, or for patients with right heart endocarditis, the nurse monitors for signs and symptoms of pulmonary infarction and infiltrates. The nurse assesses signs and symptoms of organ damage such as stroke (ie, cerebrovascular accident or brain attack), meningitis, heart failure, myocardial infarction, glomerulonephritis, and splenomegaly.

Patient care is directed toward management of infection. The patient is started on antibiotics as soon as blood cultures have been obtained. All invasive lines and wounds should be assessed daily for redness, tenderness, warmth, swelling, drainage, or other signs of infection. Patients and their families are instructed about any activity restrictions, medications, and signs and symptoms of infection. The nurse should instruct the patient and family about the need for prophylactic antibiotics before, and possibly after, dental, respiratory, gastrointestinal, or genitourinary procedures. Home care nurses supervise and monitor intravenous antibiotic therapy delivered in the home setting and educate the patient and family about prevention and health promotion. The nurse provides the patient and family with emotional support and facilitates coping strategies during the prolonged course of the infection and antibiotic treatment required. If the patient received surgical treatment, the nurse provides postoperative care and instruction.

MYOCARDITIS

Myocarditis is an inflammatory process involving the myocardium. Myocarditis can cause heart dilation, thrombi on the heart wall (mural thrombi), infiltration of circulating blood cells around the coronary vessels and between the muscle fibers, and degeneration of the muscle fibers themselves. The incidence of myocarditis is estimated to be 1 to 10 cases per 100,000 persons. The rate may be higher because the variety of clinical presentations may cause underreporting (Tang, 2001). Mortality varies with the severity of symptoms. Most patients with mild symptoms recover completely. Other patients may develop cardiomyopathy and heart failure. Patients with symptomatic heart failure and an ejection fraction of less than 45% had a 1-year mortality rate of 20% and a 4-year mortality rate of 56% (Tang, 2001).

Pathophysiology

Myocarditis usually results from a viral, bacterial, mycotic, parasitic, protozoal, or spirochetal infection. It also may occur in patients after acute systemic infections such as rheumatic fever, in those receiving immunosuppressive therapy, or in those with infective endocarditis. Myocarditis may result from an allergic reaction to pharmacologic agents used in the treatment of other diseases. It may begin in one small area and then spread throughout the myocardium. The degree of myocardial involvement determines the degree of hemodynamic effect and resulting signs and symptoms. It is theorized that dilated cardiomyopathy is a latent manifestation of myocarditis.

Clinical Manifestations

The symptoms of acute myocarditis depend on the type of infection, the degree of myocardial damage, and the capacity of the myocardium to recover. The patient may be asymptomatic, and the infection resolves on its own. The patient may develop mild to moderate symptoms and seek medical attention. The patient may also sustain sudden cardiac death or quickly develop severe congestive heart failure. The patient with mild to moderate symptoms often complains of fatigue and dyspnea, palpitations, and occasional discomfort in the chest and upper abdomen.

Assessment and Diagnostic Findings

Assessment of the patient may reveal no abnormalities; as a result, the entire illness goes unrecognized. The patient may complain of chest pain (with a subsequent cardiac catheterization demonstrating normal coronary arteries). The patient without any abnormal heart structure (at least initially) may suddenly develop dysrhythmias. If the patient has developed structural abnormalities (eg, systolic dysfunction), the clinical assessment may disclose cardiac enlargement, faint heart sounds, gallop rhythm, and a systolic murmur.

Prevention

Prevention of infectious diseases by means of appropriate immunizations (eg, influenza, hepatitis) and early treatment appears to be important in decreasing the incidence of myocarditis (Braunwald et al., 2001).

Medical Management

The patient receives specific treatment for the underlying cause if it is known (eg, penicillin for hemolytic streptococci) and is placed on bed rest to decrease the cardiac workload. Bed rest also helps to decrease myocardial damage and the complications of myocarditis. Activities, especially sports in young patients with myocarditis, should be limited for a 6-month period or at least until heart size and function have returned to normal. Physical activity is increased slowly, and the patient is instructed to report any symptoms that occur with increasing activity, such as a rapidly beating heart. The use of corticosteroids in treating myocarditis remains controversial (Braunwald et al., 2001). Nonsteroidal anti-inflammatory drugs (NSAIDs) such as aspirin and ibuprofen are not to be used during the acute phase or if the patient develops heart failure, because these medications can cause further myocardial damage. If the patient develops heart failure, management is essentially the same as for all causes of heart failure (see Chap. 30).

Nursing Management

The nurse assesses the patient's temperature to determine whether the disease is subsiding. The cardiovascular assessment focuses on signs and symptoms of heart failure and dysrhythmia. The patient experiencing dysrhythmias should receive continuous cardiac monitoring with personnel and equipment readily available to treat life-threatening dysrhythmias.

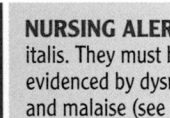

NURSING ALERT Patients with myocarditis are sensitive to digitalis. They must be closely monitored for digitalis toxicity, which is evidenced by dysrhythmia, anorexia, nausea, vomiting, headache, and malaise (see Chap. 30).

Elastic compression stockings and passive and active exercises should be used, because embolization from venous thrombosis and mural thrombi can occur.

PERICARDITIS

Pericarditis refers to an inflammation of the pericardium, the membranous sac enveloping the heart. It may be a primary illness, or it may develop in the course of a variety of medical and surgical disorders. The incidence of pericarditis varies with the cause. For example, pericarditis occurs after pericardectomy (opening of the pericardium) in 5% to 30% of patients after cardiac surgery (Beers et al., 1999). Pericarditis that occurs within 10 days to 2 months after acute myocardial infarction (Dressler's syndrome) causes 1% to 3% of all cases of pericarditis (Beers et al., 1999). Pericarditis may be acute or chronic. It may be classified by the layers of the pericardium becoming attached to each other (adhesive) or by what accumulates in the pericardial sac: serum (serous), pus (purulent), calcium deposits (calcific), clotting proteins (fibrinous), or blood (sanguinous).

Pathophysiology

The following are some of the causes underlying or associated with pericarditis:

- Idiopathic or nonspecific causes
- Infection: usually viral (eg, Coxsackie, influenza); rarely bacterial (eg, streptococci, staphylococci, meningococci, gonococci); and mycotic (fungal)
- Disorders of connective tissue: systemic lupus erythematosus, rheumatic fever, rheumatoid arthritis, polyarteritis
- Hypersensitivity states: immune reactions, medication reactions, serum sickness
- Disorders of adjacent structures: myocardial infarction, dissecting aneurysm, pleural and pulmonary disease (pneumonia)
- Neoplastic disease: caused by metastasis from lung cancer or breast cancer, leukemia, and primary (mesothelioma) neoplasms
- Radiation therapy
- Trauma: chest injury, cardiac surgery, cardiac catheterization, pacemaker implantation
- Renal failure and uremia
- Tuberculosis

Pericarditis can lead to an accumulation of fluid in the pericardial sac (pericardial effusion) and increased pressure on the heart, leading to cardiac tamponade (see Chap. 30). Frequent or prolonged episodes of pericarditis may also lead to thickening and decreased elasticity that restrict the heart's ability to fill properly with blood (constrictive pericarditis). The pericardium may become calcified, further restricting ventricular expansion during ventricular filling (diastole). With less filling, the ventricles pump out less blood, leading to decreased cardiac output and signs and symptoms of heart failure. Restricted diastolic filling may result in increased systemic venous pressure, causing peripheral edema and hepatic failure.

Clinical Manifestations

The most characteristic symptom of pericarditis is chest pain, although pain also may be located beneath the clavicle, in the neck, or in the left scapula region. The pain or discomfort usually remains fairly constant, but it may worsen with deep inspiration and when lying down or turning. It may be relieved with a forward-leaning or sitting position. The most characteristic sign of pericarditis is a friction rub. Other signs may include mild fever,

increased white blood cell count, and increased erythrocyte sedimentation rate (ESR). Dyspnea and other signs and symptoms of heart failure may occur as the result of pericardial compression due to constrictive pericarditis or cardiac tamponade.

Assessment and Diagnostic Findings

Diagnosis is most often made on the basis of the patient's history, signs, and symptoms. An echocardiogram may detect inflammation and fluid build-up, as well as indications of heart failure, and help to confirm the diagnosis. Because the pericardial sac surrounds the heart, a 12-lead ECG detects ST changes in many, if not all, leads.

Medical Management

The objectives of management are to determine the cause, administer therapy, and be alert for cardiac tamponade. When cardiac output is impaired, the patient is placed on bed rest until the fever, chest pain, and friction rub have subsided.

Analgesics and NSAIDs such as aspirin or ibuprofen may be prescribed for pain relief during the acute phase. They also hasten the reabsorption of fluid in the patient with rheumatic pericarditis. Corticosteroids (eg, prednisone) may be prescribed if the pericarditis is severe or if the patient does not respond to NSAIDs. Colchicine may also be used as an alternative medication.

Pericardiocentesis, a procedure in which some of the pericardial fluid is removed, may be performed to assist in the identification of the causative agent. It may also relieve symptoms, especially if there are signs and symptoms of heart failure. A pericardial window, a small opening made in the pericardium, may be performed to allow continuous drainage into the chest cavity. Surgical removal of the tough encasing pericardium (pericardiectomy) may be necessary to release both ventricles from the constrictive and restrictive inflammation.

Nursing Management

The nurse caring for the patient with pericarditis must be alert to the possibility of cardiac tamponade.

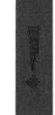

NURSING ALERT Nursing assessment skills are key to anticipating and identifying the triad of symptoms of cardiac tamponade: falling arterial pressure, rising venous pressure, and distant heart sounds.

Patients with acute pericarditis require pain management with analgesics, positioning, and psychological support. Patients experiencing chest pain often benefit from education and reassurance that the pain is not a heart attack. To minimize complications, the nurse educates and assists the patient with activity restrictions until the pain and fever subside. As the patient's condition improves, the nurse encourages gradual increases of activity. If pain, fever, or friction rub reappear, however, activity restrictions must be resumed. The nurse educates the patient and family about a healthy lifestyle to enhance the patient's immune system.

The nurse monitors the patient for heart failure. A patient who is hemodynamically unstable or experiencing congestion is treated the same as a patient with acute heart failure (see Chap. 30).

NURSING PROCESS:
THE PATIENT WITH PERICARDITIS

Assessment

The primary symptom of the patient with pericarditis is pain, which is assessed by observing and evaluating the patient in various positions. While observing the patient, the nurse tries to discover whether the pain is influenced by respiratory movements, with or without the actual passage of air; by flexion, extension, or rotation of the spine, including the neck; by movements of the shoulders and arms; by coughing; or by swallowing. Recognizing the events that precipitate or intensify pain may help establish a diagnosis and differentiate the pain of pericarditis from the pain of myocardial infarction.

A pericardial friction rub occurs when the pericardial surfaces lose their lubricating fluid because of inflammation. The rub is audible on auscultation and is synchronous with the heartbeat. However, it may be elusive and difficult to detect.

> **NURSING ALERT** A pericardial friction rub is diagnostic of pericarditis. The nurse should search diligently for the rub by placing the diaphragm of the stethoscope tightly against the thorax and auscultating the left sternal edge in the fourth intercostal space, the site where the pericardium comes into contact with the left chest wall. A pericardial friction rub has a scratching or leathery sound. The rub is louder at the end of exhalation and may be heard best with the patient sitting and leaning forward.

If there is difficulty in distinguishing a pericardial friction rub from a pleural friction rub, patients are asked to hold their breath; a pericardial friction rub will continue.

The patient's temperature is monitored frequently. Pericarditis may cause an abrupt onset of fever in a patient who has been afebrile.

Diagnosis

NURSING DIAGNOSES

Based on the assessment data, the major nursing diagnosis of the patient may include:

- Acute pain related to inflammation of the pericardium

COLLABORATIVE PROBLEMS/
POTENTIAL COMPLICATIONS

Based on the assessment data, potential complications that may develop include:

- Pericardial effusion
- Cardiac tamponade

Planning and Goals

The patient's major goals may include relief of pain and absence of complications.

Nursing Interventions

RELIEVING PAIN

Relief of pain is achieved by having the patient rest. Because sitting upright and leaning forward is the posture that tends to relieve pain, chair rest may be more comfortable. It is important to instruct the patient to restrict activity until the pain subsides. As the chest pain and friction rub abate, activities of daily living may resume gradually. If the patient is receiving medications such as analgesics, antibiotics, or corticosteroids for the pericarditis, his or her responses are monitored and recorded. If chest pain and friction rub recur, bed or chair rest resumes.

MONITORING AND MANAGING
POTENTIAL COMPLICATIONS

Pericardial Effusion. If the patient does not respond to medical management, fluid may accumulate between the pericardial linings or in the sac. This condition is called *pericardial effusion* (see Chap. 30). Fluid in the pericardial sac can constrict the myocardium and interrupt its ability to pump. Cardiac output declines with each contraction. Failure to identify and treat this problem can lead to the development of cardiac tamponade and the possibility of sudden death.

Cardiac Tamponade. The signs and symptoms of cardiac tamponade begin with falling arterial pressure. Usually, the systolic pressure falls while the diastolic pressure remains stable; hence, the pulse pressure narrows. Heart sounds may progress from sounding distant to being imperceptible. Neck vein distention and other signs of rising central venous pressure are observed. These signs and symptoms occur because, as the fluid-filled pericardial sac compresses the myocardium, blood continues to return to the heart from the periphery but cannot flow into the heart to be pumped back into the circulation.

In such situations, the nurse notifies the physician immediately and prepares to assist with pericardiocentesis (see Chap. 30). The nurse stays with the patient and continues to assess and record signs and symptoms while intervening to decrease the patient's anxiety.

Evaluation

EXPECTED PATIENT OUTCOMES

Expected patient outcomes may include:

1. Is free of pain
   a. Performs activities of daily living without pain, fatigue, or shortness of breath
   b. Temperature returns to normal range
   c. Exhibits no pericardial friction rub
2. Absence of complications
   a. Sustains blood pressure in normal range
   b. Has heart sounds that are strong and can be auscultated
   c. Shows absence of neck vein distention

 Critical Thinking Exercises

1. One of your neighbors has been diagnosed with mitral regurgitation and does not understand why antibiotics need to be taken before undergoing any dental work, including routine checkups. How would you explain the rationale for these instructions?

2. Plans for discharge from the hospital are being made for a 26-year-old man with cardiomyopathy. His 24-year-old wife says she is prepared to care for him at home; she expects that he will be unable to participate extensively in his care. Based on your knowledge about developmental tasks of 24- to 26-year-olds, how would you explain the husband's emotional and physical needs to the wife and the ways she can address these needs, as well as her own? The cardiologist has requested a consult with the transplant services; how will your plan of care change?

3. A patient recovering from heart transplantation has a short attention span, has a poor short-term memory, and cannot sleep well. The family reports the patient is speaking more rapidly than usual and is excessively excited and happy. The surgeon states the high doses of steroids are most likely the reason and expects the symptoms to diminish as the steroids are tapered. Another patient who has undergone the same surgical procedure cries frequently and has reported being overwhelmed by the variety and schedule of medications. The family has not been in to visit the patient for 2 days. How would you explain the different reactions, and how would your teaching strategies for these two patients differ?

4. You are caring for a man with pericarditis. His systolic blood pressure begins to fall, and heart sounds cannot be heard. Describe the actions you would take and why.

REFERENCES AND SELECTED READINGS

Books and Pamphlets

American Heart Association. (2001). *Heart and stroke statistical update.* Dallas, TX: American Heart Association.

Beers, M. H., Berkow, R., & Burs, M. (1999). *The Merck manual of diagnosis and therapy* (17th ed.). Whitehouse Station, NJ: Merck & Co.

Bickley, L. S., & Szilagyi, P. G. (2003). *Bates's guide to physical examination and history taking* (8th ed.). Philadelphia: Lippincott Williams & Wilkins.

Braunwald, E., Zipes, D. P., & Libby, P. (Eds.). (2001). *Heart disease: A textbook of cardiovascular medicine* (6th ed.). Philadelphia: W. B. Saunders.

Fuster, V., Alexander, R. W., O'Rourke, R. A., Roberts, R., King, S. B., III, & Wellens, H. J. J. (Eds.). (2001). *Hurst's the heart* (10th ed.). New York: McGraw-Hill.

Hudak, C. M., Gallo, B. M., & Morton, P. G. (1998). *Critical care nursing: A holistic approach* (7th ed.). Philadelphia: Lippincott-Raven.

McHale, D. J., & Carlson, K. K. (2001). *AACN procedure manual for critical care* (4th ed.). Philadelphia: W. B. Saunders.

Schakenbach, L. H. (2001). Care of the patient with a ventricular assist device. In M. Chulay & S. Wingate (eds.), *Care of the cardiovascular patient series.* Aliso Viejo, CA: American Association of Critical-Care Nurses.

Journals

Asterisks indicate nursing research articles.

Augustine, S. M. (2000). Heart transplantation. *Critical Care Nursing Clinics of North America, 12*(1), 69–77.

Baptiste, M. M. (2001). Aortic valve replacement. *RN, 64*(1), 58–64.

Bayer, A. S., Bolger, A. F., Taubert, K. A., Wilson, W., Stecklberg, J., Karchmer, A. W., et al. (1998). Diagnosis and management of infective endocarditis and its complications. *Circulation, 98*(25), 2936–2948.

Becker, C., & Petlin, A. (1999). Heart transplantation. *American Journal of Nursing, 99* (Suppl. 5), 5–14.

Berul, C., & Zevitz, M. E. (2002). Cardiomyopathy, hypertrophic. *eMedicine Journal, 3*(1). Available at: http://www.emedicine.com/ped/topic1102.htm. Accessed February 26, 2002.

Camp, D. (2000). The left ventricular assist device (LVAD). *Critical Care Nursing Clinics of North America, 12*(1), 61–68.

Canody, C. M., & Savage, L. (1999). The left ventricular assist device. *American Journal of Nursing, 99* (Suppl. 5), 15–20.

Chillcott, S. R., Atkins, P. J., & Adamson, R. M. (1998). Left ventricular assist as a viable alternative for cardiac transplantation. *Critical Care Nurse, 20*(4), 64–79.

Chin, T. K. (2001). Rheumatic heart disease. *eMedicine Journal, 2*(9). Available at: http://www.emedicine.com/ped/topic2007.htm. Accessed February 26, 2002.

Christensen, D. M. (2000). The ventricular assist device: An overview. *Nursing Clinics of North America, 35*(4), 945–959.

Dajani, A. S., Taubert, K. A., Wilson, W., Bolger, A. F., Bayer, A., Ferrieri, P., et al. (1997). Prevention of bacterial endocarditis. *Circulation, 96*(1), 358–366.

Duke, T., & Perna, J. (1999). The ventricular assist device as a bridge to cardiac transplantation. *AACN Clinical Issues, 10*(2), 217–228.

Flynn, M. B., & Bonini, S. (1999). Blunt chest trauma: Case report. *Critical Care Nurse, 19*(5), 68–77.

Fraund, S., Pethig, K., Franke, U., Wahlers, T., Harringer, W., Cremer, J., et al. (1999). Ten year survival after heart transplantation: Palliative procedure or successful long term treatment? *Heart, 82*(1), 47–51.

Freed, L. A., Levy, D., Levine, R. A., Larson, M. G., Evans, J. C., Fuller, D. L., et al. (1999). Prevalence and clinical outcome of mitral-valve prolapse. *New England Journal of Medicine, 34*(1), 1–7.

*Grady, K. L., Jalowiec, A., & White-Williams, C. (1999). Preoperative psychosocial predictors of hospital length of stay after heart transplantation. *Journal of Cardiovascular Nursing, 14*(1), 12–26.

Heijmeriks, J. A., Pourrier, S., Dassen, P., Prenger, K., & Wellens, H. J. J. (1999). Comparison of quality of life after coronary and/or valvular cardiac surgery in patients 75 years of age with younger patients. *American Journal of Cardiology, 83*(7), 1129–1132.

*Kaba, E., Thompson, D. R., & Burnard, P. (2000). Coping after heart transplantation: A descriptive study of heart transplant recipients' methods of coping. *Journal of Advanced Nursing, 32*(4), 930–936.

Kadner, A., Chen, R. H., & Adams, D. H. (2000). Heterotopic heart transplantation: Experiential development and clinical experience. *European Journal of Cardiothoracic Surgery, 7*(4), 474–481.

Kamiya, H., Yasuda, T., Nagamine, H., Sakakibara, N., Nishida, S., Kawasuji, M., et al. (2001). Surgical treatment of primary cardiac tumors: 28 years' experience in Kanazawa University Hospital. *Japan Circulation Journal, 65*(4), 315–319.

McRae, A. I., Chung, M. K., & Asher, C. R. (2001). Arrhythmogenic right ventricular cardiomyopathy: A cause of sudden death in young people. *Cleveland Clinic Journal of Medicine, 68*(5), 459–467.

Morse, C. J. (2001). Advance practice nursing in heart transplantation. *Progress in Cardiovascular Nursing, 16*(1), 21–24, 38.

Nagel, B. M., & O'Keefe, L. M. (1999). Closing in on mitral valve disease. *Nursing, 99* (Critical Care 4), 32cc1–2, 4–7.

Nauer, K. A., Schouchoff, B., & Demitras, K. (2000). Minimally invasive aortic valve surgery. *Critical Care in Nursing Quarterly, 23*(1), 66–71.

Oakley, C. (1997). Aetiology, diagnosis, investigation, and management of the cardiomyopathies. *British Medical Journal, 315*(7121), 1520–1524.

Reynan, K. (1996). Frequency of primary tumor of the heart. *American Journal Cardiology, 77*(1), 107.

Richardson, P., McKenna, W., Bristow, M., Maisch, B., Mautner, B., O'Connell, J., et al. (1996). Report of the 1995 World Health Organization/International Society and Federation of Cardiology Task Force on the Definition and Classification of Cardiomyopathies. *Circulation, 93*(5), 841–842.

Rose, E. A., Moskowitz, A. J., Packer, M., Sollano, J. A., Williams, D. L., Tierney, A. R., et al. (1999). The REMATCH trial: Rationale, design, and endpoints. Randomized evaluation of mechanical assistance for the treatment of congestive heart failure. *Annals of Thoracic Surgery, 67*(3), 723–730.

Rosenhek, R., Binder, T., Porenta, G., Lang, I., Christ, G., Schemper, M., et al. (2000). Predictors of outcome in severe, asymptomatic aortic stenosis. *New England Journal of Medicine, 343*(9), 611–617.

Rourke, T. K., Droogan, M. T., & Ohler, L. (1999). Heart transplantation: State of the art. *AACN Clinical Issues, 10*(2), 185–201.

*Savage, L. S., & Canody, C. (1999). Life with a left ventricular assist device: The patient's perspective. *American Journal of Critical Care, 8*(5), 340–343.

Scherr, K., Jensen, L., & Koshal, A. (1999). Mechanical circulatory support as a bridge to cardiac transplantation: Toward the 21st century. *American Journal of Critical Care, 8*(5), 334–339.

Schmid, M. W. (2000). Risks and complications of peripherally and centrally inserted intravenous catheters. *Critical Care Nursing Clinics of North America, 12*(2), 165–174.

*Scordo, K. A. B. (2001). Factors associated with participating in a mitral valve prolapse support group. *Heart & Lung, 30*(2), 128–137.

Shaddy, R. E. (2001). Cardiomyopathy, restrictive. *eMedicine Journal, 2*(12). Accessed February 26, 2002 from http://www.emedicine.com/ped/topic2503.htm.

Shapiro, L. M. (2001). Cardiac tumors: Diagnosis and management. *Heart, 85*(2), 218–222.

Spirito, P., Bellone, P., Harris, K., Bernabo, P., Bruzzi, P., & Maron, B. (2000). Magnitude of left ventricular hypertrophy and risk of sudden death in hypertrophic cardiomyopathy. *New England Journal of Medicine, 42*(24), 1778–1785.

Sutaria, N., Elder, A. T., & Shaw, T. R. D. (2000). Mitral balloon valvotomy for the treatment of mitral stenosis in octogenarians. *Journal of the American Geriatrics Society, 48*(8), 971–974.

Tang, W. H. T., & Young, R. H. (2001). Myocarditis. *eMedicine Journal, 2*(11). Available at: http://www.emedicine.com/med/topic1569.htm. Accessed February 26, 2002.

Thourani, V. H., Feliciano, D. V., Cooper W. A., Brady, K. M., Adams, A. B., Rozycki, G. S., et al. (1999). Penetrating cardiac trauma in an urban trauma center: A 22-year experience. *American Surgeon, 65*(9), 811–818.

Wahi, S., Haluska, B., Pasquet, A., Case, C., Rimmerman, C. M., & Marwick, T. H. (2000). Exercise echocardiography predicts development of left ventricular dysfunction in medically and surgically treated patients with asymptomatic severe aortic regurgitation. *Heart, 84*(6), 606–614.

Wall, M. J., Jr., Mattox, K. C., Chen, C. D., & Baldwin, J. C. (1997). Acute management of complex cardiac injuries. *The Journal of Trauma, 42*(5), 905–912.

RESOURCES AND WEBSITES

American Heart Association, National Center, 7272 Greenville Avenue, Dallas, TX 75231; 1-800-242-8721; http://www.americanheart.org.

Heartmates, Inc., P.O. Box 16202, Minneapolis, MN 55416; 952-929-3331; http://www.heartmates.com.

National Heart, Lung, and Blood Institute, Health Information Center, National Institutes of Health, P.O. Box 30105, Bethesda, MD 20824; 301-592-8573; http://www.nhlbi.nih.gov.

Management of Patients With Complications From Heart Disease

On completion of this chapter, the learner will be able to:

1. Describe the management of patients with chronic heart failure.
2. Use the nursing process as a framework for care of patients with heart failure.
3. Describe the management of patients with acute heart failure.
4. Develop teaching plans for patients with heart failure.
5. Describe the management of patients with cardiogenic shock.
6. Describe the management of patients with thromboembolic episodes, pericardial effusion and cardiac tamponade, and myocardial rupture.
7. Demonstrate the techniques of cardiopulmonary resuscitation.

*T*oday, the patient with heart disease can be assisted to live longer and achieve a higher quality life than even a decade ago. Through advancements in diagnostic procedures that allow earlier and more accurate diagnoses, treatment can begin well before significant debilitation occurs. Newer treatments, technologies, and pharmacotherapies are being developed rapidly. However, heart disease remains a chronic condition, and complications may develop. This chapter presents the complications most often resulting from heart diseases and the treatments provided by the health care team for these complications.

Cardiac Hemodynamics

The basic function of the heart is to pump blood. The heart's ability to pump is measured by **cardiac output (CO)**, the amount of blood pumped in 1 minute. CO is determined by measuring the heart rate (HR) and multiplying it by the **stroke volume (SV)**, which is the amount of blood pumped out of the ventricle with each contraction. CO usually is calculated using the equation $CO = HR \times SV$.

One of the factors controlling HR is the autonomic nervous system. When SV falls, the nervous system is stimulated to increase HR and thereby maintain adequate CO. SV depends on three factors: preload, afterload, and contractility.

Preload is the amount of myocardial stretch just before systole caused by the pressure created by the volume of blood within the ventricle. Like a rubber band, the ventricular muscle fibers need to be stretched (by the blood) to produce optimal ejection of blood. Too little or too much muscle fiber stretch decreases the volume of blood ejected. The major factor that determines preload is venous return, the volume of blood that enters the ventricle during diastole. Another factor that determines preload is ventricular **compliance**, which is the elasticity or amount of "give" when blood enters the ventricle. Elasticity is decreased when the muscle thickens, as in hypertrophic cardiomyopathy (see Chap. 29) or when there is increased fibrotic tissue within the ventricle. Fibrotic tissue replaces dead cells, such as after a myocardial infarction (see Chap. 28). Fibrotic tissue has little compliance, making the ventricle stiff. Given the same volume of blood, a noncompliant ventricle has a higher intraventricular pressure than a compliant one. The higher pressure increases the workload of the heart and can lead to **heart failure (HF)**.

Afterload refers to the amount of resistance to the ejection of blood from the ventricle. To eject blood, the ventricle must overcome this resistance. Afterload is inversely related to SV. The major factors that determine afterload are the diameter and distensibility of the great vessels (aorta and pulmonary artery) and the opening and competence of the semilunar valves (pulmonic and aortic valves). The more open the valves, the lower the resistance. If the patient has significant vasoconstriction, hypertension, or a narrowed opening from a stenotic valve, resistance (afterload) increases. When afterload increases, the workload of the heart must increase to overcome the resistance and eject blood.

Contractility, which refers to the force of contraction, is related to the number and status of myocardial cells. Catecholamines, released by sympathetic stimulation such as exercise or from administration of positive inotropic medications, can increase contractility and stroke volume. MI causes necrosis of some myocardial cells, shifting the workload to the remaining cells. Significant loss of myocardial cells can decrease contractility and cause HF. Afterload must be reduced by stress reduction techniques or medications to match the lower contractility.

Glossary

afterload: the amount of resistance to ejection of blood from a ventricle

anuria: urine output of less than 50 mL per 24 hours

cardiac failure: heart failure

cardiac output (CO): the amount of blood pumped out of the heart in 1 minute

compliance: the elasticity or amount of "give" when blood enters the ventricle

congestive heart failure (CHF): a fluid overload condition (congestion) that may or may not be caused by HF; often an acute presentation of HF with increased amount of fluid in the blood vessels

contractility: the force of ventricular contraction; related to the number and state of myocardial cells

diastolic heart failure: the inability of the heart to pump sufficiently because of an alteration in the ability of the heart to fill; current term used to describe a type of HF

dyspnea on exertion (DOE): shortness of breath that occurs with exertion

ejection fraction (EF): percent of blood volume in the ventricles at the end of diastole that is ejected during systole; a measurement of contractility

heart failure (HF): the inability of the heart to pump sufficient blood to meet the needs of the tissues for oxygen and nutrients; signs and symptoms of pulmonary and systemic congestion may or may not be present

left-sided heart failure (left ventricular failure): inability of the left ventricle to fill or pump (empty) sufficient blood to meet the needs of the tissues for oxygen and nutrients; traditional term used to describe patient's HF symptoms

oliguria: diminished urine output; less than 400 mL per 24 hours

orthopnea: shortness of breath when lying flat

paroxysmal nocturnal dyspnea (PND): shortness of breath that occurs suddenly during sleep

pericardiocentesis: procedure that involves surgically opening the pericardial sac

pericardiotomy: surgically created opening of the pericardium

preload: the amount of myocardial stretch just before systole caused by the pressure created by the volume of blood within a ventricle

pulmonary edema: abnormal accumulation of fluid occurring in the interstitial spaces or in the alveoli of the lungs

pulseless electrical activity (PEA): condition in which electrical activity is present but there is not an adequate pulse or blood pressure because of ineffective cardiac contraction or circulating blood volume

pulsus paradoxus: systolic blood pressure that is more than 10 mm Hg higher during exhalation than during inspiration; difference is normally less than 10 mm Hg

right-sided heart failure (right ventricular failure): inability of the right ventricle to fill or pump (empty) sufficient blood to the pulmonary circulation

stroke volume (SV): amount of blood pumped out of the ventricle with each contraction

systolic heart failure: inability of the heart to pump sufficiently because of an alteration in the ability of the heart to contract; current term used to describe a type of HF

thermodilution: method of determining cardiac output that involves injecting fluid into the pulmonary artery catheter. A thermistor measures the difference between the temperature of the fluid and the temperature of the blood ejected from the ventricle. Cardiac output is calculated from the change in temperature.

NONINVASIVE ASSESSMENT OF CARDIAC HEMODYNAMICS

Several noninvasive assessment findings can indicate cardiac hemodynamic status, although the findings do not directly correlate to preload, afterload, or contractility. Right ventricular preload may be estimated by measuring jugular venous distention. Elevated left ventricular preload may be identified by a positive hepatojugular test. Mean arterial blood pressure is a rough indicator of left ventricular afterload. Activity tolerance may be used as an indicator of overall cardiac functioning. These assessments are described in more detail later in the chapter.

Impedance cardiography (ICG) is a noninvasive method for continuous calculation of SV, CO, systemic vascular resistance, ventricular contractility, and fluid status (Turner, 2000). Electrodes are placed on the patient's chest. The electrodes are connected to a device that transmits a very small amount of alternating electric current through the chest and measures the resistance (Z) to the flow (conduction) of the current. Because the current seeks the path of least resistance and fluid is an excellent conductor, the current flows through the blood. ICG measures the volume of blood flow.

The cardiac cycle produces normal changes in blood flow volume; for example, there is more blood flow volume during systole and less blood flow volume during diastole. The changes in blood flow volume change the resistance to flow of the current, which is called electrical impedance (dZ). During systole, the higher blood flow volume causes the red blood cells to be aligned in a more parallel pattern, which makes the flow of current faster and reduces impedance. During diastole, the lower blood flow volume causes the red blood cells to be more randomly arranged, which makes the flow of current slower and increases impedance. Stroke volume is determined by comparing dZ to the changes in time (dt) (Von Rueden & Turner, 1999). The preejection period (PEP) and ventricular ejection times (VET) can be measured, which further assists in understanding the hemodynamic status of the patient. For example, a dysfunctional left ventricle requires more time to generate pressure to overcome the resistance to ejection so that the aortic valve opens (increased PEP) and has less time during which blood is ejected into the aorta (decreased VET).

INVASIVE ASSESSMENT OF CARDIAC HEMODYNAMICS

An important method for evaluating the components of SV in a hemodynamically unstable patient is the pulmonary artery (PA) catheter, which is used to obtain the hemodynamic data essential for diagnosis and treatment (see Chap. 26). Connected to a computerized transducer apparatus, the PA catheter serves as a fluid-filled conduit for detecting pressure changes within the heart. The pulsatile changes in pressure are converted into electrical signals, which are displayed as waveforms on a monitor (Fig. 30-1; Chart 30-1).

CO is measured most often by the **thermodilution** method with the thermistor port of the catheter. The port is connected to a computer that calculates CO and other cardiac parameters. In thermodilution, a specific volume of fluid that is colder than the patient's blood is injected into the proximal port (right atrium). The fluid enters the right ventricle and is then ejected into the PA. The thermistor records the temperature before and after the ejection of fluid. The change in temperature is inversely related to CO; the greater the CO, the faster the blood and fluid moves, the less time the fluid has to mix with the blood to cause a change

in temperature, and the less change in temperature detected by the thermistor.

Cardiac parameters for afterload and contractility are calculated at the same time as CO (Table 30-1). Measurements of the various pressures are made at intervals. Therapy, especially intravenous medication, is adjusted based on the assessment and diagnostic findings.

The patient with an invasive hemodynamic catheter is usually managed in an intensive care environment (see Chart 30-1) because of the need for frequent nursing assessments and interventions.

Heart Failure

HF, often referred to as **congestive heart failure (CHF)**, is the inability of the heart to pump sufficient blood to meet the needs of the tissues for oxygen and nutrients. However, the term CHF is misleading, because it indicates that patients must experience pulmonary or peripheral congestion to have HF, and it implies that patients with congestion have HF. The Agency for Health Care Policy and Research (AHCPR) HF guidelines panel (1994) defined HF as a clinical syndrome characterized by signs and symptoms of fluid overload or of inadequate tissue perfusion. These signs and symptoms result when the heart is unable to generate a CO sufficient to meet the body's demands. The HF guideline panel used the term *heart failure* because many patients with HF do not manifest pulmonary or systemic congestion. The term HF is preferred and indicates myocardial heart disease in which there is a problem with contraction of the heart (systolic dysfunction) or filling of the heart (diastolic dysfunction) and which may or may not cause pulmonary or systemic congestion. Some cases of HF are reversible, depending on the cause. Most often, HF is a life-long diagnosis that is managed with lifestyle changes and medications to prevent acute congestive episodes. CHF is usually an acute presentation of HF.

CHRONIC HEART FAILURE

As with coronary artery disease, the incidence of HF increases with age. However, the rate of coronary artery disease is decreasing and just the opposite is true for HF. Nearly 5 million people in the United States have HF, with more than one-half million new cases diagnosed each year (American Heart Association, 2001). The prevalence rate of HF among non-Hispanic whites 20 years of age or older is 2.3% for men and 1.5% for women; for non-Hispanic blacks, the rates are 3.5% and 3.1%, respectively (American Heart Association, 2001). HF is the most common reason for hospitalization of people older than age 65 and the second most common reason for visits to a physician's office. The rate of readmission to the hospital remains staggeringly high. The rise in the incidence of HF reflects the increased number of elderly and improvements in treatment of HF resulting in increased survival rates. However, the economic burden caused by HF is estimated to be more than 23 billion dollars in direct and indirect costs and is expected to increase (American Heart Association, 2001). Many hospitalizations could be prevented by improved and appropriate outpatient care. Prevention and early intervention to arrest the progression of HF are major health initiatives in the United States.

Medical management is based on the type, severity, and cause of HF. There are two types of HF, which are identified by assessment of left ventricular functioning: an alteration in ventricular filling (**diastolic heart failure**) and an alteration in ventricular contraction

(text continues on page 792)

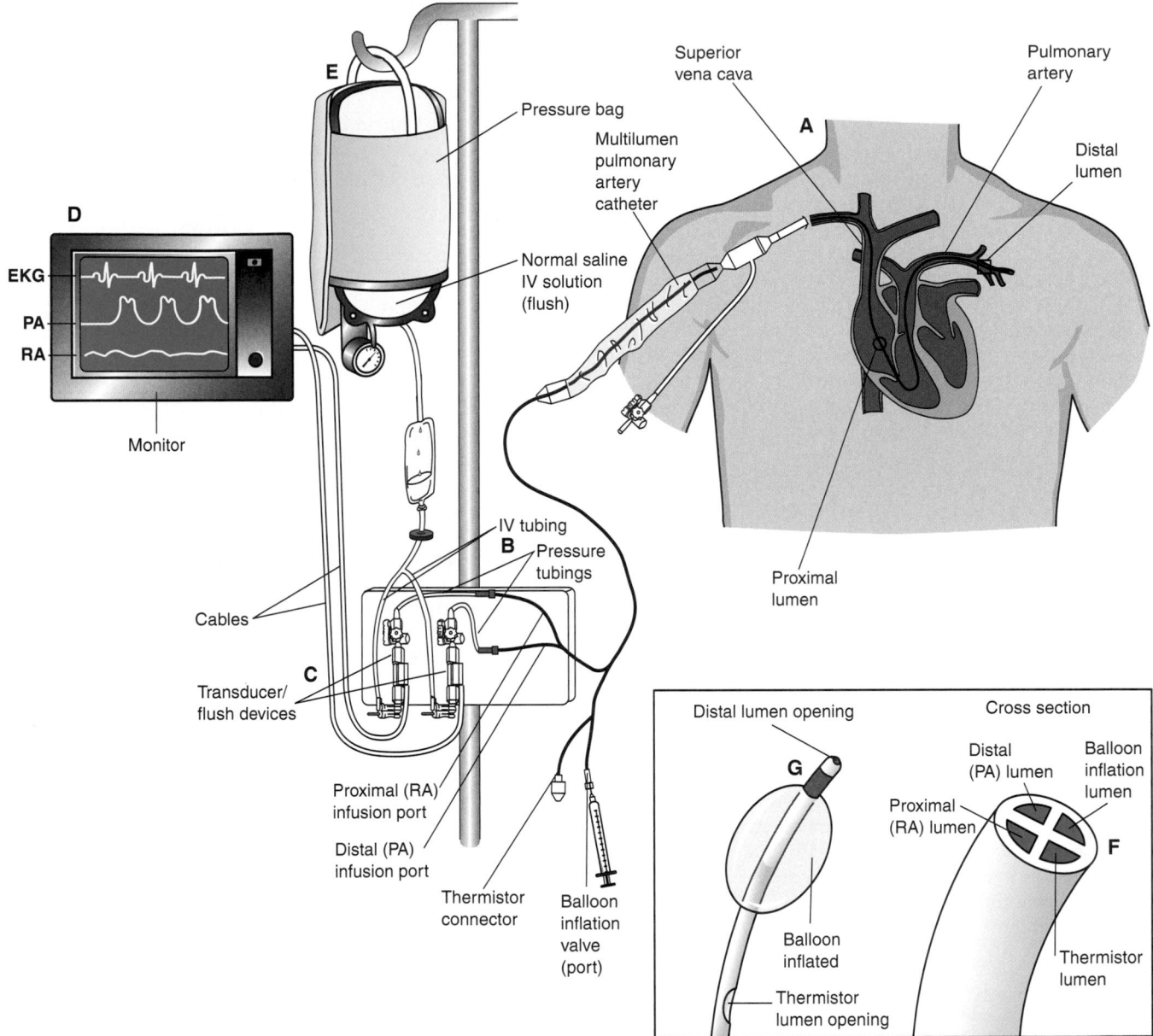

FIGURE 30-1 The pulmonary artery (PA) catheter system serves as a fluid-filled conduit for detecting pressure changes within the heart. (**A**) The PA catheter is inserted through a sheath into the superior vena cava, usually via the right internal jugular or subclavian vein. It is connected to pressure tubing (**B**) which is then connected to a transducer (**C**). The transducer detects pulsatile changes in pressure and converts them into electrical signals. These signals are converted into waveforms, which are shown on a monitor (**D**). The transducer also contains a flush device (**E**) that automatically infuses a small amount of flush fluid through the catheter to help maintain its patency. Because of the pressure that the heart generates, pressure is applied to the flush fluid to ensure that the fluid flows into the catheter and into the bloodstream and that blood does not flow back into the catheter. The PA catheter contains several lumens (**F**) with openings located at various intervals. These lumens allow for the measurement of hemodynamic pressures at different points. The proximal port is usually in the right atrium and is used to measure central venous pressure (CVP). The distal tip of the catheter rests in the pulmonary artery and measures the pulmonary artery systolic and diastolic pressures. When the balloon is inflated (**G**), the tip floats into smaller branches of the pulmonary artery until it can no longer pass, that is, until it is "wedged" in the vessel. The distal tip then records the pressure in front of it, called pulmonary artery wedge pressure (PAWP). Cardiac output is measured most often by the thermodilution method with the thermistor port. The port is connected to a computer that calculates cardiac output and other cardiac parameters.

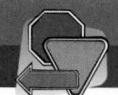

Chart 30-1

GUIDELINES FOR Hemodynamic Monitoring: Multilumen Pulmonary Artery Catheter

ACTIONS	RATIONALE/AMPLIFICATION
Preparatory Phase	
1. Explain the procedure to the patient, family, and significant others.	1. The information may assist in reducing the patient's anxiety, which may also help to limit the patient's movement during the procedure.
2. Check vital signs and apply ECG electrodes.	2. An initial assessment provides a baseline for comparison.
3. Position the patient to allow the physician access to the insertion site, decrease the risk of complications, and promote patient comfort. To ensure consistency, the angle of elevation should be documented if the patient cannot lie flat.	3. The patient is usually placed in a flat or Trendelenburg position to minimize the risk of air embolization and facilitate access.
4. Set up equipment according to manufacturer's directions.	4. Monitoring systems and setups vary according to manufacturer.
a. The pulmonary artery (PA) catheter requires pressure tubing, a transducer, a flush system, and a pressure amplifier connected to a monitoring–recording system. In addition, an IV pole and a transducer holder are usually needed.	a. The complexity of the setup requires an understanding of the equipment in use.
b. The pressure equipment is calibrated and flushed according to the manufacturer's directions.	b. Flushing the catheter system ensures patency and eliminates air bubbles.
c. The balloon is inflated with air to test for leakage.	c. Testing for leakage ensures that the balloon is intact.
5. Prepare the skin over the insertion site.	5. Decreases risk of infection at insertion site
Performance Phase (Physician Responsibility)	
1. The PA catheter is inserted through a sheath that has been placed in the internal jugular, subclavian, or any easily accessible, large-diameter vein by percutaneous puncture or venotomy. The sheath may be surrounded by a protective cover that maintains the sterility of the catheter.	1. The internal jugular vein insertion site has standard landmarks, establishes a straight route into the central venous system, and is associated with few complications. The subclavian insertion site allows the patient more mobility. It is also easier to secure the catheter from this site.
2. The catheter is advanced while observing the monitor for pressure waveforms, which indicate the placement of the tip of the catheter within the heart. Occasionally fluoroscopy is used to verify proper placement of the PA catheter.	2. Catheter placement is determined by characteristic waveforms and changes.
3. When the catheter is in the large vein, the balloon is inflated to its recommended volume.	3. The amount of air to be used is indicated on the catheter.
4. The patient's blood flow will gently pull the inflated balloon at the tip of the catheter through the right atrium and tricuspid valve into the right ventricle and into the main pulmonary artery. The monitoring equipment displays specific pressure waveforms as the catheter advances through the various chambers of the heart. These initial waveforms and pressures are recorded.	4. Watching the ECG monitor for signs of ventricular irritability as the catheter enters the right ventricle allows dysrhythmias to be reported to the physician promptly. Subsequent pressure readings are taken from this baseline.
5. The flowing blood will continue to direct the catheters more distally into the pulmonary arteries. When the catheter reaches a pulmonary vessel that is approximately the same size or slightly smaller in diameter than the inflated balloon, it will not advance any further. This is the wedge position from which pulmonary artery wedge pressure (PAWP) [pulmonary artery obstructive pressure (PAOP) or pulmonary capillary wedge pressure (PCWP)] is measured.	5. With the catheter in the wedge position, the balloon blocks the flow of blood from the right side of the heart toward the lungs. The resulting artery wedge pressure (PAWP) correlates with the mean left ventricular end-diastolic pressure.
6. The pressure is recorded with the balloon wedged in the pulmonary vascular bed. A mean capillary wedge pressure between 8 and 12 mm Hg indicates normal left ventricular function.	6. Wedge pressure is a valuable measure of cardiac function. Lower-than-normal pressure readings indicate hypovolemia. Higher-than-normal pressure readings indicate hypervolemia and/or left ventricular failure.
7. The balloon is then deflated, causing the catheter to retract spontaneously into a larger pulmonary artery. The change in the catheter tip position causes a reappearance of the pulmonary artery waveform. The pulmonary artery systolic, diastolic, and mean pressures are recorded.	7. The normal pulmonary artery systolic pressure is 15 to 30 mm Hg, and the diastolic pressure range is 10 to 15 mm Hg. The normal mean pulmonary artery pressure (average pressure in pulmonary artery throughout the entire cardiac cycle) ranges from 10 to 20 mm Hg. Elevated pulmonary pressures can indicate several clinical problems, such as pulmonary disease, mitral valve disease, and ventricular failure.

(continued)

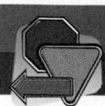

ACTIONS	RATIONALE/AMPLIFICATION
8. The protective cover is attached to the introducer and secured to the catheter. The catheter is sutured in place and a dry dressing placed over the insertion site.	8. Maintaining catheter sterility in this manner allows for the advancement and repositioning of the catheter if needed. Apply sterile dressing.
9. A chest x-ray to confirm catheter position and to serve as a baseline for future reference is obtained after catheter insertion.	9. Accurate position will assure accurate readings and prevent complications.

To Obtain a Wedge Pressure Reading

1. Inflate the balloon slowly until the pulmonary artery pressure waveform changes (indicating a wedge pressure waveform) and an increase in resistance to injection is detected. Once these changes occur, no more air is introduced. (The amount of air to cause these changes should be less than 1.5 mL.) Most cardiac monitors allow for freezing the wedge pressure waveform and its immediate printing.	1. Do not allow the catheter to remain in the wedge position. The decrease in blood flow through the pulmonary artery that occurs when wedging the catheter may cause segmental pulmonary infarction.
2. As soon as the wedge pressure is obtained, allow passive deflation of the balloon by releasing pressure on the syringe. To make sure that the syringe cannot be inflated accidentally, remove it, push the plunger to the bottom of the barrel so that it is totally empty of air, reattach it to the PA catheter, and lock it closed.	2. These are standard safety measures.

Follow-up Phase

1. Inspect the insertion site daily. Observe for signs of infection, swelling, and bleeding.	1. Careful monitoring helps prevent complications. A foreign body (catheter) in the vascular system increases the risk of sepsis.
2. In accord with protocol, record date and time of dressing change and IV tubing change. If a peripheral vessel access site is used, assess the extremity for color, temperature, capillary filling, and sensation.	2. Ischemia may occur from inadequate arterial flow.
3. Evaluate pulse.	3. Absence of a pulse may indicate occlusion of the vessel.
4. Assess for complications: pneumothorax, pulmonary ischemia or infarction (due to persistent balloon wedging from inflation or catheter migration), pulmonary artery rupture (due to overinflation of the balloon), dysrhythmias, heart block, damage to tricuspid valve, knotting of catheter within the heart or blood vessels, thromboembolus, infection, balloon rupture, hematoma at insertion site, and bleeding.	4. These are standard nursing practices.

For Removal of the Catheter

1. Explain the procedure to the patient, and make sure the balloon is not inflated.	1. An informed patient is less fearful; a deflated balloon is less likely to injure the patient's heart or blood vessels during catheter removal.
2. Place the patient in a supine position.	2. The supine position results in the least patient movement and is the best position for maintaining blood pressure and venous return.
3. Stop all IVs running through the PA catheter and turn stopcocks off.	3. This prevents fluid from infusing into tissues as the catheter is removed; it also prevents air from entering the catheter.
4. While the patient holds the breath or exhales, the catheter is withdrawn gently and continuously, without excessive force or traction; a sterile dressing is applied over the site.	4. Positive intrathoracic pressure minimizes the chance of air entering the chest and vasculature through or around the catheter. Continuous gentle traction minimizes the risk of the catheter becoming kinked, knotted, or tangled. A sterile dressing minimizes the risk of infection from the skin wound.

(systolic heart failure). An assessment of the **ejection fraction (EF)** is performed to assist in determining the type of HF. EF is the percentage of the end-diastolic blood volume in the ventricle minus the end-systolic blood volume in the ventricle divided by the end-diastolic blood volume in the ventricle—an indication of the amount of blood that was ejected and the contractile ability of the ventricle. The EF is normal in diastolic HF, whereas the EF is less than 40% in systolic HF. The severity of HF is frequently classified according to the patient's symptoms. The New York Heart Association classification is described in Table 30-2, and the causes are explained in subsequent sections of this chapter.

Pathophysiology

HF results from a variety of cardiovascular diseases but leads to some common heart abnormalities that result in decreased contraction (systole), decreased filling (diastole), or both. Significant myocardial dysfunction most often occurs before the patient experiences signs and symptoms of HF.

Systolic HF decreases the amount of blood ejected from the ventricle, which stimulates the sympathetic nervous system to release epinephrine and norepinephrine. The purpose of this initial response is to support the failing myocardium, but the continued

Table 30-1 • **Hemodynamic Parameters**

PARAMETER	RIGHT VENTRICLE	LEFT VENTRICLE
Preload		
Normal Values	CVP: 0–8 mm Hg	PAWP: 4–12 mm Hg
Afterload		
Normal Values	PVR: 20–120 dyne/sec/cm^{-5}	SVR: 800–1500 dyne/sec/cm^{-5}
Calculation	$\dfrac{\text{mean PAP} - \text{PAWP}}{\text{CO}} \times 80$	$\dfrac{\text{Mean arterial pressure} - \text{CVP}}{\text{CO}} \times 80$
Contractility		
Normal Values	Right ventricular stroke work index: 7–12 g/beat/m^2	Left ventricular stroke work index: 35–85 g/beat/m^2
Calculation	$\dfrac{(\text{PA systolic pressure} - \text{CVP}) \times \text{SV} \times 0.0136}{\text{Body Surface Area (height and weight)}}$	$\dfrac{(\text{Systolic BP} - \text{PAWP}) \times \text{SV} \times 0.0136}{\text{Body Surface Area (height and weight)}}$

BP, blood pressure; CO, cardiac output; CVP, central venous pressure; PA, pulmonary artery; PAP, pulmonary artery pressure; PAWP, pulmonary artery wedge pressure; PVR, pulmonary vascular resistance; SV, stroke volume; SVR, systemic vascular resistance.

response causes loss of beta$_1$-adrenergic receptor sites (down-regulation) and further damage to the heart muscle cells. The sympathetic stimulation and the decrease in renal perfusion by the failing heart cause the release of renin by the kidney. Renin promotes the formation of angiotensin I, a benign, inactive substance. Angiotensin-converting enzyme (ACE) in the lumen of blood vessels converts angiotensin I to angiotensin II, a vasoconstrictor that also causes the release of aldosterone. Aldosterone promotes sodium and fluid retention and stimulates the thirst center. Aldosterone causes additional detrimental effects to the myocardium and exacerbates myocardial fibrosis (Pitt et al., 1999; Weber, 2001). Angiotensin, aldosterone, and other neurohormones (eg, atrial natriuretic factor, endothelin, and prostacyclin) lead to an increase in preload and afterload, which increases stress on the ventricular wall, causing an increase in the workload of the heart.

Table 30-2 • **New York Heart Association (NYHA) Classification of Heart Failure**

CLASSIFICATION	SYMPTOMS	PROGNOSIS
I	Ordinary physical activity does not cause undue fatigue, dyspnea, palpitations, or chest pain. No pulmonary congestion or peripheral hypotension. Patient is considered asymptomatic. Usually no limitations of activities of daily living (ADLs)	Good
II	Slight limitation on ADLs. Patient reports no symptoms at rest but increased physical activity will cause symptoms. Basilar crackles and S$_3$ murmur may be detected	Good
III	Marked limitation on ADL. Patient feels comfortable at rest but less than ordinary activity will cause symptoms	Fair
IV	Symptoms of cardiac insufficiency at rest	Poor

As the heart's workload increases, contractility of the myofibrils decreases. Decreased contractility results in an increase in end-diastolic blood volume in the ventricle, stretching the myofibers and increasing the size of the ventricle (ventricular dilation). The increased size of the ventricle further increases the stress on the ventricular wall, adding to the workload of the heart. One way the heart compensates for the increased workload is to increase the thickness of the heart muscle (ventricular hypertrophy). However, the hypertrophy is not accompanied by an adequate increase in capillary blood supply, resulting in myocardial ischemia. The sympathetic-induced coronary artery vasoconstriction, increased ventricular wall stress, and decreased mitochondrial energy production also lead to myocardial ischemia. Eventually, the myocardial ischemia causes myofibril death, even in patients without coronary artery disease. The compensatory mechanisms of HF have been called the "vicious cycle of HF" because the heart does not pump sufficient blood to the body, which causes the body to stimulate the heart to work harder; the heart is unable to respond and failure becomes worse.

Diastolic HF develops because of continued increased workload on the heart, which responds by increasing the number and size of myocardial cells (ie, ventricular hypertrophy and altered myocellular functioning). These responses cause resistance to ventricular filling, which increases ventricular filling pressures despite a normal or reduced blood volume. Less blood in the ventricles causes decreased CO. The low CO and high ventricular filling pressures cause the same neurohormonal responses as described for systolic HF.

Etiology

Myocardial dysfunction is most often caused by coronary artery disease, cardiomyopathy, hypertension, or valvular disorders. Atherosclerosis of the coronary arteries is the primary cause of HF. Coronary artery disease is found in more than 60% of the patients with HF (Braunwald et al., 2001). Ischemia causes myocardial dysfunction because of resulting hypoxia and acidosis from the accumulation of lactic acid. Myocardial infarction causes focal heart muscle necrosis, the death of heart muscle cells, and a loss of contractility; the extent of the infarction correlates with the severity of HF. Revascularization of the coronary artery by a percutaneous coronary intervention or by coronary artery bypass surgery may correct the underlying cause so that HF is resolved.

Cardiomyopathy is a disease of the myocardium. There are three types: dilated, hypertrophic, and restrictive (see Chap. 29). Dilated cardiomyopathy, the most common type of cardiomyopathy, causes diffuse cellular necrosis, leading to decreased contractility (systolic failure). Dilated cardiomyopathy can be idiopathic (unknown cause), or it can result from an inflammatory process, such as myocarditis, from pregnancy, or from a cytotoxic agent, such as alcohol or adriamycin. Hypertrophic cardiomyopathy and restrictive cardiomyopathy lead to decreased distensibility and ventricular filling (diastolic failure). Usually, HF due to cardiomyopathy becomes chronic. However, cardiomyopathy and HF may resolve after the end of pregnancy or with the cessation of alcohol ingestion.

Systemic or pulmonary hypertension increases afterload (resistance to ejection), which increases the workload of the heart and leads to hypertrophy of myocardial muscle fibers; this can be considered a compensatory mechanism because it increases contractility. However, the hypertrophy may impair the heart's ability to fill properly during diastole.

Valvular heart disease is also a cause of HF. The valves ensure that blood flows in one direction. With valvular dysfunction, blood has increasing difficulty moving forward, increasing pressure within the heart and increasing cardiac workload, leading to diastolic HF. Chapter 29 discusses the effects of valvular heart disease.

Several systemic conditions contribute to the development and severity of HF, including increased metabolic rate (eg, fever, thyrotoxicosis), iron overload (eg, from hemochromatosis), hypoxia, and anemia (serum hematocrit less than 25%). All of these conditions require an increase in CO to satisfy the systemic oxygen demand. Hypoxia or anemia also may decrease the supply of oxygen to the myocardium. Cardiac dysrhythmias may cause HF, or they may be a result of HF; either way, the altered electrical stimulation impairs the myocardial contraction and decreases the overall efficiency of myocardial function. Other factors, such as acidosis (respiratory or metabolic), electrolyte abnormalities, and antiarrhythmic medications, can worsen the myocardial dysfunction.

Clinical Manifestations

The clinical manifestations produced by the different types of HF (systolic, diastolic, or both) are similar (Chart 30-2) and therefore do not assist in differentiating the types of HF. The signs and symptoms of HF are most often described in terms of the effect on the ventricles. **Left-sided heart failure (left ventricular failure)** causes different manifestations than **right-sided heart failure (right ventricular failure)**. Chronic HF produces signs and symptoms of failure of both ventricles. Although dysrhythmias (especially tachycardias, ventricular ectopic beats, or atrioventricular [AV] and ventricular conduction defects) are common in HF, they may also be a result of treatments used in HF (eg, side effect of digitalis).

LEFT-SIDED HEART FAILURE

Pulmonary congestion occurs when the left ventricle cannot pump the blood out of the ventricle to the body. The increased left ventricular end-diastolic blood volume increases the left ventricular end-diastolic pressure, which decreases blood flow from the left atrium into the left ventricle during diastole. The blood volume and pressure in the left atrium increases, which decreases blood flow from the pulmonary vessels. Pulmonary venous blood volume and pressure rise, forcing fluid from the pulmonary capillar-

Chart 30-2 • ASSESSMENT

Signs and Symptoms of Heart Failure

General
Pale, cyanotic skin (with decreased perfusion to extremities)
Dependent edema (with increased venous pressure)
Decreased activity tolerance

Cardiovascular
Apical impulse, enlarged and left lateral displacement (with cardiac enlargement)
Third heart sound (S_3)
Murmurs (with valvular dysfunction)
Tachycardia
Increased jugular venous distention (JVD)

Cerebrovascular
Lightheadness
Dizziness
Confusion

Gastrointestinal
Nausea and anorexia
Enlarged, pulsatile liver
Ascites
Hepatojugular test, increased (with increased right ventricular filling pressure)

Renal
Decreased urinary frequency during the day
Nocturia

Respiratory
Dyspnea on exertion
Orthopnea
Paroxysmal nocturnal dyspnea
Bilateral crackles that do not clear with cough

ies into the pulmonary tissues and alveoli, which impairs gas exchange. These effects of left ventricular failure have been referred to as *backward failure*. The clinical manifestations of pulmonary venous congestion include dyspnea, cough, pulmonary crackles, and lower-than-normal oxygen saturation levels. An extra heart sound, S_3, may be detected on auscultation.

Dyspnea, or shortness of breath, may be precipitated by minimal to moderate activity (**dyspnea on exertion [DOE]**); dyspnea also can occur at rest. The patient may report **orthopnea**, difficulty in breathing when lying flat. Patients with orthopnea usually prefer not to lie flat. They may need pillows to prop themselves up in bed, or they may sit in a chair and even sleep sitting up. Some patients have sudden attacks of orthopnea at night, a condition known as **paroxysmal nocturnal dyspnea (PND)**. Fluid that accumulated in the dependent extremities during the day begins to be reabsorbed into the circulating blood volume when the person lies down. Because the impaired left ventricle cannot eject the increased circulating blood volume, the pressure in the pulmonary circulation increases, causing further shifting of fluid into the alveoli. The fluid filled alveoli cannot exchange oxygen and carbon dioxide. Without sufficient oxygen, the patient experiences dyspnea and has difficulty getting an adequate amount of sleep.

The cough associated with left ventricular failure is initially dry and nonproductive. Most often, patients complain of a dry hacking cough that may be mislabeled as asthma or chronic obstructive pulmonary disease (COPD). The cough may become moist. Large quantities of frothy sputum, which is sometimes pink (blood tinged), may be produced, usually indicating severe pulmonary congestion (pulmonary edema).

Adventitious breath sounds may be heard in various lobes of the lungs. Usually, bi-basilar crackles that do not clear with coughing are detected in the early phase of left ventricular failure. As the failure worsens and pulmonary congestion increases, crackles may be auscultated throughout all lung fields. At this point, a decrease in oxygen saturation may occur.

In addition to increased pulmonary pressures that cause decreased oxygenation, the amount of blood ejected from the left ventricle may decrease, sometimes called *forward failure.* The dominant feature in HF is inadequate tissue perfusion. The diminished CO has widespread manifestations because not enough blood reaches all the tissues and organs (low perfusion) to provide the necessary oxygen. The decrease in SV can also lead to stimulation of the sympathetic nervous system, which further impedes perfusion to many organs.

Blood flow to the kidneys decreases, causing decreased perfusion and reduced urine output (**oliguria**). Renal perfusion pressure falls, which results in the release of renin from the kidney. Release of renin leads to aldosterone secretion. Aldosterone secretion causes sodium and fluid retention, which further increases intravascular volume. However, when the patient is sleeping, the cardiac workload is decreased, improving renal perfusion, which then leads to frequent urination at night (nocturia).

Decreased CO causes other symptoms. Decreased gastrointestinal perfusion causes altered digestion. Decreased brain perfusion causes dizziness, lightheadedness, confusion, restlessness, and anxiety due to decreased oxygenation and blood flow. As anxiety increases, so does dyspnea, enhancing anxiety and creating a vicious cycle. Stimulation of the sympathetic system also causes the peripheral blood vessels to constrict, so the skin appears pale or ashen and feels cool and clammy.

The decrease in the ejected ventricular volume causes the sympathetic nervous system to increase the heart rate (tachycardia), often causing the patient to complain of palpitations. The pulses become weak and thready. Without adequate CO, the body cannot respond to increased energy demands, and the patient is easily fatigued and has decreased activity tolerance. Fatigue also results from the increased energy expended in breathing and the insomnia that results from respiratory distress, coughing, and nocturia.

RIGHT-SIDED HEART FAILURE

When the right ventricle fails, congestion of the viscera and the peripheral tissues predominates. This occurs because the right side of the heart cannot eject blood and cannot accommodate all the blood that normally returns to it from the venous circulation. The increase in venous pressure leads to jugular vein distention (JVD).

The clinical manifestations that ensue include edema of the lower extremities (dependent edema), hepatomegaly (enlargement of the liver), distended jugular veins, ascites (accumulation of fluid in the peritoneal cavity), weakness, anorexia and nausea, and paradoxically, weight gain due to retention of fluid.

Edema usually affects the feet and ankles, worsening when the patient stands or dangles the legs. The swelling decreases when the patient elevates the legs. The edema can gradually progress up the legs and thighs and eventually into the external genitalia and lower trunk. Edema in the abdomen, as evidenced by increased abdominal girth, may be the only edema present. Sacral edema is not uncommon for patients who are on bed rest, because the sacral area is dependent. Pitting edema, in which

indentations in the skin remain after even slight compression with the fingertips (Fig. 30-2), is obvious only after retention of at least 4.5 kg (10 lb) of fluid (4.5 liters).

Hepatomegaly and tenderness in the right upper quadrant of the abdomen result from venous engorgement of the liver. The increased pressure may interfere with the liver's ability to perform (secondary liver dysfunction). As hepatic dysfunction progresses, pressure within the portal vessels may rise enough to force fluid into the abdominal cavity, a condition known as ascites. This collection of fluid in the abdominal cavity may increase pressure on the stomach and intestines and cause gastrointestinal distress. Hepatomegaly may also increase pressure on the diaphragm, causing respiratory distress.

Anorexia (loss of appetite) and nausea or abdominal pain results from the venous engorgement and venous stasis within the abdominal organs. The weakness that accompanies right-sided HF results from reduced CO, impaired circulation, and inadequate removal of catabolic waste products from the tissues.

Assessment and Diagnostic Findings

HF may go undetected until the patient presents with signs and symptoms of pulmonary and peripheral edema (congestion), which can lead the physician to make a preliminary diagnosis of CHF. However, the physical signs that suggest HF may also occur with other diseases, such as renal failure, liver failure, oncologic conditions, and COPD. If further assessment and evaluation are

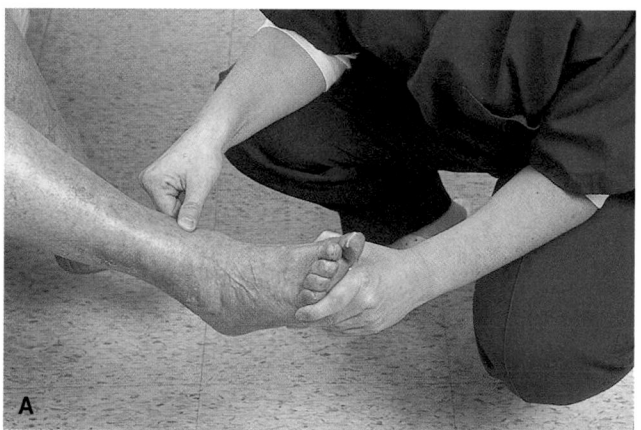

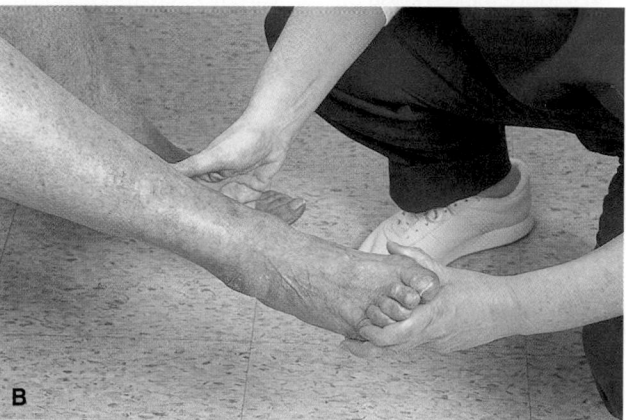

FIGURE 30-2 Example of pitting edema. (**A**) The nurse applies finger pressure to an area near the ankle. (**B**) When the pressure is released, an indentation remains in the edematous tissue. Photographs © B. Proud.

not completed, these patients may be treated for HF inappropriately. The term *congestive heart failure* (CHF) means the patient has a fluid overload condition (congestion) that may or may not be caused by HF. CHF is caused by HF when ventricular dysfunction (systolic, diastolic, or both) has been identified. Assessment of ventricular function is an essential part of the initial diagnostic workup.

An echocardiogram is usually performed to confirm the diagnosis of HF, assist in the identification of the underlying cause, and determine the patient's ejection fraction, which assists in identification of the type and severity of HF. This information may also be obtained noninvasively by radionuclide ventriculography or invasively by ventriculogram as part of a cardiac catheterization procedure. A chest x-ray and an electrocardiogram (ECG) are obtained to assist in the diagnosis and to determine the underlying cause of HF. Laboratory studies usually completed in the initial workup include serum electrolytes, blood urea nitrogen (BUN), creatinine, B-type natriuretic peptide (BNP), thyroid-stimulating hormone (TSH), a complete blood cell count (CBC), and routine urinalysis. The results of these laboratory studies assist in determining the underlying cause and in establishing a baseline from which to measure effects of treatment. Exercise testing or cardiac catheterization may be performed to determine whether coronary artery disease and cardiac ischemia are causing the HF.

Ventricular function should be determined before discharge from a hospital of patients with acute myocardial infarction (MI) who are at risk for the development of HF. Patients who are at low risk for HF are those who meet all of the following criteria: no previous myocardial infarction, inferior myocardial infarction, small (less than two to four times normal) increase in cardiac enzymes, no Q waves on the ECG, and an uncomplicated clinical course (AHCPR, 1994). Evaluation of ventricular function may also be performed for patients whose initial assessment of HF suggested noncardiac causes but who failed to respond to treatment.

Medical Management

A critical step in the management of HF is early identification and documentation of the type of HF. Medical management, especially the pharmacologic therapy, varies with the type of HF. The basic objectives in treating patients with HF are the following:

- Eliminate or reduce any etiologic contributory factors, especially those that may be reversible, such as atrial fibrillation or excessive alcohol ingestion.
- Reduce the workload on the heart by reducing afterload and preload.

Managing the patient with HF includes providing general counseling and education about sodium restriction, monitoring daily weights and other signs of fluid retention, encouraging regular exercise, and recommending avoidance of excessive fluid intake, alcohol, and smoking. Medications are prescribed based on the patient's type and severity of HF. Oxygen therapy is based on the degree of pulmonary congestion and resulting hypoxia. Some patients may need supplemental oxygen therapy only during activity. Others may require hospitalization and endotracheal intubation. If the patient has underlying coronary artery disease, coronary artery revascularization with percutaneous transluminal coronary angioplasty (PTCA) or bypass surgery (see Chap. 28) may be considered. If the patient's condition is unresponsive to advanced aggressive medical therapy, innovative therapies, including mechanical assist devices and transplantation, may be considered.

Cardiac resynchronization, involving the use of left ventricular and biventricular pacing, is a treatment for HF with electrical conduction defects. Left bundle branch block (LBBB) is frequently found in patients with systolic dysfunction. LBBB occurs when the electrical impulse, which normally depolarizes the right and left bundle branches at the same time, depolarizes the right bundle branch but not the left bundle branch. The dyssynchronous electrical stimulation of the ventricles causes the right ventricle to contract before the left ventricle, which can lead to further decreased ejection fraction (Gerber et al., 2001). Use of a pacing device (eg, Medtronic InSync), with leads placed on the inner wall of the right atrium and right ventricle and on the outer wall of the left ventricle, provides synchronized electrical stimulation to the heart. In one study, 63% of the patients who had received these devices showed improvement in clinical status, including NYHA functional class and global assessment, compared with 38% of placebo patients (Abraham, 2002).

PHARMACOLOGIC THERAPY

Several medications are indicated for systolic HF. Medications for diastolic failure depend on the underlying condition, such as hypertension (see Chap. 32) or valvular dysfunction (see Chap. 29). If the patient is in mild systolic failure, an ACE inhibitor usually is prescribed. If the patient is unable to continue an ACE inhibitor (eg, because of development of renal impairment as evidenced by elevated serum creatinine or persistent serum potassium levels of 5.5 mEq/L or above), an angiotensin II receptor blocker (ARB) or hydralazine and isosorbide dinitrate are considered as part of the treatment plan. A diuretic is added if signs of fluid overload develop. Digitalis is added to ACE inhibitors if the symptoms continue. Although previously contraindicated in HF, specific beta-blockers decrease mortality and morbidity if added to the initial medications. Spironolactone, a weak diuretic may also be added for persistent symptoms.

Angiotensin-Converting Enzyme Inhibitors. ACE inhibitors (ACE-Is) have a pivotal role in the management of HF due to systolic dysfunction. They have been found to relieve the signs and symptoms of HF and significantly decrease mortality and morbidity (when used to treat a symptomatic patient) by inhibiting neurohormonal activation (CONSENSUS Trial Study Group, 1987; SOLVD Investigators, 1992). Available as oral and intravenous medications, ACE-Is promote vasodilation and diuresis by decreasing afterload and preload. By doing so, they decrease the workload of the heart. Vasodilation reduces resistance to left ventricular ejection of blood, diminishing the heart's workload and improving ventricular emptying. In promoting diuresis, ACE-Is decrease the secretion of aldosterone, a hormone that causes the kidneys to retain sodium. ACE-Is stimulate the kidneys to excrete sodium and fluid (while retaining potassium), thereby reducing left ventricular filling pressure and decreasing pulmonary congestion. ACE-Is may be the first medication prescribed for patients in mild failure—patients with fatigue or dyspnea on exertion but without signs of fluid overload and pulmonary congestion.

Results from studies (Clement et al., 2000; NETWORK Investigators, 1998) to identify the specific dose to achieve this effect are equivocal, although one large study showed significant reductions in death and hospitalization with higher doses (Packer et al., 1999). However, it is recommended to start at a low dose and increase every 2 weeks until the optimal dose is achieved and the patient is hemodynamically stable. The final maintenance dose depends on the patient's blood pressure, fluid status, renal status, and degree of **cardiac failure**.

Patients receiving ACE-I therapy are monitored for hypotension, hypovolemia, hyponatremia, and alterations in renal function, especially if they are also receiving diuretics. When to observe for these effects and for how long depends on the onset, peak, and duration of the medication. Table 30-3 identifies several types of ACE-Is and their pharmacokinetics. Hypotension is most likely to develop from ACE-I therapy in patients older than age 75 and in those with a systolic blood pressure of 100 mm Hg or less, a serum sodium level of less than 135 mEq/L, or severe cardiac failure. Adjusting the dose or type of diuretic in response to the patient's blood pressure and renal function may allow for continued increases in the dosage of ACE-Is.

Because ACE-Is cause the kidneys to retain potassium, the patient who is also receiving a diuretic may not need to take oral potassium supplements. However, patients receiving potassium-sparing diuretics (which do not cause potassium loss with diuresis) must be carefully monitored for hyperkalemia, an increased level of potassium in the blood. Before the initiation of the ACE-I, hyperkalemic and hypovolemic states must be corrected. ACE-Is may be discontinued if the potassium remains above 5.0 mEq/L or if the serum creatinine is 3.0 mg/dL and continues to increase. Other side effects of ACE-Is include a dry, persistent cough that may not respond to cough suppressants. However, the cough could also indicate a worsening of ventricular function and failure. Rarely, the cough indicates angioedema. If angioedema affects the oropharyngeal area and impairs breathing, the ACE-I must be stopped immediately.

Angiotensin II Receptor Blockers (ARBs).

Although their action is different than that of ACE-Is, ARBs (eg, losartan [Cozaar]) have a similar hemodynamic effect as ACE-Is: lowered blood pressure and lowered systemic vascular resistance. Whereas ACE-Is block the conversion of angiotensin I to angiotensin II, ARBs block the effects of angiotensin II at the angiotensin II receptor. ACE-Is and ARBs also have similar side effects: hyperkalemia, hypotension, and renal dysfunction. ARBs are usually prescribed when patients are not able to tolerate ACE-Is.

Hydralazine and Isosorbide Dinitrate.

A combination of hydralazine (Apresoline) and isosorbide dinitrate (Dilatrate-SR, Isordil, Sorbitrate) may be another alternative for patients who cannot take ACE-Is. Nitrates (eg, isosorbide dinitrate) cause venous dilation, which reduces the amount of blood return to the heart and lowers preload. Hydralazine lowers systemic vascular resistance and left ventricular afterload. It has also been shown to help avoid the development of nitrate tolerance. As with ARBs, this combination of medications is usually used when patients are not able to tolerate ACE-Is.

Beta-Blockers.

When used with ACE-Is, beta-blockers, such as carvedilol (Coreg), metoprolol (Lopressor, Toprol), or bisoprolol (Zebeta), have been found to reduce mortality and morbidity in NYHA class II or III HF patients by reducing the cytotoxic effects from the constant stimulation of the sympathetic nervous system (Beta-Blocker Evaluation of Survival Trial [BEST] Investigators, 2001; CIBIS-II Investigators and Committees, 1999; MERIT, 1999; Packer et al., 1996; Packer et al., 2001). These agents have also been recommended for patients with asymptomatic systolic dysfunction, such as after acute myocardial infarction or revascularization to prevent the onset of symptoms of HF. However, beta-blockers may also produce many side effects, including exacerbation of HF. The side effects are most common in the initial few weeks of treatment. The most frequent side effects are dizziness, hypotension, and bradycardia. To minimize these side effects, staggering the administration of the beta-blocker with the ACE-I is recommended. Because of the side effects, beta-blockers are initiated only after stabilizing the patient and ensuring a euvolemic (normal volume) state. They are titrated slowly (every 2 weeks), with close monitoring at each increase in dose. If the patient develops symptoms during the titration phase, treatment options include increasing the diuretic, reducing the dose of ACE-I, or decreasing the dose of the beta-blocker.

An important nursing role during titration is educating the patient about the potential worsening of symptoms during the early phase of treatment, and that improvement may take several weeks. It is very important that nurses provide support to patients going through this symptom-provoking phase of treatment. Because beta-blockade can cause bronchiole constriction, a beta$_1$-selective beta-blocker (ie, one that primarily blocks the beta-adrenergic receptor sites in the heart), such as metoprolol (Lopressor, Toprol), is recommended for patients with well-controlled, mild to moderate asthma. However, these patients need to be monitored closely for increased asthma symptoms. Any type of beta-blocker is contraindicated in patients with severe or uncontrolled asthma.

Table 30-3 • Angiotensin-Converting Enzyme (ACE) Inhibitors

ACE INHIBITOR	PHARMACOKINETICS			NURSING CONSIDERATIONS
	Onset	Peak (hr)	Duration (hr)	
benazepril (Lotensin)	within 1 hr	2–4	24	Monitor blood pressure, urine output, and electrolyte levels.
captopril (Capoten)	15–60 min	1–1.5	6–12*	Monitor serum creatinine and urine creatinine clearance.
enalapril (Vasotec)	1 hr	4–6	24	Monitor for development of cough that is resistant to cough
enalaprilat (Vasotec I.V.)	15 min	1–4	6	suppressants.
fosinopril (Monopril)	within 1 hr	2–6	24	Teach patient to change positions gradually and to report
lisinopril (Prinival, Zestril)	1 hr	6	24	signs of dizziness or lethargy.
moexipril (Univasc)	1 hr	3–6	24	Instruct patient to weigh self daily and to report rapid weight
quinapril (Accupril)	within 1 hr	2–4	up to 24*	gain and significant feet and hand swelling.
ramipril (Altace)	1–2 hr	4–6	24	
trandolapril (Mavik)	within 30 min	2–4	> 8 days	

*Duration of effect is related to the dose.

Diuretics. Diuretics are medications used to increase the rate of urine production and the removal of excess extracellular fluid from the body. Of the types of diuretics prescribed for patients with edema from HF, three are most common: thiazide, loop, and potassium-sparing diuretics. These medications are classified according to their site of action in the kidney and their effects on renal electrolyte excretion and reabsorption. Thiazide diuretics, such as metolazone (Mykrox, Zaroxolyn), inhibit sodium and chloride reabsorption mainly in the early distal tubules. They also increase potassium and bicarbonate excretion. Loop diuretics, such as furosemide (Lasix), inhibit sodium and chloride reabsorption mainly in the ascending loop of Henle. Patients with signs and symptoms of fluid overload should be started on a diuretic, a thiazide for those with mild symptoms or a loop diuretic for patients with more severe symptoms or with renal insufficiency (Brater, 1998). Both types of diuretics may be used for those in severe HF

and unresponsive to a single diuretic. These medications may not be necessary if the patient responds to activity recommendations, avoidance of excessive fluid intake (<2 quarts/day), and a low-sodium diet (eg, <2 g/day).

Spironolactone (Aldactone) is a potassium-sparing diuretic that inhibits sodium reabsorption in the late distal tubule and collecting duct. It has been found to be effective in reducing mortality and morbidity in NYHA class III and IV HF patients when added to ACE-Is, loop diuretics, and digoxin. Serum creatinine and potassium levels are monitored frequently (eg, within the first week and then every 4 weeks) when this medication is first administered.

Side effects of diuretics include electrolyte imbalances, symptomatic hypotension (especially with overdiuresis), hyperuricemia (causing gout), and ototoxicity. Dosages depend on the indications, patient age, clinical signs and symptoms, and renal function. Table 30-4 lists commonly used diuretics, dosages, and pharma-

Table 30-4 • Diuretic Medications Used to Treat Heart Failure

DIURETIC	USUAL ADULT DOSE	ONSET (HR)	PEAK (HR)	DURATION (HR)
Thiazide Diuretics				
bendroflumethiazide (Naturetin)	2.5–20 mg in single or divided dose, once a day, once every other day, or once a day for 3–5 days per week	2	4	12–16
benzthiazide (Exna)	12.5–200 mg in single or divided dose	2	4–6	16–18
chlorothiazide (Diuril)	Oral: 0.25–2 g as single or divided dose; may be given on alternate days	2	4	16–18
	IV: 0.5–1 g in single or divided dose (note: avoid extravasation)	15 min	30 min	
chlorthalidone (Hygroton)	12.5–200 mg once a day, once every other day, or once a day for 3 days per week	2	2–6	24–72
hydrochlorothiazide (HydroDIURIL, Esidrix, Oretic)	12.5–200 mg as single or divided dose once a day, once every other day, or once a day for 3–5 days per week	2	4–6	12–16
hydroflumethiazide (Diucardin, Saluron)	25–200 mg as single or divided dose once a day, once every other day, or once a day for 3–5 days per week	2	4	12–16
methyclothiazide (Enduron)	2.5–10 mg once a day	2	6	24
metolazone (Zaroxolyn, Mykrox)	Zaroxolyn: 2.5–20 mg once a day Mykrox: 0.5–1 mg once a day	1	2	12–24
polythiazide (Renese)	1–4 mg once a day, once every other day, or once a day for 3–5 days per week	2	6	24–28
quinethazone (Hydromox)	25–100 mg as single or divided dose; rarely, 200 mg once a day	2	6	18–24
trichlormethiazide (Metahydrin, Naqua)	1–4 mg once or twice a day	2	6	24
Loop Diuretics				
bumetanide (Bumex)	0.5–2 mg once, twice or three times a day; may be given on alternate days or once every 3 days	30–60 min	1–2	4–6
	0.5–1 mg over 2 min; repeat every 2–3 h; a continuous infusion may be given at a rate of 1 mg/h.	5–10 min	15–30 min	½–1
ethacrynic acid (Edecrin)	50–400 mg as single or divided dose	<30 min	2	6–8
	0.5–1 mg/kg (max 100 mg) over several min; may be repeated within 2–6 h; repeat every hour in emergencies	<5 min	15–30 min	2
furosemide (Lasix)	20–600 mg as single daily dose, divided daily dose, as a dose given every other day or given once a day for 2–4 days per week	<1	1–2	6–8
	20–200 mg (max 6 mg/kg) given at a rate of 4 mg/min; after response obtained, given once or twice a day	<5 min	30 min	2
torsemide (Demadex)	5–200 mg as a daily single dose	<1	1–2	6–8
	IV and oral doses are equivalent. Give IV over 2 min.	<10 min	<1	6–8
Potassium-Sparing Diuretics				
amiloride (Midamor)	5–20 mg daily as single dose	2	6–10	24
spironolactone (Aldactone)	25–400 mg as single dose or divided up to 4 doses	24–48	48–72	48–72
triamterene (Dyrenium)	50–300 mg as single dose	2–4	6–8	12–16

cokinetic properties. Careful patient monitoring and dose adjustments are necessary to balance the effectiveness with the side effects of therapy. Diuretics greatly improve the patient's symptoms, but they do not prolong life.

Digitalis. The most commonly prescribed form of digitalis for patients with HF is digoxin (Lanoxin). The medication increases the force of myocardial contraction and slows conduction through the AV node. It improves contractility, increasing left ventricular output. The medication also enhances diuresis, which removes fluid and relieves edema. The effect of a given dose of medication depends on the state of the myocardium, electrolyte and fluid

balance, and renal and hepatic function. Although digitalis does not decrease the mortality rate, it is effective in decreasing the symptoms of systolic HF and in increasing the patient's ability to perform activities of daily living (Digitalis Investigation Group, 1997). It also has been shown to significantly decrease hospitalization rates and emergency room visits for NYHA class II and III HF patients (Uretsky et al., 1993).

A key concern associated with digitalis therapy is digitalis toxicity. Chart 30-3 summarizes the actions and uses of digitalis along with the nursing surveillance required when it is administered. The patient is observed for the effectiveness of digitalis therapy: lessening dyspnea and orthopnea, decrease in pulmonary

---

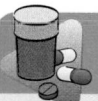

Chart 30-3 • PHARMACOLOGY
Digoxin Use and Toxicity in Heart Failure

Digoxin, a cardiac glycoside derived from digitalis, is used for patients with systolic HF, atrial fibrillation, and atrial flutter. Digoxin improves cardiac function as follows:

- Increases the force of myocardial contraction
- Slows cardiac conduction through the AV node and therefore slows the ventricular rate in instances of supraventricular dysrhythmias
- Increases cardiac output by enhancing the force of ventricular contraction
- Promotes diuresis by increasing cardiac output.

The therapeutic level is usually 0.5 to 2.0 ng/mL. Blood samples are usually obtained and analyzed to determine digitalis concentration at least 6 to 10 hours after the last dose. Toxicity may occur despite normal serum levels, and recommended dosages vary considerably.

Preparations
Digoxin
- Tablets: 0.125, 0.25, 0.5 mg (Lanoxin)
- Capsules: 0.05, 0.1, 0.2 mg (Lanoxicaps)
- Elixir: 0.05 mg/mL (Lanoxin Pediatric elixir)
- Injection: 0.25 mg/mL, 0.1 mg/mL (Lanoxin)

Digoxin Toxicity
A serious complication of digoxin therapy is toxicity. The incidence is high, and toxicity may occur even though the serum digoxin level remains within a normal range. Diagnosis of digoxin toxicity is based on the patient's clinical symptoms, which include the following:

- Fatigue, depression, malaise, anorexia, nausea, and vomiting (early effects of digitalis toxicity)
- Changes in heart rhythm: new onset of regular rhythm or new onset of irregular rhythm
- ECG changes indicating SA or AV block; new onset of irregular rhythm indicating ventricular dysrhythmias; and atrial tachycardia with block, junctional tachycardia, and ventricular tachycardia

Reversal of Toxicity
Digoxin toxicity is treated by holding the medication while monitoring the patient's symptoms and serum digoxin level. If the toxicity is severe, digoxin immune FAB (Digibind) may be prescribed. Digibind binds with digoxin and makes it unavailable for use. The Digibind dosage is based on the digoxin level and the patient's weight. Serum digoxin values are not accurate for several days after administration of Digibind because they do not differentiate between bound and unbound digoxin. Because Digibind quickly decreases the amount of available digoxin, an increase in ventricular rate due to atrial fibrillation and worsening of symptoms of HF may ensue shortly after its administration.

Nursing Considerations and Actions
1. Assess the patient's clinical response to digoxin therapy by evaluating relief of symptoms such as dyspnea, orthopnea, crackles, hepatomegaly, and peripheral edema.

2. Monitor serum potassium levels in patients receiving digoxin, especially those receiving both digoxin and diuretics. *An undetected, uncorrected potassium imbalance predisposes patients to digoxin toxicity and dysrhythmias.*

3. Assess for symptoms of electrolyte depletion: lassitude, apathy, mental confusion, anorexia, decreasing urinary output, azotemia.

4. Monitor the patient for factors that increase the risk of toxicity:
   - Oral antibiotics, quinidine, amiodarone, calcium channel blocker therapy (See Table 27-1).
   - Decreased potassium level (hypokalemia), which increases the action of digoxin and which may be caused by malnutrition, diarrhea, vomiting, or prolonged muscle wasting
   - Impaired renal function, particularly in patients age 65 and older with decreased renal clearance.

5. Before administering digoxin, it is standard nursing practice to assess apical heart rate. When the patient's rhythm is atrial fibrillation and the heart rate is less than 60, or the rhythm becomes regular, the nurse may withhold the medication and notify the physician, because these signs indicate the development of AV conduction block. Although withholding digoxin is a common practice, the medication does not need to be withheld for a heart rate of less than 60 if the patient is in sinus rhythm because digoxin does not affect sinoatrial node automaticity. Measuring the PR interval for a patient with cardiac monitoring is more important than the apical pulse in determining whether digoxin should be held.

   Note: If monitoring discloses that the patient is in sinus rhythm, the nurse monitors the patient's PR interval instead of the patient's heart rate. If the patient is in atrial fibrillation, the nurse monitors for the development of regular R-R intervals, indicating AV block.

6. Monitor for gastrointestinal side effects: anorexia, nausea, vomiting, abdominal pain and distention.

7. Monitor for neurologic side effects: headache, malaise, nightmares, forgetfulness, social withdrawal, depression, agitation, confusion, paranoia, hallucinations, decreased visual acuity, yellow or green halo around objects (especially lights), or "snowy" vision.

8. Observe for and anticipate potential drug interactions when other medications are added to the patient's regimen. This is an important step in preventing toxicity. For example, antiarrhythmic and antibiotic medications may increase the amount of digoxin available to the patient. Diuretics may decrease the amount of potassium and increase the availability of digoxin. In addition, because digoxin is eliminated by the kidneys, renal function (serum creatinine and urine creatinine clearance) are monitored carefully.

crackles on auscultation, relief of peripheral edema, weight loss, and increase in activity tolerance. The serum potassium level is measured at intervals because diuresis may have caused hypokalemia. The effect of digitalis is enhanced in the presence of hypokalemia, so digitalis toxicity may occur. Serum digoxin levels are obtained once each year or more frequently if there have been changes in the patient's medications, renal function, or symptoms.

Calcium Channel Blockers. First-generation calcium channel blockers, such as verapamil (Calan, Isoptin, Verelan), nifedipine (Adalat, Procardia), and diltiazem (Cardizem, Dilacor, Tiazac), are contraindicated in patients with systolic dysfunction, although they may be used in patients with diastolic dysfunction. Amlodipine (Norvasc) and felodipine (Plendil), dihydropyridine calcium channel blockers, cause vasodilation, reducing systemic vascular resistance. They may be used to improve symptoms especially in patients with nonischemic cardiomyopathy, although they have no effect on mortality.

Other Medications. Anticoagulants may be prescribed, especially if the patient has a history of an embolic event or atrial fibrillation or mural thrombus is present. Other medications such as antianginal medications may be given to treat the underlying cause of HF. Nonsteroidal anti-inflammatory drugs (NSAIDs), such as ibuprophen (Aleve, Advil, Motrin) should be avoided (Page & Henry, 2000). They can increase systemic vascular resistance and decrease renal perfusion, especially in the elderly. For similar reasons, use of decongestants should be avoided.

NUTRITIONAL THERAPY

A low-sodium (≤ 2 to 3 g/day) diet and avoidance of excessive amounts of fluid are usually recommended. Although it has not been shown to affect the mortality rate, this recommendation reduces fluid retention and the symptoms of peripheral and pulmonary congestion. The purpose of sodium restriction is to decrease the amount of circulating volume, which would decrease the need for the heart to pump that volume. A balance needs to be achieved between the ability of the patient to alter the diet and the amount of medications that are prescribed. Any change in diet needs to be done with consideration of good nutrition as well as the patient's likes, dislikes, and cultural food patterns.

> **NURSING ALERT** The sources of sodium should be specified in describing the regimen, rather than simply saying "low-salt" or "salt-free," and the quantity should be indicated in milligrams. Salt is not 100% sodium; there are 393 mg of sodium in 1 g (1000 mg) of salt.

Nursing Management

The nurse is responsible for administering the medications and for assessing their beneficial and detrimental effects to the patient. It is the balance of these effects that determines the type and dosage of pharmacologic therapy. Nursing actions to evaluate therapeutic effectiveness include the following:

- Keeping an intake and output record to identify a negative balance (more output than input)
- Weighing the patient daily at the same time and on the same scale, usually in the morning after urination; monitoring for a 2- to 3-lb gain in a day or 5-lb gain in week
- Auscultating lung sounds at least daily to detect an increase or decrease in pulmonary crackles

- Determining the degree of JVD
- Identifying and evaluating the severity of dependent edema
- Monitoring pulse rate and blood pressure, as well as monitoring for postural hypotension and making sure that the patient does not become hypotensive from dehydration
- Examining skin turgor and mucous membranes for signs of dehydration
- Assessing symptoms of fluid overload (eg, orthopnea, paroxysmal nocturnal dyspnea, and dyspnea on exertion) and evaluating changes

MONITORING AND MANAGING POTENTIAL COMPLICATIONS

Profuse and repeated diuresis can lead to hypokalemia (ie, potassium depletion). Signs are weak pulse, faint heart sounds, hypotension, muscle flabbiness, diminished deep tendon reflexes, and generalized weakness. Hypokalemia poses new problems for the patient with HF because it markedly weakens cardiac contractions. In patients receiving digoxin, hypokalemia can lead to digitalis toxicity. Digitalis toxicity and hypokalemia increase the likelihood of dangerous dysrhythmias (see Chart 30-3). Low levels of potassium may also indicate a low level of magnesium, which can add to the risk for dysrhythmias. Hyperkalemia may also occur, especially with the use of ACE-Is or ARBs and spironolactone.

> **NURSING ALERT** To reduce the risk for hypokalemia, the nurse advises patients to increase their dietary intake of potassium. Dried apricots, bananas, beets, figs, orange or tomato juice, peaches, and prunes (dried plums), potatoes, raisins, spinach, squash, and watermelon are good dietary sources of potassium. An oral potassium supplement (potassium chloride) may also be prescribed for patients receiving diuretic medications. If the patient is at risk for hyperkalemia, the nurse advises the patient to avoid the above products, including salt substitutes.

> **NURSING ALERT** Grapefruit (fresh and juice) is a good dietary source of potassium but has serious drug–food interactions. Patients are advised to consult their physician or pharmacist before including grapefruit in their diet.

Prolonged diuretic therapy may also produce hyponatremia (deficiency of sodium in the blood), which results in apprehension, weakness, fatigue, malaise, muscle cramps and twitching, and a rapid, thready pulse.

> **NURSING ALERT** Periodic assessment of the patient's electrolyte levels will alert health team members to hypokalemia, hypomagnesemia, and hyponatremia. Serum levels are assessed frequently when the patient starts diuretic therapy and then usually every 3 to 12 months. It is important to remember that serum potassium levels do not always indicate the total amount of potassium within the body.

Other problems associated with diuretic administration are hyperuricemia (excessive uric acid in the blood), volume depletion from excessive urination, and hyperglycemia.

Gerontologic Considerations

Several normal changes that occur with aging increase the frequency of diastolic HF: increased systolic blood pressure, increased ventricular wall thickness, increased atrial size, and increased myocardial fibrosis. Elderly people may present with atypical signs and symptoms: fatigue, weakness, and somnolence. Decreased renal function makes the elderly patient resistant to diuretics and more sensitive to changes in volume, especially with diastolic dysfunction. The administration of diuretics to elderly men requires nursing surveillance for bladder distention caused by urethral obstruction from an enlarged prostate gland. The bladder may be assessed with an ultrasound scanner, or the suprapubic area palpated for an oval mass and percussed for dullness, indicative of bladder fullness,

NURSING PROCESS: THE PATIENT WITH HEART FAILURE

Assessment

The nursing assessment for the patient with HF focuses on observing for effectiveness of therapy and for the patient's ability to understand and implement self-management strategies. Signs and symptoms of pulmonary and systemic fluid overload are recorded and reported immediately so that adjustments can be made in therapy. The nurse also explores the patient's emotional response to the diagnosis of HF, a chronic illness.

HEALTH HISTORY
The nurse explores sleep disturbances, particularly sleep suddenly interrupted by shortness of breath. The nurse also asks about the number of pillows needed for sleep (an indication of orthopnea), activities of daily living, and the activities that cause shortness of breath. The nurse also explores the patient's understanding of HF, the self-management strategies, and the desire to adhere to those strategies. The nurse helps patients to identify things that they have lost because of the diagnosis, their emotional response to that loss, and successful coping skills that they have used previously. Family and significant others are often included in these discussions.

PHYSICAL EXAMINATION
The lungs are auscultated to detect crackles and wheezes or their absence. Crackles, which are produced by the sudden opening of small airways and alveoli that have adhered together by edema and exudate, may be heard at the end of inspiration and are not cleared with coughing. They may also sound like gurgling that may clear with coughing or suctioning. The rate and depth of respirations are also documented.

The heart is auscultated for an S_3 heart sound, a sign that the heart is beginning to fail and that increased blood volume remains in the ventricle with each beat. HR and rhythm are also documented. Rapid rates indicate that SV has decreased and that the ventricle has less time to fill, producing some blood stagnation in the atria and eventually in the pulmonary bed.

JVD is also assessed; distention greater than 3 cm above the sternal angle is considered abnormal. This is an estimate, not a precise measurement, of central venous pressure.

Sensorium and level of consciousness must be evaluated. As the volume of blood ejected by the heart decreases, so does the amount of oxygen transported to the brain.

The nurse makes sure that dependent parts of the patient's body are assessed for perfusion and edema. With significant decreases in SV, there is a decrease in perfusion to the periphery, causing the skin to feel cool and appear pale or cyanotic. If the patient is sitting upright, the feet and lower legs are examined for edema; if the patient is supine in bed, the sacrum and back are assessed for edema. Fingers and hands may also become edematous.

In extreme cases of HF, the patient may develop periorbital edema, in which the eyelids may swell shut.

The liver is assessed for hepatojugular reflux. The patient is asked to breathe normally while manual pressure is applied over the right upper quadrant of the abdomen for 30 to 60 seconds. If neck vein distention increases more than 1 cm, the test finding is positive for increased venous pressure.

If the patient is hospitalized, the nurse measures output carefully to establish a baseline against which to measure the effectiveness of diuretic therapy. Intake and output records are rigorously maintained. It is important to know whether the patient has ingested more fluid than he or she has excreted (positive fluid balance), which is then correlated with a gain in weight. The patient must be monitored for oliguria (diminished urine output, <400 mL/24 hours) or **anuria** (urine output <50 mL/24 hours).

The patient is weighed daily in the hospital or at home, at the same time of day, with the same type of clothing, and on the same scale. If there is a significant change in weight (ie, 2- to 3-lb increase in a day or 5-lb increase in a week), the patient is instructed to notify the physician or adjust the medications (eg, increase the diuretic dose).

Diagnosis

NURSING DIAGNOSES
Based on the assessment data, major nursing diagnoses for the patient with HF may include the following:

- Activity intolerance (or risk for activity intolerance) related to imbalance between oxygen supply and demand because of decreased CO
- Excess fluid volume related to excess fluid or sodium intake and retention of fluid because of HF and its medical therapy
- Anxiety related to breathlessness and restlessness from inadequate oxygenation
- Powerlessness related to inability to perform role responsibilities because of chronic illness and hospitalizations
- Noncompliance related to lack of knowledge

COLLABORATIVE PROBLEMS/ POTENTIAL COMPLICATIONS
Based on the assessment data, potential complications that may develop include the following:

- Cardiogenic shock (see also Chap. 15)
- Dysrhythmias (see Chap. 27)
- Thromboembolism (see Chap. 31)
- Pericardial effusion and cardiac tamponade (see also Chap. 29)

Planning and Goals

Major goals for the patient may include promoting activity and reducing fatigue, relieving fluid overload symptoms, decreasing the incidence of anxiety or increasing the patient's ability to manage anxiety, teaching the patient about the self-care program, and encouraging the patient to verbalize his or her ability to make decisions and influence outcomes.

Nursing Interventions

PROMOTING ACTIVITY TOLERANCE
Although prolonged bed rest and even short periods of recumbency promote diuresis by improving renal perfusion, they also promote

decreased activity tolerance. Prolonged bed rest, which may be self-imposed, should be avoided because of the deconditioning effects and hazards, such as pressure ulcers (especially in edematous patients), phlebothrombosis, and pulmonary embolism. An acute event that causes severe symptoms or that requires hospitalization indicates the need for initial bed rest. Otherwise, a total of 30 minutes of physical activity three to five times each week should be encouraged (Georgiou et al., 2001). The nurse and patient can collaborate to develop a schedule that promotes pacing and prioritization of activities. The schedule should alternate activities with periods of rest and avoid having two significant energy-consuming activities occur on the same day or in immediate succession.

Before undertaking physical activity, the patient should be given the following safety guidelines:

- Begin with a few minutes of warm-up activities.
- Avoid performing physical activities outside in extreme hot, cold, or humid weather.
- Ensure that you are able to talk during the physical activity; if you are unable to do so, decrease the intensity of activity.
- Wait 2 hours after eating a meal before performing the physical activity.
- Stop the activity if severe shortness of breath, pain, or dizziness develops.
- End with cool-down activities and a cool-down period.

Because some patients may be severely debilitated, they may need to perform physical activities only 3 to 5 minutes at a time, one to four times per day. The patient then should be advised to increase the duration of the activity, then the frequency, before increasing the intensity of the activity (Meyer, 2001).

Barriers to performing an activity are identified, and methods of adjusting an activity to ensure pacing but still accomplish the task are discussed. For example, objects that need to be taken upstairs can be put in a basket at the bottom of the stairs throughout the day. At the end of the day, the person can carry the objects up the stairs all at once. Likewise, the person can carry cleaning supplies around in a basket or backpack rather than walk back and forth to obtain the items. Vegetables can be chopped or peeled while sitting at the kitchen table rather than standing at the kitchen counter. Small, frequent meals decrease the amount of energy needed for digestion while providing adequate nutrition. The nurse helps the patient to identify peak and low periods of energy and plan energy-consuming activities for peak periods. For example, the person may prepare the meals for the entire day in the morning. Pacing and prioritizing activities help maintain the patient's energy to allow participation in regular physical activity (see Chap. 28).

The patient's response to activities needs to be monitored. If the patient is hospitalized, vital signs and oxygen saturation level are monitored before, during, and immediately after an activity to identify whether they are within the desired range. Heart rate should return to baseline within 3 minutes. If the patient is at home, the degree of fatigue felt after the activity can be used as assessment of the response. If the patient tolerates the activity, short-term and long-term goals can be developed to gradually increase the intensity, duration, and frequency of activity. Referral to a cardiac rehabilitation program may be needed, especially for HF patients with recent myocardial infarction, recent open-heart surgery, or increased anxiety. A supervised program may also benefit those who need the structured environment, significant educational support, regular encouragement, and interpersonal contact.

MANAGING FLUID VOLUME

Patients with severe HF may receive intravenous diuretic therapy, but patients with less severe symptoms may receive oral diuretic medication (see Table 30-4 for a summary of common diuretics). Oral diuretics should be administered early in the morning so that diuresis does not interfere with the patient's nighttime rest. Discussing the timing of medication administration is especially important for patients, such as elderly people, who may have urinary urgency or incontinence. A single dose of a diuretic may cause the patient to excrete a large volume of fluid shortly after administration.

The nurse monitors the patient's fluid status closely—auscultating the lungs, monitoring daily body weights, and assisting the patient to adhere to a low-sodium diet by reading food labels and avoiding high-sodium foods such as canned, processed, and convenience foods (Chart 30-4). If the diet includes fluid restriction, the nurse can assist the patient to plan the fluid intake throughout the day while respecting the patient's dietary preferences. If the patient is receiving intravenous fluids, the

---

Chart 30-4 — **Facts About Dietary Sodium**

Although the major source of sodium in the average American diet is salt, many types of natural foods contain varying amounts of sodium. Even if no salt is added in cooking and if salty foods are avoided, the daily diet may still contain between 1000 and 2000 mg of sodium.

Additives in Food
Added food substances (additives), such as sodium alginate, which improves food texture; sodium benzoate, which acts as a preservative; and disodium phosphate, which improves cooking quality in certain foods, increase the sodium intake when included in the daily diet. Therefore, patients on low-sodium diets should be advised to check labels carefully for such words as "salt" or "sodium," especially on canned foods. For example, without looking at the sodium content per serving found on the nutrition labels, when given a choice between a serving of salt and vinegar potato chips and a cup of canned cream of mushroom soup, most would think that soup is lower in sodium. However, when the labels are examined, the lower sodium choice is found to be the chips. Although potato chips are *not* recommended in a low sodium diet, this example illustrates that it is important to read food labels to determine both sodium content and serving size.

Nonfood Sodium Sources
Sodium is also contained in toothpaste and municipal water. Patients on sodium-restricted diets should be cautioned against using nonprescription medications such as antacids, cough syrups, laxatives, sedatives, or salt substitutes, because these products contain sodium or excessive amounts of potassium. Over-the-counter medications should not be used without first consulting the physician.

Promoting Dietary Adherence
If patients find food unpalatable because of the dietary sodium restrictions and/or the taste disturbances caused by the medications, they may refuse to eat or to comply with the dietary regimen. For this reason, severe sodium restrictions should be avoided and the amount of medication should be balanced with the patient's ability to restrict dietary sodium. A variety of flavorings, such as lemon juice, vinegar, and herbs, may be used to improve the taste of the food and increase acceptance of the diet. The patient's food preferences should be taken into account—diet counseling and educational handouts can be geared to individual and ethnic preferences. It is very important to involve the family in the dietary teaching.

amount of fluid needs to be monitored closely, and the physician or pharmacist can be consulted about the possibility of maximizing the amount of medication in the same amount of intravenous fluid (eg, double-concentrating to decrease the fluid volume administered).

The nurse positions the patient or teaches the patient how to assume a position that shifts fluid away from the heart. The number of pillows may be increased, the head of the bed may be elevated (20- to 30-cm [8- to 10-inch] blocks may be used), or the patient may sit in a comfortable armchair. In this position, the venous return to the heart (preload) is reduced, pulmonary congestion is alleviated, and impingement of the liver on the diaphragm is minimized. The lower arms are supported with pillows to eliminate the fatigue caused by the constant pull of their weight on the shoulder muscles.

The patient who can breathe only in the upright position may sit on the side of the bed with the feet supported on a chair, the head and arms resting on an overbed table, and the lumbosacral spine supported by a pillow. If pulmonary congestion is present, positioning the patient in an armchair is advantageous, because this position favors the shift of fluid away from the lungs.

Because decreased circulation in edematous areas increases the risk of skin injury, the nurse assesses for skin breakdown and institutes preventive measures. Frequent changes of position, positioning to avoid pressure, the use of elastic compression stockings, and leg exercises may help to prevent skin injury.

CONTROLLING ANXIETY

Because patients in HF have difficulty maintaining adequate oxygenation, they are likely to be restless and anxious and feel overwhelmed by breathlessness. These symptoms tend to intensify at night. Emotional stress stimulates the sympathetic nervous system, which causes vasoconstriction, elevated arterial pressure, and increased heart rate. This sympathetic response increases the amount of work that the heart has to do. By decreasing anxiety, the patient's cardiac work also is decreased. Oxygen may be administered during an acute event to diminish the work of breathing and to increase the patient's comfort.

When the patient exhibits anxiety, the nurse takes steps to promote physical comfort and psychological support. In many cases, a family member's presence provides reassurance. To help decrease the patient's anxiety, the nurse should speak in a slow, calm, and confident manner and maintain eye contact. When necessary, the nurse should also state specific, brief directions for an activity.

After the patient is comfortable, the nurse can begin teaching ways to control anxiety and to avoid anxiety-provoking situations. The nurse explains how to use relaxation techniques and assists the patient to identify factors that contribute to anxiety. Lack of sleep may increase anxiety, which may prevent adequate rest. Other contributing factors may include misinformation, lack of information, or poor nutritional status. Promoting physical comfort, providing accurate information, and teaching the patient to perform relaxation techniques and to avoid anxiety-triggering situations may relax the patient.

> **NURSING ALERT** Cerebral hypoxia with superimposed carbon dioxide retention may be a problem in HF, causing the patient to react to sedative-hypnotic medications with confusion and increased anxiety. Hepatic congestion may slow the liver's metabolism of medication, leading to toxicity. Sedative-hypnotic medications must be administered with caution.

In cases of confusion and anxiety reactions that affect the patient's safety, the use of restraints should be avoided. Restraints are likely to be resisted, and resistance inevitably increases the cardiac workload. The patient who insists on getting out of bed at night can be seated comfortably in an armchair. As cerebral and systemic circulation improves, the degree of anxiety decreases, and the quality of sleep improves.

MINIMIZING POWERLESSNESS

Patients need to recognize that they are not helpless and that they can influence the direction of their lives and the outcomes of treatment. The nurse assesses for factors contributing to a sense of powerlessness and intervenes accordingly. Contributing factors may include lack of knowledge and lack of opportunities to make decisions, particularly if health care providers and family members behave in maternalistic or paternalistic ways. If the patient is hospitalized, hospital policies may promote standardization and limit the patient's ability to make decisions (eg, what time to have meals, take medications, prepare for bed).

Taking time to listen actively to patients often encourages them to express their concerns and ask questions. Other strategies include providing the patient with decision-making opportunities, such as when activities are to occur or where objects are to be placed, and increasing the frequency and significance of those opportunities over time; providing encouragement while identifying the patient's progress; and assisting the patient to differentiate between factors that can be controlled and those that cannot. In some cases, the nurse may want to review hospital policies and standards that tend to promote powerlessness and advocate for their elimination or change (eg, limited visiting hours, prohibition of food from home, required wearing of hospital gowns).

PROMOTING HOME AND COMMUNITY-BASED CARE

Teaching Patients Self-Care

The nurse provides patient education and involves the patient in implementing the therapeutic regimen to promote understanding and adherence to the plan. When the patient understands or believes that the diagnosis of HF can be successfully managed with lifestyle changes and medications, recurrences of acute HF lessen, unnecessary hospitalizations decrease, and life expectancy increases. Patients and their families need to be taught to follow the medication regimen as prescribed, maintain a low-sodium diet, perform and record daily weights, engage in routine physical activity, and recognize symptoms that indicate worsening HF. Although noncompliance is not well understood, interventions that may promote adherence include teaching to ensure accurate understanding. A summary of teaching points for the patient with HF is presented in Chart 30-5.

The patient and family members are supported and encouraged to ask questions so that information can be clarified and understanding enhanced. The nurse should be aware of cultural factors and adapt the teaching plan accordingly. Patients and their families need to be informed that the progression of the disease is influenced in part by choices made about health care and the decisions about following the treatment plan. They also need to be informed that health care providers are there to assist them in reaching their health care goals. Patients and family members need to make the decisions about the treatment plan, but they also need to understand the possible outcomes of those decisions. The treatment plan then will be based on what the patient wants, not just what the physician or other health care team members think is needed. Ultimately, the nurse needs to convey that monitoring symptoms and daily weights, restricting sodium intake, avoiding

Chart 30-5
Home Care Checklist ○ **The Patient With Heart Failure**

At the completion of the home care instruction, the patient or caregiver will be able to:	Patient	Caregiver
• Identify heart failure as a chronic disease that can be managed with medications and specific self-management behaviors.	✓	✓
• Take or administer medications daily, exactly as prescribed.	✓	✓
• Monitor effects of medication.	✓	✓
• Know signs and symptoms of orthostatic hypotension and how to prevent it.	✓	✓
• Weigh self daily. – Obtain weight at the same time each day (eg, every morning after urination). – Keep a record and report weight gain of ≥ 2–3 lb (0.9–1.4 kg) in 1 day or 5 lb (2.3 kg) in 1 week.	✓	
• Restrict sodium intake to 2–3 g daily: adapt diet by examining nutrition labels to check sodium content per serving; avoid canned or processed foods; eat fresh or frozen foods; consult the written diet plan and the list of permitted and restricted foods; avoid salt use; and avoid excesses in eating and drinking.	✓	✓
• Review activity program. – Participate in a daily exercise program. – Increase walking and other activities gradually, provided they do not cause unusual fatigue or dyspnea. – Conserve energies by balancing activity with rest periods. – Avoid activity in extremes of heat and cold, which increase the work of the heart. – Recognize that air conditioning may be essential in a hot, humid environment.	✓	
• Develop methods to manage stress.	✓	
• Keep regular appointments with physician or clinic.	✓	✓
• Be alert for symptoms that may indicate recurring heart failure. – Recall the symptoms experienced when illness began.	✓	✓
• Report immediately to the physician or clinic any of the following: – Gain in weight of ≥ 2–3 lb (0.9–1.4 kg) in 1 day, or 5 lb (2.3 kg) in 1 week – Loss of appetite – Unusual shortness of breath with activity – Swelling of ankles, feet, or abdomen – Persistent cough – Development of restless sleep; increase in number of pillows needed to sleep	✓	✓

excess fluids, preventing infection with influenza and pneumococcal immunizations, avoiding noxious agents (eg, alcohol, tobacco), and participating in regular exercise all aid in preventing exacerbations of HF.

Continuing Care

Depending on the patient's physical status and the availability of family assistance, a home care referral may be indicated for a patient who has been hospitalized. Elderly patients and those who have long-standing heart disease with compromised physical stamina often require assistance with the transition to home after hospitalization for an acute episode of HF. It is important for the home care nurse to assess the physical environment of the home. Suggestions for adapting the home environment to meet the patient's activity limitations are important. If stairs are the concern, the patient can plan the day's activities so that stair climbing is minimized; for some patients, a temporary bedroom may be set up on the main level of the home. The home care nurse collaborates with the patient and family to maximize the benefits of these changes.

The home care nurse also reinforces and clarifies information about dietary changes and fluid restrictions, the need to monitor symptoms and daily body weights, and the importance of obtaining follow-up health care. Assistance may be given in scheduling and keeping appointments as well. The patient is encouraged to gradually increase his or her self-care and responsibility for accomplishing the therapeutic regimen.

Evaluation

EXPECTED PATIENT OUTCOMES

Expected patient outcomes may include:

1. Demonstrates tolerance for increased activity
   a. Describes adaptive methods for usual activities
   b. Stops any activity that causes symptoms of intolerance
   c. Maintains vital signs (pulse, blood pressure, respiratory rate, and pulse oximetry) within the targeted range
   d. Identifies factors that contribute to activity intolerance and takes actions to avoid them
   e. Establishes priorities for activities
   f. Schedules activities to conserve energy and to reduce fatigue and dyspnea
2. Maintains fluid balance
   a. Exhibits decreased peripheral and sacral edema
   b. Demonstrates methods for preventing edema
3. Is less anxious
   a. Avoids situations that produce stress
   b. Sleeps comfortably at night
   c. Reports decreased stress and anxiety
4. Makes decisions regarding care and treatment
   a. States ability to influence outcomes
5. Adheres to self-care regimen
   a. Performs and records daily weights
   b. Ensures dietary intake includes no more than 2 to 3 g of sodium per day

c. Takes medications as prescribed

d. Reports any unusual symptoms or side effects

ACUTE HEART FAILURE (PULMONARY EDEMA)

Pulmonary edema is the abnormal accumulation of fluid in the lungs. The fluid may accumulate in the interstitial spaces or in the alveoli.

Pathophysiology

Pulmonary edema is an acute event that results from HF. It can occur acutely, such as with myocardial infarction, or it can occur as an exacerbation of chronic HF. Myocardial scarring as a result of ischemia can limit the ventricular distensibility and render it vulnerable to a sudden increase in workload. With increased resistance to left ventricular filling, the blood backs up into the pulmonary circulation. The patient quickly develops pulmonary edema, sometimes called flash pulmonary edema, from the blood volume overload in the lungs. Pulmonary edema can also be caused by noncardiac disorders, such as renal failure, liver failure, and oncologic conditions that cause the body to retain fluid. The left ventricle cannot handle the resulting hypervolemia, preventing blood from easily flowing from the left atrium into the left ventricle. This causes the pressure to increase in the left atrium. The increase in atrial pressure may result in an increase in pulmonary venous pressure, which produces an increase in hydrostatic pressure that forces fluid out of the pulmonary capillaries into the interstitial spaces and alveoli.

Impaired lymphatic drainage also contributes to the accumulation of fluid in the lung tissues. The fluid within the alveoli mixes with air, creating "bubbles" that are expelled from the mouth and nose, producing the classic symptom of pulmonary edema, frothy pink (blood-tinged) sputum. Because of the fluid within the alveoli, air cannot enter, and gas exchange is impaired. The result is hypoxemia, which is often severe. The onset may be preceded by premonitory symptoms of pulmonary congestion, but it also may develop quickly in the patient with a ventricle that has little reserve to meet increased oxygen needs.

In pulmonary edema, as well as in HF, preload, contractility, and afterload may be altered, thereby impairing CO. Technological advances (eg, impedance cardiography) have made it easier to implement effective pharmacologic therapy in treating acute pulmonary edema.

Clinical Manifestations

As a result of decreased cerebral oxygenation, the patient becomes increasingly restless and anxious. Along with a sudden onset of breathlessness and a sense of suffocation, the patient's hands become cold and moist, the nail beds become cyanotic (bluish), and the skin turns ashen (gray). The pulse is weak and rapid, and the neck veins are distended. Incessant coughing may occur, producing increasing quantities of mucoid sputum. As pulmonary edema progresses, the patient's anxiety and restlessness increase; the patient becomes confused, then stuporous. Breathing is rapid, noisy, and moist sounding. The patient's oxygen levels (saturation) are significantly decreased. The patient, nearly suffocated by the blood-tinged, frothy fluid filling the alveoli, is literally drowning in secretions. The situation demands immediate action.

Assessment and Diagnostic Findings

The diagnosis is made by evaluating the clinical manifestations resulting from pulmonary congestion. Most often, a chest x-ray is obtained to confirm that the pulmonary veins are engorged. Abrupt onset of signs and symptoms of left-sided HF(eg, crackles on auscultation of the lungs, flash pulmonary edema) without evidence of right-sided HF (eg, no JVD, no dependent edema) may indicate diastolic failure due to ischemia.

Prevention

Like most complications, pulmonary edema is easier to prevent than to treat. To recognize it in its early stages, the nurse auscultates the lung fields and heart sounds, measures JVD, and assesses the degree of peripheral edema and the severity of breathlessness. A dry, hacking cough; fatigue; weight gain; development or worsening of edema; and decreased activity tolerance may be early indicators of developing pulmonary edema.

In an early stage, the condition may be corrected by placing the patient in an upright position with the feet and legs dependent, eliminating overexertion, and minimizing emotional stress to reduce the left ventricular load. A re-examination of the patient's treatment regimen and the patient's understanding of and adherence to it are also needed. The long-range approach to preventing pulmonary edema must be directed at identifying its precipitating factors.

Medical Management

Clinical management of a patient with acute pulmonary edema due to HF is directed toward improving ventricular function and increasing respiratory exchange. These goals are accomplished through a combination of oxygen, medication therapies, and nursing support.

PHARMACOLOGIC THERAPY

Various treatments and medications are prescribed for pulmonary edema, among them oxygen, morphine, diuretics, and various intravenous medications.

Oxygen Therapy. Oxygen is administered in concentrations adequate to relieve hypoxemia and dyspnea. Usually, a face mask or non-rebreathing mask is initially used. If respiratory failure is severe or persists despite optimal management, endotracheal intubation and mechanical ventilation are required. The use of positive end-expiratory pressure (PEEP) is effective in reducing venous return, decreasing fluid movement from the pulmonary capillaries to the alveoli, and improving oxygenation. Oxygenation is monitored with pulse oximetry and by measurement of arterial blood gases.

Morphine. Morphine is administered intravenously in small doses (2 to 5 mg) to reduce peripheral resistance and venous return so that blood can be redistributed from the pulmonary circulation to other parts of the body. This action decreases pressure in the pulmonary capillaries and decreases seepage of fluid into the lung tissue. The effect of morphine in decreasing anxiety is also beneficial.

Diuretics. Diuretics promote the excretion of sodium and water by the kidneys. Furosemide (Lasix), for example, is administered intravenously to produce a rapid diuretic effect. Furosemide also causes vasodilation and pooling of blood in peripheral blood vessels, which reduces the amount of blood returned to the heart, even before the diuretic effect. Some physicians may prescribe bumetanide (Bumex) and metolazone (Mykrox, Zaroxolyn) in place of furosemide.

Dobutamine. Dobutamine (Dobutrex) is an intravenous medication given to patients with significant left ventricular dysfunction. A catecholamine, dobutamine stimulates the beta$_1$-adrenergic receptors. Its major action is to increase cardiac contractility. However, at higher amounts, it also increases the heart rate and the incidence of ectopic beats and tachydysrhythmias. Because it also increases AV conduction, care must be taken in patients who have underlying atrial fibrillation. A medication that protects the AV node, such as digitalis, a beta-blocker, or a calcium channel blocker, may be indicated before dobutamine therapy is initiated to prevent increased ventricular response rate.

Milrinone. Milrinone (Primacor) is a phosphodiesterase inhibitor that delays the release of calcium from intracellular reservoirs and prevents the uptake of extracellular calcium by the cells. This promotes vasodilation, decreasing preload and afterload, reducing the workload of the heart. Milrinone is administered intravenously, usually to patients who have not responded to other therapies. It is not usually used to treat patients with renal failure. The major side effects are hypotension (usually asymptomatic), gastrointestinal dysfunction, increased ventricular dysrhythmias, and decreased platelet counts. The patient's blood pressure is monitored closely.

Nesiritide. Nesiritide (Natrecor) is an intravenous medication that is indicated for acutely decompensated HF. Natriuretic peptides are produced by the myocardium as a compensatory response to increased ventricular end-diastolic pressure and myocardial wall stress and to the increased release of neurohormones (eg, norepinephrine, renin, aldosterone) that occur with HF. Nesiritide is a human B-type natriuretic peptide (BNP) made from *Escherichia coli* using recombinant technology. Human BNP binds to vascular smooth muscle and endothelial cells, causing dilation of arteries and veins and suppression of the neurohormones. The result is improved stroke volume and reduced preload and afterload (Colucci et al., 2000). This medication causes rapid improvement in the symptoms of HF and may be used with other HF medications (eg, beta-blockers, digoxin). The most common side effect is dose-related hypotension.

Nursing Management

POSITIONING THE PATIENT TO PROMOTE CIRCULATION

Proper positioning can help reduce venous return to the heart. The patient is positioned upright, preferably with the legs dangling over the side of the bed. This has the immediate effect of decreasing venous return, lowering the output of the right ventricle, and decreasing lung congestion. If the patient is unable to sit with the lower extremities dependent, the patient may be placed in an upright position in bed.

PROVIDING PSYCHOLOGICAL SUPPORT

As the ability to breathe decreases, the patient's sense of fear and anxiety rises proportionately, making the condition more severe. Reassuring the patient and providing skillful anticipatory nursing care are integral parts of the therapy. Because this patient feels a sense of impending doom and has an unstable condition, the nurse must remain with the patient. The nurse should give the patient simple, concise information in a reassuring voice about what is being done to treat the condition and the expected results. The nurse should also identify any anxiety-inducing factors (eg, a pet left alone at home, presence of an unwelcome family member at the bedside, a wallet full of money) and initiate strategies to eliminate the concern or reduce its effect.

MONITORING MEDICATIONS

The patient receiving morphine is observed for respiratory depression, hypotension, and vomiting; a morphine antagonist, such as naloxone hydrochloride (Narcan), is kept available and given to the patient who exhibits these side effects.

The patient receiving diuretic therapy may excrete a large volume of urine within minutes after a potent diuretic is administered. A bedside commode may be used to decrease the energy required by the patient and to reduce the resultant increase in cardiac workload induced by getting on and off a bedpan. If necessary, an indwelling urinary catheter may be inserted.

> **NURSING ALERT** Because of the resulting diuresis, the patient's electrolyte levels, especially potassium and sodium, need to be monitored closely. Fluid balance in some patients is very brittle; they easily become hypovolemic or hypervolemic with small changes in the amount of circulating fluid. Falling blood pressure, increasing heart rate, and decreasing urine output indicate that the circulatory system is not tolerating diuresis and that measures must be taken to reverse the fluid imbalance that has occurred. Serum creatinine is monitored to assess renal function. Men with prostatic hyperplasia must be observed for signs of urinary retention. Additional monitoring activities are discussed in Chart 30-6.

Other Complications

CARDIOGENIC SHOCK

Cardiogenic shock occurs when the heart cannot pump enough blood to supply the amount of oxygen needed by the tissues. This may occur because of one significant or multiple smaller infarctions in which more than 40% of the myocardium becomes necrotic, because of a ruptured ventricle, significant valvular dysfunction, trauma to the heart resulting in myocardial contusion, or as the end stage of HF. It also can occur with cardiac tamponade, pulmonary embolism, cardiomyopathy, and dysrhythmias.

Pathophysiology

The signs and symptoms of cardiogenic shock reflect the circular nature of the pathophysiology of HF. The degree of shock is proportional to the extent of left ventricular dysfunction. The heart muscle loses its contractile power, resulting in a marked reduction in SV and CO, which is sometimes called forward failure. The damage to the myocardium results in a decrease in CO, which reduces arterial blood pressure and tissue perfusion in the vital organs (heart, brain, lung, kidneys). Flow to the coronary arteries is reduced, resulting in decreased oxygen supply to the myocardium, which increases ischemia and further reduces the heart's ability to pump. The inadequate emptying of the ventricle also leads to increased pulmonary pressures, pulmonary congestion, and pulmonary edema, exacerbating the hypoxia, causing ischemia of vital organs, and setting a vicious cycle in motion (Fig. 30-3).

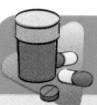

Chart 30-6 • PHARMACOLOGY
Administering and Monitoring Diuretic Therapy

When nursing care involves diuretic therapy for conditions such as pulmonary edema or heart failure, the nurse needs to administer the medication and monitor the patient's response carefully, as follows:

- Administer the diuretic at a time conducive to the patient's lifestyle; for example, early in the day to avoid nocturia.
- Give supplementary potassium with thiazide and loop diuretics as prescribed to replace potassium lost.
- Check laboratory results for electrolyte depletion, especially potassium, magnesium, and sodium; and for electrolyte elevation, especially potassium with potassium-sparing agents and calcium with thiazides.
- Monitor urine output or daily weights to identify appropriate response: intake and output balance, serum BUN and creatinine; notify the health care provider if renal impairment is suspected.
- Assess lung sounds, jugular vein distention, daily weight, and peripheral, abdominal, or sacral edema to identify need to adjust dose.
- Monitor for adverse reactions, such as nausea and gastrointestinal distress, vomiting, diarrhea, weakness, headache, fatigue, anxiety or agitation, and cardiac dysrhythmias.
- Assess for signs of volume depletion, such as postural hypotension, dizziness, imbalance, and reduced jugular venous distention (JVD).
- Monitor for glucose intolerance in patients with and without diabetes mellitus who are receiving thiazide diuretics.
- Monitor for potential ototoxicity in patients, especially those with renal failure, who are receiving a loop diuretic.
- Advise patients to avoid prolonged exposure to the sun because of the risk of photosensitivity.
- Monitor for elevated serum uric acid levels and the development of gout.
- Implement nursing actions to facilitate effect of medication, such as positioning patient upright with legs dangling.

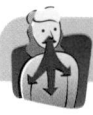

Physiology/Pathophysiology

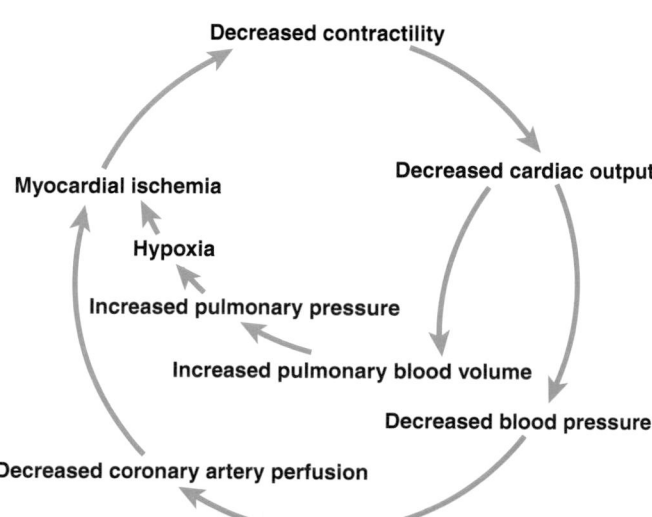

FIGURE 30-3 Pathophysiology of cardiogenic shock.

Clinical Manifestations

The classic signs of cardiogenic shock are tissue hypoperfusion manifested as cerebral hypoxia (restlessness, confusion, agitation), low blood pressure, rapid and weak pulse, cold and clammy skin, increased respiratory crackles, hypoactive bowel sounds, and decreased urinary output. Initially, arterial blood gas analysis may show respiratory alkalosis. Dysrhythmias are common and result from a decrease in oxygen to the myocardium.

Assessment and Diagnostic Findings

Use of a PA catheter to measure left ventricular pressures and CO is important in assessing the severity of the problem and planning management. The PA wedge pressure is elevated and the CO decreased as the left ventricle loses its ability to pump. The systemic vascular resistance is elevated because of the sympathetic nervous system stimulation that occurs as a compensatory response to the decrease in blood pressure. The decreased blood flow to the kidneys causes a hormonal response (ie, increased catecholamines and activation of the renin-angiotensin-aldosterone system) that causes fluid retention and further vasoconstriction. Increases in HR, circulating volume, and vasoconstriction occur to maintain circulation to the brain, heart, kidneys, and lungs, but at a cost: an increase in the workload of the heart.

The reduction in blood volume delivered to the tissues results in an increase in the amount of oxygen that is extracted from the blood that is delivered to the tissues (to try to meet the cellular demand for oxygen). The increased systemic oxygen extraction results in decreased venous (mixed and central) oxygen saturation. When the cellular oxygen needs cannot be met by the systemic oxygen delivery and the oxygen extraction, anaerobic metabolism and the resulting build up of lactic acid occur. Continuous central venous oximetry and measurement of blood lactic acid levels may assist in assessing the severity of the shock as well as the effectiveness of treatment.

Continued cellular hypoperfusion eventually results in organ failure. The patient becomes unresponsive, severe hypotension ensues, and the patient develops shallow respirations; cold, cyanotic or mottled skin; and absent bowel sounds. Arterial blood gas analysis shows metabolic acidosis, and all laboratory test results indicate organ dysfunction. Chapter 15 presents in more detail the pathophysiology and management of cardiogenic shock.

Medical Management

The major approach to treating cardiogenic shock is to correct the underlying problems, reduce any further demand on the heart, improve oxygenation, and restore tissue perfusion. For example, if the ventricular failure is the result of an acute myocardial infarction, emergency percutaneous coronary intervention may be indicated (Webb et al., 2001). Ventricular assist devices may be implanted to support the pumping action of the heart (Barron et al., 2001) (see Chap. 29). Major dysrhythmias are corrected because they may have caused or contributed to the shock. If the patient has hypervolemia, diuresis is indicated. Diuretics, vasodilators, and mechanical devices, such as filtration (continuous renal replacement therapy [CRRT]) and dialysis, have been used to reduce the circulating blood volume. If hypovolemia or low intravascular volume is suspected or detected through pressure readings, the patient is given intravenous volume expanders (eg, normal saline solution, lactated Ringer's solution, albumin) to increase the amount of circulating fluid. The patient is placed on strict bedrest to conserve energy. If the patient has hypoxemia, as detected by pulse oximetry or arterial blood gas analysis, oxygen administration is increased, often under positive pressure when regular flow is insufficient to meet tissue demands. Intubation and sedation may be necessary to maintain oxygenation. The settings for mechanical ventilation are adjusted according to the patient's oxygenation status and the need for conserving energy.

PHARMACOLOGIC THERAPY

Medication therapy is selected and guided according to CO, other cardiac parameters, and mean arterial blood pressure. Because of the decreased perfusion to the gastrointestinal system and the need to adjust the dosage quickly, most medications are administered intravenously.

Vasopressors, or pressor agents, are medications used to raise blood pressure and increase CO. Many pressor medications are catecholamines, such as norepinephrine (Levophed) and high-dose (>10 μg/kg per minute) dopamine (Intropin). Their purpose is to promote perfusion to the heart and brain, but they compromise circulation to other organs (eg, kidney). Because they also tend to increase the workload of the heart by increasing oxygen demand, they are not administered early in the cardiogenic shock process.

Diuretics and vasodilators may be administered carefully to reduce the workload of the heart as long as they do not cause worsening of the tissue hypoperfusion. Agents such as amrinone (Inocor), milrinone (Primacor), sodium nitroprusside (Nipride), and nitroglycerin (Tridil) are effective vasoactive medications that lower the volume returning to the heart, decrease blood pressure, and decrease cardiac work. They cause the arteries and veins to dilate, thereby shunting much of the intravascular volume to the periphery and causing a reduction in preload and afterload.

Positive inotropic medications are given to increase myocardial contractility. Dopamine (Intropin, given at more than 2 μg/kg per minute), dobutamine (Dobutrex), and epinephrine (Adrenalin) are catecholamines that increase contractility. Each of these can cause tachydysrhythmias because they increase automaticity with increasing dosage. Monitoring baseline HR is therefore important. As the baseline HR increases, so does the risk of developing tachydysrhythmias.

OTHER TREATMENTS

Other therapeutic modalities for cardiogenic shock include use of circulatory assist devices. The most frequently used mechanical support device is the intra-aortic balloon pump (IABP). The IABP is a catheter with an inflatable balloon at the end. The catheter is usually inserted through the femoral artery, and the balloon is positioned in the descending thoracic aorta (Fig. 30-4). IABP uses internal counterpulsation through the regular inflation and deflation of the balloon to augment the pumping action of the heart. The device inflates during diastole, increasing the pressure in the aorta during diastole and therefore increasing blood flow through the coronary and peripheral arteries. It deflates just before systole, lessening the pressure within the aorta before left ventricular contraction, decreasing the amount of resistance the heart has to overcome to eject blood and therefore decreasing the amount of work the heart must put forth to eject blood. The device is connected to a console that synchronizes the inflation and deflation of the balloon with the ECG or the arterial pressure (as indicators for systole and diastole). Hemodynamic monitoring is essential to determine the patient's response to the IABP. Other ventricular assist devices are described in Chapter 29.

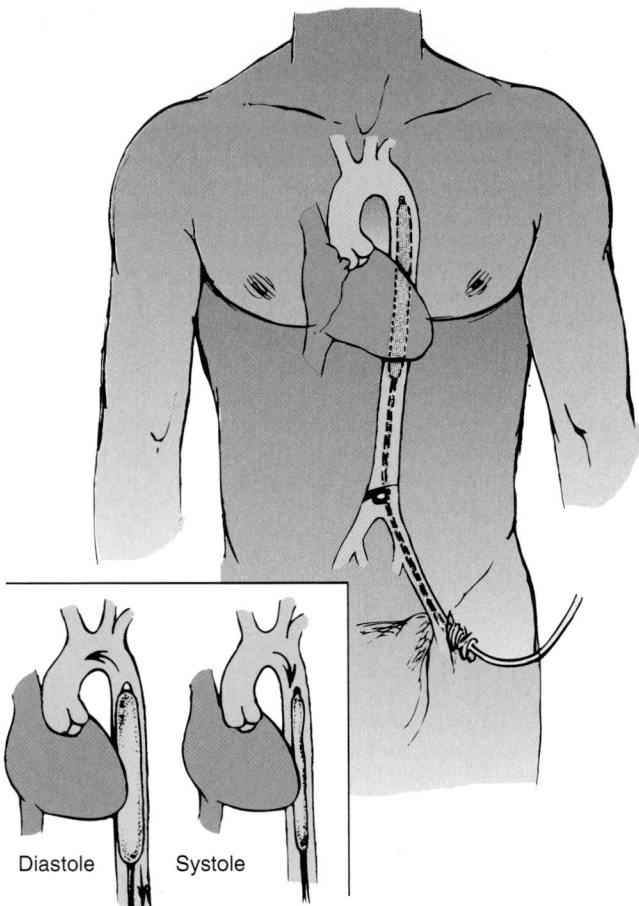

Diastole   Systole

FIGURE 30-4 The intra-aortic balloon pump (IABP) inflates at the beginning of diastole, which results in increased perfusion of the coronary and peripheral arteries; it deflates just before systole, which results in a decrease in afterload (resistance to ejection) and in the left ventricular workload.

Nursing Management

The patient in cardiogenic shock requires constant monitoring and intensive care. The critical care (intensive care) nurse must carefully assess the patient, observe the cardiac rhythm, monitor hemodynamic parameters, and record fluid intake and urinary output. The patient must be closely assessed for responses to the medical interventions and for the development of complications, which must be corrected immediately.

Because of the frequency of nursing interventions and the technology required for effective medical management, the patient is always treated in an intensive care environment. Critical care nurses are responsible for the nursing management, which includes frequent assessments and timely adjustments to medications and therapies based on the assessment data. More information about nursing management of the patient in cardiogenic shock can be found in Chapter 15.

THROMBOEMBOLISM

The decreased mobility of the patient with cardiac disease and the impaired circulation that accompany these disorders contribute to the development of intracardiac and intravascular thrombosis. Intracardiac thrombus is especially common in patients with atrial fibrillation, because the atria do not contract forcefully and blood flow slows through the atrium, increasing thrombus formation. Intracardiac thrombus is detected by an echocardiogram and treated with anticoagulants, such as heparin and warfarin (Coumadin). A part of the thrombus may become detached (embolus) and may be carried to the brain, kidneys, intestines, or lungs. The most common problem is pulmonary embolism. The symptoms of pulmonary embolism include chest pain, cyanosis, shortness of breath, rapid respirations, and hemoptysis (bloody sputum).

The pulmonary embolus may block the circulation to a part of the lung, producing an area of pulmonary infarction. Usually, there is a significant decrease in oxygenation measured by arterial blood gas analysis or pulse oximetry. Pain experienced is usually pleuritic; it increases with respiration and may subside when the patient holds the breath. Cardiac pain is usually continuous and does not vary with respirations. However, it may be difficult to differentiate by symptoms alone. The patient usually undergoes a ventilation-perfusion scan or a pulmonary arteriogram for definitive diagnosis. The treatment and care for patients with pulmonary embolism are discussed in Chapter 23.

Systemic embolism may manifest as cerebral, mesenteric, or renal infarction; an embolism can also compromise the blood supply to an extremity, which is discussed in more detail in Chapter 31. The nurse must be aware of such possible complications and be prepared to identify and report signs and symptoms.

PERICARDIAL EFFUSION AND CARDIAC TAMPONADE

Pathophysiology

Pericardial effusion refers to the accumulation of fluid in the pericardial sac. This occurrence may accompany pericarditis (see Chap. 29), advanced HF, metastatic carcinoma, cardiac surgery, trauma, or nontraumatic hemorrhage.

Normally, the pericardial sac contains less than 50 mL of fluid, which is needed to decrease friction for the beating heart. An increase in pericardial fluid raises the pressure within the pericardial sac and compresses the heart. This has the following effects:

- Increased right and left ventricular end-diastolic pressures
- Decreased venous return
- Inability of the ventricles to distend adequately and to fill

Pericardial fluid may accumulate slowly without causing noticeable symptoms. A rapidly developing effusion, however, can stretch the pericardium to its maximum size and, because of increased pericardial pressure, reduce venous return to the heart and decrease CO. The result is cardiac tamponade (compression of the heart).

Clinical Manifestations

The patient may complain of a feeling of fullness within the chest or may have substantial or ill-defined pain. The feeling of pressure in the chest may result from stretching of the pericardial sac. Because of increased pressure within the pericardium, venous pressure tends to rise, as evidenced by engorged neck veins. Other signs include shortness of breath and a drop and fluctuation in blood pressure. Systolic blood pressure that is detected during exhalation but not heard with inhalation is called **pulsus paradoxus**. The difference in systolic pressure between the point that it is heard during exhalation and the point that it is heard during inhalation is measured. Pulsus paradoxus exceeding 10 mm Hg

is abnormal. The cardinal signs of cardiac tamponade are falling systolic blood pressure, narrowing pulse pressure, rising venous pressure (increased jugular venous distention), and distant (muffled) heart sounds (Chart 30-7).

 NURSING ALERT Cardiac tamponade is a life-threatening situation, demanding immediate intervention.

Assessment and Diagnostic Findings

Pericardial effusion is detected by percussing the chest and noticing an extension of flatness across the anterior aspect of the chest. An echocardiogram may be performed to confirm the diagnosis. The clinical signs and symptoms and chest x-ray findings are usually sufficient to diagnose pericardial effusion.

Medical Management

PERICARDIOCENTESIS

If cardiac function becomes seriously impaired, **pericardiocentesis** (puncture of the pericardial sac to aspirate pericardial fluid) is performed to remove fluid from the pericardial sac. The major

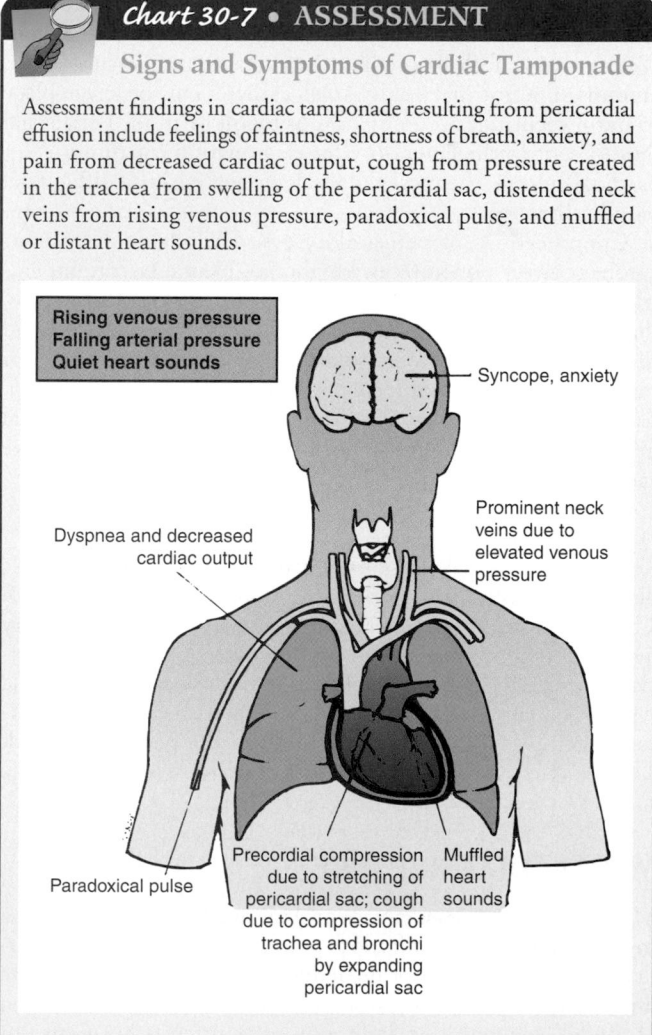

Chart 30-7 • **ASSESSMENT**

Signs and Symptoms of Cardiac Tamponade

Assessment findings in cardiac tamponade resulting from pericardial effusion include feelings of faintness, shortness of breath, anxiety, and pain from decreased cardiac output, cough from pressure created in the trachea from swelling of the pericardial sac, distended neck veins from rising venous pressure, paradoxical pulse, and muffled or distant heart sounds.

Rising venous pressure
Falling arterial pressure
Quiet heart sounds

Syncope, anxiety

Dyspnea and decreased cardiac output

Prominent neck veins due to elevated venous pressure

Paradoxical pulse

Precordial compression due to stretching of pericardial sac; cough due to compression of trachea and bronchi by expanding pericardial sac

Muffled heart sounds

goal is to prevent cardiac tamponade, which restricts normal heart action.

During the procedure, the patient is monitored by ECG and hemodynamic pressure measurements. Emergency resuscitative equipment should be readily available. The head of the bed is elevated to 45 to 60 degrees, placing the heart in proximity to the chest wall so that the needle can be inserted into the pericardial sac more easily. If a peripheral intravenous device is not already in place, one is inserted, and a slow intravenous infusion is started in case it becomes necessary to administer emergency medications or blood products.

The pericardial aspiration needle is attached to a 50-mL syringe by a three-way stopcock. Several possible sites are used for pericardial aspiration. The needle may be inserted in the angle between the left costal margin and the xiphoid, near the cardiac apex; at the fifth or sixth intercostal space at the left sternal margin; or on the right sternal margin of the fourth intercostal space. The needle is advanced slowly until it has entered the epicardium and fluid is obtained. The ECG can help determine when the needle has contacted the epicardium. The cable of a precordial lead is attached to the aspirating needle with alligator clamps; contact with the epicardium is seen by ST segment elevation on the ECG. During the procedure, drainage fluid must be checked for clotting. Although not entirely accurate, the guideline is that pericardial blood does not clot readily, whereas blood obtained from inadvertent puncture of one of the heart chambers does clot.

A resulting fall in central venous pressure and an associated rise in blood pressure after withdrawal of pericardial fluid indicate that the cardiac tamponade has been relieved. The patient almost always feels immediate relief. If there is a substantial amount of pericardial fluid, a small catheter may be left in place to drain recurrent accumulation of blood or fluid. Pericardial fluid is sent to the laboratory for examination for tumor cells, bacterial culture, chemical and serologic analysis, and differential blood cell count.

Complications of pericardiocentesis include ventricular or coronary artery puncture, dysrhythmias, pleural laceration, gastric puncture, and myocardial trauma. After pericardiocentesis, the patient's heart rhythm, blood pressure, venous pressure, and heart sounds are monitored to detect any possible recurrence of cardiac tamponade. If it recurs, repeated aspiration is necessary. Cardiac tamponade may require treatment by open pericardial drainage (pericardiotomy). The patient is ideally in an intensive care unit.

PERICARDIOTOMY

Recurrent pericardial effusions, usually associated with neoplastic diseases, may be treated by a **pericardiotomy** (pericardial window). The patient receives a general anesthetic, but cardiopulmonary bypass is seldom necessary. A portion of the pericardium is excised to permit the pericardial fluid to drain into the lymphatic system. Uncommonly, catheters are placed between the pericardium and abdominal cavity to drain the pericardial fluid. The nursing care is the same as that described for other cardiac surgery (see Chap. 28).

MYOCARDIAL RUPTURE

Myocardial rupture is a rare event. However, it can occur when a myocardial infarction, infectious process, cardiac trauma, pericardial disease, or other myocardial dysfunction weakens the cardiac muscle (eg, ventricular aneurysm) substantially. Persistent elevation of the ST segment is an indication of ventricular aneurysm. In

many cases, the result of myocardial rupture is immediate death, even if the patient undergoes immediate cardiac surgery.

CARDIAC ARREST

Cardiac arrest occurs when the heart ceases to produce an effective pulse and blood circulation. It may be caused by a cardiac electrical event, as when the HR is too fast (especially ventricular tachycardia or ventricular fibrillation) or too slow (bradycardia or AV block) or when there is no heart rate at all (asystole). Cardiac arrest may follow respiratory arrest; it may also occur when electrical activity is present but there is ineffective cardiac contraction or circulating volume, which is called **pulseless electrical activity (PEA)**. Formerly called electrical-mechanical dissociation (EMD), PEA can be caused by hypovolemia (eg, with excessive bleeding), cardiac tamponade, hypothermia, massive pulmonary embolism, medication overdoses (eg, tricyclic agents, digitalis, beta-blockers, calcium channel blockers), significant acidosis, and massive acute myocardial infarction.

Clinical Manifestations

Consciousness, pulse, and blood pressure are lost immediately. Ineffective respiratory gasping may occur. The pupils of the eyes begin dilating within 45 seconds. Seizures may or may not occur.

The risk of irreversible brain damage and death increases with every minute from the time that circulation ceases. The interval varies with the age and underlying condition of the patient. During this period, the diagnosis of cardiac arrest must be made, and measures must be taken immediately to restore circulation.

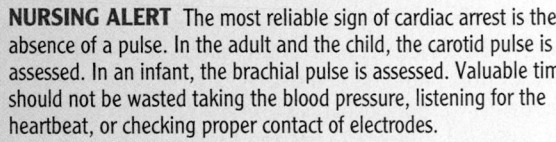

NURSING ALERT The most reliable sign of cardiac arrest is the absence of a pulse. In the adult and the child, the carotid pulse is assessed. In an infant, the brachial pulse is assessed. Valuable time should not be wasted taking the blood pressure, listening for the heartbeat, or checking proper contact of electrodes.

Emergency Management: Cardiopulmonary Resuscitation

The ABCDs of basic cardiopulmonary resuscitation (CPR) are *a*irway, *b*reathing, *c*irculation, and *d*efibrillation (Guidelines 2000 for Cardiopulmonary Resuscitation and Emergency Cardiovascular Care, 2000). Once loss of consciousness has been established, the resuscitation priority for the adult in most cases is placing a phone call to activate the code team or the emergency medical system (EMS). Exceptions to this include near drowning, drug or medication overdose, and respiratory arrest situations, for which 1 minute of CPR should be performed before activating the EMS. Because the underlying cause of arrest in an infant or child is usually respiratory, the priority is to begin CPR and then activate the EMS after 1 minute of CPR. Because the care of the pediatric patient is individualized, the following discussion on the care of a cardiac arrest patient applies only to adults.

Resuscitation consists of the following steps:

1. Airway: maintaining an open airway
2. Breathing: providing artificial ventilation by rescue breathing
3. Circulation: promoting artificial circulation by external cardiac compression
4. Defibrillation: restoring the heartbeat (see Chap. 27)

If the patient is monitored or is immediately placed on the monitor using the multifunction pads or the quick-look paddles (found on most defibrillators) and the ECG shows ventricular tachycardia or ventricular fibrillation, defibrillation rather than CPR is the treatment of choice. In this scenario, CPR is performed initially only if the defibrillator is not immediately available. The survival rate decreases by 10% for every minute that defibrillation is delayed (Guidelines, 2000). If the patient has not been defibrillated within 10 minutes, the chance of survival is close to zero. More information on defibrillation can be found in Chapter 27.

MAINTAINING AIRWAY AND BREATHING

The first step in CPR is to obtain an open airway. Any obvious material in the mouth or throat should be removed. The chin is directed up and back, or the jaw (mandible) is lifted forward. The rescuer "looks, listens, and feels" for air movement. An oropharyngeal airway is inserted if available. Two rescue ventilations over 3 to 4 seconds are provided using a bag-mask or mouth-mask device (Fig. 30-5). An obstructed airway should be suspected when the rescuer cannot give the initial ventilations, and the Heimlich maneuver or abdominal thrusts should be administered to relieve the obstruction.

If the first rescue ventilations enter easily, the patient is ventilated with 12 breaths per minute, and the open airway is maintained. Endotracheal intubation is frequently performed by a physician, nurse anesthetist, or respiratory therapist during a resuscitation procedure (also called a code) to ensure an adequate airway and ventilation. The resuscitation bag device is then connected directly to the endotracheal tube.

Because of the risk of unrecognized esophageal intubation or dislodgement of the endotracheal tube (ET), tracheal intubation must be confirmed by one technique from each of two different methods: a primary method (visualization of the ET through the vocal cords, auscultation of breath sounds in five areas on the chest, or bilateral chest expansion) and a secondary method (an esophageal detector device [such as Ambu TubeChek] or an end-tidal CO_2 detector). The end-tidal CO_2 detectors available give qualitative (yes/no) or quantitative (measurable; ie, capnometry) results. Because delivery of CO_2 is low in patients in cardiopulmonary arrest, the qualitative devices are not as accurate in detecting incorrect placement as are esophageal detector devices (EDDs). There are two main types of EDD: a bulb type and a syringe type.

The bulb is collapsed or the plunger of the syringe compressed before its attachment to the ET; each creates a suction force at the end of the ET. If the ET is in the trachea, the presence of air in the lungs and the rigid walls of the trachea allow re-inflation of the bulb or aspiration of the syringe. If the ET is in the esophagus, the suction pulls on the unsupported walls of the esophagus, causing them to collapse and preventing the bulb from re-inflating or the syringe to aspirate. A chest x-ray, which is frequently obtained after ET placement, is helpful in determining whether the ET is too high, too low, or in a main bronchus. However, a chest x-ray cannot confirm placement of an ET. The ET may be in the esophagus or the trachea and result in the same appearance on the x-ray (Guidelines, 2000). Arterial blood gas levels are measured to guide oxygen therapy.

RESTORING CIRCULATION

After performing ventilation, the carotid pulse is assessed and external cardiac compressions are provided when no pulse is detected. If a defibrillator is not yet available but a process has been put into place to obtain one, chest compressions are initiated. Compressions are performed with the patient on a firm surface, such as the floor, a cardiac board, or a meal tray. The rescuer (facing the patient's side) places the heel of one hand on the lower half of the sternum, two fingerwidths (3.8 cm [1.5 inches]) from the tip of the xiphoid and positions the other hand on top of the first hand (Fig. 30-6) (Guidelines, 2000). The fingers should not touch the chest wall.

Using the body weight while keeping the elbows straight, the rescuer presses quickly downward from the shoulder area to deliver a forceful compression to the victim's lower sternum about 3.8 to 5 cm (1.5 to 2 inches) toward the spine (Guidelines, 2000). The chest compression rate is 80 to 100 times per minute. If only one rescuer is available, the rate is two ventilations to every 15 cardiac compressions. When two rescuers are available, the first person performs the cardiac compressions, pausing after the fifth compression, when the second rescuer gives one ventilation over 1.5 to 2 seconds and at a tidal volume of less than 1 L.

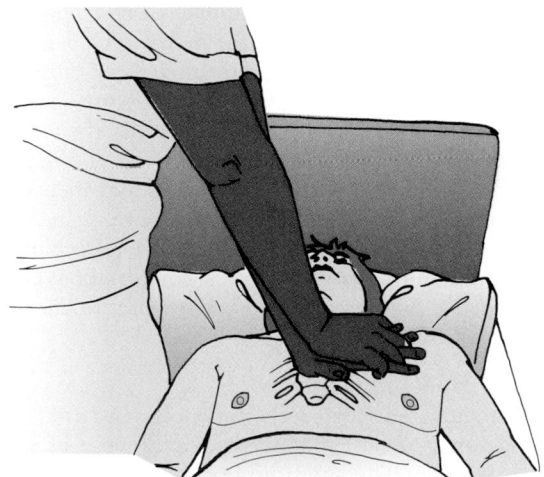

FIGURE 30-6 Chest compressions in cardiopulmonary resuscitation (CPR) are performed by placing the heel of one hand on the lower half of the sternum and the other hand on top of the first hand. Elbows are kept straight and body weight is used to apply quick, forceful compressions to the lower sternum. For the most effective hand placement and outcome, the patient's chest should be bare.

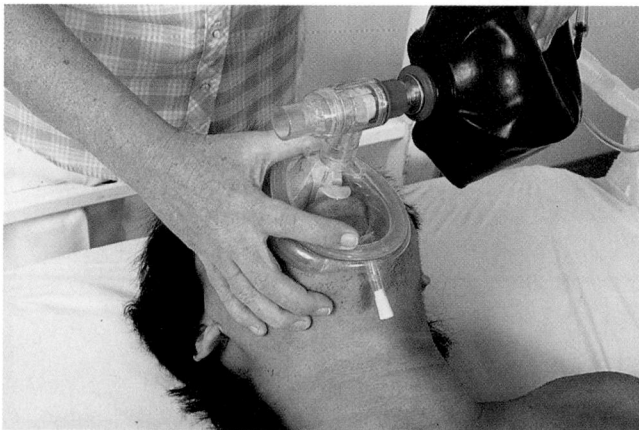

FIGURE 30-5 The chin lift and bag-and-mask technique for ventilating patients who need cardiopulmonary resuscitation.

Table 30-5 • Medications Used in Cardiopulmonary Resuscitation

AGENT AND ACTION	INDICATIONS	NURSING CONSIDERATIONS
Oxygen—improves tissue oxygenation and corrects hypoxemia	Administered to all patients with acute cardiac ischemia or suspected hypoxemia, including those with COPD	• Use 100% FiO_2 during resuscitation. • Recognize that no lung damage occurs when used for less than 24 hours. • Monitor dose by end-tidal CO_2 or pulse oximeter.
Epinephrine (Adrenalin)—increases systemic vascular resistance and blood pressure; improves coronary and cerebral perfusion and myocardial contractility	Given to patients in cardiac arrest, especially caused by asystole or pulseless electrical activity; may be given if caused by ventricular tachycardia or ventricular fibrillation	• Administer by IV push (IVP) or through the endotracheal (ET) tube. • Avoid adding to IV lines that contain alkaline solution (eg, bicarbonate).
Atropine—blocks parasympathetic action; increases SA node automaticity and AV conduction	Given to patients with symptomatic bradycardia (hemodynamically unstable, frequent premature ventricular contractions and symptoms of ischemia)	• Give rapidly as 2.0 to 2.5 mg IVP or through the ET tube. • Be aware that less than 0.5 mg in the adult can cause the heart rate to decrease to a worse bradycardia. • Monitor patient for reflexive tachycardia.
Sodium bicarbonate ($NaHCO_3$)—corrects metabolic acidosis	Given to correct metabolic acidosis that is refractory to standard advanced cardiac life support interventions (cardiopulmonary resuscitation, intubation, and respiratory management)	• Administer initial dose of 1 mEq/kg IV; then administer the dose based on the base deficit calculated from arterial blood gas values. • Recognize that to prevent development of rebound metabolic alkalosis, complete correction of acidosis is not indicated
Magnesium—promotes adequate functioning of the cellular sodium–potassium pump	Given to patients with torsades de pointes	• May give diluted over 1–2 min or intravenous push. • Monitor for hypotension, asystole, bradycardia, respiratory paralysis.
Vasopressin (Pitressin)—increases inotropic action (contraction) of the heart	An alternative to epinephrine when cardiac arrest is caused by ventricular tachycardia or ventricular fibrillation	• Give 40 U IV one time only.

When the code team or emergency medical personnel arrive, the patient is quickly assessed to determine cardiac rhythm and respiratory status, as well as possible causes for the arrest. The specific subsequent advanced life support interventions depend on the assessment results. For example, after the patient is placed on a cardiac monitor and ventricular fibrillation is detected, the patient will be defibrillated up to three times, and then CPR will be resumed. However, if asystole is detected on the monitor, CPR is resumed immediately while trying to identify the underlying cause, such as hypovolemia, hypothermia, or hypoxia. CPR may be stopped when the patient responds and begins to breathe, the rescuers are too exhausted or at risk (eg, the building is at risk of collapsing) to continue CPR, or signs of death are obvious. If the patient does not respond to therapies given during the arrest, the resuscitation effort may be stopped or "called" by the physician. The decision to terminate resuscitation is based on medical considerations and takes into account the underlying condition of the patient and the chances for survival.

FOLLOW-UP MONITORING

Once successfully resuscitated, the patient is transferred to an intensive care unit for close monitoring. Continuous ECG monitoring and frequent blood pressure assessments are essential until hemodynamic stability is reestablished. Etiologic factors that precipitated the arrest, such as metabolic or rhythm abnormalities, must be identified and treated. Possible contributing factors, such as electrolyte or acid-base imbalances, need to be identified and corrected. Selected medications, as described in Table 30-5, may be used during and after resuscitation.

Critical Thinking Exercises

1. Your patient is a 55-year-old man who was diagnosed last year with systolic HF (due to coronary artery disease) and was stabilized with lisinopril, Lasix, and metoprolol. He follows a low-sodium diet, with only an occasional indiscretion. He is complaining of a nagging cough. What are some of the possible causes for the cough? What would be key assessment factors that would help identify the cause? What medical treatments and nursing interventions would be appropriate for each of the possible causes?

2. A 77-year-old female patient was readmitted for HF for the third time in 2 months. Identify the factors that possibly contribute to her readmission and that would need to be assessed. What interventions could be implemented to prevent another readmission? Describe the interaction (ie, behaviors, words, and communication techniques) that would demonstrate the concept of partnering with the patient.

REFERENCES AND SELECTED READINGS

Books

Agency for Health Care Policy and Research. (1994). *Heart failure: Evaluation and care of patients with left-ventricular systolic dysfunction.* Clinical Practice Guideline Number 11. AHCPR Publication

No. 94-0612. Rockville, MD: Public Health Service, U.S. Department of Health and Human Services.

American Heart Association. (2001). *2001 Heart and stroke statistical update.* Dallas, TX: American Heart Association.

Bickley, L. S., & Szilagyi, P.G. (2003). *Bates's guide to physical examination and history taking* (8th ed.). Philadelphia: Lippincott Williams & Wilkins.

Braunwald, E., Zipes, D. P., & Libby, P. (2001). *Heart disease: A textbook of cardiovascular medicine* (6th ed.). Philadelphia: W. B. Saunders.

Carpenito, L. J. (1997). *Nursing diagnosis: Application to clinical practice* (7th ed.). Philadelphia: Lippincott-Raven.

Fuster, V., Alexander, R. W., & O'Rourke, R. A. (Eds.). (2001). *Hurst's the heart* (10th ed.). New York: McGraw-Hill.

Kinney, M. R., Dunbar, S. B., Brooks-Brunn, J. A., Molter, N., & Vitello-Ciccui, J. M. (1998). *AACN clinical reference for critical care nursing* (4th ed.). St. Louis: Mosby.

Murphy, J. (Ed.). (2000). *Mayo Clinic cardiology review* (2nd ed.). Philadelphia: Lippincott Williams & Wilkins.

Journals

Asterisks indicate nursing research articles.

Abraham, W. T. (2002). Multicenter InSync Randomized Clinical Evaluation (MIRACLE). Available at: http://www.acc.org/education/online/trials/acc2001/miracle.html. Accessed January 22, 2002.

Ammon, S. (2001). Managing patients with heart failure. *American Journal of Nursing, 101*(12), 34–40.

Asselin, M. E., & Cullen, H. A. (2001). What you need to know about the new ACLS guidelines: Find out about changes in algorithms and policies and how they'll affect your practice. *Nursing 2001, 31*(4), 48–50.

Barron, H. V., Every, N. R., Parsons, L. S., Angeja, B., Goldberg, R. J., & Gore, J. M., Chou, T. M., & Investigators in the National Registry of Myocardial Infarction 2. (2001). The use of intra-aortic balloon counterpulsation in patients with cardiogenic shock complicating acute myocardial infarction: Data from the National Registry of Myocardial Infarction 2. *American Heart Journal, 141*(6), 933–939.

Beckett, J. L. (1999). Endothelial dysfunction and the promise of ACE inhibitors. *American Journal of Nursing, 99*(10), 44–50.

*Bennett, S. J., Huster, G. A., Baker, S. L., Milgrom, L. B., Kirchgassner, A., Birt, J., & Pressler, M. L. (1998). Characterization of the precipitants of hospitalization for heart failure decompensation. *American Journal of Critical Care, 7*(8), 168–174.

Beta-Blocker Evaluation of Survival Trial (BEST) Investigators. (2001). A trial of the beta-blocker bucindolol in patients with advanced chronic heart failure. *New England Journal of Medicine, 344*(22), 1659–1667.

Bither, C. J., & Apple, S. (2001). Home management of the failing heart. *American Journal of Nursing, 101*(12), 41–47.

Bixby, M. B., Konick-McMahon, J., & McKenna, C. G. (2000). Applying the transitional care model to elderly patients with heart failure. *Journal of Cardiovascular Nursing, 14*(3), 53–63.

Brater, D. C. (1998). Diuretic therapy. *New England Journal of Medicine, 339*(6), 387–395.

Carelock, J., & Clark, A. P. (2001). Heart failure: Pathophysiological mechanisms. *American Journal of Nursing, 101*, 26–33.

CIBIS-II Investigators and Committees. (1999). The Cardiac Insufficiency Bisoprolol Study II (CIBIS-II): A randomized trial. *Lancet, 353*(9146), 9–13.

Clement, D. L., De Buyzere, M., Tomas, M., & Vanavermaete, G. (2000). Long-term effects of clinical outcome with low and high dose captopril in the heart insufficient patients study (CHIPS). *Acta Cardiologica, 55*(1), 1–7.

Colucci, W. S., Elkayam, U., Horton, D. P., Abraham, W. T., Bourge, R. C., Johnson, A. D., Wagoner, L. E., Givertz, M. M., Liang, C. S., Neibaur, M., Haught, W. H., & LeJemtel, T. H. (2000). Intravenous nesiritide, a natriuretic peptide, in the treatment of decompensated heart failure. Nesiritide Study Group. *New England Journal of Medicine, 343*(4), 246–253.

The CONSENSUS Trial Study Group. (1987). Effects of enalapril on mortality in severe congestive heart failure: Results of the Coopera-

tive North Scandinavian Enalapril Survival Study (CONSENSUS). *New England Journal of Medicine, 316*(23), 1429–1435.

Cook, D. M. (1993). The use of central nervous manifestations in the early detection of digitalis toxicity. *Heart & Lung, 22*(6), 477–480.

DeWald, T., Gaulden L., Beyler, M., Whellan, D., & Bowers, M. (2000). Current trends in the management of heart failure. *Nursing Clinics of North America, 35*(4), 855–875.

The Digitalis Investigation Group (DIG). (1997). The effect of digoxin on mortality and morbidity in patients with heart failure. *New England Journal of Medicine, 336*(8), 525–533.

Georgiou, D., Chen, Y., Appadoo, S., Belardinelli, R., Greene, R., Parides, M., & Glied, S. (2001). Cost-effectiveness analysis of long-term moderate exercise training in chronic heart failure. *American Journal of Cardiology, 87*(8), 984–988.

Gerber, T. C., Nishimura, R. A., Holmes, D. R., Jr., Lloyd, M. A., Zehr, K. J., Tajik, A. J., & Hayes, D. L. (2001). Left ventricular and biventricular pacing in congestive heart failure. *Mayo Clinic Proceedings, 76*(8), 803–812.

Guidelines 2000 for Cardiopulmonary Resuscitation and Emergency Cardiovascular Care: The American Heart Association in collaboration with the International Liaison Committee on Resuscitation. *Circulation, 102*(8)(Suppl. 8), I1–384.

Halm, M. A., & Penque, S. (1999). Heart disease in women. *American Journal of Nursing, 99*(4), 26–32.

*Happ, M. B., Naylor, M. D., & Roe-Prior, P. (1997). Factors contributing to rehospitalization of elderly patients with heart failure. *Journal of Cardiovascular Nursing, 11*(4), 75–84.

Hunt, S. A., Baker, D. W., Chin, M. H., Cinquegrani, M. P., Feldman, A. M., Francis, G. S., Ganiats, T. G., Goldstein, S., Gregoratos, G., Jessup, M. L., Noble, R. J., Packer, M., Silver, M. A., Stevenson, L. W., Gibbons, R. J., Antman, E. M., Alpert, J. S., Faxon, D. P., Fuster, V., Gregoratos, G., Jacobs, A. K., Hiratzka, L. F., Russell, R. O., Smith, S. C., Jr., American College of Cardiology/American Heart Association Task Force on Practice Guidelines (Committee to Revise the 1995 Guidelines for the Evaluation and Management of Heart Failure), International Society for Heart and Lung Transplantation, & Heart Failure Society of America. (2001). ACC/AHA guidelines for the evaluation and management of chronic heart failure in the adult: A report of the American College of Cardiology/American Heart Association Task Force on Practice Guidelines (Committee to Revise the 1995 Guidelines for the Evaluation and Management of Heart Failure). *Journal of the American College of Cardiology, 38*(7), 2101–2113.

*Jaarsma, T., Halfens, R., Tan, F., Abu-Saad, H., Dracup, K., & Diederiks, J. (2000). Self-care and quality of life in patients with advanced heart failure: The effect of a supportive educational intervention. *Heart & Lung, 29*(5), 319–330.

Mancini, M. E., & Kaye, W. (1999). AEDs. Changing the way you respond to cardiac arrest. *American Journal of Nursing, 99*(5), 26–30.

MERIT-HF Study Group. (1999). Effect of metoprolol CR/XL in chronic heart failure: Metoprolol CR/XL randomized intervention trial in congestive heart failure (MERIT-HF). *Lancet, 353*, 2001–2007.

Meyer, K. (2001). Exercise training in heart failure: Recommendations based on current research. *Medicine and Science in Sports and Exercise, 33*(4), 525–531.

The NETWORK Investigators. (1998). Clinical outcome with enalapril in symptomatic chronic heart failure: A dose comparison. *European Heart Journal, 19*(3), 481–489.

Packer, M. (2000). *Carvedilol improves survival in patients with advanced heart failure: Results of the COPERNICUS study.* Presented at the 4th Scientific Meeting of the Heart Failure Society of America, Boca Raton, FL, September 10–13.

Packer, M., Bristow, M. R., Cohn, J. N., Colucci, W. S., Fowler, M. B., Gilbert, E. M., & Shusterman, N. H. (1996). The effect of carvedilol on morbidity and mortality in patients with chronic heart failure. U.S. Carvedilol Heart Failure Study Group. *New England Journal of Medicine, 334*(21), 1349–1355.

Packer, M., Coats, A. J. S., Fowler, M. B., Katus, H. A., Krum, H., Mohacsi, P., Rouleau, J. L., Tendera, M., Castaigne, A., Roecker, E. B., Schultz, M. K., DeMets, D. L., & Carvedilol Prospective

Randomized Cumulative Survival Study Group. (2001). Effect of carvedilol on survival in severe chronic heart failure. *New England Journal of Medicine, 344* (22), 1651–1658.

Packer, M., Poole-Wilson, P. A., & Armstrong, P. W. (1999). Comparative effects of low and high doses of the angiotensin-converting enzyme inhibitor, lisinopril, on morbidity and mortality in chronic heart failure. ATLAS Study Group. *Circulation, 100*(23), 2312–2318.

Page, J., & Henry, D. (2000). Consumption of NSAIDs and the development of congestive heart failure in the elderly. *Archives of Internal Medicine, 160*(6), 777–784.

Pitt, B., Zannad, F., Remme, W. J., Cody, R., Castaigre, A., Perez, A., Palensky, J., & Wittes, J. (1999). The effect of spironolactone on morbidity and mortality in patients with severe heart failure. *New England Journal of Medicine, 341*(10), 709–717.

Rich, M. W., Beckham, V., Wittenberg, C., Leven, C. L., Freedland, K. E., Carney, R. M. (1995). A multidisciplinary intervention to prevent the readmission of elderly patients with congestive heart failure. *New England Journal of Medicine, 333*(18), 1190–1195.

*Riegle, B., Carlson, B., & Glaser, D. (2000). Developing and testing a clinical tool measuring self-management of heart failure. *Heart & Lung, 29*(1), 4–12.

Sanderson, J. E., Chan, S. K., Yip, G., Yeung, L. Y., Chan, K. W., Raymond, K., & Woo, K. S. (1999). Beta-blockade in heart failure: A comparison of carvedilol with metoprolol. *Journal of American College of Cardiology, 34*(5), 1522–1528.

Shamsham, F., & Mitchell, J. (2000). Essentials of the diagnosis of heart failure. *American Family Physician, 61*(5), 1319–1328.

The SOLVD Investigators. (1992). Effect of enalapril on mortality and the development of heart failure in asymptomatic patients with reduced left ventricular ejection fractions. *New England Journal of Medicine, 327*(10), 685–691.

*Ströberg, A., Broströ, A., Dahlström, U., & Fridlund, B. (1999). Factors influencing patient compliance with therapeutic regimens in chronic heart failure: A critical incident technique analysis. *Heart & Lung, 28*(5), 334–341.

*Stull, D., Starling, R., Hass, G., & Young, J. B. (1999). Becoming a patient with heart failure. *Heart & Lung, 28*(4), 284–292.

Turner, M. A. (2000). Impedance cardiography: A noninvasive way to monitor hemodynamics. *Dimensions in Critical Care Nursing, 19*(3), 2–12.

Uretsky, B. F., Young, J. B., Shahidi, F. E., Yellen, L. G., Harrison, M. C., & Jolly, M. K. (1993). Randomized study assessing the effect of digoxin withdrawal in patients with mild to moderate chronic congestive heart failure: Results of the PROVED trial. PROVED Investigative Group. *Journal of American College of Cardiology, 22*(4), 955–962.

Vasan, R. S., & Levy, K. (2000). Defining diastolic heart failure. *Circulation, 101*(17), 2118–2121.

Von Rueden, K. T., & Turner, M. (1999). Advances in continuous, noninvasive hemodynamic surveillance. *Critical Care Nursing Clinics of North America, 11*(1), 63–75.

Webb, J. G., Sanborn, T. A., Sleeper, L. A., Carere, R. G., Buller, C. E., Slater, J. N., Baran, K. W., Koller, P. T., Talley, J. D., Porway, M., Hochman, J. S., & SHOCK Investigators. (2001). Percutaneous coronary intervention for cardiogenic shock in the SHOCK Trial Registry. *American Heart Journal, 141*(6), 964–970.

Weber, K. T. (2001). Mechanisms of disease: Aldosterone in congestive heart failure. *New England Journal of Medicine, 345*(23), 1689–1697.

RESOURCES AND WEBSITES

The American College of Cardiology Heart House, 9111 Old Georgetown Road, Bethesda, MD 20814-1699; 1-800-253-4636, ext. 694 or 301-897-5400; http://www.acc.org.

American Heart Association, 7320 Greenville Ave., Dallas, TX 75231; 1-800-242-8721; http://www.americanheart.org.

Heart Failure Society of America, Court International, Suite 238-N, 2550 University Avenue West, Saint Paul, MN 55144; 651-642-1633; http://www.abouthf.org.

Heartmates, Inc., PO Box 16202, Minneapolis, MN 55416; 952-929-3331; http://www.heartmates.com.

National Heart, Lung, and Blood Institute, National Institutes of Health, Building 31, Room 5A52, Bethesda, MD 20892; 301-592-8573; http://www.nhlbi.nih.gov.

National Institute on Aging, Building 31, Room 5C27, 31 Center Drive, MSC 2292, Bethesda, MD 20892; 301-496-1752; http://www.nih.gov/nia.

Assessment and Management of Patients With Vascular Disorders and Problems of Peripheral Circulation

LEARNING OBJECTIVES ●

On completion of this chapter, the learner will be able to:

1. Identify anatomic and physiologic factors that affect peripheral blood flow and tissue oxygenation.

2. Use appropriate parameters for assessment of peripheral circulation.

3. Use the nursing process as a framework of care for patients with circulatory insufficiency of the extremities.

4. Compare the various diseases of the arteries, their causes, pathologic and physiologic changes, clinical manifestations, management, and prevention.

5. Describe the prevention and management of venous thrombosis.

6. Compare the preventive management of venous insufficiency, leg ulcers, and varicose veins.

7. Use the nursing process as a framework of care for patients with leg ulcers.

8. Describe the relationship between lymphangitis and lymphedema.

Adequate perfusion oxygenates and nourishes body tissues and depends in part on a properly functioning cardiovascular system. Adequate blood flow depends on the efficient pumping action of the heart, patent and responsive blood vessels, and adequate circulating blood volume. Nervous system activity, blood viscosity, and the metabolic needs of tissues influence the rate and adequacy of blood flow.

Anatomic and Physiologic Overview

The vascular system consists of two interdependent systems. The right side of the heart pumps blood through the lungs to the pulmonary circulation, and the left side of the heart pumps blood to all other body tissues through the systemic circulation. The blood vessels in both systems channel the blood from the heart to the tissues and back to the heart (Fig. 31-1). Contraction of the ventricles is the driving force that moves blood through the vascular systems.

Arteries distribute oxygenated blood from the left side of the heart to the tissues, whereas the veins carry deoxygenated blood from the tissues to the right side of the heart. Capillary vessels, located within the tissues, connect the arterial and venous systems and are the site of exchange of nutrients and metabolic wastes between the circulatory system and the tissues. Arterioles and venules immediately adjacent to the capillaries, together with the capillaries, make up the microcirculation.

The lymphatic system complements the function of the circulatory system. Lymphatic vessels transport lymph (a fluid similar to plasma), and tissue fluids (containing smaller proteins, cells, and cellular debris) from the interstitial space to systemic veins.

ANATOMY OF THE VASCULAR SYSTEM

Arteries and Arterioles

Arteries are thick-walled structures that carry blood from the heart to the tissues. The aorta, which has a diameter of approximately 25 mm (1 inch), gives rise to numerous branches, which divide into smaller arteries that are about 4 mm (0.16 inch) in diameter by the time they reach the tissues. Within the tissues,

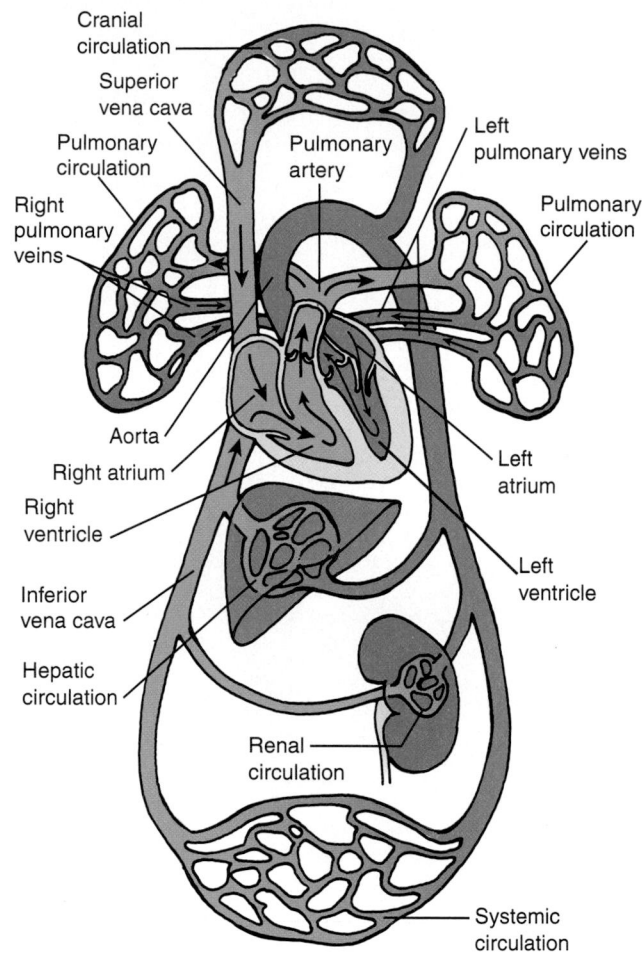

FIGURE 31-1 Systemic and pulmonary circulation. Oxygen-rich blood from the pulmonary circulation is pumped from the left heart into the aorta and the systemic arteries to the capillaries, where the exchange of nutrients and waste products takes place. The deoxygenated blood returns to the right heart by way of the systemic veins and is pumped into the pulmonary circulation. From *Stedman's Medical Dictionary* (27th ed.). (2000). Philadelphia: Lippincott Williams & Wilkins.

Glossary

anastomosis: surgical junction of two vessels

aneurysm: a localized sac or dilation of an artery formed at a weak point in the vessel wall

ankle-brachial index (ABI) or **ankle-arm index (AAI):** ratio of the ankle systolic pressure to the arm systolic pressure; an objective measurement of arterial disease that provides quantification of the degree of stenosis

angioplasty: an invasive procedure that uses a balloon-tipped catheter to dilate a stenotic area of a blood vessel

arteriosclerosis: diffuse process whereby the muscle fibers and the endothelial lining of the walls of small arteries and arterioles thicken

atherosclerosis: disease process involving the accumulation of lipids, calcium, blood components, carbohydrates, and fibrous tissue on the intimal layer of a large or medium-sized artery

bruit: sound produced by turbulent blood flow through an irregular, tortuous, stenotic, or dilated vessel

dissection: separation of the weakened elastic and fibromuscular elements in the medial layer of an artery

duplex ultrasonography: combines B-mode gray-scale imaging of tissue, organs, and blood vessels with capabilities of estimating velocity changes by use of a pulsed Doppler

intermittent claudication: a muscular, cramp-like pain in the extremities consistently reproduced with the same degree of exercise or activity and relieved by rest

international normalized ratio (INR): method of measuring anticoagulation levels, such as warfarin (Coumadin); devised to bring a universal standard to monitoring of anticoagulation achieved by oral medications

ischemia: deficient blood supply

rest pain: persistent pain in the foot or digits when the patient is resting, indicating a severe degree of arterial insufficiency

rubor: reddish blue discoloration of the extremities; indicative of severe peripheral arterial damage in vessels that remain dilated and unable to constrict

stenosis: narrowing or constriction of a vessel

the vessels divide further, diminishing to approximately 30 μm in diameter; these vessels are called arterioles.

The walls of the arteries and arterioles are composed of three layers: the intima, an inner endothelial cell layer; the media, a middle layer of smooth elastic tissue; and the adventitia, an outer layer of connective tissue. The intima, a very thin layer, provides a smooth surface for contact with the flowing blood. The media makes up most of the vessel wall in the aorta and other large arteries of the body. This layer is composed chiefly of elastic and connective tissue fibers that give the vessels considerable strength and allow them to constrict and dilate to accommodate the blood ejected from the heart (stroke volume) and maintain an even, steady flow of blood. The adventitia is a layer of connective tissue that anchors the vessel to its surroundings. There is much less elastic tissue in the smaller arteries and arterioles, and the media in these vessels is composed primarily of smooth muscle.

Smooth muscle controls the diameter of the vessels by contracting and relaxing. Chemical, hormonal, and nervous system factors influence the activity of smooth muscle. Because arterioles can alter their diameter, thereby offering resistance to blood flow, they are often referred to as *resistance vessels*. Arterioles regulate the volume and pressure in the arterial system and the rate of blood flow to the capillaries. Because of the large amount of muscle, the walls of the arteries are relatively thick, accounting for approximately 25% of the total diameter of the artery. The walls of the arterioles account for approximately 67% of the total diameter of arterioles.

The intima and the inner third of the smooth muscle layer are in such close contact with the blood that the blood vessel receives its nourishment by direct diffusion. The adventitia and the outer media layers have a limited vascular system for nourishment and require their own blood supply to meet metabolic needs.

Capillaries

Capillary walls, which lack smooth muscle and adventitia, are composed of a single layer of endothelial cells. This thin-walled structure permits rapid and efficient transport of nutrients to the cells and removal of metabolic wastes. The diameter of capillaries ranges from 5 to 10 μm; this narrow channel requires red blood cells to alter their shape to pass through these vessels. Changes in a capillary's diameter are passive and are influenced by contractile changes in the blood vessels that carry blood to and from a capillary. The capillary's diameter also changes in response to chemical stimuli. In some tissues, a cuff of smooth muscle, called the precapillary sphincter, is located at the arteriolar end of the capillary and is responsible, along with the arteriole, for controlling capillary blood flow.

Some capillary beds, such as in the fingertips, contain arteriovenous anastomoses, through which blood passes directly from the arterial to the venous system. These vessels are believed to regulate heat exchange between the body and the external environment.

The distribution of capillaries varies with the type of tissue. For example, skeletal tissue, which is metabolically active, has a denser capillary network than does cartilage, which is less active.

Veins and Venules

Capillaries join to form larger vessels called venules, which join to form veins. The venous system is therefore structurally analogous to the arterial system; venules correspond to arterioles, veins to arteries, and the vena cava to the aorta. Analogous types of vessels in the arterial and venous systems have approximately the same diameters (see Fig. 31-1).

The walls of the veins, in contrast to those of the arteries, are thinner and considerably less muscular. The wall of the average vein amounts to only 10% of the vein diameter, in contrast to 25% in the artery. The walls of a vein, like those of arteries, are composed of three layers, although these layers are not as well defined.

The thin, less muscular structure of the vein wall allows these vessels to distend more than arteries. Greater distensibility and compliance permit large volumes of blood to be stored in the veins under low pressure. For this reason, veins are referred to as *capacitance vessels*. Approximately 75% of total blood volume is contained in the veins. The sympathetic nervous system, which innervates the vein musculature, can stimulate the veins to constrict (venoconstriction), thereby reducing venous volume and increasing the volume of blood in the general circulation. Contraction of skeletal muscles in the extremities creates the primary pumping action to facilitate venous blood flow back to the heart.

Some veins, unlike arteries, are equipped with valves. In general, veins that transport blood against the force of gravity, as in the lower extremities, have one-way bicuspid valves that interrupt the column of blood to prevent blood from seeping backward as it is propelled toward the heart. Valves are composed of endothelial leaflets, the competency of which depends on the integrity of the vein wall.

Lymphatic Vessels

The lymphatic vessels are a complex network of thin-walled vessels similar to the blood capillaries. This network collects lymphatic fluid from tissues and organs and transports the fluid to the venous circulation. The lymphatic vessels converge into two main structures: the thoracic duct and the right lymphatic duct. These ducts empty into the junction of the subclavian and the internal jugular veins. The right lymphatic duct conveys lymph primarily from the right side of the head, neck, thorax, and upper arms. The thoracic duct conveys lymph from the remainder of the body. Peripheral lymphatic vessels join larger lymph vessels and pass through regional lymph nodes before entering the venous circulation. The lymph nodes play an important role in filtering foreign particles.

The lymphatic vessels are permeable to large molecules and provide the only means by which interstitial proteins can return to the venous system. With muscular contraction, lymph vessels become distorted to create spaces between the endothelial cells, allowing protein and particles to enter. Muscular contraction of the lymphatic walls and surrounding tissues aids in propelling the lymph toward the venous drainage points.

FUNCTION OF THE VASCULAR SYSTEM
Circulatory Needs of Tissues

The amount of blood flow needed by body tissues constantly changes. The percentage of blood flow received by individual organs or tissues is determined by the rate of tissue metabolism, the availability of oxygen, and the function of the tissues (Table 31-1). When metabolic requirements increase, blood vessels dilate to increase the flow of oxygen and nutrients to the tissues. When metabolic needs decrease, vessels constrict, and blood flow to the tissues decreases. Metabolic demands of tissues increase with physical activity or exercise, local heat application, fever, and infection. Reduced metabolic requirements of tissues accompany rest or decreased physical activity, local cold application, and

Table 31-1 • **Blood Flow and Oxygen Consumption for Selected Human Organs**

Organ	Organ Weight (kg)	BLOOD FLOW DURING REST		OXYGEN USAGE DURING REST	
		Organ Blood Flow (mL/min)	% Total Cardiac Output	Organ O_2 Usage (mL/min)	% Total O_2 Usage
Brain	1.4	750	14	45	18
Heart	0.3	250	5	25	10
Liver	1.5	1300	23	75	30
GI tract	2.5	1000			
Kidneys	0.3	1200	22	15	6
Muscle	35.0	1000	18	50	20
Skin	2.0	200	4	5	2
Remainder (eg, skeleton, bone marrow, fat, connective tissue)	27.0	800	14	35	14
TOTAL	70	6500	100	250	100

Folkow B., & Neil E. *Circulation.* New York: Oxford University Press.

cooling of the body. If the blood vessels fail to dilate in response to the need for increased blood flow, tissue **ischemia** (ie, deficient blood supply to a body part) results. The mechanism by which blood vessels dilate and constrict to adjust for metabolic changes ensures that normal arterial pressure is maintained.

As blood passes through tissue capillaries, oxygen is removed, and carbon dioxide is added. The amount of oxygen extracted by each tissue differs. For example, the myocardium tends to extract about 50% of the oxygen from arterial blood in one pass through its capillary bed, whereas the kidneys extract only about 7% of the oxygen from the blood that passes through them. The average amount of oxygen removed collectively by all of the body tissues is about 25%. This means that the blood in the vena cavae contains about 25% less oxygen than aortic blood. This is known as the *systemic arteriovenous oxygen difference.* The value increases when the amount of oxygen delivered to the tissues is decreased relative to their metabolic needs (see Table 31-1).

Blood Flow

Blood flow through the cardiovascular system always proceeds in the same direction: left side of the heart to the aorta, arteries, arterioles, capillaries, venules, veins, vena cavae, and right side of the heart. This unidirectional flow is caused by a pressure difference that exists between the arterial and venous systems. Because arterial pressure (approximately 100 mm Hg) is greater than venous pressure (approximately 4 mm Hg) and fluid always flows from an area of high pressure to an area of lower pressure, blood flows from the arterial to the venous system.

The pressure difference (ΔP) between the two ends of the vessel provides the impetus for the forward propulsion of blood. Impediments to blood flow offer the opposing force, which is known as resistance (R). The rate of blood flow is determined by dividing the pressure difference by the resistance:

$$\text{Flow rate} = \Delta P/R$$

This equation clearly shows that, when resistance increases, a greater driving pressure is required to maintain the same degree of flow. In the body, an increase in driving pressure is accomplished by an increase in the force of contraction of the heart. If arterial resistance is chronically elevated, the myocardium hypertrophies (enlarges) to sustain the greater contractile force.

In most long smooth blood vessels, flow is laminar or streamlined, with blood in the center of the vessel moving slightly faster than the blood near the vessel walls. Laminar flow becomes turbulent when the blood flow rate increases, when blood viscosity increases, when the diameter of the vessel becomes greater than normal, or when segments of the vessel are narrowed or constricted. Turbulent blood flow creates a sound, called a **bruit**, that can be auscultated with a stethoscope.

Blood Pressure

Chapters 26 and 32 provide more information on the physiology and measurement of blood pressure.

Capillary Filtration and Reabsorption

Fluid exchange across the capillary wall is continuous. This fluid, which has the same composition as plasma without the proteins, forms the interstitial fluid. The equilibrium between hydrostatic and osmotic forces of the blood and interstitium, as well as capillary permeability, governs the amount and direction of fluid movement across the capillary. Hydrostatic force is a driving pressure that is generated by the blood pressure. Osmotic pressure is the pulling force created by plasma proteins. Normally, the hydrostatic pressure at the arterial end of the capillary is relatively high compared with that at the venous end. This high pressure at the arterial end of the capillaries tends to drive fluid out of the capillary and into the tissue space. Osmotic pressure tends to pull fluid back into the capillary from the tissue space, but this osmotic force cannot overcome the high hydrostatic pressure at the arterial end of the capillary. At the venous end of the capillary, however, the osmotic force predominates over the low hydrostatic pressure, and there is a net reabsorption of fluid from the tissue space back into the capillary.

Except for a very small amount, fluid that is filtered out at the arterial end of the capillary bed is reabsorbed at the venous end. The excess filtered fluid enters the lymphatic circulation. These processes of filtration, reabsorption, and lymph formation aid in maintaining tissue fluid volume and removing tissue waste and debris. Under normal conditions, capillary permeability remains constant.

Under certain abnormal conditions, the fluid filtered out of the capillaries may greatly exceed the amounts reabsorbed and carried away by the lymphatic vessels. This imbalance can result from damage to capillary walls and subsequent increased permeability, obstruction of lymphatic drainage, elevation of venous pressure, or decrease in plasma protein osmotic force. The accumulation of fluid that results from these processes is known as *edema*.

Hemodynamic Resistance

The most important factor that determines resistance in the vascular system is the vessel radius. Small changes in vessel radius lead to large changes in resistance. The predominant sites of change in the caliber or width of blood vessels, and therefore in resistance, are the arterioles and the precapillary sphincter. Peripheral vascular resistance is the opposition to blood flow provided by the blood vessels. Poiseuille's law provides the method by which resistance can be calculated:

$$R = 8\theta L/\pi r^4$$

where R = resistance, r = radius of the vessel, L = length of the vessel, θ = viscosity of the blood, and $8/\pi$ = a constant. This equation shows that the resistance is proportional to the viscosity or thickness of the blood and the length of the vessel but is inversely proportional to the fourth power of the vessel radius.

Under normal conditions, blood viscosity and vessel length do not change significantly, and these factors do not usually play an important role in blood flow. A large increase in hematocrit, however, may increase blood viscosity and reduce capillary blood flow.

Peripheral Vascular Regulating Mechanisms

Because the metabolic needs of body tissues, even at rest, are continuously changing, an integrated and coordinated regulatory system is necessary so that blood flow to individual areas is maintained in proportion to the needs of that area. As might be expected, this regulatory mechanism is complex and consists of central nervous system influences, circulating hormones and chemicals, and independent activity of the arterial wall itself.

Sympathetic (adrenergic) nervous system activity, mediated by the hypothalamus, is the most important factor in regulating the caliber and therefore the blood flow of peripheral blood vessels. All vessels are innervated by the sympathetic nervous system except the capillary and precapillary sphincters. Stimulation of the sympathetic nervous system causes vasoconstriction. The neurotransmitter responsible for sympathetic vasoconstriction is norepinephrine. Sympathetic activation occurs in response to physiologic and psychological stressors. Diminution of sympathetic activity by medications or sympathectomy results in vasodilation.

Other hormonal substances affect peripheral vascular resistance. Epinephrine, released from the adrenal medulla, acts like norepinephrine in constricting peripheral blood vessels in most tissue beds. In low concentrations, however, epinephrine causes vasodilation in skeletal muscles, the heart, and the brain. Angiotensin, a potent substance formed from the interaction of renin (synthesized by the kidney) and a circulating serum protein, stimulates arterial constriction. Although the amount of angiotensin concentrated in the blood is usually small, its profound vasoconstrictor effects are important in certain abnormal states, such as heart failure and hypovolemia.

Alterations in local blood flow are influenced by various circulating substances that have vasoactive properties. Potent vasodilators include histamine, bradykinin, prostaglandin, and certain muscle metabolites. A reduction in available oxygen and nutrients and changes in local pH also affect local blood flow. Serotonin, a substance liberated from platelets that aggregate at the site of vessel wall damage, constricts arterioles. The application of heat to parts of the body surface causes local vasodilation, whereas the application of cold causes vasoconstriction.

PATHOPHYSIOLOGY OF THE VASCULAR SYSTEM

Reduced blood flow through peripheral blood vessels characterizes all peripheral vascular diseases. The physiologic effects of altered blood flow depend on the extent to which tissue demands exceed the supply of oxygen and nutrients available. If tissue needs are high, even modestly reduced blood flow may be inadequate to maintain tissue integrity. Tissues then fall prey to ischemia (deficient blood supply), become malnourished, and ultimately die if adequate blood flow is not restored.

Pump Failure

Inadequate peripheral blood flow occurs when the heart's pumping action becomes inefficient. Left ventricular failure causes an accumulation of blood in the lungs and a reduction in forward flow or cardiac output, which results in inadequate arterial blood flow to the tissues. Right ventricular failure causes systemic venous congestion and a reduction in forward flow (see Chap. 30).

Alterations in Blood and Lymphatic Vessels

Intact, patent, and responsive blood vessels are necessary to deliver adequate amounts of oxygen to tissues and to remove metabolic wastes. Arteries can become obstructed by atherosclerotic plaque, a thrombus, or an embolus. Arteries can become damaged or obstructed as a result of chemical or mechanical trauma, infections or inflammatory processes, vasospastic disorders, and congenital malformations. A sudden arterial occlusion causes profound and often irreversible tissue ischemia and tissue death. When arterial occlusions develop gradually, there is less risk for sudden tissue death because collateral circulation has an opportunity to develop and the body adapts to the decreased blood flow.

Venous blood flow can be reduced by a thrombus obstructing the vein, by incompetent venous valves, or by a reduction in the effectiveness of the pumping action of surrounding muscles. Decreased venous blood flow results in increased venous pressure, a subsequent rise in capillary hydrostatic pressure, net filtration of fluid out of the capillaries into the interstitial space, and subsequent edema. Edematous tissues cannot receive adequate nutrition from the blood and consequently are more susceptible to breakdown, injury, and infection. Obstruction of lymphatic vessels also results in edema. Lymphatic vessels can become obstructed by tumor or by damage resulting from mechanical trauma or inflammatory processes.

Gerontologic Considerations

Aging produces changes in the walls of the blood vessels that affect the transport of oxygen and nutrients to the tissues. The intima thickens as a result of cellular proliferation and fibrosis. Elastin fibers of the media become calcified, thin, and fragmented, and collagen accumulates in the intima and the media. These changes cause the vessels to stiffen, which results in increased peripheral resistance, impaired blood flow, and increased left ventricular workload.

Circulatory Insufficiency of the Extremities

Although many types of peripheral vascular diseases exist, most result in ischemia and produce some of the same symptoms: pain, skin changes, diminished pulse, and possible edema. The type and severity of symptoms depend in part on the type, stage, and extent of the disease process and on the speed with which the disorder develops. Table 31-2 highlights the distinguishing features of arterial and venous insufficiency. In this chapter, peripheral vascular disease is categorized as arterial, venous, or lymphatic disorders.

Assessment

HEALTH HISTORY AND CLINICAL MANIFESTATIONS

A description of the pain and any precipitating factors, the skin color and temperature, and the peripheral pulses are important for the diagnosis of arterial disorders.

Intermittent Claudication

A muscular, cramp-type pain in the extremities consistently reproduced with the same degree of exercise or activity and relieved by rest is experienced by patients with peripheral arterial insufficiency. Referred to as **intermittent claudication**, this pain is caused by the inability of the arterial system to provide adequate blood flow to the tissues in the face of increased demands for nutrients during exercise. As the tissues are forced to complete the energy cycle without the nutrients, muscle metabolites and lactic acid are produced. Pain is experienced as the metabolites aggravate the nerve endings of the surrounding tissue. Usually, about 50% of the arterial lumen or 75% of the cross-sectional area must be obstructed before intermittent claudication is experienced. When the patient rests and thereby decreases the metabolic needs of the muscles, the pain subsides. The progression of the arterial disease can be monitored by documenting the amount of exercise or the distance a patient can walk before pain is produced. Persistent pain in the forefoot when the patient is resting indicates a severe degree of arterial insufficiency and a critical state of ischemia. Known as **rest pain**, this discomfort is often worse at night and may interfere with sleep. This pain frequently requires that the extremity be lowered to a dependent position to improve perfusion pressure to the distal tissues.

The site of arterial disease can be deduced from the location of claudication, because pain occurs in muscle groups below the disease. As a general rule, the pain of intermittent claudication occurs one joint level below the disease process. Calf pain may accompany reduced blood flow through the superficial femoral or popliteal artery, whereas pain in the hip or buttock may result from reduced blood flow in the abdominal aorta or the common iliac or hypogastric arteries.

Changes in Skin Appearance and Temperature

Adequate blood flow warms the extremities and gives them a rosy coloring. Inadequate blood flow results in cool and pale extremities. Further reduction of blood flow to these tissues, which occurs when the extremity is elevated, for example, results in an even whiter or more blanched appearance (pallor). **Rubor**, a reddish blue discoloration of the extremities, may be observed within 20 seconds to 2 minutes after the extremity is dependent. Rubor suggests severe peripheral arterial damage in which vessels that cannot constrict remain dilated. Even with rubor, the extremity begins to turn pale with elevation. Cyanosis, a bluish tint on the skin, is manifested when the amount of oxygenated hemoglobin contained in the blood is reduced.

Additional changes resulting from a chronically reduced nutrient supply include loss of hair, brittle nails, dry or scaling skin, atrophy, and ulcerations. Edema may be apparent bilaterally or unilaterally and is related to the affected extremity's chronically dependent position because of severe rest pain. Gangrenous changes appear after prolonged, severe ischemia and represent tissue necrosis. In elderly patients who are inactive, gangrene may be the first sign of disease. These patients may have adjusted their lifestyle to accommodate the limitations imposed by the disease, and may not walk far enough to develop symptoms of claudication. Circulation is decreased, but this is not apparent to the patient until trauma occurs. At this point, gangrene develops when minimal arterial flow is impaired further by edema formation resulting from the traumatic event.

Table 31-2 • Characteristics of Arterial and Venous Insufficiency

CHARACTERISTIC	ARTERIAL	VENOUS
Pain	Intermittent claudication to sharp, unrelenting, constant	Aching, cramping
Pulses	Diminished or absent	Present, but may be difficult to palpate through edema
Skin characteristics	Dependent rubor—elevation pallor of foot, dry, shiny skin, cool-to-cold temperature, loss of hair over toes and dorsum of foot, nails thickened and ridged	Pigmentation in gaitor area (area of medial and lateral malleolus), skin thickened and tough, may be reddish blue, frequently with associated dermatitis
Ulcer characteristics		
Location	Tip of toes, toe webs, heel or other pressure areas if confined to bed	Medial malleolus; infrequently lateral malleolus or anterior tibial area
Pain	Very painful	Minimal pain if superficial or may be very painful
Depth of ulcer	Deep, often involving joint space	Superficial
Shape	Circular	Irregular border
Ulcer base	Pale to black and dry gangrene	Granulation tissue—beefy red to yellow fibrinous in chronic long-term ulcer
Leg edema	Minimal unless extremity kept in dependent position constantly to relieve pain	Moderate to severe

Pulses

Determining the presence or absence, as well as the quality, of peripheral pulses is important in assessing the status of peripheral arterial circulation (Fig. 31-2). Absence of a pulse may indicate that the site of **stenosis** (narrowing or constriction) is proximal to that location. Occlusive arterial disease impairs blood flow and can reduce or obliterate palpable pulsations in the extremities. Pulses should be palpated bilaterally and simultaneously, comparing both sides for symmetry in rate, rhythm, and quality.

Gerontologic Considerations

In elderly people, symptoms of peripheral arterial disease may be more pronounced than in younger people because of the condition's duration and coexisting chronic disease. Intermittent claudication may occur after walking only a few short blocks or after walking up a slight incline. Any prolonged pressure on the foot can cause pressure areas that become ulcerated, infected, and gangrenous. The outcomes of arterial insufficiency in the elderly person include reduced mobility and activity and a loss of independence.

Diagnostic Evaluation

In identifying and diagnosing the various abnormalities affecting the vascular structures (arteries, veins, and lymphatics), various tests may be performed.

DOPPLER ULTRASOUND FLOW STUDIES

Palpating pulses is subjective, and the examiner may mistake his or her own pulse for that of the patient. To prevent this, the examiner should use light touch and avoid using only the index finger for palpation, because this finger has the strongest arterial pulsation of all the fingers. The thumb should not be used for the same reason. When pulses cannot be reliably palpated, use of a microphone-like, hand-held Doppler ultrasound device, called a transducer or probe, may be helpful in detecting and assessing peripheral flow.

A continuous-wave (CW) Doppler ultrasound device may be used to hear (insonate) the blood flow in vessels when pulses cannot be palpated. This hand-held device emits a continuous signal through the patient's tissues. The signals are reflected by (echo off) the moving blood cells and are received by the device. The filtered-output Doppler signal is then transmitted to a loudspeaker or headphones, where it can be heard for interpretation. Because CW Doppler emits a continuous signal, all vascular structures in the path of the sound beam are insonated, and differentiating arterial from venous flow and detecting the site of a stenosis may be difficult. The depth at which blood flow can be detected by Doppler is determined by the frequency (in megahertz [MHz]) it generates. The lower the frequency, the deeper the tissue penetration; a 5- to 10-MHz probe may be used to evaluate the peripheral arteries.

To evaluate the lower extremities, the patient is placed in a supine position with the head of bed elevated 20 to 30 degrees; the legs are externally rotated, if possible, to permit adequate access to the medial malleolus. Acoustic gel is applied to the patient's skin

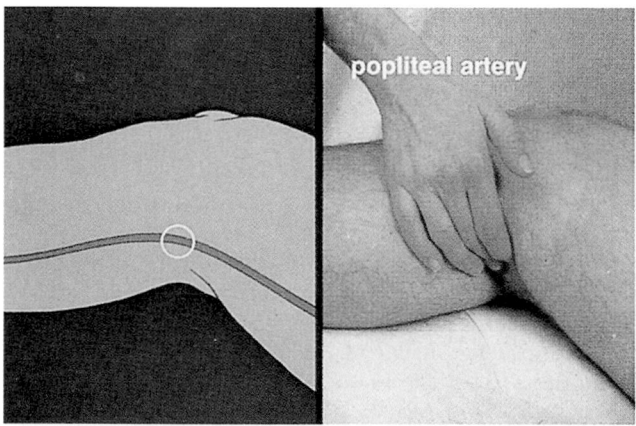

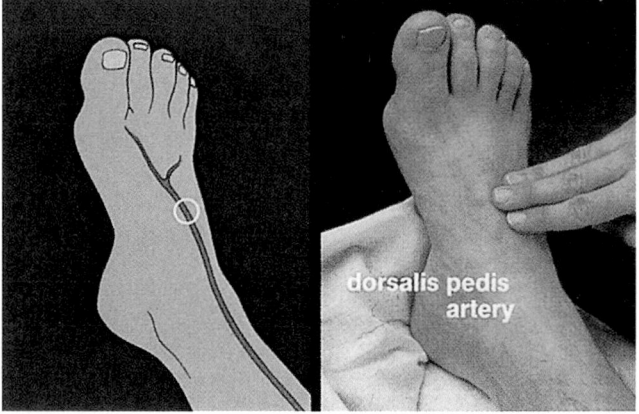

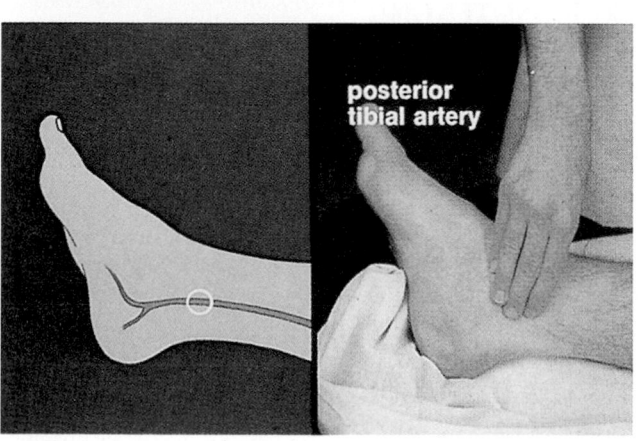

FIGURE 31-2 Assessing peripheral pulses. (*Left*) Popliteal pulse. (*Right*) Dorsalis pedis pulse. (*Bottom*) Posterior tibial pulse.

to permit uniform transmission of the ultrasound wave (electrocardiogram gel is not used because it contains sodium, which may dissolve the epoxy that covers the transducer's tip). The tip of the Doppler transducer is positioned at a 45- to 60-degree angle over the expected location of the artery and angled slowly to identify arterial blood flow. Excessive pressure is avoided because severely diseased arteries can collapse with even minimal pressure.

Because the equipment can detect blood flow in advanced arterial disease states, especially if collateral circulation has developed, identifying a signal documents only the presence of blood flow. However, it is clinically relevant to notify the primary care provider of the absence of a signal if one had been detected during a previous examination.

CW Doppler (Fig. 31-3) is more useful as a clinical tool when combined with ankle blood pressures, which are used to determine the **ankle-brachial index (ABI)**, also called the **ankle-arm index (AAI)**. The ABI is the ratio of the ankle systolic blood pressure to the arm systolic blood pressure. It is an objective indicator of arterial disease that allows the examiner to quantify the degree of stenosis. With increasing degrees of arterial narrowing, there is a progressive decrease in systolic pressure distal to the involved sites.

The first step in determining the ABI is to have the patient rest in a supine position (not seated) for at least 5 minutes. An appropriate-sized blood pressure cuff (typically, a 10-cm cuff) is applied to the patient's ankle above the malleolus. After identifying an arterial signal at the posterior tibial and dorsalis pedis arteries, the systolic ankle pressures are obtained in both feet. Diastolic pressures cannot be measured with a Doppler. If pressure in these arteries cannot be measured, pressure can be measured in the peroneal artery, which can also be assessed at the ankle (Fig. 31-4).

Doppler ultrasonography is used to measure brachial pressures in both arms. Both arms are evaluated because the patient may have an asymptomatic stenosis in the subclavian artery, causing brachial pressure on the affected side to be 20 mm Hg or more lower than systemic pressure. The abnormally low pressure should not be used for assessment.

To calculate ABI, the ankle systolic pressure for each foot is divided by the higher of the two brachial systolic pressures;

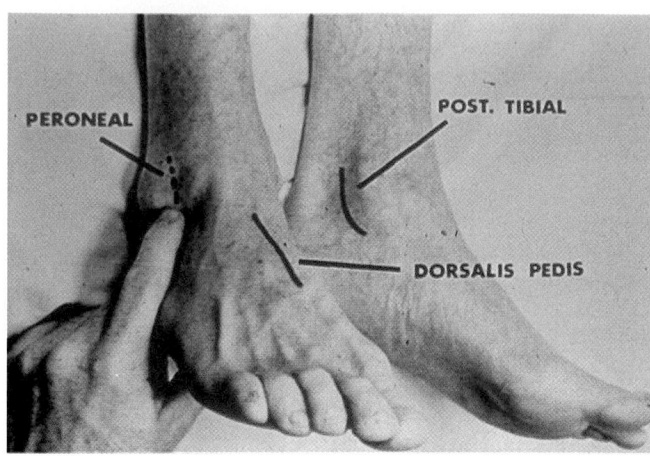

FIGURE 31-4 Location of peroneal artery; lateral malleolus. Photo reprinted with permission from Cantwell-Gab, K. (1996). Identifying chronic PAD. *American Journal of Nursing, 96*(7), 40–46.

Chart 31-1 offers more information. The ABI can be computed for a patient with the following systolic pressures:

Right brachial: 160 mm Hg
Left brachial: 120 mm Hg
Right posterior tibial: 80 mm Hg
Right dorsalis pedis: 60 mm Hg
Left posterior tibial: 100 mm Hg
Left dorsalis pedis: 120 mm Hg

The highest systolic pressure for each ankle (80 mm Hg for the right, 120 mm Hg for the left) would be divided by the highest brachial pressure (160 mm Hg).

Right: 80/160 mm Hg = 0.50 ABI
Left: 120/160 mm Hg = 0.75 ABI

In general, systolic pressure in the ankle of a healthy person is the same or slightly higher than the brachial systolic pressure, resulting in an ABI of about 1.0 (no arterial insufficiency). Patients with claudication usually have an ABI of 0.95 to 0.50 (mild to moderate insufficiency); patients with ischemic rest pain have an ABI of less than 0.50, and patients with severe ischemia or tissue loss have an ABI of 0.25 or less.

EXERCISE TESTING

Exercise testing is used to determine how long a patient can walk and to measure the ankle systolic blood pressure in response to walking. The patient walks on a treadmill at 1.5 mph with a 10% incline for a maximum of 5 minutes. Most patients can complete the test unless they have severe cardiac, pulmonary, or orthopedic problems or are physically disabled. A normal response to the test is little or no drop in ankle systolic pressure after exercise. In a patient with true claudication, however, ankle pressure drops. Combining this hemodynamic information with the walking time helps the physician determine whether intervention is necessary.

DUPLEX ULTRASONOGRAPHY

Duplex ultrasonography involves B-mode gray-scale imaging of the tissue, organs, and blood vessels (arterial and venous) and permits estimation of velocity changes by use of a pulsed Doppler

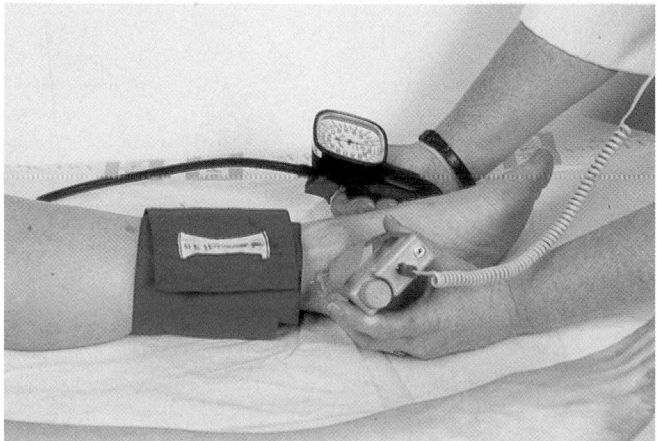

FIGURE 31-3 Continuous-wave (CW) Doppler ultrasound detects blood flow in peripheral vessels. Combined with computation of ankle or arm pressures, this diagnostic technique helps health care providers characterize the nature of peripheral vascular disease. Photo reprinted with permission from Cantwell-Gab, K. (1996). Identifying chronic PAD. *American Journal of Nursing, 96*(7), 40–46.

Chart 31-1 Avoiding Common Errors in Calculating Ankle-Brachial Index (ABI)

Take the following precautions to ensure an accurate ABI calculation:

- *Use the correctly sized blood pressure cuffs.* To obtain accurate blood pressure measurements, use a cuff with a bladder width at least 40% and length at least 80% of the limb circumference.

- *On the nursing plan of care, document the blood pressure cuff sizes used* (for example, "12-cm BP cuff used for brachial pressures; 10-cm BP cuff used for ankle pressures"). This minimizes the risk of shift-to-shift discrepancies in ABIs.

- *Use sufficient blood pressure cuff inflation.* To ensure complete closure of the artery and the most accurate measurements, inflate cuffs 20 to 30 mm Hg beyond the point at which the last arterial signal is detected.

- *Do not deflate blood pressure cuffs too rapidly.* Try to maintain a deflation rate of 2 to 4 mm Hg/second for patients without dysrhythmias and 2 mm Hg/second or slower for patients with dysrhythmias. Deflating the cuff more rapidly may miss the patient's highest pressure and result in recording an erroneous (low) blood pressure measurement.

- *Be suspicious of arterial pressures recorded at less than 40 mm Hg.* This may mean the venous signal has been mistaken for the arterial signal. If the arterial pressure, which is normally 120 mm Hg, is measured at less than 40 mm Hg, ask a colleague to double-check the findings before recording this as an arterial pressure.

- *Suspect medial calcific sclerosis anytime an ABI is 1.3 or greater or ankle pressure is more than 300 mm Hg.* Medial calcific sclerosis is associated with diabetes mellitus, chronic renal failure, and hyperparathyroidism. It produces falsely elevated ankle pressures by hardening the medra of the arteries; making the vessels noncompressible.

(From Cantwell-Gab, K. [1996]. Identifying chronic PAD. *American Journal of Nursing, 96*[1] 40–46, with permission.)

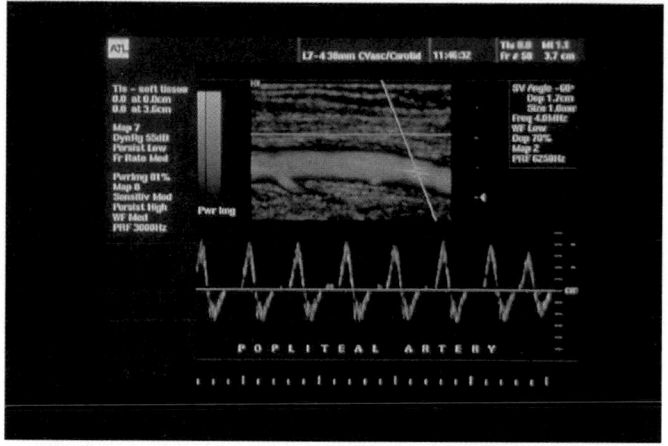

FIGURE 31-5 Color flow duplex image of popliteal artery with normal triphasic Doppler flow.

x-rays, and contrast agent usually must be injected to adequately visualize the blood vessels. Using computer software, the slicelike images are reconstructed into three-dimensional images that can be rotated and viewed from multiple angles.

COMPUTED TOMOGRAPHIC ANGIOGRAPHY

In computed tomographic angiography (CTA), a spiral CT scanner and rapid intravenous infusion of contrast agent are used to image very thin (1-mm) sections of the target area; the results are configured in three dimensions so that the image closely resembles a regular angiogram (Verta & Verta, 1998). CTA shows the aorta and main visceral arteries better than it shows smaller branch vessels. Scan times are usually between 20 and 30 seconds. The large volume of contrast agent required for CTA limits the usefulness of this study in patients with allergy to the contrast agent or with significantly impaired renal function.

MAGNETIC RESONANCE ANGIOGRAPHY

Magnetic resonance angiography is performed with a standard MRI scanner but with image-processing software specifically programmed to isolate the blood vessels. The images are reconstructed to resemble a standard angiogram, but because the images are reassembled in three dimensions, they can be rotated and viewed from multiple angles. Because no contrast agent is necessary, this study is useful in patients with poor renal function or allergy to contrast agent. Scan time is long, and motion artifacts are common, restricting the use of the test to relatively short segments of the vascular system (Verta & Verta, 1998).

ANGIOGRAPHY

An arteriogram produced by angiography may be used to confirm the diagnosis of occlusive arterial disease when considering surgery or other interventions. The procedure involves injecting a radiopaque contrast agent directly into the vascular system to visualize the vessels. The location of a vascular obstruction or an **aneurysm** (abnormal dilation of a blood vessel) and the collateral circulation can be demonstrated. Usually, patients experience a temporary sensation of warmth as the contrast agent is injected, and local irritation may occur at the injection site. Infrequently, a patient

(Fig. 31-5). Color flow techniques, which can identify vessels, may be used to shorten the examination time. The procedure helps determine the level and extent of disease and is universally employed to evaluate the venous system. The technique makes it possible to image and assess blood flow, evaluate the runoff status of the distal vessels, locate the disease (stenosis versus occlusion), and determine anatomic morphology and the hemodynamic significance of plaque causing stenosis. Duplex ultrasound findings help in planning therapy and monitoring its outcomes. Moreover, the test is noninvasive and usually requires no patient preparation. The equipment is portable, making it useful anywhere for initial diagnosis or follow-up evaluations.

COMPUTED TOMOGRAPHY

Computed tomography (CT) provides cross-sectional images of soft tissue and can identify the area of volume changes to an extremity and the compartment where changes take place. CT of a lymphedematous arm or leg, for example, demonstrates a characteristic honeycomb pattern in the subcutaneous tissue.

In spiral (also called volumetric) CT, the scan head moves circumferentially around the patient as the patient passes through the scanner, creating a series of overlapping images that are connected to one another in a continuous spiral (Verta & Verta, 1998). Scan times are short; however, the patient is exposed to

may have an immediate or delayed allergic reaction to the iodine contained in the contrast agent. Manifestations include dyspnea, nausea and vomiting, sweating, tachycardia, and numbness of the extremities. Any such reaction must be reported to the physician at once; treatment may include the administration of one or more of epinephrine (adrenaline), antihistamines, or corticosteroids. Additional risks include vessel injury, bleeding, and CVA (brain attack, stroke).

AIR PLETHYSMOGRAPHY

Named for the standardized air chambers that fit around the lower leg and that are calibrated after being filled with a standard amount of air, air plethysmography quantifies venous reflux and calf muscle pump ejection. Changes in volume are measured with the patient's legs elevated, with the patient supine and standing, and after the patient performs toe-ups (patient extends ankle while standing; stands on tip-toes). Air plethysmography provides information about venous filling time, functional venous volume, ejected volume, and residual volume. It is useful in evaluating patients with suspected valvular incompetence or chronic venous insufficiency.

CONTRAST PHLEBOGRAPHY

Also known as venography, contrast phlebography involves injecting radiographic contrast media into the venous system through a dorsal foot vein. If a thrombus exists, the x-ray image discloses an unfilled segment of vein in an otherwise completely filled vein. Injection of the contrast agent may cause a brief but painful inflammation of the vein. The test is generally performed if the patient is to undergo thrombolytic therapy, but duplex ultrasonography is now accepted as the gold standard for diagnosing venous thrombosis.

LYMPHANGIOGRAPHY

Lymphangiography affords a means of detecting lymph node involvement that results from metastatic carcinoma, lymphoma, or infection in sites that are otherwise inaccessible to the examiner except by surgery. In this test, a lymphatic vessel in each foot (or hand) is injected with contrast agent. A series of x-rays are taken at the conclusion of the injection, 24 hours later, and periodically thereafter, as indicated. The failure to identify subcutaneous lymphatic collection of contrast agent and the persistence of contrast agent in the tissue for days afterward help to confirm a diagnosis of lymphedema.

LYMPHOSCINTIGRAPHY

Lymphoscintigraphy is a reliable alternative to lymphangiography. A radioactively labeled colloid is injected subcutaneously in the second interdigital space. The extremity is then exercised to facilitate the uptake of the colloid by the lymphatic system, and serial images are obtained at preset intervals. No adverse reactions have been reported.

Management of Arterial Disorders

ARTERIOSCLEROSIS AND ATHEROSCLEROSIS

Arteriosclerosis is the most common disease of the arteries; the term means *hardening of the arteries*. It is a diffuse process whereby the muscle fibers and the endothelial lining of the walls of small arteries and arterioles become thickened. **Atherosclerosis** involves a different process, affecting the intima of the large and medium-sized arteries. These changes consist of the accumulation of lipids, calcium, blood components, carbohydrates, and fibrous tissue on the intimal layer of the artery. These accumulations are referred to as atheromas or plaques.

Although the pathologic processes of arteriosclerosis and atherosclerosis differ, rarely does one occur without the other, and the terms are often used interchangeably. Because atherosclerosis is a generalized disease of the arteries, when it is present in the extremities, atherosclerosis is usually present elsewhere in the body.

Pathophysiology

The most common direct results of atherosclerosis in arteries include narrowing (stenosis) of the lumen, obstruction by thrombosis, aneurysm, ulceration, and rupture. Its indirect results are malnutrition and the subsequent fibrosis of the organs that the sclerotic arteries supply with blood. All actively functioning tissue cells require an abundant supply of nutrients and oxygen and are sensitive to any reduction in the supply of these nutrients. If such reductions are severe and permanent, the cells undergo ischemic necrosis (death of cells due to deficient blood flow) and are replaced by fibrous tissue, which requires much less blood flow.

Atherosclerosis can develop at any point in the body, but certain sites are more vulnerable, typically bifurcation or branch areas. In the proximal lower extremity, these include the distal abdominal aorta, the common iliac arteries, the orifice of the superficial femoral and profunda femoris arteries, and the superficial femoral artery in the adductor canal. Distal to the knee, atherosclerosis occurs anywhere along the artery. There are no specific areas, such as arterial bifurcations, that are more vulnerable for atherosclerosis.

Although many theories exist about the development of atherosclerosis, no single theory fully explains the pathogenesis; however, parts of several theories have been combined into the reaction-to-injury theory. According to this theory, vascular endothelial cell injury results from prolonged hemodynamic forces, such as shearing stresses and turbulent flow, irradiation, chemical exposure, or chronic hyperlipidemia in the arterial system. Injury to the endothelium increases the aggregation of platelets and monocytes at the site of the injury. Smooth muscle cells migrate and proliferate, allowing a matrix of collagen and elastic fibers to form. It may be that there is no single cause or mechanism for the development of atherosclerosis; rather, multiple processes may be involved (Moore, 2002).

Morphologically, atherosclerotic lesions are of two types: fatty streaks and fibrous plaque. Fatty streaks are yellow and smooth, protrude slightly into the lumen of the artery, and are composed of lipids and elongated smooth muscle cells. These lesions have been found in the arteries of people of all age groups, including infants. It is not clear whether fatty streaks predispose the person to the formation of fibrous plaques or if they are reversible. They do not usually cause clinical symptoms.

The fibrous plaque characteristic of atherosclerosis is composed of smooth muscle cells, collagen fibers, plasma components, and lipids. It is white to whitish yellow and protrudes in various degrees into the arterial lumen, sometimes completely obstructing it. These plaques are found predominantly in the abdominal aorta and the coronary, popliteal, and internal carotid arteries. This plaque is believed to be an irreversible lesion (Fig. 31-6). Gradual narrowing of the arterial lumen as the disease process progresses stimulates the development of collateral circulation

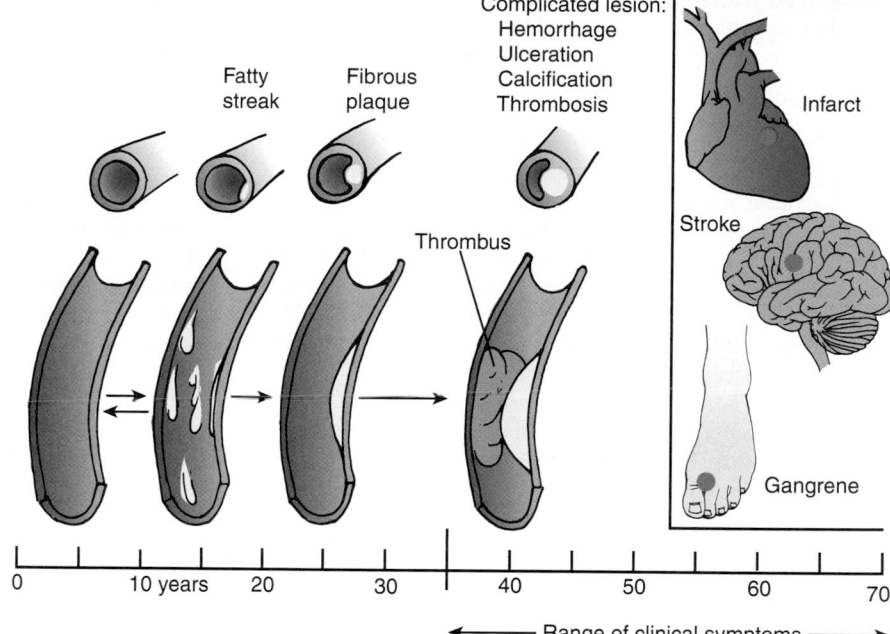

FIGURE 31-6 Schematic concept of the progression of atherosclerosis. Fatty streaks constitute one of the earliest lesions of atherosclerosis. Many fatty streaks regress, whereas others progress to fibrous plaques and eventually to atheroma, which may be complicated by hemorrhage, ulceration, calcification, or thrombosis and may produce myocardial infarction, stroke, or gangrene.

(Fig. 31-7). Collateral circulation consists of preexisting vessels that enlarge to reroute blood flow in the presence of a hemodynamically significant stenosis or occlusion. Collateral flow allows continued perfusion to the tissues beyond the arterial obstruction, but it is often inadequate to meet imposed metabolic demand, and ischemia results.

Risk Factors

Many risk factors are associated with atherosclerosis (Chart 31-2). Although it is not completely clear whether modification of these risk factors prevents the development of cardiovascular disease, evidence indicates that it may slow the disease process. Some risk factors, such as age or gender, cannot be modified. However, it is believed that genetic factors can be modified indirectly by altering other risk factors (Moore, 2002).

Tobacco use may be one of the strongest risk factors in the development of atherosclerotic lesions. Nicotine decreases blood flow to the extremities and increases heart rate and blood pressure by stimulating the sympathetic nervous system, causing vasoconstriction. It also increases the risk for clot formation by increasing the aggregation of platelets. Carbon monoxide, a toxin produced by burning tobacco, combines more readily with the hemoglobin than oxygen does, depriving the tissues of oxygen. The amount of tobacco use is directly related to the extent of the disease, and cessation of tobacco use reduces the risks. Many other factors

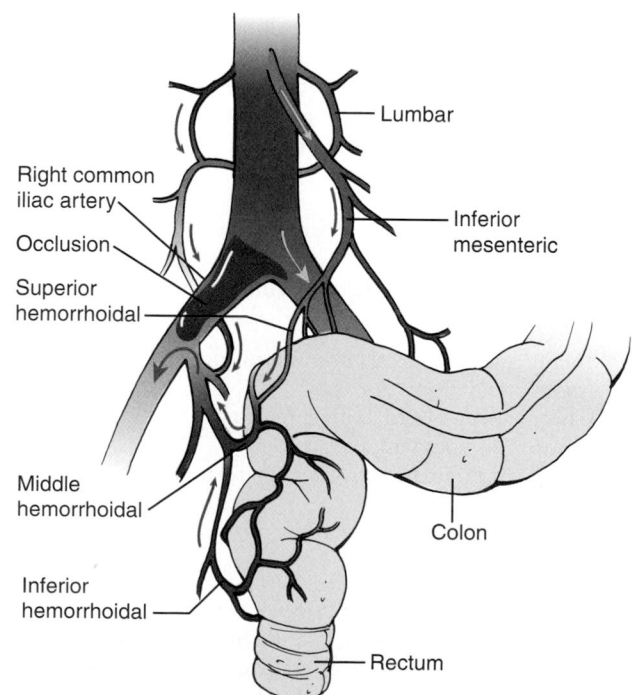

FIGURE 31-7 Development of channels for collateral blood flow in response to occlusion of the right common iliac artery and the terminal aortic bifurcation.

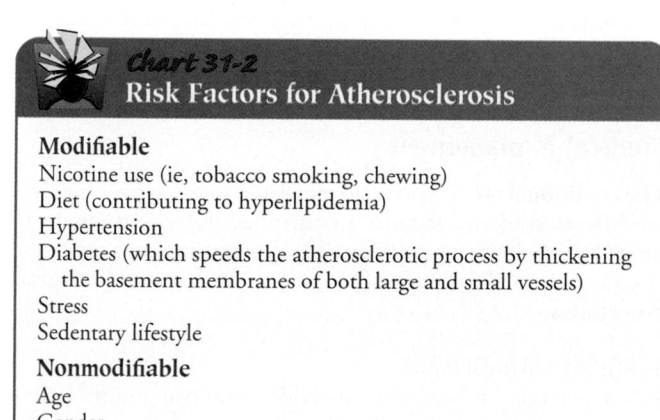

Chart 31-2
Risk Factors for Atherosclerosis

Modifiable
Nicotine use (ie, tobacco smoking, chewing)
Diet (contributing to hyperlipidemia)
Hypertension
Diabetes (which speeds the atherosclerotic process by thickening the basement membranes of both large and small vessels)
Stress
Sedentary lifestyle

Nonmodifiable
Age
Gender

such as obesity, stress, and lack of exercise have been identified as contributing to the disease process.

Prevention

Intermittent claudication is a sign of generalized atherosclerosis and may be a marker of occult coronary artery disease. Because a high-fat diet is suspected of contributing to atherosclerosis, it is reasonable to measure serum cholesterol and to begin prevention efforts. The American Heart Association recommends reducing the amount of fat ingested in a healthy diet, substituting unsaturated fats for saturated fats, and decreasing cholesterol intake to no more than 300 mg daily to reduce the risk of cardiovascular disease (Krauss et al., 2000).

Certain medications combined with dietary modification and exercise are being used to reduce blood lipid levels. There is limited evidence that these medications can alter the course of peripheral arterial disease, but they may reduce the mortality rate from cardiovascular disease. Several classes of medication are used to prevent atherosclerosis: bile acid sequestrants (cholestyramine [Questran, Prevalite] or colestipol [Colestid]), nicotinic acid (niacin, B_3, Niacor; Niaspan), statins (atorvastatin [Lipitor], lovastatin [Mevacor], pravastatin [Pravachol], simvastatin [Zocor]), fibric acids (gemfibrozil [Lopid]), and lipophilic substances (probucol). Patients receiving long-term therapy with these medications require close medical supervision. Hypertension, which may accelerate the rate at which atherosclerotic lesions form in high-pressure vessels, can lead to cerebrovascular accident (CVA; brain attack, stroke), ischemic renal disease, severe peripheral arterial disease, or coronary artery disease. Results of large, randomized studies demonstrated dramatic reductions in myocardial infarction, stroke, and cardiovascular death when blood pressure was decreased to at least 140/90 mm Hg (Moser, 1999; McAlister et al., 2001).

Although no single risk factor has been identified as the primary contributor to the development of atherosclerotic cardiovascular disease, it is clear that the greater the number of risk factors, the greater the likelihood of developing the disease. Elimination of all controllable risk factors, particularly tobacco use, is strongly recommended.

Clinical Manifestations

The clinical signs and symptoms resulting from atherosclerosis depend on the organ or tissue affected. Coronary atherosclerosis (heart disease), angina, and acute myocardial infarction are discussed in Chapter 28. Cerebrovascular diseases, including transient cerebral ischemic attacks and stroke, are discussed in Chapter 62. Atherosclerosis of the aorta, including aneurysm, and atherosclerotic lesions of the extremities are discussed later in this chapter. Renovascular disease (renal artery stenosis and end-stage renal disease), including hypertension, is discussed in Chapter 45.

Medical Management

The traditional medical management of atherosclerosis involves modification of risk factors, a controlled exercise program to improve circulation and increase the functioning capacity of the circulation, medication, and interventional or surgical graft procedures.

SURGICAL MANAGEMENT

Vascular surgical procedures are divided into two groups: inflow procedures, which provide blood supply from the aorta into the femoral artery, and outflow procedures, which provide blood sup-

ply to vessels below the femoral artery. Inflow surgical procedures are discussed with diseases of the aorta and outflow procedures with peripheral arterial occlusive disease.

RADIOLOGIC INTERVENTIONS

Several interventional radiologic techniques are important adjunctive therapies to surgical procedures. If an isolated lesion or lesions are identified during the arteriogram, **angioplasty**, also called percutaneous transluminal angioplasty (PTA), may be performed. After the patient receives a local anesthetic, a balloon-tipped catheter is maneuvered across the area of stenosis. Exactly how PTA works is controversial. Some theorize that it improves blood flow by overstretching (and thereby dilating) the elastic fibers of the nondiseased arterial segment, but most clinicians believe that the procedure widens the arterial lumen by cracking and flattening the plaque against the vessel wall (see Chap. 28). Complications from PTA include hematoma formation, embolus, **dissection** (separation of the intima) of the vessel, and bleeding. To decrease the risk of reocclusion, stents (small, mesh tubes made of nitinol, titanium, or stainless steel) may be inserted to support the walls of blood vessels and prevent collapse immediately after balloon inflation (Fig. 31-8). A variety of covered wall stents and stent-grafts may be used for short-segment stenoses. Complications associated with stent or stent-graft use include distal embolization, intimal damage (dissection), and dislodgment. The advantage of angioplasty, stents, and stent-grafts is the decreased length of hospital stay required for the treatment; many of the procedures are performed on an outpatient basis.

NURSING PROCESS: THE PATIENT WHO HAS PERIPHERAL ARTERIAL INSUFFICIENCY OF THE EXTREMITIES

Assessment

The nursing assessment includes a complete health and medication history and identification of risk factors for peripheral artery disease. Signs and symptoms detected during the nursing assessment may include claudication pain; rest pain in the forefoot; pallor, rubor, or cyanosis; weak or absent peripheral pulses; and skin breakdown or ulcerations.

Nursing Diagnosis

Based on assessment data, major nursing diagnoses for the patient may include the following:

- Ineffective peripheral tissue perfusion related to compromised circulation
- Chronic pain related to impaired ability of peripheral vessels to supply tissues with oxygen
- Risk for impaired skin integrity related to compromised circulation
- Deficient knowledge regarding self-care activities

Planning and Goals

The major goals for the patient may include increased arterial blood supply to the extremities, promotion of vasodilation, prevention of vascular compression, relief of pain, attainment or maintenance of tissue integrity, and adherence to the self-care program.

Measures used by the patient and members of the health care team to accomplish a single goal must be evaluated in terms of

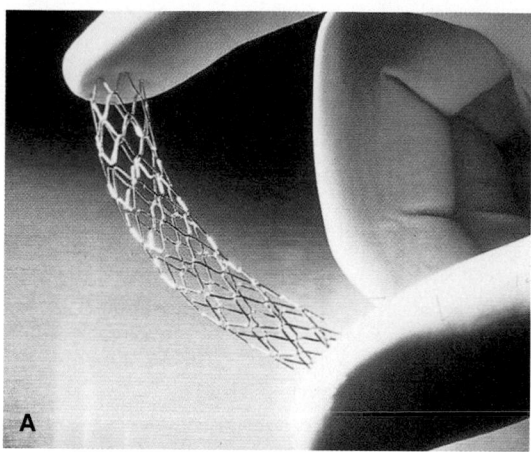
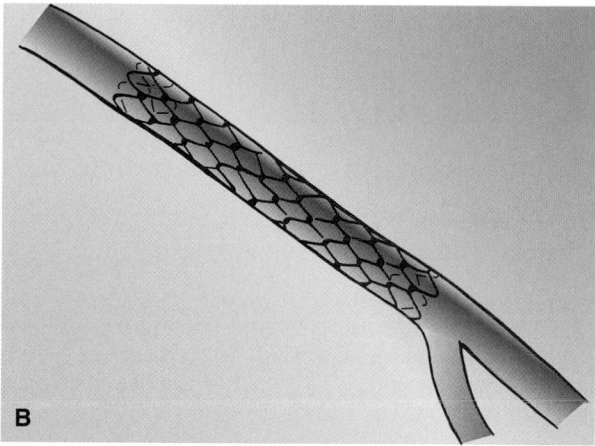

FIGURE 31-8 (**A**) Flexible stent. Courtesy of Medtronics, Peripheral Division, Santa Rosa, California. (**B**) Representation of a common iliac artery with a Wallstent (Boston Scientific).

the positive and the negative effects these measures may have on the simultaneous achievement of other goals. An overview of the care of a patient with peripheral arterial problems is provided in the Plan of Nursing Care: The Patient With Peripheral Vascular Problems.

Nursing Interventions

IMPROVING PERIPHERAL ARTERIAL CIRCULATION

Arterial blood supply to a body part can be enhanced by positioning the part below the level of the heart. For the lower extremities, this is accomplished by elevating the head of the patient's bed on 15-cm (6-inch) blocks or by having the patient use a reclining chair or sit with the feet resting on the floor.

The nurse can assist the patient with walking or other moderate or graded isometric exercises that may be prescribed to promote blood flow and encourage the development of collateral circulation. The nurse instructs the patient to walk to the point of pain, rest until pain subsides, and then resume walking so that endurance can be increased as collateral circulation develops. Pain can serve as a guide in determining the amount of exercise appropriate for an individual. The onset of pain indicates that the tissues are not receiving adequate oxygen, signaling the patient to rest before continuing activity. However, a regular exercise program can result in increased walking distance before the onset of claudication. The amount of exercise a patient can tolerate before the onset of pain is determined to provide a baseline for evaluation.

Not all patients with peripheral vascular disease should exercise. Before recommending any exercise program, the primary health care provider should be consulted. Conditions that worsen with activity include leg ulcers, cellulitis, gangrene, or acute thrombotic occlusions.

PROMOTING VASODILATION AND PREVENTING VASCULAR COMPRESSION

Arterial dilation promotes increased blood flow to the extremities and is therefore a desirable goal for patients with peripheral arterial disease. However, if the arteries are severely sclerosed, inelastic, or damaged, dilation is not possible. For this reason, measures to promote vasodilation, such as medications or surgery, may be only minimally effective.

Nursing interventions may involve applications of warmth to promote arterial flow and instructions to the patient to avoid exposure to cold temperatures, which causes vasoconstriction. Adequate clothing and warm temperatures protect the patient from chilling. If chilling occurs, a warm bath or drink is helpful.

When heat is applied directly to ischemic extremities, the temperature of the heat source must not exceed body temperature. Even at lower temperatures, burn injuries can occur in ischemic extremities. Excess heat may increase the metabolic rate of the extremities and increase the need for oxygen beyond that provided by the reduced arterial flow through the diseased artery.

> **NURSING ALERT** Patients are instructed to test the temperature of bath water and to avoid using hot-water bottles and heating pads on the extremities. Applying a heating pad to the abdomen can cause reflex vasodilation in the extremities and is safer than direct application of heat to affected extremities.

Nicotine causes vasospasm and can thereby dramatically reduce circulation to the extremities. Tobacco smoke also impairs transport and cellular use of oxygen and increases blood viscosity. Patients with arterial insufficiency who use tobacco (ie, smoke, chew) must be fully informed of the effects of nicotine on circulation and encouraged to stop using tobacco.

Emotional upsets stimulate the sympathetic nervous system, resulting in peripheral vasoconstriction. Although emotional stress is unavoidable, it can be minimized to some degree by avoiding stressful situations when possible or by consistently following a stress-management program. Counseling services or relaxation training may be indicated for people who cannot cope effectively with situational stressors.

Constrictive clothing and accessories such as tight socks, panty girdles, and shoelaces impede circulation to the extremities and promote venous stasis and therefore should be avoided. Crossing the legs should be discouraged because it compresses vessels in the legs.

RELIEVING PAIN

Frequently, the pain associated with peripheral arterial insufficiency is chronic and continuous. It limits activities, affects work and responsibilities, disturbs sleep, and alters patients' sense of well-being. Patients are often depressed, irritable, and unable to exert the energy necessary to execute prescribed therapies, making pain relief even more difficult. Analgesics such as oxycodone plus acetylsalicylic acid (Percodan) or oxycodone plus acetamin-

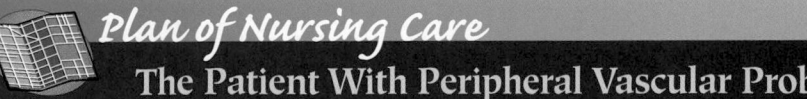

Plan of Nursing Care
The Patient With Peripheral Vascular Problems

Nursing Interventions	Rationale	Expected Outcomes

Nursing Diagnosis: Ineffective peripheral tissue perfusion related to compromised circulation
Goal: Increased arterial blood supply to extremities

1. Lower the extremities below the level of the heart (if condition is arterial in nature). 2. Encourage moderate amount of walking or graded extremity exercises.	1. Dependency of lower extremities enhances arterial blood supply. 2. Muscular exercise promotes blood flow and the development of collateral circulation.	• Extremities warm to touch • Color of extremities improved • Experiences decreased muscle pain with exercise

Goal: Decrease in venous congestion

1. Elevate extremities above heart level (if condition is venous in nature). 2. Discourage standing still or sitting for prolonged periods. 3. Encourage walking.	1. Elevation of extremities counteracts gravitational pull, promotes venous return, and prevents venous stasis. 2. Prolonged standing still or sitting promotes venous stasis. 3. Walking promotes venous return by activating the "muscle pump."	• Elevates lower extremities as prescribed • Decreased edema of extremities • Avoids prolonged standing still or sitting • Gradually increases walking time daily

Goal: Promotion of vasodilation and prevention of vascular compression

1. Maintain warm temperature and avoid chilling. 2. Discourage nicotine use. 3. Counsel in ways to avoid emotional upsets; stress management. 4. Encourage avoidance of constrictive clothing and accessories. 5. Encourage avoidance of leg crossing. 6. Administer vasodilator medications and adrenergic blocking agents as prescribed, with appropriate nursing considerations.	1. Warmth promotes arterial flow by preventing the vasoconstriction effects of chilling. 2. Nicotine causes vasospasm, which impedes peripheral circulation. 3. Emotional stress causes peripheral vasoconstriction by stimulating the sympathetic nervous system. 4. Constrictive clothing and accessories impede circulation and promote venous stasis. 5. Leg crossing causes compression of vessels with subsequent impediment of circulation, resulting in venous stasis. 6. Vasodilators relax smooth muscle; adrenergic blocking agents block the response to sympathetic nerve impulses or circulating catecholamines.	• Protects extremities from exposure to cold • Avoids nicotine • Uses stress-management program to minimize emotional upset • Avoids constricting clothing and accessories • Avoids leg crossing • Takes medication as prescribed

Nursing Diagnosis: Chronic pain related to impaired ability of peripheral vessels to supply tissues with oxygen
Goal: Relief of pain

1. Promote increased circulation. 2. Administer analgesics as prescribed, with appropriate nursing considerations.	1. Enhancement of peripheral circulation increases the oxygen supplied to the muscle and decreases the accumulation of metabolites that cause muscle spasms. 2. Analgesics help to reduce pain and allow the patient to participate in activities and exercises that promote circulation.	• Uses measures to increase arterial blood supply to extremities • Uses analgesics as prescribed

Nursing Diagnosis: Risk for impaired skin integrity related to compromised circulation
Goal: Attainment/maintenance of tissue integrity

1. Instruct in ways to avoid trauma to extremities.	1. Poorly nourished tissues are susceptible to trauma and bacterial invasion; healing of wounds is delayed or inhibited due to poor tissue perfusion.	• Inspects skin daily for evidence of injury or ulceration • Avoids trauma and irritation to skin

(continued)

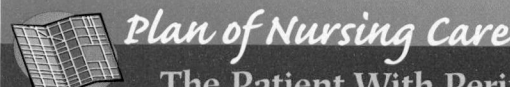

Plan of Nursing Care

The Patient With Peripheral Vascular Problems *(Continued)*

Nursing Interventions	Rationale	Expected Outcomes
2. Encourage wearing protective shoes and padding for pressure areas.	2. Protective shoes and padding prevent foot injuries and blisters.	• Wears protective shoes • Adheres to meticulous hygiene regimen • Eats a healthy diet that contains adequate protein and vitamins A and C
3. Encourage meticulous hygiene; bathing with neutral soaps, applying lotions, carefully trimming nails.	3. Neutral soaps and lotions prevent drying and cracking of skin.	
4. Caution to avoid scratching or vigorous rubbing.	4. Scratching and rubbing can cause skin abrasions and bacterial invasion.	
5. Promote good nutrition; adequate intake of vitamins A and C, protein, and zinc; control of obesity.	5. Good nutrition promotes healing and prevents tissue breakdown.	

Nursing Diagnosis: Deficient knowledge regarding self-care activities
Goal: Adherence to the self-care program

1. Include family/significant others in teaching program.	1. Adherence to the self-care program is enhanced when the patient receives support from family and from appropriate self-help groups and agencies.	• Practices frequent position changes as prescribed • Practices postural exercises as prescribed • Takes medications as prescribed • Avoids vasoconstrictors • Uses measures to prevent trauma • Uses stress management program • Accepts condition as chronic but amenable to therapies that will decrease symptoms
2. Provide written instructions about foot care, leg care, and exercise program.	2. Written instructions serve as reminder and reinforcement of information.	
3. Assist to obtain properly fitting clothing, shoes, stockings.	3. Constrictive clothing and accessories impede circulation and promote venous stasis.	
4. Refer to self-help groups as indicated, such as smoking cessation clinics, stress management, weight management, and exercise program.	4. Reducing risk factors may reduce symptoms or slow disease progression.	

ophen (Percocet) may be helpful in reducing pain to the point where the patient can participate in the therapies that can increase circulation and ultimately relieve pain more effectively.

MAINTAINING TISSUE INTEGRITY

Poorly nourished tissues are susceptible to damage and infection. When lesions develop, healing may be delayed or inhibited because of the poor blood supply to the area. Infected, nonhealing ulcerations of the extremities can be debilitating and may require prolonged and often expensive treatments. Amputation of an ischemic limb may eventually be necessary. Measures to prevent these complications must be a high priority and vigorously implemented.

Trauma to the extremities must be avoided. Advising the patient to wear sturdy, well-fitting shoes or slippers to prevent foot injury and blisters may be helpful, as may be recommending neutral soaps and body lotions to prevent drying and cracking of skin. Scratching and vigorous rubbing can abrade skin and create a site for bacterial invasion; therefore, feet should be patted dry. Stockings should be clean and dry. Fingernails and toenails should be carefully trimmed straight across and sharp corners filed to follow the contour of the nail. If nails are thick and brittle and cannot be trimmed safely, a podiatrist must be consulted. Corns and calluses need to be removed by a health care professional. Special shoe inserts may be needed to prevent calluses from recurring. All signs of blisters, ingrown toenails, infection, or other problems should be

reported to health care professionals for treatment and follow-up. Patients with diminished vision may require assistance in periodically examining the lower extremities for trauma.

Good nutrition promotes healing and prevents tissue breakdown and is therefore included in the overall therapeutic program for patients with peripheral vascular disease. Eating a well-balanced diet that contains adequate protein and vitamins is necessary for patients with arterial insufficiency. Key nutrients play specific roles in wound healing. Vitamin C is essential for collagen synthesis and capillary development. Vitamin A enhances epithelialization. Zinc is necessary for cell mitosis and cell proliferation. Obesity strains the heart, increases venous congestion, and reduces circulation; therefore, a weight-reduction plan may be necessary for some patients. A diet low in lipids may be indicated for patients with atherosclerosis.

PROMOTING HOME AND COMMUNITY-BASED CARE

The self-care program is planned with the patient so that activities that promote arterial and venous circulation, relieve pain, and promote tissue integrity are acceptable. The patient and family are helped to understand the reasons for each aspect of the program and the possible consequences of nonadherence. Long-term care of the feet and legs is of prime importance in the prevention of trauma, ulceration, and gangrene. The Plan of Nursing Care describes nursing care for patients with peripheral vascular disease. Chart 31-3 provides detailed patient instructions for foot and leg care.

Chart 31-3
Home Care Checklist • Foot and Leg Care in Peripheral Vascular Disease

At the completion of the home care instruction, the patient or caregiver will be able to:

	Patient	Caregiver
• Demonstrate daily foot bathing: Wash between toes with mild soap and lukewarm water, then rinse thoroughly and pat rather than rub dry.	✓	✓
• Recognize the dangers of thermal injury: – Wear clean, loose, soft cotton socks (they are comfortable, allow air to circulate, and will absorb moisture) – In cold weather, wear extra socks in extra-large shoes. – Avoid heating pads, whirlpools, and hot tubs. – Avoid sunburn.	✓	
• Identify safety concerns: – Inspect feet daily with a mirror for redness, dryness, cuts, blisters, etc. – Always wear soft shoes or slippers when out of bed. – Trim nails straight across after showering. – Consult podiatrist to trim nails if vision is decreased; also for care of corns, blisters, ingrown nails. – Clear pathways in house to prevent injury. – Avoid wearing thong sandals. – Use lamb's wool between toes if they overlap or rub each other.	✓	✓
• Demonstrate comfort measures: – Wear leather shoes with an extra-depth toebox. Synthetic shoes do not allow air to circulate. – If feet become dry and scaly, use cream with lanolin. Never put cream between toes. – If feet perspire, especially between toes, use powder daily and/or lamb's wool between toes to promote drying.	✓	
• Demonstrate ability to decrease risk of constricting blood vessels: – Avoid promoting circular compression around feet or knees—for example, by applying knee-high stockings or tight socks. – Do not cross legs at knees. – Stop using nicotine (ie, tobacco smoking or chewing) because nicotine causes vasoconstriction and vasospasm. – Avoid applying tight, constricting bandages. – Participate in a regular walking exercise program to stimulate circulation.	✓	
• Recognize when to seek medical attention: – Contact health care provider at the onset of skin breakdown such as abrasions, blisters, athlete's foot, or pain. – Do not use any medication on feet or legs unless prescribed. – Avoid using iodine, alcohol, corn/wart-removing compound, or adhesive products before checking with health care provider.	✓	✓

Evaluation

EXPECTED PATIENT OUTCOMES

Expected patient outcomes may include:

1. Demonstrates an increase in arterial blood supply to extremities
   a. Exhibits extremities warm to touch
   b. Has improved color of extremities (ie, free of rubor or cyanosis)
   c. Experiences decreased muscle pain with exercise
   d. Demonstrates an increase in walking distance or duration
2. Promotes vasodilation; prevents vascular compression
   a. Protects extremities from exposure to cold
   b. Avoids use of tobacco
   c. Uses stress management strategies to minimize emotional upset
   d. Wears nonconstricting clothing
   e. Avoids leg crossing
   f. Takes medication as prescribed
3. Has decrease in severity and duration of pain
4. Attains or maintains tissue integrity
   a. Avoids trauma and irritation to skin
   b. Wears protective shoes
   c. Adheres to meticulous hygienic regimen
   d. Eats a healthy diet that contains adequate protein, vitamins A and C, and zinc
   e. Performs self-care activities

PERIPHERAL ARTERIAL OCCLUSIVE DISEASE

Arterial insufficiency of the extremities is usually found in individuals older than 50 years of age, most often in men. The legs are most frequently affected; however, the upper extremities may be involved. The age of onset and the severity are influenced by the type and number of atherosclerotic risk factors (Chart 31-4). In peripheral arterial disease, obstructive lesions are predominantly confined to segments of the arterial system extending from the aorta below the renal arteries to the popliteal artery (Fig. 31-9). However, distal occlusive disease is frequently seen in patients with diabetes mellitus and in elderly patients.

Chart 31-4
Risk Factors for Peripheral Arterial Disease

Nonmodifiable	Hypertension
Age	Diet (contributing to
Gender	hyperlipidemia)
Familial predisposition	Obesity
Modifiable	Sedentary lifestyle
Nicotine use (eg, tobacco	Stress
smoking, chewing)	Diabetes mellitus

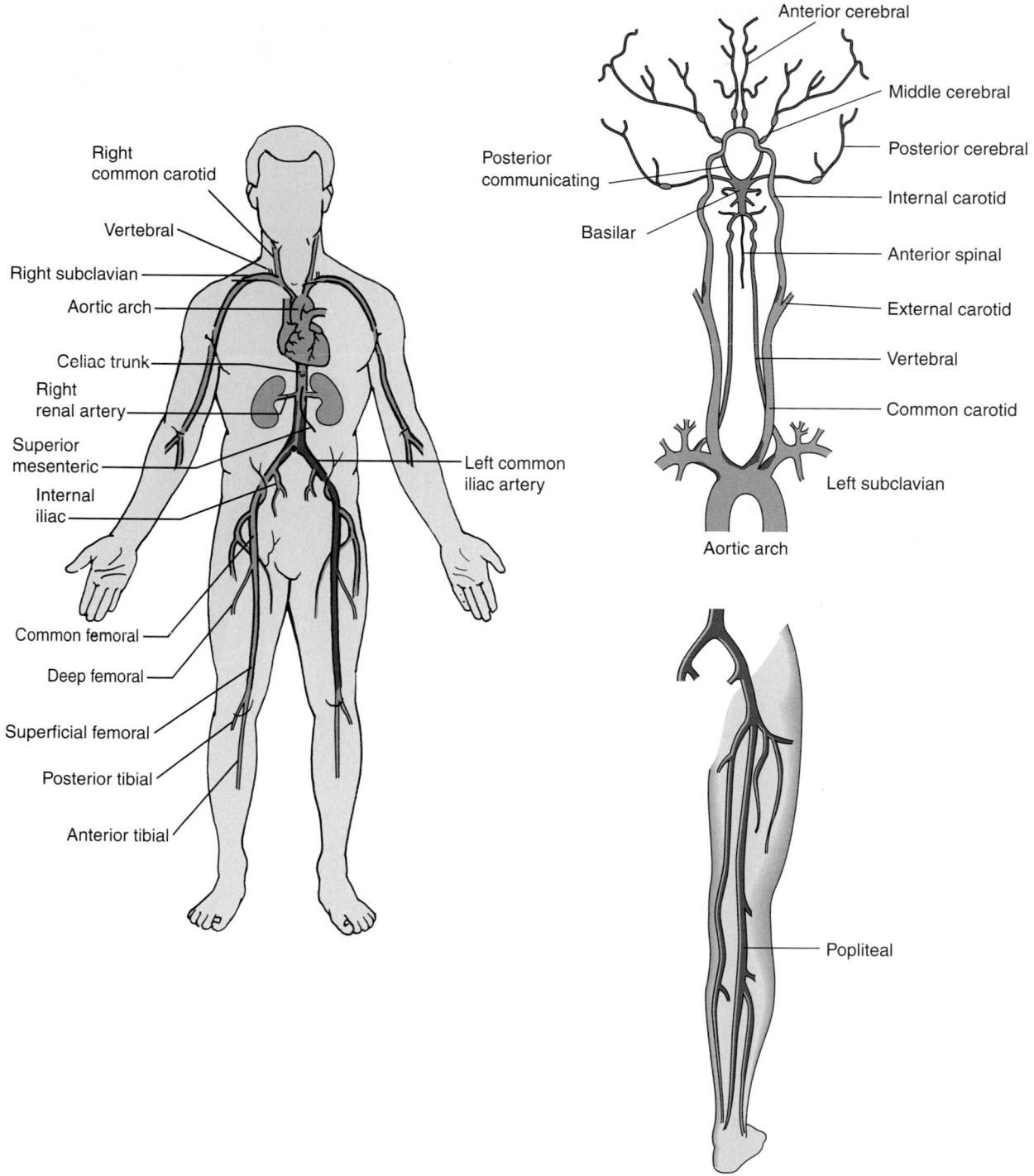

FIGURE 31-9 Common sites of atherosclerotic obstruction in major arteries.

Clinical Manifestations

The hallmark is intermittent claudication. This pain may be described as aching, cramping, fatigue, or weakness that is consistently reproduced with the same degree of exercise or activity and relieved with rest. The pain commonly occurs in muscle groups one joint level below the stenosis or occlusion. As the disease progresses, the patient may have a decreased ability to walk the same distance or may notice increased pain with ambulation. When the arterial insufficiency becomes severe, the patient begins to have rest pain. This pain is associated with critical ischemia of the distal extremity and is persistent, aching, or boring; it may be so excruciating that it is unrelieved by opioids. Ischemic rest pain is usually worse at night and often wakes the patient. Elevating the extremity or placing it in a horizontal position increases the pain, whereas placing the extremity in a dependent position reduces the pain. In bed, some patients sleep with the affected leg hanging over the side of the bed. Some patients sleep in a reclining chair in an attempt to relieve the pain.

Assessment and Diagnostic Findings

A sensation of coldness or numbness in the extremities may accompany intermittent claudication and is a result of the reduced arterial flow. When the extremity is examined, it may feel cool to the touch and look pale when elevated or ruddy and cyanotic when placed in a dependent position. Skin and nail changes, ulcerations, gangrene, and muscle atrophy may be evident. Bruits may be auscultated with a stethoscope; a bruit is the sound produced by turbulent blood flow through an irregular, tortuous, stenotic vessel or through a dilated segment of the vessel (aneurysm). Peripheral pulses may be diminished or absent.

Examining the peripheral pulses is an important part of assessing arterial occlusive disease. Unequal pulses between extremities or the absence of a normally palpable pulse is a sign of peripheral arterial disease. The femoral pulse in the groin and the posterior tibial pulse beside the medial malleolus are most easily palpated. The popliteal pulse is sometimes difficult to palpate; the location of the dorsalis pedis artery on the dorsum of the foot varies and is normally absent in about 7% of the population.

The presence, location, and extent of arterial occlusive disease are determined by a careful history of the symptoms and by physical examination. The color and temperature of the extremity are noted and the pulses palpated. The nails may be thickened and opaque, and the skin may be shiny, atrophic, and dry, with sparse hair growth. The assessment includes comparison of the right and left extremities.

The diagnosis of peripheral arterial occlusive disease may be made using CW Doppler and ankle-brachial indices (ABIs), treadmill testing for claudication, duplex ultrasonography, or other imaging studies previously described.

Medical Management

Generally, patients feel better with some type of exercise program. If this program is combined with weight reduction and cessation of tobacco use, patients often can improve their activity tolerance. Patients should not be promised that their symptoms will be relieved if they stop tobacco use, because claudication may persist, and they may lose their motivation to stop using tobacco.

PHARMACOLOGIC THERAPY

Various medications are prescribed to treat the symptoms of peripheral arterial disease. Pentoxifylline (Trental) increases erythrocyte flexibility and reduces blood viscosity, and it is therefore thought to improve the supply of oxygenated blood to the muscle. Cilostazol (Pletal) works by inhibiting platelet aggregation, inhibiting smooth muscle cell proliferation, and increasing vasodilation. Antiplatelet aggregating agents such as aspirin, ticlopidine (Ticlid), and clopidogrel (Plavix) are thought to improve circulation throughout diseased arteries or prevent intimal hyperplasia leading to stenosis.

SURGICAL MANAGEMENT

In most patients, when intermittent claudication becomes severe and disabling or when the limb is at risk for amputation because of tissue loss, vascular grafting or endarterectomy is the treatment of choice. The choice of the surgical procedure depends on the degree and location of the stenosis or occlusion. Other important considerations are the overall health of the patient and the length of the procedure that can be tolerated. It is sometimes necessary to provide the palliative therapy of primary amputation rather than an arterial bypass. If endarterectomy is performed, an incision is made into the artery, and the atheromatous obstruction is

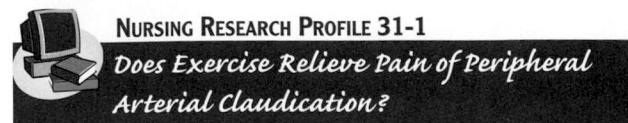

NURSING RESEARCH PROFILE 31-1
Does Exercise Relieve Pain of Peripheral Arterial Claudication?

Braun, C. M., Colucci, A. M., & Patterson, R. B. (1999). Components of an optimal exercise program for the treatment of patients with claudication. *Journal of Vascular Nursing, 17*(2), 32–36.

Purpose
Because patients with peripheral arterial claudication increasingly limit activity because of pain, they become physically deconditioned. The patients and their families report decreased quality of life (QOL) because of the activity limitations. Traditional treatment for peripheral arterial claudication has been surgical bypass. Exercise programs are beginning to be offered as treatment for patients with peripheral arterial claudication. Little is known about the effectiveness of exercise in the treatment of this patient population. This study evaluated whether a supervised exercise and education program increased pain-free walking distance and improved total fitness of patients with peripheral arterial claudication.

Study Sample and Design
This study was a retrospective review of 96 patients who had experienced symptoms of peripheral arterial claudication for longer than 3 months. Patients participated in a cardiovascular conditioning and muscle training exercise program with education classes for 12 weeks. Twenty-two patients monitored for 2 years; data were collected at 1 year and 2 years after the original 12-week program.

Findings
Patients' walking distances increased threefold after participation in the 12-week program. The average maximum distance patients were able to walk at the beginning of the program was 190 meters. After the 12-week program the average distance was 580 m. The 22 patients followed for two years had an average maximum walking distance of 882 m 1 year after the 12-week program and 731 m 2 years after the 12-week program. The researchers concluded that patients were able to maintain and continue exercising after completion of the 12-week program. Families reported improvement in general health and psychosocial behavior of the patients.

Nursing Implications
Patients with peripheral arterial claudication benefit from a supervised exercise program combined with education programs. Supervised exercise programs may enable patients with peripheral arterial claudication to increase the distance they can walk without symptoms, improve their quality of life, and avoid or delay surgical intervention.

removed. The artery is then sutured closed to restore vascular integrity (Fig. 31-10).

Bypass grafts are performed to reroute the blood flow around the stenosis or occlusion. Before bypass grafting, the surgeon determines where the distal **anastomosis** (site where the vessels are surgically joined) will be placed. The distal outflow vessel must be at least 50% patent for the graft to remain patent. A higher bypass graft patency rate is associated with keeping the length of the bypass as short as possible.

If the atherosclerotic occlusion is below the inguinal ligament in the superficial femoral artery, the surgical procedure of choice is the femoral-to-popliteal graft. This procedure is further classified as above-knee and below-knee grafts, referring to the location of the distal anastomosis.

Lower leg or ankle vessels with occlusions may also require grafts. Occasionally, the entire popliteal artery is occluded, and there is only collateral circulation. The distal anastomosis may be

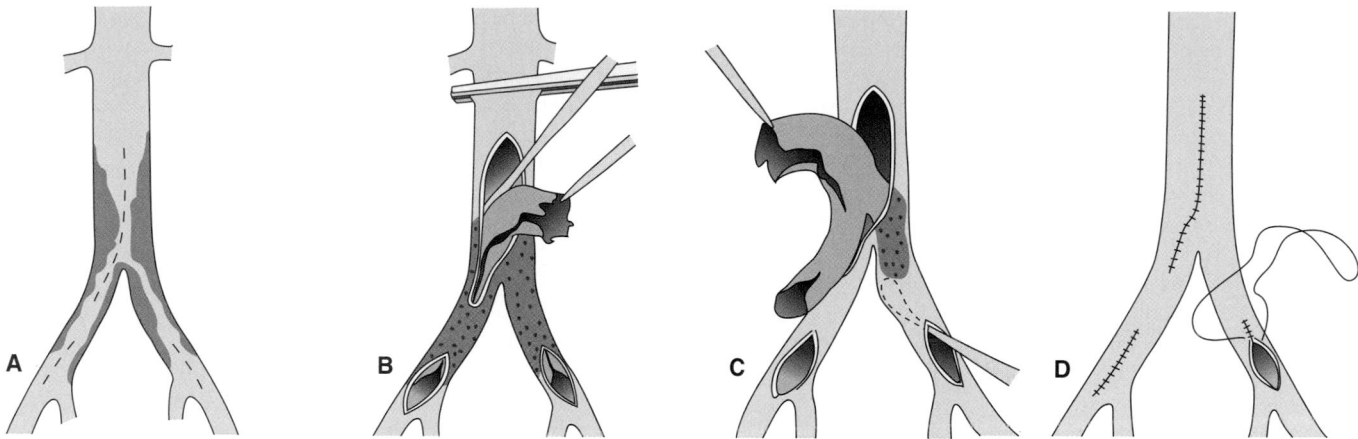

FIGURE 31-10   In an aortoiliac endarterectomy, the vascular surgeon (**A**) identifies the diseased area, (**B**) clamps off the blood supply to the vessel, (**C**) removes the plaque, and (**D**) sutures the vessel shut, after which blood flow is restored. Adapted with permission from Rutherford, R. B. (1999). *Vascular surgery: Vol. 1 and 2* (5th ed.). Philadelphia: W. B. Saunders.

made onto any of the tibial arteries (posterior tibial, anterior tibial, or peroneal arteries) or the dorsalis pedis or plantar artery. The distal anastomosis site is determined by the ease of exposure of the vessel in surgery and by which vessel provides the best flow to the distal limb. These grafts require the use of native vein to ensure patency. Native vein is autologous vein (the patient's own vein). The greater or lesser saphenous vein or a combination of one of the saphenous veins and an upper extremity vein such as the cephalic vein are used to meet the required length.

How long the graft remains patent is determined by several factors, including the size of the graft, graft location, and development of intimal hyperplasia at anastomosis sites. Bypass grafts may be synthetic or autologous vein. Several synthetic materials are available for use as a peripheral bypass graft: woven or knitted Dacron, expanded polytetrafluoroethylene (ePTFE, such as Gore-Tex or Impra), collagen-impregnated, and umbilical vein. Infection is a problem that threatens survival of the graft and almost always requires removal of the graft.

If a vein graft is the surgical choice, care must be taken in the operating room not to damage the vein after harvesting (removing the vein from the patient's body). The vein is occluded at one end and inflated with a heparinized solution to check for leakage and competency. When this is done, the graft is placed in a heparinized solution to keep it from becoming dry and brittle.

Nursing Management

MAINTAINING CIRCULATION

The primary objective in the postoperative management of patients who have undergone vascular procedures is to maintain adequate circulation through the arterial repair. Pulses, Doppler assessment, color and temperature of the extremity, capillary refill, and sensory and motor function of the affected extremities are checked, compared with those of the other extremity, and recorded every hour for the first 8 hours and then every 2 hours for 24 hours. Doppler evaluation of the vessels distal to the bypass graft should be performed for all postoperative vascular patients, because it is more sensitive than palpation for pulses. The ABI is monitored at least once every 8 hours for the first 24 hours and then once each day until discharge (not usually assessed for pedal artery bypasses). An adequate circulating blood volume should be established and maintained. Disappearance of a pulse that was present may indicate thrombotic occlusion of the graft; the surgeon is immediately notified.

MONITORING AND MANAGING POTENTIAL COMPLICATIONS

Continuous monitoring of urine output (more than 30 mL/hour), central venous pressure, mental status, and pulse rate and volume permit early recognition and treatment of fluid imbalances. Bleeding can result from the heparin administered during surgery or from an anastomotic leak. A hematoma may form as well.

Leg crossing and prolonged extremity dependency are avoided to prevent thrombosis. Edema is a normal postoperative finding; however, elevating the extremities and encouraging the patient to exercise the extremities while in bed reduces edema. Elastic compression stockings may be prescribed for some patients, but care must be taken to avoid compressing distal vessel bypass grafts. Severe edema of the extremity, pain, and decreased sensation of toes or fingers can be an indication of compartment syndrome.

PROMOTING HOME AND COMMUNITY-BASED CARE

Discharge planning includes assessing the patient's ability to manage independently. The nurse determines if the patient has a network of family and friends to assist with activities of daily living. The patient may need to be encouraged to make the lifestyle changes necessary with a chronic disease, including pain management and modifications in diet, activity, and hygiene (skin care). The nurse ensures that the patient has the knowledge and ability to assess for any postoperative complications such as infection, occlusion of the artery or graft, and decreased blood flow. The nurse assists the patient in developing a plan to stop using tobacco. The Plan of Nursing Care describes nursing care for patients with peripheral vascular disease.

UPPER EXTREMITY ARTERIAL OCCLUSIVE DISEASE

Arterial occlusions occur less frequently in the upper extremities (arms) than in the legs and cause less severe symptoms because the collateral circulation is significantly better in the arms. The arms also have less muscle mass and are not subjected to the workload of the legs.

Clinical Manifestations

Stenosis and occlusions in the upper extremity result from atherosclerosis or trauma. The stenosis usually occurs at the origin of the vessel proximal to the vertebral artery, setting up the vertebral artery as the major contributor of flow. The patient may develop a "subclavian steal" syndrome characterized by reverse flow in the vertebral and basilar artery to provide blood flow to the arm. This syndrome may cause vertebrobasilar (cerebral) symptoms. Most patients are asymptomatic; however, some report vertigo, ataxia, syncope, or bilateral visual changes.

The patient typically complains of arm fatigue and pain with exercise (forearm claudication) and inability to hold or grasp objects (eg, painting, combing hair, placing objects on shelves above the head). Some even notice difficulties driving.

Assessment and Diagnostic Findings

Assessment findings include coolness and pallor of the affected extremity, decreased capillary refill, and a difference in arm blood pressures of more than 20 mm Hg. Noninvasive studies performed to evaluate for upper extremity arterial occlusions include upper and forearm blood pressure determinations and duplex ultrasonography to identify the anatomic location of the lesion and to evaluate the hemodynamics of the blood flow. Transcranial Doppler evaluation is performed to evaluate the intracranial circulation and to detect any siphoning of blood flow from the posterior circulation to provide blood flow to the affected arm. If a surgical or interventional procedure is planned, an arteriogram may be necessary.

Medical Management

If a short, focal lesion is identified in an upper extremity artery, a PTA may be performed. If the lesion involves the subclavian artery with documented siphoning of blood flow from the intracranial circulation, several surgical procedures are available: carotid–to–subclavian artery bypass, axillary–to–axillary artery bypass, and autogenous reimplantation of the subclavian to the carotid artery.

Nursing Management

Nursing assessment involves bilateral comparison of upper arm blood pressures (obtained by stethoscope and Doppler); radial, ulnar, and brachial pulses; motor and sensory function; temperature; color changes; and capillary refill every 2 hours. Disappearance of a pulse or Doppler flow that had been present may indicate an acute occlusion of the vessel, and the physician is notified immediately.

 NURSING ALERT Before and for 24 hours after surgery, the patient's arm is kept at heart level and protected from cold, venipunctures or arterial sticks, tape, and constrictive dressings.

After surgery, the arm is kept at heart level or elevated, with the fingers at the highest level. Pulses are monitored with Doppler assessment of the arterial flow every hour for 8 hours and then every 2 hours for 24 hours. Blood pressure (obtained by stethoscope and Doppler) is also assessed every hour for 8 hours and then every 2 hours for 24 hours. Motor and sensory function, warmth, color, and capillary refill are monitored with each arterial flow (pulse) assessment.

Discharge planning includes assessing the patient's ability to manage independently. The nurse determines whether the patient has a network of family and friends to assist with activities of daily living. The patient may need to be encouraged to make the lifestyle changes necessary for a chronic disease, including pain management and modifications in diet, activity, and hygiene

(skin care). The nurse ensures that the patient has the knowledge and ability to assess for any postoperative complications such as infection, reocclusion of the artery or occlusion of the graft, and decreased blood flow. The patient is assisted in developing a plan to stop using tobacco. The Plan of Nursing Care describes nursing care for patients with peripheral vascular disease.

THROMBOANGIITIS OBLITERANS (BUERGER'S DISEASE)

Buerger's disease is characterized by recurring inflammation of the intermediate and small arteries and veins of the lower and (in rare cases) upper extremities. It results in thrombus formation and occlusion of the vessels. It is differentiated from other vessel diseases by its microscopic appearance. In contrast to atherosclerosis, Buerger's disease is believed to be an autoimmune disease that results in occlusion of distal vessels.

The cause of Buerger's disease is unknown, but it is believed to be an autoimmune vasculitis. It occurs most often in men between the ages of 20 and 35 years, and it has been reported in all races and in many areas of the world. There is considerable evidence that heavy smoking or chewing of tobacco is a causative or an aggravating factor (Frost-Rude et al., 2000). Generally, the lower extremities are affected, but arteries in the upper extremities or viscera can also be involved. Buerger's disease is generally bilateral and symmetric with focal lesions. Superficial thrombophlebitis may be present.

Gerontologic Considerations

Although this condition is different from atherosclerosis, Buerger's disease in older patients may also be followed by atherosclerosis of the larger vessels after involvement of the smaller vessels. The patient's ability to walk may be severely limited. Patients are at higher risk for nonhealing wounds because of impaired circulation.

Clinical Manifestations

Pain is the outstanding symptom of Buerger's disease. The patient complains of foot cramps, especially of the arch (instep claudication), after exercise. The pain is relieved by rest; often, a burning pain is aggravated by emotional disturbances, nicotine, or chilling. Cold sensitivity of the Raynaud type is found in one half the patients and is frequently confined to the hands. Digital rest pain is constant, and the characteristics of the pain do not change between activity and rest.

Physical signs include intense rubor (reddish blue discoloration) of the foot and absence of the pedal pulse but with normal femoral and popliteal pulses. Radial and ulnar artery pulses are absent or diminished. Various types of paresthesia may develop.

As the disease progresses, definite redness or cyanosis of the part appears when the extremity is in a dependent position. Involvement is generally bilateral, but color changes may affect only one extremity or only certain digits. Color changes may progress to ulceration, and ulceration with gangrene eventually occurs.

Assessment and Diagnostic Findings

Segmental limb blood pressures are taken to demonstrate the distal location of the lesions or occlusions. Duplex ultrasonography is used to document patency of the proximal vessels and to visualize the extent of distal disease. Contrast angiography is performed to demonstrate the diseased portion of the anatomy.

Management

The treatment of Buerger's disease is essentially the same as that for atherosclerotic peripheral arterial disease. The main objectives are to improve circulation to the extremities, prevent the progression of the disease, and protect the extremities from trauma and infection. Treatment of ulceration and gangrene is directed toward minimizing infection and conservative débridement of necrotic tissue. Tobacco use is highly detrimental, and patients are strongly advised to stop using tobacco completely. Symptoms are often relieved by cessation of smoking and other uses of tobacco.

Vasodilators are rarely prescribed because these medications cause dilation of only healthy vessels; vasodilators may divert blood away from the partially occluded vessels, making the situation worse. A regional sympathetic block or ganglionectomy may be useful in some instances to produce vasodilation and increase blood flow.

SURGICAL MANAGEMENT OF COMPLICATIONS

If gangrene of a toe develops as a result of arterial occlusive disease in the leg, it is unlikely that toe amputation or even transmetatarsal amputation will be sufficient; usually, a below-knee amputation or, occasionally, an above-knee amputation is necessary. The indications for amputation are worsening gangrene, especially if the infected area is moist, severe rest pain, or fulminating sepsis.

NURSING MANAGEMENT OF COMPLICATIONS

If an amputation is performed, immediate postoperative care includes elevating the stump for the first 24 hours to promote venous return and minimize edema. The incision is monitored for signs of hematoma (unapproximated suture line, discoloration or ruddy color changes of the skin along the suture line, tenderness with palpation, or oozing of dark blood from the suture line). The nurse assesses the fit of the elastic bandages and ensures the integrity of the wrap and continued ability to fit two fingers between layers of the wrap. Distal skin color and warmth are assessed, if accessible, and recorded. Elastic bandages are removed and reapplied as prescribed by the surgeon (eg, every 6 hours using figure-of-eight turns).

The patient may experience grief, fear, or anxiety related to loss of the limb. The patient is encouraged to discuss his or her feelings. Spiritual advisors and other health care team members are consulted as appropriate. Recovery and rehabilitation require consultation among health care providers (eg, physicians, physical and occupational therapists, prosthetists, dietitians, nurses, discharge coordinators). The patient may decide to be fitted for and learn to use a prosthetic device. Rehabilitation facilities, home care, and outpatient therapy can assist the patient to adapt to the changes in lifestyle.

Discharge planning includes assessing the patient's ability to manage independently. The patient is assisted in developing a plan to stop using tobacco and to manage pain. The patient may need to be encouraged to make the lifestyle changes necessary with a chronic disease, including modifications in diet, activity, and hygiene (skin care). The nurse determines whether the patient has a network of family and friends to assist with activities of daily living. The nurse ensures that the patient has the knowledge and ability to assess for any postoperative complications such as infection and decreased blood flow. The Plan of Nursing Care describes nursing care for patients with peripheral vascular disease.

AORTITIS

The aorta, which is the main trunk of the arterial system, is divided into the ascending aorta (5 cm [2 inches] in diameter, contained in the pericardium), the aortic arch (extending upward, backward, and downward), and the descending aorta. The thoracic aorta is above the diaphragm; the abdominal aorta is below the diaphragm. The abdominal aorta is further designated as suprarenal (above renal artery level), perirenal level (at renal artery level), and infrarenal (below renal artery level).

Aortitis is inflammation of the aorta, particularly of the aortic arch. Two types are known to occur: Takayasu's disease and syphilitic aortitis. Takayasu's disease, or occlusive thromboaortopathy, is uncommon; today, syphilitic aortitis is rare.

Takayasu's disease, a chronic inflammatory disease of the aortic arch and its branches, primarily affects young or middle-aged women and is more common in those of Asian descent. It is nonatherosclerotic; the exact pathologic mechanism is unknown but thought to be immune complex mediated. It progresses from a systemic inflammation with localized arteritis to end-organ ischemia because of large vessel stenosis or obstruction. Magnetic resonance angiography, CT, duplex ultrasonography, or arteriography is used to diagnose and evaluate the lesions, which are typically long, smooth areas of narrowing with or without aneurysms. In the early stages, the disease may respond to corticosteroids, and patients may benefit from the addition of cytotoxic immunosuppressive agents (Strider et al., 1996). Selective PTA and surgical revascularization may be performed after suppression of the systemic vascular inflammation.

AORTOILIAC DISEASE

If collateral circulation has developed, patients with a stenosis or occlusion of the aortoiliac segment may be asymptomatic, or they may complain of buttock or low back discomfort associated with walking. Men may experience impotence. These patients may have decreased or absent femoral pulses.

Medical Management

The treatment of aortoiliac disease is essentially the same as that for atherosclerotic peripheral arterial occlusive disease. The surgical procedure of choice is the aortobiiliac graft. If possible, the distal anastomosis is made to the iliac artery, and the entire surgical procedure can be performed within the abdomen. If the iliac vessels are diseased, the distal anastomosis is made to the femoral arteries (aortobifemoral graft). Bifurcated woven or knitted Dacron grafts are preferred for this surgical procedure.

Nursing Management

Preoperative assessment, in addition to the standard parameters (see Chap. 18), includes evaluating the brachial, radial, ulnar, femoral, posterior tibial, and dorsalis pedis pulses to establish a baseline for follow-up after arterial lines are placed and postoperatively. Patient teaching includes an overview of the procedure to be performed, the preparation for surgery, and the anticipated postoperative plan of care. Sights, sounds, and sensations that the patient may experience are discussed.

Postoperative care includes monitoring for signs of thrombosis in arteries distal to the surgical site. The nurse assesses color and temperature of the extremity, capillary refill time, sensory and motor function, and pulses by palpation and Doppler every hour for the first 8 hours and then every 2 hours for the first

24 hours. Any dusky or bluish discoloration, coolness, capillary refill time greater than 3 seconds, decrease in sensory or motor function, or decrease in pulse quality are reported immediately to the physician.

Postoperative care also includes monitoring for urine output greater than or equal to 30 mL/hour. Renal function may be impaired as a result of hypoperfusion from hypotension, involvement of the renal arteries during the surgical procedure, hypovolemia, or embolization of the renal artery or renal parenchyma. Vital signs, pain, and intake and output are monitored with the pulse and extremity assessments. Results of laboratory tests are monitored and reported to the physician. Abdominal assessment for bowel sounds and paralytic ileus is performed at least every 8 hours. Bowel sounds may not return before the third postoperative day. The absence of bowel sounds, absence of flatus, and abdominal distention are indications of paralytic ileus. Manual manipulation of the bowel during surgery may have caused bruising, resulting in decreased peristalsis. Nasogastric suction may be necessary to decompress the bowel until peristalsis returns. A liquid bowel movement before the third postoperative day may indicate bowel ischemia, which may occur when the mesenteric blood supply (celiac, superior mesenteric, or inferior mesenteric arteries) is occluded. Ischemic bowel usually causes increased pain and an elevated white blood cell count (20,000 to 30,000 cells/mm³).

AORTIC ANEURYSM

An aneurysm is a localized sac or dilation formed at a weak point in the wall of the aorta (Fig. 31-11). It may be classified by its shape or form. The most common forms of aneurysms are saccular or fusiform. A saccular aneurysm projects from one side of the vessel only. If an entire arterial segment becomes dilated, a fusiform aneurysm develops. Very small aneurysms due to localized infection are called mycotic aneurysms.

Historically, the cause of abdominal aortic aneurysm, the most common type of degenerative aneurysm, has been attributed to atherosclerotic changes in the aorta. Other causes of aneurysm formation are listed in Chart 31-5. Aneurysms are serious because they can rupture, leading to hemorrhage and death.

Chart 31-5 — **Etiologic Classification of Arterial Aneurysms**

Congenital: Primary connective tissue disorders (Marfan's syndrome, Ehlers-Danlos syndrome) and other diseases (focal medial agenesis, tuberous sclerosis, Turner's syndrome, Menkes' syndrome)
Mechanical (hemodynamic): Poststenotic and arteriovenous fistula and amputation-related
Traumatic (pseudoaneurysms): Penetrating arterial injuries, blunt arterial injuries, pseudoaneurysms
Inflammatory (noninfectious): Associated with arteritis (Takayasu's disease, giant cell arteritis, systemic lupus erythematosus, Behçet's syndrome, Kawasaki's disease) and periarterial inflammation (ie, pancreatitis)
Infectious (mycotic): Bacterial, fungal, spirochetal infections
Pregnancy-related degenerative: Nonspecific, inflammatory variant
Anastomotic (postarteriotomy) and graft aneurysms: Infection, arterial wall failure, suture failure, graft failure

Adapted with permission from Rutherford, R. B. (1999). *Vascular surgery* (Vols. 1 and 2, 5th ed.). Philadelphia: W. B. Saunders.

THORACIC AORTIC ANEURYSM

Approximately 85% of all cases of thoracic aortic aneurysm are caused by atherosclerosis. They occur most frequently in men between the ages 40 and 70 years. The thoracic area is the most common site for a dissecting aneurysm. About one third of patients with thoracic aneurysms die of rupture of the aneurysm (Rutherford, 1999).

Clinical Manifestations

Symptoms are variable and depend on how rapidly the aneurysm dilates and how the pulsating mass affects surrounding intrathoracic structures. Some patients are asymptomatic. In most cases, pain is the most prominent symptom. The pain is usually constant and boring but may occur only when the person is supine.

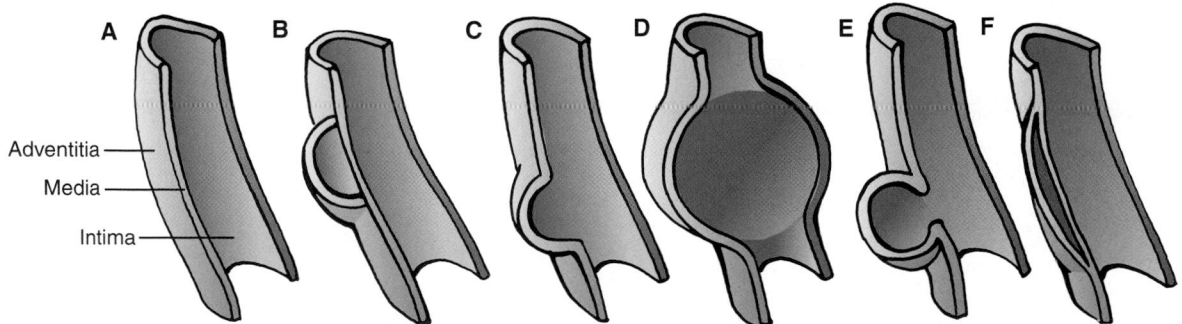

FIGURE 31-11 Characteristics of arterial aneurysm. (**A**) Normal artery. (**B**) False aneurysm—actually a pulsating hematoma. The clot and connective tissue are outside the arterial wall. (**C**) True aneurysm. One, two, or all three layers of the artery may be involved. (**D**) Fusiform aneurysm—symmetric, spindle-shaped expansion of entire circumference of involved vessel. (**E**) Saccular aneurysm—a bulbous protrusion of one side of the arterial wall. (**F**) Dissecting aneurysm—this usually is a hematoma that splits the layers of the arterial wall.

Other conspicuous symptoms are dyspnea, the result of pressure of the sac against the trachea, a main bronchus, or the lung itself; cough, frequently paroxysmal and with a brassy quality; hoarseness, stridor, or weakness or complete loss of the voice (aphonia), resulting from pressure against the left recurrent laryngeal nerve; and dysphagia (difficulty in swallowing) due to impingement on the esophagus by the aneurysm.

Assessment and Diagnostic Findings

When large veins in the chest are compressed by the aneurysm, the superficial veins of the chest, neck, or arms become dilated, and edematous areas on the chest wall and cyanosis are often evident. Pressure against the cervical sympathetic chain can result in unequal pupils. Diagnosis of a thoracic aortic aneurysm is principally made by chest x-ray, transesophageal echocardiography, and CT.

Medical Management

In most cases, an aneurysm is treated by surgical repair. General measures such as controlling blood pressure and correcting risk factors may be helpful. It is important to control blood pressure in patients with dissecting aneurysms. Systolic pressure is maintained at about 100 to 120 mm Hg with antihypertensive medications (eg, hydralazine hydrochloride [Hydralazine], esmolol hydrochloride [Brevibloc] or another beta-blocker such as atenolol [Tenormin] or timolol maleate [Timoptic]). Pulsatile flow is reduced by medications that reduce cardiac contractility (eg, pro-

pranolol [Inderal]). The goal of surgery is to repair the aneurysm and restore vascular continuity with a vascular graft (Fig. 31-12). Intensive monitoring is usually required after this type of surgery, and the patient is cared for in the critical care unit. Repair of thoracic aneurysms using endovascular grafts implanted (deployed) percutaneously in an interventional laboratory (eg, cardiac catheterization laboratory) may decrease postoperative recovery time and decrease complications compared with traditional surgical techniques.

ABDOMINAL AORTIC ANEURYSM

The most common cause of abdominal aortic aneurysm is atherosclerosis. The condition, which is more common among Caucasians, affects men four times more often than women and is most prevalent in elderly patients (Rutherford, 1999). Most of these aneurysms occur below the renal arteries (infrarenal aneurysms). Untreated, the eventual outcome may be rupture and death.

Pathophysiology

All aneurysms involve a damaged media layer of the vessel. This may be caused by congenital weakness, trauma, or disease. After an aneurysm develops, it tends to enlarge. Risk factors include genetic predisposition, smoking (or other tobacco use), and hypertension; more than one half of patients with aneurysms have hypertension.

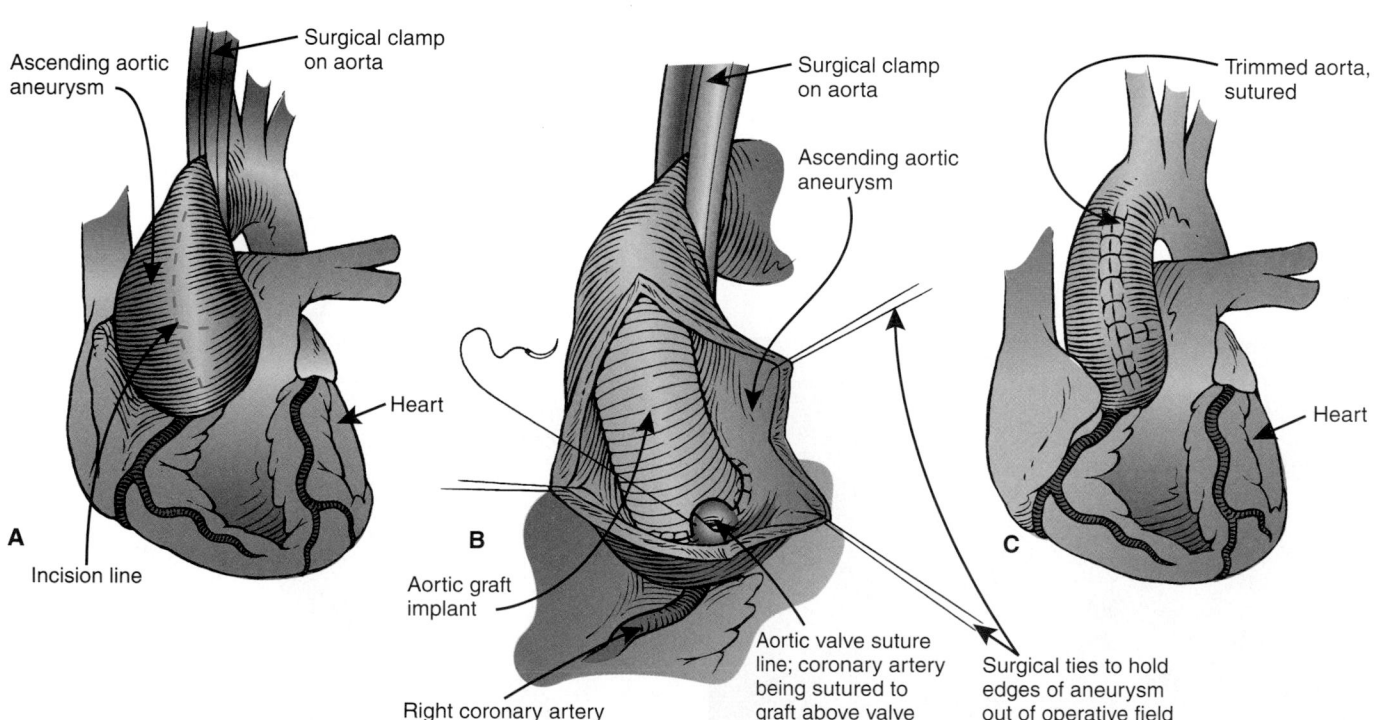

FIGURE 31-12 Repair of an ascending aortic aneurysm and aortic valve replacement. (**A**) Incision into aortic aneurysm. (**B**) Aortic valve replacement with aortic graft implant to repair ascending aortic aneurysm. (**C**) Aortic aneurysm trimmed and closed over graft.

Clinical Manifestations

About two fifths of patients with abdominal aortic aneurysms have symptoms; the remainder do not. Some patients complain that they can feel their heart beating in their abdomen when lying down, or they may say they feel an abdominal mass or abdominal throbbing. If the abdominal aortic aneurysm is associated with thrombus, a major vessel may be occluded or smaller distal occlusions may result from emboli. A small cholesterol, platelet, or fibrin emboli may lodge in the interosseous or digital arteries, causing blue toes.

Assessment and Diagnostic Findings

The most important diagnostic indication of an abdominal aortic aneurysm is a pulsatile mass in the middle and upper abdomen. About 80% of these aneurysms can be palpated. A systolic bruit may be heard over the mass. Duplex ultrasonography or CT is used to determine the size, length, and location of the aneurysm (Fig. 31-13). When the aneurysm is small, ultrasonography is conducted at 6-month intervals until the aneurysm reaches a size at which surgery to prevent rupture is of more benefit than the possible complications of a surgical procedure. Some aneurysms remain stable over many years of observation.

 ### Gerontologic Considerations

Most abdominal aneurysms occur in patients between the ages of 60 and 90 years. Rupture is likely with coexisting hypertension and with aneurysms wider than 6 cm. In most cases at this point, the chances of rupture are greater than the chance of death during surgical repair. If the elderly patient is considered at moderate risk for complications related to surgery or anesthesia, the aneurysm is not repaired until it is at least 5 cm (2 inches) wide.

Medical Management

An expanding or enlarging abdominal aneurysm is likely to rupture. Surgery is the treatment of choice for abdominal aneurysms wider than 5 cm (2 inches) wide or those that are enlarging.

SURGICAL MANAGEMENT

The standard treatment for abdominal aortic aneurysm repair has been open surgical repair of the aneurysm by resecting the vessel and sewing a bypass graft in place. The mortality rate associated with elective aneurysm repair, a major surgical procedure, is reported to be 1% to 4%. The prognosis for a patient with a ruptured aneurysm is poor, and surgery is performed immediately (Rutherford, 1999).

An alternative for treating an infrarenal abdominal aortic aneurysm is endovascular grafting. Endovascular grafting involves the transluminal placement and attachment of a sutureless aortic graft prosthesis across an aneurysm (Fig. 31-14). This procedure can be performed under local or regional anesthesia. Endovascular grafting of abdominal aortic aneurysms may be performed if the patient's abdominal aorta and iliac arteries are not extremely tortuous and if the aneurysm does not begin at the level of the renal arteries. Clinical trials are evaluating endograft treatment of abdominal aortic aneurysms at or above the level of the renal arteries and the thoracic aorta. Potential complications include bleeding, hematoma, or wound infection at the femoral insertion site; distal ischemia or embolization; dissection or perforation of the aorta; graft thrombosis; graft infection; break of the attachment system; graft migration; proximal or distal graft leaks; delayed rupture; and bowel ischemia.

Nursing Management

Before surgery, nursing assessment is guided by anticipating a rupture and by recognizing that the patient may have cardiovascular, cerebral, pulmonary, and renal impairment from atherosclerosis. The functional capacity of all organ systems should be assessed. Medical therapies designed to stabilize physiologic function should be promptly implemented.

Signs of impending rupture include severe back pain or abdominal pain, which may be persistent or intermittent and is often

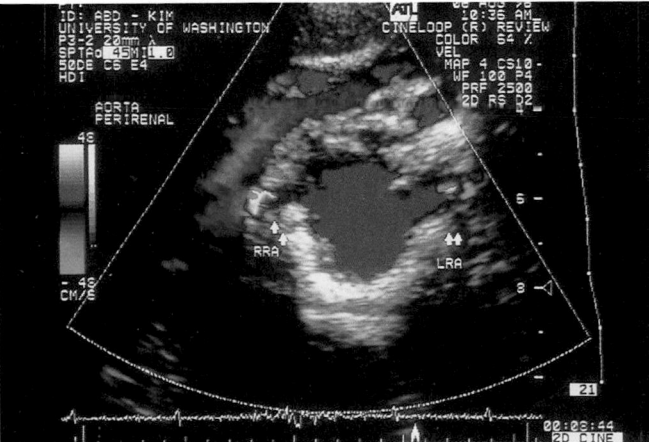

FIGURE 31-13 Duplex ultrasonic image of abdominal aortic aneurysm at the perirenal level. Cross-sectional image documents the location of right and left renal arteries.

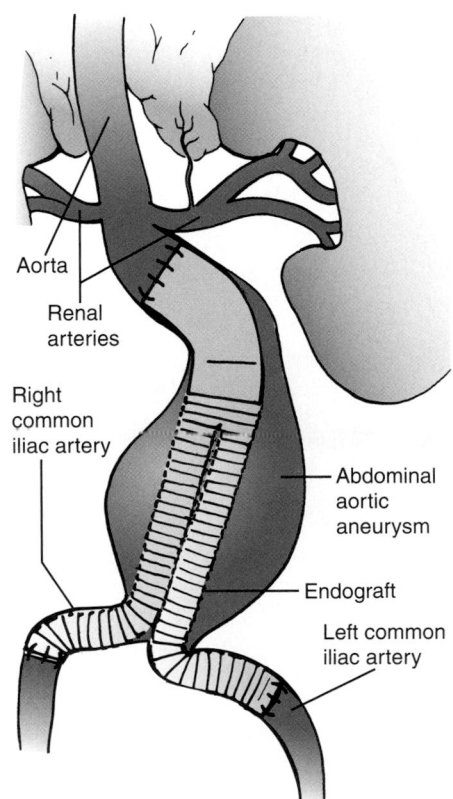

FIGURE 31-14 Ancure Endograft repair of an abdominal aortic aneurysm.

localized in the middle or lower abdomen to the left of the midline. Low back pain may also be present because of pressure of the aneurysm on the lumbar nerves. This is a serious symptom, usually indicating that the aneurysm is expanding rapidly and is about to rupture. Indications of a rupturing abdominal aortic aneurysm include constant, intense back pain; falling blood pressure; and decreasing hematocrit. Rupture into the peritoneal cavity is rapidly fatal. A retroperitoneal rupture of an aneurysm may result in hematomas in the scrotum, perineum, flank, or penis. Signs of heart failure or a loud bruit may suggest a rupture into the vena cava. Rupture into the vena cava results in the higher-pressure arterial blood entering the lower-pressure venous system and causing turbulence, which is heard as a bruit. The high blood pressure and increased blood volume returning to the right heart from the vena cava may cause the right heart to fail. The overall surgical mortality rate associated with a ruptured aneurysm is 50% to 75%.

Postoperative care requires intense monitoring of pulmonary, cardiovascular, renal, and neurologic status. Possible complications of surgery include arterial occlusion, hemorrhage, infection, ischemic bowel, renal failure, and impotence.

DISSECTING AORTA

Occasionally, in an aorta diseased by arteriosclerosis, a tear develops in the intima or the media degenerates, resulting in a dissection (see Fig. 31-11).

Pathophysiology

Arterial dissections (separations) are commonly associated with poorly controlled hypertension; they are three times more common in men than in women and occur most commonly in the 50- to 70-year-old age group (Rutherford, 1999). Dissection is caused by rupture in the intimal layer. A rupture may occur through adventitia or into the lumen through the intima, allowing blood to reenter the main channel and resulting in chronic dissection or occlusion of branches of the aorta.

As the separation progresses, the arteries branching from the involved area of the aorta shear and occlude. The tear occurs most commonly in the region of the aortic arch, with the highest mortality rate associated with ascending aortic dissection. The dissection of the aorta may progress backward in the direction of the heart, obstructing the openings to the coronary arteries or producing hemopericardium (effusion of blood into the pericardial sac) or aortic insufficiency, or it may extend in the opposite direction, causing occlusion of the arteries supplying the gastrointestinal tract, kidneys, spinal cord, and legs.

Clinical Manifestations

Onset of symptoms is usually sudden. Severe and persistent pain, described as tearing or ripping, may be reported. The pain is in the anterior chest or back and extends to shoulders, epigastric area, or abdomen. Aortic dissection may be mistaken for an acute myocardial infarction, which could confuse the clinical picture and initial treatment. Cardiovascular, neurologic, and gastrointestinal symptoms are responsible for other clinical manifestations, depending on the location and extent of the dissection. The patient may appear pale. Sweating and tachycardia may be detected. Blood pressure may be elevated or markedly different from one arm to the other if dissection involves the orifice of the subclavian artery on one side. Because of the variable clinical picture associated with this condition, early diagnosis is usually difficult.

Assessment and Diagnostic Findings

Arteriography, CT, transesophageal echocardiography, duplex ultrasonography, and magnetic resonance imaging aid in the diagnosis.

Medical Management

Medical or surgical treatment of a dissecting aneurysm depends on the type of dissection present and follows the general principles outlined for the treatment of thoracic aortic aneurysms.

Nursing Management

A patient with a dissecting aorta requires the same nursing care as a patient with an aortic aneurysm requiring surgical intervention, as described earlier in this chapter. Interventions described in the Plan of Nursing Care are also appropriate.

OTHER ANEURYSMS

Aneurysms may also arise in the peripheral vessels, most often as a result of atherosclerosis. These may involve such vessels as the subclavian artery, renal artery, femoral artery, or (most frequently) popliteal artery. Between 50% and 60% of popliteal aneurysms are bilateral and may be associated with abdominal aortic aneurysms.

The aneurysm produces a pulsating mass and disturbs peripheral circulation distal to it. Pain and swelling develop because of pressure on adjacent nerves and veins. Diagnosis is made by duplex ultrasonography and CT to determine the size, length, and extent of the aneurysm. Arteriography may be performed to evaluate the level of proximal and distal involvement.

Surgical repair is performed with replacement grafts or endovascular repair using a stent-graft or wall graft, which is a Dacron or PTFE (polytetrafluoroethylene) graft with external structures made from a variety of materials (nitinol, titanium, stainless steel) for additional support.

Nursing Management

The patient who has had an endovascular repair must lie supine for 6 hours; the head of the bed may be elevated up to 45 degrees after 2 hours. The patient needs to use a bedpan or urinal while on bed rest, or a Foley catheter may be used. Vital signs and Doppler assessment of peripheral pulses are performed every 15 minutes for four times, then every 30 minutes for four times, then every hour for four times, and then as directed by the physician or unit standards. The catheterization site is assessed when vital signs and pulses are monitored. The nurse assesses for bleeding, swelling, pain, and hematoma formation. Any changes in vital signs, pulse quality, bleeding, swelling, pain, or hematoma are reported to the physician. The physician is also notified of persistent coughing, sneezing, vomiting, or systolic blood pressure above 180 mm Hg because of the increased risk for hemorrhage. Most patients are able to resume their preprocedure diet and are encouraged to drink fluids. An intravenous infusion may be continued until the patient is able to drink normally. Fluids are important to maintain blood flow through the arterial repair site and to assist the kidneys with excreting intravenous contrast agent and other medications used during the procedure. Six hours after the procedure, the patient may be able to roll side to side and may be able to ambulate with assistance to the bathroom. After the patient is able to take adequate fluids orally, the intravenous infusion may be discontinued and the intravenous access converted to a saline lock.

ARTERIAL EMBOLISM AND ARTERIAL THROMBOSIS

Acute vascular occlusion may be caused by an embolus or acute thrombosis. Acute arterial occlusions may result from iatrogenic injury, which can occur during insertion of invasive catheters such as those used for arteriography, PTA or stent placement, or an intra-aortic balloon pump. Other causes include trauma from a fracture, crush injury, and penetrating wounds that disrupt the arterial intima. The accurate diagnosis of an arterial occlusion as embolic or thrombotic in origin is necessary to initiate appropriate treatment.

Pathophysiology

Arterial emboli arise most commonly from thrombi that develop in the chambers of the heart as a result of atrial fibrillation, myocardial infarction, infective endocarditis, or chronic heart failure. These thrombi become detached and are carried from the left side of the heart into the arterial system, where they lodge in and obstruct an artery that is smaller than the embolus. Emboli may also develop in advanced aortic atherosclerosis because the atheromatous plaques ulcerate or become rough. Acute thrombosis frequently occurs in patients with preexisting ischemic symptoms.

Clinical Manifestations

The symptoms of arterial emboli depend primarily on the size of the embolus, the organ involved, and the state of the collateral vessels. The immediate effect is cessation of distal blood flow. The blockage can progress above and below the obstruction. Secondary vasospasm can contribute to the ischemia. The embolus can fragment or break apart, resulting in occlusion of distal vessels. Emboli tend to lodge at arterial bifurcations and areas narrowed by atherosclerosis. Cerebral, mesenteric, renal, and coronary arteries are often involved in addition to the large arteries of the extremities.

The symptoms of acute arterial embolism in extremities with poor collateral flow are acute, severe pain and a gradual loss of sensory and motor function. The six *P*s associated with acute arterial embolism are pain, pallor, pulselessness, paresthesia, poikilothermia (coldness), and paralysis. Eventually, superficial veins may collapse because of decreased blood flow to the extremity. The part of the extremity below the occlusion is markedly colder and paler than the part above the occlusion because of ischemia.

Arterial thrombosis can also acutely occlude an artery. A thrombosis is a slowly developing clot that usually occurs where the arterial wall has become damaged, generally as a result of atherosclerosis. Thrombi may also develop in an arterial aneurysm. The manifestations of an acute thrombotic arterial occlusion are similar to those described for embolic occlusion. However, treatment is more difficult with a thrombus because the arterial occlusion has occurred in a degenerated vessel and requires more extensive reconstructive surgery to restore flow than is required with an embolic event.

Assessment and Diagnostic Findings

An arterial embolus is usually diagnosed on the basis of the sudden nature of the onset of symptoms and an apparent source for the embolus. Two-dimensional echocardiography or transesophageal echocardiography, chest x-ray, and electrocardiography may reveal underlying cardiac disease. Noninvasive duplex and Doppler ultrasonography can determine the presence and extent of underlying atherosclerosis, and arteriography may be performed.

Medical Management

Management of arterial thrombosis depends on its cause. Management of acute embolic occlusion usually requires surgery because time is of the essence. Because the onset of the event is acute, collateral circulation has not developed, and the patient quickly moves through the list of six *P*s to paralysis, which is the most advanced stage. Heparin therapy is initiated immediately to prevent further development of emboli and to hamper the extension of existing thrombi. Typically, an initial bolus of 5,000 to 10,000 units is administered intravenously, followed by a continuous infusion of 1,000 units per hour until the patient is able to undergo surgery.

SURGICAL MANAGEMENT

Emergency embolectomy is the procedure of choice only if the involved extremity is viable (Fig. 31-15). Arterial emboli are usually treated by insertion of an embolectomy catheter. The catheter is passed through a groin incision into the affected artery and advanced past the occlusion. The balloon is inflated with sterile saline solution, and the thrombus is extracted as the catheter is withdrawn. This procedure involves incising the vessel and removing the clot.

PHARMACOLOGIC THERAPY

When the patient has collateral circulation, treatment may include intravenous anticoagulation with heparin, which can prevent the thrombus from spreading and reduce muscle necrosis. The use of intra-arterial thrombolytic medications helps to dissolve the embolus. Fibrin-specific thrombolytic medications (eg, tissue plasminogen activator [t-PA, alteplase, Activase] and single-chain urokinase-type plasminogen activator [scu-PA, pro-urokinase]) avoid systemic depletion of circulating fibrinogen and plasminogen, which prevents the development of systemic fibrinolysis.

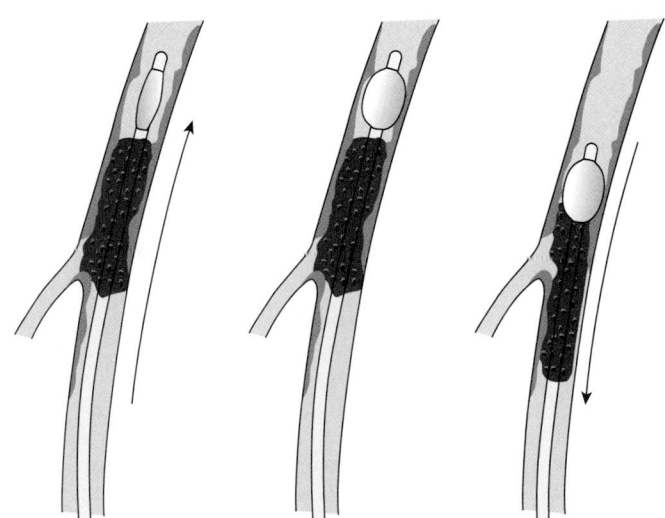

FIGURE 31-15 Extraction of an embolus by balloon-tipped embolectomy catheter. The deflated balloon-tipped catheter is advanced past the embolus, inflated and then gently withdrawn, carrying the embolic material with it. Adapted with permission from Rutherford, R. B. (1999). *Vascular surgery: Vol. 1 and 2* (5th ed.). Philadelphia: W. B. Saunders.

Other thrombolytic medications are reteplase (r-PA, Retavase), tenecteplase (TNKase), and staphylokinase (Moore, 2002). Although these agents differ in their pharmacokinetics, they are administered in a similar manner. A catheter is advanced under x-ray visualization to the clot, and the thrombolytic agent is infused.

Thrombolytic therapy should not be used when there are known contraindications to therapy or when the extremity cannot tolerate the several additional hours of ischemia that it takes for the agent to lyse (disintegrate) the clot. Contraindications to thrombolytic therapy include active internal bleeding, CVA (brain attack, stroke), recent major surgery, uncontrolled hypertension, and pregnancy.

Nursing Management

Before surgery, the patient remains on bed rest with the extremity level or slightly dependent (15 degrees). The affected part is kept at room temperature and protected from trauma. Heating and cooling pads are contraindicated because ischemic extremities are easily traumatized by alterations in temperature. If possible, tape and electrocardiogram electrodes should not be used on the extremity; sheepskin and foot cradles are used to protect the leg from mechanical trauma.

If the patient is treated with thrombolytic therapy, she or he is accurately weighed in kilograms, and the dose of thrombolytic therapy is determined based on the patient's weight. The patient is admitted to a critical care unit for continuous monitoring. Vital signs are taken every 15 minutes for 2 hours, then every 30 minutes for the next 6 hours, and then every hour for 16 hours. Bleeding is the most common side effect of thrombolytic therapy, and the patient is closely monitored for any signs of bleeding. The nurse also minimizes the number of punctures for inserting intravenous lines, avoids intramuscular injections, prevents any possible tissue trauma, and applies pressure at least twice as long as usual after any puncture that is performed. If t-PA is used for the treatment, heparin is usually administered to prevent another thrombus from forming at the site of the lesion. The t-PA activates plasminogen on the thrombus more than circulating plasminogen, but it does not decrease the clotting factors as much as other thrombolytic therapies, so patients receiving t-PA are able to make new thrombi more easily than with some of the other thrombolytics.

During the postoperative period, the nurse collaborates with the surgeon about the patient's appropriate activity level based on the patient's condition. Generally, every effort is made to encourage the patient to move the leg to stimulate circulation and prevent stasis. Anticoagulant therapy may be continued after surgery to prevent thrombosis of the affected artery and to diminish the development of subsequent thrombi at the initiating site. The nurse assesses for evidence of local and systemic hemorrhage, including mental status changes, which can occur when anticoagulants are administered. Pulses, Doppler signals, ABI, and motor and sensory function are assessed every hour for the first 24 hours, because significant changes may indicate reocclusion. Metabolic abnormalities, renal failure, and compartment syndrome may be complications after an acute arterial occlusion.

RAYNAUD'S DISEASE

Raynaud's disease is a form of intermittent arteriolar vasoconstriction that results in coldness, pain, and pallor of the fingertips or toes. The cause is unknown, although many patients with the disease seem to have immunologic disorders. Symptoms may result from a defect in basal heat production that eventually decreases the ability of cutaneous vessels to dilate. Episodes may be triggered by emotional factors or by unusual sensitivity to cold. The disease is most common in women between 16 and 40 years of age, and it occurs more frequently in cold climates and during the winter.

The term *Raynaud's phenomenon* is used to refer to localized, intermittent episodes of vasoconstriction of small arteries of the feet and hands that cause color and temperature changes. Generally unilateral and affecting only one or two digits, the phenomenon is always associated with underlying systemic disease. It may occur with scleroderma, systemic lupus erythematosus, rheumatoid arthritis, obstructive arterial disease, or trauma.

The prognosis for Raynaud's disease varies; some patients slowly improve, some become progressively worse, and others show no change. Ulceration and gangrene are rare; however, chronic disease may cause atrophy of the skin and muscles. With appropriate patient teaching and lifestyle modifications, the disorder is generally benign and self-limiting.

Clinical Manifestations

The classic clinical picture reveals pallor brought on by sudden vasoconstriction. The skin then becomes bluish (cyanotic) due to pooling of deoxygenated blood during vasospasm. As a result of exaggerated reflow (hyperemia) due to vasodilation, a red color is produced (rubor) when oxygenated blood returns to the digits after the vasospasm stops. The characteristic sequence of color change of Raynaud's phenomenon is described as white, blue, and red. Numbness, tingling, and burning pain occur as the color changes. The involvement tends to be bilateral and symmetric.

Medical Management

Avoiding the particular stimuli (eg, cold, tobacco) that provoke vasoconstriction is a primary factor in controlling Raynaud's disease. Calcium channel blockers may be effective in relieving symptoms. Studies indicate that nifedipine (Procardia, Adalat) is an effective calcium channel blocker for treating an acute episode of vasospasm (Kaufman et al., 1996). Sympathectomy (interrupting the sympathetic nerves by removing the sympathetic ganglia or dividing their branches) may help some patients.

Nursing Management

The nurse teaches patients to avoid situations that may be stressful or unsafe. Stress management classes may be helpful. Exposure to cold must be minimized, and in areas where the fall and winter months are cold, the patient should remain indoors as much as possible and wear layers of clothing when outdoors. Hats and mittens or gloves should be worn at all times when outside. Fabrics specially designed for cold climates (eg, Thinsulate) are recommended. Patients should warm up their vehicles before getting in so that they can avoid touching a cold steering wheel or door handle, which could elicit an attack. During summer, a sweater should be available when entering air-conditioned rooms.

Concerns about serious complications, such as gangrene and amputation, are common among patients. However, these consequences are uncommon. Patients should avoid all forms of nicotine; the nicotine gum or patches used to help people quit smoking may induce attacks.

Patients should be careful about safety. Sharp objects should be handled carefully to avoid injuring the fingers. Patients should be informed about the postural hypotension that may result from medications, such as calcium channel blockers, used to treat Raynaud's disease. The nurse also discusses safety precautions related to alcohol, exercise, and hot weather.

Management of Venous Disorders

VENOUS THROMBOSIS, DEEP VEIN THROMBOSIS (DVT), THROMBOPHLEBITIS, AND PHLEBOTHROMBOSIS

Although the terms *venous thrombosis, deep vein thrombosis (DVT), thrombophlebitis,* and *phlebothrombosis* do not necessarily reflect identical disease processes, for clinical purposes, they are often used interchangeably.

Pathophysiology

Superficial veins, such as the greater saphenous, lesser saphenous, cephalic, basilic, and external jugular veins, are thick-walled muscular structures that lie just under the skin. Deep veins are thin walled and have less muscle in the media. They run parallel to arteries and bear the same names as the arteries. Deep and superficial veins have valves that permit unidirectional flow back to the heart. The valves lie at the base of a segment of the vein that is expanded into a sinus. This arrangement permits the valves to open without coming into contact with the wall of the vein, permitting rapid closure when the blood starts to flow backward. Other kinds of veins are known as perforating veins. These vessels have valves that allow one-way blood flow from the superficial system to the deep system.

Although the exact cause of venous thrombosis remains unclear, three factors, known as Virchow's triad, are believed to play a significant role in its development: stasis of blood (venous stasis), vessel wall injury, and altered blood coagulation (Chart 31-6). At least two of the factors seem to be necessary for thrombosis to occur. Venous stasis occurs when blood flow is reduced, as in heart failure or shock; when veins are dilated, as with some medication therapies; and when skeletal muscle contraction is reduced, as in immobility, paralysis of the extremities, or anesthesia. Moreover, bed rest reduces blood flow in the legs by at least 50%. Damage to the intimal lining of blood vessels creates a site for clot formation. Direct trauma to the vessels, as with fractures or dislocation, diseases of the veins, and chemical irritation of the vein from intravenous medications or solutions, can damage veins. Increased blood coagulability occurs most commonly in patients who have been abruptly withdrawn from anticoagulant medications. Oral contraceptive use and several blood dyscrasias (abnormalities) also can lead to hypercoagulability.

Formation of a thrombus frequently accompanies thrombophlebitis, which is an inflammation of the vein walls. When a thrombus develops initially in the veins as a result of stasis or hypercoagulability but without inflammation, the process is referred to as phlebothrombosis. Venous thrombosis can occur in any vein but occurs more in the veins of the lower extremities. The superficial and deep veins of the extremities may be affected.

Upper extremity venous thrombosis is not as common as lower extremity thrombosis. However, upper extremity venous thrombosis is more common in patients with intravenous catheters or in patients with an underlying disease that causes hypercoagulability. Internal trauma to the vessels may result from pacemaker leads, chemotherapy ports, dialysis catheters, or parenteral nutri-

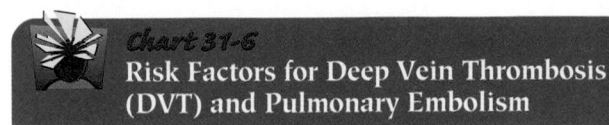

Chart 31-6

Risk Factors for Deep Vein Thrombosis (DVT) and Pulmonary Embolism

Endothelial damage
  Trauma
  Surgery
  Pacing wires
  Central venous catheters
  Dialysis access catheters
  Local vein damage
  Repetitive motion injury
Venous stasis
  Bed rest or immobilization
  Obesity
  History of varicosities
  Spinal cord injury
  Age (>65 yr)
Coagulopathy
Cancer
Pregnancy
Oral contraceptive use
Presence of congenital proteins C and S
Presence of anticardiolipin antibody
Antithrombin III deficiency
Polycythemia
Septicemia

tion lines. The lumen of the vein may be decreased as a result of the catheter or from external compression, such as by neoplasms or an extra cervical rib. Effort thrombosis of the upper extremity is caused by repetitive motion, such as experienced by competitive swimmers, tennis players, and construction workers, that irritates the vessel wall, causing inflammation and subsequent thrombosis.

Venous thrombi are aggregates of platelets attached to the vein wall, along with a tail-like appendage containing fibrin, white blood cells, and many red blood cells. The "tail" can grow or can propagate in the direction of blood flow as successive layers of the thrombus form. A propagating venous thrombosis is dangerous because parts of the thrombus can break off and produce an embolic occlusion of the pulmonary blood vessels. Fragmentation of the thrombus can occur spontaneously as it dissolves naturally, or it can occur in association with an elevation in venous pressure, as occurs when a person stands suddenly or engages in muscular activity after prolonged inactivity. After an episode of acute deep vein thrombosis, recanalization of the lumen typically occurs. The time required for complete recanalization is an important determinant of venous valvular incompetence, which is one complication of venous thrombosis (Meissner et al., 2000). Other complications of venous thrombosis are listed in Chart 31-7.

Clinical Manifestations

A major problem associated with recognizing deep vein thrombosis is that the signs and symptoms are nonspecific. The exception is phlegmasia cerulea dolens (massive iliofemoral venous thrombosis), in which the entire extremity becomes massively swollen, tense, painful, and cool to the touch. Despite this variability, clinical signs should always be investigated.

DEEP VEINS

With obstruction of the deep veins comes edema and swelling of the extremity because the outflow of venous blood is inhibited.

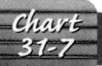

The amount of swelling can be determined by measuring the circumference of the affected extremity at various levels with a tape measure and comparing one extremity with the other at the same level to determine size differences. If both extremities are swollen, a size difference may be difficult to detect. The affected extremity may feel warmer than the unaffected extremity, and the superficial veins may appear more prominent.

Tenderness, which usually occurs later, is produced by inflammation of the vein wall and can be detected by gently palpating the affected extremity. Homans' sign (pain in the calf after the foot is sharply dorsiflexed) is not specific for deep vein thrombosis because it can be elicited in any painful condition of the calf. In some cases, signs of a pulmonary embolus are the first indication of deep vein thrombosis.

SUPERFICIAL VEINS

Thrombosis of superficial veins produces pain or tenderness, redness, and warmth in the involved area. The risk of the superficial venous thrombi becoming dislodged or fragmenting into emboli is very low because most of them dissolve spontaneously. This condition can be treated at home with bed rest, elevation of the leg, analgesics, and possibly anti-inflammatory medication.

Assessment and Diagnostic Findings

Careful assessment is invaluable in detecting early signs of venous disorders of the lower extremities. Patients with a history of varicose veins, hypercoagulation, neoplastic disease, cardiovascular disease, or recent major surgery or injury are at high risk. Other patients at high risk include those who are obese or elderly and women taking oral contraceptives.

When performing the nursing assessment, key concerns include limb pain, a feeling of heaviness, functional impairment, ankle engorgement, and edema; differences in leg circumference bilaterally from thigh to ankle; increase in the surface temperature of the leg, particularly the calf or ankle; and areas of tenderness or superficial thrombosis (ie, cordlike venous segment). Homans' sign (pain in the calf as the foot is sharply dorsiflexed) has been used historically to assess for DVT. It is not a reliable or valid sign for DVT and has no clinical value in the assessment of a patient for DVT.

Prevention

Venous thrombosis, thrombophlebitis, and DVT can be prevented, especially if patients who are considered at high risk are identified and preventive measures are instituted without delay.

Preventive measures include the application of elastic compression stockings, the use of intermittent pneumatic compression devices, and special body positioning and exercise (discussed later in the section on nursing management). A further method to prevent venous thrombosis in surgical patients is administration of subcutaneous unfractionated or low molecular weight heparin.

Medical Management

The objectives of treatment for deep vein thrombosis are to prevent the thrombus from growing and fragmenting (risking pulmonary embolism) and to prevent recurrent thromboemboli. Anticoagulant therapy (administration of a medication to delay the clotting time of blood, prevent the formation of a thrombus in postoperative patients, and forestall the extension of a thrombus after it has formed) can meet these objectives, although anticoagulants cannot dissolve a thrombus that has already formed.

ANTICOAGULATION THERAPY

Measures for preventing or reducing blood clotting within the vascular system are indicated in patients with thrombophlebitis, recurrent embolus formation, and persistent leg edema from heart failure. They are also indicated in elderly patients with a hip fracture that may result in lengthy immobilization.

Unfractionated Heparin. Unfractionated heparin (heparin) is administered subcutaneously to prevent development of deep vein thrombosis, or by intermittent intravenous infusion or continuous infusion for 5 to 7 days to prevent the extension of a thrombus and the development of new thrombi. Oral anticoagulants, such as warfarin (Coumadin), are administered with heparin therapy. Medication dosage is regulated by monitoring the partial thromboplastin time, the **international normalized ratio** (INR), and the platelet count.

Low-Molecular-Weight Heparin. Subcutaneous low-molecular-weight heparin (LMWH) is an effective treatment for some cases of deep vein thrombosis. It has a longer half-life than unfractionated heparin, so doses can be given in one or two subcutaneous injections each day. Doses are adjusted according to weight. LMWH prevents the extension of a thrombus and development of new thrombi and is associated with fewer bleeding complications than unfractionated heparin. Because there are several preparations, the dosing schedule must be based on the product used and the protocol at each institution. The cost is higher than for unfractionated heparin; however, LMWH may be used safely in pregnant women, and the patients may be more mobile and have an improved quality of life.

Thrombolytic Therapy. Unlike the heparins, thrombolytic (fibrinolytic) therapy causes the thrombus to lyse and dissolve in 50% of patients. Thrombolytic therapy (eg, tissue plasminogen activator [t-PA, alteplase, Activase], reteplase [r-PA, Retavase], tenecteplase [TNKase], staphylokinase, urokinase, streptokinase) is given within the first 3 days after acute thrombosis. Therapy initiated beyond 5 days after the onset of symptoms is significantly less effective (Moore, 2002). The advantages of thrombolytic therapy include less long-term damage to the venous valves and a reduced incidence of postthrombotic syndrome and chronic venous insufficiency. However, thrombolytic therapy results in approximately a threefold greater incidence of bleeding than heparin. If bleeding occurs and cannot be stopped, the thrombolytic agent is discontinued.

SURGICAL MANAGEMENT

Surgery is necessary for deep vein thrombosis when anticoagulant or thrombolytic therapy is contraindicated (Chart 31-8), the danger of pulmonary embolism is extreme, or the venous drainage is so severely compromised that permanent damage to the extremity will probably result. A thrombectomy (removal of the thrombosis) is the procedure of choice. A vena cava filter may be placed at the time of the thrombectomy; this filter traps large emboli and prevents pulmonary emboli (see Chap. 23).

Nursing Management

If the patient is receiving anticoagulant therapy, the nurse must frequently monitor the partial thromboplastin time, prothrombin time, hemoglobin and hematocrit values, platelet count, and fibrinogen level. Close observation is also required to detect bleeding; if bleeding occurs, it must be reported immediately and anticoagulant therapy discontinued.

ASSESSING AND MONITORING ANTICOAGULANT THERAPY

To prevent inadvertent infusion of large volumes of heparin, which could cause hemorrhage, continuous intravenous infusion by electronic infusion device is the preferred method of administering unfractionated heparin. Dosage calculations are based on the patient's weight, and any possible bleeding tendencies are detected by a pretreatment clotting profile. If renal insufficiency exists, lower doses of heparin are required. Periodic coagulation tests and hematocrit levels are obtained. Heparin is in the effective, or therapeutic, range when the partial thromboplastin time is 1.5 times the control.

Intermittent intravenous injection is another means of administering heparin; a dilute solution of heparin is administered every 4 hours. Administration may be facilitated by using a heparin lock, an intravenous catheter or a small, butterfly-type scalp vein needle with an injection site at the end of the tubing.

Oral anticoagulants, such as warfarin, are monitored by the prothrombin time or INR. Because their effect is delayed for 3 to 5 days, they are usually administered with heparin until desired anticoagulation has been achieved (ie, when the prothrombin time is 1.5 to 2 times normal or the INR is 2.0 to 3.0).

MONITORING AND MANAGING POTENTIAL COMPLICATIONS

Bleeding. The principal complication of anticoagulant therapy is spontaneous bleeding anywhere in the body. Bleeding from the kidneys is detected by microscopic examination of the urine and is often the first sign of anticoagulant toxicity from excessive dosage. Bruises, nosebleeds, and bleeding gums are also early signs. To reverse the effects of heparin promptly, intravenous injections of protamine sulfate may be administered. Reversing the effects of warfarin, a coumarin derivative, is more difficult, but effective measures that may be prescribed include vitamin K and possibly transfusion of fresh frozen plasma.

Thrombocytopenia. Another complication of therapy may be heparin-induced thrombocytopenia (decrease in platelets), which may develop in patients who receive heparin for more than 5 days or on readministration after a brief interruption of heparin therapy. Beginning warfarin concomitantly with heparin can provide a stable INR or prothrombin time by day 5 of heparin treatment.

The use of LMWH is less frequently associated with heparin-induced thrombocytopenia. The thrombocytopenia is thought to result from an immunologic mechanism that causes aggregation of platelets. This serious complication results in thromboembolic manifestations, and the prognosis is extremely guarded.

Prevention of thrombocytopenia depends on regular monitoring of platelet counts. Early signs of thrombocytopenia are a falling platelet count to less than 100,000/mL, a decrease in platelet count exceeding 25% at one time, the need for increasing doses of heparin to maintain the therapeutic level, thromboembolic or hemorrhagic complications, and a history of heparin sensitivity (Stevens, 2000). If thrombocytopenia does occur, platelet aggregation studies are conducted, the heparin is discontinued, and protamine sulfate is administered to reverse heparin's effects.

Drug Interactions. Because oral anticoagulants interact with many other medications and herbal and nutritional supplements, close monitoring of the patient's medication schedule is necessary. Medications and supplements that potentiate oral anticoagulants include salicylates, anabolic steroids, chloral hydrate, glucagon, chloramphenicol, neomycin, quinidine, phenylbutazone (Butazolidin), coenzyme Q10, dong quai, garlic, gingko, ginseng, green tea, and vitamin E; those that decrease the anticoagulant effect include phenytoin, barbiturates, diuretics, estrogen, and vitamin C. It is advisable to identify medication interactions for patients taking specific oral anticoagulants. Contraindications to anticoagulant therapy are summarized in Chart 31-8.

PROVIDING COMFORT

Bed rest, elevation of the affected extremity, elastic compression stockings, and analgesics for pain relief are adjuncts to therapy. They help to improve circulation and increase comfort. Depending on the extent and location of a venous thrombosis, bed rest may be required for 5 to 7 days after diagnosis. This is approximately the time necessary for the thrombus to adhere to the vein wall, preventing embolization.

Warm, moist packs applied to the affected extremity reduce the discomfort associated with deep vein thrombosis, as do mild analgesics prescribed for pain control. When the patient begins to ambulate, elastic compression stockings are used. Walking is

---

Chart 31-8 • PHARMACOLOGY
Contraindications to Anticoagulation Therapy

Lack of patient cooperation
Bleeding from the following systems:
  Gastrointestinal
  Genitourinary
  Respiratory
  Reproductive
Hemorrhagic blood dyscrasias
Aneurysms
Severe trauma
Alcoholism
Recent or impending surgery of:
  Eye
  Spinal cord
  Brain
Severe hepatic or renal disease
Recent cerebrovascular hemorrhage
Infections
Open ulcerative wounds
Occupations that involve a significant hazard for injury
Recent delivery of a baby

better than standing or sitting for long periods. Bed exercises, such as dorsiflexion of the foot, are also recommended.

APPLYING ELASTIC COMPRESSION STOCKINGS

Elastic compression stockings usually are prescribed for patients with venous insufficiency. These stockings exert a sustained, evenly distributed pressure over the entire surface of the calves, reducing the caliber of the superficial veins in the legs and resulting in increased flow in the deeper veins. The stockings may be knee-high, thigh-high, or panty hose. Thigh-high stockings are difficult for the patient to wear, because they have a tendency to roll down. The roll of the stocking further restricts blood flow rather than the stocking providing evenly distributed pressure over the thigh.

> **NURSING ALERT** Any type of stocking, including the elastic type, can inadvertently become a tourniquet if applied incorrectly (ie, rolled tightly at the top). In such instances, the stockings produce stasis rather than prevent it. For ambulatory patients, elastic compression stockings are removed at night and reapplied before the legs are lowered from the bed to the floor in the morning.

When the stockings are off, the skin is inspected for signs of irritation, and the calves are examined for possible tenderness. Any skin changes or signs of tenderness are reported. Stockings are contraindicated in patients with severe pitting edema because they can produce severe pitting at the knee.

Gerontologic Considerations

Because of decreased strength and manual dexterity, elderly patients may be unable to apply elastic compression stockings properly. If such is the case, a family member or friend should be taught to assist the patient to apply the stockings so that they do not cause undue pressure on any part of the feet or legs.

USING INTERMITTENT PNEUMATIC COMPRESSION DEVICES

These devices can be used with elastic compression stockings to prevent deep vein thrombosis. They consist of an electric controller that is attached by air hoses to plastic knee-high or thigh-high sleeves. The leg sleeves are divided into compartments, which sequentially fill to apply pressure to the ankle, calf, and thigh at 35 to 55 mm Hg of pressure. These devices can increase blood velocity beyond that produced by the stockings. Nursing measures include ensuring that prescribed pressures are not exceeded and assessing for patient comfort.

POSITIONING THE BODY AND ENCOURAGING EXERCISE

When the patient is on bed rest, the feet and lower legs should be elevated periodically above the level of the heart. This position allows the superficial and tibial veins to empty rapidly and to remain collapsed. Active and passive leg exercises, particularly those involving calf muscles, should be performed to increase venous flow. Early ambulation is most effective in preventing venous stasis. Deep-breathing exercises are beneficial because they produce increased negative pressure in the thorax, which assists in emptying the large veins. Once ambulatory, patients are instructed to avoid sitting for more than 2 hours at a time. The goal is to walk at least 10 minutes every 1 to 2 hours. Patients are also instructed to perform active and passive leg exercises when they are not able to ambulate as frequently as necessary, such as during long car, train, and plane trips.

PROMOTING HOME AND COMMUNITY-BASED CARE

In addition to teaching the patient how to apply elastic compression stockings and explaining the importance of elevating the legs and exercising adequately, the nurse teaches about the medication, its purpose, and the need to take the correct amount at the specific times prescribed (Chart 31-9). The patient should also be aware that blood tests are scheduled periodically to determine whether a change in medication or dosage is required. If the patient fails to adhere to the therapeutic regimen, continuation of the medication therapy should be questioned. A person who refuses to discontinue the use of alcohol should not receive anticoagulants because chronic alcohol use decreases their effectiveness. In patients with liver problems, the potential for bleeding may be exacerbated by anticoagulant therapy.

CHRONIC VENOUS INSUFFICIENCY

Venous insufficiency results from obstruction of the venous valves in the legs or a reflux of blood back through the valves. Superficial and deep leg veins can be involved. Resultant venous hypertension can occur whenever there has been a prolonged increase in venous pressure, such as occurs with deep venous thrombosis. Because the walls of veins are thinner and more elastic than

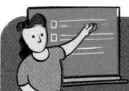

Chart 31-9 • PATIENT EDUCATION
Taking Anticoagulant Medications

- Take the anticoagulant at the same time each day, usually between 8:00 and 9:00 AM.
- Wear or carry identification indicating the anticoagulant being taken.
- Keep all appointments for blood tests.
- Because other medications affect the action of the anticoagulant, do not take any of the following medications or supplements without consulting with the primary health care provider: vitamins, cold medicines, antibiotics, aspirin, mineral oil, and anti-inflammatory agents, such as ibuprofen (Motrin) and similar medications or herbal or nutritional supplements. The primary health care provider should be contacted before taking any over-the-counter drugs.
- Avoid alcohol, because it may change the body's response to an anticoagulant.
- Avoid food fads, crash diets, or marked changes in eating habits.
- Do not take warfarin (Coumadin) unless directed.
- Do not stop taking Coumadin (when prescribed) unless directed.
- When seeking treatment from physician, a dentist, a podiatrist, or another health care provider, be sure to inform the caregiver that you are taking an anticoagulant.
- Contact your primary health care provider before having dental work or elective surgery.
- If any of the following signs appear, report them immediately to the primary health care provider:
  Faintness, dizziness, or increased weakness
  Severe headaches or abdominal pain
  Reddish or brownish urine
  Any bleeding—for example, cuts that do not stop bleeding
  Bruises that enlarge, nosebleeds, or unusual bleeding from any part of the body
  Red or black bowel movements
  Rash
- Avoid injury that can cause bleeding.
- For women: Notify the primary health care provider if you suspect pregnancy.

the walls of arteries, they distend readily when venous pressure is consistently elevated. In this state, leaflets of the venous valves are stretched and prevented from closing completely, allowing a backflow or reflux of blood in the veins. Duplex ultrasonography confirms the obstruction and identifies the level of valvular incompetence.

Clinical Manifestations

When the valves in the deep veins become incompetent after a thrombus has formed, postthrombotic syndrome may develop (Fig. 31-16). This disorder is characterized by chronic venous stasis, resulting in edema, altered pigmentation, pain, and stasis dermatitis. The patient may notice the symptoms less in the morning and more in the evening. Obstruction or poor calf muscle pumping in addition to valvular reflux must be present for the development of severe postthrombotic syndrome, which includes stasis ulceration (Caps et al., 1999). Superficial veins may be dilated. The disorder is long-standing, difficult to treat, and often disabling.

Stasis ulcers develop as a result of the rupture of small skin veins and subsequent ulcerations. When these vessels rupture, red blood cells escape into surrounding tissues and then degenerate, leaving a brownish discoloration of the tissues. The pigmentation and ulcerations usually occur in the lower part of the extremity, in the area of the medial malleolus of the ankle. The skin becomes dry, cracks, and itches; subcutaneous tissues fibrose and atrophy. The risk of injury and infection of the extremities is increased.

Complications

Venous ulceration is the most serious complication of chronic venous insufficiency and can be associated with other conditions affecting the circulation of the lower extremities. Cellulitis or dermatitis may complicate the care of chronic venous insufficiency and venous ulcerations.

Management

Management of the patient with venous insufficiency is directed at reducing venous stasis and preventing ulcerations. Measures that increase venous blood flow are antigravity activities, such as elevating the leg, and compression of superficial veins with elastic compression stockings.

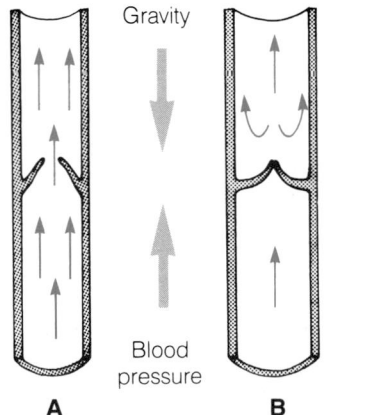
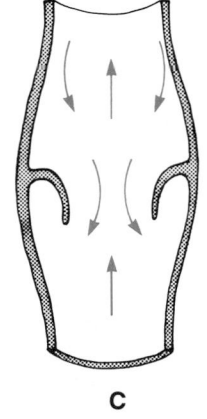

FIGURE 31-16 Competent valves showing blood flow patterns when the valve is open (**A**) and closed (**B**), allowing blood to flow against gravity. (**C**) With faulty or incompetent valves, the blood is unable to move toward the heart.

Elevating the legs decreases edema, promotes venous return, and provides symptomatic relief. The legs should be elevated frequently throughout the day (at least 15 to 30 minutes every 2 hours). At night, the patient should sleep with the foot of the bed elevated about 15 cm (6 inches). Prolonged sitting or standing still is detrimental; walking should be encouraged. When sitting, the patient should avoid placing pressure on the popliteal spaces, as occurs when crossing the legs or sitting with the legs dangling over the side of the bed. Constricting garments such as panty girdles or tight socks should be avoided.

Compression of the legs with elastic compression stockings reduces the pooling of venous blood and enhances venous return to the heart. Elastic compression stockings are recommended for people with venous insufficiency. The stocking should fit so that pressure is greater at the foot and ankle and then gradually declines to a lesser pressure at the knee or groin. If the top of the stocking is too tight or becomes twisted, a tourniquet effect is created, which worsens venous pooling. Stockings should be applied after the legs have been elevated for a period, when the amount of blood in the leg veins is at its lowest.

Extremities with venous insufficiency must be carefully protected from trauma; the skin is kept clean, dry, and soft. Signs of ulceration are immediately reported to the health care provider for treatment and follow-up.

LEG ULCERS

A leg ulcer is an excavation of the skin surface that occurs when inflamed necrotic tissue sloughs off. About 75% of all leg ulcers result from chronic venous insufficiency. Lesions due to arterial insufficiency account for approximately 20%; the remaining 5% are caused by burns, sickle cell anemia, and other factors (Gloviczki & Yao, 2001).

Pathophysiology

Inadequate exchange of oxygen and other nutrients in the tissue is the metabolic abnormality that underlies the development of leg ulcers. When cellular metabolism cannot maintain energy balance, cell death (necrosis) results. Alterations in blood vessels at the arterial, capillary, and venous levels may affect cellular processes and lead to the formation of ulcers.

Clinical Manifestations

The clinical appearance and associated characteristics of leg ulcers are determined by the cause of the ulcer. Most ulcers, especially in an elderly patient, have more than one cause. The symptoms depend on whether the problem is arterial or venous in origin (see Table 31-2). The severity of the symptoms depends on the extent and duration of the vascular insufficiency. The ulcer itself appears as an open, inflamed sore. The area may be draining or covered by eschar (dark, hard crust).

ARTERIAL ULCERS

Chronic arterial disease is characterized by intermittent claudication, which is pain caused by activity and relieved after a few minutes of rest. The patient may also complain of digital or forefoot pain at rest. If the onset of arterial occlusion is acute, ischemic pain is unrelenting and rarely relieved even with opioid analgesics. Typically, arterial ulcers are small, circular, deep ulcerations on the tips of toes or in the web spaces between toes. Ulcers often occur on the medial side of the hallux or lateral fifth toe and may be caused by a combination of ischemia and pressure (Fig. 31-17).

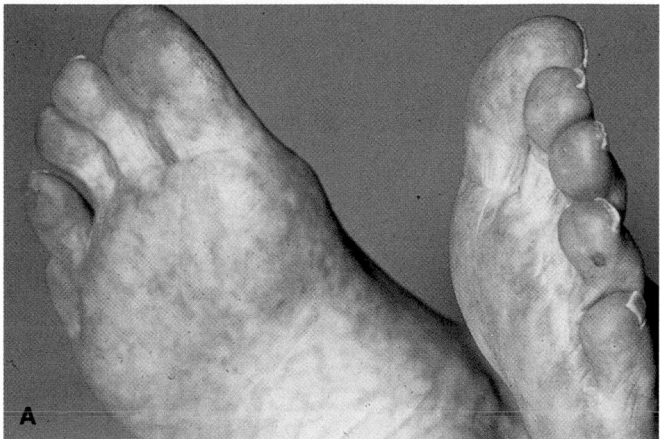

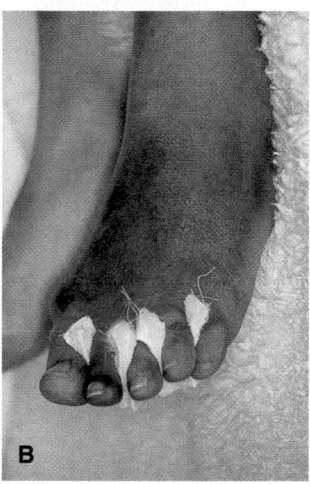
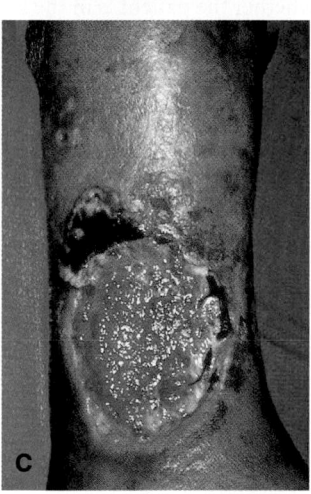

FIGURE 31-17 (**A**) Ulcers resulting from arterial emboli. (**B**) Gangrene of the toes resulting from severe arterial ischemia. (**C**) Ulcer from venous stasis.

Arterial insufficiency may result in gangrene of the toe (digital gangrene), which usually is caused by trauma. The toe is stubbed and then turns black (see Fig. 31-17). Usually, patients with this problem are elderly people without adequate circulation to provide revascularization. Débridement is contraindicated in these instances. Although the toe is gangrenous, it is dry. Managing dry gangrene is preferable to débriding the toe and causing an open wound that will not heal because of insufficient circulation. If the toe were to be amputated, the lack of adequate circulation would prevent healing and might make further amputation necessary—a below-knee or an above-knee amputation. A higher-level amputation in the elderly could result in a loss of independence and possibly institutional care. Dry gangrene of the toe in an elderly person with poor circulation is usually left undisturbed. The nurse keeps the toe clean and dry until it separates (without creating an open wound).

VENOUS ULCERS

Chronic venous insufficiency is characterized by pain described as aching or heaviness. The foot and ankle may be edematous. Ulcerations are in the area of the medial or lateral malleolus (gaiter area) and are typically large, superficial, and highly exudative. Venous hypertension causes extravasation of blood, which discolors the gaiter area (see Fig. 31-17). Patients with neuropathy frequently have ulcerations on the side of the foot over the metatarsal heads. These ulcers are painless and are described in further detail in Chapter 41.

Assessment and Diagnostic Findings

Because ulcers have many causes, the cause of each ulcer needs to be identified so appropriate therapy can be prescribed. The history of the condition is important in determining venous or arterial insufficiency. The pulses of the lower extremities (femoral, popliteal, posterior tibial, and dorsalis pedis) are carefully examined. More conclusive diagnostic aids are Doppler and duplex ultrasound studies, arteriography, and venography. Cultures of the ulcer bed may be necessary to determine whether the infecting agent is the primary cause of the ulcer.

Medical Management

Patients with ulcers can be effectively managed by advanced practice nurses or certified wound care nurses in collaboration with physicians. All ulcers have the potential to become infected.

PHARMACOLOGIC THERAPY

Antibiotic therapy is prescribed when the ulcer is infected; the specific antibiotic is selected on the basis of culture and sensitivity test results. Oral antibiotics usually are prescribed because topical antibiotics have not proven to be effective for leg ulcers.

DÉBRIDEMENT

To promote healing, the wound is kept clean of drainage and necrotic tissue. The usual method is to flush the area with normal saline solution. If this is unsuccessful, débridement may be necessary. Débridement is the removal of nonviable tissue from wounds. Removing the dead tissue is important, particularly in instances of infection. Débridement can be accomplished by several different methods:

- Sharp surgical débridement is the fastest method and can be performed by a physician, skilled advanced practice nurse, or certified wound care nurse in collaboration with the physician.
- Nonselective débridement can be accomplished by applying isotonic saline dressings of fine-mesh gauze to the ulcer. When the dressing dries, it is removed (dry), along with the debris adhering to the gauze. Pain management is usually necessary.
- Enzymatic débridement with the application of enzyme ointments may be prescribed to treat the ulcer. The ointment is applied to the lesion but not to normal surrounding skin. Most enzymatic ointments are covered with saline-soaked gauze that has been thoroughly wrung out. A dry gauze dressing and a loose bandage are then applied. The enzymatic ointment is discontinued when the necrotic tissue has been débrided and an appropriate wound dressing is applied.
- Débriding agents can be used. Dextranomer (Debrisan) beads are small, highly porous, spherical beads (0.1 to 0.3 mm in diameter) that can absorb wound secretions. Bacteria and the products of tissue necrosis and protein degradation are absorbed into the bead layer. When the beads are saturated, they take on a grayish yellow color, at which point their cleansing action stops. They are then flushed from the wound with normal saline, and a fresh layer is applied.
- Calcium alginate dressings can also be used for débridement when absorption of exudate is needed. These dressings are changed when the exudate seeps through the cover dressing or at least every 7 days. The dressing can also be used on areas that are bleeding, because the material helps stop the bleeding. As the dry fibers absorb exudate, they become a gel that is painlessly removed from the ulcer bed. Calcium alginate dressings should not be used on dry or nonexudative wounds.

TOPICAL THERAPY

A variety of topical agents can be used in conjunction with cleansing and débridement therapies to promote healing of leg ulcers. The goals of treatment are to remove devitalized tissue and to keep the ulcer clean and moist while healing takes place. The treatment should not destroy developing tissue. For topical treatments to be successful, adequate nutritional therapy must be maintained.

WOUND DRESSING

After the circulatory status has been assessed and determined to be adequate for healing (ABI of more than 0.5), surgical dressings can be used to promote a moist environment. The simplest method is to use a wound contact material (eg, Tegapore) next to the wound bed and cover it with gauze. Tegapore maintains a moist environment, can be left in place for several days, and does not disrupt the capillary bed when removed for evaluation. Hydrocolloids (eg, Comfeel, DuoDerm CGF, Restore, Tegasorb) are also available options to promote granulation tissue and re-epithelialization. They also provide a barrier for protection because they adhere to the wound bed and surrounding tissue. However, deep wounds and infected wounds are often more appropriately treated with other dressings.

Knowledge deficit, frustration, fear, and depression can result in the patient's and family's decreased compliance with the prescribed therapy; therefore, patient and family education is necessary before beginning and throughout the wound care program.

STIMULATED HEALING

Tissue-engineered human skin equivalent along with therapeutic compression has been developed by Apligraf; it is a skin product cultured from human dermal fibroblasts and keratinocytes. When applied, it seems to react to factors in the wound and may interact with the patient's cells to stimulate the production of growth factors. Application is not difficult, no suturing is involved, and the procedure is painless.

NURSING PROCESS:
THE PATIENT WHO HAS LEG ULCERS

Assessment

A careful nursing history and assessment of symptoms are important. The extent and type of pain are carefully assessed, as are the appearance and temperature of the skin of both legs. The quality of all peripheral pulses is assessed, and comparisons are made of the pulses in both legs. The legs are checked for edema. If the extremity is edematous, the degree of edema is determined. Any limitation of mobility and activity that results from the vascular insufficiency is identified. The patient's nutritional status is assessed, and a history of diabetes, collagen disease, or varicose veins is obtained.

Diagnosis

NURSING DIAGNOSES

Based on the assessment data, major nursing diagnoses for the patient may include:

- Impaired skin integrity related to vascular insufficiency
- Impaired physical mobility related to activity restrictions of the therapeutic regimen and pain
- Imbalanced nutrition: less than body requirements, related to increased need for nutrients that promote wound healing

COLLABORATIVE PROBLEMS/POTENTIAL COMPLICATIONS

Based on the assessment data, potential complications that may develop include:

- Infection
- Gangrene

Planning and Goals

The major goals for the patient may include restoration of skin integrity, improved physical mobility, adequate nutrition, and absence of complications.

Nursing Interventions

The nursing challenge in caring for these patients is great, whether the patient is in the hospital, in a long-term care facility, or at home. The physical problem is often a long-term one that causes a substantial drain on the patient's physical, emotional, and economic resources.

RESTORING SKIN INTEGRITY

To promote wound healing, measures are used to keep the area clean. Cleansing requires very gentle handling, a mild soap, and lukewarm water. Positioning of the legs depends on whether the ulcer is of arterial or venous origin. If there is arterial insufficiency, the patient should be referred to be evaluated for vascular reconstruction. If there is venous insufficiency, dependent edema can be avoided by elevating the lower extremities. A decrease in edema promotes the exchange of cellular nutrients and waste products in the area of the ulcer, promoting healing.

Avoiding trauma to the lower extremities is imperative in promoting skin integrity. Protective boots may be used (eg, the Rooke Vascular boot, Lunax Boot, Bunny Boot); they are soft and provide warmth and protection from injury. If the patient is on bed rest, it is important to relieve pressure on the heels to prevent pressure ulcerations. When the patient is in bed, a bed cradle can be used to relieve pressure from bed linens and to prevent anything from touching the legs. When the patient is ambulatory, all obstacles are moved from the patient's path so that the patient's legs will not be bumped. Heating pads, hot-water bottles, or hot baths are avoided. Heat increases the oxygen demands and thus the blood flow demands of the tissue, which in this case are already compromised. The patient with diabetes mellitus suffers from neuropathy with decreased sensation, and heating pads may produce injury before the patient is aware of being burned.

IMPROVING PHYSICAL MOBILITY

Generally, physical activity is initially restricted to promote healing. When infection resolves and healing begins, ambulation should resume gradually and progressively. Activity promotes arterial flow and venous return and is encouraged after the acute phase of the ulcer process. Until full activity resumes, the patient is encouraged to move about when in bed, to turn from side to side frequently, and to exercise the upper extremities to maintain muscle tone and strength. Meanwhile, diversional activities that interest the patient are encouraged. Consultation with an occupational therapist may be helpful if a prolonged period of limited mobility and activity is anticipated.

If pain limits the patient's activity, analgesics may be prescribed by the physician. The pain of peripheral vascular disease, whether it is arterial or venous, is typically chronic. Analgesics may be taken before scheduled activities to help the patient participate more comfortably.

PROMOTING ADEQUATE NUTRITION

Nutritional deficiencies are determined from the patient's report of usual dietary intake. Alterations in the diet are made to remedy these deficiencies. A diet that is high in protein, vitamins C and A, iron, and zinc is encouraged in an attempt to promote healing.

Many patients with peripheral vascular disease are elderly. Their caloric intake may need to be adjusted because of their decreased metabolic rate and level of activity. Particular consideration should also be given to their iron intake, because many elderly people are anemic.

After a diet plan has been developed that meets the patient's nutritional needs and promotes healing, diet instruction is provided to the patient and family. The nurse and patient design the diet plan to be compatible with the lifestyle and preferences of the patient and family.

PROMOTING HOME AND COMMUNITY-BASED CARE

The self-care program is planned with the patient so that activities to promote arterial and venous circulation, relieve pain, and promote tissue integrity will be used. Reasons for each aspect of the program are explained to the patient and family. Leg ulcers are often chronic and difficult to heal; they frequently recur, even when patients rigorously follow the plan of care. Long-term care of the feet and legs to promote healing of wounds and prevent recurrence of ulcerations is the primary goal. Leg ulcers increase the patient's risk for infection, may be painful, and limit mobility, necessitating life-style changes. Participation of family members and home-health providers may be necessary for treatments such as dressing changes, reassessments, and evaluation of the plan of care. Regular follow-up with a primary health care provider is necessary.

Evaluation

EXPECTED PATIENT OUTCOMES

Expected patient outcomes may include:

1. Demonstrates restored skin integrity
   a. Exhibits absence of inflammation
   b. Exhibits absence of drainage; negative wound culture
   c. Avoids trauma to the legs
2. Increases physical mobility
   a. Progresses gradually to optimal level of activity
   b. Reports that pain does not impede activity
3. Attains adequate nutrition
   a. Selects foods high in protein, vitamins, iron, and zinc
   b. Discusses with family members dietary modifications that need to be made at home
   c. Plans, with the family, a diet that is nutritionally sound

VARICOSE VEINS

Varicose veins (varicosities) are abnormally dilated, tortuous, superficial veins caused by incompetent venous valves (see Fig. 31-16). Most commonly, this condition occurs in the lower extremities, the saphenous veins, or the lower trunk; however, it can occur elsewhere in the body, such as esophageal varices (see Chap. 39).

It is estimated that varicose veins occur in up to 60% of the adult population in the United States, with an increased incidence correlated with increased age (Johnson, 1997). The condition is most common in women and in people whose occupations require prolonged standing, such as salespeople, hair stylists, teach-

ers, nurses, ancillary medical personnel, and construction workers. A hereditary weakness of the vein wall may contribute to the development of varicosities, and it is not uncommon to see this condition occur in several members of the same family. Varicose veins are rare before puberty. Pregnancy may cause varicosities. The leg veins dilate during pregnancy because of hormonal effects related to distensibility, increased pressure by the gravid uterus, and increased blood volume which all contribute to the development of varicose veins (Johnson, 1997).

Pathophysiology

Varicose veins may be considered primary (without involvement of deep veins) or secondary (resulting from obstruction of deep veins). A reflux of venous blood in the veins results in venous stasis. If only the superficial veins are affected, the person may have no symptoms but may be troubled by the appearance of the dilated veins.

Clinical Manifestations

Symptoms, if present, may take the form of dull aches, muscle cramps, and increased muscle fatigue in the lower legs. Ankle edema and a feeling of heaviness of the legs may occur. Nocturnal cramps are common. When deep venous obstruction results in varicose veins, patients may develop the signs and symptoms of chronic venous insufficiency: edema, pain, pigmentation, and ulcerations. Susceptibility to injury and infection is increased.

Assessment and Diagnostic Findings

Diagnostic tests for varicose veins include the duplex scan, which documents the anatomic site of reflux and provides a quantitative measure of the severity of valvular reflux. Air plethysmography measures the changes in venous blood volume. Venography is not routinely performed to evaluate for valvular reflux. When it is used, however, it involves injecting an x-ray contrast agent into the leg veins so that the vein anatomy can be visualized by x-ray studies during various leg movements.

Prevention

The patient should avoid activities that cause venous stasis, such as wearing tight socks or a constricting panty girdle, crossing the legs at the thighs, and sitting or standing for long periods. Changing position frequently, elevating the legs when they are tired, and getting up to walk for several minutes of every hour promote circulation. The patient should be encouraged to walk 1 or 2 miles each day if there are no contraindications. Walking up the stairs rather than using the elevator or escalator is helpful in promoting circulation. Swimming is also good exercise for the legs.

Elastic compression stockings, especially knee-high stockings, are useful. Patients are more likely to use knee-high stockings than thigh-high stockings. The overweight patient should be encouraged to begin a weight-reduction plan.

Medical Management

Surgery for varicose veins requires that the deep veins be patent and functional. The saphenous vein is ligated and divided. The vein is ligated high in the groin, where the saphenous vein meets the femoral vein. Additionally, the vein may be removed (stripped). After the vein is ligated, an incision is made in the ankle, and a metal or plastic wire is passed the full length of the vein to the point of ligation. The wire is then withdrawn, pulling (removing, "stripping") the vein as it is removed (Fig. 31-18). Pressure and elevation keep bleeding at a minimum during surgery.

SCLEROTHERAPY

In sclerotherapy, a chemical is injected into the vein, irritating the venous endothelium and producing localized phlebitis and fibrosis, thereby obliterating the lumen of the vein. This treatment may be performed alone for small varicosities or may follow vein ligation or stripping. Sclerosing is palliative rather than curative. After the sclerosing agent is injected, elastic compression bandages are applied to the leg and are worn for approximately 5 days. The health care provider who performed sclerotherapy removes the first bandages. Elastic compression stockings are then worn for an additional 5 weeks.

After sclerotherapy, patients are encouraged to perform walking activities as prescribed to maintain blood flow in the leg. Walking enhances dilution of the sclerosing agent.

Nursing Management

Surgery can be performed in an outpatient setting, or patients can be admitted to the hospital on the day of surgery and discharged the next day, but nursing measures are the same as if the patient were hospitalized. Bed rest is maintained for 24 hours, after which the patient begins walking every 2 hours for 5 to 10 minutes. Elastic compression stockings are used to maintain compression of the leg. They are worn continuously for about 1 week after vein stripping. The nurse assists the patient to perform exercises and move the legs. The foot of the bed should be elevated. Standing still and sitting are discouraged.

PROMOTING COMFORT AND UNDERSTANDING

Analgesics are prescribed to help patients move affected extremities more comfortably. Dressings are inspected for bleeding, particularly at the groin, where the risk of bleeding is greatest. The nurse is alert for reported sensations of "pins and needles." Hyper-

sensitivity to touch in the involved extremity may indicate a temporary or permanent nerve injury resulting from surgery, because the saphenous vein and nerve are close to each other in the leg.

Usually, the patient may shower after the first 24 hours. The patient is instructed to dry the incisions well with a clean towel using a patting technique rather than rubbing. Application of skin lotion is to be avoided until the incisions are completely healed to decrease the chance of developing an infection.

If the patient underwent sclerotherapy, a burning sensation in the injected leg may be experienced for 1 or 2 days. The nurse may encourage the use of a mild analgesic (eg, propoxyphene napsylate and acetaminophen [Darvocet N], oxycodone and acetaminophen [Percocet], oxycodone and acetylsalicylic acid [Percodan]) as prescribed by a physician or nurse practitioner and walking to provide relief.

PROMOTING HOME AND COMMUNITY-BASED CARE

Patients require long-term elastic support of the leg after discharge, and plans are made to obtain adequate supplies of elastic compression stockings or bandages as appropriate. Exercises of the legs are necessary; the development of an individualized plan requires consultation with the patient and the health care team.

Cellulitis

Pathophysiology and Clinical Manifestations

Cellulitis is the most common infectious cause of limb swelling. Cellulitis can occur as a single isolated event or a series of recurrent events. It is often misdiagnosed, usually as recurrent thrombophlebitis or chronic venous insufficiency. Cellulitis occurs when an entry point through normal skin barriers allows bacteria to enter and release their toxins in the subcutaneous tissues. The acute onset of swelling, localized redness, and pain is frequently associated with systemic signs of fever, chills, and sweating. The redness may not be uniform and often skips areas. Regional lymph nodes may also be tender and enlarged.

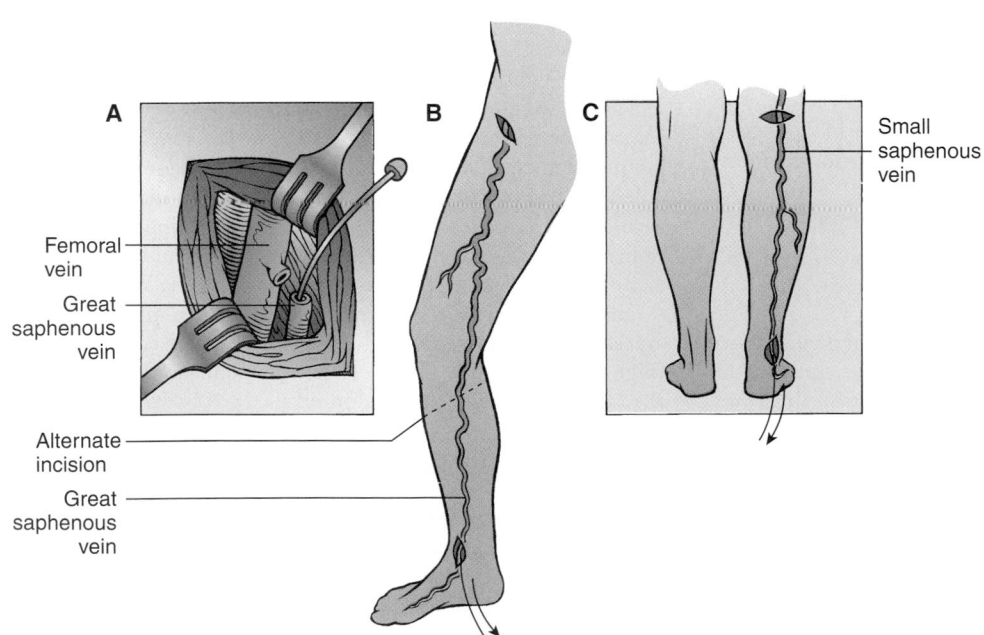

A

Femoral vein

Great saphenous vein

Alternate incision

Great saphenous vein

B

C

Small saphenous vein

FIGURE 31-18 Ligation and stripping of the great and the small saphenous veins. (**A**) The tributaries of the saphenous vein have been ligated at the saphenofemoral junction. (**B**) The vein stripper has been inserted from the ankle superiorly to the groin. The vein is removed ("stripped") from above downward. A number of alternate incisions may be needed to remove separate varicose masses. (**C**) The small saphenous vein is stripped from its junction with the popliteal vein to a point posterior to the lateral malleolus.

Medical Management

Mild cases of cellulitis can be treated on an outpatient basis with oral antibiotic therapy. If the cellulitis is severe, the patient is hospitalized and treated with intravenous antibiotics for at least 7 to 14 days. The key to preventing recurrent episodes of cellulitis lies in adequate antibiotic therapy for the initial event and in identifying the site of the bacterial entry. The most commonly overlooked areas are the cracks and fissures that occur in the skin between the toes. Other possible locations are drug use injection sites, contusions, abrasions, ulcerations, ingrown toenails, and hangnails.

Nursing Management

The patient is instructed to elevate the affected area above heart level and apply warm, moist packs to the site every 2 to 4 hours. Individuals with sensory and circulatory deficits, such as diabetes and paralysis, should use caution when applying warm packs because burns may occur; it is advisable to use a thermometer or have a caregiver ensure that the temperature is not more than lukewarm. Education should focus on preventing a recurrent episode. The patient with peripheral vascular disease or diabetes mellitus should receive education or re-education about skin and foot care.

Management of Lymphatic Disorders

The lymphatic system consists of a set of vessels that spread throughout most of the body. These vessels start as lymph capillaries that drain unabsorbed plasma from the interstitial spaces (spaces between the cells). The lymphatic capillaries unite to form the lymph vessels, which pass through the lymph nodes and then empty into the large thoracic duct that joins the jugular vein on the left side of the neck.

The fluid drained from the interstitial space by the lymphatic system is called lymph. The flow of lymph depends on the intrinsic contractions of the lymph vessels, the contraction of muscles, respiratory movements, and gravity. The lymphatic system of the abdominal cavity maintains a steady flow of digested fatty food (chyle) from the intestinal mucosa to the thoracic duct. In other parts of the body, the lymphatic system's function is regional; the lymphatic vessels of the head, for example, empty into clusters of lymph nodes located in the neck, and those of the extremities empty into nodes of the axillae and the groin.

LYMPHANGITIS AND LYMPHADENITIS

Lymphangitis is an acute inflammation of the lymphatic channels. It arises most commonly from a focus of infection in an extremity. Usually, the infectious organism is a hemolytic *Streptococcus*. The characteristic red streaks that extend up the arm or the leg from an infected wound outline the course of the lymphatic vessels as they drain.

The lymph nodes located along the course of the lymphatic channels also become enlarged, red, and tender (acute lymphadenitis). They can also become necrotic and form an abscess (suppurative lymphadenitis). The nodes involved most often are those in the groin, axilla, or cervical region.

Because these infections are nearly always caused by organisms that are sensitive to antibiotics, it is unusual to see abscess formation. Recurrent episodes of lymphangitis are often associated with progressive lymphedema. After acute attacks, an elastic compres-

sion stocking or sleeve should be worn on the affected extremity for several months to prevent long-term edema.

LYMPHEDEMA AND ELEPHANTIASIS

Lymphedemas are classified as primary (congenital malformations) or secondary (acquired obstructions). Tissue swelling occurs in the extremities because of an increased quantity of lymph that results from obstruction of lymphatic vessels. It is especially marked when the extremity is in a dependent position. Initially, the edema is soft, pitting, and relieved by treatment. As the condition progresses, the edema becomes firm, nonpitting, and unresponsive to treatment. The most common type is congenital lymphedema (lymphedema praecox), which is caused by hypoplasia of the lymphatic system of the lower extremity. This disorder is usually seen in women and first appears between ages 15 and 25.

The obstruction may be in the lymph nodes and the lymphatic vessels. Sometimes, it is seen in the arm after an axillary node dissection (eg, for breast cancer) and in the leg in association with varicose veins or chronic thrombophlebitis. In the latter case, the lymphatic obstruction usually is caused by chronic lymphangitis. Lymphatic obstruction caused by a parasite (filaria) is seen frequently in the tropics. When chronic swelling is present, there may be frequent bouts of acute infection characterized by high fever and chills and increased residual edema after the inflammation has resolved. These lead to chronic fibrosis, thickening of the subcutaneous tissues, and hypertrophy of the skin. This condition, in which chronic swelling of the extremity recedes only slightly with elevation, is referred to as elephantiasis.

Medical Management

The goal of therapy is to reduce and control the edema and prevent infection. Active and passive exercises assist in moving lymphatic fluid into the bloodstream. External compression devices milk the fluid proximally from the foot to the hip or from the hand to the axilla. When the patient is ambulatory, custom-fitted elastic compression stockings or sleeves are worn; those with the highest compression strength (exceeding 40 mm Hg) are required. When the leg is affected, strict bed rest with the leg elevated may aid in mobilizing the fluids.

PHARMACOLOGIC THERAPY

As initial therapy, the diuretic furosemide (Lasix) is prescribed as needed to prevent the fluid overload that can result from the mobilization of extracellular fluid. Diuretics have also been used palliatively for lymphedema in conjunction with elevating the leg and wearing elastic compression stockings or sleeves. However, the use of diuretics alone has little benefit because their main action is to limit capillary filtration by decreasing the circulating blood volume. If lymphangitis or cellulitis is present, antibiotic therapy is initiated. The patient is taught to inspect the skin for evidence of infection.

SURGICAL MANAGEMENT

Surgery is performed if the edema is severe and uncontrolled by medical therapy, if mobility is severely compromised, or if infection persists. One surgical approach involves the excision of the affected subcutaneous tissue and fascia, with skin grafting to cover the defect. Another procedure involves the surgical relocation of superficial lymphatic vessels into the deep lymphatic system by means of a buried dermal flap to provide a conduit for lymphatic drainage.

Nursing Management

After surgery, the management of skin grafts and flaps is the same as when these therapies are used for other conditions. Prophylactic antibiotics may be prescribed for 5 to 7 days. Constant elevation of the affected extremity and observations for complications are essential. Complications may include flap necrosis, hematoma or abscess under the flap, and cellulitis. The nurse instructs the patient or caregiver to inspect the dressing daily. Unusual drainage or any inflammation around the wound margin may suggest infection and should be reported to the physician. The patient is informed that there may be a loss of sensation in the skin graft area. The patient is also instructed to avoid the application of heating pads or exposure to sun to prevent burns or trauma to the area.

Critical Thinking Exercises

1. Your patient has been diagnosed with an enlarging abdominal aortic aneurysm (AAA). The physician gives the patient two surgical options: repair of the AAA using an endovascular graft or open surgical repair. What factors would you include in discussing the surgical options, post-operative care, continuing care, and home care? If the patient is taking warfarin (Coumadin) for atrial fibrillation and insulin for diabetes, how would you incorporate these factors into the plan of care?

2. Your 96-year-old patient presents with a 1-year history of experiencing symptoms of claudication after walking four or five blocks. The patient lives alone, six blocks from the local shopping area, and no longer drives a vehicle. The patient does not wish to undergo surgery at this time and wants to continue living at his current location. What options would you discuss with the patient? If this patient also had a nonhealing foot wound and had smoked two packs of cigarettes each day for the past 80 years, how would your plan of care change?

3. Your patient has been diagnosed with deep vein thrombosis of a calf. The physician gives the patient two treatment options: hospitalization with intravenous sodium heparin therapy or home treatment with LMWH. What factors would you include in discussing the treatment options with the patient?

REFERENCES AND SELECTED READINGS

Books

Bickley, L. S., & Szilagyi, P. G. (2003). *Bates' guide to physical examination and history taking* (8th ed.). Philadelphia: Lippincott Williams & Wilkins.

Bullock, B., & Henze R. (1999). *Focus on pathophysiology* (4th ed.). Philadelphia: Lippincott Williams & Wilkins.

Coleman, R. W., Hirsch, J., Marder, V. J., Clowes, A. W., George, J. N. (2000). *Hemostasis and thrombosis: Basic principles and clinical practice* (4th ed.). Philadelphia: Lippincott Williams & Wilkins.

Fahey, V. (1999). *Vascular nursing* (3rd ed.). Philadelphia: W. B. Saunders.

Gloviczki, P., & Yao, J. T. (2001). *Handbook of venous disorders—Guidelines of the American Venous Forum* (2nd ed.). New York: Oxford University Press.

Guyton, A., & Hall, J. (2000). *Textbook of medical physiology* (10th ed.). Philadelphia: W. B. Saunders.

Haimovici, H. (1996). *Vascular surgery principles and techniques* (4th ed.). Cambridge, MA: Blackwell Science.

Jarvis, C. (1999). *Physical examination and health assessment* (3rd ed.). Philadelphia: W. B. Saunders.

Lynn-McHale, D. J. (2000). *AACN procedure manual for critical care nurses* (4th ed.). St. Louis: Mosby.

Moore, W. S. (2002). *Vascular surgery: A comprehensive review* (6th ed.). Philadelphia: W. B. Saunders.

Parodi, J. C., Veith, F. J., & Marin, M. (1999). *Endovascular grafting techniques.* Baltimore: Williams & Wilkins.

Rutherford, R. B. (1999). *Vascular surgery* (5th ed., Vols. I and II). Philadelphia: W. B. Saunders.

Strandness, D. E. (2002). *Duplex scanning in vascular disorders* (3rd ed.). Philadelphia: Lippincott Williams & Wilkins.

White, R. A., & Fogarty, T. J. (1999). *Peripheral endovascular interventions* (2nd ed.). New York: Singer-Verlag.

Yao, J. T. & Pearce, W. H. (1999). *Practical vascular surgery.* Stamford, CT: Appleton & Lange.

Journals

Beckey, N. P. (1999). Outpatient management of patients on warfarin. *Lippincott's Primary Care Practice, 3*(3), 280–289.

Berdejo, G. L., Lyon, R. T., Ohki, T., Sanchez, L. A., Wain, R. A., del Valle, W. N., et al. (1998). Color duplex ultrasound evaluation of transluminally placed endovascular grafts for aneurysm repair. *Journal of Vascular Technology, 22*(4), 201–207.

Bryant, J. L., & Turkoski, B. B. (1999). Relieving intermittent claudication: A nursing approach. *Journal of Vascular Nursing, 16*(4), 81–85.

Caps, M. T., Meissner, M. H., Tullis, M. J., Polissar, N. L., Manzo, R. A., Zierler, B. K., et al. (1999). Venous thrombus stability during acute phase of therapy. *Vascular Medicine, 4*(1), 9–14.

Finkelmeier, B. A. (1997). Dissection of the aorta: A clinical update. *Journal of Vascular Nursing, 15*(3), 88–93.

Frost-Rude, J. A., Nunnelee, J. D., & Spaner, S. (2000). Buerger's disease. *Journal of Vascular Nursing, 18*(4), 128–130.

Gramse, C. A., Hingorani, A., & Ascher, E. (2001). Postoperative anticoagulation in vascular surgery: Part 1. A retrospective comparison of clinical outcomes for unfractionated heparin versus low-molecular-weight heparin. *Journal of Vascular Nursing, 19*(2), 42–49.

Hirsch, A. T., Criqui, M. H., Treat-Jacobson, D., Regensteiner, J. G., Creager, M. A., Olin, J. W., et al. (2001). Peripheral arterial disease detection, awareness, and treatment in primary care. *Journal of the American Medical Association, 286*(11), 1317–1324.

Johnson, M. T. (1997). Treatment and prevention of varicose veins. *Journal of Vascular Nursing, 15*(3), 97–103.

Kaufman, M. W., & All, A. C. (1996). Raynaud's disease: Patient education as a primary nursing intervention. *Journal of Vascular Nursing, 14*(2), 34–39.

Kowallek, D. L., & DePalma, R. G. (1997). Venous ulceration: Active approaches to treatment. *Journal of Vascular Nursing, 15*(2), 50–57.

Krauss, R. M., Eckel, R. H., Howard, B., Appel, L. J., Daniels, S. R., Deckelbaum, R. J., et al. (2000). AHA dietary guidelines. Revision 2000: A statement for healthcare professionals from the Nutrition Committee of the American Heart Association. *Circulation, 102*(18), 2284–2299.

Lacey, K. O. (1996). Subclavian steal syndrome: A review. *Journal of Vascular Nursing, 14*(1), 1–7.

Lombardo, K. M. (1997). Endovascular grafting of abdominal aortic aneurysms. *Journal of Vascular Nursing, 15*(3), 83–87.

Mawhorter, S. D. (2000). Nonhealing cellulitis in a 54-year-old man with diabetes mellitus. *Cleveland Clinic Journal of Medicine, 67*(1), 21–24.

McAlister, F. A., Levine, M., Zarnke, K. B., Campbell, N., Lewanczuk, R., Leenen, F., et al. (2001). The 2000 Canadian recommendations for the management of hypertension: Part 1. Therapy. *Canadian Journal of Cardiology, 17*(5), 543–559.

Meissner, M. H., Caps, M. T., Zierler, B. F., Bergelin, R. O., Manzo, R. A., Stradnes, D. E., Jr. (2000). Deep venous thrombosis and superficial venous reflux. *Journal of Vascular Surgery, 32*(1), 48–56.

Moser, M. (1999). World Health Organization-International Society of Hypertension guidelines for the management of hypertension—Do these differ from the U.S. recommendations? Which guidelines should the practicing physician follow? *Journal of Clinical Hypertension, 1,* 48–54.

O'Connor, C. M. (2001). Raynaud's phenomenon. *Journal of Vascular Nursing, 19*(3), 87–92.

Phillips, L. (2000). Putting a damper on cellulitis. *Nursing, 30*(12), 52–53.

Rudolph, D. (2001). Standards of care for venous leg ulcers: Compression therapy and moist wound healing. *Journal of Vascular Nursing, 19*(1), 20–27.

Stevens, S. L. (2000). Heparin-induced thrombocytopenia. *Journal of Vascular Nursing, 18*(2), 54–58.

Strider, D., Robinson, T., Guarini, J., Ivey, J. (1996). Challenges with Takayasu's arteritis: A case study. *Journal of Vascular Nursing, 14*(1), 12–17.

Verta, K. F., & Verta, M. J. (1998). Alternative imaging techniques in vascular surgery. *Journal of Vascular Nursing, 16*(4), 78–83.

Vogeley, C. L., & Coeling, H. (2000). Prevention of venous ulceration by use of compression after deep vein thrombosis. *Journal of Vascular Nursing, 18*(4), 123–127.

Zierler, R. E. (1999). Vascular surgery without arteriography: use of Duplex ultrasound. *Cardiovascular Surgery, 7*(1), 74–82.

RESOURCES AND WEBSITES

Agency for Healthcare Research and Quality, Public Health Service, U.S. Department of Health and Human Services, National Guideline Clearinghouse, P.O. Box 8547, Silver Spring, MD 20907; 1-800-358-9295; http://www.ahrq.gov and http://www.guideline.gov.

American Venous Forum, 13 Elm Street, Manchester, MA 01944; 978-526-8330; http://www.venous-info.com.

National Heart, Lung, and Blood Institute, Health Information Center, P.O. Box 30105, Bethesda, MD 20824-0105; 301-592-8573; http://www.nhlbi.nih.gov.

Society for Vascular Surgery, 13 Elm Street, Manchester, MA 01944-1314; 978-526-8330; http://www.vascularweb.org.

Society of Vascular Nursing, 7794 Grow Drive, Pensacola, FL 32514; 888-536-4786; http://www.svnnet.org.

Society of Vascular Ultrasound, 4601 Presidents Drive, Suite 260, Lanham, MD 20706-4831; 301-459-7550; http://www.svtnet.org.

Vascular Disease Foundation, 3333 S. Wadsworth Boulevard, #B104-37, Lakewood, CO 80227; 1-866-723-4636; http://www.vdf.org.

Assessment and Management of Patients With Hypertension

On completion of this chapter, the learner will be able to:

1. Define blood pressure and identify risk factors for hypertension.
2. Explain the difference between normal blood pressure and hypertension and discuss the significance of hypertension.
3. Describe the treatment approach for hypertension, including lifestyle changes and medication therapy.
4. Use the nursing process as a framework for care of the patient with hypertension.
5. Describe the necessity for immediate treatment of hypertensive crisis.

Blood pressure is the product of cardiac output multiplied by peripheral resistance. Cardiac output is the product of the heart rate multiplied by the stroke volume. In normal circulation, pressure is exerted by the flow of blood through the heart and blood vessels. High blood pressure, known as hypertension, can result from a change in cardiac output, a change in peripheral resistance, or both. The medications used for treating hypertension decrease peripheral resistance, blood volume, or the strength and rate of myocardial contraction.

Hypertension Defined

Hypertension is defined as a systolic blood pressure greater than 140 mm Hg and a diastolic pressure greater than 90 mm Hg based on the average of two or more correct blood pressure measurements taken during two or more contacts with a health care provider (Chobanian et al., 2003). Table 32-1 shows the classification of blood pressure established by the Seventh Report of the Joint National Committee on Prevention, Detection, Evaluation, and Treatment of High Blood Pressure (JNC 7) in 2003. The categories of blood pressure from normal to stage 2 hypertension are designed to emphasize the direct relationship between the risk of morbidity and mortality from increasing levels of blood pressure and the specific levels of both the systolic and diastolic blood pressures. The higher either the systolic or diastolic pressure, the greater the risk (Lewington, Clarke, Qizilbash, Peto, & Collins, 2002).

JNC 7 defines a blood pressure of <120/<80 mm Hg as normal; 120–139/80–89 mm Hg as prehypertension; and then, as shown in Table 32-1, two stages of hypertension. The term "stage" was used specifically to define the two levels of hypertension so that, as with cancer progression, the public and health care professionals would be aware that sustained elevations in blood pressure are associated with increased risks to health. The JNC 7 introduced the new category, prehypertension, into the categorization of blood pressure levels to emphasize the growing awareness that persons whose blood pressure begins to rise above 120/80 mm Hg are likely to progress to definite hypertension. To prevent or delay progression to hypertension, the JNC 7 Committee hopes that health care providers will encourage persons with blood pressures in the prehypertension category to begin lifestyle modifications such as nutritional changes and exercise. The JNC 7 report recommends that persons with hypertension be treated with medications and be evaluated by their health care provider about every month until their blood pressure goal is reached, and about every 3 to 6 months thereafter. Persons with higher levels of blood pressure (Stage 2) or other complicating conditions need to be evaluated more frequently.

Primary Hypertension

Between 21% and 36% of the adult population in the United States has hypertension (Hajjar & Kotchen, 2003). Of this population, between 90% and 95% have **primary hypertension**, meaning that the reason for the elevation in blood pressure cannot be identified. The remaining 5% to 10% of this group have high blood pressure related to specific causes, such as narrowing of the renal arteries, renal parenchymal disease, hyperaldosteronism (mineralocorticoid hypertension) certain medications, pregnancy, and coarctation of the aorta (Kaplan, 2001). **Secondary hypertension** is the term used to signify high blood pressure from an identified cause. Table 32-2 lists the most frequent causes of secondary hypertension.

Hypertension is sometimes called "the silent killer" because people who have it are often symptom free. In a national survey (1999 to 2000), 31% of people who had pressures exceeding 140/90 mm Hg were unaware of their elevated blood pressure (Hajjar & Kotchen, 2003). Once identified, elevated blood pressure should be monitored at regular intervals because hypertension is a lifelong condition.

Hypertension often accompanies risk factors for atherosclerotic heart disease, such as **dyslipidemia** (abnormal blood fat levels) and diabetes mellitus. The incidence of hypertension is higher in the southeastern United States, particularly among African Americans. Cigarette smoking does not cause high blood pressure; however, if a person with hypertension smokes, his or her risk of dying from heart disease or related disorders increases significantly.

High blood pressure can be viewed in three ways: as a sign, a risk factor for atherosclerotic cardiovascular disease, or a disease. As a sign, nurses and other health care professionals use blood pressure to monitor a patient's clinical status. Elevated pressure may indicate an excessive dose of vasoconstrictive medication or other problems. As a risk factor, hypertension contributes to the rate at which atherosclerotic plaque accumulates within arterial walls. As a disease, hypertension is a major contributor to death from cardiac, renal, and peripheral vascular disease.

Prolonged blood pressure elevation eventually damages blood vessels throughout the body, particularly in target organs such as the heart, kidneys, brain, and eyes. The usual consequences of prolonged, uncontrolled hypertension are myocardial infarction, heart failure, renal failure, strokes, and impaired vision. The left ventricle of the heart may become enlarged (left ventricular hypertrophy) as it works to pump blood against the elevated pressure. An echocardiogram is the recommended method of determining whether hypertrophy (enlargement) has occurred.

Pathophysiology

Although the precise cause for most cases of hypertension cannot be identified, it is understood that hypertension is a multifactorial

Glossary

dyslipidemia: abnormally high or low blood lipid levels

hypertensive emergency: a situation in which blood pressure must be lowered immediately to prevent damage to target organs

hypertensive urgency: a situation in which blood pressure must be lowered within a few hours to prevent damage to target organs

JNC 7: Seventh Joint National Committee on the Prevention, Detection, Evaluation and Treatment of High Blood Pressure; committee established to study and make recommendations about hypertension in the United States. Findings and recommendations of JNC 7 are contained in an extensive report published in 2003.

monotherapy: medication therapy with a single medication

primary hypertension: also called essential hypertension; denotes high blood pressure from an unidentified cause

rebound hypertension: pressure that is controlled with therapy and that becomes uncontrolled (abnormally high) with the discontinuation of therapy

secondary hypertension: high blood pressure from an identified cause, such as renal disease

Table 32-1 • Classification and Management of Blood Pressure for Adults*

BP CLASSIFICATION	SBP* (MMHG)	DBP* (MMHG)	LIFESTYLE MODIFICATION	INITIAL DRUG THERAPY	
				Without Compelling Indication	With Compelling Indications (See Table 8)
Normal	<120	and <80	Encourage		
Prehypertension	120–139	or 80–89	Yes	No antihypertensive drug indicated.	Drug(s) for compelling indications.‡
Stage 1 Hypertension	140–159	or 90–99	Yes	Thiazide-type diuretics for most. May consider ACEI, ARB, BB, CCB, or combination.	Drug(s) for the compelling indications.‡ Other antihypertensive drugs (diuretics, ACEI, ARB, BB, CCB) as needed.
Stage 2 Hypertension	≥160	or ≥100	Yes	Two-drug combination for most† (usually thiazide-type diuretic and ACEI or ARB or BB or CCB).	

DBP, diastolic blood pressure; SBP, systolic blood pressure.
Drug abbreviations: ACEI, angiotensin converting enzyme inhibitor; ARB, angiotensin receptor blocker; BB, beta-blocker; CCB, calcium channel blocker.
*Treatment determined by highest BP category.
†Initial combined therapy should be used cautiously in those at risk for orthostatic hypotension.
‡Treat patients with chronic kidney disease or diabetes to BP goal of <130/80 mmHg.
From the Seventh Report of the Joint National Committee on Prevention, Detection, Evaluation, and Treatment of High Blood Pressure. (2003). *JAMA, 289*(19), 2560–2572.

condition. Because hypertension is a sign, it is most likely to have many causes, just as fever has many causes. For hypertension to occur, there must be a change in one or more factors affecting peripheral resistance or cardiac output (some of these factors are outlined in Figure 32-1). In addition, there must also be a problem with the control systems that monitor or regulate pressure. Single gene mutations have been identified for a few rare types of hypertension, but most types of high blood pressure are thought to be polygenic (mutations in more than one gene) (Dominiczak et al., 2000).

Several hypotheses about the pathophysiologic bases of elevated blood pressure are associated with the concept of hypertension as a multifactorial condition. Given the overlap among these hypotheses, it is likely that aspects of all of them will eventually prove correct. Hypertension may be caused by one or more of the following:

- Increased sympathetic nervous system activity related to dysfunction of the autonomic nervous system
- Increased renal reabsorption of sodium, chloride, and water related to a genetic variation in the pathways by which the kidneys handle sodium
- Increased activity of the renin-angiotensin-aldosterone system, resulting in expansion of extracellular fluid volume and increased systemic vascular resistance
- Decreased vasodilation of the arterioles related to dysfunction of the vascular endothelium

Table 32-2 • Identifiable Causes of Hypertension

Sleep apnea
Drug-induced or related causes
Chronic kidney disease
Primary aldosteronism
Renovascular disease
Chronic steroid therapy and Cushing's syndrome
Pheochromocytoma
Coarctation of the aorta
Thyroid or parathyroid disease

From the Seventh Report of the Joint National Committee on Prevention, Detection, Evaluation, and Treatment of High Blood Pressure. (2003). *JAMA, 289*(19), 2560–2572.

- Resistance to insulin action, which may be a common factor linking hypertension, type 2 diabetes mellitus, hypertriglyceridemia, obesity, and glucose intolerance

 Gerontologic Considerations

Structural and functional changes in the heart and blood vessels contribute to increases in blood pressure that occur with age. The changes include accumulation of atherosclerotic plaque, fragmentation of arterial elastins, increased collagen deposits, and impaired vasodilation. The result of these changes is a decrease in the elasticity of the major blood vessels. Consequently, the aorta and large arteries are less able to accommodate the volume of blood pumped out by the heart (stroke volume), and the energy that would have stretched the vessels instead elevates the systolic blood pressure. Isolated systolic hypertension is more common in older adults.

Clinical Manifestations

Physical examination may reveal no abnormalities other than high blood pressure. Occasionally, retinal changes such as hemorrhages, exudates (fluid accumulation), arteriolar narrowing, and cotton-wool spots (small infarctions) occur. In severe hypertension, papilledema (swelling of the optic disc) may be seen. People with hypertension can be asymptomatic and remain so for many years. However, when specific signs and symptoms appear, they usually indicate vascular damage, with specific manifestations related to the organs served by the involved vessels. Coronary artery disease with angina or myocardial infarction is a common consequence of hypertension. Left ventricular hypertrophy occurs in response to the increased workload placed on the ventricle as it contracts against higher systemic pressure. When heart damage is extensive, heart failure ensues. Pathologic changes in the kidneys (indicated by increased blood urea nitrogen [BUN] and creatinine levels) may manifest as nocturia. Cerebrovascular involvement may lead to a stroke or transient ischemic attack (TIA), manifested by alterations in vision or speech, dizziness, weakness, a sudden fall, or temporary paralysis on one side (hemiplegia). Cerebral infarctions account for most of the strokes and TIAs in patients with hypertension.

Physiology/Pathophysiology

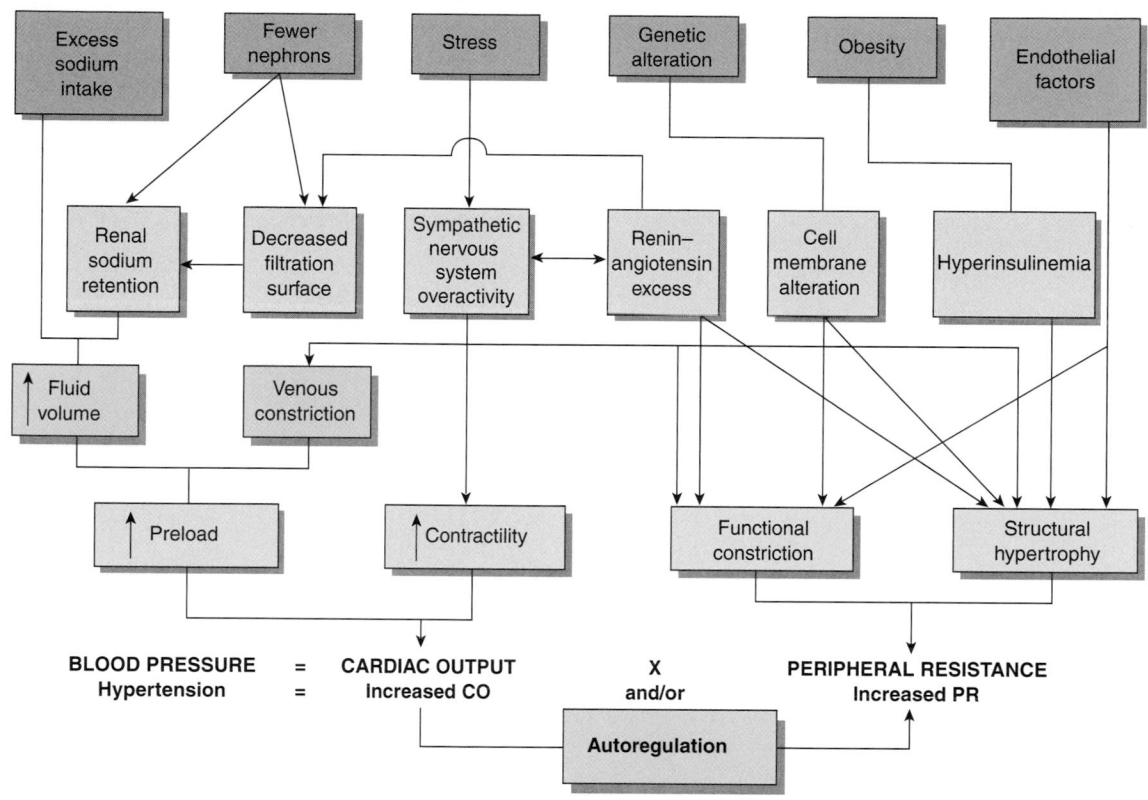

FIGURE 32-1 Factors involved in control of blood pressure, which is cardiac output multiplied by peripheral resistance. Adapted from Kaplan, N. M., Lieberman, E., & Neal, W. (2002). *Kaplan's clinical hypertension* (8th ed.). Philadelphia: Lippincott Williams & Wilkins.

Assessment and Diagnostic Evaluation

A thorough health history and physical examination are necessary. The retinas are examined, and laboratory studies are performed to assess possible target organ damage. Routine laboratory tests include urinalysis, blood chemistry (ie, analysis of sodium, potassium, creatinine, fasting glucose, and total and high-density lipoprotein [HDL] cholesterol levels), and a 12-lead electrocardiogram. Left ventricular hypertrophy can be assessed by echocardiography. Renal damage may be suggested by elevations in BUN and creatinine levels or by microalbuminuria or macroalbuminuria. Additional studies, such as creatinine clearance, renin level, urine tests, and 24-hour urine protein, may be performed.

A risk factor assessment, as advocated by the JNC 7, is needed to classify and guide treatment of hypertensive people at risk for cardiovascular damage. Risk factors and cardiovascular problems related to hypertension are presented in Chart 32-1.

Medical Management

The goal of hypertension treatment is to prevent death and complications by achieving and maintaining the arterial blood pressure at 140/90 mm Hg or lower. The JNC 7 (2003) specified a lower goal pressure of 130/80 mm Hg for people with diabetes mellitus or chronic kidney disease, defined as (1) a reduced glomerular filtration rate resulting in a serum creatinine >1.3 mg/dL in women or >1.5 mg/dL in men, or (2) an albuminuria

of >300 mg/day. The optimal management plan is inexpensive, simple, and causes the least possible disruption in the patient's life.

The management options for hypertension are summarized in Table 32-3, which lists recommended lifestyle modifications, and in the treatment algorithm issued by the JNC 7 (2003) (Fig. 32-2). The clinician uses the algorithm with the risk factor assessment data and the patient's blood pressure category to choose the initial and subsequent treatment plans for patients. Research findings demonstrate that weight loss, reduced alcohol and sodium intake, and regular physical activity are effective lifestyle adaptations to reduce blood pressure (Appel et al., 1997; Cushman et al., 1998; Hagberg et al., 2000; Sacks et al., 2001). Studies show that diets high in fruits, vegetables, and low-fat diary products can prevent the development of hypertension and can lower elevated pressures. Table 32-4 delineates the Dietary Approaches to Stop Hypertension (DASH) diet.

PHARMACOLOGIC THERAPY

For patients with uncomplicated hypertension and no specific indications for another medication, the recommended initial medications include diuretics, beta-blockers, or both. Patients are first given low doses of medication. If blood pressure does not fall to less than 140/90 mm Hg, the dose is increased gradually, and additional medications are included as necessary to achieve control. Table 32-5 describes the various pharmacologic agents used in

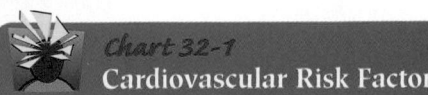

Chart 32-1

Cardiovascular Risk Factors

Major Risk Factors
- Hypertension*
- Cigarette smoking
- Obesity* (body mass index ≥30 kg/m²)
- Physical inactivity
- Dyslipidemia*
- Diabetes mellitus*
- Microalbuminuria or estimated GFR <60 mL/min
- Age (older than 55 for men, 65 for women)
- Family history of premature cardiovascular disease (men under age 55 or women under age 65)

Target Organ Damage

Heart
- Left ventricular hypertrophy
- Angina or prior myocardial infarction
- Prior coronary revascularization
- Heart failure

Brain
- Stroke or transient ischemic attack

Chronic kidney disease

Peripheral arterial disease

Retinopathy

GFR, glomerular filtration rate.

*Components of the metabolic syndrome.

Adapted from the Seventh Report of the Joint National Committee on the Prevention, Detection, Evaluation, and Treatment of High Blood Pressure. (2003). *JAMA, 289*(19), 2560–2572.

treating hypertension. When the blood pressure has been less than 140/90 mm Hg for at least 1 year, gradual reduction of the types and doses of medication is recommended. To promote compliance, clinicians try to prescribe the simplest treatment schedule possible, ideally one pill once each day.

 Gerontologic Considerations

Hypertension, particularly elevated systolic blood pressure in persons over age 50, increases the risk of death and complications (JNC 7, 2003). Treatment reduces this risk. Like younger patients, elderly patients should begin treatment with lifestyle modifications. If medications are needed to achieve the blood pressure goal of less than 140/90 mm Hg, the starting dose should be one-half that used in younger patients.

NURSING PROCESS: THE PATIENT WITH HYPERTENSION

Assessment

When hypertension is initially detected, nursing assessment involves carefully monitoring the blood pressure at frequent intervals and then, after diagnosis, at routinely scheduled intervals. The American Heart Association and the American Society of Hypertension have defined the standards for blood pressure measurement, including conditions required before measurements are made, equipment specifications, and techniques for measuring blood pressure to obtain accurate and reliable readings (Chart 32-2) (American Society of Hypertension, 1992; Perloff et al., 1993). When the patient begins an antihypertensive treatment regimen, blood pressure assessments are needed to determine the effectiveness of medication therapy and to detect any changes in blood pressure that indicate the need for a change in the treatment plan.

A complete history is obtained to assess for symptoms that indicate target organ damage (whether other body systems have been affected by the elevated blood pressure). Such symptoms may include anginal pain; shortness of breath; alterations in speech, vision, or balance; nosebleeds; headaches; dizziness; or nocturia.

During the physical examination, the nurse must also pay specific attention to the rate, rhythm, and character of the apical and peripheral pulses to detect effects of hypertension on the

Table 32-3 • Lifestyle Modifications to Manage Hypertension*†

MODIFICATION	RECOMMENDATION	APPROXIMATE SBP REDUCTION (RANGE)
Weight reduction	Maintain normal body weight (body mass index 18.5–24.9 kg/m²).	5–20 mm Hg/ 10 kg weight loss
Adopt DASH eating plan	Consume a diet rich in fruits, vegetables, and low-fat dairy products with a reduced content of saturated and total fat.	8–14 mm Hg
Dietary sodium reduction	Reduce dietary sodium intake to no more than 100 mmol per day (2.4 g sodium or 6 g sodium chloride).	2–8 mm Hg
Physical activity	Engage in regular aerobic physical activity such as brisk walking (at least 30 min per day, most days of the week).	4–9 mm Hg
Moderation of alcohol consumption	Limit consumption to no more than 2 drinks (1 oz or 30 mL ethanol; e.g., 24 oz beer, 10 oz wine, or 3 oz 80-proof whiskey) per day in most men and to no more than 1 drink per day in women and lighter-weight persons.	2–4 mm Hg

DASH, Dietary Approaches to Stop Hypertension.

*For overall cardiovascular risk reduction, stop smoking.

†The effects of implementing these modifications are dose and time dependent, and could be greater for some individuals.

From the Seventh Report of the Joint National Committee on Prevention, Detection, Evaluation, and Treatment of High Blood Pressure. (2003). *JAMA, 289*(19), 2560–2572.

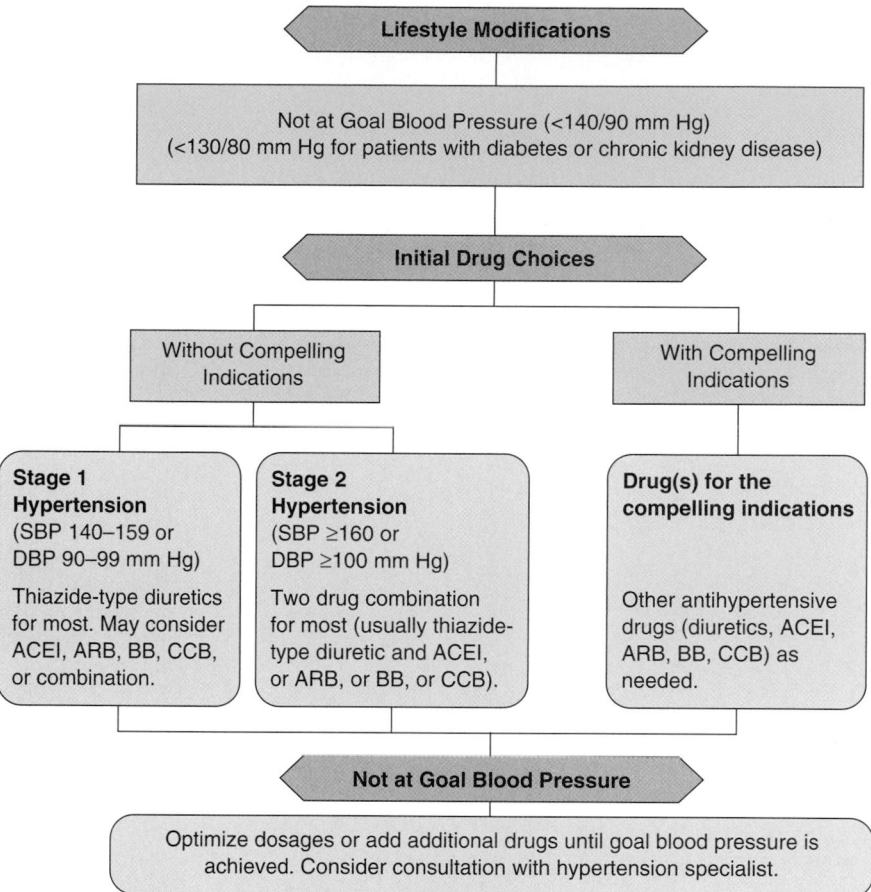

FIGURE 32-2 Algorithm for treatment of hypertension. Treatment begins with lifestyle modifications and continues with various medication regimens. Adapted from the Seventh Report of the Joint National Committee on Prevention, Detection, Evaluation, and Treatment of High Blood Pressure. (2003). *JAMA, 289*(19), 2560–2572.

heart and blood vessels. A thorough assessment can yield valuable information about the extent to which the hypertension has affected the body and about any other personal, social, or financial factors related to the condition.

Diagnosis

NURSING DIAGNOSES
Based on the assessment data, nursing diagnoses for the patient may include the following:

- Deficient knowledge regarding the relation between the treatment regimen and control of the disease process
- Noncompliance with therapeutic regimen related to side effects of prescribed therapy

COLLABORATIVE PROBLEMS/POTENTIAL COMPLICATIONS
Based on the assessment data, potential complications that may develop include the following:

- Left ventricular hypertrophy
- Myocardial infarction
- Heart failure
- TIAs
- Cerebrovascular accident (stroke or brain attack)
- Renal insufficiency and failure
- Retinal hemorrhage

Planning and Goals

The major goals for the patient include understanding of the disease process and its treatment, participation in a self-care program, and absence of complications.

Nursing Interventions

The objective of nursing care for hypertensive patients focuses on lowering and controlling the blood pressure without adverse effects and without undue cost. To achieve these goals, the nurse must

(text continues on page 864)

Table 32-4 • The DASH (Dietary Approaches to Stop Hypertension) Diet*

FOOD GROUP	NO. SERVINGS PER DAY
Grains and grain products	7–8
Vegetables	4–5
Fruits	4–5
Lowfat or fat-free dairy foods	2–3
Meat, fish, and poultry	2 or fewer
Nuts, seeds, and dry beans	4–5 weekly

*Based on 2000 calories per day.
Source: www.nhlbi.nih.gov/health/public/heart/hbp/dash/new_dash.pdf

Table 32-5 • **Medication Therapy for Hypertension**

MEDICATIONS	MAJOR ACTION	ADVANTAGES AND CONTRAINDICATIONS	EFFECTS AND NURSING CONSIDERATIONS
Purpose: To maintain blood pressure within normal ranges by the simplest and safest means possible with the fewest side effects for each individual patient			
Diuretics and Related Drugs			
Thiazide Diuretics chlorothiazide (Diuril) chlorthalidone (Hygroton) hydrochlorothiazide (Microzide, HydroDiuril) indapamide (Lozol) metolazone (Mykrox, Zaroxolyn) polythiazide (Renese) quinethazone (Hydromox)	Decrease of blood volume, renal blood flow, and cardiac output Depletion of extracellular fluid Negative sodium balance (from natriuresis), mild hypokalemia Directly affect vascular smooth muscle	Relatively inexpensive Effective orally Effective during long-term administration Mild side effects Enhance other antihypertensive medications Counter sodium retention effect of other antihypertensive medications *Contraindications:* Gout, known sensitivity to sulfonamide-derived medications, severely impaired kidney function and history of hyponatremia	Side effects include dry mouth, thirst, weakness, drowsiness, lethargy, muscle aches, muscular fatigue, tachycardia, GI disturbance. Postural hypotension may be potentiated by alcohol, barbiturates, opioids, or hot weather. Because thiazides cause loss of sodium, potassium, and magnesium, monitor for signs of electrolyte imbalance. Encourage intake of potassium-rich foods (eg, fruits). *Gerontological Considerations:* Risk of postural hypotension is significant because of volume depletion; measure blood pressure in three positions; caution patient to rise slowly.
Loop Diuretics bumetanide (Bumex) furosemide (Lasix) torsemide (Demadex)	Volume depletion Blocks reabsorption of sodium, chloride, and water in kidney	Action rapid Potent Used when thiazides fail or patient needs rapid diuresis *Contraindications:* Same as for thiazides	Volume depletion is rapid—profound diuresis can occur. Electrolyte depletion—replacement is required. Thirst, nausea, vomiting, skin rash, postural hypotension. Sweet taste noted; oral and gastric burning. *Gerontologic Considerations:* Same as for thiazides.
Potassium-Sparing Diuretics amiloride (Midamor) triamterene (Dyrenium)	Acts on distal tubule independently of aldosterone	Triamterene causes retention of potassium. *Contraindications:* Renal disease, azotemia, severe hepatic disease, hyperkalemia	Drowsiness, lethargy, headache—decrease dosage. Monitor for hyperkalemia if given with ACE inhibitor. Diarrhea and other GI symptoms—administer medication after meals. Skin eruptions, urticaria Mental confusion, ataxia (with triamterene)—dosage may need to be reduced. Gynecomastia (not for triamterene)

(continued)

Table 32-5 • **Medication Therapy for Hypertension** (Continued)

MEDICATIONS	MAJOR ACTION	ADVANTAGES AND CONTRAINDICATIONS	EFFECTS AND NURSING CONSIDERATIONS
Aldosterone Receptor Blockers eplerenone (Inspra) spironolactone (Aldactone)	Competitive inhibitors of aldosterone binding	Indicated for persons with history of myocardial infarction or symptomatic ventricular dysfunction. Spironolactone is effective in treating hypertension accompanying primary aldosteronism. Spironolactone causes retention of potassium. Contraindicated in persons with hyperkalemia and impaired renal function. Eplerenone contraindicated in diabetes mellitus with micoralbuminuria.	Monitor patients carefully for hyperkalemia if given with an ACE inhibitor Avoid use of potassium supplements or salt substitutes. Teach patients signs and symptoms of hyperkalemia
Central Alpha₂ Agonists and Other Centrally Acting Medications clonidine hydrochloride (Catapres) clonidine patch (Catapres-TTS)	Exact mode of action not understood, but acts through the central nervous system, apparently through centrally mediated alpha-adrenergic stimulation in the brain, producing blood pressure reduction	Little or no orthostatic effect. Moderately potent, and sometimes is effective when other medications fail to lower blood pressure. *Contraindications:* Severe coronary artery disease, pregnancy, children	Most common side effects are dry mouth, drowsiness, sedation, and occasional headaches and fatigue. Anorexia, malaise, and vomiting with mild disturbance of liver function have been reported. Rebound or withdrawal hypertension is relatively common; monitor blood pressure when stopping medication.
guanfacine (Tenex)	Stimulates central alpha-2 adrenergic receptors	Reduces heart rate and causes vasodilation. Serious adverse reactions are uncommon. Use with caution in persons with diminished liver function, recent myocardial infarction, or known cardiovascular disease.	Common side effects include dry mouth, dizziness, sleepiness, fatigue, headache, constipation, and impotence.
methyldopa (Aldomet)	Dopa-decarboxylase inhibitor; displaces norepinephrine from storage sites	Drug of choice for pregnant women with hypertension Useful in patients with renal failure or prostatism Does not decrease cardiac output or renal blood flow Does not induce oliguria *Contraindications:* Liver disease	Drowsiness, dizziness Dry mouth; nasal stuffiness (troublesome at first but then tends to disappear) Hemolytic anemia (a hypersensitization reaction)—positive Coombs' test *Gerontologic Considerations:* May produce mental and behavioral changes in the elderly.
reserpine (Serpasil)	Impairs synthesis and re-uptake of norepinephrine	Slows pulse, which counteracts tachycardia of hydralazine *Contraindications:* History of depression, psychosis, obesity, chronic sinusitis, peptic ulcer	May cause severe depression; report manifestations, as this may require that drug be omitted. Nasal stuffiness, which may require nasal vasoconstrictor. Increases appetite—therefore, weight control may be difficult. Recurrence of peptic ulcer—administer with meals or milk. *Gerontologic Considerations:* Depression and postural hypotension common in elderly

(continued)

Table 32-5 • **Medication Therapy for Hypertension** (Continued)

MEDICATIONS	MAJOR ACTION	ADVANTAGES AND CONTRAINDICATIONS	EFFECTS AND NURSING CONSIDERATIONS
Beta-Blockers atenolol (Tenormin) betaxolol (Kerlone) bisoprolol (Zebeta) metoprolol (Lopressor) metoprolol extended release (Toprol XL) nadolol (Corgard) propranolol (Inderal) propranolol long-acting (Inderal LA) timolol (Blocadren)	Block the sympathetic nervous system (beta-adrenergic receptors), especially the sympathetics to the heart, producing a slower heart rate and lowered blood pressure	Reduces pulse rate in patients with tachycardia and blood pressure elevation Indicated for patients who also have stable angina pectoris or have had a myocardial infarction. *Contraindications:* Bronchial asthma, allergic rhinitis, right ventricular failure from pulmonary hypertension, congestive heart failure, depression, diabetes mellitus, dyslipidemia, heart block, peripheral vascular disease, heart rate under 60 bpm	Mental depression manifested by insomnia, lassitude, weakness, and fatigue. Lightheadedness and occasional nausea, vomiting, and epigastric distress Check heart rate before giving. *Gerontologic Considerations:* Risk of toxicity is increased for elderly patients with decreased renal and liver function. Take blood pressure in three positions and observe for hypotension.
Beta-blockers With Intrinsic Sympathomimetic Activity acebutolol (Sectral) penbutolol (Levatrol) pindolol (Visken)	Block both cardiac beta$_1$- and beta$_2$-receptors. Also have antiarrhythmic activity by slowing atrioventricular conduction.	Contraindicated in heart failure, cardiac shock, or heart block. Use with caution if hepatic or renal impairment or failure.	May cause fatigue, dizziness, or lightheadedness Caution patients not to stop taking without consulting care giver as rebound hypertension can occur. Check heart rate before giving.
Alpha$_1$ Blocker doxazosin (Cardura) prazosin hydrochloride (Minipress) terazosin (Hytrin)	Peripheral vasodilator acting directly on the blood vessel; similar to hydralazine	Acts directly on the blood vessel and is an effective agent in patients with adverse reactions to hydralazine *Contraindications:* Angina pectoris and coronary artery disease. Induces tachycardia if not preceded by administration of propranolol and a diuretic.	Occasional vomiting and diarrhea, urinary frequency, and cardiovascular collapse, especially if given in addition to hydralazine without lowering the dose of the latter. Patients occasionally experience drowsiness, lack of energy, and weakness.
Combined Alpha and Beta Blockers carvedilol (Coreg) labetalol hydrochloride (Normodyne, Trandate)	Blocks alpha- and beta-adrenergic receptors; causes peripheral dilation and decreases peripheral vascular resistance	Fast-acting No decrease in renal blood flow *Contraindications:* Asthma, cardiogenic shock, severe tachycardia, heart block	Orthostatic hypotension, tachycardia
Vasodilators fenoldopam mesylate	Stimulates dopamine and alpha$_2$ adrenergic receptors	Given intravenously for hypertensive emergencies. Use with caution in persons with glaucoma, recent stroke (brain attack), asthma, hypokalemia, or diminished liver function.	Headache, flushing, hypotension, sweating, tachycardia caused by vasodilation Observe for local reactions at the injection site.
hydralazine hydrochloride (Apresoline)	Decreases peripheral resistance but concurrently elevates cardiac output Acts directly on smooth muscle of blood vessels	Not used as initial therapy; used in combination with other medications. Used also in pregnancy-induced hypertension *Contraindications:* Angina or coronary disease, congestive heart failure, hypersensitivity	Headache, tachycardia, flushing, and dyspnea may occur—can be prevented by pretreating with reserpine. Peripheral edema may require diuretics. May produce lupus erythematosus-like syndrome
minoxidil (Loniten)	Direct vasodilating action on arteriolar vessels, causing decreased peripheral vascular resistance; reduces systolic and diastolic pressures	Hypotensive effect more pronounced than with hydralazine No effect on vasomotor reflexes so does not cause postural hypotension *Contraindications:* Pheochromocytoma	Tachycardia, angina pectoris, ECG changes, edema Take blood pressure and apical pulse before administration. Monitor intake and output and daily weights. Causes hirsutism

(continued)

Table 32-5 • **Medication Therapy for Hypertension** (Continued)

MEDICATIONS	MAJOR ACTION	ADVANTAGES AND CONTRAINDICATIONS	EFFECTS AND NURSING CONSIDERATIONS
sodium nitroprusside (Nipride, Nitropress) nitroglycerin (Nitro-Bid IV, Tridil) diazoxide (Hyperstat)	Peripheral vasodilation by relaxation of smooth muscle	Fast-acting Used only in hypertensive emergencies *Contraindications:* Sepsis, azotemia, high intracranial pressure.	Dizziness, headache, nausea, edema, tachycardia, palpitations. Can cause thiocyanate and cyanide intoxication.
Angiotensin-Converting Enzyme (ACE) Inhibitors benazepril (Lotensin) captopril (Capoten) enalapril (Vasotec) enalaprilat (Vasotec IV) lisinopril (Prinivil, Zestril) moexipril (Univasc) perindopril (Aceon) quinapril (Accupril) ramipril (Altace) trandolapril (Mavik)	Inhibit conversion of angiotensin I to angiotensin II Lower total peripheral resistance	Fewer cardiovascular side effects Can be used with thiazide diuretic and digitalis Hypotension can be reversed by fluid replacement. *Contraindications:* Renal impairment, pregnancy	*Gerontologic Considerations:* Require reduced dosages and the addition of loop diuretics when there is renal dysfunction
Angiotensin II Antagonists candesartan (Atacand) eprosartan (Teveten) irbesartan (Avapro) losartan (Cozaar) olmesartan (Benicar) telmisartan (Micardis) valsartan (Diovan)	Block the effects of angiotensin II at the receptor Reduce peripheral resistance	Minimal side effects *Contraindications:* Pregnancy, renovascular disease	Monitor for hypokalemia
Calcium Channel blockers *Nondihydropyridines* diltiazem hydrochloride (Cardizem SR, Cardizem CD, Dilacor XR, Tiazac) diltiazem long-acting (Cardizem LA)	Inhibits calcium ion influx Reduces cardiac afterload	Inhibits coronary artery spasm not controlled by beta-blockers or nitrates *Contraindications:* Sick sinus syndrome; AV block; hypotension; heart failure	Do not discontinue suddenly. Observe for hypotension. Report irregular heartbeat, dizziness, edema. Instruct on regular dental care because of potential gingivitis.
verapamil immediate release (Calan, Isoptin) verapamil long-acting (Calan SR, Isoptin SR) verapamil-Coer (Covera HS, Verelan PM)	Inhibits calcium ion influx Slows velocity of conduction of cardiac impulse	Effective antiarrhythmic Rapid IV onset Blocks SA and AV node channels *Contraindications:* Sinus or AV node disease; severe heart failure; severe hypotension	Administer on empty stomach or before meal. Do not discontinue suddenly. Depression may subside when medication is discontinued. To relieve headaches, reduce noise, monitor electrolytes. Decrease dose for patients with liver or renal failure.
Dihydropyridines amlodipine (Norvasc) felodipine (Plendil) isradipine (DynaCirc CR) nicardipine sustained release (Cardene SR) nifedipine long-acting (Adalat CC, Procardia XL) nisoldipine (Sular)	Inhibit calcium ion influx across membranes Vasodilating effects on coronary and peripheral arteriole Decrease cardiac work and energy consumption, increase delivery of oxygen to myocardium	Rapid action Effective by oral or sublingual route No tendency to slow SA nodal activity or prolong AV node conduction Isolated systolic hypertension *Contraindications:* None (except heart failure for nifedipine)	Administer on empty stomach. Use with caution in diabetic patients. Small frequent meals if nausea. Muscle cramps, joint stiffness, sexual difficulties may disappear when dose decreased. Report irregular heartbeat, constipation, shortness of breath, edema. May cause dizziness.

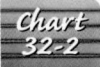

Chart 32-2 Measuring Blood Pressure

Instructions for Patient
- Avoid smoking cigarettes or drinking caffeine for 30 minutes before blood pressure is measured.
- Sit quietly for 5 minutes before the reading.
- Sit comfortably with the forearm supported at heart level on a firm surface, with both feet on the ground; avoid talking during measurement.

Equipment for Practitioner
- Mercury sphygmomanometer, recently calibrated aneroid manometer, or validated electronic device
- Choose from several cuffs of different size so that rubber bladder width is at least 40% and length at least 80% of the arm circumference

Equipment for Patient at Home
- Automatic or semiautomatic device with digital display of readings

Procedure
Assessment is based on the average of at least two readings. (If two readings differ by more than 5 mm Hg, additional readings are taken and an average reading is calculated from the results.)

Conclusion
Inform patient of the numeric blood pressure value and what it means. Emphasize the need for periodic reassessment, and encourage patients who measure blood pressure at home to keep a written record of readings.

---

support and teach the patient to adhere to the treatment regimen by implementing necessary lifestyle changes, taking medications as prescribed, and scheduling regular follow-up appointments with the health care provider to monitor progress or identify and treat any complications of disease or therapy.

INCREASING KNOWLEDGE
The patient needs to understand the disease process and how lifestyle changes and medications can control hypertension. The nurse needs to emphasize the concept of controlling hypertension rather than curing it. The nurse can encourage the patient to consult a dietitian to help develop a plan for weight loss. The program usually consists of restricting sodium and fat intake, increasing intake of fruits and vegetables, and implementing regular physical activity. Explaining that it takes 2 to 3 months for the taste buds to adapt to changes in salt intake may help the patient adjust to reduced salt intake. The patient should be advised to limit alcohol intake (see Table 32-3 for specific recommendations), and tobacco should be avoided—not because smoking is related to hypertension, but because anyone with high blood pressure is already at increased risk for heart disease, and smoking amplifies this risk. Support groups for weight control, smoking cessation, and stress reduction may be beneficial for some patients; others can benefit from the support of family and friends. The nurse assists the patient to develop and adhere to an appropriate exercise regimen, because regular activity is a significant factor in weight reduction and a blood pressure–reducing intervention in the absence of any loss in weight (JNC 7, 2003).

PROMOTING HOME AND COMMUNITY-BASED CARE
Blood pressure screenings with the sole purpose of case finding are not recommended by the National High Blood Pressure Education Program because approximately 70% of persons with hypertension are already aware of their blood pressure levels (JNC 7, 2003). If asked to participate in a blood pressure screening, the nurse should be sure that proper blood pressure measurement technique is being used (see Chart 32-2), that the manometers used are calibrated (Perloff et al., 1993), and that provision has been made to provide follow-up for any person identified as having an elevated blood pressure. Adequate time should also be allowed to teach people what the blood pressure numbers mean. Each person should be given a written record of his or her blood pressure at the screening.

Teaching Patients Self-Care
The therapeutic regimen is the responsibility of the patient in collaboration with the health care provider. Education about high blood pressure and how to manage it, including medications, lifestyle changes of diet, weight control, and exercise (see Table 32-3), setting goal blood pressures, and assistance with social support, can help the patient achieve blood pressure control. Involving family members in education programs enables them to support the patient's efforts to control hypertension. The American Heart Association and the National Heart Lung and Blood Institute provide printed and electronic patient education materials.

Written information about the expected effects and side effects of medications is important. When side effects occur, patients need to understand the importance of reporting them and to whom they should be reported. Patients need to be informed that **rebound hypertension** can occur if antihypertensive medications are suddenly stopped. Female and male patients should be informed that some medications, such as beta-blockers, may cause sexual dysfunction and that, if a problem with sexual function or satisfaction occurs, other medications are available. The nurse can encourage and teach patients to measure their blood pressure at home. This practice involves patients in their own care and emphasizes the fact that failing to take medications may result in an identifiable rise in blood pressure. Patients need to know that blood pressure varies continuously and that the range within which their pressure varies should be monitored.

Continuing Care
Regular follow-up care is imperative so that the disease process can be assessed and treated, depending on whether control or progression is found. A history and physical examination should be completed at each clinic visit. The history should include all data that pertain to any potential problem, specifically medication-related problems such as postural (orthostatic) hypotension (experienced as dizziness or lightheadedness).

Deviation from the therapeutic program is a significant problem for people with hypertension and other chronic conditions requiring lifetime management. It is estimated that 50% discontinue their medications within 1 year of beginning to take them. Blood pressure control is achieved by only 34% (JNC 7, 2003). However, when patients actively participate in self-care, including self-monitoring of blood pressure and diet, compliance increases—possibly because patients receive immediate feedback and have a greater sense of control.

Considerable effort is required by patients with hypertension to adhere to recommended lifestyle modifications and to take regularly prescribed medications. The effort needed to follow the therapeutic plan may seem unreasonable to some, particularly when they have no symptoms without medications but do have side effects with medications. The recommended lifestyle changes are listed in Table 32-3. Continued education and encouragement are usually needed to enable patients to formulate an acceptable plan that helps them live with their hypertension and adhere to the treatment plan. Compromises may have to be made about some aspects of therapy to achieve success in higher-priority goals. The nurse can assist with behavior change by supporting patients in making small changes with each visit that move them toward their goals. Another important factor is following up at each visit to see how the patient has progressed with the plans made at the prior visit. If the patient has had difficulty with a particular aspect of the plan, the patient and nurse can work together to develop an alternative or modification to the plan that the patient believes will be more successful.

MONITORING AND MANAGING POTENTIAL COMPLICATIONS

Symptoms suggesting that hypertension is progressing to the extent that target organ damage is occurring must be detected early so that appropriate treatment can be initiated accordingly. When the patient returns for follow-up care, all body systems must be assessed to detect any evidence of vascular damage. Examining the eyes with an ophthalmoscope is particularly important because retinal blood vessel damage indicates similar damage elsewhere in the vascular system. The patient is questioned about blurred vision, spots in front of the eyes, and diminished visual acuity. The heart, nervous system, and kidneys are also carefully assessed and examined. Any significant findings are promptly reported to determine whether additional diagnostic studies are required. Based on the findings, medications may be changed to improve blood pressure control.

Gerontologic Considerations

Compliance with the therapeutic program may be more difficult for elderly people. The medication regimen can be difficult to remember, and the expense can be a problem. **Monotherapy** (treatment with a single agent), if appropriate, may simplify the medication regimen and make it less expensive. Special care must be taken to ensure that the elderly patient understands the regimen and can see and read instructions, open the medication container, and get the prescription refilled. The elderly person's family or caregivers should be included in the teaching program so that they can understand the patient's needs, encourage adherence to the treatment plan, and know when and whom to call if problems arise or information is needed.

> **NURSING ALERT** The patient and caregivers should be cautioned that antihypertensive medications can cause hypotension. Low blood pressure or postural hypotension should be reported immediately. Because elderly people have impaired cardiovascular reflexes, they are often more sensitive than younger people to the extracellular volume depletion caused by diuretic therapy and to the sympathetic inhibition caused by adrenergic antagonists. The nurse teaches patients to change positions slowly when moving from a lying or sitting position to a standing position. The nurse also counsels elderly patients to use supportive devices such as hand rails and walkers when necessary to prevent falls that could result from dizziness.

Evaluation

EXPECTED PATIENT OUTCOMES

Expected patient outcomes may include the following:

1. Maintains adequate tissue perfusion
   a. Maintains blood pressure at less than 140/90 mm Hg (or less than 130/80 mm Hg for persons with diabetes mellitus or chronic kidney disease) with lifestyle modifications, medications, or both
   b. Demonstrates no symptoms of angina, palpitations, or vision changes
   c. Has stable BUN and serum creatinine levels

   d. Has palpable peripheral pulses
2. Complies with the self-care program
   a. Adheres to the dietary regimen as prescribed: reduces calorie, sodium, and fat intake; increases fruit and vegetable intake
   b. Exercises regularly
   c. Takes medications as prescribed and reports any side effects
   d. Measures blood pressure routinely
   e. Abstains from tobacco and excessive alcohol intake
   f. Keeps follow-up appointments
3. Has no complications
   a. Reports no changes in vision
   b. Exhibits no retinal damage on vision testing
   c. Maintains pulse rate and rhythm and respiratory rate within normal ranges
   d. Reports no dyspnea or edema
   e. Maintains urine output consistent with intake
   f. Has renal function test results within normal range
   g. Demonstrates no motor, speech, or sensory deficits
   h. Reports no headaches, dizziness, weakness, changes in gait, or falls

Hypertensive Crises

There are two hypertensive crises that require nursing intervention: hypertensive emergency and hypertensive urgency. Hypertensive emergencies and urgencies may occur in patients whose hypertension has been poorly controlled or in those who have abruptly discontinued their medications. Once the hypertensive crisis has been managed, a complete evaluation is performed to review the patient's ongoing treatment plan and strategies to minimize the occurrence of subsequent hypertensive crises.

HYPERTENSIVE EMERGENCY

Hypertensive emergency is a situation in which blood pressure must be lowered immediately (not necessarily to less than 140/90 mm Hg) to halt or prevent damage to the target organs. Conditions associated with hypertensive emergency include acute myocardial infarction, dissecting aortic aneurysm, and intracranial hemorrhage. Hypertensive emergencies are acute, life-threatening blood pressure elevations that require prompt treatment in an intensive care setting because of the serious target organ damage that may occur. The medications of choice in hypertensive emergencies are those that have an immediate effect. Intravenous vasodilators, including sodium nitroprusside (Nipride, Nitropress), nicardipine hydrochloride (Cardene), fenoldopam mesylate (Corlopam), enalaprilat (Vasotec I.V.), and nitroglycerin (Nitro-Bid IV, Tridil), have an immediate action that is short lived (minutes to 4 hours), and they are therefore used as the initial treatment. Table 32-5 provides for more information about these medications.

HYPERTENSIVE URGENCY

Hypertensive urgency is a situation in which blood pressure must be lowered within a few hours. Severe perioperative hypertension is considered a hypertensive urgency. Hypertensive urgencies are managed with oral doses of fast-acting agents such as loop diuretics (bumetanide [Bumex], furosemide [Lasix]), beta-blockers propranolol (Inderal), metoprolol (Lopressor), nadolol (Corgard), angiotensin-converting enzyme inhibitors (benazepril [Lotensin], captopril [Capoten], enalapril [Vasotec]), calcium antagonists (diltiazem [Cardizem], verapamil [Isoptin SR, Calan SR, Covera HS]), or alpha₂-agonists, such as clonidine (Catapres) and guanfacine (Tenex) (see Table 32-5).

Extremely close hemodynamic monitoring of the patient's blood pressure and cardiovascular status is required during treatment of hypertensive emergencies and urgencies. The exact frequency of monitoring is a matter of clinical judgment and varies with the patient's condition. The nurse may think that taking vital signs every 5 minutes is appropriate if the blood pressure is changing rapidly or may check vital signs at 15 or 30 minutes intervals if the situation is more stable. A precipitous drop in blood pressure can occur, which would require immediate action to restore blood pressure to an acceptable level.

Critical Thinking Exercises

1. You are a nursing student assigned to a hypertension clinic. One of the patients is a 58-year-old telemarketer. During the physical assessment, the patient, who is 5 feet 6 inches tall and weighs 180 lb, asks you what he can do to reduce his blood pressure. How would you answer this patient's question? Identify what additional data you need to consider before you answer the patient's question. How would your assessment and plan change if the patient also had degenerative arthritis of his knees?

2. You are a home care nurse. One of your patients is an elderly man who lives alone and who has hypertension along with other health problems, including heart failure and atrial fibrillation. During a home visit, you learn that he has difficulty taking his medications as directed. What questions come to mind as you consider the situation? How will you direct your assessment to identify factors contributing to this problem? Using the factors identified, develop a sample follow-up home care teaching plan for this patient.

REFERENCES AND SELECTED READINGS

Books

Braunwald, E., Zipes, D. P., & Libby, P. (Eds.) (2001). *Heart disease: A textbook of cardiovascular medicine.* (6th ed.) Philadelphia: W. B. Saunders.

Kaplan, N. (2002). *Clinical hypertension* (8th ed.). Philadelphia: Lippincott Williams & Wilkins.

Journals

American Society of Hypertension. (1992). Recommendations for routine blood pressure measurement by indirect cuff sphygmomanometry. *American Journal of Hypertension, 5* (4, Pt. 1), 207–209.

Appel, L. J., Moore, T. J., Obarzanek, E., Vollmer, W. M., Svetkey, L. P., Sacks, F. M., et al. (1997). A clinical trial of the effects of dietary patterns on blood pressure. *New England Journal of Medicine, 336*(16), 1117–1124.

Burnier, M., & Brunner, H. R. (2000). Angiotensin II receptor antagonists. *Lancet, 355*(9204), 637–645.

Chase, S. L. (2000). Hypertensive crisis. *RN, 63*(6), 62–68.

Chobanian, A. V., Bakris, G. L., Black, H. R., Cushman, W. C., Green, L. A., Izzo, J. L., Jr., et al. (2003). The Seventh Report of the Joint National Committee on Prevention, Detection, Evaluation, and Treatment of High Blood Pressure: The JNC 7 report (Erratum in: *JAMA, 2003 Jul 9; 290*[2]:197). *JAMA, 289*(19), 2560–2572.

Cushman, W. C., Cutler, J. A., Hanna, E., Bingham, S. F., Follmann, D., Harford, T., et al. (1998). Prevention and treatment of hypertension study (PATHS): Effects of an alcohol treatment program on blood pressure. *Archives of Internal Medicine, 158*(11), 1197–1207.

Dominiczak, A. F., Negrin, D. C., Clark, J. S., Brosnan, M. J., McBride, M. W., & Alexander, M. Y. (2000). Genes and hypertension: From gene mapping in experimental models to vascular gene transfer strategies. *Hypertension, 35* (1, Pt. 2), 164–172.

Gress, T. W., Nieto, F. J., Shahar, E., Wofford, M. R., & Brancati, F. L. (2000). Hypertension and antihypertensive therapy as risk factors for type 2 diabetes mellitus. *New England Journal of Medicine, 342*(13), 905–912.

Gus, M., Fuchs, F. D., Pimentel, M., Rosa, D., Melo, A. G., & Moreira, L. B. (2001). Behavior of ambulatory blood pressure surrounding episodes of headache in mildly hypertensive patients. *Archives of Internal Medicine, 161*(2), 252–255.

Hagberg, J. M., Park, J. J., & Brown, M. D. (2000). The role of exercise training in the treatment of hypertension: An update. *Sports Medicine, 30*(3), 193–206.

Hajjar, I., & Kotchen, T. A. (2003). Trends in prevalence, awareness, treatment, and control of hypertension in the United States, 1988–2000. *JAMA, 290*(2), 199–206.

Lewington, S., Clarke, R., Qizilbash, N., Peto, R., & Collins, R. (2002). Age-specific relevance of usual blood pressure to vascular mortality: A meta-analysis of individual data for one million adults in 61 prospective studies. *Lancet, 360*(9349), 1903–1913.

McAlister, F. A., & Straus, S. E. (2001). Evidence based treatment of hypertension. Measurement of blood pressure: An evidence based review. *British Medical Journal, 322*(7291), 908–911.

Miller, N. H., Hill, M., Kottke, T., & Ockene, I. S. (1997). The multi-level compliance challenge: Recommendations for a call to action. A statement for healthcare professionals. *Circulation, 95*(4), 1085–1090.

Neal, B., MacMahon, S., & Chapman, N. (2000). Effects of ACE inhibitors, calcium antagonists, and other blood-pressure-lowering drugs: Results of prospectively designed overviews of randomised trials. Blood Pressure Lowering Treatment Trialists' Collaboration. *Lancet, 356*(9246), 1955–1964.

Perloff, D., Grim, C., Flack, J., Frohlich, E. D., Hill, M., McDonald, M., et al. (1993). Human blood pressure determination by sphygmomanometry. *Circulation, 88*, (5, Pt. 1), 2460–2467.

Perry, H. M., Jr., Davis, B. R., Price, T. R., Applegate, W. B., Fields, W. S., Guralnik, J. M., et al. (2000). Effect of treating isolated systolic hypertension on the risk of developing various types and subtypes of stroke: The Systolic Hypertension in the Elderly Program (SHEP). *Journal of the American Medical Association, 284*(4), 465–471.

Pickering, T. G. (1999). Contempo 1999: Advances in the treatment of hypertension. *Journal of the American Medical Association, 281*(2), 114–116.

Sacks, F. M., Svetkey, L. P., Vollmer, W. M., Appel, L. J., Bray, G. A., Harsha, D., et al. (2001). Effects on blood pressure of reduced dietary sodium and the dietary approaches to stop hypertension (DASH) diet. *New England Journal of Medicine, 344*(1), 3–10.

RESOURCES AND WEBSITES

American Heart Association National Center, 7272 Greenville Ave., Dallas, TX 75231-4596; 1-214-373-6300; fax, 1-214-706-1191; http://www.americanheart.org/hbp/.

Centers for Disease Control and Prevention (CDC), 600 Clifton Rd., Atlanta, GA 30333; cardiovascular health program: 1-404-639-3534 or 1-800-311-3435; http://www.cdc.gov/nccdphp/cvd/.

Heart and Stroke Foundation of Canada, 222 Queen St., Suite 1402, Ottawa, Ontario K1P5V9, 1-613-569-4361; fax, 1-613-569-3278; http://www.heartandstroke.ca/.

National Heart, Lung, and Blood Institute, NHLBI Information Center, P.O. Box 30105, Bethesda, MD 20824-0105; Health Information: High Blood Pressure Information, http://www.nhlbi.nih.gov/health/public/heart/index.html.

World Health Association (WHO), Avenue Appia 20, 1211 Geneva 27 Switzerland; cardiovascular diseases: http://www.who.int/ncd/cvd/index.htm.

Assessment and Management of Patients With Hematologic Disorders

On completion of this chapter, the learner will be able to:

1. Describe the process of hematopoiesis.
2. Describe the processes involved in maintaining hemostasis.
3. Differentiate between the hypoproliferative and the hemolytic anemias and compare and contrast the physiologic mechanisms, clinical manifestations, medical management, and nursing interventions for each.
4. Use the nursing process as a framework for care of patients with anemia.
5. Compare the leukemias, their incidence, physiologic alterations, clinical manifestations, management, and prognosis.
6. Use the nursing process as a framework for care of patients with acute leukemia.
7. Use the nursing process as a framework for care of patients with lymphoma or multiple myeloma.
8. Use the nursing process as a framework for care of patients with bleeding disorders.
9. Identify therapies for blood disorders, including the nursing implications for the administration of blood and blood components.

*U*nlike many other body systems, the hematologic system truly encompasses the entire human body. Patients with hematologic disorders can be quite challenging to nurses because they often have significant abnormalities in blood tests but few or no symptoms. It is therefore imperative that nurses have a good understanding of the pathophysiology of the patient's condition and can make a thorough assessment that relies heavily on the interpretation of laboratory tests. It is equally important for the nurse to anticipate potential patient needs and to target nursing interventions accordingly. Because it is so important to the understanding of most hematologic diseases, a basic appreciation of blood cells and bone marrow function is necessary.

Anatomic and Physiologic Overview

The hematologic system consists of the blood and the sites where blood is produced, including the bone marrow and the **reticuloendothelial system (RES)**. Blood is a specialized organ that differs from other organs in that it exists in a fluid state. Blood is

Glossary

absolute neutrophil count (ANC): a mathematical calculation of the actual number of neutrophils in the circulation, derived from the total WBCs and the percentage of neutrophils counted in a microscope's visual field; provides a rough indication of infection risk

anemia: decreased RBC count

anergy: diminished reactivity to antigens (transient or complete)

angiogenesis: formation of new blood vessels, such as in a healing wound or in a malignant tumor

angular cheilosis: cracking sore at corner of mouth

aplasia: lack of cellular development (eg, of cells within the bone marrow)

apoptosis: complex process of programmed cell death

band cell: slightly immature neutrophil

blast cell: primitive WBC

cytokines: hormones produced by leukocytes that are vital to regulation of hematopoiesis, apoptosis, and immune responses

D-dimer: test that measures fibrin breakdown; considered to be more specific than fibrin degradation products in the diagnosis of disseminated intravascular coagulation (DIC)

differentiation: development of functions and characteristics that are different from those of the parent stem cell

dysplasia: abnormal development (eg, of blood cells); size, shape and appearance of cells are altered

ecchymosis: bruise

erythrocyte: see RBC

erythrocyte sedimentation rate (ESR): laboratory test that measures the rate of settling of RBCs; elevation is indicative of inflammation; also called the "sed rate"

erythroid cells: broad term used in reference to any cell that is or will become a mature RBC

erythropoiesis: process of formation of RBCs

erythropoietin: hormone produced primarily by the kidney; necessary for erythropoiesis

fibrin: filamentous protein; basis of thrombus and blood clot

fibrinogen: protein converted into fibrin to form thrombus and clot

granulocyte: granulated WBC (neutrophil, eosinophil, basophil); sometimes used synonymously with neutrophil

granulocytopenia: fewer than normal granulocytes

hematocrit: percentage of total blood volume consisting of RBCs

hematopoiesis: complex process of the formation and maturation of blood cells

hemoglobin: iron-containing protein of RBCs; delivers oxygen to tissues

hemolysis: destruction of RBCs; can occur within or outside of the vasculature

hemosiderin: iron-containing pigment derived from breakdown of hemoglobin

hemostasis: intricate balance between clot formation and clot dissolution

histiocytes: cells present in all loose connective tissue, capable of phagocytosis; part of the RES

hyperplasia: abnormally increased proliferation of normal cells

hypochromia: pallor within the RBC caused by decreased hemoglobin content

left shift, or **shift to the left:** increased release of immature forms of WBCs from the bone marrow in response to need

leukocyte: see WBC

leukemia: uncontrolled proliferation of WBCs, often immature

leukopenia: less than normal amount of WBCs in circulation

lymphoid: pertaining to lymphocytes

lymphocyte: form of WBC involved in immune functions

lysis: destruction of cells

macrocytosis: larger than normal RBCs

macrophage: cells of the RES that are capable of phagocytosis

mast cell: cells found in connective tissue involved in defense of the body and coagulation

microcytosis: smaller than normal RBCs

monocyte: large WBC that becomes a macrophage when it leaves the circulation and moves into body tissues

myeloid: pertaining to nonlymphoid blood cells that differentiate into RBCs, platelets, monocytes and macrophages, neutrophils, eosinophils, basophils, and mast cells

myelopoiesis: formation and maturation of cells derived from myeloid stem cell

neutropenia: lower than normal number of neutrophils

neutrophil: fully mature WBC capable of phagocytosis; primary defense against bacterial infection

normochromic: normal RBC color, indicating normal amount of hemoglobin

normocytic: normal size of RBC

nucleated RBCs: immature form of RBC; portion of nucleus remains within the red cell; not normally seen in circulating blood

oxyhemoglobin: combined form of oxygen and hemoglobin; found in arterial blood

pancytopenia: abnormal decrease in WBCs, RBCs, and platelets

petechiae: tiny capillary hemorrhages

phagocytosis: process of ingestion and digestion of bacteria

plasma: liquid portion of blood

plasminogen: protein that is converted to plasmin to dissolve thrombi and clots

platelet: thrombocyte; a cellular component of blood involved in blood coagulation

poikilocytosis: variation in shape of RBCs

polycythemia: excess RBCs

RBC: red blood cell, erythrocyte; a cellular component of blood involved in the transport of oxygen and carbon dioxide

red blood cell: see RBC

reticulocytes: slightly immature RBCs, usually only 1% of total circulating RBCs

reticuloendothelial system (RES): complex system of cells throughout body capable of phagocytosis

serum: portion of blood remaining after coagulation occurs

stem cell: primitive cell, capable of self-replication and differentiation into myeloid or lymphoid stem cell

thrombin: enzyme necessary to convert fibrinogen into fibrin clot

thrombocyte: see platelet

thrombocytopenia: lower than normal platelet count

thrombocytosis: higher than normal platelet count

WBC: white blood cells, leukocytes; cellular components of blood involved in defense of the body; subtypes include neutrophils, eosinophils, basophils, monocytes, and lymphocytes

white blood cell: see WBC

composed of plasma and various types of cells. **Plasma** is the fluid portion of blood; it contains various proteins, such as albumin, globulin, **fibrinogen**, and other factors necessary for clotting, as well as electrolytes, waste products, and nutrients. About 55% of blood volume is plasma.

BLOOD

The cellular component of blood consists of three primary cell types (Table 33-1): **RBCs (red blood cells or erythrocytes)**, **WBCs (white blood cells or leukocytes)**, and **platelets (thrombocytes)**. These cellular components of blood normally make up 40% to 45% of the blood volume. Because most blood cells have a short life span, the need for the body to replenish its supply of cells is continuous; this process is termed **hematopoiesis.** The primary site for hematopoiesis is the bone marrow. During embryonic development and in other conditions, the liver and spleen may also be involved.

Under normal conditions, the adult bone marrow produces about 175 billion RBCs, 70 billion **neutrophils** (mature form of a WBC), and 175 billion platelets each day. When the body needs more blood cells, as in infection (when WBCs are needed to fight the invading pathogen) or in bleeding (when more RBCs are required), the marrow increases its production of the cells required. Thus, under normal conditions, the marrow responds to increased demand and releases adequate numbers of cells into the circulation.

The volume of blood in humans is approximately 7% to 10% of the normal body weight and amounts to 5 to 6 L. Circulating through the vascular system and serving as a link between body organs, the blood carries oxygen absorbed from the lungs and nutri-

ents absorbed from the gastrointestinal tract to the body cells for cellular metabolism. Blood also carries waste products produced by cellular metabolism to the lungs, skin, liver, and kidneys, where they are transformed and eliminated from the body. Blood also carries hormones, antibodies, and other substances to their sites of action or use.

To function, blood must remain in its normally fluid state. Because blood is fluid, the danger always exists that trauma can lead to loss of blood from the vascular system. To prevent this, an intricate clotting mechanism is activated when necessary to seal any leak in the blood vessels. Excessive clotting is equally dangerous, because it can obstruct blood flow to vital tissues. To prevent this, the body has a fibrinolytic mechanism that eventually dissolves clots (thrombi) formed within blood vessels. The balance between these two systems, clot (thrombus) formation and clot (thrombus) dissolution or fibrinolysis, is called **hemostasis**.

BONE MARROW

The bone marrow is the site of hematopoiesis, or blood cell formation (Fig. 33-1). In a child all skeletal bones are involved, but as the child ages marrow activity decreases. By adulthood, marrow activity is usually limited to the pelvis, ribs, vertebrae, and sternum.

Marrow is one of the largest organs of the body, making up 4% to 5% of total body weight. It consists of islands of cellular components (red marrow) separated by fat (yellow marrow). As the adult ages, the proportion of active marrow is gradually replaced by fat; however, in the healthy person, the fat can again be replaced by active marrow when more blood cell production is required. In adults with disease that causes marrow destruction, fibrosis, or scarring, the liver and spleen can also resume production of blood cells by a process known as extramedullary hematopoiesis.

The marrow is highly vascular. Within it are primitive cells called **stem cells**. The stem cells have the ability to self-replicate, thereby ensuring a continuous supply of stem cells throughout the life cycle. When stimulated to do so, stem cells can begin a process of **differentiation** into either **myeloid** or **lymphoid** stem cells. These stem cells are committed to produce specific types of blood cells. Lymphoid stem cells produce either T or B **lymphocytes**. Myeloid stem cells differentiate into three broad cell types: RBCs, WBCs, and platelets. Thus, with the exception of lymphocytes, all blood cells are derived from the myeloid stem cell. A defect in the myeloid stem cell can cause problems not only with WBC production but also with RBC and platelet production. The entire process of hematopoiesis is highly complex. Research has identified many of the complex mechanisms involved, often at the molecular level. A thorough description of these processes is beyond the scope of this textbook; however, some mechanisms against which a specific treatment is targeted are briefly described in the relevant disease-specific sections of this chapter.

BLOOD CELLS

Red Blood Cells (RBCs)

The normal RBC is a biconcave disk that resembles a soft ball compressed between two fingers (Fig. 33-2). It has a diameter of about 8 μm and is so flexible that it can pass easily through capillaries that may be as small as 2.8 μm in diameter. The RBC membrane is so thin that gases, such as oxygen and carbon dioxide, can easily diffuse across it; the disk shape provides a large surface area that facilitates the absorption and release of oxygen molecules.

Table 33-1 • **Blood Cells**

CELL TYPE	MAJOR FUNCTION
WBC (Leukocyte)	Fights infection
Neutrophil	Essential in preventing or limiting bacterial infection via phagocytosis; average life span is 2 to 4 h
Monocyte	Enters tissue as macrophage; highly phagocytic, especially against fungus; immune surveillance
Eosinophil	Involved in allergic reactions (neutralizes histamine); digests foreign proteins
Basophil	Contains histamine; integral part of hypersensitivity reactions
Lymphocyte	Integral component of immune system
T lymphocyte	Responsible for cell-mediated immunity; recognizes material as "foreign" (surveillance system)
B lymphocyte	Responsible for humoral immunity; many mature into plasma cells to form antibodies
Plasma cell	Secretes immunoglobulin (Ig, antibody); most mature form of B lymphocyte
RBC (Erythrocyte)	Carries hemoglobin to provide oxygen to tissues; average life span is 120 days
Platelet (Thrombocyte)	Fragment of megakaryocyte, not really a cell; provides basis for coagulation to occur; maintains hemostasis; average life span is 10 days

Physiology/Pathophysiology

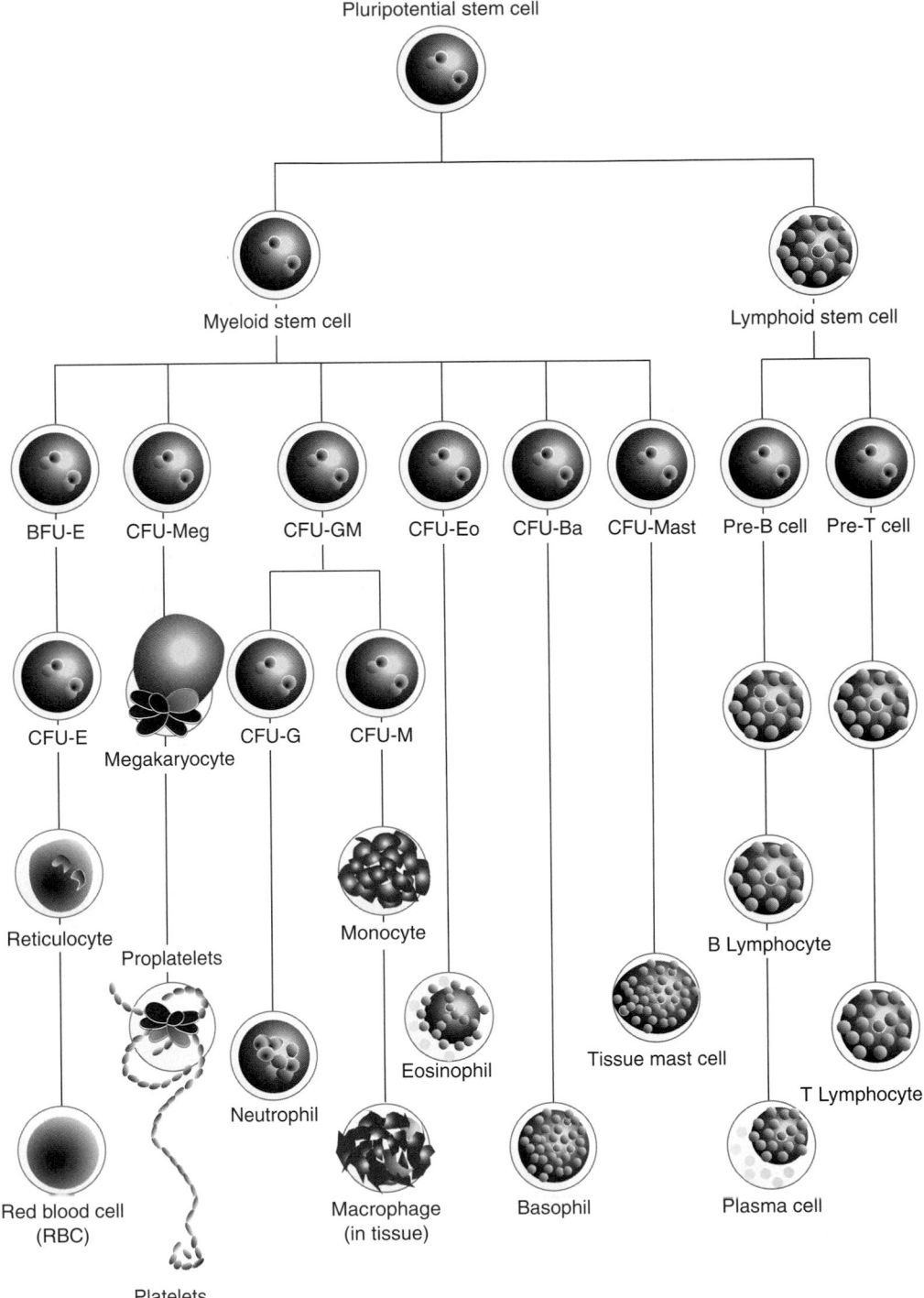

FIGURE 33-1 Hematopoiesis. Uncommitted (pluripotent) stem cells can differentiate into myeloid or lymphoid stem cells. These stem cells then undergo a complex process of differentiation and maturation into normal cells that are released into the circulation. The myeloid stem cell is responsible not only for all nonlymphoid white blood cells (WBCs) but also for the production of red blood cells (RBCs) and platelets. Each step of the differentiation process depends in part on the presence of specific growth factors for each cell type. When the stem cells are dysfunctional, they may respond inadequately to the need for more cells, or they may respond excessively, sometimes uncontrollably, as in leukemia. Adapted from Amgen, Inc., 1995, Thousand Oaks, CA.

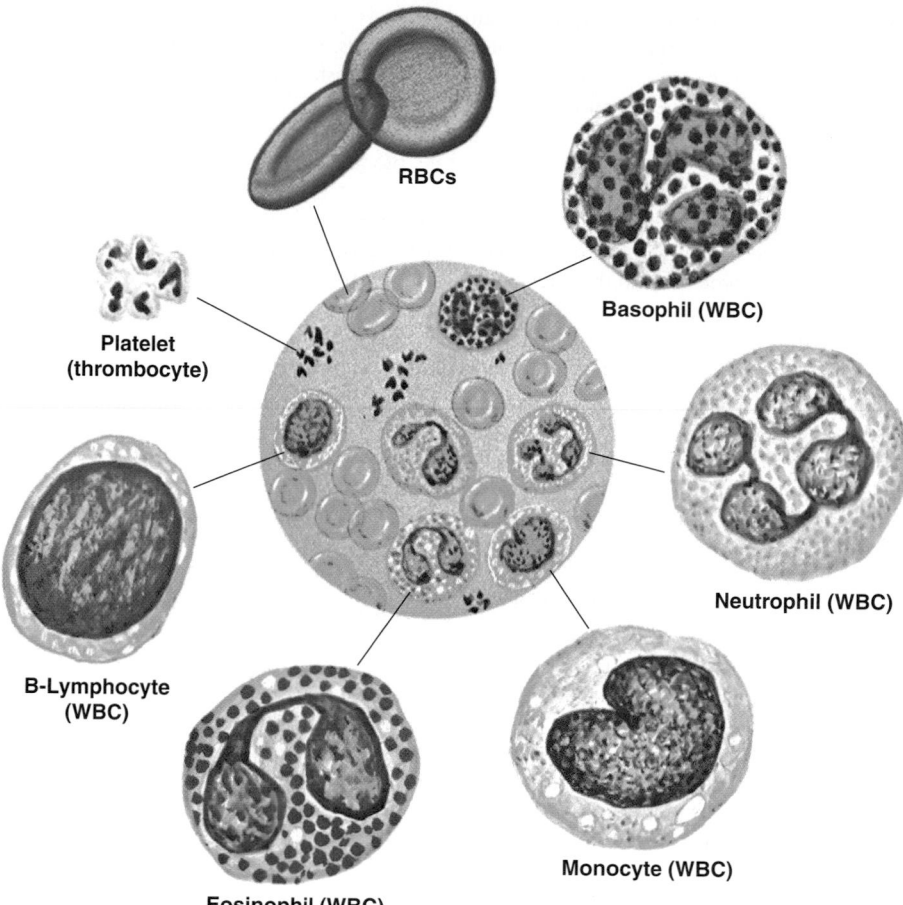

RBCs

Basophil (WBC)

Platelet
(thrombocyte)

Neutrophil (WBC)

B-Lymphocyte
(WBC)

Monocyte (WBC)

Eosinophil (WBC)

FIGURE 33-2 Normal types of blood cells.

Mature RBCs consist primarily of **hemoglobin**, which contains iron and makes up 95% of the cell mass. RBCs have no nuclei, and they have many fewer metabolic enzymes than do most other cells. The presence of a large amount of hemoglobin enables the RBC to perform its principal function, the transport of oxygen between the lungs and tissues. Occasionally the marrow releases slightly immature forms of RBCs, called **reticulocytes**, into the circulation. This occurs as a normal response to an increased demand for RBCs (as in bleeding) or in some disease states.

The oxygen-carrying hemoglobin molecule is made up of four subunits, each containing a heme portion attached to a globin chain. Iron is present in the heme component of the molecule. An important property of heme is its ability to bind to oxygen loosely and reversibly. Oxygen readily binds to hemoglobin in the lungs and is carried as **oxyhemoglobin** in arterial blood. Oxyhemoglobin is a brighter red than hemoglobin that does not contain oxygen (reduced hemoglobin), which is why arterial blood is a brighter red than venous blood. The oxygen readily dissociates (detaches) from hemoglobin in the tissues, where the oxygen is needed for cellular metabolism. In venous blood, hemoglobin combines with hydrogen ions produced by cellular metabolism and thus buffers excessive acid. Whole blood normally contains about 15 g of hemoglobin per 100 mL of blood.

ERYTHROPOIESIS

Erythroblasts arise from the primitive myeloid stem cells in bone marrow. The erythroblast is a nucleated cell that, in the process of maturing within the bone marrow, accumulates hemoglobin and gradually loses its nucleus. At this stage, the cell is known as a reticulocyte. Further maturation into an RBC entails the loss of the dark-staining material and slight shrinkage. The mature RBC is then released into the circulation. Under conditions of rapid **erythropoiesis** (RBC production), reticulocytes and other immature cells (eg, **nucleated RBCs**) may be released prematurely into the circulation.

Differentiation of the primitive myeloid stem cell of the marrow into an erythroblast is stimulated by **erythropoietin**, a hormone produced primarily by the kidney. If the kidney detects low levels of oxygen (as would occur in **anemia**, in which fewer RBCs are available to bind oxygen, or in people living at high altitudes), the release of erythropoietin is increased. The increased erythropoietin then stimulates the marrow to increase production of RBCs. The entire process typically takes 5 days.

For normal RBC production, the bone marrow also requires iron, vitamin B_{12}, folic acid, pyridoxine (vitamin B_6), protein, and other factors. A deficiency of these factors during erythropoiesis can result in decreased RBC production and anemia.

Iron Stores and Metabolism. The average daily diet in the United States contains 10 to 15 mg of elemental iron; normally 0.5 to 1 mg of ingested iron is absorbed from the small intestine. The rate of iron absorption is regulated by the amount of iron already stored in the body and by the rate of RBC production. Additional amounts of iron, up to 2 mg daily, must be absorbed by women to replace blood lost during menstruation. Total body iron content in the average adult is approximately 3 g, most of which is present in hemoglobin or in one of its breakdown products. Iron is stored in the small intestine as ferritin and in reticuloendothelial cells. When required, the iron is released into the plasma, binds to transferrin, and is transported into the membranes of the normoblasts (RBC precursor cells) within the marrow, where it is incorporated into hemoglobin. Iron is lost in the feces, either in bile, blood, or mucosal cells from the intestine.

The concentration of iron in blood is normally about 75 to 175 μg/dL (13 to 31 μmol/L) for men and 65 to 165 μg/dL (11 to 29 μmol/L) for women. With iron deficiency, bone marrow iron stores are rapidly depleted; hemoglobin synthesis is depressed, and the RBCs produced by the marrow are small and low in hemoglobin. Iron deficiency in the adult generally indicates that blood has been lost from the body (eg, from bleeding in the gastrointestinal tract or heavy menstrual flow). In the adult, lack of dietary iron is rarely the sole cause of iron deficiency anemia. The source of iron deficiency should be investigated promptly, because iron deficiency in an adult may be a sign of bleeding in the gastrointestinal tract or colon cancer.

Vitamin B₁₂ and Folic Acid Metabolism. Vitamin B_{12} and folic acid are required for the synthesis of DNA in many tissues, but deficiencies of either of these vitamins have the greatest effect on erythropoiesis. Both vitamin B_{12} and folic acid are derived from the diet. Folic acid is absorbed in the proximal small intestine, but only small amounts are stored within the body. If the diet is deficient in folic acid, stores within the body quickly become depleted. Because vitamin B_{12} is found only in foods of animal origin, strict vegetarians may ingest little B_{12}. Vitamin B_{12} combines with intrinsic factor produced in the stomach. The vitamin B_{12}–intrinsic factor complex is absorbed in the distal ileum. People who have had a partial or total gastrectomy may have limited amounts of intrinsic factor, and therefore the absorption of B_{12} may be diminished. The effects of either decreased absorption or decreased intake of B_{12} are not apparent for 2 to 4 years.

Vitamin B_{12} and folic acid deficiencies are characterized by the production of abnormally large RBCs called megaloblasts. Because these cells are abnormal, many are sequestered (trapped) while still in the bone marrow, and their rate of release is decreased. Some of these cells actually die in the marrow before they can be released into the circulation. This results in megaloblastic anemia.

RED BLOOD CELL DESTRUCTION

The average life span of a normal circulating RBC is 120 days. Aged RBCs lose their elasticity and become trapped in small blood vessels, particularly in the spleen. They are removed from the blood by the reticuloendothelial cells, particularly in the liver and the spleen. As the RBCs are destroyed, their hemoglobin is largely recycled. Some hemoglobin also breaks down to form bilirubin and is secreted in the bile. Most of the iron is recycled to form new hemoglobin molecules within the bone marrow; small amounts are lost daily in the feces and urine and monthly in menstrual flow.

White Blood Cells (WBCs)

Leukocytes are divided into two general categories: granulocytes and lymphocytes. In normal blood, the total leukocyte count is 5,000 to 10,000 cells per cubic millimeter. Of these, approximately 60% to 70% are granulocytes and 30% to 40% are lymphocytes. Primarily, WBCs protect the body against infection and tissue injury.

GRANULOCYTES

Granulocytes are defined by the presence of granules in the cytoplasm of the cell. Granulocytes are divided into three main subgroups, which are characterized by the staining properties of these granules (see Fig. 33-2). Eosinophils have bright-red granules in their cytoplasm, whereas the granules in basophils stain deep blue. The third and by far the most numerous cell in this class is the neutrophil, with granules that stain a pink to violet hue. Neutrophils are also called polymorphonuclear neutrophils (PMNs, or polys) or segmented neutrophils (segs).

The nucleus of the mature neutrophil has multiple lobes (usually two to five) that are connected by thin filaments of nuclear material, a "segmented" nucleus; it is usually twice the size of an RBC. The somewhat less mature granulocyte has a single-lobed, elongated nucleus and is called a **band cell**. Ordinarily, band cells account for only a small percentage of circulating granulocytes, although their percentage can increase greatly under conditions in which neutrophil production increases, such as infection. An increased number of band cells is sometimes called a "**left shift**" or "**shift to the left.**" (Traditionally, the diagram of neutrophil maturation shows the stem cell on the left with progressive maturation stages toward the right, ending with a fully mature neutrophil on the right side. A shift to the left indicates that more immature cells are present in the blood than normally occurs.)

Granulocyte production from the myeloid stem cell pool results in the gradual differentiation of these cells from a myeloid **blast cell** into a fully mature neutrophil. The process, called **myelopoiesis**, is highly complex and depends on many factors. These factors, including specific **cytokines** such as growth factors, are normally present within the marrow itself. As the blast cell matures, the cytoplasm of the cell changes in color (from blue to violet) and granules begin to form with the cytoplasm. The shape of the nucleus also changes. The entire process of maturation and differentiation takes about 10 days (see Fig. 33-1). Once the neutrophil is released into the circulation from the marrow, it stays there for only about 6 hours before it migrates into the body tissues to perform its function of **phagocytosis** (ingestion and digestion of bacteria and particles) (Fig. 33-3). Here, neutrophils last no more than 1 to 2 days before they die. The number of circulating granulocytes found in the healthy person is relatively constant, but in infection large numbers of these cells are rapidly released into the circulation.

MONONUCLEAR WHITE BLOOD CELLS (AGRANULOCYTES)

Monocytes. **Monocytes** (also called mononuclear leukocytes) are WBCs with a single-lobed nucleus and a granule-free cytoplasm—hence the term *agranulocyte*. In normal adult blood, monocytes account for approximately 5% of the total WBCs. Monocytes are the largest of the WBCs. Produced by the bone marrow, they remain in the circulation for a short time before entering the tissues and transforming into **macrophages**. Macrophages are particularly active in the spleen, liver, peritoneum, and the alveoli of the lungs.

Lymphocytes. Mature lymphocytes are small cells with scanty cytoplasm. Immature lymphocytes are produced in the marrow from the lymphoid stem cells. A second major source of production is the cortex of the thymus. Cells derived from the thymus are known as T lymphocytes (or T cells); those derived from the marrow can also be T cells but are more commonly B lymphocytes (or B cells). Lymphocytes complete their differentiation and maturation primarily in the lymph nodes and in the lymphoid tissue of the intestine and spleen after exposure to a specific antigen. Mature lymphocytes are antigen-specific cells.

Physiology/Pathophysiology

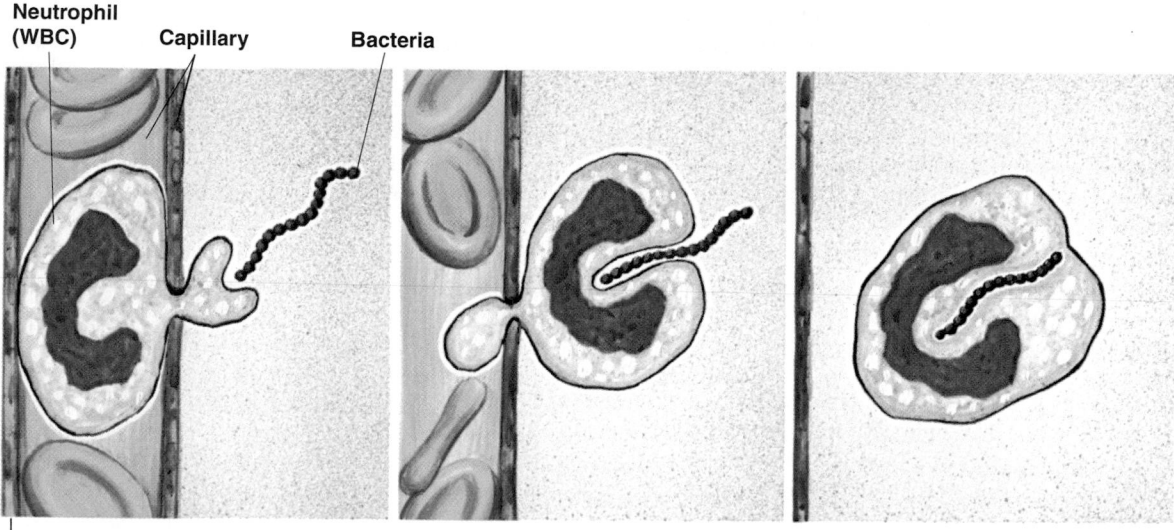

Neutrophil
(WBC)   Capillary   Bacteria

Endothelial cell

FIGURE 33-3 Phagocytosis. When foreign matter (such as bacteria or dead tissue) comes in contact with the cell membrane of the neutrophil, the membrane surrounds and pinches off the area, leaving the membrane intact. Thus, the engulfed material is left in a vacuole within the neutrophil, where enzymes within the cell destroy the foreign material.

FUNCTION OF WHITE BLOOD CELLS

WBCs protect the body from invasion by bacteria and other foreign entities. The major function of neutrophils is phagocytosis (see Fig. 33-3). Neutrophils arrive at the site within 1 hour after the onset of an inflammatory reaction and initiate phagocytosis, but they are short-lived. An influx of monocytes follows; these cells continue their phagocytic activities for long periods as macrophages. This process constitutes a second line of defense for the body against inflammation and infection. Although neutrophils can often work adequately against bacteria without the need for excessive involvement with macrophages, macrophages are particularly effective against fungi and viruses. Macrophages also digest senescent (aging or aged) blood cells, such as RBCs, primarily within the spleen.

The primary function of lymphocytes is to produce substances that aid in attacking foreign material. One group of lymphocytes (T lymphocytes) kills foreign cells directly or releases a variety of lymphokines, substances that enhance the activity of phagocytic cells. T lymphocytes are responsible for delayed allergic reactions, rejection of foreign tissue (eg, transplanted organs), and destruction of tumor cells. This process is known as *cellular immunity*. The other group of lymphocytes (B lymphocytes) is capable of differentiating into plasma cells. Plasma cells, in turn, produce immunoglobulin (Ig), or antibodies, which are protein molecules that destroy foreign material by several mechanisms. This process is known as *humoral immunity*.

Eosinophils and basophils function in hypersensitivity reactions. Eosinophils are important in the phagocytosis of parasites. The increase in eosinophil levels in allergic states indicates that these cells are involved in the hypersensitivity reaction; their function there is to neutralize histamine. Basophils produce and store histamine as well as other substances involved in hypersensitivity reactions. The release of these substances provokes allergic reactions.

Platelets (Thrombocytes)

Platelets, or thrombocytes, are not actually cells. Rather, they are granular fragments of giant cells in the bone marrow called megakaryocytes. Platelet production in the marrow is regulated in part by the hormone thrombopoietin, which stimulates the production and differentiation of megakaryocytes from the myeloid stem cell.

Platelets play an essential role in the control of bleeding. They circulate freely in the blood in an inactive state, where they nurture the endothelium of the blood vessels, maintaining the integrity of the vessel. When vascular injury does occur, platelets collect at the site and are activated. They adhere to the site of injury and to each other, forming a platelet plug that temporarily stops bleeding. Substances released from platelet granules activate coagulation factors in the blood plasma and initiate the formation of a stable clot composed of **fibrin**, a filamentous protein. Platelets have a normal life span of 7 to 10 days.

PLASMA AND PLASMA PROTEINS

After cellular elements are removed from blood, the remaining liquid portion is called plasma. More than 90% of plasma is water. The remainder consists primarily of plasma proteins, clotting factors (particularly fibrinogen), and small amounts of other substances such as nutrients, enzymes, waste products, and gases. If plasma is allowed to clot, the remaining fluid is called **serum**. Serum has essentially the same composition as plasma, except that fibrinogen and several clotting factors have been removed in the clotting process.

Plasma proteins consist primarily of albumin and globulins. The globulins can be separated into three main fractions—alpha, beta, and gamma—each of which consists of distinct proteins that have different functions. Important proteins in the alpha and beta fractions are the transport globulins and the clotting factors that are made in the liver. The transport globulins carry various substances in bound form around the circulation. For example, thyroid-binding globulin carries thyroxin, and transferrin carries iron. The clotting factors, including fibrinogen, remain in an inactive form in the blood plasma until activated by the clotting cascade. The gamma globulin fraction refers to the immunoglobulins, or antibodies. These proteins are produced by the well-differentiated lymphocytes and plasma cells. The actual fractionation of the globulins can be seen on a specific laboratory test (serum protein electrophoresis).

Albumin is particularly important for the maintenance of fluid balance within the vascular system. Capillary walls are impermeable to albumin, so its presence in the plasma creates an osmotic force that keeps fluid within the vascular space. Albumin, which is produced by the liver, has the capacity to bind to several substances that are transported in plasma (eg, certain medications, bilirubin, some hormones). People with poor hepatic function may have low concentrations of albumin, with a resultant decrease in osmotic pressure and the development of edema.

RETICULOENDOTHELIAL SYSTEM (RES)

The RES is composed of special tissue macrophages, which are derived from monocytes. When released from the marrow, monocytes spend a short time in the circulation (about 24 hours) and then enter the body tissues. Within the tissues, the monocytes continue to differentiate into cells called macrophages, which can survive for months. Macrophages have a variety of important functions. They defend the body against foreign invaders (ie, bacteria and other pathogens) via phagocytosis. They remove old or damaged cells from the circulation. They stimulate the inflammatory process and present antigen to the immune system (see Chapter 50). Macrophages give rise to tissue **histiocytes**, including Kupffer cells of the liver, peritoneal macrophages, alveolar macrophages, and other components of the RES. Thus, the RES is a component of many other organs within the body, particularly the spleen, lymph nodes, lung, and liver.

The spleen is the site of activity for most macrophages. Most of the spleen (75%) is made of red pulp; here the blood enters the venous sinuses through capillaries that are surrounded by macrophages. Within the red pulp are tiny aggregates of white pulp, consisting of B and T lymphocytes. The spleen sequesters newly released reticulocytes from the marrow, removing nuclear fragments and other materials (eg, denatured hemoglobin, iron) before the now fully mature RBC returns to the circulation. Although a minority of RBCs (less than 5%) is pooled in the spleen, a significant proportion of platelets (20%–40%) is pooled here. If the spleen is enlarged, a greater proportion of RBCs and platelets can be sequestered. The spleen is a major source of hematopoiesis in fetal life. It can resume hematopoiesis later in adulthood if necessary (eg, in bone marrow fibrosis). The spleen has important immunologic functions as well. It forms a substance that promotes the phagocytosis of neutrophils; it also forms the antibody IgM after exposure to antigen.

HEMOSTASIS

Hemostasis is the process of preventing blood loss from intact vessels and of stopping bleeding from a severed vessel. The prevention of blood loss from intact vessels requires adequate numbers of functional platelets. Platelets nurture the endothelium

and thereby maintain the structural integrity of the vessel wall. Two processes are involved in arresting bleeding: primary and secondary hemostasis.

In primary hemostasis, the severed blood vessel constricts. Circulating platelets aggregate at the site and adhere to the vessel and to one another. An unstable hemostatic plug is formed. For the coagulation process to be correctly activated, circulating inactive coagulation factors must be converted to active forms. This process occurs on the surface of the aggregated platelets at the site of vessel injury. The end result is the formation of fibrin, which reinforces the platelet plug and anchors it to the injury site. This process is termed secondary hemostasis (Fig. 33-4). The process of blood coagulation is highly complex. It can be activated by the intrinsic or the extrinsic pathway. Both pathways are needed for maintenance of normal hemostasis.

Many factors are involved in the reaction cascade that forms fibrin. When tissue is injured, the extrinsic pathway is activated by the release from the tissue of a substance called thromboplastin. As the result of a series of reactions, prothrombin is converted to **thrombin**, which in turn catalyzes the conversion of fibrinogen to fibrin. Clotting by the intrinsic pathway is activated when the collagen that lines blood vessels is exposed. Clotting factors are activated sequentially until, as with the extrinsic pathway, fibrin is ultimately formed. Although the intrinsic pathway is slower, this sequence is probably most often responsible for clotting in vivo.

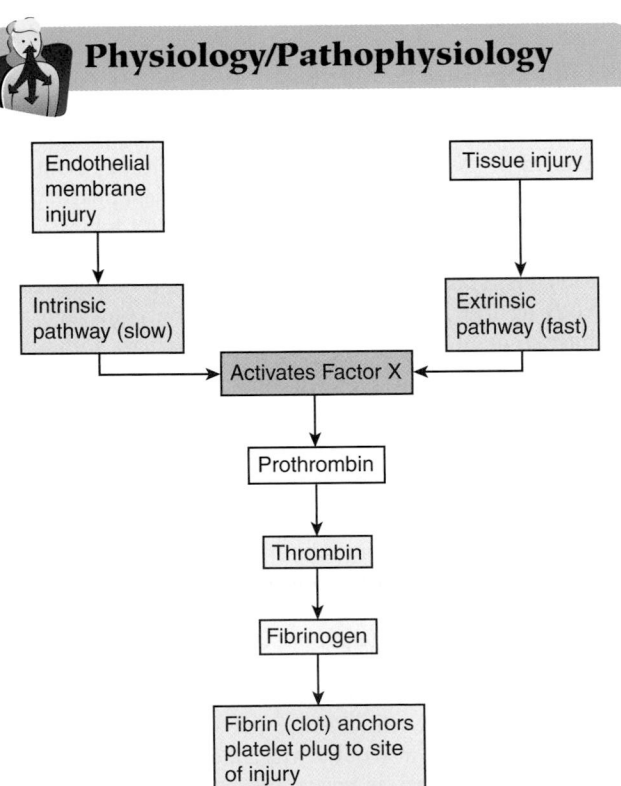

Physiology/Pathophysiology

FIGURE 33-4 Secondary hemostasis. Based on the type of stimulus (injury to the endothelial membrane of a blood vessel or a tissue), one of two clotting pathways is initiated. The end result from either pathway is the conversion of prothrombin to thrombin. Thrombin is necessary for fibrinogen to be converted into fibrin, the stabilizing protein that anchors the fragile platelet plug to the site of injury to prevent further bleeding and permit the injured vessel or site to heal.

As the injured vessel is repaired and again covered with endothelial cells, the fibrin clot is no longer needed. The fibrin is digested via two systems: the plasma fibrinolytic system and the cellular fibrinolytic system. The substance **plasminogen** is required to lyse (break down) the fibrin. Plasminogen, which is present in all body fluids, circulates with fibrinogen and is therefore incorporated into the fibrin clot as it forms. When the clot is no longer needed (eg, after an injured blood vessel has healed), the plasminogen is activated to form plasmin. Plasmin digests the fibrinogen and fibrin. The breakdown particles of the clot (fibrin degradation products) are released into the circulation. Through this system, clots are dissolved as tissue is repaired, and the vascular system returns to its normal baseline state.

PATHOPHYSIOLOGY OF THE HEMATOLOGIC SYSTEM

Most hematologic diseases reflect a defect in the hematopoietic, hemostatic, or RES systems. The defect can be quantitative (eg, increased or decreased production of cells), qualitative (eg, the cells that are produced are defective in their normal functional capacity), or both.

Gerontologic Considerations

In elderly patients, a common problem is decreased ability of the bone marrow to respond to the body's need for blood cells (RBCs, WBCs, and platelets). This inability is a result of many factors, including diminished production of the growth factors necessary for hematopoiesis by stromal cells within the marrow or a diminished response to the growth factors (in the case of erythropoietin). When an elderly person needs more blood cells (eg, WBCs in infection, RBCs in anemia), the bone marrow may not be able to increase production of these cells adequately. **Leukopenia** (a decreased number of circulating WBCs) or anemia can result. In the elderly, the bone marrow may be more susceptible to the myelosuppressive effects of medications.

Anemia is the most common hematologic condition affecting elderly patients; with each successive decade of life, the incidence of anemia increases. Anemia frequently results from iron deficiency (in the case of blood loss) or from a nutritional deficiency, particularly folate or B_{12} deficiency or protein-calorie malnutrition; it may also result from inflammation or chronic disease. Management of the disorder varies depending on the etiology. Therefore, it is important to identify the cause of the anemia rather than to consider it an inevitable consequence of aging. Elderly people with concurrent cardiac or pulmonary problems may not tolerate anemia very well, and a prompt, thorough evaluation is warranted.

Assessment and Diagnostic Findings

Many hematologic conditions cause few symptoms. Therefore, the use of extensive laboratory tests is often required to diagnose a hematologic disorder. For most hematologic conditions, continued monitoring via specific blood tests is required because it is very important to assess for changes in test results over time.

HEMATOLOGIC STUDIES

The most common tests used are the complete blood count (CBC) and the peripheral blood smear (Table 33-2). The CBC identifies the total number of blood cells (WBCs, RBCs, and platelets) as well as the hemoglobin, **hematocrit** (percentage of blood consisting of RBCs), and RBC indices. Because cellular morphology (shape and appearance of the cells) is particularly important in most hematologic disorders, the physician needs to examine the blood cells involved. This process is referred to as the manual examination of the peripheral smear, which may be part of the CBC. In this test, a drop of blood is spread on a glass slide, stained, and examined under a microscope. The shape and size of the RBCs and platelets as well as the actual appearance of the WBCs provides useful information in identifying hematologic conditions. Blood for the CBC is typically obtained by venipuncture.

BONE MARROW ASPIRATION AND BIOPSY

The bone marrow aspiration and biopsy are crucial when additional information is needed to assess how an individual's blood cells are being formed and to assess the quantity and quality of each type of cell produced within the marrow. These tests are also used to document infection or tumor within the marrow.

Normal bone marrow is in a semifluid state and can be aspirated through a special large needle. In adults, bone marrow is usually aspirated from the iliac crest and occasionally from the sternum. The aspirate provides only a sample of cells. Aspirate alone may be adequate for evaluating certain conditions, such as anemia. However, when more information is required, a biopsy is also performed. Biopsy samples are taken from the posterior iliac crest; occasionally, an anterior approach is required. A marrow biopsy shows the architecture of the bone marrow as well as its degree of cellularity.

Most patients need no more preparation than a careful explanation of the procedure, but for some very anxious patients, an antianxiety agent may be useful. It is always important for the physician or nurse to describe and explain to the patient the procedure and the sensations that will be experienced. The risks, benefits, and alternatives are also discussed. A signed informed consent is needed before the procedure is performed.

Before aspiration, the skin is cleansed as for any minor surgery, using aseptic technique. Then a small area is anesthetized with a local anesthetic through the skin and subcutaneous tissue to the periosteum of the bone. It is not possible to anesthetize the bone itself. The bone marrow needle is introduced with a stylet in place. When the needle is felt to go through the outer cortex of bone and enter the marrow cavity, the stylet is removed, a syringe is attached, and a small volume (0.5 mL) of blood and marrow is aspirated. Patients typically feel a pressure sensation as the needle is advanced into position. The actual aspiration always causes sharp but brief pain, resulting from the suction exerted as the marrow is aspirated into the syringe; the patient should be forewarned about this. Taking deep breaths or using relaxation techniques often helps ease the discomfort.

If a bone marrow biopsy is necessary, it is best performed after the aspiration and in a slightly different location, because the marrow structure may be altered after aspiration. A special biopsy needle is used. Because these needles are large, the skin is punctured first with a surgical blade to make a 3- or 4-mm incision. The biopsy needle is advanced well into the marrow cavity. When the needle is properly positioned, a portion of marrow is cored out, using a twisting or gentle rocking motion to free the sample and permit its removal within the biopsy needle. Patients feel a pressure sensation but should not feel actual pain. The nurse should instruct the patient to inform the physician if pain occurs so that additional anesthetic can be administered.

The major hazard of either bone marrow aspiration or biopsy is a slight risk of bleeding and infection. The bleeding risk is somewhat increased if the patient's platelet count is low or if the patient has been taking a medication (eg, aspirin) that alters platelet func-

Table 33-2 • **Frequently Used Laboratory Tests in Hematology**

TEST	NORMAL RANGE	DESCRIPTION	INDICATIONS/COMMENTS
Complete blood count (CBC)		General survey of bone marrow function; evaluates all three cell lines (WBCs, RBCs, platelets)	Important to note changes over time; many hematologic conditions show changes in CBC long before patient becomes symptomatic
Red blood cells (RBCs)	M: $4.7–6.1 \times 10^6$ F: $4.2–5.4 \times 10^6$	Carries hemoglobin; survival time, 120 days	
Hemoglobin (Hgb)	M: 13.5–17.5 g/dL F: 11.5–15.5 g/dL	Delivers O_2 through circulation to body tissues and returns CO_2 from tissues to lungs	Decreased in anemia; increased in polycythemia
Hematocrit (Hct)	M: 40–52% F: 36–48%	Indicates relative proportions of plasma and RBCs (volume of RBCs/L whole blood)	Usually three times the Hgb
Mean corpuscular volume (MCV)	81–96 μm^3	Indicates size of RBCs; very useful in differentiating types of anemia	If <80, cells are microcytic; if >100, cells are macrocytic
Mean corpuscular hemoglobin concentration (MCHC)	33–36 g/dL	Average concentration of Hgb in RBCs; independent of cell size	
Red cell distribution width (RDW)	11–14.5%	Measures degree of variation in size of RBCs	
Reticulocyte count	0.5–1.5%	Measure of marrow production of erythrocytes; 1% of RBC mass is produced daily (to replace the 1% of old cells that die)	Indicates marrow's response to anemia (when anemia is present, reticulocyte level should rise)
White blood cells (WBCs)	4,500–11,000/mm³	Total WBC count	
Differential	Percentages of various types of WBCs	% of cell type × total WBC = absolute number of that cell type	Left shift: bone marrow ↑ production of WBCs; more immature forms released into the bloodstream
Neutrophils	40–75% (2,500–7,500/mm³)	Essential in preventing/limiting bacterial infection; average life span: 2–4 hr	If >8,000: infection, some inflammatory states, stress, steroids, other drugs, myeloproliferative disease Absolute neutrophil count (ANC) <500: increased risk for infection; ANC <100: infection certain (if neutropenia persists)
Lymphocytes	20–50% (1,500–5,500/mm³)	Integral component of immune system	<1,500: lymphopenia; >4,000: lymphocytosis; increased in convalescent phase after bacterial or viral infection, lymphoproliferative disease
Monocytes	1–10% (100–800/mm³)	Enter tissue as macrophages; phagocytosis	Increased in acute and chronic infection, inflammation, some myeloproliferative disorders, chronic myelomonocytic leukemia (CMML)
Eosinophils	0–6% (0–440/mm³)	Involved in allergic reactions (neutralizes histamine); digest foreign proteins	Increased in allergic states, medications, parasites, chronic myeloid leukemia (CML), metastatic/necrotic tumors
Basophils	0–2% (0–200/mm³)	Contain histamine; integral part of hypersensitivity reactions	Increase is very rare (CML)
Platelets	150,000–400,000/mm³	Total number of platelets in circulation; average life span, 7–10 days	Thrombocytopenia: <20,000/mm³, serious; <10,000/mm³, potentially life-threatening

(continued)

Table 33-2 • **Frequently Used Laboratory Tests in Hematology** (Continued)

TEST	NORMAL RANGE	DESCRIPTION	INDICATIONS/COMMENTS
Prothrombin time (PT)	Varies (compare with control), 11–12.5 sec	Measure time elapsed until clot forms; measures extrinsic and common pathways	Increased in liver disease, disseminated intravascular coagulation (DIC), obstructive biliary disease, clotting factor depletion, warfarin (Coumadin) use
International normalized ratio (INR)	1.0 Standard warfarin (Coumadin) treatment, 2.0–3.0 INR; high-dose warfarin (Coumadin) treatment, 3.0–4.5 INR	A standard method of measuring PT independent of the thromboplastin reagent used in the test; calculated by dividing the PT result by the mean normal PT	Increased with anticoagulant excess and conditions that cause increased PT; decreased with insufficient anticoagulant and conditions that cause decreased PT
Partial thromboplastin time (PTT)	Varies (compare with control), 25–35 sec	Surface active agent added to plasma; measures time elapsed until clot forms; measures intrinsic and common pathways	Increased in clotting factor depletion, DIC, liver disease, biliary obstruction, circulating anticoagulants (heparin)
Thrombin time (TT)	Varies (compare with control), 8–11 sec	Tests conversion of fibrinogen to fibrin	Time to clot is inversely proportional to fibrinogen level
Fibrinogen	170–340 mg/100 mL	Measurement of fibrinogen concentration within plasma available for conversion to fibrin clot	Decreased in bleeding disorders, pregnancy, malignancy, inflammatory disease
D-dimer	0–0.5μg/mL	Measures the amount of fragments of fibrin when it is lysed (broken down); useful for distinguishing fibrinolysis from fibrinogenolysis	Increased with fibrinolytic activity, rheumatoid arthritis, ovarian cancer (with increased CA 125)
Fibrin degradation products (FDP)	<10 μg/mL	Byproduct of fibrinolysis	>40 μg/mL indicates DIC

tion. After the marrow sample is obtained, pressure is applied to the site for several minutes. The site is then covered with a sterile dressing. Most patients have no discomfort after a bone marrow aspiration, but the site of a biopsy may ache for 1 or 2 days. Warm tub baths and use of a mild analgesic (eg, acetaminophen) may be useful. Aspirin-containing analgesics should be avoided because they can aggravate or potentiate any bleeding that may occur.

Management of Hematologic Disorders

Commonly encountered blood disorders are anemia, polycythemia, leukopenia and **neutropenia**, leukocytosis, lymphoma, myeloma, **leukemia**, and various bleeding and coagulation disorders. Nursing management of patients with these disorders requires skillful assessment and monitoring as well as meticulous care and teaching to prevent deterioration and complications.

ANEMIA

Anemia, per se, is not a specific disease state but a sign of an underlying disorder. It is by far the most common hematologic condition. Anemia, a condition in which the hemoglobin concentration is lower than normal, reflects the presence of fewer than normal RBCs within the circulation. As a result, the amount of oxygen delivered to body tissues is also diminished.

There are many different kinds of anemia (Table 33-3), but all can be classified into three broad etiologic categories:

- Loss of RBCs—occurs with bleeding, potentially from any major source, such as the gastrointestinal tract, the uterus, the nose, or a wound
- Decreased production of RBCs—can be caused by a deficiency in cofactors (including folic acid, vitamin B_{12}, and iron) required for erythropoiesis; RBC production may also be reduced if the bone marrow is suppressed (eg, by tumor, medications, toxins) or is inadequately stimulated because of a lack of erythropoietin (as occurs in chronic renal disease).
- Increased destruction of RBCs—may occur because of an overactive RES (including hypersplenism) or because the bone marrow produces abnormal RBCs that are then destroyed by the RES (eg, sickle cell anemia).

A conclusion as to whether the anemia is caused by destruction or by inadequate production of RBCs usually can be reached on the basis of the following factors:

- The marrow's ability to respond to the decreased RBCs (as evidenced by an increased reticulocyte count in the circulating blood)
- The degree to which young RBCs proliferate in the bone marrow and the manner in which they mature (as observed on bone marrow biopsy)
- The presence or absence of end products of RBC destruction within the circulation (eg, increased bilirubin level, decreased haptoglobin level)

Table 33-3 • Classification of Anemias

TYPE OF ANEMIA	LABORATORY FINDINGS
Hypoproliferative (Resulting From Defective RBC Production)	
Iron deficiency	Decreased reticulocytes, iron, ferritin, iron saturation, MCV; increased TIBC
Vitamin B₁₂ deficiency (megaloblastic)	Decreased vitamin B₁₂ level; increased MCV
Folate deficiency	Decreased folate level; increased MCV
Decreased erythropoietin production (eg, from renal dysfunction)	Decreased erythropoietin level; normal MCV and MCH; increased creatinine level
Cancer/inflammation	Normal MCV, MCH, normal or decreased erythropoietin level; increased % of iron saturation, ferritin level; decreased iron; TIBC
Bleeding (Resulting From RBC Loss)	
Bleeding from gastrointestinal tract, menorrhagia (excessive menstrual flow), epistaxis (nosebleed), trauma	Increased reticulocyte level; normal Hgb and Hct if measured soon after bleeding starts, but levels decrease thereafter; normal MCV initially but later decreases; decreased ferritin and iron levels (later)
Hemolytic (Resulting From RBC Destruction)	
Altered erythropoiesis (sickle cell anemia, thalassemia, other hemoglobinopathies)	Decreased MCV; fragmented RBCs; increased reticulocyte level
Hypersplenism (hemolysis)	Increased MCV
Drug-induced anemia	Increased spherocyte level
Autoimmune anemia	Increased spherocyte level
Mechanical heart valve–related anemia	Fragmented red cells

Hct, hematocrit; Hgb, hemoglobin concentration; MCH, mean corpuscular hemoglobin; MCV, mean corpuscular volume; RBCs, red blood cells; TIBC, total iron binding capacity.

Classification of Anemias

Anemia may be classified in several ways. The physiologic approach is to determine whether the deficiency in RBCs is caused by a defect in their production (hypoproliferative anemia), by their destruction (hemolytic anemia), or by their loss (bleeding).

In the hypoproliferative anemias, RBCs usually survive normally, but the marrow cannot produce adequate numbers of these cells. The decreased production is reflected in a low reticulocyte count. Inadequate production of RBCs may result from marrow damage due to medications or chemicals (eg, chloramphenicol, benzene) or from a lack of factors necessary for RBC formation (eg, iron, vitamin B₁₂, folic acid, erythropoietin).

Hemolytic anemias stem from premature destruction of RBCs, which results in a liberation of hemoglobin from the RBC into the plasma. The increased RBC destruction results in tissue hypoxia, which in turn stimulates erythropoietin production. This increased production is reflected in an increased reticulocyte count, as the bone marrow responds to the loss of RBCs. The released hemoglobin is converted in large part to bilirubin; therefore, the bilirubin concentration rises. **Hemolysis** can result from an abnormality within the RBC itself (eg, sickle cell anemia, glucose-6-phosphate

dehydrogenase [G-6-PD] deficiency) or within the plasma (eg, immune hemolytic anemias), or from direct injury to the RBC within the circulation (eg, hemolysis caused by mechanical heart valve). Chart 33-1 identifies the causes of hemolytic anemia.

Clinical Manifestations

Aside from the severity of the anemia itself, several factors influence the development of anemia-associated symptoms:

- The speed with which the anemia has developed
- The duration of the anemia (ie, its chronicity)
- The metabolic requirements of the individual
- Other concurrent disorders or disabilities (eg, cardiopulmonary disease)
- Special complications or concomitant features of the condition that produced the anemia

In general, the more rapidly an anemia develops, the more severe its symptoms. An otherwise healthy person can often tolerate as much as a 50% gradual reduction in hemoglobin without pronounced symptoms or significant incapacity, whereas the rapid loss of as little as 30% may precipitate profound vascular collapse in the same individual. A person who has been anemic for a very long time, with hemoglobin levels between 9 and 11 g/dL, usually has few or no symptoms other than slight tachycardia on exertion and fatigue.

Chart 33-1 — Causes of Hemolytic Anemias

Inherited Hemolytic Anemia
Abnormal hemoglobin
   Sickle cell anemia*
   Thalassemia*
Red blood cell membrane abnormality
   Hereditary spherocytosis*
   Hereditary elliptocytosis
   Acanthocytosis
   Stomatocytosis
Enzyme deficiencies
   Glucose-6-phosphate dehydrogenase (G-6-PD) deficiency*

Acquired Hemolytic Anemia
Antibody-related
   Iso-antibody/transfusion reaction*
   Autoimmune hemolytic anemia (AIHA)*
   Cold agglutinin disease*
Not antibody-related
   Red blood cell membrane defects
   Paroxysmal nocturnal hemoglobinuria (PNH)
   Liver disease
   Uremia
   Trauma
   Mechanical heart valve
   Microangiopathic hemolytic anemia
   Infection
      Bacterial
      Parasitic
   Disseminated intravascular coagulation (DIC)*
   Toxins
   Hypersplenism*

*Discussed in text.

Patients who customarily are very active or who have significant demands on their lives (eg, a single, working mother of small children) are more likely to have symptoms, and those symptoms are more likely to be pronounced than in a more sedentary person. A patient with hypothyroidism with decreased oxygen needs may be completely asymptomatic, without tachycardia or increased cardiac output, at a hemoglobin level of 10 g/dL. Similarly, patients with coexistent cardiac, vascular, or pulmonary disease may develop more pronounced symptoms of anemia (eg, dyspnea, chest pain, muscle pain or cramping) at a higher hemoglobin level than those without these concurrent health problems.

Finally, some anemic disorders are complicated by various other abnormalities that do not result from the anemia but are inherently associated with these particular diseases. These abnormalities may give rise to symptoms that completely overshadow those of the anemia, as in the painful crises of sickle cell anemia.

Assessment and Diagnostic Findings

A variety of hematologic studies are performed to determine the type and cause of the anemia. In an initial evaluation, the hemoglobin, hematocrit, reticulocyte count, and RBC indices, particularly the mean corpuscular volume (MCV), are particularly useful. Iron studies (serum iron level, total iron-binding capacity [TIBC], percent saturation, and ferritin), as well as serum vitamin B_{12} and folate levels, are also frequently obtained. Other tests include haptoglobin and erythropoietin levels. The remaining CBC values are useful in determining whether the anemia is an isolated problem or part of another hematologic condition, such as leukemia or myelodysplastic syndrome (MDS). Bone marrow aspiration may be performed. In addition, other diagnostic studies may be performed to determine the presence of underlying chronic illness, such as malignancy, and the source of any blood loss, such as polyps or ulcers within the gastrointestinal tract.

Complications

General complications of severe anemia include heart failure, paresthesias, and confusion. At any given level of anemia, patients with underlying heart disease are far more likely to have angina or symptoms of heart failure than those without heart disease. Complications associated with specific types of anemia are included in the description of each type.

Medical Management

Management of anemia is directed toward correcting or controlling the cause of the anemia; if the anemia is severe, the RBCs that are lost or destroyed may be replaced with a transfusion of packed RBCs (PRBCs). The management of the various types of anemia is covered in the discussions that follow.

NURSING PROCESS: THE PATIENT WITH ANEMIA

Assessment

The health history and physical examination provide important data about the type of anemia involved, the extent and type of symptoms it produces, and the impact of those symptoms on the patient's life. Weakness, fatigue, and general malaise are common, as are pallor of the skin and mucous membranes (sclera, oral mucosa).

Jaundice may be present in patients with megaloblastic anemia or hemolytic anemia. The tongue may be smooth and red (in iron deficiency anemia) or beefy red and sore (in megaloblastic anemia); the corners of the mouth may be ulcerated (**angular cheilosis**) in both types of anemia. Individuals with iron deficiency anemia may crave ice, starch, or dirt (known as pica); their nails may be brittle, ridged, and concave.

The health history should include a medication history, because some medications can depress bone marrow activity or interfere with folate metabolism. An accurate history of alcohol intake, including the amount and duration, should be obtained. Family history is important, because certain anemias are inherited. Athletic endeavors should be assessed, because extreme exercise can decrease erythropoiesis and RBC survival in some athletes.

A nutritional assessment is important, because it may indicate deficiencies in essential nutrients such as iron, vitamin B_{12}, and folic acid. Children of indigent families may be at higher risk for anemia because of nutritional deficiencies. Strict vegetarians are also at risk for megaloblastic types of anemia if they do not supplement their diet with vitamin B_{12}.

Cardiac status should be carefully assessed. When the hemoglobin level is low, the heart attempts to compensate by pumping faster and harder in an effort to deliver more blood to hypoxic tissue. This increased cardiac workload can result in such symptoms as tachycardia, palpitations, dyspnea, dizziness, orthopnea, and exertional dyspnea. Heart failure may eventually develop, as evidenced by an enlarged heart (cardiomegaly) and liver (hepatomegaly) and by peripheral edema.

Assessment of the gastrointestinal system may disclose complaints of nausea, vomiting (with specific questions as to the appearance of any emesis [eg, looks like "coffee grounds"]), melena or dark stools, diarrhea, anorexia, and glossitis (inflammation of the tongue). Stools should be tested for occult blood. Women should be questioned about their menstrual periods (eg, excessive menstrual flow, other vaginal bleeding) and the use of iron supplements during pregnancy.

The neurologic examination is also important because of the effect of pernicious anemia on the central and peripheral nervous systems. Assessment should include the presence and extent of peripheral numbness and paresthesias, ataxia, poor coordination, and confusion. Finally, it is important to monitor relevant laboratory test results and to note any changes over time.

Diagnosis

NURSING DIAGNOSES

Based on the assessment data, major nursing diagnoses for the anemic patient may include:

- Activity intolerance related to weakness, fatigue, and general malaise
- Imbalanced nutrition, less than body requirements, related to inadequate intake of essential nutrients
- Ineffective tissue perfusion related to inadequate blood volume or hematocrit
- Noncompliance with prescribed therapy

COLLABORATIVE PROBLEMS/ POTENTIAL COMPLICATIONS

Based on the assessment data, potential complications that may develop include:

- Heart failure
- Paresthesias
- Confusion

Planning and Goals

The major goals for the patient may include increased tolerance of normal activity, attainment or maintenance of adequate nutrition, maintenance of adequate tissue perfusion, compliance with prescribed therapy, and absence of complications.

Nursing Interventions

MANAGING FATIGUE

The most frequent symptom and complication of anemia is fatigue. This distressing symptom is too often minimized by health care providers. Fatigue is often the symptom that has the greatest negative impact on the individual's level of functioning and consequent quality of life. Patients describe the fatigue from anemia as oppressive. Fatigue can be significant, yet the anemia may not be severe enough to warrant transfusion. Fatigue can interfere with an individual's ability to work, both inside and outside the home. It can harm relationships with family and friends. Patients often lose interest in hobbies and activities, including sexual activity. The distress from fatigue is often related to an individual's responsibilities and life demands as well as the amount of assistance and support received from others.

Nursing interventions can focus on assisting the patient to prioritize activities and to establish a balance between activity and rest that is realistic and feasible from the patient's perspective. Patients with chronic anemia need to maintain some physical activity and exercise to prevent the deconditioning that results from inactivity.

MAINTAINING ADEQUATE NUTRITION

Inadequate intake of essential nutrients, such as iron, vitamin B_{12}, folic acid, and protein can cause some anemias. The symptoms associated with anemia (eg, fatigue, anorexia) can in turn interfere with maintaining adequate nutrition. A healthy diet should be encouraged. Because alcohol interferes with the utilization of essential nutrients, the nurse should advise the patient to avoid alcoholic beverages or to limit their intake and should provide the rationale for this recommendation. Dietary teaching sessions should be individualized, including cultural aspects related to food preferences and food preparation. The involvement of family members enhances compliance with dietary recommendations. Dietary supplements (eg, vitamins, iron, folate, protein) may be prescribed as well.

Equally important, the patient and family must understand the role of nutritional supplements in the proper context, because many forms of anemia are not the result of a nutritional deficiency. In such cases, excessive intake of nutritional supplements will not improve the anemia. A potential problem in individuals with chronic transfusion requirements occurs with the indiscriminate use of iron. Unless an aggressive program of chelation therapy is implemented, these individuals are at risk for iron overload from their transfusions alone. The addition of an iron supplement only exacerbates the situation.

MAINTAINING ADEQUATE PERFUSION

Patients with acute blood loss or severe hemolysis may have decreased tissue perfusion from decreased blood volume or reduced circulating RBCs (decreased hematocrit). Lost volume is replaced with transfusions or intravenous fluids, based on the symptoms and the laboratory findings. Supplemental oxygen may be necessary, but it is rarely needed on a long-term basis unless there is underlying severe cardiac or pulmonary disease as well. The nurse monitors vital signs closely; other medications, such as antihypertensive agents, may need to be adjusted or withheld.

PROMOTING COMPLIANCE WITH PRESCRIBED THERAPY

For patients with anemia, medications or nutritional supplements are often prescribed to alleviate or correct the condition. These patients need to understand the purpose of the medication, how to take the medication and over what time period, and how to manage any side effects of therapy. To enhance compliance, the nurse can assist patients in developing ways to incorporate the therapeutic plan into their lives, rather than merely giving the patient a list of instructions. For example, many patients have difficulty taking iron supplements because of related gastrointestinal effects. Rather than seeking assistance from a health care provider in managing the problem, some of these patients simply stop taking the iron.

Abruptly stopping some medications can have serious consequences, as in the case of high-dose corticosteroids to manage hemolytic anemias. Some medications, such as growth factors, are extremely expensive. Patients receiving these medications may need assistance with obtaining needed insurance coverage or with exploring alternatives for obtaining these medications.

MONITORING AND MANAGING POTENTIAL COMPLICATIONS

A significant complication of anemia is heart failure from chronic diminished blood volume and the heart's compensatory effort to increase cardiac output. Patients with anemia should be assessed for signs and symptoms of heart failure. A serial record of body weights can be more useful than a record of dietary intake and output, because the intake and output measurements may not be accurate. In the case of fluid retention resulting from heart failure, diuretics may be required.

In megaloblastic forms of anemia, the significant potential complications are neurologic. A neurologic assessment should be performed for patients with known or suspected megaloblastic anemia. Patients may initially complain of paresthesias in their lower extremities. These paresthesias are usually manifested as numbness and tingling on the bottom of the foot, and they gradually progress. As the anemia progresses and damage to the spinal cord occurs, other signs become apparent. Position and vibration sense may be diminished; difficulty maintaining balance is not uncommon, and some patients have gait disturbances as well. Initially mild but gradually progressive confusion may develop.

Evaluation

EXPECTED PATIENT OUTCOMES

Expected patient outcomes may include:

1. Tolerates activity at a safe and acceptable level
   a. Follows a progressive plan of rest, activity, and exercise
   b. Prioritizes activities
   c. Paces activities according to energy level
2. Attains and maintains adequate nutrition
   a. Eats a healthy diet
   b. Develops meal plan that promotes optimal nutrition
   c. Maintains adequate amounts of iron, vitamins, and protein from diet or supplements
   d. Adheres to nutritional supplement therapy when prescribed
   e. Verbalizes understanding of rationale for using recommended nutritional supplements
   f. Verbalizes understanding of rationale for avoiding non-recommended nutritional supplements
3. Maintains adequate perfusion
   a. Has vital signs within baseline for patient

   b. Has pulse oximetry (arterial oxygenation) value within normal limits
4. Absence of complications
   a. Avoids or limits activities that cause dyspnea, palpitations, dizziness, or tachycardia
   b. Uses rest and comfort measures to alleviate dyspnea
   c. Has vital signs within baseline for patient
   d. Has no signs of increasing fluid retention (eg, peripheral edema, decreased urine output, neck vein distention)
   e. Remains oriented to time, place, and situation
   f. Ambulates safely, using assistive devices as necessary
   g. Remains free of injury
   h. Verbalizes understanding of importance of serial CBC measurements
   i. Maintains safe home environment; obtains assistance as necessary.

Hypoproliferative Anemias

IRON DEFICIENCY ANEMIA

Iron deficiency anemia typically results when the intake of dietary iron is inadequate for hemoglobin synthesis. The body can store about one fourth to one third of its iron, and it is not until those stores are depleted that iron deficiency anemia actually begins to develop. Iron deficiency anemia is the most common type of anemia in all age groups, and it is the most common anemia in the world. More than 500 million people are affected, more commonly in underdeveloped countries, where inadequate iron stores can result from inadequate intake of iron (seen with vegetarian diets) or from blood loss (eg, from intestinal hookworm). Iron deficiency is also common in the United States. In children, adolescents, and pregnant women, the cause is typically inadequate iron in the diet to keep up with increased growth. However, for most adults with iron deficiency anemia, the cause is blood loss. In fact, in adults, the cause of iron deficiency anemia should be considered to be bleeding until proven otherwise.

The most common cause of iron deficiency in men and postmenopausal women is bleeding (from ulcers, gastritis, inflammatory bowel disease, or gastrointestinal tumors). The most common cause of iron deficiency anemia in premenopausal women is menorrhagia (excessive menstrual bleeding) and pregnancy with inadequate iron supplementation. Patients with chronic alcoholism often have chronic blood loss from the gastrointestinal tract, which causes iron loss and eventual anemia. Other causes include iron malabsorption, as is seen after gastrectomy or with celiac disease.

Clinical Manifestations

Patients with iron deficiency primarily have the symptoms of anemia. If the deficiency is severe or prolonged, they may also have a smooth, sore tongue, brittle and ridged nails, and angular cheilosis (an ulceration of the corner of the mouth). These signs subside after iron-replacement therapy. The health history may be significant for multiple pregnancies, gastrointestinal bleeding, and pica (a craving for unusual substances, such as ice, clay, or laundry starch).

Assessment and Diagnostic Findings

The most definitive method of establishing the diagnosis of iron deficiency anemia is bone marrow aspiration. The aspirate is stained to detect iron, which is at a low level or even absent. However, few patients with suspected iron deficiency anemia undergo bone marrow aspiration. In many patients, the diagnosis can be

established with other tests, particularly in patients with a history of conditions that predispose them to this type of anemia.

There is a strong correlation between laboratory values measuring iron stores and levels of hemoglobin. After the iron stores are depleted (as reflected by low serum ferritin levels), the hemoglobin level falls. The diminished iron stores cause small RBCs. Therefore, as the anemia progresses, the MCV, which measures the size of the RBC, also decreases. Hematocrit and RBC levels are also low in relation to the hemoglobin level. Other laboratory tests that measure iron stores are useful but are not as consistent indicators as a low ferritin level, which reflects low iron stores. Typically, patients with iron deficiency anemia have a low serum iron level and an elevated TIBC, which measures the transport protein supplying the marrow with iron as needed (also referred to as transferrin). However, other disease states, such as infection and inflammatory conditions, can also cause a low serum iron level and TIBC with an elevated ferritin level. Therefore, the most reliable laboratory findings in evaluating iron deficiency anemia are the ferritin and hemoglobin values.

Medical Management

Except in the case of pregnancy, the cause of iron deficiency should be investigated. Anemia may be a sign of a curable gastrointestinal cancer or of uterine fibroid tumors. Stool specimens should be tested for occult blood. People 50 years of age or older should have a colonoscopy, endoscopy, or x-ray examination of the gastrointestinal tract to detect ulcerations, gastritis, polyps, or cancer. Several oral iron preparations—ferrous sulfate, ferrous gluconate, and ferrous fumarate—are available for treating iron deficiency anemia. The hemoglobin level may increase in only a few weeks, and the anemia can be corrected in a few months. Iron store replenishment takes much longer, so it is important that the patient continue taking the iron for as long as 6 to 12 months.

In some cases, oral iron is poorly absorbed or poorly tolerated, or iron supplementation is needed in large amounts. In these situations, intravenous or intramuscular administration of iron dextran may be needed. Before parenteral administration of a full dose, a small test dose should be administered to avoid the risk of anaphylaxis with either intravenous or intramuscular injections. Emergency medications (eg, epinephrine) should be close at hand. If no signs of allergic reaction have occurred after 30 minutes, the remaining dose of iron may be administered. Several doses are required to replenish the patient's iron stores.

Nursing Management

Preventive education is important, because iron deficiency anemia is common in menstruating and pregnant women. Food sources high in iron include organ meats (beef or calf's liver, chicken liver), other meats, beans (black, pinto, and garbanzo), leafy green vegetables, raisins, and molasses. Taking iron-rich foods with a source of vitamin C enhances the absorption of iron.

The nurse helps the patient select a healthy diet. Nutritional counseling can be provided for those whose usual diet is inadequate. Patients with a history of eating fad diets or strict vegetarian diets are counseled that such diets often contain inadequate amounts of absorbable iron. The nurse encourages patients to continue iron therapy as long as it is prescribed, although they may no longer feel fatigued.

Because iron is best absorbed on an empty stomach, patients should be advised to take the supplement an hour before meals. Most patients can use the less expensive, more standard forms of ferrous sulfate. Tablets with enteric coating may be poorly

absorbed and should be avoided. Other patients have difficulty taking iron supplements because of gastrointestinal side effects (primarily constipation, but also cramping, nausea, and vomiting). Some iron formulations are designed to limit gastrointestinal side effects by the addition of a stool softener or use of sustained-release formulations to limit nausea or gastritis. Specific patient teaching aids, such as the accompanying patient education guide (Chart 33-2), can assist patients with the use of iron supplements.

If taking iron on an empty stomach causes gastric distress, the patient may need to take the iron supplement with meals. However, doing so diminishes iron absorption by as much as 50%, thus prolonging the time required to replenish iron stores. Antacids or dairy products should not be taken with iron, because they greatly diminish the absorption of iron. Polysaccharide iron complex forms that have less gastrointestinal toxicity are also available, but they are more expensive.

Liquid forms of iron that cause less gastrointestinal distress are available. However, they can stain the teeth; patients should be instructed to take this medication through a straw, to rinse the mouth with water, and to practice good oral hygiene after taking this medication. Finally, patients should be informed that iron salts may color the stool dark green or black. However, iron replacement therapy does not cause a false-positive result on stool analyses for occult blood.

Intramuscular supplementation is used infrequently. The volume of iron required may be excessive. The intramuscular injection causes some local pain and can stain the skin. These side effects are minimized by using the Z-track technique for administering iron dextran deep into the gluteus maximus muscle (buttock). Avoid vigorously rubbing the injection site after the injection. Because of the problems with intramuscular administration, the intravenous route is preferred for administration of iron dextran.

ANEMIAS IN RENAL DISEASE

The degree of anemia in patients with end-stage renal disease varies greatly, but in general patients do not become significantly anemic until the serum creatinine level exceeds 3 mg/100 mL. The symptoms of anemia are often the most disturbing of the patient's symptoms. The hematocrit usually falls to between 20% and 30%, although in rare cases it may fall to less than 15%. The RBCs appear normal on the peripheral smear.

This anemia is caused by both a mild shortening of RBC life span and a deficiency of erythropoietin (necessary for erythro-

poiesis). As renal function decreases, erythropoietin, which is produced by the kidney, also decreases. Because erythropoietin is also produced outside the kidney, some erythropoiesis does continue, even in patients whose kidneys have been removed. However, the amount is small and the degree of erythropoiesis is inadequate.

Patients undergoing long-term hemodialysis lose blood into the dialyzer and therefore may become iron deficient. Folic acid deficiency develops because this vitamin passes into the dialysate. Therefore, patients who receive hemodialysis and who are anemic should be evaluated for iron and folate deficiency and treated appropriately.

The availability of recombinant erythropoietin (epoetin alfa [Epogen, Procrit]) has dramatically altered the management of anemia in end-stage renal disease by decreasing the need for RBC transfusion, with its associated risks. Erythropoietin, in combination with oral iron supplements, can raise and maintain hematocrit levels to between 33% and 38%. This treatment has been successful with dialysis patients. Many patients report decreased fatigue, increased energy, increased feelings of well-being, improved exercise tolerance, better tolerance of dialysis treatments, and improved quality of life. Hypertension is the most serious side effect in this patient population when the hematocrit rapidly increases to a high level. Therefore, the hematocrit should be checked frequently when a patient with renal disease begins erythropoietin therapy. The dose of erythropoietin (epoetin alfa) should be titrated to the hematocrit. In some patients, the elevated hematocrit and associated hypertension may necessitate antihypertensive therapy.

ANEMIA OF CHRONIC DISEASE

The term "anemia of chronic disease" is a misnomer in that only the chronic diseases of inflammation, infection, and malignancy cause this type of anemia. Many chronic inflammatory diseases are associated with a **normochromic**, **normocytic** anemia (ie, the RBCs are normal in color and size). These disorders include rheumatoid arthritis; severe, chronic infections; and many cancers. It is therefore imperative that the "chronic disease" be diagnosed when this form of anemia is identified so that it can be appropriately managed.

The anemia is usually mild to moderate and nonprogressive. It develops gradually over 6 to 8 weeks and then stabilizes at a hematocrit seldom less than 25%. The hemoglobin level rarely falls below 9 g/dL, and the bone marrow has normal cellularity with increased stores of iron as the iron is diverted from the serum (and thus is unavailable as a growth factor for invading pathogens). Erythropoietin levels are low, perhaps because of decreased production, and iron use is blocked by **erythroid cells** (cells that are or will become mature RBCs). A moderate shortening of RBC survival also occurs.

Most of these patients have few symptoms and do not require treatment for the anemia. With successful treatment of the underlying disorder, the bone marrow iron is used to make RBCs and the hemoglobin level rises.

APLASTIC ANEMIA

Aplastic anemia is a rather rare disease caused by a decrease in or damage to marrow stem cells, damage to the microenvironment within the marrow, and replacement of the marrow with fat. It results in bone marrow **aplasia** (markedly reduced hematopoiesis). Therefore, in addition to severe anemia, significant neutropenia and thrombocytopenia (a deficiency of platelets) are also seen.

Pathophysiology

Aplastic anemia can be congenital or acquired, but most cases are idiopathic (ie, without apparent cause). Infections and pregnancy can trigger it, or it may be caused by certain medications, chemicals, or radiation damage (Chart 33-3). Agents that regularly produce marrow aplasia include benzene and benzene derivatives (eg, airplane glue). Certain toxic materials, such as inorganic arsenic and several pesticides (including DDT, which is no longer used or available in the United States), have also been implicated as potential causes. Various medications have been associated with aplastic anemia.

Clinical Manifestations

The manifestations of aplastic anemia are often insidious. Complications resulting from bone marrow failure may occur before

---

Chart 33-3

Substances Associated With Aplastic Anemia

Analgesics
Antiseizure agents (mephenytoin, triethadione*)
Antihistamines
Antimicrobials*
Antineoplastic agents (alkylating agents, antitumor antibiotics, antimetabolites)
Antithyroid medications
Benzene*
Chloramphenicol*
Gold compounds*
Heavy metals
Hypoglycemic agents
Insecticides
Organic arsenicals*
Phenylbutazone*
Phenothiazines
Sulfonamides*
Sedatives

---

*Most common.

---

the diagnosis is established. Typical complications are infection and symptoms of anemia (eg, fatigue, pallor, dyspnea). Purpura (bruising) may develop later and should trigger a CBC and hematologic evaluation if these were not performed initially. If the patient has had repeated throat infections, cervical lymphadenopathy may be seen. Other lymphadenopathies and splenomegaly sometimes occur. Retinal hemorrhages are common.

Assessment and Diagnostic Findings

In many situations, aplastic anemia occurs when a medication or chemical is ingested in toxic amounts. However, in a few people, it develops after a medication has been taken at the recommended dosage. This may be considered an idiosyncratic reaction in those who are highly susceptible, possibly caused by a genetic defect in the medication biotransformation or elimination process. A bone marrow aspirate shows an extremely hypoplastic or even aplastic (very few to no cells) marrow replaced with fat.

Medical Management

It is presumed that the lymphocytes of patients with aplastic anemia destroy the stem cells and consequently impair the production of RBCs, WBCs, and platelets. Despite its severity, aplastic anemia can be successfully treated in most people. Potentially, those who are younger than 60 years of age, who are otherwise healthy, and who have a compatible donor can be cured of the disease by a bone marrow transplantation (BMT) or peripheral blood stem cell transplantation (PBSCT). In others, the disease can be managed with immunosuppressive therapy. A combination of antithymocyte globulin and cyclosporine is used most commonly. Immunosuppressants prevent the patient's lymphocytes from destroying the stem cells. If relapse occurs (ie, the patient becomes pancytopenic again), reinstitution of the same immunologic agents may induce another remission. Corticosteroids are not very useful as an immunosuppressive agent, because patients with aplastic anemia appear particularly susceptible to the development of bone complications from corticosteroids (ie, aseptic necrosis of the head of the femur).

Supportive therapy plays a major role in the management of aplastic anemia. Any offending agent is discontinued. The patient is supported with transfusions of RBCs and platelets as necessary. Death usually is caused by hemorrhage or infection.

Nursing Management

Patients with aplastic anemia are vulnerable to problems related to RBC, WBC, and platelet deficiencies. They should be assessed carefully for signs of infection and bleeding. Specific interventions are delineated in the sections on neutropenia and thrombocytopenia.

MEGALOBLASTIC ANEMIAS

In the anemias caused by deficiencies of vitamin B_{12} or folic acid, identical bone marrow and peripheral blood changes occur, because both vitamins are essential for normal DNA synthesis. In either anemia, the RBCs that are produced are abnormally large and are called megaloblastic RBCs. Other cells derived from the myeloid stem cell (nonlymphoid WBCs, platelets) are also abnormal. A bone marrow analysis reveals **hyperplasia** (abnormal increase in the number of cells), and the precursor erythroid and myeloid cells are large and bizarre in appearance. Many of these abnormal RBCs and myeloid cells are destroyed within the marrow, however, so the mature cells that do leave the marrow are actually fewer in number. Thus, **pancytopenia** (a decrease in all myeloid-derived cells) can develop. In an advanced situation, the hemoglobin value may be as low as 4 to 5 g/dL, the WBC count 2,000 to 3,000/mm^3, and the platelet count less than 50,000/mm^3. Those cells that are released into the circulation are often abnormally shaped. The neutrophils are hypersegmented. The platelets may be abnormally large. The RBCs are abnormally shaped, and the shapes may vary widely (**poikilocytosis**). Because the RBCs are very large, the MCV is very high, usually exceeding 110 μm^3.

Pathophysiology

FOLIC ACID DEFICIENCY

Folic acid, a vitamin that is necessary for normal RBC production, is stored as compounds referred to as folates. The folate stores in the body are much smaller than those of vitamin B$_{12}$, and they are quickly depleted when the dietary intake of folate is deficient (within 4 months). Folate is found in green vegetables and liver. Folate deficiency occurs in people who rarely eat uncooked vegetables. Alcohol increases folic acid requirements, and, at the same time, patients with alcoholism usually have a diet that is deficient in the vitamin. Folic acid requirements are also increased in patients with chronic hemolytic anemias and in women who are pregnant, because the need for RBC production is increased in these conditions. Some patients with malabsorptive diseases of the small bowel, such as sprue, may not absorb folic acid normally.

VITAMIN B$_{12}$ DEFICIENCY

A deficiency of vitamin B$_{12}$ can occur in several ways. Inadequate dietary intake is rare but can develop in strict vegetarians who consume no meat or dairy products. Faulty absorption from the gastrointestinal tract is more common. This occurs in conditions such as Crohn's disease, or after ileal resection or gastrectomy. Another cause is the absence of intrinsic factor, as in pernicious anemia. Intrinsic factor is normally secreted by cells within the gastric mucosa; normally it binds with the dietary vitamin B$_{12}$ and travels with it to the ileum, where the vitamin is absorbed. Without intrinsic factor, orally consumed vitamin B$_{12}$ cannot be absorbed, and RBC production is eventually diminished. Even if adequate vitamin B$_{12}$ and intrinsic factor are present, a deficiency may occur if disease involving the ileum or pancreas impairs absorption. Pernicious anemia, which tends to run in families, is primarily a disorder of adults, particularly the elderly. The abnormality is in the gastric mucosa: the stomach wall atrophies and fails to secrete intrinsic factor. Therefore, the absorption of vitamin B$_{12}$ is significantly impaired.

The body normally has large stores of vitamin B$_{12}$, so years may pass before the deficiency results in anemia. Because the body compensates so well, the anemia can be severe before the patient becomes symptomatic. For unknown reasons, patients with pernicious anemia have a higher incidence of gastric cancer than the general population; these patients should have endoscopies at regular intervals (every 1 to 2 years) to screen for early gastric cancer.

Clinical Manifestations

Symptoms of folic acid and vitamin B$_{12}$ deficiencies are similar, and the two anemias may coexist. However, the neurologic manifestations of vitamin B$_{12}$ deficiency do not occur with folic acid deficiency, and they persist if B$_{12}$ is not replaced. Therefore, careful distinction between the two anemias must be made. Serum levels of both vitamins can be measured. In the case of folic acid deficiency, even small amounts of folate will increase the serum folate level, sometimes to normal. Measuring the amount of folate within the RBC itself (red cell folate) is therefore a more sensitive test in determining true folate deficiency.

After the body stores of vitamin B$_{12}$ are depleted, patients may begin to show signs of the anemia. However, because the onset and progression of the anemia are so gradual, the body can compensate very well until the anemia is severe, so that the typical manifestations of anemia (weakness, listlessness, fatigue) may not be apparent initially. The hematologic effects of deficiency are accompanied by effects on other organ systems, particularly the gastrointestinal tract and nervous system. Patients with pernicious anemia develop a smooth, sore, red tongue and mild diarrhea. They are extremely pale, particularly in the mucous membranes. They may become confused; more often they have paresthesias in the extremities (particularly numbness and tingling in the feet and lower legs). They may have difficulty maintaining their balance because of damage to the spinal cord, and they also lose position sense (proprioception). These symptoms are progressive, although the course of illness may be marked by spontaneous partial remissions and exacerbations. Without treatment, patients can die after several years, usually from heart failure secondary to anemia.

Assessment and Diagnostic Findings

The classic method of determining the cause of vitamin B$_{12}$ deficiency is the Schilling test, in which the patient receives a small oral dose of radioactive vitamin B$_{12}$, followed in a few hours by a large, nonradioactive parenteral dose of vitamin B$_{12}$ (this aids in renal excretion of the radioactive dose). If the oral vitamin is absorbed, more than 8% will be excreted in the urine within 24 hours; therefore, if no radioactivity is present in the urine (ie, the radioactive vitamin B$_{12}$ stays within the gastrointestinal tract), the cause is gastrointestinal malabsorption of the vitamin B$_{12}$. Conversely, if the urine is radioactive, the cause of the deficiency is not ileal disease or pernicious anemia. Later, the same procedure is repeated, but this time intrinsic factor is added to the oral radioactive vitamin B$_{12}$. If radioactivity is now detected in the urine (ie, the B$_{12}$ was absorbed from the gastrointestinal tract in the presence of intrinsic factor), the diagnosis of pernicious anemia can be made. The Schilling test is useful only if the urine collections are complete; therefore, the nurse must promote the patient's understanding and ability to comply with this collection.

Another useful, easier test is the intrinsic factor antibody test. A positive test indicates the presence of antibodies that bind the vitamin B$_{12}$–intrinsic factor complex and prevent it from binding to receptors in the ileum, thus preventing its absorption. Unfortunately, this test is not specific for pernicious anemia alone, but it can aid in the diagnosis.

Medical Management

Folate deficiency is treated by increasing the amount of folic acid in the diet and administering 1 mg of folic acid daily. Folic acid is administered intramuscularly only for people with malabsorption problems. With the exception of the vitamins administered during pregnancy, most proprietary vitamin preparations do not contain folic acid, so it must be administered as a separate tablet. After the hemoglobin level returns to normal, the folic acid replacement can be stopped. However, patients with alcoholism should continue receiving folic acid as long as they continue alcohol consumption.

Vitamin B_{12} deficiency is treated by vitamin B_{12} replacement. Vegetarians can prevent or treat deficiency with oral supplements through vitamins or fortified soy milk. When, as is more common, the deficiency is due to defective absorption or absence of intrinsic factor, replacement is by monthly intramuscular injections of vitamin B_{12}, usually at a dose of 1000 µg. The reticulocyte count rises within 1 week, and in several weeks the blood counts are all normal. The tongue improves in several days. However, the neurologic manifestations require more time for recovery; if there is severe neuropathy, the patient may never recover fully. To prevent recurrence of pernicious anemia, vitamin B_{12} therapy must be continued for life.

> **NURSING ALERT** Even when the anemia is severe, RBC transfusions should not be used because the patient's body has compensated over time by expanding the total blood volume. Administration of blood transfusions to such patients, particularly those who are elderly or who have cardiac dysfunction, can precipitate pulmonary edema. If transfusions are required, the RBCs should be transfused slowly, with careful attention to signs and symptoms of fluid overload.

Nursing Management

Assessment of patients who have or are at risk for megaloblastic anemia includes inspection of the skin and mucous membranes. Mild jaundice may be apparent and is best seen in the sclera without using fluorescent lights. Vitiligo (patchy loss of skin pigmentation) and premature graying of the hair are often seen in patients with pernicious anemia. The tongue is smooth, red, and sore. Because of the neurologic complications associated with these anemias, a careful neurologic assessment is important, including tests of position and vibration sense.

PROMOTING HOME AND COMMUNITY-BASED CARE

The nurse needs to pay particular attention to ambulation and should assess the patient's gait and stability as well as the need for assistive devices (eg, canes, walkers) and for assistance in managing daily activities. Of particular concern is ensuring safety when position sense, coordination, and gait are affected. Physical and occupational therapy referrals may be needed.

If sensation is altered, patients need to be instructed to avoid excessive heat and cold.

Because mouth and tongue soreness may restrict nutritional intake, the nurse can advise patients and families to prepare bland, soft foods and to eat small amounts frequently. The nurse also may explain that other nutritional deficiencies, such as alcohol-induced anemia, can induce neurologic problems.

Patients must also be taught about the chronicity of their disorder and the necessity for monthly vitamin B_{12} injections even in the absence of symptoms. Many patients can be taught to self-administer their injections. The gastric atrophy associated with pernicious anemia increases the risk of gastric carcinoma, so these patients need to understand that ongoing medical follow-up and screening are important.

MYELODYSPLASTIC SYNDROMES (MDS)

The MDS are a group of disorders of the myeloid stem cell that cause **dysplasia** (abnormal development) in one or more types of cell lines. The most common feature of MDS—dysplasia of the RBCs—is manifested as a macrocytic anemia; however, the WBCs (myeloid cells, particularly neutrophils) and platelets can also be affected. Although the bone marrow is actually hypercellular, many of the cells within it die before being released into the circulation. Therefore, the number of affected cells in the circulation is typically lower than normal. In addition to the quantitative defect (ie, fewer cells than normal), there is also a qualitative defect: the cells are not as functional as normal. The neutrophils have diminished ability to destroy bacteria by phagocytosis; platelets are less able to aggregate and are less adhesive than usual. The result of these qualitative defects is an increased risk for infection and bleeding, even when the actual number of circulating cells may not be excessively low. A significant proportion of MDS cases evolve into acute myeloid leukemia (AML); this type of leukemia tends to be nonresponsive to standard therapy.

Primary MDS tends to be a disease of the elderly; more than 80% of patients with MDS are older than 60 years of age. Secondary MDS may occur at any age and results from prior toxic exposure to chemicals, including chemotherapeutic medications (particularly alkylating agents). Secondary MDS tends to have a poorer prognosis than does primary MDS.

Clinical Manifestations

The manifestations of MDS can vary widely. Many patients are asymptomatic, with the illness being discovered incidentally when a CBC is performed for other purposes. Other patients have profound symptoms and complications from the illness. Fatigue is often present, at varying levels. Neutrophil dysfunction renders the person at risk for infection; recurrent pneumonias are not uncommon. Because platelet function can also be altered, bleeding can occur. These problems may persist in a fairly steady state for months, even years. They may also progress over time; as the dysplasia evolves into a leukemic state, the complications increase in severity.

Assessment and Diagnostic Findings

The CBC typically reveals a macrocytic anemia; WBC and platelet counts may be diminished as well. Serum erythropoietin levels may be inappropriately low, as is the reticulocyte count. As the disease evolves into AML, more immature blast cells are noted on the CBC.

Medical Management

With the exception of allogeneic bone marrow transplantation (BMT), there is no known cure for MDS. Chemotherapy has been used, particularly in patients with more aggressive forms of the illness, typically with disappointing results (Deeg & Applebaum, 2000; Beran, 2000). However, patients with mild cytopenias (low blood counts) actually require no therapy. For most patients with MDS, transfusions of RBCs are required to control the anemia and its symptoms. These patients can develop significant problems with iron overload from the repeated transfusions; this problem can be diminished with prompt initiation of chelation therapy to remove the excess iron (see Nursing Management). In some patients, the use of erythropoietin can be successful in reducing the need for transfusions and their attendant complications. Some patients may also require ongoing platelet transfusions to prevent significant bleeding. Infections need to be managed aggressively and promptly. Administration of growth factors, particularly granulocyte colony-stimulating factor (G-CSF), erythropoietin, or both, has been successful in increasing neutrophils and diminishing anemia in certain patients; however, these agents are expensive and the effect is lost if the medications are stopped. Because MDS tend to occur in elderly people, other chronic conditions may limit treatment options. Secondary MDS and MDS that evolve into AML tend to be much more refractory to conventional therapy for leukemia.

Nursing Management

Caring for patients with MDS can be challenging because the illness is unpredictable. As with other hematologic conditions, some patients (especially those with no symptoms) have difficulty perceiving that they have a serious illness that can place them at risk for life-threatening complications. At the other extreme, many patients have tremendous difficulty coping with the uncertain trajectory of the illness and fear that the illness will evolve into AML at a time when they are feeling very well physically.

Patients with MDS need extensive instruction about infection risk, measures to avoid it, signs and symptoms of developing infection, and appropriate actions to initiate should such symptoms occur. Instruction should also be given regarding the risk for bleeding. Patients with MDS who are hospitalized may require neutropenic precautions.

Laboratory values need to be monitored closely to anticipate the need for transfusion and to determine response to treatment with growth factors. Patients with chronic transfusion requirements usually benefit from a vascular access device for this purpose. Patients receiving growth factors or chelation therapy must be educated about these medications, their side effects, and administration techniques.

Chelation therapy is a process that is used to remove excess iron acquired from chronic transfusions. Iron is bound to a substance, the chelating agent, and then excreted in the urine. Oral forms of chelating agents have not been successful (due to either diminished efficacy or excessive toxicity). Chelation therapy is most effective as a subcutaneous infusion administered over 8 to 12 hours; most patients prefer to do this at night. Because chelation therapy removes only a small amount of iron with each treatment, patients with chronic transfusion requirements (and iron overload) need to continue chelation therapy as long as the iron overload exists, potentially for the rest of their lives. Patients who are embarking on chelation therapy must be highly motivated and need instruction in the subcutaneous infusion technique, infusion pump maintenance, and side effect management. Local erythema at the injection site is the most common reaction and typically requires no intervention. Patients should have baseline and annual auditory and eye examinations, because hearing loss and visual changes can occur with treatment.

Hemolytic Anemias

In hemolytic anemias, the RBCs have a shortened life span; thus, the number of RBCs in circulation is reduced. Fewer RBCs result in decreased available oxygen, causing hypoxia, which in turn stimulates an increase in erythropoietin release from the kidney. The erythropoietin stimulates the bone marrow to compensate by producing new RBCs and releasing some of them into the circulation somewhat prematurely as reticulocytes. If the RBC destruction persists, the hemoglobin is broken down excessively; about 80% of the heme is converted to bilirubin, conjugated in the liver, and excreted in the bile.

The mechanism of RBC destruction varies, but all types of hemolytic anemia share certain laboratory features: the reticulocyte count is elevated, the fraction of indirect (unconjugated) bilirubin is increased, and the supply of haptoglobin (a binding protein for free hemoglobin) is depleted as more hemoglobin is released. As a result, the plasma haptoglobin level is low. If the marrow cannot compensate to replace the RBCs (indicated by a decreased reticulocyte count), the anemia will progress.

Hemolytic anemia has various forms. Among the inherited forms are sickle cell anemia, thalassemia and thalassemia major, G-6-PD deficiency, and hereditary spherocytosis. Acquired forms include autoimmune hemolytic anemia, nonimmune-mediated paroxysmal nocturnal hemoglobinuria, microangiopathic hemolytic anemia, and heart valve hemolysis, as well as anemias associated with hypersplenism.

SICKLE CELL ANEMIA

Sickle cell anemia is a severe hemolytic anemia that results from inheritance of the sickle hemoglobin gene. This gene causes the hemoglobin molecule to be defective. The sickle hemoglobin (HbS) acquires a crystal-like formation when exposed to low oxygen tension. The oxygen level in venous blood can be low enough to cause this change; consequently, the RBC containing HbS loses its round, very pliable, biconcave disk shape and becomes deformed, rigid, and sickle-shaped (Fig. 33-5). These long, rigid RBCs can adhere to the endothelium of small vessels; when they pile up against each other, blood flow to a region or an organ may be reduced (Hoffman, et al., 2000). If ischemia or infarction results, the patient may have pain, swelling, and fever. The sickling process takes time; if the RBC is again exposed to adequate amounts of oxygen (eg, when it travels through the pulmonary circulation) before the membrane becomes too rigid, it can revert to a normal shape. For this reason, the "sickling crises" are intermittent. Cold can aggravate

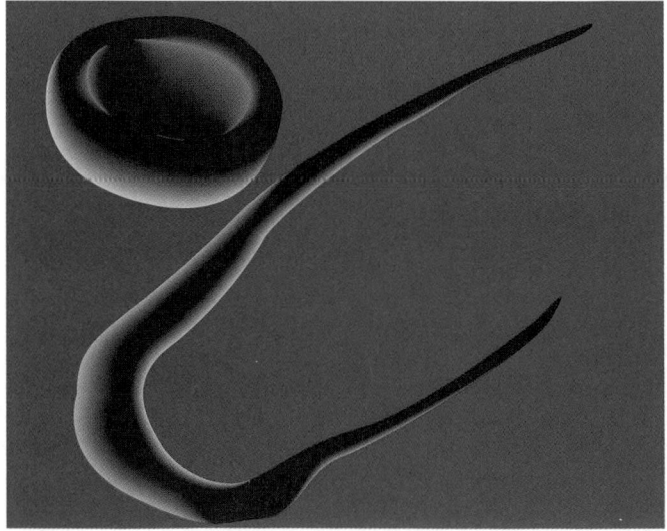

FIGURE 33-5 A normal red blood cell (*upper left*) and a sickled red blood cell.

the sickling process, because vasoconstriction slows the blood flow. Oxygen delivery can also be impaired by an increased blood viscosity, with or without occlusion due to adhesion of sickled cells; in this situation, the effects are seen in larger vessels, such as arterioles.

The *HbS* gene is inherited in people of African descent and to a lesser extent in people from the Middle East, the Mediterranean area, and aboriginal tribes in India. Sickle cell anemia is the most severe form of sickle cell disease. Less severe forms include sickle cell hemoglobin C (SC) disease, sickle cell hemoglobin D (SD) disease, and sickle cell beta-thalassemia. The clinical manifestations and management are the same as for sickle cell anemia. The term *sickle cell trait* refers to the carrier state for SC diseases; it is the most benign type of SC disease, in that less than 50% of the hemoglobin within an RBC is HbS. However, in terms of genetic counseling, it is still an important condition. If two people with sickle cell trait have children, the children may inherit two abnormal genes. These children will produce only HbS and therefore will have sickle cell anemia.

Clinical Manifestations

Symptoms of sickle cell anemia vary and are only somewhat based on the amount of HbS. Symptoms and complications result from chronic hemolysis or thrombosis. The sickled RBCs have a shortened life span. Patients are always anemic, usually with hemoglobin values of 7 to 10 g/dL. Jaundice is characteristic and is usually obvious in the sclerae. The bone marrow expands in childhood in a compensatory effort to offset the anemia, sometimes leading to enlargement of the bones of the face and skull. The chronic anemia is associated with tachycardia, cardiac murmurs, and often an enlarged heart (cardiomegaly). Dysrhythmias and heart failure may occur in adults.

Virtually any organ may be affected by thrombosis, but the primary sites involve those areas with slowed circulation, such as the spleen, lungs, and central nervous system. All the tissues and organs are constantly vulnerable to microcirculatory interruptions by the sickling process and therefore are susceptible to hypoxic damage or true ischemic necrosis. Patients with sickle cell anemia are unusually susceptible to infection, particularly pneumonia and osteomyelitis. Complications of sickle cell anemia include infection, stroke, renal failure, impotence, heart failure, and pulmonary hypertension. Table 33-4 summarizes the complications resulting from sickle cell anemia.

SICKLE CELL CRISIS

There are three types of sickle cell crisis in the adult population. The most common is the very painful *sickle crisis,* which results from tissue hypoxia and necrosis due to inadequate blood flow to a specific region of tissue or organ. *Aplastic crisis* results from infection with the human parvovirus. The hemoglobin level falls rapidly and the marrow cannot compensate, as evidenced by an absence of reticulocytes. *Sequestration crisis* results when other organs pool the sickled cells. Although the spleen is the most common organ responsible for sequestration in children, by 10 years of age most children with sickle cell anemia have had a splenic infarction and the spleen is then no longer functional (autosplenectomy). In adults, the common organs involved in sequestration are the liver and, more seriously, the lungs.

ACUTE CHEST SYNDROME

Acute chest syndrome is manifested by a rapidly falling hemoglobin level, tachycardia, fever, and bilateral infiltrates seen on the chest x-ray. These signs often mimic infection; in fact, recent studies have identified infection as a major cause of acute chest syndrome (Vichinsky, et al., 2000). Another common cause is pulmonary fat embolism. Increased secretory phospholipase A_2

Table 33-4 • Summary of Complications in Sickle Cell Anemia*

ORGAN INVOLVED	MECHANISMS*	ASSESSMENT FINDINGS	SIGNS AND SYMPTOMS
Spleen	Primary site of sickling → infarctions → ↓ phagocytic function of macrophages	Autosplenectomy; ↑ infection (esp. pneumonia, osteomyelitis)	Abdominal pain; fever, signs of infection
Lungs	Infection	Pulmonary infiltrate	Chest pain; dyspnea
	Infarction → ↑ pulmonary pressure → pulmonary hypertension	↑ sPLA$_2$[†]	
Central Nervous System	Infarction	CVA (cerebral vascular accident, brain attack)	Weakness (if severe); learning difficulties (if mild)
Kidney	Sickling → damage to renal medulla	Hematuria; inability to concentrate urine; renal failure	Dehydration
Heart	Anemia	Tachycardia; cardiomegaly → heart failure	Weakness, fatigue, dyspnea
Bone	↑ Erythroid production	Widening of medullary spaces and cortical thinning	Ache
	Infarction of bone	Osteosclerosis → avascular necrosis	Bone pain, especially hips
Liver	Hemolysis	Jaundice and gallstone formation; hepatomegaly	Abdominal pain
Skin and peripheral vasculature	↑ Viscosity/stasis → infarction → skin ulcers	Skin ulcers; ↓ wound healing	Pain
Eye	Infarction	Scarring, hemorrhage, retinal detachment	↓ Vision; blindness
Penis	Sickling	Priapism → impotence	Pain, impotence

* Problems encountered in sickle cell anemia vary and are the result of a variety of mechanisms, as depicted in this table. Common physical findings and symptoms are also variable.
[†] sPLA$_2$: Secretory phospholipase A_2, a laboratory test that can predict impending acute chest syndrome (see text).

concentration has been identified as a predictor of impending acute chest syndrome; the increased amounts of free fatty acids can cause increased permeability of the pulmonary endothelium and leakage of the pulmonary capillaries. Although this syndrome is potentially lethal, prompt intervention can result in a favorable outcome.

Assessment and Diagnostic Findings

The patient with sickle cell trait usually has a normal hemoglobin level, a normal hematocrit, and a normal blood smear. In contrast, the patient with sickle cell anemia has a low hematocrit and sickled cells on the smear. The diagnosis is confirmed by hemoglobin electrophoresis.

Prognosis

Patients with sickle cell anemia are usually diagnosed in childhood, because they become anemic in infancy and begin to have sickle cell crises at 1 or 2 years of age. Some children die in the first years of life, typically from infection, but the use of antibiotics and parent teaching have greatly improved the outcomes for these children. However, with current management strategies, the average life expectancy is still suboptimal, at 42 years. Young adults are often forced to live with multiple, often severe, complications from their disease. In some patients, the symptoms and complications diminish by 30 years of age; these patients live into the sixth decade or longer. At this time, there is no way to predict which patients will fall into this subgroup.

Medical Management

Treatment for sickle cell anemia is the focus of continued research (Steinberg, 1999). Many trials of medications that have antisickling properties are being conducted, as is research using antiadhesion treatment for vasoocclusive crises. However, aside from the equally important aggressive management of symptoms and complications, currently there are only three primary treatment modalities for sickle cell diseases: BMT, hydroxyurea, and long-term RBC transfusion.

BMT offers the potential for cure for this disease. However, this treatment modality is available to only a small subset of the patient population, because of either the lack of a compatible donor or the severe organ (eg, renal, liver, lung) damage already present in the patient.

PHARMACOLOGIC THERAPY

Hydroxyurea (Hydrea), a chemotherapy agent, has been shown to be effective in increasing hemoglobin F levels in patients with sickle cell anemia, thereby decreasing the permanent formation of sickled cells. Patients who receive hydroxyurea appear to have fewer painful episodes of sickle cell crisis, a lower incidence of acute chest syndrome, and less need for transfusions (Ferster et al., 2001). However, whether hydroxyurea can prevent or reverse actual organ damage remains unknown. Side effects of hydroxyurea include chronic suppression of WBC formation, teratogenesis, and potential for later development of a malignancy. Patient response to the medication varies significantly. The incidence and severity of side effects are also highly variable within a dose range. Some patients have toxicity when receiving a very small dose (5 mg/kg per day), whereas others have little toxicity with a much higher dose (35 mg/kg per day). More research is needed to identify specific patient subgroups that are more likely to respond to this medication.

TRANSFUSION THERAPY

Chronic transfusions with RBCs have been shown to be highly effective in several situations: in an acute exacerbation of anemia (eg, aplastic crisis), in the prevention of severe complications from anesthesia and surgery, and in improving the response to infection (when it results in exacerbated anemia) (Ohene-Frempong, 2001). Chronic transfusions have also been shown to be effective in diminishing episodes of sickle cell crisis in pregnant women; however, these transfusions have not been shown to improve fetal survival. Transfusion therapy may be effective in preventing complications from sickle cell disease. Although controversial, some data support the use of chronic transfusions in patients with cerebral ischemic injury (as seen on magnetic resonance imaging [MRI] or Doppler studies) to prevent more severe injury (eg, CVA). More than 50% of asymptomatic patients have some cerebral ischemia documented by MRI. In a recent study (Adams, 2000), chronic transfusion with RBCs resulted in a 90% reduction of stroke in children at risk for this complication, as demonstrated by elevated blood viscosity on transcranial Doppler ultrasonography. Transfusions may also be useful in the management of severe cases of acute chest syndrome.

The risk of complications from transfusion is important to consider. These risks include iron overload, which necessitates chronic chelation therapy (see MDS Nursing Management); poor venous access, which necessitates a vascular access device (and its attendant risk for infection or thrombosis); infections (hepatitis, human immunodeficiency virus [HIV]); and alloimmunization from repeated transfusions. Another complication from transfusion is the increased viscosity of blood before the concentration of hemoglobin S is reduced. Exchange transfusion (in which the patient's own blood is removed and replaced via transfusion) may be performed to diminish the risk of increasing the viscosity excessively; the objective is to reduce the hematocrit to less than 30%, with transfusions supplying more than 80% of the patient's blood volume. Finally, it is important to consider the significant financial cost of an aggressive transfusion and chelation program.

Patients with sickle cell anemia require daily folic acid replacements to maintain the supply required for increased erythropoiesis from hemolysis. Infections must be treated promptly with appropriate antibiotics; infection remains a major cause of death in these patients.

Acute chest syndrome is managed by prompt initiation of antibiotic therapy. Incentive spirometry has been shown to decrease the incidence of pulmonary complications significantly. In severe cases, bronchoscopy may be required to identify the source of pulmonary disease. Fluid restriction may be more beneficial than aggressive hydration. Corticosteroids may also be useful. Transfusions reverse the hypoxia and decrease the level of secretory phospholipase A_2. Pulmonary function should be monitored regularly to detect pulmonary hypertension early, when therapy (hydroxyurea, transfusions, or transplantation) may have a positive impact.

Because repeated blood transfusions are necessary, patients may develop multiple autoantibodies, making cross-matching difficult. In this patient population, a hemolytic transfusion reaction (see later discussion) may mimic the signs and symptoms of a sickle cell crisis. The classic distinguishing factor is that, with a hemolytic transfusion reaction, the patient becomes more anemic after being transfused. These patients need very close observation. Further transfusion is avoided if possible until the hemolytic process abates. If possible, the patient is supported with corticosteroids (Prednisone), intravenous immunoglobulin (IVIG; Gammagard, Sandoglobulin, Venoglobulin), and erythropoietin (Epogen, Procrit).

SUPPORTIVE THERAPY

Supportive care is equally important. A significant issue is pain management. The incidence of painful sickle cell crises is highly variable; many patients have pain on a daily basis. The severity of the pain may not be enough to cause the patient to seek assistance from health care providers but severe enough to interfere with the ability to work and function within the family. Acute pain episodes tend to be self-limited, lasting hours to days. If the patient cannot manage the pain at home, intervention is frequently sought in the acute care setting, usually at an urgent care facility or emergency department. Adequate hydration is important during a painful sickling episode. Oral hydration is acceptable if the patient can maintain adequate amounts of fluids; intravenous hydration with dextrose 5% in water (D_5W) or dextrose 5% in 0.25 normal saline solution (3 L/m²/24 hours) is usually required for sickle crisis. Supplemental oxygen may also be needed.

The use of medication to relieve pain is important (see Chap. 13 for a discussion of pain management). Aspirin is very useful in diminishing mild to moderate pain; it also diminishes inflammation and potential thrombosis (due to its ability to diminish platelet adhesion). Nonsteroidal anti-inflammatory drugs (NSAIDs) are useful for moderate pain or in combination with opioid analgesics. Although no tolerance develops with NSAIDs, a "ceiling effect" does develop whereby an increase in dosage does not increase analgesia. NSAID use must be carefully monitored, because these medications can precipitate renal dysfunction. When opioid analgesics are used, morphine is the medication of choice for acute pain. Patient-controlled analgesia is frequently used.

Chronic pain increases in incidence as the patient ages. Here, the pain is caused by complications from the sickling, such as avascular necrosis of the hip. With chronic pain management, the principal goal is to maximize functioning; pain may not be completely eliminated without sacrificing function. This concept may be difficult for patients to accept; they may need repeated explanations and support from nonjudgmental health care providers. Nonpharmacologic approaches to pain management are crucial in this setting. Examples include physical and occupational therapy, physiotherapy (including the use of heat, massage, and exercise), cognitive and behavioral intervention (including distraction, relaxation, and motivational therapy), and support groups.

Working with patients who have multiple episodes of severe pain can be challenging. It is important for health care providers to realize that patients with sickle cell disease must face a lifelong experience with severe and unpredictable pain. Such pain is disruptive to the person's level of functioning, including social functioning, and may result in a feeling of helplessness. Patients with inadequate social support systems may have more difficulty coping with chronic pain.

NURSING PROCESS:
THE PATIENT WITH SICKLE CELL CRISIS

Patients in sickle cell crisis should be assessed for factors that could have precipitated the crisis, such as symptoms of infection or dehydration, or situations that promote fatigue or emotional stress.

Assessment

Patients are asked to recall factors that seemed to precipitate previous crises and measures they use to prevent and manage crises. Pain levels should always be monitored; a pain-rating scale, such as a 0-to-10 scale, best accomplishes this. The quality of the pain (eg, sharp, dull, burning), the frequency of the pain (constant versus intermittent), and factors that aggravate or alleviate the pain are included in this assessment. If a sickle cell crisis is suspected, the nurse needs to determine whether the pain currently experienced is the same as or different than the pain typically encountered in crisis.

Because the sickling process can interrupt circulation in any tissue or organ, with resultant hypoxia and ischemia, a careful assessment of all body systems is necessary. Particular emphasis is placed on assessing for pain, swelling, and fever. All joint areas are carefully examined for pain and swelling. The abdomen is assessed for pain and tenderness because of the possibility of splenic infarction.

The respiratory system must be assessed carefully, including auscultation of breath sounds, measurement of oxygen saturation levels, and signs of cardiac failure, such as the presence and extent of dependent edema, an increased point of maximal impulse, and cardiomegaly (as seen on chest x-ray). The patient should be assessed for signs of dehydration by a history of fluid intake and careful examination of mucous membranes, skin turgor, urine output, and serum creatinine and blood urea nitrogen values.

A careful neurologic examination is important to elicit symptoms of cerebral hypoxia. However, ischemic findings on MRI or Doppler studies may significantly precede the findings on the physical examination. MRI and Doppler studies are used for early diagnosis and may be more beneficial to improve patient outcome, because therapy can be initiated more promptly.

Because patients with sickle cell anemia are so susceptible to infections, they are assessed for the presence of any infectious process. Particular attention is given to examination of the chest, long bones, and femoral head, because pneumonia and osteomyelitis are especially common. Leg ulcers, which may be infected and are slow to heal, are common.

The extent of anemia (as measured by the hemoglobin level and the hematocrit) and the ability of the marrow to replenish RBCs (as measured by the reticulocyte count) should be monitored and compared with the patient's baseline values. The patient's current and past history of medical management should also be assessed, particularly chronic transfusion therapy, hydroxyurea use, and prior treatment for infection.

Diagnosis

NURSING DIAGNOSES

Based on the assessment data, major nursing diagnoses for the patient with sickle cell crisis may include:

- Acute pain related to tissue hypoxia due to agglutination of sickled cells within blood vessels
- Risk for infection
- Risk for powerlessness related to illness-induced helplessness
- Deficient knowledge regarding sickle crisis prevention

COLLABORATIVE PROBLEMS/
POTENTIAL COMPLICATIONS

Based on the assessment data, potential complications may include:

- Hypoxia, ischemia, infection, and poor wound healing leading to skin breakdown and ulcers
- Dehydration
- Cerebrovascular accident (CVA, brain attack, stroke)
- Anemia
- Renal dysfunction
- Heart failure, pulmonary hypertension, and acute chest syndrome
- Impotence
- Poor compliance
- Substance abuse related to poorly managed chronic pain

Planning and Goals

The major goals for the patient are relief of pain, decreased incidence of crisis, enhanced sense of self-esteem and power, and absence of complications.

Nursing Interventions

MANAGING PAIN

Acute pain during a sickle cell crisis can be severe and unpredictable. The patient's subjective description and rating of pain on a pain scale must guide the use of analgesics, which are valuable in controlling the acute pain of a sickle crisis. Any joint that is acutely swollen should be supported and elevated until the swelling diminishes. Relaxation techniques, breathing exercises, and distraction are helpful for some patients. After the acute painful episode has diminished, aggressive measures should be implemented to preserve function. Physical therapy, whirlpool baths, and transcutaneous nerve stimulation are examples of such modalities.

PREVENTING AND MANAGING INFECTION

Nursing care focuses on monitoring the patient for signs and symptoms of infection. Prescribed antibiotics should be initiated promptly, and the patient should be assessed for signs of dehydration. If the patient is to take prescribed oral antibiotics at home, he or she must understand the need to complete the entire course of antibiotic therapy and must be able to identify a feasible administration schedule.

PROMOTING COPING SKILLS

This illness, because of its acute exacerbations that often result in chronic health problems, frequently leaves the patient feeling powerless and with decreased self-esteem. These feelings can be exacerbated by inadequate pain management. The patient's ability to use normal coping resources of physical strength, psychological stamina, and positive self-esteem is dramatically diminished. Enhancing pain management can be extremely useful in establishing a therapeutic relationship based on mutual trust. Nursing care that focuses on the patient's strengths rather than deficits can enhance effective coping skills. Providing the patient with opportunities to make decisions about daily care may increase the patient's feelings of control.

MINIMIZING DEFICIENT KNOWLEDGE

Patients with sickle cell anemia benefit from understanding what situations can precipitate a sickle cell crisis and the steps they can take to prevent or diminish such crises. Keeping warm and maintaining adequate hydration can be very effective in diminishing the occurrence and severity of attacks. Avoiding stressful situations is more challenging. Group education may be more effective if it is carried out by members of the community who are from the same ethnic group as those with the disease.

MONITORING AND MANAGING POTENTIAL COMPLICATIONS

Management measures for many of the potential complications were delineated in previous sections. Other measures follow.

Leg Ulcers

Leg ulcers require careful management and protection from trauma and contamination. Referral to a wound care specialist may facilitate healing and assist with prevention. If leg ulcers fail to heal, skin grafting may be necessary. Scrupulous aseptic technique is warranted to prevent nosocomial infections.

Priapism Leading to Impotence

Male patients may develop sudden, painful episodes of priapism (persistent penile erection). The patient is taught to empty his bladder at the onset of the attack, exercise, and take a warm bath. If an episode persists longer than 3 hours, medical attention is recommended. Repeated episodes may lead to extensive vascular thrombosis, resulting in impotence.

Chronic Pain and Substance Abuse

Many patients have considerable difficulty coping with chronic pain and repeated episodes of sickle crisis. Those who feel they have little control over their health and the physical complications that result from this illness may find it difficult to understand the importance of complying with a prescribed treatment plan. Being nonjudgmental and actively seeking involvement from the patient in establishing a treatment plan are useful strategies.

Some patients with sickle cell anemia develop problems with substance abuse. For many, this abuse results from inadequate management of acute pain during episodes of crisis. Some clinicians suggest that abuse may result from prescribing inadequate amounts of opioid analgesics for an inadequate time. The patient's pain may never be adequately relieved, promoting mistrust of the health care system and (from the patient's perspective) the need to seek care from a variety of sources when the pain is not severe. This cycle is best managed by prevention. Receiving care from a single provider over time is much more beneficial than receiving care from rotating physicians and staff in an emergency department. When crises do arise, the staff in the emergency department should be in contact with the patient's primary health care provider so that optimal management can be achieved. Once the pattern of substance abuse is established, it is very difficult to manage, but continuity of care and establishing written contracts with the patient can be useful management strategies.

PROMOTING HOME AND COMMUNITY-BASED CARE

Teaching Patients Self-Care

Because patients with sickle cell anemia are typically diagnosed as children, parents participate in the initial education. Based on the parents' education, literacy, socioeconomic level, and interest, teaching focuses on the disease process (including some pathophysiology), treatment, and the assessment and monitoring skills for potential complications. As the child ages, educational interventions prepare the child to assume more responsibility for self-care.

Vascular access device management and chelation therapy can be taught to most families. Follow-up and care for patients with vascular access devices may also need to be provided by nurses in an outpatient facility or by a home care agency.

Continuing Care

The illness trajectory of sickle cell anemia is highly varied, with unpredictable episodes of complications and crises. Care is often provided on an emergency basis, especially for some patients with pain management problems (see previous section). Nurses in all settings used by this patient population need to communicate regularly with each other. Patients need to learn which parameters are important for them to monitor and how to monitor them. Parameters should also be given as to when to seek urgent care.

Evaluation

EXPECTED PATIENT OUTCOMES

Expected patient outcomes may include:

1. Control of pain
   a. Acute pain is controlled with analgesics
   b. Uses relaxation techniques, breathing exercises, distraction to help relieve pain
2. Is free of infection
   a. Has normal temperature
   b. Shows WBC count within normal range (5,000 to 10,000/mm^3)
   c. Identifies importance of continuing antibiotics at home (if applicable)
3. Expresses improved sense of control
   a. Participates in goal setting and in planning and implementing daily activities
   b. Participates in decisions about care
4. Increases knowledge about disease process
   a. Identifies situations and factors that can precipitate sickle cell crisis
   b. Describes lifestyle changes needed to prevent crisis
   c. Describes the importance of warmth, adequate hydration, and prevention of infection in preventing crisis
5. Absence of complications

THALASSEMIA

The thalassemias are a group of hereditary disorders associated with defective hemoglobin-chain synthesis. These anemias occur worldwide, but the highest prevalence is found in people of Mediterranean, African, and Southeast Asian ancestry (Hoffman et al., 2000). Thalassemias are characterized by **hypochromia** (an abnormal decrease in the hemoglobin content of RBCs), extreme **microcytosis** (smaller-than-normal RBCs), destruction of blood elements (hemolysis), and variable degrees of anemia.

In thalassemia, the production of one or more globulin chains within the hemoglobin molecule is reduced. When this occurs, the imbalance in the configuration of the hemoglobin causes it to precipitate in the erythroid precursors or the RBCs themselves. This increases the rigidity of the RBCs and thus the premature destruction of these cells.

The thalassemias are classified into two major groups according to the globin chain diminished: alpha and beta. The alpha-thalassemias occur mainly in people from Asia and the Middle East; the beta-thalassemias are most prevalent in Mediterranean populations but also occur in people from the Middle East or Asia. The alpha-thalassemias are milder than the beta forms and often occur without symptoms. The RBCs are extremely microcytic, but the anemia, if present, is mild.

The severity of beta-thalassemia varies depending on the extent to which the hemoglobin chains are affected. Patients with mild forms have a microcytosis and mild anemia. If left untreated, severe beta-thalassemia (thalassemia major, or Cooley's anemia) can be fatal within the first few years of life. If it is treated with regular transfusion of RBCs, patients may survive into their 20s and 30s. Patient teaching during the reproductive years should include pre-conception counseling about the risk of congenital thalassemia major.

Thalassemia Major

Thalassemia major (Cooley's anemia) is characterized by severe anemia, marked hemolysis, and ineffective erythropoiesis (production of RBCs). With early regular transfusion therapy, growth and development through childhood are facilitated. Organ dysfunction due to iron overload results from the excessive amounts of iron obtained through the RBC transfusions. Regular chelation therapy (eg, via subcutaneous deferoxamine) has reduced the complications of iron overload and prolonged the life of these patients. This disease is potentially curable by BMT if the procedure can be performed before damage to the liver occurs (ie, during childhood).

GLUCOSE-6-PHOSPHATE DEHYDROGENASE DEFICIENCY

The abnormality in this disorder is in the G-6-PD gene; this gene produces an enzyme within the RBC that is essential for membrane stability. A few patients have inherited an enzyme so defective that they have a chronic hemolytic anemia; however, the most common type of defect results in hemolysis only when the RBCs are stressed by certain situations, such as fever or the use of certain medications. The disorder came to the attention of researchers during World War II, when some soldiers developed hemolysis while taking primaquine, an antimalarial agent. African Americans and people of Greek or Italian origin are those primarily affected by this disorder. The type of deficiency found in the Mediterranean population is more severe than that in the African Caribbean population, resulting in greater hemolysis and sometimes in life-threatening anemia. All types of G-6-PD deficiency are inherited as X-linked defects; therefore, many more men are at risk than women. In the United States, about 12% of African American males are affected. The deficiency is also common in those of Asian ancestry and in certain Jewish populations.

Medications that have hemolytic effects for people with G-6-PD deficiency are oxidant drugs. These medications include antimalarial agents (eg, chloroquine [Aralen]), sulfonamides (eg, trimethoprim and sulfamethoxazole [Septra]), nitrofurantoin (eg, Macrodantin), common coal tar analgesics (including aspirin in high doses), thiazide diuretics (eg, hydrochlorothiazide [Hydro-DIURIL], chlorothiazide [Diuril]), oral hypoglycemic agents (eg, glyburide [Micronase], metformin [Glucophage]), chloramphenicol (Chloromycetin), and vitamin K (phytonadione [Aqua-Mephyton]). In affected people, a severe hemolytic episode can result from ingestion of fava beans.

Clinical Manifestations

Patients are asymptomatic and have normal hemoglobin levels and reticulocyte counts most of the time. However, several days after exposure to an offending medication, they may develop pallor, jaundice, and hemoglobinuria (hemoglobin in the urine). The reticulocyte count rises, and symptoms of hemolysis develop. Special stains of the peripheral blood may then disclose Heinz bodies (degraded hemoglobin) within the RBCs. Hemolysis is often mild and self-limited. However, in the more severe Mediterranean type of G-6-PD deficiency, spontaneous recovery may not occur and transfusions may be necessary.

Assessment and Diagnostic Findings

The diagnosis is made by a screening test or by a quantitative assay of G-6-PD.

Medical Management

The treatment is to stop the offending medication. Transfusion is necessary only in the severe hemolytic state, which is more commonly seen in the Mediterranean variety of G-6-PD deficiency.

Nursing Management

The patient should be educated about the disease and given a list of medications to avoid. If hemolysis does develop, nursing interventions are the same as for hemolysis from other causes.

HEREDITARY SPHEROCYTOSIS

Hereditary spherocytosis is a relatively common (1 in 5,000 people) hemolytic anemia characterized by an abnormal permeability of the RBC membrane; this permits the cells to change into a spherical shape. These RBCs are destroyed prematurely in the spleen. The severity of this hemolytic anemia varies; jaundice can be intermittent, and splenomegaly (enlarged spleen) also can occur. Surgical removal of the spleen is the principal treatment for this disorder.

IMMUNE HEMOLYTIC ANEMIA

Hemolytic anemias can result from exposure of the RBC to antibodies. Alloantibodies (ie, antibodies against the host, or "self") result from the immunization of an individual with foreign antigens (eg, the immunization of an Rh-negative person with Rh-positive blood). Alloantibodies tend to be large (IgM type) and cause immediate destruction of the sensitized RBCs, either within the blood vessel (intravascular hemolysis) or within the liver. The most common type of alloimmune hemolytic anemia in adults results from a hemolytic transfusion reaction.

Autoantibodies are developed by an individual for varying reasons. In many instances, the person's immune system is dysfunctional, so that it falsely recognizes its own RBCs as foreign and produces antibodies against them. This mechanism is seen in people with chronic lymphocytic leukemia (CLL). Another mechanism is a deficiency in suppressor lymphocytes, which normally prevent antibody formation against a person's own antigens. Autoantibodies tend to be of the IgG type. The RBCs are sequestered in the spleen and destroyed by the macrophages outside the blood vessel (extravascular hemolysis).

Autoimmune hemolytic anemias can be classified based on the body temperature involved when the antibodies react with the RBC antigen. Warm-body antibodies bind to RBCs most actively in warm conditions (37°C); cold-body antibodies react in cold (0°C). Most autoimmune hemolytic anemias are the warm-body type. Autoimmune hemolytic anemia is associated with other disorders in most cases (eg, medication exposure, lymphoma, CLL, other malignancy, collagen vascular disease, autoimmune disease, infection). In idiopathic autoimmune hemolytic states, the reason why the immune system produces the antibodies is not known. All ages and both genders are equally vulnerable to this form, whereas the incidence of secondary forms is greater in people older than 45 years of age and in females.

Clinical Manifestations

Clinical manifestations can vary, and they usually reflect the degree of anemia. The hemolysis may be very mild, so that the patient's marrow compensates adequately and the patient is asymptomatic. At the other extreme, the hemolysis can be so severe that the resul-

tant anemia is life-threatening. Most patients complain of fatigue and dizziness. Splenomegaly is the most common physical finding, occurring in more than 80% of patients; hepatomegaly, lymphadenopathy, and jaundice are also common.

Assessment and Diagnostic Findings

The laboratory tests show a low hemoglobin level and hematocrit, most often with an accompanying increase in the reticulocyte count. RBCs appear abnormal; spherocytes are common. The serum bilirubin level is elevated, and if the hemolysis is severe, the haptoglobin level is low or absent. The Coombs test (also referred to as the direct antiglobulin test [DAT]), which detects antibodies on the surface of RBCs, shows a positive result.

Medical Management

Any possibly offending medication should be immediately discontinued. The treatment consists of high doses of corticosteroids (1 mg/kg per day) until hemolysis decreases. Corticosteroids decrease the macrophage's ability to clear the antibody-coated RBCs. If the hemoglobin level returns toward normal, usually after several weeks, the corticosteroid dose can be lowered or, in some cases, tapered and discontinued. However, corticosteroids rarely produce a lasting remission. In severe cases, blood transfusions may be required. Because the antibody may react with all possible donor cells, careful blood typing is necessary, and the transfusion should be administered slowly and cautiously.

Splenectomy (removal of the spleen) removes the major site of RBC destruction; therefore, splenectomy may be performed if corticosteroids do not produce a remission. If neither corticosteroid therapy nor splenectomy is successful, immunosuppressive agents may be administered. The two immunosuppressive agents most frequently used are cyclophosphamide (eg, Cytoxan), which has a more rapid effect but more toxicity, or azathioprine (Imuran), which has a less rapid effect but less toxicity. The synthetic androgen danazol (eg, Cyclomen, Danocrine) can be useful in some patients, particularly in combination with corticosteroids. The mechanism for this success is unclear. If corticosteroids or immunosuppressive agents are used, the taper must be very gradual to prevent a rebound "hyperimmune" response and exacerbation of the hemolysis. Immunoglobulin administration is effective in about one third of patients, but the effect is transient and the medication is expensive. Transfusions may be necessary if the anemia is severe; it may be extremely difficult to cross-match samples of available units of RBCs with that of the patient.

For patients with cold-antibody hemolytic anemia, treatment may not be required, other than to advise the patient to keep warm; relocation to a warm climate may be necessary.

Nursing Management

Patients may have great difficulty understanding the pathologic mechanisms underlying the disease and need repeated explanations in terms they can understand. Patients who have had a splenectomy should be vaccinated against pneumococcal infections (Pneumovax) and informed that they are permanently at greater risk for infection. Patients receiving long-term corticosteroid therapy, particularly those with concurrent diabetes or hypertension, need careful monitoring. They must understand the need for this medication and the importance of never abruptly discontinuing it. A written explanation and a tapering schedule should be provided, and adjustments based on hemoglobin levels should be emphasized. Similar teaching should be provided when immunosuppressive agents are used. Corticosteroid therapy is not without significant risk, and patients need to be monitored closely for complications. The short- and long-term complications of corticosteroid therapy are presented in Chart 33-4 and in Chap. 42.

> **NURSING ALERT** It can be difficult to cross-match blood when antibodies are present. If imperfectly cross-matched RBCs must be transfused, the nurse begins the infusion very slowly (10 to 15 mL over 20 to 30 minutes) and monitors the patient very closely for signs and symptoms of a hemolytic transfusion reaction.

HEREDITARY HEMOCHROMATOSIS

Hemochromatosis is a genetic condition in which iron is abnormally (excessively) absorbed from the gastrointestinal tract. The excessive iron is deposited in various organs, particularly the liver, myocardium, testes, thyroid, and pancreas. Eventually, the affected organs become dysfunctional. The actual incidence of hemochromatosis is unknown; however, hereditary hemochromatosis is diagnosed in 0.5% of the population in the United States (ie, 1 million people). Recent data suggest that this defect may be a common cause of diabetes (Schechter, et al., 2000). Because of their natural loss of iron through menses, women are less affected than men.

Because the accumulation of iron in body organs occurs gradually, there often is no evidence of tissue injury until middle age. Symptoms of weakness, lethargy, arthralgia, weight loss, and loss of libido are common. The skin may be hyperpigmented with melanin deposits (occasionally **hemosiderin**, an iron-containing pigment) and appears bronze in color. Cardiac dysrhythmias and cardiomyopathy can occur, with resulting dyspnea and edema. Endocrine dysfunction is manifested as hypothyroidism, diabetes mellitus, and hypogonadism (testicular atrophy, diminished libido, and impotence). A significant effect of hemochromatosis is the

---

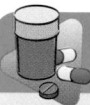

Chart 33-4 • PHARMACOLOGY
Complications Associated with Corticosteroid Therapy

Whenever a patient begins a course of corticosteroid therapy, the potential for complications is great. Dosing regimens vary widely, depending on the underlying hematologic condition and the patient's response to the medication. For example, several chemotherapy protocols include high doses of corticosteroids for a period of several days. After that time, the medication is stopped abruptly without tapering the dosage. In other conditions, such as idiopathic thrombocytopenic purpura or hemolytic anemias, the corticosteroids are very carefully tapered to prevent a flare up of the underlying disease. With the exception of patients with preexisting conditions such as diabetes, hypertension, and osteoporosis, it is difficult to predict which complications will occur in a given patient. Patients who receive high doses of corticosteroids for longer than a few weeks should be screened for symptoms related to the potential complications listed here. If at all possible, patients who require long-term corticosteroid use should be switched to an alternate-day dosing schedule; this method may diminish the severity of complications that arise.

Short-Term Complications
Fluid and Electrolyte Complications
Fluid retention
Sodium retention
Potassium loss
Hypokalemic alkalosis
Hypertension

Endocrine Complications
Decreased carbohydrate tolerance
Diabetes mellitus
Uncontrolled glucose levels in diabetes mellitus

Neurologic Complications
Headache

Musculoskeletal Complications
Muscle weakness

Psychologic Complications
Depression
Euphoria
Mood swings
Insomnia
Psychosis

Long-Term Complications
Endocrine Complications
Decreased adrenocortical activity
Decreased ability to respond to stress
Decreased carbohydrate tolerance
Decreased growth rate (children)
Cushingoid state
Menstrual irregularities
Increased sweating

Metabolic Complications
Protein catabolism causing negative nitrogen balance

Gastrointestinal Complications
Gastritis
Ulcerative esophagitis
Peptic ulcer
Pancreatitis

Musculoskeletal Complications
Decreased muscle mass
Osteoporosis
Vertebral compression fracture
Pathologic fracture
Aseptic necrosis of femoral and humeral heads

Neurologic Complications
Vertigo
Increased intracranial pressure
Seizures

Ophthalmic Complications
Cataract formation
Glaucoma
Exophthalmos

Dermatologic Complications
Impaired wound healing
Ecchymoses
Increased skin fragility
Decreased skin thickness
Petechiae

Immunologic Complications
Decreased response to infection
Masked signs of early stages of infection
Suppressed reaction to skin tests
Increased risk for opportunistic infection (eg, *Pneumocystis*, herpes zoster)

development of hepatocellular carcinoma in one third of those affected. CBC values are typically normal. The most useful laboratory findings are an elevated serum iron level and high transferrin saturation (more than 60% in men, more than 50% in women). The definitive diagnostic test is a liver biopsy. Recently, a mutation in the *HFE* gene has been shown to occur in most patients with hereditary hemochromatosis (Gochee & Powell, 2001). Patients who are homozygous for the gene are at high risk for development of the disorder.

Medical Management

Therapy involves the removal of excess iron via therapeutic phlebotomy (removal of whole blood from a vein). Each unit of blood removed results in a decrease of 200–250 mg of iron. The objective typically is to reduce the serum ferritin to less than 50 μg/L and the transferrin saturation to 35% or less. To achieve this, a frequent phlebotomy schedule is required (1 to 2 units weekly), with a gradual reduction in frequency of phlebotomies over a 1- to 3-year period. After 1 to 3 years, the frequency of phlebotomy can be reduced to 1 unit of blood every several months to prevent reaccumulation of iron deposits. Removal of excess iron appears to diminish the severity of diabetes and skin hyperpigmentation; cardiac function also tends to improve.

Nursing Management

Patients with hemochromatosis often believe that it is important to limit their dietary intake of iron, although this management method has been shown to be very ineffective and need not be encouraged. However, it is important for these patients to avoid any additional insults to the liver, such as alcohol abuse. Serial screening tests for hepatoma are important; alpha-fetoprotein is used for this purpose. Other body systems should be monitored for signs of organ dysfunction, particularly the endocrine and cardiac systems. These systems should also be screened routinely for dysfunction so that appropriate management can be implemented quickly. Because patients with hemochromatosis require frequent phlebotomies, problems with venous access are common. Patients who are heterozygous for the *HFE* do not develop the disease but need to be counseled that they can transmit the gene to their children.

The Polycythemias

Polycythemia refers to an increased volume of RBCs. It is a term used when the hematocrit is elevated (to more than 55% in males, more than 50% in females). Dehydration (decreased volume of plasma) can cause an elevated hematocrit, but not typically to the level to be considered polycythemia. Polycythemia is classified as either primary or secondary.

POLYCYTHEMIA VERA

Polycythemia vera, or primary polycythemia, is a proliferative disorder in which the myeloid stem cells seem to have escaped normal control mechanisms. The bone marrow is hypercellular, and the RBC, WBC, and platelet counts in the peripheral blood are elevated. However, the RBC elevation is predominant; the hematocrit can exceed 60%. This phase can last for an extended period (10 years or longer). The spleen resumes its embryonic function of hematopoiesis and enlarges. Over time, the bone marrow may become fibrotic, with a resultant inability to produce as many cells

("burnt out" or spent phase). The disease evolves into myeloid metaplasia with myelofibrosis or AML in a significant proportion of patients; this form of AML is usually refractory to standard treatments (Hoffman, et al., 2000). The median survival time exceeds 15 years (Gruppo Italiano Studio Policitemia, 1995).

Clinical Manifestations

Patients typically have a ruddy complexion and splenomegaly (enlarged spleen). The symptoms result from the increased blood volume (headache, dizziness, tinnitus, fatigue, paresthesias, and blurred vision) or from increased blood viscosity (angina, claudication, dyspnea, and thrombophlebitis), particularly if the patient has atherosclerotic blood vessels. Another common and bothersome problem is generalized pruritus, which may be caused by histamine release due to the increased number of basophils. Erythromelalgia, a burning sensation in the fingers and toes, may be reported and is only partially relieved by cooling.

Assessment and Diagnostic Findings

Diagnosis is made by finding an elevated RBC mass (a nuclear medicine procedure), a normal oxygen saturation level, and an enlarged spleen. Other factors useful in establishing the diagnosis include elevated WBC and platelet counts. The erythropoietin level is not as low as would be expected with an elevated hematocrit; it is normal or only slightly low. Causes of secondary erythrocytosis should not be present (see later discussion).

Complications

Patients with polycythemia vera are at increased risk for thromboses resulting in a CVA (brain attack, stroke) or heart attack (MI); thrombotic complications are the most frequent cause of death. Bleeding is also a complication, possibly due to the fact that the platelets (often very large) are somewhat dysfunctional. The bleeding can be significant and can occur in the form of nosebleeds, ulcers, and frank gastrointestinal bleeding.

Medical Management

The objective of management is to reduce the high blood cell mass. Phlebotomy is an important part of therapy and can be performed repeatedly to keep the hematocrit within normal range. This is achieved by removing enough blood (initially 500 mL once or twice weekly) to deplete the patient's iron stores, thereby rendering the patient iron deficient and consequently unable to continue to manufacture RBCs excessively. Patients need to be instructed to avoid iron supplements, including those within multivitamin supplements. If the patient has an elevated uric acid concentration, allopurinol (Zyloprim) is used to prevent gouty attacks. Antihistamines are not particularly effective in controlling itching. If the patient develops ischemic symptoms, dipyridamole (eg, Persantine) is sometimes used. Radioactive phosphorus (^{32}P) or chemotherapeutic agents (eg, hydroxyurea [Hydrea]) can be used to suppress marrow function, but they may increase the risk for leukemia. Patients receiving hydroxyurea appear to have a lower incidence of thrombotic complications; this may result from a more controlled platelet count. The use of aspirin to prevent thrombotic complications is controversial. Low-dose aspirin is frequently used in patients with cardiovascular disease, but even this dose is often avoided in patients with prior bleeding, especially bleeding from the gastrointestinal tract. Aspirin is also useful in diminishing pain associated with erythromelalgia. Anagrelide (Agrylin) inhibits platelet aggregation and can also be useful in controlling the thrombocytosis associated with polycythemia vera. Interferon alfa-2b (Intron-A) has also been studied, but it may be difficult for patients to tolerate due to the frequent side effects experienced (Tefferi et al., 2000; Lengfelder, Berger, & Hehlmann, 2000).

Nursing Management

The nurse's role is primarily that of educator. Risk factors for thrombotic complications should be assessed, and patients should be instructed regarding the signs and symptoms of thrombosis. Patients with a history of bleeding are usually advised to avoid aspirin and aspirin-containing medications, because these medications alter platelet function. Minimizing alcohol intake should also be emphasized to further diminish any risk for bleeding. For pruritus, the nurse may recommend bathing in tepid or cool water, along with applications of cocoa butter–based lotions and bath products.

SECONDARY POLYCYTHEMIA

Secondary polycythemia is caused by excessive production of erythropoietin. This may occur in response to a reduced amount of oxygen, which acts as a hypoxic stimulus, as in cigarette smoking, chronic obstructive pulmonary disease, or cyanotic heart disease, or in nonpathologic conditions such as high altitude. It can also result from certain hemoglobinopathies in which the hemoglobin has an abnormally high affinity for oxygen (eg, hemoglobin Chesapeake). Secondary polycythemia can also occur from neoplasms (eg, renal cell carcinoma) that stimulate erythropoietin production.

Medical Management

Management of secondary polycythemia may not be necessary; when it is, it involves treating the primary conditions. If the cause cannot be corrected (eg, by treating the renal cell carcinoma or improving pulmonary function), therapeutic phlebotomy may be necessary in symptomatic patients to reduce blood viscosity and volume.

Leukopenia and Neutropenia

Leukopenia, a condition in which there are fewer WBCs than normal, results from neutropenia (diminished neutrophils) or lymphopenia (diminished lymphocytes). Even if other types of WBCs (eg, monocytes, basophils) are diminished, their numbers are too few to reduce the total WBC count significantly. Lymphopenia (lymphocytes less than 1,500/mm³) can result from ionizing radiation, long-term use of corticosteroids, uremia, some neoplasms (eg, breast and lung cancers, advanced Hodgkin's disease), and some protein-losing enteropathies (in which the lymphocytes within the intestines are lost).

NEUTROPENIA

Neutropenia (neutrophils less than 2,000/mm³) results from decreased production of neutrophils or increased destruction of these cells (Chart 33-5). Neutrophils are essential in preventing and limiting bacterial infection. A patient with neutropenia is at increased risk for infection, both exogenous and endogenous (the gastro-

intestinal tract and skin are common endogenous sources). The risk for infection is based not only on the severity of the neutropenia (low neutrophil count), but also on the duration of the neutropenia. The actual number of neutrophils, known as the **absolute neutrophil count (ANC)**, is determined by a simple mathematical calculation using data obtained from the CBC and differential test (Chart 33-6). The risk of infection increases proportionately with the decrease in neutrophil count. The risk is significant when the ANC is less than 1000, is high when it is less than 500, and is almost certain when it is less than 100. The risk

Chart 33-5 Causes of Neutropenia

Decreased Production of Neutrophils
- Aplastic anemia, due to medications or toxins
- Metastatic cancer, lymphoma, leukemia
- Myelodysplastic syndromes
- Chemotherapy
- Radiation therapy

Ineffective Granulocytopoiesis
- Megaloblastic anemia

Increased Destruction of Neutrophils
- Hypersplenism
- Medication-induced*
- Immunologic disease (eg, systemic lupus erythematosus [SLE])
- Viral disease (eg, infectious hepatitis, mononucleosis)
- Bacterial infections

*Formation of antibody to medication, leading to a rapid decrease in neutrophils.

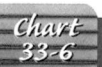

Chart 33-6 Calculating the Absolute Neutrophil Count (ANC)

$$ANC = \frac{\text{Total WBC count} \times (\% \text{ neutrophils} + \% \text{ bands})}{100}$$

Normally, the neutrophil count is greater than 2000/mm³. The actual (or absolute) neutrophil count (ANC) is calculated using the above formula.

For example, if the total white blood cell (WBC) count is 3000/mm³ with 72% neutrophils and 3% bands, the ANC would be calculated as follows:

$$ANC = \frac{3000\,(72 + 3)}{100} = 2250$$

This result is not indicative of neutropenia, because the ANC is greater than 2000 despite the low total WBC count (3000/mm³).

Conversely, in the following example, neutropenia is evident despite a normal WBC count (5500/mm³) with 8% neutrophils and 0% bands:

$$ANC = \frac{5500\,(8 + 0)}{100} = 440$$

Here, the ANC is severely low (440) despite the normal total WBC count (5500/mm³).

When evaluating neutropenia, it is important to calculate the ANC and not to rely solely on the total WBCs and percentage of neutrophils alone.

of developing infection increases with the length of time during which neutropenia persists, even if it is fairly mild. Conversely, even a severe neutropenia may not result in infection if the duration of the neutropenia is brief, as is often seen after chemotherapy (Chart 33-7).

Clinical Manifestations

There are no definite symptoms of neutropenia until the patient becomes infected. Routine CBC with differential tests, such as those obtained after chemotherapy treatment, can reveal neutropenia before the onset of infection.

Medical Management

Treatment of the neutropenia varies depending on its cause. If the neutropenia is medication induced, the offending agent needs to be stopped, if possible. Treatment of an underlying neoplasm can temporarily make the neutropenia worse, but with bone marrow recovery treatment may improve it. Corticosteroids may be used if the cause is an immunologic disorder. The use of growth factors such as G-CSF or granulocyte/macrophage colony-stimulating factor (GM-CSF) can be effective in increasing neutrophil production when the cause of the neutropenia is decreased production. Withholding or reducing the dose of chemotherapy or radiation therapy may be required when the neutropenia is caused by these treatments; however, in the case of potentially curative therapy, administration of growth factor is considered to be preferable, so that the maximum antitumor effect can be achieved. Should the neutropenia be accompanied by fever, the patient is automatically considered to be infected and usually is admitted to the hospital. Cultures of blood, urine, and sputum should be obtained, as well as a chest x-ray. To ensure adequate therapy against the invading infectious organisms, broad-spectrum antibiotics are initiated as soon as the samples for culture are obtained, although the medications may be changed after culture and sensitivity results become available.

Nursing Management

Nurses in all settings have a crucial role in assessing the severity of neutropenia and in preventing and managing infectious complications. Patient teaching is equally important, particularly in the outpatient setting, so that the patient can implement appropriate self-care measures and know when and how to seek medical care (Chart 33-8). Patients at risk for neutropenia should have blood drawn for CBCs; the frequency is based on the suspected severity and duration of the neutropenia. Nurses need to be able to calculate the ANC (see Chart 33-6) and to assess the severity of neutropenia and the risk for infection. Chart 33-9 identifies nursing interventions related to neutropenia.

Leukocytosis and the Leukemias

The term *leukocytosis* refers to an increased level of WBCs in the circulation. Typically, only one specific cell type is increased. Usually, because the proportions of several types of WBCs are small (eg, eosinophils, basophils, monocytes), only an increase in neutrophils or lymphocytes can be great enough to elevate the total WBC count. Although leukocytosis can be a normal response to increased need (eg, in acute infection), the elevation in WBCs should decrease as the need decreases. A prolonged or progressively increasing elevation in WBCs is abnormal and should be evaluated. A significant cause for persistent leukocytosis is malignancy.

Hematopoiesis is characterized by a rapid, continuous turnover of cells. Normally, production of specific blood cells

---

Chart 33-7

Risk Factors for Development of Infection and Bleeding in Patients with Hematologic Disorders

Risk for Infection

Severity of neutropenia: Risk of infection is proportional to duration and severity of neutropenia

Duration of neutropenia: Increased duration leads to increased risk of infection

Nutritional status: Decreased protein stores lead to decreased immune response and anergy

Deconditioning: Decreased mobility leads to decreased respiratory effort, leading to increased pooling of secretions

Lymphocytopenia; disorders of lymphoid system (chronic lymphocytic leukemia [CLL], lymphoma, myeloma): Decreased cell-mediated and humoral immunity

Invasive procedures: Break in skin integrity leads to increased opportunity for organisms to enter blood system

Hypogammaglobulinemia: Decreased antibody formation

Poor hygiene: Increased organisms on skin, mucous membranes

Poor dentition; mucositis: Decreased endothelial integrity leads to increased opportunity for organisms to enter blood system

Antibiotic therapy: Increased risk for superinfection, often fungal

Certain medications: See text

Risk for Bleeding

Severity of thrombocytopenia: Risk increases when platelet count decreases; usually not a significant risk until platelet count is lower than 20,000/mm³; lower than 50,000/mm³ when invasive procedure performed

Duration of thrombocytopenia: Risk increases when duration increases (eg, risk is less when duration is transient after chemotherapy than when duration is permanent with poor marrow production)

Sepsis: Mechanism unknown; appears to cause increased platelet consumption

Increased intracranial pressure: Increased blood pressure leads to rupture of blood vessels

Liver dysfunction: Decreased synthesis of clotting factors

Renal dysfunction: Decreased platelet function

Dysproteinemia: Protein coats surface of platelet, leading to decreased platelet function; protein causes increased viscosity, which leads to increased stretching of capillaries and thus increased bleeding

Alcohol abuse: Suppressive effect on marrow leads to decreased platelet production, decreased platelet function; decreased liver function, resulting in decreased production of clotting factors

Splenomegaly: Increased platelet destruction; spleen traps circulating platelets

Concurrent medications: See text

Chart 33-8
Home Care Checklist • The Patient at Risk for Infection

At the completion of the home care instruction, the patient or caregiver will be able to:	Patient	Caregiver
• Describe consequences of alterations in neutrophils, lymphocytes, immunoglobulins, or their sources.	✓	✓
• Verbalize the rationale for being at risk for infection.	✓	✓
• Identify signs and symptoms of infection.	✓	✓
• Demonstrate how to monitor for signs of infection.	✓	✓
• Describe to whom, how, and when to report signs of infection.	✓	✓
• Identify appropriate behaviors to take to prevent infection: – Maintain good hand hygiene technique, total body hygiene, and skin integrity. – Avoid fresh flowers, plants, garden work (soil), bird cages, and litter boxes. – Avoid fresh salads and unpeeled fruits or vegetables. – Maintain a high-calorie, high-protein diet, with fluid intake of 3,000 mL (unless fluids are restricted). – Avoid people with infections, crowds. – Perform deep breathing, use incentive spirometer every 4 hr while awake. – Provide adequate lubrication with gentle vaginal manipulation during sexual intercourse; avoid anal intercourse.	✓	✓
• Describe appropriate actions to take should infection occur.	✓	✓

from their stem cell precursors is carefully regulated according to the body's needs. If the mechanisms that control the production of these cells are disrupted, the cells can proliferate to an excessive, potentially dangerous degree. Hematopoietic malignancies are often classified according to the cells involved. **Leukemia**, literally "white blood," is a neoplastic proliferation of one particular cell type (granulocytes, monocytes, lymphocytes, or megakaryocytes). The defect originates in the hematopoietic stem cell, the myeloid, or the lymphoid stem cell. The lymphomas are neoplasms of lymphoid tissue, usually derived from B lymphocytes. Multiple myeloma is a malignancy of the most mature form of B lymphocyte, the plasma cell.

The common feature of the leukemias is an unregulated proliferation of WBCs in the bone marrow. In acute forms (or late stages of chronic forms), the proliferation of leukemic cells leaves little room for normal cell production. There can also be a proliferation of cells in the liver and spleen (extramedullary hematopoiesis). With acute forms, there can be infiltration of other organs, such as the meninges, lymph nodes, gums, and skin. The cause of leukemia is not fully known, but there is some evidence that genetic influence and viral pathogenesis may be involved. Bone marrow damage from radiation exposure or from chemicals such as benzene and alkylating agents (eg, melphalan [Alkeran]) can cause leukemia.

The leukemias are commonly classified according to the stem cell line involved, either lymphoid or myeloid. They are also classified as either acute or chronic, based on the time it takes for symptoms to evolve and the phase of cell development that is halted (ie, with few WBCs differentiating beyond that phase).

In acute leukemia, the onset of symptoms is abrupt, often occurring within a few weeks. WBC development is halted at the blast phase, so that most WBCs are undifferentiated or are blasts. Acute leukemia progresses very rapidly; death occurs within weeks to months without aggressive treatment. In chronic leukemia, symptoms evolve over a period of months to years, and the majority of WBCs produced are mature. Chronic leukemia progresses more slowly; the disease trajectory can extend for years.

ACUTE MYELOID LEUKEMIA (AML)

AML results from a defect in the hematopoietic stem cell that differentiates into all myeloid cells: monocytes, granulocytes (neutrophils, basophils, eosinophils), erythrocytes, and platelets. All age groups are affected; the incidence rises with age, with a peak incidence at age 60 years. AML is the most common nonlymphocytic leukemia.

The prognosis is highly variable and is not consistently based on patient or disease variables. Patients with AML have a potentially curable disease. However, patients who are older or have a more undifferentiated form of AML tend to have a worse prognosis. Those who have preexisting MDS or who had previously received alkylating agents for cancer (secondary AML) have a much worse prognosis; the leukemia tends to be more resistant to treatment, resulting in a much shorter duration of remission. With treatment, these patients survive an average of less than 1 year, with death usually a result of infection or hemorrhage. Patients receiving supportive care also usually survive less than 1 year, dying from infection or bleeding.

Clinical Manifestations

Most of the signs and symptoms evolve from insufficient production of normal blood cells. Fever and infection result from neutropenia, weakness and fatigue from anemia, and bleeding tendencies from thrombocytopenia. The proliferation of leukemic cells within organs leads to a variety of additional symptoms: pain from an enlarged liver or spleen, hyperplasia of the gums, and bone pain from expansion of marrow.

Assessment and Diagnostic Findings

The disorder develops without warning, with symptoms occurring over a period of weeks to months. CBC results show a decrease in both erythrocytes and platelets. Although the total leukocyte count can be low, normal, or high, the percentage of normal cells is usually vastly decreased. A bone marrow analysis shows an ex-

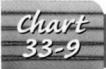

Chart 33-9 Neutropenia Precautions

Nursing Diagnosis
Risk for infection secondary to impaired immunoincompetence due to:

- Diminished neutrophil count (see below) secondary to bone marrow invasion or hypocellularity secondary to medications
- Dysfunctional neutrophils (eg, secondary to myelodysplastic syndrome [MDS])
- Dysfunctional or diminished lymphocytes
- Hypogammaglobulinemia
- Diminished immune response or anergy
- Malnutrition
- Surgery or invasive procedures
- Antibiotic therapy (increased risk for superimposed infection)
  - Neutropenic, infected patients often do *not* exhibit the classic signs of inflammation/infection (ie, redness, cloudiness of any drainage); the only initial sign may be fever (and it often occurs later in the infectious process with neutropenia).
  - Skin and mucous membranes are the body's first line of defense against infection; loss of endothelial cell integrity allows organisms to enter the blood and lymph systems.

Assessment
Patient
Assess the following areas thoroughly every shift or visit (with spot checks throughout shift if hospitalized) and notify physician of any signs of infection or worsening of status:

- *Skin:* Check for tenderness, edema, breaks in skin integrity, moisture, drainage, lesions (especially under breasts, axillae, groin, skin folds, bony prominences, perineum); check all puncture sites (eg, intravenous sites) for signs and symptoms of inflammation/infection.
- *Oral mucosa:* Check for moisture, lesions, color (check palate, tongue, buccal mucosa, gums, lips, oropharynx).
- *Respiratory:* Check for presence of cough, sore throat; auscultate breath sounds.
- *Gastrointestinal:* Check for abdominal discomfort/distention, nausea, change in bowel pattern; auscultate bowel sounds.
- *Genitourinary:* Check for dysuria, urgency, frequency; check urine for color, clarity, odor.
- *Neurologic:* Check for complaints of headache, neck stiffness, visual disturbances; assess level of consciousness, orientation, behavior.
- *Temperature:* Check every 4 hr or every visit; call primary health care provider if temperature is >38°C (>101°F), fever is unresponsive to acetaminophen, or patient shows a decline in hemodynamic status.

Diagnostic Studies
- Monitor complete blood count (CBC) and differential daily (especially absolute neutrophil count [ANC], lymphocyte count).
- Call physician if ANC is <1,000, significantly different from previous count, or whenever patient becomes symptomatic (eg, febrile).
- Monitor globulin, albumin, total protein levels.
- Monitor all culture and sensitivity reports.
- Monitor radiology reports.

Nursing Interventions
Environment and Staff
- **Thorough hand hygiene must be done by everyone before entering patient's room each and every time.**

- Allow no one with a cold or sore throat to care for the patient or to enter room, or come in contact with patient at home.
- Care for neutropenic patients before caring for other patients (as much as possible).
- Use private room for patient if ANC is <1,000.
- Allow no fresh flowers (stagnant water).
- Change water in containers every shift (include O_2 humidification systems every 24 hr).
- Ensure room is cleaned daily.

Dietary
- Provide low microbial diet.
- Eliminate fresh salads and unpeeled fresh fruits or vegetables.

Patient
- Avoid suppositories, enemas, rectal temperatures.
- Practice deep breathing (with incentive spirometer) every 4 hr while awake.
- Ambulate; wear high-efficiency particulate air (HEPA) filter mask if neutropenia is severe.
- Prevent skin dryness with water-soluble lubricants, especially in high-risk areas (eg, lips, corners of mouth, elbows, feet, bony prominences).

Hygiene
- Provide meticulous total body hygiene daily (preferably with antimicrobial solution), including perineal care after every bowel movement.
- Provide thorough oral hygiene after meals and every 4 hr while awake; warm saline, or salt and soda solution, is effective; avoid use of lemon-glycerine swabs, commercial mouthwashes, and hydrogen peroxide.

Intravenous (IV) Therapy
- Do not use plastic cannulas for peripheral IVs when ANC is <500 (if possible per agency); a central vascular access device is preferred for long-term or intensive IV therapy.
- Inspect IV sites every shift; monitor closely for any discomfort; erythema may not be present.
- Maintain meticulous IV site care.
- Cleanse skin with antimicrobial solution before venipuncture (unless patient is allergic).
- Moisture-vapor–permeable dressings are permissible with strict adherence to institutional protocol.
- Change IV tubing per institution policy, using aseptic technique.
- Administer antimicrobial agents on time.

Expected Patient Outcomes
- Patient demonstrates an absence of infection as evidenced by an absence of fever, chills, inflammation, drainage, cough, dyspnea, sore throat, dysuria, or urinary frequency.
- Patient demonstrates an absence of infection as evidenced by the presence of vital signs within normal limits, including intact neurologic status and intact skin.

Duration of Evaluation
Until patient is no longer neutropenic and any infection is resolved.

---

cess of immature blast cells (more than 30%). AML can be further classified into seven different subgroups, based on cytogenetics, histology, and morphology (appearance) of the blasts. The actual prognosis varies somewhat between subgroups, but the clinical course and treatment differ substantially with only one subtype, acute promyelocytic leukemia (APL, or AML-M3). Patients with this leukemia often have significantly more problems with bleed-

ing, in that they have underlying coagulopathy and a higher incidence of disseminated intravascular coagulation (DIC).

Complications

Complications of AML include bleeding and infection, the major causes of death. The risk of bleeding correlates with the level of platelet deficiency (thrombocytopenia). The low platelet count can result in **ecchymoses** (bruises) and **petechiae** (pinpoint red or purple hemorrhagic spots on the skin). Major hemorrhages also may develop when the platelet count drops to less than 10,000/mm³. The most common sites of bleeding are gastrointestinal, pulmonary, and intracranial. For undetermined reasons, fever and infection also increase the likelihood of bleeding.

Because of the lack of mature and normal granulocytes, patients with leukemia are always threatened by infection. The likelihood of infection increases with the degree and duration of neutropenia; neutrophil counts that persist at less than 100/mm³ make the chances of systemic infection extremely high. As the duration of severe neutropenia increases, the patient's risk for developing fungal infection also increases.

Medical Management

The overall objective of treatment is to achieve complete remission, in which there is no detectable evidence of residual leukemia remaining in the bone marrow. Attempts are made to achieve remission by the aggressive administration of chemotherapy, called induction therapy, which usually requires hospitalization for several weeks. Induction therapy typically involves high doses of cytarabine (Cytosar, Ara-C) and daunorubicin (DaunoXome) or mitoxantrone (Novantrone) or idarubicin (Idamycin); sometimes etoposide (VP-16, VePesid) is added to the regimen. The choice of agents is based on the patient's physical status and history of prior antineoplastic treatment.

The aim of induction therapy is to eradicate the leukemic cells, but this is often accompanied by the eradication of normal types of myeloid cells. Thus, the patient becomes severely neutropenic (an ANC of 0 is not uncommon), anemic, and thrombocytopenic (a platelet count of less than 10,000/mm³ is common). During this time, the patient is typically very ill, with bacterial, fungal, and occasionally viral infections, bleeding, and severe mucositis, which causes diarrhea and a marked decline in the ability to maintain adequate nutrition. Supportive care consists of administering blood products (RBCs and platelets) and promptly treating infections. The use of granulocytic growth factors, either G-CSF (filgrastim [Neupogen]) or GM-CSF (sargramostim [Leukine]), can shorten the period of significant neutropenia by stimulating the bone marrow to produce leukocytes more quickly; these agents do not appear to increase the risk of producing more leukemic cells.

When the patient has recovered from the induction therapy (ie, the WBC and platelet counts have returned to normal and any infection has resolved), the patient typically receives consolidation therapy (postremission therapy). The goal of consolidation therapy is to eliminate any residual leukemia cells that are not clinically detectable, thereby diminishing the chance for recurrence. Multiple treatment cycles of various agents are used, usually containing some form of cytarabine (eg, Cytosar, Ara-C). Frequently, the patient receives one cycle of treatment that is almost the same, if not identical, to the induction treatment but uses lower dosages (therefore resulting in less toxicity).

Despite the aggressive use of chemotherapy, the likelihood of remaining in remission for a prolonged period is not great. About 70% of patients with AML experience a relapse (Hiddemann & Buchner, 2001). A recent study of long-term survival of patients with AML found that only 11% survived 10 years or longer (Micallef et al., 2001).

Another aggressive treatment option is bone marrow transplantation (BMT) or peripheral blood stem cell transplantation (PBSCT). When a suitable tissue match can be obtained, the patient embarks on an even more aggressive regimen of chemotherapy (sometimes in combination with radiation therapy), with the treatment goal of destroying the hematopoietic function of the patient's bone marrow. The patient is then "rescued" with the infusion of the donor stem cells to reinitiate blood cell production. Patients who undergo PBSCT transplantation have a significant risk for problems with infection, potential graft-versus-host disease (in which the donor's lymphocytes [graft] recognize the patient's body as "foreign" and set up reactions to attack the "foreign" host), and other complications. PBSCT has been shown to cure AML in 25% to 50% of patients who are at high risk for relapse or who have relapsed (Radich & Sievers, 2000).

Recent advances in understanding of the molecular biology of myeloid blast cells have resulted in a new therapeutic option. After the uncommitted stem cell differentiates into a myeloid stem cell, it expresses a specific antigen on the cell surface, called CD33. It appears that 90% of blast cells found in AML express CD33; normal hematopoietic stem cells do not express this antigen (Radich & Sievers, 2000). Armed with that discovery, researchers developed a monoclonal antibody to target cells with the CD33 antigen. The anti-CD33 antibody is linked to a potent antitumor antibiotic, calicheamicin; this medication is called gemtuzumab ozogamicin (Mylotarg). When administered, the anti-CD33 antibody binds to cells with CD33 antigens, and the calicheamicin causes cell death. Normal myeloid and megakaryocyte precursors have the CD33 antigen, so the Mylotarg destroys them. Patients develop severe neutropenia and thrombocytopenia after receiving this medication. Nonetheless, Mylotarg shows promise as an effective agent against AML. In elderly patients, it appears to be somewhat less toxic than conventional induction therapy regimens.

Another important option for the patient to consider is supportive care alone. In fact, supportive care may be the only option if the patient has significant comorbidity, such as extremely poor cardiac, pulmonary, renal, or hepatic function. In such cases, aggressive antileukemia therapy is not used; occasionally, hydroxyurea (eg, Hydrea) may be used briefly to control the increase of blast cells. Patients are more commonly supported with antimicrobial therapy and transfusions as needed. This treatment approach provides the patient with some additional time at home; however, death frequently occurs within months, typically from infection or bleeding.

COMPLICATIONS OF TREATMENT

The massive leukemic cell destruction from chemotherapy results in release of electrolytes and fluids within the cell into the systemic circulation. Increases in uric acid levels, potassium, and phosphate are seen; this process is referred to as tumor **lysis** syndrome (see Chap. 16). The increased uric acid and phosphorus levels make patients vulnerable to renal stone formation and renal colic, which can progress to acute renal failure. Hyperkalemia and hypocalcemia can lead to cardiac dysrhythmias, hypotension, neuromuscular effects such as muscle cramps, weakness, spasm/tetany, confusion, and seizure. Patients require a high fluid intake, alkalization of the urine, and prophylaxis with allopurinol to prevent crystallization of uric acid and subsequent stone formation. Gastrointestinal problems may result from the infiltration of abnormal leukocytes into the abdominal organs and from the toxicity of the chemotherapeutic agents. Anorexia, nausea, vomiting, diarrhea, and severe mucositis are common. Because of the profound myelosuppressive effects of chemotherapy, significant neutropenia and thrombocytopenia typically result in serious infection and increased risk for bleeding.

Nursing Management

Nursing management of the patient with acute leukemia is discussed at the end of the leukemia section in this chapter.

CHRONIC MYELOID LEUKEMIA (CML)

Chronic myeloid leukemia (CML) arises from a mutation in the myeloid stem cell. Normal myeloid cells continue to be produced, but there is a preference for immature (blast) forms. Therefore, a wide spectrum of cell types exists within the blood, from blast forms through mature neutrophils. Because there is an uncontrolled proliferation of cells, the marrow expands into the cavities of long bones (eg, the femur), and cells are also formed in the liver and spleen (extramedullary hematopoiesis), resulting in enlargement of these organs that is sometimes painful. In 90% to 95% of patients with CML, a section of DNA is found to be missing from chromosome 22 (the Philadelphia chromosome [Ph1]); it is, in fact, translocated onto chromosome 9. The specific location of these changes is on the *BCR* gene of chromosome 22 and the *ABL* gene of chromosome 9. When these two genes fuse (*BCR-ABL* gene), they produce an abnormal protein (a tyrosine kinase protein) that causes WBCs to divide rapidly. This *BCR-ABL* gene is present in virtually all patients with this disease. CML is uncommon in people younger than 20 years of age, but the incidence increases with age (median age, 40 to 50 years).

Patients diagnosed with CML in the chronic phase have an overall median life expectancy of 3 to 5 years. During that time, they have very few symptoms and complications from the disease itself. Problems with infections and bleeding are rare. However, once the disease transforms to the acute phase (blast crisis), the overall survival time rarely exceeds several months.

Clinical Manifestations

The clinical picture of CML varies. Many patients are asymptomatic, and leukocytosis is detected by a CBC performed for some other reason. The WBC count commonly exceeds 100,000/mm³. Patients with extremely high WBC counts may be somewhat short of breath or slightly confused due to decreased capillary perfusion to the lungs and brain from leukostasis (the excessive amount of WBCs inhibits blood flow through the capillaries). Patients may complain of an enlarged, tender spleen. The liver may also be enlarged. Some patients have somewhat insidious symptoms, such as malaise, anorexia, and weight loss. Lymphadenopathy is rare. There are three stages in CML: chronic, transformation, and accelerated or blast crisis. Patients have more symptoms and complications as the disease progresses.

Medical Management

Advances in understanding of the pathology of CML at a molecular level have led to dramatic changes in its medical management. An oral formulation of a tyrosine kinase inhibitor, imatinib mesylate (Gleevec) works by blocking signals within the leukemia cells that express the *BCR-ABL* protein, thus preventing a series of chemical reactions that cause the cell to grow and divide (Tennant, 2001; Goldman & Melo, 2001). Gleevec appears to be more useful in the chronic phase of the illness. In clinical trials, it has been generally well tolerated. Antacids and grapefruit juice may limit drug absorption, and large doses of acetaminophen can cause hep-

atotoxicity. The long-term effects of Gleevec, its impact on survival, and the optimal length of treatment are being determined.

Conventional therapy depends on the stage of disease. In the chronic phase, the expected outcome is correction of the chromosomal abnormality (ie, conversion of the malignant stem cell population back to normal). Agents that have been used successfully for this purpose are interferon-alfa (Roferon-A) and cytosine, often in combination. These agents are administered daily as subcutaneous injections. This therapy is not benign; many patients cannot tolerate the profound fatigue, depression, anorexia, mucositis, and inability to concentrate. A less aggressive therapeutic approach focuses on reducing the WBC count to a more normal level, but does not alter cytogenetic changes. This goal can be achieved by using oral chemotherapeutic agents, typically hydroxyurea (eg, Hydrea) or busulfan (eg, Myleran). In the case of an extreme leukocytosis at diagnosis (eg, WBC count higher than 300,000/mm³), a more emergent treatment may be required. In this instance, leukopheresis (in which the patient's blood is removed and separated, with the leukocytes withdrawn, and the remaining blood returned to the patient) can temporarily reduce the number of WBCs. An anthracycline chemotherapeutic agent (eg, daunomycin) may also be used to bring the WBC count down quickly to a safer level, where more conservative therapy can be instituted.

The transformation phase can be insidious, but it marks the process of evolution (or transformation) to the acute form of leukemia (blast crisis). In the transformation phase, the patient may complain of bone pain and may report fevers (without any obvious sign of infection) and weight loss. Even with chemotherapy, the spleen may continue to enlarge. The patient may become more anemic and thrombocytopenic; an increased basophil level is detected by the CBC. Despite its being a myeloid stem cell disease, CML will transform in up to 25% of patients to resemble not AML, but acute lymphoid leukemia (ALL), with lymphoid-appearing blasts (Derderian et al., 1993). Transformation into the acute phase can be gradual or rapid.

In the more acute form of leukemia (blast crisis), treatment may resemble induction therapy for acute leukemia, using the same medications as for AML or ALL. Patients whose disease evolves into a "lymphoid" blast crisis are more likely to be able to reenter a chronic phase after induction therapy. For those whose disease evolves into AML, therapy is largely ineffective in achieving a second chronic phase. Life-threatening infections and bleeding occur frequently in this phase. CML is a disease that can potentially be cured with BMT or PBSCT. Patients who receive such transplants while still in the chronic phase of the illness tend to have a greater chance for cure than those who receive them in the acute phase. The transplantation procedure may now be considered for otherwise healthy patients who are younger than 70 years of age.

ACUTE LYMPHOCYTIC LEUKEMIA (ALL)

ALL results from an uncontrolled proliferation of immature cells (lymphoblasts) derived from the lymphoid stem cell. The cell of origin is the precursor to the B lymphocyte in approximately 75% of ALL cases; T-lymphocyte ALL occurs in approximately 25% of ALL cases. The *BCR-ABL* translocation (see earlier discussion) is found in 20% of ALL blast cells. ALL is most common in young children, with boys affected more often than girls; the peak incidence is 4 years of age. After age 15 years, ALL is relatively uncommon. Increasing age appears to be associated with diminished survival (Nachman, 1999). Because of improvements in therapy for ALL, more than 80% of children survive at least

5 years. Even if relapse occurs, resumption of induction therapy can often achieve a second complete remission. Moreover, BMT may be successful even after a second relapse.

Clinical Manifestations

Immature lymphocytes proliferate in the marrow and crowd the development of normal myeloid cells. As a result, normal hematopoiesis is inhibited, resulting in reduced numbers of leukocytes, erythrocytes, and platelets. Leukocyte counts may be either low or high, but there is always a high proportion of immature cells. Manifestations of leukemic cell infiltration into other organs are more common with ALL than with other forms of leukemia and include pain from an enlarged liver or spleen, bone pain, and headache and vomiting (because of meningeal involvement).

Medical Management

The expected outcome of treatment is complete remission. Lymphoid blast cells are typically very sensitive to corticosteroids and to vinca alkaloids; therefore, these medications are an integral part of the initial induction therapy. Because ALL frequently invades the central nervous system, prophylaxis with cranial irradiation or intrathecal chemotherapy (eg, methotrexate [Folex]) or both is an integral part of the treatment plan.

Treatment protocols for ALL tend to be complex, using a wide variety of chemotherapeutic agents. They often include a maintenance phase, when lower doses of medications are given for up to 3 years. Despite the complexity, treatment can be provided in the outpatient setting in some circumstances until severe complications develop.

Infections are common, especially viral infections. The use of corticosteroids to treat ALL increases the patient's susceptibility to infection. Patients with ALL tend to have a better response to treatment than patients with AML do. BMT or PBSCT offers a chance for prolonged remission or even cure if the illness recurs after therapy.

Nursing Management

Nursing management of the patient with acute leukemia is discussed at the end of the leukemia section in this chapter.

CHRONIC LYMPHOCYTIC LEUKEMIA (CLL)

CLL is a common malignancy of older adults; two thirds of all patients are older than 60 years of age at diagnosis. It is the most common form of leukemia in the United States and Europe, affecting more than 120,000 people, but is rarely seen in Asia. The average survival time for patients with CLL ranges from 14 years (early stage) to 2.5 years (late stage).

Pathophysiology

CLL typically derives from a malignant clone of B lymphocytes (T-lymphocyte CLL is rare). In contrast to the acute forms of leukemia, most of the leukemia cells in CLL are fully mature. It appears that these cells can escape **apoptosis** (programmed cell death), with the result being an excessive accumulation of the cells in the marrow and circulation. The antigen CD52 is prevalent on the surface of many of these leukemic B cells. The disease is classified into three or four stages (two classification systems are

in use). In the early stage, an elevated lymphocyte count is seen and can exceed 100,000/mm³. Because the lymphocytes are small, they can easily travel through the small capillaries within the circulation, and the pulmonary and cerebral complications of leukocytosis (as seen with myeloid leukemias) typically are not found in CLL.

Lymphadenopathy occurs as the lymphocytes are trapped within the lymph nodes. The nodes can become very large and are sometimes painful. Hepatomegaly and splenomegaly then develop.

In later stages, anemia and thrombocytopenia may develop. Treatment is typically initiated in the later stages; earlier treatment does not appear to increase survival. Autoimmune complications can also occur at any stage, as either autoimmune hemolytic anemia or idiopathic thrombocytopenic purpura (ITP). In the autoimmune process, the RES destroys the body's own RBCs or platelets.

Clinical Manifestations

Many patients are asymptomatic and are diagnosed incidentally during routine physical examinations or during the course of treatment for another disease. An increased lymphocyte count (lymphocytosis) is always present. The RBC and platelet counts may be normal or, in later stages of the illness, decreased. Enlargement of lymph nodes (lymphadenopathy) is common; it can be severe and sometimes painful. The spleen can also be enlarged (splenomegaly).

Patients with CLL can develop "B symptoms," a constellation of symptoms including fevers, drenching sweating (especially at night), and unintentional weight loss. These patients have defects in their humoral and cell-mediated immune systems; therefore, infections are common. The defect in cellular immunity is evidenced by an absent or decreased reaction to skin sensitivity tests (eg, *Candida*, mumps), which is known as **anergy**. Problems with life-threatening infections are common. Viral infections, such as herpes zoster, can become widely disseminated.

Medical Management

In early stages, CLL may require no treatment. When symptoms are severe (drenching night sweats, painful lymphadenopathy), or when the disease progresses to later stages (with resultant anemia and thrombocytopenia), chemotherapy with corticosteroids and chlorambucil (Leukeran) is often used. Other useful agents include cyclophosphamide (eg, Cytoxan), vincristine (eg, Oncovin), and doxorubicin (eg, Adriamycin). A significant number of patients who do not respond to these medications have achieved remission with fludarabine (Fludara), and this medication is increasingly being used as front-line therapy. The major side effect of fludarabine is prolonged bone marrow suppression, manifested by prolonged periods of neutropenia, lymphopenia, and thrombocytopenia. Patients are then at risk for such infections as *Pneumocystis carinii, Listeria,* mycobacteria, herpes viruses, and cytomegalovirus (CMV). The monoclonal antibody rituximab (Rituxan) also has efficacy in CLL therapy. It is often used in combination with other chemotherapeutic medications. Research has shown that the monoclonal antibody alemtuzumab (Campath) targets the CD52 antigen commonly found on CLL cells and that it is effective in clearing the marrow and circulation of these cells without affecting the stem cells. Because CD52 is present on both B and T lymphocytes, patients receiving alemtuzumab are at significant risk for infection; prophylactic use of antiviral agents and antibiotics (eg, trimethoprim and sulfamethoxazole [Septra]) is important and needs to continue for a minimum of 2 months after the patient stops treatment. Because bacterial infections are common in patients with CLL, intravenous treatment with immunoglobulin may be given to selected patients.

NURSING PROCESS:
THE PATIENT WITH ACUTE LEUKEMIA

Assessment

Although the clinical picture varies with the type of leukemia involved as well as the treatment implemented, the health history may reveal a range of subtle symptoms reported by the patient before the problem is manifested by findings on physical examination. Weakness and fatigue are common manifestations, not only of the leukemia but also of the resulting complications of anemia and infection. If the patient is hospitalized, the assessments should be performed daily, or more frequently as warranted. Because the physical findings may be subtle initially, a thorough, systematic assessment incorporating all body systems is essential. For example, a dry cough, mild dyspnea, and diminished breath sounds may indicate a pulmonary infection. However, the infection may not be seen initially on the chest x-ray. The lack of neutrophils delays the inflammatory response against the pulmonary infection, and it is the inflammatory response that causes the x-ray changes. The platelet count can become dangerously low, leaving the patient at risk for significant bleeding. The specific body system assessments are delineated in the neutropenic precautions and bleeding precautions, found in Charts 33-9 and 33-10, respectively. When serial assessments are performed, current findings are compared with previous findings to evaluate improvement or worsening.

The nurse also must closely monitor the results of laboratory studies. Flow sheets and spreadsheets are particularly useful in

---

Chart 33-10   Bleeding Precautions

Nursing Diagnosis

Potential bleeding* and injury secondary to thrombocytopenia/altered coagulation due to:
- Malignant invasion in bone marrow
- Bone marrow suppression resulting from chemotherapy (particularly alkylators, antitumor antibiotics, antimetabolites) and radiation therapy
- Hypersplenism
- Disseminated intravascular coagulation (DIC)
- Altered coagulation

Assessment

Patient

Assess the following areas thoroughly every shift or visit (with spot checks throughout the shift if patient is hospitalized), and notify physician if there is new onset of the following and/or worsening of status:
- *Integument:* Petechiae (usually located on trunk, thighs), ecchymoses or hematomas, conjunctival hemorrhages, bleeding gums, bleeding at puncture sites (venipuncture, lumbar puncture, bone marrow)
- *Cardiovascular:* Hypotension, tachycardia, complaints of dizziness, epistaxis
- *Pulmonary:* Respiratory distress, tachypnea
- *Gastrointestinal:* Hemoptysis, abdominal distention, rectal bleeding
- *Genitourinary:* Vaginal or urethral bleeding
- *Neurologic:* Headache, blurred vision, mental status changes

Laboratory Tests

- Monitor complete blood count (CBC), platelets daily (at least); coagulation panel.
- Notify physician if platelet count is <10,000/mm³ or if count has changed significantly from previous count (including coagulation), or whenever patient becomes symptomatic.
- Ensure patient's blood was human leukocyte antigen (HLA) typed before transfusions or chemotherapy begins if admitted for induction therapy (eg, for acute leukemia).
- Obtain 1-hour posttransfusion platelet count if warranted.
- Test all urine, emesis, stools for occult blood.

Nursing Interventions

Prevent Complications

- Avoid aspirin and aspirin-containing medications or other medications known to inhibit platelet function, if possible.
- Do not give intramuscular injections.
- Do not insert indwelling catheters.
- Take no rectal temperatures; do not give suppositories, enemas.
- Use stool softeners, oral laxatives to prevent constipation.
- Use smallest possible needles when performing venipuncture.
- Apply pressure to venipuncture sites for 5 min or until bleeding has stopped.
- Permit no flossing of teeth and no commercial mouthwashes.
- Use only soft-bristled toothbrush for mouth care.
- Use only toothettes for mouth care if platelet count is <10,000/mm³, or if gums bleed.
- Lubricate lips with water-soluble lubricant every 2 hr while awake.
- Avoid suctioning if at all possible; if unavoidable, use only gentle suctioning.
- Discourage vigorous coughing or blowing of the nose.
- Use only electric razor for shaving.
- Pad side rails as needed.
- Prevent falls by ambulating with patient as necessary.

Control Bleeding

- Apply direct pressure.
- For epistaxis, position patient in high Fowler's position; apply ice pack to back of neck and direct pressure to nose.
- Notify physician for prolonged bleeding (eg, unable to stop within 10 min).
- Administer platelets, fresh frozen plasma, packed red blood cells, as prescribed.

Evaluation and Expected Patient Outcomes

- Patient demonstrates an absence of bleeding as evidenced by absence of spontaneous petechiae, ecchymoses, epistaxis, hemoptysis, bleeding gums, conjunctival hemorrhage, vaginal bleeding, hematuria, guaiac positive stool, blurred vision, orthostatic hypotension, and prolonged bleeding from puncture sites.
- Patient demonstrates an absence of bleeding as evidenced by the presence of vital signs within normal limits and intact neurologic status.

---

*Serious hemorrhage is unusual in mildly thrombocytopenic patients in absence of local lesions (peptic ulcer, bleeding from hemorrhoids, cystitis).

tracking the WBC count, ANC, hematocrit, platelet, and creatinine levels, hepatic function tests, and electrolyte levels. Culture results need to be reported immediately so that appropriate antimicrobial therapy can begin or be modified.

Diagnosis

NURSING DIAGNOSES

Based on the assessment data, major nursing diagnoses for the patient with acute leukemia may include:

- Risk for infection and bleeding
- Risk for impaired skin integrity related to toxic effects of chemotherapy, alteration in nutrition, and impaired mobility
- Impaired gas exchange
- Impaired mucous membranes due to changes in epithelial lining of the gastrointestinal tract from chemotherapy or prolonged use of antimicrobial medications
- Imbalanced nutrition, less than body requirements, related to hypermetabolic state, anorexia, mucositis, pain, and nausea
- Acute pain and discomfort related to mucositis, WBC infiltration of systemic tissues, fever, and infection
- Hyperthermia related to tumor lysis and infection
- Fatigue and activity intolerance related to anemia and infection
- Impaired physical mobility due to anemia and protective isolation
- Risk for excess fluid volume related to renal dysfunction, hypoproteinemia, need for multiple intravenous medications and blood products
- Diarrhea due to altered gastrointestinal flora, mucosal denudation
- Risk for deficient fluid volume related to potential for diarrhea, bleeding, infection, and increased metabolic rate
- Self-care deficit due to fatigue, malaise, and protective isolation
- Anxiety due to knowledge deficit and uncertain future
- Disturbed body image related to change in appearance, function, and roles
- Grieving related to anticipatory loss and altered role functioning
- Potential for spiritual distress
- Deficient knowledge about disease process, treatment, complication management, and self-care measures

COLLABORATIVE PROBLEMS/ POTENTIAL COMPLICATIONS

Based on the assessment data, potential complications that may develop include:

- Infection
- Bleeding
- Renal dysfunction
- Tumor lysis syndrome
- Nutritional depletion
- Mucositis

Planning and Goals

The major goals for the patient may include absence of complications and pain, attainment and maintenance of adequate nutrition, activity tolerance, ability for self-care and to cope with the diagnosis and prognosis, positive body image, and an understanding of the disease process and its treatment.

Nursing Interventions

PREVENTING OR MANAGING INFECTION AND BLEEDING

The nursing interventions related to diminishing the risk for infection and for bleeding are delineated in Charts 33-9 and 33-10.

MANAGING MUCOSITIS

Although emphasis is placed on the oral mucosa, it is important to realize that the entire gastrointestinal mucosa can be altered, not only by the effects of chemotherapy but also from prolonged administration of antibiotics. Assessment of the oral mucosa must be thorough; therefore, dentures must be removed. Areas to assess include the palate, buccal mucosa, tongue, gums, lips, oropharynx, and the area under the tongue. In addition to identifying and describing lesions, the color and moisture of the mucosa should be noted.

Oral hygiene is very important to diminish the bacteria within the mouth, maintain moisture, and provide comfort. Soft-bristled toothbrushes should be used until the neutrophil and platelet counts become very low; at that time, sponge-tipped applicators should be substituted. Lemon-glycerin swabs and commercial mouthwashes should never be used because the glycerin and alcohol within them are extremely drying to the tissues. Simple rinses with saline (or saline and baking soda) solutions are inexpensive but effective in cleaning and moistening the oral mucosa. Because the risk of yeast or fungal infection in the mouth is great, other medications are often prescribed, such as chlorhexidine rinses (eg, Peridex) or clotrimazole troches (eg, Mycelex). The nurse reminds the patient about the importance of these medications to enhance adherence to the therapeutic regimen. Chlorhexidine rinses may discolor the teeth.

To diminish perineal–rectal complications, it is important to cleanse the perineal–rectal area thoroughly after each bowel movement. Women are instructed to cleanse the perineum from front to back. Sitz baths are a comfortable method of cleansing; the perineal–anal region and buttocks must be carefully dried afterward to minimize the chance of excoriation. Stool softeners should be used to increase the moisture of bowel movements; however, the stool texture must be monitored so that the softeners can be decreased or stopped if the stool becomes too loose.

IMPROVING NUTRITIONAL INTAKE

The disease process can increase, and sepsis further increases, the patient's metabolic rate and nutritional requirements. Nutritional intake is often reduced because of pain and discomfort associated with stomatitis. Mouth care before and after meals and administration of analgesics before eating can help increase intake. If oral anesthetics are used, the patient must be warned to chew with extreme care to avoid inadvertently biting the tongue or buccal mucosa.

Nausea should not be a major contributing factor, because recent advances in antiemetic therapy are highly effective. However, nausea can result from antimicrobial therapy, so some antiemetic therapy may still be required after the chemotherapy has been completed.

Small, frequent feedings of foods that are soft in texture and moderate in temperature may be better tolerated. Low-microbial diets are typically prescribed (avoiding uncooked fruits or vegetables and those without a peelable skin). Nutritional supplements are frequently used. Daily body weights (as well as intake and output measurements) are useful in monitoring fluid status.

Calorie counts are useful, as are more formal nutritional assessments. Parenteral nutrition is often required to maintain adequate nutrition.

EASING PAIN AND DISCOMFORT

Recurrent fevers are common in acute leukemia; at times, they are accompanied by shaking chills, which can be severe (rigors). Myalgias and arthralgias can result. Acetaminophen is typically given to decrease fever, but it does so by increasing diaphoresis. Sponging with cool water may be useful, but cold water or ice packs should be avoided because the heat cannot dissipate from constricted blood vessels. Bedclothes need frequent changing as well. Gentle back and shoulder massage may provide comfort.

Stomatitis can also cause significant discomfort. In addition to oral hygiene practices, patient-controlled analgesia can be effective in controlling the pain (see Chap. 13).

Because patients with acute leukemia require hospitalization for extensive nursing care (either during induction or consolidation therapy or during resultant complications), sleep deprivation frequently results. Nurses need to implement creative strategies that permit uninterrupted sleep for at least a few hours while still administering necessary medications on time.

With the exception of severe mucositis, less pain is associated with acute leukemia than with many other forms of cancer. However, the amount of psychologic suffering that the patient must endure can be immense. Patients greatly benefit from active listening.

DECREASING FATIGUE AND DECONDITIONING

Fatigue is a common and oppressive problem. Nursing interventions should focus on assisting the patient to establish a balance between activity and rest. Patients with acute leukemia need to maintain some physical activity and exercise to prevent the deconditioning that results from inactivity. Use of a high-efficiency particulate air (HEPA) filter mask can permit the patient to ambulate outside the room despite severe neutropenia. Although many patients lack the motivation to use them, stationary bicycles within the room can also be used. At a minimum, patients should be encouraged to sit up in a chair while awake rather than staying in bed; even this simple activity can improve the patient's tidal volume and enhance circulation. Physical therapy can also be beneficial.

MAINTAINING FLUID AND ELECTROLYTE BALANCE

Febrile episodes, bleeding, and inadequate or overly aggressive fluid replacement can alter the patient's fluid status. Similarly, persistent diarrhea, vomiting, and long-term use of certain antimicrobial agents can cause significant deficits in electrolytes. Intake and output need to be measured accurately, and daily weights should also be monitored. The patient should be assessed for signs of dehydration as well as fluid overload, with particular attention to pulmonary status and the development of dependent edema. Laboratory test results, particularly electrolytes, blood urea nitrogen, creatinine, and hematocrit, should be monitored and compared with previous results. Replacement of electrolytes, particularly potassium and magnesium, is commonly required. Patients receiving amphotericin or certain antibiotics are at increased risk for electrolyte depletion.

IMPROVING SELF-CARE

Because hygiene measures are so important in this patient population, they must be performed by the nurse when the patient cannot do so. However, the patient should be encouraged to do as much as possible, to preserve mobility and function as well as self-esteem. Patients may have negative feelings, even disgust that they can no longer care for themselves. Empathetic listening is helpful, as is realistic reassurance that these deficits are temporary. As the patient recovers, it is important to assist him or her to resume more self-care. Patients are usually discharged from the hospital with a central vascular access device (eg, Hickman catheter, PICC), and most patients can care for the catheter with adequate instruction and practice under observation.

MANAGING ANXIETY AND GRIEF

Being diagnosed with acute leukemia can be extremely frightening. In many instances, the need to begin treatment is emergent, and patients have little time to process the fact that they have the illness before making decisions about therapy. Providing emotional support and discussing the uncertain future are crucial. The nurse also needs to assess how much information patients want to have regarding the illness, its treatment, and potential complications. This desire should be reassessed at intervals, because needs and interest in information change throughout the course of the disease and treatment. Priorities must be identified so that procedures, assessments, and self-care expectations are adequately explained even to those who do not wish extensive information.

Many patients become depressed and begin to grieve for the losses they feel, such as normal family functioning, professional roles and responsibilities, and social roles, as well as physical functioning. Nurses can assist patients to identify the source of the grief and encourage them to allow time to adjust to the major life changes produced by the illness. Role restructuring, in both family and professional life, may be required. Again, when possible, permitting patients to identify options and to take time making significant decisions regarding such restructuring is helpful.

Discharge from the hospital can also provoke anxiety. Although most patients are extremely eager to go home, they may lack confidence in their ability to manage potential complications and to resume their normal activity. Close communication between nurses across care settings can reassure patients that they will not be abandoned.

ENCOURAGING SPIRITUAL WELL-BEING

Because acute leukemia is a serious, potentially life-threatening illness, the nurse may offer support to enhance the patient's spiritual well-being. The patient's spiritual and religious practices should be assessed and pastoral services offered. Throughout the patient's illness, it is important that the nurse assist the patient to maintain hope. However, that hope should be realistic and will certainly change over the course of the illness. For example, the patient may initially hope to be cured, but with repeated relapses and a change to terminal care the same patient may hope for a quiet, dignified death.

MONITORING AND MANAGING POTENTIAL COMPLICATIONS

Nursing interventions for potential complications were described previously.

PROMOTING HOME AND COMMUNITY-BASED CARE

Teaching Patients Self-Care

Most patients cope better when they have an understanding of what is happening to them. Based on their education, literacy level, and interest, teaching of patient and family should focus on the disease (including some pathophysiology), its treatment, and certainly the significant risk for infection and bleeding (Charts 33-8 and 33-11) that results.

Management of a vascular access device can be taught to most patients or family members. Follow-up and care for the devices may also need to be provided by nurses in an outpatient facility or by a home care agency or a health care provider.

Continuing Care. Shortened hospital stays and outpatient care have significantly altered care for patients with acute leukemia. In many instances, when the patient is clinically stable but still requires parenteral antibiotics or blood products, these procedures can be performed in an outpatient setting. Nurses in these various settings must communicate regularly. Patients need to learn which parameters are important for them to monitor, and how to monitor them. Specific instructions need to be given as to when the patient should seek care from the physician or a health care provider.

Patients and their families need to have a clear understanding of the disease and the prognosis. The nurse acts as an advocate to ensure that this information is provided. When patients no longer respond to therapy, it is important to respect their choices about treatment, including measures to prolong life and other end-of-life measures. Advance directives and living wills provide patients with some measure of control during terminal illness.

Many patients in this stage still choose to be cared for at home, and families often need support when considering this option. Coordination of home care services and instruction can help to alleviate anxiety about managing the patient's care in the home. As the patient becomes weaker, the caregivers must assume more of the patient's care. In addition, caregivers often need to be encouraged to take care of themselves, allowing time for rest and accepting emotional support. Hospice staff can assist in providing respite for family members as well as care for the patient. Patients and families also need assistance to cope with changes in their roles and responsibilities. Anticipatory grieving is an essential task during this time (see Chap. 17).

In patients with acute leukemia, death typically occurs from infection or bleeding. Family members need to have information about these complications and the measures to take should either occur. Many family members cannot cope with the care required when a patient begins to bleed actively. It is important to delineate alternatives to keeping the patient at home. Should another option be sought, family members who may feel guilty that they could not keep the patient at home will require support from the nurse.

Evaluation

EXPECTED PATIENT OUTCOMES

Expected patient outcomes may include:

1. Shows no evidence of infection
2. Experiences no bleeding
3. Has intact oral mucous membranes
   a. Participates in oral hygiene regimen
   b. Reports no discomfort in mouth
4. Attains optimal level of nutrition
   a. Maintains weight with increased food and fluid intake
   b. Maintains adequate protein stores (albumin)
5. Reports satisfaction with pain and discomfort levels
6. Has less fatigue and increased activity
7. Maintains fluid and electrolyte balance
8. Participates in self-care
9. Copes with anxiety and grief
   a. Discusses concerns and fears
   b. Uses stress management strategies appropriately
   c. Participates in decisions regarding end-of-life care
10. Absence of complications

AGNOGENIC MYELOID METAPLASIA (AMM)

Agnogenic myeloid metaplasia (AMM), also known as myelofibrosis, is a chronic myeloproliferative disorder that arises from neoplastic transformation of an early hematopoietic stem cell. The disease is characterized by marrow fibrosis or scarring, splenomegaly, extramedullary hematopoiesis (typically spleen, liver, or both), leukocytosis and thrombocytosis, and anemia. Some patients have suppressed WBC and platelet counts as well as anemia (pancytopenia). Patients with AMM have increased **angiogenesis** (formation of new blood vessels) within the marrow. Early forms of blood cells (including nucleated RBCs and megakaryocyte fragments) are frequently found in the circulation. AMM is a disease of the elderly, with a median age at diagnosis of 60 to 65 years. Survival time varies from as little as 1 year to more than 30 years; the average is 4 to 5 years (Anderson, Hamblin, & Traynor, 1999). Heart failure, complications of marrow failure, and transformation to AML are the common causes of death.

Chart 33-11

Home Care Checklist • The Patient at Risk for Bleeding

At the completion of the home care instruction, the patient or caregiver will be able to:	Patient	Caregiver
• Describe the source and function of platelets and clotting factors.	✓	✓
• Verbalize the rationale for being at risk for bleeding.	✓	✓
• Identify medications and other substances to avoid (eg, aspirin-containing medications, alcohol).	✓	✓
• Demonstrate how to monitor for signs of bleeding.	✓	✓
• Describe to whom, how, and when to report signs of bleeding.	✓	✓
• Notify health care professional before having dental work.	✓	✓
• Describe appropriate ways to prevent bleeding (avoid use of suppositories, enemas, tampons; avoid constipation, vigorous sexual intercourse, anal sex; use only electric razor for shaving and a soft-bristled toothbrush for teeth).	✓	✓
• Demonstrate appropriate actions to take should bleeding occur.	✓	✓

Medical Management

Medical management is directed toward palliation, reducing symptoms related to cytopenias, splenomegaly, and hypermetabolic state. Although one third of anemic patients respond to the combination of an androgen plus a corticosteroid, the primary treatment remains RBC transfusion. Because of the prolonged requirement for RBC transfusion, iron overload is a common problem. Iron chelation therapy should be initiated for those individuals in whom survival is expected to exceed a few years (Anderson, Hamblin, & Traynor, 1999). Hydroxyurea is often used to control high WBC and platelet counts and to reduce the size of the spleen. Splenic irradiation or splenectomy may also be used to control the massive splenomegaly that can develop. However, both modalities render the patient at significant risk for development of infection. BMT or PBSCT may be a useful treatment modality in younger, otherwise healthy individuals.

Nursing Management

The extent of splenomegaly can be profound in patients with AMM, with enlargement of the spleen that extends to the pelvic rim. This condition is extremely uncomfortable to the patient and can severely limit nutritional intake. Analgesics are often ineffective. Methods to reduce the spleen's size are usually more effective in controlling pain. Splenomegaly, coupled with a hypermetabolic state, results in weight loss (often severe) and muscle wasting. Patients benefit from very small, frequent meals of foods that are high in calories and protein. Weakness, fatigue, and altered body image are other significant problems. Energy conservation methods and active listening are important nursing interventions. Patients need to be educated about signs and symptoms of infection as well as appropriate interventions when an infection is suspected.

The Lymphomas

The lymphomas are neoplasms of cells of lymphoid origin. These tumors usually start in lymph nodes but can involve lymphoid tissue in the spleen, the gastrointestinal tract (eg, the wall of the stomach), the liver, or the bone marrow. They are often classified according to the degree of cell differentiation and the origin of the predominant malignant cell. Lymphomas can be broadly classified into two categories: Hodgkin's disease and non-Hodgkin's lymphoma (NHL).

HODGKIN'S DISEASE

Hodgkin's disease is a relatively rare malignancy that has an impressive cure rate. It is somewhat more common in men than women and has two peaks of incidence: one in the early 20s and the other after 50 years of age. Unlike other lymphomas, Hodgkin's disease is unicentric in origin in that it initiates in a single node. The disease spreads by contiguous extension along the lymphatic system. The cause of Hodgkin's disease is unknown, but a viral etiology is suspected. In fact, fragments of the Epstein-Barr virus have been found in 40% to 50% of patients; this occurs more commonly in the younger patient population (Weiss, 2000). There is a familial pattern associated with Hodgkin's disease: first-degree relatives have a higher-than-normal frequency of the disease. There is no increased incidence documented for non-blood relatives (eg, spouses).

The malignant cell of Hodgkin's disease is the Reed-Sternberg cell, a gigantic tumor cell that is morphologically unique and is thought to be of immature lymphoid origin. It is the pathologic hallmark and essential diagnostic criterion for Hodgkin's disease. However, the tumor is very heterogeneous and may actually contain few Reed-Sternberg cells. Repeated biopsies may be required to establish the diagnosis.

Hodgkin's disease is customarily classified into five subgroups based on pathologic analyses that reflect the natural history of the malignancy and suggest the prognosis. For example, when lymphocytes predominate, with few Reed-Sternberg cells and minimal involvement of the lymph nodes, the prognosis is much more favorable than when the lymphocyte count is low and the lymph nodes are virtually replaced by tumor cells of the most primitive type. The majority of patients with Hodgkin's disease have the types currently designated "nodular sclerosis" or "mixed cellularity." The nodular sclerosis type tends to occur more often in young women, at an earlier stage but with a worse prognosis than the mixed cellularity subgroup, which occurs more commonly in men and causes more constitutional symptoms but has a better prognosis.

Clinical Manifestations

Hodgkin's disease usually begins as a painless enlargement of one or more lymph nodes on one side of the neck. The individual nodes are painless and firm but not hard. The most common sites for lymphadenopathy are the cervical, supraclavicular, and mediastinal nodes; involvement of the iliac or inguinal nodes or spleen is much less common. A mediastinal mass may be seen on chest x-ray; occasionally, the mass is large enough to compress the trachea and cause dyspnea. Pruritus is common; it can be extremely distressing, and the cause is unknown. Approximately 20% of patients experience brief but severe pain after drinking alcohol (Cavalli, 1998). The pain is usually at the site of the Hodgkin's disease; again, the cause is unknown.

All organs are vulnerable to invasion by Hodgkin's disease. The symptoms result from compression of organs by the tumor, such as cough and pulmonary effusion (from pulmonary infiltrates), jaundice (from hepatic involvement or bile duct obstruction), abdominal pain (from splenomegaly or retroperitoneal adenopathy), or bone pain (from skeletal involvement). Herpes zoster infections are common. A cluster of constitutional symptoms has important prognostic implications. Referred to as "B symptoms," they include fever (without chills), drenching sweats (particularly at night), and unintentional weight loss of more than 10%. "B symptoms" are found in 40% of patients and are more common in advanced disease.

A mild anemia is the most common hematologic finding. The WBC count may be elevated or decreased. The platelet count is typically normal, unless the tumor has invaded the bone marrow, suppressing hematopoiesis. The **erythrocyte sedimentation rate (ESR)** and the serum copper level are used by some clinicians to assess disease activity. Patients with Hodgkin's disease have impaired cellular immunity, as evidenced by an absent or decreased reaction to skin sensitivity tests (eg, *Candida*, mumps).

Assessment and Diagnostic Findings

Because many manifestations are similar to those occurring with infection, diagnostic studies are performed to rule out an infectious origin for the disease. The diagnosis is made by means of an excisional lymph node biopsy and the finding of the Reed-Sternberg cell. Once the diagnosis is confirmed and the histologic type is established, it is necessary to assess the extent of the disease, a process referred to as staging.

During the health history, the nurse should assess for any "B symptoms." Physical examination requires a careful, systematic evaluation of the lymph node chains, as well as the size of the spleen and liver. A chest x-ray and a CT scan of the chest, abdomen, and pelvis are crucial to identify the extent of lymphadenopathy within these regions. Laboratory tests include CBC, platelet count, ESR, and liver and renal function studies. A bone marrow biopsy is performed if there are signs of marrow involvement, and some physicians routinely perform bilateral biopsies. Bone scans may be performed to identify any involvement in these areas. A staging laparotomy and lymphangiography are no longer considered mandatory, primarily because of the accuracy of CT.

Medical Management

The general intent in treating Hodgkin's disease, regardless of stage, is cure. Treatment is determined primarily by the stage of the disease, not the histologic type; however, extensive research is ongoing to target treatment regimens to histologic subtypes or prognostic features. Traditionally, early Hodgkin's disease was treated by a staging laparotomy followed by radiation therapy. Recent data show improved results and decreased complications with a short course (2 to 4 months) of chemotherapy followed by radiation therapy in certain subsets of early-stage disease (IA and IIA); patients with early-stage disease and good prognostic features may receive radiation therapy alone (Hoppe et al., 2000). Combination chemotherapy, for example with doxorubicin (eg, Adriamycin), bleomycin (eg, Blenoxane), vinblastine (eg, Velban), and dacarbazine (eg, DTIC), referred to as ABVD, is now the standard treatment for more advanced disease (stages III and IV and all B stages).

Radiation therapy is still very useful for patients with extensive adenopathy (often termed bulky disease). In this group, residual disease often persists after the chemotherapy treatment is finished; radiation therapy to the areas of remaining adenopathy has been shown to improve survival.

Even when Hodgkin's disease does recur, the use of high doses of chemotherapeutic agents, followed by autologous BMT or stem cell transplantation (PBSCT), can be very effective in controlling the disease and extending survival time.

Long-Term Complications of Therapy

Much is now known about the long-term effects of chemotherapy and radiation therapy, primarily from the large numbers of people who were cured of Hodgkin's disease by these treatments. The various complications of treatment are listed in Chart 33-12. Risk factors for other cancers should be assessed, and long-term surveillance is crucial. The potential development of a second malignancy is obviously of concern to patients, and this potential should be addressed with the patient when treatment decisions are made. However, it is important to consider that Hodgkin's disease is curable. Revised treatment approaches are aimed at diminishing the risk for complications without sacrificing the potential for cure.

NON-HODGKIN'S LYMPHOMAS (NHLs)

The NHLs are a heterogeneous group of cancers that originate from the neoplastic growth of lymphoid tissue. As in CLL, the neoplastic cells are thought to arise from a single clone of lymphocytes; however, in NHL, the cells may vary morphologically. Most NHLs involve malignant B lymphocytes; only 5% involve T lymphocytes. In contrast to Hodgkin's disease, the lymphoid tissues involved are largely infiltrated with malignant cells. The spread of these ma-

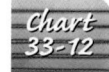

Chart 33-12   **Potential Long-Term Complications of Therapy for Hodgkin's Disease**

Immune dysfunction
Herpes infections (zoster and varicella)
Pneumococcal sepsis
Acute myeloid leukemia (AML)
Myelodysplastic syndromes (MDS)
Non-Hodgkin's lymphoma
Solid tumors
Thyroid cancer
Thymic hyperplasia
Hypothyroidism
Pericarditis (acute or chronic)
Cardiomyopathy
Pneumonitis (acute or chronic)
Avascular necrosis
Growth retardation
Infertility
Impotence
Dental caries

lignant lymphoid cells occurs unpredictably, and true localized disease is uncommon. Lymph nodes from multiple sites may be infiltrated, as may sites outside the lymphoid system (extranodal tissue).

The incidence of NHL has increased dramatically over the past decade; it is now the fourth most common type of cancer diagnosed in the United States and the fifth most common cause of cancer death (Greenlee, Hill-Horton, Murray, & Thun, 2001; Zelenetz et al., 2000). The incidence increases with each decade of life; the average age at diagnosis is 50 to 60 years. Although no common etiologic factor has been identified, there is an increased incidence of NHL in people with immunodeficiencies or autoimmune disorders, viral infections (including Epstein-Barr virus and HIV), or exposure to pesticides, solvents, or dyes. Prognosis varies greatly among the various types of NHL. Long-term survival (more than 10 years) is commonly achieved in low-grade, localized lymphomas. Even with aggressive disease forms, cure is possible in at least one third of patients who receive aggressive treatment.

Clinical Manifestations

Symptoms are highly variable, reflecting the diverse nature of these diseases. With early-stage disease, or with the types that are considered more indolent, symptoms may be virtually absent or very minor, and the illness typically is not diagnosed until it progresses to a later stage, when the patient is more symptomatic. At these stages (III or IV), lymphadenopathy is noticeable. One third of patients have "B symptoms" (recurrent fever, drenching night sweats, and unintentional weight loss of 10% or more).

Assessment and Diagnostic Findings

The actual diagnosis of NHL is categorized into a highly complex classification system based on histopathology, immunophenotyping, and cytogenetic analyses of the malignant cells. The specific histopathologic type of the disease has important prognostic implications. Treatment also varies and is based on these features. Indolent (less aggressive) types tend to have small cells and are distributed in a follicular pattern. Aggressive types tend to have large or immature cells distributed through the nodes in a diffuse pattern. Staging, also an important factor, is typically based on data obtained from CT scans, bone marrow biopsies, and occasionally cerebrospinal fluid analysis. The stage is based on the site of disease and its spread to other sites. For example, in stage I disease, only one area of involvement is detected; thus, stage I disease is highly localized and may respond well to localized therapy (eg, radiation therapy). In contrast, stage IV disease is detected in at least one extranodal site. Although low-grade lymphomas may not require treatment until the disease progresses to a later stage, historically they have also been relatively unresponsive to treatment in that most therapeutic modalities did not improve overall survival. More aggressive types of NHL (eg, lymphoblastic lymphoma, Burkitt's lymphoma) require prompt initiation of chemotherapy; however, these types tend to be more responsive to treatment.

Medical Management

Treatment is based on the actual classification of disease, the stage of disease, prior treatment (if any), and the patient's ability to tolerate therapy. If the disease is not an aggressive form and is truly localized, radiation alone may be the treatment of choice. With aggressive types of NHL, aggressive combinations of chemotherapeutic agents are given even in early stages. More intermediate forms are commonly treated with combination chemotherapy and radiation therapy for stage I and II disease. The biologic agent interferon has been approved for the treatment of follicular low-grade lymphomas, and an antibody to CD20, rituximab (Rituxan), has been effective in achieving partial responses in patients with recurrent low-grade lymphoma. Studies of this agent in combination with conventional chemotherapy have demonstrated an improvement in survival as well (Coiffier, 2002; Emmanouilides et al., 2000; Petryk & Grossbard, 2000). Central nervous system involvement is also common with some aggressive forms of NHL; in this situation, cranial radiation or intrathecal chemotherapy is used in addition to systemic chemotherapy. Treatment after relapse is controversial. BMT or PBSCT may be considered for patients younger than 60 years of age (See Chap. 16).

Nursing Management

Most of the care for patients with Hodgkin's disease or NHL is performed in the outpatient setting, unless complications occur (eg, infection, respiratory compromise due to mediastinal mass). For patients who require treatment, chemotherapy and radiation therapy are most commonly used. Chemotherapy causes systemic side effects (eg, myelosuppression, nausea, hair loss, risk for infection), whereas the side effects from radiation therapy are specific to the area being irradiated. For example, patients receiving abdominal radiation therapy may experience nausea and diarrhea but not hair loss. Regardless of the type of treatment, all patients may experience fatigue.

The risk of infection is significant for these patients, not only from treatment-related myelosuppression but also from the defective immune response that results from the disease itself. Patients need to be taught to minimize the risks for infection, to recognize signs of possible infection, and to contact the health care professional should such signs develop (see Chart 33-8).

Many lymphomas can be cured with current treatments. However, as survival rates increase, the incidence of second malignancies, particularly AML or MDS, also increases. Therefore, survivors should be screened regularly for the development of second malignancies.

Lymphoma is a highly complex constellation of diseases. When caring for the patient with lymphoma, it is extremely important to know the specific disease type, stage of disease, treatment history, and current treatment plan.

MULTIPLE MYELOMA

Multiple myeloma is a malignant disease of the most mature form of B lymphocyte, the plasma cell. It is not classified as a lymphoma. Plasma cells secrete immunoglobulins, proteins necessary for antibody production to fight infection.

Pathophysiology

In myeloma, the malignant plasma cells produce an increased amount of a specific immunoglobulin that is nonfunctional. Functional types of immunoglobulin are still produced by nonmalignant plasma cells, but in lower-than-normal quantity. The specific immunoglobulin secreted by the myeloma cells is detectable in the blood or urine and is referred to as the monoclonal protein, or M protein. This protein serves as a useful marker to monitor the extent of disease and the patient's response to therapy. It is measured by serum or urine protein electrophoresis. Moreover, the patient's total protein level is typically elevated, again due to the production of M protein. Malignant plasma cells also secrete certain substances to stimulate the creation of new blood vessels to enhance the growth of these clusters of plasma cells; this process is referred to as angiogenesis. Occasionally the plasma cells infiltrate other tissue, in which case they are referred to as plasmacytomas. Plasmacytomas can occur in the sinuses, spinal cord, and soft tissues. Median survival time is 3 to 5 years. Death usually results from infection.

Clinical Manifestations

The classic presenting symptom of multiple myeloma is bone pain, usually in the back or ribs. Bone pain is reported by two thirds of all patients at diagnosis. Unlike arthritic pain, the bone pain associated with myeloma increases with movement and decreases with rest; patients may report that they have less pain on awakening but the pain intensity increases during the day. In myeloma, a substance secreted by the plasma cells, osteoclast activating factor, as well as other substances (eg, interleukin-6 [IL-6]) are involved in stimulating osteoclasts. Both mechanisms appear to be involved in the process of bone breakdown. Thus, lytic lesions as well as osteoporosis may be seen on bone x-rays. (They are not well visualized on bone scans.) The bone destruction can be severe enough to cause fractures, including spinal fractures, which can impinge on the spinal cord and result in spinal cord compression. It is this bone destruction that causes significant pain.

 NURSING ALERT Any elderly patient whose chief complaint is back pain, and who has an elevated total protein level, should be evaluated for possible myeloma.

If the bone destruction is fairly extensive, excessive ionized calcium is lost from the bone and enters the serum; patients may therefore become hypercalcemic (frequently manifested by excessive thirst, dehydration, constipation, altered mental status, confusion, and perhaps coma). Renal failure may also be seen; the configuration of the circulating immunoglobulin molecule (particularly the shape of lambda light chains) can damage the renal tubules.

As more and more malignant plasma cells are produced, the marrow has less space for RBC production, and the patient can become anemic. This anemia is also caused to a great extent by a diminished production of erythropoietin (a glycoprotein necessary for RBC production) by the kidney. Patients may complain of fatigue and weakness due to the anemia. In the late stage of the disease, a reduced number of WBCs and platelets may also be seen because the bone marrow is infiltrated by malignant plasma cells.

When plasma cells secrete excessive amounts of immunoglobulin, particularly IgA, the serum viscosity can be elevated. Hyperviscosity may be manifested by bleeding from the nose or mouth, headache, blurred vision, paresthesias, or heart failure.

Assessment and Diagnostic Findings

Finding an elevated monoclonal protein spike in the serum (via serum protein electrophoresis) or urine (via urine protein electrophoresis) or light chain in the urine (sometimes referred to as Bence Jones protein) is considered to be a major criterion in the diagnosis of multiple myeloma. The presence of lytic bone lesions on x-ray aids in the diagnosis, as does the presence of anemia or hypercalcemia. The diagnosis of myeloma can be confirmed by bone marrow biopsy; the presence of sheets of plasma cells is the hallmark diagnostic criterion. Because the infiltration of the marrow by these malignant plasma cells is not uniform, the extent of plasma cells may not be increased in a given sample (a false-negative result).

Gerontologic Considerations

The incidence of multiple myeloma increases with age; the disease rarely occurs in patients younger than 40 years of age. Because of the increasing older population, more patients are seeking treatment for this disease. BMT or PBSCT is an option that can prolong remission and potentially cure some patients. However, it is unavailable to most because of age limitations. Back pain, which is often a presenting symptom in this disease, should be closely investigated in elderly patients.

Medical Management

There is no cure for multiple myeloma. Even BMT or PBSCT is considered by most authorities to extend remission rather than provide a cure. However, for many patients, it is possible to control the illness and maintain their level of functioning quite well for several years or longer. Chemotherapy is the primary treatment; corticosteroids, particularly dexamethasone (Decadron), are especially effective and are often combined with other agents (such as melphalan (eg, Alkeran), cyclophosphamide (eg, Cytoxan), doxorubicin (eg, Adriamycin), vincristine (eg, Oncovin), and BCNU (eg, Carmustine).

Radiation therapy is very useful in strengthening the bone at a specific lesion, particularly one at risk for bone fracture or spinal cord compression. It is also useful in relieving bone pain and reducing the size of plasma cell tumors that occur outside the skeletal system. However, because it is a nonsystemic form of treatment, it does not diminish the source of the bone conditions (ie, the production of malignant plasma cells). Therefore, radiation therapy is typically used with systemic treatment such as chemotherapy.

The biologic agent alpha-interferon has been used successfully to maintain remission in selected types of myeloma, particularly IgA type; however, its role in prolonging survival is controversial. Newer forms of bisphosphonates, such as pamidronate (Aredia) and zoledronic acid (Zometa), have been shown to strengthen bone

in this disease (by diminishing the secretion of osteoclast activating factor) (Berenson, 2001), controlling bone pain and potentially preventing bone fracture. They are also effective in managing and preventing hypercalcemia. Some evidence suggests that bisphosphonates may actually have activity against the myeloma cells themselves by inhibiting a growth factor necessary for myeloma cell survival (Berenson, 2001) (see later discussion).

When patients manifest signs and symptoms of hyperviscosity, plasmapheresis may be used to lower the immunoglobulin level. Symptoms may be more useful than serum viscosity levels in determining the need for this intervention.

Recent advances in the understanding of the process of angiogenesis have resulted in new therapeutic options. The sedative thalidomide (Thalomid), initially used as an antiemetic, has significant antimyeloma effects. It inhibits cytokines necessary for new vascular generation, such as vascular endothelial growth factor (VEGF), and for myeloma cell growth and survival, such as IL-6 and tumor necrosis factor (TNF), by boosting the body's immune response against the tumor and by creating favorable conditions for apoptosis (programmed cell death) of the myeloma cells. Thalidomide is effective in refractory myeloma and in "smoldering" disease states, and may prevent progression to a more active state. Thalidomide is not a typical chemotherapeutic agent and has a unique side effect profile. Fatigue, dizziness, constipation, rash, and peripheral neuropathy are commonly encountered; myelosuppression is not (Goldman, 2001). Thalidomide is contraindicated in pregnancy because of associated severe birth defects.

Nursing Management

Pain management is very important in this patient population. NSAIDs can be very useful for mild pain, or in combination with opioid analgesics. However, care needs to be taken, because NSAIDs can cause renal dysfunction. Patients need to be educated about activity restrictions (eg, lifting no more than 10 pounds, use of proper body mechanics). Braces are occasionally needed to provide support to the spinal column.

Patients also need to be instructed about the signs and symptoms of hypercalcemia. Maintaining mobility and hydration is important to diminish exacerbations of this complication; however, the primary cause is the disease itself. Renal function should also be monitored closely. Renal failure can become severe, and dialysis may be needed. Maintaining high urine output (3 L/day) can be very useful in preventing this complication.

Because antibody production is impaired, infections, particularly bacterial infections, are common and can be life-threatening. Patients need to be instructed in appropriate infection prevention measures (see Chart 33-8) and should be advised to contact their health care provider immediately if they have a fever or other signs and symptoms of infection. Patients should receive Pneumovax and flu vaccines. Prophylactic antibiotics are sometimes used. Intravenous immune globulin (IVIG) can be useful for patients with recurrent infections.

Bleeding Disorders

Normal hemostatic mechanisms can control bleeding from vessels and prevent spontaneous bleeding. The bleeding vessel constricts and platelets aggregate at the site, forming an unstable hemostatic plug. Circulating coagulation factors are activated on the surface of these aggregated platelets, forming fibrin, which anchors the platelet plug to the site of injury.

The failure of normal hemostatic mechanisms can result in bleeding, which is severe at times. This bleeding is commonly provoked by trauma, but in certain circumstances it can occur spontaneously. When the source is platelet or coagulation factor abnormalities, the site of spontaneous bleeding can be anywhere in the body. When the defect is caused by vascular abnormalities, the site of bleeding may be more localized. Some patients have defects in more than one hemostatic mechanism simultaneously.

In a variety of situations, the bone marrow may be stimulated to increase platelet production (thrombopoiesis). The increased production may be a reactive response, as in a compensatory response to significant bleeding, or a more general response to increase hematopoiesis, as in iron deficiency anemia. Sometimes, the increase in platelets does not result from increased production but from a loss in platelet pooling within the spleen. The spleen typically holds about one third of the circulating platelets at any time. If the spleen is lost (eg, splenectomy), the platelet reservoir is also lost, and an abnormally high amount of platelets enter the circulation. In time, the rate of thrombopoiesis slows to reestablish a more normal platelet level.

Clinical Manifestations

Signs and symptoms of bleeding disorders vary depending on the type of defect. A careful history and physical examination can be very useful in determining the source of the hemostatic defect. Abnormalities of the vascular system give rise to local bleeding, usually into the skin. Because platelets are primarily responsible for stopping bleeding from small vessels, patients with platelet defects develop petechiae, often in clusters; these are seen on the skin and mucous membranes but also occur throughout the body. Bleeding from platelet disorders can be severe. Unless the platelet disorder is severe, bleeding can often be stopped promptly when local pressure is applied; it does not typically recur when the pressure is released.

In contrast, coagulation factor defects do not tend to cause superficial bleeding, because the primary hemostatic mechanisms are still intact. Instead, bleeding occurs deeper within the body (eg, subcutaneous or intramuscular hematomas, hemorrhage into joint spaces). External bleeding diminishes very slowly when local pressure is applied; it often recurs several hours after pressure is removed. For example, severe bleeding may start several hours after a tooth extraction. Risk factors for bleeding are provided in Chart 33-7.

Medical Management

Management varies based on the underlying cause of the bleeding disorder. If bleeding is significant, transfusions of blood products are indicated. The specific blood product used is determined by the underlying defect. In specific situations in which fibrinolysis is excessive, hemostatic agents such as aminocaproic acid (Amicar) can be used to inhibit this process. This agent must be used with caution, because excessive inhibition of fibrinolysis can result in thrombosis.

Nursing Management

Patients who have bleeding disorders or who have the potential for development of such disorders as a result of disease or therapeutic agents must be taught to observe themselves carefully and frequently for bleeding. They need to understand the importance of avoiding activities that increase the risk of bleeding, such as

contact sports. The skin is observed for petechiae and ecchymoses (bruises) and the nose and gums for bleeding. Hospitalized patients may be monitored for bleeding by testing all drainage and excreta (feces, urine, emesis, and gastric drainage) for occult as well as obvious blood. Outpatients are often given fecal occult blood screening cards to detect occult blood in stools.

PRIMARY THROMBOCYTHEMIA

Primary thrombocythemia (also called essential thrombocythemia [ET]) is a stem cell disorder within the bone marrow. A marked increase in platelet production occurs, with the platelet count consistently greater than 600,000/mm³. Platelet size may be abnormal, but platelet survival is typically normal. Occasionally, the platelet increase is accompanied by an increase in RBCs or WBCs or both; however, these cells are not increased to the extent that they are in polycythemia vera, CML, or myelofibrosis. Although the exact cause is unknown, primary thrombocythemia is similar to other myeloproliferative disorders, particularly polycythemia vera. Unlike the other myeloproliferative disorders, however, it rarely evolves into acute leukemia.

Clinical Manifestations

Many patients with primary thrombocythemia are asymptomatic; the illness is diagnosed as the result of finding an elevated platelet count on a CBC. Symptoms, when they do occur, result primarily from hemorrhage or vasoocclusion in the microvasculature. Symptoms may occur more when the platelet count exceeds 1 million/mm³. However, symptoms do not always correlate with the extent to which the platelet count is elevated. Thrombosis is common and can be either arterial or venous; major thromboses occur in 15% to 40% of these patients (Jantunen et al., 2001). Because these platelets can be dysfunctional, minor or major hemorrhage can also occur. Bleeding from the mucous membranes of the nose and mouth is common, and significant gastrointestinal bleeding is also possible. Bleeding typically does not occur until the platelet count exceeds 1 million/mm³.

Vasoocclusive manifestations are most frequently seen in the form of erythromelalgia. The toxic effects of platelet substances include painful burning, warmth, and redness in a localized distal area of the extremities. Neurologic manifestations may also be seen, such as numbness, tingling, and visual disturbance; these occlusive manifestations can progress to stroke and seizure and, less commonly, to myocardial infarction. The spleen may be enlarged, but usually not to a significant extent.

Assessment and Diagnostic Findings

The diagnosis of primary thrombocythemia is made by ruling out other potential disorders. Iron deficiency should be excluded, because a reactive increase in the platelet count often accompanies this deficiency. The myeloproliferative disorders (CML, polycythemia vera) should also be excluded. Examination of the CBC shows markedly abnormal platelets. Analysis of the bone marrow (by aspiration and biopsy) shows a marked increase in megakaryocytes (platelet precursors) and is useful in excluding CML as a possible cause for the elevated platelet count. The disease, which affects men and women equally, tends to occur in late middle age. The median survival time exceeds 10 years.

No data reliably predict the development of complications. Risk factors for the development of thrombotic complications are age greater than 65 years, prior thrombotic events, and long duration of thrombocytosis. Major bleeding tends to occur when the platelet count is very high.

Medical Management

The management of primary thrombocythemia is highly controversial. The risk of significant thrombotic or hemorrhagic complications may not be increased until the platelet count exceeds 1 million/mm³ (Briere & Guilmin, 2001). A careful assessment of other risk factors, such as history of peripheral vascular disease, history of tobacco use, atherosclerosis, and prior thrombotic events, should be used in making the decision as to when to initiate therapy. In younger patients with no risk factors, low-dose aspirin therapy may be sufficient to prevent thrombotic complications; however, the use of aspirin can increase the risk for hemorrhagic complications and may be considered a contraindication in patients with a history of gastrointestinal bleeding. The neurologic symptoms (eg, headache and erythromelalgia) and visual symptoms of primary thrombocytopenia can be relieved by low-dose aspirin.

More aggressive measures may be required in older patients and in those with concurrent risk factors. Hydroxyurea (eg, Hydrea), a chemotherapeutic medication, is effective in lowering the platelet count. It is taken orally and causes minimal side effects other than dose-related leukopenia. However, its potential for leukogenesis is in question. The medication anagrelide (Agrylin) is more specific in lowering the platelet count than is hydroxyurea, but it has more side effects. Severe headaches cause many patients to stop taking the medication. Tachycardia and chest pain may also occur, and anagrelide is contraindicated in patients with concurrent cardiac problems. Interferon-alfa-2b (eg, Intron-A) has been shown to lower platelet counts by an unknown mechanism. The medication is administered subcutaneously at varying frequency, commonly three times per week. Significant side effects, such as fatigue, weakness, memory defects, dizziness, anemia, and liver dysfunction, limit its usefulness.

Rarely, the occlusive symptoms are so great that the platelet count must be reduced immediately. Platelet pheresis (see later discussion) can reduce the amount of circulating platelets, but only transiently. The extent by which symptoms and complications (eg, thromboses) are reduced remains unclear.

Nursing Management

Patients with primary thrombocythemia need to be instructed about the accompanying risks of hemorrhage and thrombosis. Patients should be informed about signs and symptoms of thrombosis, particularly the neurologic manifestations, such as visual changes, numbness, tingling, and weakness. Risk factors for thrombosis should be assessed, and measures to diminish risk factors (particularly cessation of tobacco use) should be encouraged. Patients receiving aspirin therapy should be informed about the increased risk for bleeding. Patients who are at risk for bleeding should be instructed about medications that can alter platelet function, such as aspirin, NSAIDs, and alcohol. Patients receiving interferon therapy should be taught to self-administer the medication and manage side effects.

SECONDARY THROMBOCYTOSIS

Increased platelet production is the primary mechanism of secondary, or reactive, **thrombocytosis**. The platelet count is above

normal, but, in contrast to primary thrombocythemia, an increase above 1 million/mm³ is rare. Platelet function is normal; the platelet survival time is normal or decreased. Symptoms associated with hemorrhage or thrombosis are rare. Many disorders can cause a reactive increase in platelets, including chronic inflammatory disorders, iron deficiency, malignant disease, acute hemorrhage, and splenectomy (see previous discussion of primary thrombocythemia). Treatment is aimed at the underlying disorder. With successful management, the platelet count usually returns to normal.

THROMBOCYTOPENIA

Thrombocytopenia (low platelet level) can result from various factors: decreased production of platelets within the bone marrow, increased destruction of platelets, or increased consumption of platelets. Causes and treatments are summarized in Table 33-5.

Clinical Manifestations

Bleeding and petechiae usually do not occur with platelet counts greater than 50,000/mm³, although excessive bleeding can follow surgery or other trauma. When the platelet count drops below

Table 33-5 • **Causes and Management of Thrombocytopenia**

CAUSE	MANAGEMENT
Decreased Production	
Hematologic malignancy, especially acute leukemias	Treat leukemia; platelet transfusion
Myelodysplastic syndromes (MDS): metastatic involvement of bone marrow from solid tumors	Treat MDS; platelet transfusion
	Treat solid tumor
Aplastic anemia	Treat underlying condition
Megaloblastic anemia	Treat underlying anemia
Toxins	Remove toxin
Medications	Stop medication
Infection (esp. septicemia, viral infection, tuberculosis)	Treat infection
Alcohol	Refrain from alcohol consumption
Chemotherapy	Delay or decrease dose; growth factor; platelet transfusion
Increased Destruction	
Due to Antibodies	Treat condition
Idiopathic thrombocytopenic purpura	
Lupus erythematosus	
Malignant lymphoma	
Chronic lymphocytic leukemia (CLL)	Treat CLL and/or treat as ITP
Medications	Stop medication
Due to Infection	Treat infection
Bacteremia	
Postviral infection	
Sequestration of platelets in an enlarged spleen	If thrombocytopenia is severe, splenectomy may be needed
Increased Consumption	
Disseminated intravascular coagulation (DIC)	Treat underlying condition triggering DIC; administer heparin, EACA, blood products

20,000/mm³, petechiae can appear, along with nose and gingival bleeding, excessive menstrual bleeding, and excessive bleeding after surgery or dental extractions. When the platelet count is less than 5000/mm³, spontaneous, potentially fatal central nervous system or gastrointestinal hemorrhage can occur. If the platelets are dysfunctional due to disease (eg, MDS) or medications (eg, aspirin), the risk of bleeding may be much greater even when the actual platelet count is not significantly reduced.

Assessment and Diagnostic Findings

A platelet deficiency that results from decreased production (eg, leukemia, MDS) can usually be diagnosed by examining the bone marrow via aspiration and biopsy. When platelet destruction is the cause of thrombocytopenia, the marrow shows increased megakaryocytes (the cells from which the platelets originate) and normal or even increased platelet production as the body attempts to compensate for the decreased platelets in circulation. Another cause of thrombocytopenia is sequestration. Approximately one third of the circulating platelets are within the spleen, and a greatly enlarged spleen results in increased sequestration of platelets.

Medical Management

The management for secondary thrombocytopenia is usually treatment of the underlying disease. If platelet production is impaired, platelet transfusions may raise the platelet count and stop bleeding or prevent spontaneous hemorrhage. If excessive platelet destruction occurs, transfused platelets will also be destroyed, and the platelet count will not rise. The most common cause of excessive platelet destruction is ITP (see the following discussion). In some instances splenectomy can be a useful therapeutic intervention, but often it is not a therapeutic option, for example in patients in whom the enlarged spleen is due to portal hypertension related to excessive alcohol consumption.

Nursing Management

The interventions for a patient with thrombocytopenia are delineated in Chart 33-10.

IDIOPATHIC THROMBOCYTOPENIC PURPURA (ITP)

ITP is a disease that affects people of all ages, but it is more common among children and young women. There are two forms of ITP: acute and chronic. The acute form, which occurs predominately in children, often appears 1 to 6 weeks after a viral illness. This form is self-limited; remission often occurs spontaneously within 6 months. Occasionally, corticosteroids are needed for a brief time. Chronic ITP is often diagnosed by exclusion of other causes of thrombocytopenia.

Pathophysiology

Although the precise cause remains unknown, viral infections sometimes precede ITP in children. Occasionally medications such as sulfa drugs can induce ITP. Other conditions, such as systemic lupus erythematosus (SLE) or pregnancy, can also induce ITP. Anti-platelet autoantibodies that bind to the patient's platelets are found in the blood of patients with ITP. When the platelets are bound by the antibodies, the RES or tissue macrophage system ingests the platelets, destroying them. The body attempts to compensate for this destruction by increasing platelet production within the marrow.

Clinical Manifestations

Many patients have no symptoms, and the low platelet count (often less than 20,000/mm³, and less than 5000/mm³ is not uncommon) is an incidental finding. Common physical manifestations are easy bruising, heavy menses, and petechiae on the extremities or trunk. Patients with simple bruising or petechiae ("dry purpura") tend to have fewer complications from bleeding than those with bleeding from mucosal surfaces, such as the gastrointestinal tract (including the mouth) and pulmonary system (eg, hemoptysis), which is termed "wet purpura." Patients with wet purpura have a greater risk for intracranial bleeding than do those with dry purpura. Despite low platelet counts, the platelets are young and very functional. They adhere to endothelial surfaces and to one another, so spontaneous bleeding does not always occur.

Assessment and Diagnostic Findings

Patients may have an isolated decrease in platelets (less than 20,000/mm³ is common), but they may also have an increase in megakaryocytes (platelet precursors) within the marrow, as detected on bone marrow aspirate.

Medical Management

The primary goal of treatment is a safe platelet count. Because the risk of bleeding typically does not increase until the platelet count is lower than 10,000/mm³, a patient whose count exceeds 30,000 to 50,000/mm³ may be carefully observed without additional intervention. However, if the count is lower than 20,000/mm³, or if bleeding occurs, the goal is to improve the patient's platelet count, rather than to cure the disease. Treatment for ITP usually requires several approaches. If the patient is taking a medication that is known to cause ITP (eg, quinine, sulfa-containing medications), that medication must be stopped immediately. The mainstay of short-term therapy is the use of immunosuppressive agents. The immunosuppressants block the binding receptors on macrophages so that the platelets are not destroyed. Prednisone is the agent typically used (at a dose of 1 mg/kg), and it is effective in about 75% of patients. Cyclophosphamide (eg, Cytoxan) and azathioprine (Imuran) can also be used, and dexamethasone (eg, Decadron) may be effective. Platelet counts rise within a few days after institution of corticosteroid therapy; this effect takes longer with azathioprine. Because of the associated side effects, patients cannot take high doses of corticosteroids indefinitely. It is not unusual for the platelet count to drop once the corticosteroid dose is tapered. Some patients can be successfully maintained on low doses of prednisone (eg, 2.5 to 10 mg every other day).

Intravenous immune globulin (IVIG) is also commonly used to treat ITP. It is effective in binding the receptors on the macrophages; however, high doses (1 g/kg for 2 days) are required, and the drug is very expensive. Splenectomy is an alternative treatment but results in a normal platelet count only 50% of the time; however, many patients can maintain a "safe" platelet count of more than 30,000/mm³ after removal of the spleen. Even those who do respond to splenectomy may have recurrences of severe thrombocytopenia months or years later. Patients who have splenectomy are permanently at risk for sepsis; these patients should receive Pneumovax, *Haemophilus influenzae* B, and meningococcal vaccines, preferably 2 to 3 weeks before the splenectomy is performed. Pneumovax vaccine should be repeated at 5- to 10-year intervals.

Other options for management include use of the chemotherapy agent vincristine (Oncovin). Vincristine appears to work by blocking the receptors on the macrophages and therefore inhibiting platelet destruction; it may also stimulate thrombopoiesis. Some data support the efficacy of certain monoclonal antibodies (eg, rituximab) in increasing platelet counts, but more research is needed (Stasi, Pagano, Stipa, & Amadori, 2001; Saleh et al., 2000).

Another approach to the management of chronic ITP involves the use of anti-D (eg, WinRho) in patients who are Rh(D)-positive. The actual mechanism of action is unknown. One theory is that the anti-D binds to the patient's RBCs, which are in turn destroyed by the body's macrophages. While the macrophages destroy the anti-D/RBC complex, they are not able to destroy platelets. Anti-D produces a transient decreased hematocrit and increased platelet count in many, but not all, patients with ITP. Anti-D appears to be most effective in children with ITP and least effective in patients who have undergone splenectomy.

Despite the extremely low platelet count, platelet transfusions are usually avoided. Transfusions tend to be ineffective because the patient's anti-platelet antibodies bind with the transfused platelets, causing them to be destroyed. Platelet counts can actually drop after platelet transfusion. Occasionally, transfusion of platelets may protect against catastrophic bleeding in patients with severe wet purpura. Epsilon-aminocaproic acid (EACA; Amicar) may be useful for patients with significant mucosal bleeding refractory to other treatments.

Nursing Management

Nursing care for these patients should include an assessment of the patient's life style to determine the risk of bleeding from activity. A careful medication history should also be obtained, including use of over-the-counter medications, herbs, and nutritional supplements. The nurse must be alert for sulfa-containing medications and medications that alter platelet function (eg, medications that contain aspirin or other NSAIDs). The nurse should assess for any history of recent viral illness and reports of headache or visual disturbances (which could be initial symptoms of intracranial bleeding). Patients who are admitted to the hospital with wet purpura and low platelet counts should have a neurologic assessment incorporated into their routine vital sign measurements. No intramuscular injections or rectal medications should be administered, and rectal temperature measurements should not be performed, because they can stimulate bleeding.

Patient teaching should address signs of exacerbation of disease (petechiae, ecchymoses); how to contact appropriate health care personnel; the name and type of medication inducing ITP (if appropriate); current medical treatment (medications, tapering schedule if relevant, side effects); and the frequency of monitoring the platelet count. Patients should be instructed to avoid all agents that interfere with platelet function. The patient should avoid constipation, the Valsalva maneuver (eg, straining at stool), and flossing of the teeth. Electric razors should be used for shaving, and soft-bristled toothbrushes should replace stiff-bristled ones. Patients should also be counseled to refrain from vigorous sexual intercourse when the platelet count is less than 10,000/mm³. Patients who are receiving chronic corticosteroids are at risk for

complications including osteoporosis, proximal muscle wasting, cataract formation, and dental caries (see Chart 33-4). Bone mineral density should be monitored, and these patients may benefit from calcium and vitamin D supplementation and bisphosphonate therapy to prevent significant bone disease.

PLATELET DEFECTS

Quantitative platelet defects are relatively common (thrombocytopenia), but qualitative defects can also occur. With qualitative defects, the number of platelets may be normal, but the platelets do not function normally. Platelet function is most commonly evaluated by the bleeding time; however, this test is a crude measurement at best.

An important functional platelet disorder is that induced by aspirin. Even small amounts of aspirin reduce normal platelet aggregation, and the prolonged bleeding time lasts for several days after aspirin ingestion. Although this does not cause bleeding in most people, patients with a coagulation disorder (eg, hemophilia) or thrombocytopenia can have significant bleeding after taking aspirin, particularly if invasive procedures or trauma has occurred.

NSAIDs can also inhibit platelet function, but the effect is not as prolonged as with aspirin (about 5 days versus 7 to 10 days). Other causes of platelet dysfunction include end-stage renal disease, possibly from metabolic products affecting platelet function; MDS; multiple myeloma (due to abnormal protein interfering with platelet function); cardiopulmonary bypass; and other medications and substances (Chart 33-13).

Clinical Manifestations

Bleeding may be mild or severe. Its extent is not necessarily correlated with the platelet count or with tests that measure coagulation (prothrombin time [PT], partial thromboplastin time [PTT]). Ecchymoses are common, particularly on the extremities. Patients with platelet dysfunction may be at risk for significant bleeding after trauma or invasive procedures (eg, biopsy, dental extraction).

Medical Management

If the platelet dysfunction is caused by medication, use of the offending medication should be stopped, if possible, particularly when bleeding occurs. If platelet dysfunction is marked, bleeding can often be prevented by transfusion of normal platelets before invasive procedures. Amniocaproic acid (EACA; Amicar) may be required to prevent significant bleeding after such procedures.

Nursing Management

Patients with significant platelet dysfunction need to be instructed to avoid agents that can diminish platelet function, such as certain over-the-counter medications, herbs, nutritional supplements, and alcohol. They also need to be assisted to serve as their own advocates and to inform their health care providers (including dentists) of the underlying condition before any invasive procedure is performed, so that appropriate steps can be initiated to diminish the risk of bleeding. Bleeding precautions should be initiated as appropriate (see Chart 33-10).

HEMOPHILIA

Two inherited bleeding disorders—hemophilia A and hemophilia B—are clinically indistinguishable, although they can be distinguished by laboratory tests. Hemophilia A is caused by a

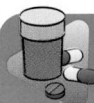

Chart 33-13 • PHARMACOLOGY
Medications and Substances That Impair Platelet Function

Anesthetic Agents
Local anesthetics
Halothane

Antibiotics
Beta-lactam antibiotics
    Penicillins
    Cephalosporins
Nitrofurantoin
Sulfonylureas

Anticoagulation Agents
Heparin
Fibrinolytic agents

Anti-inflammatory Agents (Nonsteroidal)
Aspirin
Ibuprofen
Naproxen

Antineoplastic Agents
BCNU
Daunorubicin
Mithramycin

Cardiovascular Drugs
Beta-blockers
Calcium channel blockers
Isosorbide
Nitroglycerine
Nitroprusside
Quinidine

Medications That Increase Platelet CAMP
Dipyridamole
Prostacycline
Theophylline

Food and Food Additives
Caffeine
Chinese black tree fungus
Clove
Cumin
Ethanol
Fish oils
Garlic
Onion extract
Turmeric

Plasma Expanders
Dextrans
Hydroxyethyl starch

Psychotropic Agents
Tricyclic antidepressants
Phenothiazines

Miscellaneous
Antihistamines
Clofibrate
Furosemide
Heroin
Contrast agents
Ticlopidine
Vitamin E

Herbal Supplements
Feverfew
Ginger
Gingko
Ginseng
Kava kava

genetic defect that results in deficient or defective factor VIII; hemophilia B (also called Christmas disease) stems from a genetic defect that causes deficient or defective factor IX. Hemophilia is a relatively rare disease; hemophilia A, which occurs in 1 of every 10,000 births, is three times more common than hemophilia B. Both types of hemophilia are inherited as X-linked traits, so almost all affected people are males; females can be carriers but are almost always asymptomatic. The disease is recognized in early childhood, usually in the toddler age group. However, patients with mild hemophilia may not be diagnosed until they experience severe trauma (eg, a high-school football injury) or surgery. Hemophilia occurs in all ethnic groups.

Clinical Manifestations

The disease, which can be severe, is manifested by hemorrhages into various parts of the body. Hemorrhage can occur even after minimal trauma. The frequency and severity of the bleeding depend on the degree of factor deficiency as well as the intensity of the precipitating trauma. For example, patients who have a mild factor VIII deficiency (ie, 6% to 50% of normal levels) rarely develop hemorrhage spontaneously; hemorrhage tends to occur

secondary to trauma. In contrast, spontaneous hemorrhages, particularly hemarthroses and hematomas, can frequently occur in patients with severe factor VIII deficiency (ie, less than 1% of normal levels). These patients require frequent factor replacement therapy.

About 75% of all bleeding in patients with hemophilia occurs into joints. The most commonly affected joints are the knees, elbows, ankles, shoulders, wrists, and hips. Patients often note pain in a joint before they are aware of swelling and limitation of motion. Recurrent joint hemorrhages can result in damage so severe that chronic pain or ankylosis (fixation) of the joint occurs. Many patients with severe factor deficiency are crippled by the joint damage before they become adults. Hematomas can be superficial or deep hemorrhages into muscle or subcutaneous tissue. With severe factor deficiency, they can occur without known trauma and progressively extend in all directions. When the hematomas occur within muscle, particularly in the extremities, peripheral nerves can be compressed. Over time, this compression results in decreased sensation, weakness, and atrophy of the area involved. Spontaneous hematuria and gastrointestinal bleeding can occur. Bleeding is also common in other mucous membranes, such as the nasal passages. The most dangerous site of hemorrhage is in the head (intracranial or extracranial). Any head trauma requires prompt evaluation and treatment. Surgical procedures typically result in excessive bleeding at the surgical site. Because clot formation is poor, wound healing is also poor. Such bleeding is most commonly associated with dental extraction.

Medical Management

In the past, the only treatment for hemophilia was infusion of fresh frozen plasma, which had to be administered in such large quantities that patients experienced fluid volume overload. Now factor VIII and factor IX concentrates are available to all blood banks. Recombinant forms of these factors have been made available and may diminish the use of factor concentrates. Patients are given concentrates when they are actively bleeding or as a preventive measure before traumatic procedures (eg, lumbar puncture, dental extraction, surgery). The patient and family are taught how to administer the concentrate intravenously at home at the first sign of bleeding. It is crucial to initiate treatment as soon as possible so that bleeding complications can be avoided. A few patients eventually develop antibodies to the concentrates, so their factor levels cannot be increased. Treatment of this problem is extremely difficult and often unsuccessful.

Aminocaproic acid (EACA; Amicar) is a fibrinolytic enzyme inhibitor that can slow the dissolution of blood clots that do form; it is very effective as an adjunctive measure after oral surgery. It is also useful in treating mucosal bleeding. Another agent, desmopressin (eg, DDAVP), induces a transient rise in factor VIII levels; the mechanism for this response is unknown. In patients with mild forms of hemophilia A, desmopressin is extremely useful, significantly reducing the amount of blood products required. However, desmopressin is not effective in patients with severe factor VIII deficiency.

Nursing Management

Most patients with hemophilia are diagnosed as children. They often require assistance in coping with the condition because it is chronic, places restrictions on their lives, and is an inherited disorder that can be passed to future generations. From childhood, patients are helped to accept themselves and the disease and to identify the positive aspects of their lives. They are encouraged to be self-sufficient and to maintain independence by preventing unnecessary trauma that can cause acute bleeding episodes and temporarily interfere with normal activities. As they work through their feelings about the condition and progress to accepting it, they can assume more and more responsibility for maintaining optimal health.

Patients with mild factor deficiency may not be diagnosed until adulthood if they do not experience significant trauma or surgery as children. These patients need extensive teaching about activity restrictions and self-care measures to diminish the chance of hemorrhage and complications of bleeding. The nurse should emphasize safety at home and in the workplace.

Patients with hemophilia are instructed to avoid any agents that interfere with platelet aggregation, such as aspirin, NSAIDs, herbs, nutritional supplements, and alcohol. This restriction applies to over-the-counter medications such as cold remedies. Dental hygiene is very important as a preventive measure because dental extractions are so hazardous. Applying pressure may be sufficient to control bleeding resulting from minor trauma if the factor deficiency is not severe. Nasal packing should be avoided, because bleeding frequently resumes when the packing is removed. Splints and other orthopedic devices may be useful in patients with joint or muscle hemorrhages. All injections should be avoided; invasive procedures (eg, endoscopy, lumbar puncture) should be minimized or performed after administration of appropriate factor replacement. Patients with hemophilia should be encouraged to carry or wear medical identification.

During hemorrhagic episodes, the extent of bleeding must be assessed carefully. Patients who are at risk for significant compromise (eg, bleeding into the respiratory tract or brain) warrant close observation and systematic assessment for emergent complications (eg, respiratory distress, altered level of consciousness). If the patient has had recent surgery, the nurse frequently and carefully assesses the surgical site for bleeding. Frequent vital sign monitoring is needed until the nurse is certain that there is no excessive postoperative bleeding.

Analgesics are commonly required to alleviate the pain associated with hematomas and hemorrhage into joints. Many patients report that warm baths promote relaxation, improve mobility, and lessen pain. However, during bleeding episodes, heat, which can accentuate bleeding, is avoided; applications of cold are used instead.

Although recent technology (ie, the formulation of heat-solvent or detergent-treated factor concentrates) has rendered factor VIII and IX preparations free from viruses such as HIV and hepatitis, many patients have already been exposed to these infections. These patients and their families may need assistance in coping with the diagnosis and the consequences of these infections.

Between 15% and 50% of patients with hemophilia A and between 1% and 3% of patients with hemophilia B develop antibodies (inhibitors) to factor concentrates, complicating factor replacement management (Lusher, 2000; White, Greenwood, Escobar, & Frelinger, 2000). These patients may require plasmapheresis or concurrent immunosuppressive therapy, particularly in the setting of significant bleeding. Patients with severe factor deficiency should be screened for antibodies, particularly before major surgery.

VON WILLEBRAND'S DISEASE

Von Willebrand's disease, a common bleeding disorder affecting males and females equally, is usually inherited as a dominant trait. The disease is caused by a deficiency of von Willebrand factor (vWF), which is necessary for factor VIII activity. vWF is also nec-

essary for platelet adhesion at the site of vascular injury. Although synthesis of factor VIII is normal, its half-life is shortened; therefore, factor VIII levels commonly are mildly low (15% to 50% of normal).

Clinical Manifestations

Patients commonly have nosebleeds, excessively heavy menses, bleeding from cuts, and postoperative bleeding, although they do not suffer from massive soft tissue or joint hemorrhages. As the laboratory values fluctuate, so does the bleeding. For example, a careful history of prior bleeding may show little problem with postoperative bleeding on one occasion but significant bleeding from a dental extraction at another time.

Assessment and Diagnostic Findings

Laboratory test results show a normal platelet count but prolonged bleeding time and slightly prolonged PTT. These defects are not static, and laboratory test results can vary widely within the same patient over time.

Medical Management

Both the factor deficiency and the platelet impairment can be corrected by administration of cryoprecipitate, which contains factor VIII, fibrinogen, and factor XIII (or fresh frozen plasma, if cryoprecipitate is unavailable). Replacement continues for several days to ensure correction of the factor VIII deficiency; up to 7 to 10 days of treatment may be necessary after major surgery. Desmopressin (DDAVP), a synthetic vasopressin analog, can be used to prevent bleeding associated with dental or surgical procedures or to manage mild bleeding after surgery. Desmopressin provides a transient increase in factor VIII coagulant activity and may also correct the bleeding time. It can be administered as an intravenous infusion or intranasally. With major surgery or invasive procedures, both desmopressin and cryoprecipitate may be needed to prevent hemorrhage.

Acquired Coagulation Disorders

LIVER DISEASE

With the exception of factor VIII, most blood coagulation factors are synthesized in the liver. Therefore, hepatic dysfunction (due to cirrhosis, tumor, or hepatitis; see Chap. 39) can result in diminished amounts of the factors needed to maintain coagulation and hemostasis. Prolongation of the PT, unless it is caused by vitamin K deficiency, may indicate severe hepatic dysfunction. Although minor bleeding is common (eg, ecchymoses), these patients are also at risk for significant bleeding, related especially to trauma or surgery. Transfusion of fresh frozen plasma may be required to replace clotting factors and to prevent or stop bleeding. Patients may also have life-threatening hemorrhage from peptic ulcers or esophageal varices. In these cases, replacement with fresh frozen plasma, PRBCs, and platelets is usually required.

VITAMIN K DEFICIENCY

The synthesis of many coagulation factors depends on vitamin K. Vitamin K deficiency is typical in malnourished patients, and some antibiotics decrease the intestinal flora that produce vitamin K, depleting vitamin K stores. Administration of vitamin K (phytonadione [eg, Mephyton], either orally or as a subcutaneous injection) can correct the deficiency quickly; adequate synthesis of coagulation factors is reflected by normalization of the PT.

COMPLICATIONS OF ANTICOAGULANT THERAPY

Anticoagulants are used in the treatment or prevention of thrombosis. These agents, particularly warfarin or heparin, can result in bleeding. If the PT or PTT is longer than desired and bleeding has not occurred, the medication can be stopped or the dose decreased. Vitamin K is administered for warfarin toxicity. Protamine sulfate is rarely needed for heparin toxicity, because the half-life of heparin is very short. With significant bleeding, fresh frozen plasma replaces the vitamin K–dependent coagulation factors. Other complications of anticoagulant therapy are discussed in Chapter 31.

DISSEMINATED INTRAVASCULAR COAGULATION (DIC)

DIC is not a disease but a sign of an underlying condition. DIC may be triggered by sepsis, trauma, cancer, shock, abruptio placentae, toxins, or allergic reactions (Chart 33-14). It is potentially life-threatening.

Pathophysiology

In DIC, the normal hemostatic mechanisms are altered so that a massive amount of tiny clots forms in the microcirculation. Initially, the coagulation time is normal. However, as the platelets and clotting factors are consumed to form the microthrombi, coagulation fails. Thus, the paradoxical result of excessive clotting is bleeding. The clinical manifestations of DIC are reflected in the organs, which are affected either by excessive clot formation (with resultant ischemia to all or part of the organ) or by bleeding. The bleeding is characterized by low platelet and fibrinogen levels; prolonged PT, PTT, and thrombin time; and elevated fibrin degradation products (**D-dimers**) (Table 33-6).

The mortality rate can exceed 80% of patients who develop DIC. Identification of patients who are at risk for DIC and recognition of the early clinical manifestations of this syndrome can result in earlier medical intervention, which may improve the prognosis. However, the primary prognostic factor is the ability to treat the underlying condition that precipitated DIC.

Clinical Manifestations

Patients with DIC may bleed from mucous membranes, venipuncture sites, and the gastrointestinal and urinary tracts. The bleeding can range from minimal occult internal bleeding to profuse hem-

orrhage from all orifices. Patients may also develop organ dysfunction, such as renal failure and pulmonary and multifocal central nervous system infarctions as a result of microthromboses, macrothromboses, or hemorrhages.

During the initial process of DIC, the patient may have no new symptoms, the only manifestation being a progressive decrease in the platelet count. As the thrombosis becomes more extensive, the patient exhibits signs and symptoms of thrombosis in the organs involved. Then, as the clotting factors and platelets are consumed to form these thrombi, bleeding occurs. Initially the bleeding is subtle, but it can develop into frank hemorrhage. Signs and symptoms depend on the organs involved and are listed in Table 33-7.

Medical Management

The most important management issue is treating the underlying cause of the DIC. Until the cause is controlled, the mechanism for DIC will persist. A second goal is to correct the secondary effects of tissue ischemia by improving oxygenation, replacing fluids, correcting electrolyte imbalances, and administering vasopressor medications. If serious hemorrhage occurs, the depleted coagulation factors and platelets may be replaced to reestablish the potential for normal hemostasis and thereby diminish bleeding. Cryoprecipitate is given to replace fibrinogen and factors V and VII; fresh frozen plasma is administered to replace other coagulation factors.

A controversial method to interrupt the thrombosis process is the use of heparin infusion. Heparin may inhibit the formation of microthrombi and thus permit perfusion of the organs (skin, kidneys, or brain) to resume. Heparin is typically reserved for the patient in whom thrombotic manifestations predominate or in whom extensive blood component replacement fails to halt the hemorrhage or increase fibrinogen and other clotting levels. When heparin is administered, bleeding may actually worsen initially until the thrombotic process is interrupted. Consumed platelets and clotting factors need to be replaced. The effectiveness of heparin can best be determined by observing for normalization of the plasma fibrinogen concentration and diminishing signs of bleeding.

NURSING PROCESS: THE PATIENT WITH DISSEMINATED INTRAVASCULAR COAGULATION (DIC)

Assessment

Nurses need to be aware of patients who are at risk for DIC. Sepsis and acute promyelocytic leukemia are the most common causes of DIC. Patients need to be assessed thoroughly and frequently for signs and symptoms of thrombi and bleeding and monitored for any progression of these signs (see Table 33-7).

Diagnosis

NURSING DIAGNOSES

Based on the assessment data, major nursing diagnoses for the patient with DIC may include the following:

- Risk for deficient fluid volume related to bleeding
- Risk for impaired skin integrity related to ischemia or bleeding
- Potential for excess fluid volume related to excessive blood/factor component replacement
- Ineffective tissue perfusion related to microthrombi
- Anxiety and fear of the unknown and possible death

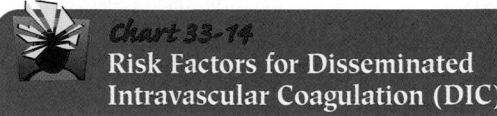

Chart 33-14

Risk Factors for Disseminated Intravascular Coagulation (DIC)

Sepsis
Obstetric complications
Acute hemolysis (eg, transfusion reaction)
Trauma
Shock
Cancer (especially prostate cancer and acute promyelocytic leukemia)
Allergic reactions

Table 33-6 • **Laboratory Values Commonly Found in Disseminated Intravascular Coagulation (DIC)***

TEST	FUNCTION EVALUATED	NORMAL RANGE	CHANGES IN DIC
Platelet count	Platelet number	150,000–450,000/mm³	↓
Prothrombin time (PT)	Extrinsic pathway	11–12.5 sec	↑
Partial thromboplastin time (PTT)	Intrinsic pathway	23–35 sec	↑
Thrombin time (TT)	Clot formation	8–11 sec	↑
Fibrinogen	Amount available for coagulation	170–340 mg/dL	↓
D-dimer	Local fibrinolysis	0–250 ng/mL	↑
Fibrin degradation products (FDPs)	Fibrinolysis	0–5 µg/mL	↑
Euglobulin clot lysis	Fibrinolytic activity	≥2 hours	≤1 hour

*Because DIC is a dynamic condition, the laboratory values measured will change over time. Therefore, a progressive increase or decrease in a given laboratory value is likely to be more important than the actual value of a test at a single point in time.

COLLABORATIVE PROBLEMS/ POTENTIAL COMPLICATIONS

Collaborative problems include the clinical conditions that precipitated the DIC. Based on the assessment data, potential complications may include:

- Renal failure
- Gangrene
- Pulmonary embolism or hemorrhage
- Altered level of consciousness
- Acute respiratory distress syndrome
- Stroke

Planning and Goals

Major patient goals include maintenance of hemodynamic status, maintenance of intact skin and oral mucosa, mainte-nance of fluid balance, maintenance of tissue perfusion, en-hanced coping, and absence of complications (see Plan of Nurs-ing Care).

Nursing Interventions

See Plan of Nursing Care: The Patient with Disseminated In-travascular Coagulation.

MONITORING AND MANAGING POTENTIAL COMPLICATIONS

Despite aggressive measures, the lack of renal perfusion may result in acute renal failure, sometimes necessitating dialysis. Placement of a large-bore dialysis catheter is extremely hazardous in this patient population and should be accompanied by adequate platelet and plasma transfusions.

Table 33-7 • **Recognizing Thrombosis and Bleeding in Disseminated Intravascular Coagulation (DIC)***

SYSTEM	SIGNS AND SYMPTOMS OF MICROVASCULAR THROMBOSIS	SIGNS AND SYMPTOMS OF MICROVASCULAR AND FRANK BLEEDING
Integumentary system (skin)	↓ Temperature, sensation; ↑ pain; cyanosis in extremities, nose, earlobes; focal ischemia, superficial gangrene	Petechiae, including periorbital and oral mucosa; bleed-ing: gums, oozing from wounds, previous injection sites, around catheters (IVs, tracheostomies); epistaxis; diffuse ecchymoses; subcutaneous hemorrhage; joint pain
Circulatory system	↓ Pulses; capillary filling time > 3 sec	Tachycardia
Respiratory system	Hypoxia (secondary to clot in lung); dyspnea; chest pain with deep inspiration; ↓ breath sounds over areas of large embolism	High-pitched bronchial breath sounds; tachypnea; ↑ consolidation; signs and symptoms of acute respiratory distress syndrome
Gastrointestinal system	Gastric pain; "heartburn"	Hematemesis (heme⊕† NG output) melana (heme⊕ stools → tarry stools → bright-red blood from rec-tum) retroperitoneal bleeding (abdomen firm and tender to palpation; distended; ↑ abdominal girth)
Renal system	↓ Urine output; ↑ creatinine, ↑ blood urea nitrogen	Hematuria
Neurologic system	↓ Alertness and orientation; ↓ pupillary reaction; ↓ response to commands; ↓ strength and movement ability	Anxiety; restlessness; ↓ mentation, altered level of con-sciousness; headache; visual disturbances; conjunctival hemorrhage

*Note: Signs of microvascular thrombosis are the result of an inappropriate activation of the coagulation system, causing thrombotic occlusion of small vessels within all body organs. As the clotting factors and platelets are consumed, signs of microvascular bleeding appear. This bleed-ing can quickly extend into frank hemorrhage. Treatment must be aimed at the disorder underlying the DIC; otherwise, the stimulus for the syndrome will persist.
†*heme*⊕, positive for hemoglobin

Nursing Interventions	Rationale	Expected Outcomes

Nursing Diagnosis: Potential for fluid volume deficit related to bleeding
Goals: Hemodynamic status maintained; urine output ≥30 mL/hr

1. Avoid procedures/activities that can increase intracranial pressure (eg, coughing, straining to have a bowel movement).	1. Prevents intracranial bleeding.	• Level of consciousness (LOC) stable • CVP 5–12 cm H₂O, systolic BP ≥70 mm Hg • Urine output ≥30 mL/hour • Decreased bleeding • Decreased oozing • Decreased ecchymoses • Amenorrhea • Absence of oral and bronchial bleeding • Oral mucosa clean, moist, intact • Absence of bleeding

2. Monitor vital signs closely, including neurologic checks:
  a. Monitor hemodynamics
  b. Monitor abdominal girth
  c. Monitor urine output
	2. Identifies signs of hemorrhage/shock quickly.	

3. Avoid medications that interfere with platelet function if possible (eg, ASA, NSAIDs, beta-lactam antibiotics).	3. Decreases problems with platelet aggregation and adhesion.	
4. Avoid rectal probes, rectal medications.	4. Decreases chance for rectal bleeding.	
5. Avoid IM injections.	5. Decreases chance for intramuscular bleeding.	

6. Monitor amount of external bleeding carefully
  a. Monitor number of dressings, % of dressing saturated; time to saturate a dressing is more objective than "dressing saturated a moderate amount."
  b. Monitor suction output, all excreta
  c. Monitor pad counts in menstruating females.
  d. Females may receive progesterone to prevent menses.
	6.
	
	  a. Provides accurate, objective assessment of extent of bleeding.
	
	  b. Identifies presence of or quantifies extent of bleeding.
	  c. Quantifies extent of bleeding
	
	  d. Decreases chance for gynecologic source of hemorrhage.	

7. Use low pressure with any suctioning needed.	7. Prevents excessive trauma that could cause bleeding.	

8. Administer oral hygiene carefully.
  a. Avoid lemon-glycerine swabs, hydrogen peroxide, commercial mouthwashes.
  b. Use sponge-tipped swabs, salt/baking soda (bicarbonate of soda) mouth rinses.
	8. Prevents excessive trauma that could cause bleeding. Glycerin and alcohol (in commercial mouthwashes) will dry mucosa, increasing risk for bleeding.	

9. Avoid dislodging any clots, including those around IV sites and injection sites.	9. Prevents excessive bleeding at sites.	

Nursing Diagnosis: Potential for impaired skin integrity secondary to ischemia or bleeding
Goals: Skin integrity remains intact; oral mucosa remains intact

1. Assess skin, with particular attention to bony prominences, skin folds.	1. Prompt identification of any area at risk for skin breakdown or showing early signs of breakdown can facilitate prompt intervention and thus prevent complications.	• Skin integrity remains intact; skin is warm, and of normal color • Oral mucosa is intact, pink, moist, without bleeding
2. Reposition carefully; use pressure-reducing mattress.	2–4. Meticulous skin care and use of measures to prevent pressure on bony prominences decrease the risk of skin trauma.	
3. Perform careful skin care every 2 hr, emphasizing dependent areas, all bony prominences, perineum.		
4. Use lamb's wool between digits, around ears, as needed.		
5. Use prolonged pressure after injection or procedure when such measures must be performed (at least 5 min)	5. Initial platelet plug is very unstable and easily dislodged, which can lead to increased bleeding.	
6. Administer oral hygiene carefully (see above).	6. Meticulous care to decreased trauma, bleeding, and risk of infection.	

(continued)

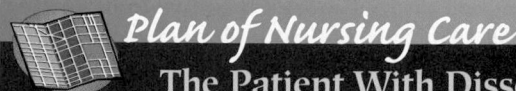

Plan of Nursing Care

The Patient With Disseminated Intravascular Coagulation (DIC) *(Continued)*

Nursing Interventions	Rationale	Expected Outcomes

Nursing Diagnosis: Potential for fluid volume excess
Goals: Absence of edema; absence of rales; intake not greater than output

1. Auscultate breath sounds every 2–4 hr.	1. Crackles can develop quickly.	• Breath sounds clear
2. Monitor extent of edema	2. Fluid may extend beyond intravascular system.	• Absence of edema • Intake does not exceed output
3. Monitor volume of IVs, blood products; decrease volume of IV medications if possible.	3. Helps prevent fluid overload.	• Weight stable
4. Administer diuretics as prescribed	4. Decreases fluid volume.	

Nursing Diagnosis: Potential for diminished tissue perfusion secondary to microthrombi
Goals: Neurologic status remains intact; absence of hypoxemia; peripheral pulses remain intact; skin integrity remains intact; urine output remains ≥30 mL/hr

1. Assess neurologic, pulmonary, integumentary systems.	1. Initial signs of thrombosis can be subtle.	• Arterial blood gases, O_2 saturation, pulse oximetry, LOC within normal limits.
2. Monitor response to heparin therapy.	2. Response to heparin is most accurately reflected in fibrinogen level.	• Breath sounds clear
3. Assess extent of bleeding.	3. Objective measurements of all sites of bleeding are crucial to accurately assess extent of blood loss.	• Absence of edema • Intake does not exceed output
4. Monitor fibrinogen levels.	4. Response to heparin is most accurately reflected in fibrinogen level.	• Weight stable
5. Stop ∈-aminocaproic acid (EACA) if symptoms of thrombosis occur (see Table 33-7).	5. EACA should be used only in setting of extensive hemorrhage not responding to replacement therapy.	

Nursing Diagnosis: Potential for fear of unknown and possible death
Goals: Fears verbalized/identified; realistic hope maintained

1. Identify previous coping mechanisms, if possible: a. Encourage patient to use them as appropriate.	1. Identifying previous stressful situations can aid in recall of successful coping mechanisms.	• Previously used coping strategies identified and tried, to extent patient is able to do so • Patient indicates understanding of procedures and situation as condition permits
2. Explain all procedures and rationale for these in terms patient and family can understand.	2. Decreased knowledge and uncertainty can increase anxiety.	
3. Assist family in supporting patient.	3. Family can be useful in assisting patient to use coping strategies and to maintain hope.	
4. Use services from behavioral medicine, chaplain as needed.	4. Additional professional intervention may be necessary, particularly if previous coping mechanisms are maladaptive or ineffective. Spiritual dimension should be supported.	

Evaluation

See the Plan of Nursing Care for evaluation and expected outcomes for the patient with DIC.

THROMBOTIC DISORDERS

As in many bleeding disorders, several conditions can alter the balance within the normal hemostasis process and cause excessive thrombosis. Abnormalities that predispose a person to thrombotic events include decreased clotting inhibitors within the circulation (which enhances coagulation), altered hepatic function (which may decrease production of clotting factors or clearance of activated coagulation factors), lack of fibrinolytic enzymes, and tortuous vessels (which promote platelet aggregation). Thrombosis can be caused by more than one predisposing factor. Several conditions can result from thrombosis, such as myocardial infarction (see Chap. 28), cerebral vascular accident

(CVA, brain attack, or stroke; see Chap. 62), and peripheral arterial occlusion (see Chap. 31). Several inherited or acquired deficiency conditions, including hyperhomocystinemia, antithrombin III (AT III) deficiency, Protein C deficiency, activated Protein C (APC) resistance, factor V Leiden, and Protein S deficiency can predispose a patient to repeated episodes of thrombosis; they are referred to as hypercoagulable states or thrombophilia. Table 33-8 delineates these disorders, their abnormal laboratory values, and the need for family testing.

Thrombosis requires anticoagulation therapy. The duration of therapy varies with the location and extent of the thrombosis, precipitating events (eg, trauma, immobilization), and concurrent risk factors (eg, use of oral contraceptives, tortuous blood vessels, history of thrombotic events).

HYPERHOMOCYSTINEMIA

Increased plasma levels of homocystine are a significant risk factor not only for venous thrombosis (eg, deep venous thrombosis [DVT], pulmonary embolism) but also for arterial thrombosis (eg, stroke, myocardial infarction). This disorder can be heredi-

tary, or it can result from a nutritional deficiency of folic acid and, to a lesser extent, of vitamin B_{12} and B_6, because these vitamins are cofactors in homocystine metabolism. For unknown reasons, people who are elderly, have renal failure, or smoke tobacco may also have elevated levels of homocystine in the absence of nutritional deficiencies of these vitamins. Although a simple fasting measurement of plasma homocystine can serve as a useful screening test, people with heterozygous defects in this gene and those who are vitamin B_6 deficient may have normal or minimally elevated levels. A much more sensitive method involves obtaining a second measurement 4 hours after the patient consumes methionine; the prevalence of hyperhomocystinemia is twice as great when this method is used. In hyperhomocystinemia, the endothelial lining of the vessel walls is denuded; this can precipitate unnecessary thrombus formation. Recent studies have determined that this disorder is much more common than previously thought. In a long-term epidemiologic study on nurses' health (Rimm et al., 1998), women who used dietary supplements with folic acid and vitamin B_6 were found to have a lower incidence of thrombotic conditions such as DVT. Patients who are found to have hyperhomocystinemia should receive folic acid, B_6, and/or B_{12} supplements and should be instructed in the rationale for their use to enhance compliance.

ANTITHROMBIN III DEFICIENCY

Antithrombin is a protein that inhibits thrombin and certain coagulation factors. AT III deficiency is a common hereditary condition that can cause venous thrombosis, particularly when the level is less than 60% of normal. Patients with AT III deficiency can develop venous thrombosis as young adults; by 50 years of age, two thirds of patients with AT III deficiency have developed a venous thrombosis. The most common sites for thrombosis are the deep veins of the leg and the mesentery. Recurrent thrombosis often occurs. There is an increased resistance to heparin anticoagulation, so these patients may require greater amounts of heparin to achieve adequate anticoagulation. Patients with AT III deficiency should be encouraged to have their family members tested for the deficiency.

PROTEIN C DEFICIENCY

Protein C is an enzyme that, when activated, inhibits coagulation. When levels of Protein C are deficient, the risk of thrombosis increases, and thrombosis can often occur spontaneously. Protein C deficiency is at least as prevalent as AT III deficiency, and people who are Protein C–deficient can develop thrombosis early in life, as early as 15 years of age. Warfarin-induced skin necrosis is a rare but significant complication of anticoagulation management in patients with Protein C deficiency (Hoffman et al., 2000). This complication appears to result from progressive thrombosis in the capillaries within the skin; the extent of the necrosis can be extreme.

ACTIVATED PROTEIN C RESISTANCE AND FACTOR V LEIDEN MUTATION

Activated protein C (APC) resistance is a common condition that can occur with other hypercoagulable states. APC is an anticoagulant, and resistance to APC increases the risk for venous thrombosis. A molecular defect in the factor V gene has been identified in

Table 33-8 • Hypercoagulable States	
DISORDER	**ABNORMAL LABORATORY VALUE***
Inherited Disorders (Family Testing Necessary)	
Hyperhomocysteinemia	Homocystine ↑ after methionine load
Antithrombin III (AT III) deficiency	AT III ↓
Protein C deficiency	Protein C activity ↓ (must be measured off warfarin [Coumadin])
Activated protein C (APC) resistance	Must be measured off anticoagulant; <2× prolongation of PTT when APC added. Patients with APC resistance have a smaller increase in clotting time than normal (ie, the prolongation of clotting time is less than normal).
Factor V Leiden	Positive
Protein S deficiency	Protein S activity ↓; must be measured off warfarin (Coumadin)
Dysfibrinogenemia	↑ thrombin time; ↑ reptilase time; ↓ functional fibrinogen; often requires special fibrinogen assays
Acquired Disorders (Family Testing Unnecessary)	
Anticardiolipin antibody	Positive
Cancer	
Lupus anticoagulant	Positive
Hyperhomocysteinemia	Homocystine ↑ after methionine load
AT III Deficiency	AT III ↓
Paroxysmal nocturnal hemoglobinuria	+ Hamm's test; acid hemolysis
Myeloproliferative disorders	Varied, depending on disorder
Nephrotic syndrome	Varied, depending on disorder
Cancer chemotherapy	Varied, depending on disorder

*Protein C and Protein S are vitamin K–dependent proteins. Warfarin (Coumadin) interferes with the hepatic synthesis of vitamin K-dependent factors, which may decrease levels of Protein C or Protein S; therefore, Protein C and Protein S should be measured while the patient is off warfarin.

most (90%) of those with APC resistance; this defect is called factor V Leiden mutation. It has been identified as the most common cause of inherited hypercoagulability in Caucasians, but its incidence appears to be much lower in other ethnic groups. Factor V Leiden mutation synergistically increases the risk for thrombosis in patients with other risk factors (eg, use of oral contraceptives, hyperhomocystinemia, increased age). It does not appear that the use of postmenopausal hormone therapy in women increases the risk for thrombotic events as does the use of oral contraceptives; the dose of estrogen in the former situation is much lower than in the latter. People who are homozygous for the factor V Leiden mutation are at extremely high risk for thrombosis.

PROTEIN S DEFICIENCY

Protein S is another natural anticoagulant normally produced in the liver. APC requires Protein S to inactivate certain clotting factors. When the level of Protein S is deficient, this inactivation process is diminished, and the risk for thrombosis can be increased. Like patients with Protein C deficiency, those with Protein S deficiency have a greater risk for recurrent venous thrombosis at a young age, as young as 15 years.

ACQUIRED THROMBOPHILIA

Antibodies to phospholipids are common, acquired causes for thrombophilia (hypercoagulable states). The most common antibodies present against phospholipids are either lupus or anticardiolipin antibodies. Both of these antibodies can be transient, resulting from infection or certain medications. Most thrombotic events are venous, but arterial thrombosis can occur in up to one third of the cases. Patients who persistently test positive for either antibody and who have had a thrombotic event are at significant risk for recurrent thrombosis (greater than 50%). Recurrent thromboses tend to be of the same type—that is, venous thrombosis after an initial venous thrombosis, arterial thrombosis after an initial arterial thrombosis.

Another common acquired cause for thrombophilia is cancer. Specific types of stomach, pancreatic, lung, and ovarian cancers are most commonly associated with thrombophilia. The type of thrombosis that results is unusual. Rather than deep vein thrombosis or pulmonary embolism, the thrombosis occurs in unusual sites, such as the portal, hepatic, or renal vein or the inferior vena cava. Migratory superficial thrombophlebitis or nonbacterial thrombotic endocarditis can also occur. In these patients, anticoagulation can be difficult to manage in that the thrombosis can progress despite standard amounts of anticoagulation.

Medical Management

The primary method of treating thrombotic disorders is anticoagulation. However, in thrombophilic conditions, when to treat (prophylaxis or not) and how long to treat (lifelong or not) can be controversial. Anticoagulation therapy is not without risks; the most significant risk is bleeding. Risks of anticoagulation therapy are identified in Chapter 31. The most common anticoagulant medications are identified in the following section.

PHARMACOLOGIC THERAPY

Along with administering anticoagulant therapy, concerns include minimizing any risk factors that predispose a patient to thrombosis. When risk factors (eg, immobility after surgery, pregnancy) cannot be avoided, prophylactic anticoagulation may be necessary.

Unfractionated Heparin Therapy. Heparin is a naturally occurring anticoagulant that enhances AT III and inhibits platelet function. To prevent thrombosis, heparin is typically given as a subcutaneous injection, two or three times daily. To treat thrombosis, heparin is usually administered intravenously. The therapeutic effect of heparin is monitored by serial measurements of the activated partial prothrombin time; the dose is adjusted to maintain the range at 1.5 to 2.5 times the laboratory control. Oral forms are being evaluated, but their absorption remains variable (Money & York, 2001).

A significant potential complication of heparin-based therapy is heparin-induced thrombocytopenia (HIT). Antibodies are formed within the body against the heparin complex. The actual incidence of HIT is unknown, but it is thought to occur in as many as 5% of patients receiving heparin (Kelton, 1999). Whereas most patients remain asymptomatic, a significant proportion of those individuals with serologic HIT develop actual thrombocytopenia. A decline in platelet count typically develops after 5 to 8 days of heparin therapy, and the platelets can drop significantly, although in most instances the level stays higher than 50,000/mm^3. These patients are at increased risk for thrombosis, either venous or arterial, and the thrombosis can range from DVT to myocardial infarction, CVA (brain attack, stroke), and ischemic damage to an extremity necessitating amputation. The risk for development of HIT appears to be increased when heparin is used at higher concentrations (ie, therapeutic versus prophylactic dosage) and with preexisting comorbidity, such as underlying cardiac disease.

Low-Molecular-Weight Heparin Therapy. Low molecular-weight heparin (LMWH; eg, Dalteparin, Enoxaparin) is a special form of heparin that has a more selective effect on coagulation. Based on its biochemical properties, LMWH has a longer half-life and a less variable anticoagulant response than does standard heparin. These differences permit LMWH to be safely administered only once or twice daily, without the need for laboratory monitoring for dose adjustments. The incidence of HIT is much lower when LMWH is used. In certain conditions, the use of LMWH has allowed anticoagulation therapy to be moved entirely to the outpatient setting. Many cases of uncomplicated DVT are being managed outside the hospital setting. LMWH is also being increasingly used as "bridge therapy" when patients receiving anticoagulation therapy (warfarin) require an invasive procedure (eg, biopsy, surgery). In this situation, warfarin is stopped and LMWH is used in its place until the procedure is completed. After the procedure, warfarin therapy is resumed. LMWH is discontinued after a therapeutic level of warfarin is achieved.

Warfarin (Coumadin) Therapy. Coumarin anticoagulants (warfarin; eg, Coumadin) are antagonists of vitamin K and therefore interfere with the synthesis of vitamin K–dependent clotting factors. Coumarin anticoagulants bind to albumin, are metabolized in the liver, and have an extremely long half-life. Typically, a patient is initially treated with both heparin (either the unfractionated form or LMWH) and warfarin. When the international normalized ratio (INR) reaches the desired therapeutic range, the heparin is stopped. The dosage required to maintain the therapeutic range (typically using an INR of 2.0 to 3.0) varies widely among patients and even within the same patient. Frequent monitoring of the INR is extremely important so that the dosage of warfarin can be adjusted as needed. Warfarin is affected by many medications; consultation with a pharmacist is important to assess the extent to which concurrently administered medications, herbs, and nutritional supplements may interact with warfarin. It is also affected by many foods, so patients need dietary instruction and may benefit from consultation with a dietitian when receiving warfarin therapy. See Chart 33-15 for a listing of agents that interact with warfarin.

Nursing Management

Patients with thrombotic disorders should avoid activities that promote circulatory stasis (eg, immobility, crossing the legs). Exercise, especially ambulation, should be performed frequently throughout the day, particularly during long trips by car or plane.

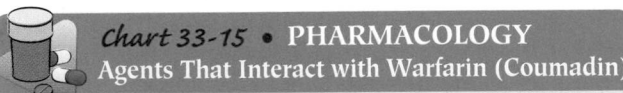

Chart 33-15 • PHARMACOLOGY
Agents That Interact with Warfarin (Coumadin)

Although warfarin (Coumadin), an anticoagulant medication, is commonly used to treat and prevent thrombosis, many drug–drug and drug–food interactions are associated with its use. A careful medication history (including over-the-counter medications, herbs, and other substances, such as vitamins and minerals) is important when oral anticoagulation therapy is prescribed. Consultation with a pharmacist is recommended to assess the extent to which concurrent medications may affect the anticoagulant and for appropriate dosage adjustments. The following list contains a few examples of agents that interact with warfarin.

Agents That Inhibit Warfarin Function

Barbiturates	Glutethimide
Carbamazepine	Griseofulvin
Cholestyramine	Haloperidol
Corticosteroids	Oral contraceptives
Digitalis	Phenytoin
Estrogens	Rifampin
Ethanol	Spironolactone

Agents That Potentiate Warfarin Function

Acetaminophen	Vitamin C (in very large doses)
Allopurinol	Vitamin E (in very large doses)
Amiodarone	Isoniazid
Anabolic steroids	Mefenamic acid
Anti-inflammatory agents	Methotrexate
Antimalarial agents	Metronidazole
Aspirin	Oral hypoglycemic agents
Broad-spectrum antibiotics	Oxyphenbutazone
Chloral hydrate	Phenytoin
Chloramphenicol	Probenecid
Cimetidine	Propylthiouracil
Colchicine	Quinidine
Clofibrate	Quinine
Chlorpromazine	Salicylates
Danazol	Sulfinpyrazone
Disulfiram	Sulfonamides (long-acting)
Ethacrynic acid	Thyroxine
Feprazone	Triclofos
Herbal medicines:	Tricyclic antidepressants
feverfew, garlic, gingko, ginseng	

Medications that alter platelet aggregation, such as low-strength aspirin, may be prescribed. Some patients require life-long therapy with anticoagulants such as warfarin (eg, Coumadin).

Patients with thrombotic disorders, particularly those with thrombophilia, should be assessed for concurrent risk factors for thrombosis and should avoid concomitant risk factors if possible. For example, use of tobacco and nicotine products exacerbates the problem and should be avoided.

Just as for other conditions, patients with thrombotic disorders, particularly thrombophilia, should know the name of their specific condition and understand its significance. In many instances, younger patients with thrombophilia may not require prophylactic anticoagulation; however, with concomitant risk factors (eg, pregnancy), increasing age, or subsequent thrombotic events, prophylactic or lifelong anticoagulation therapy may be required. Being able to provide the health care provider with an accurate health history can be extremely useful and can help guide the selection of appropriate therapeutic interventions. Patients with hereditary disorders should be encouraged to have their siblings and children tested for the disorder.

When patients with thrombotic disorders are hospitalized, frequent assessments should be performed for signs and symptoms of beginning thrombus formation, particularly in the legs (DVT) and lungs (pulmonary embolism). Ambulation or range-of-motion exercises as well as the use of elastic compression stockings should be initiated promptly to decrease stasis. Prophylactic anticoagulants are commonly prescribed.

Therapies for Blood Disorders

SPLENECTOMY

The surgical removal of the spleen (splenectomy) is sometimes necessary after trauma to the abdomen. Because the spleen is very vascular, severe hemorrhage can result if the spleen is ruptured. Under such circumstances, splenectomy becomes an emergency procedure.

Splenectomy is also a possible treatment for other hematologic disorders. For example, an enlarged spleen may be the site of excessive destruction of blood cells. If the destruction is life-threatening, surgery may be lifesaving. This is the case in autoimmune hemolytic anemia or ITP when these disorders do not respond to more conservative measures, such as corticosteroid therapy. Some patients with severe anemia due to inherited RBC defects (eg, thalassemia) may also benefit from splenectomy.

In general, the mortality rate after splenectomy is low. Laparoscopic splenectomy can be used in selected patients, with a resultant decrease in the postoperative morbidity rate. Complications that may result from surgery are atelectasis, pneumonia, abdominal distention, and abscess formation. Although young children are at the highest risk after splenectomy, all age groups are vulnerable to overwhelming lethal infections and should receive Pneumovax before undergoing this surgical procedure, if possible.

Patients are instructed to seek prompt medical attention if even relatively minor symptoms of infection occur. Often, patients with high platelet counts have even higher counts after splenectomy—more than 1 million/mm³—which can predispose them to serious thrombotic or hemorrhagic problems. This increase is, however, transient.

THERAPEUTIC APHERESIS

Apheresis is a Greek word meaning separation. In therapeutic apheresis (or pheresis), blood is taken from the patient and passed through a centrifuge, where a specific component is separated from the blood and removed (Table 33-9). The remaining blood is then returned to the patient. The entire system is closed, so the risk of bacterial contamination is extremely low. When platelets or WBCs are removed, the decrease in these cells within the circulation is temporary. However, the temporary decrease provides a window of time until suppressive medications (eg, chemotherapy) can have therapeutic effects. Sometimes plasma is removed rather than blood cells—typically so that specific, abnormal proteins within the plasma will be transiently lowered until a long-term therapy can be initiated.

Apheresis is also used to obtain larger amounts of platelets from a donor than can be provided from a single unit of whole blood. A unit of platelets obtained in this way is equivalent to six to eight units of platelets obtained from six to eight separate donors via standard blood donation methods. Platelet donors can have their platelets apheresed as often as every 14 days. WBCs can be obtained similarly, typically after the donor has received growth factors (G-CSF, GM-CSF) to stimulate the formation of additional WBCs and thereby increase the WBC count. The use of these growth factors also stimulates the release of stem cells within the circulation. Apheresis is used to harvest these stem cells (typically over a period of several days) for use in PBSCT (peripheral blood stem cell transplant; see Chap. 16).

THERAPEUTIC PHLEBOTOMY

Therapeutic phlebotomy is the removal of a certain amount of blood under controlled conditions. Patients with elevated hematocrits (eg, those with polycythemia vera) or excessive iron absorption (eg, hemochromatosis) can usually be managed by periodically removing 1 unit (about 500 mL) of whole blood. Eventually this process can produce iron deficiency, leaving the patient unable to produce as many RBCs. The actual procedure for therapeutic phlebotomy is similar to that for blood donation (see later discussion).

BLOOD AND BLOOD COMPONENT THERAPY

A single unit of whole blood contains 450 mL of blood and 50 mL of an anticoagulant. A unit of whole blood can be processed and dispensed for administration. However, it is more appropriate, economical, and practical to separate that unit of whole blood into its primary components: RBCs, platelets, and plasma (WBCs are rarely used; see later discussion). Because the plasma is removed, a unit of RBCs (packed RBCs, PRBCs) is very concentrated (hematocrit, approximately 70%). Each component must be processed and stored differently to maximize the longevity of the viable cells and factors within it; each individual blood component has a different storage life. PRBCs are stored at 4°C. With special preservatives, they can be stored safely for up to 42 days before they must be discarded. In contrast, platelets must be stored at room temperature because they cannot withstand cold temperatures, and they last for only 5 days before they must be discarded. To prevent clumping, platelets are gently agitated while stored. Plasma is immediately frozen to maintain the activity of the clotting factors within; it lasts for 1 year if it remains frozen. Plasma can be further pooled and processed into blood derivatives, such as albumin, immune globulin, factor VIII, and factor IX. Table 33-10 describes each blood component and how it is commonly used.

SPECIAL PREPARATIONS

Factor VIII concentrate (antihemophilic factor) is a lyophilized, freeze-dried concentrate of pooled fractionated human plasma. It is used in treating hemophilia A. Factor IX concentrate (prothrombin complex) is similarly prepared and contains factors II,

Table 33-9 • **Types of Apheresis***

PROCEDURE	PURPOSE	EXAMPLES OF CLINICAL USE
Platelet pheresis	Remove platelets	Extreme thrombocytosis, essential thrombocythemia (temporary measure); single-donor platelets transfusion
Leukapheresis	Remove WBCs (can be specific to neutrophils or lymphocytes)	Extreme leukocytosis (eg, AML, CML) (very temporary measure); harvest WBCs for transfusion
Erythrocytapheresis (RBC exchange)	Remove RBCs	RBC dyscrasias (eg, sickle cell disease); RBCs replaced via transfusion
Plasmapheresis (plasma exchange)	Remove plasma proteins	Hyperviscosity syndromes; treatment for some renal and neurologic diseases (eg, Goodpasture's syndrome, Guillain-Barré)
Stem cell harvest	Remove circulating stem cells	Transplantation (donor harvest or autologous)

*Therapeutic apheresis can be used to treat a wide variety of conditions. When it is used to treat a disease that causes an increase in a specific cell type with a short life in circulation (ie, WBCs, platelets), the reduction in those cells is temporary. However, this temporary reduction permits a margin of safety while waiting for a longer-lasting treatment modality (eg, chemotherapy) to take effect. Apheresis can also be used to obtain stem cells for transplantation, either from a matched donor (allogenic) or from the patient (autologous).
AML, acute myeloid leukemia; CML, chronic myeloid leukemia; RBC, red blood cell; WBC, white blood cell.

Table 33-10 • **Blood and Blood Components Commonly Used in Transfusion Therapy***

	COMPOSITION	INDICATIONS AND CONSIDERATIONS
Whole blood	Cells and plasma, hematocrit about 40%	Volume replacement and oxygen-carrying capacity; usually used only in significant bleeding (>25% blood volume lost)
Packed red blood cells (PRBCs)	RBCs with little plasma (hematocrit about 75%); some platelets and WBCs remain	↑ RBC mass Symptomatic anemia: platelets in the unit are not functional; WBCs in the unit may cause reaction and are not functional
Platelets—random	Platelets (5.5×10^{10} platelets/unit) Plasma; some RBCs, WBCs	Bleeding due to severe ↓ platelets Prevent bleeding when platelets <5,000–10,000/mm³ Survival ↓ in presence of fever, chills, infection Repeated treatment → ↓ survival due to alloimmunization
Platelets—single donor	Platelets (3×10^{11} platelets/unit) 1 unit is equivalent to 6–8 units of random platelets	Used for repeated treatment: ↓ alloimmunization risk by limiting exposure to multiple donors
Plasma (FFP)	Plasma; all coagulation factors Complement	Bleeding in patients with coagulation factor deficiencies; plasmapheresis
Granulocytes (pheresed)	Neutrophils (>1×10^{10}/unit); lymphocytes; some RBCs and platelets	Severe neutropenia in selected patients; controversial
Lymphocytes (WBCs) (apheresed)	Lymphocytes (number varies)	Stimulate graft-versus-disease effect
Cryoprecipitate	Fibrinogen ≥150 mg/bag, AHF (VIII:C) 80–110 units/bag, von Willebrand factor; fibronectin	von Willebrand's disease Hypofibrinoginemia Hemophilia A
Antihemophilic factor (AHF)	Factor VIII	Hemophilia A
Factor IX concentrate	Factor IX	Hemophilia B (Christmas disease)
Factor IX complex	Factor II, VII, IX, X	Hereditary factor VII, IX, X deficiency; Hemophilia A with factor VII inhibitors
Albumin	Albumin 5%, 25%	Hypoproteinemia; burns; volume expansion by 5% to ↑ blood volume; 25% → ↓ hematocrit
Intravenous gamma globulin	IgG antibodies	Hypogammaglobulinemia (in CLL, recurrent infections); ITP; primary immunodeficiency states
Antithrombin III concentrate (AT III)	AT III (trace amounts of other plasma proteins)	AT III deficiency with or at risk for thrombosis

* The composition of each type of blood component is described as well as the most common indications for using a given blood component. RBCs, platelets, and fresh frozen plasma are the blood products most commonly used. When transfusing these blood products, it is important to realize that the individual product is always "contaminated" with very small amounts of other blood products (eg, WBCs mixed in a unit of platelets). This contamination can cause some difficulties, particularly isosensitization, in certain patients.
AHF, antihemophilic factor; CLL, chronic lymphocytic leukemia; ITP, idiopathic thrombopenic purpura.

VII, IX, and X. It is used primarily for treatment of factor IX deficiency (hemophilia B). Factor IX concentrate is also useful in treating congenital factor VII and factor X deficiencies.

Plasma albumin is a large protein molecule that usually stays within vessels and is a major contributor to plasma oncotic pressure. This protein is used to expand the blood volume of patients in hypovolemic shock and, rarely, to increase the concentration of circulating albumin in patients with hypoalbuminemia.

Immune globulin is a concentrated solution of the antibody IgG; it contains very little IgA or IgM. It is prepared from large pools of plasma. The intravenous form (IVIG) is used in various clinical situations to replace inadequate amounts of IgG in patients who are at risk for recurrent bacterial infection (eg, those with CLL, those receiving BMT or PBSCT). IVIG, in contrast to all other fractions of human blood, cells, or plasma, are able to survive being subjected to heating at 60°C (140°F) for 10 hours to free them of viral contaminants.

Procuring Blood and Blood Products

BLOOD DONATION

To protect both the donor and the recipients, all prospective donors are examined and interviewed before they are allowed to donate their blood. The intent of the interview is to assess the general health status of the donor and to identify risk factors that might harm a recipient of the donor's blood. Donors should be in good health and without any of the following:

- A history of viral hepatitis at any time in the past, or a history of close contact with a hepatitis or dialysis patient within 6 months
- A history of receiving a blood transfusion or an infusion of any blood derivative (other than serum albumin) within 6 months
- A history of untreated syphilis or malaria, because these diseases can be transmitted by transfusion even years later. A

person who has been free of symptoms and off therapy for 3 years after malaria may be a donor.

- A history or evidence of drug abuse in which substances were self-injected, because many intravenous/injection drug users are hepatitis carriers and because the risk for human immunodeficiency virus (HIV) is high in this group
- A history of possible exposure to HIV; the population at risk includes people who engage in anal sex, people with multiple sexual partners, intravenous/injection drug users, sexual partners of people at risk for HIV, and people with hemophilia
- A skin infection, because of the possibility of contaminating the phlebotomy needle, and subsequently the blood itself
- A history of recent asthma, urticaria, or allergy to medications, because hypersensitivity can be transferred passively to the recipient
- Pregnancy within 6 months, because of the nutritional demands of pregnancy on the mother
- A history of tooth extraction or oral surgery within 72 hours, because such procedures are frequently associated with transient bacteremia
- A history of exposure to infectious disease within the past 3 weeks, because of the risk of transmission to the recipient
- Recent immunizations, because of the risk of transmitting live organisms (2-week waiting period for live, attenuated organisms; 1 month for rubella; 1 year for rabies)
- A history of recent tattoo, because of the risk of blood-borne infections (eg, hepatitis, HIV)
- Cancer, because of the uncertainty about transmission of the disease
- A history of whole blood donation within the past 56 days

Potential donors should be asked whether they have consumed any aspirin or aspirin-containing medications within the past 3 days. Although aspirin use does not render the donor ineligible, the platelets obtained would be dysfunctional and therefore not useful. Aspirin does not affect the RBCs or plasma obtained from the donor.

All donors are expected to meet the following minimal requirements:

- Body weight should exceed 50 kg (110 pounds) for a standard 450-mL donation. Donors weighing less than 50 kg donate proportionately less blood. People younger than 17 years of age are disqualified from donation.
- The oral temperature should not exceed 37.5°C (99.6°F).
- The pulse rate should be regular and between 50 and 100 beats per minute.
- The systolic arterial pressure should be 90 to 180 mm Hg, and the diastolic pressure should be 50 to 100 mm Hg.
- The hemoglobin level should be at least 12.5 g/dL for women and 13.5 g/dL for men.

Directed Donation

At times, friends and family of a patient wish to donate blood for that person. These blood donations are termed directed donations. These donations are not any safer than those provided by random donors, because directed donors may not be as willing to identify themselves as having a history of any of the risk factors that disqualify a person from donating blood.

Standard Donation

Phlebotomy consists of venipuncture and blood withdrawal. Standard precautions are used. Donors are placed in a semi-recumbent position. The skin over the antecubital fossa is carefully cleansed with an antiseptic preparation, a tourniquet is applied, and venipuncture is performed. Withdrawal of 450 mL of blood usually takes less than 15 minutes. After the needle is removed, donors are asked to hold the involved arm straight up, and firm pressure is applied with sterile gauze for 2 or 3 minutes or until bleeding stops. A firm bandage is then applied. Donors remain recumbent until they feel able to sit up, usually within a few minutes. Donors who experience weakness or faintness should rest for a longer period. Donors then receive food and fluids and are asked to remain another 15 minutes.

Donors are instructed to leave the dressing on and to avoid heavy lifting for several hours, to avoid smoking for 1 hour, to avoid drinking alcoholic beverages for 3 hours, to increase fluid intake for 2 days, and to eat healthy meals for 2 weeks. Specimens from this donated blood are tested to detect infections and to identify the specific blood type (see later discussion).

Autologous Donation

A patient's own blood may be collected for future transfusion; this method is useful for many elective surgeries where the potential need for transfusion is high (eg, orthopedic surgery). Preoperative donations are ideally collected 4 to 6 weeks before surgery. Iron supplements are prescribed during this period to prevent depletion of iron stores. Occasionally, erythropoietin (epoetin-alfa [eg, Epogen, Procrit]) is given to stimulate erythropoiesis to ensure that the donor's hematocrit remains high enough to be eligible for donation. Typically, 1 unit of blood is drawn each week; the number of units obtained varies with the type of surgical procedure to be performed (ie, the amount of blood anticipated to be transfused). Phlebotomies are not performed within 72 hours of surgery. Individual blood components can also be collected.

The primary advantage of autologous transfusions is the prevention of viral infections from another person's blood. Other advantages include safe transfusion for patients with a history of transfusion reactions, prevention of alloimmunization, and avoidance of complications in patients with alloantibodies. The policy of the American Red Cross requires autologous blood to be transfused only to the donor. If the blood is not required, it can be frozen until the donor needs it in the future (for up to 10 years). The blood is never returned to the general donor supply of blood products to be used by someone else.

The disadvantage of autologous donation is that it may be performed even when the likelihood that the anticipated procedure will necessitate a transfusion is small. Needless autologous donation is expensive, takes time, and uses resources inappropriately. Moreover, in an emergency situation, the autologous units available may be inadequate, and the patient may still require additional units from the general donor supply.

Contraindications to donation of blood for autologous transfusion are acute infection, severely debilitating chronic disease, hemoglobin level less than 11 g/dL, hematocrit less than 33%, unstable angina, and acute cardiovascular or cerebrovascular disease. A history of poorly controlled epilepsy may be considered a contraindication in some centers. Patients with cancer may donate for themselves.

Intraoperative Blood Salvage

This transfusion method provides replacement for patients who are unable to donate before surgery and for those undergoing vascular, orthopedic, or thoracic surgery. During a surgical procedure, blood lost into a sterile cavity (eg, hip joint) is suctioned into a cell-saver machine. The RBCs are washed, often with saline solution, and then returned to the patient as an intravenous infusion. Salvaged blood cannot be stored, because bacteria cannot be completely removed from the blood.

Hemodilution

This transfusion method is initiated before or after induction of anesthesia. About 1 or 2 units of blood are removed from the patient through a venous or arterial line and simultaneously replaced with a colloid or crystalloid solution. The blood obtained is then reinfused after surgery (Kreimeier & Messmer, 2002). The advantage of this method is that the patient loses fewer RBCs during surgery, because the added intravenous solutions dilute the concentration of RBCs and lower the hematocrit. Patients who are at risk for myocardial injury, however, should not be further stressed by hemodilution.

COMPLICATIONS OF BLOOD DONATION

Excessive bleeding at the donor's venipuncture site is sometimes caused by a bleeding disorder in the donor but more often results from a technique error: laceration of the vein, excessive tourniquet pressure, or failure to apply enough pressure after the needle is withdrawn.

Fainting is common after blood donation and may be related to emotional factors, a vasovagal reaction, or prolonged fasting before donation. Because of the loss of blood volume, hypotension and syncope may occur when the donor assumes an erect position. A donor who appears pale or complains of faintness should immediately lie down or sit with head lowered below the knees; he or she should be observed for another 30 minutes.

Anginal chest pain may be precipitated in patients with unsuspected coronary artery disease. Seizures can occur in donors with epilepsy, although the incidence is very low. Both angina and seizures require further medical evaluation.

Many people have the misconception that donating blood can cause AIDS and other infections. Potential donors need to be educated that the equipment used in donation is sterile, a closed system, and not reusable; they are at no risk for acquiring such infections from donating blood.

BLOOD PROCESSING

Samples of the unit of blood are always taken immediately after donation so that the blood can be typed and tested. Each donation is tested for antibodies to HIV 1 and 2, hepatitis B core antibody (anti-HBc), hepatitis C virus (HCV), and human T-cell lymphotropic virus, type I (anti-HTLV-I/II). The blood is also tested for hepatitis B surface antigen (HbsAG) and for syphilis. Negative reactions are required for the blood to be used, and each unit of blood is labeled to certify the results. A new testing method, using nucleic acid amplification testing (NAT), has increased the ability to detect the presence of HCV and HIV infection, because it directly tests for genomic nucleic acids of the virus itself, rather than for the presence of antibod-

ies to the virus (Korman, Leparc & Benson, 2001). This testing significantly shortens the "window" of inability to detect HIV and HCV from a donated unit, further ensuring the safety of the blood. Blood is also screened for CMV; if it tests positive for CMV, it can still be used, except in recipients who are negative for CMV and who are immunocompromised (eg, BMT or PBSCT recipients).

Equally important to viral testing is accurate determination of the blood type. More than 200 antigens have been identified on the surface of RBC membranes. Of these, the most important for safe transfusion are the ABO and Rh systems. The ABO system identifies which sugars are present on the membrane of an individual's RBCs: A, B, both A and B, or neither A nor B (type O). To prevent a significant reaction, the same type of RBCs should be transfused. Previously, it was thought that in an emergency situation in which the patient's blood type was not known, type O blood could be safely transfused. This practice is no longer advised by the American Red Cross.

The Rh antigen (also called D) is present on the surface of RBCs in 85% of the population (Rh-positive). Those who lack the D antigen are called Rh-negative. RBCs are routinely tested for the D antigen as well as ABO. Patients should receive PRBCs with a compatible Rh type.

TRANSFUSION

Administration of blood and blood components requires knowledge of correct administration techniques and possible complications. It is very important to be familiar with the agency's policies and procedures for transfusion therapy. Methods for transfusing blood components are presented in Charts 33-16 and 33-17. Potential complications of transfusion follow.

Setting

Although most blood transfusions are performed in the acute care setting, patients with chronic transfusion requirements often can receive transfusions in other settings. Free-standing infusion centers, ambulatory care clinics, a physician's office, and even the home may be appropriate settings for transfusion. Typically, patients who need chronic transfusions but are otherwise stable physically are appropriate candidates for outpatient therapy. Verification and administration of the blood product are performed much as in a hospital setting. Although most blood products can be transfused in the outpatient setting, the home is typically limited to transfusions of PRBCs and factor components (eg, factor VIII for patients with hemophilia).

Pretransfusion Assessment

PATIENT HISTORY

Patient history is an important component of the pretransfusion assessment to determine the history of previous transfusions as well as previous reactions to transfusion. The history should include the type of reaction, its manifestations, the interventions required, and whether any preventive interventions were used in subsequent transfusions. It is important to assess the number of pregnancies a woman has had, because a high number can increase her risk for reaction due to antibodies developed from exposure to fetal circulation. Other concurrent health problems should also be noted, with careful attention to cardiac, pulmonary, and vascular disease.

Chart 33-16 Transfusion of Packed Red Blood Cells (PRBCs)

Preprocedure
1. Confirm that the transfusion has been prescribed.
2. Check that patient's blood has been typed and cross-matched.
3. Verify that patient has signed a written consent form per institution policy.
4. Explain the procedure to the patient. Instruct patient in signs and symptoms of transfusion reaction (itching, hives, swelling, shortness of breath, fever, chills).
5. Take patient's temperature, pulse, respiration, and blood pressure to establish a baseline for comparing vital signs during transfusion.
6. Use hand hygiene and wear gloves in accordance with Standard Precautions.
7. Use a 20-gauge or larger needle for placement in a large vein. Use special tubing that contains a blood filter to screen out fibrin clots and other particulate matter. Do not vent the blood container.

Procedure
1. Obtain the PRBCs from the blood bank *after* the intravenous line is started. (Institution policy may limit release to only 1 unit at a time.)
2. Double-check the labels with another nurse or physician to make sure that the ABO group and Rh type agree with the compatibility record. Check to see that the number and type on the donor blood label and on the patient's chart are correct. Check the patient's identification by asking the patient's name and checking the identification wristband.
3. Check the blood for gas bubbles and any unusual color or cloudiness. (Gas bubbles may indicate bacterial growth. Abnormal color or cloudiness may be a sign of hemolysis.)

4. Make sure PRBC transfusion is initiated within 30 min after removal of the PRBCs from the blood bank refrigerator.
5. For first 15 minutes, run the transfusion slowly—no faster than 5 mL/min. Observe the patient carefully for adverse effects. If no adverse effects occur during the first 15 min, increase the flow rate unless the patient is at high risk for circulatory overload.
6. Monitor closely for 15–30 min to detect signs of reaction. Monitor vital signs at regular intervals per institution policy; compare results with baseline measurements. Increase frequency of measurements based on patient's condition. Observe the patient frequently throughout the transfusion for any signs of adverse reaction, including restlessness, hives, nausea, vomiting, torso or back pain, shortness of breath, flushing, hematuria, fever, or chills. Should any adverse reaction occur, stop infusion immediately, notify physician, and follow the agency's transfusion reaction standard.
7. Note that administration time does not exceed 4 hr because of the increased risk for bacterial proliferation.
8. Be alert for signs of adverse reactions: circulatory overload, sepsis, febrile reaction, allergic reaction, and acute hemolytic reaction.
9. Change blood tubing after every 2 units transfused, to decrease chance of bacterial contamination.

Postprocedure
1. Obtain vital signs and compare with baseline measurements.
2. Dispose of used materials properly.
3. Document procedure in patient's medical record, including patient assessment findings and tolerance to procedure.
4. Monitor patient for response to and effectiveness of the procedure.

Note: Never add medications to blood or blood products; if blood is too thick to run freely, normal saline may be added to the unit. If blood must be warmed, use an in-line blood warmer with a monitoring system.

Chart 33-17 Transfusion of Platelets or Fresh Frozen Plasma (FFP)

Preprocedure
1. Confirm that the transfusion has been prescribed.
2. Verify that patient has signed a written consent form per institution policy.
3. Explain the procedure to the patient. Instruct patient in signs and symptoms of transfusion reaction (itching, hives, swelling, shortness of breath, fever, chills).
4. Take patient's temperature, pulse, respiration, and blood pressure to establish a baseline for comparing vital signs during transfusion.
5. Use hand hygiene and wear gloves in accordance with Standard Precautions.
6. Use a 22-gauge or larger needle for placement in a large vein, if possible. Use appropriate tubing per institution policy (platelets often require different tubing from that used for other blood products).

Procedure
1. Obtain the platelets or FFP from the blood bank (only *after* the intravenous line is started.)
2. Double-check the labels with another nurse or physician to make sure that the ABO group matches the compatibility record (not usually necessary for platelets; here only if compatible platelets are ordered). Check to see that the number and type on the donor blood label and on the patient's chart are correct. Check the patient's identification by asking the patient's name and checking the identification wristband.
3. Check the blood product for any unusual color or clumps (excessive redness indicates contamination with larger amounts of red blood cells).

4. Make sure platelets or FFP units are administered immediately after they are obtained.
5. Infuse each unit as fast as patient can tolerate to diminish platelet clumping during administration. Observe the patient carefully for adverse effects, including circulatory overload. Decrease rate of infusion if necessary.
6. Observe the patient closely throughout the transfusion for any signs of adverse reaction, including restlessness, hives, nausea, vomiting, torso or back pain, shortness of breath, flushing, hematuria, fever, or chills. Should any adverse reaction occur, stop infusion immediately, notify physician, and follow the agency's transfusion reaction standard.
7. Monitor vital signs at end of transfusion per institution policy; compare results with baseline measurements.
8. Flush line with saline after transfusion to remove blood component from tubing.

Postprocedure
1. Obtain vital signs and compare with baseline measurements.
2. Dispose of used materials properly.
3. Document procedure in patient's medical record, including patient assessment findings and tolerance to procedure.
4. Monitor patient for response to and effectiveness of procedure. A platelet count may be ordered 1 hr after platelet transfusion to facilitate this evaluation.

Note: FFP requires ABO but not Rh compatibility. Platelets are not typically cross-matched for ABO compatibility. Never add medications to blood or blood products.

PHYSICAL ASSESSMENT

A systematic physical assessment and measurement of baseline vital signs are important before transfusing any blood product. The respiratory system should be assessed, including careful auscultation of the lungs and for use of accessory muscles. Cardiac system assessment should include careful inspection for any edema as well as other signs of cardiac failure (eg, jugular venous distention). The skin should be observed for rashes, petechiae, and ecchymoses. The sclera should be examined for icterus. In the event of a possible transfusion reaction, a comparison of findings can help differentiate between types of reactions.

Patient Teaching

Reviewing the signs and symptoms of a potential transfusion reaction is crucial for patients who have not received a transfusion before. Even for those patients who have received prior transfusions, a brief review of signs and symptoms of potential transfusion reactions is advised. Signs and symptoms of a possible reaction include fever, chills, respiratory distress, low back pain, nausea, pain at the intravenous site, or anything "unusual." Although a thorough review is very important, it is also important to reassure the patient that the blood is carefully tested against the patient's own blood (cross-matched) to diminish the likelihood of any untoward reaction. Such assurance can be extremely beneficial in allaying anxiety. Similarly, it can be useful to mention again the very low possibility of contracting HIV from the transfusion; this fear persists among many people.

Transfusion Complications

Any patient who receives a blood transfusion may develop complications from that transfusion. When explaining the reasons for the transfusion, it is important to include the risks and benefits and what to expect during and after the transfusion. Patients must be informed that the supply of blood is not completely risk-free although it has been tested carefully. Nursing management is directed toward preventing complications, promptly recognizing complications if they develop, and promptly initiating measures to control any complications that occur. The following sections describe the most common or potentially severe transfusion-related complications.

FEBRILE, NONHEMOLYTIC REACTION

The nonhemolytic reaction, caused by antibodies to donor WBCs that are still present in the unit of blood or blood component, is the most common type of transfusion reaction, accounting for more than 90% of reactions. It occurs more frequently in patients who have had previous transfusions (exposure to multiple antigens from previous blood products) and in Rh-negative women who have borne Rh-positive children (exposure to an Rh-positive fetus raises antibody levels in the mother). These reactions occur in 1% of PRBC transfusions and 20% of platelet transfusions. More than 10% of patients with a chronic transfusion requirement develop this type of reaction.

NURSING RESEARCH PROFILE 33-1
Perspectives of Recipients of Blood Transfusions

Fitzgerald, M., Hodgkinson, B., & Thorp, D. (1999). Blood transfusion from the recipient's perspective. *Journal of Clinical Nursing 8(5),* 593–600.

Purpose

The process of informed consent requires that information be provided to the patient before consent and implies that a dialogue between the patient and physicians and nurses occurs during this process. This study stemmed from previous studies examining transfusion practices in a large teaching hospital in Australia; the studies revealed that little is known about how much patients understood about the transfusion process. The purpose of this study was to more closely examine the meaning of patients' experiences with blood transfusions.

Study Sample and Design

The study design employed interpretive phenomenology, a qualitative analysis process that allowed researchers to identify meanings that may have been hidden in common actions. A convenience sample of 19 patients was interviewed; subjects were asked to discuss their experience of receiving a blood transfusion, beginning with the time they were told about it. Subjects received transfusions for a variety of clinical conditions, primarily surgery, cancer, and emergency situations. The interviews were tape recorded and transcribed verbatim. The data were analyzed and themes were identified.

Findings

Three broad themes were identified and more closely analyzed: information regarding the transfusion, reaction to receiving a transfusion, and care received during the transfusion. The focus of many of the interviews was on the information process. Physicians' explanations regarding the purpose of the transfusion were typically brief and were focused on providing factual information, particularly before the patient's signing of the consent for the procedure. Nurses' explanations continued as the procedure progressed but tended to focus only on potential reactions. Neither physicians nor nurses tended to encourage the patient to express his or her concerns, nor sought information from the patient. Few patients could actually recall any of the factual information presented to them. Fear of infection, particularly human immunodeficiency virus (HIV) infection, was present but was not excessive. Subjects verbalized understanding that the risk of acquiring HIV from their transfusion was very remote. Most subjects were told that the transfusion would make them feel better; in reality (and likely due to the severity of their illness/injury) such was not the case. Beyond the initial procedure by the nurse of double-checking the blood product for transfusion against the patient's identity and hanging the blood, patients did not notice any difference in the nursing care they received during the transfusion.

Nursing Implications

Findings from this study have important implications for nurses, particularly concerning the information process. Despite the focus of both physicians and nurses on providing information, patients demonstrated that they did not comprehend it well. Informational needs vary, as do learning styles. It is crucial that nurses assess their patients' level of understanding about the entire transfusion process. Not having the opportunity to deliberate on the information provided and to express concern was a common theme from the study subjects. Nurses need to make the time for patients to express their concerns and verbalize their feelings. This need exists not only for those receiving their first transfusion but also for those who have long-term transfusion requirements.

The diagnosis of a febrile, nonhemolytic reaction is made by excluding other potential causes, such as a hemolytic reaction or bacterial contamination of the blood product. The signs and symptoms of a febrile, nonhemolytic transfusion reaction are chills (absent to severe) followed by fever (more than 1°C elevation). The fever typically begins within 2 hours after the transfusion is begun. Although not life-threatening, the fever and particularly the chills and muscle stiffness can be frightening to the patient.

These reactions can be diminished, even prevented, by further depleting the blood component of donor WBCs; this is accomplished by a leukocyte reduction filter. The blood product may be filtered during processing, which achieves better results but is more expensive, or during the actual transfusion by adding the filter to the blood administration tubing. Antipyretics can be given to prevent fever, but routine premedication is not advised because it can mask the beginning of a more serious transfusion reaction.

ACUTE HEMOLYTIC REACTION

The most dangerous, and potentially life threatening, type of transfusion reaction occurs when the donor blood is incompatible with that of the recipient. Antibodies already present in the recipient's plasma rapidly combine with antigens on donor RBCs, and the RBCs are hemolyzed (destroyed) in the circulation (intravascular hemolysis). The most rapid hemolysis occurs in ABO incompatibility. This reaction can occur after transfusion of as little as 10 mL of RBCs. Rh incompatibility often causes a less severe reaction. The most common causes of acute hemolytic reaction are errors in blood component labeling and patient identification that result in the administration of an ABO-incompatible transfusion.

Symptoms consist of fever, chills, low back pain, nausea, chest tightness, dyspnea, and anxiety. As the RBCs are destroyed, the hemoglobin is released from the cells and excreted by the kidneys; therefore, hemoglobin is present in the urine (hemoglobinuria). Hypotension, bronchospasm, and vascular collapse may result. Diminished renal perfusion results in acute renal failure, and DIC may also occur.

The reaction must be recognized promptly and the transfusion discontinued immediately. Blood and urine specimens must be obtained and analyzed for evidence of hemolysis. Treatment goals include maintaining blood volume and renal perfusion and preventing and managing DIC.

Acute hemolytic transfusion reactions are preventable. Meticulous attention to detail in labeling blood samples and blood components and identifying the recipient cannot be overemphasized.

ALLERGIC REACTION

Some patients may develop urticaria (hives) or generalized itching during a transfusion. The cause of these reactions is thought to be a sensitivity reaction to a plasma protein within the blood component being transfused. Symptoms of an allergic reaction are urticaria, itching, and flushing. The reactions are usually mild and respond to antihistamines. If the symptoms resolve after administration of an antihistamine (eg, diphenhydramine [eg, Benadryl]), the transfusion may be resumed. Rarely, the allergic reaction is severe, with bronchospasm, laryngeal edema, and shock. These reactions are managed with epinephrine, corticosteroids, and pressor support, if necessary.

Giving the patient antihistamines before the transfusion may prevent future reactions. For severe reactions, future blood components are washed to remove any remaining plasma proteins. Leukocyte filters are not useful, because the offending plasma proteins can pass through the filter.

CIRCULATORY OVERLOAD

If too much blood infuses too quickly, hypervolemia can occur. This condition can be aggravated in patients who already have increased circulatory volume (eg, those with heart failure). PRBCs are safer to use than whole blood. If the administration rate is sufficiently slow, circulatory overload may be prevented. For patients who are at risk for, or already in, circulatory overload, diuretics are administered after the transfusion or between units of PRBCs. Patients receiving fresh frozen plasma or even platelets may also develop circulatory overload. The infusion rate of these blood components must also be titrated to the patient's tolerance.

Signs of circulatory overload include dyspnea, orthopnea, tachycardia, and sudden anxiety. Neck vein distention, crackles at the base of the lungs, and a rise in blood pressure can also occur. If the transfusion is continued, pulmonary edema can develop, as manifested by severe dyspnea and coughing of pink, frothy sputum.

If fluid overload is mild, the transfusion can often be continued after slowing the rate of infusion and administering diuretics. However, if the overload is severe, the patient is placed in an upright position with the feet in a dependent position, the transfusion is discontinued, and the physician is notified. The intravenous line is kept patent with a very slow infusion of normal saline solution or a saline or heparin lock device to maintain access to the vein in case intravenous medications are necessary. Oxygen and morphine may be needed for severe dyspnea.

BACTERIAL CONTAMINATION

The incidence of bacterial contamination of blood components is very low; however, administration of contaminated products puts the patient at great risk. Contamination can occur at any point during procurement or processing. Many bacteria cannot survive in the cold temperatures used to store PRBCs (platelets are at greater risk for contamination because they are stored at room temperature), but some organisms can survive cold temperatures.

Preventive measures include meticulous care in the procurement and processing of blood components. When PRBCs or whole blood is transfused, it should be administered within a 4-hour period, because warm room temperatures promote bacterial growth. A contaminated unit of blood product may appear normal, or it may have an abnormal color.

The signs of bacterial contamination are fever, chills, and hypotension. These signs may not occur until the transfusion is complete, occasionally not until several hours after the transfusion. If the condition is not treated immediately with fluids and broad-spectrum antibiotics, shock can occur. Even with aggressive management, including vasopressor support, the mortality rate is high.

As soon as the reaction is recognized, any remaining transfusion is discontinued and the intravenous line is kept open with normal saline solution. The physician and the blood bank are notified, and the blood container is returned to the blood bank for testing and culture. Septicemia is treated with intravenous fluids and antibiotics; corticosteroids and vasopressors also may be necessary.

TRANSFUSION-RELATED ACUTE LUNG INJURY

This is a potentially fatal, idiosyncratic reaction that occurs in fewer than 1 in 5000 transfusions. Plasma antibodies (usually in the donor's plasma) that are present in the blood component stimulate the recipient's WBCs; aggregates of these WBCs form and occlude the microvasculature within the lungs. This lung injury is manifested as pulmonary edema; it can occur within 4 hours after the transfusion.

Signs and symptoms include fever, chills, acute respiratory distress (in the absence of other signs of left ventricular failure, such as elevated central venous pressure), and bilateral pulmonary infiltrates. Aggressive supportive therapy (oxygen, intubation, diuretics) may prevent death.

DELAYED HEMOLYTIC REACTION

Delayed hemolytic reactions usually occur within 14 days after transfusion, when the level of antibody has been increased to the extent that a reaction can occur. The hemolysis of the RBCs is extravascular, via the RES, and occurs gradually.

Signs and symptoms of a delayed hemolytic reaction are fever, anemia, increased bilirubin level, decreased or absent haptoglobin, and possibly jaundice. Rarely is there hemoglobinuria. Generally, these reactions are not dangerous, but it is useful to recognize them, because subsequent transfusions with blood products containing these antibodies may cause a more severe hemolytic reaction. However, recognition is also difficult, because the patient may not be in a health care setting to be tested for this reaction, and even if the patient is hospitalized, the reaction may be too mild to be recognized clinically. Because the amount of antibody present can be too low to detect, it is difficult to prevent delayed hemolytic reactions. The reaction is usually mild and requires no intervention.

DISEASES TRANSMITTED BY BLOOD TRANSFUSION

Despite the advances in donor screening and blood testing, certain diseases can still be transmitted by transfusion of blood components. The diseases in Chart 33-18 are examples of this phenomenon.

COMPLICATIONS OF LONG-TERM TRANSFUSION THERAPY

The complications that have been described represent a real risk for any patient any time a unit of blood is administered. However, patients with long-term transfusion therapy (eg, those with MDS, thalassemia, sickle cell anemia) are at greater risk for infection transmission and for becoming more sensitized to donor antigens, simply because they are exposed to more units of blood and, consequently, more donors. Iron overload is a complication unique to those individuals with long-term PRBC transfusions. A summary of complications associated with long-term transfusion therapy is depicted in Table 33-11.

Iron Overload. One unit of PRBCs contains 250 mg of iron. Patients with chronic transfusion requirements can quickly acquire more iron than they can use, leading to iron overload. Over time, the excess iron deposits in the tissues and can cause

---

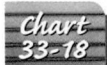

Chart 33-18 **Diseases Transmitted by Blood Transfusion**

Hepatitis (Viral Hepatitis B, C)
- Greater risk from pooled blood products and blood of paid donors than from volunteer donors
- Screening test detects most hepatitis B and C
- Transmittal risk estimated at 1:10,000

AIDS (HIV and HTLV)
- Donated blood screened for antibodies to HIV
- Transmittal risk estimated at 1:670,000
- People with high-risk behaviors (multiple sex partners, anal sex, intravenous/injection drug use) and people with signs and symptoms that suggest AIDS should not donate blood

Cytomegalovirus (CMV)
- Transmittal risk greater for premature newborns with CMV antibody-negative mothers and for immunocompromised recipients who are CMV-negative (eg, those with acute leukemia, organ or tissue transplant recipients).
- Blood products rendered "leukocyte-reduced" help reduce transmission of virus.

Graft-Versus-Host Disease (GVHD)
- Occurs only in severely immunocompromised recipients (eg, Hodgkin's disease, bone marrow transplantation).
- Transfused lymphocytes engraft in recipient and attack host lymphocytes or body tissues; signs and symptoms are fever, diffuse reddened skin rash, nausea, vomiting, diarrhea.
- Preventive measures include irradiating blood products to inactivate donor lymphocytes (no known radiation risks to transfusion recipient) and processing donor blood with leukocyte reduction filters.

Creutzfeldt-Jakob Disease (CJD)
- Rare, fatal disease causing irreversible brain damage
- No evidence of transmittal by transfusion, but hemophiliacs and others are concerned that transmittal is possible
- All blood donors must be screened for positive family history of CJD.
- Potential donors who spent 6 months or more in the United Kingdom (or Europe) from 1980 to 1996 cannot donate blood; blood products from a donor who develops CJD are recalled.

---

organ damage, particularly in the liver, heart, testes, and pancreas. Promptly initiating a program of iron chelation therapy (eg, with deferoxamine [Desferal]) can prevent end-organ damage from iron toxicity (Giardina & Grady, 1995).

NURSING MANAGEMENT FOR TRANSFUSION REACTIONS

If a transfusion reaction is suspected, the transfusion must be immediately stopped and the physician notified. A thorough patient assessment is crucial, because many complications have similar signs and symptoms. The following steps are taken to determine the type and severity of the reaction:

- Stop the transfusion. Maintain the intravenous line with normal saline solution through new intravenous tubing, administered at a slow rate.
- Assess the patient carefully. Compare the vital signs with those from the baseline assessment. Assess the patient's respiratory status carefully. Note the presence of adventitious breath sounds, use of accessory muscles, extent of dyspnea

Table 33-11 • Common Complications Resulting from Long-Term PRBC Transfusion Therapy*

	MANIFESTATION	MANAGEMENT
Infection	Hepatitis (B,C)	May immunize against hepatitis B; give alpha-interferon for hepatitis C; monitor hepatic function
	Cytomegalovirus (CMV)	WBC filters to protect against CMV
Iron overload	Heart failure	Prevent by chelation therapy
	Endocrine failure (diabetes, hypothyroidism, hypoparathyroidism, hypogonadism)	
Transfusion reaction	Sensitization	Diminish by RBC phenotyping, using WBC-filtered products
	Febrile reactions	Diminish by using WBC-filtered products

* Patients with long-term transfusion therapy requirements are at risk not only for the transfusion reactions discussed in the text but also for the complications noted above. In many cases, the use of WBC-filtered (eg, leukocyte-poor) blood products is standard for patients who receive long-term PRBC transfusion therapy. An aggressive chelation program initiated early in the course of therapy can prevent problems with iron overload.
PRBC, packed red blood cells; WBC, white blood cell; RBC, red blood cell.

(if any), and changes in mental status, including anxiety and confusion. Note any chills, diaphoresis, complaints of back pain, urticaria, and jugular vein distention.

- Notify the physician of the assessment findings, and implement any orders obtained. Continue to monitor the patient's vital signs and respiratory, cardiovascular, and renal status.
- Notify the blood bank that a suspected transfusion reaction has occurred.
- Send the blood container and tubing to the blood bank for repeat typing and culture. The identifying tags and numbers are verified.

If a hemolytic transfusion reaction or bacterial infection is suspected, the nurse should do the following:

- Obtain appropriate blood specimens from the patient.
- Collect a urine sample as soon as possible for a hemoglobin determination.
- Document the reaction, according to the institution's policy.

PHARMACOLOGIC ALTERNATIVES TO BLOOD TRANSFUSIONS

Pharmacologic agents to stimulate production of one or more types of blood cells by the marrow are commonly used. Chart 33-19 presents examples of such pharmacologic agents.

Researchers continue to seek a blood substitute that is practical and safe. Blood substitutes previously tried have not been successful. However, newer blood substitutes focus solely on oxygen delivery, as an RBC substitute (Rabinovici, 2001). Current blood substitutes in clinical trials have distinct advantages and disadvantages compared with human RBCs. They are manufactured hemoglobin solutions that can be sterilized without destroying the blood substitute. They require no refrigeration and appear to have a long shelf-life (possibly 1 year, versus little more than 1 month for PRBCs). Perhaps more importantly, they require no cross-matching, because there is no RBC membrane to interact with antibodies in the recipient's serum. The most significant disadvantage stems from the blood substitutes extremely short life within human circulation—approximately 1 day, instead of the 30-day life span of a conventionally transfused RBC. Therefore, the use of these products would likely be limited to situations in which the need is short-term (eg, surgery, trauma). Finally, the blood substitutes are likely to be extremely expensive.

PERIPHERAL BLOOD STEM CELL TRANSPLANTATION (PBSCT) AND BONE MARROW TRANSPLANTATION (BMT)

PBSCT and BMT are therapeutic modalities that offer the possibility of cure for some patients with hematologic disorders such as severe aplastic anemia, some forms of leukemia, and thalassemia. Because most hematologic disease states arise from some form of bone marrow dysfunction, an autologous transplantation (receiving one's own stem cells) is not as common an option as is allogeneic transplantation. A patient receives intensive chemotherapy (sometimes with radiation therapy as well), with the goal being complete ablation of the patient's bone marrow. Stem cells from the donor (ideally, from a matched sibling), or actual marrow from the donor, is then infused into the patient using a process similar to an RBC transfusion. The stem cells travel to the marrow and slowly begin the process of resuming hematopoiesis. The advantage of autotransplantation is the reduced likelihood of complications and mortality; however, the risk of relapse is also higher.

A relatively new strategy is based on transplantation for adoptive cell therapy using certain immune mechanisms derived from the donor's lymphocytes (Slavin et al., 2001; Margolis, Borrello, & Flinn, 2000). In nonmyeloablative stem cell or marrow transplantation, also referred to as a "minitransplant," the conditioning regimen involves much less myelosuppression than in conventional regimens, rendering the patient immunosuppressed but for a shorter period of time. Consequently, the procedure is less toxic to the patient, and there is a significant decrease in morbidity.

After the deconditioning regimen (ie, during the time the patient is immunosuppressed), the allotransplantation is performed, using either marrow or stem cells. The goal is for the donor's lymphocytes to react against any residual malignant cells within the patient and destroy them. This process is typically augmented by

Chart 33-19 | Pharmacologic Alternatives to Blood Transfusions

Growth Factors

Recombinant technology has provided a means to produce hematopoietic growth factors necessary for the production of blood cells within the bone marrow. By increasing the body's production of blood cells, transfusions and complications resulting from diminished blood cells (eg, infection from neutropenia or transfusions) may be avoided. However, the successful use of growth factors requires functional bone marrow.

Erythropoietin

Erythropoietin (epoetin alpha [eg, Epogen, Procrit]) is an effective alternative treatment for patients with chronic anemia secondary to diminished levels of erythropoietin, as in chronic renal disease. This medication stimulates erythropoiesis. It also has been used for patients who are anemic from chemotherapy or zidovudine (AZT) therapy and for those who have diseases involving bone marrow suppression, such as myelodysplastic syndrome (MDS). The use of erythropoietin can also enable a patient to donate several units of blood for future use (eg, preoperative autologous donation). The medication can be administered intravenously or subcutaneously, although plasma levels are better sustained with the subcutaneous route. Side effects are rare, but erythropoietin can cause or exacerbate hypertension. If the anemia is corrected too quickly or is overcorrected, the elevated hematocrit can cause headache and, potentially, seizures. These adverse effects are rare except for patients with renal failure. Serial complete blood counts (CBCs) should be performed to evaluate the response to the medication. The dose and frequency of administration are titrated to the hematocrit.

Granulocyte-Colony Stimulating Factor (G-CSF)

G-CSF (filgrastim [Neupogen]) is a cytokine that stimulates the proliferation and differentiation of myeloid stem cells; a rapid increase in neutrophils is seen within the circulation. G-CSF is effective in improving transient but severe neutropenia after chemotherapy or in some forms of MDS. It is particularly useful in preventing bacterial infections that would be likely to occur with neutropenia. G-CSF is administered subcutaneously on a daily basis. The primary side effect is bone pain; this probably reflects the increase in hematopoiesis within the marrow. Serial CBCs should be performed to evaluate the response to the medication and to ensure that the rise in white blood cells is not excessive. The effect of G-CSF on myelopoiesis is short; the neutrophil count drops once the medication is stopped.

Granulocyte-Macrophage Colony Stimulating Factor (GM-CSF)

GM-CSF (sargramostim [Leukine]) is a cytokine that is naturally produced by a variety of cells, including monocytes and endothelial cells. It works either directly or synergistically with other growth factors to stimulate myelopoiesis. GM-CSF is not as specific to neutrophils as is G-CSF; thus, an increase in erythroid (RBC) and megakaryocytic (platelet) production may also be seen. GM-CSF serves the same purpose as G-CSF. However, it may have a greater effect on macrophage function and therefore may be more useful against fungal infections, whereas G-CSF may be better used to fight bacterial infections. GM-CSF is also administered subcutaneously. Side effects include bone pain, fevers, and myalgias.

Thrombopoietin

Thrombopoietin (TPO) is a cytokine that is necessary for the proliferation of megakaryocytes and subsequent platelet formation. Clinical studies have demonstrated efficacy of TPO in the setting of chemotherapy-induced thrombocytopenia with few side effects (Vadhan-Raj, 2000). Further studies are ongoing to assess the efficacy of TPO in other, more chronic conditions associated with thrombocytopenia (Kuter, 2000).

---

infusion of the donor's lymphocytes as well (referred to as donor lymphocyte infusion, or DLI). If relapse occurs, repeated DLI has been effective in reestablishing remission in many patients. This approach has great promise, particularly in the setting of hematologic malignancy, and may provide a mechanism to increase the utility of transplantation for more patients than is possible with conventional methods.

Success of transplantation depends on tissue compatibility and the patient's tolerance of the immunosuppression that results from the ablative therapy. Patients require intensive nursing care that is directed toward preventing infection and assessing for early signs and symptoms of complications. One common complication involves the formation of lymphocytes that respond to their new host (ie, the patient) as foreign and mount a reaction against the body. This process, known as graft-versus-host disease (GVHD), can involve the skin, gastrointestinal tract, and liver and can be life-threatening. In hematologic malignancies, some GVHD is actually desirable in that the donor lymphocytes can also mount a reaction against any lingering tumor cells; this process is referred to as graft-versus-malignancy. GVHD is a significant complication in nonmyeloablative transplantation therapy, as well as in conventional allotransplantation. Late complications (occurring more than 100 days after transplantation) are frequent; these patients, particularly those who receive an allogeneic transplant, require careful follow-up for years after transplantation. (See Chap. 16 for further information on GVHD.)

Critical Thinking Exercises

1. You are working in a hematology-oncology clinic. The laboratory reports a critical study result for one of your patients with CLL: the reticulocyte count is 25%. What other laboratory results would be important to review or consider? The patient is profoundly anemic; does this support your original thinking and problem solving? What medical treatment orders would you anticipate? What nursing interventions would be appropriate?

2. You are caring for a young adult patient who has had repeated hospitalizations for sickle cell crisis. What factors should be assessed to determine the patient's education, coping, and pain management needs? What is important for the patient's discharge plan?

3. You are caring for a patient diagnosed with leukemia. The family members are very concerned about the patient's risk for infection at home. What assessments will assist you to determine the patient's risk of developing an infection at home? What instructions should you give about decreasing the risks for infection? How would you alter your interventions if the family members are not fluent in English?

4. You are caring for a patient who is septic and is now receiving a transfusion of 2 units of PRBCs. The patient's temperature spikes to 38.5°C after half of the second unit has been transfused. What are the possible causes of the fever? What are the appropriate nursing interventions?

REFERENCES AND SELECTED READINGS

Books

Abrams, A. C. (2001). *Clinical drug therapy: Rationales for nursing practice.* Philadelphia: Lippincott Williams & Wilkins.

American Association of Blood Banks. (2002). *Blood transfusion therapy: A physician's handbook* (7th ed.). Bethesda, MD: Author.

Anderson, K. C., & Ness, P. M. (Eds.). (2000). *Scientific basis of transfusion medicine: Implications for clinical practice.* Philadelphia: W. B. Saunders.

Blumenthal, M., Goldberg, A., & Brinkman, J. (Eds.). (2000). *Herbal medicine.* Newton, MA: Integrative Medicine Communications.

Hoffman, R., Benz, E. J., Shattil, S. J., Furie, B., Cohen, H. J., Silberstein, L. E., et al. (Eds.). (2000). *Hematology: Basic principles and practice* (3rd ed.). New York: Churchill Livingstone.

Lee, G., Foerster, J., Lukens, J., Paraskevas, F., Rogers, G. (1999). *Wintrobe's clinical hematology* (10th ed.). Baltimore: Williams & Wilkins.

Mintz, P. D. (Ed.). (1999). *Transfusion therapy: Clinical principles and practice.* Bethesda, MD: American Association of Blood Banks Press.

Rieger, P. T. (Ed.). (2001). *Biotherapy: A comprehensive overview* (2nd ed.). Boston: Jones and Bartlett.

Schechter, G., Berliner, N., & Telen, M. J. (Eds.). (2000). *Hematology 2000.* [Monograph]. San Francisco: American Society of Hematology Educational Program Book.

Schechter, G., Hoffman, R., & Schrier, S. (Eds.). (1999). *Hematology.* [Monograph]. New Orleans: American Society of Hematology Educational Program Book.

Skeel, R. (Ed.). (1999). *Handbook of cancer chemotherapy* (5th ed.). Philadelphia: Lippincott Williams & Wilkins.

Westphal, R. G. (1996). *Handbook of transfusion medicine* (3rd ed.). Washington, DC: American Red Cross Blood Services.

Wilkes, G. M., Ingwersen, K., & Barton-Burke, M. (2000). *2000 Oncology nursing drug handbook.* Boston: Jones and Bartlett.

Winningham, M. L., & Barton-Burke, M. (Eds.). (2000). *Fatigue in cancer: A multidimensional approach.* Boston: Jones and Bartlett.

Journals

Asterisks indicate nursing research articles.

Aaronson, L. S., Teel, C. S., Cassmeyer, V., Neuberger, G. B., Pallikkathayil, L., Pierce, J., Press, A. N., Williams, P. D., & Wingate, A. (1999). Defining and measuring fatigue. *Image: The Journal of Nursing Scholarship, 31*(1), 45–50.

Adams, R. J. (2000). Lessons from the Stroke Prevention Trial in Sickle Cell Anemia (STOP) study. *Journal of Child Neurology, 15*(5), 344–349.

Alcoser, P. W., & Burchetts, S. (1999). Bone marrow transplantation: Immune system suppression and reconstitution. *American Journal of Nursing, 99*(6), 26–30.

Anderson, K., Hamblin, T. J., & Traynor, A. (1999). Management of multiple myeloma today. *Seminars in Hematology, 36,* (1 Suppl. 3), 3–8.

Andrews, N. C. (1999). Disorders of iron metabolism. *New England Journal of Medicine, 341*(26), 1986–1995.

Applebaum, F. R., Baer, M. R., Carabisi, M. H., Coutre, S. E., Erba, H. P., Estey, E., Glenn, M. J., Kraut, E. H., Maslak, P., Millenson, M., Miller, C. B., Saba, H. I., Stone, R., & Tallman, M. S.; National Comprehensive Cancer Network. (2000). NCCN practice guidelines for acute myelogenous leukemia. *Oncology, 14*(11A), 53–61.

*Baker, F., Zabora, J., Pollard, A., & Wingard, J. (1999). Reintegration after bone marrow transplantation. *Cancer Practice, 7*(4), 190–197.

Barbui, T., & Finazzi, G. (1999). Clinical parameters for determining when and when not to treat essential thrombocytopenia. *Seminars in Hematology, 36* (1, Suppl. 2), 14–18.

Bensinger, W., Martin, P. J., Storer, B., Clift, R., Forman, S. J., Negrin, R., Kashyap, A., Flowers, M. E., Lilleby, K., Chauncey, T. R., Storb, R., & Appelbaum, F. R. (2001). Transplantation of bone marrow as compared with peripheral-blood cells from HLA-identical relatives in patients with hematologic cancers. *New England Journal of Medicine, 344*(3), 175–181.

Beran, M. (2000). Intensive chemotherapy for patients with high-risk myelodysplastic syndrome. *International Journal of Hematology, 72*(2), 139–150.

Berman, E., Clift, R. A., Copelan, E. A., Emanuel, P. D., Erba, H. P., Glenn, M. J., Greenberg, P. L., Jones, R. J., O'Brien, S., Saba, H. I., Schilder, R., Snyder, D. S., Soiffer, R. J., Tallman, M. S., Wetzler, M., Ravansi-Kashani, F., Kantarjian, H., & Talpaz, M. (2000). NCCN practice guidelines for chronic myelogenous leukemia. *Oncology, 14*(11A), 229–240.

Berenson, J. (2001). New advances in the biology and treatment of myeloma bone disease. *Seminars in Hematology, 38*(2, Suppl. 3), 15–20.

Bick, R. L. (1999). Low molecular weight heparins in the outpatient management of venous thromboembolism. *Seminars in Thrombosis and Hemostasis, 25* (Suppl. 3), 97–99.

Bradbury, M., & Cruickshank, J. P. (2000). Blood transfusion: Crucial steps in maintaining safe practice. *British Journal of Nursing, 9*(3), 134–138.

Briere, J., & Guilmin, F. (2001). Management of patients with essential thrombocythemia: Current concepts and perspectives. *Pathologie-biologie, 49*(2), 178–183.

Brown, P. (2001). Transfusion medicine and spongiform encephalopathy. *Transfusion, 41*(4), 433–436.

Burney, K. (2000). Tips for timely management of febrile neutropenia. *Oncology Nursing Forum, 27*(4), 617–618.

Carella, A. M., Cavaliere, M., Lerma, E., Ferrara, R., Tedeschi, L., Romanelli, A., Vinci, M., Pinotti, G., Lambelet, P., Loni, C., Verdiani, S., De Stefano, F., Valbonesi, M., & Corsetti, M. T. (2000). Autografting followed by nonmyeloablative immunosuppressive chemotherapy and allogeneic peripheral-blood hematopoietic stem-cell transplantation as treatment of resistant Hodgkin's disease and non-Hodgkin's lymphoma. *Journal of Clinical Oncology, 18*(23), 3918–3924.

Carella, A. M., Giralt, S., & Slavin, S. (2000). Low intensity regimens with allogeneic hematopoietic stem cell transplantation as treatment of hematologic neoplasia. *Haematologica, 85*(3), 304–313.

Cassileth, P. A., Harrington, D. P., Appelbaum, F., Lazarus, H. M., Rowe, J. M., Paietta, E., Willman, C., Hurd, D. D., Bennett, J. M., Blume, K. G., Head, D. R., & Wiernik, P. H. (1998). Chemotherapy compared with autologous or allogeneic bone marrow transplantation in the management of acute myeloid leukemia in first remission. *New England Journal of Medicine, 339*(23), 1649–1656.

Cavalli, F. (1998). Rare syndromes in Hodgkin's disease. *Annals of Oncology, 9* (Suppl. 5), S109–S113.

Cervantes, F. (2001). Prognostic factors and current practice in treatment of myelofibrosis with myeloid metaplasia: An update anno 2000. *Pathologie-biologie, 49*(2), 148–152.

Champlin, R., Khouri, I., Kornblau, S., Molidrem, J., & Giralt, S. (1999). Reinventing bone marrow transplantation: Nonmyeloablative preparative regimens and induction of graft vs malignancy effect. *Oncology, 13*(5), 621–628.

Cheson, B., Horning, S., Coiffier, B., Shipp, M., Fisher, R., Conners, J., Lister, T., Vose, J., Grillo-Lopez, A., Hagenbeek, A., Cabanillas, F., Klippensten, D., Hiddemann, W., Castellino, R., Harris, N., Armitage, J., Carter, W., Hoppe, R., & Canellos, G. (1999). Report of an international workshop to standardize response criteria for non-Hodgkin's lymphomas. *Journal of Clinical Oncology, 17*(4), 1244–1253.

Coiffer, B. (2002). Rituximab in the treatment of diffuse large B-cell lymphomas. *Seminars in Oncology, 29*(1, Suppl. 2), 30–35.

Corwin, E. J. (2000). Understanding cytokines. Part I: Physiology and mechanisms of action. *Biologic Research for Nursing, 2*(1), 30–40.

Corwin, E. J. (2000). Understanding cytokines. Part II: Implications for nursing research and practice. *Biologic Research for Nursing, 2*(1), 41–48.

Creteur, J., Sibbald, W., & Vincent, J. L. (2000). Hemoglobin solutions: Not just red blood cell substitutes. *Critical Care Medicine, 28*(8), 3025–3034.

Derderian, P. M., Kantarjian, H. M., Talpaz, M., O'Brien, S., Cork, A., Estey, E., Pierce, S., & Keating, M. (1993). Chronic myelogenous leukemia in the lymphoid blastic phase: Characteristics, treatment response, and prognosis. *American Journal of Medicine, 94*(1), 69–74.

Deagle, J., & Kelaher, N. (1999). Deep-vein thrombosis: The shift to outpatient care. *Nursing Times, 95*(46), 48–49.

*de Carvalho, E. C., Goncalves, P. G., Bontempo, A. M., & Sloer, V. (2000). Interpersonal needs expressed by patients during bone marrow transplantation. *Cancer Nursing, 23*(6), 462–467.

Deeg, H. J., & Applebaum, F. R. (2000). Hematopoietic stem cell transplantation in patients with myelodysplastic syndrome. *Leukemia Research, 24*(8), 653–663.

Delmore, B. A., Hansen, D., Mooney, K. A., Paplanus, L. M., & Sutton, P. R. (2000). An anticoagulation pathway for quality management. *Applied Nursing Research, 13*(2), 105–110.

Druker, B., Talpaz, M., Resta, D., Peng, B., Buchdinger, E., Ford., J., Lydon, N., Kantargian, H., Capdeville, R., Ohno-Jones, S., & Sawyers, C. L. (2001). Efficacy and safety of a specific inhibitor of the BCR-ABL tyrosine kinase in chronic myeloid leukemia. *New England Journal of Medicine, 344*(14), 1031–1037.

*Duquette-Petersen, L., Francis, M., Dohnalek, L., Skinner, R., & Dudas, P. (1999). The role of protective clothing in infection prevention in patients undergoing autologous bone marrow transplantation. *Oncology Nursing Forum, 26*(8), 1319–1324.

Elalamy, I., Lecrubier, C., Horellou, M. H., Conard, J., & Samama, M. M. (2000). Heparin-induced thrombocytopenia: Laboratory diagnosis and management. *Annals of Medicine, 32*, (Suppl. 1), 60–67.

Ely, E. W., & Bernard, G. R. (1999). Transfusions in critically ill patients. *New England Journal of Medicine, 340*(6), 467–468.

Emmanouilides, C., Rosen, P., Telatar, M., Malone, R., Bosserman, L., Menco, H., Patel, R., Barstis, J., & Grody, W. (2000). Excellent tolerance of rituximab when given after mitoxantrone/cyclophosphamide: An effective and safe combination for indolent non-Hodgkin's lymphoma. *Clinical Lymphoma, 1*(2), 146–151.

Engstrom, C. A., & Sarkodee-Adoo, C. (1998). The molecular biology of lymphoma. *Seminars in Oncology Nursing, 14*(4), 256–261.

Fareed, J., Hoppensteadt, D. A., & Bick, R. L. (2000). An update on heparins at the beginning of the new millennium. *Seminars in Thrombosis and Hemostasis, 26* (Suppl. 1), 5–21.

Ferster, A., Tahriri, P., Vermylen, C., Sturbois, G., Corazza, F., Fondu, P., Devalck, C., Dresse, M., Feremans, W., Hunninck, K., Toppet, M., Philippet, P., Van Geet, C., & Sariban, E. (2001). Five years of experience with hydroxyurea in children and young adults with sickle cell disease. *Blood, 97*(11), 3628–3632.

*Fitzgerald, M., Hodgkinson, B., & Thorp, D. (1999). Blood transfusion from the recipient's perspective. *Journal of Clinical Nursing, 8*(5), 593–600.

George, J. N., Kojouri, K., Perdue, J. J., & Vesely, S. K. (2000). Management of patients with chronic, refractory idiopathic thrombocytopenic purpura. *Seminars in Hematology, 37*(3), 290–298.

Giardina, P. J., & Grady, R. W. (1995). Chelation therapy in beta-thalassemia: The benefits and limitations of desferrioxamine. *Seminars in Hematology, 32*(4), 304–312.

Gilbert, H. S. (1999). Historical perspective on the treatment of essential thrombocythemia and polycythemia vera. *Seminars in Hematology, 36* (1, Suppl. 2), 19–22.

Gobel, B. H. (1999). Disseminated intravascular coagulation. *Seminars in Oncology Nursing, 15*(3), 174–182.

Gochee, P. A., & Powell, L. W. (2001). What's new in hemochromatosis. *Current Opinion in Hematology, 8*(2), 98–104.

Goldman, D. A. (2001). Thalidomide use: Past history and current implications for practice. *Oncology Nursing Forum, 28*(3), 471–477.

Goldman, J., & Melo, J. (2001). Targeting the BCR-ABL tyrosine kinase in chronic myeloid leukemia. *New England Journal of Medicine, 344*(14), 1084–1086.

Gorman, K. (1999). Sickle cell disease. *American Journal of Nursing, 99*(3), 38–43.

Greenberg, P., Baer, M., Bennett, J., Bloomfield, C., Deeg, H., J., Erba, H. P., et al. (2000). NCCN practice guidelines for myelodysplastic syndromes, Version 2000. In *The Complete Library of NCCN Guidelines* [CD-ROM]. Rockledge, PA. National Comprehensive Cancer Network.

Greenlee, R. T., Hill-Harmon, M., Murray, T., & Thun, M. (2001). Cancer statistics, 2001. *CA: A Cancer Journal for Clinicians, 51*(1), 15–36.

Gruppo Italiano Studio Policitemia (GISP). (1995). Polycythemia vera: The natural history of 1213 patients followed over 20 years. *Annals of Internal Medicine, 123*(9), 656–664.

Hainsworth, J., Burris, H., Morrissey, L., Litchy, S., Scullin, D., Bearden, J., Richards, P., & Greco, F. (2000). Rituximab monoclonal antibody as initial systemic therapy for patients with low-grade non-Hodgkin lymphoma. *Blood, 95*(10), 3052–3056.

Hays, K., & McCartney, S. (1998). Nursing care of the patient with chronic lymphocytic leukemia. *Seminars in Oncology, 25*(1), 75–79.

Heaney, M. L., & Golde, D. W. (1999). Myelodysplasia. *New England Journal of Medicine, 340*(21), 1649–1660.

Hiddemann, W., & Buchner, T. (2001). Current status and perspectives of therapy for acute myeloid leukemia. *Seminars in Hematology, 38* (3, Suppl. 6), 3–9.

Hoelzer, D., & Gokbuget, N. (2000). New approaches to acute lymphoblastic leukemia in adults: Where do we go? *Seminars in Oncology, 27*(5), 540–559.

Hu, K., & Yahalom, J. (2000). Radiotherapy in the management of plasma cell tumors. *Oncology, 14*(1), 101–108.

Huffstutler, S. Y. (2000). Adult anemia. *Advance for Nurse Practitioners, 8*(3), 89–91.

Jantunen, R., Juvonen, E., Ikkala, E., Okansen, K., Antilla, P., & Ruutu, T. (2001). The predictive value of vascular risk factors and gender for the development of thrombotic complications in essential thrombocythemia. *Annals of Hematology, 80*(2), 74–78.

Josting, A., & Diehl, V. (2001). Early-stage Hodgkin's disease. *Current Oncology Reports, 3*(3), 279–284.

Kanis, J. A., & McCloskey, E. V. (2000). Bisphosphonates in multiple myeloma. *Cancer, 88* (12, Suppl.), 3022–3032.

Kelton, J. G. (1999). The clinical management of heparin-induced thrombocytopenia. *Seminars in Hematology, 36*, (1 Suppl. 1), 17–21.

Kelton, J. G., & Bussel, J. B. (2000). Idiopathic immune thrombocytopenic purpura: An update. *Seminars in Hematology, 37*(3), 219–221.

Korman, M. T., Leparc, G., & Benson, K. (2001). Nucleic acid amplification testing: The new infectious disease testing method for donor blood. Available at: http://www.moffitt.usf.edu/pubs/ccj/v6n5/dept5.htm. Accessed June 28, 2001.

Kornblith, A. B., Herndon, J. E. II, Silverman, L. R., Demakos, E. P., Holland, J. F., et al. (1998). The impact of 5-azacytidine on the quality of life of patients with myelodysplastic syndrome (MDS) treated in a randomized phase III trial of the cancer and leukemia group B (CALGB). *Proceedings of the American Society of Clinical Oncology, 17*, Abstract 189.

Kosits, C., & Callaghan M. (2000). Rituximab: A new monoclonal antibody therapy for non-Hodgkin's lymphoma. *Oncology Nursing Forum, 27*(1), 51–59.

Kreimeier, U., & Messmer, K. (2002). Perioperative hemodilution. *Transfusions and Apheresis Science, 27*(1), 59–72.

Kuter, D. J. (2000) Future directions with platelet growth factors. *Seminars in Hematology, 37*(2, Suppl. 4), 41–49.

Lengfelder, E., Berger, U., & Hehlmann, R. (2002). Interferon alpha in the treatment of polycythemia vera. *Annals of Hematology, 79*(3), 103–109.

Loney, M., & Chernecky, C. (2000). Anemia. *Oncology Nursing Forum, 27*(6), 951–962.

Lusher, J. M. (2000). Inhibitor antibodies to factor VIII and factor IX: Management. *Seminars in Thrombosis and Hemostasis, 26*(2), 179–188.

Major, P., Lortholary, A., Hon, J., Abdi, E., Mills, G., Menssen, H. D., Yunus, F., Bell, R., Body, J., Quebe-Fehling, E., & Seaman, J. (2001). Zolendronic acid is superior to pamidronate in the treatment of tumor-induced hypercalcemia: A pooled analysis of two randomized, controlled clinical trials. *Journal of Clinical Oncology, 19*(2), 558–567.

Marcaccio, M. J. (2000). Laparoscopic splenectomy in chronic idiopathic thrombocytopenic purpura. *Seminars in Hematology, 37*(3), 267–274.

Margolis, J., Borrello, I., & Flynn, I. W. (2000). New approaches to treating malignancies with stem cell transplantation. *Seminars in Oncology, 27*(5), 524–530.

McCullough, J. (2000). Current issues with platelet transfusion in patients with cancer. *Seminars in Hematology, 37* (2, Suppl. 4), 3–10.

Micallef, I. N., Rohatiner, A. Z., Carter, M., Boyle, M., Slater, S., Amess, J. A., & Lister, T. A. (2001). Long-term outcome of patients surviving for more than ten years following treatment for acute leukemia. *British Journal of Haematology, 113*(2), 443–445.

Michiels, J. J., Barbui, T., Finazzi, G., Fuchtman, S. M., Kutti, J., Rain, J. D., et al. (2000). Diagnosis and treatment of polycythemia vera and possible future study designs of the PVSG. *Leukemia and Lymphoma, 36*(3–4), 239–253.

Mitka, M. (2001). FDA wants more restrictions on donated blood. *Journal of the American Medical Association, 286*(4), 408.

Money, S. R., & York, J. W. (2001). Development of oral heparin therapy for prophylaxis and treatment of deep venous thrombosis. *Cardiovascular Surgery, 9*(3), 211–218.

Murphy, S. (1999). Diagnostic criteria and prognosis in polycythemia vera and essential thrombocythemia. *Seminars in Hematology, 36* (1, Suppl. 2), 9–13.

NCCN practice guidelines for Hodgkin's disease. National Comprehensive Cancer Network. *Oncology, 13*(5A), 78–110.

Ohene-Frempong, K. (2001). Indications for red cell transfusion in sickle cell disease. *Seminars in Hematology, 38* (1, Suppl. 1), 5–13.

O'Rourke, M. E., & High, K. (2000). Diagnosing graft versus host disease. *Clinical Journal of Oncology Nursing, 4*(1), 47–48.

Osterbor, A. (2000). The role of recombinant human erythropoietin in the management of anaemic cancer patients: Focus on haematological malignancies. *Medical Oncology, 17* (Suppl 1), S17–S22.

Patt, J., & Morrison, S. (2001). National Cancer Institute resources for patients and their caregivers. *Cancer Practice, 9*(5), 257–261.

*Pederson, C., & Parren, L. (1999). Pain in adult recipients of blood or marrow transplant. *Cancer Nursing, 22*(6), 397–407.

Petrykk, M., & Grossbard, M. L. (2000). Rituximab therapy of B-cell neoplasms. *Clinical Lymphoma, 1*(3), 186–194.

Rabinovici, R. (2001). The status of hemoglobin-based red cell substitutes. *Israel Medical Association Journal, 3*(9), 691–697.

Radich, J., & Sievers, E. (2000). New developments in the treatment of acute myeloid leukemia. *Oncology, 14*(11A), 125–131.

Reed, W., Walker, P., Haddix, T., & Perkins, H. A. (2000). Acute anemic events in sickle cell disease. *Transfusion, 40*(3), 267–273.

Rimm, E. B., Willett, W. C., Hu, F. B., Sampson, L., Colditz, G. A., Manson, J. E., Hennekens, C., & Stampfer, M. J. (1998). Folate and vitamin B$_6$ from diet and supplements in relation to risk of coronary heart disease among women. *Journal of the American Medical Association, 279*(5), 359–364.

Rust, D., Simpson, J., & Lister, J. (2000). Nutritional issues in patients with severe neutropenia. *Seminars in Oncology Nursing, 16*(16), 152–162.

Saleh, M. N., Gutheil, J., Moore, M., Bunch, P. W., Butler, J., Kunkel, L., Grillo-Lopez, A. J., & LoBuglio, A. F. (2000). A pilot study of the anti-CD20 monoclonal antibody rituximab in patients with refractory immune thrombocytopenia. *Seminars in Oncology, 27* (6, Suppl. 12), 99–103.

Scaradavou, A. (2000). Splenectomy-sparing, long-term maintenance with anti-D for chronic immune (idiopathic) thrombocytopenic purpura: The New York Hospital experience. *Seminars in Hematology, 37* (1, Suppl. 1), 42–44.

Seligsohn, U., & Lubetsky, A. (2001). Genetic susceptibility to venous thrombosis. *New England Journal of Medicine, 344*(16), 1222–1231.

Shapiro, A. D. (2000). Platelet function disorders. *Haemophilia, 6* (Suppl. 1), 120–127.

Shelton, B. K. (1999). Sepsis. *Seminars in Oncology Nursing, 15*(3), 209–221.

Sievers, E., Appelbaum, F., Speilberger, R. T., Forman, S., Flowers, D., Smith, F., Shannon-Dorcy, K., Berger, M. S., & Bernstein, I. D. (1999). Selective ablation of acute myeloid leukemia using antibody-targeted chemotherapy: A phase I study of anti-CD33 calicheamicin immunoconjugate. *Blood, 93*(11), 3678–3684.

Silverstein, M. R., & Tefferi, A. (1999). Treatment of essential thrombocythemia with anagrelide. *Seminars in Hematology, 36* (1, Suppl. 2), 23–25.

Singhal, S., Mehta, J., Desikan, R., Ayers, D., Roberson, P., Eddlemon, P., Munshi, N., Anaissie, E., Wilson, C., Dhodapkar, M., Zeddis, J., & Barlogie, B. (1999). Antitumor activity of thalidomide in refractory multiple myeloma. *New England Journal of Medicine, 341*(21), 1565–1571.

Slavin, S., Or, R., Aker, M., Shapira, M. Y., Panigrahi, S., Symeonidis, A., Cividalli, G., & Nagler, A. (2001). Nonmyeloablative stem cell transplantation for the treatment of cancer and life-threatening nonmalignant disorders: Past accomplishments and future goals. *Cancer Chemotherapy and Pharmacology, 48* (Suppl. 1), S79–S84.

*Smith, L. H., & Besser, S. G. (2000). Dietary restrictions for patients with neutropenia: A survey of institutional practices. *Oncology Nursing Forum, 27*(3), 515–520.

Stampfer, M. J., Hu, F. B., Manson, J. E., Rimm, E. B., & Willett, W. C. (2000). Primary prevention of coronary heart disease in women through diet and lifestyle. *New England Journal of Medicine, 343*(1), 16–22.

Stasi, R., Pagano, A., Stipa, E., & Amadori, S. (2001). Rituximab chimeric anti-CD20 monoclonal antibody treatment for adults with chronic idiopathic thrombocytopenic purpura. *Blood, 98*(4), 952–957.

Steinberg, M. H. (1999). Management of sickle cell disease. *New England Journal of Medicine, 340*(13), 1021–1030.

Tefferi, A., Fonseca, R., Pereira, D. L., & Hoagland, H. C. (2001). A long-term retrospective study of young women with essential thrombocythemia. *Mayo Clinic Proceedings, 76*(1), 22–28.

Tefferi, A., Solberg, L. A., & Silverstein, M. N. (2000). A clinical update in polycythemia vera and essential thrombocythemia. *American Journal of Medicine, 109*(2), 141–149.

Tennant, L. (2001). Chronic myelogenous leukemia: An overview. *Clinical Journal of Oncology Nursing, 5*(5), 218–219.

Terpos, E., Palermos, J., Tsinos, K., Anargyrou, K., Viniou, N., Papassavas, P., Meletis, J., & Yataganas, X. (2000). Effect of pamidronate administration on markers of bone turnover and disease activity in multiple myeloma. *European Journal of Haematology, 65*(5), 331–336.

Tesch, H., Sieber, M., & Diehl, V. (2001). Treatment of advanced stage Hodgkin's disease. *Oncology, 60*(2), 101–109.

Thomas, M. L. (1998). Anemia and quality of life in cancer patients: Impact of transfusion and erythropoeitin. *Medical Oncology, 15* (Suppl. 1), S13–S18.

Thomas, M. L. (1998). Quality of life and psychsocial adjustment in patients with myelodysplastic syndromes. *Leukemia Research, 22* (Suppl. 1), S41–S47.

Traynor, A. E., & Noga, S. J. (2001). NCCN: multiple myeloma. *Cancer Control, 8* (6, Suppl. 2), 78–87.

Vadhan-Raj, S. (2000). Clinical experience with recombinant human thrombopoietin in chemotherapy-induced thrombocytopenia. *Seminars in Hematology, 37* (2, Suppl. 4), 28–34.

Viale, P. H. (1999). Management of thromboembolism in patients with cancer. *Oncology Nursing Forum, 26*(10), 1625–1632.

Vichinsky, E. P., Neumayr, L. D., Earles, A. N., Williams, R., Lennett, E. T., Dean, D. D., Nickerson, B., Orringer, E., McKie, V., Bellevue, R., Daeschner, C., & Manci, E. A. (2000). Causes and outcomes of the acute chest syndrome in sickle cell disease. National Acute Chest Syndrome Study Group. *New England Journal of Medicine, 342*(25), 1855–1865.

Wazny, L. D., & Ariano, R. E. (2000). Evaluation and management of drug-induced thrombocytopenia in the acutely ill patient. *Pharmacotherapy, 20*(3), 292–307.

Weiss, L. M. (2000). Epstein-Barr virus and Hodgkin's disease. *Current Oncology Reports 2*(2), 199–204.

White, G. C., Greenwood, R., Escobar, M., & Frelinger, J. A. (2000). Hemophilia factor VIII therapy: Immunological tolerance. *Haematologica, 85* (10, Suppl.), 113–116.

Young, N. S. (2000). Hematopoietic cell destruction by immune mechanisms in acquired aplastic anemia. *Seminars in Hematology, 37*(1), 3–14.

Young, N. S. (1999). Acquired aplastic anemia. *Journal of the American Medical Association, 282*(3), 271–278.

Zaidi, A. A., & Vesole, D. H. (2001). Multiple myeloma: An old disease with new hope for the future. *CA: A Cancer Journal for Clinicians, 51*(5), 273–285.

Zelenetz, A., & Hoppe, R. T. (2001). NCCN: Non-Hodgkin's lymphomas. *Cancer Control, 8*(6, Suppl. 2), 102–113.

RESOURCES AND WEBSITES

Alternative Medicine Foundation, Inc., 5411 W. Cedar Lane, Suite 205-A, Bethesda, MD 20814; 301-340-1960; http://www.amfoundation.org.

American Association of Blood Banks (AABB), 8101 Glenbrook Road, Bethesda, MD 20814-2749; 301-907-6977; http://www.aabb.org.

American Cancer Society, 1599 Clifton Rd., N.E., Atlanta, GA 30329; 800-227-2345; http://www.cancer.org.

American Hemochromatosis Society, 777 E. Atlantic Ave., PMB Z-363, Delray Beach, FL 33483-5352; 1-888-655-4766; http://www.americanhs.org.

American Pain Society, 4700 W. Lake Ave., Glenview, IL 60025; 1-847-375-4715; http://www.ampainsoc.org.

American Red Cross, 1730 E Street NW, Washington, DC 20006; 1-202-639-3520; http://www.redcross.org.

Aplastic Anemia and MDS International Foundation, PO Box 613, Annapolis, MD 21404; 1-800-747-2820; http://www.aplastic.org.

Blood and Marrow Transplant Newsletter, 1985 Spruce Ave., Highland Park, IL 60036.

International Myeloma Foundation, 12650 Riverside Drive, Suite 206, North Hollywood, CA 91607; 1-800-452-2873; http://www.myeloma.org.

Leukemia and Lymphoma Society, 1311 Mamaroneck Ave. White Plains, NY 10605; 1-800-955-4572 http://www.leukemialymphoma.org.

Myelodysplastic Syndromes Foundation, PO Box 477, 464 Main St., Crosswicks, NJ 08515; 1-800-637-0839; http://www.mds-foundation.org.

National Association of Vascular Access Networks, 11417 S. 700 East, Suite 205, Draper, UT 84020; 888-576-2826; http://www.navannet.org.

National Cancer Institute Cancer Information Service, 31 Center Drive, MSC 2580, Building 31, Room 10A16, Bethesda, MD 20892-2580; 1-800-4-CANCER; http://www.nci.nih.gov.

National Hemophilia Foundation, 116 W. 32nd St., 11th Floor, New York, NY 10001; 800-424-2634; http://www.hemophilia.org.

National Marrow Donor Program, Suite 500, 3001 Broadway St. N.E., Minneapolis, MN 55413; 800-627-7692; http://www.marrow.org.

Office of Dietary Supplements, National Institutes of Health, 6100 Executive Blvd., Rm 3B0l, MSC 7517, Bethesda, Maryland 20892-7517; 301-435-2920; http://ods.od.nih.gov.

Oncology Nursing Society, 501 Holiday Dr., Pittsburgh, PA 15220-2749; http://www.ons.org.

Sickle Cell Disease Association of America, Inc., 200 Corporate Pointe, Suite 495, Culver City, CA 90230-8727; http://www.sicklecelldisease.org.

Digestive and Gastrointestinal Function

Mr. Sullivan is a 32-year-old man who has had several episodes of bloody diarrhea with severe cramping, nausea, and vomiting after attending a party 12 hours earlier where he drank eggnog and ate foods from a buffet table. His temperature is 103°F, heart rate 108, respiratory rate 20, and BP 118/80. Because he is a kidney transplant recipient and is on immunosuppressive medications, he is admitted to the hospital; his diagnosis is salmonellosis. The concept map illustrates the relationships that exist among the nursing diagnoses, interventions, and outcomes for one of Mr. Sullivan's clinical problems.

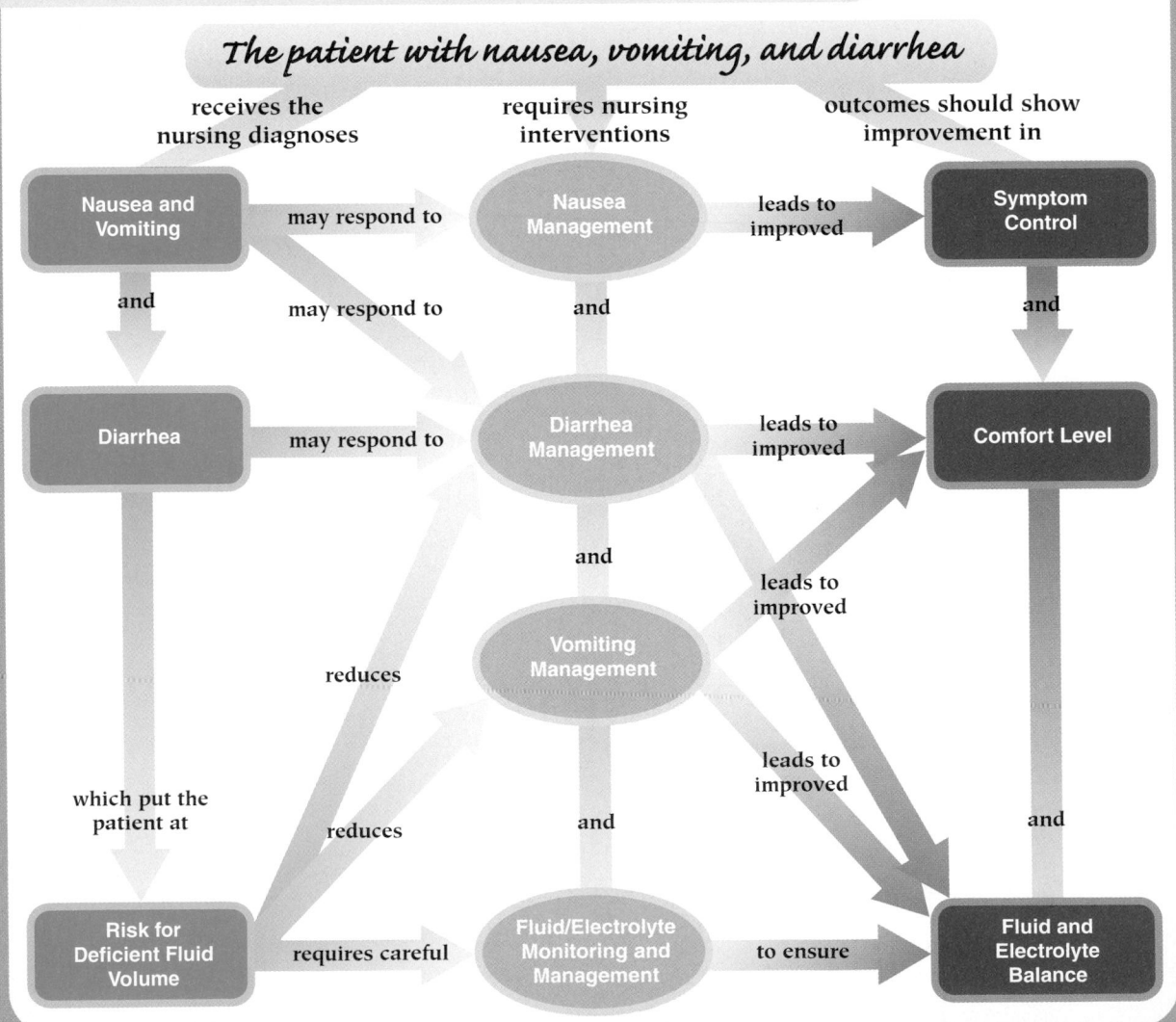

The patient with nausea, vomiting, and diarrhea

Nursing Classifications and Languages

NANDA
Nursing Diagnoses

Nausea—Unpleasant wavelike sensation in the back of the throat, epigastrium, or throughout the abdomen that may or may not lead to vomiting

Diarrhea—Passage of loose, unformed stools

Risk for Deficient Fluid Volume—Risk for decreased intravascular, interstitial, and/or intracellular fluid. This refers to dehydration, water loss alone, without change in sodium.

NIC
Nursing Interventions*

Nausea Management—Prevention and alleviation of nausea

Diarrhea Management—Management and alleviation of diarrhea

Vomiting Management—Prevention and alleviation of vomiting

Fluid/Electrolyte Monitoring and Management—Collection and analysis of patient data to regulate fluid balance, and regulation and prevention of complications from altered fluid and/or electrolyte levels

NOC
Nursing Outcomes†

Return to functional baseline status, stabilization of, or improvement in

Symptom Control—Personal actions to minimize perceived adverse changes in physical functioning

Comfort Level—Extent of physical and psychological ease

Fluid/Electrolyte Balance—Balance of water and electrolytes in the intracellular and extracellular compartments of the body

NANDA, North American Nursing Diagnosis Association; NIC, Nursing Interventions Classification; NOC, Nursing Outcomes Classification

*Iowa Intervention Project © 2000. In McCloskey, J. C., & Bulechek, G. M. (2000). *Nursing interventions classification (NIC)* (3rd ed.). St. Louis: Mosby.

†Iowa Outcomes Project © 2000. In Johnson, M., Maas, M., & Moorhead, S. (2000). *Nursing outcomes classification (NOC)* (3rd ed.). St. Louis: Mosby.

Assessment of Digestive and Gastrointestinal Function

On completion of this chapter, the learner will be able to:

1. Describe the structure and function of the organs of the gastrointestinal tract.

2. Describe the mechanical and chemical processes involved in digesting and absorbing foods and eliminating waste products.

3. Use assessment parameters appropriate for determining the status of gastrointestinal function.

4. Describe the appropriate preparation, teaching, and follow-up care for patients who are undergoing diagnostic testing of the gastrointestinal tract.

Anatomic and Physiologic Overview

ANATOMY OF THE GASTROINTESTINAL TRACT

The GI tract is a 23- to 26-foot-long pathway that extends from the **mouth** through the esophagus, stomach, and intestines to the anus (Fig. 34-1). The **esophagus** is located in the mediastinum in the thoracic cavity, anterior to the spine and posterior to the trachea and heart. This collapsible tube, which is about 25 cm (10 inches) in length, becomes distended when food passes through it. It passes through the diaphragm at an opening called the diaphragmatic hiatus.

The remaining portion of the GI tract is located within the peritoneal cavity. The **stomach** is situated in the upper portion of the abdomen to the left of the midline, just under the left diaphragm. It is a distensible pouch with a capacity of approximately 1500 mL. The inlet to the stomach is called the esophagogastric junction; it is surrounded by a ring of smooth muscle called the lower esophageal sphincter (or cardiac sphincter), which, on contraction, closes off the stomach from the esophagus. The stomach can be divided into four anatomic regions: the cardia (entrance), fundus, body, and pylorus (outlet). Circular smooth muscle in the wall of the pylorus forms the pyloric sphincter and controls the opening between the stomach and the small intestine.

The **small intestine** is the longest segment of the GI tract, accounting for about two thirds of the total length. It folds back and forth on itself, providing approximately 7000 cm of surface area for secretion and **absorption,** the process by which nutrients enter the bloodstream through the intestinal walls. The small intestine is divided into three anatomic parts: the upper part, called the duodenum; the middle part, called the jejunum; and the lower part, called the ileum. The common bile duct, which allows for the passage of both bile and pancreatic secretions, empties into the duodenum at the ampulla of Vater. The junction between the small and large intestine, the cecum, is located in the right lower portion of the abdomen. The ileocecal valve is located at this junction. It controls the passage of intestinal contents into the large intestine and prevents reflux of bacteria into the small intestine. The vermiform appendix is located near this junction.

The **large intestine** consists of an ascending segment on the right side of the abdomen, a transverse segment that extends from right to left in the upper abdomen, and a descending segment on the left side of the abdomen. The terminal portion of the large intestine consists of two parts: the sigmoid colon and the rectum. The rectum is continuous with the **anus.** A network of striated muscle that forms both the internal and the external anal sphincters regulates the anal outlet.

The GI tract receives blood from arteries that originate along the entire length of the thoracic and abdominal aorta. Of particular importance are the gastric artery and the superior and inferior mesenteric arteries. Oxygen and nutrients are supplied to the stomach by the gastric artery and to the intestine by the mesenteric arteries (Fig. 34-2). Blood is drained from these organs by veins that merge with others in the abdomen to form a large vessel called the portal vein. Nutrient-rich blood is then carried to the liver. The blood flow to the GI tract is about 20% of the total cardiac output and increases significantly after eating.

Both the sympathetic and parasympathetic portions of the autonomic nervous system innervate the GI tract. In general, sympathetic nerves exert an inhibitory effect on the GI tract, decreasing gastric secretion and motility and causing the sphincters and blood vessels to constrict. Parasympathetic nerve stimulation causes peristalsis and increases secretory activities. The sphincters relax under the influence of parasympathetic stimulation. The only portions of the tract that are under voluntary control are the upper esophagus and the external anal sphincter.

FUNCTION OF THE DIGESTIVE SYSTEM

All cells of the body require nutrients. These nutrients are derived from the intake of food that contains proteins, fats, carbohydrates, vitamins and minerals, and cellulose fibers and other vegetable matter of no nutritional value. The primary digestive functions of the GI tract are the following:

- To break down food particles into the molecular form for digestion

---

Glossary

absorption: phase of the digestive process that occurs when small molecules, vitamins, and minerals pass through the walls of the small and large intestine and into the bloodstream

amylase: an enzyme that aids in the digestion of starch

anus: last section of the GI tract; outlet for waste products from the system

chyme: mixture of food with saliva, salivary enzymes, and gastric secretions that is produced as the food passes through the mouth, esophagus, and stomach

digestion: phase of the digestive process that occurs when digestive enzymes and secretions mix with ingested food and when proteins, fats, and sugars are broken down into their component smaller molecules

elimination: phase of digestive process that occurs after digestion and absorption, when waste products are evacuated from the body

esophagus: collapsible tube connecting the mouth to the stomach, through which food passes as it is ingested

fibroscopy (gastrointestinal): intubation of a part of the GI system with a flexible, lighted tube to assist in diagnosis and treatment of diseases of that area

hydrochloric acid: acid secreted by the glands in the stomach; mixes with chyme to break it down into absorbable molecules and to aid in the destruction of bacteria

ingestion: phase of the digestive process that occurs when food is taken into the GI tract via the mouth and esophagus

intrinsic factor: a gastric secretion that combines with vitamin B_{12} so that the vitamin can be absorbed

large intestine: the portion of the GI tract into which waste material from the small intestine passes as absorption continues and elimination begins; consists of several parts—ascending segment, transverse segment, descending segment, sigmoid colon, and rectum

lipase: an enzyme that aids in the digestion of fats

mouth: first portion of the GI tract, through which food is ingested

pepsin: a gastric enzyme that is important in protein digestion

small intestine: longest portion of the GI tract, consisting of three parts—duodenum, jejunum, and ileum—through which food mixed with all secretions and enzymes passes as it continues to be digested and begins to be absorbed into the bloodstream

stomach: distensible pouch into which the food bolus passes to be digested by gastric enzymes

trypsin: enzyme that aids in the digestion of protein

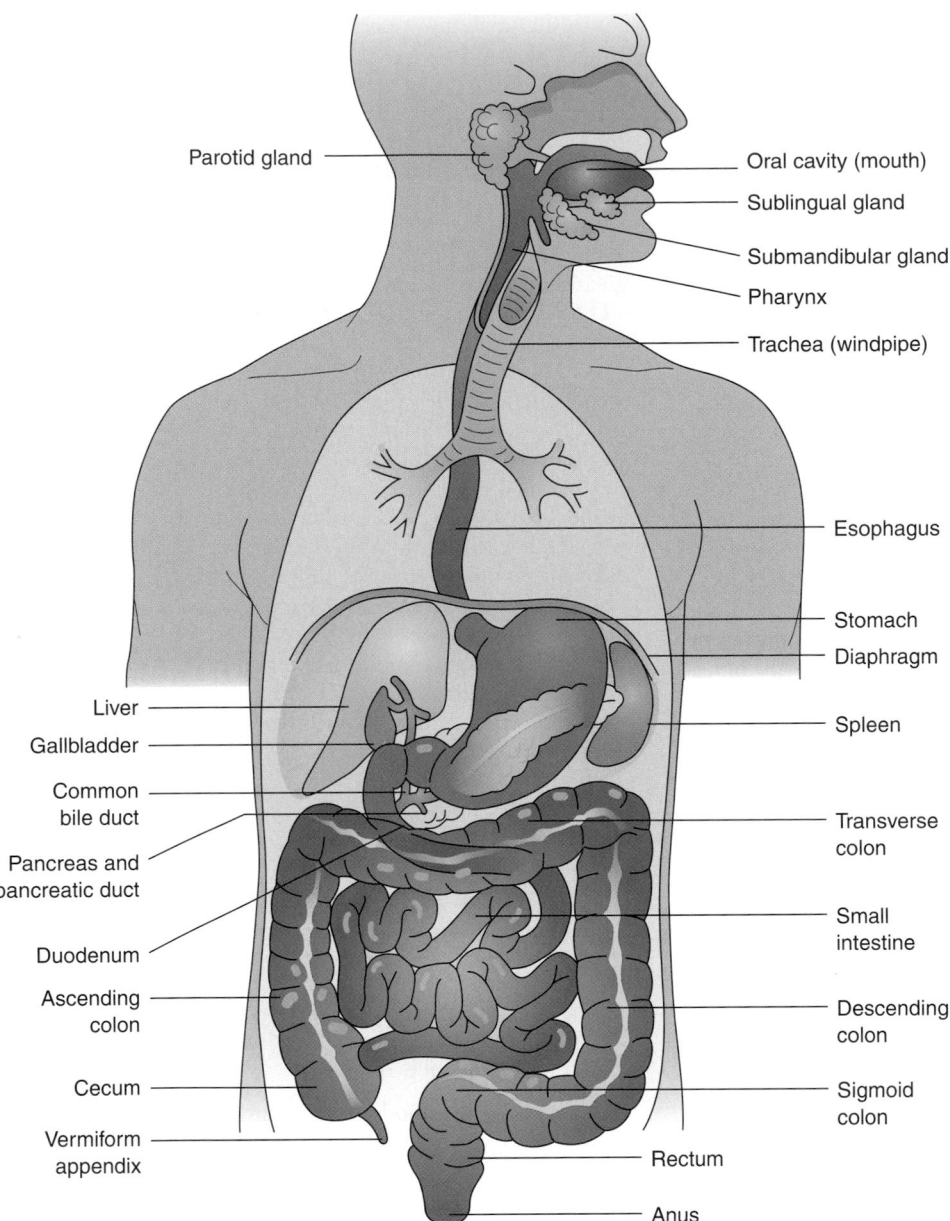

Parotid gland

Oral cavity (mouth)

Sublingual gland

Submandibular gland

Pharynx

Trachea (windpipe)

Esophagus

Stomach

Diaphragm

Liver

Gallbladder

Spleen

Common
bile duct

Pancreas and
pancreatic duct

Transverse
colon

Duodenum

Small
intestine

Ascending
colon

Descending
colon

Cecum

Sigmoid
colon

Vermiform
appendix

Rectum

Anus

FIGURE 34-1 Organs of the digestive system and associated structures.

- To absorb into the bloodstream the small molecules produced by **digestion**
- To eliminate undigested and unabsorbed foodstuffs and other waste products from the body

After food is ingested, it is propelled through the GI tract, coming into contact with a wide variety of secretions that aid in its digestion, absorption, or **elimination** from the GI tract.

Chewing and Swallowing

The process of digestion begins with the act of chewing, in which food is broken down into small particles that can be swallowed and mixed with digestive enzymes. Eating—or even the sight, smell, or taste of food—can cause reflex salivation. Saliva is secreted from three pairs of glands: the parotid, the submaxillary, and the sublingual glands. Approximately 1.5 L of saliva is se-

creted daily. Saliva is the first secretion that comes in contact with food. Saliva contains the enzyme ptyalin, or salivary amylase, which begins the digestion of starches (Table 34-1). Saliva also contains mucus and water, which help to lubricate the food as it is chewed, thereby facilitating swallowing.

Swallowing begins as a voluntary act that is regulated by a swallowing center in the medulla oblongata of the central nervous system. As food is swallowed, the epiglottis moves to cover the tracheal opening and prevent aspiration of food into the lungs. Swallowing, which propels the bolus of food into the upper esophagus, thus ends as a reflex action. The smooth muscle in the wall of the esophagus contracts in a rhythmic sequence from the upper esophagus toward the stomach to propel the bolus of food along the tract. During this process of esophageal peristalsis, the lower esophageal sphincter relaxes and permits the bolus of food to enter the stomach. Subsequently, the lower esophageal sphincter closes tightly to prevent reflux of stomach contents into the esophagus.

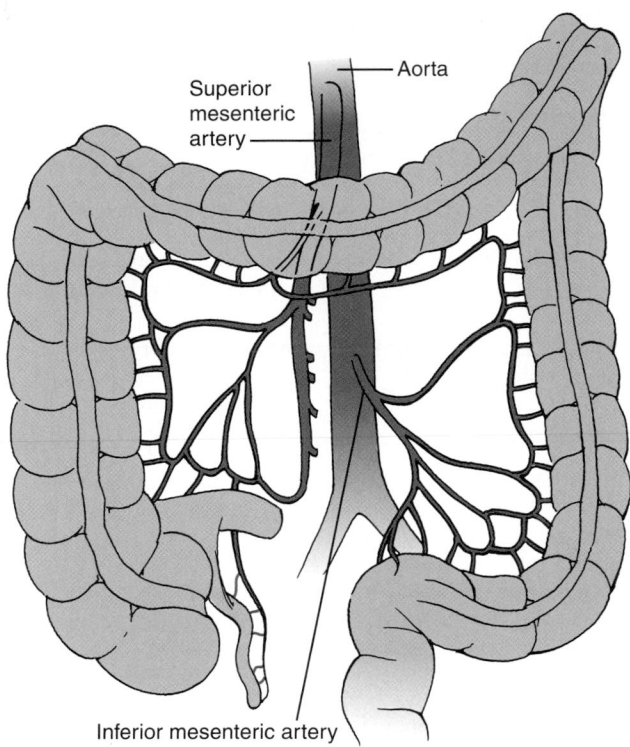

FIGURE 34-2 Anatomy and blood supply of the large intestine.

Gastric Function

The stomach stores and mixes the food with secretions. It secretes a highly acidic fluid in response to the presence or anticipated **ingestion** of food. This fluid, which may have a pH as low as 1, derives its acidity from the **hydrochloric acid** (HCl) secreted by the

glands of the stomach. The function of this gastric secretion is two-fold: to break down food into more absorbable components and to aid in the destruction of most ingested bacteria. The stomach can produce about 2.4 L per day of these gastric secretions. Gastric secretions also contain the enzyme **pepsin**, which is important for initiating protein digestion. **Intrinsic factor** is also secreted by the gastric mucosa. This compound combines with dietary vitamin B_{12} so that the vitamin can be absorbed in the ileum. In the absence of intrinsic factor, vitamin B_{12} cannot be absorbed and pernicious anemia results (see Chapter 33).

Peristaltic contractions in the stomach propel its contents toward the pylorus. Because large food particles cannot pass through the pyloric sphincter, they are churned back into the body of the stomach. In this way, food in the stomach is agitated mechanically and broken down into smaller particles. Food remains in the stomach for a variable length of time, from a half-hour to several hours, depending on the size of food particles, the composition of the meal, and other factors. Peristalsis in the stomach and contractions of the pyloric sphincter allow the partially digested food to enter the small intestine at a rate that permits efficient absorption of nutrients. This food mixed with gastric secretions is called **chyme**. Hormones, neuroregulators, and local regulators found in the gastric secretions control the rate of gastric secretions and influence gastric motility (Table 34-2).

Small Intestine Function

The digestive process continues in the duodenum. Secretions in the duodenum come from the accessory digestive organs—the pancreas, liver, and gallbladder—and the glands in the wall of the intestine itself. These secretions contain digestive enzymes and bile. Pancreatic secretions have an alkaline pH because of high concentrations of bicarbonate. This neutralizes the acid entering the duodenum from the stomach. The pancreas also secretes digestive enzymes, including **trypsin**, which aids in digesting protein; **amylase**, which aids in digesting starch; and **lipase**, which

Table 34-1 • The Major Digestive Enzymes and Secretions

ENZYME/SECRETION	ENZYME SOURCE	DIGESTIVE ACTION
Action of Enzymes That Digest Carbohydrates		
Ptyalin (salivary amylase)	Salivary glands	Starch→dextrin, maltose, glucose
Amylase	Pancreas and intestinal mucosa	Starch→dextrin, maltose, glucose
		Dextrin→maltose, glucose
Maltase	Intestinal mucosa	Maltose→glucose
Sucrase	Intestinal mucosa	Sucrose→glucose, fructose
Lactase	Intestinal mucosa	Lactose→glucose, galactose
Action of Enzymes/Secretions That Digest Protein		
Pepsin	Gastric mucosa	Protein→polypeptides
Trypsin	Pancreas	Proteins and polypeptides→polypeptides, dipeptides, amino acids
Aminopeptidase	Intestinal mucosa	Polypeptides→dipeptides, amino acids
Dipeptidase	Intestinal mucosa	Dipeptides→amino acids
Hydrochloric acid	Gastric mucosa	Protein→polypeptides, amino acids
Action of Enzymes That Digest Fat (Triglyceride)		
Pharyngeal lipase	Pharynx mucosa	Triglycerides→fatty acids, diglycerides, monoglycerides
Steapsin	Gastric mucosa	Triglycerides→fatty acids, diglycerides, monoglycerides
Pancreatic lipase	Pancreas	Triglycerides→fatty acids, diglycerides, monoglycerides
Bile	Liver and gallbladder	Fat emulsification

Table 34-2 • **The Major Gastrointestinal Regulatory Substances**

SUBSTANCE	STIMULUS FOR PRODUCTION	TARGET TISSUE	EFFECT ON SECRETIONS	EFFECT ON MOTILITY
Neuroregulators				
Acetylcholine	Sight, smell, chewing food, stomach distention	Gastric glands, other secretory glands, gastric and intestinal muscle	Increased gastric acid	Generally increased; decreased sphincter tone
Norepinephrine	Stress, other various stimuli	Secretory glands, gastric and intestinal muscle	Generally inhibitory	Generally decreased; increased sphincter tone
Hormonal Regulators				
Gastrin	Stomach distention with food	Gastric glands	Increased secretion of gastric juice, which is rich in HCl	Increased motility of stomach, decreased time required for gastric emptying. Relaxation of ileocecal sphincter. Excitation of colon. Constriction of gastro-esophageal sphincter
Cholecystokinin	Fat in duodenum	Gallbladder	Release of bile into duodenum	
		Pancreas	Increased production of enzyme-rich pancreatic secretions	
		Stomach	Inhibits gastric secretion somewhat	
Secretin	pH of chyme in duodenum below 4–5	Stomach	Inhibits gastric secretion somewhat	Inhibits stomach contractions
		Pancreas	Increased production of bicarbonate-rich pancreatic juice	
Local Regulator				
Histamine	Unclear; substances in food	Gastric glands	Increased gastric acid production	

aids in digesting fats. Bile (secreted by the liver and stored in the gallbladder) aids in emulsifying ingested fats, making them easier to digest and absorb.

The intestinal glands secrete mucus, hormones, electrolytes, and enzymes. The mucus coats the cells and protects the mucosa from injury by HCl. Hormones, neuroregulators, and local regulators found in these intestinal secretions control the rate of intestinal secretions and also influence GI motility. Intestinal secretions total approximately 1 L/day of pancreatic juice, 0.5 L/day of bile, and 3 L/day of secretions from the glands of the small intestine. Tables 34-1 and 34-2 summarize the actions of digestive enzymes and GI regulatory substances.

Two types of contractions occur regularly in the small intestine: segmentation contractions and intestinal peristalsis. *Segmentation contractions* produce mixing waves that move the intestinal contents back and forth in a churning motion. *Intestinal peristalsis* propels the contents of the small intestine toward the colon. Both movements are stimulated by the presence of chyme.

Food, initially ingested in the form of fats, proteins, and carbohydrates, is broken down into absorbable particles (constituent nutrients) by the process of digestion. Carbohydrates are broken down into disaccharides (eg, sucrose, maltose, galactose) and monosaccharides (eg, glucose, fructose). Glucose is the major carbohydrate that the tissue cells use as fuel. Proteins are broken down into amino acids and peptides. Ingested fats are emulsified into monoglycerides and fatty acids. These smaller molecules are then ready to be absorbed. Chyme stays in the small intestine for 3 to 6 hours, allowing for continued breakdown and absorption of nutrients.

Small, finger-like projections called villi are present throughout the entire intestine and function to produce digestive enzymes as well as to absorb nutrients. Absorption is the primary function of the small intestine. Vitamins and minerals are not digested but rather absorbed essentially unchanged. Absorption begins in the jejunum and is accomplished by both active transport and diffusion across the intestinal wall into the circulation. Absorption of different nutrients takes place at different locations in the small intestine. Iron and calcium absorption takes place in the duodenum. Fats, proteins, carbohydrates, sodium, and chloride are absorbed in the jejunum. Vitamin B_{12} and bile salts are absorbed in the ileum. Magnesium, phosphate, and potassium are absorbed throughout the small intestine (Society of Gastroenterologic Nursing and Associates, 1998).

Colonic Function

Within 4 hours after eating, residual waste material passes into the terminal ileum and passes slowly into the proximal portion of the colon through the ileocecal valve. This valve, which is normally closed, helps prevent colonic contents from refluxing into the small intestine. With each peristaltic wave of the small intestine, the valve opens briefly and permits some of the contents to pass into the colon.

Bacteria make up a major component of the contents of the large intestine. They assist in completing the breakdown of waste material, especially of undigested or unabsorbed proteins and bile salts. Two types of colonic secretions are added to the residual material: an electrolyte solution and mucus. The electrolyte solution is chiefly a bicarbonate solution that acts to neutralize the end products formed by the colonic bacterial action. The mucus protects the colonic mucosa from the interluminal contents and also provides adherence for the fecal mass.

Slow, weak peristaltic activity moves the colonic contents slowly along the tract. This slow transport allows efficient reabsorption of water and electrolytes, which is the primary purpose of the colon. Intermittent strong peristaltic waves propel the contents for considerable distances. This generally occurs after another meal is eaten, when intestine-stimulating hormones are released. The waste materials from a meal eventually reach and distend the rectum, usually in about 12 hours. As much as one fourth of the waste materials from a meal may still be in the rectum 3 days after the meal was ingested.

Waste Products of Digestion

Feces consist of undigested foodstuffs, inorganic materials, water, and bacteria. Fecal matter is about 75% fluid and 25% solid material. The composition is relatively unaffected by alterations in diet, because a large portion of the fecal mass is of nondietary origin, derived from the secretions of the GI tract. The brown color of the feces results from the breakdown of bile by the intestinal bacteria. Chemicals formed by intestinal bacteria (especially indole and skatole) are responsible in large part for the fecal odor. Gases formed contain methane, hydrogen sulfide, and ammonia, among others. The GI tract normally contains approximately 150 mL of these gases, which are either absorbed into the portal circulation and detoxified by the liver or expelled from the rectum as flatus.

Elimination of stool begins with distention of the rectum, which reflexively initiates contractions of the rectal musculature and relaxes the normally closed internal anal sphincter. The internal sphincter is controlled by the autonomic nervous system; the external sphincter is under the conscious control of the cerebral cortex. During defecation, the external anal sphincter voluntarily relaxes to allow colonic contents to be expelled. Normally, the external anal sphincter is maintained in a state of tonic contraction. Thus, defecation is seen to be a spinal reflex (involving the parasympathetic nerve fibers) that can be inhibited voluntarily by keeping the external anal sphincter closed. Contracting the abdominal muscles (straining) facilitates emptying of the colon. The average frequency of defecation in humans is once daily, but the frequency varies among individuals.

Assessment

HEALTH HISTORY AND CLINICAL MANIFESTATIONS

The nurse begins by taking a complete history, focusing on symptoms common to GI dysfunction. These symptoms include pain, indigestion, intestinal gas, nausea and vomiting, hematemesis, and changes in bowel habits and stool characteristics. Information about any previous GI disease is important. The nurse notes past and current medication use and any previous treatment or surgery. Information pertaining to medications is of particular interest because medications are a frequent cause of GI symptoms. The nurse takes a dietary history to assess nutritional status. Questioning about the use of tobacco and alcohol includes details about type and amount. The nurse and patient discuss changes in appetite or eating patterns and any examples of unexplained weight gain or loss over the past year. The nurse also assesses the stool characteristics. The nurse records all abnormal findings and reports them to the physician. It is important to include in the history questions about psychosocial, spiritual, or cultural factors that may be affecting the patient.

Pain

Pain can be a major symptom of GI disease. The character, duration, pattern, frequency, location, distribution of referred pain (Fig. 34-3), and time of the pain vary greatly depending on the underlying cause. Other factors, such as meals, rest, defecation, and vascular disorders, may directly affect this pain.

Indigestion

Upper abdominal discomfort or distress associated with eating (commonly called *indigestion*) is the most common symptom of patients with GI dysfunction. The basis for this abdominal distress may be the patient's own gastric peristaltic movements. Bowel movements may or may not relieve the pain. Indigestion can result from disturbed nervous system control of the stomach

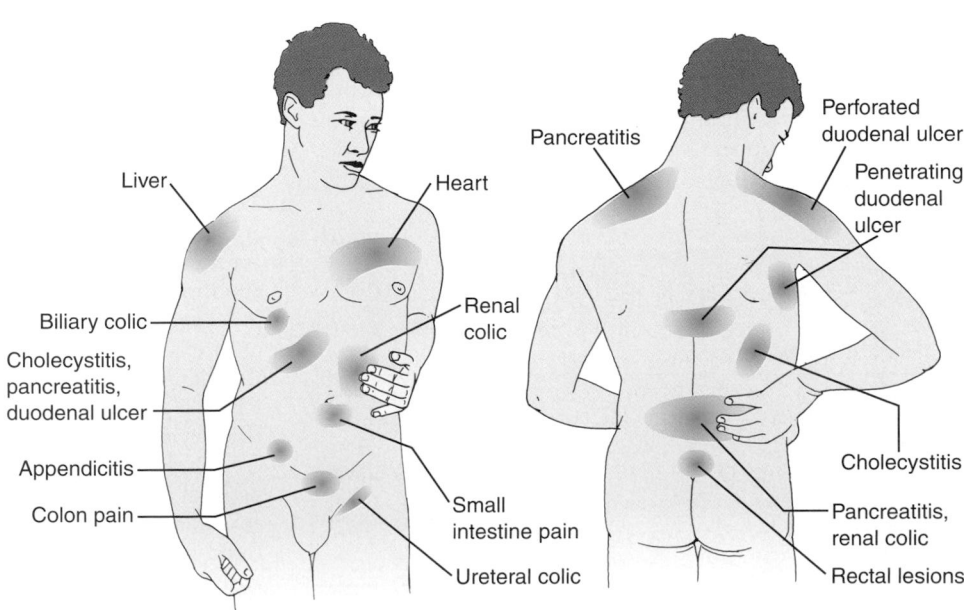

FIGURE 34-3 Common sites of referred abdominal pain.

or from a disorder in the GI tract or elsewhere in the body. Fatty foods tend to cause the most discomfort, because they remain in the stomach longer than proteins or carbohydrates do. Coarse vegetables and highly seasoned foods can also cause considerable distress.

Intestinal Gas

The accumulation of gas in the GI tract may result in belching (the expulsion of gas from the stomach through the mouth) or flatulence (the expulsion of gas from the rectum). It is through belching that swallowed air is expelled quickly when it reaches the stomach. Usually, gases in the small intestine pass into the colon and are released as flatus. Patients often complain of bloating, distention, or being "full of gas." Excessive flatulence may be a symptom of gallbladder disease or food intolerance.

Nausea and Vomiting

Vomiting is another major symptom of GI disease. Vomiting is usually preceded by nausea, which can be triggered by odors, activity, or food intake. The emesis, or vomitus, may vary in color and content. It may contain undigested food particles or blood (hematemesis). When vomiting occurs soon after hemorrhage, the emesis is bright red. If blood has been retained in the stomach, it takes on a coffee-ground appearance because of the action of the digestive enzymes.

Change in Bowel Habits and Stool Characteristics

Changes in bowel habits may signal colon disease. Diarrhea (an abnormal increase in the frequency and liquidity of the stool or in daily stool weight or volume) commonly occurs when the contents move so rapidly through the intestine and colon that there is inadequate time for the GI secretions to be absorbed. Diarrhea is sometimes associated with abdominal pain or cramping and nausea or vomiting. Constipation (a decrease in the frequency of stool, or stools that are hard, dry, and of smaller volume than normal) may be associated with anal discomfort and rectal bleeding. See Chapter 38 for further discussion of diarrhea and constipation.

The characteristics of the stool can vary greatly. Stool is normally light to dark brown. However, many circumstances, including the ingestion of certain foods and medications, can change the appearance of stool (Table 34-3). Blood in the stool can present in various ways and must be investigated. If blood is shed in sufficient quantities into the upper GI tract, it produces a tarry-black color

(melena). Blood entering the lower portion of the GI tract or passing rapidly through it will appear bright or dark red. Lower rectal or anal bleeding is suspected if there is streaking of blood on the surface of the stool or if blood is noted on toilet tissue. Other common abnormalities in stool characteristics that the patient may describe during the health history include the following:

- Bulky, greasy, foamy stools that are foul in odor; stool color is gray, with a silvery sheen
- Light gray or clay-colored stool, caused by the absence of urobilin
- Stool with mucus threads or pus that may be visible on gross inspection of the stool
- Small, dry, rock-hard masses called scybala; sometimes streaked with blood from rectal trauma as they pass through the rectum
- Loose, watery stool that may or may not be streaked with blood

PHYSICAL ASSESSMENT

The physical examination includes assessment of the mouth, abdomen, and rectum. The mouth, tongue, buccal mucosa, teeth, and gums are inspected, and ulcers, nodules, swelling, discoloration, and inflammation are noted. People with dentures should remove them during this part of the examination to allow good visualization.

The patient lies supine with knees flexed slightly for inspection, auscultation, palpation, and percussion of the abdomen (Fig. 34-4). The nurse performs inspection first, noting skin changes and scars from previous surgery. It also is important to note the contour and symmetry of the abdomen, to identify any localized bulging, distention, or peristaltic waves.

The nurse performs auscultation before percussion and palpation (which can increase intestinal motility and thereby change bowel sounds) and notes the character, location, and frequency of bowel sounds. The nurse assesses bowel sounds in all four quadrants using the diaphragm of the stethoscope; the high-pitched and gurgling sounds can be heard best in this manner. It is important to document the frequency of the sounds, using the terms *normal* (sounds heard about every 5 to 20 seconds), *hypoactive* (one or two sounds in 2 minutes), *hyperactive* (5 to 6 sounds heard in less than 30 seconds), or *absent* (no sounds in 3 to 5 minutes).

The nurse notes tympany or dullness during percussion. Use of light palpation is appropriate for identifying areas of tenderness or swelling; the nurse may use deep palpation to identify masses in any of the four quadrants. If the patient identifies any area of discomfort, the nurse can assess for rebound tenderness. To elicit rebound tenderness, the nurse exerts pressure over the area and then releases it quickly. It is important to note any pain experienced on withdrawal of the pressure. The nurse notes any abnormal finding in relation to the surface landmarks (xiphoid process, costal margins, anterior iliac spine, and symphysis pubis) or in relation to the four quadrants commonly used to describe the abdomen (right upper quadrant, RUQ; right lower quadrant, RLQ; left upper quadrant, LUQ; and left lower quadrant, LLQ) (Bickley & Hoekelman, 1999).

The final part of the examination is inspection of the anal and perineal area. The nurse should inspect and palpate areas of excoriation or rash, fissures or fistula openings, or external hemorrhoids. A digital rectal examination can be performed to note any areas of tenderness or mass.

Table 34-3 • Foods and Medications That Alter Stool Color

ALTERING SUBSTANCE	COLOR
Meat protein	Dark brown
Spinach	Green
Carrots and beets	Red
Cocoa	Dark red or brown
Senna	Yellow
Bismuth, iron, licorice, and charcoal	Black
Barium	Milky white

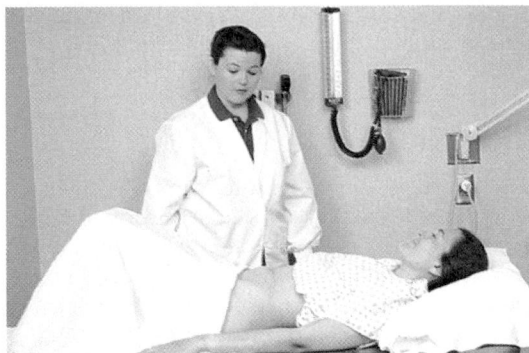

Inspecting the abdomen

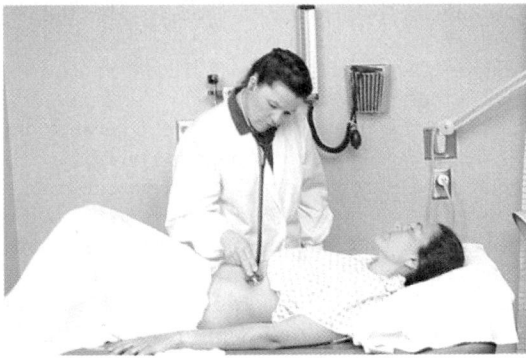

Auscultating the abdomen

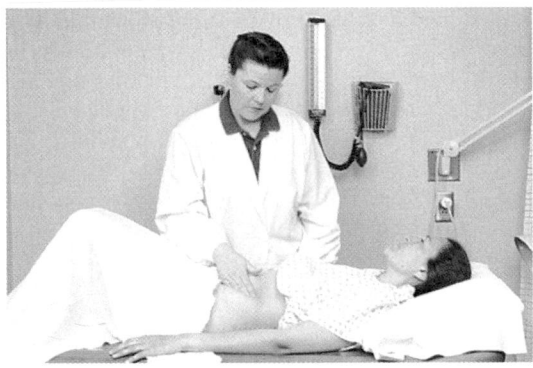

Palpating the abdomen

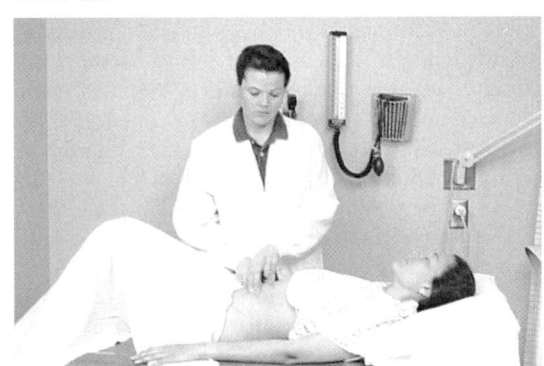

Percussing the abdomen

FIGURE 34-4 Examination of the abdomen includes inspection, auscultation, palpation, and percussion.

Diagnostic Evaluation

Blood tests are ordered initially. Common blood tests include complete blood count (CBC), carcinoembryonic antigen (CEA), liver function tests, serum cholesterol, and triglycerides. Test findings may reveal alterations in basal metabolic function and may indicate the severity of a disorder.

Many other modalities are available for diagnostic assessment of the GI tract. The majority of these tests and procedures are performed on an outpatient basis in special units designed for this purpose (eg, endoscopy or GI laboratory). The nurse supports and educates patients who are undergoing diagnostic evaluation, whether in an inpatient or an outpatient setting. Patients who require such tests frequently are anxious, elderly, or debilitated. The preparation for many of these studies includes fasting, the use of laxatives or enemas, and ingestion or injection of a contrast agent or a radiopaque dye. These preparatory measures are poorly tolerated by weak and many elderly patients and have the potential to cause fluid and electrolyte imbalances. If further assessment or treatment is needed after any outpatient procedure, the patient may be admitted to the hospital.

Specific nursing interventions for each test are provided later in this chapter. General nursing interventions for the patient who is having GI diagnostic assessment include the following:

- Providing general information about a healthy diet and the nutritional factors that can cause GI disturbances; after a diagnosis has been confirmed, the nurse provides information about specific nutrients that should be included in the diet

- Providing needed information about the test and the activities required of the patient
- Providing instructions about postprocedure care and activity restrictions
- Alleviating anxiety
- Helping the patient cope with discomfort
- Encouraging family members or others to offer emotional support to the patient during the diagnostic testing
- Assessing for adequate hydration before, during, and immediately after the procedure, and providing education about maintenance of hydration

STOOL TESTS

Basic examination of the stool includes inspecting the specimen for consistency and color and testing for occult (not visible) blood. Special tests, including tests for fecal urobilinogen, fat, nitrogen, parasites, pathogens, food residues, and other substances, require that the specimen be sent to the laboratory.

Stool samples are usually collected on a random basis unless a quantitative study (eg, fecal fat, urobilinogen) is to be performed. Random specimens should be sent promptly to the laboratory for analysis. The quantitative 24- to 72-hour collections must be kept refrigerated until they are taken to the laboratory. Some stool collections require the patient to follow a special diet or to refrain from taking certain medications before the collection. It is important to follow test guidelines closely for accurate results.

Fecal occult blood testing is one of the most commonly performed stool tests. It can be useful in initial screening for several disorders. It tests only for the presence of blood, so other follow-up testing is required. It is most frequently used in cancer screening programs and for early cancer detection (Chart 34-1). The test can be performed at the bedside, in the laboratory, or at home. It tests for heme, the iron-containing portion of the hemoglobin molecule that is altered during transit through the intestines.

Probably the most widely used occult blood test is the Hematest. It is inexpensive and noninvasive, and it carries no risk to the patient. It should not, however, be performed when there is hemorrhoidal bleeding. The test can be performed at home as well as in the doctor's office. The patient provides a stool specimen, and the physician smears it on a dry, guaiac-impregnated paper slide. If the test is done at home, the patient mails the slide to the physician in an envelope provided for that purpose. The stool specimen is then examined for occult blood. Serial 3- to 6-day testing is recommended. The test is not perfect, because certain factors interfere with its sensitivity and specificity. False-positive results may occur if the patient has eaten rare meat, liver, poultry, turnips, broccoli, cauliflower, melons, salmon, sardines, or horseradish within 7 days before testing. Medications that can cause gastric irritation, such as aspirin, ibuprofen, indomethacin, colchicine, corticosteroids, cancer chemotherapeutic agents, and anticoagulants, may also cause false-positive results. Extensive research has demonstrated that therapeutic doses of iron preparations do not cause false-positive results. Ingestion of vitamin C from supplements or foods can cause false-negative results. Therefore, a careful assessment of the patient's diet and medication regimen is essential to reduce incorrect interpretation of results (Ahmed, 2000).

Other occult blood tests that may yield more specific and more sensitive readings include Hematest II SENSA and HemoQuant. Immunologic tests are more specific to human hemoglobin and decrease the problem of dietary interference. Hemoporphyrin assays detect the broadest range of blood derivatives, but a strict dietary protocol is essential. Immunochemical tests using anti-human antibodies that are extremely sensitive to human hemoglobin are also available.

BREATH TESTS

The *hydrogen breath test* was developed to evaluate carbohydrate absorption. It also is used to aid in the diagnosis of bacterial overgrowth in the intestine and short bowel syndrome. This test determines the amount of hydrogen expelled in the breath after it has been produced in the colon (on contact of galactose with fermenting bacteria) and absorbed into the blood.

Urea breath tests detect the presence of *Helicobacter pylori,* the bacteria that can live in the mucosal lining of the stomach and cause peptic ulcer disease. The patient takes a capsule of carbon-labeled urea and then provides a breath sample 10 to 20 minutes later. Because *H. pylori* metabolizes urea rapidly, the labeled carbon is absorbed quickly; it can then be measured as carbon dioxide in the expired breath to determine whether *H. pylori* is present. The patient is instructed to avoid antibiotics or loperamide (Pepto-Bismol) for 1 month before the test; sucralfate (Carafate) and omeprazole (Prilosec) for 1 week before the test; and cimetidine (Tagamet), famotidine (Pepcid), ranitidine (Zantac), and nizatidine (Axid) for 24 hours before urea breath testing. *H. pylori* also can be detected by assessing serum antibody levels.

ABDOMINAL ULTRASONOGRAPHY

Ultrasonography is a noninvasive diagnostic technique in which high-frequency sound waves are passed into internal body structures and the ultrasonic echoes are recorded on an oscilloscope as they strike tissues of different densities. During abdominal ultrasonography, an image of the abdominal organs and structures is produced on the oscilloscope. This procedure is generally used to indicate the size and configuration of abdominal structures. It is particularly useful in the detection of cholelithiasis, cholecystitis, and appendicitis. Most recently this technique has proven useful in diagnosing acute colonic diverticulitis.

Advantages of abdominal ultrasonography are that it requires no ionizing radiation, there are no noticeable side effects, and it is relatively inexpensive. One disadvantage is that it cannot be used to examine structures that lie behind bony tissue, because bone prevents sound waves from passing to deeper structures. Gas and fluid in the abdomen or air in the lungs also prevent transmission of ultrasound.

Endoscopic ultrasonography (EUS) is a specialized enteroscopic procedure that aids in the diagnosis of GI disorders by providing direct imaging of a target area. A small high-frequency ultrasonic transducer is mounted at the tip of the fiberoptic scope so that a transintestinal study can be completed. This procedure gives results with better quality resolution and definition than regular ultrasound imaging. It helps in staging of a tumor, including size, spread, and whether the tumor is operable. It is useful in evaluating transmural changes in the bowel wall that occur in ulcerative colitis. Intestinal gas, bone, and thick layers of adipose tissue (all of which hamper conventional ultrasonography) are not problems when this technique is used.

Nursing Interventions

The patient fasts for 8 to 12 hours before the test to decrease the amount of gas in the bowel. If gallbladder studies are being performed, the patient should eat a fat-free meal the evening before

---

Chart 34-1

Health Promotion: Guidelines for Colorectal Cancer Screening

For adults older than 50 years of age, one of the screening approaches below should be followed:

If low-to-average risk (asymptomatic):
- Digital rectal examination annually
- Fecal occult blood testing annually

AND
- Flexible sigmoidoscopy every 5 years

If moderate risk (colorectal cancer in family members):
- Digital rectal examination annually
- Fecal occult blood testing annually

AND
- Colonoscopy every 5–10 years (if there is a history of polypectomy, colonoscopy in 1 year and then every 5 years)

If high risk (family history of hereditary disease or inflammatory bowel disease):
- Digital rectal examination annually
- Fecal occult blood testing annually
- Flexible sigmoidoscopy every 1–2 years

OR
- Colonoscopy every 1–2 years
- Genetic testing

From Pontieri-Lewis, V. (2000). Colorectal cancer. *MedSurg Nursing, 9,* 9–15, 20.

the test. If barium studies are to be performed, the nurse should make sure they are scheduled after this test; otherwise, the barium will interfere with the transmission of the sound waves.

DNA TESTING

Researchers have refined methods for genetic risk assessment, preclinical diagnosis, and prenatal diagnosis to identify persons who are at risk for certain GI disorders (eg, gastric cancer, lactose deficiency, inflammatory bowel disease, colon cancer). In some cases, DNA testing allows practitioners to prevent (or minimize) disease, by intervening before its onset, and to improve therapy. Persons who are identified as at risk for certain GI disorders may choose to undergo genetic counseling to learn about the disease; to understand options for preventing and treating the disease; and to receive support in coping with the situation (Yamada, 1999). Persons at risk for colon cancer often are targeted for DNA testing because it can provide a head start on this preventable cancer.

IMAGING STUDIES

Imaging studies include x-ray and contrast studies, computed tomography (CT) scans, magnetic resonance imaging (MRI), and scintigraphy (radionuclide imaging).

Upper Gastrointestinal Tract Study

X-rays can delineate the entire GI tract after the introduction of a contrast agent. A radiopaque liquid (eg, barium sulfate) is commonly used. The patient ingests this tasteless, odorless, nongranular, and completely insoluble (hence, not absorbable) powder in the form of a thick or thin aqueous suspension for the purpose of studying the upper GI tract (upper GI series or barium swallow). The upper GI series enables the examiner to detect or exclude anatomic or functional derangement of the upper GI organs or sphincters. It also aids in the diagnosis of ulcers, varices, tumors, regional enteritis, and malabsorption syndromes. The procedure may be extended to examine the duodenum and small bowel (small bowel follow-through).

The patient swallows barium under direct fluoroscopic examination. As the barium descends into the stomach, the position, patency, and caliber of the esophagus are visualized, enabling the examiner to detect or exclude any anatomic or functional derangement of that organ. Fluoroscopic examination next extends to the stomach as its lumen fills with barium, allowing observation of stomach motility, thickness of the gastric wall, the mucosal pattern, patency of the pyloric valve, and the anatomy of the duodenum. Multiple x-ray films are obtained during the procedure, and additional images may be taken at intervals for up to

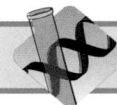

GENETICS IN NURSING PRACTICE—Digestive and Gastrointestinal Disorders

SELECTED DIGESTIVE AND GASTROINTESTINAL DISORDERS INFLUENCED BY GENETIC FACTORS
- Cleft lip and/or palate
- Familial adenomatous polyposis
- Hereditary nonpolyposis colorectal cancer (HNPCC)
- Hirschsprung disease (aganglionic megacolon)
- Inflammatory bowel disease (eg, Crohn's disease)
- Pyloric stenosis

NURSING ASSESSMENTS
FAMILY HISTORY ASSESSMENT
- Careful family history assessment for other family members with a similar condition (eg, cleft lip/palate, pyloric stenosis)
- Assess for other family members in several generations with early-onset colorectal cancer
- Inquire about other family members with inflammatory bowel disease
- Assess family history for other cancers (eg, endometrial, ovarian, renal)

PHYSICAL ASSESSMENT
Assess for presence of other clinical symptoms:
- With clefting—congenital heart defect, mental retardation, other birth defects suggestive of a genetic syndrome
- With familial adenomatous polyposis—congenital hypertrophy of retinal pigment epithelium (CHRPE)

MANAGEMENT ISSUES SPECIFIC TO GENETICS
- Inquire whether any affected family member has had DNA mutation testing

- If indicated, refer for further genetic counseling and evaluation so that family members can discuss inheritance, risk to other family members, availability of genetic testing, and gene-based interventions
- Offer appropriate genetics information and resources
- Assess patients' understanding of genetics information
- Provide support to families with newly diagnosed genetics-related digestive disorders
- Participate in management and coordination of care for patients with genetic conditions and for those who are predisposed to develop or pass on a genetic condition

GENETICS RESOURCES
Genetic Alliance—a directory of support groups for patients and families with genetic conditions; http://www.geneticalliance.org.

American Cancer Society—offers general information about cancer and support resources for families; http://www.cancer.org.

Gene Clinics—a listing of common genetic disorders with up-to-date clinical summaries, genetic counseling and testing information; http://www.geneclinics.org.

National Organization of Rare Disorders—a directory of support groups and information for patients and families with rare genetic disorders; http://www.rarediseases.org.

National Cancer Institute—current information about cancer research, treatment, resources for health providers, individuals, and families; http://www.nci.nih.gov.

Online Mendelian Inheritance in Man (OMIM)—a complete listing of inherited genetic conditions; http://www.ncbi.nlm.nih.gov/omim/stats/html.

24 hours to evaluate the rate of gastric emptying. Small bowel x-rays taken while the barium is passing through that area allow for observation of the motility of the small bowel. Obstructions, ileitis, and diverticula can be detected if present.

Variations of the upper GI study include double-contrast studies and enteroclysis. The double-contrast method of examining the upper GI tract involves administration of a thick barium suspension to outline the stomach and esophageal wall, after which tablets that release carbon dioxide in the presence of water are given. This technique has the advantage of showing the esophagus and stomach in finer detail, permitting signs of early superficial neoplasms to be noted.

Enteroclysis is a very detailed, double-contrast study of the entire small intestine that involves the continuous infusion, through a duodenal tube, of 500 to 1000 mL of a thin barium sulfate suspension. Methylcellulose is then infused into the small intestine through the tube. The barium and methylcellulose fill the intestinal loops and are observed continuously by fluoroscopy and viewed at frequent intervals as they progress through the jejunum and the ileum. This process (even with normal motility) can take up to 6 hours. The procedure aids in the diagnosis of partial small-bowel obstructions or diverticula.

NURSING INTERVENTIONS

The patient may need to maintain a low-residue diet for several days before the test. He or she should receive nothing by mouth after midnight before the test. The physician may prescribe a laxative to clean out the intestinal tract. Because smoking can stimulate gastric motility, the nurse discourages the patient from smoking on the morning before the examination. In addition, the nurse withholds all medications.

Follow-up care is needed after any of the upper GI procedures to ensure that the patient has completely eliminated the ingested barium. Fluids must be increased to facilitate evacuation of stool and barium. The nurse monitors the patient's stools until they return to their normal color (the barium will look like clay). A laxative or enema may be needed.

Lower Gastrointestinal Tract Study

When barium is instilled rectally to visualize the lower GI tract, the procedure is called a barium enema. The purpose of a barium enema is to detect the presence of polyps, tumors, and other lesions of the large intestine and to demonstrate any abnormal anatomy or malfunction of the bowel.

The radiopaque substance is instilled rectally in the radiology department during fluoroscopy. If the patient has been prepared adequately and the colon has been evacuated completely, the contour of the entire colon, including the cecum and appendix (if patent), is clearly visible and the motility of each portion may be observed readily. The procedure usually takes about 15 to 30 minutes, during which time x-ray images are taken.

Other means for visualizing the colon include double-contrast studies and a water-soluble contrast study. A double-contrast or air-contrast barium enema involves the instillation of a thicker barium solution, followed by the instillation of air. The patient may feel some cramping or discomfort with this process. This test provides a contrast between the air-filled lumen and the barium-coated mucosa, allowing easier detection of smaller lesions.

If active inflammatory disease, fistulas, or perforation of the colon is suspected, a water-soluble iodinated contrast agent (eg, Gastrografin) can be used. The procedure is the same as for a barium enema; however, the patient must be assessed for allergy to iodine or contrast agent. The contrast agent is eliminated readily after the procedure, so there is no need for postprocedure laxatives. Some diarrhea may occur in a few patients until the contrast agent has been totally eliminated.

NURSING INTERVENTIONS

Preparing the patient includes emptying and cleansing the lower bowel. This often necessitates a low-residue diet 1 to 2 days before the test (the preparation required by different radiology departments may vary); a clear liquid diet and a laxative the evening before; nothing by mouth after midnight; and cleansing enemas until returns are clear the following morning. The nurse should make sure that barium enemas are scheduled before any upper GI studies. If the patient has active inflammatory disease of the colon, enemas are contraindicated. Barium enema also is contraindicated in patients with signs of perforation or obstruction; instead, a water-soluble contrast study may be performed in these situations. Active GI bleeding may prohibit the use of laxatives and enemas.

The nurse administers an enema or laxative after these tests to facilitate barium removal. Increasing fluid intake also will assist in eliminating the barium. As with any barium study, the nurse monitors the patient for complete elimination of the barium.

Computed Tomography

CT provides cross-sectional images of abdominal organs and structures. Multiple x-ray images are taken from many different angles, digitized in the computer, reconstructed, and then viewed on a computer monitor. Indications for abdominal CT scanning are diseases of the liver, spleen, kidney, pancreas, and pelvic organs. CT is a valuable tool for detecting and localizing many inflammatory conditions in the colon, such as appendicitis, diverticulitis, regional enteritis, and ulcerative colitis. Because the adequacy of detail in the test depends on the presence of fat, this diagnostic tool is not useful for very thin, cachectic patients. The procedure is completely painless, but radiation doses are considerable. Because a scanning time of 5 seconds is required, motion artifacts produced by heartbeat and respiration cannot be avoided, resulting in pictures that are less than clear.

New, continuous-motion (helical or spiral), three-dimensional CT scans have been developed that provide very detailed pictures of the GI organs and vasculature (Yamada, 1999). Colonography can be completed in minutes. It involves inserting a thin, straw-like tube into the colon and inflating the bowel with air to generate a computer image of the intestine. There is little discomfort, and sedation is not needed.

NURSING INTERVENTIONS

The patient should not eat or drink for 6 to 8 hours before the test. The practitioner may prescribe an intravenous or oral contrast agent. Therefore, the nurse should question the patient about contrast dye allergies. If barium studies are to be performed, it is important to schedule them after CT scanning, so as not to interfere with imaging.

Magnetic Resonance Imaging

MRI is used in gastroenterology to supplement ultrasonography and CT scanning. It is a noninvasive technique that uses magnetic fields and radio waves to produce an image of the area being studied. The use of oral contrast agents to enhance the image has increased the application of this technique for the diagnosis of GI diseases. It is useful in evaluating abdominal soft tissues as well as blood vessels, abscesses, fistulas, neoplasms, and other sources of bleeding.

The physiologic artifacts of heartbeat, respiration, and peristalsis may create a less-than-clear image. Newer, fast-imaging MRI techniques help to eliminate these physiologic motion artifacts. MRI is contraindicated for patients with permanent pacemakers, artificial heart valves and defibrillators, implanted insulin pumps, or implanted transcutaneous electrical nerve stimulation devices, because the magnetic field could cause malfunction. MRI is also contraindicated for patients with internal metal devices (eg, aneurysm clips) or intraocular metallic fragments.

NURSING INTERVENTIONS

The patient should not eat or drink for 6 to 8 hours before the test. Before the test, the patient must remove all jewelry and other metals. The patient lies in a machine that constructs an image based on the magnetic field created between the machine and the structures scanned. The entire procedure takes 30 to 90 minutes.

It is important to warn patients that the close-fitting scanners used in many MRI facilities may induce feelings of claustrophobia and that the machine will make a knocking sound during the procedure. Open MRIs that are less close-fitting eliminate the claustrophobia that many patients experience.

Scintigraphy

Scintigraphy (radionuclide testing) relies on the use of radioactive isotopes (ie, technetium, iodine, and indium) to reveal displaced anatomic structures, changes in organ size, and the presence of neoplasms or other focal lesions, such as cysts or abscesses.

Scintigraphic scanning is also used to measure the uptake of tagged red blood cells and leukocytes. Tagging of red blood cells and leukocytes by injection of a radionuclide is performed to define areas of inflammation, abscess, blood loss, or neoplasm. A sample of blood is removed, mixed with a radioactive substance, and reinjected into the patient. Abnormal concentrations of blood cells are then detected at 24- and 48-hour intervals.

Gastrointestinal Motility Studies

Radionuclide testing also is used to assess gastric emptying and colonic transit time. For gastric emptying studies, the liquid and solid components of a meal are tagged with radionuclide markers. After the patient ingests the meal, the patient is positioned under a scintiscanner, which measures the rate of passage of the radioactive substance out of the stomach. This is useful in diagnosing disorders of gastric motility. Radionuclide evaluation of gastric emptying is now preferred over intubation methods because it gives more defined results (Phillips & Wingate, 1998). This procedure is helpful for evaluating any functional cause of gastric emptying, but its most common clinical uses at this time are in the evaluation of diabetic gastroparesis and of the rapid emptying process in the dumping syndrome.

Colonic transit studies are used to evaluate colonic motility instances of chronic constipation and obstructive defecation syndromes. This is usually an outpatient study. The patient is given a capsule containing 20 radionuclide markers and instructions to follow a regular diet and normal daily activities. Abdominal x-rays are taken every 24 hours until all markers are passed. This process usually takes 4 to 5 days, but in the presence of severe constipation it may take as long as 10 days. People with chronic diarrhea may be evaluated at 8-hour intervals. The amount of time it takes for the radioactive material to move through the colon indicates colonic motility.

ENDOSCOPIC PROCEDURES

Endoscopic procedures used in GI tract assessment include fibroscopy/esophagogastroduodenoscopy, anoscopy, proctoscopy, sigmoidoscopy, colonoscopy, small-bowel enteroscopy, and endoscopy through ostomy.

Upper Gastrointestinal Fibroscopy/ Esophagogastroduodenoscopy

Fiberscopes are flexible scopes equipped with fiberoptic lenses. **Fibroscopy** of the upper GI tract allows direct visualization of the esophageal, gastric, and duodenal mucosa through a lighted endoscope (gastroscope) (Fig. 34-5). This procedure,

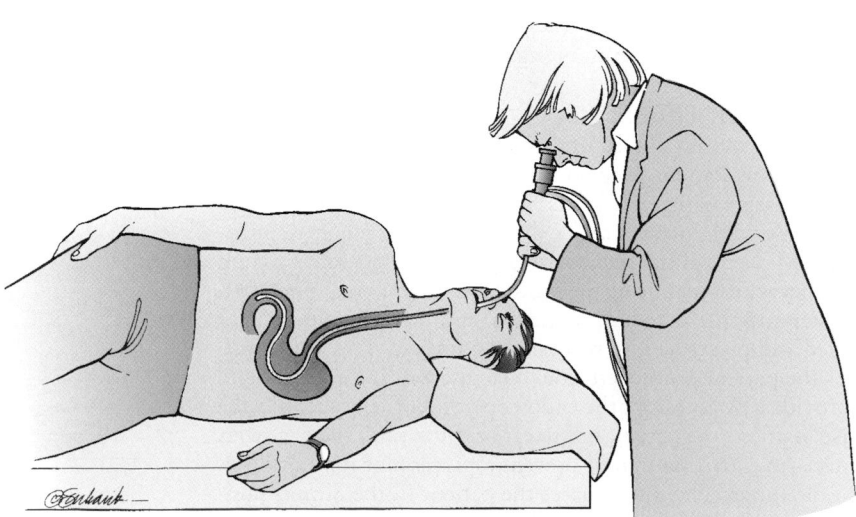

FIGURE 34-5 Patient undergoing gastroscopy.

called esophagogastroduodenoscopy (EGD), is especially valuable when esophageal, gastric, or duodenal abnormalities or inflammatory, neoplastic, or infectious processes are suspected. This procedure also can be used to evaluate esophageal and gastric motility and to collect secretions and tissue specimens for further analysis.

The gastroenterologist views the GI tract through a viewing lens and can take still or video photographs through the scope to document findings. Electronic video endoscopes also are available that attach directly to a video processor, converting the electronic signals into pictures on a television screen. This allows larger and continuous viewing capabilities, as well as the simultaneous recording of the procedure.

Side-viewing flexible scopes are used to visualize the common bile duct and the pancreatic and hepatic ducts through the ampulla of Vater in the duodenum. This procedure, called endoscopic retrograde cholangiopancreatography (ERCP), uses the endoscope in combination with radiographic techniques to view the ductal structures of the biliary tract. ERCP is helpful in evaluating jaundice, pancreatitis, pancreatic tumors, common duct stones, and biliary tract disease. ERCP is described further in Chapter 40.

Upper GI fibroscopy also can be a therapeutic procedure when it is combined with other procedures. Therapeutic endoscopy can be used to remove common bile duct stones, dilate strictures, and treat gastric bleeding and esophageal varices. Laser-compatible scopes can be used to provide laser therapy for upper GI neoplasms. Sclerosing solutions can be injected through the scope in an attempt to control upper GI bleeding.

After the patient is sedated, the endoscope is lubricated with a water-soluble lubricant and passed smoothly and slowly along the back of the mouth and down into the esophagus. The gastroenterologist views the gastric wall and the sphincters, and then advances the endoscope into the duodenum for further examination. Biopsy forceps to obtain tissue specimens or cytology brushes to obtain cells for microscopic study can be passed through the scope. The procedure usually takes about 30 minutes.

The patient may experience nausea, gagging, or choking. Use of topical anesthetics and moderate sedation makes it important to monitor and maintain the oral airway during and after the procedure. Finger or ear oximeters are used to monitor oxygen saturation, and supplemental oxygen may be used if needed. Emergency equipment must be readily available. Precautions must be taken to protect the scope, because the fiberoptic bundles can be broken if the scope is bent at an acute angle. The patient wears a mouth guard to keep from biting the scope.

NURSING INTERVENTIONS

The patient should not eat or drink for 6 to 12 hours before the examination. Patient preparation includes helping the patient spray or gargle with a local anesthetic, and administering midazolam (Versed) intravenously just before the scope is introduced. Midazolam is a sedative that provides moderate sedation and relieves anxiety during the procedure. The nurse also may administer atropine to reduce secretions, and may give glucagon, if needed and prescribed, to relax smooth muscle. The nurse positions the patient on the left side to facilitate saliva drainage and to provide easy access for the endoscope. After the procedure, the nurse instructs the patient not to eat or drink until the gag reflex returns (in 1 to 2 hours), to prevent aspiration of food or fluids into the lungs. The nurse places the patient in the Simms position until he or she is awake and then places the patient in the semi-Fowler's position until ready for discharge. After gastroscopy,

assessment by the nurse includes observing for signs of perforation, such as pain, bleeding, unusual difficulty swallowing, and an elevated temperature. The nurse monitors the pulse and blood pressure for changes that can occur with sedation. The nurse can test the gag reflex by placing a tongue blade onto the back of the throat to see whether gagging occurs. After the patient's gag reflex has returned, the nurse can offer lozenges, saline gargle, and oral analgesics to relieve minor throat discomfort. Patients who were sedated for the procedure must stay on bed rest until fully alert. After moderate sedation, the patient must be accompanied and transported home if the procedure was performed on an outpatient basis. The nurse instructs the patient not to drive for 10 to 12 hours if sedation was used.

Anoscopy, Proctoscopy, and Sigmoidoscopy

The lower portion of the colon also can be viewed directly to evaluate rectal bleeding, acute or chronic diarrhea, or change in bowel patterns and to observe for ulceration, fissures, abscesses, tumors, polyps, or other pathologic processes. Rigid or flexible fiberoptic scopes can be used. The anoscope is a rigid scope that is used to examine the anus and lower rectum. Proctoscopes and sigmoidoscopes are rigid scopes that are used to inspect the rectum and the sigmoid colon.

Flexible scopes have largely replaced the rigid scopes for routine examinations. The flexible fiberoptic sigmoidoscope (Fig. 34-6) permits the colon to be examined up to 40 to 50 cm (16 to 20 inches) from the anus, much more than the 25 cm (10 inches) that can be visualized with the rigid sigmoidoscope. The flexible scope has many of the same capabilities as the scopes used for the upper GI study, including the use of still or video images to document findings.

For rigid scope procedures, the patient assumes the knee-chest position at the edge of the bed or the examining table. With the back inclined at about a 45-degree angle, the patient is properly positioned for the introduction of an anoscope, proctoscope, or

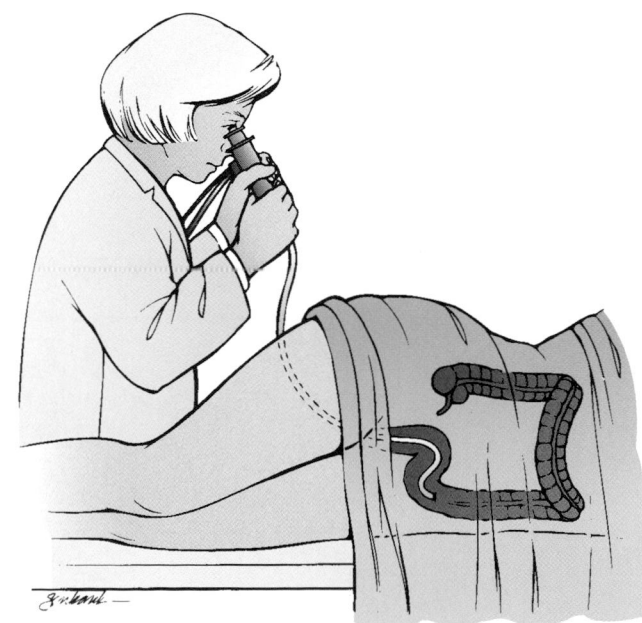

FIGURE 34-6 Flexible fiberoptic sigmoidoscopy. The flexible scope is advanced past the proximal sigmoid and then into the descending colon.

sigmoidoscope. During the examination, it is important to keep the patient informed about the progress of the examination and to explain that the pressure exerted by the instrument will create the urge to have a bowel movement.

For flexible scope procedures, the patient assumes a comfortable position on the left side with the right leg bent and placed anteriorly. Again, it is important to keep the patient informed throughout the examination and to explain the sensations associated with the examination. Biopsies and polypectomies can be performed during this procedure. Biopsy is performed with small biting forceps introduced through the endoscope; one or more small pieces of tissue may be removed. If rectal or sigmoid polyps are present, they may be removed with a wire snare, which is used to grasp the pedicle, or stalk. An electrocoagulating current is then used to sever the polyp and prevent bleeding. It is extremely important that all excised tissue be placed immediately in moist gauze or in an appropriate receptacle, labeled correctly, and delivered without delay to the pathology laboratory for examination.

NURSING INTERVENTIONS

These examinations require only limited bowel preparation, including a warm tap water or Fleet's enema until returns are clear. Dietary restrictions usually are not necessary, and sedation usually is not required. During the procedure, the nurse monitors vital signs, skin color and temperature, pain tolerance, and vagal response (Society of Gastroenterologic Nursing and Associates, 2000). After the procedure, the nurse monitors the patient for rectal bleeding and signs of intestinal perforation (ie, fever, rectal drainage, abdominal distention, and pain). On completion of the examination, the patient can resume regular activities and dietary practices.

Fiberoptic Colonoscopy

Direct visual inspection of the colon to the cecum is possible by means of a flexible fiberoptic colonoscope (Fig. 34-7). These scopes have the same capabilities as those used for esophagogastro-

duodenoscopy; however, they are larger in diameter and longer. Still and video recordings can be used to document the procedure and findings.

This procedure is used commonly as a diagnostic aid and screening device. It is most frequently used for cancer screening (see Chart 34-1) and for surveillance in patients with previous colon cancer or polyps. In addition, tissue biopsies can be obtained as needed, and polyps can be removed and evaluated. Other uses of colonoscopy include the evaluation of patients with diarrhea of unknown cause, occult bleeding, or anemia; further study of abnormalities detected on barium enema; and diagnosis, clarification, and determination of the extent of inflammatory or other bowel disease.

Therapeutically, the procedure can be used to remove all visible polyps with a special snare and cautery through the colonoscope. Many colon cancers begin with adenomatous polyps of the colon; therefore, one goal of colonoscopic polypectomy is early detection and prevention of colorectal cancer. This procedure also can be used to treat areas of bleeding or stricture. Use of bipolar and unipolar coagulators, use of heater probes, and injections of sclerosing agents or vasoconstrictors are all possible during this procedure. Laser-compatible scopes provide laser therapy for bleeding lesions or colonic neoplasms. Bowel decompression can also be completed during the procedure.

Colonoscopy is performed while the patient is lying on the left side with the legs drawn up toward the chest. The patient's position may be changed during the test to facilitate advancement of the scope. The procedure usually takes about 1 hour. Discomfort may result from instillation of air to expand the colon or from insertion and moving of the scope. Biopsy forceps or a cytology brush may be passed through the scope to obtain specimens for histology and cytology examinations. Potential complications of colonoscopy include cardiac dysrhythmias and respiratory depression resulting from the medications administered, vasovagal reactions, and circulatory overload or hypotension resulting from overhydration or underhydration during bowel preparation. Therefore, it is important to monitor the patient's cardiac and respiratory function continuously. Oxygen saturation is monitored with a

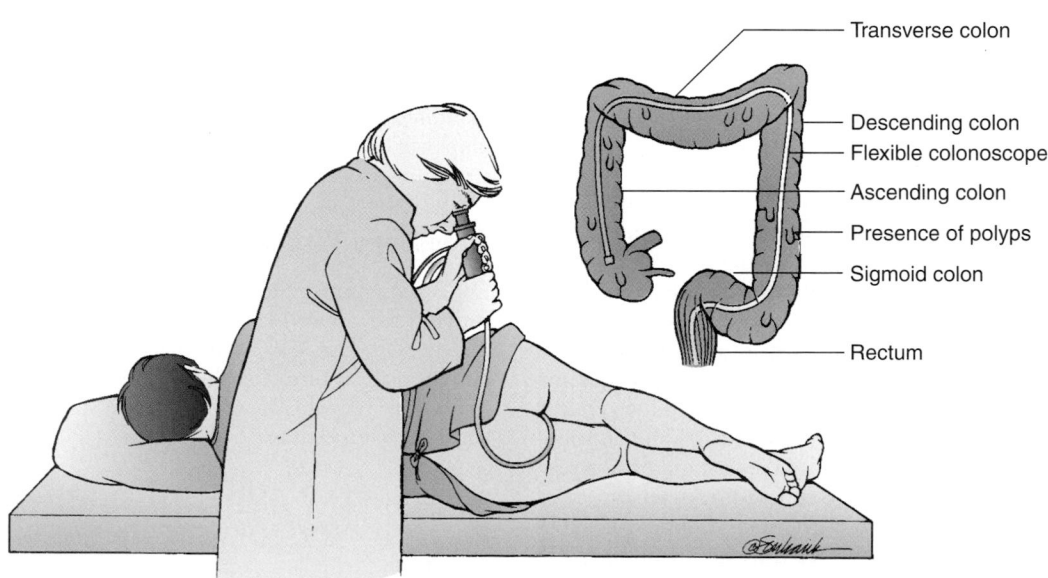

FIGURE 34-7 Colonoscopy. The flexible scope is passed through the rectum and sigmoid colon into the descending, transverse, and ascending colon.

finger or ear oximeter. Supplemental oxygen should be used as necessary.

NURSING INTERVENTIONS

The success of the procedure depends on how well the colon is prepared. Adequate colon cleansing provides optimal visualization and decreases the time needed for the procedure. First, the patient should limit the intake of liquids for 24 to 72 hours before the examination. Then, cleansing of the colon can be accomplished in various ways. The physician may prescribe a laxative for two nights before the examination and a Fleet's or saline enema until the return runs clear the morning of the test. More frequently, however, polyethylene glycol electrolyte lavage solutions (Golytely, Colyte, NuLytely) are used as intestinal lavages for effective cleansing of the bowel. The patient maintains a clear liquid diet starting at noon the day before the procedure. Then the patient ingests lavage solutions orally at intervals over 3 to 4 hours. If necessary, the nurse can give this solution through a feeding tube if the patient is unable to swallow. Patients with a colostomy can receive this same bowel preparation. With the use of lavage solutions, bowel cleansing is fast (rectal effluent is clear in about 4 hours) and is tolerated fairly well by most patients. Side effects of the electrolyte solutions include nausea, bloating, cramps or abdominal fullness, fluid and electrolyte imbalance, and hypothermia (patients are often told to drink the preparation as cold as possible to make it more palatable). The side effects are especially problematic for elderly patients, and sometimes they have difficulty ingesting the required volume of solution. The use of lavage solutions is contraindicated in patients with intestinal obstruction or inflammatory bowel disease.

Additional nursing actions include the following:

- Instructing the patient not to take routine medications when the lavage solution is ingested; the medications will not be digested and therefore will be ineffective
- Advising the diabetic patient to consult with his or her physician about medication adjustment to prevent hyperglycemia or hypoglycemia resulting from dietary modifications required in preparation for the test
- Instructing all patients, especially the elderly, to maintain adequate fluid, electrolyte, and caloric intake while undergoing bowel cleansing

Special precautions must be taken for some patients. Implantable defibrillators and pacemakers are at high risk for malfunction if electrosurgical procedures (ie, polypectomy) are performed in conjunction with colonoscopy. A cardiologist should be consulted before the test is performed, and the defibrillator should be turned off. These patients require careful cardiac monitoring during the procedure. Colonoscopy cannot be performed if there is a suspected or documented colon perforation, acute severe diverticulitis, or fulminant colitis. Therapeutic colonoscopy may be contraindicated in patients with coagulopathies and in those receiving anticoagulation therapy, because of the high risk for excessive bleeding during and after the procedure. Nonsteroidal anti-inflammatory agents (NSAIDs), aspirin, ticlopidine, and pentoxifylline must be discontinued before the test and for 2 weeks after the procedure. Patients taking coumadin or heparin must consult the physician for specific instructions. Those with prosthetic heart valves or a history of endocarditis require prophylactic antibiotics before the procedure.

Informed consent is obtained before the test. The patient receives nothing by mouth (NPO) after midnight before the test,

but most medications can be taken with a small amount of water; the physician should be consulted about medication use. Before the examination, the nurse may administer intravenously an opioid analgesic or a sedative (eg, midazolam) to provide moderate sedation and relieve anxiety during the procedure. Glucagon may be used, if needed, to relax the colonic musculature and to reduce spasm during the test. Elderly or debilitated patients may require a reduced dosage of these medications to decrease the risks of oversedation and cardiopulmonary complications.

During the procedure, the nurse monitors for changes in oxygen saturation, vital signs, color and temperature of the skin, level of consciousness, abdominal distention, vagal response, and pain intensity. After the procedure, patients who were sedated are maintained on bed rest until fully alert. Some will have abdominal cramps caused by increased peristalsis stimulated by the air insufflated into the bowel during the procedure. Immediately after the test, the nurse observes the patient for signs and symptoms of bowel perforation (eg, rectal bleeding, abdominal pain or distention, fever, focal peritoneal signs). If midazolam was used, the nurse explains its amnesic effects. It is important to provide written instructions, because the patient may be unable to recall verbal information. If the procedure is performed on an outpatient basis, someone must accompany and transport the patient home. After a therapeutic procedure, the nurse instructs the patient to report any bleeding to the physician.

Small-Bowel Enteroscopy

Technology for the use of the small-caliber transnasal endoscope to allow direct inspection of the wall of the small intestine continues to be developed. Two methods are being used at this time: the "push" and the "pull" endoscope methods. The "pull" endoscope is very long and flexible and has a balloon at its tip. When inflated, the balloon tip advances the scope by peristalsis through the small intestine. Reglan may be administered intravenously to assist passage. This procedure takes up to 10 hours to complete. The patient may be kept in the recovery area or sent home during this period. Once the scope has entered the distal ileum, the balloon is deflated and the tube is retracted slowly while the endoscopist examines the intestinal wall. "Push" endoscopes have been designed to be smaller in caliber and longer in length, while still allowing the use of biopsy forceps and probes (Lightdale, 2000). These two methods are especially useful in the evaluation of patients who have continued bleeding even after extensive diagnostic testing has identified no other problem area. They can also be used when biopsy of the small bowel is needed to diagnose malabsorption syndromes.

Endoscopy Through Ostomy

Endoscopy using a flexible endoscope through an ostomy stoma is useful for visualizing a segment of the small or large intestine. It may be indicated to evaluate an anastomosis, to screen for recurrent disease, or to visualize and treat bleeding in a segment of the bowel. Nursing interventions are similar to those for other endoscopic procedures.

MANOMETRY AND ELECTROPHYSIOLOGIC STUDIES

Manometry and electrophysiologic studies are methods for evaluating patients with GI motility disorders. The manometry test measures changes in intraluminal pressures and the coordination of muscle activity in the GI tract. The pressures can be recorded manually, on a physiograph, or on a computer.

Esophageal manometry is used to detect motility disorders of the esophagus and the lower esophageal sphincter. Patients must refrain from eating or drinking for 8 to 12 hours before the test. Medications that could have a direct affect on motility (eg, calcium channel blockers, anticholinergic agents, sedatives) are withheld for 24 to 48 hours. A pressure-sensitive catheter is inserted through the nose and is connected to a transducer and a video recorder. The patient then swallows small amounts of water while the resultant pressure changes are recorded.

Gastroduodenal, small-intestine, and colonic manometry are used to evaluate delayed gastric emptying and gastric and intestinal motility disorders such as irritable bowel syndrome or atonic colon. This is often an ambulatory outpatient procedure lasting 24 to 72 hours. Anorectal manometry measures the resting tone of the internal anal sphincter and the contractibility of the external anal sphincter. It is helpful in evaluating patients with chronic constipation or fecal incontinence and is useful in biofeedback for the treatment of fecal incontinence. It can be performed in conjunction with rectal sensory functioning tests. Phospho-Soda or a saline cleansing enema is administered 1 hour before the test. Positioning for the test is either the prone or the lateral position.

A rectal sensory function test is used to evaluate rectal sensory function and neuropathy. A catheter and balloon are passed into the rectum, and the balloon is inflated until the patient feels distention. Then the tone and pressure of the rectum and anal sphincter are measured. The results are especially helpful in the evaluation of patients with chronic constipation, diarrhea, or incontinence.

Electrogastrography, an electrophysiologic study, also may be performed to assess gastric motility disturbances. Electrodes are placed over the abdomen, and gastric electrical activity is recorded for up to 24 hours. Patients may exhibit rapid, slow, or irregular waveform activity. Electrogastrography can be useful in detecting motor or nerve dysfunction in the stomach.

Defecography

Defecography measures anorectal function. Very thick barium paste is instilled into the rectum, and then fluoroscopy is performed to assess the function of the rectum and anal sphincter while the patient attempts to expel the barium. The test requires no preparation. The use of scintigraphic techniques to measure rectal emptying of radioisotope-labeled artificial stool can provide more quantitative information.

Electromyographic (EMG) studies can supplement anorectal manometry to measure the integrity and function of the anal sphincters in an effort to treat functional bowel incontinence and constipation.

GASTRIC ANALYSIS, GASTRIC ACID STIMULATION TEST, AND pH MONITORING

Analysis of the gastric juice yields information about the secretory activity of the gastric mucosa and the presence or degree of gastric retention in patients thought to have pyloric or duodenal obstruction. It is also useful for diagnosing diseases such as Zollinger-Ellison syndrome.

The patient is kept NPO for 8 to 12 hours before the procedure. Any medications that affect gastric secretions are withheld for 24 to 48 hours before the test. Smoking is not allowed on the morning before the test, because it increases gastric secretions. A small nasogastric tube with a catheter tip marked at various points is inserted through the nose. When the tube is at a point slightly less than 50 cm (21 inches) distant, it should be within the stomach, lying along the greater curvature. Once in place, the tube is secured to the patient's cheek and the patient is placed in a semi-reclining position. The entire stomach contents are aspirated by gentle suction into a syringe, and gastric samples are collected every 15 minutes for the next hour.

The gastric acid stimulation test usually is performed in conjunction with gastric analysis. Histamine or pentagastrin is administered subcutaneously to stimulate gastric secretions. It is important to inform the patient that this injection may produce a flushed feeling. The nurse monitors blood pressure and pulse frequently to detect hypotension. Gastric specimens are collected after the injection every 15 minutes for 1 hour and are labeled to indicate the time of specimen collection after histamine injection. The volume and pH of the specimen are measured. In certain instances, cytologic study by the Papanicolaou technique may be used to determine the presence or absence of malignant cells. Enzyme analysis of the gastric juice may be indicated.

Important diagnostic information to be gained from gastric analysis includes the ability of the mucosa to secrete HCl. This ability is altered in various disease states, including

- Pernicious anemia—patients with this disease secrete no acid under basal conditions or after stimulation
- Severe chronic atrophic gastritis or gastric cancer—patients with these diseases secrete little or no acid
- Peptic ulcer—patients with peptic ulcers secrete some acid
- Duodenal ulcers—patients with duodenal ulcers usually secrete an excess amount of acid

Esophageal reflux of gastric acid may be diagnosed by ambulatory pH monitoring. The patient is NPO for 6 hours before the test, and all medications affecting gastric secretions are withheld for 24 to 36 hours before the test. A probe that measures pH is placed through the nose and into position about 5 inches above the lower esophageal sphincter. It is connected to an external recording device and is worn for 24 hours while the patient continues his or her normal daily activities. The end result is a computer analysis and graphic display of the results. This test allows for the direct correlation between chest pain and reflux episodes (Wolfe, 2000).

A Bernstein test may be performed to evaluate complaints of acid-related chest or epigastric pain. HCl is instilled through a small feeding tube positioned in the esophagus. This is done to try to elicit reported chest pain. Resultant signs and symptoms are compared with the usual symptoms the patient reports. However, since the advent of ambulatory pH monitoring, this previously popular evaluation tool is used infrequently (Wolfe, 2000).

LAPAROSCOPY (PERITONEOSCOPY)

Laparoscopy can be used for the diagnosis of GI disease. This procedure is performed through a small incision in the abdominal wall. Special fiberoptic laparoscopes allow direct visualization of the organs and structures within the abdomen, permitting visualization and identification of any growths, anomalies, and inflammatory processes. In addition, biopsy samples can be taken from the structures and organs as necessary. This procedure can be used to evaluate peritoneal disease, chronic abdominal pain, abdominal masses, and gallbladder and liver disease. However, laparoscopy has not become an important diagnostic modality in patients with acute abdominal pain, because less invasive tools (ie, CT and MRI) are readily available (Wolfe, 2000). Laparoscopy usually requires general anesthesia and sometimes requires that the stomach and bowel be decompressed. Gas (usually carbon dioxide) is insufflated into the peritoneal cavity to create a working space for visualization. One of the most positive benefits of this procedure is that after visualization of a problem, excision (eg, removal of the gallbladder) can then be performed at the same time, if appropriate.

Pathophysiologic and Psychological Considerations

Abnormalities of the GI tract are numerous and represent every type of major pathology that can affect other organ systems, including bleeding, perforation, obstruction, inflammation, and cancer. Congenital, inflammatory, infectious, traumatic, and neoplastic lesions have been encountered in every portion, and at every site, along the length of the GI tract. As with all other organ systems, the GI tract is subject to circulatory disturbances, faulty nervous system control, and aging.

Apart from the many organic diseases to which the GI tract is susceptible, there are many extrinsic factors that can interfere with its normal function and produce symptoms. Stress and anxiety, for example, often find their chief expression in indigestion, anorexia, or motor disturbances of the intestines, sometimes producing constipation or diarrhea. In addition to the state of mental health, physical factors such as fatigue and an inadequate or abruptly changed dietary intake can markedly affect the GI tract. When assessing and instructing the patient, the nurse should consider the variety of mental and physical factors that affect the function of the GI tract.

 Gerontologic Considerations

Normal physiologic changes of the GI system that occur with aging are identified in the accompanying Gerontologic Considerations box. The nurse should carefully assess and monitor signs and symptoms related to these changes. Age-related changes in the mouth include loss of teeth, diminished number of taste buds, decreased production of saliva, and atrophy of gingival tissue. These changes cause difficulty in chewing and swallowing. Changes in the esophagus include decreased muscle tone and weakness in the lower esophageal sphincter, leading to reflux and heartburn.

Decreased gastric motility leads to delayed gastric emptying. Atrophy of the mucosa causes a decrease in HCl production, and this can lead to food intolerances, malabsorption, or decrease in vitamin B_{12} absorption. Changes in the small and large intestine are evidenced largely by decreased motility and decreased transit time, which lead to complaints of indigestion and constipation. Other changes lead to decreased absorption of nutrients (dextrose, fats, calcium, and iron) in the large intestine. The nerve supply to the anal sphincter is sometimes impaired, causing fecal incontinence (Luekenotte, 2000).

Gerontologic Considerations
Age-Related Changes of the Gastrointestinal System

Oral Cavity and Pharynx
- Injury/loss or decay of teeth
- Atrophy of taste buds
- Decreased saliva production
- Reduced ptyalin and amylase in saliva

Esophagus
- Decreased motility and emptying
- Weakened gag reflex
- Decreased resting pressure of lower esophageal sphincter

Stomach
- Degeneration and atrophy of gastric mucosal surfaces with decreased production of HCl
- Decreased secretion of gastric acids and most digestive enzymes
- Decreased motility and emptying

Small Intestine
- Atrophy of muscle and mucosal surfaces
- Thinning of villi and epithelial cells

Large Intestine
- Decrease in mucus secretion
- Decrease in elasticity of rectal wall
- Decreased tone of internal anal sphincter
- Slower and duller nerve impulses in rectal area

 Critical Thinking Exercises

1. You are caring for a 24-year-old male patient who was admitted for acute abdominal pain. He has just arrived from the emergency room and is being scheduled for tests this afternoon. What laboratory tests would you expect to be ordered? He is scheduled for a CT and ultrasound in 2 hours. What preparation is needed for these tests? What preprocedure education is needed?

2. A 58-year-old patient assigned to you this morning has just left to go to the Endoscopy Suite, where she will undergo a colonoscopy. You know that your patient will receive moderate sedation during the procedure and that she will be returned to your care once she is fully alert. What should you anticipate in the course of recovery for your patient after the colonoscopy? What medications might be used for the moderate sedation, and what effects of those medications would you expect to see during the recovery period? Describe the potential complications that could occur and what you will monitor. What are the goals for care during this period?

REFERENCES AND SELECTED READINGS
Books
Bickley, L. S., & Hoekelman, R. A. (2003). *Bates' guide to physical examination and history taking* (8th ed.). Philadelphia: Lippincott Williams & Wilkins.

Castell, D. (1999). *The esophagus* (3rd ed.). Philadelphia: Lippincott Williams & Wilkins.

Grendell, J., et al. (Eds.). (1996). *Current diagnosis and treatment in gastroenterology.* Stamford, CT: Appleton & Lange.

Keeffe, E. (Ed.) . (1998). *Atlas of gastrointestinal endoscopy.* New York: McGraw-Hill Professional.

Kirsner, J. (Ed.). (2000). *Inflammatory bowel disease* (5th ed.). Philadelphia: W. B. Saunders.

Levine, M. (Ed.). (2000). *Double contrast gastrointestinal radiology.* Philadelphia: W. B. Saunders.

Luekenotte, A. (2000). *Gerontologic nursing* (2nd ed.). St. Louis: Mosby.

Phillips, S., & Wingate, D. (1998). Functional disorders of the gut. New York: Churchill-Livingstone.

Rosenthal, M. (1999). *The gastrointestinal sourcebook.* Los Angeles: Lowell House.

Society of Gastroenterologic Nursing and Associates. (1998). *Core curriculum* (2nd ed.), St. Louis: Mosby.

Wolfe, M. (Ed) (2000). *Therapy of digestive disorders.* Philadelphia: W. B. Saunders.

Yamada, T. (1998). *Atlas of gastroenterology* (2nd ed.). Philadelphia: Lippincott-Raven.

Yamada, T. (Ed.). (1999). *Textbook of gastroenterology* (3rd ed.). Philadelphia: Lippincott Williams & Wilkins.

Journals

Ahmed, D. (2000). Hidden factors in occult blood testing. *American Journal of Nursing, 100*(2), 25.

Anonymous. (2000). SGNA guideline for nursing care of patients during sedation and analgesia in the GI endoscopy setting. *Gastroenterology Nursing, 23*(3), 125–129.

Forsberg, F. (1999). Advances in ultrasound contrast techniques. *Applied Radiology (Supplement), 16,* 5–10.

Gavaghan, M. (1999). Anatomy and physiology of the esophagus. *AORN J, 69*(2), 370, 372, 374.

Glaser, Y. (2001). Colorectal cancer screening: New directions, evolving guidelines. *Patient Care, 35*(4), 24–30, 33–34.

Heflin, M. (2001). Cancer screening in the elderly. *Hospital Practice, 36*(3), 61–69.

Lightdale, C. (2000). Small bowel endoscopy. *Gastrointestinal Endoscopy, 9*(1), 101–108.

Lessick, M. (2001). Advances in genetic testing for cancer risk. *MedSurg Nursing, 10*(3), 123–127.

O'Hanlon-Nichols, T. (1998). Basic assessment series: Gastrointestinal system. *American Journal of Nursing, 98*(4), 48–53.

Pontieri-Lewis, V. (2000). Colorectal cancer. *MedSurg Nursing, 9*(1), 9–15, 20.

Staff, D., & Shaker, R. (2001). Aging and the gastrointestinal tract. *Disease a Month, 47*(3), 69–104.

Management of Patients With Oral and Esophageal Disorders

LEARNING OBJECTIVES

On completion of this chapter, the learner will be able to:

1. Use the nursing process as a framework for care of patients with conditions of the oral cavity.

2. Describe the relationship of dental hygiene and dental problems to nutrition.

3. Describe the nursing management of patients with abnormalities of the lips, gums, teeth, mouth, and salivary glands.

4. Use the nursing process as a framework for care of patients with cancer of the oral cavity.

5. Identify the physical and psychosocial long-term needs of patients with oral cancer.

6. Use the nursing process as a framework for care of patients undergoing neck dissection.

7. Use the nursing process as a framework for care of patients with conditions of the esophagus.

8. Describe the various conditions of the esophagus and their clinical manifestations and management.

*B*ecause digestion normally begins in the mouth, adequate nutrition is related to good dental health and the general condition of the mouth. Any discomfort or adverse condition in the oral cavity can affect a person's nutritional status. Changes in the oral cavity may influence the type and amount of food ingested as well as the degree to which food particles are properly mixed with salivary enzymes. Disease of the mouth or tongue can interfere with speech and thus affect communication and self-image. Esophageal problems related to swallowing can also adversely affect food and fluid intake, thereby jeopardizing general health and well-being. Given the close relationship between adequate nutritional intake and the structures of the upper gastrointestinal tract (lips, mouth, teeth, pharynx, esophagus), health teaching can help prevent disorders associated with these structures.

The oral cavity, which includes the lips, mouth, and gums, is subject to many disorders and diseases. Table 35-1 reviews common abnormalities, their possible causes, and nursing management. As identified in a report by the U.S. Surgeon General in 2000, oral health is a very important component of a person's physical and psychological sense of well-being. Severe periodontal disease affects approximately 14% of adults 45 to 64 years of age and 23% of adults 65 to 74 years of age (US Department of Health and Human Services, 2000).

Disorders of the Teeth

DENTAL PLAQUE AND CARIES

Tooth decay is an erosive process that begins with the action of bacteria on fermentable carbohydrates in the mouth, which produces acids that dissolve tooth enamel. The extent of damage to the teeth depends on the following:

- The presence of dental plaque
- The strength of the acids and the ability of the saliva to neutralize them
- The length of time the acids are in contact with the teeth
- The susceptibility of the teeth to decay

Dental plaque is a gluey, gelatin-like substance that adheres to the teeth. The initial action that causes damage to a tooth occurs under dental plaque.

Dental decay begins with a small hole, usually in a fissure (a break in the tooth's enamel) or in an area that is hard to clean. Left unchecked, the affected area penetrates the enamel into the dentin. Because dentin is not as hard as enamel, decay progresses more rapidly and in time reaches the pulp. When the blood, lymph vessels, and nerves are exposed, they become infected and an abscess may form, either within the tooth or at the tip of the root. Soreness and pain usually occur with an abscess. As the in-

fection continues, the patient's face may swell, and there may be pulsating pain. The dentist can determine by x-ray studies the extent of damage and the type of treatment needed. Treatment for dental caries includes fillings, dental implants, and extractions. If treatment is not successful, the tooth may need to be extracted. In general, dental decay is associated with young people, but older adults are subject to decay as well, particularly from drug-induced or age-related oral dryness (see the accompanying Gerontologic Considerations box).

Prevention

Measures used to prevent and control dental caries include practicing effective mouth care, reducing the intake of starches and sugars (refined carbohydrates), applying fluoride to the teeth or drinking fluoridated water, refraining from smoking, controlling diabetes, and using pit and fissure sealants (Chart 35-1).

MOUTH CARE

Healthy teeth must be conscientiously and effectively cleaned on a daily basis. Brushing and flossing are particularly effective in mechanically breaking up the bacterial plaque that collects around teeth.

Normal mastication (chewing) and the normal flow of saliva also aid greatly in keeping the teeth clean. Because many ill patients do not eat adequate amounts of food, they produce less saliva, which in turn reduces this natural tooth cleaning process. The nurse may need to assume the responsibility for brushing the patient's teeth. In any case, merely wiping the patient's mouth and teeth with a swab is ineffective. The most effective method is mechanical cleansing (brushing). If brushing is impossible, it is better to wipe the teeth with a gauze pad, then have the patient swish an antiseptic mouthwash several times before expectorating into an emesis basin. A soft-bristled toothbrush is more effective than a sponge or foam stick. The lips may be coated with a water-soluble gel to prevent drying.

DIET

Dental caries may be prevented by decreasing the amount of sugar and starch in the diet. Patients who snack should be encouraged to choose less cariogenic alternatives, such as fruits, vegetables, nuts, cheeses, or plain yogurt.

FLUORIDATION

Fluoridation of public water supplies has been found to decrease dental caries. Some areas of the country have natural fluoridation; other communities have added fluoride to public water supplies. Fluoridation may be achieved also by having a dentist apply a concentrated gel or solution to the teeth, adding fluoride to home

Glossary

achalasia: absent or ineffective peristalsis (wavelike contraction) of the distal esophagus accompanied by failure of the esophageal sphincter to relax in response to swallowing

dysphagia: difficulty swallowing

gastroesophageal reflux: back-flow of gastric or duodenal contents into the esophagus

hernia: protrusion of an organ or part of an organ through the wall of the cavity that normally contains it

lithotripsy: use of shock waves to break up or disintegrate stones

odynophagia: pain on swallowing

parotitis: inflammation of the parotid gland

pyrosis: heartburn

periapical abscess: abscessed tooth

sialadenitis: inflammation of the salivary glands

stomatitis: inflammation of the oral mucosa

temporomandibular disorders: a group of conditions that cause pain or dysfunction of the temporomandibular joint (TMJ) and surrounding structures

xerostomia: dry mouth

Table 35-1 • **Disorders of the Lips, Mouth, and Gums**

CONDITION	SIGNS AND SYMPTOMS	POSSIBLE CAUSES AND SEQUELAE	NURSING CONSIDERATIONS
Abnormalities of the Lips			
Actinic cheilitis	Irritation of lips associated with scaling, crusty, fissure; white overgrowth of horny layer of epidermis (hyperkeratosis) Considered a premalignant squamous cell skin cancer	Exposure to sun; more common in fair-skinned people and in those whose occupations involve sun exposure, such as farmers May lead to squamous cell cancer	Teach patient importance of protecting lips from the sun by using protective ointment such as sun block Instruct patient to have a periodic checkup by physician
Herpes simplex 1 (cold sore or fever blister)	Symptoms may be delayed up to 20 days after exposure; singular or clustered painful vesicles that may rupture	An opportunistic infection; frequently seen in immunosuppressed patients; very contagious May recur with menstruation, fever, or sun exposure	Use acyclovir or zovirax ointment or systemic medications as prescribed Administer analgesics as prescribed Instruct patient to avoid irritating foods
Chancre	Reddened circumscribed lesion that ulcerates and becomes crusted	Primary lesion of syphilis; very contagious	Comfort measures: cold soaks to lip, mouth care Administer antibiotics as prescribed Instruct patient regarding contagion
Contact dermatitis	Red area or rash; itching	Allergic reaction to lipstick, cosmetic ointments, or toothpaste	Instruct patient to avoid possible causes Administer corticosteroids as prescribed
Abnormalities of the Mouth			
Leukoplakia	White patches; may be hyperkeratotic; usually in buccal mucosa; usually painless	Fewer than 2% are malignant, but may progress to cancer Common among tobacco users	Instruct patient to see a physician if leukoplakia persists longer than 2 weeks Eliminate risk factors, such as tobacco
Hairy leukoplakia	White patches with rough hair-like projections; typically found on lateral border of the tongue	Possibly viral; smoking and use of tobacco Often seen in people who are HIV positive	Instruct patient to see a physician if condition persists longer than 2 weeks
Lichen planus	White papules at the intersection of a network of interlacing lesions; usually ulcerated and painful	Recurrences are common May lead to a malignant process Unknown cause	Apply topical corticosteroids such as fluocinolone acetonide oral base gel Avoid foods that irritate Administer corticosteroids systemically or intralesionally as prescribed Instruct the patient of need for follow-up if condition is chronic
Candidiasis (moniliasis/thrush)	Cheesy white plaque that looks like milk curds; when rubbed off, it leaves an erythematous and often bleeding base	*Candida albicans* fungus; predisposing factors include diabetes, antibiotic therapy, and immunosuppression	Antifungal medications such as nystatin (Mycostatin), Amphotericin B, clotrimazole, or ketoconazole may be prescribed; these may be taken in pill form or as a suspension; when used as a suspension, instruct the patient to swish vigorously for at least 1 minute and then swallow
Aphthous stomatitis (canker sore)	Shallow ulcer with a white or yellow center and red border; seen on the inner side of the lip and cheek or on the tongue; it begins with a burning or tingling sensation and slight swelling; painful; usually lasts 7–10 days and heals without a scar	Associated with emotional or mental stress, fatigue, hormonal factors, minor trauma (such as biting), allergies, acidic foods and juices, and dietary deficiencies Associated with HIV infection May recur	Instruct the patient in comfort measures, such as saline rinses, and a soft or bland diet Antibiotics or corticosteroids may be prescribed
Nicotine stomatitis (smoker's patch)	Two stages—begins as a red stomatitis; over time the tongue and mouth become covered with a creamy, thick, white mucous membrane, which may slough, leaving a beefy red base	Chronic irritation by tobacco	Cessation of tobacco use; if condition exists for longer than 2 weeks a physician should be consulted and a biopsy may be needed

(continued)

Table 35-1 • **Disorders of the Lips, Mouth, and Gums** (Continued)

CONDITION	SIGNS AND SYMPTOMS	POSSIBLE CAUSES AND SEQUELAE	NURSING CONSIDERATIONS
Krythoplakia	Red patch on the oral mucous membrane	Nonspecific inflammation; more frequently seen in the elderly	
Kaposi's sarcoma	Appears first on the oral mucosa as a red, purple, or blue lesion; may be singular or multiple; may be flat or raised	HIV infection	Instruct patient regarding side effects of planned treatment
Abnormalities of the Gums			
Gingivitis	Painful, inflamed, swollen gums; usually the gums bleed in response to light contact	Poor oral hygiene: food debris, bacterial plaque, and calculus (tartar) accumulate; the gums may also swell in response to normal processes such as puberty and pregnancy	Teach patient proper oral hygiene; see Preventive Oral Hygiene chart
Necrotizing gingivitis (trench mouth)	Gray-white pseudomembranous ulcerations affecting the edges of the gums, mucosa of the mouth, tonsils, and pharynx; foul breath; painful, bleeding gums; swallowing and talking are painful	Poor oral hygiene; bacterial infection, inadequate rest, overwork, emotional stress, smoking, and poor nutrition may contribute to development	Teach patient proper oral hygiene; see Preventive Oral Hygiene chart Irrigate with 2% to 3% hydrogen peroxide or normal saline solution Avoid irritants such as smoking and spicy foods
Herpetic gingivostomatitis	Burning sensation with the appearance of small vesicles 24–48 hours later; vesicles may rupture, forming sore, shallow ulcers covered with a gray membrane	Herpes simplex virus; occurs most frequently in people who are immunosuppressed; may occur in other infectious processes such as streptococcal pneumonia, meningococcal meningitis, and malaria	Apply topical anesthetics as prescribed; may need opioids if pain is severe Saline or 2% to 3% hydrogen peroxide irrigations Antiviral agents such as acyclovir may be prescribed
Periodontitis	Little discomfort at onset; may have bleeding, infection, gum recession, and loosening of teeth; later in the disease tooth loss may occur	May result from untreated gingivitis Poor or inadequate dental hygiene and inadequate diet contribute to development	Instruct patient in proper oral hygiene Instruct patient to consult a dentist

water supplies, using fluoridated toothpaste or mouth rinse, or using sodium fluoride tablets, drops, or lozenges.

PIT AND FISSURE SEALANTS
The occlusal surfaces of the teeth have pits and fissures, areas that are prone to caries. Some dentists apply a special coating to fill and

Gerontologic Considerations
Oral Problems

Many medications taken by the elderly cause dry mouth, which is uncomfortable, impairs communication, and increases the risk of oral infection. These medications include the following:
- Diuretics
- Antihypertensive medications
- Anti-inflammatory agents
- Antidepressant medications

Poor dentition can exacerbate problems of aging, such as
- Decreased food intake
- Loss of appetite
- Social isolation
- Increased susceptibility to systemic infection (from periodontal disease)
- Trauma to the oral cavity secondary to thinner, less vascular oral mucous membranes

seal these areas from potential exposure to cariogenic processes. These sealants last up to 7 years.

DENTOALVEOLAR ABSCESS OR PERIAPICAL ABSCESS

Periapical abscess, more commonly referred to as an abscessed tooth, involves the collection of pus in the apical dental periosteum (fibrous membrane supporting the tooth structure) and

Chart 35-1 • PATIENT EDUCATION
Preventive Oral Hygiene

- Brush teeth using a soft toothbrush at least two times daily. Hold toothbrush at a 45-degree angle between the brush and the gums and teeth. A small brush is better than a large brush. Gums and tongue surface should be brushed.
- Floss at least once daily.
- Use an antiplaque mouth rinse.
- Visit a dentist at least every 6 months, or when you have a chipped tooth, a lost filling, an oral sore that persists longer than 2 weeks, or a toothache.
- Avoid alcohol and tobacco products, including smokeless tobacco.
- Maintain adequate nutrition and avoid sweets.
- Replace toothbrush at first signs of wear, usually every 2 months.

the tissue surrounding the apex of the tooth (where it is suspended in the jaw bone). The abscess has two forms: acute and chronic. Acute periapical abscess is usually secondary to a suppurative pulpitis (a pus-producing inflammation of the dental pulp) that arises from an infection extending from dental caries. The infection of the dental pulp extends through the apical foramen of the tooth to form an abscess around the apex.

Chronic dentoalveolar abscess is a slowly progressive infectious process. It differs from the acute form in that the process may progress to a fully formed abscess without the patient's knowing it. The infection eventually leads to a "blind dental abscess," which is really a periapical granuloma. It may enlarge to as much as 1 cm in diameter. It is often discovered on x-ray films and is treated by extraction or root canal therapy, often with apicectomy (excision of the apex of the tooth root).

Clinical Manifestations

The abscess produces a dull, gnawing, continuous pain, often with a surrounding cellulitis and edema of the adjacent facial structures, and mobility of the involved tooth. The gum opposite the apex of the tooth is usually swollen on the cheek side. Swelling and cellulitis of the facial structures may make it difficult for the patient to open the mouth. In well-developed abscesses, there may be a systemic reaction, fever, and malaise.

Management

In the early stages of an infection, a dentist or dental surgeon may perform a needle aspiration or drill an opening into the pulp chamber to relieve tension and pain and to provide drainage. Usually, the infection will have progressed to a periapical abscess. Drainage is provided by an incision through the gingiva down to the jawbone. Pus (purulent material) escapes under pressure. This procedure is commonly performed in the dentist's office, but it may be performed in an outpatient surgery center or a same-day surgery department. After the inflammatory reaction has subsided, the tooth may be extracted or root canal therapy performed. Antibiotics may be prescribed.

Nursing Management

The nurse assesses the patient for bleeding after treatment and instructs the patient to use a warm saline or warm water mouth rinse to keep the area clean. The patient is also instructed to take antibiotics and analgesics as prescribed, to advance from a liquid diet to a soft diet as tolerated, and to keep follow-up appointments.

MALOCCLUSION

Malocclusion is a misalignment of the teeth of the upper and lower dental arcs when the jaws are closed. Malocclusion can be inherited or acquired (from thumb-sucking, trauma, or some medical conditions). Malocclusion makes the teeth difficult to clean and can lead to decay, gum disease, and excess wear on supporting bone and gum tissues. About 50% of the population has some form of malocclusion. Correction of malocclusion requires an orthodontist with special training, a patient who is motivated and cooperative, and adequate time. Most treatments begin when the patient has shed the last primary tooth and the last permanent successor has erupted, usually at about 12 or 13 years of age, but treatment may occur in adulthood. Preventive orthodontics may be started at age 5 years if malocclusion is diagnosed early. The need for teeth straightening in adolescence is reduced if preventive orthodontics is started with the primary teeth.

Management

People with malocclusion have an obviously misaligned bite or crooked, crowded, widely spaced, or protruding teeth. To realign the teeth, the orthodontist gradually forces the teeth into a new location by using wires or plastic bands (braces). These devices may be unattractive, but this psychological burden must be overcome if good results are to be achieved. In the final phase of treatment, a retaining device is worn for several hours each day to support the tissues as they adjust to the new alignment of the teeth.

Nursing Management

The patient must practice meticulous oral hygiene, and the nurse encourages the patient to persist in this important part of the treatment. An adolescent undergoing orthodontic correction who is admitted to the hospital for some other problem may have to be reminded to continue wearing the retainer (if it does not interfere with the problem requiring hospitalization).

Disorders of the Jaw

Abnormal conditions affecting the mandible (jaw) and of the temporomandibular joint (which connects the mandible to the temporal bone at the side of the head in front of the ear) include congenital malformation, fracture, chronic dislocation, cancer, and syndromes characterized by pain and limited motion. Temporomandibular disorders and jaw surgery (a treatment common in many structural abnormalities or cancer of the jaw) are presented in this section.

TEMPOROMANDIBULAR DISORDERS

Temporomandibular disorders are categorized as follows (National Oral Health Information Clearinghouse, 2000):

- Myofascial pain—a discomfort in the muscles controlling jaw function and in neck and shoulder muscles
- Internal derangement of the joint—a dislocated jaw, a displaced disc, or an injured condyle
- Degenerative joint disease—rheumatoid arthritis or osteoarthritis in the jaw joint

Diagnosis and treatment of temporomandibular disorders remain somewhat ambiguous, but the condition is thought to affect about 10 million people in the United States. Misalignment of the joints in the jaw and other problems associated with the ligaments and muscles of mastication are thought to result in tissue damage and muscle tenderness. Suggested causes include arthritis of the jaw, head injury, trauma or injury to the jaw or joint, stress, and malocclusion (although research does not support malocclusion as a cause).

Clinical Manifestations

Patients have pain ranging from a dull ache to throbbing, debilitating pain that can radiate to the ears, teeth, neck muscles, and facial sinuses. They often have restricted jaw motion and locking of the jaw. They may hear clicking and grating noises, and chewing and swallowing may be difficult. Depression may occur in response to these symptoms.

Assessment and Diagnostic Findings

Diagnosis is based on the patient's subjective symptoms of pain, limitations in range of motion, dysphagia, difficulty chewing, difficulty with speech, or hearing difficulties. Magnetic resonance imaging, x-ray studies, and an arthrogram may be performed.

Management

Although some practitioners think the role of stress in temporomandibular joint (TMJ) disorders is overrated, patient education in stress management may be helpful (to reduce grinding and clenching of teeth). Patients may also benefit from range-of-motion exercises. Pain management measures may include nonsteroidal anti-inflammatory drugs (NSAIDs), with the possible addition of opioids, muscle relaxants, or mild antidepressants. Occasionally, a bite plate or splint (plastic guard worn over the upper and lower teeth) may be worn to protect teeth from grinding; however, this is a short-term therapy. Conservative and reversible treatment is recommended. If irreversible surgical options are recommended, the patient is encouraged to seek a second opinion.

SURGICAL MANAGEMENT

Correction of mandibular structural abnormalities may require surgery involving repositioning or reconstruction of the jaw. Simple fractures of the mandible without displacement, resulting from a blow on the chin, and planned surgical interventions, as in the correction of long or short jaw syndrome, may require treatment by these means. Jaw reconstruction may be necessary in the aftermath of trauma from a severe injury or cancer, both of which can cause tissue and bone loss.

Mandibular fractures are usually closed fractures. Rigid plate fixation (insertion of metal plates and screws into the bone to approximate and stabilize the bone) is the current treatment of choice in many cases of mandibular fracture and in some mandibular reconstructive surgery procedures. Bone grafting may be performed to replace structural defects using bones from the patient's own ilium, ribs, or cranial sites. Rib tissue may also be harvested from cadaver donors.

Nursing Management

The patient who has had rigid fixation should be instructed not to chew food in the first 1 to 4 weeks after surgery. A liquid diet is recommended, and dietary counseling should be obtained to ensure optimal caloric and protein intake.

PROMOTING HOME AND COMMUNITY-BASED CARE

The patient needs specific guidelines for mouth care and feeding. Any irritated areas in the mouth should be reported to the physician. The importance of keeping scheduled appointments for assessing the stability of the fixation appliance is emphasized.

Consultation with a dietitian may be indicated so that the patient and family can learn about foods that are high in essential nutrients and ways in which these foods can be prepared so that they can be consumed through a straw or spoon, while remaining palatable. Nutritional supplements may be recommended.

Disorders of the Salivary Glands

The salivary glands consist of the parotid glands, one on each side of the face below the ear; the submandibular and sublingual glands, both in the floor of the mouth; and the buccal gland, beneath the lips. About 1200 mL of saliva are produced daily. The glands' primary functions are lubrication, protection against harmful bacteria, and digestion.

PAROTITIS

Parotitis (inflammation of the parotid gland) is the most common inflammatory condition of the salivary glands, although inflammation can occur in the other salivary glands as well. Mumps (epidemic parotitis), a communicable disease caused by viral infection and most commonly affecting children, is an inflammation of a salivary gland, usually the parotid.

Elderly, acutely ill, or debilitated people with decreased salivary flow from general dehydration or medications are at high risk for parotitis. The infecting organisms travel from the mouth through the salivary duct. The organism is usually *Staphylococcus aureus* (except in mumps). The onset of this complication is sudden, with an exacerbation of both the fever and the symptoms of the primary condition. The gland swells and becomes tense and tender. The patient feels pain in the ear, and swollen glands interfere with swallowing. The swelling increases rapidly, and the overlying skin soon becomes red and shiny.

Preventive measures are essential and include advising the patient to have necessary dental work performed before surgery. In addition, maintaining adequate nutritional and fluid intake, good oral hygiene, and discontinuing medications (eg, tranquilizers, diuretics) that can diminish salivation may help prevent the condition. If parotitis occurs, antibiotic therapy is necessary. Analgesics may also be prescribed to control pain. If antibiotic therapy is not effective, the gland may need to be drained by a surgical procedure known as parotidectomy. This procedure may be necessary to treat chronic parotitis.

SIALADENITIS

Sialadenitis (inflammation of the salivary glands) may be caused by dehydration, radiation therapy, stress, malnutrition, salivary gland calculi (stones), or improper oral hygiene. The inflammation is associated with infection by *S. aureus, Streptococcus viridans,* or pneumococcus. In hospitalized or institutionalized patients the infecting organism may be methicillin-resistant *S. aureus* (MRSA) (McQuone, 1999). Symptoms include pain, swelling, and purulent discharge. Antibiotics are used to treat infections. Massage, hydration, and corticosteroids frequently cure the problem. Chronic sialadenitis with uncontrolled pain is treated by surgical drainage of the gland or excision of the gland and its duct.

SALIVARY CALCULUS (SIALOLITHIASIS)

Sialolithiasis, or salivary calculi (stones), usually occurs in the submandibular gland. Salivary gland ultrasonography or sialography (x-ray studies filmed after the injection of a radiopaque substance into the duct) may be required to demonstrate obstruction of the duct by stenosis. Salivary calculi are formed mainly from calcium phosphate. If located within the gland, the calculi are irregular and vary in diameter from 3 to 30 mm. Calculi in the duct are small and oval.

Calculi within the salivary gland itself cause no symptoms unless infection arises; however, a calculus that obstructs the gland's duct causes sudden, local, and often colicky pain, which is abruptly relieved by a gush of saliva. This characteristic symptom is often disclosed in the patient's health history. On physical assessment, the gland is swollen and quite tender, the stone itself can be palpable, and its shadow may be seen on x-ray films.

The calculus can be extracted fairly easily from the duct in the mouth. Sometimes, enlargement of the ductal orifice permits the stone to pass spontaneously. Occasionally **lithotripsy**, a procedure that uses shock waves to disintegrate the stone, may be used instead of surgical extraction for parotid stones and smaller submandibular stones. Lithotripsy requires no anesthesia, sedation, or analgesia. Side effects can include local hemorrhage and swelling. Surgery may be necessary to remove the gland if symptoms and calculi recur repeatedly.

NEOPLASMS

Although they are uncommon, neoplasms (tumors or growths) of almost any type may develop in the salivary gland. Tumors occur more often in the parotid gland. The incidence of salivary gland tumors is similar in men and women. Risk factors include prior exposure to radiation to the head and neck. Diagnosis is based on the health history and physical examination and the results of fine needle aspiration biopsy.

Management of salivary gland tumors evokes controversy, but the common procedure involves partial excision of the gland, along with all of the tumor and a wide margin of surrounding tissue. Dissection is carefully performed to preserve the seventh cranial nerve (facial nerve), although it may not be possible to preserve the nerve if the tumor is extensive. If the tumor is malignant, radiation therapy may follow surgery. Radiation therapy alone may be a treatment choice for tumors that are thought to be contained or if there is risk of facial nerve damage from surgical intervention. Chemotherapy is usually used for palliative purposes. Local recurrences are common, and the recurrent growth usually is more aggressive than the original. It has also been observed that patients with salivary gland tumors have an increased incidence of second primary cancers (Bull, 2001).

Cancer of the Oral Cavity

Cancers of the oral cavity, which can occur in any part of the mouth or throat, are curable if discovered early. These cancers are associated with the use of alcohol and tobacco. The combination of alcohol and tobacco seems to have a synergistic carcinogenic effect. About 95% of cases of oral cancer occur in people older than 40 years of age, but the incidence is increasing in men younger than age 30 because of the use of smokeless tobacco, especially snuff (Centers for Disease Control and Prevention, 2002).

Cancer of the oral cavity accounts for less than 2% of all cancer deaths in the United States. Men are afflicted more often than women; however, the incidence of oral cancer in women is increasing, possibly because they use tobacco and alcohol more frequently than they did in the past. The 5-year survival rate for cancer of the oral cavity and pharynx is 55% for whites and 33% for African Americans. Of the 7400 annual deaths from oral cancer, the distribution by site is estimated as follows: tongue, 1700; mouth, 2000; pharynx, 2100; other, 1600 (American Cancer Society, Cancer Facts and Figures, 2002).

Chronic irritation by a warm pipestem or prolonged exposure to the sun and wind may predispose a person to lip cancer. Predisposing factors for other oral cancers are exposure to tobacco (including smokeless tobacco), ingestion of alcohol, dietary deficiency, and ingestion of smoked meats.

Pathophysiology

Malignancies of the oral cavity are usually squamous cell cancers. Any area of the oropharynx can be a site for malignant growths, but the lips, the lateral aspects of the tongue, and the floor of the mouth are most commonly affected.

Clinical Manifestations

Many oral cancers produce few or no symptoms in the early stages. Later, the most frequent symptom is a painless sore or mass that will not heal. A typical lesion in oral cancer is a painless indurated (hardened) ulcer with raised edges. Tissue from any ulcer of the oral cavity that does not heal in 2 weeks should be examined through biopsy. As the cancer progresses, the patient may complain of tenderness; difficulty in chewing, swallowing, or speaking; coughing of blood-tinged sputum; or enlarged cervical lymph nodes.

Assessment and Diagnostic Findings

Diagnostic evaluation consists of an oral examination as well as an assessment of the cervical lymph nodes to detect possible metastases. Biopsies are performed on suspicious lesions (those that have not healed in 2 weeks). High-risk areas include the buccal mucosa and gingiva for people who use snuff or smoke cigars or pipes. For those who smoke cigarettes and drink alcohol, high-risk areas include the floor of the mouth, the ventrolateral tongue, and the soft palate complex (soft palate, anterior and posterior tonsillar area, uvula, and the area behind the molar and tongue junction).

Medical Management

Management varies with the nature of the lesion, the preference of the physician, and patient choice. Surgical resection, radiation therapy, chemotherapy, or a combination of these therapies may be effective.

In cancer of the lip, small lesions are usually excised liberally; larger lesions involving more than one third of the lip may be more appropriately treated by radiation therapy because of superior cosmetic results. The choice depends on the extent of the lesion and what is necessary to cure the patient while preserving the best appearance. Tumors larger than 4 cm often recur.

Cancer of the tongue may be treated with radiation therapy and chemotherapy to preserve organ function and maintain quality of life. A combination of radioactive interstitial implants (surgical implantation of a radioactive source into the tissue adjacent to or at the tumor site) and external beam radiation may be used. If the cancer has spread to the lymph nodes, the surgeon may perform a neck dissection. Surgical treatments leave a less functional tongue; surgical procedures include hemiglossectomy (surgical removal of half of the tongue) and total glossectomy (removal of the tongue).

Often cancer of the oral cavity has metastasized through the extensive lymphatic channel in the neck region (Fig. 35-1), requiring a neck dissection and reconstructive surgery of the oral

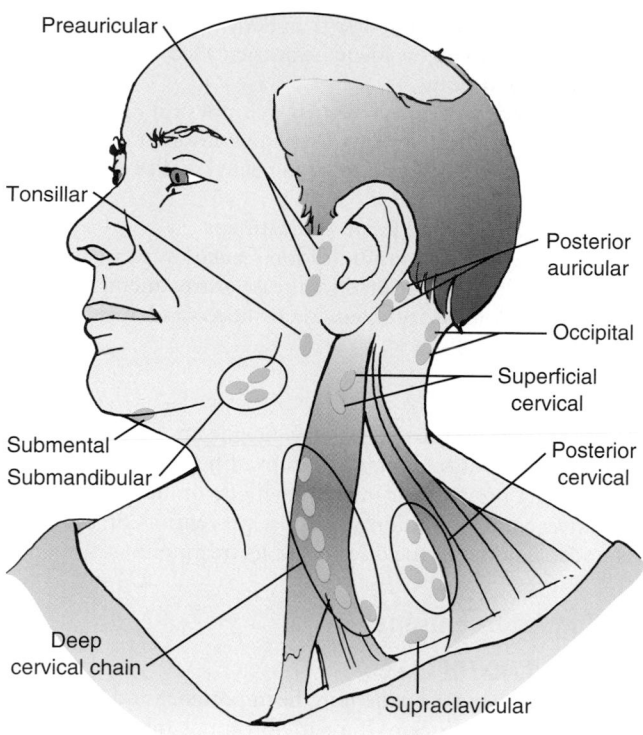

FIGURE 35-1 Lymphatic drainage of the head and neck.

cavity. A common reconstructive technique involves use of a radial forearm free flap (a thin layer of skin from the forearm along with the radial artery).

Nursing Management

The nurse assesses the patient's nutritional status preoperatively, and a dietary consultation may be necessary. The patient may require enteral (through the intestine) or parenteral (intravenous) feedings before and after surgery to maintain adequate nutrition. If a radial graft is to be performed, an Allen test on the donor arm must be performed to ensure that the ulnar artery is patent and can provide blood flow to the hand after removal of the radial artery. The Allen test is performed by asking the patient to make a fist and then manually compressing the ulnar artery. The patient is then asked to open the hand into a relaxed, slightly flexed position. The palm will be pale. Pressure on the ulnar artery is released. If the ulnar artery is patent, the palm will flush within about 3 to 5 seconds.

Postoperatively, the nurse assesses for a patent airway. The patient may be unable to manage oral secretions, making suctioning necessary. If grafting was included in the surgery, suctioning must be performed with care to prevent damage to the graft. The graft is assessed postoperatively for viability. Although color should be assessed (white may indicate arterial occlusion, and blue mottling may indicate venous congestion), it can be difficult to assess the graft by looking into the mouth. A Doppler ultrasound device may be used to locate the radial pulse at the graft site and to assess graft perfusion.

NURSING PROCESS: THE PATIENT WITH CONDITIONS OF THE ORAL CAVITY

Assessment

Obtaining a health history allows the nurse to determine the patient's learning needs concerning preventive oral hygiene and to identify symptoms requiring medical evaluation. The history includes questions about the patient's normal brushing and flossing routine; frequency of dental visits; awareness of any lesions or irritated areas in the mouth, tongue, or throat; recent history of sore throat or bloody sputum; discomfort caused by certain foods; daily food intake; use of alcohol and tobacco, including smokeless chewing tobacco; and the need to wear dentures or a partial plate. For more information about dentures, see the accompanying Gerontologic Considerations box.

A careful physical assessment follows the health history. Both the internal and the external structures of the mouth and throat are inspected and palpated. Dentures and partial plates are removed to ensure a thorough inspection of the mouth. In general, the examination can be accomplished by using a bright light source (penlight) and a tongue depressor. Gloves are worn to palpate the tongue and any abnormalities.

LIPS

The examination begins with inspection of the lips for moisture, hydration, color, texture, symmetry, and the presence of ulcerations or fissures. The lips should be moist, pink, smooth, and symmetric. The patient is instructed to open the mouth wide; a tongue blade is then inserted to expose the buccal mucosa for an assessment of color and lesions. Stensen's duct of each parotid gland is visible as a small red dot in the buccal mucosa next to the upper molars.

GUMS

The gums are inspected for inflammation, bleeding, retraction, and discoloration. The odor of the breath is also noted. The hard palate is examined for color and shape.

TONGUE

The dorsum (back) of the tongue is inspected for texture, color, and lesions. A thin white coat and large, vallate papillae in a "V" formation on the distal portion of the dorsum of the tongue are

Gerontologic Considerations
Denture Care

Many older adults wear dentures. Mouth care and regular checkups remain part of the denture-wearing older adult's health promotion activities.

- Brush dentures twice a day.
- Remove dentures at night and soak them in water or a denture product. (Never put dentures in hot water, because they may warp.)
- Rinse mouth with warm salt water in the morning, after meals, and at bedtime.
- Clean well under partial dentures, where food particles tend to get caught.
- Consume nonsticky foods that have been cut into small pieces; chew slowly.
- See dentist regularly to assess and readjust fit.

normal findings. The patient is instructed to protrude the tongue and move it laterally. This provides the examiner with an opportunity to estimate the tongue's size as well as its symmetry and strength (to assess the integrity of the 12th cranial nerve [hypoglossal]).

Further inspection of the ventral surface of the tongue and the floor of the mouth is accomplished by asking the patient to touch the roof of the mouth with the tip of the tongue. Any lesions of the mucosa or any abnormalities involving the frenulum or superficial veins on the undersurface of the tongue are assessed for location, size, color, and pain. This is a common area for oral cancer, which presents as a white or red plaque, an indurated ulcer, or a warty growth.

A tongue blade is used to depress the tongue for adequate visualization of the pharynx. It is pressed firmly beyond the midpoint of the tongue; proper placement avoids a gagging response. The patient is told to tip the head back, open the mouth wide, take a deep breath, and say "ah." Often this flattens the posterior tongue and briefly allows a full view of the tonsils, uvula, and posterior pharynx (Fig. 35-2). These structures are inspected for color, symmetry, and evidence of exudate, ulceration, or enlargement. Normally, the uvula and soft palate rise symmetrically with a deep inspiration or "ah"; this indicates an intact vagus nerve (10th cranial nerve).

A complete assessment of the oral cavity is essential because many disorders, such as cancer, diabetes, and immunosuppressive conditions resulting from medication therapy or AIDS, may be manifested by changes in the oral cavity. The neck is examined for enlarged lymph nodes (adenopathy).

Nursing Diagnoses

Based on all the assessment data, major nursing diagnoses may include the following:

- Impaired oral mucous membrane related to a pathologic condition, infection, or chemical or mechanical trauma (eg, medications, ill-fitting dentures)

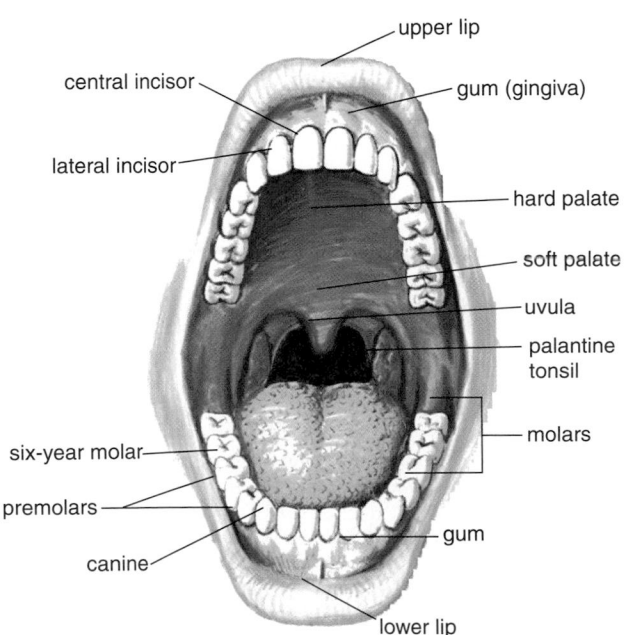

- Imbalanced nutrition, less than body requirements, related to inability to ingest adequate nutrients secondary to oral or dental conditions
- Disturbed body image related to a physical change in appearance resulting from a disease condition or its treatment
- Fear of pain and social isolation related to disease or change in physical appearance
- Pain related to oral lesion or treatment
- Impaired verbal communication related to treatment
- Risk for infection related to disease or treatment
- Deficient knowledge about disease process and treatment plan

Planning and Goals

The major goals for the patient may include improved condition of the oral mucous membrane, improved nutritional intake, attainment of a positive self-image, relief of pain, identification of alternative communication methods, prevention of infection, and understanding of the disease and its treatment.

Nursing Interventions

PROMOTING MOUTH CARE

The nurse instructs the patient in the importance and techniques of preventive mouth care. If a patient cannot tolerate brushing or flossing, an irrigating solution of 1 teaspoon of baking soda to 8 ounces of warm water, half-strength hydrogen peroxide, or normal saline solution is recommended. The nurse reinforces the need to perform oral care and provides such care to patients who are unable to provide it for themselves.

If a bacterial or fungal infection is present, the nurse administers the appropriate medications and instructs the patient in how to administer the medications at home. The nurse monitors the patient's physical and psychological response to treatment.

Xerostomia, dryness of the mouth, is a frequent sequela of oral cancer, particularly when the salivary glands have been exposed to radiation or major surgery. It is also seen in patients who are receiving psychopharmacologic agents, patients with HIV infection, and patients who cannot close the mouth and as a result become mouth-breathers. To minimize this problem, the patient is advised to avoid dry, bulky, and irritating foods and fluids, as well as alcohol and tobacco. The patient is also encouraged to increase intake of fluids (when not contraindicated) and to use a humidifier during sleep. The use of synthetic saliva, a moisturizing antibacterial gel such as Oral Balance, or a saliva production stimulant such as Salagen may be helpful.

Stomatitis, or mucositis, which involves inflammation and breakdown of the oral mucosa, is often a side effect of chemotherapy or radiation therapy. Prophylactic mouth care is started when the patient begins receiving treatment; however, mucositis may become so severe that a break in treatment is necessary. If a patient receiving radiation therapy has poor dentition, extraction of the teeth before radiation treatment in the oral cavity is often initiated to prevent infection. Many radiation therapy centers recommend the use of fluoride treatments for patients receiving radiation to the head and neck.

ENSURING ADEQUATE FOOD AND FLUID INTAKE

The patient's weight, age, and level of activity are recorded to determine whether nutritional intake is adequate. A daily calorie count may be necessary to determine the exact quantity of food and fluid ingested. The frequency and pattern of eating are recorded to determine whether any psychosocial or physiologic factors are

FIGURE 35-2 Structures of the mouth, including the tongue and palate.

Chart 35-2
Home Care Checklist • **The Patient With an Oral Condition**

At the completion of the home care instruction, the patient or caregiver will be able to:

	Patient	Caregiver
• Demonstrate use of suction equipment if indicated.	✓	✓
• State rationale for humidification.	✓	✓
• State foods necessary to meet caloric needs and dietary needs (ie, change in consistency, seasoning limitations, supplements).	✓	✓
• Demonstrate oral hygiene.	✓	✓
• Demonstrate care of incision.	✓	✓
• State when next medical/dental follow-up appointment will be scheduled.	✓	✓

affecting ingestion. The nurse recommends changes in the consistency of foods and the frequency of eating, based on the disorder and the patient's preferences. Consultation with a dietitian can be helpful. The goal is to help the patient attain and maintain desirable body weight and level of energy, as well as to promote the healing of tissue.

SUPPORTING A POSITIVE SELF-IMAGE

A patient who has a disfiguring oral condition or has undergone disfiguring surgery may experience an alteration in self-image. The patient is encouraged to verbalize the perceived change in body appearance and to realistically discuss actual changes or losses. The nurse offers support while the patient verbalizes fears and negative feelings (withdrawal, depression, anger). The nurse listens attentively and determines whether the patient's needs are primarily psychosocial or cognitive-perceptual. This determination will help the nurse to individualize a plan of care. The patient's strengths, achievements, and positive attributes are reinforced.

The nurse should determine the patient's anxieties concerning relationships with others. Referral to support groups, a psychiatric liaison nurse, a social worker, or a spiritual advisor may be useful in helping the patient to cope with anxieties and fears. Emphasizing that the patient's worth is not diminished by a physical change in a body part can be a helpful approach. The patient's progress toward development of positive self-esteem is documented. The nurse should be alert to signs of grieving and should record emotional changes. By providing acceptance and support, the nurse encourages the patient to verbalize feelings.

MINIMIZING PAIN AND DISCOMFORT

Oral lesions can be painful. Strategies to reduce pain and discomfort include avoiding foods that are spicy, hot, or hard (eg, pretzels, nuts). The patient is instructed about mouth care. It may be necessary to provide the patient with an analgesic such as viscous lidocaine (Xylocaine Viscous 2%) or opioids, as prescribed. The nurse can reduce the patient's fear of pain by providing information about pain control methods.

PROMOTING EFFECTIVE COMMUNICATION

Verbal communication may be impaired by radical surgery for oral cancer. It is therefore vital to assess the patient's ability to communicate in writing before surgery. Pen and paper are provided postoperatively to patients who can use them to communicate. A communication board with commonly used words or pictures is obtained preoperatively and given after surgery to patients who cannot write so that they may point to needed items. A speech therapist is also consulted postoperatively.

PREVENTING INFECTION

Leukopenia (a decrease in white blood cells) may result from radiation, chemotherapy, AIDS, and some medications used to treat HIV infection. Leukopenia reduces defense mechanisms, increasing the risk for infections. Malnutrition, which is also common among these patients, may further decrease resistance to infection. If the patient has diabetes, the risk of infection is further increased.

Laboratory results should be evaluated frequently and the patient's temperature checked every 4 to 8 hours for an elevation that may indicate infection. Visitors who might transmit microorganisms are prohibited because the patient's immunologic system is depressed. Sensitive skin tissues are protected from trauma to maintain skin integrity and prevent infection. Aseptic technique is necessary when changing dressings. Desquamation (shedding of the epidermis) is a reaction to radiation therapy that causes dryness and itching and can lead to a break in skin integrity and subsequent infection.

As described earlier, adequate nutrition is helpful in preventing infection. Signs of wound infection (redness, swelling, drainage, tenderness) are reported to the physician. Antibiotics may be prescribed prophylactically.

PROMOTING HOME AND COMMUNITY-BASED CARE

Teaching Patients Self-Care

The patient who is recovering from treatment of an oral condition is instructed about mouth care, nutrition, prevention of infection, and signs and symptoms of complications (Chart 35-2). Methods of preparing nutritious foods that are seasoned according to the patient's preference and at the preferred temperature are explained. For some patients, it may be more convenient to use commercial baby foods than to prepare liquid and soft diets. The patient who cannot take foods orally may receive enteral or parenteral nutrition; the administration of these feedings is explained and demonstrated to the patient and the care provider.

For patients with cancer, instructions are provided in the use and care of any prostheses. The importance of keeping dressings clean is emphasized, as is the need for conscientious oral hygiene.

Continuing Care

The need for ongoing care in the home depends on the patient's condition. The patient, the family members or others responsible for home care, the nurse, and other health care professionals (eg, speech therapist, nutritionist, psychologist) work together to prepare an individual plan of care.

If suctioning of the mouth or tracheostomy tube is required, the necessary equipment is obtained and the patient and care providers are taught how to use it. Considerations include the control of odors and humidification of the home to keep secretions moist. The patient and the care providers are taught how to assess for obstruction, hemorrhage, and infection and what actions to take if they occur. The home care nurse may provide physical care, monitor for changes in the patient's physical status (eg, skin integrity, nutritional status, respiratory function), and assess the adequacy of pain control measures. The nurse also assesses the patient's and family's ability to manage incisions, drains, and feeding tubes and the use of recommended strategies for communication. The ability of the patient and family to accept physical, psychological, and role changes is assessed and addressed.

Follow-up visits to the physician are important to monitor the patient's condition and to determine the need for modifications in treatment and general care. The nurse reinforces instructions in an effort to promote the patient's self-care and comfort.

Because patients and their family members and health care providers tend to focus on the most obvious needs and issues, the nurse reminds the patient and family about the importance of continuing health promotion and screening practices. Those patients who have not been involved in these practices in the past are educated about their importance and are referred to appropriate health care providers.

Evaluation

EXPECTED PATIENT OUTCOMES

Expected patient outcomes may include:

1. Shows evidence of intact oral mucous membranes
   a. Is free of pain and discomfort in the oral cavity
   b. Has no visible alteration in membrane integrity
   c. Identifies and avoids foods that are irritating (eg, nuts, pretzels, spicy foods)
   d. Describes measures that are necessary for preventive mouth care
   e. Complies with medication regimen
   f. Limits or avoids use of alcohol and tobacco (including smokeless tobacco)
2. Attains and maintains desirable body weight
3. Has a positive self-image
   a. Verbalizes anxieties
   b. Is able to accept change in appearance and modify self-concept accordingly
4. Attains an acceptable level of comfort
   a. Verbalizes that pain is absent or under control
   b. Avoids foods and liquids that cause discomfort
   c. Adheres to medication regimen
5. Has decreased fears related to pain, isolation, and the inability to cope
   a. Accepts that pain will be managed if not eliminated
   b. Freely expresses fears and concerns
6. Is free of infection
   a. Exhibits normal laboratory values
   b. Is afebrile
   c. Performs oral hygiene after every meal and at bedtime
7. Acquires information about disease process and course of treatment

Neck Dissection

Malignancies of the head and neck include those of the oral cavity, oropharynx, hypopharynx, nasopharynx, nasal cavity, paranasal sinus, and larynx (Fig. 35-3). (Laryngeal cancer is

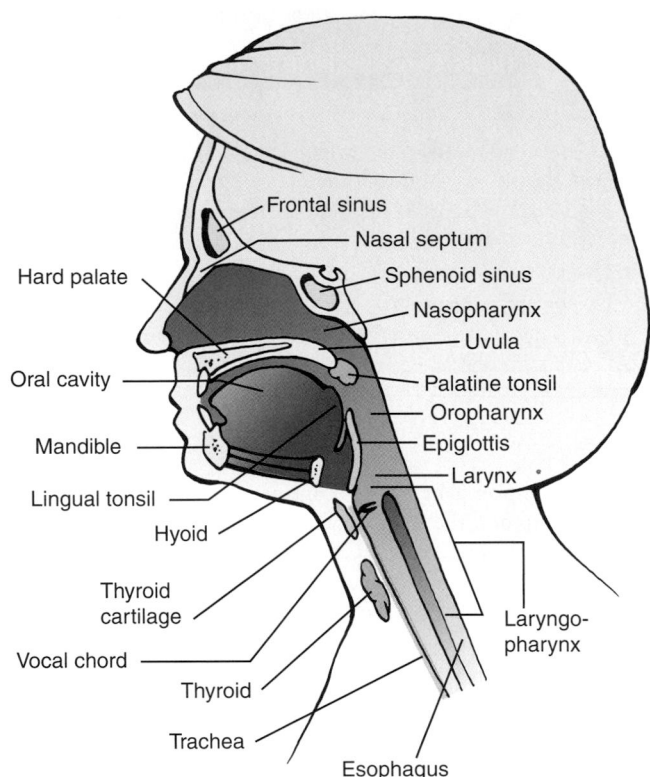

FIGURE 35-3 Anatomy of the head and neck.

presented in Chapter 22.) These cancers account for fewer than 5% of all cancers. Depending on the location and stage, treatment may consist of radiation therapy, chemotherapy, surgery, or a combination of these modalities. Deaths from malignancies of the head and neck are primarily attributable not to recurrence at the primary site but to local-regional metastasis to the cervical lymph nodes in the neck. This often occurs by way of the lymphatics before the primary lesion has been treated. This local-regional metastasis is not amenable to surgical resection and responds poorly to chemotherapy and radiation therapy.

A radical neck dissection involves removal of all cervical lymph nodes from the mandible to the clavicle and removal of the sternocleidomastoid muscle, internal jugular vein, and spinal accessory muscle on one side of the neck. The associated morbidities include shoulder drop and poor cosmesis (visible neck depression). Modified radical neck dissection, which preserves one or more of the nonlymphatic structures, is used more often. A selective neck dissection (in comparison to a radical dissection) preserves one or more of the lymph node groups, the internal jugular vein, the sternocleidomastoid muscle, and the spinal accessory nerve (Fig. 35-4).

Reconstructive techniques may be performed with a variety of grafts. A cutaneous flap (skin and subcutaneous tissue), such as the deltopectoral flap, may be used. A more frequently used graft for head and neck reconstruction is a myocutaneous flap (subcutaneous tissue, muscle and skin). The pectoralis major muscle is usually used. A microvascular free flap may be used for large defects. This involves the transfer of muscle, skin, or bone with an artery and vein to the area of reconstruction, using microinstrumentation. Areas used for a free flap include the scapula, the radial area of the forearm, or the fibula. The fibula, which provides a larger bone area, may be used if mandibular reconstruction is involved.

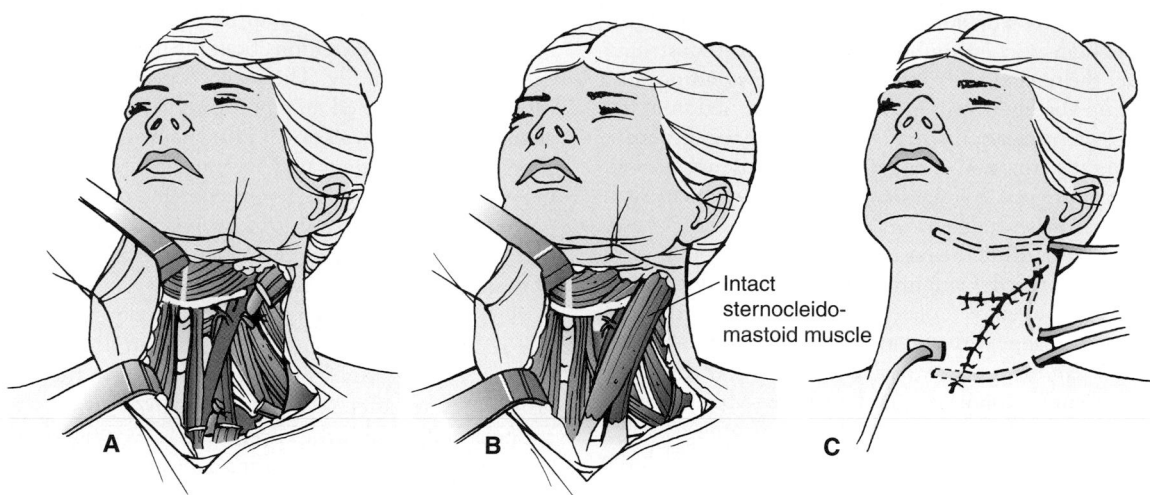

FIGURE 35-4 (**A**) A classic radical neck dissection in which the sternocleidomastoid and smaller muscles are removed. All tissue is removed, from the ramus of the jaw to the clavicle. The jugular vein has also been removed. The selective neck dissection (**B**) is similar but preserves the sternocleidomastoid muscle, internal jugular vein, and spinal accessory nerve. The wound is closed (**C**), and portable suction drainage tubes are in place.

Intact sternocleido-mastoid muscle

NURSING PROCESS:
THE PATIENT UNDERGOING
A NECK DISSECTION

Assessment

Preoperatively, the patient's physical and psychological preparation for major surgery is assessed, along with his or her knowledge of the preoperative and postoperative procedures. Postoperatively, the patient is assessed for complications such as altered respiratory status, wound infection, and hemorrhage. As healing occurs, neck range of motion is assessed to determine whether there has been a decrease in range of motion due to nerve or muscle damage.

Diagnosis

NURSING DIAGNOSES
Based on all the assessment data, major nursing diagnoses may include the following:

- Deficient knowledge about preoperative and postoperative procedures
- Ineffective airway clearance related to obstruction by mucus, hemorrhage, or edema
- Acute pain related to surgical incision
- Risk for infection related to surgical intervention secondary to decreased nutritional status, or immunosuppression from chemotherapy or radiation therapy
- Impaired tissue integrity secondary to surgery and grafting
- Imbalanced nutrition, less than body requirements, related to disease process or treatment
- Situational low self-esteem related to diagnosis or prognosis
- Impaired verbal communication secondary to surgical resection
- Impaired physical mobility secondary to nerve injury

COLLABORATIVE PROBLEMS/
POTENTIAL COMPLICATIONS
Potential postoperative complications that may develop include the following:

- Hemorrhage
- Chyle fistula
- Nerve injury

Planning and Goals

The major goals for the patient include participation in the treatment plan, maintenance of respiratory status, absence of infection, viability of the graft, maintenance of adequate intake of food and fluids, effective coping strategies, attainment of comfort, effective communication, and absence of complications.

Nursing Interventions

PROVIDING PREOPERATIVE PATIENT EDUCATION
Before surgery, the patient should be informed about the nature and extent of the surgery, and what the postoperative period will be like. The patient is encouraged to ask questions and to express concerns about the upcoming surgery and the expected results. During this exchange, the nurse has an opportunity to assess the patient's coping abilities, answer questions, and develop a plan for offering assistance. A sense of mutual understanding and rapport will make the postoperative experience less traumatic for the patient. The patient's expressions of concern, anxieties, and fears can guide the nurse in providing support postoperatively.

PROVIDING GENERAL POSTOPERATIVE CARE
The general postoperative nursing interventions are similar to those presented in Chapter 20. For the patient who has had extensive neck surgery, specific postoperative interventions include maintenance of a patent airway and continuous assessment of respiratory status, wound care and oral hygiene, maintenance of adequate nutrition, and observation for hemorrhage or nerve injury.

MAINTAINING THE AIRWAY
After the endotracheal tube or airway has been removed and the effects of the anesthesia have worn off, the patient may be placed in Fowler's position to facilitate breathing and promote comfort. This position also increases lymphatic and venous drainage, facilitates swallowing, and decreases venous pressure on the skin flaps.

In the immediate postoperative period, the nurse assesses for stridor (coarse, high-pitched sound on inspiration) by listening frequently over the trachea with a stethoscope. This finding must be reported immediately because it indicates obstruction of the airway. Signs of respiratory distress, such as dyspnea, cyanosis, changes in mental status, and changes in vital signs, are assessed because they may suggest edema, hemorrhage, inadequate oxygenation, or inadequate drainage.

Pneumonia may occur in the postoperative phase if pulmonary secretions are not removed. Coughing and deep breathing are encouraged to aid in the removal of secretions. The patient should assume a sitting position, with the nurse supporting the neck so that the patient can bring up excessive secretions. If this is ineffective, the patient's respiratory tract may have to be suctioned. Care is taken to protect the suture lines during suctioning. If a tracheostomy tube is in place, suctioning is performed through the tube. The patient may also be instructed on use of Yankauer suction (tonsil tip suction) to remove oral secretions. Temperature should not be taken orally.

RELIEVING PAIN

Pain and the patient's fear of pain are assessed and managed. Patients with head and neck cancer often report less pain than patients with other types of cancer; however, the nurse needs to be aware that each person's pain experience is individual. The nurse administers analgesics as prescribed and assesses their effectiveness.

PROVIDING WOUND CARE

Wound drainage tubes are usually inserted during surgery to prevent the collection of fluid subcutaneously. The drainage tubes are connected to portable suction device (eg, Jackson-Pratt), and the container is emptied periodically. Between 80 and 120 mL of serosanguineous secretions may drain over the first 24 hours. Excessive drainage may be indicative of a chyle fistula or hemorrhage (see later discussion). If dressings are present, they may need to be reinforced from time to time. Dressings are observed for evidence of hemorrhage and constriction, which impairs respiration and perfusion of the graft. The graft is assessed for color and temperature, and for the presence of a pulse if applicable, to determine viability. The graft should be pale pink and warm to the touch. The surgical incisions are also assessed for infection, which is reported immediately. Prophylactic antibiotics may be prescribed.

MAINTAINING ADEQUATE NUTRITION

Nutritional status is assessed preoperatively; early intervention to correct nutritional imbalances may decrease the risk of postoperative complications. Frequently, nutrition is less than optimal because of inadequate intake, and the patient often requires enteral or parenteral supplements preoperatively to attain a positive nitrogen balance. This therapy may need to be continued postoperatively if the patient cannot take enough nutrients by mouth. Supplements (eg, Ensure, Sustacal) that are nutritionally dense may help reestablish a positive nitrogen balance. They may be taken enterally by mouth, by nasogastric feeding tube, or by gastrostomy feeding tube. (See the Plan of Nursing Care for further discussion.)

The patient who is able to chew may take food by mouth; the level of the patient's chewing ability will determine whether some diet modification (eg, soft, pureed, or liquid foods) is necessary. Food preferences should also be discussed with the patient. Oral care before eating may enhance the patient's appetite, and oral care after eating is important to prevent infection and dental caries. Most patients are able to maintain and gain weight.

SUPPORTING COPING MEASURES

Preoperatively, information about the planned surgery is given to the patient and family. The psychological postoperative nursing intervention is aimed at supporting the patient who has had a change in body image or who has major concerns regarding the prognosis. The patient may have difficulty communicating and may be concerned about his or her ability to breathe and swallow normally. The nurse enlists the support of family or friends in encouraging and reassuring the patient that adjusting to the results of this surgery will take time.

The person who has had extensive neck surgery often is sensitive about his or her appearance. This can occur when the operative area is covered by bulky dressings, when the incision line is visible, or later after healing has occurred but the appearance of the neck and possibly the lower face has been significantly altered. If the nurse accepts the patient's appearance and expresses a positive, optimistic attitude, the patient is more likely to be encouraged. The patient also needs an opportunity to express concerns regarding the success of the surgery and the prognosis. The American Cancer Society may be a resource to provide a volunteer to meet with the patient either preoperatively or postoperatively.

People with cancer of the head and neck frequently have used alcohol or tobacco before surgery; postoperatively, the patient is encouraged to abstain from these substances. Alternative methods of coping need to be explored. A referral to Alcoholics Anonymous may be appropriate.

PROMOTING EFFECTIVE COMMUNICATION

If a laryngectomy was performed, the nurse explores other methods of communicating with the patient and obtains a consultation with a speech/language therapist. Alternatives to verbal communication may include use of a pencil and paper or pointing to needed items on a picture pad. Alternative speech techniques, such as an electrolarynx (a mechanical device held against the neck) or esophageal speech, may be taught by a speech/language therapist.

MAINTAINING PHYSICAL MOBILITY

Excision of muscles and nerves results in weakness at the shoulder that can cause shoulder drop, a forward curvature of the shoulder. Many problems can be avoided with a conscientious exercise program. These exercises are usually begun after the drains have been removed and the neck incision is sufficiently healed. The purpose of the exercises depicted in Figure 35-5 is to promote maximal shoulder function and neck motion after surgery. Physical therapists and occupational therapists can assist patients in performing these exercises.

MONITORING AND MANAGING POTENTIAL COMPLICATIONS

Hemorrhage

Hemorrhage may occur from carotid artery rupture as a result of necrosis of the graft or damage to the artery itself from tumor or infection. The following measures are indicated:

- Vital signs are assessed. Tachycardia, tachypnea, and hypotension may indicate hemorrhage and impending hypovolemic shock.
- The patient is instructed to avoid the Valsalva maneuver to prevent stress on the graft and carotid artery.
- Signs of impending rupture, such as high epigastric pain or discomfort, are reported.

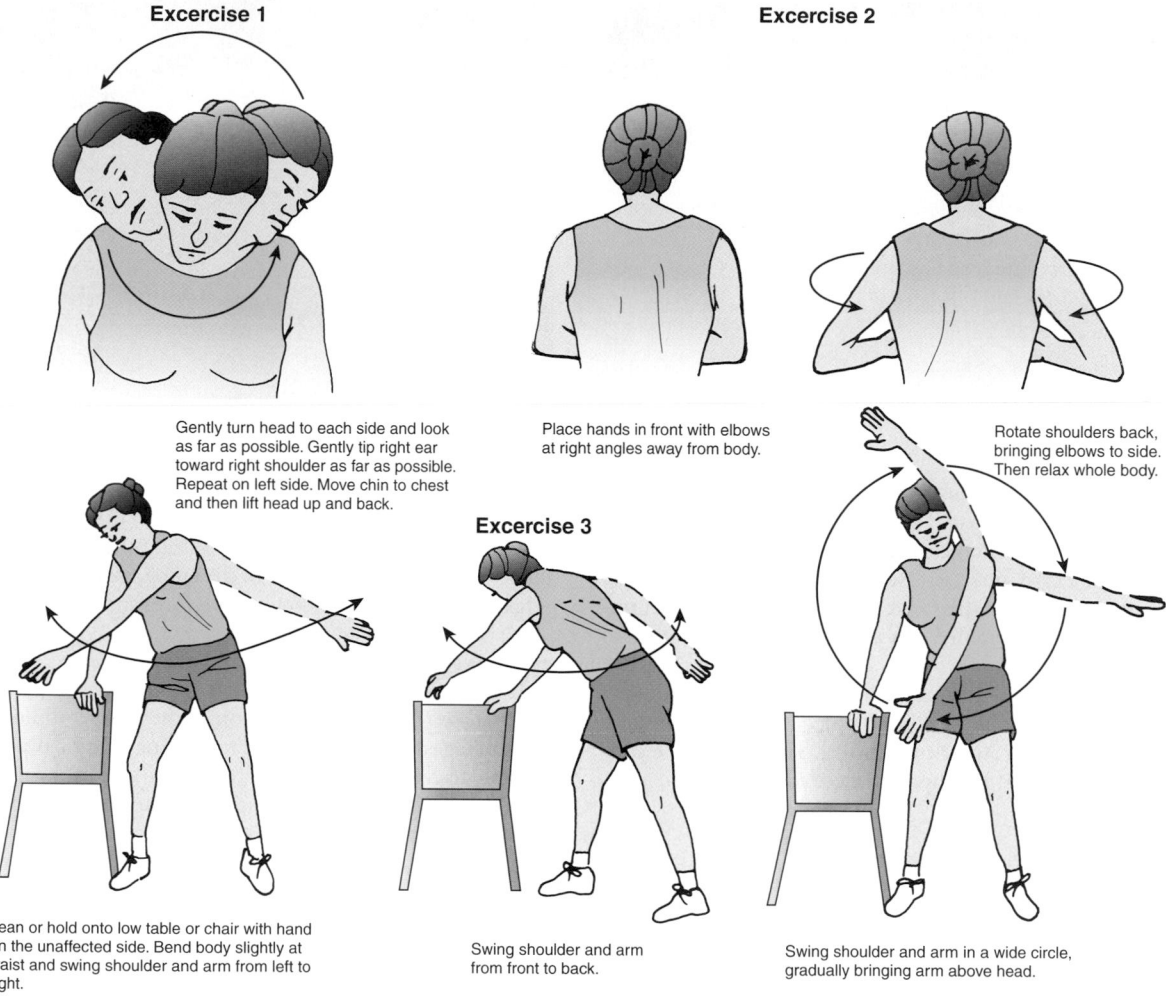

Excercise 1

Gently turn head to each side and look as far as possible. Gently tip right ear toward right shoulder as far as possible. Repeat on left side. Move chin to chest and then lift head up and back.

Excercise 2

Place hands in front with elbows at right angles away from body.

Rotate shoulders back, bringing elbows to side. Then relax whole body.

Excercise 3

Lean or hold onto low table or chair with hand on the unaffected side. Bend body slightly at waist and swing shoulder and arm from left to right.

Swing shoulder and arm from front to back.

Swing shoulder and arm in a wide circle, gradually bringing arm above head.

FIGURE 35-5 Three rehabilitation exercises after head and neck surgery. The objective is to regain maximum shoulder function and neck motion after neck surgery. From *Exercise for Radical Neck Surgery Patients.* Head and Neck Service, Department of Surgery, Memorial Hospital, New York, NY.

- Dressings and wound drainage are observed for excessive bleeding.
- If hemorrhage occurs, assistance is summoned immediately.
- Hemorrhage requires the continuous application of pressure to the bleeding site or major associated vessel.
- Although some advocate placing the patient in modified Trendelenburg position to maintain blood pressure, others recommend that the head of the patient's bed be elevated to maintain airway patency and prevent aspiration.
- A controlled, calm manner will allay the patient's anxiety.
- The surgeon is notified immediately, because a vascular or ligature tear requires surgical intervention.

Chyle Fistula

A chyle fistula (milk-like drainage from the thoracic duct into the thoracic cavity) may develop as a result of damage to the thoracic duct during surgery. The diagnosis is made if there is excess drainage which has a 3% fat content and a specific gravity of 1.012 or greater. Treatment of a small leak (500 mL or less) includes application of a pressure dressing and a diet of medium-chain fatty acids or parenteral nutrition. Surgical intervention to repair the damaged duct is necessary for larger leaks.

Nerve Injury

Nerve injury can occur if the cervical plexus or spinal accessory nerves are severed during surgery. Because lower facial paralysis may occur as a result of injury to the facial nerve, this complication is observed for and reported. Likewise, if the superior laryngeal nerve is damaged, the patient may have difficulty swallowing liquids and food because of the partial lack of sensation of the glottis. Speech therapy may be indicated to assist with the problems related to nerve injury.

PROMOTING HOME AND COMMUNITY-BASED CARE

Teaching Patients Self-Care

The patient and care provider will require instructions about management of the wound, the dressing, and any drains that remain in place. Patients who require oral suctioning or who have a tracheostomy may be very anxious about their care at home; the transition to home can be eased if the care provider is given several opportunities to demonstrate the ability to meet the patient's needs (Chart 35-3).

If the patient cannot take food by mouth, detailed instructions and demonstration of enteral or parenteral feedings will be required. Education in techniques of effective oral hygiene is also important.

Chart 35-3

Home Care Checklist • Recovering From Neck Surgery

At the completion of the home care instruction, the patient or caregiver will be able to:	Patient	Caregiver
• Demonstrate use of suction equipment.	✓	✓
• State rationale for humidification.	✓	✓
• State dietary modifications needed to meet caloric needs.	✓	✓
• Demonstrate enteral or parenteral feeding techniques.	✓	✓
• Demonstrate care of incision and drains.	✓	✓
• State when next checkup is needed.	✓	✓
• Demonstrate exercises.	✓	
• Identify available support groups.	✓	✓

Continuing Care

A referral for home care nursing may be necessary in the early period after discharge. The nurse will assess healing, ensure that feedings are being administered properly, and detect any complications. The home care nurse assesses the patient's adjustment to changes in physical appearance and status, ability to communicate, and ability to eat normally. Physical and speech therapy also may be continued at home.

The patient is given information regarding local support groups such as "I Can Cope" or "New Voice Club," if indicated. The local chapter of the American Cancer Society may be contacted for information and equipment needed for the patient.

Evaluation

EXPECTED PATIENT OUTCOMES

Expected patient outcomes may include:

1. Discusses expected course of treatment
2. Demonstrates good respiratory exchange
   a. Lungs are clear to auscultation
   b. Breathes easily with no shortness of breath
   c. Demonstrates ability to use suction effectively
3. Remains free of infection
   a. Maintains normal laboratory values
   b. Is afebrile
4. Graft is pink and warm to touch
5. Maintains adequate intake of foods and fluids
   a. Accepts altered route of feeding
   b. Is well hydrated
   c. Maintains or gains weight
6. Demonstrates ability to cope
   a. Discusses emotional responses to the diagnosis
   b. Attends support group meetings
7. Verbalizes comfort
8. Attains maximal mobility
   a. Adheres to physical therapy exercises
   b. Attains maximal range of motion

The Plan of Nursing Care presents an overview of the care of a patient undergoing a neck dissection.

Disorders of the Esophagus

The esophagus is a mucus-lined, muscular tube that carries food from the mouth to the stomach. It begins at the base of the pharynx and ends about 4 cm below the diaphragm. Its ability to transport food and fluid is facilitated by two sphincters. The upper esophageal sphincter, also called the hypopharyngeal sphincter, is located at the junction of the pharynx and the esophagus. The lower esophageal sphincter, also called the gastroesophageal sphincter, is located at the junction of the esophagus and the stomach. An incompetent lower esophageal sphincter allows reflux (backward flow) of gastric contents. There is no serosal layer of the esophagus; therefore, if surgery is necessary, it is more difficult to perform suturing or anastomosis.

DYSPHAGIA

Dysphagia (difficulty swallowing) is the most common symptom of esophageal disease. This symptom may vary from an uncomfortable feeling that a bolus of food is caught in the upper esophagus (before it eventually passes into the stomach) to acute pain on swallowing (**odynophagia**). Obstruction of food (solid and soft) and even liquids may occur anywhere along the esophagus. Often the patient can indicate that the problem is located in the upper, middle, or lower third of the esophagus.

There are many pathologic conditions of the esophagus, including motility disorders (achalasia, diffuse spasm), gastroesophageal reflux, hiatal hernias, diverticula, perforation, foreign bodies, chemical burns, benign tumors, and carcinoma.

ACHALASIA

Achalasia is absent or ineffective peristalsis of the distal esophagus, accompanied by failure of the esophageal sphincter to relax in response to swallowing. Narrowing of the esophagus just above the stomach results in a gradually increasing dilation of the esophagus in the upper chest. Achalasia may progress slowly and occurs most often in people 40 years of age or older.

Clinical Manifestations

The primary symptom of achalasia is difficulty in swallowing both liquids and solids. The patient has a sensation of food sticking in the lower portion of the esophagus. As the condition progresses, food is commonly regurgitated, either spontaneously or intentionally by the patient to relieve the discomfort produced by prolonged distention of the esophagus by food that will not pass into the stomach. The patient may also complain of chest pain and heartburn (**pyrosis**). Pain may or may not be associated with eating. There may be secondary pulmonary complications from aspiration of gastric contents.

Assessment and Diagnostic Findings

X-ray studies show esophageal dilation above the narrowing at the gastroesophageal junction. Barium swallow, computed tomography

(text continues on page 975)

Plan of Nursing Care

The Patient Who Has Undergone Neck Dissection

Nursing Interventions	Rationale	Expected Outcomes

Nursing Diagnosis: Ineffective airway clearance related to obstruction secondary to edema, hemorrhage, or inadequate wound drainage

Goal: Maintenance of normal respiratory function

Nursing Interventions	Rationale	Expected Outcomes
1. Place the patient in Fowler's position.	1. Fowler's position facilitates expansion of the lungs because the diaphragm is pulled downward and the abdominal viscera are pulled away from the lungs. Breathing is promoted. This position also increases lymphatic and venous drainage, decreases swallowing, and decreases venous pressure on the graft. Regurgitation and aspiration of stomach contents are prevented postoperatively.	• Achieves a normal respiratory rate • Breathes comfortably • Avoids use of accessory muscles of respiration • Maintains vital signs within normal range • Shows evidence of normal breath sounds • Coughs effectively • Maintains a patent airway • Does not develop a mucus plug
2. Monitor vital signs according to postoperative routine.	2. Edema, hemorrhage, or inadequate drainage will alter heart rate and respirations. Tachypnea and restlessness may indicate respiratory distress.	
3. Auscultate breath sounds as needed. In the immediate postoperative period, place the stethoscope over the trachea to assess for stridor.	3. Abnormal breath sounds may indicate ineffective ventilation, decreased perfusion, and fluid accumulation. Stridor, a harsh, high-pitched sound primarily heard on inspiration, indicates airway obstruction.	
4. Encourage deep breathing and coughing. Place the patient in a sitting position and support the neck area with both hands.	4. Deep breathing before coughing promotes expansion of the airways and a more forceful cough. The coughing mechanism assists airway cilia with removal of secretions. Splinting the incision during coughing reduces strain and promotes the expulsion of secretions by allowing deeper inspirations.	
5. Suction the airway as needed using sterile technique and a soft catheter.	5. Suctioning assists in removal of secretions that the patient may be unable to cough up, thereby assisting with maintaining a patent airway.	
6. Provide humidified air or oxygen if the patient has a tracheostomy.	6. Keeps secretions thin.	

Nursing Diagnosis: Risk for infection

Goal: Absence of infection

Nursing Interventions	Rationale	Expected Outcomes
1. Instruct the patient in preoperative and postoperative oral hygiene using slightly alkaline solutions such as 8 oz of water mixed with 1 teaspoon of baking soda, or normal saline solution, every 4 hours.	1. Oral care decreases oral bacteria, thereby decreasing the risk of bacterial infection postoperatively. Hydrogen peroxide should not be used, because it may break down fresh granulation tissue.	• Patient performs oral hygiene preoperatively and postoperatively every 4 hours • Mouth remains clean • Wound drains less than 200 mL of serosanguineous drainage on the first postoperative day
2. Monitor wound suction drainage.	2. Suction drainage negates the need for pressure dressings because the skin flaps are pulled down tightly. Drainage should be 80–120 mL of serosanguineous secretions for the first 24 hours; then the secretions should decrease daily. Continuous bloody drainage indicates small vessel oozing.	• No hematoma at skin graft • Serosanguineous drainage is within normal limits • Dressing remains intact with no constriction of airway or blood flow • Wound and surrounding skin remain clean and free of infection • Patient is afebrile with normal respirations and a normal heart rate • Patient is alert and aware of surroundings

(continued)

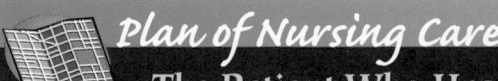

Plan of Nursing Care

The Patient Who Has Undergone Neck Dissection *(Continued)*

Nursing Interventions	Rationale	Expected Outcomes
3. Note drainage quantity and odor.	3. Purulent, malodorous drainage indicates an infection. Drainage greater than 300 mL in the first 24 hours is considered abnormal.	
4. Assess condition of dressing and reinforce pressure dressings as needed. Assess for any possible constrictions that would affect respirations or decrease blood flow to graft.	4. If portable wound suction is not used, pressure dressings may be applied to obliterate dead spaces and provide immobilization. These dressings are reinforced, not changed, as needed.	
5. Use aseptic technique to cleanse skin around the drains; change the dressings as ordered by surgeon (usually the second through fifth postoperative days).	5. Aseptic technique prevents wound contamination. Sterile saline effectively cleans the skin around the drains.	
6. Monitor vital signs. Assess for symptoms of infection: chills, diaphoresis, altered level of consciousness.	6. An elevated temperature, tachypnea, and tachycardia may indicate an infection.	

Nursing Diagnosis: Impaired skin integrity
Goal: Maintenance of intact skin and viability of graft

1. Assess condition of graft for viability.	1. Cyanotic, cool graft indicates possible necrosis. (Pale graft indicates arterial thrombosis; purple graft indicates venous congestion.)	• Graft is pale pink in color and warm to touch • Tissue blanches to gentle touch • Graft has pulse via Doppler ultrasound
2. Assess wound for signs and symptoms of infection.	2. Infected wound interferes with healing and threatens the viability of the graft.	• Patient does not have wound infection

Nursing Diagnosis: Imbalanced nutrition, less than body requirements, related to anorexia and dysphagia

Goal: Attainment/maintenance of adequate nutrition

1. Assess nutritional status preoperatively, consult with dietitian.	1. Poor nutritional status preoperatively impairs wound healing and increases potential for infection.	• Does not have weight loss greater than 10% of body weight. (If weight loss is greater than 10%, supplements are given to maintain/increase weight and obtain positive nitrogen balance.)
2. Administer tube feedings as prescribed. Keep head of bed elevated during feeding to prevent aspiration. Monitor for signs of tracheoesophageal fistula (feeding in tracheal secretions).	2. A nasogastric tube may be in place for several days to administer enteral feedings.	• Tolerates tube feedings • No signs of aspiration • No sign of fistula
3. Provide oral hygiene before and after meals.	3. Oral hygiene enhances appetite.	• Expresses a desire for food
4. Assist with oral intake: 　a. Offer easily chewed foods; mash or blenderize if necessary. 　b. Suggest that the head be tilted to the unaffected side when swallowing. 　c. Inquire whether privacy is desired when eating. 　d. Provide altered eating utensils as needed.	4. Soft-textured foods facilitate swallowing. Passage of food may be tolerated better when the head is tilted to the unaffected side. Self-feeding difficulties may cause embarrassment and interfere with intake quantity.	• Swallows food easily • Is comfortable eating alone or with others

(continued)

Plan of Nursing Care

The Patient Who Has Undergone Neck Dissection *(Continued)*

Nursing Interventions	Rationale	Expected Outcomes

Nursing Diagnosis: Situational low self-esteem and body image related to changes in appearance and alterations in communication

Goal: Attainment of positive self-image

Nursing Interventions	Rationale	Expected Outcomes

1. Assist the patient to communicate effectively:
  a. Provide materials for writing messages.
  b. Make certain that the call bell is readily accessible.
  c. Develop nonverbal ways to communicate (eg, finger-tapping, sign language, sign board).
  d. Consult speech/language therapist.
	1. Temporary hoarseness is common after neck surgery. A tracheostomy may be performed, and verbal communication may not be possible. Communication with head movement may be impossible because of incisional pain and need to maintain position of neck for graft. A speech/language therapist may assist with other forms of communication, such as esophageal speech or electrolarynx.	• Recognizes that hoarseness is temporary
		• Develops alternative forms of communication
		• Willingly conveys fears and concerns
		• Accepts prognosis with realistic limitations
		• Accepts support as offered
		• Absence of facial paralysis
		• Absence of drooling and dysphagia
		• Maintains normal shoulder function
		• Verbalizes methods to enhance physical appearance

2. Encourage verbalization of fears:
  a. Provide time to listen.
  b. Project a positive, optimistic attitude.
  c. Reinforce reality.
  d. Collaborate with family members to elicit their support and encouragement.
  e. Consult support groups such as New Voice Club through the American Cancer Society.
	2. Listening conveys acceptance and encourages further verbalization. An optimistic approach conveys interest and hope. Honesty will promote a trusting relationship. This includes confirming cosmetic and functional limitations. Family members or significant others can provide valuable support to the patient.	

3. Observe for facial paralysis.	3. Injury to facial nerve will cause lower facial paralysis.	
4. Observe for excessive drooling.	4. Damage to the hypoglossal nerve will result in excessive drooling and decreased ability to swallow.	
5. Check for normal shoulder position and function.	5. Damage to the spinal accessory nerve will result in drooping of the shoulder. Rehabilitation exercises are begun after the incision is healed.	
6. Provide information on clothing/cosmetics to deemphasize physical defects (offer information on "Look Good, Feel Better" program through American Cancer Society).	6. Physical appearance may be enhanced through use of cosmetics or clothing.	

(CT) of the esophagus, and endoscopy may be used for diagnosis; however, the diagnosis is confirmed by manometry, a process in which the esophageal pressure is measured by a radiologist or gastroenterologist.

Management

The patient should be instructed to eat slowly and to drink fluids with meals. As a temporary measure, calcium channel blockers and nitrates have been used to decrease esophageal pressure and improve swallowing. Injection of botulinum toxin (Botox) to quadrants of the esophagus via endoscopy has been helpful because it inhibits the contraction of smooth muscle. Periodic injections are required to maintain remission. If these methods are unsuccessful, pneumatic (forceful) dilation or surgical separation of the muscle fibers may be recommended (Streeter, 1999; Annese et al., 2000).

Achalasia may be treated conservatively by pneumatic dilation to stretch the narrowed area of the esophagus (Fig. 35-6). Pneumatic dilation has a high success rate. Although perforation is a potential complication, its incidence is low. The procedure can be painful; therefore, moderate sedation in the form of an analgesic or tranquilizer, or both, is administered for the treatment. The patient is monitored for perforation. Complaints of abdominal tenderness and fever may be indications of perforation (see later discussion).

Achalasia may be treated surgically by esophagomyotomy (Fig. 35-7). The procedure usually is performed laparoscopically, either with a complete lower esophageal sphincter myotomy and an antireflux procedure (see later discussion of fundoplasty), or without an antireflux procedure. The esophageal muscle fibers are separated to relieve the lower esophageal stricture. Although patients with a history of achalasia have a slightly higher incidence of esophageal cancer, long-term follow-up with esophagoscopy for early detection has not proved beneficial.

DIFFUSE SPASM

Diffuse spasm is a motor disorder of the esophagus. The cause is unknown, but stressful situations can produce contractions of the

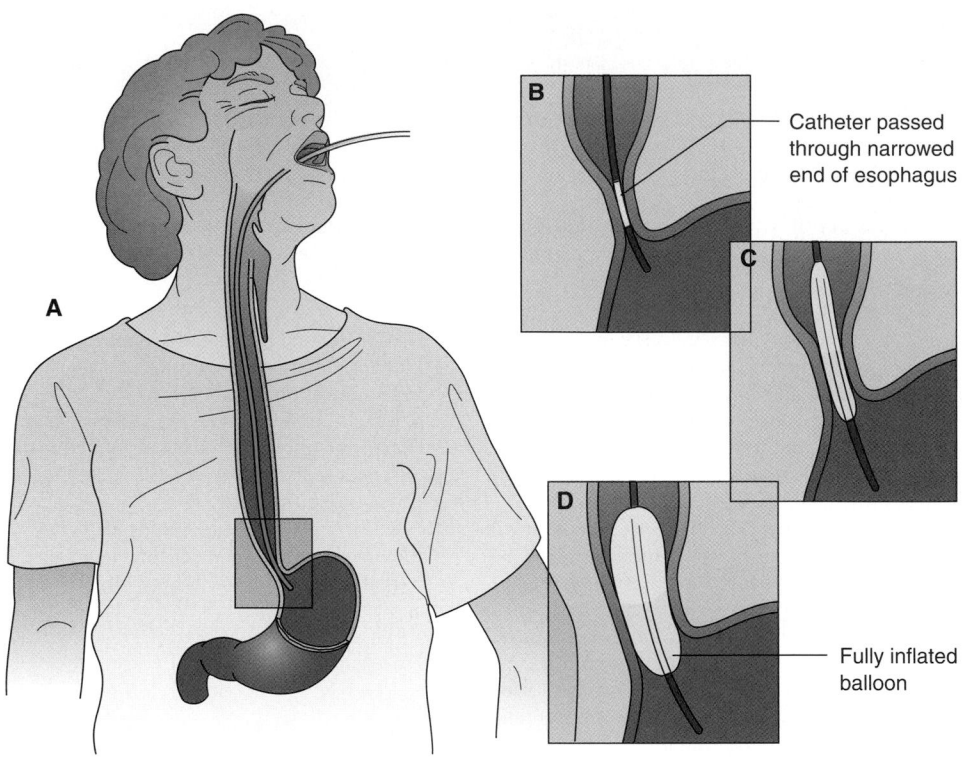

Catheter passed through narrowed end of esophagus

Fully inflated balloon

FIGURE 35-6 Treatment of achalasia by the conservative approach. (**A–C**) The dilator is passed, guided by a previously inserted guidewire. (**D**) When the balloon is in proper position, it is distended by pressure sufficient to dilate the narrowed area of the esophagus.

esophagus. It is more common in women and usually manifests in middle age.

Clinical Manifestations

Diffuse spasm is characterized by difficulty or pain on swallowing (dysphagia, odynophagia) and by chest pain similar to that of coronary artery spasm.

Assessment and Diagnostic Findings

Esophageal manometry, which measures the motility of the esophagus and the pressure within the esophagus, indicates that simultaneous contractions of the esophagus occur irregularly. Diagnostic x-ray studies after ingestion of barium show separate areas of spasm.

Management

Conservative therapy includes administration of sedatives and long-acting nitrates to relieve pain. Calcium channel blockers have also been used to manage diffuse spasm. Small, frequent feedings and a soft diet are usually recommended to decrease the esophageal pressure and irritation that lead to spasm. Dilation performed by bougienage (use of progressively sized flexible dilators), pneumatic dilation, or esophagomyotomy may be necessary if the pain becomes intolerable.

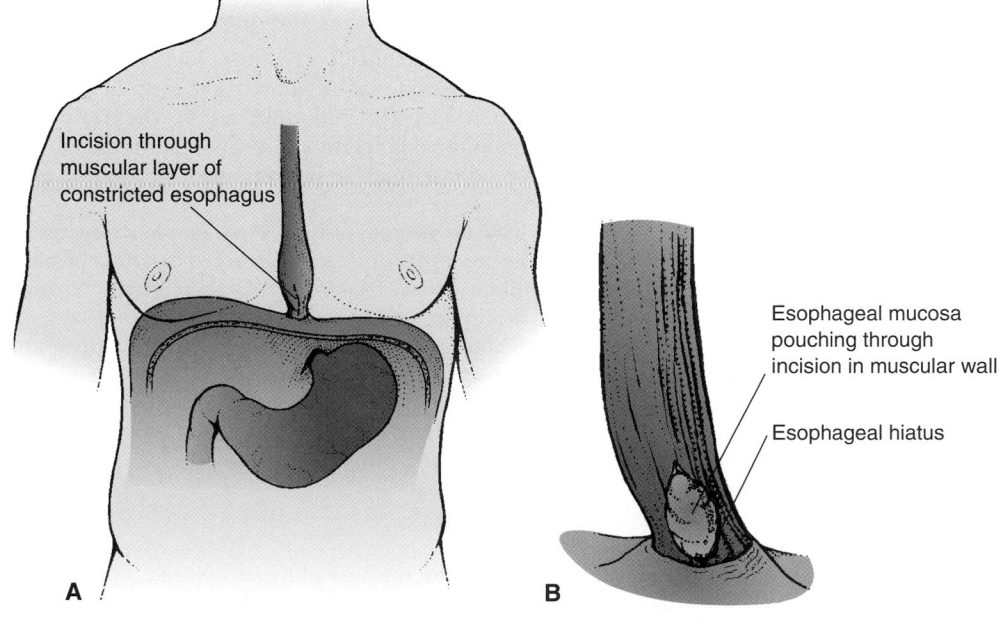

Incision through muscular layer of constricted esophagus

Esophageal mucosa pouching through incision in muscular wall

Esophageal hiatus

FIGURE 35-7 Treatment of achalasia: esophagomyotomy. (**A**) The esophagus is approached via thoracotomy from the front, on the left side. An incision is made through the muscularis of the esophagus extending about 1 cm into the gastric area. (**B**) The incision is large enough to allow a pouching of the esophageal mucosa. Separation of the muscular fibers relieves the narrowing at the lower end of the esophagus and permits the patient to swallow normally again.

HIATAL HERNIA

The esophagus enters the abdomen through an opening in the diaphragm and empties at its lower end into the upper part of the stomach. Normally, the opening in the diaphragm encircles the esophagus tightly, and the stomach lies completely within the abdomen. In a condition known as hiatus (or hiatal) **hernia**, the opening in the diaphragm through which the esophagus passes becomes enlarged, and part of the upper stomach tends to move up into the lower portion of the thorax. Hiatal hernia occurs more often in women than men. There are two types of hiatal hernias: sliding and paraesophageal. Sliding, or type I, hiatal hernia occurs when the upper stomach and the gastroesophageal junction (GEJ) are displaced upward and slide in and out of the thorax (Fig. 35-8A). About 90% of patients with esophageal hiatal hernia have a sliding hernia. A paraesophageal hernia occurs when all or part of the stomach pushes through the diaphragm beside the esophagus (see Fig. 35-8B). Paraesophageal hernias may be further classified as types II, III, or IV, depending on the extent of herniation, with type IV having the greatest herniation.

Clinical Manifestations

The patient with a sliding hernia may have heartburn, regurgitation, and dysphagia, but at least 50% of patients are asymptomatic. Sliding hiatal hernia is often implicated in reflux. The patient with a paraesophageal hernia usually feels a sense of fullness after eating or may be asymptomatic. Reflux usually does not occur, because the gastroesophageal sphincter is intact. The complications of hemorrhage, obstruction, and strangulation can occur with any type of hernia.

Assessment and Diagnostic Findings

Diagnosis is confirmed by x-ray studies, barium swallow, and fluoroscopy.

Management

Management for an axial hernia includes frequent, small feedings that can pass easily through the esophagus. The patient is advised not to recline for 1 hour after eating, to prevent reflux or movement of the hernia, and to elevate the head of the bed on 4- to 8-inch (10- to 20-cm) blocks to prevent the hernia from sliding upward. Surgery is indicated in about 15% of patients. Medical and surgical management of a paraesophageal hernia is similar to that for gastroesophageal reflux; however, paraesophageal hernias may require emergency surgery to correct torsion (twisting) of the stomach or other body organ that leads to restriction of blood flow to that area.

DIVERTICULUM

A diverticulum is an outpouching of mucosa and submucosa that protrudes through a weak portion of the musculature. Diverticula may occur in one of the three areas of the esophagus—the pharyngoesophageal or upper area of the esophagus, the midesophageal area, or the epiphrenic or lower area of the esophagus—or they may occur along the border of the esophagus intramurally.

The most common type of diverticulum, which is found three times more frequently in men than in women, is Zenker's diverticulum (also known as pharyngoesophageal pulsion diverticulum or a pharyngeal pouch). It occurs posteriorly through the cricopharyngeal muscle in the midline of the neck. It is usually seen in people older than 60 years of age. Other types of diverticula include midesophageal, epiphrenic, and intramural diverticula.

Midesophageal diverticula are uncommon. Symptoms are less acute, and usually the condition does not require surgery. Epiphrenic diverticula are usually larger diverticula in the lower esophagus just above the diaphragm. They are thought to be related to the improper functioning of the lower esophageal sphincter or to motor disorders of the esophagus. Intramural diverticulosis is the occurrence of numerous small diverticula associated with a stricture in the upper esophagus.

Clinical Manifestations

Symptoms experienced by the patient with a pharyngoesophageal pulsion diverticulum include difficulty swallowing, fullness in the neck, belching, regurgitation of undigested food, and gurgling

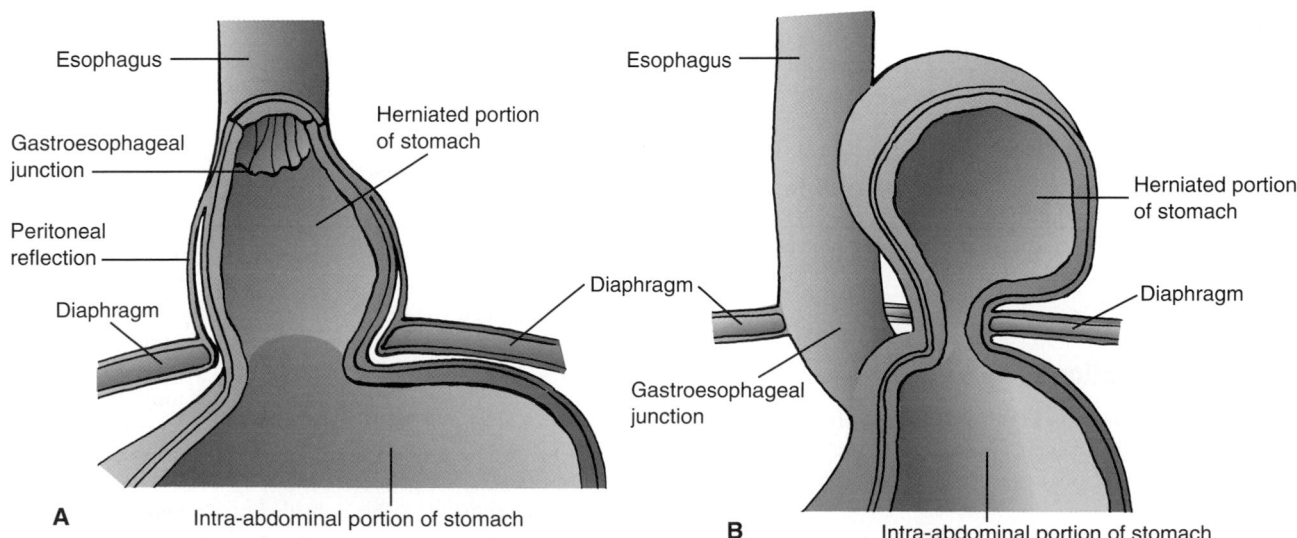

FIGURE 35-8 Sliding esophageal and paraesophageal hernias. (**A**) Sliding esophageal hernia. The upper stomach and cardioesophageal junction have moved upward and slide in and out of the thorax. (**B**) Paraesophageal hernia. All or part of the stomach pushes through the diaphragm next to the gastroesophageal junction.

noises after eating. The diverticulum, or pouch, becomes filled with food or liquid. When the patient assumes a recumbent position, undigested food is regurgitated, and coughing may be caused by irritation of the trachea. Halitosis and a sour taste in the mouth are also common because of the decomposition of food retained in the diverticulum.

Symptoms produced by midesophageal diverticula are less acute. One third of patients with epiphrenic diverticula are asymptomatic, and the remaining two thirds complain of dysphagia and chest pain. Dysphagia is the most common complaint of patients with intramural diverticulosis.

Assessment and Diagnostic Findings

A barium swallow may be performed to determine the exact nature and location of a diverticulum. Manometric studies are often performed for patients with epiphrenic diverticula to rule out a motor disorder. Esophagoscopy usually is contraindicated because of the danger of perforation of the diverticulum, with resulting mediastinitis (inflammation of the organs and tissues that separate the lungs). Blind insertion of a nasogastric tube should be avoided.

Management

Because pharyngoesophageal pulsion diverticulum is progressive, the only means of cure is surgical removal of the diverticulum. During surgery, care is taken to avoid trauma to the common carotid artery and internal jugular veins. The sac is dissected free and amputated flush with the esophageal wall. In addition to a diverticulectomy, a myotomy of the cricopharyngeal muscle is often performed to relieve spasticity of the musculature, which otherwise seems to contribute to a continuation of the previous symptoms. Postoperatively, the patient may have a nasogastric tube inserted at the time of surgery. The surgical incision must be observed for evidence of leakage from the esophagus and a developing fistula. Food and fluids are withheld until x-ray studies show no leakage at the surgical site. The diet begins with liquids and progresses as tolerated.

Surgery is indicated for epiphrenic and midesophageal diverticula only if the symptoms are troublesome and becoming worse. Treatment consists of a diverticulectomy and long myotomy. Intramural diverticula usually regress after the esophageal stricture is dilated.

PERFORATION

The esophagus is not an uncommon site of injury. Perforation may result from stab or bullet wounds of the neck or chest, trauma from motor vehicle crash, caustic injury from a chemical burn (described later), or inadvertent puncture by a surgical instrument during examination or dilation.

Clinical Manifestations

The patient has persistent pain followed by dysphagia. Infection, fever, leukocytosis, and severe hypotension may be noted. In some instances, signs of pneumothorax are observed.

Assessment and Diagnostic Findings

Diagnostic x-ray studies and fluoroscopy are used to identify the site of the injury.

Management

Because of the high risk of infection, broad-spectrum antibiotic therapy is initiated. A nasogastric tube is inserted to provide suction and to reduce the amount of gastric juice that can reflux into the esophagus and mediastinum. Nothing is given by mouth; nutritional needs are met by parenteral nutrition. Parenteral nutrition is preferred to gastrostomy because the latter might cause reflux into the esophagus.

Surgery may be necessary to close the wound, and postoperative nutritional support then becomes a primary concern. Depending on the incision site and the nature of surgery, the postoperative nursing management is similar to that for patients who have had thoracic or abdominal surgery.

FOREIGN BODIES

Many swallowed foreign bodies pass through the gastrointestinal tract without the need for medical intervention. However, some swallowed foreign bodies (eg, dentures, fish bones, pins, small batteries, items containing mercury or lead) may injure the esophagus or obstruct its lumen and must be removed. Pain and dysphagia may be present, and dyspnea may occur as a result of pressure on the trachea. The foreign body may be identified by x-ray film. Perforation may have occurred (see earlier discussion).

Glucagon, because of its relaxing effect on the esophageal muscle, may be injected intramuscularly. An endoscope (with a covered hood or overtube) may be used to remove the impacting food or object from the esophagus. A mixture consisting of sodium bicarbonate and tartaric acid may be used to increase intraluminal pressure by the formation of a gas. Caution must be used with this treatment because there is risk of perforation.

CHEMICAL BURNS

Chemical burns of the esophagus may be caused by undissolved medications in the esophagus. This occurs more frequently in the elderly than it does among the general adult population. A chemical burn may also occur after swallowing of a battery, which may release caustic alkaline. Chemical burns of the esophagus occur most often when a patient, either intentionally or unintentionally, swallows a strong acid or base (eg, lye). This patient is emotionally distraught as well as in acute physical pain. An acute chemical burn of the esophagus may be accompanied by severe burns of the lips, mouth, and pharynx, with pain on swallowing. There may be difficulty in breathing due to either edema of the throat or a collection of mucus in the pharynx.

The patient, who may be profoundly toxic, febrile, and in shock, is treated immediately for shock, pain, and respiratory distress. Esophagoscopy and barium swallow are performed as soon as possible to determine the extent and severity of damage. The patient is given nothing by mouth, and intravenous fluids are administered. A nasogastric tube may be inserted by the physician. Vomiting and gastric lavage are avoided to prevent further exposure of the esophagus to the caustic agent. The use of corticosteroids to reduce inflammation and minimize subsequent scarring and stricture formation is of questionable value. The value of the prophylactic use of antibiotics for these patients has also been questioned; however, these treatments continue to be prescribed (Schaffer & Herbert, 2000).

After the acute phase has subsided, the patient may need nutritional support via enteral or parenteral feedings. The patient may require further treatment to prevent or manage strictures of the esophagus. Dilation by bougienage may be sufficient, but dilation treatment may need to be repeated periodically. (In bougienage, cylindrical rubber tubes of different sizes, called bougies, are advanced into the esophagus via the oral cavity. Progressively larger bougies are used to dilate the esophagus. The procedure usually is performed in the endoscopy suite or clinic by the gastroenterologist.) For strictures that do not respond to dilation, surgical management is necessary. Reconstruction may be accomplished by esophagectomy and colon interposition to replace the portion of esophagus removed.

GASTROESOPHAGEAL REFLUX DISEASE

Some degree of **gastroesophageal reflux** (back-flow of gastric or duodenal contents into the esophagus) is normal in both adults and children. Excessive reflux may occur because of an incompetent lower esophageal sphincter, pyloric stenosis, or a motility disorder. The incidence of reflux seems to increase with aging.

Clinical Manifestations

Symptoms of gastroesophageal reflux disease (GERD) may include pyrosis (burning sensation in the esophagus), dyspepsia (indigestion), regurgitation, dysphagia or odynophagia (difficulty swallowing, pain on swallowing), hypersalivation, and esophagitis. The symptoms may mimic those of a heart attack. The patient's history aids in obtaining an accurate diagnosis.

Assessment and Diagnostic Findings

Diagnostic testing may include an endoscopy or barium swallow to evaluate damage to the esophageal mucosa. Ambulatory 12- to 36-hour esophageal pH monitoring is used to evaluate the degree of acid reflux. Bilirubin monitoring (Bilitec) is used to measure bile reflux patterns. Exposure to bile can cause mucosal damage (Aronson, 2000; Stein et al., 1999).

Management

Management begins with teaching the patient to avoid situations that decrease lower esophageal sphincter pressure or cause esophageal irritation. The patient is instructed to eat a low-fat diet; to avoid caffeine, tobacco, beer, milk, foods containing peppermint or spearmint, and carbonated beverages; to avoid eating or drinking 2 hours before bedtime; to maintain normal body weight; to avoid tight-fitting clothes; to elevate the head of the bed on 6- to 8-inch (15- to 20-cm) blocks; and to elevate the upper body on pillows. If reflux persists, the patient may be given medications such as antacids or histamine receptor blockers. Proton pump inhibitors (medications that decrease the release of gastric acid, such as lansoprazole [Prevacid] or rabeprazole [Aciphex]) may be used; however, there is concern that these products may increase intragastric bacterial growth and the risk for infection. In addition, the patient may receive prokinetic agents, which accelerate gastric emptying. These agents include bethanechol (Urecholine), domperidone (Motilium), and metoclopramide (Reglan). Metoclopramide has central nervous system complications with long-term use. The use of pectin-based products is now being studied (Aronson, 2000).

If medical management is unsuccessful, surgical intervention may be necessary. Surgical management involves a fundoplication (wrapping of a portion of the gastric fundus around the sphincter area of the esophagus). Fundoplication may be performed by laparoscopy.

BARRETT'S ESOPHAGUS

It is believed that long-standing untreated GERD may result in a condition known as Barrett's esophagus. This has been identi-

fied as a precancerous condition that, if left untreated, can result in adenocarcinoma of the esophagus, which has a poor prognosis. It is more common among middle-aged white men; however, the incidence is increasing among women and among African Americans.

Clinical Manifestations

The patient complains of symptoms of GERD, notably frequent heartburn. The heartburn is a result of reflux, which eventually causes changes in the cells lining the lower esophagus. The patient may also complain of symptoms related to peptic ulcers or esophageal stricture, or both.

Assessment and Diagnostic Findings

An esophagogastroduodenoscopy (EGD) is performed. This usually reveals an esophageal lining that is red rather than pink. Biopsies are taken, and the cells resemble those of the intestine.

Management

Monitoring varies depending on the amount of cell changes. Some physicians may recommend a repeat EGD in 6 to 12 months if there are minor cell changes. Medical and surgical management is similar to that for GERD. Because this is a condition that is increasing in incidence, research is underway to determine the best monitoring and surgical interventions (Mueller et al., 2000; Stein et al., 1999).

BENIGN TUMORS OF THE ESOPHAGUS

Benign tumors can arise anywhere along the esophagus. The most common lesion is a leiomyoma (tumor of the smooth muscle), which can occlude the lumen of the esophagus. Most benign tumors are asymptomatic and are distinguished from cancerous lesions by a biopsy. Small lesions are excised during esophagoscopy; lesions that occur within the wall of the esophagus may require treatment via a thoracotomy.

CANCER OF THE ESOPHAGUS

In the United States, carcinoma of the esophagus occurs more than three times as often in men as in women. It is seen more frequently in African Americans than in Caucasians and usually occurs in the fifth decade of life. Cancer of the esophagus has a much higher incidence in other parts of the world, including China and northern Iran (Greenlee, 2001; Castell & Richter, 1999).

Chronic irritation is a risk factor for esophageal cancer. In the United States, cancer of the esophagus has been associated with ingestion of alcohol and with the use of tobacco. There seems to be an association between GERD and adenocarcinoma of the esophagus. People with Barrett's esophagus (which is caused by chronic irritation of mucous membranes due to reflux of gastric and duodenal contents) have a higher incidence of esophageal cancer (Stein, 1999).

Pathophysiology

Esophageal cancer is usually of the squamous cell epidermoid type; however, the incidence of adenocarcinoma of the esophagus is increasing in the United States. Tumor cells may spread beneath the esophageal mucosa or directly into, through, and beyond the muscle layers into the lymphatics. In the latter stages, obstruction of the esophagus is noted, with possible perforation into the mediastinum and erosion into the great vessels.

Clinical Manifestations

Many patients have an advanced ulcerated lesion of the esophagus before symptoms are manifested. Symptoms include dysphagia, initially with solid foods and eventually with liquids; a sensation of a mass in the throat; painful swallowing; substernal pain or fullness; and, later, regurgitation of undigested food with foul breath and hiccups. The patient first becomes aware of intermittent and increasing difficulty in swallowing. As the tumor progresses and the obstruction becomes more complete, even liquids cannot pass into the stomach. Regurgitation of food and saliva occurs, hemorrhage may take place, and progressive loss of weight and strength occurs from starvation. Later symptoms include substernal pain, persistent hiccup, respiratory difficulty, and foul breath. The delay between the onset of early symptoms and the time when the patient seeks medical advice is often 12 to 18 months. Anyone with swallowing difficulties should be encouraged to consult a physician immediately.

Assessment and Diagnostic Findings

Although new endoscopic techniques are being studied for screening and diagnosis of esophageal cancer, currently diagnosis is confirmed most often by EGD with biopsy and brushings. Bronchoscopy usually is performed, especially in tumors of the middle and the upper third of the esophagus, to determine whether the trachea has been affected and to help determine whether the lesion can be removed. Endoscopic ultrasound or mediastinoscopy is used to determine whether the cancer has spread to the nodes and other mediastinal structures. Cancer of the lower end of the esophagus may be caused by adenocarcinoma of the stomach that extends upward into the esophagus.

Medical Management

If esophageal cancer is found at an early stage, treatment goals may be directed toward cure; however, it is often found in late stages, making relief of symptoms the only reasonable goal of therapy. Treatment may include surgery, radiation, chemotherapy, or a combination of these modalities, depending on the extent of the disease.

Standard surgical management includes a total resection of the esophagus (esophagectomy) with removal of the tumor plus a wide tumor-free margin of the esophagus and the lymph nodes in the area. The surgical approach may be through the thorax or the abdomen, depending on the location of the tumor. When tumors occur in the cervical or upper thoracic area, esophageal continuity may be maintained by free jejunal graft transfer, in which the tumor is removed and the area is replaced with a portion of the jejunum (Fig. 35-9). A segment of the colon may be used, or the stomach can be elevated into the chest and the proximal section of the esophagus anastomosed to the stomach.

Tumors of the lower thoracic esophagus are more amenable to surgery than are tumors located higher in the esophagus, and gastrointestinal tract integrity is maintained by anastomosing the lower esophagus to the stomach.

Surgical resection of the esophagus has a relatively high mortality rate because of infection, pulmonary complications, or leakage through the anastomosis. Postoperatively, the patient will have a nasogastric tube in place that should not be manipulated. The patient is given nothing by mouth until x-ray studies confirm that the anastomosis is secure and not leaking.

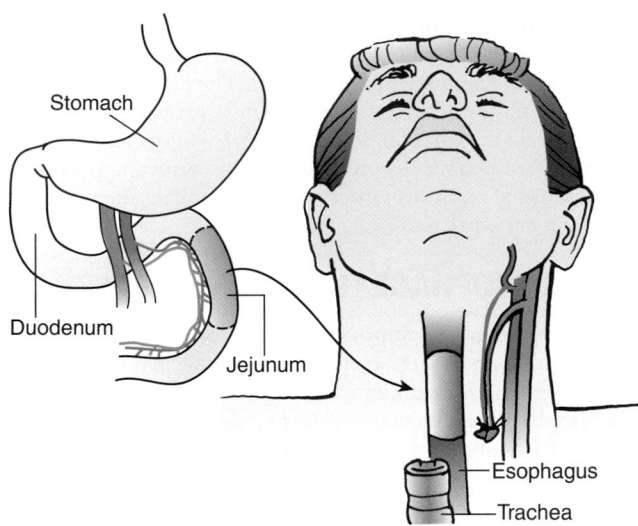

FIGURE 35-9 Esophageal reconstruction with free jejunal transfer. A portion of the jejunum is grafted between the esophagus and pharynx to replace the abnormal portion of the esophagus. The vascular structures are also anastomosed. A portion of the graft may be externalized through the neck wound to evaluate graft viability.

Preoperative radiation therapy or chemotherapy, or both, may be used; however, treatment is based on type of cell, tumor spread, and patient condition.

Palliative treatment may be necessary to keep the esophagus open, to assist with nutrition, and to control saliva. Palliation may be accomplished with dilation of the esophagus, laser therapy, placement of an endoprosthesis (stent), radiation, or chemotherapy. Because the ideal method of treating esophageal cancer has not yet been found, treatment is individually determined.

Nursing Management

Intervention is directed toward improving the patient's nutritional and physical condition in preparation for surgery, radiation therapy, or chemotherapy. A program to promote weight gain based on a high-calorie and high-protein diet, in liquid or soft form, is provided if adequate food can be taken by mouth. If this is not possible, parenteral or enteral nutrition is initiated. Nutritional status is monitored throughout treatment. The patient is informed about the nature of the postoperative equipment that will be used, including that required for closed chest drainage, nasogastric suction, parenteral fluid therapy, and gastric intubation. Immediate postoperative care is similar to that provided for patients undergoing thoracic surgery. After recovering from the effects of anesthesia, the patient is placed in a low Fowler's position, and later in a Fowler's position, to assist in preventing reflux of gastric secretions. The patient is observed carefully for regurgitation and dyspnea. A common postoperative complication is aspiration pneumonia. The patient's temperature is monitored to detect any elevation that may indicate aspiration or seepage of fluid through the operative site into the mediastinum.

If jejunal grafting has been performed, the nurse checks for graft viability hourly for at least the first 12 hours. To make the graft visible, the surgeon usually brings a portion of the jejunum to the exterior neck by way of a small incision. Moist gauze covers the external portion of the graft. The gauze is removed briefly to assess the graft for color and to assess for the presence of a pulse by means of Doppler ultrasonography.

If an endoprosthesis has been placed or an anastomosis has been performed, a functioning continuum will exist between the throat and the stomach. Immediately after surgery, the nasogastric tube should be marked for position, and the physician is notified if displacement occurs. The nurse does not attempt to reinsert a displaced nasogastric tube, because damage to the anastomosis may occur. The nasogastric tube is removed 5 to 7 days after surgery, and a barium swallow is performed to assess for any anastomotic leak before the patient is allowed to eat.

Once feeding begins, the nurse encourages the patient to swallow small sips of water and, later, small amounts of pureed food. When the patient is able to increase food intake to an adequate amount, parenteral fluids are discontinued. If an endoprosthesis is used, it may easily become obstructed if food is not chewed sufficiently. After each meal, the patient remains upright for at least 2 hours to allow the food to move through the gastrointestinal tract. It is a challenge to encourage the patient to eat, because appetite is usually poor. Family involvement and home-cooked favorite foods may help the patient to eat. Antacids may help those with gastric distress.

If radiation is part of the therapy, the patient's appetite is further depressed and esophagitis may occur, causing pain when food is eaten. Liquid supplements may be more easily tolerated.

Often, in either the preoperative or the postoperative period, an obstructed or nearly obstructed esophagus causes difficulty with excess saliva, so that drooling becomes a problem. Oral suction may be used if the patient is unable to handle oral secretions, or a wick-type gauze may be placed at the corner of the mouth to direct secretions to a dressing or emesis basin. The possibility that the patient may aspirate saliva into the tracheobronchial tree and develop pneumonia is of great concern.

When the patient is ready to go home, the family is instructed about how to promote nutrition, what observations to make, what measures to take if complications occur, how to keep the patient comfortable, and how to obtain needed physical and emotional support.

NURSING PROCESS: THE PATIENT WITH A CONDITION OF THE ESOPHAGUS

Assessment

Emergency conditions of the esophagus (perforation, chemical burns) usually occur in the home or away from medical help and require emergency medical care. The patient is treated for shock and respiratory distress and transported as quickly as possible to a medical facility. Foreign bodies in the esophagus do not pose an immediate threat to life unless pressure is exerted on the trachea, resulting in dyspnea or interfering with respiration, or unless there is leakage of caustic alkali from a battery. Educating the public to prevent inadvertent swallowing of foreign bodies or corrosive agents is a major health issue.

For nonemergency symptoms, a complete health history may reveal the nature of the esophageal disorder. The nurse asks about the patient's appetite. Has it remained the same, increased, or decreased? Is there any discomfort with swallowing? If so, does it occur only with certain foods? Is it associated with pain? Does a change in position affect the discomfort? The patient is asked to describe the pain. Does anything aggravate it? Are there any other symptoms that occur regularly, such as regurgitation, nocturnal regurgitation, eructation (belching), heartburn, substernal pressure, a sensation that food is sticking in the throat, a feeling of becoming full after eating a small amount of food, nausea, vom-

iting, or weight loss? Are the symptoms aggravated by emotional upset? If the patient reports any of these symptoms, the nurse asks about the time of their occurrence, their relationship to eating, and factors that relieve or aggravate them (eg, position change, belching, antacids, vomiting).

This history also includes questions about past or present causative factors, such as infections and chemical, mechanical, or physical irritants; the degree to which alcohol and tobacco are used; and the amount of daily food intake. The nurse determines whether the patient appears emaciated and auscultates the patient's chest to determine whether pulmonary complications exist.

Nursing Diagnosis

Based on the assessment data, the nursing diagnoses may include the following:

- Imbalanced nutrition, less than body requirements, related to difficulty swallowing
- Risk for aspiration related to difficulty swallowing or to tube feeding
- Acute pain related to difficulty swallowing, ingestion of an abrasive agent, tumor, or frequent episodes of gastric reflux
- Deficient knowledge about the esophageal disorder, diagnostic studies, medical management, surgical intervention, and rehabilitation

Planning and Goals

The major goals for the patient may include attainment of adequate nutritional intake, avoidance of respiratory compromise from aspiration, relief of pain, and increased knowledge level.

Nursing Interventions

ENCOURAGING ADEQUATE NUTRITIONAL INTAKE
The patient is encouraged to eat slowly and to chew all food thoroughly so that it can pass easily into the stomach. Small, frequent feedings of nonirritating foods are recommended to promote digestion and to prevent tissue irritation. Sometimes liquid swallowed with food helps the food pass through the esophagus. Food should be prepared in an appealing manner to help stimulate the appetite. Irritants such as tobacco and alcohol should be avoided. A baseline weight is obtained, and daily weights are recorded. The patient's intake of nutrients is assessed.

DECREASING RISK OF ASPIRATION
The patient who has difficulty swallowing or difficulty handling secretions should be kept in at least a semi-Fowler's position to decrease the risk of aspiration. The patient can be instructed in the use of oral suction to decrease the risk of aspiration further.

RELIEVING PAIN
Small, frequent feedings are recommended, because large quantities of food overload the stomach and promote gastric reflux. The patient is advised to avoid any activities that increase pain, and to remain upright for 1 to 4 hours after each meal to prevent reflux. The head of the bed should be placed on 4- to 8-inch (10- to 20-cm) blocks. Eating before bedtime is discouraged.

The patient is advised that excessive use of over-the-counter antacids can cause rebound acidity. Antacid use should be directed by the primary care provider, who can recommend the daily, safe dose needed to neutralize gastric juices and prevent esophageal

Chart 35-4

Home Care Checklist • **The Patient With an Esophageal Condition**

At the completion of the home care instruction, the patient or caregiver will be able to:	Patient	Caregiver
• Demonstrate use of suction equipment.	✓	✓
• State dietary modifications needed to meet caloric needs.	✓	✓
• Demonstrate enteral or parenteral feeding techniques.	✓	✓
• Demonstrate care of incision if indicated.	✓	✓
• State when next checkup is needed.	✓	✓
• Identify available support groups.	✓	✓

irritation. Histamine$_2$ antagonists are administered as prescribed to decrease gastric acid irritation.

PROVIDING PATIENT EDUCATION

The patient is prepared physically and psychologically for diagnostic tests, treatments, and possible surgical intervention. The principal nursing interventions include reassuring the patient and discussing the procedures and their purposes. Some disorders of the esophagus evolve over time, whereas others are the result of trauma (eg, chemical burns, perforation). In instances of trauma, the emotional and physical preparation for treatment is more difficult because of the short time available and the circumstances of the injury. Treatment interventions must be evaluated continually; the patient is given sufficient information to participate in care and diagnostic tests. If endoscopic diagnostic methods are used, the patient is instructed regarding the moderate sedation that will be used during the procedure. If procedures are being performed on an outpatient basis with the use of moderate sedation, the patient is instructed to have someone available to drive him or her home after the procedure. If surgery is required, immediate and long-term evaluation is similar to that for a patient undergoing thoracic surgery.

PROMOTING HOME AND COMMUNITY-BASED CARE

Teaching Patients Self-Care

The self-care required of the patient depends on the nature of the disorder and on the surgery or treatment measures used (eg, diet, positioning, medications). If an ongoing condition exists, the nurse helps the patient plan for needed physical and psychological adjustments and for follow-up care (Chart 35-4).

Special equipment, such as suction or enteral or parenteral feeding devices, may be required. The patient may need assistance in planning meals, using medications as prescribed, and resuming activities. Education about nutritional requirements and how to measure the adequacy of nutrition is important. Elderly and debilitated patients in particular often need assistance and education in ways to adjust to their limitations and to resume activities that are important to them.

Continuing Care

Patients with chronic esophageal conditions require an individualized approach to their management at home. Foods may need to be prepared in a special way (blenderized foods, soft foods), and the patient may need to eat more frequently (eg, four to six small servings per day). The medication schedule is adjusted to the patient's daily activities as much as possible. Analgesic medications and antacids can usually be taken as needed every 3 to 4 hours.

Postoperative home health care focuses on nutritional support, management of pain, and respiratory function. Some patients are discharged from the hospital with enteral feeding by means of a gastrostomy or jejunostomy tube or parenteral nutrition. The patient and care provider need specific instructions regarding management of the equipment and treatments. Home care visits by a nurse may be necessary to assess the patient's care and the care provider's ability to provide the necessary care. (See Chapter 36 for more information about parenteral nutrition and management of the patient with a gastrostomy.) For some patients, a multidisciplinary team comprising a dietitian, a social worker, and family members is helpful. Hospice care is appropriate for some patients.

Evaluation

EXPECTED PATIENT OUTCOMES

Expected patient outcomes may include:

1. Achieves an adequate nutritional intake
   a. Eats small, frequent meals
   b. Drinks water with small servings of food
   c. Avoids irritants (alcohol, tobacco, very hot beverages)
   d. Maintains desired weight
2. Does not aspirate or develop pneumonia
   a. Maintains upright position during feeding
   b. Uses oral suction equipment effectively
3. Is free of pain or able to control pain within a tolerable level
   a. Avoids large meals and irritating foods
   b. Takes medications as prescribed and with adequate fluids (at least 4 ounces), and remains upright for at least 10 minutes after taking medications
   c. Maintains an upright position after meals for 1 to 4 hours
   d. Reports that there is less eructation and chest pain
4. Increases knowledge level of esophageal condition, treatment, and prognosis
   a. States cause of condition
   b. Discusses rationale for medical or surgical management and diet or medication regimen
   c. Describes treatment program
   d. Practices preventive measures so injuries are avoided

Critical Thinking Exercises

1. You are interviewing a patient in the medical clinic. The patient is complaining of difficulty swallowing as well as indigestion. Describe how you would continue to assess this patient to obtain the additional information that is needed. Identify the various factors that may be causing this patient's symptoms.

2. You are caring for two postoperative patients. One patient is being treated for cancer of the mouth, the other for cancer of the esophagus. How will the nutritional care of these two patients differ? Describe the communication needs and psychosocial needs of these patients.

REFERENCES AND SELECTED READINGS

Books

Bickley, L. S., & Hoekelman, R. A. (2003). *Bates' guide to physical examination and history taking* (8th ed.). Philadelphia: Lippincott Williams & Wilkins.

Brandt, L. J. (Ed.). (1999). *Clinical practice of gastroenterology* (Vols. I & II). Philadelphia: Churchill-Livingstone.

Castell, D. O., & Richter, J. E. (1999). *The esophagus* (3rd ed.). Philadelphia: Lippincott Williams & Wilkins.

DeVita, V. T., Hellman, S., & Rosenberg, S. A. (Eds.). (2001). *Cancer: Principles and practice of oncology* (6th ed.). Philadelphia: Lippincott Williams & Wilkins.

Fonseca, R. J. (Ed.). (2000). *Oral and maxillofacial surgery.* Philadelphia: W. B. Saunders.

Garber, T. M. (Ed.). (2000). *Orthodontics: Current principles and techniques.* St. Louis: Mosby.

Harris, N. O., & Garcia-Godoy, F. (1999). *Primary preventive dentistry* (5th ed.). Norwalk, CT: Appleton & Lange.

Harrison, L. B., et al. (1999). *Head and neck cancer: A multidisciplinary approach.* Philadelphia: Lippincott Williams & Wilkins.

McEvoy, G. R. (Ed.). (2000). *American Hospital Formulary Service.* Bethesda, MD: American Society of Health-System Pharmacists.

Murray, J. (1999). *Manual of dysphagia assessment in adults.* San Diego: Singular Publishing.

Pappas, T. N., et al. (1999). *Atlas of laparoscopic surgery* (2nd ed.). Norwalk, CT: Appleton & Lange.

Proffit, W. R. (2000). *Contemporary orthodontics.* St. Louis: Mosby.

U.S. Department of Health and Human Services. (2000). *Oral health in America: A report of the surgeon general. Executive summary.* Rockville, MD: National Institutes of Dental and Craniofacial Research, National Institutes of Health.

Yamada, T. (Ed.). (1999). *Textbook of gastroenterology* (3rd ed., Vols. I & II). Philadelphia: Lippincott Williams & Wilkins.

Journals

Conditions and Cancer of the Oral Cavity

Bull, P. D. (2001). Salivary gland stones: Diagnosis and treatment. *Hospital Medicine, 62*(7), 396–399.

Greenlee, R. T. (2001). Cancer statistics, 2001. *CA Cancer Journal for Clinicians, 51*(1), 15–36.

Kimata, Y., et al. (2000). Postoperative complications and functional results after total glossectomy with microvascular reconstruction. *Plastic Reconstructive Surgery, 106*(5), 1028–1035.

Lingstrom, P., et al. (2000). Food starches and dental caries. *Critical Reviews in Oral Biology and Medicine, 11*(3), 366–380.

McQuone, S. J. (1999). Acute viral and bacterial infections of the salivary glands. *Otolaryngology Clinics of North America, 32*(5), 793–811.

Reimers, M., et al. (2000). Results after shock wave lithotripsy for salivary gland stones. *Schweizerische Medizinishe Wochenschrift, 125,* 122s–126s.

Rethman, J. (2000). Trends in preventive care: Caries risk assessment and indications for sealants. *Journal of the American Dental Association, 131,* (Suppl.), 8S–12S.

Rice, D. H. (1999a). Chronic inflammatory disorders of the salivary glands. *Otolaryngology Clinics of North America, 32*(5), 813–818.

Rice, D. H. (1999b). Noninflammatory, non-neoplastic disorders of the salivary gland. *Otolaryngology Clinics of North America, 32*(5), 835–843.

Sessons, D. G., et al. (2000). Analysis of treatment results for floor-of-mouth cancer. *Laryngoscope, 110*(10 Pt. 1), 1764–1772.

Villarrel, P. M., et al. (2000). Study of mandibular repair using quantitative radiodensitometry: A comparison between maxillomandibular and rigid internal fixation. *Journal of Oral and Maxillofacial Surgery, 58,* 776–781.

Wright, E. F. (2000). Referred craniofacial pain patterns in patients with temporomandibular disorder. *Journal of the American Dental Association, 131*(9), 1307–1315.

Conditions and Treatment of the Esophagus

Annese, V., et al. (2000). A multicenter randomized study of intrasphincteric botulism toxin in patients with oesophageal achalasia. *Gut, 46,* 597–600.

Aronson, B. S. (2000). Applying clinical practice guidelines to a patient with complicated gastroesophageal reflux disease. *Gastroenterology Nursing, 23*(4), 143–147.

Bowrey, D. J. (2000). Laparoscopic esophageal surgery. *Surgical Clinics of North America, 80*(4), 1213–1242.

Frenken, M. (2001). Best palliation in esophageal cancer: Surgery, stenting, radiation therapy. *Diseases of the Esophagus, 14*(2), 120–123.

Heath, E. I., et al. (2000). Adenocarcinoma of the esophagus: Risk factors and prevention. *Oncology, 14*(2), 507–514.

Hirano, I. (1999). Pathophysiology of achalasia. *Current Gastroenterology Report, 1*(3), 198–202.

Mueller, J., et al. (2000). Malignant progression in Barrett's esophagus: Pathology and biology. *Recent Results in Cancer Research, 155,* 29–41.

Nguyen, N. T., et al. (2000). Laparoscopy or thoracoscopy for achalasia. *Seminars in Thoracic and Cardiovascular Surgery, 12*(3), 201–205.

Para, M. Epidemiology of esophageal cancer, especially adenocarcinoma of the esophagus and esophagogastric junction. *Recent Results in Cancer Research, 155,* 1–14.

Schaffer, S. B., & Herbert, A. F. (2000). Caustic ingestion. *Journal of the Louisiana State Medical Society, 152*(12), 590–596.

Stein, H. J., et al. (2000). Malignant degeneration of Barrett's esophagus: Clinical point options. *Recent Results in Cancer Research, 155,* 42–53.

Stein, H. J., et al. (1999). Bile acids as components of the duodenogastric refluate: Detection, relationship to bilirubin, mechanism of injury, and clinical relevance. *Hepatogastroenterology, 46,* 66–73.

Streeter, B. L. (1999). Botulinum toxin: A case study. *Gastroenterology Nursing, 22*(2), 59–61.

Vaezi, M. F., & Shay, S. S. (2001). New techniques in measuring nonacidic esophageal reflux. *Seminars in Thoracic Cardiovascular Surgery, 13*(3), 255–264.

Conditions and Treatment of the Head and Neck

Richards, B. L., & Spiro, J. D. (2000). Controlling advanced neck disease: Efficacy of neck dissection and radiotherapy. *Laryngoscope, 110*(7), 1124–1127.

Talmi, Y. P., et al. (2000). Pain in the neck after neck dissection. *Otolaryngology Head and Neck Surgery, 123*(3), 302–306.

Weymuller, E. A. (2000). Quality of life in patient with head and neck cancer: Lessons learned from 549 prospectively evaluate patients. *Archives of Otolaryngology Head and Neck Surgery, 126*(3), 329–335.

RESOURCES AND WEBSITES

American Cancer Society, 1599 Clifton Rd. NE, Atlanta, GA 30329; 1-800-ACS-2345; http://www.cancer.org.

American Dental Association, 211 E. Chicago Ave., Chicago, IL 60611; 312-440-2806; http://www.ada.org.

Centers for Disease Control and Prevention, 1600 Clifton Rd., Atlanta, GA 30333; 404-639-7000; http://www.cdc.gov/health.

National Institute of Dental and Craniofacial Research, National Institutes of Health, 900 Rockville Pike, Bethesda, MD 20892; 301-496-4261; http://www.nidr.nih.gov.

National Oral Health Information Clearinghouse, 1 NOHIC Way, Bethesda, MD 20892-3500; 1-301-402-7364; http://www.nohic.nider.nih.gov.

Gastrointestinal Intubation and Special Nutritional Modalities

LEARNING OBJECTIVES ●

On completion of this chapter, the learner will be able to:

1. Describe the purposes and types of GI intubation.
2. Discuss nursing management of the patient who has a nasogastric or nasoenteric tube.
3. Use the nursing process as a framework for care of the patient receiving an enteral feeding.
4. Explain the preoperative and postoperative care of the patient with a gastrostomy.
5. Use the nursing process as a framework for care of the patient with a gastrostomy.
6. Identify the purposes and uses of parenteral nutrition.
7. Use the nursing process as a framework for care of the patient receiving parenteral nutrition.
8. Describe the nursing measures used to prevent complications from parenteral nutrition.

*T*his chapter presents several topics related to gastrointestinal (GI) intubation. Nursing management topics relate to managing the care of patients with nasogastric (NG) and nasoenteric tubes and gastrostomies, providing tube feedings, and teaching points related to home health care and nutritional therapy. In addition, parenteral nutrition is presented, including general indications for this nutritional modality and nursing care of patients receiving these support measures.

Gastrointestinal Intubation

GI intubation is the insertion of a rubber or plastic tube into the stomach, the **duodenum** (first section of the small intestine), or the intestine. The tube may be inserted through the mouth, the nose, or the abdominal wall. The tubes can be short, medium, or long, depending on their intended use; **nasogastric (NG) tubes** are short, **nasoduodenal tubes** are of medium length, and nasoenteric tubes are long. GI intubation may be performed for the following reasons:

- To decompress the stomach and remove gas and fluid
- To lavage the stomach and remove ingested toxins
- To diagnose disorders of GI motility and other disorders
- To administer medications and feedings
- To treat an obstruction
- To compress a bleeding site
- To aspirate gastric contents for analysis

A variety of tubes are used for decompression, aspiration, and lavage. The Sengstaken-Blakemore tube is a type of NG tube used to treat bleeding esophageal varices (see Chapter 39). Orogastric tubes are large-bore tubes with wide proximal outlets for removal of particles of ingested substances (eg, pills); they are primarily used in emergency departments. Various other tubes are used to administer feedings and medications. The tubes are made of various materials (rubber, polyurethane, silicone), and they vary in length

(90 cm to 3 m [3 to 10 ft]), in size (6 to 18 French [Fr]), in purpose, and in placement in the GI tract (stomach, duodenum, jejunum) (Table 36-1). Any solution administered through a tube is either poured through a syringe or delivered by a drip mechanism regulated by gravity or by an electric pump. **Aspiration** (suctioning) to remove gas and fluids is accomplished with the use of a syringe, an electric suction machine, or a wall suction outlet.

SHORT TUBES

An NG tube or short tube is introduced through the nose into the stomach, often before or during esophageal or stomach surgery. Commonly used short tubes include the Levin tube and the gastric sump tube. Short tubes are used in adults primarily to remove fluid and gas from the upper GI tract or to obtain a specimen of gastric contents for laboratory studies. They are occasionally used for the short-term (3 to 4 weeks) administration of medications or feedings.

Levin Tube

The Levin tube has a single lumen (the hollow part of the tube), ranges from 14 to 18 Fr in size, and is made of plastic or rubber with openings near its tip. It is 125 cm (50 in) long. Circular markings at specific points on the tube serve as guides for insertion. A marking is made on the tube to indicate the midpoint. The tube is advanced cautiously until this marking reaches the patient's nostril, suggesting that the tube is in the stomach. Placement is checked by observing the characteristics of the aspirate and by testing the **pH** (which varies according to the source of the aspirate). Seeing the tube on an x-ray study is the only sure way to verify its location. The Levin tube is connected to low intermittent suction (30 to 40 mm Hg). Intermittent suction is used to avoid erosion or tearing of the stomach lining, which can result from constant adherence of the tube's lumen to the mucosal lining of the stomach.

Glossary

antireflux valve: valve that prevents return or backward flow of fluid

aspiration: breathing of fluids or foods into the trachea and lungs; removal of substance by suction

bolus: a feeding administered into the stomach in large amounts and at designated intervals

central venous access device (CVAD): a device designed and used for long-term administration of medications and fluids into central veins

cyclic feeding: periodic feeding/infusion given over a short period (8 to 12 hours)

decompression (intestinal): removal of intestinal contents to prevent gas and fluid from distending the coils of the intestine

dumping syndrome: rapid emptying of the stomach contents into the small intestine; characterized by sweating and weakness

duodenum: the first part of the small intestine, which connects with the pylorus of the stomach and extends to the jejunum

feeding tube: tube through which nutritional products, water, and other fluids can be introduced into the GI tract

gastrostomy: surgical creation of an opening into the stomach for the purpose of administering foods and fluids

irrigation: flushing of the tube with water or other fluids to clear it

jejunum: second portion of the small intestine, extending from the duodenum to the ileum

low-profile gastrostomy device (LPGD, G-button): an enteral feeding access device that is flush with the skin and is used for long-term feeding

nasoduodenal tube: tube inserted through the nose into the beginning of the small intestine (duodenum)

nasogastric (NG) tube: tube inserted through the nose into the stomach

nasojejunal tube: tube inserted through the nose into the second portion of the small intestine (jejunum)

osmolality: ionic concentration of fluid

osmosis: passage of solvent through a semipermeable membrane; the solvent, usually water, passes through the membrane from a region of low concentration of solute to that of a higher concentration of solute

parenteral nutrition: method of supplying nutrients to the body by an intravenous route

percutaneous endoscopic gastrostomy (PEG): an endoscopic procedure for placing a permanent feeding tube into the stomach

peristalsis: wavelike movement that occurs involuntarily in the alimentary canal

pH: the degree of acidity or alkalinity of a substance or solution

peripherally inserted central catheter (PICC): a device used for intermediate-term intravenous therapy

stoma: artificially created opening between a body cavity (eg, intestine) and the body surface

total nutrient admixture: an admixture of lipid emulsions, proteins, carbohydrates, electrolytes, vitamins, trace minerals, and water

Table 36-1 • **Nasogastric, Nasoenteric, and Feeding Tubes**

TUBE TYPE	LENGTH (CM)	SIZE (FRENCH)	LUMEN	OTHER CHARACTERISTICS
Nasogastric Tubes				
Levin (plastic or rubber)	125	14–18	Single	Circular markings at intervals along the tube serve as guidelines for insertion
Gastric sump or Salem (plastic)	120	12–18	Double	Smaller lumen acts as a vent
Moss	90	12–16	Triple	Contains both a gastric decompression lumen and a duodenal lumen for postoperative feedings
Sengstaken-Blakemore (rubber)			Triple	Two lumens are used to inflate the gastric and esophageal balloons
Nasoenteric Decompression Tubes				
Miller-Abbott (rubber)	300	12–18	Double	One lumen uses mercury, water, saline, or air for balloon inflation
Harris	180	14, 16	Single	Mercury-weighted tip (or may use water as a weight)
Cantor (rubber)	300	16	Single	Mercury-weighted bag (or may use water as a weight)
Baker (plastic)	270	16	Double	One lumen is used for balloon inflation
Nasoenteric Feeding Tubes				
Dobbhoff or EnteraFlo (polyurethane or silicone rubber)	160–175	8–12	Single	Tungsten-weighted tip, radiopaque, stylet

Gastric Sump

The gastric sump (Salem) tube is a radiopaque, clear plastic, double-lumen NG tube used to decompress the stomach and keep it empty. It is 120 cm (48 in) long and is passed into the stomach in the same way as the Levin tube. The inner, smaller tube vents the larger suction-drainage tube to the atmosphere by means of an opening at the distal end of the tube. The sump tube can protect gastric suture lines because, when used properly, it maintains the force of suction at the drainage openings, or outlets, at less than 25 mm Hg, the level of capillary fragility. The small vent tube (known as the blue pigtail) controls this action. These tubes are connected to low continuous suction. The suction lumen is irrigated as prescribed to maintain patency.

To prevent reflux of gastric contents through the vent lumen (blue pigtail), the vent lumen is kept above the patient's waist; otherwise it will act as a siphon. A one-way **antireflux valve** seated in the blue pigtail prevents the reflux of gastric contents out the vent lumen (Fig. 36-1). The valve is removed after irrigation of the suction lumen, and 20 mL of air is injected to reestablish a buffer of air between the gastric contents and the valve.

MEDIUM TUBES

Medium-length nasoenteric tubes are used for feeding. Feeding tubes placed in the duodenum are 160 cm (60 in) long; feeding tubes placed in the **jejunum** (portion of the small intestine adjacent to the duodenum) are 175 cm (66 in) long. They can be inserted at the time of surgery or before surgery, by interventional radiologists assisted by fluoroscopy or at the bedside. If the tube is inserted at the bedside, placement is verified by radiography.

After insertion, the tip of the tube will initially be in the stomach; it usually takes 24 hours for the tube to pass through the stomach and into the intestines.

 NURSING ALERT Having the patient lie on the right side facilitates passage, because gravity and peristaltic motion will move the weighted tube into the duodenum.

Polyurethane or silicone rubber feeding tubes have narrow diameters (6 to 12 Fr) and tungsten tips (rather than mercury-filled bags); some have a water-activated lubricant that makes it easier to insert the tube. The tubing may kink when a stylet is not used, particularly if the patient is uncooperative or unable to swallow. Feeding tubes with a stylet are inserted with caution in patients who are predisposed to esophageal puncture, such as elderly and frail patients with thin tissues. These tubes are advanced in the same way as an NG tube; that is, with the patient in Fowler's position. If this is not feasible, the patient is placed on the right side.

LONG TUBES

A long nasoenteric tube is introduced through the nose and passed through the esophagus and stomach into the intestinal tract. It is used to aspirate intestinal contents so that gas and fluid do not distend the intestine; this is called **decompression**. Three major nasoenteric tubes used for aspiration and decompression are the Miller-Abbott tube, the Harris tube, and the Cantor tube. These tubes are used to relieve obstruction of the small intestine. They are also used prophylactically; they may be inserted the night before GI surgery to prevent postoperative obstruction.

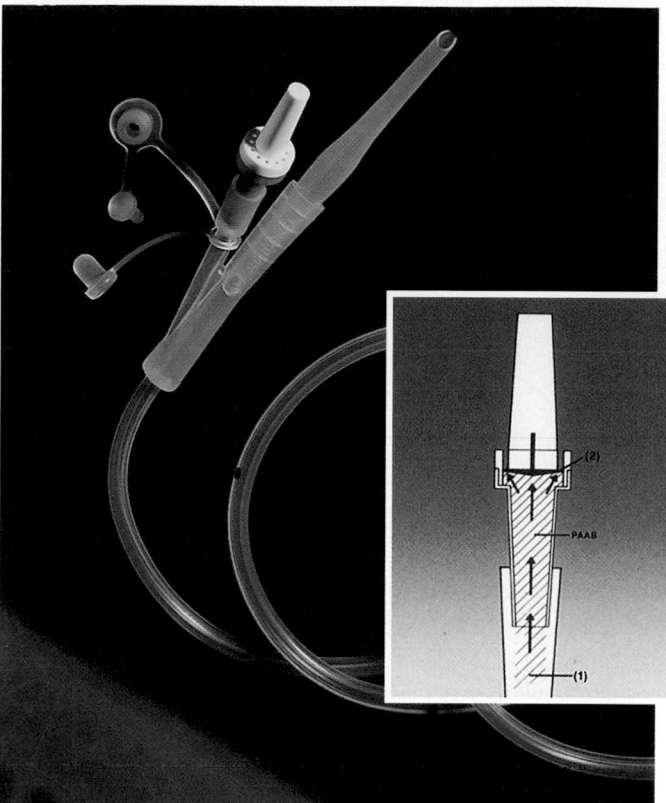

FIGURE 36-1 Gastric sump tube (Salem) equipped with a one-way antireflux valve that allows air to enter and prevents gastric contents from escaping. The antireflux valve is designed with a pressure activated air buffer (PAAB). The buffer is activated (1) and the valve closes (2) when pressure from gastric contents enters the tubing. Argyle Silicone Salem Sump Tube with preattached Argyle Salem Sump Anti-Reflux Valve courtesy of Sherwood Medical, St. Louis, Missouri.

Because **peristalsis** is either stopped or slowed for 24 to 48 hours after surgery as a result of anesthesia and visceral manipulation, NG or nasoenteric suction is used to evacuate fluids and flatus so that vomiting is prevented, tension is reduced along the incision line, and obstruction is prevented. Usually, the tube remains in place until peristalsis returns, as evidenced by the resumption of bowel sounds and the passage of flatus.

Miller-Abbott Tube

The Miller-Abbott tube is a double-lumen rubber tube that is 300 cm (10 ft) long and 12, 14, 16, or 18 Fr in size. One lumen is used to introduce mercury, water, or saline into the balloon at the end of the tube for weighting of the tube; the other lumen is used for aspiration. Before the tube is inserted, the balloon should be tested and its capacity measured; then it should be deflated completely. The tube should be lubricated sparingly and chilled well (chilling causes the tube to become stiff and facilitates its passage) before the tip is inserted through the patient's nose. Markings on the tube indicate the distance it has been passed. Before removal, the balloon at the end of the lumen must be completely deflated.

Harris Tube

The Harris tube is a single-lumen (14 Fr), mercury-weighted tube of about 180 cm (6 ft). This tube has a metal tip that is lu-bricated and introduced through the nose. The mercury-weighted bag follows. The weight of the mercury promotes the passage of the bag by gravity. This tube is used solely for suction and **irrigation**. Usually, a Y-tube is attached to the end of the Harris tube. The suction is applied to one side of the Y and the other side is clamped, except when irrigation of the tube is being performed.

Cantor Tube

The Cantor tube is 300 cm (10 ft) long and has a 16-Fr lumen. Its distinguishing feature is that it is larger than the other long tubes. It has a 4- or 5-mL bag at the extreme end of the rubber tubing; mercury, water or saline is introduced into this bag to weight the tube. Before the tube is inserted, the bag is wrapped around the tube. After the tube is lubricated, it is advanced through the nose and into the esophagus (Fig. 36-2). The patient assumes a sitting position and may be offered sips of water to facilitate passage of the tube. Fluoroscopy helps to verify that the tube has passed into the duodenum.

NURSING MANAGEMENT OF PATIENTS UNDERGOING NASOGASTRIC OR NASOENTERIC INTUBATION

Nursing interventions include the following:

- Instructing the patient about the purpose of the tube and the procedure required for inserting and advancing it
- Describing the sensations to be expected during tube insertion
- Inserting the NG tube and assisting with insertion of the nasoenteric tube
- Confirming the placement of the NG tube
- Advancing the nasoenteric tube
- Monitoring the patient and maintaining tube function
- Providing oral and nasal hygiene and care
- Monitoring for potential complications
- Removing the tube

Providing Instruction

Before the patient is intubated, the nurse explains the purpose of the tube; this information may assist the patient to be cooperative and tolerant of what is often an unpleasant procedure. The general activities related to inserting the tube are then reviewed, including the fact that the patient may have to breathe through the mouth and that the procedure may cause gagging until the tube has passed the area of the gag reflex.

Inserting the Tube

Before inserting the tube, the clinician determines how much tubing will be needed to reach the stomach or the small intestine. A mark is made on the tube to indicate the desired length. This length is determined by measuring the distance from the tip of the nose to the earlobe, and from the earlobe to the xiphoid process, then adding 6 inches for NG placement or 8 to 10 inches for intestinal placement (Fig. 36-3).

While the tube is being inserted, the patient usually sits upright with a towel spread bib-fashion over the chest. Tissue wipes are made available. Privacy and adequate light are provided. The physician may swab the nostril and spray the oropharynx with

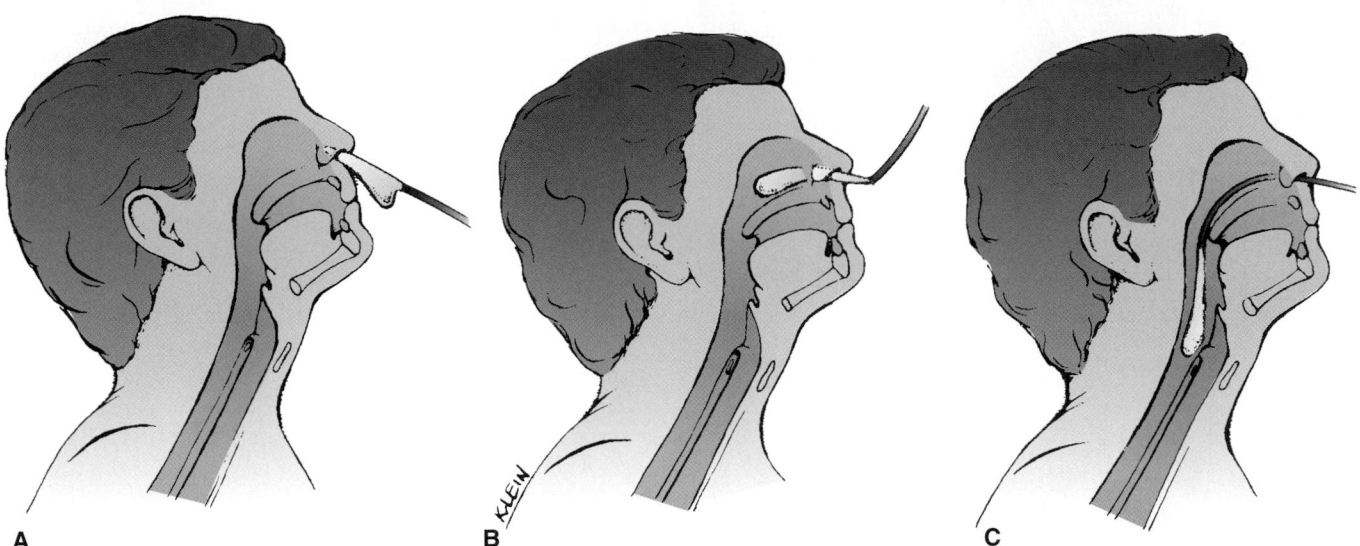

FIGURE 36-2 Passage of Cantor tube. (**A**) Tube with weighted bag (mercury, water, normal saline solution) is introduced through the nose. (**B**) After the weighted bag has entered the nostril, the catheter is tilted upward (head can also be tilted slightly upward) to facilitate gravity pull on the weighted bag. (**C**) The weight of the mercury (or water or normal saline solution) pulls the bag downward.

1. Mark the nasogastric tube at a point 50 cm from the distal tip; call this point 'A'.

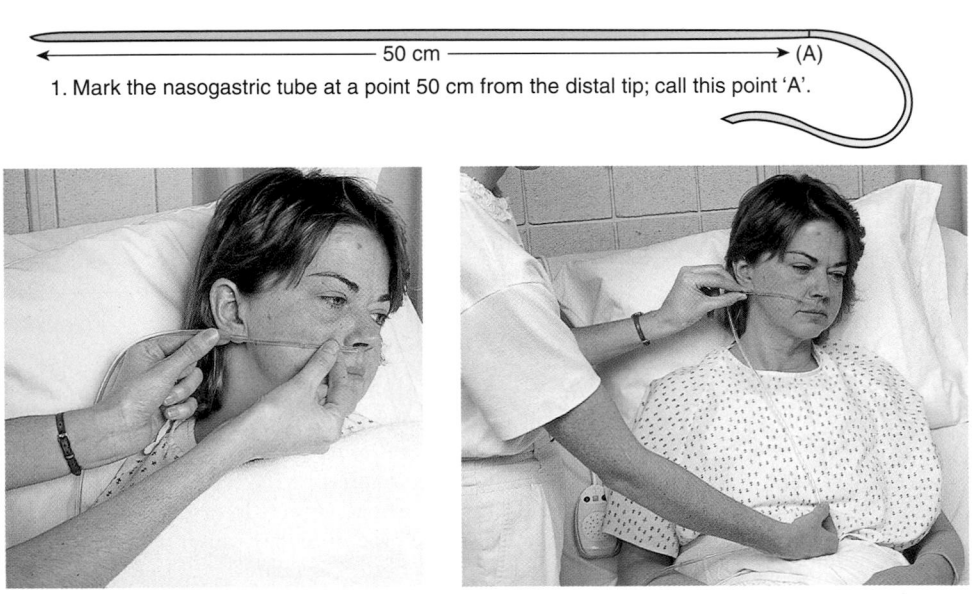

Measuring distance from nostril to tip of earlobe.

Measuring distance from earlobe to tip of xiphoid process.

2. Have the patient sit in a neutral position with head facing forward. Place the distal tip of the tubing at the tip of the patient's nose (N); extend tube to the tragus (tip) of the ear (E), and then extend the tube straight down to the tip of the xiphoid (X). Mark this point 'B' on the tubing.

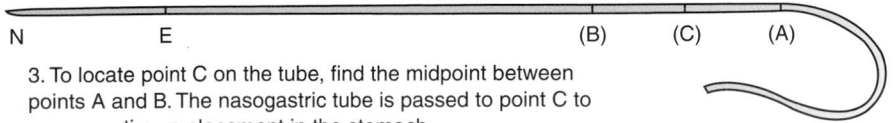

3. To locate point C on the tube, find the midpoint between points A and B. The nasogastric tube is passed to point C to ensure optimum placement in the stomach.

FIGURE 36-3 Measuring length of nasogastric tube for placement into stomach.

Cetacaine (tetracaine/benzocaine) to numb the nasal passage and suppress the gag reflex. This makes the entire procedure more tolerable. Having the patient gargle with a liquid anesthetic or hold ice chips in the mouth for a few minutes can have the same effect. Encouraging the patient to breathe through the mouth or to pant often helps, as does swallowing water, if permitted.

A polyurethane tube may need to be warmed to make it more pliable. To make the tube easier to insert, it should be lubricated with a water-soluble substance (K-Y jelly) unless it has a dry coating called hydromer, which, when moistened, provides its own lubrication. The nurse wears gloves during the procedure.

The patient is placed in Fowler's position, and the nostrils are inspected for any obstruction. The more patent nostril is selected for use. The tip of the patient's nose is tilted, and the tube is aligned to enter the nostril. When the tube reaches the nasopharynx, the patient is instructed to lower the head slightly and to begin to swallow as the tube is advanced. The patient may also sip water through a straw to facilitate advancement of the tube. The oropharynx is inspected to ensure that the tube has not coiled in the pharynx or mouth.

Confirming Placement

To ensure patient safety, it is essential to confirm that the tube has been placed correctly, particularly because tubes may be accidentally inserted in the lungs, which may be undetected in high-risk patients. Examples of high-risk patients are those with a decreased level of consciousness, confused mental state, poor or absent cough and gag reflexes, or agitation during insertion. Presence of an endotracheal tube and recent removal of an endotracheal tube also increase the risk for inadvertent placement of the tube in the lung (Metheny, 1998). Initially, an x-ray study should confirm tube placement. However, each time liquids or medications are administered, and once a shift for continuous feedings, the tube must be checked to ensure that it remains properly placed. The traditional recommendation has been to inject air through the tube while auscultating the epigastric area with a stethoscope to detect air insufflations. However, studies indicate that this auscultatory method is not accurate in determining whether the tube has been inserted into the stomach, intestines, or respiratory tract (Metheny et al., 1999). Instead of the auscultation method, a combination of three methods is recommended:

- Measurement of tube length
- Visual assessment of aspirate
- pH measurement of aspirate

After the tube is inserted, the exposed portion of the tube is measured and the length is documented. The nurse measures the exposed tube length every shift and compares it with the original measurement. An increase in the length of exposed tube may indicate dislodgement, or a leaking or ruptured balloon if the tube has a balloon.

Visual assessment of the color of the aspirate may help identify tube placement. Metheny et al. (1994) found that gastric aspirate is most frequently cloudy and green, tan or off-white, or bloody or brown. Intestinal aspirate is primarily clear and yellow to bile-colored. Pleural fluid is usually pale yellow and serous, and tracheobronchial secretions are usually tan or off-white mucus. Researchers suggest that the appearance of the aspirate may be helpful in distinguishing between gastric and intestinal placement but is of little value in ruling out respiratory placement. This method is less helpful when the patient is receiving continuous feedings, because aspirate often looks like the formula that is used for the feeding (Metheny & Titler, 2001).

Determining the pH of the tube aspirate is a more accurate method of confirming tube placement. The pH method can also be used to monitor the advancement of the tube into the small intestines. The pH of gastric aspirate is acidic (1 to 5). The pH of intestinal aspirate is approximately 6 or greater, and the pH of respiratory aspirate is more alkaline (7 or greater). pH testing is best suited for distinguishing between gastric and intestinal placement. A pH sensor enteral tube is available which does not require fluid aspirate to obtain pH values; it can be useful in distinguishing gastric from small bowel placement of the tube. The pH method is less helpful with continuous feedings, because tube feedings have a pH value of 6.6 and neutralize the GI pH (Metheny & Titler, 2001). For more information, see Nursing Research Profile 36-1.

Using gastric aspiration as a means of verifying that the NG tube has been placed correctly may be a problem because of the characteristic properties and diameter of the tubes. Studies suggest that aspiration may be performed more easily with polyurethane tubes and tubes with a size 10 Fr diameter. Metheny et al. (1993) recommended the following steps if problems occur with aspiration of fluid from small-bore feeding tubes:

1. Insufflate 20 mL of air through the tube with a large syringe (30 to 60 mL).
2. Pull back on the plunger.
3. If step 2 is ineffective, insufflate another 20 mL of air and replace the large syringe with a smaller one (12 mL); attempt to aspirate.
4. If the measure is still ineffective, repeat step 3.
5. Change the patient's position and attempt to aspirate.

Securing the Tube

After the correct position of the tip has been confirmed, the NG tube is secured to the nose (Fig. 36-4). A liquid skin barrier should be applied to the skin where the NG tube will be secured. The prepared area is covered with a strip of hypoallergenic tape or Op-site; the tube is then placed over the tape and secured with a second piece of tape. The nasoenteric tube can be secured by taping it to the forehead (see Fig. 36-4). This keeps the tube from dislodging when the patient moves but still allows it to pass into the intestine. Instead of tape, a feeding tube attachment device (Hollister) can be used to secure the tube. This device adheres to the nose and uses an adjustable clip to hold the tube in place (Fig. 36-5). After the nasoenteric tube has progressed into the intestine (after approximately 24 hours), the tube may be taped in place.

Advancing the Nasoenteric Decompression Tube

After the tube has passed through the pyloric sphincter, it may be advanced 5 to 7.5 cm (2 to 3 in) every hour. To enable gravity and peristalsis to assist in the passage of the tube, the patient is generally asked to lie in the following positions in this order: on the right side for 2 hours, on the back for 2 hours, and then on the left side for 2 hours. Ambulation, if possible, also helps advance the tube. If the tube is advanced too rapidly, it will curl and kink in the stomach. The tube is irrigated with normal saline solution every 6 to 8 hours to prevent blockage.

NURSING RESEARCH PROFILE 36-1

Assessment of Feeding Tube Location

Metheny, N. A., Smith, L., & Stewart, B. J. (2000). Development of a reliable and valid bedside test for bilirubin and its utility for improving prediction of feeding tube location. *Nursing Research, 49,* 302–309.

Purpose

Although a wide variety of methods have been used to assess feeding tube location at the bedside, pH testing of aspirate has been found to be the most reliable in differentiating between gastric and respiratory placement of the tube and between gastric and intestinal placement of the tube. However, it is not reliable in distinguishing intestinal from respiratory fluids, because both of these fluids are alkaline. One new method that is being studied to distinguish these fluids is testing the tube aspirate for bilirubin, which is normally found in intestinal fluids but not in respiratory fluids.

The purposes of this study were (1) to assess the validity of a visual bilirubin teststrip used with a colorimetric visual bilirubin (VBIL) scale to predict laboratory bilirubin values, (2) to evaluate the interrater reliability of staff nurses using the visual bilirubin test strip and VBIL scale, and (3) to evaluate the ability of the visual bilirubin test strip and VBIL scale in combination with pH testing to predict feeding tube placement in the respiratory tract, stomach, or intestine.

Study Sample and Design

Concurrent pH and bilirubin testing was conducted on 631 GI specimens obtained from adult, acutely ill patients with newly inserted feeding tubes; the testing was done within 5 minutes of x-ray studies obtained to confirm tube placement. Also, 225 respiratory specimens were tested. A teststrip and VBIL scale as well as laboratory assay were used to measure bilirubin. A pH meter and pH teststrips were used to measure pH. Results were read by research assistants and staff nurses, who were blinded to (unaware of) the source or type of specimens. These readings were compared with the x-ray results.

Findings

There was a high correlation (0.93) between the readings made from the VBIL scale and the laboratory bilirubin assay. A pH reading greater than 5 and a bilirubin reading lower than 5 mg/dL accurately identified 100% of the respiratory specimens. A pH of 5 or less and a bilirubin concentration lower than 5 mg/dL accurately identified 98% of the gastric specimens. Approximately 88% of the specimens with a pH greater than 5 and a bilirubin value of 5 mg/dL or higher were intestinal specimens.

Nursing Implications

Use of the VBIL scale and bilirubin test strip has the potential for greatly improving the accuracy of determining feeding tube placement at the bedside. However, before its approval by the U.S. Food and Drug Administration for this purpose, further refinements are required to make sure that the most accurate readings can be made. Until such approval, nurses must rely on the auscultatory method, pH measurements, and observations of the patient's physical status to determine tube placement. Any question about correct tube placement should be investigated, and placement should be confirmed by x-ray studies whenever indicated.

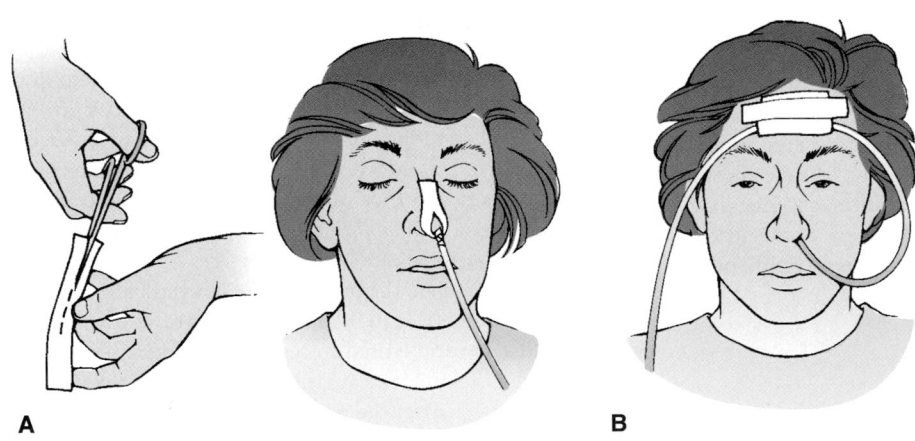

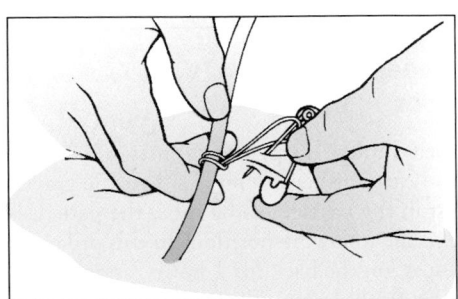

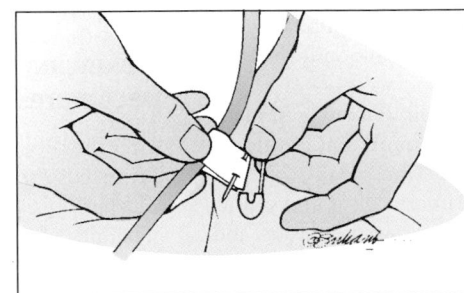

A   **B**   **C**   **D**

FIGURE 36-4 Securing NG and naso-enteric tubes. (**A**) The NG tube is secured to the nose with tape to prevent injury to the nasopharyngeal passages. (**B**) Tape is placed on the forehead and the nasoenteric tube is taped to it, thereby allowing the tube to be advanced until desired placement is achieved. (**C, D**) Secure tubing to the patient's gown with either an elastic band or tape attached to a safety pin to prevent tension on the line during movement of the patient.

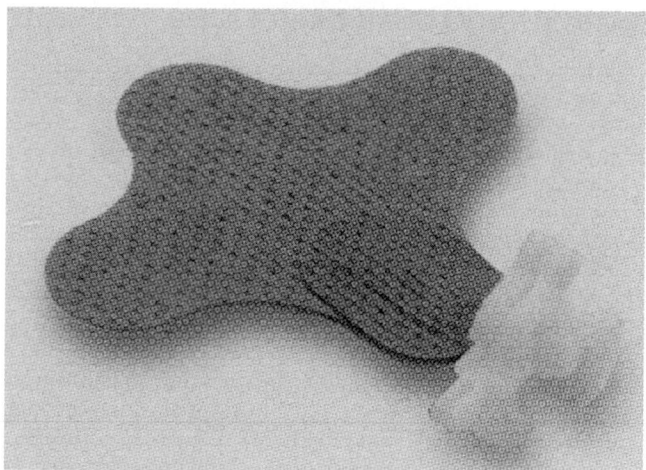

FIGURE 36-5 Feeding tube attachment device. Courtesy of Hollister, Incorporated.

Monitoring the Patient and Maintaining Tube Function

If the NG tube is used for decompression, it is attached to intermittent low suction. If it is used for enteral nutrition, the end of the tube is plugged between feedings. The nurse confirms tube placement before any fluids or medications are instilled and once a shift for continuous feedings. Displacement of the tube may be caused by tension on the tube (when the patient moves around in the bed or room), coughing, tracheal or nasotracheal suctioning, or airway intubation. If the NG tube is removed inadvertently in a patient who has undergone esophageal or gastric surgery, it is replaced by the physician, usually under fluoroscopy to avoid trauma to the suture line.

It is important to keep an accurate record of all fluid intake, feedings, and irrigation. To maintain patency, the tube is irrigated every 4 to 6 hours with normal saline to avoid electrolyte loss through gastric drainage. If an automatic flush enteral pump is used, the flushing schedule may be altered. The nurse records the amount, color, and type of all drainage every 8 hours.

When double- or triple-lumen tubes are used, each lumen is labeled according to its intended use: aspiration, feeding, or balloon inflation. To avoid tension on the tube, the portion of the tube from the nose to the drainage unit is fixed in position, either with a safety pin or with adhesive tape loops that are pinned to the patient's pajamas or gown. The tube must be looped loosely to prevent tension and dislodgement (see Fig. 36-4).

Providing Oral and Nasal Hygiene

Regular and conscientious oral and nasal hygiene is a vital part of patient care, because the tube causes discomfort and pressure and may be in place for several days. Moistened cotton-tipped swabs can be used to clean the nose, followed by cleansing with a water-soluble lubricant. Frequent mouth care is comforting for the patient. The nasal tape is changed every 2 to 3 days, and the nose is inspected for skin irritation. If the nasal and pharyngeal mucosa are

excessively dry, steam or cool vapor inhalations may be beneficial. Throat lozenges, an ice collar, chewing gum, or sucking on hard candies (if permitted), and frequent movement also assist in relieving patient discomfort. These activities keep the mucous membranes moist and help prevent inflammation of the parotid glands.

Monitoring and Managing Potential Complications

Patients with NG or nasoenteric intubation are susceptible to a variety of problems, including fluid volume deficit, pulmonary complications, and tube-related irritations. These potential complications require careful ongoing assessment.

Symptoms of fluid volume deficit include dry skin and mucous membranes, decreased urinary output, lethargy, and decreased body temperature. Assessment of fluid volume deficit involves maintaining an accurate record of intake and output. This includes measuring NG drainage, fluid instilled by irrigation of the NG tube, water taken by mouth, vomitus, water administered with tube feedings, and intravenous (IV) fluids. Laboratory values, particularly blood urea nitrogen and creatinine, are monitored. The nurse assesses 24-hour fluid balance and reports negative fluid balance, increased NG output, interruption of IV therapy, or any other disturbance in fluid intake or output.

Pulmonary complications from NG intubation occur because coughing and clearing of the pharynx are impaired, because gas buildup can irritate the phrenic nerve, and because tubes may become dislodged, retracting the distal end above the esophagogastric sphincter. Medications (antacids, simethicone, and metoclopramide) are administered to decrease potential problems. Signs and symptoms of complications include coughing during the administration of foods or medications, difficulty clearing the airway, tachypnea, and fever. Assessment includes regular auscultation of lung sounds and routine assessment of vital signs. It is important to encourage the patient to cough and to take deep breaths regularly. The nurse also carefully confirms the proper placement of the tube before instilling any fluids or medications.

Irritation of the mucous membranes is a common complication of NG intubation. The nostrils, oral mucosa, esophagus, and trachea are susceptible to irritation and necrosis. Visible areas are inspected frequently, and the adequacy of hydration is assessed. When providing oral hygiene, the nurse carefully inspects the mucous membranes for signs of irritation or excessive dryness. The nurse palpates the area around the parotid glands to detect any tenderness or enlarged nodes, indicating parotitis, and observes for any skin or mucous membrane irritation or necrosis. In addition, it is important to assess the patient for esophagitis and tracheitis; symptoms include sore throat and hoarseness.

Removing the Tube

Before removing a tube, the nurse may intermittently clamp and unclamp the NG tube for a trial period of 24 hours to ensure that the patient does not experience nausea, vomiting, or distention. Before the tube is removed, it is flushed with 10 mL of normal saline to ensure that it is free of debris and away from the gastric lining; then the balloon (if present) is deflated. Gloves are worn to remove the tube. The tube is withdrawn gently and slowly for 15 to 20 cm (6 to 8 in) until the tip reaches the esophagus; the remainder is withdrawn rapidly from the nostril. A nasointestinal tube is withdrawn at intervals of 10 minutes until the end reaches the esophagus. If the tube does not come out easily, force should not be used, and the problem should be reported to the physician. As the tube is withdrawn, it is concealed in a towel, because the sight of it may be unpleasant to the patient. After the tube is removed, the nurse provides oral hygiene.

Tube Feedings With Nasogastric and Nasoenteric Devices

Tube feedings are given to meet nutritional requirements when oral intake is inadequate or not possible and the GI tract is functioning normally. Tube feedings have several advantages over parenteral nutrition: they are low in cost, safe, well tolerated by the patient, and easy to use both in extended care facilities and in the patient's home. Tube feedings have other advantages:

- They preserve GI integrity by delivery of nutrients and medications (antacids, simethicone, and metoclopramide) intraluminally
- They preserve the normal sequence of intestinal and hepatic metabolism
- They maintain fat metabolism and lipoprotein synthesis
- They maintain normal insulin/glucagon ratios

Tube feedings are delivered to the stomach (in the case of NG intubation or gastrostomy) or to the distal duodenum or proximal jejunum (in the case of nasoduodenal or **nasojejunal tube** feeding). Nasoduodenal or nasojejunal feeding is indicated when the esophagus and stomach need to be bypassed or when the patient is at risk for **aspiration** (breathing fluids or foods into the trachea and lungs). For long-term feedings (longer than 4 weeks), nasoduodenal, gastrostomy, or jejunostomy tubes are preferred for administration of medications or food. The numerous conditions requiring enteral nutrition are summarized in Table 36-2.

OSMOSIS AND OSMOLALITY

Osmolality is an important consideration for patients receiving tube feedings through the duodenum or jejunum, because feeding formulas with a high osmolality may lead to undesirable effects, such as dumping syndrome (described below).

Fluid balance is maintained by **osmosis**, the process by which water moves through membranes from a dilute solution of lower **osmolality** (ionic concentration) to a more concentrated solution of higher osmolality until both solutions are of nearly equal osmolality. The osmolality of normal body fluids is approximately 300 mOsm/kg. The body attempts to keep the osmolality of the contents of the stomach and intestines at approximately this level.

Highly concentrated solutions and certain foods can upset the normal fluid balance in the body. Individual amino acids and carbohydrates are small particles that have great osmotic effect. Proteins are extremely large particles and therefore have less osmotic effect. Fats are not water-soluble and do not enter into a solution in water; thus, they have no osmotic effect. Electrolytes, such as sodium and potassium, are comparatively small particles; they have a great effect on osmolality and consequently on the patient's ability to tolerate a given solution.

When a concentrated solution of high osmolality is taken in large amounts, water will move to the stomach and intestines from fluid surrounding the organs and the vascular compartment. The patient has a feeling of fullness, nausea, and diarrhea; this causes dehydration, hypotension, and tachycardia, collectively termed the **dumping syndrome**. Starting with a more dilute solution and increasing the concentration over several days can generally alleviate this problem. Patients vary in the degree to which they tolerate the effects of high osmolality; usually debilitated patients are more sensitive. The nurse needs to be knowledgeable about the osmolality of the patient's formula and needs to observe for and take steps to prevent undesired effects.

TUBE FEEDING FORMULAS

The choice of formula to be delivered by tube feeding is influenced by the status of the GI tract and the nutritional needs of

---

Table 36-2 • Conditions Requiring Enteral Therapy

CONDITION OR NEED	EXAMPLES
Preoperative bowel preparation	—
Gastrointestinal problems	Fistula, short-bowel syndrome, mild pancreatitis, Crohn's disease, ulcerative colitis, nonspecific maldigestion or malabsorption
Cancer therapy	Radiation, chemotherapy
Convalescent care	Surgery, injury, severe illness
Coma, semiconsciousness*	Stroke, head injury, neurologic disorder, neoplasm
Hypermetabolic conditions	Burns, trauma, multiple fractures, sepsis, AIDS, organ transplantation
Alcoholism, chronic depression, anorexia nervosa*	Chronic illness, psychiatric or neurologic disorder
Debilitation*	Disease or injury
Maxillofacial or cervical surgery	Disease or injury
Oropharyngeal or esophageal paralysis*	Disease or injury, neoplasm, inflammation, trauma, respiratory failure

*Because some of these patients are at risk for regurgitating or vomiting and aspirating administered formula, each condition must be considered individually.

the patient. The formula characteristics evaluated include chemical composition of the nutrient source (protein, carbohydrates, fat), caloric density, osmolality, residue, bacteriologic safety, vitamins, minerals, and cost.

Various major formula types for tube feedings are available commercially. Blenderized formulas can be made by the patient's family or obtained in a ready-to-use form that is carefully prepared according to directions. Commercially prepared polymeric formulas (formulas with high molecular weight) are composed of protein, carbohydrates, and fats in a high-molecular-weight form (Boost Plus, TwoCal HN, Isosource). Chemically defined formulas contain predigested and easy-to-absorb nutrients (Osmolite HN). Modular products contain only one major nutrient, such as protein (Promote). Disease-specific formulas are available for various conditions, such as renal failure (Nepro), severe chronic obstructive pulmonary disease (Pulmocare). Nepro is high in calories and low in electrolytes. It is ideal for patients who require electrolyte and fluid restriction. Pulmocare is high in fat and low in carbohydrates. Its high density (1.5 calories/mL) is ideal for patients who require fluid restriction, and it is also designed to reduce carbon dioxide production. Fiber has also been added to formulas (Jevity) in an attempt to decrease the occurrence of diarrhea. Some feedings are given as supplements, and others are designed to meet the patient's total nutritional needs. Dietitians collaborate with physicians and nurses in determining the best formula for the individual patient.

> **NURSING ALERT** Commercial formulas frequently present problems because the composition is fixed and some patients are not able to tolerate certain ingredients, such as sodium, protein, or potassium. Modular products may be substituted, and the critical constituents of sodium, potassium, and fat can be added. Attention is given to including all essential minerals and vitamins. Total intake of calories, nutrients, and fluids must be assessed when there is a reduction in total intake or excessive dilution of feedings.

TUBE FEEDING ADMINISTRATION METHODS

Many patients do not tolerate NG and nasoenteric tube feedings well. Often a medium- or fine-bore Silastic nasoenteric tube is tolerated better than a plastic or rubber tube. The finer-bore tube requires a finely dispersed formula to ensure that the patency of the tube is maintained. For long-term tube feeding therapy, a gastrostomy or jejunostomy tube is used (see later discussion).

The tube feeding method chosen depends on the location of the tube, patient tolerance, convenience, and cost. Intermittent bolus feedings are administered into the stomach (usually by gastrostomy tube) in large amounts at designated intervals and may be given 4 to 8 times per day. The intermittent gravity drip is another method for administering tube feedings into the stomach and is commonly used when the patient is at home. In this instance, the tube feeding is administered over 30 minutes at designated intervals. Both of these tube-feeding methods are practical and inexpensive. However, the feedings delivered at variable rates may be poorly tolerated and time-consuming.

The continuous infusion method is used when feedings are administered into the small intestine. This method is preferred for patients who are at risk for aspiration or who tolerate the tube feedings poorly. The feedings are given continuously at a constant rate by means of a pump. The continuous tube feeding method, which requires a pump device, decreases abdominal distention, gastric residuals, and the risk of aspiration. However, pumps are expensive, and they permit the patient less flexibility than intermittent feedings do.

An alternative to the continuous infusion method is **cyclic feeding**. The infusion is given at a faster rate over a shorter time (usually 8 to 12 hours). Feeding may be infused at night to avoid interrupting the patient's lifestyle. Cyclic continuous infusions may be appropriate for patients who are being weaned from tube feedings to an oral diet, as a supplement for a patient who cannot eat enough, and for patients at home who need daytime hours free from the pump.

Tube feeding solutions vary in terms of required preparation, consistency, and the number of calories and supplemental vitamins they contain. The choice of solution depends on the size and location of the tube, the patient's nutrient needs, the type of nutritional supplement, the method of delivery, and the convenience for the patient at home. A wide variety of containers, feeding tubes and catheters, delivery systems, and pumps are available for use with tube feedings.

NURSING PROCESS: THE PATIENT RECEIVING A TUBE FEEDING

Assessment

A preliminary assessment of the patient who requires a tube feeding includes several considerations, as well as the family's need for information:

- What is the patient's nutritional status, as judged by current physical appearance, dietary history, and recent weight loss?
- Are there any existing chronic illnesses or factors that will increase metabolic demands on the body (eg, surgical stress, fever)?
- What is the patient's hydration status? What are the electrolyte levels?
- Is the patient's digestive tract functioning?
- Are the kidneys functioning normally?
- Are fluid requirements (ie, 30 to 40 mL/kg body weight) being met?
- What medications and other therapies is the patient receiving that may affect digestive intake and function of the digestive system?
- Does the dietary prescription fulfill the patient's needs?

In addition, a more elaborate assessment is performed for patients who require extensive nutritional therapy. A team that includes the nurse, physician, and dietitian conducts this assessment. In addition to the history and physical examination (which includes anthropometric measurements), nutritional assessment consists of recording any weight change; determining albumin, prealbumin, and transferrin levels and total lymphocyte count; testing for the delayed hypersensitivity reaction; and evaluating muscle function. (See Chapter 5 for a detailed description of nutritional assessment.)

Diagnosis

NURSING DIAGNOSES

Based on the assessment data, the major nursing diagnoses may include the following:

- Imbalanced nutrition, less than body requirements, related to inadequate intake of nutrients
- Risk for diarrhea related to the dumping syndrome or to tube feeding intolerance
- Risk for ineffective airway clearance related to aspiration of tube feeding
- Risk for deficient fluid volume related to hypertonic dehydration
- Risk for ineffective coping related to discomfort imposed by the presence of the NG or nasoenteric tube
- Risk for ineffective therapeutic regimen management
- Deficient knowledge about home tube feeding regimen

COLLABORATIVE PROBLEMS/ POTENTIAL COMPLICATIONS

Complications of NG and nasoenteric tube feeding therapy are classified into three types—GI, mechanical, and metabolic. Table 36-3 lists complications, possible causes, and appropriate interventions.

Planning and Goals

The major goals for the patient may include nutritional balance, normal bowel elimination pattern, reduced risk of aspiration, adequate hydration, individual coping, knowledge and skill in self-care, and prevention of complications.

Nursing Interventions

MAINTAINING FEEDING EQUIPMENT AND NUTRITIONAL BALANCE

The temperature and volume of the feeding, the flow rate, and the total fluid intake are important factors to be considered when tube feedings are administered. The schedule of tube feedings, including the correct quantity and frequency, is maintained. The nurse must carefully monitor the drip rate and avoid administering fluids too rapidly.

Feedings are administered by gravity (drip), bolus, or continuous controlled pump (mL/hour or drops/hour). Gravity feedings are placed above the level of the stomach, with the speed of administration determined by gravity. **Bolus** feedings are given in large volumes (300 to 400 mL every 4 to 6 hours). Continuous feeding is the preferred method; delivery of the feeding in small amounts over long periods reduces the incidence of aspiration, distention, nausea, vomiting, and diarrhea. Continuous administration rates of about 100 to 150 mL/hour (2400 to 3600 calories/day) are effective in inducing positive nitrogen balance and progressive weight gain without producing abdominal cramps and diarrhea. If the feeding is intermittent, 200 to 350 mL is given in 10 to 15 minutes. Enteral pumps are mechanical devices that control the delivery rate of feeding formula (Fig. 36-6). Pumps allow for a constant flow rate and can infuse a viscous formula through a small-diameter feeding tube. These pumps are relatively heavy and must be attached to an IV pole. For home use, there are portable lightweight enteral pumps available that weigh about 4 pounds and are easy to handle. An enteral pump is available with an automatic water flush system. In addition to administering the feeding formula, these pumps provide hourly water flushes that are designed to prevent clogged feeding tubes (Petnicki, 1998).

Residual gastric content is measured before each intermittent feeding and every 4 to 8 hours during continuous feedings. (This aspirated fluid is readministered to the patient.) The research findings of McClave et al. (1992) indicated that, if the amount of aspirated gastric content is greater than or equal to 200 mL for NG tubes or if residual volumes are greater than or equal to 100 mL for gastrostomy tubes, tube feeding intolerance should be considered. Tube feedings may be continued with close monitoring of gastric residual volume, radiographic studies, and the patient's physical status. If excessive residual volumes occur twice, the nurse notifies the physician.

Maintaining tube function is an ongoing responsibility of the nurse, patient, or primary caregiver. To ensure patency and to decrease the chance of bacterial growth, crusting, or occlusion of the tube, 20 to 30 mL of water is administered in each of the following instances:

- Before and after each dose of medication and each tube feeding
- After checking for gastric residuals and gastric pH
- Every 4 to 6 hours with continuous feedings
- If the tube feeding is discontinued for any reason

PROVIDING MEDICATIONS BY TUBE

When different types of medications are administered, each type is given separately, using a bolus method that is compatible with the medication's preparation (Table 36-4). The tube is flushed with 20 to 30 mL of water after each dose. If a liquid form of a medication is not available and the medication can be crushed, it must first be reduced to a fine powder or the tube will become clogged. Devices are available (eg, Handicrush Irrigation Syringe by Nestle) that crush and dissolve tablets with water (Fig. 36-7). Medications are not mixed with each other or with the feeding formula. When small-bore feeding tubes for continuous infusion are irrigated after medication administration, a 30-mL or larger syringe is used, because the pressure generated by smaller syringes could rupture the tube.

MAINTAINING FEEDING REGIMENS AND DELIVERY SYSTEMS

Tube feeding formula is delivered to patients by either an open or a closed system. The open system comes in cans or as a powder and may be mixed with water. The feeding container (which is hung on a pole) and the tubing used with the open system are changed—usually every 24 to 72 hours. To avoid bacterial contamination, the amount of feeding formula in the bag should never exceed what is expected to be infused in 4 hours.

Closed delivery systems use a prefilled, sterile container that is spiked with enteral tubing. The bag holding the feeding formula for the closed system can be hung safely for 24 to 48 hours.

The tube-feeding regimen must be assessed frequently to evaluate its effectiveness and avoid complications (Chart 36-1).

MAINTAINING NORMAL BOWEL ELIMINATION PATTERN

Patients receiving NG or nasoenteric tube feedings commonly have diarrhea (watery stools occurring three or more times in 24 hours). Pasty, unformed stool is expected with enteral therapy, because many formulas have little or no residue. The dumping syndrome also leads to diarrhea, but to confirm dumping syndrome as the cause of diarrhea other possible causes must be ruled out, among them the following:

Table 36-3 • **Complications of Enteral Therapy**

COMPLICATIONS	CAUSES	SELECTED NURSING INTERVENTIONS
Gastrointestinal		
Diarrhea (most common)	Hyperosmolar feedings Rapid infusion/bolus feedings Bacteria-contaminated feedings Lactase deficiency Medications/antibiotic therapy Decreased serum osmolality level Food allergies Cold formula	Assess fluid balance and electrolyte levels; report findings Assess rate of infusion and temperature of formula Implement changes in tube feeding formula or rate Replace formula every 4 hours; change tube feeding container and tubing daily
Nausea/vomiting	Change in rate Hyperosmolar formula Inadequate gastric emptying	Check residuals; if ≥ 200 mL for NG or >100 mL for gastrostomy, continue feeding and recheck; report if residual is still high Review medications
Gas/bloating/cramping	Air in tube	Keep tubing free of air
Dumping syndrome	Bolus feedings/rapid rate	Check fiber and water content; report findings
	Cold formula	Check rate and temperature of formula
Constipation	High milk (lactose) content Lack of fiber Inadequate fluid intake/dehydration	Check fiber and water content; report findings
Mechanical		
Aspiration pneumonia	Improper tube placement Vomiting and aspirated tube feeding Flat in bed Use of large tube	Implement reliable method for checking small-bore enteral tube placement (ie, measuring length of exposed tube) Keep head of bed elevated 30 degrees continuously
Tube displacement	Excessive coughing/vomitus Tension on the tube or unsecured tube Tracheal suctioning Airway intubation	Check tube placement before administering feeding
Tube obstruction	Inadequate flushing/formula rate	Follow policy for flushing of tube and for crushing medications
Residue	Inadequate crushing of medications and flushing after administration	Obtain liquid medications when possible Flush feeding tube before and after medication administration
Nasopharyngeal irritation	Tube position/improper taping Use of large tubes	Tape tube to prevent pressure on nares Assess nasopharyngeal mucous membranes every 4 hours
Metabolic		
Hyperglycemia	Glucose intolerance High carbohydrate content of the feeding	Check blood glucose levels periodically
Dehydration and azotemia (excessive urea in the blood)	Hyperosmolar feedings with insufficient fluid intake	Report signs and symptoms of dehydration Implement changes in tube feeding formula, rate, or ratio to water
Tube feeding syndrome	Excessive urea from high-protein mixture and formulas lacking fat Dehydration	Implement changes in tube feeding formula, rate, or ratio to water

• Zinc deficiency—Adding 15 mg of zinc to the tube feeding every 24 hours is recommended to maintain a normal serum level of 50 to 150 fg/dL (7.65 to 22.95 fmol/L)
• Contaminated formula
• Malnutrition—A decrease in the intestinal absorptive area resulting from malnutrition can cause diarrhea
• Medication therapy—Antibiotics, such as clindamycin (Cleocin) and lincomycin (Lincocin); antiarrhythmics, such as quinidine and propranolol (Inderal); and aminophylline, theophylline, and digitalis have been found to increase the frequency of diarrhea in some patients

The dumping syndrome results from rapid distention of the jejunum when hypertonic solutions are administered quickly (over 10 to 20 minutes). Foods high in carbohydrates and electrolytes draw extracellular fluid from the vascular system into the jejunum so that dilution and absorption can occur. Measures for managing the GI symptoms (diarrhea, nausea) associated with the dumping syndrome are presented in Chart 36-2.

REDUCING THE RISK OF ASPIRATION

Aspiration pneumonia occurs when stomach contents or enteral feedings are regurgitated and aspirated, or when an NG tube is improperly positioned and feedings are instilled into the pharynx or the trachea. Nasoenteric tubes, especially those that provide for gastric and esophageal or duodenal decompression, have helped decrease the frequency of regurgitation and aspiration.

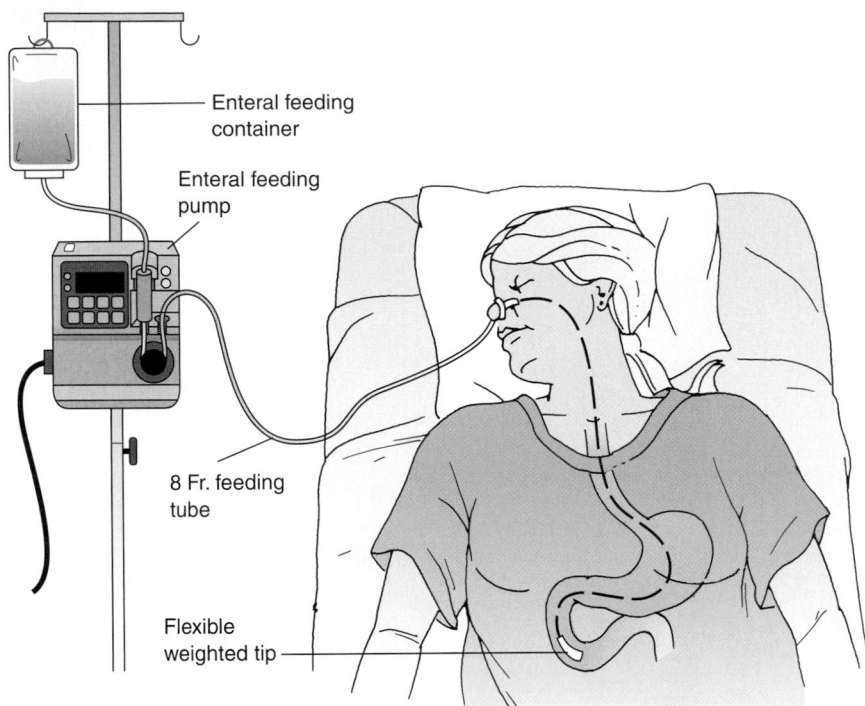

Enteral feeding
container

Enteral feeding
pump

8 Fr. feeding
tube

Flexible
weighted tip

FIGURE 36-6 Nasoenteric tube feeding by continuous controlled pump.

To prevent aspiration, the nurse must establish the correct tube feeding placement before every feeding, each time medications are administered, and once every shift if the tube feeding is continuous. Feedings and medications should always be given with the patient in the proper position to prevent regurgitation. To reduce the risk of reflux and pulmonary aspiration, the semi-Fowler's position is necessary for an NG feeding, with the patient's head elevated at least 30 to 45 degrees. This position is maintained at least 1 hour after completion of an intermittent tube feeding and is maintained at all times for patients receiving continuous tube feedings. Another prevention strategy is to monitor residual volumes (Edwards & Metheny, 2000).

If aspiration is suspected, the feeding is stopped immediately, the pharynx and trachea are suctioned, and the patient is placed on the right side with the head of the bed down. The physician is notified immediately.

MAINTAINING ADEQUATE HYDRATION

The nurse carefully monitors hydration because, in many cases, the patient cannot communicate the need for water. Water (at least 2 L/day) is given every 4 to 6 hours and after feedings to prevent hypertonic dehydration. At the beginning of administration, the feeding is diluted to at least half-strength and not more than 50 to 100 mL is given at a time, or 40 to 60 mL/hour is given in continuous drip administration. This gradual administration helps the patient to develop tolerance, especially for hyperosmolar solutions. Key nursing interventions include observing for signs of dehydration (dry mucous membranes, thirst, decreased urine output); administering water routinely and as needed; and monitoring intake, output, and fluid balance (24-hour intake versus output).

Table 36-4 • Preparing Medication for Delivery by Feeding Tube

MEDICATION FORM	PREPARATION
Liquid	None
Simple compressed tablets	Crush and dissolve in water
Buccal or sublingual tablets	Administer as prescribed
Soft gelatin capsules filled with liquid	Make an opening in capsule and squeeze out contents
Enteric-coated tablets	Do not crush; change in form is required
Timed-release tablets	Do not crush tablets because doing so may release too much drug too quickly (overdose); check with pharmacist for alternative formulation
Timed-release capsules or sustained-release capsules	Some can be opened and contents added to tube-feeding formula; *always* check with pharmacist before doing this

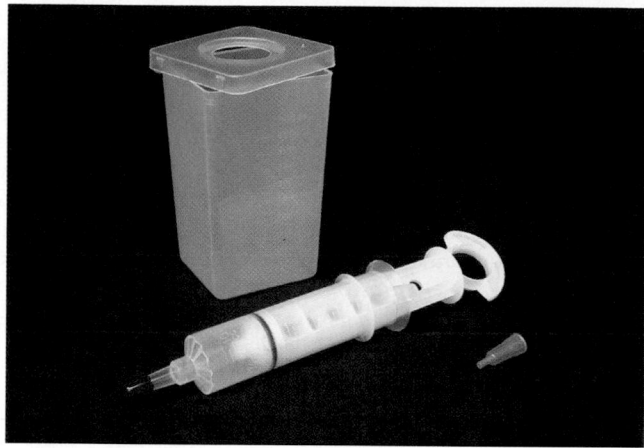

FIGURE 36-7 The Pill Crusher™ Syringe (from Welcon, Inc.) crushes medications to a fine powder and then allows them to be administered to persons with feeding tubes. The Pill Crusher™ is also used to irrigate the feeding tube and assists in hydrating the patient. Courtesy of Welcon, Inc., Fort Worth, TX (www.welcon.com).

PROMOTING COPING ABILITY

The psychosocial goal of nursing care is to support and encourage the patient to accept physical changes and to convey hope that daily progressive improvement is possible. If the patient is having difficulty adjusting to the treatment, the nurse intervenes

---

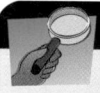

Chart 36-1 • ASSESSMENT

Measures for Assessing Tube Feeding Regimens

The following nursing measures may be implemented when assessing the effectiveness and safety of tube feeding:

1. Assess tube placement, patient's position (head of bed elevated 30 to 45 degrees), and formula flow rate.
2. Determine the patient's ability to tolerate the formula. Observe for fullness, bloating, distention, urticaria, nausea, vomiting, and stool pattern and character.
3. Check clinical responses, as noted in laboratory findings (blood urea nitrogen, serum protein, prealbumin, electrolytes, renal function, hemoglobin, hematocrit).
4. Observe for signs of dehydration (dry mucous membranes, thirst, decreased urine output).
5. Record the amount of formula actually taken in by the patient.
6. Report an elevated blood glucose level, decreased urinary output, sudden weight gain, and periorbital or dependent edema.
7. Replace any formula administered by an open system every 4 hours with fresh formula. Formula should be at room temperature or cool (not cold).
8. Change tube feeding container and tubing every 24 to 72 hours.
9. Assess residual volume before each feeding or, in the case of continuous feedings, every 4 hours. Return the aspirate to the stomach.
10. Monitor intake and output.
11. Weigh the patient twice weekly.
12. Consult the dietitian regularly.

Chart 36-2 **Preventing Symptoms of Dumping Syndrome**

The following strategies may help prevent some of the uncomfortable symptoms of dumping syndrome related to tube feeding:

- Slow the formula instillation rate to provide time for carbohydrates and electrolytes to be diluted.
- Administer feedings at room temperature, because temperature extremes stimulate peristalsis.
- Administer feeding by continuous drip (if tolerated) rather than by bolus, to prevent sudden distention of the intestine.
- Advise the patient to remain in semi-Fowler's position for 1 hour after the feeding; this position prolongs intestinal transit time by decreasing the effect of gravity.
- Instill the minimal amount of water needed to flush the tubing before and after a feeding, because fluid given with a feeding increases intestinal transit time.

---

by encouraging self-care (eg, recording daily weight and intake and output), within the parameters of the patient's activity level. In addition, the nurse reinforces an optimistic approach by identifying signs and symptoms that indicate progress (daily weight gain, electrolyte balance, absence of nausea and diarrhea).

PROMOTING HOME AND COMMUNITY-BASED CARE

Teaching Patients Self-Care

Patients who require long-term tube feedings in the home care setting have conditions such as obstruction of the upper GI tract, malabsorption syndrome, surgery of the GI tract or of the head or neck region, or decreased level of consciousness. For a patient to be considered for tube feeding at home, the following criteria must be met: The patient must be medically stable and must have successfully completed a tube feeding trial (tolerated 70% of feeding). In addition, the patient must be capable of self-care or have a caregiver who is willing to assume the responsibility, and the patient or caregiver must have access to supplies and interest in learning how to administer tube feedings at home.

Preparation of the patient for home administration of enteral feedings begins while the patient is still hospitalized. Ideally, the nurse teaches while administering the feedings so that the patient can observe the mechanics of the procedure, participate in the procedure, ask questions, and express any concerns. Before discharge, the nurse provides information about the equipment needed, formula purchase and storage, and administration of the feedings (frequency, quantity, rate of instillation).

Family members who will be active in the patient's home care are encouraged to participate in all teaching sessions. Available printed information about the equipment, the formula, and the procedure is reviewed. The nurse encourages the patient and caregiver to learn to use the equipment with the supervision of the nurse. Arrangements are made for the caregiver to obtain the equipment and formula and have it ready for use before the patient's discharge.

Continuing Care

Referral to a home care agency is important so that a nurse can arrange to be present to supervise and provide support during the first feeding at home. Further visits will depend on the skill and comfort of the patient or caregiver in administering the feedings.

During all visits, the nurse monitors the patient's physical status (weight, vital signs, activity level) and the ability of the patient and family to administer the tube feedings correctly. In addition, the nurse assesses for any complications (dumping syndrome, nausea or vomiting, weight loss, lethargy, confusion, excessive thirst). The patient or caregiver is encouraged to keep a diary to record times and amounts of feedings and any symptoms that occur. The nurse reviews the diary with the patient and caregiver during home visits.

Evaluation

EXPECTED PATIENT OUTCOMES

Expected patient outcomes may include the following:

1. Attains or maintains nutritional balance
   a. Has a positive nitrogen balance
   b. Maintains laboratory values within normal limits (ie, blood urea nitrogen, hemoglobin, hematocrit, prealbumin, serum protein)
   c. Attains or maintains hydration of body tissue
   d. Attains or maintains desired body weight
2. Is free of episodes of diarrhea
   a. Has fewer than three watery stools a day
   b. Does not have a bowel movement after a bolus feeding
   c. States that there is no intestinal cramping
   d. Has normal bowel sounds
3. Avoids aspiration
   a. Lungs are clear to auscultation
   b. Exhibits normal heart rate and respirations
4. Attains or maintains hydration of body tissue
   a. Has a balanced intake and output every 24 hours
   b. Does not have dry skin or dry mucous membranes
5. Copes effectively with tube feeding regimen
6. Demonstrates skill in managing tube feeding regimen
7. Experiences no complications
   a. Has no GI disturbances
   b. Tube remains intact and patent for duration of therapy
   c. Maintains metabolic balance within normal limits

Gastrostomy

A **gastrostomy** is a surgical procedure in which an opening is created into the stomach for the purpose of administering foods and fluids. In some instances, a gastrostomy is preferred for prolonged nutrition (greater then 3 to 4 weeks)—for example, in the elderly or debilitated patient. Gastrostomy is also preferred over NG feedings in the comatose patient because the gastroesophageal sphincter remains intact. Regurgitation and aspiration are less likely to occur with a gastrostomy than with NG feedings.

Different types of feeding gastrostomies may be used, including the Stamm (temporary and permanent), Janeway (permanent), and percutaneous endoscopic gastrostomy (temporary) systems. The Stamm and Janeway gastrostomies require either an upper abdominal midline incision or a left upper quadrant transverse incision. The Stamm procedure requires the use of concentric purse-string sutures to secure the tube to the anterior gastric wall. To create the gastrostomy, an exit wound is created in the left upper abdomen. The Janeway procedure necessitates the creation of a tunnel (called a gastric tube) that is brought out through the abdomen to form a permanent **stoma**.

A **percutaneous endoscopic gastrostomy (PEG)** is a procedure that requires the services of two physicians (or a physician and a nurse with specialty skills). After administering a local anesthetic, one physician inserts a cannula into the stomach through an abdominal incision and then threads a nonabsorbable suture through the cannula; the second physician looks through an endoscope that has been passed into the upper GI tract and uses the endoscopic snare to grasp the end of the suture and guide it up through the patient's mouth. The suture is knotted to the dilator tip at the end of the PEG tube. The endoscopist then advances the dilator tip through the patient's mouth while the first physician pulls the suture through the cannula site. The attached PEG tube is guided down the esophagus, into the stomach, and out through the abdominal incision (Fig. 36-8A). The mushroom catheter tip and internal crossbar secure the tube against the stomach wall. An external crossbar or bumper keeps the catheter

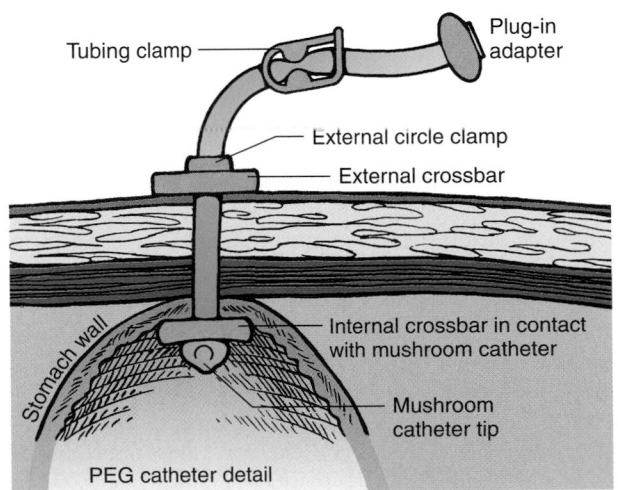

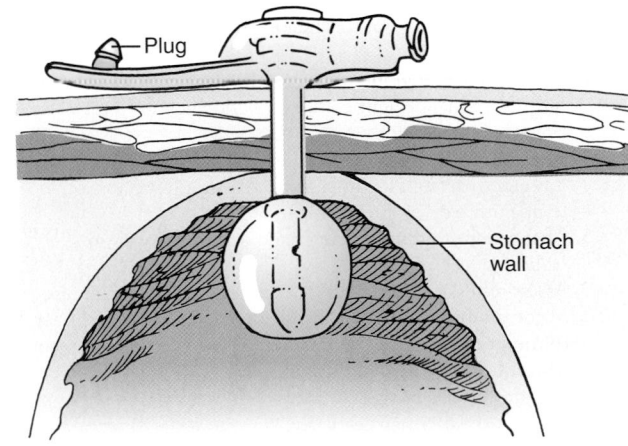

FIGURE 36-8 (**A**) A detail of the abdomen and the PEG tube, showing catheter fixation. (**B**) A detail of the abdomen and the nonobturated LPGD, showing balloon fixation.

in place. A tubing adaptor is in place between feedings, and a clamp or plug is used to close or open the tubing. If an endoscope is unable to pass through the esophagus, then the gastrostomy can be performed under x-ray guidance through the abdominal wall. This procedure is known as fluoroscopically guided percutaneous gastrostomy, or FGPG (Johnson, 1997).

The initial PEG device can be removed and replaced once the tract is well established (10 to 14 days after insertion). Replacement of the PEG device is indicated to provide long-term nutritional support, to replace a clotted or migrated tube, or to enhance patient comfort. The PEG replacement device should be fitted securely to the stoma to prevent leakage of gastric acid and is maintained in place through traction between the internal and anchoring devices.

An alternative to the PEG device is a **low-profile gastrostomy device (LPGD)** (see Fig. 36-8B). The LPGD may be inserted 3 to 6 months after initial gastrostomy tube placement. These devices are inserted flush with the skin; they eliminate the possibility of tube migration and obstruction and have antireflux valves to prevent gastric reflux. Two types of devices may be used—obturated or nonobturated. The obturated devices (G-button) have a dome tip that acts as an internal stabilizer. A major drawback is the need for a physician to obturate (insert a tube that is larger than the actual stoma). The nonobturated device (MIC-KEY) has an external skin disk and is inserted into the stoma without force; a balloon is inflated to secure placement. A nurse in the home setting can insert these devices easily. The drawbacks of both types of LPGDs are the inability to check residual volumes (one-way valve) and the need for a special adaptor to connect the device to the feeding container.

Patients with severe gastroesophageal reflux are at risk for aspiration pneumonia and therefore are not candidates for a gastrostomy. A jejunostomy is preferred, or jejunal feeding through a nasojejunal tube may be recommended.

NURSING PROCESS:
THE PATIENT WITH A GASTROSTOMY

Assessment

The focus of the preoperative assessment is to determine the patient's ability both to understand and to cope with the impending surgical experience. The nurse evaluates the patient's ability to adjust to a change in body image and to participate in self-care, along with the patient's and the family's psychological status.

The purpose of the operative procedure is explained so that the patient will have a better understanding of the expected postoperative course. The patient needs to know that the result of this surgery is to bypass the mouth and esophagus so that liquid feedings can be administered directly into the stomach by means of a rubber or plastic tube or a prosthesis. If the prosthesis is to be permanent, the patient should be made aware of this. Psychologically, this is often difficult for the patient to accept. If the procedure is being performed to relieve discomfort, prolonged vomiting, debilitation, or an inability to eat, the patient may find it more acceptable.

The nurse evaluates the patient's skin condition and determines whether a delay in healing may be anticipated because of a systemic disorder (eg, diabetes mellitus, cancer).

In the postoperative period, the patient's fluid and nutritional needs are assessed to ensure proper intake of food and fluids. The nurse inspects the tube for proper maintenance and the incision for signs of infection. At the same time, the nurse evaluates the patient's response to the change in body image and the patient's understanding of the feeding methods. Interventions are identified to help the patient cope with the tube and learn self-care measures.

Diagnosis

NURSING DIAGNOSES

Based on the assessment data, the major nursing diagnoses in the postoperative period may include the following:

- Imbalanced nutrition, less than body requirements, related to enteral feeding problems
- Risk for infection related to presence of wound and tube
- Risk for impaired skin integrity at tube site
- Ineffective coping related to inability to eat normally
- Disturbed body image related to presence of tube
- Risk for ineffective therapeutic regimen management related to knowledge deficit about home care and the feeding procedure

COLLABORATIVE PROBLEMS/
POTENTIAL COMPLICATIONS

Potential complications that may develop include the following:

- Wound infection, cellulitis, and abdominal wall abscess
- GI bleeding
- Premature removal of the tube

Planning and Goals

The major goals for the patient may include attaining an optimal level of nutrition, preventing infection, maintaining skin integrity, enhancing coping, adjusting to changes in body image, acquiring knowledge of and skill in self-care, and preventing complications.

Nursing Interventions

MEETING NUTRITIONAL NEEDS

The first fluid nourishment is administered soon after surgery and usually consists of tap water and 10% glucose. At first, only 30 to 60 mL (1 to 2 oz) is given at one time, but the amount is increased gradually. By the second day, 180 to 240 mL (6 to 8 oz) may be given at one time, provided it is tolerated and no leakage of fluid occurs around the tube. Water and milk can be instilled after 24 hours for a permanent gastrostomy. High-calorie liquids are added gradually. In some settings, during the early postoperative period the nurse aspirates gastric secretions and reinstills them after adding enough feeding solution to bring the volume to the desired total. By this method, gastric dilation is avoided.

Blenderized foods are added gradually to clear liquids until a full diet is achieved. Powdered feedings that are easily liquefied are commercially available. The patient who receives blenderized tube feedings typically is not forced to give up usual dietary patterns, which may prove to be psychologically more acceptable. In addition, near-normal bowel function is promoted because the fiber and residue are similar to that of a normal diet. Intake of milk is avoided in patients with lactase deficiency.

PROVIDING TUBE CARE AND PREVENTING INFECTION

A small dressing can be applied over the tube outlet, and the gastrostomy tube can be held in place by a thin strip of adhesive tape that is first placed around the tube and then firmly attached to the abdomen. The dressing protects the skin around the incision from seepage of gastric acid and spillage of feedings.

The nurse verifies the tube's placement, assesses residuals, and rotates the tube or stabilizing disk once daily to prevent skin breakdown. Some gastrostomy tubes have balloons that are inflated with water to anchor the tube in the stomach. The adequacy of balloon inflation is checked weekly by deflating the balloon using a Luer-tip syringe.

PROVIDING SKIN CARE

The skin surrounding a gastrostomy requires special care because it may become irritated from the enzymatic action of gastric juices that leak around the tube. Left untreated, the skin becomes macerated, red, raw, and painful. The nurse washes the area around the tube with soap and water daily, removes any encrustation with saline solution, rinses the area well with water, and pats it dry. Once the stoma heals and drainage ceases, a dressing is not required. A long-term gastrostomy may require a special dressing or stabilization device to protect the skin around the tube from gastric secretions and to help secure the tube in place (Fig. 36-9).

Skin at the exit site is evaluated daily for signs of breakdown, irritation, excoriation, and the presence of drainage or gastric leakage. The nurse encourages the patient and family members to participate in this inspection and in hygiene activities. If skin problems do occur, an enterostomal therapist or wound care specialist can be of assistance.

ENHANCING BODY IMAGE

The patient with a gastrostomy has experienced a major assault to body image. Eating, a physiologic and social function, can no longer be taken for granted. The patient is also aware that gastrostomy as a therapeutic intervention is performed only in the presence of a major, chronic, or perhaps terminal illness.

Calm discussion of the purposes and routines of gastrostomy feeding can help keep the patient from feeling overwhelmed. Talking with a person who has had a gastrostomy can also help the patient to accept the expected changes. Adjusting to a change in body image takes time and requires family support and acceptance. Evaluating the existing family support system is necessary. One family member may emerge as the primary support person.

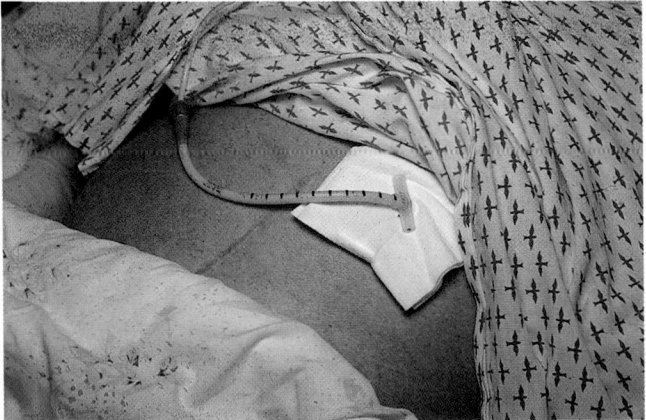

FIGURE 36-9 Protection at the gastrostomy site. A PEG tube may be protected by a dressing that allows access to the tube but covers the exit site. Typically the tube is stabilized with tape over the dressing. From Craven, R., & Hirnle, C. (2002). *Fundamentals of nursing: Human health and function* (4th ed.). Philadelphia: Lippincott Williams & Wilkins.

MONITORING AND MANAGING POTENTIAL COMPLICATIONS

During the postoperative course, the nurse monitors the patient for potential complications. The most common complications are wound infection and other wound problems, including cellulitis at the wound site and abscesses in the abdominal wall. Because many patients who receive tube feedings are debilitated and have compromised nutritional status, any signs of infections are promptly reported to the physician so that appropriate antibiotic therapy can be instituted.

Bleeding from the insertion site in the stomach may also occur. The nurse closely monitors the patient's vital signs and observes all drainage from the operative site, vomitus, and stool for evidence of bleeding. Any signs of bleeding are reported promptly.

Premature removal of the tube, whether it is done inadvertently by the patient or by the caregiver, is another complication. If the tube is removed prematurely, the skin is cleansed and a sterile dressing is applied; the nurse immediately notifies the physician. The tract will close within 4 to 6 hours if the tube is not replaced promptly.

PROMOTING HOME AND COMMUNITY-BASED CARE

Teaching Patients Self-Care

The patient who is to receive gastrostomy tube feedings in the home setting must be capable of, and responsible for, administering the tube feedings or have a caregiver who is able to do so. There must also be the physical, financial, and social resources to maintain care.

The nurse assesses the patient's level of knowledge, interest in learning about the tube feeding, and ability to understand and apply the information before providing detailed instructions about how to prepare the formula and manage the tube feeding. Written materials for patients and caregivers are designed to outline the care instructions. To facilitate self-care, the nurse encourages the patient to participate in the tube feedings during hospitalization and to establish as normal a routine as possible.

Demonstration of the tube feeding begins by showing the patient how to check for residual gastric contents before the feeding. The patient then learns how to check and maintain the patency of the tube by administering room-temperature water before and after the feeding. This will establish patency before the feeding and then clear the tube of food particles, which could decompose if allowed to remain in the tube. All feedings are given at room temperature or near body temperature.

For a bolus feeding, the nurse shows the patient how to introduce the liquid into the catheter by using a funnel or the barrel of a syringe. The receptacle is tilted to allow air to escape while the liquid is being instilled initially. As the funnel or syringe fills with liquid, the feeding is allowed to flow into the stomach by gravity by holding the barrel or syringe perpendicular to the abdomen (Fig. 36-10). Raising or lowering the receptacle to no higher than 45 cm (18 in) above the abdominal wall regulates the rate of flow.

A bolus feeding of 300 to 500 mL usually is given for each meal and requires 10 to 15 minutes to complete. The amount is often determined by the patient's reaction. If the patient feels full, it may be desirable to give smaller amounts more frequently.

The patient and caregiver must understand that keeping the head of the bed elevated for at least 1 hour after feeding facilitates digestion and decreases the risk for aspiration. Any obstruction requires that the feeding be stopped and the physician notified.

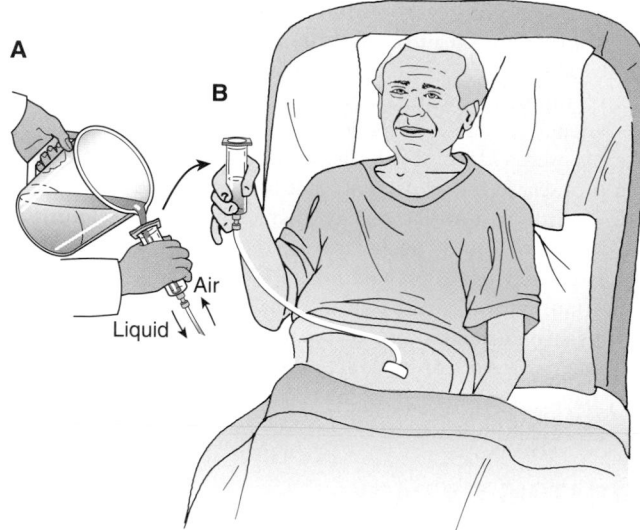

A **B**

Air

Liquid

FIGURE 36-10 Bolus gastrostomy feeding by gravity. (**A**) Feeding is instilled at an angle so that air does not enter the stomach. (**B**) Syringe is raised perpendicular to the abdomen so that feeding can enter by gravity.

The patient or caregiver is instructed to flush the tube with 30 mL of water after each bolus or medication administration, and otherwise to flush the tube daily to keep it patent. Adaptors are available that can be secured to the end of the tube to create a "Y" site for ease of flushing or medication delivery. The flushing equipment is cleaned with warm, soapy water and rinsed after each use.

The patient and caregiver are made aware that the tube is marked at skin level to provide the patient a baseline for later comparison. They are advised to monitor the tube's length and to notify the physician or home care nurse if the segment of the tube outside the body becomes shorter or longer.

If the patient is to use an intermittent or continuous-pressure feeding pump at home, instruction in the use of the particular type of pump is essential. Most feeding pumps have built-in alarms that signal when the bag is empty, when the battery is low, or when an occlusion is present. The patient and caregiver need to be aware of these alarms and how to troubleshoot the pump.

Continuing Care

Referral to a home care agency is important to ensure initial supervision and support for the patient and caregiver. The home care nurse assesses the patient's status and progress and evaluates the techniques that are used in administering the tube feeding. Further instruction and supervision in the home setting may be required to help the patient and caregiver adapt to a physical environment and equipment that are different from the hospital setting. The nurse also reviews with the patient and caregiver information about complications to report (eg, dumping syndrome, nausea and vomiting, infection of the skin at the insertion site of the tube).

The home care nurse assists the patient and family in establishing as normal a routine as possible. Some patients will want to experience a sensation of normal eating and are advised that they can try smelling, tasting, and chewing small amounts of food before taking their tube feedings. This stimulates the flow of salivary and gastric secretions and may give some sensation of a normal meal. The chewed food can then be deposited by the patient into a funnel or syringe attached to the gastrostomy tube for ad-

ministration into the stomach. The patient or caregiver is encouraged to keep a diary to record the times and amounts of feedings and any symptoms that occur. The nurse reviews the diary during home visits. When the tube is to be replaced, the patient or caregiver must be taught how to do this.

Evaluation

EXPECTED PATIENT OUTCOMES

Expected patient outcomes may include the following:

1. Achieves an adequate intake of nutrients
   a. Tolerates quantity and frequency of tube feedings
   b. Has 50 mL or less of residual gastric content before each feeding
   c. Has no diarrhea
   d. Maintains or gains weight
   e. Has normal electrolyte values
2. Is free from infection and skin breakdown
   a. Is afebrile
   b. Has no drainage from the incision
   c. Demonstrates intact skin surrounding the exit site
   d. Inspects exit site twice a day
3. Adjusts to change in body image
   a. Is able to discuss expected changes
   b. Verbalizes concerns
   c. Asks to speak with someone who has experienced this procedure
4. Demonstrates skill in managing feeding regimen
   a. Helps prepare prescribed formula or blenderized food
   b. Handles equipment competently
   c. Helps administer the feeding or does so independently
   d. Demonstrates how to maintain tube patency
   e. Cleans tubing as needed
   f. Keeps an accurate record of intake
   g. Can remove and reinsert the tube as appropriate and needed for feedings
5. Avoids complications
   a. Exhibits adequate wound healing
   b. Has no abnormal bleeding from puncture site
   c. Tube remains intact for the duration of therapy

Parenteral Nutrition

Parenteral nutrition (PN) is a method of providing nutrients to the body by an IV route. It is a very complex admixture of individual chemicals combined in a single container. The components of a PN admixture are proteins, carbohydrates, fats, electrolytes, vitamins, trace minerals, and sterile water. The goals of PN are to improve nutritional status, establish a positive nitrogen balance, maintain muscle mass, promote weight gain, and enhance the healing process.

ESTABLISHING POSITIVE NITROGEN BALANCE

When a patient's intake of protein and nutrients is significantly less than that required by the body to meet energy expenditures, a state of negative nitrogen balance results. In response, the body begins to convert the protein found in muscles into carbohydrates to be used to meet energy needs. The result is muscle wasting, weight loss, fatigue, and, if left uncorrected, death.

The average postoperative adult patient requires approximately 1500 calories per day to keep the body from using its own store of protein. Traditional IV fluids do not provide sufficient calories or nitrogen to meet the body's daily requirements. PN solutions, which supply nutrients such as dextrose, amino acids, electrolytes, vitamins, minerals, and fat emulsions, provide enough calories and nitrogen to meet the patient's daily nutritional needs. In general, PN can provide 30 to 35 kcal/kg of body weight and 1.0 to 1.5 g of protein/kg of body weight (Rombeau & Rolandelli, 2000).

The patient with fever, trauma, burns, major surgery, or hypermetabolic disease may require up to 10,000 additional calories daily. The volume of fluid necessary to provide these calories would surpass fluid tolerance and lead to pulmonary edema or heart failure. To provide the required calories in small volume, it is necessary to increase the concentration of nutrients and use a route of administration (ie, a large, high-flow vein [subclavian vein]) that will rapidly dilute incoming nutrients to the proper levels of body tolerance.

When highly concentrated glucose is administered, caloric requirements are satisfied and the body uses amino acids for protein synthesis rather than for energy. Additional potassium is added to the solution to maintain proper electrolyte balance and to transport glucose and amino acids across cell membranes. To prevent deficiencies and fulfill requirements for tissue synthesis, other elements, such as calcium, phosphorus, magnesium, and sodium chloride, are added (Rombeau & Rolandelli, 2000).

CLINICAL INDICATIONS

The indications for PN include a 10% deficit in body weight (compared with preillness weight), an inability to take oral food or fluids within 7 days after surgery, and hypercatabolic situations such as major infection with fever. In both the home and hospital setting, PN is indicated in the following situations:

- The patient's intake is insufficient to maintain an anabolic state (eg, severe burns, malnutrition, short bowel syndrome, AIDS, sepsis, cancer).
- The patient's ability to ingest food orally or by tube is impaired (eg, paralytic ileus, Crohn's disease with obstruction, postradiation enteritis, severe hyperemesis gravidarum in pregnancy).
- The patient is not interested in or is unwilling to ingest adequate nutrients (eg, anorexia nervosa, postoperative elderly patients).
- The underlying medical condition precludes being fed orally or by tube (eg, acute pancreatitis, high enterocutaneous fistula).
- Preoperative and postoperative nutritional needs are prolonged (eg, extensive bowel surgery).

FORMULAS

A total of 2 to 3 L of solution is administered over a 24-hour period using a filter (1.2-micron particulate filter). Before administration, the PN infusion must be inspected for clarity and any precipitate. The label is compared with the physician's order, noting the expiration date. Fat emulsions (Intralipid) may be infused simultaneously with PN through a Y-connector close to the infusion site. Fat emulsions should not be filtered. Before administration, the fat emulsion solution is inspected for frothiness, separation, or oily appearance. Usually 500 mL of a 10% emulsion is administered over 4 to 6 hours, one to three times a week. Fat emulsions can provide up to 30% of the total daily calorie intake.

Lipid emulsions can be admixed with other components of PN to create a **total nutrient admixture** (TNA). TNA is commonly called a "three-in-one" formulation. All the parenteral nutrient components are mixed in one container and administered to the patient over a 24-hour period. A special final filter (1.5 micron filter) is used with this solution. Before administration, the solution is observed for oil droplets that have separated from the solution, forming a noticeable layer (cracking of lipid emulsion); such a solution should be discarded. Advantages of the TNA over PN are cost savings in preparation and equipment, decreased risk of contamination, decreased risk of catheter contamination, decreased pharmacy preparation time, less nursing time, and increased patient convenience and satisfaction. Ideally, the pharmacist, nutritionist, and physician collaborate to determine the specific formula needed.

INITIATING THERAPY

PN solutions are initiated slowly and advanced gradually each day to the desired rate, as the patient's fluid and glucose tolerance permits. The patient's laboratory test results and response to PN therapy are monitored on an ongoing basis by the nutritional support team. Standing orders are initiated for weighing the patient; monitoring intake, output, and blood glucose; and baseline and periodic monitoring of complete blood count, platelet count, and chemistry panel, including serum carbon dioxide, magnesium, phosphorus, triglycerides, and prealbumin. A 24-hour urine nitrogen determination may be performed for analysis of nitrogen balance. In most hospitals, the physician prescribes PN solutions on a daily standard PN order form. The formulation of the PN solutions is calculated carefully each day to meet the complete nutritional needs of the individual patient.

ADMINISTRATION METHODS

Various vascular access devices are used to administer PN solutions in clinical practice. PN may be administered by either peripheral or central IV lines, depending on the patient's condition and the anticipated length of therapy.

Peripheral Method

To supplement oral intake when complete bowel rest is not indicated and NG or nasoenteric suction is not required, a peripheral parenteral nutrition (PPN) formula may be prescribed. PPN is administered through a peripheral vein; this is possible because the solution is less hypertonic than PN solution. PPN formulas are not nutritionally complete. Protein and dextrose are limited. Dextrose concentrations of more than 10% should not be administered through peripheral veins because they irritate the intima (innermost walls) of small veins, causing chemical phlebitis. Lipids are administered simultaneously to buffer the PPN and to protect the peripheral vein from irritation. The usual length of therapy using PPN is 5 to 7 days (Hamilton, 2000).

Central Method

Because PN solutions have five or six times the solute concentration of blood (and exert an osmotic pressure of about 2000 mOsm/L), they are injurious to the intima of peripheral veins. Therefore, to prevent phlebitis and other venous complications, these solutions are administered into the vascular system through a catheter inserted into a high-flow, large blood vessel (the subclavian vein). Concentrated solutions are then very rapidly diluted to isotonic levels by the blood in this vessel.

Four types of **central venous access devices (CVAD)** are available—nontunneled (or percutaneous) central catheters, peripherally inserted central catheters, tunneled catheters, and implanted ports. Whenever one of these catheters is inserted, catheter tip placement should be confirmed by x-ray studies before PN therapy is initiated. The optimal position is the midproximal third of the superior vena cava.

NONTUNNELED CENTRAL CATHETERS

Nontunneled central catheters are used for short-term (less than 30 days) IV therapy in the acute care, long-term care, and home care settings. The physician inserts these catheters. Examples of nontunneled central catheters are Vas Cath, Percutaneous Subclavian, and Hohn catheters. The subclavian vein is the most common vessel used, because the subclavian area provides a stable insertion site to which the catheter can be anchored, allows the patient freedom of movement, and provides easy access to the dressing site. The jugular or femoral vein also may be used. Single-, double-, and triple-lumen central catheters are available for central lines. To ensure accessibility, a triple-lumen subclavian catheter should be used, because it offers three ports for various uses (Fig. 36-11). The 16-gauge distal lumen can be used to infuse blood or other viscous fluids. The 18-gauge middle lumen is reserved for PN infusion. The 18-gauge proximal port can be used for administration of blood or medications. A port not being used for fluid administration can be used for obtaining blood specimens if indicated.

If a single-lumen central catheter is used for administering PN, various restrictions apply. Blood cannot be drawn from the catheter and medications cannot be administered through it, because the medication may be incompatible with the components of the nutritional solution (insulin is an exception). If medications must be given, they must be infused through a separate peripheral IV line, not by piggyback into the PN line. Transfusions of blood products also cannot be given through the main line, because red cells may possibly coat the lumen of the catheter, thereby reducing the flow of the nutritional solution.

PERIPHERALLY INSERTED CENTRAL CATHETERS

Peripherally inserted central catheters (PICC) are used for intermediate-term (3 to 12 months) IV therapy in the hospital, long-term care, or home setting. These catheters may be inserted at the bedside or in the outpatient setting by a specially trained nurse. The basilic or cephalic vein is accessed through the antecubital space, and the catheter is threaded to a designated location, depending on the type of solution to be infused (superior vena cava for PN). Taking of blood pressure and blood specimens from the extremity with the PICC is avoided (see Chapter 14).

TUNNELED CENTRAL CATHETERS

Tunneled central catheters are for long-term use and may remain in place for many years. These catheters are cuffed and can have single or double lumens; examples are the Hickman, Groshong, and Permacath. These catheters are inserted surgically. They are threaded under the skin (reducing the risk of ascending infection) to the subclavian vein, and the distal end of the catheter is advanced into the superior vena cava 2 to 3 cm above the junction with the right atrium (see Chapter 16).

IMPLANTED PORTS

Implanted ports are also used for long-term home IV therapy; examples include the Port-A-Cath, Mediport, Hickman Port, and P.A.S. Port. Instead of exiting from the skin, as do the Hickman and Groshong catheters, the end of the catheter is attached to a small chamber that is placed in a subcutaneous pocket, either on the anterior chest wall or on the forearm. The subcutaneous port requires minimal care and allows the patient complete freedom

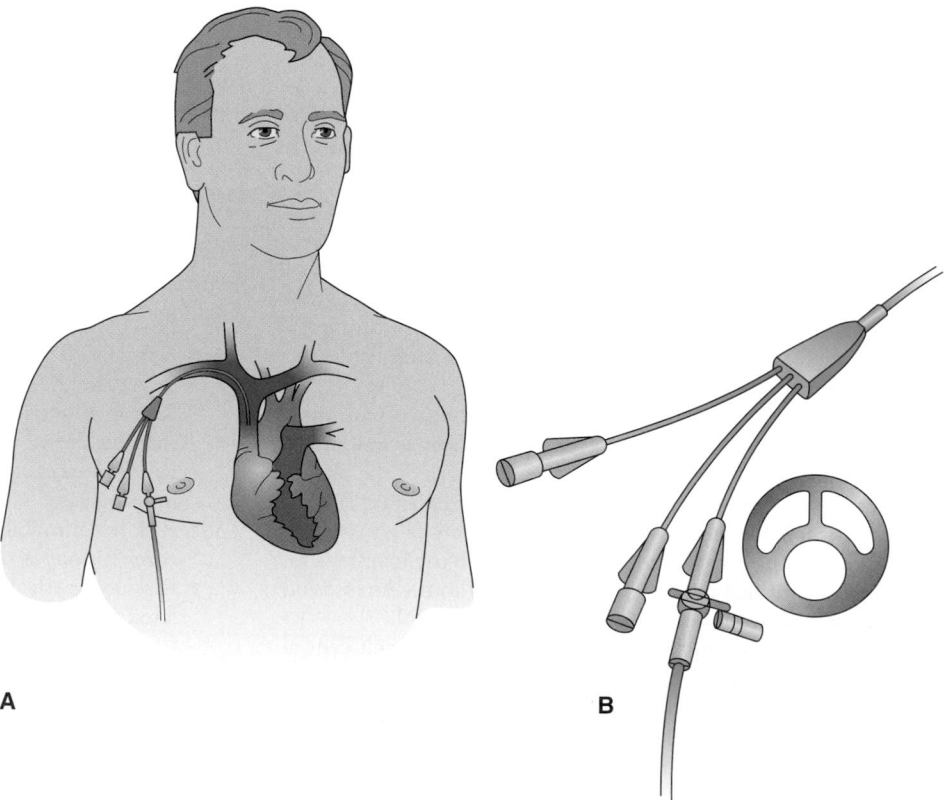

FIGURE 36-11 Subclavian triple-lumen catheter used for parenteral nutrition and other adjunctive therapy. **(A)** The catheter is threaded through the subclavian vein into the vena cava. **(B)** Each lumen is an avenue for solution administration. The lumens are secured with threaded needleless adapters or Luer-lock caps when the device is not in use.

A

B

of activity. Implanted ports are more expensive than the external catheters, and access requires passing a special needle (Huber-tipped) through the skin into the chamber to initiate IV therapy (see Chapter 16). Taking of blood pressure and blood specimens from the extremity with the port system is avoided.

NONTUNNELED CENTRAL CATHETER INSERTION

The procedure is explained so that the patient understands the importance of not touching the catheter insertion site and is aware of what to expect during the insertion procedure. To insert the catheter, the patient is placed supine, in head-low position (to produce dilation of neck and shoulder vessels, which makes entry easier and prevents air embolus). The area is shaved if necessary, and the skin is prepared with acetone and alcohol to remove surface oils. Final skin preparation includes cleaning with tincture of 2% iodine or chlorhexidine. To afford maximal accuracy in the placement of the catheter, the patient is instructed to turn the head away from the site of venipuncture and to remain motionless while the catheter is inserted and the wound is dressed.

The preferred insertion route is the subclavian vein, which leads into the superior vena cava. The external jugular route can be used, but usually only in emergency situations. Because a non-tunneled central catheter is always a potential source of serious infection, the site should be changed every 4 weeks or as recommended by the Centers for Disease Control and Prevention.

Sterile drapes are applied to the upper chest. The patient may be asked to wear a facemask to prevent the spread of micro-organisms. Procaine or lidocaine is injected to anesthetize the skin and underlying tissues. The target area is the inferior border at the midpoint of the clavicle. A large-bore needle on a syringe is inserted and moved parallel to and beneath the clavicle until it enters the vein. The syringe is then detached and a radiopaque catheter is inserted through the needle into the vein.

When the catheter is positioned, the needle is withdrawn and the hub of the catheter is attached to the IV tubing. Until the syringe is detached from the needle and the catheter is inserted, the patient may be asked to perform the Valsalva maneuver. (To do this, the patient is instructed to take a deep breath, hold it, and bear down with mouth closed. Compression of the abdomen may also accomplish the maneuver.) The Valsalva maneuver is performed to produce a positive phase in central venous pressure, to lessen the possibility of air being drawn into the circulatory system (air embolism). The physician sutures the catheter to the skin to avoid inadvertent removal.

The catheter insertion site is swabbed with either tincture of 2% iodine or a chlorhexidine solution. A gauze or transparent dressing is applied using strict sterile technique. An isotonic IV solution, such as dextrose 5% in water (D_5W), is administered to keep the vein patent.

The position of the tip of the catheter is checked with fluoroscopy to confirm its location in the superior vena cava and to rule out a pneumothorax resulting from puncture of the pleura. Once the catheter position is confirmed, the prescribed PN solution is started. The initial rate of infusion is usually 50 mL/hour, and the rate is gradually increased to the maintenance rate or predetermined dose (eg, 100 to 125 mL/hour). An infusion pump is always used for administration of PN or PPN.

An injection site cap is attached to the end of each central catheter lumen, creating a closed system. IV infusion tubing is connected to the insertion site cap of the central catheter with a threaded needleless adapter or Luer-lock device. Each lumen is labeled according to location (proximal, middle, distal). To ensure patency, all lumens are flushed with a diluted heparin flush initially, daily when not in use, after each intermittent infusion, after blood drawing, and whenever an infusion is disconnected. Force is never used to flush the catheter. If resistance is met, aspiration may be effective in cleansing the lumen; if this is not effective, the physician is notified. Low-dose t-PA (alteplase) may be prescribed to dissolve a clot or fibrin sheath. If attempts to clear the lumen are ineffective, the lumen is labeled as "clotted off."

DISCONTINUING PARENTERAL NUTRITION

The PN solution is discontinued gradually to allow the patient to adjust to decreased levels of glucose. After administration of the PN solution is terminated, isotonic glucose is administered for several hours to protect against rebound hypoglycemia. Providing oral carbohydrates will shorten the tapering time. Specific symptoms of rebound hypoglycemia include weakness, faintness, sweating, shakiness, feeling cold, confusion, and increased heart rate. Once all IV therapy is completed, the nurse (with a physician's order) removes the nontunneled central venous catheter or PICC and applies an occlusive dressing to the exit site. Tunneled catheters and implanted ports are removed by the physician.

In cases of serious illness when death is imminent, some patients or families may request that PN be discontinued. This difficult issue poses many ethical questions, some of which are discussed in Chart 36-3.

NURSING PROCESS: THE PATIENT RECEIVING PARENTERAL NUTRITION

Assessment

The nurse assists in identifying patients who may be candidates for PN. Indicators include any significant weight loss (10% or more of usual weight), a decrease in oral food intake for more than 1 week, any significant sign of protein loss (serum albumin levels less than 3.2 g/dL [32 g/L], muscle wasting, decreased tissue healing, or abnormal urea nitrogen excretion), and persistent vomiting and diarrhea. The nurse carefully monitors the patient's hydration, electrolyte levels, and calorie intake.

Diagnosis

NURSING DIAGNOSES

Based on the assessment data, the major nursing diagnoses may include the following:

- Imbalanced nutrition, less than body requirements, related to inadequate oral intake of nutrients
- Risk for infection related to contamination of the central catheter site or infusion line
- Risk for excess or deficient fluid volume related to altered infusion rate
- Risk for immobility related to fear that the catheter will become dislodged or occluded
- Risk for ineffective therapeutic regimen management related to knowledge deficit about home PN therapy

COLLABORATIVE PROBLEMS/ POTENTIAL COMPLICATIONS

The most common complications are pneumothorax, air embolism, a clotted or displaced catheter, sepsis, hyperglycemia, rebound hypoglycemia, and fluid overload. These problems

Is It Ethical to Withhold or Withdraw Nutrition and Hydration?

Situation

It is generally agreed that patients (or their designated decision makers) can refuse life-saving treatment, particularly if the means of treatment are extraordinary (eg, ventilators, dialysis machines, extracorporeal oxygenators). Extraordinary means include medications, treatments, and procedures that can be obtained only at excessive cost, pain, or inconvenience and offer no reasonable hope of benefit. Nutrition and hydration therapy, however, are perceived as ordinary means by many.

Ordinary means are those medications, treatments, and procedures that offer a reasonable hope of benefit and can be obtained without excessive expense, pain, or inconvenience. Additionally, withdrawing or withholding nutrition and hydration can in and of itself cause death. Thus, some have argued that nutrition and hydration should always be provided to every patient, regardless of the patient's preference or condition.

Dilemma

The patient's desire to have nutrition or hydration withdrawn or withheld may conflict with the reluctance of others to harm the patient by withdrawing the food and water needed for survival (autonomy versus nonmaleficence).

Discussion

- What arguments would you offer against the withholding and withdrawing of nutrition and hydration?
- What arguments would you offer in favor of withholding and withdrawing of nutrition and hydration?
- Are foods and fluids always "ordinary means," or are there instances in which they might be considered "extraordinary"? Support your answer.

Answer the above questions using as an example a patient in a persistent vegetative state (ie, unable to express his or her wishes).

---

and the associated collaborative interventions are described in Table 36-5.

Planning and Goals

The major goals for the patient may include optimal level of nutrition, absence of infection, adequate fluid volume, optimal level of activity (within individual limitations), knowledge of and skill in self-care, and prevention of complications.

Nursing Interventions

MAINTAINING OPTIMAL NUTRITION

A continuous, uniform infusion of PN solution over a 24-hour period is desired. In some cases, however (eg, home care patients), cyclic PN may be appropriate. With cyclic PN, there is a set time during a 24-hour period when PN is infused and a set time when it is not. The time periods for infusion are sufficient to meet the patient's nutritional and pharmacologic needs. Ideally, cyclic PN is infused over an 8- to 10-hour period during the night.

The patient is weighed daily (this may be decreased to two or three times per week), at the same time of the day under the same conditions for accurate comparison. Under the PN regimen (without additional energy expenditure), a satisfactory weight

gain is usually achieved. It is important to keep accurate intake and output records and calculations of fluid balance. A calorie count is kept of any oral nutrients. Trace elements (copper, zinc, chromium, manganese, and selenium) are included in PN solutions and are individualized for each patient. The PN solutions are prescribed daily by the physician on a standard PN order form based on laboratory values and patient tolerance.

PREVENTING INFECTION

The high glucose content of PN solutions makes these solutions ideal culture media for bacterial and fungal growth, and CVADs provide a port of entry. *Candida albicans* is the most common infectious organism. Other infectious organisms include *Staphylococcus aureus, Staphylococcus epidermidis,* and *Klebsiella pneumoniae.* Meticulous technique is essential to prevent infection.

The primary sources of microorganisms for catheter-related infections are the skin and the catheter hub. The catheter site is covered with an occlusive gauze dressing that is usually changed every other day. Alternatively, a transparent dressing may be used and changed weekly. The Centers for Disease Control and Prevention recommends changing dressings for CVADs only if they are damp, bloody, loose, or soiled. The dressings are changed using sterile technique. The nurse and patient wear masks during dressing changes to reduce the possibility of airborne contamination. The area is checked for leakage, bloody drainage, a kinked catheter, and skin reactions such as inflammation, redness, swelling, tenderness, or purulent drainage. The nurse puts on sterile gloves and cleanses the area with tincture of 2% iodine or a chlorhexidine solution on a sterile gauze. The site is cleaned thoroughly using circular motion from the site outward approximately 3 inches. This is repeated two times. This is followed with the same cleaning procedure using 2 × 2-inch gauze pads moistened with sterile water or saline solution (alcohol is used to remove iodine). Next the catheter lumens are cleaned from the exit site to the distal end with an alcohol wipe. The insertion site is covered with an occlusive gauze pad or transparent dressing centered over the area.

The advantages of using a transparent dressing over the gauze pad are that it allows frequent examination of the catheter site without changing the dressing, it adheres well, and it is more comfortable for the patient. When an extension set is used with a central catheter, it is considered an extension of the catheter itself. It is not routinely changed with dressing or tubing changes. The connection (hub) between the catheter and extension tubing is secured with adhesive tape to prevent separation and exposure to air. Main-line IV tubing and filters are changed every 72 to 96 hours, and all connections are taped securely to avoid breaks in the integrity of the system. The dressing and tubing are labeled with the date, time of insertion, time of dressing change, and initials of the person who carried out the procedure; this information is also documented in the medical record.

The catheter is another major source of colonization and infection. Antiseptic-impregnated central venous catheters are new devices that reduce catheter colonization by coating of the catheter surfaces with antimicrobial agents. Two types are available, one coated with chlorhexidine/silver sulfadiazine and the other with minocycline/rifampin (Hanna et al., 2001).

MAINTAINING FLUID BALANCE

An infusion pump is necessary for PN to maintain an accurate rate of administration. A designated rate is set in milliliters per hour, and the rate checked every 30 to 60 minutes. An alarm signals a problem. The infusion rate should not be increased or decreased

Table 36-5 • **Complications of Parenteral Nutrition**

COMPLICATION	CAUSE	NURSING ACTIONS AND COLLABORATIVE INTERVENTIONS
Pneumothorax	Improper catheter placement and inadvertent puncture of the pleura	Place patient in Fowler's position. Offer reassurance. Monitor vital signs. Prepare for thoracentesis or chest tube insertion.
Air embolism	Disconnected tubing	Tape all tubing connection sites securely. Replace tubing immediately and notify physician.
	Cap missing from port	Replace cap and notify physician.
	Blocked segment of vascular system	Turn patient on left side and place in the head-low position. Notify physician.
Clotted catheter line	Inadequate/infrequent heparin flushes Disruption of infusion	Administer heparin flush in unused lines twice a day. Monitor infusion rate hourly and inspect the integrity of the line. On *rare* occasions, flush with urokinase as prescribed.
Catheter displacement and contamination	Excessive movement, possibly with a nonsecured catheter	Stop the infusion and notify the physician.
	Separation of tubing and contamination	Tape all tubing connection sites. Avoid interrupting the main line or piggybacking other lines.
Sepsis	Separation of dressings	Reinforce or change dressing quickly using aseptic technique.
	Contaminated solution	Discard. Notify pharmacist.
	Infection at insertion site of catheter	Notify physician. Monitor vital signs every 4 hours. Catheter site is changed every 4 weeks.
Hyperglycemia	Glucose intolerance	Monitor glucose levels (blood and urine). Monitor urine output. Observe for stupor, confusion, lethargy. Notify physician; the addition of insulin to the PN solution may be prescribed.
Fluid overload	Fluid infusing rapidly	Decrease infusion rate, use infusion pump. Monitor vital signs. Notify physician. Treat respiratory distress by sitting patient upright and administering oxygen as needed, if prescribed.
Rebound hypoglycemia	Feedings stopped too abruptly	Monitor for symptoms (weakness, tremors, diaphoresis, headache, hunger, and apprehension); notify physician. Gradually wean patient from PN.

to compensate for fluids that have infused too quickly or too slowly. If the solution runs out, 10% dextrose and water is infused until the next PN solution is available from the pharmacy.

If the rate is too rapid, hyperosmolar diuresis occurs (excess sugar will be excreted), which, if severe enough, can cause intractable seizures, coma, and death. Symptoms of rapid hypertonic fluid intake include headache, nausea, fever, chills, and increasing lethargy.

If the flow rate is too slow, the patient does not get the maximal benefit of calories and nitrogen. Intake and output are recorded every 8 hours so that fluid imbalance can be readily detected. The patient is weighed two or three times a week; in ideal situations, the patient will show neither weight loss nor significant weight gain. The nurse assesses for signs of dehydration (eg, thirst, decreased skin turgor, decreased central venous pressure) and reports these findings to the physician immediately. It is es-

sential to monitor blood glucose levels, because hyperglycemia can cause diuresis and excessive fluid loss.

ENCOURAGING ACTIVITY

Activities and ambulation are encouraged when the patient is physically capable. With a catheter in the subclavian vein, the patient is free to move the extremities and should be encouraged to maintain good muscle tone. If applicable, the teaching and exercise program initiated in the occupational and physical therapy departments should be reinforced.

PROMOTING HOME AND COMMUNITY-BASED CARE

Teaching Patients Self-Care

Successful home PN requires teaching the patient and family specialized skills using an intensive training program and follow-up

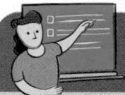

Chart 36-4 • PATIENT EDUCATION
Teaching Patients About Home Parenteral Nutrition

An effective home care teaching program prepares the patient to manage the appropriate form of PN: how to store solutions, set up the infusion, flush the line with heparin, change the dressings, and troubleshoot for problems. The most common complication is sepsis. Strict aseptic technique is taught for hand hygiene, handling equipment, changing the dressing, and preparing the solution.

Troubleshooting Mechanical Difficulties
Mechanical problems usually arise from technical complications in the infusion pump or catheter site. The patient needs to know how to measure the length of the external portion of the catheter; this measurement is used as a comparison if the line is pulled or if dislodgement is suspected. The patient also needs to know how to recognize catheter problems (eg, leakage, loose cap, blood clot, dislodgement) and should receive a list of instructions explaining what to do for each problem.

Recognizing Metabolic Complications
The patient is given a list of symptoms that indicate metabolic complications (neuropathies, mentation changes, diarrhea, nausea, skin changes, decreased urine output) and directions on how to contact the home health care nurse or physician if any of these complications occurs. The patient is instructed to have weekly serum chemistry and hematology tests as well.

Obtaining Psychosocial Support
The psychosocial aspects of home PN are as important as the physiologic and technical concerns. Patients must cope with the loss of eating and with changes in lifestyle brought on by sleep disturbances (frequent urination during infusions, usually two or three times during the night).

Major psychosocial reactions include depression, anger, withdrawal, anxiety, and impaired self-image. A successful home parenteral nutrition program depends on the patient's and family's motivation, emotional stability, and technical competence. Patients and families need to know which support groups are available in the community to help them cope with the transition and to minimize disruption of lifestyle.

---

supervision in the home. This is accomplished through a team effort. The financial costs of such programs, although high, are less than those incurred in a hospital. Initiation of a home program may be the only way the patient can be discharged from the hospital.

Ideal candidates for home PN are those patients who have a reasonable life expectancy after return home, have only a limited number of medical illnesses other than the one that has resulted in the need for PN, and are highly motivated and fairly self-sufficient. In addition, ability to learn, availability of family interest and support, adequate finances, and the physical plan of the home are factors that must be assessed when the decision for home PN is made.

Home health care agencies sponsoring home PN programs have developed teaching brochures for every aspect of the treatment, including catheter and dressing care, use of an infusion pump, administration of fat emulsions, and instillation of heparin flushes. Teaching begins in the hospital and continues in the home or in an ambulatory infusion center.

Continuing Care
The home care nurse should be aware that the average patient needs about 2 weeks of instruction and reinforcement. For more information about home patient education, see Charts 36-4 and 36-5.

Evaluation

EXPECTED PATIENT OUTCOMES
Expected patient outcomes may include the following:

1. Attains or maintains nutritional balance
2. Is free of infection at the catheter site
    a. Is afebrile
    b. Has no purulent drainage from the catheter insertion site
    c. Has intact IV line
3. Is hydrated, as evidenced by good skin turgor
4. Achieves an optimal level of activity, within limitations
5. Demonstrates skill in managing PN regimen

Chart 36-5
Home Care Checklist • The Patient Receiving Parenteral Nutrition

At the completion of the home care instruction, the patient or caregiver will be able to:	Patient	Caregiver
• Discuss goal and purpose of PN therapy	✓	✓
• Discuss basic components of PN solution.	✓	✓
• List emergency phone numbers.	✓	✓
• Demonstrate how to handle PN solutions and medications correctly.	✓	✓
• Demonstrate how to operate infusion pump.	✓	✓
• Demonstrate how to prime tubing and filter.	✓	✓
• Demonstrate how to connect and disconnect PN infusion.	✓	✓
• Demonstrate how to perform catheter dressing changes.	✓	✓
• Demonstrate how to heparinize central line.	✓	✓
• Identify possible PN complications and interventions.	✓	✓

6. Prevents complications
   a. Maintains proper catheter and equipment function
   b. Has no symptoms of sepsis
   c. Maintains metabolic balance within normal limits
   d. Shows improved and stabilized nutritional status

Critical Thinking Exercises

1. You are caring for a patient with an NG feeding tube. Before administering the patient's tube feeding, you explain to the patient that you will be checking to make sure the tube is placed correctly. The patient responds that she is accustomed to this and that the other nurses "check the tube by placing the end of it in a cup of water;" the patient also states that the nurses then "put air in the tube and use a stethoscope to listen for bubbles in my stomach." How would you respond to the patient? What research findings guide your actions in confirming the placement of the tube? What follow-up actions would you take to ensure that there is consistency among the nursing staff in the procedure used for confirmation of tube placement?

2. A patient who is receiving gastrostomy tube feedings is to be discharged from the hospital to return home within the next few days. Several family members are to be taught how to administer the tube feedings. What are the learning priorities that should be accomplished before the patient is discharged? What assessment parameters should be used to determine whether the family has the necessary resources for providing care for the patient at home?

3. A patient who had major abdominal surgery 1 week ago and who has developed a paralytic ileus is to begin receiving PN. What explanation would you give to this patient about the benefits of PN and the procedure for its administration? How would you alter your plan of care to include assessment for complications of PN? What assessment would you conduct to determine whether the patient is a candidate for home PN therapy?

REFERENCES AND SELECTED READINGS

Books

American Society of Parenteral and Enteral Nutrition (ASPEN). (1998). *The A.S.P.E.N. Nutrition Support Practice Manual.* Silver Spring, MD: Author.

Brandt, L. J., & Daum, F. (Eds.). (1999). *Clinical practice of gastroenterology.* New York: Churchill-Livingstone.

Domkowski, K. (Ed.). (1998). *Gastroenterology nursing: A core curriculum* (2nd ed.). St. Louis: Mosby–Year Book.

Guenter, P., & Silkroski, M. (2001). *Tube Feeding: Practical guidelines and nursing protocols.* Gaithersburg, MD: Aspen.

Hamilton, H. (2000). *Total parenteral nutrition: A practical guide for nurses.* New York: Churchill-Livingstone.

Hankins, J., Lonsway, R. A. W., Hedrick, C., et al. (Eds.). (2001). *Infusion therapy in clinical practice* (2nd ed.). Philadelphia: W. B. Saunders.

Rombeau, J. L., & Rolandelli, R. (Eds.). (2000). *Clinical nutrition: Parenteral nutrition* (3rd ed.). Philadelphia: W. B. Saunders.

Yamada, T., Alpers, D. H., & Laine, L. (Eds.). (1999). *Textbook of gastroenterology.* Philadelphia: Lippincott Williams & Wilkins.

Weinstein, S. (Ed.). (2001). *Plumer's principles & practice of intravenous therapy.* Philadelphia: Lippincott Williams & Wilkins.

Journals

Asterisks indicate nursing research articles.

Gastrostomies

Bowers, S. (1996). Tubes: A nurse's guide to enteral feeding devices. *MedSurg Nursing, 5*(5), 313–325.

Johnson, M. S. (1997). Radiologic placement of gastrostomy tubes. *Nutrition in Clinical Practice, 12*(1), S20–S22.

O'Brien, B., Davis, S., & Erwin-Toth, P. (1999). G-tube site care: A practical guide. *RN, 62*(2), 52–56.

*Smarszez, R. M. (2000). Microbial contamination of low-profile balloon gastrostomy extension tubes and three cleaning methods. *Nutrition in Clinical Practice, 15*(3), 138–142.

Thompson, L. (1995). Percutaneous endoscopic gastrostomy. *Nursing '95, 25*(4), 62–63.

Nasogastric and Nasoenteric Intubation and Feeding

Bowers, S. (1999). Nutrition support for malnourished, acutely ill adults. *MedSurg Nursing, 8*(3), 145–166.

Case, K. O., Cuddy, P. G., & McGurk, E. P. D. (2000). Nutrition support in the critically ill patient. *Critical Care Nursing Quarterly, 22*(4), 75–89.

Edwards, S. J., & Metheny, N. A. (2000). Measurement of gastric residual volume: State of the science. *MedSurg, 9*(1), 125–128.

Fellows, L. S., Miller, R. H., Frederickson, M., et al. (2000). Evidence-based practice for enteral feedings: Aspiration prevention strategies, bedside detection, and practice change. *MedSurg, 9*(1), 27–31.

Livingston, A., Seamons, C., & Dalton, T. (2000). If the gut works use it. *Nursing Management, 7*(2), 39–42.

*McClave, S. A., Snider, H. L., & Lowen, C. C., et al. (1992). Use of residual volume as a marker for enteral feeding intolerance: Prospective blinded comparison with physical examination and radiographic findings. *Journal of Parenteral and Enteral Nutrition, 16*(2), 99–105.

Metheny, N. A. (1998). Detection of improperly positioned feeding tubes. *Journal of Health Care Risk Management, 18*(3), 37–45.

*Metheny, N. A., Dettenmeier, P., Hampton, K., et al. (1990a). Detection of inadvertent respiratory placement of small-bore feeding tubes: A report of 10 cases. *Heart and Lung, 19*(6), 631–638.

*Metheny, N. A., McSweeney, M., Wehrle, M. A., et al. (1990b). Effectiveness of the auscultatory method in predicting feeding tube location. *Nursing Research, 39*(5), 262–267.

*Metheny, N. A., Reed, L., Berglund, B., et al. (1994). Visual characteristics of aspirates from feeding tubes as a method for predicting tube location. *Nursing Research, 43*(5), 282–287.

*Metheny, N. A., Reed, L., Worseck, M., et al. (1993). How to aspirate fluid from small-bore feeding tubes. *American Journal of Nursing, 93*(5), 86–88.

*Metheny, N. A., Smith, L., & Stewart, B. J., et al. (2000). Development of a reliable and valid bedside test for bilirubin and its utility for improving prediction of feeding tube location. *Nursing Research, 49*(6), 302–309.

*Metheny, N. A., Stewart, B. J., Smith, L, et al. (1999). pH and concentration of bilirubin in feeding tube aspirates as predictors of tube placement. *Nursing Research, 48*(3), 189–197.

*Metheny, N. A., & Titler, M. G. (2001). Assessing placement of feeding tubes. *American Journal of Nursing, 101*(5), 36–46.

*Metheny, N. A., Wehrle, M. A., Wiersema, L., et al. (1998). Testing feeding tube placement: Auscultation vs. pH method. *American Journal of Nursing, 98*(5), 37–43.

Mitchell, J. F. (2000). Oral dosage forms that should not be crushed: 2000 update. *Hospital Pharmacy, 35*(5), 553–567.

Petnicki, P. J. (1998). Cost savings and improved patient care with the use of a flush enteral feeding pump. Proceedings of the Third Annual Ross Enteral Device Conference, Winston-Salem, NC, September 19–21, 1997. *Nutrition in Clinical Practice, 13,* (3 Suppl. l), s39–s41, s50–s51.

Trujillo, E. B., Robinson, M. K., & Jacobs, D. O. (2001). Nutrition: Feeding critically ill patients. Current concepts. *Critical Care Nurse, 21*(4), 60–71.

Parenteral Nutrition

*Collin, G. R. (1999). Decreasing catheter colonization through the use of an antiseptic-impregnated catheter. *Clinical Investigations in Critical Care, 111*(6), 1632–1639.

Driscoll, M., Buckenmyer, C., Spirk, M., et al. (1997). Inserting and maintaining peripherally inserted central catheters. *MedSurg Nursing, 6*(6), 350–358.

Griffiths, V. R., & Philpot, P. (2002). Peripherally inserted central catheters (PICCs): Do they have a role in the care of the critically ill patient? *Intensive and Critical Care Nursing 18*(1), 37–47.

Hanna, H., Darouicher, R., & Raad, I. (2001). New approaches for prevention of intravascular catheter-related infections. *Infections in Medicine, 18*(9), 38–48.

Masoorli, S., & Angeles, T. (2002). Getting a line on CVAD: Central vascular access devices. *Nursing 02, 32*(4), 36–45.

McConnell, E. A. (2001). Clinical do's and don'ts: Administering total parenteral nutrition. *Nursing 01, 31*(7), 17.

Moureau, N. (2001). Preventing complications with vascular access devices. *Nursing 01, 31*(7), 52–54.

*Norwood, S. (2000). The safety of prolonging the use of central catheters: A prospective analysis of the effects of using antiseptic-bonded catheters with daily site care. *Critical Care Medicine, 28*(5), 1376–1382.

RESOURCES AND WEBSITES

American Cancer Society, 1599 Clifton Rd. N.E., Atlanta, GA 30329; 1-404-320-3333; http://www.cancer.org.

American Society for Clinical Nutrition, 9650 Rockville Pike, Bethesda, MD 20814-3998; http://www.faseb.org/assn.

American Society for Gastrointestinal Endoscopy, 13 Elm St., Manchester, MA 01944; http://www.asge.org.

American Society of Parenteral and Enteral Nutrition (ASPEN), 8630 Fenton St., #412, Silver Spring, MD 20910-3805; http://www.nutritioncare.org.

Oley Foundation for Home Parenteral and Enteral Nutrition, 214 Hun Memorial, A-23, New Scotland Ave., Albany, NY 12208; http://www.wizvax.net/oleyfdn.

Society of Gastroenterology Nurses & Associates, Inc., 140 North Michigan Ave., Chicago, IL, 60611-4267; 800-245-7462; in Illinois, 312-321-5165; http://www.sgna.org.

Management of Patients With Gastric and Duodenal Disorders

On completion of this chapter, the learner will be able to:

1. Compare the etiology, clinical manifestations, and management of acute gastritis, chronic gastritis, and peptic ulcer.

2. Use the nursing process as a framework for care of patients with gastritis.

3. Use the nursing process as a framework for care of patients with peptic ulcer.

4. Describe the dietary, pharmacologic, and surgical treatment of peptic ulcer.

5. Describe the nursing management of patients who undergo surgical procedures to treat obesity.

6. Use the nursing process as a framework for care of patients with gastric cancer.

7. Use the nursing process as a framework for care of patients undergoing gastric surgery.

8. Identify the complications of gastric surgery and their prevention and management.

9. Describe the home health care needs of the patient who has had gastric surgery.

*A*n individual's nutritional status depends not only on the type and amount of intake but also on the functioning of the gastric and intestinal portions of the gastrointestinal (GI) system. This chapter describes disorders of the stomach and duodenum and their treatment.

Gastritis

Gastritis (inflammation of the **gastric** or stomach mucosa) is a common GI problem. Gastritis may be acute, lasting several hours to a few days, or chronic, resulting from repeated exposure to irritating agents or recurring episodes of acute gastritis.

Acute gastritis is often caused by dietary indiscretion—the person eats food that is contaminated with disease-causing microorganisms or that is irritating or too highly seasoned. Other causes of acute gastritis include overuse of aspirin and other nonsteroidal anti-inflammatory drugs (NSAIDs), excessive alcohol intake, bile reflux, and radiation therapy. A more severe form of acute gastritis is caused by the ingestion of strong acid or alkali, which may cause the mucosa to become gangrenous or to perforate. Scarring can occur, resulting in pyloric obstruction. Gastritis also may be the first sign of an acute systemic infection.

Chronic gastritis and prolonged inflammation of the stomach may be caused by either benign or malignant ulcers of the stomach or by the bacteria *Helicobacter pylori*. Chronic gastritis is sometimes associated with autoimmune diseases such as pernicious anemia; dietary factors such as caffeine; the use of medications, especially NSAIDs; alcohol; smoking; or reflux of intestinal contents into the stomach.

Pathophysiology

In gastritis, the gastric mucous membrane becomes edematous and hyperemic (congested with fluid and blood) and undergoes superficial erosion (Fig. 37-1). It secretes a scanty amount of gastric juice, containing very little acid but much mucus. Superficial ulceration may occur and can lead to hemorrhage.

Clinical Manifestations

The patient with acute gastritis may have abdominal discomfort, headache, lassitude, nausea, anorexia, vomiting, and hiccuping. Some patients, however, have no symptoms. The patient with chronic gastritis may complain of anorexia, heartburn after eating, belching, a sour taste in the mouth, or nausea and vomiting. Patients with chronic gastritis from vitamin deficiency usually have evidence of malabsorption of vitamin B_{12} caused by antibodies against intrinsic factor.

Assessment and Diagnostic Findings

Gastritis is sometimes associated with achlorhydria or hypochlorhydria (absence or low levels of hydrochloric acid [HCl]) or with hyperchlorhydria (high levels of HCl). Diagnosis can be determined by endoscopy, upper GI radiographic studies, and histologic examination of a tissue specimen obtained by biopsy. In addition to biopsy, other diagnostic measures for detecting *H. pylori* include serologic testing for antibodies against the *H. pylori* antigen, a 1-minute ultrarapid urease test, and a breath test.

Medical Management

The gastric mucosa is capable of repairing itself after a bout of gastritis. As a rule, the patient recovers in about 1 day, although the appetite may be diminished for an additional 2 or 3 days. Acute gastritis is also managed by instructing the patient to refrain from alcohol and food until symptoms subside. After the patient can take nourishment by mouth, a nonirritating diet is recommended. If the symptoms persist, fluids may need to be administered parenterally. If bleeding is present, management is similar to the procedures used for upper GI tract hemorrhage (discussed later in this chapter).

If gastritis is caused by ingestion of strong acids or alkalis, treatment consists of diluting and neutralizing the offending agent. To neutralize acids, common antacids (eg, aluminum hydroxide) are used; to neutralize an alkali, diluted lemon juice or diluted vinegar is used. If corrosion is extensive or severe, emetics and lavage are avoided because of the danger of perforation and damage to the esophagus.

Therapy is supportive and may include nasogastric (NG) intubation, analgesic agents and sedatives, antacids, and intravenous (IV) fluids. Fiberoptic endoscopy may be necessary. In extreme cases, emergency surgery may be required to remove gangrenous or perforated tissue. Gastrojejunostomy or gastric resection may be necessary to treat pyloric obstruction, a narrowing of the pyloric orifice.

Chronic gastritis is managed by modifying the patient's diet, promoting rest, reducing stress, and initiating pharmacotherapy. *H. pylori* may be treated with antibiotics (eg, tetracycline or amoxicillin, combined with clarithromycin) and a proton pump inhibitor (eg, lansoprazole [Prevacid]), and possibly bismuth salts (Pepto-Bismol) (Table 37-1). Research is being conducted to develop a vaccine against *H. pylori* (Alsahli et al., 2001).

NURSING PROCESS: THE PATIENT WITH GASTRITIS

Assessment

When obtaining the history, the nurse asks about the patient's presenting signs and symptoms. Does the patient have heartburn, indigestion, nausea, or vomiting? Do the symptoms occur

---

Glossary

antrectomy: removal of the pyloric (antrum) portion of the stomach with anastomosis (surgical connection) to the duodenum (gastroduodenostomy or Billroth I) or anastomosis to the jejunum (gastrojejunostomy or Billroth II)

dumping syndrome: physiologic response to rapid emptying of gastric contents into the jejunum, manifested by nausea, weakness, sweating, palpitations, syncope, and possibly diarrhea; occurs in patients who have had partial gastrectomy and gastrojejunostomy

duodenum: first portion of the small intestine, between the stomach and the jejunum

gastric: refers to the stomach

gastritis: inflammation of the stomach

hematemesis: vomiting of blood

melena: tarry or black stools; indicative of blood in stools

morbid obesity: 100 pounds or more over ideal body weight

pyloroplasty: surgical procedure to increase the opening of the pyloric orifice

pylorus: opening between the stomach and the duodenum

pyrosis: heartburn

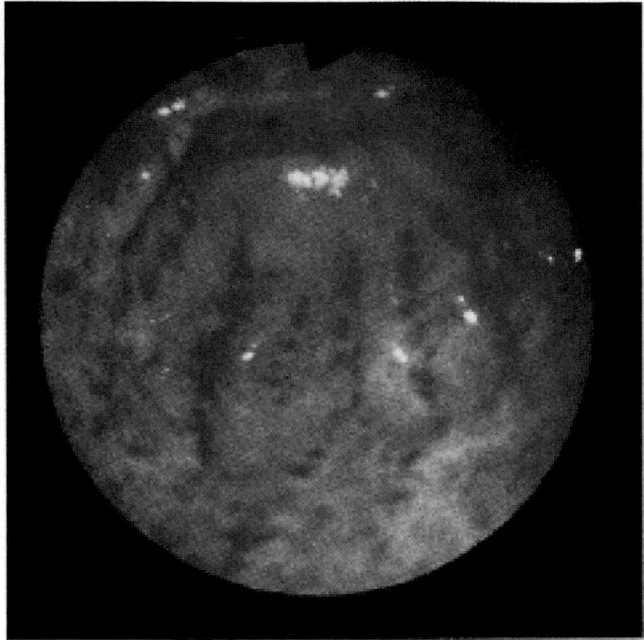
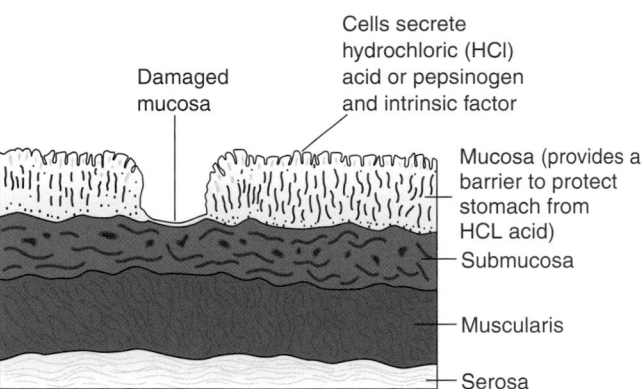

FIGURE 37-1 Endoscopic view of erosive gastritis (*left*). Damage from irritants (*right*) results in increased intracellular pH, impaired enzyme function, disrupted cellular structures, ischemia, vascular stasis, and tissue death. From Porth, C. (2002). *Pathophysiology: Concepts of altered health states* (6th ed.). Philadelphia: Lippincott Williams & Wilkins.

at any specific time of the day, before or after meals, after ingesting spicy or irritating foods, or after the ingestion of certain drugs or alcohol? Has there been recent weight gain or loss? Are the symptoms related to anxiety, stress, allergies, eating or drinking too much, or eating too quickly? How are the symptoms relieved? Is there a history of previous gastric disease or surgery? A diet history plus a 72-hour dietary recall (a list of everything the patient ate and drank in the last 72 hours) may be helpful.

A thorough history is important because it helps the nurse to identify whether known dietary excesses or other indiscretions are associated with the current symptoms, whether others in the patient's environment have similar symptoms, whether the patient is vomiting blood, and whether any known caustic element has been ingested. The nurse also identifies the duration of the current symptoms, any methods used by the patient to treat these symptoms, and whether the methods are effective. Signs to note during the physical examination include abdominal tenderness, dehydration, and evidence of any systemic disorder that might be responsible for the symptoms of gastritis.

Nursing Diagnoses

Based on the assessment data, the patient's major nursing diagnoses may include the following:

- Anxiety related to treatment
- Imbalanced nutrition, less than body requirements, related to inadequate intake of nutrients
- Risk for imbalanced fluid volume related to insufficient fluid intake and excessive fluid loss subsequent to vomiting
- Deficient knowledge about dietary management and disease process
- Acute pain related to irritated stomach mucosa

Planning and Goals

The major goals for the patient may include reduced anxiety, avoidance of irritating foods, adequate intake of nutrients, maintenance of fluid balance, increased awareness of dietary management, and relief of pain.

Nursing Interventions

REDUCING ANXIETY

If the patient has ingested acids or alkalis, emergency measures may be needed. The nurse offers supportive therapy to the patient and family during treatment and after the ingested acid or alkali has been neutralized or diluted. In some cases, the nurse may need to prepare the patient for additional diagnostic studies (endoscopy) or surgery. The patient usually feels anxious about the pain and the treatment modalities. The nurse uses a calm approach to assess the patient and to answer all questions as completely as possible. It is important to explain all procedures and treatments according to the patient's level of understanding.

PROMOTING OPTIMAL NUTRITION

For acute gastritis, the nurse provides physical and emotional support and helps the patient manage the symptoms, which may include nausea, vomiting, heartburn, and fatigue. The patient should take no foods or fluids by mouth—possibly for days—until the acute symptoms subside, thus allowing the gastric mucosa to heal. If IV therapy is necessary, the nurse monitors it regularly, along with serum electrolyte values. After the symptoms subside, the nurse can offer the patient ice chips followed by clear liquids. Introducing solid food as soon as possible will provide oral nutrition, decrease the need for IV therapy, and minimize irritation to the gastric mucosa. As food is introduced, the nurse evaluates and reports any symptoms that suggest a repeat episode of gastritis.

Table 37-1 • **Pharmacologic Therapy for Peptic Ulcer Disease and Gastritis**

PHARMACOLOGIC AGENT	MAJOR ACTION	NURSING CONSIDERATIONS
Antibiotics and Bismuth Salts		
Tetracycline (plus metronidazole, proton pump inhibitor, and bismuth salts)	Exerts bacteriostatic effects to eradicate *Helicobacter pylori* bacteria in the gastric mucosa	May cause photosensitivity reaction; warn patient to use sunscreen. Use with caution in patients with renal or hepatic impairment. Milk or dairy products may reduce medication effectiveness.
Amoxicillin (plus clarithromycin and proton pump inhibitor such as omeprazole [Prilosec])	A bactericidal antibiotic that assists with eradicating *H. pylori* bacteria in the gastric mucosa	May cause diarrhea. Do not use in patients allergic to penicillin.
Metronidazole (Flagyl); use with clarithromycin and proton pump inhibitor	An amebocide that assists with eradicating *H. pylori* bacteria in the gastric mucosa	Administer with meals to decrease GI distress. Administer with other antibiotics and proton pump inhibitors.
Clarithromycin (Biaxin); use with proton pump inhibitor and amoxicillin	Exerts bactericidal effects to eradicate *H. pylori* bacteria in the gastric mucosa	May cause GI upset.
Bismuth subsalicylate (Pepto-Bismol); use with antibiotics	Suppresses *H. pylori* bacteria in the gastric mucosa and assists with healing of mucosal lesions	Given concurrently with antibiotics to cure *H. pylori* infection. Should be taken on an empty stomach.
Histamine 2 (H₂) Receptor Antagonists		
Cimetidine (Tagamet)	Inhibits acid secretion by blocking the action of histamine on the histamine receptors of the parietal cells in the stomach	Least expensive of the H₂ receptor antagonists. May cause confusion, agitation, or coma in the elderly or those with renal or hepatic insufficiency. Long-term use may cause gynecomastia, impotence, and diarrhea.
Ranitidine (Zantac)	Inhibits acid secretion by blocking the action of the histamine on the histamine receptors of the parietal cells in the stomach	Prolonged drug half-life in patients with renal and hepatic insufficiency. Causes fewer side effects than cimetidine. Rarely causes constipation, diarrhea, dizziness, and depression.
Famotidine (Pepcid)	Inhibits acid secretion by blocking the action of histamine on the histamine receptors on the parietal cells in the stomach	Best choice for critically ill patient because it is known to have least risk of interaction with other medications. (It is unclear whether other H₂ receptor antagonists are as safe as famotidine.) Does not alter medication metabolism in the liver. Prolonged half-life in patients with renal insufficiency. Short-term relief for gastroesophageal reflux. Dilute before IV injection. Rarely causes constipation or diarrhea.
Nizantidine (Axid)	Inhibits acid secretion by blocking the action of histamine on the histamine receptors on the parietal cells in the stomach	Used for duodenal ulcers. Prolonged half-life in patients with renal insufficiency. Rarely causes sweating, increased liver enzymes, nausea, urticaria.
Proton (Gastric Acid) Pump Inhibitor		
Omeprazole (Prilosec)	Decreases gastric acid secretion by slowing the hydrogen-potassium adenosine triphosphatase (H+, K+-ATPase) pump on the surface of the parietal cells	Long-term use may cause gastric tumors and bacterial invasion. May cause diarrhea, additional pain, and nausea.
Lansoprazole (Prevacid)	Decreases gastric acid secretion by slowing the H+, K+-ATPase pump on the surface of the parietal cells.	A delayed-release capsule that is to be swallowed whole and taken before meals.
Rabeprazole (Aciphex)	Decreases gastric acid secretion by slowing the H+, K+-ATPase pump on the surface of the parietal cells	A delayed-release tablet; swallow whole.

(continued)

Table 37-1 • **Pharmacologic Therapy for Peptic Ulcer Disease and Gastritis** (Continued)

PHARMACOLOGIC AGENT	MAJOR ACTION	NURSING CONSIDERATIONS
Cytoprotective Medications		
Misoprostol (Cytotec)	A synthetic prostaglandin; protects the gastric mucosa from ulcerogenic agents; also increases mucus production and bicarbonate levels	Used as a preventive medication (to prevent ulceration in patients using NSAIDs). Administer with food. May cause diarrhea and cramping (including uterine cramping).
Sucralfate (Carafate)	In the presence of gastric acid, sucralfate creates a viscous substance that forms a protective layer at the site of the ulcer and prevents digestion by pepsin	May cause constipation or nausea. Approved for duodenal—*not gastric*—ulcers.

The nurse discourages the intake of caffeinated beverages, because caffeine is a central nervous system stimulant that increases gastric activity and pepsin secretion. It also is important to discourage alcohol use. Discouraging cigarette smoking is important because nicotine reduces the secretion of pancreatic bicarbonate and thus inhibits the neutralization of gastric acid in the duodenum (Eastwood, 1997). When appropriate, the nurse refers the patient for alcohol counseling and smoking cessation programs.

PROMOTING FLUID BALANCE

Daily fluid intake and output are monitored to detect early signs of dehydration (minimal urine output of 30 mL/hour, minimal intake of 1.5 L/day). If food and fluids are withheld, IV fluids (3 L/day) usually are prescribed and a record of fluid intake plus caloric value (1 L of 5% dextrose in water = 170 calories of carbohydrate) needs to be maintained. Electrolyte values (sodium, potassium, chloride) are assessed every 24 hours to detect imbalance.

The nurse must always be alert for any indicators of hemorrhagic gastritis, which include **hematemesis** (vomiting of blood), tachycardia, and hypotension. If these occur, the physician is notified and the patient's vital signs are monitored as the patient's condition warrants. Guidelines for managing upper GI tract bleeding are discussed later in this chapter.

RELIEVING PAIN

Measures to help relieve pain include instructing the patient to avoid foods and beverages that may be irritating to the gastric mucosa (described earlier) and instructing the patient about using medications to relieve chronic gastritis. To follow up, the nurse assesses the patient's level of pain and the extent of comfort attained from the use of medications and avoidance of irritating substances.

PROMOTING HOME AND COMMUNITY-BASED CARE

Teaching Patients Self-Care

The nurse evaluates the patient's knowledge about gastritis and develops an individualized teaching plan that includes information about stress management, diet, and medications (Chart 37-1). Dietary instructions take into account the patient's daily caloric needs, food preferences, and pattern of eating. The nurse and patient review foods and other substances to be avoided (eg, spicy, irritating, or highly seasoned foods; caffeine; nicotine; alcohol). Consultation with a dietitian may be recommended.

Providing information about prescribed antibiotics, bismuth salts, medications to decrease gastric secretion, and medications to protect mucosal cells from gastric secretions can help the patient recover and prevent recurrence. Patients with pernicious anemia need information about long-term vitamin B$_{12}$ injections; the nurse may instruct a family member about administering these injections or make arrangements for the patient to receive the injections from a health care provider. Finally, the nurse emphasizes the importance of keeping follow-up appointments with health care providers.

Evaluation

EXPECTED PATIENT OUTCOMES

Expected patient outcomes may include the following:

1. Exhibits less anxiety
2. Avoids eating irritating foods or drinking caffeinated beverages or alcohol
3. Maintains fluid balance
   a. Has intake of at least 1.5 L daily
   b. Drinks six to eight glasses of water daily

Chart 37-1
Home Care Checklist • **The Patient With Gastritis**

At the completion of the home care instruction, the patient or caregiver will be able to:	Patient	Caregiver
• Identify foods and other substances that may cause gastritis.	✓	✓
• Describe medication regimen to follow.	✓	✓
• State need for vitamin B$_{12}$ injections if patient has pernicious anemia.	✓	✓

c. Has a urinary output of about 1 L daily
d. Displays adequate skin turgor
4. Adheres to medical regimen
   a. Selects nonirritating foods and beverages
   b. Takes medications as prescribed
5. Maintains appropriate weight
6. Reports less pain

Gastric and Duodenal Ulcers

A peptic ulcer is an excavation (hollowed-out area) that forms in the mucosal wall of the stomach, in the **pylorus** (opening between stomach and duodenum), in the **duodenum** (first part of small intestine), or in the esophagus. A peptic ulcer is frequently referred to as a gastric, duodenal, or esophageal ulcer, depending on its location, or as peptic ulcer disease. Erosion of a circumscribed area of mucous membrane is the cause (Fig. 37-2). This erosion may extend as deeply as the muscle layers or through the muscle to the peritoneum. Peptic ulcers are more likely to be in the duodenum than in the stomach. As a rule they occur alone, but they may occur in multiples. Chronic gastric ulcers tend to occur in the lesser curvature of the stomach, near the pylorus. Table 37-2 compares the features of gastric and duodenal ulcers.

Peptic ulcer disease occurs with the greatest frequency in people between the ages of 40 and 60 years. It is relatively uncommon in women of childbearing age, but it has been observed in children and even in infants. After menopause, the incidence of peptic ulcers in women is almost equal to that in men. Peptic ulcers in the body of the stomach can occur without excessive acid secretion.

Table 37-2 • Comparing Duodenal and Gastric Ulcers	
DUODENAL ULCER	GASTRIC ULCER
Incidence	
Age 30–60	Usually 50 and over
Male: female = 2–3:1	Male: female = 1:1
80% of peptic ulcers are duodenal	15% of peptic ulcers are gastric
Signs, Symptoms, and Clinical Findings	
Hypersecretion of stomach acid (HCl)	Normal—hyposecretion of stomach acid (HCl)
May have weight gain	Weight loss may occur
Pain occurs 2–3 hours after a meal; often awakened between 1–2 AM; ingestion of food relieves pain	Pain occurs ½ to 1 hour after a meal; rarely occurs at night; may be relieved by vomiting; ingestion of food does not help, sometimes increases pain
Vomiting uncommon	Vomiting common
Hemorrhage less likely than with gastric ulcer, but if present melena more common than hematemesis	Hemorrhage more likely to occur than with duodenal ulcer; hematemesis more common than melena
More likely to perforate than gastric ulcers	
Malignancy Possibility	
Rare	Occasionally
Risk Factors	
H. pylori, alcohol, smoking, cirrhosis, stress	*H. pylori*, gastritis, alcohol, smoking, use of NSAIDs, stress

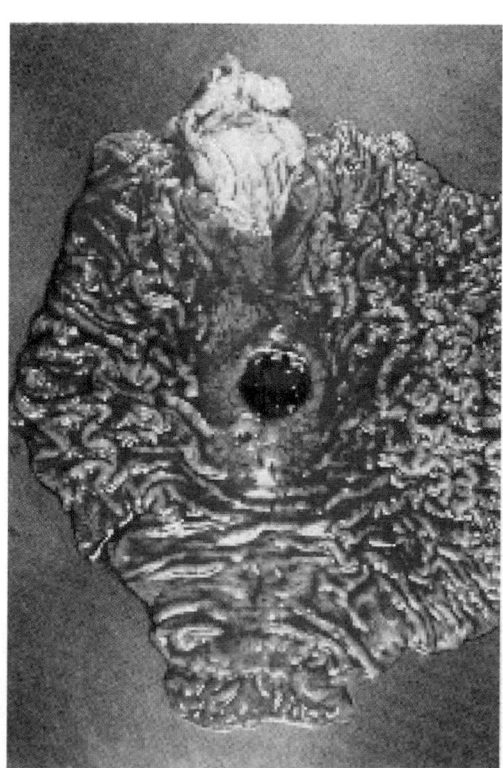

FIGURE 37-2 Deep peptic ulcer. From Porth, C. (2002). *Pathophysiology: Concepts of altered health states* (6th ed). Philadelphia: Lippincott Williams & Wilkins.

In the past, stress and anxiety were thought to be causes of ulcers. Research has identified that peptic ulcers result from infection with the gram-negative bacteria *H. pylori* (Tytgat, 2000). However, ulcers do seem to develop more commonly in people who are tense; whether this is a contributing factor to the condition is uncertain. In addition, excessive secretion of HCl in the stomach may contribute to the formation of gastric ulcers, and stress may be associated with its increased secretion. The ingestion of milk and caffeinated beverages, smoking, and alcohol also may increase HCl secretion.

Familial tendency may be a significant predisposing factor. A further genetic link is noted in the finding that people with blood type O are more susceptible to peptic ulcers than are those with blood type A, B, or AB. There also is an association between duodenal ulcers and chronic pulmonary disease or chronic renal disease. Other predisposing factors associated with peptic ulcer include chronic use of NSAIDs, alcohol ingestion, and excessive smoking.

Rarely, ulcers are caused by excessive amounts of the hormone gastrin, produced by tumors. This Zollinger-Ellison syndrome (ZES) consists of severe peptic ulcers, extreme gastric hyperacidity, and gastrin-secreting benign or malignant tumors of the pancreas. Stress ulcers, which are clinically different from peptic ulcers, are ulcerations in the mucosa that can occur in the gastroduodenal area. Stress ulcers may occur in patients who are exposed to stressful conditions. Esophageal ulcers occur as a result of the backward flow of HCl from the stomach into the esophagus (gastroesophageal reflux disease [GERD]).

Pathophysiology

Peptic ulcers occur mainly in the gastroduodenal mucosa because this tissue cannot withstand the digestive action of gastric acid (HCl) and pepsin. The erosion is caused by the increased concentration or activity of acid-pepsin, or by decreased resistance of the mucosa. A damaged mucosa cannot secrete enough mucus to act as a barrier against HCl. The use of NSAIDs inhibits the secretion of mucus that protects the mucosa. Patients with duodenal ulcer disease secrete more acid than normal, whereas patients with gastric ulcer tend to secrete normal or decreased levels of acid.

ZES is suspected when a patient has several peptic ulcers or an ulcer that is resistant to standard medical therapy. It is identified by the following findings: hypersecretion of gastric juice, duodenal ulcers, and gastrinomas (islet cell tumors) in the pancreas. Ninety percent of tumors are found in the "gastric triangle," which encompasses the cystic and common bile ducts, the second and third portions of the duodenum, and the neck and body of the pancreas. Approximately one third of gastrinomas are malignant. Diarrhea and steatorrhea (unabsorbed fat in the stool) may be evident. The patient may have coexisting parathyroid adenomas or hyperplasia and may therefore exhibit signs of hypercalcemia. The most common complaint is epigastric pain. *H. pylori* is not a risk factor for ZES.

Stress ulcer is the term given to the acute mucosal ulceration of the duodenal or gastric area that occurs after physiologically stressful events, such as burns, shock, severe sepsis, and multiple organ traumas. These ulcers are most common in ventilator-dependent patients after trauma or surgery. Fiberoptic endoscopy within 24 hours after injury reveals shallow erosions of the stomach wall; by 72 hours, multiple gastric erosions are observed. As the stressful condition continues, the ulcers spread. When the patient recovers, the lesions are reversed. This pattern is typical of stress ulceration.

Differences of opinion exist as to the actual cause of mucosal ulceration in stress ulcers. Usually, it is preceded by shock; this leads to decreased gastric mucosal blood flow and to reflux of duodenal contents into the stomach. In addition, large quantities of pepsin are released. The combination of ischemia, acid, and pepsin creates an ideal climate for ulceration.

Stress ulcers should be distinguished from Cushing's ulcers and Curling's ulcers, two other types of gastric ulcers. Cushing's ulcers are common in patients with trauma to the brain. They may occur in the esophagus, stomach, or duodenum and are usually deeper and more penetrating than stress ulcers. Curling's ulcer is frequently observed about 72 hours after extensive burns and involves the antrum of the stomach or the duodenum.

Clinical Manifestations

Symptoms of an ulcer may last for a few days, weeks, or months and may disappear only to reappear, often without an identifiable cause. Many people have symptomless ulcers, and in 20% to 30% perforation or hemorrhage may occur without any preceding manifestations.

As a rule, the patient with an ulcer complains of dull, gnawing pain or a burning sensation in the midepigastrium or in the back. It is believed that the pain occurs when the increased acid content of the stomach and duodenum erodes the lesion and stimulates the exposed nerve endings. Another theory suggests that contact of the lesion with acid stimulates a local reflex mechanism that initiates contraction of the adjacent smooth muscle. Pain is usually relieved by eating, because food neutralizes the acid, or by taking alkali; however, once the stomach has emptied or the alkali's effect has decreased, the pain returns. Sharply localized tenderness can be elicited by applying gentle pressure to the epigastrium at or slightly to the right of the midline.

Other symptoms include **pyrosis** (heartburn), vomiting, constipation or diarrhea, and bleeding. Pyrosis is a burning sensation in the esophagus and stomach that moves up to the mouth. Heartburn is often accompanied by sour eructation, or burping, which is common when the patient's stomach is empty.

Although vomiting is rare in uncomplicated duodenal ulcer, it may be a symptom of a peptic ulcer complication. It results from obstruction of the pyloric orifice, caused by either muscular spasm of the pylorus or mechanical obstruction from scarring or acute swelling of the inflamed mucous membrane adjacent to the ulcer. Vomiting may or may not be preceded by nausea; usually it follows a bout of severe pain and bloating, which is relieved by ejection of the gastric contents. Emesis often contains undigested food eaten many hours earlier. Constipation or diarrhea can occur, probably as a result of diet and medications.

Fifteen percent of patients with gastric ulcers experience bleeding. Patients may present with GI bleeding as evidenced by the passage of tarry stools. A small portion of patients who bleed from an acute ulcer have had no previous digestive complaints, but they develop symptoms thereafter (Yamada, 1999).

Assessment and Diagnostic Findings

A physical examination may reveal pain, epigastric tenderness, or abdominal distention. A barium study of the upper GI tract may show an ulcer; however, endoscopy is the preferred diagnostic procedure because it allows direct visualization of inflammatory changes, ulcers, and lesions. Through endoscopy, a biopsy of the gastric mucosa and of any suspicious lesions can be obtained. Endoscopy may reveal lesions that are not evident on x-ray studies because of their size or location.

Stools may be tested periodically until they are negative for occult blood. Gastric secretory studies are of value in diagnosing achlorhydria and ZES. *H. pylori* infection may be determined by biopsy and histology with culture. There is also a breath test that detects *H. pylori,* as well as a serologic test for antibodies to the *H. pylori* antigen. Pain that is relieved by ingesting food or antacids and absence of pain on arising are also highly suggestive of an ulcer.

Medical Management

Once the diagnosis is established, the patient is informed that the problem can be controlled. Recurrence may develop; however, peptic ulcers treated with antibiotics to eradicate *H. pylori* have a lower recurrence rate than those not treated with antibiotics. The goals are to eradicate *H. pylori* and to manage gastric acidity. Methods used include medications, lifestyle changes, and surgical intervention.

PHARMACOLOGIC THERAPY

Currently, the most commonly used therapy in the treatment of ulcers is a combination of antibiotics, proton pump inhibitors, and bismuth salts that suppresses or eradicates *H. pylori;* histamine 2 (H_2) receptor antagonists and proton pump inhibitors are used to treat NSAID-induced and other ulcers not associated with *H. pylori* ulcers. Table 37-1 provides details about pharmacologic treatment.

The patient is advised to adhere to the medication regimen to ensure complete healing of the ulcer. Because most patients become symptom-free within a week, it becomes a nursing responsibility to stress the importance of following the prescribed regimen so that the healing process can continue uninterrupted and the return of chronic ulcer symptoms can be prevented. Rest, sedatives, and tranquilizers may add to the patient's comfort and are prescribed as needed. Maintenance dosages of H_2 receptor antagonists are usually recommended for 1 year.

For patients with ZES, hypersecretion of acid may be controlled with high doses of H_2 receptor antagonists. These patients may require twice the normal dose, and dosages usually need to be increased with prolonged use. Octreotide (Sandostatin), a medication that suppresses gastrin levels, also may be prescribed.

Patients at risk for stress ulcers may be treated prophylactically with IV H_2 receptor antagonists and cytoprotective agents (e.g., misoprostol, sucralfate) because of the risk for upper GI tract hemorrhage. Frequent gastric aspiration is performed to allow monitoring of gastric secretion pH.

STRESS REDUCTION AND REST

Reducing environmental stress requires physical and psychological modifications on the patient's part as well as the aid and cooperation of family members and significant others. The patient may need help in identifying situations that are stressful or exhausting. A rushed lifestyle and an irregular schedule may aggravate symptoms and interfere with regular meals taken in relaxed settings and with the regular administration of medications. The patient may benefit from regular rest periods during the day, at least during the acute phase of the disease. Biofeedback, hypnosis, or behavior modification may be helpful.

SMOKING CESSATION

Studies have shown that smoking decreases the secretion of bicarbonate from the pancreas into the duodenum, resulting in increased acidity of the duodenum. Research indicates that continuing to smoke cigarettes may significantly inhibit ulcer repair. Therefore, the patient is strongly encouraged to stop smoking. Smoking cessation support groups and other smoking cessation approaches are helpful for many patients (Eastwood, 1997).

DIETARY MODIFICATION

The intent of dietary modification for patients with peptic ulcers is to avoid oversecretion of acid and hypermotility in the GI tract. These can be minimized by avoiding extremes of temperature and overstimulation from consumption of meat extracts, alcohol, coffee (including decaffeinated coffee, which also stimulates acid secretion) and other caffeinated beverages, and diets rich in milk and cream (which stimulate acid secretion). In addition, an effort is made to neutralize acid by eating three regular meals a day. Small, frequent feedings are not necessary as long as an antacid or a histamine blocker is taken. Diet compatibility becomes an individual matter: the patient eats foods that can be tolerated and avoids those that produce pain.

SURGICAL MANAGEMENT

The introduction of antibiotics to eradicate *H. pylori* and of H_2 receptor antagonists as treatment for ulcers has greatly reduced the need for surgical interventions. However, surgery is usually recommended for patients with intractable ulcers (those that fail to heal after 12 to 16 weeks of medical treatment), life-threatening hemorrhage, perforation, or obstruction, and for those with ZES not responding to medications (Yamada, 1999). Surgical procedures include vagotomy, with or without pyloroplasty, and the Billroth I and Billroth II procedures (Table 37-3; see also the section on gastric surgery later in this chapter). Patients who need ulcer surgery may have had a long illness. They may be discouraged and have had interruptions in their work role and pressures in their family life.

FOLLOW-UP CARE

Recurrence within 1 year may be prevented with the prophylactic use of H_2 receptor antagonists given at a reduced dose. Not all patients require maintenance therapy; it may be prescribed only for those with two or three recurrences per year, those who have had a complication such as bleeding or outlet obstruction, or those who are candidates for gastric surgery but are at too high a risk for surgery. The likelihood of recurrence is reduced if the patient avoids smoking, coffee (including decaffeinated coffee) and other caffeinated beverages, alcohol, and ulcerogenic medications (eg, NSAIDs).

NURSING PROCESS: THE PATIENT WITH ULCER DISEASE

Assessment

The nurse asks the patient to describe the pain and the methods used to relieve it (e.g., food, antacids). The patient usually describes peptic ulcer pain as burning or gnawing; it occurs about 2 hours after a meal and frequently awakens the patient between midnight and 3 AM. Taking antacids, eating, or vomiting often relieves the pain. If the patient reports a recent history of vomiting, the nurse determines how often emesis has occurred and notes important characteristics of the vomitus: Is it bright red, does it resemble coffee grounds, or is there undigested food from previous meals? Has the patient noted any bloody or tarry stools?

The nurse also asks the patient to list his or her usual food intake for a 72-hour period and to describe food habits (e.g., speed of eating, regularity of meals, preference for spicy foods, use of seasonings, use of caffeinated beverages and decaffeinated coffee). Lifestyle and habits are a concern as well. Does the patient use irritating substances? For example, does he or she smoke cigarettes? If yes, how many? Does the patient ingest alcohol? If yes, how much and how often? Are NSAIDs used? The nurse inquires about the patient's level of anxiety and his or her perception of current stressors. How does the patient express anger or cope with stressful situations? Is the patient experiencing occupational stress or problems within the family? Is there a family history of ulcer disease?

The nurse assesses vital signs and reports tachycardia and hypotension, which may indicate anemia from GI bleeding. The stool is tested for occult blood, and a physical examination, including palpation of the abdomen for localized tenderness, is performed as well.

Diagnosis

NURSING DIAGNOSES

Based on the assessment data, the patient's nursing diagnoses may include the following:

- Acute pain related to the effect of gastric acid secretion on damaged tissue
- Anxiety related to coping with an acute disease
- Imbalanced nutrition related to changes in diet
- Deficient knowledge about prevention of symptoms and management of the condition

Table 37-3 • **Surgical Procedures for Peptic Ulcer Disease**

OPERATION	DESCRIPTION	COMMENTS
Vagotomy 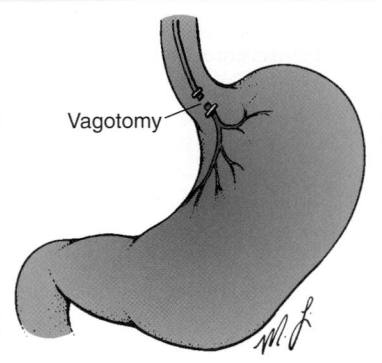	Severing of the vagus nerve. Decreases gastric acid by diminishing cholinergic stimulation to the parietal cells, making them less responsive to gastrin. May be done via open surgical approach, laparoscopy, or thoracoscopy	May be performed to reduce gastric acid secretion. A drainage type of procedure (see pyloroplasty) is usually performed to assist with gastric emptying (because there is total denervation of the stomach). Some patients experience problems with feeling of fullness, dumping syndrome, diarrhea, and gastritis.
Truncal vagotomy	Severs the right and left vagus nerves as they enter the stomach at the distal part of the esophagus.	This type of vagotomy is most commonly used to decrease acid secretions and reduce gastric and intestinal motility. Recurrence rate of ulcer is 10%–15%.
Selective vagotomy	Severs vagal innervation to the stomach but maintains innervation to the rest of the abdominal organs.	
Proximal (parietal cell) gastric vagotomy without drainage	Denervates acid-secreting parietal cells but preserves vagal innervation to the gastric antrum and pylorus.	No dumping syndrome. No need for drainage procedure. Recurrence rate of ulcer is 10%–15%.
Pyloroplasty 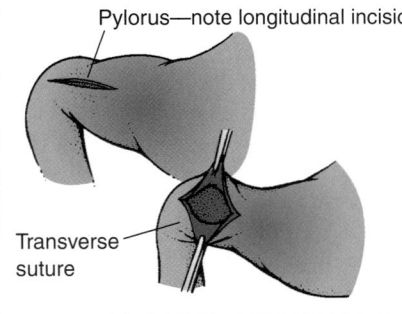	A surgical procedure in which a longitudinal incision is made into the pylorus and transversely sutured closed to enlarge the outlet and relax the muscle	Usually accompanies truncal and selective vagotomies, which produce delayed gastric emptying due to decreased innervation.
Antrectomy Billroth I (Gastroduodenostomy) 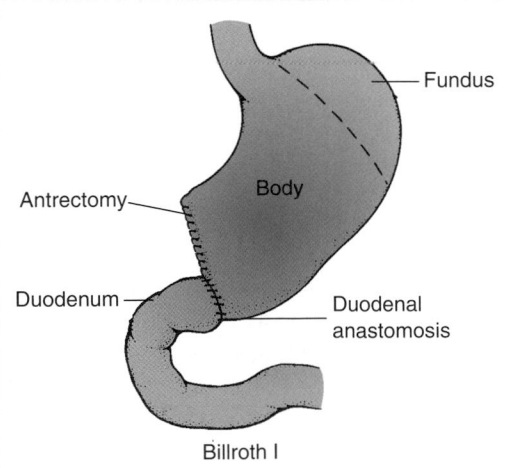	Removal of the lower portion of the antrum of the stomach (which contains the cells that secrete gastrin) as well as a small portion of the duodenum and pylorus. The remaining segment is anastomosed to the duodenum (Billroth I) or to the jejunum (Billroth II)	May be performed in conjunction with a truncal vagotomy. The patient may have problems with feeling of fullness, dumping syndrome, and diarrhea. Recurrence rate of ulcer is <1%.

(continued)

Table 37-3 • **Surgical Procedures for Peptic Ulcer Disease** (Continued)

OPERATION	DESCRIPTION	COMMENTS
Billroth II (Gastrojejunostomy) 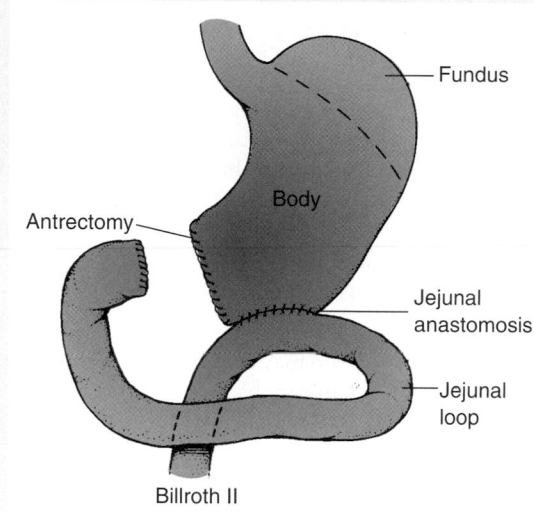		
Subtotal gastrectomy with Billroth I or II anastomosis	Removal of distal third of stomach; anastomosis with duodenum or jejunum. Removes gastrin-producing cells in the antrum and part of the parietal cells.	Dumping syndrome, anemia, malabsorption, weight loss. Recurrence rate of ulcer is 10%–15%.

COLLABORATIVE PROBLEMS/ POTENTIAL COMPLICATIONS

Potential complications may include the following:

- Hemorrhage
- Perforation
- Penetration
- Pyloric obstruction (gastric outlet obstruction)

Planning and Goals

The goals for the patient may include relief of pain, reduced anxiety, maintenance of nutritional requirements, knowledge about the management and prevention of ulcer recurrence, and absence of complications.

Nursing Interventions

RELIEVING PAIN

Pain relief can be achieved with prescribed medications. The patient should avoid aspirin, foods and beverages that contain caffeine, and decaffeinated coffee, and meals should be eaten at regularly paced intervals in a relaxed setting. Some patients benefit from learning relaxation techniques to help manage stress and pain and to enhance smoking cessation efforts.

REDUCING ANXIETY

The nurse assesses the patient's level of anxiety. Patients with peptic ulcers are usually anxious, but their anxiety is not always obvious. Appropriate information is provided at the patient's level of understanding, all questions are answered, and the patient is encouraged to express fears openly. Explaining diagnostic tests and administering medications on schedule also help to reduce anxiety. The nurse interacts with the patient in a relaxed manner, helps identify stressors, and explains various coping techniques

and relaxation methods, such as biofeedback, hypnosis, or behavior modification. The patient's family is also encouraged to participate in care and to provide emotional support.

MAINTAINING OPTIMAL NUTRITIONAL STATUS

The nurse assesses the patient for malnutrition and weight loss. After recovery from an acute phase of peptic ulcer disease, the patient is advised about the importance of complying with the medication regimen and dietary restrictions.

MONITORING AND MANAGING POTENTIAL COMPLICATIONS

Hemorrhage

Gastritis and hemorrhage from peptic ulcer are the two most common causes of upper GI tract bleeding (which may also occur with esophageal varices, as discussed in Chapter 39). Hemorrhage, the most common complication, occurs in about 15% of patients with peptic ulcers (Yamada, 1999). The site of bleeding is usually the distal portion of the duodenum. Bleeding may be manifested by hematemesis or **melena** (tarry stools). The vomited blood can be bright red, or it can have a "coffee grounds" appearance (which is dark) from the oxidation of hemoglobin to methemoglobin. When the hemorrhage is large (2000 to 3000 mL), most of the blood is vomited. Because large quantities of blood may be lost quickly, immediate correction of blood loss may be required to prevent hemorrhagic shock. When the hemorrhage is small, much or all of the blood is passed in the stools, which will appear tarry black because of the digested hemoglobin. Management depends on the amount of blood lost and the rate of bleeding.

The nurse assesses the patient for faintness or dizziness and nausea, which may precede or accompany bleeding. It is important to monitor vital signs frequently and to evaluate the patient for tachycardia, hypotension, and tachypnea. Other nursing interventions include monitoring the hemoglobin and hematocrit, testing the stool for gross or occult blood, and recording hourly urinary output to detect anuria or oliguria (absence or decreased urine production).

Many times the bleeding from a peptic ulcer stops spontaneously; however, the incidence of recurrent bleeding is high. Because bleeding can be fatal, the cause and severity of the hemorrhage must be identified quickly and the blood loss treated to prevent hemorrhagic shock. Management of upper GI tract bleeding consists of quickly determining the amount of blood lost and the rate of bleeding, rapidly replacing the blood that has been lost, stopping the bleeding, stabilizing the patient, and diagnosing and treating the cause. Related nursing and collaborative interventions include the following:

- Inserting a peripheral IV line for the infusion of saline or lactated Ringer's solution and blood products. The nurse may need to assist with the placement of a pulmonary artery catheter for hemodynamic monitoring. Blood component therapy is initiated if there are signs of shock (eg, tachycardia, sweating, coldness of the extremities).
- Monitoring the hemoglobin and hematocrit to assist in evaluating blood loss
- Inserting an NG tube to distinguish fresh blood from "coffee grounds" material, to aid in the removal of clots and acid, to prevent nausea and vomiting, and to provide a means of monitoring further bleeding
- Administering a room-temperature lavage of saline solution or water. This is controversial; some authorities recommend using ice lavage (Yamada, 1999).
- Inserting an indwelling urinary catheter and monitoring urinary output
- Monitoring vital signs and oxygen saturation and administering oxygen therapy
- Placing the patient in the recumbent position with the legs elevated to prevent hypotension; or, to prevent aspiration from vomiting, placing the patient on the left side
- Treating hemorrhagic shock (described in Chapter 15)

If bleeding cannot be managed by the measures described, other treatment modalities may be used. Transendoscopic coagulation by laser, heat probe, medication, a sclerosing agent, or a combination of these therapies can halt bleeding and make surgical intervention unnecessary. There is much debate regarding how soon endoscopy should be performed. Some believe that endoscopy should be performed in the first 24 hours after hemorrhage has been stabilized. Others believe that endoscopy may be performed during acute bleeding, as long as the esophageal or gastric area can be visualized (blood may decrease visibility) (Yamada, 1999).

For those who are unable to undergo surgery, selective embolization may be used. This procedure involves forcing emboli of autologous blood clots with or without Gelfoam (absorbable gelatin sponge) through a catheter in the artery to a point above the bleeding lesion. A radiologist performs this procedure.

Rebleeding may occur and often warrants surgical intervention. The nurse monitors the patient carefully so that bleeding can be detected quickly. Signs of bleeding include tachycardia, tachypnea, hypotension, mental confusion, thirst, and oliguria. If bleeding recurs within 48 hours after medical therapy has begun, or if more than 6 to 10 units of blood are required within 24 hours to maintain blood volume, the patient is likely to require surgery. Some physicians recommend surgical intervention if a patient hemorrhages three times. Other criteria for surgery are the patient's age (massive hemorrhaging is three times more likely to be fatal in those older than 60 years of age); a history of chronic duodenal ulcer; and

a coincidental gastric ulcer (Yamada, 1999). The area of the ulcer is removed or the bleeding vessels are ligated. Many patients also undergo procedures (eg, vagotomy and pyloroplasty, gastrectomy) aimed at controlling the underlying cause of the ulcers (see Table 37-3).

Perforation and Penetration

Perforation is the erosion of the ulcer through the gastric serosa into the peritoneal cavity without warning. It is an abdominal catastrophe and requires immediate surgery. Penetration is erosion of the ulcer through the gastric serosa into adjacent structures such as the pancreas, biliary tract, or gastrohepatic omentum. Symptoms of penetration include back and epigastric pain not relieved by medications that were effective in the past. Like perforation, penetration usually requires surgical intervention.

Signs and symptoms of perforation include the following:

- Sudden, severe upper abdominal pain (persisting and increasing in intensity); pain may be referred to the shoulders, especially the right shoulder, because of irritation of the phrenic nerve in the diaphragm.
- Vomiting and collapse (fainting)
- Extremely tender and rigid (boardlike) abdomen
- Hypotension and tachycardia, indicating shock

Because chemical peritonitis develops within a few hours after perforation and is followed by bacterial peritonitis, the perforation must be closed as quickly as possible. In a few patients, it may be deemed safe and advisable to perform surgery for the ulcer disease in addition to suturing the perforation.

Postoperatively, the stomach contents are drained by means of an NG tube. The nurse monitors fluid and electrolyte balance and assesses the patient for peritonitis or localized infection (increased temperature, abdominal pain, paralytic ileus, increased or absent bowel sounds, abdominal distention). Antibiotic therapy is administered parenterally as prescribed.

Pyloric Obstruction

Pyloric obstruction, also called gastric outlet obstruction (GOO), occurs when the area distal to the pyloric sphincter becomes scarred and stenosed from spasm or edema or from scar tissue that forms when an ulcer alternately heals and breaks down. The patient has nausea and vomiting, constipation, epigastric fullness, anorexia, and, later, weight loss.

In treating the patient with pyloric obstruction, the first consideration is to insert an NG tube to decompress the stomach. Confirmation that obstruction is the cause of the discomfort is accomplished by assessing the amount of fluid aspirated from the NG tube. A residual of more than 400 mL strongly suggests obstruction. Usually an upper GI study or endoscopy is performed to confirm gastric outlet obstruction. Decompression of the stomach and management of extracellular fluid volume and electrolyte balances may improve the patient's condition and avert the need for surgical intervention. A balloon dilatation of the pylorus via endoscopy may be beneficial. If the obstruction is unrelieved by medical management, surgery (in the form of a vagotomy and **antrectomy** or gastrojejunostomy and vagotomy) may be required.

PROMOTING HOME AND COMMUNITY-BASED CARE

Teaching Patients Self-Care

To manage ulcer disease successfully, the patient is instructed about the factors that will help or aggravate the condition (Chart 37-2). The nurse reviews information about medications to be taken at

Chart 37-2
Home Care Checklist • The Patient With Peptic Ulcer Disease

At the completion of the home care instruction, the patient or caregiver will be able to:	Patient	Caregiver
• State the medication regimen and importance of complying with medication schedule.	✓	✓
• State dietary restrictions and foods that may exacerbate condition (caffeine products, milk).	✓	✓
• Identify smoking cessation groups.	✓	
• Identify methods to reduce stress.	✓	✓
• State signs and symptoms of complications:	✓	✓
Hemorrhage—cool skin, confusion, increased heart rate, labored breathing, blood in stool		
Penetration and perforation—severe abdominal pain, rigid and tender abdomen, vomiting, elevated temperature, increased heart rate		
Pyloric obstruction—nausea and vomiting, distended abdomen, abdominal pain		
• State need for follow-up medical care.	✓	✓

home, including name, dosage, frequency, and possible side effects, stressing the importance of continuing to take medications even after signs and symptoms have decreased or subsided. Then the patient is instructed to avoid certain medications and foods that exacerbate symptoms as well as substances that have acid-producing potential (eg, alcohol; caffeinated beverages such as coffee, tea, and colas). It is important to counsel the patient to eat meals at regular times and in a relaxed setting, and to avoid overeating. If relevant, the nurse also informs the patient about the irritant effects of smoking on the ulcer and provides information about smoking cessation programs.

> **NURSING ALERT** The nurse reviews with the patient and family the signs and symptoms of complications to be reported. They include hemorrhage (cool skin, confusion, increased heart rate, labored breathing, and blood in the stool); penetration and perforation (severe abdominal pain, rigid and tender abdomen, vomiting, elevated temperature, and increased heart rate); and pyloric obstruction (nausea, vomiting, distended abdomen, and abdominal pain).

The nurse reinforces the importance of follow-up care for approximately 1 year, the need to report recurrence of symptoms, and the need for treating possible problems that occur after surgery, such as intolerance to dairy products and sweet foods.

Evaluation

EXPECTED PATIENT OUTCOMES
Expected patient outcomes may include the following:

1. Reports freedom from pain between meals
2. Feels less anxiety by avoiding stress
3. Complies with therapeutic regimen
   a. Avoids irritating foods and beverages
   b. Eats regularly scheduled meals
   c. Takes prescribed medications as scheduled
   d. Uses coping mechanisms to deal with stress
4. Maintains weight
5. Is free of complications

Morbid Obesity

One in three Americans is 20% or more over his or her ideal body weight (U.S. Department of Health and Human Services, 2001). **Morbid obesity** is the term applied to people who are more than

two times their ideal body weight or whose body mass index (BMI) exceeds 30 kg/m². (See Chapter 5.)

Another definition of morbid obesity is body weight that is more than 100 pounds greater than the ideal body weight (Monteforte & Turkelson, 2000). Patients with morbid obesity are at higher risk for health complications, such as cardiovascular disease, arthritis, asthma, bronchitis, and diabetes. They frequently suffer from low self-esteem, impaired body image, and depression.

Medical Management

Conservative management consists of placing the person on a weight loss diet in conjunction with behavioral modification and exercise; however, diet therapy is usually unsuccessful. There is a belief that depression may be a contributing factor to weight gain, and treatment of the depression with bupropion hydrochloride (Wellbutrin) may be helpful (Wangsness, 2000). Some physicians recommend acupuncture and hypnosis before recommending surgery.

PHARMACOLOGIC MANAGEMENT
Several medications have recently been approved for obesity. They include sibutramine HCl (Meridia) and orlistat (Xenical). By inhibiting the reuptake of serotonin and norepinephrine, sibutramine decreases appetite. Orlistat reduces caloric intake by binding to gastric and pancreatic lipase to prevent digestion of fats. Both medications require a physician's prescription. Sibutramine may increase blood pressure and should not be taken by people with a history of coronary artery disease, angina pectoris, dysrhythmias, or kidney disease; by those taking antidepressants or monoamine oxidase inhibitors; or by pregnant or nursing women. Side effects may include dry mouth, insomnia, headache, increased sweating, and increased heart rate. Side effects of orlistat may include increased bowel movements, gas with oily discharge, decreased food absorption, decreased bile flow, and decreased absorption of some vitamins. A multivitamin is usually recommended for patients taking orlistat. Women who are pregnant or nursing should not take orlistat (Hussar, 2000).

SURGICAL MANAGEMENT
Bariatric surgery, or surgery for morbid obesity, is performed only after other nonsurgical attempts at weight control have failed. The first surgical procedure to treat morbid obesity was the jejunoileal bypass. This procedure, which resulted in significant

complications, has been largely replaced by gastric restriction procedures. Gastric bypass and vertical banded gastroplasty are the current operations of choice. These procedures may be performed laparoscopically or by an open surgical technique.

In gastric bypass surgery, the proximal segment of the stomach is transected to form a small pouch with a small gastroenterostomy stoma. The Roux-en-Y gastric bypass is the recommended procedure for long-term weight loss. In this procedure, a horizontal row of staples creates a stomach pouch with a 1-cm stoma that is anastomosed with a portion of distal jejunum, creating a gastroenterostomy. The transected proximal portion of the jejunum is anastomosed to the distal jejunum (Fig. 37-3A).

In vertical banded gastroplasty, a double row of staples is applied vertically along the lesser curvature of the stomach, beginning at the angle of His. A small stoma is created at the end of the staples by adding a circle of staples or a band of polypropylene mesh or silicone tubing (see Fig. 37-3B).

After weight loss, the patient may need surgical intervention for body contouring. This may include lipoplasty to remove fat deposits or a panniculectomy to remove excess abdominal skinfolds.

Nursing Management

Nursing management focuses on care of the patient after surgery. General postoperative nursing care is similar to that for a patient recovering from a gastric resection, but with attention given to the risks of complications associated with morbid obesity. Complications that may occur in the immediate postoperative period include peritonitis, stomal obstruction, stomal ulcers, atelectasis and pneumonia, thromboembolism, and metabolic imbalances resulting from prolonged vomiting and diarrhea. After bowel sounds have returned and oral intake is resumed, the nurse provides six

small feedings consisting of a total of 600 to 800 calories per day and encourages fluid intake to prevent dehydration.

Patients are usually discharged in 4 to 5 days with detailed dietary instructions. The nurse instructs patients to report excessive thirst or concentrated urine, both of which are indications of dehydration. Psychosocial interventions are also essential for these patients. Efforts are directed toward helping them modify their eating behaviors and cope with changes in body image. The nurse explains that noncompliance by eating too much or too fast or eating high-calorie liquid and soft foods results in vomiting and painful esophageal distention. The nurse discusses dietary instructions before discharge and schedules monthly outpatient visits. Long-term side effects may include increased risk of gallstones, nutritional deficiencies, and potential to regain weight.

Gastric Cancer

The incidence of cancer of the stomach continues to decrease in the United States; however, it still accounts for 12,400 deaths annually (American Cancer Society, 2002). Most of these deaths occur in people older than 40 years of age, but they occasionally occur in younger people. Men have a higher incidence of gastric cancers than women do. The incidence of gastric cancer is much greater in Japan, which has instituted mass screening programs for earlier diagnosis. Diet appears to be a significant factor. A diet high in smoked foods and low in fruits and vegetables may increase the risk of gastric cancer. Other factors related to the incidence of gastric cancer include chronic inflammation of the stomach, pernicious anemia, achlorhydria, gastric ulcers, *H. pylori* infection, and genetics. The prognosis is poor, because most patients have metastases at the time of diagnosis (Greenlee, 2001).

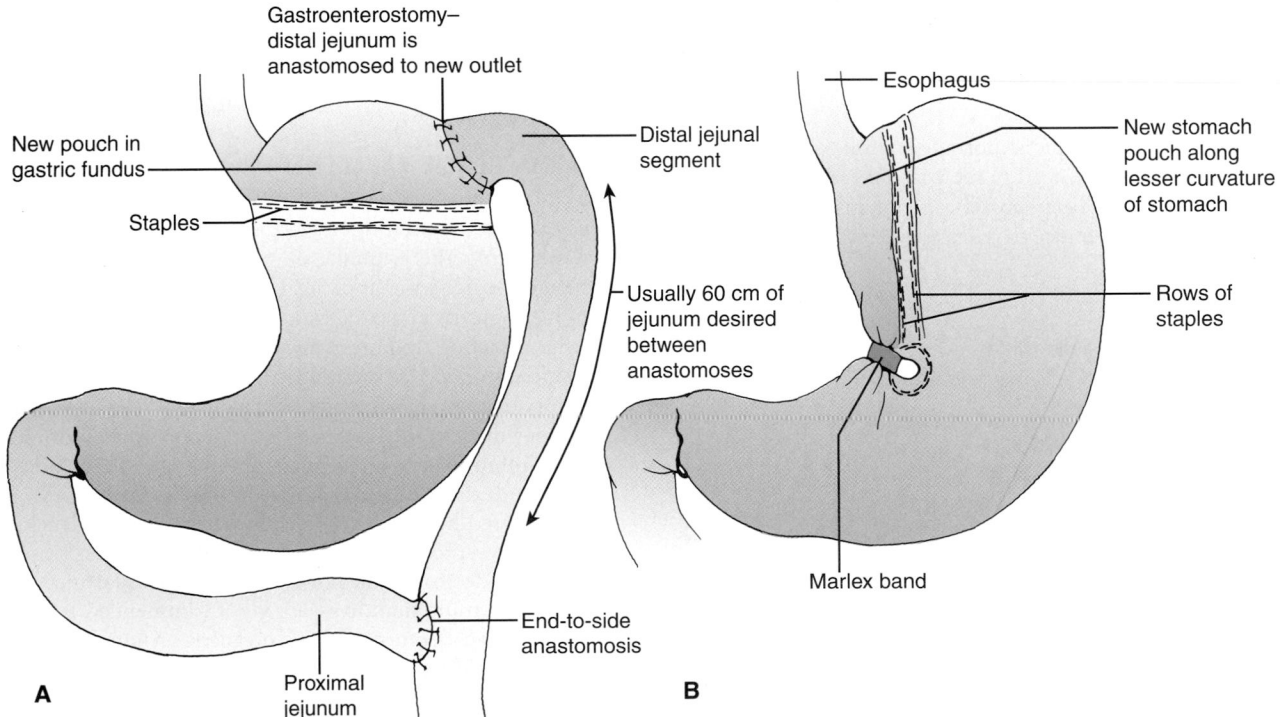

FIGURE 37-3 Surgical procedures for morbid obesity. **(A)** Gastric bypass with roux-en-Y. A horizontal row of staples creates a pouch with a capacity of 50 mL or less. The proximal jejunum is transected and the distal end anastomosed to the new pouch. The proximal segment is anastomosed to the jejunum. **(B)** Vertical banded gastroplasty. A vertical row of staples along the lesser curvature of the stomach creates a new, smaller stomach pouch of 10 to 15 mL.

Pathophysiology

Most gastric cancers are adenocarcinomas and can occur in any portion of the stomach. The tumor infiltrates the surrounding mucosa, penetrating the wall of the stomach and adjacent organs and structures. The liver, pancreas, esophagus, and duodenum are often affected at the time of diagnosis. Metastasis through lymph to the peritoneal cavity occurs later in the disease.

Clinical Manifestations

In the early stages of gastric cancer, symptoms may be absent. Early symptoms are seldom definitive because most gastric tumors begin on the lesser curvature, where they cause little disturbance of gastric functions. Some studies show that early symptoms, such as pain relieved with antacids, resemble those of benign ulcers. Symptoms of progressive disease may include anorexia, dyspepsia (indigestion), weight loss, abdominal pain, constipation, anemia, and nausea and vomiting.

Assessment and Diagnostic Findings

Usually the physical examination is not helpful in detecting cancer because most gastric tumors are not palpable. Ascites may be apparent if the cancer cells have metastasized to the liver. Endoscopy for biopsy and cytologic washings is the usual diagnostic study, and a barium x-ray examination of the upper GI tract may also be performed. Because metastasis often occurs before warning signs develop, a computed tomography (CT) scan, bone scan, and liver scan are valuable in determining the extent of metastasis. A complete x-ray examination of the GI tract should be performed when any person older than 40 years of age has had indigestion (dyspepsia) of more than 4 weeks' duration.

Medical Management

There is no successful treatment for gastric carcinoma except removal of the tumor. If the tumor can be removed while it is still localized to the stomach, the patient can be cured. If the tumor has spread beyond the area that can be excised, cure is impossible. Palliative rather than radical surgery is performed if there is metastasis to other vital organs, such as the liver. In many of these patients, effective palliation to prevent discomfort caused by obstruction or dysphagia may be obtained by resection of the tumor (see Gastric Surgery).

If a radical subtotal gastrectomy is performed, the stump of the stomach is anastomosed to the jejunum, as in the gastrectomy for ulcer. When a total gastrectomy is performed, GI continuity is restored by means of an anastomosis between the ends of the esophagus and the jejunum.

If surgical treatment does not offer cure, treatment with chemotherapy may offer further control of the disease or palliation. Commonly used chemotherapeutic medications include cisplatin, irinotecan, or a combination of 5-fluorouracil, doxorubicin (Adriamycin), and mitomycin-C. Some studies are being conducted on the use of chemotherapy before surgery. Radiation therapy also may be used for palliation. Assessment of tumor markers (blood analysis for antigens indicative of colon cancer) such as carcinoembryonic antigen, CA 19-9, and CA 50 may help determine the effectiveness of treatment. If these values were elevated before treatment, they should decrease if the tumor is responding to the treatment (Bobbio-Pallavicini et al., 2001; Kerby & Heslin, 1999).

NURSING PROCESS:
THE PATIENT WITH GASTRIC CANCER

Assessment

The nurse elicits a dietary history from the patient, focusing on recent nutritional intake and status. Has the patient lost weight? If so, how much and over what period of time? Can the patient tolerate a full diet? If not, what foods can he or she eat? What other changes in eating habits have occurred? Does the patient have an appetite? Is the patient in pain? Do foods, antacids, or medications relieve the pain, make no difference, or worsen the pain? Is there a history of infection with *H. pylori* bacteria? Other health information to obtain includes the patient's smoking and alcohol history and the family history (any first- or second-degree relatives with gastric or other cancer). A psychosocial assessment, including questions about social support, individual and family coping skills, and financial resources, will help the nurse plan for care in acute and community settings.

After the interview, the nurse performs a complete physical examination, carefully assesses the patient's abdomen for tenderness or masses, and also palpates and percusses to detect ascites.

Nursing Diagnosis

Based on the assessment data, the patient's major nursing diagnoses may include the following:

- Anxiety related to the disease and anticipated treatment
- Imbalanced nutrition, less than body requirements, related to anorexia
- Pain related to tumor mass
- Anticipatory grieving related to the diagnosis of cancer
- Deficient knowledge regarding self-care activities

Planning and Goals

The major goals for the patient may include reduced anxiety, optimal nutrition, relief of pain, and adjustment to the diagnosis and anticipated lifestyle changes.

Nursing Interventions

REDUCING ANXIETY

A relaxed, nonthreatening atmosphere is provided so that patient can express fears, concerns, and possibly anger about the diagnosis and prognosis. The nurse encourages the family in their efforts to support the patient, offering reassurance and supporting positive coping measures. The nurse advises the patient about any procedures and treatments so that the patient knows what to expect. The nurse also may suggest talking with a support person (eg, spiritual advisor), if the patient desires.

PROMOTING OPTIMAL NUTRITION

The nurse encourages the patient to eat small, frequent portions of nonirritating foods to decrease gastric irritation. Food supplements should be high in calories, as well as vitamins A and C and iron, to enhance tissue repair. If the patient is unable to eat adequately to meet nutritional requirements, parenteral nutrition may be necessary. Because the patient may develop dumping syndrome when enteral feeding resumes after gastric resection, the nurse explains ways to prevent and manage it (six small feedings daily that are low in carbohydrates and sugar; fluids between meals rather than with meals) and informs the patient that symptoms often resolve after several months. If a total gastrectomy is performed, parenteral vitamin B_{12} will be required indefinitely, because dietary vitamin B_{12} is absorbed in the stomach. The nurse monitors the IV therapy and nutritional status and records intake, output, and daily weights to ensure that the patient is maintaining or gaining weight. The nurse assesses for signs of dehydration (thirst, dry mucous membranes, poor skin turgor, tachycardia, decreased urine output) and reviews the results of daily laboratory studies to note any metabolic abnormalities (sodium, potassium, glucose, blood urea nitrogen). Antiemetics are administered as prescribed.

RELIEVING PAIN

The nurse administers analgesics as prescribed. A continuous infusion of an opioid may be necessary for severe pain. The nurse assesses the frequency, intensity, and duration of the pain to determine the effectiveness of the analgesic being administered. The nurse works with the patient to manage pain by suggesting nonpharmacologic methods for pain relief, such as position changes, imagery, distraction, relaxation exercises (using relaxation audiotapes), backrubs, massage, and periods of rest and relaxation.

PROVIDING PSYCHOSOCIAL SUPPORT

The nurse helps the patient express fears, concerns, and grief about the diagnosis. It is important to answer the patient's questions honestly and to encourage the patient to participate in treatment decisions. Some patients mourn the loss of a body part and perceive their surgery as a type of mutilation. Some express disbelief and need time and support to accept the diagnosis.

The nurse offers emotional support and involves family members and significant others whenever possible. This includes recognizing mood swings and defense mechanisms (eg, denial, rationalization, displacement, regression) and reassuring the patient and family members that emotional responses are normal and expected. The services of clergy, psychiatric clinical nurse specialists, psychologists, social workers, and psychiatrists are made available, if needed. The nurse projects an empathetic attitude and spends time with the patient. Most patients will begin to participate in self-care activities after they have acknowledged their loss.

PROMOTING HOME AND COMMUNITY-BASED CARE

Teaching Patients Self-Care

Self-care activities will depend on the mode of treatment used—surgery, chemotherapy, radiation, or palliative care. Patient and family teaching will include information about diet and nutrition, treatment regimens, activity and lifestyle changes, pain management, and possible complications (Chart 37-3). Consul-

tation with a dietitian is essential to determine how the patient's nutritional needs can best be met at home. The nurse teaches the patient or care provider about administration of enteral or parenteral nutrition. If chemotherapy or radiation is prescribed, the nurse provides explanations to the patient and family about what to expect, including the length of treatments, the expected side effects (eg, nausea, vomiting, anorexia, fatigue, neutropenia), and the need for transportation to appointments for treatment. Psychological counseling may also be helpful.

Continuing Care

The need for ongoing care in the home will depend on the patient's condition and treatment. The home care nurse reinforces nutritional counseling and supervises the administration of any enteral or parenteral feedings; the patient or family member must become skillful in administering the feedings and in detecting and preventing untoward effects or complications related to the feedings (see Chapter 36 to review management of enteral and parenteral feedings). The nurse teaches the patient or a family member to record the patient's daily intake, output, and weight and explains strategies to manage pain, nausea, vomiting, or other symptoms. The nurse also teaches the patient or caregiver to recognize and report signs and symptoms of complications that require medical attention, such as bleeding, obstruction, perforation, or any symptoms that become progressively worse. It is important to explain the chemotherapy or radiation therapy regimen. The patient and family need to know about the care that will be needed during and after treatments (see Chapter 16). Because the prognosis for gastric cancer is so poor, the nurse may need to assist the patient and family with decisions regarding end-of-life care. Referral to hospice may be warranted.

Evaluation

EXPECTED PATIENT OUTCOMES

Expected patient outcomes may include the following:

1. Reports less anxiety
   a. Expresses fears and concerns about surgery
   b. Seeks emotional support
2. Attains optimal nutrition
   a. Eats small, frequent meals high in calories, iron, and vitamins A and C
   b. Complies with enteral or parenteral nutrition as needed
3. Has less pain
4. Performs self-care activities and adjusts to lifestyle changes
   a. Resumes normal activities within 3 months
   b. Alternates periods of rest and activity
   c. Manages tube feedings

Chart 37-3

Home Care Checklist • The Patient With Gastric Cancer

At the completion of the home care instruction, the patient or caregiver will be able to:	Patient	Caregiver
• Demonstrate safe management of enteral or parenteral feedings, if applicable.	✓	✓
• Describes dietary restrictions.	✓	✓
• Identifies potential side effects of chemotherapy or radiation therapy, if applicable	✓	✓
• Identifies signs and symptoms of wound infection.	✓	✓
• State signs and symptoms of obstruction or perforation.	✓	✓
• Describes follow-up needs.	✓	✓

Gastric Surgery

Gastric surgery may be performed on patients with peptic ulcers who have life-threatening hemorrhage, obstruction, perforation, or penetration or whose condition does not respond to medication. It also may be indicated for patients with gastric cancer or trauma. Surgical procedures include a vagotomy and **pyloroplasty** (disconnecting nerves that stimulate acid secretion and opening the pylorus), a partial gastrectomy, and a total gastrectomy (removal of the stomach) with either an end-to-end or an end-to-side esophagojejunal anastomosis (see Table 37-3).

NURSING PROCESS: THE PATIENT UNDERGOING GASTRIC SURGERY

Assessment

Before surgery, the nurse assesses the patient's and family's knowledge of preoperative and postoperative surgical routines and the rationale for surgery. The nurse also assesses the patient's nutritional status: Has the patient lost weight? How much? Over how much time? Does the patient have nausea and vomiting? Has the patient had hematemesis? The nurse assesses for the presence of bowel sounds and palpates the abdomen to detect masses or tenderness.

After surgery, the nurse assesses the patient for complications secondary to the surgical intervention, such as hemorrhage, infection, abdominal distention, or decreased nutritional status. (See Chapters 20 and 25.)

Diagnosis

NURSING DIAGNOSES
Based on the assessment data, the patient's major nursing diagnoses may include the following:

- Anxiety related to surgical intervention
- Acute pain related to surgical incision
- Deficient knowledge about surgical procedures and postoperative course
- Imbalanced nutrition, less than body requirements, related to poor nutrition before surgery and altered GI system after surgery

COLLABORATIVE PROBLEMS/POTENTIAL COMPLICATIONS
In addition to the complications to which all postoperative patients are subject, the patient undergoing gastric surgery is at increased risk for:

- Hemorrhage
- Dietary deficiencies
- Bile reflux
- Dumping syndrome

Planning and Goals

The major goals for the patient undergoing gastric surgery may include reduced anxiety, increased knowledge and understanding about the surgical procedure and postoperative course, optimal nutrition and management of the complications that can interfere with nutrition, relief of pain, avoidance of hemorrhage and steatorrhea, and enhanced self-care skills at home. General postoperative care for the patient who has received general anesthesia, as discussed in Chapter 20, should be followed.

Nursing Interventions

REDUCING ANXIETY
An important part of the preoperative nursing care involves allaying the patient's fears and anxieties about the impending surgery and its implications. The nurse encourages the patient to express feelings and answers the patient's and family's questions. If the patient has an acute obstruction, a perforated bowel, or an active GI hemorrhage, adequate psychological preparation may not be possible. In this event, the nurse caring for the patient after surgery should anticipate the concerns, fears, and questions that are likely to surface and should be available for support and further explanations.

RELIEVING PAIN
After surgery, analgesics may be administered as prescribed to relieve pain and discomfort. It is important to avoid sedating the patient so as not to impair his or her ability to perform pulmonary care activities (deep breathing and coughing) and to ambulate. The nurse assesses the effectiveness of analgesic intervention. Positioning the patient in a Fowler's position promotes comfort and allows emptying of the stomach after a partial gastrectomy.

The nurse maintains functioning of the NG tube to prevent distention and resultant pain and damage to the suture line. Normally, the amount of NG drainage after a total gastrectomy is small.

INCREASING KNOWLEDGE
The nurse explains routine preoperative and postoperative activities to the patient, which include preoperative medications, NG intubation, IV fluids, abdominal dressings, and pulmonary care. These explanations need to be reinforced after surgery, especially if the patient had emergency surgery.

RESUMING ENTERAL INTAKE
The patient's nutritional status is evaluated before surgery, because many patients with gastric cancer are malnourished and may require preoperative enteral or, more often, parenteral nutrition (see Chapter 36). After surgery, parenteral nutrition may be continued to meet caloric needs, to replace fluids lost through drainage and vomitus, and to support the patient metabolically until oral intake is adequate.

After the return of bowel sounds and removal of the NG tube, the nurse may give fluids, followed by food in small portions. The nurse adds foods gradually until the patient is able to eat six small meals a day and drink 120 mL of fluid between meals. The key to increasing the dietary content is to offer food and fluids gradually as tolerated and to recognize that each patient's tolerance is different.

RECOGNIZING OBSTACLES TO ADEQUATE NUTRITION

Dysphagia and Gastric Retention
Dysphagia may occur in patients who have had truncal vagotomy, a surgical procedure that can result in trauma to the lower esophagus. Gastric retention may be evidenced by abdominal distention, nausea, and vomiting. Regurgitation may also occur if the patient has eaten too much or too quickly. It also may indicate that edema along the suture line is preventing fluids and food from moving into the intestinal tract. If gastric retention occurs, it may be necessary to reinstate NG suction; pressure must be low to avoid disrupting the suture line.

Bile Reflux
Bile reflux gastritis and esophagitis may occur with the removal of the pylorus, which acts as a barrier to the reflux of duodenal contents. Burning epigastric pain and vomiting of bilious material manifest this condition. Eating or vomiting does not relieve the

situation. Agents that bind with bile acid, such as cholestyramine (Questran), may be helpful. Aluminum hydroxide gel (an antacid) and metoclopramide hydrochloride (Reglan) have been used with some success.

Dumping Syndrome

The term **dumping syndrome** refers to an unpleasant set of vasomotor and GI symptoms that sometimes occur in patients who have had gastric surgery or a form of vagotomy. It may be the mechanical result of surgery in which a small gastric remnant is connected to the jejunum through a large opening. Foods high in carbohydrates and electrolytes must be diluted in the jejunum before absorption can take place, but the passage of food from the stomach remnant into the jejunum is too rapid to allow this to happen. The symptoms that occur are probably a result of rapid distention of the jejunal loop anastomosed to the stomach. The hypertonic intestinal contents draw extracellular fluid from the circulating blood volume into the jejunum to dilute the high concentration of electrolytes and sugars. The ingestion of fluid at mealtime is another factor that causes the stomach contents to empty rapidly into the jejunum.

Early symptoms include a sensation of fullness, weakness, faintness, dizziness, palpitations, diaphoresis, cramping pains, and diarrhea. Later, there is a rapid elevation of blood glucose, followed by increased insulin secretion. This results in a reactive hypoglycemia, which also is unpleasant for the patient. Vasomotor symptoms that occur 10 to 90 minutes after eating are pallor, perspiration, palpitations, headache, and feelings of warmth, dizziness, and even drowsiness. Anorexia may also be a result of the dumping syndrome.

Steatorrhea also may occur in the patient with gastric surgery. It is partially the result of rapid gastric emptying, which prevents adequate mixing with pancreatic and biliary secretions. In mild cases, reducing the intake of fat and administering an antimotility medication can control steatorrhea.

Vitamin and Mineral Deficiencies

Other dietary deficiencies the nurse should be aware of include malabsorption of organic iron, which may require supplementation with oral or parenteral iron, and a low serum level of vitamin B_{12}, which may require supplementation by the intramuscular route. Total gastrectomy results in lack of intrinsic factor, a gastric secretion required for the absorption of vitamin B_{12} from the GI tract. Unless this vitamin is supplied by parenteral injection after gastrectomy, the patient inevitably will suffer vitamin B_{12} deficiency, which eventually leads to a condition identical to pernicious anemia. All manifestations of pernicious anemia, including macrocytic anemia and combined system disease, may be expected to develop within a period of 5 years or less; they progress in severity thereafter and, in the absence of therapy, are fatal. This complication is avoided by the regular monthly intramuscular injection of 100 to 1000 μg (usual dose is 300 μg) of vitamin B_{12}.

This regimen should be started without delay after gastrectomy. Weight loss is a common long-term problem because the patient experiences early fullness, which suppresses the appetite.

TEACHING DIETARY SELF-MANAGEMENT

Because the patient may experience any of the described conditions affecting nutrition, nursing intervention includes proper dietary instruction. The following teaching points are emphasized:

- To delay stomach emptying, the patient should assume a low Fowler's position during mealtime, and after the meal the patient should lie down for 20 to 30 minutes.
- Antispasmodics, as prescribed, also may aid in delaying the emptying of the stomach.
- Fluid intake with meals is discouraged; instead, fluids may be consumed up to 1 hour before or 1 hour after mealtime.
- Meals should contain more dry items than liquid items.
- The patient can eat fat as tolerated but should keep carbohydrate intake low and avoid concentrated sources of carbohydrates.
- The patient should eat smaller but more frequent meals.
- Dietary supplements of vitamins and medium-chain triglycerides and injections of vitamin B_{12} and iron may be prescribed.

The nurse also gives instructions regarding enteral or parenteral supplementation if it is needed.

MONITORING AND MANAGING POTENTIAL COMPLICATIONS

Occasionally hemorrhage complicates gastric surgery. The patient has the usual signs of rapid blood loss and shock (see Chapter 15) and may vomit considerable amounts of bright red blood. The nurse assesses NG drainage for type and amount; some bloody drainage for the first 12 hours is expected, but excessive bleeding should be reported. The nurse also assesses the abdominal dressing for bleeding. Because this situation is upsetting to the patient and family, the nurse should remain calm. The nurse performs emergency measures, such as NG lavage and administration of blood and blood products.

PROMOTING HOME AND COMMUNITY-BASED CARE

Teaching Patients Self-Care

Nurse-patient teaching stems from the assessment of the patient's physical and psychological readiness to participate in self-care. The nurse provides information about nutrition, enteral or parenteral nutrition if required, nutritional supplements, pain management, and the symptoms of dumping syndrome and measures to use to prevent or minimize these symptoms (Chart 37-4). It is important to emphasize the continued need for vitamin B_{12} injections.

Chart 37-4
Home Care Checklist • The Patient With Gastric Resection

At the completion of the home care instruction, the patient or caregiver will be able to:	Patient	Caregiver
• Demonstrate enteral or parenteral feedings as applicable.	✓	✓
• State necessary dietary changes.	✓	✓
• Identify available support groups.	✓	✓
• Explain medication regimen.	✓	✓
• Identify signs and symptoms of complications	✓	✓

Continuing Care

Both the patient and the family can benefit from a team approach to discharge planning. The team members include the home care nurse, physician, dietitian, social worker, patient and family; written instructions about meals, activities, medications, and follow-up care are helpful. The home care nurse supervises the administration of any enteral or parenteral feedings, emphasizing information about detection and prevention of untoward effects or complications related to the feedings. Information about community support groups is provided to the patient and family.

Evaluation

EXPECTED PATIENT OUTCOMES

Expected patient outcomes may include:

1. Reports decreased anxiety; expresses fears and concerns about surgery
2. Demonstrates knowledge regarding postoperative course by discussing the surgical procedure and postoperative course
3. Attains optimal nutrition
   a. Maintains a reasonable weight
   b. Does not have excessive diarrhea
   c. Tolerates 6 small meals a day
   d. Does not experience dysphagia, gastric retention, bile reflux, dumping syndrome, or vitamin and mineral deficiencies
4. Attains optimal level of comfort
5. Has no evidence of hemorrhage

Critical Thinking Exercises

1. You are working in the office of a gastroenterologist. You have a patient coming in today with symptoms of a peptic ulcer. What questions will you ask the patient, and what types of teaching regimen do you anticipate you will need to review with this patient?

2. You are caring for a patient who is to have a gastrectomy to treat gastric cancer. What nutritional needs do you anticipate for this patient preoperatively, immediately postoperatively, and after discharge from the hospital?

3. Your 45-year-old patient who weighs 375 pounds has had gastric bypass to treat morbid obesity. Describe the preoperative interventions for this patient. How would you modify your interventions if the patient had diabetes? If he had angina?

REFERENCES AND SELECTED READINGS

Books

American Cancer Society. (2002). *Cancer facts and figures*. Atlanta: Author.

Brandt, L. J. (Ed.). (1999). *Clinical practice of gastroenterology* (Vols. I & II). Philadelphia: Churchill-Livingstone.

DeVita, V. T., Hellman, S., & Rosenberg, S. A. (Eds.). (1997). *Cancer: Principles and practice of oncology* (5th ed.). Philadelphia: Lippincott-Raven.

McEvoy, G. R. (Ed.). (2000). *American hospital formulary service*. Bethesda, MD: American Society of Health-System Pharmacists.

Pappas, T. N., et al. (1999). *Atlas of laparoscopic surgery* (2nd ed.). Norwalk, CT: Appleton & Lange.

Porth, C. (2002). *Pathophysiology: Concepts of altered health states* (6th ed.). Philadelphia: Lippincott Williams & Wilkins.

Townsend, C. M. Jr. (Ed.). (2001). *Textbook of surgery* (7th ed.). Philadelphia: W. B. Saunders.

U.S. Department of Health and Human Services. (2001). *The surgeon general's call to action to prevent and decrease overweight and obesity*. Rockville, MD: Author.

Wolfe, M. M. (2000). *Therapy of digestive disorders*. Philadelphia: W. B. Saunders.

Yamada, T. (1999). *Textbook of gastroenterology* (3rd ed., Vols. I & II). Philadelphia: Lippincott Williams & Wilkins.

Journals

Gastric Cancer

Bobbio-Pallavicini, E., et al. (2001). Cisplatin, mitomycin-C, 5-fluorouracil and leucovorin combination chemotherapy (L-FCM) in locally advanced unresectable or metastatic gastric carcinoma: A phase-II study. *Oncology Reports, 8*(1), 167–171.

Greenlee, R. T. (2001). Cancer statistics, 2001. *CA: A Cancer Journal for Clinicians, 5*(1), 15–16.

Hanazaki, K., et al. (2000). Postoperative chemotherapy in elderly patients with advanced cancer. *Hepatogastroenterology, 47*(36), 1761–1764.

Kerby, J. D., & Heslin, M. J. (1999). Gastric cancer. *Current Treatment Options in Gastroenterology, 2*(3), 163–170.

La Veccha, J. C., & Franceschi, S. (2000). Nutrition and gastric cancer. *Canadian Journal of Gastroenterology, 14,* (Suppl D), 51D–54D.

Stucky-Marshall, L. S. (1999). New agents in gastrointestinal malignancies. Part 1: Irinotecan in clinical practice. *Cancer Nursing, 22*(3), 212–219.

Morbid Obesity

Davila-Cervantes, A, et al. (2000). Open vs laparoscopic vertical banded gastroplasty: A case control study with a 1-year follow-up. *Obesity Surgery 2000, 10*(5), 409–412.

Hussar, D. A. (1999). New drugs 1999: Part II. *Nursing 99, 29*(2), 45–51.

Hussar, D. A. (2000). New drugs 2000: Part I. *Nursing 00, 30*(1), 50–62.

Monteforte M. J., & Turkelson, C. M. (2000). Bariatric surgery for morbid obesity. *Obesity Surgery, 10*(5), 391–401.

Schirmer, B. D. (2000). Laparoscopic bariatric surgery. *Surgical Clinics of North America, 80*(4), 1253–1267.

Wangsness, M. (2000). Pharmacological treatment of obesity: Past, present and future. *Minnesota Medicine, 83*(11), 21–26.

Weiss, D. (2000). How to help your patients lose weight: Current therapy for obesity. *Cleveland Clinic Journal of Medicine, 67*(10), 739, 743–746, 749–754.

Peptic Ulcers and Gastritis

Alsahli, M., et al. (2001). Vaccines: An ongoing promise? *Digestive Diseases, 19*(2), 148–157.

Axon, A. T. (2000). Treatment of *Helicobacter pylori:* An overview. *Alimentary Pharmacology and Therapeutics, 14* (Suppl. 3), 1–6.

Beehrie, D. M., & Evans, D. (1999). A review of NSAID complications: Gastrointestinal and more. *Primary Care Practice, 3*(3), 305–315.

Eastwood, G. L. (1997). Is smoking still important in the pathogenesis of peptic ulcer disease? *Journal of Clinical Gastroenterology, 25* (Suppl. 1), S1–S7.

McManus, T. J. (2000). *Helicobacter pylori:* An emerging infectious disease. *Nurse Practitioner, 25*(8), 40–50.

Tytgat, G. (2000). *Helicobacter pylori:* Past, present and future. *Journal of Gastroenterology and Hepatology, 15* (Suppl.) G30–G33.

Weart, C. W. (2000). Peptic ulcer disease: Let's help cure it. *Journal of the American Pharmaceutical Association, 40*(4), 560–561.

RESOURCES AND WEBSITES

American Cancer Society, 1599 Clifton Rd., N.E., Atlanta, GA 30329; 1-800-ACS-2345; http://www.cancer.org.

American Gastroenterological Association, 7910 Woodmont Ave., Seventh Floor, Bethesda, MD 20814; http://www.gastro.org.

Management of Patients With Intestinal and Rectal Disorders

LEARNING OBJECTIVES ●

On completion of this chapter, the learner will be able to:

1. Identify the health care teaching needs of patients with constipation or diarrhea.
2. Compare the conditions of malabsorption with regard to their pathophysiology, clinical manifestations, and management.
3. Use the nursing process as a framework for care of patients with diverticulitis.
4. Compare regional enteritis and ulcerative colitis with regard to their pathophysiology, clinical manifestations, diagnostic evaluation, and medical, surgical, and nursing management.
5. Use the nursing process as a framework for care of the patient with an inflammatory bowel disease.
6. Describe the responsibilities of the nurse in meeting the needs of the patient with an ileostomy.
7. Describe the various types of intestinal obstructions and their management.
8. Use the nursing process as a framework for care of the patient with cancer of the colon or rectum.
9. Use the nursing process as a framework for care of the patient with an anorectal condition.

*D*iseases of the gastrointestinal (GI) tract account for about 10% of the total burden of illness in the United States. They account for more than 50 million office visits annually and nearly 10 million hospital admissions. GI diseases probably cost the American public up to $100 billion yearly and account for 10% of all deaths each year (Goldman & Bennett, 2000). The types of diseases and disorders that affect the lower GI tract are many and varied.

In all age groups, a fast-paced lifestyle, high levels of stress, irregular eating habits, insufficient intake of fiber and water, and lack of daily exercise contribute to GI problems. Nurses can have an impact on these chronic problems by identifying behavior patterns that put patients at risk, by educating the public about prevention and management, and by helping those affected to improve their condition and prevent complications.

Abnormalities of Fecal Elimination

Changes in patterns of fecal elimination are symptoms of functional disorders or disease of the GI tract. The most common changes seen are constipation, diarrhea, and fecal incontinence. The nurse should be aware of the possible causes and therapeutic management of these problems and of nursing management techniques. Education is important for patients with these abnormalities.

CONSTIPATION

Constipation is a term used to describe an abnormal infrequency or irregularity of defecation, abnormal hardening of stools that makes their passage difficult and sometimes painful, a decrease in stool volume, or retention of stool in the rectum for a prolonged period. Any variation from normal habits may be considered a problem.

Constipation can be caused by certain medications (ie, tranquilizers, anticholinergics, antidepressants, antihypertensives, opioids, antacids with aluminum, and iron); rectal or anal disorders (eg, hemorrhoids, fissures); obstruction (eg, cancer of the bowel); metabolic, neurologic, and neuromuscular conditions (eg, diabetes mellitus, Hirschsprung's disease, Parkinson's disease, multiple sclerosis); endocrine disorders (eg, hypothyroidism, pheochromocytoma); lead poisoning; and connective tissue disorders (eg, scleroderma, lupus erythematosus). Constipation is a major problem for patients taking opioids for chronic pain. Diseases of the colon commonly associated with constipa-

tion are irritable bowel syndrome (IBS) and diverticular disease. Constipation can also occur with an acute disease process in the abdomen (eg, appendicitis).

Other causes include weakness, immobility, debility, fatigue, and an inability to increase intra-abdominal pressure to facilitate the passage of stools, as occurs with emphysema. Many people develop constipation because they do not take the time to defecate or they ignore the urge to defecate. In the United States, constipation is also a result of dietary habits (ie, low consumption of fiber and inadequate fluid intake), lack of regular exercise, and a stress-filled life.

Perceived constipation can also be a problem. This subjective problem occurs when an individual's bowel elimination pattern is not consistent with what he or she perceives as normal. Chronic laxative use is attributed to this problem and is a major health concern in the United States, especially among the elderly population.

Pathophysiology

The pathophysiology of constipation is poorly understood, but it is thought to include interference with one of three major functions of the colon: mucosal transport (ie, mucosal secretions facilitate the movement of colon contents), myoelectric activity (ie, mixing of the rectal mass and propulsive actions), or the processes of defecation. Any of the causative factors previously identified can interfere with any of these three processes.

The urge to defecate is stimulated normally by rectal distention, which initiates a series of four actions: stimulation of the inhibitory rectoanal reflex, relaxation of the internal sphincter muscle, relaxation of the external sphincter muscle and muscles in the pelvic region, and increased intra-abdominal pressure. Interference with any of these processes can lead to constipation.

If all organic causes are eliminated, idiopathic constipation is diagnosed. If the urge to defecate is ignored, the rectal mucous membrane and musculature become insensitive to the presence of fecal masses, and consequently, a stronger stimulus is required to produce the necessary peristaltic rush for defecation. The initial effect of fecal retention is to produce irritability of the colon, which at this stage frequently goes into spasm, especially after meals, giving rise to colicky midabdominal or low abdominal pains. After several years of this process, the colon loses muscular tone and becomes essentially unresponsive to normal stimuli. Atony or decreased muscle tone occurs with aging. This also leads to constipation because the stool is retained for longer periods.

Glossary

appendicitis: infectious and inflammatory process of the appendix creating acute abdominal pain and nausea

azotorrhea: excess of nitrogenous matter in the feces or urine

colostomy: surgical opening into the colon by means of a stoma to allow drainage of bowel contents; one type of fecal diversion

diverticulitis: inflammation of a diverticulum from obstruction (by fecal matter), resulting in abscess formation

diverticulosis: presence of a number of diverticula in the intestine; common in middle age

diverticulum: saclike outpouching of the lining of the bowel protruding through the muscle of the intestinal wall, usually caused by high intraluminal pressure

hemorrhoids: dilated portions of the anal veins; can occur internal or external to the anal sphincter

ileostomy: surgical opening into the ileum by means of a stoma to allow drainage of bowel contents; one type of fecal diversion

inflammatory bowel disease: group of chronic disorders (most common are ulcerative colitis and regional enteritis [Crohn's disease]) that result in inflamma-

tion or ulceration (or both) of the bowel lining, associated with abdominal pain, diarrhea, fever, and weight loss

irritable bowel syndrome: functional disorder that affects frequency of defecation and consistency of stool; associated with crampy abdominal pain and bloating

malabsorption: impaired transport across the mucosa

peritonitis: inflammation of the lining of the abdominal cavity, usually as a result of a bacterial infection of an area in the GI tract with leakage of contents into the abdominal cavity

Clinical Manifestations

Clinical manifestations include abdominal distention, borborygmus (ie, gurgling or rumbling sound caused by passage of gas through the intestine), pain and pressure, decreased appetite, headache, fatigue, indigestion, a sensation of incomplete emptying, straining at stool, and the elimination of small-volume, hard, dry stools.

Assessment and Diagnostic Findings

Chronic constipation is usually considered idiopathic, but secondary causes should be excluded. In patients with severe, intractable constipation, further diagnostic testing is needed (Wong, 1999). The diagnosis of constipation is based on results of the patient's history, physical examination, possibly a barium enema or sigmoidoscopy, and stool testing for occult blood. These tests are completed to determine whether this symptom results from spasm or narrowing of the bowel. Anorectal manometry (ie, pressure studies) may be performed to determine malfunction of the muscle and sphincter. Defecography and bowel transit studies can also assist in the diagnosis (see Chap. 34).

Complications

Complications of constipation include hypertension, fecal impaction, hemorrhoids and fissures, and megacolon. Increased arterial pressure can occur with defecation. Straining at stool, which results in the Valsalva maneuver (ie, forcibly exhaling with the glottis closed), has a striking effect on arterial blood pressure. During active straining, the flow of venous blood in the chest is temporarily impeded because of increased intrathoracic pressure. This pressure tends to collapse the large veins in the chest. The atria and the ventricles receive less blood, and consequently less is delivered by the systolic contractions of the left ventricle. The cardiac output is decreased, and there is a transient drop in arterial pressure. Almost immediately after this period of hypotension, a rise in arterial pressure occurs; the pressure is elevated momentarily to a point far exceeding the original level (ie, rebound phenomenon). In patients with hypertension, this compensatory reaction may be exaggerated greatly, and the peaks of pressure attained may be dangerously high—sufficient to rupture a major artery in the brain or elsewhere.

Fecal impaction occurs when an accumulated mass of dry feces cannot be expelled. The mass may be palpable on digital examination, may produce pressure on the colonic mucosa that results in ulcer formation, and frequently may cause seepage of liquid stools.

Hemorrhoids and anal fissures can develop as a result of constipation. **Hemorrhoids** develop as a result of perianal vascular congestion caused by straining. Anal fissures may result from the passage of the hard stool through the anus, tearing the lining of the anal canal.

Megacolon is a dilated and atonic colon caused by a fecal mass that obstructs the passage of colon contents. Symptoms include constipation, liquid fecal incontinence, and abdominal distention. Megacolon can lead to perforation of the bowel.

Gerontologic Considerations

Physician visits for constipation are more frequent by individuals 65 years of age or older (Yamada et al., 1999). Elderly people report problems with constipation five times more frequently than younger people. A number of factors contribute to this increased frequency. People who have loose-fitting dentures or have lost their teeth have difficulty chewing and frequently choose soft, processed foods that are low in fiber. Convenience foods, also low in fiber, are widely used by those who have lost interest in eating. Some older people reduce their fluid intake if they are not eating regular meals. Lack of exercise and prolonged bed rest also contribute to constipation by decreasing abdominal muscle tone and intestinal motility as well as anal sphincter tone. Nerve impulses are dulled, and there is decreased sensation to defecate. Many older people who overuse laxatives in an attempt to have a daily bowel movement become dependent on them.

Medical Management

Treatment is aimed at the underlying cause of constipation and includes education, bowel habit training, increased fiber and fluid intake, and judicious use of laxatives. Management may also include discontinuing laxative abuse. Routine exercise to strengthen abdominal muscles is encouraged. Biofeedback is a technique that can be used to help patients learn to relax the sphincter mechanism to expel stool. Daily addition to the diet of 6 to 12 teaspoonfuls of unprocessed bran is recommended, especially for the treatment of constipation in the elderly. If laxative use is necessary, one of the following may be prescribed: bulk-forming agents, saline and osmotic agents, lubricants, stimulants, or fecal softeners. The physiologic action and patient education information related to these laxatives are identified in Table 38-1. Enemas and rectal suppositories are generally not recommended for constipation and should be reserved for the treatment of impaction or for preparing the bowel for surgery or diagnostic procedures. If long-term laxative use is necessary, a bulk-forming agent may be prescribed in combination with an osmotic laxative.

Doctors prescribe the use of specific medications to enhance colonic transit by increasing propulsive motor activity. Further studies are being carried out on cholinergic agents (eg, bethanechol), cholinesterase inhibitors (eg, neostigmine), and prokinetic agents (eg, metoclopramide) to determine the role these agents can play in treating constipation (Yamada et al., 1999).

Nursing Management

The nurse elicits information about the onset and duration of constipation, current and past elimination patterns, the patient's expectation of normal bowel elimination, and lifestyle information (eg, exercise and activity level, occupation, food and fluid intake, and stress level) during the health history interview. Past medical and surgical history, current medications, and laxative and enema use are important, as is information about the sensation of rectal pressure or fullness, abdominal pain, excessive straining at defecation, and flatulence.

Patient education and health promotion are important functions of the nurse (Chart 38-1). After the health history is obtained, the nurse sets specific goals for teaching. Goals for the patient include restoring or maintaining a regular pattern of elimination, ensuring adequate intake of fluids and high-fiber foods, learning about methods to avoid constipation, relieving anxiety about bowel elimination patterns, and avoiding complications.

DIARRHEA

Diarrhea is increased frequency of bowel movements (more than three per day), increased amount of stool (more than 200 g per day), and altered consistency (ie, looseness) of stool. It is usually associated with urgency, perianal discomfort, incontinence, or a combination of these factors. Any condition that causes increased intestinal secretions, decreased mucosal absorption, or altered

Table 38-1 • **Laxatives: Classification, Agent, Action, and Patient Education**

CLASSIFICATION	SAMPLE AGENT	ACTION	PATIENT EDUCATION
Bulk forming	Psyllium hydrophilic mucilloid (Metamucil)	Polysaccharides and cellulose derivatives mix with intestinal fluids, swell, and stimulate peristalsis.	Take with 8 oz water and follow with 8 oz water; do not take dry. Report abdominal distention or unusual amount of flatulence.
Saline agent	Magnesium hydroxide (Milk of Magnesia)	Nonabsorbable magnesium ions alter stool consistency by drawing water into the intestines by osmosis; peristalsis is stimulated. Action occurs within 2 h.	The liquid preparation is more effective than the tablet form. Only short-term use is recommended because of toxicity (CNS or neuromuscular depression, electrolyte imbalance). Magnesium laxatives should not be taken by patients with renal insufficiency.
Lubricant	Mineral oil	Nonabsorbable hydrocarbons soften fecal matter by lubricating the intestinal mucosa; the passage of stool is facilitated. Action occurs within 6–8 h.	Do not take with meals, because mineral oils can impair the absorption of fat-soluble vitamins and delay gastric emptying. Swallow carefully, because drops of oil that gain access to the pharynx can produce a lipid pneumonia.
Stimulant	Bisacodyl (Dulcolax)	Irritates the colon epithelium by stimulating sensory nerve endings and increasing mucosal secretions. Action occurs within 6–8 h.	Catharsis may cause fluid and electrolyte imbalance, especially in the elderly. Tablets should be swallowed, not crushed or chewed. Avoid milk or antacids within 1 hour of taking the medication, because the enteric coating may dissolve prematurely.
Fecal softener	Dioctyl sodium sulfosuccinate (Colace)	Hydrates the stool by its surfactant action on the colonic epithelium (increases the wetting efficiency of intestinal water); aqueous and fatty substances are mixed. Does not exert a laxative action.	Can be used safely by patients who should avoid straining (cardiac patients, patients with anorectal disorders).
Osmotic agent	Polyethylene glycol and electrolytes (Colyte)	Cleanses colon rapidly and induces diarrhea.	This is a large-volume product. It takes time to consume it safely. It can cause considerable nausea and bloating.

motility can produce diarrhea. Irritable bowel syndrome (IBS), inflammatory bowel disease (IBD), and lactose intolerance are frequently the underlying disease processes that cause diarrhea (Stone et al., 1999).

Diarrhea can be acute or chronic. Acute diarrhea is most often associated with infection and is usually self-limiting; chronic diarrhea persists for a longer period and may return sporadically. Diarrhea can be caused by certain medications (eg, thyroid hormone replacement, stool softeners and laxatives, antibiotics, chemotherapy, antacids), certain tube feeding formulas, metabolic and endocrine disorders (eg, diabetes, Addison's disease, thyrotoxicosis), and viral or bacterial infectious processes (eg, dysentery, shigellosis, food poisoning). Other disease processes associated with diarrhea are nutritional and malabsorptive disorders (eg, celiac disease), anal sphincter defect, Zollinger-Ellison syndrome, paralytic ileus, intestinal obstruction, and acquired immunodeficiency syndrome (AIDS).

Pathophysiology

Types of diarrhea include secretory, osmotic, and mixed diarrhea. Secretory diarrhea is usually high-volume diarrhea and is caused by increased production and secretion of water and electrolytes by the intestinal mucosa into the intestinal lumen. Osmotic diarrhea occurs when water is pulled into the intestines by the osmotic pressure of unabsorbed particles, slowing the reabsorption of water. Mixed diarrhea is caused by increased peristalsis (usually from IBD) and a combination of increased secretion and decreased absorption in the bowel. The physiology of diarrhea related to infection is discussed in Chapter 70.

Clinical Manifestations

In addition to the increased frequency and fluid content of stools, the patient usually has abdominal cramps, distention, intestinal rumbling (ie, borborygmus), anorexia, and thirst. Painful spasmodic

---

Chart 38-1
Health Promotion: Preventing Constipation

- Describe the physiology of defecation.
- Emphasize the importance of heeding the urge to defecate.
- Discuss normal variations in patterns of defecation.
- Teach how to establish a bowel routine, and explain that having a regular time for defecation (eg, best time is after breakfast) may aid in initiating the reflex.
- Provide dietary information; suggest eating high-residue, high-fiber foods, adding bran daily (must be introduced gradually), and increasing fluid intake (unless contraindicated).
- Explain how an exercise regimen, increased ambulation, and abdominal muscle toning will increase muscle strength and help propel colon contents.
- Describe abdominal toning exercises (contracting abdominal muscles 4 times daily and leg-to-chest lifts 10 to 20 times each day).
- Explain that the normal position (semisquatting) maximizes use of abdominal muscles and force of gravity.

contractions of the anus and ineffectual straining (ie, tenesmus) may occur with defecation. Other symptoms depend on the cause and severity of the diarrhea but are related to dehydration and to fluid and electrolyte imbalances.

Watery stools are characteristic of small bowel disease, whereas loose, semisolid stools are associated more often with disorders of the colon. Voluminous, greasy stools suggest intestinal malabsorption, and the presence of mucus and pus in the stools suggests inflammatory enteritis or colitis. Oil droplets on the toilet water are almost always diagnostic of pancreatic insufficiency. Nocturnal diarrhea may be a manifestation of diabetic neuropathy.

Assessment and Diagnostic Findings

When the cause of the diarrhea is not obvious, the following diagnostic tests may be performed: complete blood cell count, chemical profile, urinalysis, routine stool examination, and stool examinations for infectious or parasitic organisms, bacterial toxins, blood, fat, and electrolytes. Endoscopy or barium enema may assist in identifying the cause.

Complications

Complications of diarrhea include the potential for cardiac dysrhythmias because of significant fluid and electrolyte loss (especially loss of potassium). Urinary output of less than 30 mL per hour for 2 to 3 consecutive hours, muscle weakness, paresthesia, hypotension, anorexia, and drowsiness with a potassium level of less than 3.0 mEq/L (3 mmol/L) must be reported. Decreased potassium levels cause cardiac dysrhythmias (ie, atrial and ventricular tachycardia, ventricular fibrillation, and premature ventricular contractions) that can lead to death.

Medical Management

Primary management is directed at controlling symptoms, preventing complications, and eliminating or treating the underlying disease. Certain medications (eg, antibiotics, anti-inflammatory agents) may reduce the severity of the diarrhea and treat the underlying disease.

Nursing Management

The nurse's role includes assessing and monitoring the characteristics and pattern of diarrhea. A health history addresses the patient's medication therapy, medical and surgical history, and dietary patterns and intake. Reports of recent exposure to an acute illness or recent travel to another geographic area are important. Assessment includes abdominal auscultation and palpation for abdominal tenderness. Inspection of the abdomen and mucous membranes and skin is important to determine hydration status. Stool samples are obtained for testing.

During an episode of acute diarrhea, the nurse encourages bed rest and intake of liquids and foods low in bulk until the acute attack subsides. When food intake is tolerated, the nurse recommends a bland diet of semisolid and solid foods. The patient should avoid caffeine, carbonated beverages, and very hot and very cold foods, because they stimulate intestinal motility. It may be necessary to restrict milk products, fat, whole-grain products, fresh fruits, and vegetables for several days. The nurse administers antidiarrheal medications such as diphenoxylate (Lomotil) and loperamide (Imodium) as prescribed. Intravenous fluid therapy may be necessary for rapid rehydration, especially for the elderly and those with preexisting GI conditions (eg, IBD). It is important to closely monitor serum electrolyte levels. The nurse immediately reports evidence of dysrhythmias or a change in the level of consciousness.

> **NURSING ALERT** Elderly persons can become dehydrated quickly and develop low potassium levels (ie, hypokalemia) as a result of diarrhea. The older person taking digitalis must be aware of how quickly dehydration and hypokalemia can occur with diarrhea. The nurse instructs this person to recognize the signs of hypokalemia, because low levels of potassium intensify the action of digitalis, which can lead to digitalis toxicity.

The perianal area may become excoriated because diarrheal stool contains digestive enzymes that can irritate the skin. The patient should follow a perianal skin care routine to decrease irritation and excoriation. It is important to use skin sealants and moisture barriers as needed. The older person's skin is very sensitive because of decreased turgor and reduced subcutaneous fat layers.

FECAL INCONTINENCE

The term *fecal incontinence* describes the involuntary passage of stool from the rectum. Several factors influence fecal continence—the ability of the rectum to sense and accommodate stool, the amount and consistency of stool, the integrity of the anal sphincters and musculature, and rectal motility.

Pathophysiology

Fecal incontinence can result from trauma (eg, after surgical procedures involving the rectum), a neurologic disorder (eg, stroke, multiple sclerosis, diabetic neuropathy, dementia), inflammation, infection, radiation treatment, fecal impaction, pelvic floor relaxation, laxative abuse, medications, or advancing age (ie, weakness or loss of anal or rectal muscle tone). It is an embarrassing and socially incapacitating problem that requires a many-tiered approach to treatment and much adaptation on the patient's part.

Clinical Manifestations

Patients may have minor soiling, occasional urgency and loss of control, or complete incontinence. Patients may also experience poor control of flatus, diarrhea, or constipation.

Assessment and Diagnostic Findings

Diagnostic studies are necessary because the treatment of fecal incontinence depends on the cause. A rectal examination and other endoscopic examinations such as a flexible sigmoidoscopy are performed to rule out tumors, inflammation, or fissures. X-ray studies such as barium enema, computed tomography (CT) scans, anorectal manometry, and transit studies may be helpful in identifying alterations in intestinal mucosa and muscle tone or in detecting other structural or functional problems.

Medical Management

Although there is no known cause or cure for fecal incontinence, specific management techniques can help the patient achieve a better quality of life. If fecal incontinence is related to diarrhea, the incontinence may disappear when diarrhea is successfully treated. Fecal incontinence is frequently a symptom of a fecal impaction. After the impaction is removed and the rectum is cleansed, normal functioning of the anorectal area can resume. If the fecal incontinence is related to a more permanent condition, other treatments are initiated. Biofeedback therapy can be of assistance if the problem is decreased sensory awareness or sphincter control. Bowel training programs can also be effective. Surgical procedures include surgical reconstruction, sphincter repair, or fecal diversion.

Nursing Management

The nurse takes a thorough health history, including information about previous surgical procedures, chronic illnesses, bowel habits and problems, and current medication regimen. The nurse also completes an examination of the rectal area.

The nurse initiates a bowel-training program that involves setting a schedule to establish bowel regularity. The goal is to assist the patient to achieve fecal continence. If this is not possible, the goal should be to manage the problem so the person can have predictable, planned elimination (Stone et al., 1999). Sometimes, it is necessary to use suppositories to stimulate the anal reflex. After the patient has achieved a regular schedule, the suppository can be discontinued. Biofeedback can be used in conjunction with these therapies to help the patient improve sphincter contractility and rectal sensitivity.

Fecal incontinence can also cause problems with perineal skin integrity. Maintaining skin integrity is a priority, especially in the debilitated or elderly patient. Incontinence briefs, although helpful in containing the fecal material, allow for increased skin contact with the feces and may cause excoriation of the skin. The nurse encourages and teaches meticulous skin hygiene.

Continence sometimes cannot be achieved, and the nurse assists the patient and family to accept and cope with this chronic situation. The patient can use fecal incontinence devices, which include external collection devices and internal drainage systems. External devices are special pouches that are drainable. They are attached to a synthetic adhesive skin barrier specially designed to conform to the buttocks. Internal drainage systems can be used to eliminate fecal skin contact and are especially useful when there is extensive excoriation or skin breakdown. A large catheter is inserted into the rectum and is connected to a drainage system.

IRRITABLE BOWEL SYNDROME

IBS is one of the most common GI problems. Approximately one in six otherwise healthy persons report classic symptoms of IBS (Wolfe, 2000). It occurs more commonly in women than in men, and the cause is still unknown. Although no anatomic or biochemical abnormalities have been found that explain the common symptoms, various factors are associated with the syndrome: heredity, psychological stress or conditions such as depression and anxiety, a diet high in fat and stimulating or irritating foods, alcohol consumption, and smoking. The small intestine has become a focus of investigation as an additional site of dysmotility in IBS, and cluster contractions in the jejunum and ileum are being studied (Wolfe, 2000). The diagnosis is made only after tests have been completed that prove the absence of structural or other disorders.

Pathophysiology

IBS results from a functional disorder of intestinal motility. The change in motility may be related to the neurologic regulatory system, infection or irritation, or a vascular or metabolic disturbance. The peristaltic waves are affected at specific segments of the intestine and in the intensity with which they propel the fecal matter forward. There is no evidence of inflammation or tissue changes in the intestinal mucosa.

Clinical Manifestations

There is a wide variability in symptom presentation. Symptoms range in intensity and duration from mild and infrequent to severe and continuous. The primary symptom is an alteration in bowel patterns—constipation, diarrhea, or a combination of both. Pain, bloating, and abdominal distention often accompany this change in bowel pattern. The abdominal pain is sometimes precipitated by eating and is frequently relieved by defecation.

Assessment and Diagnostic Findings

A definite diagnosis of IBS requires tests that prove the absence of structural or other disorders. Stool studies, contrast x-ray studies, and proctoscopy may be performed to rule out other colon diseases. Barium enema and colonoscopy may reveal spasm, distention, or mucus accumulation in the intestine (Fig. 38-1). Manometry and electromyography are used to study intraluminal pressure changes generated by spasticity.

Medical Management

The goals of treatment are aimed at relieving abdominal pain, controlling the diarrhea or constipation, and reducing stress. Restriction and then gradual reintroduction of foods that are possibly irritating may help determine what types of food are acting as irritants (eg, beans, caffeinated products, fried foods, alcohol, spicy foods). A healthy, high-fiber diet is prescribed to help control the diarrhea and constipation. Exercise can assist in reducing anxiety and increasing intestinal motility. Patients often find it helpful to participate in a stress reduction or behavior-modification program.

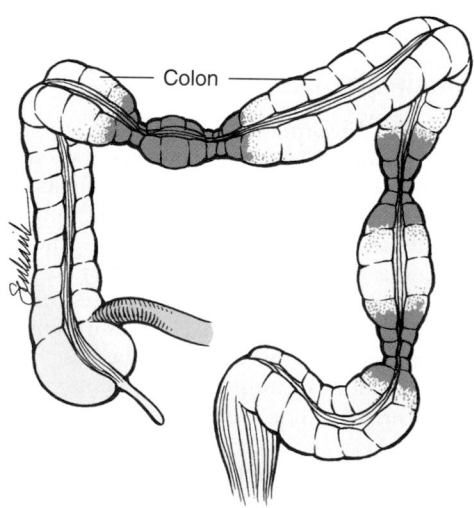

Colon

FIGURE 38-1 In IBS, the spastic contractions of the bowel can be seen in x-ray contrast studies.

Hydrophilic colloids (ie, bulk) and antidiarrheal agents (eg, loperamide) may be given to control the diarrhea and fecal urgency. Antidepressants can assist in treating underlying anxiety and depression. Anticholinergics and calcium channel blockers decrease smooth muscle spasm, decreasing cramping and constipation.

Nursing Management

The nurse's role is to provide patient and family education. The nurse emphasizes teaching and reinforces good dietary habits. The patient is encouraged to eat at regular times and to chew food slowly and thoroughly. The patient should understand that, although adequate fluid intake is necessary, fluid should not be taken with meals because this results in abdominal distention. Alcohol use and cigarette smoking are discouraged.

CONDITIONS OF MALABSORPTION

Malabsorption is the inability of the digestive system to absorb one or more of the major vitamins (especially vitamin B_{12}), minerals (ie, iron and calcium), and nutrients (ie, carbohydrates, fats, and proteins). Interruptions in the complex digestive process may occur anywhere in the digestive system and cause decreased absorption. Diseases of the small intestine are the most common cause of malabsorption.

Pathophysiology

The conditions that cause malabsorption can be grouped into the following categories:

- Mucosal (transport) disorders causing generalized malabsorption (eg, celiac sprue, regional enteritis, radiation enteritis)
- Infectious diseases causing generalized malabsorption (eg, small bowel bacterial overgrowth, tropical sprue, Whipple's disease)
- Luminal problems causing malabsorption (eg, bile acid deficiency, Zollinger-Ellison syndrome, pancreatic insufficiency)
- Postoperative malabsorption (eg, after gastric or intestinal resection)
- Disorders that cause malabsorption of specific nutrients (eg, disaccharidase deficiency leading to lactose intolerance)

Table 38-2 lists the clinical and pathologic aspects of malabsorptive diseases.

Clinical Manifestations

The hallmarks of malabsorption syndrome from any cause are diarrhea or frequent, loose, bulky, foul-smelling stools that have increased fat content and are often grayish. Patients often have associated abdominal distention, pain, increased flatus, weakness, weight loss, and a decreased sense of well-being. The chief result of malabsorption is malnutrition, manifested by weight loss and other signs of vitamin and mineral deficiency (eg, easy bruising, osteoporosis, anemia). Patients with a malabsorption syndrome, if untreated, become weak and emaciated because of starvation and dehydration. Failure to absorb the fat-soluble vitamins A, D, and K causes a corresponding avitaminosis.

Assessment and Diagnostic Findings

Several diagnostic tests may be prescribed, including stool studies for quantitative and qualitative fat analysis, lactose tolerance tests, D-xylose absorption tests, and Schilling tests. The hydrogen breath test that is used to evaluate carbohydrate absorption (see Chap. 34) is performed if carbohydrate malabsorption is suspected. Endoscopy with biopsy of the mucosa is the best diagnostic tool. Biopsy of the small intestine is performed to assay enzyme activity or to identify infection or destruction of mucosa. Ultrasound studies, CT scans, and x-ray findings can reveal pancreatic or intestinal tumors that may be the cause. A complete blood cell count is used to detect anemia. Pancreatic function tests can assist in the diagnosis of specific disorders.

Medical Management

Intervention is aimed at avoiding dietary substances that aggravate malabsorption and at supplementing nutrients that have been lost. Common supplements are water-soluble vitamins (eg, B_{12}, folic acid), fat-soluble vitamins (ie, A, D, and K), and minerals (eg, calcium, iron). Primary disease states may be managed surgically or nonsurgically. Dietary therapy is aimed at reducing gluten intake in patients with celiac sprue. Folic acid supplements are prescribed for patients with tropical sprue. Antibiotics (eg, tetracycline, ampicillin) are sometimes needed in the treatment of tropical sprue and bacterial overgrowth syndromes. Antidiarrheal agents may be used to decrease intestinal spasms. Parenteral fluids may be necessary to treat dehydration.

Nursing Management

The nurse provides patient and family education regarding diet and the use of nutritional supplements (Chart 38-2). It is important to monitor patients with diarrhea for fluid and electrolyte imbalances. The nurse conducts ongoing assessments to determine if the clinical manifestations related to the nutritional deficits have abated. Patient education includes information about the risk of osteoporosis related to malabsorption of calcium.

Acute Inflammatory Intestinal Disorders

Any part of the lower GI tract is susceptible to acute inflammation caused by bacterial, viral, or fungal infection. Two such situations are appendicitis and diverticulitis. These two conditions can lead to **peritonitis**, an inflammatory process within the abdomen.

APPENDICITIS

The appendix is a small, finger-like appendage about 10 cm (4 in) long that is attached to the cecum just below the ileocecal valve. The appendix fills with food and empties regularly into the cecum. Because it empties inefficiently and its lumen is small, the appendix is prone to obstruction and is particularly vulnerable to infection (ie, appendicitis).

Appendicitis, the most common cause of acute abdomen in the United States, is the most common reason for emergency abdominal surgery. About 7% of the population will have appendicitis at some time in their lives; males are affected more than females, and teenagers more than adults. Although it can occur at any age, it occurs most frequently between the ages of 10 and 30 years (Yamada et al., 1999).

Pathophysiology

The appendix becomes inflamed and edematous as a result of either becoming kinked or occluded by a fecalith (ie, hardened mass of stool), tumor, or foreign body. The inflammatory process

Table 38-2 • **Characteristics of Diseases of Malabsorption**

DISEASES/DISORDERS	PHYSIOLOGIC PATHOLOGY	CLINICAL FEATURES
Gastric resection with gastrojejunostomy	Decreased pancreatic stimulation because of duodenal bypass; poor mixing of food, bile, pancreatic enzymes; decreased intrinsic factor	Weight loss, moderate steatorrhea, anemia (combination of iron deficiency, vitamin B_{12} malabsorption, folate deficiency)
Pancreatic insufficiency (chronic pancreatitis, pancreatic carcinoma, pancreatic resection, cystic fibrosis)	Reduced intraluminal pancreatic enzyme activity, with maldigestion of lipids and proteins	History of abdominal pain followed by weight loss; marked steatorrhea, **azotorrhea** (excess of nitrogenous matter in the feces or urine); also frequent glucose intolerance (70% in pancreatic insufficiency)
Ileal dysfunction (resection or disease)	Loss of ileal absorbing surface leads to reduced bile-salt pool size and reduced vitamin B_{12} absorption; bile in colon inhibits fluid absorption	Diarrhea, weight loss with steatorrhea, especially when greater than 100 cm resection, decreased vitamin B_{12} absorption
Stasis syndromes (surgical strictures, blind loops, enteric fistulas, multiple jejunal diverticula, scleroderma)	Overgrowth of intraluminal intestinal bacteria, especially anaerobic organisms, to greater than 10^6/mL results in deconjugation of bile salts, leading to decreased effective bile-salt pool size, also bacterial utilization of vitamin B_{12}	Weight loss, steatorrhea; low vitamin B_{12} absorption; may have low D-xylose absorption
Zollinger-Ellison syndrome	Hyperacidity in duodenum inactivates pancreatic enzymes	Ulcer diathesis, steatorrhea
Lactose intolerance	Deficiency of intestinal lactase results in high concentration of intraluminal lactose with osmotic diarrhea	Varied degrees of diarrhea and cramps after ingestion of lactose-containing foods; positive lactose intolerance test, decreased intestinal lactase
Celiac disease (gluten enteropathy)	Toxic response to a gluten fraction by surface epithelium results in destruction of absorbing surface	Weight loss, diarrhea, bloating, anemia (low iron, folate), osteomalacia, steatorrhea, azotorrhea, low D-xylose absorption; folate and iron malabsorption
Tropical sprue	Unknown toxic factor results in mucosal inflammation, partial villous atrophy	Weight loss, diarrhea, anemia (low folate, vitamin B_{12}); steatorrhea; low D-xylose absorption, low vitamin B_{12} absorption
Whipple's disease	Bacterial invasion of intestinal mucosa	Arthritis, hyperpigmentation, lymphadenopathy, serous effusions, fever, weight loss; steatorrhea, azotorrhea
Certain parasitic diseases (giardiasis, strongyloidiasis, coccidiosis, capillariasis)	Damage to or invasion of surface mucosa	Diarrhea, weight loss; steatorrhea; organism may be seen on jejunal biopsy or recovered in stool
Immunoglobulinopathy	Decreased local intestinal defenses, lymphoid hyperplasia, lymphopenia	Frequent association with *Giardia*: hypogammaglobulinemia or isolated IgA deficiency

increases intraluminal pressure, initiating a progressively severe, generalized or upper abdominal pain that becomes localized in the right lower quadrant of the abdomen within a few hours. Eventually, the inflamed appendix fills with pus.

Clinical Manifestations

Vague epigastric or periumbilical pain progresses to right lower quadrant pain and is usually accompanied by a low-grade fever and nausea and sometimes by vomiting. Loss of appetite is common. Local tenderness is elicited at McBurney's point when pressure is applied (Fig. 38-2). Rebound tenderness (ie, production or intensification of pain when pressure is released) may be present. The extent of tenderness and muscle spasm and the existence of constipation or diarrhea depend not so much on the severity of the appendiceal infection as on the location of the appendix. If the appendix curls around behind the cecum, pain and tenderness may be felt in the lumbar region. If its tip is in the pelvis, these signs may be elicited only on rectal examination. Pain on

defecation suggests that the tip of the appendix is resting against the rectum; pain on urination suggests that the tip is near the bladder or impinges on the ureter. Some rigidity of the lower portion of the right rectus muscle may occur. Rovsing's sign may be elicited by palpating the left lower quadrant; this paradoxically causes pain to be felt in the right lower quadrant (see Fig. 38-2). If the appendix has ruptured, the pain becomes more diffuse; abdominal distention develops as a result of paralytic ileus, and the patient's condition worsens.

Constipation can also occur with an acute process such as appendicitis. Laxatives administered in this instance may produce perforation of the inflamed appendix. In general, a laxative or cathartic should never be given while the person has fever, nausea, or pain.

Assessment and Diagnostic Findings

Diagnosis is based on results of a complete physical examination and on laboratory and x-ray findings. The complete blood cell count demonstrates an elevated white blood cell count. The leukocyte

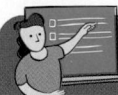

count may exceed 10,000 cells/mm³, and the neutrophil count may exceed 75%. Abdominal x-ray films, ultrasound studies, and CT scans may reveal a right lower quadrant density or localized distention of the bowel.

Complications

The major complication of appendicitis is perforation of the appendix, which can lead to peritonitis or an abscess. The incidence of perforation is 10% to 32%. The incidence is higher in young children and the elderly. Perforation generally occurs 24 hours after the onset of pain. Symptoms include a fever of 37.7°C (100°F) or higher, a toxic appearance, and continued abdominal pain or tenderness.

Gerontologic Considerations

Acute appendicitis does not occur frequently in the elderly population. Classic signs and symptoms are altered and may vary greatly. Pain may be absent or minimal. Symptoms may be vague, suggesting bowel obstruction or another process. Fever and leukocytosis may not be present. As a result, diagnosis and prompt treatment may be delayed, causing potential complications and mortality. The patient may have no symptoms until the appendix ruptures. The incidence of perforated appendix is higher in the elderly population because many of these patients do not seek health care as quickly as younger patients.

Medical Management

Surgery is indicated if appendicitis is diagnosed. To correct or prevent fluid and electrolyte imbalance and dehydration, antibiotics and intravenous fluids are administered until surgery is performed. Analgesics can be administered after the diagnosis is made. Appendectomy (ie, surgical removal of the appendix) is performed as soon as possible to decrease the risk of perforation. It may be performed under a general or spinal anesthetic with a low abdominal incision or by laparoscopy.

Nursing Management

Goals include relieving pain, preventing fluid volume deficit, reducing anxiety, eliminating infection from the potential or actual disruption of the GI tract, maintaining skin integrity, and attaining optimal nutrition.

The nurse prepares the patient for surgery, which includes an intravenous infusion to replace fluid loss and promote adequate renal function and antibiotic therapy to prevent infection. If there is evidence or likelihood of paralytic ileus, a nasogastric tube is inserted. An enema is not administered because it can lead to perforation.

After surgery, the nurse places the patient in a semi-Fowler position. This position reduces the tension on the incision and abdominal organs, helping to reduce pain. An opioid, usually morphine sulfate, is prescribed to relieve pain. When tolerated, oral fluids are administered. Any patient who was dehydrated before surgery receives intravenous fluids. Food is provided as desired and tolerated on the day of surgery.

The patient may be discharged on the day of surgery if the temperature is within normal limits, there is no undue discomfort in the operative area, and the appendectomy was uncomplicated. Discharge teaching for the patient and family is imperative. The nurse instructs the patient to make an appointment to have the surgeon remove the sutures between the fifth and seventh days after surgery. Incision care and activity guidelines are discussed; normal activity can usually be resumed within 2 to 4 weeks.

If there is a possibility of peritonitis, a drain is left in place at the area of the incision. Patients at risk for this complication may be kept in the hospital for several days and are monitored carefully for signs of intestinal obstruction or secondary hemorrhage. Secondary abscesses may form in the pelvis, under the diaphragm, or

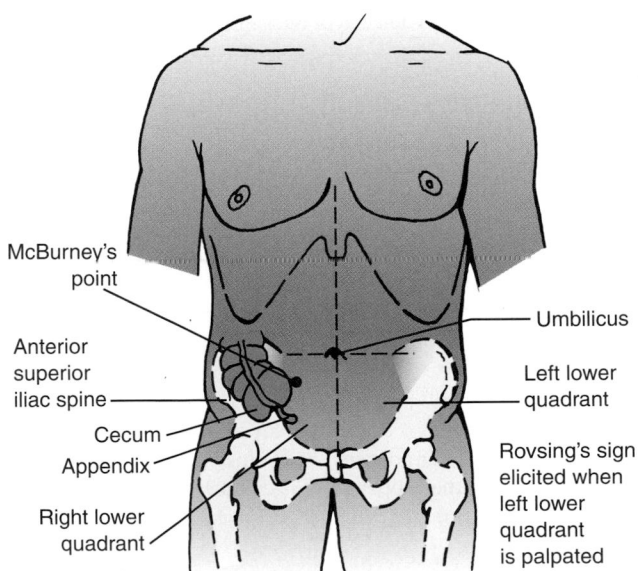

FIGURE 38-2 When the appendix is inflamed, tenderness can be noted in the right lower quadrant at McBurney's point, which is between the umbilicus and the anterior superior iliac spine. Rovsing's sign is pain felt in the right lower quadrant after the left lower quadrant has been palpated.

in the liver, elevating the temperature and pulse rate and increasing the leukocyte count.

When the patient is ready for discharge, the nurse teaches the patient and family to care for the incision and perform dressing changes and irrigations as prescribed. A home care nurse may be needed to assist with this care and to monitor the patient for complications and wound healing. Other potential complications of appendectomy are listed in Table 38-3.

DIVERTICULAR DISEASE

A **diverticulum** is a saclike outpouching of the lining of the bowel that extends through a defect in the muscle layer. Diverticula may occur anywhere along the GI tract. **Diverticulosis** exists when multiple diverticula are present without inflammation or symptoms. Diverticular disease of the colon is very common in developed countries, and its prevalence increases with age. More than 35% of Americans older than 60 years of age have diverticulosis. The incidence increases to 50% among those in the ninth decade of life (Keighley, 1999). **Diverticulitis** results when food and bacteria retained in a diverticulum produce infection and inflammation that can impede drainage and lead to perforation or abscess formation. Diverticulitis is most common (95%) in the sigmoid colon. Approximately 20% of patients with diverticulosis have diverticulitis at some point. A congenital predisposition is suspected when the disorder occurs in those younger than 40 years of age. A low intake of dietary fiber is considered a predisposing factor, but the exact cause is unknown. Diverticulitis may occur in acute attacks or may persist as a continuing, smoldering infection. Most patients remain entirely asymptomatic. The symptoms manifested generally result from its potential complications—abscesses, fistulas, obstruction, and hemorrhage.

Pathophysiology

A diverticulum forms when the mucosa and submucosal layers of the colon herniate through the muscular wall because of high intraluminal pressure, low volume in the colon (ie, fiber-deficient contents), and decreased muscle strength in the colon wall (ie, muscular hypertrophy from hardened fecal masses). Bowel contents can accumulate in the diverticulum and decompose, causing inflammation and infection. A diverticulum can become obstructed and then inflamed if the obstruction continues. The inflammation tends to spread to the surrounding bowel wall, giving rise to irritability and spasticity of the colon (ie, diverticulitis). Abscesses develop and may eventually perforate, leading to peritonitis and erosion of the blood vessels (arterial) with bleeding.

Clinical Manifestations

Chronic constipation often precedes the development of diverticulosis by many years. Frequently, no problematic symptoms occur with diverticulosis. Signs of acute diverticulosis are bowel irregularity and intervals of diarrhea, abrupt onset of crampy pain in the left lower quadrant of the abdomen, and a low-grade fever. The patient may have nausea and anorexia, and some bloating or abdominal distention may occur. With repeated local inflammation of the diverticula, the large bowel may narrow with fibrotic strictures, leading to cramps, narrow stools, and increased constipation. Weakness, fatigue, and anorexia are common symptoms. With acute diverticulosis, the patient reports mild to severe pain in the lower left quadrant. The condition, if untreated, can lead to septicemia.

Assessment and Diagnostic Findings

A CT scan is the procedure of choice and can reveal abscesses. Abdominal x-ray findings may demonstrate free air under the diaphragm if a perforation has occurred from the diverticulitis. Diverticulosis may be diagnosed using barium enema, which shows narrowing of the colon and thickened muscle layers. If there are symptoms of peritoneal irritation and when the diagnosis is diverticulitis, barium enema is contraindicated because of the potential for perforation.

A colonoscopy may be performed if there is no acute diverticulitis or after resolution of an acute episode to visualize the colon, determine the extent of the disease, and rule out other conditions. Laboratory tests that assist in diagnosis include a complete blood cell count, revealing an elevated leukocyte count, and elevated sedimentation rate.

Table 38-3 • **Potential Complications and Nursing Interventions After Appendectomy**

COMPLICATION	NURSING INTERVENTIONS
Peritonitis	Observe for abdominal tenderness, fever, vomiting, abdominal rigidity, and tachycardia. Employ constant nasogastric suction. Correct dehydration as prescribed. Administer antibiotic agents as prescribed.
Pelvic abscess	Evaluate for anorexia, chills, fever, and diaphoresis. Observe for diarrhea, which may indicate pelvic abscess. Prepare patient for rectal examination. Prepare patient for surgical drainage procedure.
Subphrenic abscess (abscess under the diaphragm)	Assess patient for chills, fever, and diaphoresis. Prepare for x-ray examination. Prepare for surgical drainage of abscess.
Ileus (paralytic and mechanical)	Assess for bowel sounds. Employ nasogastric intubation and suction. Replace fluids and electrolytes by intravenous route as prescribed. Prepare for surgery, if diagnosis of mechanical ileus is established.

Complications

Complications of diverticulitis include peritonitis, abscess formation, and bleeding. If an abscess develops, the associated findings are tenderness, a palpable mass, fever, and leukocytosis. An inflamed diverticulum that perforates results in abdominal pain localized over the involved segment, usually the sigmoid; local abscess or peritonitis follows. Abdominal pain, a rigid boardlike abdomen, loss of bowel sounds, and signs and symptoms of shock occur with peritonitis. Noninflamed or slightly inflamed diverticula may erode areas adjacent to arterial branches, causing massive rectal bleeding.

 ## Gerontologic Considerations

The incidence of diverticular disease increases with age because of degeneration and structural changes in the circular muscle layers of the colon and because of cellular hypertrophy. The symptoms are less pronounced in the elderly than in other adults. The elderly may not have abdominal pain until infection occurs. They may delay reporting symptoms because they fear surgery or are afraid that they may have cancer. Blood in the stool is overlooked frequently, especially in the elderly, because of a failure to examine the stool or the inability to see changes because of diminished vision.

Medical Management

DIETARY AND MEDICATION MANAGEMENT

Diverticulitis can usually be treated on an outpatient basis with diet and medicine therapy. When symptoms occur, rest, analgesics, and antispasmodics are recommended. Initially, the diet is clear liquid until the inflammation subsides; then, a high-fiber, low-fat diet is recommended. This type of diet helps to increase stool volume, decrease colonic transit time, and reduce intraluminal pressure. Antibiotics are prescribed for 7 to 10 days. A bulk-forming laxative also is prescribed.

In acute cases of diverticulitis with significant symptoms, hospitalization is required. Hospitalization is often indicated for those who are elderly, immunocompromised, or taking corticosteroids. Withholding oral intake, administering intravenous fluids, and instituting nasogastric suctioning if vomiting or distention occurs rests the bowel. Broad-spectrum antibiotics are prescribed for 7 to 10 days. An opioid is prescribed for pain relief; morphine is not used because it increases segmentation and intraluminal pressures. Oral intake is increased as symptoms subside. A low-fiber diet may be necessary until signs of infection decrease.

Antispasmodics such as propantheline bromide (Pro-Banthine) and oxyphencyclimine (Daricon) may be prescribed. Normal stools can be achieved by using bulk preparations (Metamucil) or stool softeners (Colace), by instilling warm oil into the rectum, or by inserting an evacuant suppository (Dulcolax). Such a prophylactic plan can reduce the bacterial flora of the bowel, diminish the bulk of the stool, and soften the fecal mass so that it moves more easily through the area of inflammatory obstruction.

SURGICAL MANAGEMENT

Although acute diverticulitis usually subsides with medical management, immediate surgical intervention is necessary if complications (eg, perforation, peritonitis, abscess formation, hemorrhage, obstruction) occur. Alternatively, when the acute episode of diverticulitis resolves, surgery may be recommended to prevent repeated episodes. Two types of surgery are considered:

- One-stage resection in which the inflamed area is removed and a primary end-to-end anastomosis is completed

- Multiple-staged procedures for complications such as obstruction or perforation (Fig. 38-3)

The type of surgery performed depends on the extent of complications found during surgery. When possible, the area of diverticulitis is resected and the remaining bowel is joined end to end (ie, primary resection and end-to-end anastomosis). This is performed through traditional surgical or laparoscopically assisted colectomy. A two-stage resection may be performed in which the diseased colon is resected (as in a one-stage procedure) but no anastomosis is performed; both ends of the bowel are brought out onto the abdomen as stomas. This "double-barrel" colostomy is then reanastomosed in a later procedure. Fecal diversion procedures are discussed later in this chapter.

NURSING PROCESS:
THE PATIENT WITH DIVERTICULITIS

Assessment

During the health history, the nurse asks the patient about the onset and duration of pain and about past and present elimination patterns. The nurse reviews dietary habits to determine fiber intake and asks the patient about straining at stool, history of constipation with periods of diarrhea, tenesmus (ie, spasms of the anal sphincter with pain and persistent urge to defecate), abdominal bloating, and distention.

Assessment includes auscultation for the presence and character of bowel sounds and palpation for lower left quadrant pain, tenderness, or firm mass. The stool is inspected for pus, mucus, or blood. It is important to monitor temperature, pulse, and blood pressure for abnormal variations.

Diagnosis

NURSING DIAGNOSES

Based on the assessment data, the nursing diagnoses may include the following:

- Constipation related to narrowing of the colon from thickened muscular segments and strictures
- Acute pain related to inflammation and infection

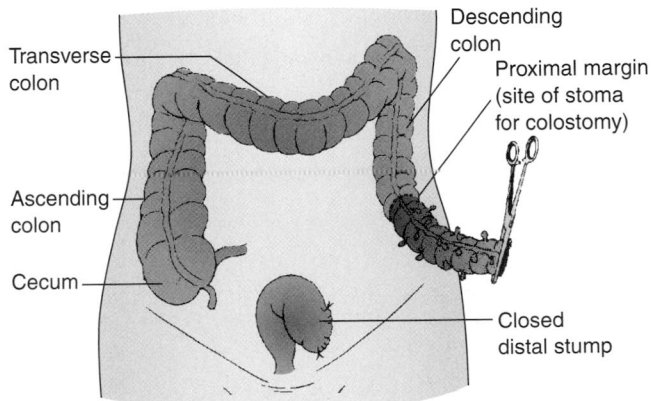

FIGURE 38-3 The Hartmann procedure for diverticulitis: primary resection for diverticulitis of the colon. The affected segment (*clamp attached*) has been divided at its distal end. In a primary anastomosis, the proximal margin (*dotted line*) is transected and the bowel attached end-to-end. In a two-stage procedure, a colostomy is constructed at the proximal margin with the distal stump oversewn (Hartmann procedure, as shown) or brought to the outer surface as a mucous fistula. The second stage consists of colostomy takedown and anastomosis.

COLLABORATIVE PROBLEMS/ POTENTIAL COMPLICATIONS

Potential complications that may develop include the following:

- Peritonitis
- Abscess formation
- Bleeding

Planning and Goals

The major goals for the patient may include attainment and maintenance of normal elimination patterns, pain relief, and absence of complications.

Nursing Interventions

MAINTAINING NORMAL ELIMINATION PATTERNS

The nurse recommends a fluid intake of 2 L per day (within limits of the patient's cardiac and renal reserve) and suggests foods that are soft but have increased fiber to increase the bulk of the stool and facilitate peristalsis, thereby promoting defecation. An individualized exercise program is encouraged to improve abdominal muscle tone. It is important to review the patient's daily routine to establish a schedule for meals and a set time for defecation and to assist in identifying habits that may have suppressed the urge to defecate. The nurse encourages daily intake of bulk laxatives such as Metamucil, which helps to propel feces through the colon. Stool softeners are administered as prescribed to decrease straining at stool, which decreases intestinal pressure. Oil retention enemas may be prescribed to soften the stool, making it easier to pass.

RELIEVING PAIN

Analgesics (eg, meperidine) to relieve the pain of diverticulitis and antispasmodic agents to decrease intestinal spasm are administered as prescribed. The nurse records the intensity, duration, and location of pain to determine if the inflammatory process worsens or subsides.

MONITORING AND MANAGING POTENTIAL COMPLICATIONS

The major nursing focus is to prevent complications by identifying patients at risk and managing their symptoms as needed. The nurse assesses for the following signs of perforation:

- Increased abdominal pain and tenderness accompanied by abdominal rigidity
- Elevated white blood cell count
- Elevated sedimentation rate
- Increased temperature
- Tachycardia
- Hypotension

Perforation is a surgical emergency. The clinical manifestations of perforation and peritonitis and the care of the patient with peritonitis are presented in the next section. The nurse monitors vital signs and urine output and administers intravenous fluids to replace volume loss as needed.

HOME AND COMMUNITY-BASED CARE

Because patients and their family members and health care providers tend to focus on the most obvious needs and issues, the nurse reminds the patient and family about the importance of continuing health promotion and screening practices. The nurse educates patients who have not been involved in these practices in the past about their importance and refers the patients to appropriate health care providers.

Evaluation

EXPECTED PATIENT OUTCOMES

Expected patient outcomes may include the following:

1. Attains a normal pattern of elimination
   a. Reports less abdominal cramping and pain
   b. Reports the passage of soft, formed stool without pain
   c. Adds unprocessed bran to foods
   d. Drinks at least 10 glasses of fluid each day (if fluid intake is tolerated)
   e. Exercises daily
2. Reports decreased pain
   a. Requests analgesics as needed
   b. Adheres to a low-fiber diet during acute episodes
3. Recovers without complications
   a. Is afebrile
   b. Has normal blood pressure
   c. Has a soft, nontender abdomen with normal bowel sounds
   d. Maintains adequate urine output
   e. Has no blood in the stool

PERITONITIS

Peritonitis is inflammation of the peritoneum, the serous membrane lining the abdominal cavity and covering the viscera. Usually, it is a result of bacterial infection; the organisms come from diseases of the GI tract or, in women, from the internal reproductive organs. Peritonitis can also result from external sources such as injury or trauma (eg, gunshot wound, stab wound) or an inflammation that extends from an organ outside the peritoneal area, such as the kidney. The most common bacteria implicated are *Escherichia coli, Klebsiella, Proteus,* and *Pseudomonas.* Inflammation and paralytic ileus are the direct effects of the infection. Other common causes of peritonitis are appendicitis, perforated ulcer, diverticulitis, and bowel perforation (Fig. 38-4). Peritonitis may also be associated with abdominal surgical procedures and peritoneal dialysis.

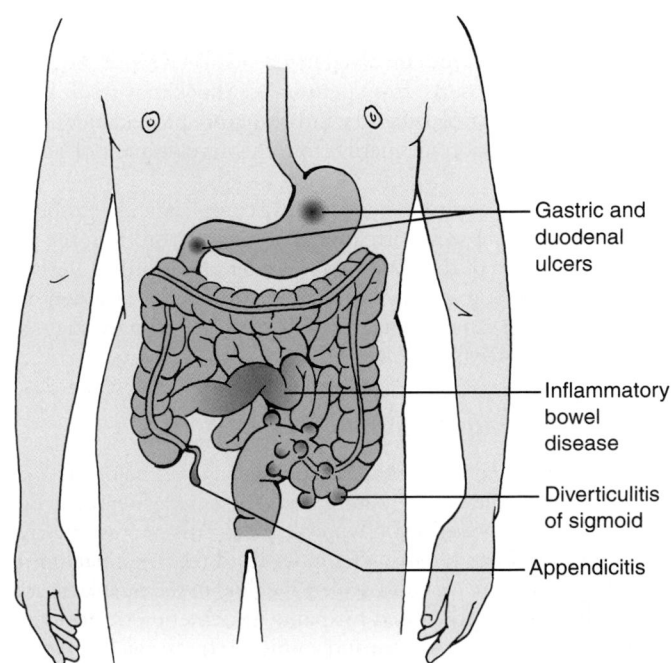

FIGURE 38-4 Common gastrointestinal causes of peritonitis.

Gastric and duodenal ulcers

Inflammatory bowel disease

Diverticulitis of sigmoid

Appendicitis

Pathophysiology

Peritonitis is caused by leakage of contents from abdominal organs into the abdominal cavity, usually as a result of inflammation, infection, ischemia, trauma, or tumor perforation. Bacterial proliferation occurs. Edema of the tissues results, and exudation of fluid develops in a short time. Fluid in the peritoneal cavity becomes turbid with increasing amounts of protein, white blood cells, cellular debris, and blood. The immediate response of the intestinal tract is hypermotility, soon followed by paralytic ileus with an accumulation of air and fluid in the bowel.

Clinical Manifestations

Symptoms depend on the location and extent of the inflammation. The early clinical manifestations of peritonitis frequently are the symptoms of the disorder causing the condition. At first, a diffuse type of pain is felt. The pain tends to become constant, localized, and more intense near the site of the inflammation. Movement usually aggravates it. The affected area of the abdomen becomes extremely tender and distended, and the muscles become rigid. Rebound tenderness and paralytic ileus may be present. Usually, nausea and vomiting occur and peristalsis is diminished. The temperature and pulse rate increase, and there is almost always an elevation of the leukocyte count.

Assessment and Diagnostic Findings

The leukocyte count is elevated. The hemoglobin and hematocrit levels may be low if blood loss has occurred. Serum electrolyte studies may reveal altered levels of potassium, sodium, and chloride.

An abdominal x-ray is obtained, and findings may show air and fluid levels as well as distended bowel loops. A CT scan of the abdomen may show abscess formation. Peritoneal aspiration and culture and sensitivity studies of the aspirated fluid may reveal infection and identify the causative organisms.

Complications

Frequently, the inflammation is not localized and the whole abdominal cavity becomes involved in a generalized sepsis. Sepsis is the major cause of death from peritonitis. Shock may result from septicemia or hypovolemia. The inflammatory process may cause intestinal obstruction, primarily from the development of bowel adhesions.

The two most common postoperative complications are wound evisceration and abscess formation. Any suggestion from the patient that an area of the abdomen is tender or painful or "feels as if something just gave way" must be reported. The sudden occurrence of serosanguineous wound drainage strongly suggests wound dehiscence (see Chap. 20).

Medical Management

Fluid, colloid, and electrolyte replacement is the major focus of medical management. The administration of several liters of an isotonic solution is prescribed. Hypovolemia occurs because massive amounts of fluid and electrolytes move from the intestinal lumen into the peritoneal cavity and deplete the fluid in the vascular space.

Analgesics are prescribed for pain. Antiemetics are administered as prescribed for nausea and vomiting. Intestinal intubation and suction assist in relieving abdominal distention and in promoting intestinal function. Fluid in the abdominal cavity can cause pressure that restricts expansion of the lungs and causes respiratory distress. Oxygen therapy by nasal cannula or mask can promote adequate oxygenation, but airway intubation and ventilatory assistance occasionally are required.

Massive antibiotic therapy is usually initiated early in the treatment of peritonitis. Large doses of a broad-spectrum antibiotic are administered intravenously until the specific organism causing the infection is identified and the appropriate antibiotic therapy can be initiated.

Surgical objectives include removing the infected material and correcting the cause. Surgical treatment is directed toward excision (ie, appendix), resection with or without anastomosis (ie, intestine), repair (ie, perforation), and drainage (ie, abscess). With extensive sepsis, a fecal diversion may need to be created.

Nursing Management

Ongoing assessment of pain, vital signs, GI function, and fluid and electrolyte balance is important. The nurse reports the nature of the pain, its location in the abdomen, and any shifts in location. Administering analgesic medication and positioning the patient for comfort are helpful in decreasing pain. The patient is placed on the side with knees flexed; this position decreases tension on the abdominal organs. Accurate recording of all intake and output and central venous pressure assists in calculating fluid replacement. The nurse administers and monitors closely intravenous fluids.

Signs that indicate that peritonitis is subsiding include a decrease in temperature and pulse rate, softening of the abdomen, return of peristaltic sounds, passing of flatus, and bowel movements. The nurse increases fluid and food intake gradually and reduces parenteral fluids as prescribed. A worsening clinical condition may indicate a complication, and the nurse must prepare the patient for emergency surgery.

Drains are frequently inserted during the surgical procedure, and the nurse must observe and record the character of the drainage postoperatively. Care must be taken when moving and turning the patient to prevent the drains from being dislodged. It is also important for the nurse to prepare the patient and family for discharge by teaching the patient to care for the incision and drains if the patient will be sent home with the drains still in place.

Inflammatory Bowel Disease

The term **inflammatory bowel disease** refers to two chronic inflammatory GI disorders: regional enteritis (ie, Crohn's disease or granulomatous colitis) and ulcerative colitis. Both disorders have striking similarities but also several differences. Table 38-4 compares regional enteritis and ulcerative colitis.

The incidence of IBD in the United States has increased in the past century; 10,000 to 15,000 new cases occur annually (Yamada et al., 1999). In the past, a higher rate was observed among Caucasians in general and the Jewish population in particular. Data now indicate a higher risk for African Americans and a lower risk for Jewish people, and women appear to be at higher risk than before. People between the ages of 10 and 30 are at greatest risk.

Despite vast amounts of research, the cause of IBD is still unknown. Researchers think it is triggered by environmental agents such as pesticides, food additives, tobacco, and radiation (Kirsner & Shorter, 2000). Nonsteroidal anti-inflammatory drugs have been found to exacerbate IBD. Allergies and immune disorders have also been suggested as causes. Abnormal response to dietary

Table 38-4 • **Comparison of Regional Enteritis and Ulcerative Colitis**

FACTOR	REGIONAL ENTERITIS	ULCERATIVE COLITIS
Course	Prolonged, variable	Exacerbations, remissions
Pathology		
Early	Transmural thickening	Mucosal ulceration
Late	Deep, penetrating granulomas	Mucosal minute ulceration
Clinical Manifestations		
Location	Ileum, right colon (usually)	Rectum, left colon
Bleeding	Usually not, but may occur	Common—severe
Perianal involvement	Common	Rare—mild
Fistulas	Common	Rare
Rectal involvement	About 20%	Almost 100%
Diarrhea	Less severe	Severe
Diagnostic Study Findings		
Radiography	Regional, discontinuous lesions	Diffuse involvement
	Narrowing of colon	No narrowing of colon
	Thickening of bowel wall	No mucosal edema
	Mucosal edema	Stenosis rare
	Stenosis, fistulas	Shortening of colon
Sigmoidoscopy	May be unremarkable unless accompanied by perianal fistulas	Abnormal inflamed mucosa
Colonoscopy	Distinct ulcerations separated by relatively normal mucosa in right colon	Friable mucosa with pseudopolyps or ulcers in left colon
Therapeutic Management	Corticosteroids, sulfonamides (sulfasalazine [Azulfidine])	Corticosteroids, sulfonamides; sulfasalazine useful in preventing recurrence
	Antibiotics	Bulk hydrophilic agents
	Parenteral nutrition	Antibiotics
	Partial or complete colectomy, with ileostomy or anastomosis	Proctocolectomy, with ileostomy
	Rectum can be preserved in some patients	Rectum can be preserved in only a few patients "cured" by colectomy
	Recurrence common	
Systemic Complications	Small bowel obstruction	Toxic megacolon
	Right-sided hydronephrosis	Perforation
	Nephrolithiasis	Hemorrhage
	Cholelithiasis	Malignant neoplasms
	Arthritis	Pyelonephritis
	Retinitis, iritis	Nephrolithiasis
	Erythema nodosum	Cholangiocarcinoma
		Arthritis
		Retinitis, iritis
		Erythema nodosum

or bacterial antigens has been studied extensively, and genetic factors also are being studied. There is a high prevalence of coexistent IBS, which complicates the overall symptom presentation.

REGIONAL ENTERITIS (CROHN'S DISEASE)

Regional enteritis commonly occurs in adolescents or young adults but can appear at any time of life. It is more common in women, and it occurs frequently in the older population (between the ages of 50 and 80). It can occur anywhere along the GI tract, but the most common areas are the distal ileum and colon. The incidence of Crohn's disease has risen over the past 30 years. Crohn's disease is seen two times more often in patients who smoke than in nonsmokers (Rose, 1998).

Pathophysiology

Regional enteritis is a subacute and chronic inflammation that extends through all layers (ie, transmural lesion) of the bowel wall from the intestinal mucosa. It is characterized by periods of remissions and exacerbations. The disease process begins with edema and thickening of the mucosa. Ulcers begin to appear on the inflamed mucosa. These lesions are not in continuous contact with one another and are separated by normal tissue. Fistulas, fissures, and abscesses form as the inflammation extends into the peritoneum. Granulomas occur in one half of patients. In advanced cases, the intestinal mucosa has a cobblestone appearance. As the disease advances, the bowel wall thickens and becomes fibrotic, and the intestinal lumen narrows. Diseased bowel loops sometimes adhere to other loops surrounding them.

Clinical Manifestations

In regional enteritis, the onset of symptoms is usually insidious, with prominent lower right quadrant abdominal pain and diarrhea unrelieved by defecation. Scar tissue and the formation of granulomas interfere with the ability of the intestine to transport products of the upper intestinal digestion through the constricted lumen, resulting in crampy abdominal pains. There is abdominal tenderness and spasm. Because eating stimulates intestinal peristalsis, the crampy pains occur after meals. To avoid these bouts of crampy pain, the patient tends to limit food intake, reducing the amounts and types of food to such a degree that normal nutritional requirements are not met. The result is weight loss, malnutrition, and secondary anemia. Ulcers in the membranous lining of the intestine and other inflammatory changes result in a weeping, swollen intestine that continually empties an irritating discharge into the colon. Disrupted absorption causes chronic diarrhea and nutritional deficits. The result is a person who is thin and emaciated from inadequate food intake and constant fluid loss. In some patients, the inflamed intestine may perforate, leading to intra-abdominal and anal abscesses. Fever and leukocytosis occur. Chronic symptoms include diarrhea, abdominal pain, steatorrhea, anorexia, weight loss, and nutritional deficiencies.

Abscesses, fistulas, and fissures are common. Symptoms extend beyond the GI tract and commonly include joint involvement (eg, arthritis), skin lesions (eg, erythema nodosum), ocular disorders (eg, conjunctivitis), and oral ulcers. The clinical course and symptoms can vary; in some patients, periods of remission and exacerbation occur, but in others, the disease follows a fulminating course.

Assessment and Diagnostic Findings

A proctosigmoidoscopic examination is usually performed initially to determine whether the rectosigmoid area is inflamed. A stool examination is also performed; the result may be positive for occult blood and steatorrhea (ie, excessive fat in the feces). The most conclusive diagnostic aid for regional enteritis is a barium study of the upper GI tract that shows the classic "string sign" on an x-ray film of the terminal ileum, indicating the constriction of a segment of intestine. Endoscopy and intestinal biopsy may be used for confirmation of the diagnosis. A barium enema may show ulcerations (the cobblestone appearance described earlier), fissures, and fistulas. A CT scan may show bowel wall thickening and fistula tracts.

A complete blood cell count is performed to assess hematocrit and hemoglobin levels (usually decreased) and the white blood cell count (may be elevated). The sedimentation rate is usually elevated. Albumin and protein levels may be decreased, indicating malnutrition.

Complications

Complications of regional enteritis include intestinal obstruction or stricture formation, perianal disease, fluid and electrolyte imbalances, malnutrition from malabsorption, and fistula and abscess formation. A fistula is an abnormal communication between two body structures, either internal (ie, between two structures) or external (ie, between an internal structure and the outside surface of the body). The most common type of small bowel fistula that results from regional enteritis is the enterocutaneous fistula (ie, between the small bowel and the skin). Abscesses can be the result of an internal fistula tract into an area that results in fluid accumulation and infection. Patients with regional enteritis are also at increased risk for colon cancer.

ULCERATIVE COLITIS

Ulcerative colitis is a recurrent ulcerative and inflammatory disease of the mucosal and submucosal layers of the colon and rectum. The incidence of ulcerative colitis is highest in Caucasians and people of Jewish heritage (Yamada et al., 1999). The peak incidence is between 30 and 50 years of age. It is a serious disease, accompanied by systemic complications and a high mortality rate. Eventually, 10% to 15% of the patients develop carcinoma of the colon.

Pathophysiology

Ulcerative colitis affects the superficial mucosa of the colon and is characterized by multiple ulcerations, diffuse inflammations, and desquamation or shedding of the colonic epithelium. Bleeding occurs as a result of the ulcerations. The mucosa becomes edematous and inflamed. The lesions are contiguous, occurring one after the other. Abscesses form, and infiltrate is seen in the mucosa and submucosa with clumps of neutrophils in the crypt lumens (ie, crypt abscesses). The disease process usually begins in the rectum and spreads proximally to involve the entire colon. Eventually, the bowel narrows, shortens, and thickens because of muscular hypertrophy and fat deposits.

Clinical Manifestations

The clinical course is usually one of exacerbations and remissions. The predominant symptoms of ulcerative colitis are diarrhea, lower left quadrant abdominal pain, intermittent tenesmus, and rectal bleeding. The bleeding may be mild or severe, and pallor results. The patient may have anorexia, weight loss, fever, vomiting, and dehydration, as well as cramping, the feeling of an urgent need to defecate, and the passage of 10 to 20 liquid stools each day. The disease is classified as mild, severe, or fulminant, depending on the severity of the symptoms. Hypocalcemia and anemia frequently develop. Rebound tenderness may occur in the right lower quadrant. Extraintestinal symptoms include skin lesions (eg, erythema nodosum), eye lesions (eg, uveitis), joint abnormalities (eg, arthritis), and liver disease.

Assessment and Diagnostic Findings

The patient should be assessed for tachycardia, hypotension, tachypnea, fever, and pallor. Other assessments include the level of hydration and nutritional status. The abdomen should be examined for characteristics of bowel sounds, distention, and tenderness. These findings assist in determining the severity of the disease.

The stool is positive for blood, and laboratory test results reveal a low hematocrit and hemoglobin concentration in addition to an elevated white blood cell count, low albumin levels, and an electrolyte imbalance. Abdominal x-ray studies are useful for determining the cause of symptoms. Free air in the peritoneum and bowel dilation or obstruction should be excluded as a source of the presenting symptoms. Sigmoidoscopy or colonoscopy and barium enema are valuable in distinguishing this condition from other diseases of the colon with similar symptoms. A barium enema may show mucosal irregularities, focal strictures or fistulas, shortening of the colon, and dilation of bowel loops. Endoscopy may reveal friable, inflamed mucosa with exudate and ulcerations. This procedure assists in defining the extent and severity of the disease. CT scanning, magnetic resonance imaging, and ultrasound can identify abscesses and perirectal involvement. Leukocyte scanning (see Chap. 34) is useful when severe colitis prohibits the use of endoscopy to determine the extent of inflammation.

Careful stool examination for parasites and other microbes is performed to rule out dysentery caused by common intestinal organisms, especially *Entamoeba histolytica* and *Clostridium difficile*.

Complications

Complications of ulcerative colitis include toxic megacolon, perforation, and bleeding as a result of ulceration, vascular engorgement, and highly vascular granulation tissue. In toxic megacolon, the inflammatory process extends into the muscularis, inhibiting its ability to contract and resulting in colonic distention. Symptoms include fever, abdominal pain and distention, vomiting, and fatigue. Colonic perforation from toxic megacolon is associated with a high mortality rate (15% to 50%) (Grendell et al., 1998). If the patient with toxic megacolon does not respond within 24 to 48 hours to medical management with nasogastric suction, intravenous fluids with electrolytes, corticosteroids, and antibiotics, surgery is required. Total colectomy is indicated. For many patients, surgery becomes necessary to relieve the effects of the disease and to treat these serious complications; an ileostomy usually is performed. The surgical procedures involved and the care of patients with this type of fecal diversion are discussed later in this chapter.

Patients with IBD also have a significantly increased risk of osteoporotic fractures due to decreased bone mineral density. Corticosteroid therapy may also contribute to the diminished bone mass.

Medical Management of Chronic Inflammatory Bowel Disease

Medical treatment for regional enteritis and ulcerative colitis is aimed at reducing inflammation, suppressing inappropriate immune responses, providing rest for a diseased bowel so that healing may take place, improving quality of life, and preventing or minimizing complications.

Most patients maintain long-term well-being interspersed with short intervals of illness (Hanauer, 2001). Management depends on the disease location, severity, and complications.

NUTRITIONAL THERAPY

Oral fluids and a low-residue, high-protein, high-calorie diet with supplemental vitamin therapy and iron replacement are prescribed to meet nutritional needs, reduce inflammation, and control pain and diarrhea. Fluid and electrolyte imbalances from dehydration caused by diarrhea are corrected by intravenous therapy as necessary if the patient is hospitalized or by oral supplementation if the patient can be managed at home. Any foods that exacerbate diarrhea are avoided. Milk may contribute to diarrhea in those with lactose intolerance. Cold foods and smoking are avoided because

both increase intestinal motility. Parenteral nutrition may be indicated.

PHARMACOLOGIC THERAPY

Sedatives and antidiarrheal and antiperistaltic medications are used to minimize peristalsis to rest the inflamed bowel. They are continued until the patient's stools approach normal frequency and consistency.

Aminosalicylate formulations such as sulfasalazine (Azulfidine) are often effective for mild or moderate inflammation and are used to prevent or reduce recurrences in long-term maintenance regimens. Newer sulfa-free aminosalicylates (eg, mesalamine [Asacol, Pentasa]) have been developed and shown effective in preventing and treating recurrence of inflammation (Wolfe, 2000). Antibiotics are used for secondary infections, particularly for purulent complications such as abscesses, perforation, and peritonitis.

Corticosteroids are used to treat severe and fulminant disease. These corticosteroids (eg, prednisone) can be administered orally in outpatient treatment or parenterally in hospitalized patients. Topical (ie, rectal administration) corticosteroids are also widely used in the treatment of distal colon disease. When the dosage of corticosteroids is reduced or stopped, the symptoms of disease may return. If corticosteroids are continued, adverse sequelae such as hypertension, fluid retention, cataracts, hirsutism (ie, abnormal hair growth), adrenal suppression, and loss of bone density may develop.

Immunomodulators (eg, azathioprene [Imuran], 6-mercaptopurine, methotrexate, cyclosporin) have been used to alter the immune response (Wolfe, 2000). The exact mechanism of action of these medications in treating IBD is unknown. They are used for patients with severe disease who have failed other therapies. These medications are useful in maintenance regimens to prevent relapses. Newer biologic therapies are being studied, and it is hoped that they will lead to improvement in the treatment of patients with chronically active disease (Yamada et al., 1999).

SURGICAL MANAGEMENT

When nonsurgical measures fail to relieve the severe symptoms of IBD, surgery may be recommended. The most common indications for surgery are medically intractable disease, poor quality of life, or complications from the disease or medical therapy (Wolfe, 2000).

More than one half of all patients with regional enteritis require surgery at some point. Recurrence of inflammation and disease after surgery in regional enteritis is inevitable. The rate of recurrence after surgery is 20% to 40% in the first 5 years. Patients younger than 25 years of age have the highest recurrence rate. Surgery for regional enteritis is indicated for refractory disease or complications (Wolfe, 2000). The procedure of choice is a total colectomy and ileostomy.

A newer surgical procedure developed for patients with severe regional enteritis is intestinal transplant. This technique is now available to children and to young and middle-age adults who have lost intestinal function from disease. Although not a cure, this procedure may eventually provide improvement in quality of life for some who are terminally ill. The technical and immunologic problems with this procedure remain formidable, and the costs and mortality rates remain high (Wolfe, 2000).

Approximately 15% to 20% of patients with ulcerative colitis require surgical intervention (Tierney et al., 2000). Indications for surgery include lack of improvement and continued deterioration, profuse bleeding, perforation, stricture formation, and cancer. Surgical excision usually improves quality of life.

Proctocolectomy with ileostomy (ie, complete excision of colon, rectum, and anus) is recommended when the rectum is severely involved.

One type of surgical technique that can be helpful is strictureplasty, in which the blocked or narrowed section of the bowel is widened, leaving the bowel intact. If a lesion can be delineated in regional enteritis or if a complication has occurred, the lesion is resected, and the remaining portions of the bowel are anastomosed. Surgical removal of up to 50% of the small bowel usually can be tolerated. Other types of surgical procedures, known as fecal diversions, are discussed later in this chapter.

Total Colectomy With Ileostomy. An **ileostomy**, the surgical creation of an opening into the ileum or small intestine (usually by means of an ileal stoma on the abdominal wall), is commonly performed after a total colectomy (ie, excision of the entire colon). It allows for drainage of fecal matter (ie, effluent) from the ileum to the outside of the body. The drainage is very mushy and occurs at frequent intervals. Nursing management of the patient with an ileostomy is discussed in a later section of this chapter.

Total Colectomy With Continent Ileostomy. Another procedure involves the removal of the entire colon and creation of the continent ileal reservoir (ie, Kock pouch). This procedure eliminates the need for an external fecal collection bag. Approximately 30 cm of the distal ileum is reconstructed to form a reservoir with a nipple valve that is created by pulling a portion of the terminal ileal loop back into the ileum. GI effluent can accumulate in the pouch for several hours and then be removed by means of a catheter inserted through the nipple valve. The major problem with the Kock pouch is malfunction of the nipple valve, which occurs in about 20% of the patients (Yamada et al., 1999).

Total Colectomy With Ileoanal Anastomosis. A total colectomy with ileoanal anastomosis is another surgical procedure that eliminates the need for a permanent ileostomy. It establishes an ileal reservoir, and anal sphincter control of elimination is retained. The procedure involves connecting a portion of the ileum to the anus (ie, ileoanal anastomosis) in conjunction with removal of the colon and the rectal mucosa (ie, total abdominal colectomy and mucosal proctectomy) (Fig. 38-5). A temporary diverting loop ileostomy is constructed at the time of surgery and closed about 3 months later.

With ileoanal anastomosis, the diseased colon and rectum are removed, voluntary defecation is maintained, and anal continence is preserved. The ileal reservoir decreases the number of bowel movements by 50%, from approximately 14 to 20 per day to 7 to 10 per day. Nighttime elimination is gradually reduced to one bowel movement. Complications of ileoanal anastomosis include irritation of the perianal skin from leakage of fecal contents, stricture formation at the anastomosis site, and small bowel obstruction.

Nursing Management

Nursing management of patients with IBD may be medical, surgical, or both. Patients in the community setting or those recently diagnosed may primarily require education about diet and medications and referral to support groups. Hospitalized patients with long-standing or severe disease also require careful monitoring, parenteral nutrition, fluid replacement, and possibly emergent surgery. The surgical procedures may involve a fecal diversion,

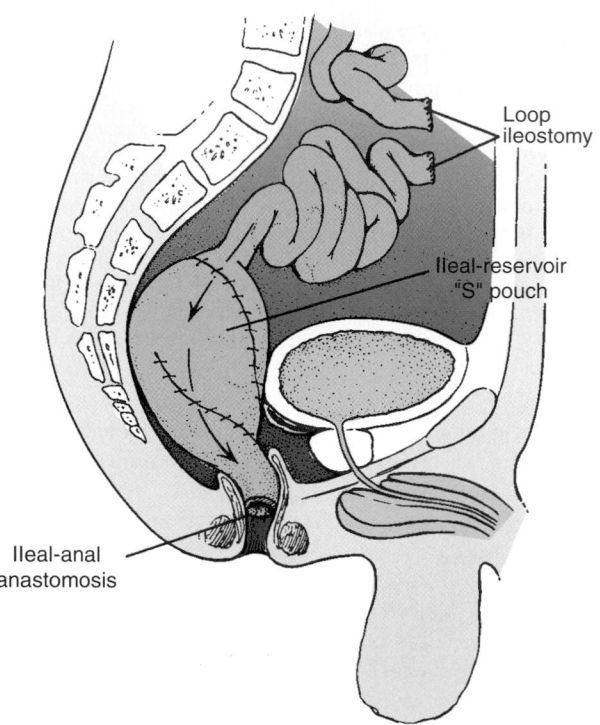

FIGURE 38-5 A mucosal proctectomy precedes anastomosis of the ileal reservoir. A temporary loop ileostomy diverts effluent for several months.

with attendant needs for physical care, emotional support, and extensive teaching about management of the ostomy.

NURSING PROCESS: MANAGEMENT OF THE PATIENT WITH INFLAMMATORY BOWEL DISEASE

Assessment

The nurse takes a health history to identify the onset, duration, and characteristics of abdominal pain; the presence of diarrhea or fecal urgency, straining at stool (tenesmus), nausea, anorexia, or weight loss; and family history of IBD. It is important to discuss dietary patterns, including the amounts of alcohol, caffeine, and nicotine containing products used daily and weekly. The nurse asks about patterns of bowel elimination, including character, frequency, and presence of blood, pus, fat, or mucus. It is important to note allergies and food intolerance, especially milk (lactose) intolerance. The patient may identify sleep disturbances if diarrhea or pain occurs at night.

Assessment includes auscultating the abdomen for bowel sounds and their characteristics; palpating the abdomen for distention, tenderness, or pain; and inspecting the skin for evidence of fistula tracts or symptoms of dehydration. The stool is inspected for blood and mucus.

With regional enteritis, pain is usually localized in the right lower quadrant, where hyperactive bowel sounds can be heard because of borborygmus and increased peristalsis. Abdominal tenderness is noticed on palpation. The most prominent symptom is intermittent pain that occurs with diarrhea but does not decrease after defecation. Pain in the periumbilical region usually indicates involvement of the terminal ileum. With ulcerative colitis, the abdomen may be distended, and rebound tenderness may be present. Rectal bleeding is a significant sign.

Diagnosis

NURSING DIAGNOSES

Based on the assessment data, the nursing diagnoses may include the following:

- Diarrhea related to the inflammatory process
- Acute pain related to increased peristalsis and GI inflammation
- Deficient fluid volume deficit related to anorexia, nausea, and diarrhea
- Imbalanced nutrition, less than body requirements, related to dietary restrictions, nausea, and malabsorption
- Activity intolerance related to fatigue
- Anxiety related to impending surgery
- Ineffective coping related to repeated episodes of diarrhea
- Risk for impaired skin integrity related to malnutrition and diarrhea
- Risk for ineffective therapeutic regimen management related to insufficient knowledge concerning the process and management of the disease

COLLABORATIVE PROBLEMS/ POTENTIAL COMPLICATIONS

Potential complications that may develop include the following:

- Electrolyte imbalance
- Cardiac dysrhythmia related to electrolyte depletion
- GI bleeding with fluid volume loss
- Perforation of the bowel

Planning and Goals

The major goals for the patient include attainment of normal bowel elimination patterns, relief of abdominal pain and cramping, prevention of fluid volume deficit, maintenance of optimal nutrition and weight, avoidance of fatigue, reducing anxiety, promoting effective coping, absence of skin breakdown, learning about the disease process and therapeutic regimen, and avoidance of complications.

Nursing Interventions

MAINTAINING NORMAL ELIMINATION PATTERNS

The nurse determines if there is a relationship between diarrhea and certain foods, activity, or emotional stress. Identifying precipitating factors, the frequency of bowel movements, and the character, consistency, and amount of stool passed is important. The nurse provides ready access to a bathroom, commode, or bedpan and keeps the environment clean and odor free. It is important to administer antidiarrheal medications as prescribed, to record the frequency and consistency of stools after therapy is initiated, and to encourage bed rest to decrease peristalsis.

RELIEVING PAIN

The character of the pain is described as dull, burning, or crampy. Asking about its onset is relevant. Does it occur before or after meals, during the night, or before elimination? Is the pattern constant or intermittent? Is it relieved with medications? The nurse administers anticholinergic medications as prescribed 30 minutes before a meal to decrease intestinal motility and administers analgesics as prescribed for pain. Position changes, local application of heat (as prescribed), diversional activities, and the prevention of fatigue also are helpful for reducing pain.

MAINTAINING FLUID INTAKE

To detect fluid volume deficit, the nurse keeps an accurate record of oral and intravenous fluids and maintains a record of output (ie, urine, liquid stool, vomitus, and wound or fistula drainage). The nurse monitors daily weights for fluid gains or losses and assesses the patient for signs of fluid volume deficit (ie, dry skin and mucous membranes, decreased skin turgor, oliguria, exhaustion, decreased temperature, increased hematocrit, elevated urine specific gravity, and hypotension). It is important to encourage oral intake of fluids and to monitor the intravenous flow rate. The nurse initiates measures to decrease diarrhea (eg, dietary restrictions, stress reduction, antidiarrheal agents).

MAINTAINING OPTIMAL NUTRITION

Parenteral nutrition (PN) is used when the symptoms of IBD are severe. With PN, the nurse maintains an accurate record of fluid intake and output as well as the patient's daily weight. The patient should gain 0.5 kg daily during PN therapy. Because PN is very high in glucose and can cause hyperglycemia, blood glucose levels are monitored every 6 hours. Elemental feedings high in protein and low in fat and residue are instituted after PN therapy because they are digested primarily in the jejunum, do not stimulate intestinal secretions, and allow the bowel to rest. The nurse notes intolerance if the patient exhibits nausea, vomiting, diarrhea, or abdominal distention.

If oral foods are tolerated, small, frequent, low-residue feedings are given to avoid overdistending the stomach and stimulating peristalsis. It is important for the patient to restrict activity to conserve energy, reduce peristalsis, and reduce calorie requirements.

PROMOTING REST

The nurse recommends intermittent rest periods during the day and schedules or restricts activities to conserve energy and reduce the metabolic rate. It is important to encourage activity within the limits of the patient's capacity. The nurse suggests bed rest for a patient who is febrile, has frequent diarrheal stools, or is bleeding. The patient on bed rest should perform active exercises to maintain muscle tone and prevent thromboembolic complications. If the patient is unable to perform these active exercises, the nurse performs passive exercises and joint range of motion. Activity restrictions are modified as needed on a day-to-day basis.

REDUCING ANXIETY

Rapport can be established by being attentive and displaying a calm, confident manner. The nurse allows time for the patient to ask questions and express feelings. Careful listening and sensitivity to nonverbal indicators of anxiety (eg, restlessness, tense facial expressions) are helpful. The patient may be emotionally labile because of the consequences of the disease; the nurse tailors information about possible impending surgery to the patient's level of understanding and desire for detail. If surgery is planned, pictures and illustrations help to explain the surgical procedure and help the patient to visualize what a stoma looks like.

ENHANCING COPING MEASURES

Because the patient may feel isolated, helpless, and out of control, understanding and emotional support are essential. The patient may respond to stress in a variety of ways that may alienate others, including anger, denial, and social self-isolation.

The nurse needs to recognize that the patient's behavior may be affected by a number of factors unrelated to inherent emotional characteristics. Any patient suffering the discomforts of frequent bowel movements and rectal soreness is anxious, discouraged, and depressed. It is important to develop a relationship with the patient that supports all attempts to cope with these stresses. It is also important to communicate that the patient's feelings are understood by encouraging the patient to talk and express his or her feelings and to discuss any concerns. Stress reduction measures that may be used include relaxation techniques, visualization, breathing exercises, and biofeedback. Professional counseling may be needed to help the patient and family manage issues associated with chronic illness.

PREVENTING SKIN BREAKDOWN

The nurse examines the patient's skin frequently, especially the perianal skin. Perianal care, including the use of a skin barrier, is important after each bowel movement. The nurse gives immediate attention to reddened or irritated areas over a bony prominence and uses pressure-relieving devices to prevent skin breakdown. Consultation with a wound care specialist or enterostomal therapist is often helpful.

MONITORING AND MANAGING POTENTIAL COMPLICATIONS

Serum electrolyte levels are monitored daily, and electrolyte replacements are administered as prescribed. It is important to report evidence of dysrhythmias or change in level of consciousness immediately.

The nurse closely monitors rectal bleeding and administers blood component therapy and volume expanders as prescribed to prevent hypovolemia. It is important to monitor the blood pressure for hypotension and to obtain coagulation and hematocrit and hemoglobin profiles frequently. Vitamin K may be prescribed to increase clotting factors.

The nurse closely monitors the patient for indications of perforation (ie, acute increase in abdominal pain, rigid abdomen, vomiting, or hypotension) and obstruction and toxic megacolon (ie, abdominal distention, decreased or absent bowel sounds, change in mental status, fever, tachycardia, hypotension, dehydration, and electrolyte imbalances).

PROMOTING HOME AND COMMUNITY-BASED CARE

Teaching Patients Self-Care

The nurse assesses the patient's understanding of the disease process and his or her need for additional information about medical management (eg, medications, diet) and surgical interventions. The nurse provides information about nutritional management; a bland, low-residue, high-protein, high-calorie, and high-vitamin diet relieves symptoms and decreases diarrhea. It is important to provide the rationale for the use of corticosteroids and anti-inflammatory, antibacterial, antidiarrheal, and antispasmodic medications. The nurse emphasizes the importance of taking medications as prescribed and not abruptly discontinuing them (especially corticosteroids) to avoid development of serious medical problems (Chart 38-3). The nurse reviews ileostomy care as necessary (see Nursing Management of the Patient with an Ileostomy). Patient education information can be obtained from the National Foundation for Ileitis and Colitis.

Continuing Care

Patients with chronic inflammatory disease are managed at home with follow-up care by their physician or through an outpatient clinic. Those whose nutritional status is compromised and who are receiving PN need home care nursing to ensure that their nutritional requirements are being met and that they or their caregivers can follow through with the instructions for PN. Patients who are medically managed need to understand that their disease can be controlled and that they can lead a healthy life between exacerbations. Control implies management based on an understanding of the disease and its treatment. Patients in the home setting need information about their medications (ie, name, dose, side effects, and frequency of administration) and need to take medications on schedule. Medication reminders such as containers that separate pills according to day and time or daily checklists are helpful.

During a flare-up, the nurse encourages patients to rest as needed and to modify activities according to their energy levels. Patients should limit tasks that impose strain on the lower abdominal muscles. They should sleep in a room close to the bathroom because of the frequent diarrhea (10 to 20 times per day); quick access to a toilet helps alleviate the worry of embarrassment if an accident occurs. Room deodorizers help control odors.

Dietary modifications can control but not cure the disease; the nurse recommends a low-residue, high-protein, high-calorie diet, especially during an acute phase. It is important to encourage patients to keep a record of the foods that irritate the bowel and to eliminate them from the diet and to remind patients to drink at least eight glasses of water each day.

Chart 38-3

Home Care Checklist • Managing Inflammatory Bowel Disease

At the completion of the home care instruction, the patient or caregiver will be able to:	Patient	Caregiver
• Verbalize an understanding of the disease process.	✓	✓
• Discuss nutritional management: bland, low-residue, high-protein, high-vitamin diet; identify foods to include and foods to be avoided.	✓	✓
• Describe medication regimen; identify medications by name, use, route, and frequency.	✓	✓
• Identify measures to be used to treat exacerbation of symptoms, to include rest, dietary modifications, medications.	✓	✓
• Identify measures to be used to promote fluid and electrolyte balance during acute exacerbations	✓	✓
• Demonstrate management of PN therapy, if applicable; identifies possible complications and interventions	✓	✓
• Incorporate stress reduction measures into life-style	✓	

The prolonged nature of the disease has an impact on the patient and often strains his or her family life and financial resources as well. Family support is vital; however, some family members may be resentful, guilty, and tired and feel unable to continue coping with the emotional demands of the illness and the physical demands of caring for another. Some patients with IBD do not socialize for fear of being embarrassed. Many prefer to eat alone. Because they have lost control over elimination, they may fear losing control over other aspects of their lives. They need time to express their fears and frustrations. Individual and family counseling may be helpful.

Evaluation

EXPECTED PATIENT OUTCOMES

Expected patient outcomes may include the following:

1. Reports a decrease in the frequency of diarrhea stools
   a. Complies with dietary restrictions; maintains bed rest
   b. Takes medications as prescribed
2. Has reduced pain
3. Maintains fluid volume balance
   a. Drinks 1 to 2 L of oral fluids daily
   b. Has a normal body temperature
   c. Displays adequate skin turgor and moist mucous membranes
4. Attains optimal nutrition; tolerates small, frequent feedings without diarrhea
5. Avoids fatigue
   a. Rests periodically during the day
   b. Adheres to activity restrictions
6. Is less anxious
7. Copes successfully with diagnosis
   a. Expresses feelings freely
   b. Uses appropriate stress reduction behaviors
8. Maintains skin integrity
   a. Cleans perianal skin after defecation
   b. Uses lotion or ointment as skin barrier
9. Acquires an understanding of the disease process
   a. Modifies diet appropriately to decrease diarrhea
   b. Adheres to medication regimen
10. Recovers without complications
    a. Maintains electrolytes within normal ranges
    b. Maintains normal sinus or baseline cardiac rhythm
    c. Maintains fluid balance
    d. Experiences no perforation or rectal bleeding

NURSING MANAGEMENT OF THE PATIENT REQUIRING AN ILEOSTOMY

Some patients with IBD eventually require permanent fecal diversion with creation of an ileostomy to manage symptoms and to treat or prevent complications. The Plan of Nursing Care 38-1 summarizes care for the patient requiring an ostomy.

Providing Preoperative Care

A period of preparation with intensive replacement of fluid, blood, and protein is necessary before surgery is performed. Antibiotics may be prescribed. If the patient has been taking corticosteroids, they will be continued during the surgical phase to prevent steroid-induced adrenal insufficiency. Usually, the patient is given a low-residue diet, provided in frequent, small feedings. All other preoperative measures are similar to those for general

abdominal surgery. The abdomen is marked for the proper placement of the stoma by the surgeon or the enterostomal therapist. Care is taken to ensure that the ostomy stoma is conveniently placed—usually in the right lower quadrant about 2 inches below the waist, in an area away from previous scars, bony prominence, skin folds, or fistulas.

The patient must have a thorough understanding of the surgery to be performed and what to expect after surgery. Information about an ileostomy is presented to the patient by means of written materials, models, and discussion. Preoperative teaching includes management of drainage from the stoma, the nature of drainage, and the need for nasogastric intubation, parenteral fluids, and possibly perineal packing.

Providing Postoperative Care

General abdominal surgery wound care is required. The nurse observes the stoma for color and size. It should be pink to bright red and shiny. For the traditional ileostomy, a temporary plastic bag with adhesive facing is placed over the ileostomy and firmly pressed onto surrounding skin. The nurse monitors the ileostomy for fecal drainage, which should begin about 72 hours after surgery. The drainage is a continuous liquid from the small intestine because the stoma does not have a controlling sphincter. The contents drain into the plastic bag and are thus kept from coming into contact with the skin. They are collected and measured when the bag becomes full. If a continent ileal reservoir was created, as described for the Kock pouch, continuous drainage is provided by an indwelling reservoir catheter for 2 to 3 weeks after surgery. This allows the suture lines to heal.

As with other patients undergoing abdominal surgery, the nurse encourages those with an ileostomy to engage in early ambulation. It is important to administer prescribed pain medications as required.

Because these patients lose much fluid in the early postoperative period, an accurate record of fluid intake, urinary output, and fecal discharge is necessary to help gauge the fluid needs of the patient. There may be 1000 to 2000 mL of fluid lost each day in addition to expected fluid loss through urine, perspiration, respiration, and other sources. With this loss, sodium and potassium are depleted. The nurse monitors laboratory values and administers electrolyte replacements as prescribed. Intravenous fluids are administered to replace fluid losses for 4 to 5 days.

Nasogastric suction is also a part of immediate postoperative care, with the tube requiring frequent irrigation, as prescribed. The purpose of nasogastric suction is to prevent a buildup of gastric contents. After the tube is removed, the nurse offers sips of clear liquids and gradually progresses the diet. It is important to immediately report nausea and abdominal distention, which may indicate obstruction.

By the end of the first week, rectal packing is removed. Because this procedure may be uncomfortable, the nurse may administer an analgesic an hour before it is performed. After the packing is removed, the perineum is irrigated two or three times daily until full healing takes place.

PROVIDING EMOTIONAL SUPPORT

The patient understandably may think that everyone is aware of the ileostomy and may view the stoma as a mutilation compared with other abdominal incisions that heal and are hidden. Because

(text continues on page 1050)

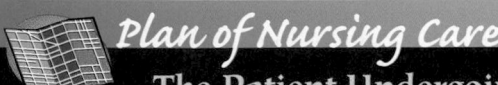

Plan of Nursing Care
The Patient Undergoing Ostomy Surgery

Nursing Interventions	Rationale	Expected Outcomes

Nursing Diagnosis: Deficient knowledge about the surgical procedure and preoperative preparation
Goal: Understands the surgical process and the necessary preoperative preparations

Preoperative Care

1. Ascertain whether the patient has had a previous surgical experience and ask for recollections of positive and negative impressions.

2. Determine what information the surgeon gave the patient and family and whether it was understood. Clarify and elaborate as necessary. Determine whether the stoma is permanent or temporary. Be aware of the patient's prognosis if carcinoma exists.

3. Use pictures or drawings to illustrate the location and appearance of the surgical wounds (abdominal, perineal) and the stoma if the patient is receptive.

4. Explain that oral/parenteral antimicrobials will be administered to cleanse the bowel preoperatively. Mechanical cleansing may also be required.

5. Assist the patient during nasogastric/nasoenteric intubation. Measure drainage from the tube.

Rationale:

1. Fear of a repeated negative experience increases anxiety. Talking about the experience with a nurse helps clarify misconceptions and helps the patient ventilate any repressed emotions. Positive experiences are reinforced.

2. Clarification prevents misunderstandings and alleviates anxiety. A positive affect may be more difficult to project if the ostomy is permanent or the prognosis poor.

3. Knowledge, for some, alleviates anxiety because fear of the unknown is decreased. Others choose not to know because it makes them more anxious.

4. Antimicrobials and mechanical cleansing reduce intestinal bacterial flora.

5. Nasoenteral intubation is used for decompression and drainage of gastrointestinal contents before surgery.

Expected Outcomes:

- Expresses anxieties and fears about the surgical process
- Projects a positive attitude toward the surgical procedure
- Repeats in own words information given by the surgeon
- Identifies normal anatomy and physiology of gastrointestinal tract and how it will be altered; can point to expected location of abdominal wound and stoma; describes stoma appearance and size
- Adheres to "bowel prep" regimen of antimicrobials or mechanical cleansing
- Tolerates the presence of nasogastric/nasoenteric tube

Nursing Diagnosis: Disturbed body image
Goal: Attainment of a positive self-concept

1. Encourage the patient to verbalize feelings about the stoma. Offer to be present when the stoma is first viewed and touched.

2. Suggest that the spouse or significant other view the stoma.

3. Offer counseling, if desired.

4. Arrange for a visit with an ostomate.

Rationale:

1. Free expression of feelings allows the patient the opportunity to verbalize and identify concerns. Expressed concerns can be therapeutically addressed by health care team members.

2. Helps patient to overcome fears about partner's response.

3. Provides opportunity for additional support.

4. Ostomates can offer support and share mutual feelings and experiences.

Expected Outcomes:

- Freely expresses concerns
- Accepts support
- Seeks help as needed
- States is willing to talk with an ostomate

Nursing Diagnosis: Anxiety related to the loss of bowel control
Goal: Reduction of anxiety

Postoperative Care

1. Provide information about expected bowel function:
   a. Characteristics of effluent
   b. Frequency of discharge

2. Teach the patient how to prepare the appliance for an adequate fit.

Rationale:

1. Emotional adjustment is facilitated if adequate information is provided at the level of the learner.

2. Adequate fit is necessary for successful use of the appliance.

Expected Outcomes:

- Expresses interest in learning about altered bowel function
- Handles equipment correctly
- Changes the appliance unassisted
- Irrigates colostomy successfully
- Progresses toward a regular schedule of elimination

(continued)

Plan of Nursing Care
The Patient Undergoing Ostomy Surgery *(Continued)*

Nursing Interventions	Rationale	Expected Outcomes
a. Choose the drainage appliance that will provide a secure fit around the stoma. Measure the stoma size with a measuring guide provided by the ostomy manufacturer and compare with the opening on the pouch. About 3-mm (⅛-in) clearance should be provided around the stoma.	a. The appliance opening should be larger than the stoma for an adequate fit. Available brands come in different sizes to fit the stoma. Adjustments are made as necessary.	
b. Remove any plastic covering that protects the appliance adhesive. *Note:* The pouch is applied by pressing the adhesive for 30 s to the skin or skin barrier.	b. The appliance is ready to apply directly to the skin or skin protector.	
3. Demonstrate how to change the appliance before leakage occurs. Be aware that the elderly person may have diminished vision and difficulty handling equipment.	3. Manipulation of the appliance is a learned motor skill that requires practice and positive reinforcement.	
4. When appropriate, demonstrate how to irrigate the colostomy (usually on the 4th–5th day). Recommend that irrigation be performed at a consistent time, depending on the type of colostomy.	4. Colostomy irrigation is used to regulate the passage of fecal material; alternatively the bowel can be allowed to evacuate naturally.	

Nursing Diagnosis: Risk for impaired skin integrity related to irritation of the peristomal skin by the effluent
Goal: Maintenance of skin integrity

1. Provide information about signs and symptoms of irritated or inflamed skin. Use pictures if possible.	1. Peristomal skin should be slightly pink without abrasions and similar to that of the entire abdomen.	• Describes appearance of healthy skin
2. Teach patient how to cleanse the peristomal skin gently.	2. Mild friction with warm water and a gentle soap cleanses the skin and minimizes irritation and possible abrasions. Patting the skin dry prevents tissue trauma.	• Correctly cleanses the skin • Successfully applies a skin barrier • Gently removes the drainage appliance without skin damage • Demonstrates intact skin around the colostomy stoma
3. Demonstrate how to apply a skin barrier (powder, gel, paste, wafer).	3. Skin barriers protect the peristomal skin from enzymes and bacteria.	
4. Demonstrate how to remove the pouch.	4. Gently separate adhesive from the skin to avoid irritation. Never pull!	

Nursing Diagnosis: Potential imbalanced nutrition, less than body requirements, related to avoidance of foods that may cause GI discomfort
Goal: Achievement of an optimal nutritional intake

1. Conduct a complete nutritional assessment to identify any foods that may increase peristalsis by irritating the bowel.	1. Patients react differently to certain foods because of individual sensitivity.	• Modifies diet to avoid offensive foods yet maintains adequate nutritional intake
2. Advise the patient to avoid food products with a cellulose or hemicellulose base (nuts, seeds).	2. Cellulose food products are the nondigestible residue of plant foods. They hold water, provide bulk, and stimulate elimination.	• Avoids foods such as peanuts • Modifies intake of certain fruits
3. Recommend moderation in intake of certain irritating fruits such as prunes, grapes, and bananas.	3. These fruits tend to increase the quantity of effluent.	

(continued)

Plan of Nursing Care

The Patient Undergoing Ostomy Surgery (Continued)

Nursing Interventions	Rationale	Expected Outcomes
Nursing Diagnosis: Sexual dysfunction related to altered body image **Goal:** Attainment of satisfactory sexual performance		
1. Encourage the patient to verbalize concerns and fears. The sexual partner is welcomed to participate in the discussion.	1. Expressed needs help the therapist develop a plan of care.	• Expresses fears and concerns
2. Recommend alternative sexual positions.	2. Avoid patient embarrassment with the visual appearance of the stoma. Avoid peristomal skin irritation secondary to friction.	• Discusses alternative sexual positions
3. Seek assistance from a sexual therapist, enterostomal therapist, or advanced practice nurse.	3. Some patients need professional sexual counseling.	• Accepts services of a professional counselor
Nursing Diagnosis: Risk for deficient fluid volume related to anorexia and vomiting and increased loss of fluids and electrolytes from GI tract **Goal:** Attainment of fluid balance		
1. Estimate fluid intake and output: a. Strict intake and output	1. Provides indication of fluid balance. a. An early indicator of fluid imbalance is a daily, significant difference between intake and output. The average person ingests (food, fluids) and loses (urine, feces, lungs) about 2 L of fluid every 24 h.	• Maintains fluid balance
b. Daily weights	b. A gain/loss of 1 L of fluid is reflected in a body weight change of 2.2 lb.	
2. Assess serum and urinary values of sodium and potassium.	2. Sodium is the major electrolyte regulating water balance. Vomiting results in decreased urinary and serum sodium levels. Urinary sodium values, in contrast to serum values, reflect early, sensitive changes in sodium balance. Sodium works in conjunction with potassium, which is also decreased with vomiting. A significant deficiency in potassium is associated with a decrease in intracellular potassium bicarbonate, which leads to acidosis and compensatory hyperventilation.	• Maintains normal serum and urinary values for sodium and potassium
3. Observe and record skin turgor and the appearance of the tongue.	3. Adequate hydration is reflected by the skin's ability to return to its normal shape after being grasped between the fingers. *Note:* In the older person, it is normal for the return to be delayed. Changes in the mucous membrane covering the tongue are accurate and early indicators of hydration status.	• Normal skin turgor • Surface of tongue is pink, with a moist mucous membrane

there is loss of a body part and a major change in anatomy, the patient often goes through the various phases of grieving—shock, disbelief, denial, rejection, anger, and restitution. Nursing support through these phases is important, and understanding of the patient's emotional outlook in each instance should determine the approach taken. For example, teaching may be ineffective until the patient is ready to learn. Concern about body image may lead to questions related to family relationships, sexual function, and for women, the ability to become pregnant and to deliver a baby normally. Patients need to know that someone understands and cares about them. A calm, nonjudgmental attitude exhibited by the nurse aids in gaining the patient's confidence. It is important to recognize the dependency needs of these patients. Their prolonged illness can make them irritable, anxious, and depressed. The nurse can coordinate patient care through meetings attended by consultants such as the physician, psychologist, psychiatrist, social worker, enterostomal therapist, and dietitian. The team approach is important in facilitating the often complex care of this patient.

Conversely, a surgical procedure to create an ileostomy can produce dramatic positive changes in patients who have suffered from IBD for several years. After the continuous discomfort of the disease has decreased and patients learn how to take care of the ileostomy, they often develop a more positive outlook. Until they progress to this phase, an empathetic and tolerant approach by the nurse plays an important part in recovery. The sooner the patient masters the physical care of the ileostomy, the sooner he or she will psychologically accept it.

The support of other ostomates is also helpful. The United Ostomy Association is dedicated to the rehabilitation of ostomates. This organization gives patients useful information about living with an ostomy through an educational program of literature, lectures, and exhibits. Local associations offer visiting services by qualified members who provide hope and rehabilitation services to new ostomy patients. Hospitals and other health care agencies may have an enterostomal therapy nurse on staff who can serve as a valuable resource person for the ileostomy patient.

MANAGING SKIN AND STOMA CARE

The patient with a traditional ileostomy cannot establish regular bowel habits because the contents of the ileum are fluid and are discharged continuously. The patient must wear a pouch at all times. Stomal size and pouch size vary initially; the stoma should be rechecked 3 weeks after surgery, when the edema has subsided. The final size and type of appliance is selected in 3 months, after the patient's weight has stabilized, and the stoma shrinks to a stable shape.

The location and length of the stoma are significant in the management of the ileostomy by the patient. The surgeon positions the stoma as close to the midline as possible and at a location where even an obese patient with a protruding abdomen can care for it easily. Usually, the ileostomy stoma is about 2.5 cm (1 in) long, which makes it convenient for the attachment of an appliance.

Skin excoriation around the stoma can be a persistent problem. Peristomal skin integrity may be compromised by several factors, such as an allergic reaction to the ostomy appliance, skin barrier, or paste; chemical irritation from the effluent; mechanical injury from the removal of the appliance; and possible infection. If irritation and yeast growth occur, nystatin powder (Mycostatin) is dusted lightly on the peristomal skin.

CHANGING AN APPLIANCE

A regular schedule for changing the pouch before leakage occurs must be established for those with a traditional ileostomy. The patient can be taught to change the pouch in a manner similar to that described in Chart 38-4.

The amount of time a person can keep the appliance sealed to the body surface depends on the location of the stoma and on body structure. The usual wearing time is 5 to 7 days. The appliance is emptied every 4 to 6 hours or at the same time the patient empties the bladder. An emptying spout at the bottom of the appliance is closed with a special clip made for this purpose.

Most pouches are disposable and odor-proof. Foods such as spinach and parsley act as deodorizers in the intestinal tract; foods that cause odors include cabbage, onions, and fish. Bismuth subcarbonate tablets, which may be prescribed and taken by mouth three or four times each day, are effective in reducing odor. A stool thickener, such as diphenoxylate (Lomotil), can also be prescribed and taken orally to assist in odor control.

IRRIGATING A CONTINENT ILEOSTOMY

For a continent ileostomy (ie, Kock pouch), the nurse teaches the patient to drain the pouch, as described in Chart 38-5. A catheter is inserted into the reservoir to drain the fluid. The length of time between drainage periods is gradually increased until the reservoir needs to be drained only every 4 to 6 hours and irrigated once each day. A pouch is not necessary; instead, most patients wear a small dressing over the opening.

When the fecal discharge is thick, water can be injected through the catheter to loosen and soften it. The consistency of the effluent is affected by food intake. At first, drainage is only 60 to 80 mL, but as time goes on, the amount increases significantly. The internal Kock pouch stretches, eventually accommodating 500 to 1000 mL. The patient learns to use the sensation of pressure in the pouch as a gauge to determine how often the pouch should be drained.

MANAGING DIETARY AND FLUID NEEDS

A low-residue diet is followed for the first 6 to 8 weeks. Strained fruits and vegetables are given. These foods are important sources of vitamins A and C. Later, there are few dietary restrictions, except for avoiding foods that are high in fiber or hard-to-digest kernels, such as celery, popcorn, corn, poppy seeds, caraway seeds, and coconut. Foods are reintroduced one at a time. The nurse assesses the patient's tolerance for these foods and reminds him or her to chew food thoroughly.

Fluids may be a problem during the summer, when fluid lost through perspiration adds to the fluid loss through the ileostomy. Fluids such as Gatorade are helpful in maintaining the electrolyte balance. If the fecal discharge is too watery, fibrous foods (eg, whole-grain cereals, fresh fruit skins, beans, corn, nuts) are restricted. If the effluent is excessively dry, salt intake is increased. Increased intake of water or fluid does not increase the effluent, because excess water is excreted in the urine.

PREVENTING COMPLICATIONS

Monitoring for complications is an ongoing activity for the patient with an ileostomy. Minor complications occur in about 40% of patients who have an ileostomy; less than 20% of the complications require surgical intervention (Kirsner & Shorter, 2000).

Common complications include skin irritation, diarrhea, stomal stenosis, urinary calculi, and cholelithiasis. Peristomal skin irritation, the most common complication of an ileostomy, results from leakage of effluent. A pouch that does not fit well is often the cause. The nurse or an enterostomal therapist adjusts the pouch and skin barriers are applied. Diarrhea, manifested by very irritating effluent that rapidly fills the pouch (every hour or sooner), can quickly lead to dehydration and electrolyte losses. Supplemental water, sodium, and potassium are administered to prevent hypovolemia and hypokalemia. Antidiarrheal agents are administered. Stenosis is caused by circular scar tissue that forms at the stoma site. The scar tissue must be surgically released. Urinary calculi occur in about 10% of ileostomy patients because of dehydration from decreased fluid intake. Intense lower abdominal pain that radiates to the legs, hematuria, and signs of dehydration indicate that the urine should be strained. Fluid intake is encouraged. Sometimes, small stones are passed during urination; otherwise, treatment is necessary to crush or remove the calculi (see Chap. 45).

Cholelithiasis (ie, gallstones) occurs three times more commonly in patients with an ileostomy than in the general population

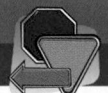

Chart 38-4

GUIDELINES FOR Changing an Ostomy Appliance

Changing an ileostomy appliance is necessary to prevent leakage (the bag is usually changed every 5 to 7 days), to allow for examination of the skin around the stoma, and to assist in controlling odor if this becomes a problem. The appliance should be changed at any time that the patient complains of burning or itching under the disk or pain in the area of the stoma; routine changes should be performed early in the morning before breakfast or 2 to 4 hours after a meal, when the bowel is least active.

NURSING ACTION	RATIONALE

1. Promote patient comfort and involvement in the procedure.
   a. Have the patient assume a relaxed position.
   b. Provide privacy.
   c. Explain details of the procedure.
   d. Expose the ileostomy area; remove the ileostomy belt (if worn).
	1. Providing a relaxed atmosphere and adequate explanations help the patient to become an active participant in the procedure.

2. Remove the appliance.
   a. Have the patient sit on the toilet or on a chair facing the toilet. A patient who prefers to stand should face the toilet.
   b. The appliance (pouch) can be removed by gently pushing the skin away from the adhesive.
	2. These positions facilitate disposal or drainage.

Selected Ostomy Pouches and Accessories

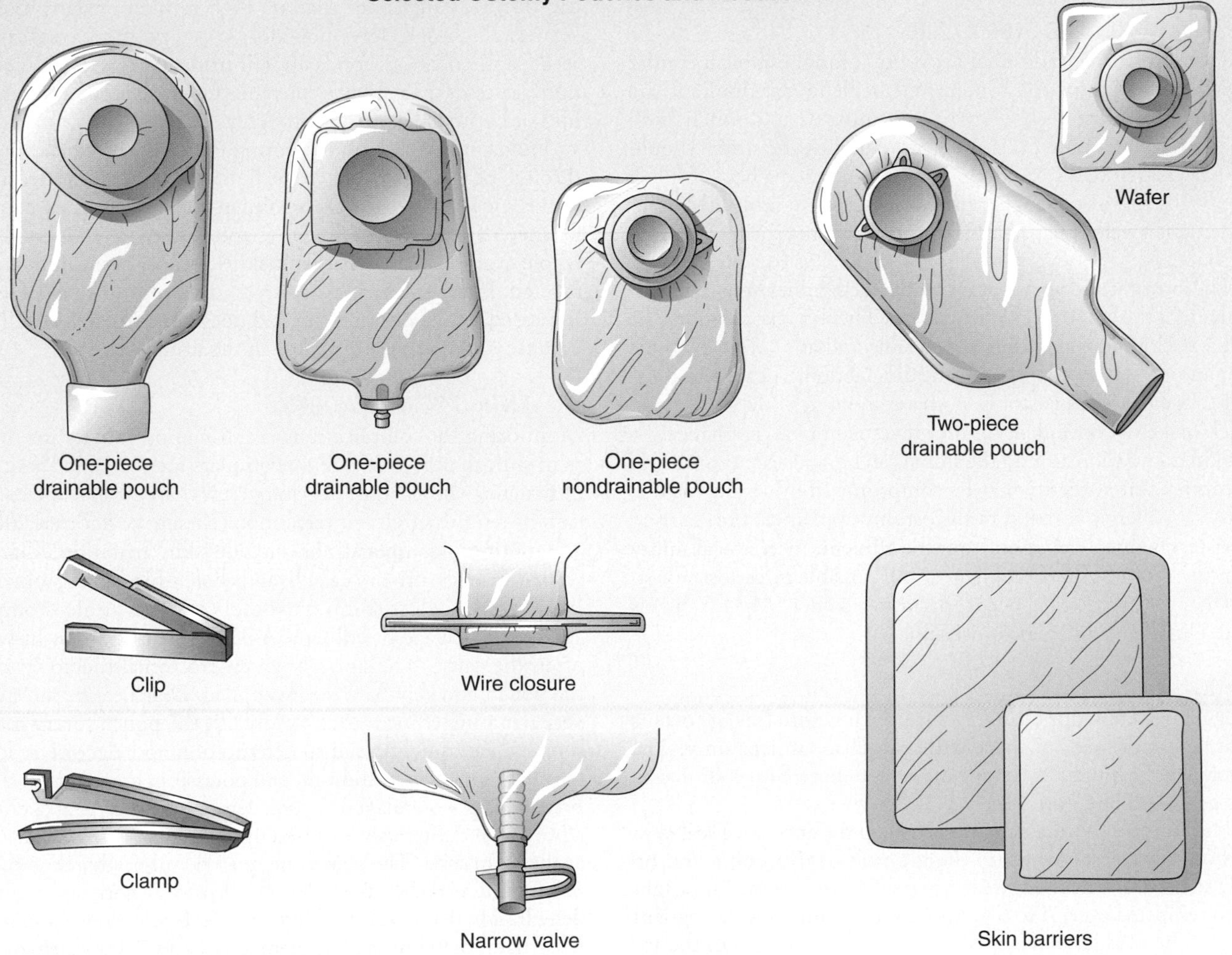

One-piece drainable pouch

One-piece drainable pouch

One-piece nondrainable pouch

Two-piece drainable pouch

Wafer

Clip

Wire closure

Clamp

Narrow valve

Skin barriers

(continued)

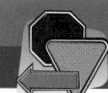

Chart 38-4

GUIDELINES FOR Changing an Ostomy Appliance (Continued)

NURSING ACTION	RATIONALE

3. Cleanse the skin:
  a. Wash the skin gently with a soft cloth moistened with tepid water and mild soap; the patient may prefer to bathe before putting on a clean appliance.
  b. Rinse and dry the skin thoroughly after cleansing.
4. Apply appliance (when there is *no* skin irritation):
  a. An appropriate skin barrier is applied to the peristomal skin before the appliance is applied.
  b. Remove cover from adherent surface of disk of disposable plastic appliance and apply directly to the skin.
  c. Press firmly in place for 30 s to ensure adherence.
	3. The patient may shower with or without the pouch.
	  a. Micropore or waterproof tape applied to the sides of the faceplate will keep it secure during bathing.
	
	  b. Moisture or soap residue will interfere with appliance adhesion.
	4. Many appliances have a built-in skin barrier. The skin should be thoroughly dried before applying the appliance.
	
	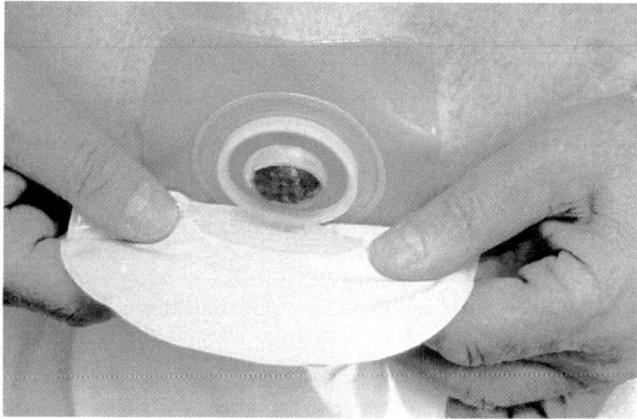
	Pressing the appliance into place. Courtesy of Convatec, a Squibb Company.

5. Apply appliance (when there is skin irritation):
  a. Cleanse the skin thoroughly but gently; pat dry.
  b. Apply Kenalog spray; blot excess moisture with a cotton pledget and dust lightly with nystatin (Mycostatin) powder.
 	
OR
 	
  Apply as an alternative a wafer of Stomahesive (Squibb), which is commercially available. The stomal opening should be cut the same size as the stoma; use a cutting guide (supplied with Stomahesive). The wafer is applied directly to the skin.
  c. Another alternative is to moisten a karaya gum washer and apply when it is tacky. If the skin is moist, karaya powder may be applied first and any excess dusted off gently.
  d. The pouch is then applied to the treated skin.
6. Check the pouch bottom for closure; use the rubber band or clip provided.
	5.
	  a. To remove debris.
	  b. The corticosteroid preparation (Kenalog) helps to decrease inflammation. The antifungal agent (nystatin) treats those types of infections that are common around stomas. A prescription is required for either medication.
	
	  Stomahesive is a substance that facilitates healing of excoriated skin. It adheres well even to moist, irritated skin.
	
	  c. Karaya also facilitates skin healing. Tackiness promotes adherence.
	
	  d. This will allow skin to heal while the appliance is in place.
	6. Proper closure controls leakage.

because of changes in the absorption of bile acids that occur postoperatively. Spasm of the gallbladder causes severe upper right abdominal pain that can radiate to the back and right shoulder (see Chap. 40).

PROMOTING HOME AND COMMUNITY-BASED CARE

Teaching Patients Self-Care

The spouse and family should be familiar with the adjustment that will be necessary when the patient returns home. They need to know why it is necessary for the patient to occupy the bathroom for 10 minutes or more at certain times of the day and why certain equipment is needed. Their understanding is necessary to reduce tension; a relaxed patient tends to have fewer problems. Visits from an enterostomal therapy nurse may be arranged to ensure that the patient is progressing as expected and to provide additional guidance and teaching as needed.

The patient needs to know the commercial name of the pouch to be used so that he or she can obtain a ready supply and should have information about obtaining other supplies. The names and contact information of the local enterostomal therapy nurse and local self-help groups are often helpful. Any special restrictions on driving or working also need to be reviewed. The nurse teaches the patient about common postoperative complications and how to recognize and report them (Chart 38-6).

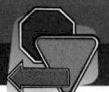

Chart 38-5

GUIDELINES FOR Draining a Continent Ileostomy (Kock Pouch)

A continent ileostomy is the surgical creation of a pouch of small intestine that can serve as an internal receptacle for fecal discharge; a nipple valve is constructed at the outlet. Postoperatively, a catheter extends from the stoma and is attached to a closed drainage suction system. To ensure patency of the catheter, usually every 3 hours 10 to 20 mL of normal saline is instilled gently into the pouch; return flow is not aspirated but is allowed to drain by gravity.

After approximately 2 weeks, when the healing process has progressed to the point at which the catheter is removed from the stoma, the patient is taught to drain the pouch. The equipment required includes a catheter, tissues, water-soluble lubricant, gauze squares, a syringe, irrigating solution in a bowl, and an emesis or receiving basin.

The following procedure is used to drain the pouch; the patient is helped to participate in this procedure to learn to perform it unassisted.

NURSING ACTION	RATIONALE
1. Lubricate the catheter and gently insert it about 5 cm (2 in), at which point some resistance may be felt at the valve or nipple.	1. When gentle pressure is used, the catheter usually will enter the pouch.
2. If there is much resistance, fill a syringe with 20 mL of air or water and inject it through the catheter, while still exerting some pressure on the catheter.	2. This will permit the catheter to enter the pouch.
3. Place the other end of the catheter in a drainage basin held below the level of the stoma. Later this process can be carried out at the toilet with drainage delivered into the toilet bowl.	3. Gravity facilitates drainage. Drainage may include flatus as well as effluent.
4. After drainage, the catheter is removed and the area around the stoma is gently washed with warm water. Pat dry and apply an absorbent pad over the stoma. Fasten the pad with hypoallergenic tape.	4. The entire procedure requires about 5 to 10 min; at first it is performed every 3 h. The time between procedures is gradually lengthened to three times daily.

Intestinal Obstruction

Intestinal obstruction exists when blockage prevents the normal flow of intestinal contents through the intestinal tract. Two types of processes can impede this flow.

- *Mechanical obstruction:* An intraluminal obstruction or a mural obstruction from pressure on the intestinal walls occurs. Examples are intussusception, polypoid tumors and neoplasms, stenosis, strictures, adhesions, hernias, and abscesses.
- *Functional obstruction:* The intestinal musculature cannot propel the contents along the bowel. Examples are amyloidosis, muscular dystrophy, endocrine disorders such as diabetes mellitus, or neurologic disorders such as Parkinson's

disease. The blockage also can be temporary and the result of the manipulation of the bowel during surgery.

The obstruction can be partial or complete. Its severity depends on the region of bowel affected, the degree to which the lumen is occluded, and especially the degree to which the vascular supply to the bowel wall is disturbed.

Most bowel obstructions occur in the small intestine. Adhesions are the most common cause of small bowel obstruction, followed by hernias and neoplasms. Other causes include intussusception, volvulus (ie, twisting of the bowel), and paralytic ileus. About 15% of intestinal obstructions occur in the large bowel; most of these are found in the sigmoid colon (Wolfe, 2000). The most common causes are carcinoma, diverticulitis, inflammatory bowel disorders, and benign tumors. Table 38-5 and Figure 38-6 list mechanical causes of obstruction and describe how they occur.

Chart 38-6

Home Care Checklist ○ Managing Ostomy Care

At the completion of the home care instruction, the patient or caregiver will be able to:	Patient	Caregiver
• Demonstrate ostomy care, including wound cleansing, irrigation, and appliance changing.	✓	✓
• Describe the importance of maintaining peristomal skin integrity.	✓	✓
• Identify sources for obtaining additional dressing and appliance supplies.	✓	✓
• Identify dietary restrictions (foods that can cause diarrhea and constipation).	✓	✓
• Identify measures to be used to promote fluid and electrolyte balance	✓	✓
• Describe medication regimen: identify medications by name, use, route, and frequency.	✓	✓
• Describe potential complications and necessary actions to be taken if complications occur.	✓	✓
• Identify how to contact enterostomal therapist or home health nurse.	✓	✓

Table 38-5 • Mechanical Causes of Intestinal Obstruction

CAUSE	COURSE OF EVENTS	RESULT
Adhesions	Loops of intestine become adherent to areas that heal slowly or scar after abdominal surgery.	After surgery, adhesions produce a kinking of an intestinal loop.
Intussusception	One part of the intestine slips into another part located below it (like a telescope shortening).	The intestinal lumen becomes narrowed.
Volvulus	Bowel twists and turns on itself.	Intestinal lumen becomes obstructed. Gas and fluid accumulate in the trapped bowel.
Hernia	Protrusion of intestine through a weakened area in the abdominal muscle or wall.	Intestinal flow may be completely obstructed. Blood flow to the area may be obstructed as well.
Tumor	A tumor that exists within the wall of the intestine extends into the intestinal lumen, or a tumor outside the intestine causes pressure on the wall of the intestine.	Intestinal lumen becomes partially obstructed; if the tumor is not removed, complete obstruction results.

SMALL BOWEL OBSTRUCTION

Pathophysiology

Intestinal contents, fluid, and gas accumulate above the intestinal obstruction. The abdominal distention and retention of fluid reduce the absorption of fluids and stimulate more gastric secretion. With increasing distention, pressure within the intestinal lumen increases, causing a decrease in venous and arteriolar capillary pressure. This causes edema, congestion, necrosis, and eventual rupture or perforation of the intestinal wall, with resultant peritonitis.

Reflux vomiting may be caused by abdominal distention. Vomiting results in a loss of hydrogen ions and potassium from the stomach, leading to a reduction of chlorides and potassium in the blood and to metabolic alkalosis. Dehydration and acidosis develop from loss of water and sodium. With acute fluid losses, hypovolemic shock may occur.

Clinical Manifestations

The initial symptom is usually crampy pain that is wavelike and colicky. The patient may pass blood and mucus, but no fecal matter and no flatus. Vomiting occurs. If the obstruction is complete, the peristaltic waves initially become extremely vigorous and eventually assume a reverse direction, with the intestinal contents propelled toward the mouth instead of toward the rectum. If the

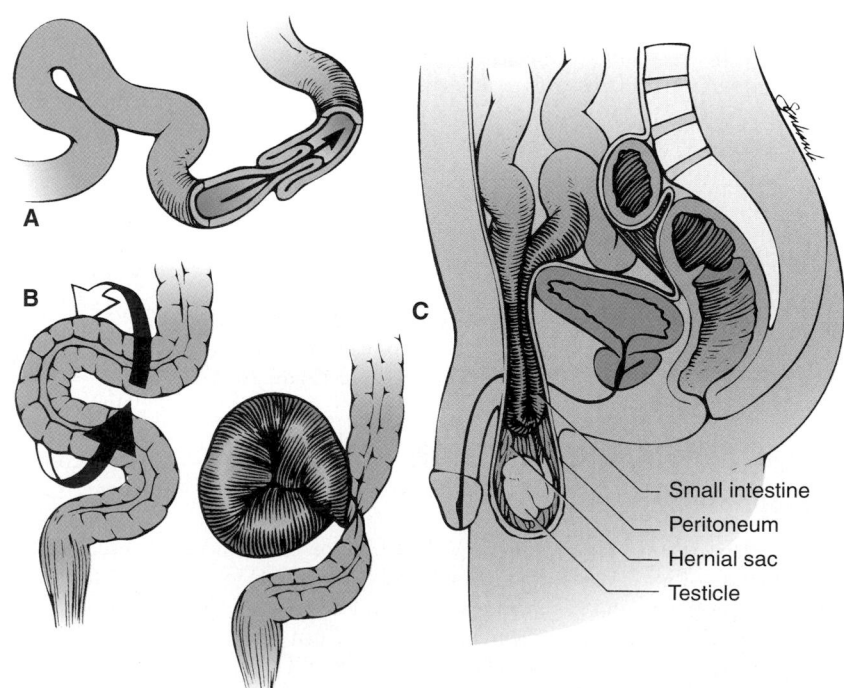

FIGURE 38-6 Three causes of intestinal obstruction. (**A**) Intussusception invagination or shortening of the colon caused by the movement of one segment of bowel into another. (**B**) Volvulus of the sigmoid colon; the twist is counterclockwise in most cases. Note the edematous bowel. (**C**) Hernia (inguinal). The sac of the hernia is a continuation of the peritoneum of the abdomen. The hernial contents are intestine, omentum, or other abdominal contents that pass through the hernial opening into the hernial sac.

Small intestine
Peritoneum
Hernial sac
Testicle

A

B

C

obstruction is in the ileum, fecal vomiting takes place. First, the patient vomits the stomach contents, then the bile-stained contents of the duodenum and the jejunum, and finally, with each paroxysm of pain, the darker, fecal-like contents of the ileum. The unmistakable signs of dehydration become evident: intense thirst, drowsiness, generalized malaise, aching, and a parched tongue and mucous membranes. The abdomen becomes distended. The lower the obstruction is in the GI tract, the more marked the abdominal distention. If the obstruction continues uncorrected, hypovolemic shock occurs from dehydration and loss of plasma volume.

Assessment and Diagnostic Findings

Diagnosis is based on the symptoms described previously and on x-ray findings. Abdominal x-ray studies show abnormal quantities of gas, fluid, or both in the bowel. Laboratory studies (ie, electrolyte studies and a complete blood cell count) reveal a picture of dehydration, loss of plasma volume, and possible infection.

Medical Management

Decompression of the bowel through a nasogastric or small bowel tube (see Chap. 36) is successful in most cases. When the bowel is completely obstructed, the possibility of strangulation warrants surgical intervention. Before surgery, intravenous therapy is necessary to replace the depleted water, sodium, chloride, and potassium.

The surgical treatment of intestinal obstruction depends largely on the cause of the obstruction. In the most common causes of obstruction, such as hernia and adhesions, the surgical procedure involves repairing the hernia or dividing the adhesion to which the intestine is attached. In some instances, the portion of affected bowel may be removed and an anastomosis performed. The complexity of the surgical procedure for intestinal obstruction depends on the duration of the obstruction and the condition of the intestine.

Nursing Management

Nursing management of the nonsurgical patient with a small bowel obstruction includes maintaining the function of the nasogastric tube, assessing and measuring the nasogastric output, assessing for fluid and electrolyte imbalance, monitoring nutritional status, and assessing improvement (eg, return of normal bowel sounds, decreased abdominal distention, subjective improvement in abdominal pain and tenderness, passage of flatus or stool). The nurse reports discrepancies in intake and output, worsening of pain or abdominal distention, and increased nasogastric output. If the patient's condition does not improve, the nurse prepares him or her for surgery. The exact nature of the surgery depends on the cause of the obstruction. Nursing care of the patient after surgical repair of a small bowel obstruction is similar to that for other abdominal surgeries (see Chap. 20).

LARGE BOWEL OBSTRUCTION

Pathophysiology

As in small bowel obstruction, large bowel obstruction results in an accumulation of intestinal contents, fluid, and gas proximal to the obstruction. Obstruction in the large bowel can lead to severe distention and perforation unless some gas and fluid can flow back through the ileal valve. Large bowel obstruction, even if complete, may be undramatic if the blood supply to the colon is not disturbed.

If the blood supply is cut off, however, intestinal strangulation and necrosis (ie, tissue death) occur; this condition is life threatening. In the large intestine, dehydration occurs more slowly than in the small intestine because the colon can absorb its fluid contents and can distend to a size considerably beyond its normal full capacity.

Clinical Manifestations

Large bowel obstruction differs clinically from small bowel obstruction in that the symptoms develop and progress relatively slowly. In patients with obstruction in the sigmoid colon or the rectum, constipation may be the only symptom for days. Eventually, the abdomen becomes markedly distended, loops of large bowel become visibly outlined through the abdominal wall, and the patient has crampy lower abdominal pain. Finally, fecal vomiting develops. Symptoms of shock may occur.

Assessment and Diagnostic Findings

Diagnosis is based on symptoms and on x-ray studies. Abdominal x-ray studies (flat and upright) show a distended colon. Barium studies are contraindicated.

Medical Management

A colonoscopy may be performed to untwist and decompress the bowel. A cecostomy, in which a surgical opening is made into the cecum, may be performed for patients who are poor surgical risks and urgently need relief from the obstruction. The procedure provides an outlet for releasing gas and a small amount of drainage. A rectal tube may be used to decompress an area that is lower in the bowel. The usual treatment, however, is surgical resection to remove the obstructing lesion. A temporary or permanent colostomy may be necessary. An ileoanal anastomosis may be performed if it is necessary to remove the entire large colon.

Nursing Management

The nurse's role is to monitor the patient for symptoms that indicate that the intestinal obstruction is worsening and to provide emotional support and comfort. The nurse administers intravenous fluids and electrolytes as prescribed. If the patient's condition does not respond to nonsurgical treatment, the nurse prepares the patient for surgery. This preparation includes preoperative teaching as the patient's condition indicates. After surgery, general abdominal wound care and routine postoperative nursing care are provided.

COLORECTAL CANCER

Tumors of the colon and rectum are relatively common; the colorectal area (the colon and rectum combined) is now the third most common site of new cancer cases and deaths in the United States. Colorectal cancer is a disease of Western cultures; there were an estimated 148,300 new cases and 56,000 deaths from the disease in 2002 (American Cancer Society, 2002).

The incidence increases with age (the incidence is highest for people older than 85 years of age) and is higher for people with a family history of colon cancer and those with IBD or polyps. The exact cause of colon and rectal cancer is still unknown, but risk factors have been identified (Chart 38-7).

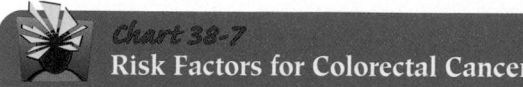

Risk Factors for Colorectal Cancer

Increasing age
Family history of colon cancer or polyps
Previous colon cancer or adenomatous polyps
History of inflammatory bowel disease
High-fat, high-protein (with high intake of beef), low-fiber diet
Genital cancer or breast cancer (in women)

The distribution of cancer sites throughout the colon is shown in Figure 38-7 (Goldman, & Bennett, 2000). Changes in this distribution have occurred in recent years. The incidence of cancer in the sigmoid and rectal areas has decreased, whereas the incidence of cancer in the cecum, ascending, and descending colon has increased.

Improved screening strategies have helped to reduce the number of deaths in recent years. Of the more than 148,000 people diagnosed each year, fewer than half that number die annually (Beyers et al., 2001). Early diagnosis and prompt treatment could save almost three of every four people with colorectal cancer. If the disease is detected and treated at an early stage, the 5-year survival rate is 90%, but only 34% of colorectal cancers are found at an early stage. Survival rates after late diagnosis are very low. Most people are asymptomatic for long periods and seek health care only when they notice a change in bowel habits or rectal bleeding. Prevention and early screening are key to detection and reduction of mortality rates.

Pathophysiology

Cancer of the colon and rectum is predominantly (95%) adenocarcinoma (ie, arising from the epithelial lining of the intestine). It may start as a benign polyp but may become malignant, invade and destroy normal tissues, and extend into surrounding structures. Cancer cells may break away from the primary tumor and spread to other parts of the body (most often to the liver).

Clinical Manifestations

The symptoms are greatly determined by the location of the cancer, the stage of the disease, and the function of the intestinal segment in which it is located. The most common presenting symptom is a change in bowel habits. The passage of blood in the stools is the second most common symptom. Symptoms may also include unexplained anemia, anorexia, weight loss, and fatigue.

The symptoms most commonly associated with right-sided lesions are dull abdominal pain and melena (ie, black, tarry stools). The symptoms most commonly associated with left-sided lesions are those associated with obstruction (ie, abdominal pain and cramping, narrowing stools, constipation, and distention), as well as bright red blood in the stool. Symptoms associated with rectal lesions are tenesmus (ie, ineffective, painful straining at stool), rectal pain, the feeling of incomplete evacuation after a bowel movement, alternating constipation and diarrhea, and bloody stool.

Assessment and Diagnostic Findings

Along with an abdominal and rectal examination, the most important diagnostic procedures for cancer of the colon are fecal occult blood testing, barium enema, proctosigmoidoscopy, and colonoscopy (see Chap. 34). As many as 60% of colorectal cancer cases can be identified by sigmoidoscopy with biopsy or cytology smears (Yamada et al., 1999).

Carcinoembryonic antigen (CEA) studies may also be performed. Although CEA may not be a highly reliable indicator in diagnosing colon cancer because not all lesions secrete CEA, studies show that CEA levels are reliable in predicting prognosis. With complete excision of the tumor, the elevated levels of CEA should return to normal within 48 hours. Elevations of CEA at a later date suggest recurrence (Yamada et al., 1999).

Complications

Tumor growth may cause partial or complete bowel obstruction. Extension of the tumor and ulceration into the surrounding blood vessels results in hemorrhage. Perforation, abscess formation, peritonitis, sepsis, and shock may occur.

🍂 Gerontologic Considerations

The incidence of carcinoma of the colon and rectum increases with age. These cancers are considered common malignancies in advanced age. Only prostate cancer and lung cancer in men exceed colorectal cancer. Among women, only breast cancer exceeds the incidence of colorectal cancer (Lueckenotte, 2000). Symptoms are often insidious. Cancer patients usually report fatigue, which is caused primarily by iron-deficiency anemia. In early stages, minor changes in bowel patterns and occasional bleeding may occur. The later symptoms most commonly reported by the elderly are abdominal pain, obstruction, tenesmus, and rectal bleeding.

Colon cancer in the elderly has been closely associated with dietary carcinogens. Lack of fiber is a major causative factor because the passage of feces through the intestinal tract is prolonged, which extends exposure to possible carcinogens. Excess fat is believed to alter bacterial flora and convert steroids into compounds that have carcinogenic properties.

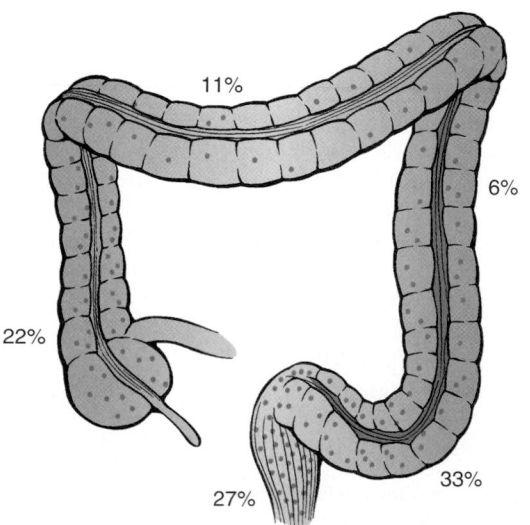
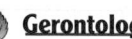

FIGURE 38-7 Percentage distribution of cancer sites in the colon and rectum.

Medical Management

The patient with symptoms of intestinal obstruction is treated with intravenous fluids and nasogastric suction. If there has been significant bleeding, blood component therapy may be required.

Treatment for colorectal cancer depends on the stage of the disease (Chart 38-8) and consists of surgery to remove the tumor, supportive therapy, and adjuvant therapy. Data demonstrate delays in tumor recurrence and increases in survival time for patients who receive some form of adjuvant therapy—chemotherapy, radiation therapy, immunotherapy, or multimodality therapy.

ADJUVANT THERAPY

The standard adjuvant therapy administered to patients with Dukes' class C colon cancer is the 5-fluorouracil plus levamisole regimen (Wolfe, 2000). Patients with Dukes' class B or C rectal cancer are given 5-fluorouracil and high doses of pelvic irradiation. Mitomycin is also used. Radiation therapy is used before, during, and after surgery to shrink the tumor, to achieve better results from surgery, and to reduce the risk of recurrence. For inoperative or unresectable tumors, irradiation is used to provide significant relief from symptoms. Intracavity and implantable devices are used to deliver radiation to the site. The response to adjuvant therapy varies.

SURGICAL MANAGEMENT

Surgery is the primary treatment for most colon and rectal cancers. It may be curative or palliative. Advances in surgical techniques can enable the patient with cancer to have sphincter-saving devices that restore continuity of the GI tract (Tierney et al., 2000). The type of surgery recommended depends on the location and size of the tumor. Cancers limited to one site can be removed through the colonoscope. Laparoscopic colotomy with polypectomy minimizes the extent of surgery needed in some cases. A laparoscope is used as a guide in making an incision into the colon; the tumor mass is then excised. Use of the neodymium/yttrium-aluminum-garnet (Nd:YAG) laser has proved effective with some lesions as well. Bowel resection is indicated for most class A lesions and all class B and C lesions. Surgery is sometimes recommended for class D colon cancer, but the goal of surgery in this instance is

palliative; if the tumor has spread and involves surrounding vital structures, it is considered nonresectable.

Surgical procedures include the following:

- Segmental resection with anastomosis (ie, removal of the tumor and portions of the bowel on either side of the growth, as well as the blood vessels and lymphatic nodes) (Fig. 38-8).
- Abdominoperineal resection with permanent sigmoid colostomy (ie, removal of the tumor and a portion of the sigmoid and all of the rectum and anal sphincter) (Fig. 38-9).
- Temporary colostomy followed by segmental resection and anastomosis and subsequent reanastomosis of the colostomy, allowing initial bowel decompression and bowel preparation before resection
- Permanent colostomy or ileostomy for palliation of unresectable obstructing lesions
- Construction of a coloanal reservoir called a colonic J pouch is performed in two steps. A temporary loop ileostomy is constructed to divert intestinal flow, and the newly constructed J pouch (made from 6 to 10 cm of colon) is reattached to the anal stump. About 3 months after the initial stage, the ileostomy is reversed, and intestinal continuity is restored. The anal sphincter and therefore continence are preserved.

A **colostomy** is the surgical creation of an opening (ie, stoma) into the colon. It can be created as a temporary or permanent fecal diversion. It allows the drainage or evacuation of colon contents to the outside of the body. The consistency of the drainage is related to the placement of the colostomy, which is dictated by the location of the tumor and the extent of invasion into surrounding tissues (Fig. 38-10). With improved surgical techniques, colostomies are performed on fewer than one third of patients with colorectal cancer.

 Gerontologic Considerations

The elderly are at increased risk for complications after surgery and may have difficulty managing colostomy care. They may have decreased vision, impaired hearing, and difficulty with fine motor coordination. It may be helpful for the patient to handle ostomy equipment and simulate cleaning the peristomal skin and irrigating the stoma before surgery. Skin care is a major concern in the elderly ostomate because of the skin changes that occur with aging—the epithelial and subcutaneous fatty layers become thin, and the skin is irritated easily. To prevent skin breakdown, special attention is paid to skin cleansing and the proper fit of an appliance. Arteriosclerosis causes decreased blood flow to the wound and stoma site. As a result, transport of nutrients is delayed, and healing time may be prolonged. Some patients have delayed elimination after irrigation because of decreased peristalsis and mucus production. Most patients require 6 months before they feel comfortable with their ostomy care.

NURSING PROCESS:
THE PATIENT WITH COLORECTAL CANCER

Assessment

The nurse completes a health history to obtain information about fatigue, abdominal or rectal pain (eg, location, frequency, duration, association with eating or defecation), past and present elimination patterns, and characteristics of stool (eg, color, odor,

---

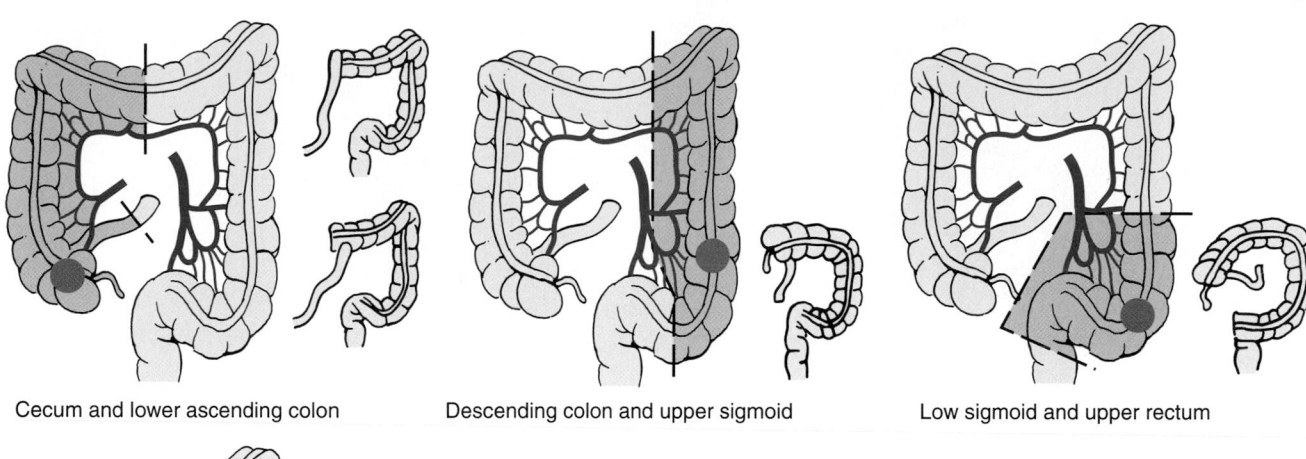

Cecum and lower ascending colon   Descending colon and upper sigmoid   Low sigmoid and upper rectum

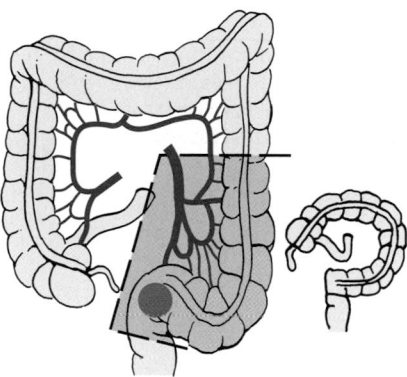

Rectal sigmoid resection

FIGURE 38-8 Examples of areas where cancer can occur, the area that is removed, and how the anastomosis is performed (*small diagrams*).

consistency, presence of blood or mucus). Additional information includes a history of IBD or colorectal polyps, a family history of colorectal disease, and current medication therapy. The nurse identifies dietary habits, including fat and fiber intake, as well as amounts of alcohol consumed. The nurse describes and documents a history of weight loss.

Assessment includes auscultating the abdomen for bowel sounds and palpating the abdomen for areas of tenderness, distention, and solid masses. Stool specimens are inspected for character and presence of blood.

Diagnosis

NURSING DIAGNOSES

Based on the assessment data, the major nursing diagnoses may include the following:

- Imbalanced nutrition, less than body requirements, related to nausea and anorexia
- Risk for deficient fluid volume related to vomiting and dehydration
- Anxiety related to impending surgery and the diagnosis of cancer
- Risk for ineffective therapeutic regimen management related to knowledge deficit concerning the diagnosis, the surgical procedure, and self-care after discharge
- Impaired skin integrity related to the surgical incisions (abdominal and perianal), the formation of a stoma, and frequent fecal contamination of peristomal skin
- Disturbed body image related to colostomy

- Ineffective sexuality patterns related to presence of ostomy and changes in body image and self-concept

COLLABORATIVE PROBLEMS/ POTENTIAL COMPLICATIONS

Potential complications that may develop include the following:

- Intraperitoneal infection
- Complete large bowel obstruction
- GI bleeding
- Bowel perforation
- Peritonitis, abscess, and sepsis

Planning and Goals

The major goals for the patient may include attainment of optimal level of nutrition; maintenance of fluid and electrolyte balance; reduction of anxiety; learning about the diagnosis, surgical procedure, and self-care after discharge; maintenance of optimal tissue healing; protection of peristomal skin; learning how to irrigate the colostomy and change the appliance; expressing feelings and concerns about the colostomy and the impact on himself or herself; and avoidance of complications.

PREPARING THE PATIENT FOR SURGERY

The patient anticipating surgery for colorectal cancer has many concerns, needs, and fears. He or she may be physically debilitated and emotionally distraught with concern about lifestyle changes after surgery, prognosis, ability to perform in established roles, and finances. Priorities for nursing care include preparing

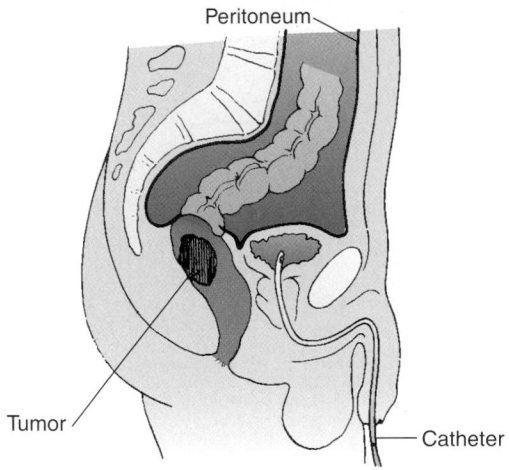

1. Prior to surgery. Note tumor in rectum.

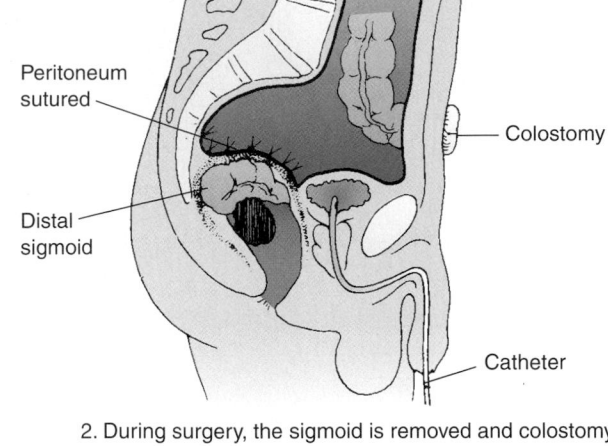

2. During surgery, the sigmoid is removed and colostomy established. The distal bowel has been dissected free to a point below the pelvic peritoneum, which is sutured over the closed end of the distal sigmoid and rectum.

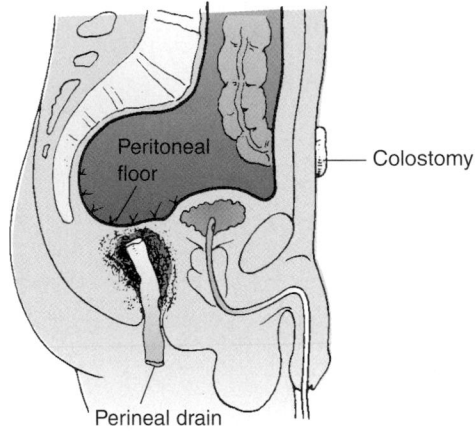

3. Perineal resection includes removal of the rectum and free portion of the sigmoid from below. A perineal drain is inserted.

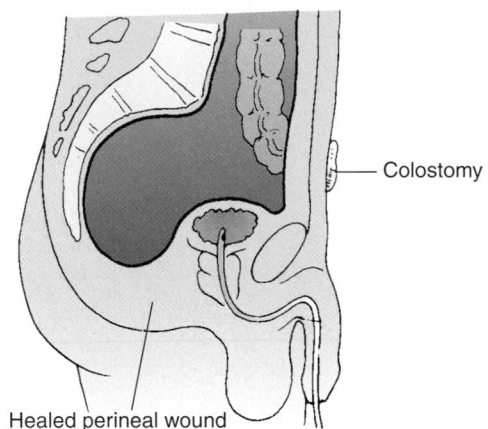

4. The final result after healing. Note healed perineal wound and the permanent colostomy.

FIGURE 38-9 Abdominoperineal resection for carcinoma of the rectum.

the patient physically for surgery, providing information about postoperative care, including stoma care if a colostomy is to be created, and supporting the patient and family emotionally.

Physical preparation for surgery involves building the patient's stamina in the days preceding surgery and cleansing and sterilizing the bowel the day before surgery. If the patient's condition permits, the nurse recommends a diet high in calories, protein, and carbohydrates and low in residue for several days before surgery to provide adequate nutrition and minimize cramping by decreasing excessive peristalsis. A full-liquid diet may be prescribed 24 to 48 hours before surgery to decrease bulk. If the patient is hospitalized in the days preceding surgery, PN may be required to replace depleted nutrients, vitamins, and minerals. In some instances, PN may be given at home before surgery. Antibiotics such as sulfonamides, neomycin, and cephalexin are administered the day before surgery to reduce intestinal bacteria. The bowel is cleansed with laxatives, enemas, or colonic irrigations the evening before and the morning of surgery.

For the patient who is very ill and hospitalized, the nurse measures and records intake and output, including vomitus, to provide an accurate record of fluid balance. The patient's intake of oral food and fluids may be restricted to prevent vomiting. The

nurse administers antiemetics as prescribed. Full or clear liquids may be tolerated, or the patient may be allowed nothing by mouth. A nasogastric tube may be inserted to drain accumulated fluids and prevent abdominal distention. The nurse monitors the abdomen for increasing distention, loss of bowel sounds, and pain or rigidity, which may indicate obstruction or perforation. It also is important to monitor intravenous fluids and electrolytes. Monitoring serum electrolyte levels can detect the hypokalemia and hyponatremia that occur with GI fluid loss. The nurse observes for signs of hypovolemia (eg, tachycardia, hypotension, decreased pulse volume), assesses hydration status, and reports decreased skin turgor, dry mucous membranes, and concentrated urine.

The nurse assesses the patient's knowledge about the diagnosis, prognosis, surgical procedure, and expected level of functioning after surgery. It is important to include information about the physical preparation for surgery, the expected appearance and care of the wound, the technique of ostomy care (if applicable), dietary restrictions, pain control, and medication management in the teaching plan (see Plan of Nursing Care 38-1). If the patient will be admitted the day of surgery, the physician's office may arrange for the patient to be seen by an enterostomal therapist in the days preceding surgery. The ther-

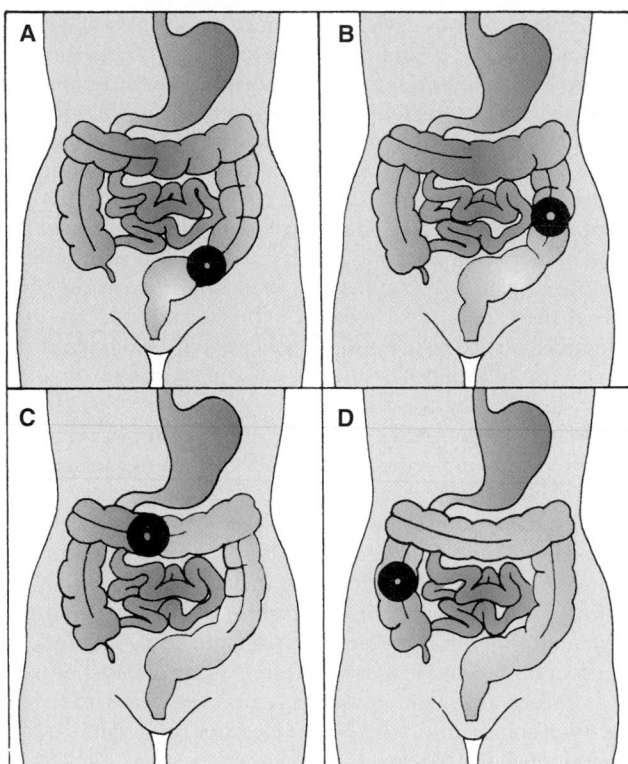

FIGURE 38-10 A diagrammatic representation of the placement of permanent colostomies. The nature of the discharge varies with the site. Shaded areas show sections of bowel removed. With a sigmoid colostomy (**A**) the feces are solid. With a descending colostomy (**B**) the feces are semimushy. With a transverse colostomy (**C**) the feces are mushy. With an ascending colostomy (**D**) the feces are fluid.

apist helps determine the optimal site for the stoma and provides teaching about care. If the patient is hospitalized before the day of surgery, the staff enterostomal therapist is involved in the preoperative teaching. All procedures are explained in language the patient understands.

PROVIDING EMOTIONAL SUPPORT

Patients anticipating bowel surgery for colorectal cancer may be very anxious. They may grieve about the diagnosis, the impending surgery, and possible permanent colostomy. Patients undergoing surgery for a temporary colostomy may express fears and concerns similar to those of a person with a permanent stoma. All members of the health care team, including the enterostomal therapy nurse, should be available for assistance and support. The nurse's role is to assess the patient's anxiety level and coping mechanisms and suggest methods for reducing anxiety such as deep-breathing exercises and visualizing a successful recovery from surgery and cancer. Other supportive measures include providing privacy and teaching relaxation techniques to the patient. Time is set aside to listen to the patient who wishes to talk, cry, or ask questions. The nurse can arrange a meeting with a spiritual advisor if the patient desires or with the physicians if the patient wishes to discuss the treatment or prognosis. To promote patient comfort, the nurse projects a relaxed, professional, and empathetic attitude. See Nursing Research Profile 38-1 about the importance of spiritual well-being for patients with colorectal cancer.

The patient undergoing a colostomy may find the anticipated changes in body image and lifestyle profoundly disturbing. Because the stoma is located on the abdomen, the patient may think that everyone will be aware of the ostomy. The nurse helps reduce this fear by presenting facts about the surgical procedure and the creation and management of the ostomy. If the patient is receptive, the nurse can use diagrams, photographs, and appliances to explain and clarify. Because the patient is experiencing emotional stress, the nurse may need to repeat some of the information. The nurse provides time for the patient and family to ask questions; the nurse's acceptance and understanding of the patient's concerns and feelings convey a caring, competent attitude that promotes confidence and cooperation. Consultation with an enterostomal therapist during the preoperative period can be extremely helpful, as can speaking with a person who is successfully managing a colostomy. The United Ostomy Association provides useful information about living with an ostomy through literature, lectures, and exhibits. Visiting services by qualified members and rehabilitation services for new ostomy patients are provided.

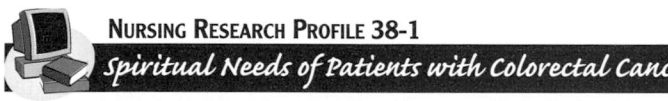

NURSING RESEARCH PROFILE 38-1
Spiritual Needs of Patients with Colorectal Cancer

Fernsler, J., Klemm, P., & Miller, M. (1999). Spiritual well-being and demands of illness in people with colorectal cancer. *Cancer Nursing, 22*(2), 134–140.

Purpose
Patients with colorectal cancer must be assisted in coping with the demands of the illness and its treatment. Using the Demands of Illness Inventory (DOI) and the Spiritual Well-Being Scale (SWBS), the authors of this descriptive study looked closely at the events that individuals experience in response to a cancer diagnosis and attempted to determine whether those events relate to spiritual well-being. The purpose of the study was to identify the demands of the illness and determine their relationship to spiritual well-being.

Study Sample and Findings
The sample for this study consisted of 121 respondents to questionnaires who were at least 21 years old and had been treated for colon, rectal, or anal cancer. Two thirds of the respondents reported a Christian affiliation. Results showed that the illness exerted the greatest demands (highest DOI scores) on those in the youngest age group

(21–45 years) and on those with terminal illness. These respondents also reported lower levels of spiritual well-being.

Subjects who reported significantly lower ($p < .05$) DOI levels related to their physical symptoms, monitoring symptoms, and treatment issues also reported higher levels of spiritual well-being.

Nursing Implications
Nurses who care for cancer patients must be aware of the intense illness-related demands placed on their patients, especially on those in the younger age range and those with a terminal diagnosis. Nurses should explore interventions to assist patients in coping with these demands, especially interventions to enhance the patients' spiritual resources.

This study had several limitations. All responses were self-reported, and measures were taken at only one point in time. Other studies need to be conducted to determine whether the findings can be generalized.

PROVIDING POSTOPERATIVE CARE

Postoperative nursing care for patients undergoing colon resection or colostomy is similar to nursing care for any abdominal surgery patient (see Chap. 20), including pain management during the immediate postoperative period. The nurse also monitors the patient for complications such as leakage from the site of the anastomosis, prolapse of the stoma, perforation, stoma retraction, fecal impaction, skin irritation, and pulmonary complications associated with abdominal surgery. The nurse assesses the abdomen for returning peristalsis and assesses the initial stool characteristics. It is important to help patients with a colostomy out of bed on the first postoperative day and encourage them to begin participating in managing the colostomy.

MAINTAINING OPTIMAL NUTRITION

The nurse teaches all patients undergoing surgery for colorectal cancer about the health benefits to be derived from consuming a healthy diet. The diet is individualized as long as it is well balanced and does not cause diarrhea or constipation. The return to normal diet is rapid.

A complete nutritional assessment is important for patients with a colostomy. The patient avoids foods that cause excessive odor and gas, including foods in the cabbage family, eggs, fish, beans, and high-cellulose products such as peanuts. It is important to determine whether the elimination of specific foods is causing any nutritional deficiency. Nonirritating foods are substituted for those that are restricted so that deficiencies are corrected. The nurse advises the patient to experiment with an irritating food several times before restricting it, because an initial sensitivity may decrease with time. The nurse can help the patient identify any foods or fluids that may be causing diarrhea, such as fruits, high-fiber foods, soda, coffee, tea, or carbonated beverages. Paregoric, bismuth subgallate, bismuth subcarbonate, or diphenoxylate with atropine (Lomotil) help control the diarrhea. For constipation, prune or apple juice or a mild laxative is effective. The nurse suggests fluid intake of at least 2 L of fluid per day.

PROVIDING WOUND CARE

The nurse frequently examines the abdominal dressing during the first 24 hours after surgery to detect signs of hemorrhage. It is important to help the patient splint the abdominal incision during coughing and deep breathing to lessen tension on the edges of the incision. The nurse monitors temperature, pulse, and respiratory rate for elevations, which may indicate an infectious process. If the patient has a colostomy, the stoma is examined for swelling (slight edema from surgical manipulation is normal), color (a healthy stoma is pink or red), discharge (a small amount of oozing is normal), and bleeding (an abnormal sign).

If the malignancy has been removed using the perineal route, the perineal wound is observed for signs of hemorrhage. This wound may contain a drain or packing, which is removed gradually. Bits of tissue may slough off for a week. This process is hastened by mechanical irrigation of the wound or with sitz baths performed two or three times each day initially. The condition of the perineal wound and any bleeding, infection, or necrosis are documented.

MONITORING AND MANAGING COMPLICATIONS

The patient is observed for signs and symptoms of complications. It is important to frequently assess the abdomen, including decreasing or changing bowel sounds and increasing abdominal girth, to detect bowel obstruction. The nurse monitors vital signs for increased temperature, pulse, and respirations and for de-creased blood pressure, which may indicate an intra-abdominal infectious process. It is important to report rectal bleeding immediately because it indicates hemorrhage. The nurse monitors hematocrit and hemoglobin levels and administers blood component therapy as prescribed. Any abrupt change in abdominal pain is reported promptly. Elevated white blood cell counts and temperature or symptoms of shock are reported because they may indicate sepsis. The nurse administers antibiotics as prescribed.

Pulmonary complications are always a concern with abdominal surgery; patients older than 50 years of age are at risk, especially if they are or have been receiving sedatives or are being maintained on bed rest for a prolonged period. Two primary pulmonary complications are pneumonia and atelectasis. Frequent activity (eg, turning the patient from side to side every 2 hours), deep breathing, coughing, and early ambulation can reduce the risks for these complications. Table 38-6 lists possible postoperative complications.

The incidence of complications related to the colostomy is about one half that seen with an ileostomy. Some common complications are prolapse of the stoma (usually from obesity), perforation (from improper stoma irrigation), stoma retraction, fecal impaction, and skin irritation. Leakage from an anastomotic site can occur if the remaining bowel segments are diseased or weakened. Leakage from an intestinal anastomosis causes abdominal distention and rigidity, temperature elevation, and signs of shock. Surgical repair is necessary.

REMOVING AND APPLYING THE COLOSTOMY APPLIANCE

The colostomy begins to function 3 to 6 days after surgery. The nurse manages the colostomy and teaches the patient about its care until the patient can take over. The nurse teaches skin care and how to apply and remove the drainage pouch. Care of the peristomal skin is an ongoing concern because excoriation or ulceration can develop quickly. The presence of such irritation makes adhering the ostomy appliance difficult, and adhering the ostomy appliance to irritated skin can worsen the skin condition. The effluent discharge and the degree to which it is irritating vary with the type of ostomy. With a transverse colostomy, the stool is soft and mushy and irritating to the skin. With a descending or sigmoid colostomy, the stool is fairly solid and less irritating to the skin. Other skin problems include yeast infections and allergic dermatitis.

If the patient wants to bathe or shower before putting on the clean appliance, micropore tape applied to the sides of the pouch will keep it secure during bathing. To remove the appliance, the patient assumes a comfortable sitting or standing position and gently pushes the skin down from the faceplate while pulling the pouch up and away from the stoma. Gentle pressure prevents the skin from being traumatized and any liquid fecal contents from spilling out. The nurse advises the patient to protect the peristomal skin by then washing the area gently with a moist, soft cloth and a mild soap. Soap acts as a mild abrasive agent to remove enzyme residue from fecal spillage. The patient should remove any excess skin barrier. While the skin is being cleansed, a gauze dressing can cover the stoma, or a vaginal tampon can be inserted gently to absorb excess drainage. After cleansing, the patient pats the skin completely dry with a gauze pad, taking care not to rub the area. The patient can lightly dust nystatin (Mycostatin) powder on the peristomal skin if irritation or yeast growth is present.

Smoothly applying the drainage appliance for a secure fit requires practice and a well-fitting appliance. Patients can choose from a wide variety of appliances, depending on their individual

Table 38-6 • **Potential Complications and Nursing Interventions After Intestinal Surgery**

COMPLICATION	NURSING INTERVENTIONS
Paralytic ileus	Initiate or continue nasogastric intubation as prescribed.
	Prepare patient for x-ray study.
	Ensure adequate fluid and electrolyte replacement.
	Administer prescribed antibiotics if patient has symptoms of peritonitis.
Mechanical obstruction	Assess patient for intermittent colicky pain, nausea, and vomiting.
Intra-abdominal Septic Conditions	
Peritonitis	Evaluate patient for nausea, hiccups, chills, spiking fever, tachycardia.
	Administer antibiotics as prescribed.
	Prepare patient for drainage procedure.
	Administer parenteral fluid and electrolyte therapy as prescribed.
	Prepare patient for surgery if condition deteriorates.
Abscess formation	Administer antibiotics as prescribed.
	Apply warm compresses as prescribed.
	Prepare for surgical drainage.
Surgical Wound Complications	
Infection	Monitor temperature; report temperature elevation.
	Observe for redness, tenderness, and pain around wound.
	Assist in establishing local drainage.
	Obtain specimen of drainage material for culture and sensitivity studies.
Wound disruption	Observe for sudden appearance of profuse serous drainage from wound.
	Cover wound area with sterile towels held in place with binder.
	Prepare patient immediately for surgery.
Intraperitoneal infection and abdominal wound infection	Monitor for evidence of constant or generalized abdominal pain, rapid pulse, and elevation of temperature.
	Prepare for tube decompression of bowel.
	Administer fluids and electrolytes by IV route as prescribed.
	Administer antibiotics as prescribed.
Anastomotic Complications	
Dehiscence of anastomosis	Prepare patient for surgery.
Fistulas	Assist in bowel decompression.
	Administer parenteral fluids as prescribed to correct fluid and electrolyte deficits.

needs. The stoma is measured to determine the correct size for the pouch; the pouch opening should be about 0.3 cm (⅛ in) larger than the stoma. After the skin is cleansed according to the previously described procedure, the patient applies the peristomal skin barrier (ie, wafer, paste, or powder). Mild skin irritation may require dusting the skin with karaya or Stomahesive powder before attaching the pouch. The patient removes the backing from the adherent surface of the appliance, and places the bag down over the stoma for 30 seconds. The patient empties or changes the drainage appliance when it is one-third to one-fourth full so that the weight of its contents does not cause the appliance to separate from the adhesive disk and spill the contents. Most appliances are disposable and odor resistant; commercially prepared deodorizers are available.

For some patients, colostomy appliances are not always necessary. As soon as the patient has learned a routine for evacuation, bags may be dispensed with, and a closed ostomy appliance or a simple dressing of disposable tissue (often covered with plastic wrap) is used, held in place by an elastic belt. Except for gas and a slight amount of mucus, nothing escapes from the colostomy opening between irrigations. Colostomy plugs that expand on insertion to prevent passage of flatus and feces are available.

IRRIGATING THE COLOSTOMY

The purpose of irrigating a colostomy is to empty the colon of gas, mucus, and feces so that the patient can go about social and business activities without fear of fecal drainage. A stoma does not have voluntary muscular control and may empty at irregular intervals. Regulating the passage of fecal material is achieved by irrigating the colostomy or allowing the bowel to evacuate naturally without irrigations. The choice often depends on the individual and the type of the colostomy. By irrigating the stoma at a regular time, there is less gas and retention of the irrigant. The time for irrigating the colostomy should be consistent with the schedule the person will follow after leaving the hospital. Chart 38-9 delineates the irrigating procedure.

SUPPORTING A POSITIVE BODY IMAGE

The patient is encouraged to verbalize feelings and concerns about altered body image and to discuss the surgery and the stoma (if one was created). A supportive environment and a supportive attitude on the nurse's part are crucial in promoting the patient's adaptation to the changes brought about by the surgery. If applicable, the patient must learn colostomy care and begin to plan for incorporating stoma care into daily life. The nurse helps the patient overcome aversion to the stoma or fear

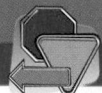

Chart 38-9

GUIDELINES FOR Irrigating a Colostomy

A colostomy is irrigated to empty the colon of feces, gas, or mucus, cleanse the lower intestinal tract, and establish a regular pattern of evacuation so that normal life activities may be pursued. A suitable time for the irrigation is selected that is compatible with the patient's posthospital pattern of activity (preferably after a meal). Irrigation should be performed at the same time each day.

Before the procedure, the patient sits on a chair in front of the toilet or on the toilet itself. An irrigating reservoir containing 500 to 1500 mL of lukewarm tapwater is hung 45 to 50 cm (18 to 20 in) above the stoma (shoulder height when the patient is seated). The dressing or pouch is removed. The following procedure is used; the patient is helped to participate in the procedure to learn to perform it unassisted.

NURSING ACTION	RATIONALE
1. Apply an irrigating sleeve or sheath to the stoma. Place the end in the commode.	1. This helps to control odor and splashing and allows feces and water to flow directly into the commode.

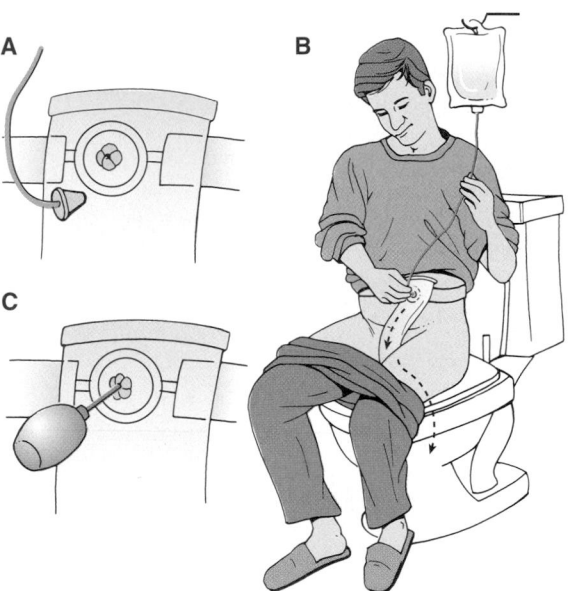

Colostomy irrigation. (**A**) Irrigating catheter has a cone attachment to prevent injury to stomal tissue. (**B**) Irrigating fluid is instilled with sleeve in place. Drainage contents empty into toilet. (**C**) The bulb syringe method can be used to stimulate fecal drainage. Note that a portion of the hard nozzle is removed and a catheter attached to minimize stomal irritation.

2. Allow some of the solution to flow through the tubing and catheter/cone.	2. Air bubbles in the setup are released so that air is not introduced into the colon, which would cause crampy pain.
3. Lubricate the catheter/cone and gently insert it into the stoma. Insert the catheter no more than 8 cm (3 in). Hold the shield/cone gently, but firmly, against the stoma to prevent backflow of water.	3. Lubrication permits ease of insertion of the catheter/cone.
4. If the catheter does not advance easily, allow water to flow slowly while advancing catheter. *Never force the catheter!*	4. A slow rate of flow helps to relax the bowel and facilitates passage of the catheter.
5. Allow tepid fluid to enter the colon slowly. If cramping occurs, clamp off the tubing and allow the patient to rest before progressing. Water should flow in over a 5- to 10-minute period.	5. Painful cramps usually are caused by too rapid a flow or by too much solution; 300 mL of fluid may be all that is needed to stimulate evacuation. Volume may be increased with subsequent irrigations to 500, 1000, or 1500 mL as needed by the patient for effective results.
6. Hold the shield/cone in place 10 seconds after the water has been instilled; then gently remove it.	
7. Allow 10 to 15 minutes for most of the return; then dry the bottom of the sleeve/sheath and attach it to the top, or apply the appropriate clamp to the bottom of the sleeve.	7. Most of the water, feces, and flatus will be expelled in 10 to 15 minutes.
8. Leave the sleeve/sheath in place for 30 to 45 minutes while the patient gets up and moves around.	8. Ambulation stimulates peristalsis and completion of the irrigation return.
9. Cleanse the area with a mild soap and water; pat the area dry.	9. Cleanliness and dryness will provide the patient with hours of comfort.
10. Replace the colostomy dressing or appliance.	10. The patient should use an appliance until the colostomy is sufficiently controlled. A dressing may be all that is needed.

of self-injury by providing care and teaching in an open, accepting manner and by encouraging the patient to talk about his or her feelings about the stoma.

DISCUSSING SEXUALITY ISSUES

The nurse encourages the patient to discuss feelings about sexuality and sexual function. Some patients may initiate questions about sexual activity directly or give indirect clues about their fears. Some may view the surgery as mutilating and a threat to their sexuality; some fear impotence. Others may express worry about odor or leakage from the pouch during sexual activity. Although the appliance presents no deterrent to sexual activity, some patients wear silk or cotton covers and smaller pouches during sex. Alternative sexual positions are recommended, as well as alternative methods of stimulation to satisfy sexual drives. The nurse assesses the patient's needs and attempts to identify specific concerns. If the nurse is uncomfortable with this or if the patient's concerns seem complex, it is appropriate for the nurse to seek assistance from an enterostomal therapy nurse, sex counselor or therapist, or advanced practice nurse.

PROMOTING HOME AND COMMUNITY-BASED CARE

Teaching Patients Self-Care

Patient education and discharge planning require the combined efforts of the physician, nurse, enterostomal therapist, social worker, and dietitian. Patients are given specific information, individualized to their needs, about ostomy care and signs and symptoms of potential complications. Dietary instructions are essential to help patients identify and eliminate irritating foods that can cause diarrhea or constipation. It is important to teach patients about their prescribed medications (ie, action, purpose, and possible side effects).

The nurse reviews treatments (eg, irrigations, wound cleansing) and dressing changes and encourages the family to participate. Because the hospital stay is short, the patient may not be able to become proficient in stoma care techniques before discharge. Many patients need referral to a home care agency and the telephone number of the local chapter of the American Cancer Society. The home care nurse goes to the home to provide further care and teaching and to assess how well the patient and family are adjusting to the colostomy. The home environment is assessed for adequacy of resources that allow the patient to accomplish self-care. A family member may assume responsibility for purchasing the equipment and supplies needed at home.

Patients need very specific directions about when to call the physician. They need to know which complications require prompt attention (ie, bleeding, abdominal distention and rigidity, diarrhea, fever, wound drainage, and disruption of suture line). If radiation therapy is planned, the possible side effects (ie, anorexia, vomiting, diarrhea, and exhaustion) are reviewed.

Continuing Care

Ongoing care of the patient with cancer and a colostomy often extends well beyond the initial hospital stay. Home care nurses manage ostomy follow-up care, manage the assessment and care of the debilitated patient, and coordinate adjuvant therapy. The home care visits also provide the nurse with opportunities to assess the patient's physical and emotional status and the patient's and family's ability to carry out recommended management strategies. Visits from an enterostomal therapy nurse are available to the patient and family as they learn to care for the ostomy and work through their feelings about it, the diagnosis of cancer, and the

future. Some patients are interested in and can benefit from involvement in an ostomy support group.

Evaluation

EXPECTED PATIENT OUTCOMES

Expected patient outcomes may include the following:

1. Consumes a healthy diet
   a. Avoids foods and fluids that cause diarrhea
   b. Substitutes nonirritating foods and fluids for those that are restricted
2. Maintains fluid balance
   a. Experiences no vomiting or diarrhea
   b. Experiences no signs or symptoms of dehydration
3. Feels less anxious
   a. Expresses concerns and fears freely
   b. Uses coping measures to manage stress
4. Acquires information about diagnosis, surgical procedure, preoperative preparation, and self-care after discharge
   a. Discusses the diagnosis, surgical procedure, and postoperative self-care
   b. Demonstrates techniques of ostomy care
5. Maintains clean incision, stoma, and perineal wound
6. Expresses feelings and concerns about self
   a. Gradually increases participation in stoma and peristomal skin care
   b. Discusses feelings related to changed appearance
7. Discusses sexuality in relation to ostomy and to changes in body image
8. Recovers without complications
   a. Is afebrile
   b. Regains normal bowel activity
   c. Exhibits no signs and symptoms of perforation or bleeding

POLYPS OF THE COLON AND RECTUM

A polyp is a mass of tissue that protrudes into the lumen of the bowel. Polyps can occur anywhere in the intestinal tract and rectum. They can be classified as neoplastic (ie, adenomas and carcinomas) or non-neoplastic (ie, mucosal and hyperplastic). Non-neoplastic polyps, which are benign epithelial growths, are common in the Western world. They occur more commonly in the large intestine than in the small intestine. Although most polyps do not develop into invasive neoplasms, they must be identified and followed closely. Adenomatous polyps are more common in men. The proportion of these polyps arising in the proximal part of the colon increases with age (after 40 years of age). Prevalence rates vary from 25% to 60%, depending on age. Non-neoplastic polyps occur in 80% of the population, and their frequency increases with age (Wolfe, 2000).

Clinical manifestations depend on the size of the polyp and the amount of pressure it exerts on intestinal tissue. The most common symptom is rectal bleeding. Lower abdominal pain may also occur. If the polyp is large enough, symptoms of obstruction occur. The diagnosis is based on history and digital rectal examination, barium enema studies, sigmoidoscopy, or colonoscopy.

After a polyp is identified, it should be removed. There are several methods: colonoscopy with the use of special equipment (ie, biopsy forceps and snares), laparoscopy, or colonoscopic excision with laparoscopic visualization. The latter technique enables immediate detection of potential problems and allows laparoscopic resection and repair of the major complications of perforation and bleeding that may occur with polypectomy. Microscopic examination of the polyp then identifies the type of polyp and indicates what further surgery is required.

Diseases of the Anorectum

Anorectal disorders are common, and more than one half of the population will experience one at some time during their lives (Yamada et al., 1999). Patients with anorectal disorders seek medical care primarily because of pain, rectal bleeding, or change in bowel habits. Other common complaints are protrusion of hemorrhoids, anal discharge, perianal itching, swelling, anal tenderness, stenosis, and ulceration. Constipation results from delaying defecation because of anorectal pain.

There has been a steady increase in the frequency of sexually transmitted diseases in recent decades, leading to the identification of new anorectal syndromes. The prevalence of these conditions is increasing. These syndromes include venereal infections such as syphilis, gonorrhea, herpes, chlamydia, and candidiasis, and they are most commonly seen in male homosexuals who practice anorectal intercourse (Wolfe, 2000).

ANORECTAL ABSCESS

An anorectal abscess is caused by obstruction of an anal gland, resulting in retrograde infection. People with regional enteritis or immunosuppressive conditions such as AIDS are particularly susceptible to these infections. Many of these abscesses result in fistulas.

An abscess may occur in a variety of spaces in and around the rectum. It often contains a quantity of foul-smelling pus and is painful. If the abscess is superficial, swelling, redness, and tenderness are observed. A deeper abscess may result in toxic symptoms, lower abdominal pain, and fever.

Palliative therapy consists of sitz baths and analgesics. However, prompt surgical treatment to incise and drain the abscess is the treatment of choice. When a deeper infection exists with the possibility of a fistula, the fistulous tract must be excised. If possible, the fistula is excised when the abscess is incised and drained, or a second procedure to do so may be necessary. The wound may be packed with gauze and allowed to heal by granulation.

ANAL FISTULA

An anal fistula is a tiny, tubular, fibrous tract that extends into the anal canal from an opening located beside the anus (Fig. 38-11A). Fistulas usually result from an infection. They may also develop from trauma, fissures, or regional enteritis. Pus or stool may leak constantly from the cutaneous opening. Other symptoms may be the passage of flatus or feces from the vagina or bladder, depending on the fistula tract. Untreated fistulas may cause systemic infection with related symptoms.

Surgery is always recommended, because few fistulas heal spontaneously. A fistulectomy (ie, excision of the fistulous tract) is the recommended surgical procedure. The lower bowel is evacuated thoroughly with several prescribed enemas. During surgery, the sinus tract is identified by inserting a probe into it or by injecting the tract with methylene blue solution. The fistula is dissected out or laid open by an incision from its rectal opening to its outlet. The wound is packed with gauze.

ANAL FISSURE

An anal fissure is a longitudinal tear or ulceration in the lining of the anal canal (see Fig. 38-11B). Fissures are usually caused by the trauma of passing a large, firm stool or from persistent tightening of the anal canal because of stress and anxiety (leading to constipation). Other causes include childbirth, trauma, and overuse of laxatives.

Extremely painful defecation, burning, and bleeding characterize fissures. Most of these fissures heal if treated by conservative measures, which include stool softeners and bulk agents, an increase in water intake, sitz baths, and emollient suppositories. A suppository combining an anesthetic with a corticosteroid helps relieve the discomfort. Anal dilation under anesthesia may be required.

If fissures do not respond to conservative treatment, surgery is indicated. The procedure considered by most surgeons to be the procedure of choice is the lateral internal sphincterotomy with excision of the fissure; the success rate is 90% to 95% (Keighley & Williams, 1999).

HEMORRHOIDS

Hemorrhoids are dilated portions of veins in the anal canal. They are very common. By the age of 50, about 50% of people have hemorrhoids to some extent (Corman, 1998). Shearing of the

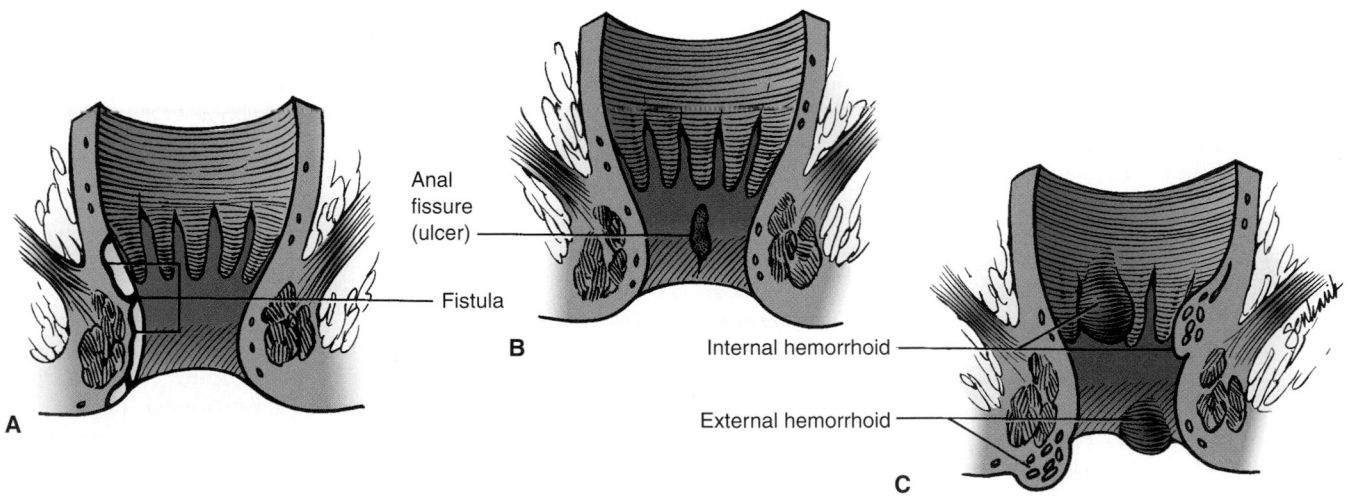

FIGURE 38-11 Various types of anal lesions. (**A**) Fistula. (**B**) Fissure. (**C**) External and internal hemorrhoids.

mucosa during defecation results in the sliding of the structures in the wall of the anal canal, including the hemorrhoidal and vascular tissues. Increased pressure in the hemorrhoidal tissue due to pregnancy may initiate hemorrhoids or aggravate existing ones. Hemorrhoids are classified as one of two types. Those above the internal sphincter are called internal hemorrhoids, and those appearing outside the external sphincter are called external hemorrhoids (see Fig. 38-11C).

Hemorrhoids cause itching and pain and are the most common cause of bright red bleeding with defecation. External hemorrhoids are associated with severe pain from the inflammation and edema caused by thrombosis (ie, clotting of blood within the hemorrhoid). This may lead to ischemia of the area and eventual necrosis. Internal hemorrhoids are not usually painful until they bleed or prolapse when they become enlarged.

Hemorrhoid symptoms and discomfort can be relieved by good personal hygiene and by avoiding excessive straining during defecation. A high-residue diet that contains fruit and bran along with an increased fluid intake may be all the treatment that is necessary to promote the passage of soft, bulky stools to prevent straining. If this treatment is not successful, the addition of hydrophilic bulk-forming agents such as psyllium and mucilloid may help. Warm compresses, sitz baths, analgesic ointments and suppositories, astringents (eg, witch hazel), and bed rest allow the engorgement to subside.

There are several types of nonsurgical treatments for hemorrhoids. Infrared photocoagulation, bipolar diathermy, and laser therapy are newer techniques that are used to affix the mucosa to the underlying muscle. Injecting sclerosing solutions is also effective for small, bleeding hemorrhoids. These procedures help prevent prolapse.

A conservative surgical treatment of internal hemorrhoids is the rubber-band ligation procedure. The hemorrhoid is visualized through the anoscope, and its proximal portion above the mucocutaneous lines is grasped with an instrument. A small rubber band is then slipped over the hemorrhoid. Tissue distal to the rubber band becomes necrotic after several days and sloughs off. Fibrosis occurs; the result is that the lower anal mucosa is drawn up and adheres to the underlying muscle. Although this treatment has been satisfactory for some patients, it has proven painful for others and may cause secondary hemorrhage. It has been known to cause perianal infection.

Cryosurgical hemorrhoidectomy, another method for removing hemorrhoids, involves freezing the hemorrhoid for a sufficient time to cause necrosis. Although it is relatively painless, this procedure is not widely used because the discharge is very foul smelling and wound healing is prolonged. The Nd:YAG laser is useful in excising hemorrhoids, particularly external hemorrhoidal tags. The treatment is quick and relatively painless. Hemorrhage and abscess are rare postoperative complications.

The previously described methods of treating hemorrhoids are not effective for advanced thrombosed veins, which must be treated by more extensive surgery. Hemorrhoidectomy, or surgical excision, can be performed to remove all the redundant tissue involved in the process. During surgery, the rectal sphincter is usually dilated digitally and the hemorrhoids are removed with a clamp and cautery or are ligated and then excised. After the operative procedures are completed, a small tube may be inserted through the sphincter to permit the escape of flatus and blood; pieces of Gelfoam or Oxycel gauze may be placed over the anal wounds.

SEXUALLY TRANSMITTED ANORECTAL DISEASES

Three infectious syndromes that are related to sexually transmitted diseases have been identified. Proctitis involves the rectum. It is commonly associated with recent anal-receptive intercourse with an infected partner. Symptoms include a mucopurulent discharge or bleeding, pain in the area, and diarrhea. The pathogens most frequently involved are *Neisseria gonorrheae* (53%), *Chlamydia* (20%), herpes simplex virus (18%), and *Treponema pallidum* (9%) (Yamada et al., 1999). Proctocolitis involves the rectum and lowest portion of the descending colon. Symptoms are similar to proctitis but may also include watery or bloody diarrhea, cramps, pain, and bloating. Enteritis involves more of the descending colon, and symptoms include watery, bloody diarrhea; abdominal pain; and weight loss. The most common pathogens causing enteritis are *E. histolytica, Giardia lamblia, Shigella,* and *Campylobacter* (Wolfe, 2000).

Sigmoidoscopy is performed to identify portions of the anorectum involved. Samples are taken with rectal swabs, and cultures are obtained to identify the pathogens involved. The treatment of choice for bacterial infections is antibiotics (ie, cefixime, doxycycline, and penicillin). Acyclovir is given to those with viral infections. Infections from *E. histolytica* and *G. lamblia* are treated with antiamebic therapy (ie, metronidazole). Ciprofloxacin is an effective treatment for *Shigella.* Antibiotics of choice for *Campylobacter* infection are erythromycin and ciprofloxacin.

PILONIDAL SINUS OR CYST

A pilonidal sinus or cyst is found in the intergluteal cleft on the posterior surface of the lower sacrum (Fig. 38-12). Current theories suggest that it results from local trauma that causes the pen-

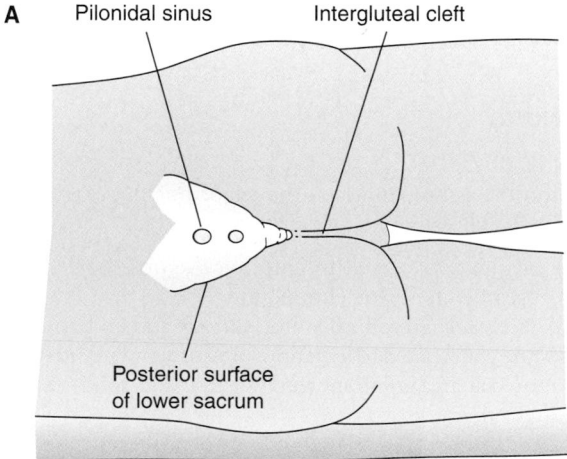

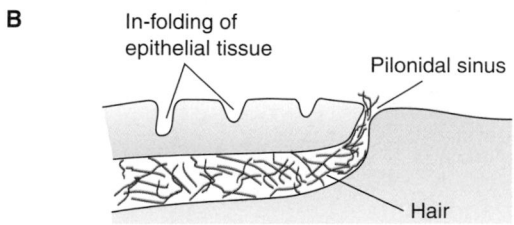

FIGURE 38-12 (**A**) Pilonidal sinus on lower sacrum about 5 cm (2 in) above the anus in the intergluteal cleft. (**B**) Note: Hair particles emerge from the sinus tract and localized indentations (pits) can appear on the skin near the sinus openings.

etration of hairs into the epithelium and subcutaneous tissue (Yamada et al., 1999). It may also be formed congenitally by an infolding of epithelial tissue beneath the skin, which may communicate with the skin surface through one or several small sinus openings. Hair frequently is seen protruding from these openings, and this gives the cyst its name, *pilonidal* (ie, a nest of hair). The cysts rarely cause symptoms until adolescence or early adult life, when infection produces an irritating drainage or an abscess. Perspiration and friction easily irritate this area.

In the early stages of the inflammation, the infection may be controlled by antibiotic therapy, but after an abscess has formed, surgery is indicated. The abscess is incised and drained under local anesthesia. After the acute process resolves, further surgery is performed to excise the cyst and the secondary sinus tracts. The wound is allowed to heal by granulation. Gauze dressings are placed in the wound to keep its edges separated while healing occurs.

NURSING PROCESS: THE PATIENT WITH AN ANORECTAL CONDITION

Assessment

The nurse takes a health history to determine the presence and characteristics of itching, burning, or pain. Does it occur during bowel movements? How long does it last? Is any abdominal pain associated with it? Does any bleeding occur from the rectum? How much? How frequently? Is it bright red? Is there any other discharge, such as mucus or pus? Other questions relate to elimination patterns and laxative use, diet history (including fiber intake), the amount of exercise, activity levels, and occupation (especially one that involves prolonged sitting or standing). Assessment also includes inspection of the stool for blood or mucus and the perianal area for hemorrhoids, fissures, irritation, or pus.

Diagnosis

NURSING DIAGNOSES

Based on the assessment data, the major nursing diagnoses may include the following:

- Constipation related to ignoring the urge to defecate because of pain during elimination
- Anxiety related to impending surgery and embarrassment
- Acute pain related to irritation, pressure, and sensitivity in the anorectal area from anorectal disease and sphincter spasms after surgery
- Urinary retention related to postoperative reflex spasm and fear of pain
- Risk for ineffective therapeutic regimen management

COLLABORATIVE PROBLEMS/ POTENTIAL COMPLICATIONS

- Hemorrhage

Planning and Goals

The major goals for the patient may include adequate elimination patterns, reduction of anxiety, pain relief, promotion of urinary elimination, managing the therapeutic regimen, and absence of complications.

Nursing Interventions

RELIEVING CONSTIPATION

The nurse encourages intake of at least 2 L of water daily to provide adequate hydration and recommends high-fiber foods to promote bulk in the stool and to make it easier to pass fecal matter through the rectum. Bulk laxatives such as Metamucil and stool softeners are administered as prescribed. The patient is advised to set aside a time for moving the bowels and to heed the urge to defecate as promptly as possible. It may be helpful to have the patient perform relaxation exercises before defecating to relax the abdominal and perineal muscles, which may be constricted or in spasm. Administering an analgesic before a bowel movement is beneficial.

REDUCING ANXIETY

Patients facing rectal surgery may be upset and irritable because of discomfort, pain, and embarrassment. The nurse identifies specific psychosocial needs and individualizes the plan of care. The nurse maintains the patient's privacy while providing care and by limiting visitors, if the patient desires. Soiled dressings are removed from the room promptly to prevent unpleasant odors; room deodorizers may be needed if dressings are foul smelling.

RELIEVING PAIN

During the first 24 hours after rectal surgery, painful spasms of the sphincter and perineal muscles may occur. Control of pain is a prime consideration. The patient is encouraged to assume a comfortable position. Flotation pads under the buttocks when sitting help to decrease the pain, as may ice and analgesic ointments. Warm compresses may promote circulation and soothe irritated tissues. Sitz baths taken three or four times each day can relieve soreness and pain by relaxing sphincter spasm. Twenty-four hours after surgery, topical anesthetic agents may be beneficial in relieving local irritation and soreness. Medications may include topical anesthetics (ie, suppositories), astringents, antiseptics, tranquilizers, and antiemetics. Patients are more compliant and less apprehensive if they are free of pain.

Wet dressings saturated with equal parts of cold water and witch hazel help relieve edema. When wet compresses are being used continuously, the petrolatum is applied around the anal area to prevent skin maceration. The patient is instructed to assume a prone position at intervals because this position promotes dependent drainage of edematous fluid.

PROMOTING URINARY ELIMINATION

Voiding may be a problem after surgery because of a reflex spasm of the sphincter at the outlet of the bladder and a certain amount of muscle guarding from apprehension and pain. The nurse tries all methods to encourage voluntary voiding (ie, increasing fluid intake, listening to running water, and dripping water over the urinary meatus) before resorting to catheterization. After rectal surgery, urinary output is closely monitored.

MONITORING AND MANAGING COMPLICATIONS

The operative site is examined frequently for rectal bleeding. The nurse assesses the patient for systemic indicators of excessive bleeding (ie, tachycardia, hypotension, restlessness, and thirst). After hemorrhoidectomy, hemorrhage may occur from the veins that were cut. If a tube has been inserted through the sphincter after surgery, evidence of bleeding may be visible on the dressings. If bleeding is obvious, direct pressure is applied to the area, and the physician is notified. It is important to avoid using moist heat because it encourages vessel dilation and bleeding.

PROMOTING HOME AND COMMUNITY-BASED CARE

Teaching Patients Self-Care

Most patients with anorectal conditions are not hospitalized. Those who have surgical procedures to correct the condition often are discharged directly from the outpatient surgical center. If they are hospitalized, it is for a short time, usually only 24 hours. Patient teaching is essential to facilitate recovery at home.

The nurse instructs the patient to keep the perianal area as clean as possible by gently cleansing with warm water and then drying with absorbent cotton wipes. The patient avoids rubbing the area with toilet tissue. Instructions are provided about how to take a sitz bath and how to test the temperature of the water. Sitz baths may be given in the bathtub or plastic sitz bath unit three or four times each day. Sitz baths should follow each bowel movement for 1 to 2 weeks after surgery. The nurse encourages the patient to respond quickly to the urge to defecate to prevent constipation. The diet is modified to increase fluids and fiber. Moderate exercise is encouraged, and the patient is taught about the prescribed diet, the significance of proper eating habits and exercise, and the laxatives that can be taken safely.

Evaluation

EXPECTED PATIENT OUTCOMES

Expected patient outcomes may include the following:

1. Attains a normal pattern of elimination
   a. Sets aside a time for defecation, usually after a meal or at bedtime
   b. Responds to the urge to defecate and takes the time to sit on the toilet and try to defecate
   c. Uses relaxation exercises as needed
   d. Increases fluid intake to 2 L per day
   e. Adds high-fiber foods to diet
   f. Reports passage of soft, formed stools
   g. Reports decreased abdominal discomfort
2. Is less anxious
3. Has less pain
   a. Modifies body position and activities to minimize pain and discomfort
   b. Applies warmth or cold to anorectal area
   c. Takes sitz baths four times each day
4. Voids without difficulty
5. Adheres to the therapeutic regimen
   a. Keeps perianal area dry
   b. Eats bulk-forming foods
   c. Has a soft, formed stool on a regular basis
6. Exhibits no evidence of complications
   a. Has a clean incision
   b. Has normal vital signs
   c. Shows no signs of hemorrhage

Critical Thinking Exercises

1. You are caring for an elderly man who was just admitted to the hospital. He complains that he has had pain throughout his abdomen for the past 2 days. He states that his bowel patterns have changed recently and that he has not had a bowel movement in 4 days. He has not eaten since yesterday. He states he has no appetite and that he is concerned because he has type 2 diabetes mellitus. When you complete your initial nursing assessment, you notice that his abdomen is distended and rigid and that bowel sounds are absent throughout all fields. Analyze these findings, indicate what you think the possible causes may be, and explain the actions you would take and why. Explain how this man's diagnosis of diabetes mellitus affects his plan of nursing care and his medical management.

2. During a conversation with a neighbor, you learn that she has recently seen her doctor and that she has been diagnosed with IBS. She asks you to help her understand this process and to explain the reason for the dietary restrictions her doctor has given her. Her doctor also prescribed a laxative and an antidepressant. She explains the amount of stress she has been under at work. Identify the facts that you know about this process and how the actions of the doctor would help in this situation. What will you tell your neighbor?

3. You are caring for a patient who has been diagnosed with colon cancer. He recently underwent a colonoscopy where the growth was detected in the lower portion of the descending colon. The patient is scheduled for a colon resection. You know that he will return from surgery with a sigmoid colostomy. What will you need to do during the preoperative period to prepare your patient for this surgery? What will be the nursing diagnoses and related interventions that are a priority during the immediate postoperative period? Explain how you would meet the postoperative emotional and health education needs of the patient with a colostomy.

4. You are assigned to a general medical clinic. Two patients with inflammatory bowel disease arrive for their appointments. One of the patients, a 52-year-old woman, has recently been diagnosed with Crohn's disease. The other patient, a 21-year-old woman, was diagnosed with ulcerative colitis at 15 years of age and has had an ileostomy since the age of 19 years. Compare the two disease processes in terms of their pathophysiology, clinical manifestations, course of the illness, and therapeutic management. What similarities and differences would you expect to find in the nutritional and pharmacologic therapies for these two patients? What assessment parameters would you use to identify the psychosocial needs of each of these patients.

REFERENCES AND SELECTED READINGS

Books

American Cancer Society. (2002). *Cancer Facts and Figures 2002.* Atlanta, Georgia: Author.

Bernard, L. (1999). *Colorectal cancer.* Atlanta: American Cancer Society.

Brandt, L., & Daum, F. (1999). *Clinical practice of gastroenterology.* New York: Churchill-Livingstone.

Bruce, F. (1997). *Nursing in gastroenterology.* Philadelphia: W. B. Saunders.

Corman, M. (1998). *Colon and rectal surgery* (4th ed.). Philadelphia: Lippincott-Raven.

Eliopoulos, C. (1999). *Manual of gerontological nursing* (2nd ed.). St. Louis: Mosby.

Goldman, L., & Bennett, J. C. (2000). *Cecil textbook of medicine* (21st ed.). Philadelphia: W. B. Saunders.

Greene, F. L., Page, D. L., Fleming, I. D., et al. (2002). *AJCC Cancer Staging Manual.* New York: Springer-Verlag.

Grendell. J., et al. (Eds.). (1998). *Current diagnosis and treatment in gastroenterology.* Stamford, CT: Appleton & Lange.

Kirsner, J., & Shorter, R. (2000). *Inflammatory bowel disease* (5th ed.), Philadelphia: W. B. Saunders.

Keighley, M., & Willaims, N. S. (1999). *Surgery of the anus, rectum and colon* (2nd ed.). Philadelphia: W. B. Saunders.

Lipsky, M. S. (2000). *Gastrointestinal problems.* Philadelphia: Lippincott Williams & Wilkins.

Lueckenotte, A. (2000). *Gerontologic nursing.* St. Louis: Mosby.

Ming, S. (Ed.). (1998). *Pathology of the gastrointestinal tract* (2nd ed.). Baltimore: Williams & Wilkins.

Phillips, S. (1998). *Functional disorders of the gut.* London: Churchill-Livingstone.

Rose, S. (1998). *Gastrointestinal and hepatobiliary physiology.* Madison, WI: Fena Creek Publishers.

Society of Gastroenterology Nurses and Associates. (1998). *Gastroenterology nursing: A core curriculum* (2nd ed.). St. Louis: Mosby.

Stone, J., et al. (1999). *Clinical gerontological nursing* (2nd ed.). Philadelphia: W. B. Saunders.

Tierney, L., et al. (Eds.). (2000). *Current medical diagnosis and treatment.* New York: Lange Medical Books.

Williams, N. (Ed.). (1996). *Colorectal cancer.* New York: Churchill-Livingstone.

Wolfe, M. (Ed.). (2000). *Therapy of digestive disorders.* Philadelphia: W. B. Saunders.

Yamada, T., Alpers, D. H., Owyang, C., Powell, D. W., Silverstein, F., Hasler, W. L., & Traber, P. G. (Eds.). (1998). *Handbook of gastroenterology.* Philadelphia: Lippincott Williams & Wilkins.

Yamada, T., Alpers, D. H., Laine, L., Owyang, C., & Powell, D. W. (Eds.). (1999). *Textbook of gastroenterology* (3rd ed.). Philadelphia: Lippincott Williams & Wilkins.

Journals

General

Andersson, R. E., Olaison, G., Tysk, C., & Ekbom, A. (2001). Appendectomy and protection against ulcerative colitis. *New England Journal of Medicine, 344*(11), 808–814.

Creason, N., & Sparks, D. (2000). Fecal impaction: A review. *Nursing Diagnosis, 11*(1), 15–23.

Cox, J. A., Rogers, M. A., & Cox, S. D. (2001). Treating benign colon disorders using laparoscopic colectomy. *AORN Journal, 73*(2), 377–382, 384–389, 391.

Ebert, E. (2001). Maldigestion and malabsorption. *Disease of the Month, 4*(2), 45–68.

Gauf, C. L. (2000). Diagnosing appendicitis across the life span. *Journal of the American Academy of Nurse Practitioners, 12*(4), 129–133.

Hyde, C. (2000). Diverticular disease. *Nursing Standard, 14*(51), 38–42.

Madick, S. S. (2001). Perioperative care of the patient with Zenker's diverticulum. *AORN Journal, 73*(5), 904–913.

McConnell, E. A., (1999). Myths and facts about lactose intolerance. *Nursing, 29*(3), 71.

Murphy-Ende, K. (2000). Bowel obstruction. *Clinical Journal of Oncology Nursing, 4*(6), 291–293.

Murphy-Ende, K. (2001). Palliation of gastrointestinal obstructive disorders. *Nursing Clinics of North America, 36*(4) 761–768.

Posarra, V. H. (1999). Recognizing the various presentations of appendicitis. *Nurse Practitioner, 24*(8), 42, 44, 49, 52–53.

Scheidler, M. & Giannella, R. (2001). Practical management of acute diarrhea. *Hospital Practice, 36*(2), 49–56.

Waldman, A. R. (2001). Bowel obstruction. *Clinical Journal of Oncology Nursing, 5*(6), 281–281, 286.

Whitehead, W. E., Wald, A., Norton, N. J. (2001). Treatment options for fecal incontinence. *Diseases of the Colon and Rectum, 44*(1), 131–142.

Wong, P. W. (1999). How to deal with chronic constipation. *Postgraduate Medicine, 106*(6), 199–200, 203–204, 207–210.

Cancer of the Colon and Rectum

Anderson, J. (2000). Review of recommendations for colorectal screening. *Geriatrics, 55*(2), 67–73.

Baker, D. (2001). Current surgical management of colorectal cancer. *Nursing Clinic of North America, 36*(3), 579–592.

Beyers, T. (2001). Colorectal cancer screening: New directions, evolving guidelines. *Patient Care, 35*(4), 24–34.

Burrer, C. V., & Bauer, S. M. (2000). Insights into genetic testing for colon cancer: The nurse practitioner role. *Clinical Excellence for Nurse Practitioners, 4*(6), 349–355.

Dest, V. M. (2000). Colorectal cancer. *RN, 63*(3), 54–59.

Greenberg, M. J. (2001). Screening for colorectal cancer. *New England Journal of Medicine, 345*(25), 1851–1852.

Longo, W. E. & Johnson, F. E. (2002). The preoperative assessment and postoperative surveillance of patients with colon and rectal cancer. *Surgical Clinic of North America, 8*(5) 1091–1098.

Olsen, S. J. & Zawacki, K. (2000). Hereditary colorectal cancer. *Nursing Clinics of North America, 35*(3), 671–685.

Pontieri-Lewis, V. (2000). Colorectal cancer: Prevention and screening. *Medsurg Nursing, 9*(1) 9–15.

Rothenberger, D. (2000). Colorectal cancer. *Surgical Oncology Clinics of North America, 9*(4), 665–730.

Rudy, D. & Zdon, M. (2000). Update on colorectal cancer. *American Family Physician, 61*(6), 1759–1770, 1773–1774.

Sarna, L. & Chang, B. I. (2000). Colon cancer screening among older women caregivers. *Cancer Nursing, 23*(2), 109–116.

Stefanik, D. (2000). Colon cancer. *American Journal of Nursing 100*(Suppl. 4), 36–40.

Young, M. (2000) Caring for patients with coloanal reservoirs for rectal cancer. *Medsurg Nursing, 9*(4), 193–197.

Inflammatory Bowel Disease

Alpers, D. (2001). Is irritable bowel syndrome more than just a gastrointestinal problem? *American Journal of Gastroenterology, 96*(6), 943–949.

Blackington, E. (2000). Irritable bowel syndrome; an update on treatment options. *Advanced Nurse Practitioner, 8*(10), 41–70.

Brown, M. (1999). Inflammatory bowel disease. *Primary Care, 26*(1), 41–70.

Colwell, J. C. & Gray, M. (2001). What functional outcomes and complications should be taught to the patient with ulcerative colitis or familial adenomatous polyposis who undergoes ileal pouch anal anastomosis? *Journal of Wound Ostomy Continence Nursing, 28*(4), 184–189.

Dudley-Brown, S. (2002). Prevention of psychological distress in persons with inflammatory bowel disease. *Issues in Mental Health Nursing, 23*(4), 403–422.

Hanauer, S. (2001). Management of Crohn's disease in adults. *American Journal of Gastroenterology, 96*(3), 635–644.

Heitkemper, M. (2001). Irritable bowel syndrome. *American Journal of Nursing, 101*(1), 26–34.

Joachim, G. (2000). Responses of people with inflammatory bowel disease to foods consumed. *Gastroenterology Nursing, 23*(4), 160–167.

*Joachim, G. (2002). An assessment of social support in people with inflammatory bowel disease. *Gastroenterology Nursing, 25*(6), 246–252.

Kefalides, P. T. & Hanauer, S. B. (2002). Ulcerative colitis: diagnosis and management. *Hospital Physician, 38*(6), 53–63.

Klonowski, E. (1999). The patient with Crohn's disease. *RN, 62*(3), 32–37.

Licht, H. (2000). Irritable bowel syndrome: Diagnostic criteria. *Postgraduate Nursing, 107*(3), 203–207.

Lombardi, D. A., Feller, E. R., & Shah, S. A. (2002). Medical management of inflammatory bowel disease in the new millennium. *Comprehensive Therapy, 28*(1), 39–49.

*Mukherjee, S., Sloper, P., & Turnbull, A. (2002). An insight into the experiences of parents with inflammatory bowel disease. *Journal of Advanced Nursing, 37*(4), 355–353.

Parascandolo, M. E. (2001). Multiple ostomy complications in a patient with Crohn's disease: A case study. *Journal of Wound Ostomy Continence Nursing, 28*(5), 236–241.

Rayhorn, N. (1999). Understanding inflammatory bowel disease. *Nursing, 29*(12), 57–61.

Rayhorn, N. & Rayhorn, D. J. (2002). An in-depth look at inflammatory bowel disease. *Nursing, 32*(7), 36–45.

Rayhorn, N. & Rayhorn, D. J. (2002). Inflammatory bowel disease: Symptoms in the bowel and beyond. *Nurse Practitioner, 27*(11), 13–27.

*Smith, G. D., Watson, R., & Palmer, K. R. (2002). Inflammatory bowel disease: Developing a short disease specific scale to measure health related quality of life. *International Journal of Nursing Studies, 39*(6), 583–590.

Smith, G. D., Watson, R., Roger, D., McRorie, E., et. al. (2002). Impact of a nurse-led counselling service on quality of life in patients with inflammatory bowel disease. *Journal of Advanced Nursing, 38*(2), 152–160.

Tung, J. K. & Warner, A. S. (2002). Colonic inflammatory bowel disease. Medical therapies for colonic Crohn's disease and ulcerative colitis. *Postgraduate Medicine, 112*(5), 45–48.

Ostomy

Ball, E. M. (2000). Ostomy guide. Part one. A practical ostomy guide. *RN, 63*(11), 61–66.

Ball, E. M. (2000). Ostomy guide. Part two. A teaching guide for continent ileostomy. *RN, 63*(12), 35–38, 40.

Bryant, D. (2000). Photo guide: Changing an ostomy appliance. *Nursing, 30*(11), 51–53.

Floruta, C. V. (2001). Dietary choices of people with ostomies. *Journal of Wound Ostomy Continence Nursing, 28*(1), 28–31.

Haugen, V. & Loehner, D. (2001). *Journal of Wound Ostomy Continence Nursing, 28*(4), 219–222.

Hocevar, B. J. & Remzi, F. (2001). The ileal pouch anal anastomosis: Past, present, and future. *Journal of Wound Ostomy Continence Nursing, 28*(1), 32–36.

Schultz, J. M. (2002). Preparing the patient for colostomy care: A lesson well learned. *Ostomy Wound Management, 48*(10), 22–25.

Taylor, P. (2001). Choosing the right stoma appliance for an ileostomy. *Community Nurse, 6*(12), 33–4.

RESOURCES AND WEBSITES

American Cancer Society, 1599 Clifton Rd., N.E., Atlanta, GA 30329; 1-800-277-2345; http://www.cancer.org.

Colon Cancer Alliance, 175 Ninth Ave., New York, NY 10011; 1-212-627-7451; http://www.ccalliance.org.

Crohn's & Colitis Foundation of America, 386 Park Avenue South, New York, NY 10016-8804; 1-800-932-2423; http://www.ccfa.org.

International Foundation for Functional Gastrointestinal Disorders, P.O. Box 17864, Milwaukee, WI 17864; 1-888-964-2001; http://www.iffgd.org.

Intestinal Disease Foundation, Inc., 1323 Forbes Ave., Suite 200, Pittsburgh, PA 15219; 1-412-261-5888; Ischorr@aol.com.

National Association for Continence, P.O. Box 544, Union, SC 29379; 1-803-585-8789; http://www.nafc.org/site2/index.html.

National Foundation for Ileitis and Colitis, 295 Madison Ave., New York, NY 10017; 1-212-685-3440.

STOP Colon/Rectal Cancer Foundation, P.O. Box 1616, Barrington, IL 60010; 1-312-782-4828; http://www.coloncancerprevention.org.

United Ostomy Association, 19772 MacArthur Blvd., Suite 200, Irvine, CA 92612-2405; 1-800-826-0826; http://www.uoa.org.

Index

Letters following page numbers indicate the following: c – chart, f – figure, t – table.

Q

R

Sheehan's syndrome. *See* Postpartum pituitary necrosis
Shift to the left, 872
 definition of, 868
Shigella
 and diarrheal diseases, 2129–2130
 incubation period of, 2116t
 transmission of, 2116t
Shingles, 1416, 2122. *See also* Herpes zoster
 distribution of, 1651f
Shock
 after thoracic surgery, 636
 anaphylactic, 296, 311–312
  medical management of, 311
  nursing management of, 311–312
  risk factors for, 309c
 anxiety in, reducing, 300, 308–309
 blood circulation in, 298, 298f
 burns and, 1712–1714, 1717c
 cardiogenic, 296, 306–309, 439, 806–808
  assessment in, 807
  clinical manifestations of, 306, 807
  coronary versus non-coronary, 306, 306c
  diagnosis of, 807
  first-line treatment of, 307
  fluid replacement in, 308
  hemodynamic monitoring in, 307, 308
  mechanical assist devices for, 308
  medical management of, 306–308, 807–808
  nursing management of, 308–309, 808
  oxygenation in, 307
  pain control in, 307
  pathophysiology of, 306, 306f, 806, 807f
  pharmacologic therapy in, 307–308, 808
  postoperative, 439
  prevention of, 308
  risk factors for, 306, 306c
  safety and comfort in, enhancing, 308–309
 cardiovascular problems in, 300
 cellular effects of, 296, 297f
 circulatory (distributive), 296, 309–312. *See also* Shock, anaphylactic; Shock, neurogenic; Shock, septic
  pathophysiology of, 309, 309f
  types of, 309
 classification of, 296
 clinical findings in, 299, 299c, 300–301
 complications of, prevention of, 301
 conditions precipitating, 296–298
 definition of, 296
 diarrheal diseases and, 2131–2132
 ectopic pregnancy and, 1405
 electrical, injury caused by, 91
 family members of patient with, supporting, 301, 302
 fluid redistribution in, 305, 305f
 fluid replacement in, 302–305, 305t, 306
  complications of, 303
 fracture and, 2083
 gastrointestinal problems in, 300–301
 hematologic problems in, 301
 hemorrhagic, prostatectomy and, 1506
 hepatic problems in, 300
 home and community-based care for, 313
 hypovolemic, 258, 296, 304–306
  blood replacement in, 305, 306, 2156
  clinical findings in, 304
  ectopic pregnancy and, 1405
  emergency management of, 2156
  fluid redistribution in, 305, 305f
  fluid replacement in, 304–305, 305t, 306, 2156
  medical management of, 304–305
  nursing management of, 305, 2156
  orthopedic surgery and, 2042, 2043
  oxygen therapy in, 306
  pathophysiology of, 304, 304f
  pharmacologic therapy for, 305
  postoperative, 438–439
  risk factors for, 304, 304c
  signs and symptoms of, 2155c
 in kidney surgery, 1299
 management of
  general strategies for, 302
  in postanesthesia care, 438–440
 medical management of, 303, 303t
  in compensatory stage, 299
  in irreversible stage, 301
  in progressive stage, 301
 neurogenic, 311, 1929–1930
  medical management of, 311
  nursing management of, 311
  postoperative, 438–439
  risk factors for, 309c
 neurologic problems in, 300
 nursing management of
  in compensatory stage, 299–300
  in irreversible stage, 302
  in progressive stage, 301

 nutritional support in, 303–304
 pathophysiology of, 296–298
  in progressive stage, 300
 patient positioning in, 305, 305f
 pelvic fracture and, 2091
 in pneumonia, 528–529, 531
 renal problems in, 300
 respiratory problems in, 300
 rest and comfort in, promoting, 301
 safety in, promoting, 300
 self-care in, patient teaching about, 313
 septic, 296, 309–311. *See also* Toxic shock syndrome
  in cancer patient, 357
  hyperdynamic phase of, 310
  hypodynamic phase of, 310
  immunotherapy for, 310
  infectious diseases and, 2143c
  medical management of, 310
  microbiology of, 309–310
  nursing management of, 310–311
  nutritional support in, 310
  pharmacologic therapy for, 310
  risk factors for, 309, 309c
 significance of, 296
 signs and symptoms of, 2153
 signs of, 439
 and skin color, 1647t
 spinal, 1929–1930
 stage of, 298–302
  compensatory, 299–300, 299c
  irreversible, 299c, 301–302
  progressive, 299c, 300–301
 tissue perfusion in, monitoring, 299
 in trauma patient, 558
 treatment of, 2083
 vascular response to, 296–297
Shock lung, 300
Short arm cast, 2018
Short bones, 2003
Short leg cast, 2018
Short tubes, 985–986
Shoulder
 adduction, ischemic stroke and, 1896, 1897f
 healing of, 2052, 2052c
 pain in, ischemic stroke and, 1898
 subluxation of, ischemic stroke and, 1898
Shoulder-hand syndrome, ischemic stroke and, 1898
Shoulder spica cast, 2018
Shunt(s), respiratory, low ventilation–perfusion ratio and, 467–468, 469f
SIADH. *See* Syndrome of inappropriate antidiuretic hormone
Sialadenitis, 963
 definition of, 959
Sialolithiasis, 963–964
Sibutramine HCl (Meridia), 1021
Sickle cell anemia, 886–891
 acute chest syndrome of, 887–888
 carrier testing for, 133t, 138
 clinical manifestations of, 887
 complications of, 887, 887t, 889, 890
 diagnosis of, 888
 expected outcomes in, 891
 genetics of, 127, 130t
 genetic testing in, 133t
 medical management of, 888–889
 pain in, 219c
 pharmacologic therapy for, 888
 prognosis for, 888
 supportive therapy for, 889
 transfusion therapy for, 888
Sickle cell crisis, 887
 aplastic crisis type, 887
 complications of, 889
 nursing diagnoses related to, 889
 nursing interventions for, 890–891
 nursing process with, 889–891
 sequestration crisis type, 887
 sickle crisis type, 887
Sickle cell disease. *See* Sickle cell anemia
Sickle cell trait, 887
Sidelying position, 166c
Sighted-guide techniques, 1756
Sigmoid colon, 942f
 adenocarcinoma of, in ureterosigmoidostomy, 1353
Sigmoidoscopy, 952–953
 flexible fiberoptic, 952, 952f
 nursing interventions in, 952–953
Sildenafil citrate (Viagra), 194
 for erectile dysfunction, 1491, 1492t
 patient education about, 1493c
 use after prostate cancer, 1497
Silent thyroiditis, 1226
Silent unit, 469f
Silicone breast implants, 1479
 and breast cancer, 1459

Silicosis, 553
Silver nitrate, for burns, 1720t
Silver sulfadiazine (Silvadene), for burns, 1720, 1720t
Simmonds' disease. *See* Panhypopituitarism
Simple fracture, 2081c
Simplex chronicus, 1426, 1426c
Sims-Huhner test, 1400–1401
Sims' position, for pelvic examination, 1378
SIMV. *See* Synchronized intermittent mandatory ventilation
Simvastatin (Zocor), 826
 as lipid-lowering agent, 717, 718t
Sinex long-lasting. *See* Oxymetazoline hydrochloride
Single-chain urokinase-type plasminogen activator, 840–841
Single-lumen central catheter(s), 1003
Single nucleotide polymorphisms, 128
 genetic testing for, 137
Single-photon emission computed tomography, 673, 674, 1822, 1843
 nursing interventions for, 1843
Sin nombre virus, 2127–2128
 incubation period of, 2116t
 transmission of, 2116t
Sinoatrial node, 649–650, 649f, 651, 683
 definition of, 647
Sinography, in intraperitoneal injury, 2159
Sinus(es)
 dural, 1826
 frontal, 968f
 paranasal
  anatomy of, 463–465f
  infection of. *See* Sinusitis
  physical examination of, 475–476f, 496
 pilonidal, 1067, 1067f
 sphenoid, 968f
Sinus arrhythmia, 690f, 1286–1290
Sinus bradycardia, 688f, 1285–1288
Sinusitis
 acute, 495–497
  assessment in, 496
  causative organisms in, 495
  clinical manifestations of, 495
  complications of, 496
  diagnosis of, 496
  medical management of, 496–497
 chronic, 497–498
  assessment in, 497
  clinical manifestations of, 497
  complications of, 497
  diagnosis of, 497
  medical management of, 497
  pathophysiology of, 497
  surgical management of, 497–498
 definition of, 493
 nasal obstruction and, 505
 nursing interventions for, 501–502
 pathophysiology of, 493, 494f, 495, 497
 self-care in, patient teaching about, 497, 498
 in upper airway infection, 502
Sinusoidal harmonic acceleration, 1797
Sinus rhythm, 683
 definition of, 683
 ECG criteria for, 687, 688f
Sinus tachycardia, 688, 689f
Sirolimus, for kidney transplantation, 1336
Sitting, with crutches, 172
Sixth Joint National Committee on the Prevention, Detection, Evaluation, and Treatment of High Blood Pressure (JNC VI), 855, 857
Six-year molar, 966f
SJS. *See* Stevens-Johnson syndrome
Skeletal reduction, for spinal cord injury, 1929, 1929f
Skeletal system
 function of, 2003–2005
 structure of, 2003–2005
Skeletal tongs, for traction, 1929, 1929f
Skeletal traction, 2026, 2027f, 2028–2029
 and exercise, 2029
 neurovascular status in, 2029
 nursing interventions for, 2028–2029
 pin site care in, 2029
 skin breakdown in, 2028–2029
 for spinal cord injury, 1929, 1929f
Skene's duct cysts, 1426
Skilled nursing facilities, 199
Skin. *See also* Integumentary system
 anatomy of, 1639–1642, 1640f
 appearance of, changes in, in arterial disease, 820
 bacterial infections of, 1668–1670
 benign tumors of, 1686–1687
 biopsy of, 1652
 blistering diseases of, 1681–1686
  nursing process for, 1683–1684
 breakdown
  amputation and, 2108–2109
  hip fracture and, 2095